5TH EDITION

ESSENTIALS of Pediatric Nursing

5TH EDITION

ESSENTIALS of Pediatric Nursing

Terri Kyle, DNP, APRN, CPNP, CNE
Professor of Nursing
RN to BSN, MSN Coordinator
AdventHealth University
Orlando, Florida

Susan Carman, MSN, MBA
Professor of Nursing
Most recently, Edison Community College
Fort Myers, Florida

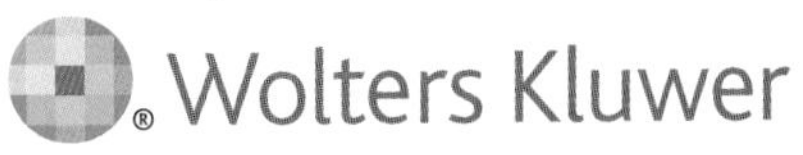

Philadelphia • Baltimore • New York • London
Buenos Aires • Hong Kong • Sydney • Tokyo

Vice President and Publisher: Julie K. Stegman
Director of Nursing Education and Practice Content: Jamie Blum
Acquisitions Editor: Jodi Rhomberg
Associate Director of Nursing Education and Practice Content: Staci Wolfson
Development Editor: Rachel Lucke
Editorial Coordinator: Erin E. Hernandez
Marketing Manager: Wendy Mears
Editorial Assistant: Sara Thul
Manager, Graphic Arts & Design: Stephen Druding
Art Director, Illustration: Jennifer Clements
Senior Production Project Manager: Catherine Ott
Manufacturing Coordinator: Margie Orzech
Prepress Vendor: S4Carlisle Publishing Services

Fifth Edition

9 8 7 6 5 4 3 2 1

Printed in the United States of America

Library of Congress Cataloging-in-Publication Data available upon request from publisher.

ISBN-13: 978-1-9752-3614-4

Library of Congress Control Number: 2024913624

shop.lww.com

As always, I remain motivated by nursing students to seek innovative learning methods for the development of clinical judgment in child health nursing. This book is dedicated to my precious family, my dedicated husband John, my outstanding children Christian and Caitlin, and my amazing granddaughters Sophia and Chloe who continue to inspire me on a daily basis; I am forever grateful for their ongoing faith in and support of me. To Sue Carman, thank you for your ongoing encouragement, dedication, and continual presence, and patience.

—TERRI KYLE

This book continues to be dedicated to the children of the world and the wonderful nurses who care for them. They inspire me to become a better nurse, educator, and person. It is the major impact nurses have on the health of children and their families that drives me to find the best methods to teach clinical judgment in order to provide the very best pediatric nurses that our children deserve. This book is also dedicated to my loving and supportive husband, Chris, without whom I could not have reached this accomplishment; and my four beautiful girls, Grace, Ella, Lily, and Maya, who have allowed me to learn first-hand about growth and development and who truly amaze me each and every day. I would also like to dedicate this to my parents, Lene and Kishor Patel, who always taught me I could do whatever I put my mind to. To Terri Kyle, thank you for this opportunity, your endless support, and your incredible vision.

—SUSAN CARMAN

ACKNOWLEDGMENTS

The thrilling and challenging experience of authoring this textbook would not have been possible without the tremendous support of the Wolters Kluwer family. In particular, we want to thank Michelle McIlvain (former regional sales manager) for initially querying about this idea, Michael Kerns (acquisitions editor) for his support of our direction for the book, and Jodi Rhomberg for continuing this support and her dedication. We would like to express our continued gratitude to Sarah Kyle (development editor) for her clarity, organizational skills, and attention to detail in prior editions and to Staci Wolfson (current development editor) for her dedication, continual support, and meticulous thorough editing. Thank you to Stephen Druding (design coordinator), Jennifer Clements (art director), and the entire art team for the beautiful illustrations, as well as Erin E. Hernandez (editorial coordinator), Sara Thul (editorial assistant), Catherine Ott (production project manager), Margie Orzech (manufacturing coordinator), and the production team at S4Carlisle Publishing Services for their diligent efforts. Special thanks to Amy Gellerman (producer), Gus Freedman (photographer), Newton-Wellesley Hospital pediatric department, and Boston Shriners Hospital for the beautiful photography they contributed. We continue to appreciate the assistance of contributors on the first edition, including Kathie Aduddell, Barbara Browning, Myra Carmon, Kim Hamilton Conn, Carol Holz, Maeve Howett, Randall Johnson, Kathy Ordelt, Marie Oren-Sosebee, Maggie Payne-Orton, and Gayle Wetzel. We would also like to thank all of the pediatric nurses who contributed their wealth of knowledge and expertise to developing content for this book. This would not have been possible without all of you.

ABOUT THE AUTHORS

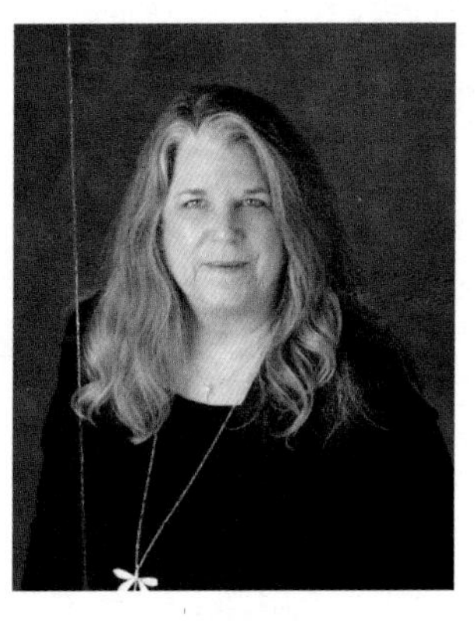

TERRI KYLE

Terri Kyle earned a Bachelor of Science in Nursing from the University of North Carolina at Chapel Hill and a Master of Science in Nursing from Emory University in Atlanta, Georgia. Terri received her Doctorate of Nursing Practice in Educational Leadership from American Sentinel University. She is a certified pediatric nurse practitioner and certified nurse educator. Practicing pediatric nursing for over 40 years, Terri has had the opportunity to serve children and their families in a variety of diverse settings.

She has experience in inpatient pediatrics in pediatric and neonatal intensive care units, newborn nursery, specialized pediatric units, and community hospitals. She has worked as a pediatric nurse practitioner in pediatric specialty clinics and primary care. She has been involved in teaching nursing for over 32 years with experience in both undergraduate and graduate nursing education. Terri delights in providing innovative leadership to nursing educators and their students. She is a fellow in the National Association of Pediatric Nurse Practitioners and a member of Sigma Theta Tau International Honor Society of Nursing, the National League for Nursing, and the Society of Pediatric Nurses.

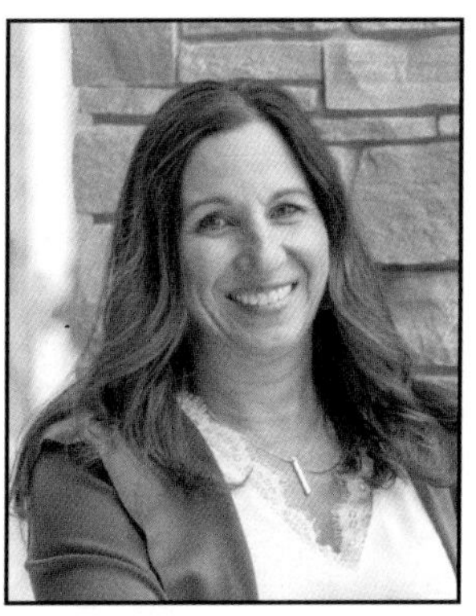

SUSAN CARMAN

Susan Carman earned a Bachelor of Science in Nursing from the University of Wisconsin–Madison and a Master of Science in Nursing and Master in Business Administration from the University of Colorado–Denver. As a pediatric nurse for over 25 years, Susan has had the opportunity to care for children in a variety of diverse settings and in many of the major children's hospitals throughout the United States. She also has provided volunteer nursing care in a variety of settings including the Dominican Republic and India. She has been involved in teaching nursing for the past 20 years and enjoys watching students transform into competent nurses with strong clinical judgment.

PREFACE

Continuing in the contemporary educational climate, reduced class time is being devoted to specialty courses like pediatric nursing. Therefore, it remains important for nursing educators to focus on key concepts, rather than attempting to cover everything within a specific topic. *Essentials of Pediatric Nursing* was written to direct students to an understanding of critical concepts related to pediatric nursing. Rather than repeating medical–surgical content that the student has already mastered, the text builds upon the student's prior knowledge. The text presents the important differences when caring for children as compared to caring for adults.

The main objectives of the fifth edition of *Essentials of Pediatric Nursing* are to provide student nurses with the foundation needed for high-quality nursing care of children and their families as well as the ability to utilize clinical judgment within various health care environments. The book covers a broad scope of topics, placing emphasis on common issues and pediatric-specific content, including atraumatic care, critical to providing patient and family-centered care. Simpler and broader concepts are mastered first, then students are able to progress to problem-solving in more complex situations.

Reflecting the importance of the nursing process, the steps of assessment, nursing analysis, goal setting with outcome identification, and specific, applicable interventions are provided in the early section of the chapters. This Clinical Judgment and the Nursing Process section provides the student with the general approach needed to care for a child with health alterations specific to that chapter.

Utilizing the nursing process, a concept-based approach provides relevant information in a concise and nonredundant manner. Focusing on conceptual learning provides a time-efficient instructional method for nursing educators and fosters the development of critical thinking in nursing students. Complex critical thinking leads to the development of clinical judgment, which may be applied in various health care environments. This approach is supported by many of the book's features, such as the recurring features, Unfolding Case Studies, Clinical Reasoning Alerts, and Thinking About Development.

ORGANIZATION

Each chapter of *Essentials of Pediatric Nursing* focuses on a different aspect of pediatric nursing care. The book is divided into four units, beginning with general concepts related to pediatric nursing and followed by expected growth and development and specifics related to caring for children. The fourth unit focuses on nursing management of alterations in children's health.

Unit I: Foundations of Pediatric Nursing

Unit I presents the foundational material the nursing student needs to understand how nursing care of the child differs from that of the adult. The unit provides information about general concepts relating to child health. Perspectives on pediatric nursing, the nursing process, and factors influencing child health are key concepts covered in this unit.

Unit II: Health Promotion of the Growing Child and Family

Unit II provides information related to growth and development expectations of the well child from the newborn period through adolescence. Though not exhaustive in nature, this unit provides a broad knowledge base related to normal growth and development that the nurse can draw upon in any situation. Common concerns related to growth and development and child/family education are included in each age-specific chapter.

Unit III: Working With Children and Families

Unit III covers broad concepts that provide the foundation for providing nursing care to children. Rather than reiterating all aspects of nursing care, this unit focuses on specific details needed to provide nursing care for children. The family-centered approach, atraumatic care, communication, and teaching children and families are key concepts in this unit. Additional topics covered in this unit include anticipatory guidance and routine well-child care (including immunizations and safety), health assessment, nursing care of the child in diverse settings, concerns common to special needs children, pediatric variations in nursing procedures, and pain management in children.

Unit IV: Nursing Care of the Child With a Health Disorder

Unit IV focuses on children's responses to health disorders. This unit provides comprehensive coverage of illnesses affecting children. It is arranged according to broad topics of disorders organized with a conceptual and body systems approach and also includes infectious, genetic, and mental health disorders as well as pediatric emergencies. Each chapter follows a similar format to facilitate presentation of the information as well as reduce repetition. The chapter begins with an overview of variations in pediatric anatomy and physiology, followed by the nursing process for the particular concept. Nursing analysis identifies the patient issue and identified outcomes, and nursing interventions with rationale are included. This approach provides a general framework for addressing alterations in the concept. The nursing process information may then be utilized to develop an individualized nursing care plan or concept map.

RECURRING FEATURES

To provide the student and educator with an exciting and user-friendly text, a number of recurring features have been developed.

Key Terms

Each chapter includes a list of key terms considered to be vital to understanding the content in the chapter. Each key term appears in boldface, with the definition included in the text. Phonetic spellings are provided for terms that may be new or difficult to pronounce.

Learning Objectives

The provision of learning objectives for each chapter helps to guide the student toward prioritizing information for learning. The objectives also provide a method for the student to evaluate understanding of the presented material.

Words of Wisdom

Each chapter opens with inspiring Words of Wisdom (WOW) that set the tone for the chapter. The WOW statements offer students helpful, motivating, or interesting statements that stimulate thinking about children and their families.

Case Studies

Real-life scenarios present relevant child and family information that is intended to improve the student's clinical reasoning skills. Questions throughout the chapter about the scenarios provide an opportunity for the student to critically evaluate the appropriate course of action.

Clinical Reasoning Alert

The Clinical Reasoning Alert promotes critical thinking in the nursing process on information key to clinical reasoning.

Unfolding Patient Stories

Unfolding Patient Stories, written by the National League for Nursing, are an engaging way to begin meaningful conversations in the classroom. These vignettes, which appear at the end of select chapters, feature patients from Wolters Kluwer's vSim for Nursing | Pediatric (codeveloped by Laerdal Medical) and DocuCare products; however, each Unfolding Patient Story in the book stands alone, not requiring purchase of these products.

Atraumatic Care

These highlights, located throughout the book, provide tips for providing atraumatic care to children in particular situations relating to the topic being discussed.

Take Note!

The *Take Note!* feature draws the student's attention to points of critical emphasis throughout the chapter. This feature is often used to stress vitally important information.

Consider This!

In every chapter, the student is asked to *Consider This!* These first-person narratives engage the student in real-life scenarios experienced by their patients. The personal accounts evoke empathy and help the student to perfect caregiving skills. Each box ends with an opportunity for further contemplation, encouraging the student to think critically about the scenario.

Thinking About Development

The content featured in these boxes will encourage students to think critically about special developmental concerns relating to the topic being discussed.

Healthy People 2030

Throughout the textbook, Healthy People 2030 objectives related to children's health and well-being are outlined in box format. Nursing implications or guidance related to working toward achievement of these objectives is provided. These objectives reflect the Healthy People 2030 guidelines.

Evidence-Based Practice

Throughout the chapters, pertinent questions addressed by current research have been highlighted into Evidence-Based Practice boxes, which discuss recent evidence-based research findings and provide recommendations for nurses.

Teaching Guidelines

Teaching Guidelines, presented in most of the chapters, serve as valuable health education tools. These guidelines raise the student's awareness, provide timely and accurate information, and are designed to ensure the student's preparation for educating children and their families about various issues.

Drug Guides

The Drug Guide tables summarize information about commonly used medications. The actions, indications, and significant nursing implications presented assist the student in providing optimum care to children and their families.

Common Laboratory and Diagnostic Tests

The Common Laboratory and Diagnostic Tests tables in each chapter of Unit IV provide the student with a general understanding of how a broad range of disorders is diagnosed. Rather than reading the information repeatedly throughout the narrative, the student is then able to refer to the table as needed.

Common Medical Treatments

The Common Medical Treatments tables in each chapter of Unit IV provide the student with a broad awareness of how a common group of disorders is treated either medically or surgically. The table serves as a reference point for common medical treatments.

Comparison Charts

These charts compare two or more disorders or other easily confused concepts. They serve to provide an explanation clarifying the concepts for the student.

Nursing Procedures

Step-by-step nursing procedures provide a clear explanation of pediatric variations to facilitate competent performance.

Concept Mastery Alerts

Concept Mastery Alerts clarify pediatric nursing concepts to improve the reader's understanding of potentially confusing topics as identified by Misconception Alerts in Lippincott's Adaptive Learning Powered by PrepU. Data from thousands of actual students using this program in courses across the United States identified common misconceptions for the authors to clarify in this new feature.

Dosage Calculation Box

This box provides a dosage calculation example in each of the alteration/disorder chapters. Reiteration of the significance of accurate dosage calculation assists the student with mastery of this critical concept.

Key Concepts

At the end of each chapter, Key Concepts provide a quick review of essential chapter elements. These bulleted lists help the student focus on the important aspects of the chapter.

Tables, Boxes, Illustrations, and Photographs

Tables and boxes are included throughout the chapters to summarize key content areas. Beautiful illustrations and photographs help the student to visualize the content. These features allow the student to quickly and easily access information.

References

References that were used in the development of the text are provided at the end of each chapter. The listings allow the student to further pursue topics of interest.

Developing Clinical Judgment

This section located at the end of each chapter assists the student with the development of clinical judgment through:

- **Practicing for NCLEX**—these NCLEX-RN style questions test the student's ability to utilize critical thinking in the application of the nursing process to chapter material. The questions are styled similarly to the national licensing examination. Next-Gen NCLEX-RN style questions are also included in most chapters.
- **Dosage Calculation Questions**—these problems test the student's ability to accurately determine medication dosages particular to children.
- **Critical Thinking Exercises**—these exercises serve to stimulate the student to incorporate the current material with previously learned concepts and reach a satisfactory conclusion. The exercises encourage students to think critically, problem solve, and consider their own perspective on given topics.
- **Study Activities**—these activities promote student participation in the learning process. This section encourages increased interaction/learning via clinical, online, and community activities.
- **Answers**—answers to the Developing Clinical Judgment questions are provided to instructors on thePoint®.

A NOTE ABOUT THE LANGUAGE USED IN THIS BOOK

Wolters Kluwer recognizes that people have a diverse range of identities, and we are committed to using inclusive and nonbiased language in our content. In line with the principles of nursing, we strive not to define people by their diagnoses, but to recognize their personhood first and foremost, using as much as possible the language diverse groups use to define themselves, and including only information that is relevant to nursing care.

We strive to better address the unique perspectives, complex challenges, and lived experiences of diverse populations traditionally underrepresented in health literature. When describing or referencing populations discussed in research studies, we will adhere to the identities presented in those studies to maintain fidelity to the evidence presented by the study investigators. We follow best practices of language set forth by *the Publication Manual of the American Psychological Association, 7th edition*, but acknowledge that language evolves rapidly, and we will update the language used in future editions of this book as necessary.

INSTRUCTOR'S RESOURCES

Tools to assist instructors with teaching the course are available through thePoint®, upon adoption of this text.

- An **E-Book** on thePoint® gives you access to the book's full text and images online.
- A **Test Generator** lets you put together exclusive new tests from a bank containing **hundreds of questions** to help you in assessing your students' understanding of the material. Test questions link to chapter learning objectives.
- **PowerPoint presentations** with **Guided Lecture Notes** provide an easy way for you to integrate the textbook with your students' classroom experience, either via slide shows or handouts. Multiple choice and true/false questions are integrated into the presentations to promote class participation and allow you to use i-clicker technology.
- An **Image Bank** lets you use the photographs and illustrations from this textbook in your PowerPoint slides or as you see fit in your course.
- An **AACN Essentials map** relates the textbook content to the current AACN Essentials.
- A sample **Syllabus** provides guidance for structuring your pediatric nursing course.
- **Journal Articles,** updated for the new edition, offer access to current research available in Wolters Kluwer journals.

Contact your sales representative or check out LWW.com/Nursing for more details and ordering information.

Lippincott CoursePoint+

This text is also available for sale in the ***Lippincott CoursePoint+*** version.

Lippincott® CoursePoint+ is an integrated, digital curriculum solution for nursing education that provides a completely interactive experience geared to help students understand, retain, and apply their course knowledge and be prepared for practice. The time-tested, easy-to-use, and trusted solution includes engaging learning tools, evidence-based practice, case studies, and in-depth reporting to meet students where they are in their learning, combined with the most trusted nursing education content on the market to help prepare students for practice. This easy-to-use digital learning solution of *Lippincott® CoursePoint+*, combined with unmatched support, gives instructors and students everything they need for course and curriculum success!

Lippincott® CoursePoint+ includes the following:

- Leading content provides a variety of learning tools to engage students of all learning styles.
- A personalized learning approach gives students the content and tools they need at the moment they need it, giving them data for more focused remediation and helping to boost their confidence and competence.
- Powerful tools, including varying levels of case studies, interactive learning activities, and adaptive learning powered by PrepU, help students learn the critical thinking and clinical judgment skills to help them become practice-ready nurses.
- Preparation for Practice tools improve student competence, confidence, and success in transitioning to practice.
  - vSim® for Nursing: Codeveloped by Laerdal Medical and Wolters Kluwer, vSim® for Nursing simulates real nursing scenarios and allows students to interact with virtual patients in a safe, online environment.
  - Lippincott® Advisor for Education: With over 8500 entries covering the latest evidence-based content and drug information, Lippincott® Advisor for Education provides students with the most up-to-date information possible, while giving them valuable experience with the same point-of-care content they will encounter in practice.
- Unparalleled reporting provides in-depth dashboards with several data points to track student progress and help identify strengths and weaknesses.
- Unmatched support includes training coaches, product trainers, and nursing education consultants to help educators and students implement CoursePoint with ease.

CONTENTS IN BRIEF

CONTENTS

UNIT I

Foundations of Pediatric Nursing

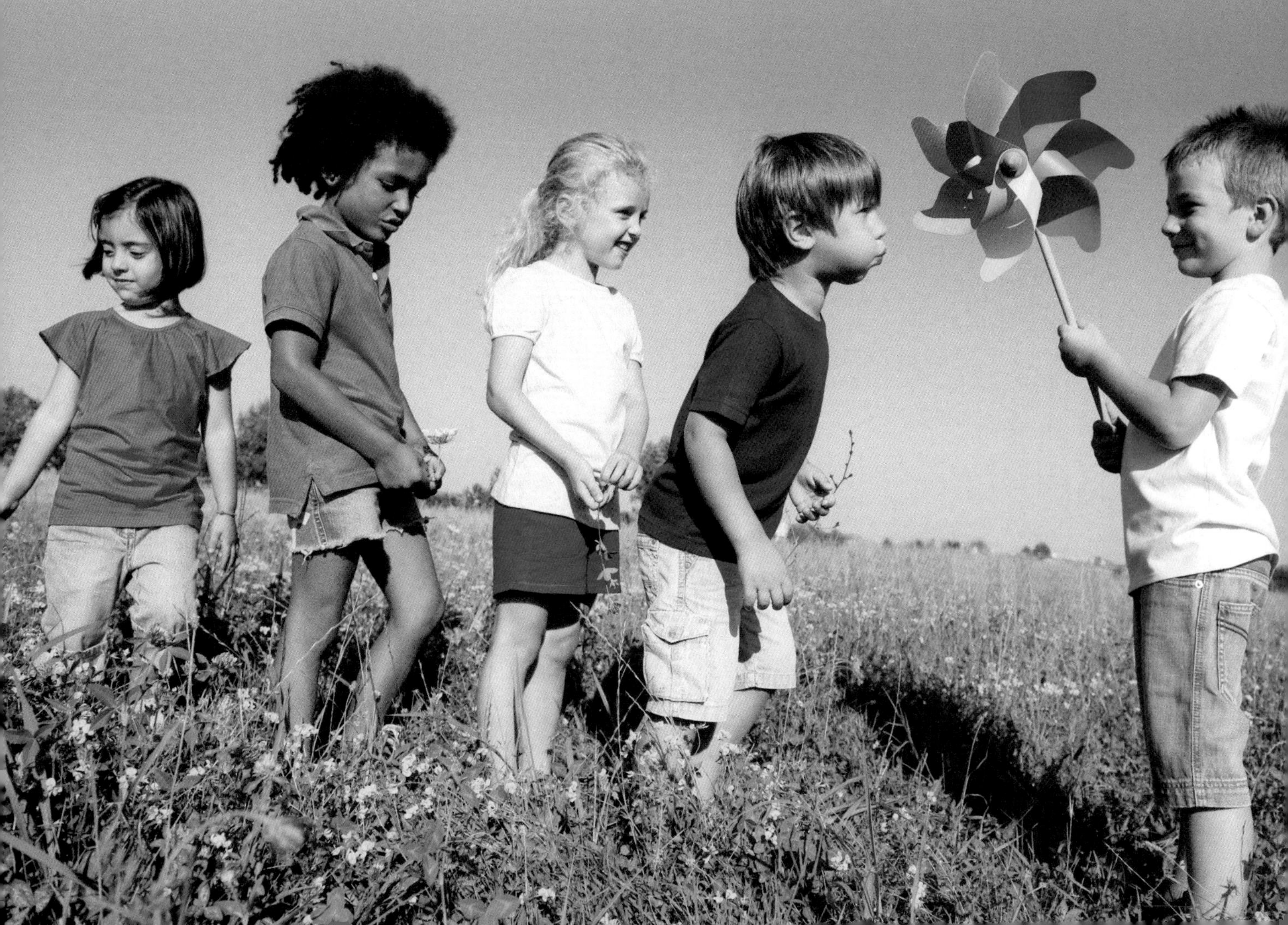

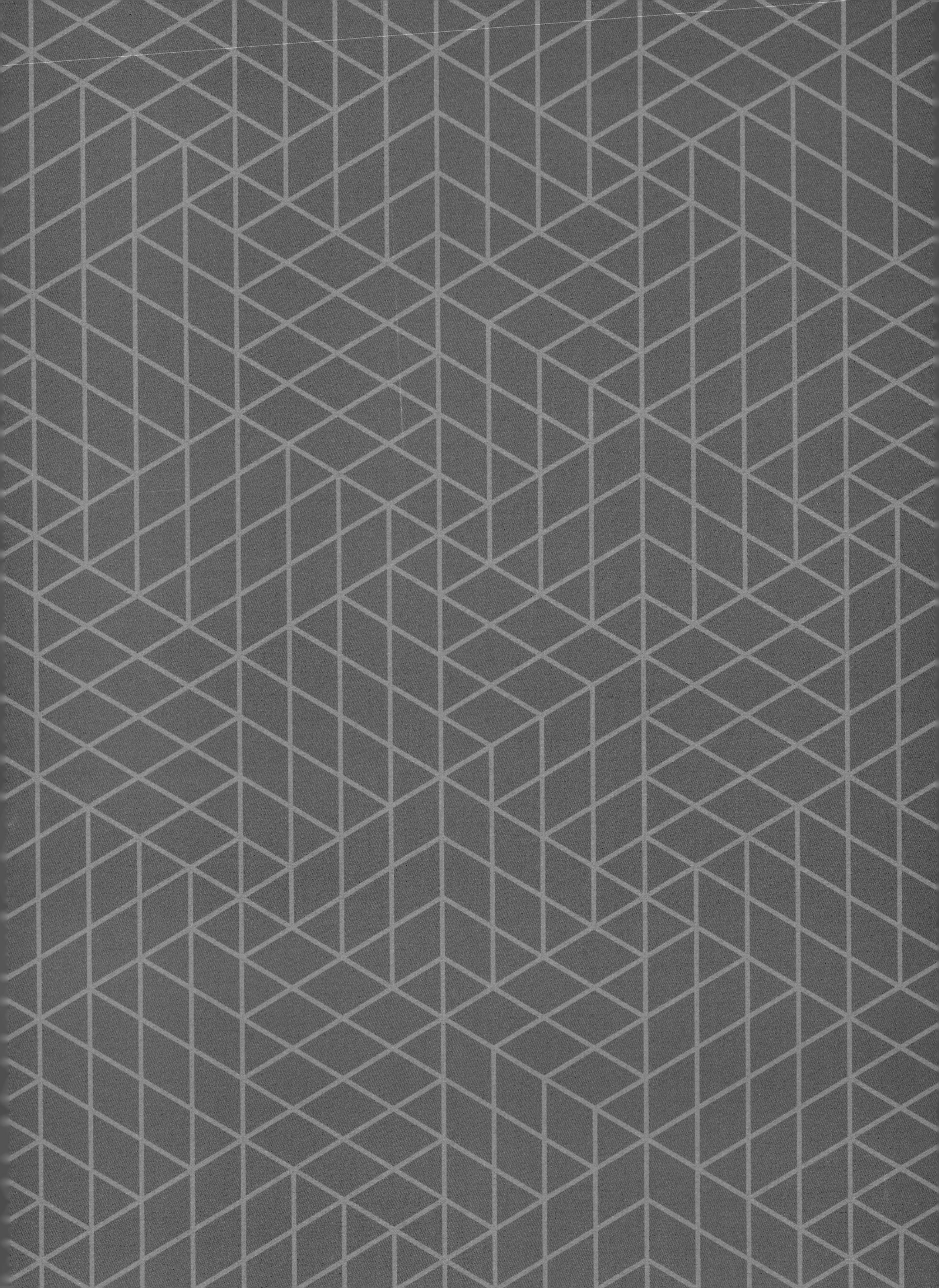

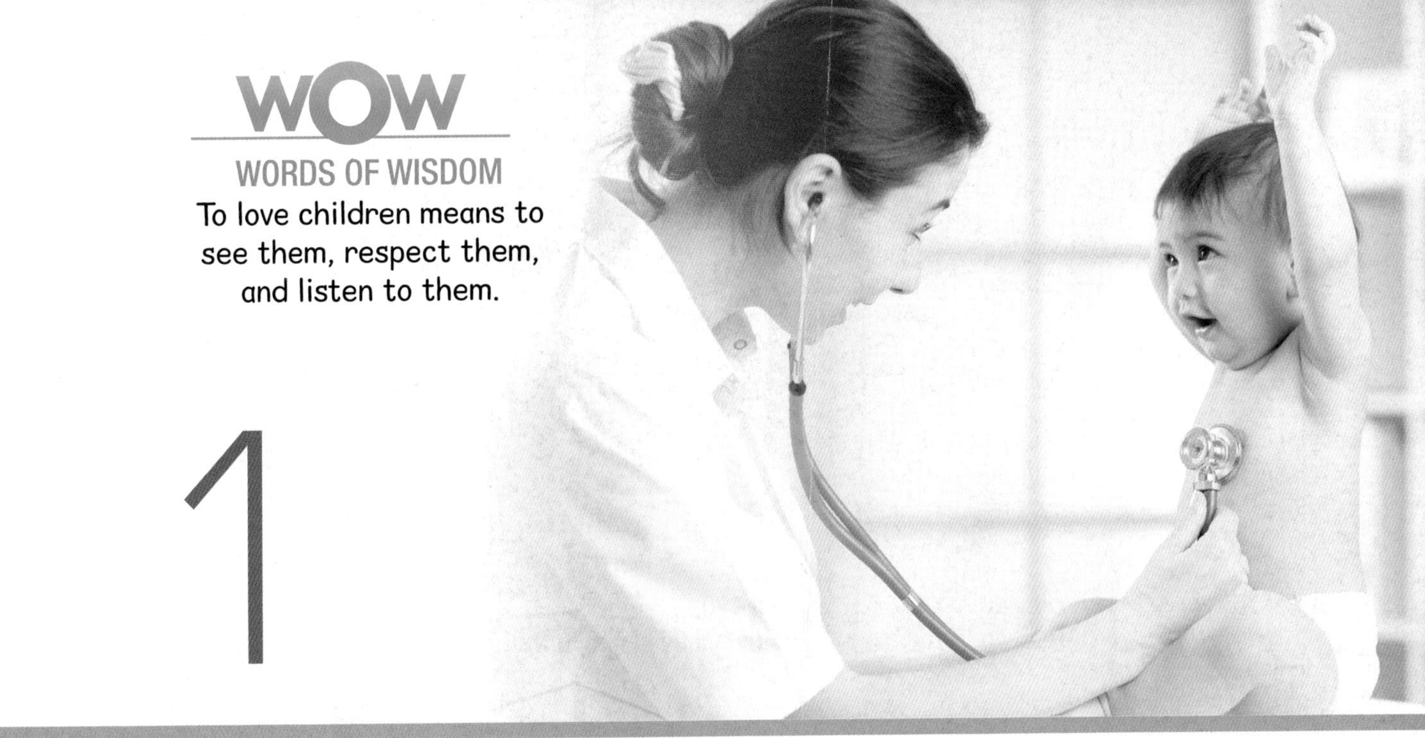
WOW
WORDS OF WISDOM
To love children means to see them, respect them, and listen to them.
1

Introduction to Child Health and Pediatric Nursing

KEY TERMS

assent

do not attempt resuscitation (DNAR) order

emancipated minor

informed consent

mature minor

morbidity

mortality

nursing process

standard of care

LEARNING OBJECTIVES

Upon completion of the chapter, you will be able to:

1. Discuss different methods of measuring child health.
2. Discuss the philosophy of pediatric nursing care.
3. Identify the major roles and functions of pediatric nursing, including the scope of practice and the professional standards for pediatric nurses.
4. Explain the components of the nursing process as they relate to nursing practice for children and their families.
5. Identify ethical concepts related to providing nursing care to children and their families.
6. Describe legal issues related to caring for children and their families.

Isabelle Romano is a 6-year-old with cerebral palsy. She was born at 28 weeks' gestation and is currently admitted to the hospital due to difficulty breathing secondary to pneumonia. Her parents are very active in her care. Isabelle lives at home with her parents and two brothers, Sergio and Tito. Consider how your role as a nurse can affect this family.

INTRODUCTION

Children are the future of our society. Their overall health has improved, and rates of death and illness in some areas have decreased, but we still must focus on children's health both in the United States and globally. Habits and practices established in childhood have profound effects on health and illness throughout life. As a society, creating a population that cares about children and promotes preventive and quality health care and positive lifestyle choices is crucial. Pediatric nurses play a major role in this task. They are often "in the trenches" advocating on various issues, drawing attention to the importance of health care for children, encouraging focus on education and prevention, and assisting families who lack resources or access to health care. This chapter provides an overview of child health, an introduction to pediatric nursing, and a discussion of ethical and legal issues related to caring for children.

CHILD HEALTH

Children are a gift to this world, and as such, it is society's responsibility to nurture and care for them. In the past, health was defined simply as the absence of disease; health was measured by monitoring the mortality and morbidity of a group. Over the past century, however, the focus of health has shifted to disease prevention, health promotion, and wellness. The World Health Organization (WHO, 2022) defines health as "a state of complete physical, mental, and social well-being, and not merely the absence of disease or infirmity."

The History of Child Health and Child Health Care

In past centuries in the United States, the health of the country was poorer than it is today; mortality rates were high, and life expectancy was short. When a large number of people immigrating from Europe settled in eastern American cities, infectious diseases were rampant due to crowded living conditions, inadequate and unsafe food (e.g., contaminated milk), lack of childhood immunizations, and harsh working conditions (including child labor). Devastating epidemics of smallpox, diphtheria, scarlet fever, and measles hit children the hardest. During this period, the prevalent view was that children were a commodity; their role was to increase the population and share in the work to be done. This view has changed over the years. Public schools were established, and the court system began viewing children as minors. The health of children began to receive more and more attention.

As the end of the 19th century neared, doctors and scientists gained a better understanding of the root causes of illness. This knowledge helped fuel public health efforts, such as the campaign for safe milk supply, which led to pasteurizing milk and to dispensing free milk in some cities (Maternal and Child Health Bureau [MCHB], Health Resources and Services Administration [HRSA], U.S. Department of Health and Human Services, n.d.). Compulsory vaccination programs began during this time. In the late 1800s, some states mandated smallpox vaccination as a condition of school attendance. These public health efforts led to a decrease in infant and child deaths (MCHB, HRSA, U.S. Department of Health and Human Services, n.d.).

In the late 19th and early 20th centuries, cities became healthier places to live due to urban public health improvements, such as sanitation services, treated municipal water, and improvements in hygiene (MCHB, HRSA, U.S. Department of Health and Human Services, n.d.). The threat of childhood diseases such as diphtheria, cholera, polio, and yellow fever began to take less of a toll on children (MCHB, HRSA, U.S. Department of Health and Human Services, n.d.). The turn of the 20th century brought new knowledge about nutrition, sanitation, bacteriology, pharmacology, medication, and psychology. Penicillin, corticosteroids, and increased numbers of vaccines, which were developed during this time, assisted with the fight against communicable diseases. Thus, by the end of the 20th century, unintentional injuries surpassed disease as the leading cause of death for children older than 1 year (Guyer et al., 2000).

By the end of the 1990s, technologic advances had significantly affected all aspects of health care. These trends have led to increased survival rates in children. However, many children who survive illnesses that were previously considered fatal are left with chronic disabilities. For example, before the 1960s, extremely premature infants did not survive because of the immaturity of their lungs. The use of medications to foster lung development has increased survival rates in premature infants, but many of these children are faced with chronic illnesses such as chronic lung disease (bronchopulmonary dysplasia), retinopathy of prematurity, cerebral palsy, and neurodevelopmental impairments (Mandy, 2022, 2023). This increased survival has resulted in a significant increase in chronic illness relative to acute illness as a cause of hospitalization and mortality (Mandy, 2023).

The beginning of the 21st century has brought tremendous improvements in technology and biomedicine. This has created a trend toward earlier diagnosis and treatment of disorders and diseases. Remarkable progress has been made linking genetics and pathophysiologic processes. Gene therapy holds the promise of correcting genetic disease before birth as research continues to progress in this area. In 2019, the Food and Drug Administration (FDA) approved an intravenous gene therapy construct for spinal muscular atrophy (FDA, 2019). In addition, many genetic defects are being identified so that counseling and treatment may occur early. Advancements in diagnostic technology and treatment methods continue to improve child health. For example, less invasive ways to administer insulin, such as inhaled insulin, have been FDA approved for adults and are currently being studied for use in children ages 4 to 18 (U.S. National Library of Medicine, ClinicalTrials.gov, 2022).

In addition to improvement in technology and biomedicine, a number of national and international organizations have been formed in recent years to protect children's rights both in the United States and worldwide. These organizations focus on such issues as violence and abuse, child labor and soldiering, juvenile justice, child immigrants, orphaned children, and children who are abandoned or experiencing homelessness—all of which have a negative impact on children's health. A child whose rights are restored and upheld has an improved opportunity for growth, development, education, and health.

The gains in child health have been huge, but unfortunately, these gains are not shared equally among all children. Certain health concerns, such as poor nutrition, higher weight, lead poisoning, and asthma, affect children from families with lower incomes at higher rates and with greater severity than those from higher-income families (American Academy of Pediatrics, Council on Community Pediatrics, 2016, reaffirmed 2021). Unintentional injuries continue to be the leading cause of death in children older than 1 year, but children's health remains threatened by illnesses and other health-related conditions in the 21st century (Centers for Disease Control and Prevention [CDC]/National Center for Health Statistics [NCHS], 2022c). Higher weight, environmental toxins, allergies, drug use, child abuse and neglect, and mental illnesses are among some of the key issues that endanger children's health today.

Federal Legislation Affecting Child Health

Numerous federal programs have had a major impact on child health. President Theodore Roosevelt began the crusade to assist children and their families, especially those with lower incomes. The establishment of the Children's Bureau in 1912 began a period of studying economic and social factors related to infant mortality, infant care in rural areas, and other factors related to children's health. The goal of these legislative efforts was to improve the standards of health care. These actions demonstrate the value society has placed on the welfare of children. Table 1.1 lists several significant pieces of federal legislation and describes their impact on children's health.

TABLE 1.1 • Milestones in Federal Programs in Support of Children's Health

Date	Action	Impact
1909	First White House Conference on Care of Dependent Children (convened by President Theodore Roosevelt)	Addressed the poor working and living conditions of many children in the United States; aimed at improving the lives of children
1912/1913	U.S. Children's Bureau	Established the first governmental agency to oversee children's health and environmental conditions, with its purpose being to research and report all issues pertaining to all children's well-being and to assist states and local government in preventing child abuse and neglect
1921	Maternity and Infancy (Sheppard–Towner) Act	Provided grants to states to establish maternal and child health divisions in state health departments
1930	White House Conference on Child Welfare Standards	Produced the Children's Charter, documenting the child's need for health, education, welfare, and protection
1935	The Social Security Act	Established federal–state partnership and provided Aid to Dependent Families and Children (ADFC), maternal and child health services, and child welfare services
1946	National School Lunch Program	Provides nutritious, well-balanced lunches to children each day at school for free or a low cost; also provides meal supplements for children in after-school care and nutrition programs for children experiencing homelessness
1962	National Institute of Child Health and Human Development (NICHD)	Supported and performed research on child, maternal, adult, and family health issues
1964	Head Start	Provides child development programs to pregnant people, families, and children from birth to age 5 with the overarching goal of increasing school readiness for children from families with low incomes
1965	Medicaid Program under Title XIX of Social Security Act; special programs such as Child Health Assessment Program	Provided state block grants to reduce financial barriers to health care for people with low incomes and special services to pregnant people, young children, and people with disabilities

(continued)

TABLE 1.1 • Milestones in Federal Programs in Support of Children's Health (*continued*)

Date	Action	Impact
1966/1974	Women, Infants, Children (WIC) program	Provided nutritional supplementation and education to families with low incomes; pregnant, postpartum, and lactating people; and infants and children up to age 5
1968	Expansion of National School Lunch Act	Provided food for school-age children from families with low incomes year-round along with those in day care and Head Start programs
1969	U.S. Children's Bureau moved to Department of Health, Education, and Welfare (HEW)	Established greater presence for these programs
1972	Head Start to serve children with disabilities	Mandated that at least 10% of the children enrolled in Head Start must have disabilities
1975	Education for All Handicapped Children Act (Public Law 94-142)	Established federally mandated special education in public schools
	Title XX Social Services	Provided block grants to day care, emergency shelters, counseling, family planning, and other services for children
1976	The Supplemental Security Income (SSI) Disabled Children's Program	Provided cash to children with disabilities from families with low incomes to help manage health care costs
1981	Alcohol, Drug Abuse, and Mental Health Services Block Grants	Began funding services for children and adolescents with mental health issues
1986	Education for All Handicapped Children Act amendments (Public Law 99-457)	Established federal funding for states to create statewide, comprehensive, coordinated, and multidisciplinary early-intervention services for infants and toddlers with disabilities
1990	Omnibus Budget Reconciliation Act	Extended Medicaid coverage to all children (6–18 years) with family incomes below 133% of the federal poverty threshold
1990	Bright Futures	Provided a comprehensive set of child health supervision guidelines for health professionals, families, and communities as well as training for these groups to work toward optimal child health
1991	Healthy Start	Community-based program that provides services to at-risk childbearing people from preconception to postpartum to help reduce infant mortality
1993	Family and Medical Leave Act (FMLA)	Allows eligible employees to take up to 12 weeks of unpaid leave from their jobs every year to care for newborns or newly adopted children or of children, parents, or spouses who have serious health conditions; employee can return to previous job or a comparable job with the same conditions
1995	Early Head Start Program	Federally funded community-based program for families with low incomes focused on child development
1997	Children's Health Insurance Program (CHIP) (formerly known as State Children's Health Insurance Program [SCHIP])	Offers federal assistance to state-based health insurance for families with low incomes who are not eligible for Medicaid but cannot afford private insurance
2000	Children's Health Act	Led to increased research and treatment of children's health issues, such as autism, asthma, epilepsy, and oral health
2002	No Child Left Behind Act	Aimed at ensuring all children in all classrooms received research-based curricula, well-prepared teachers, and safe learning environments
2006	Combating Autism Act	Led to increasing autism awareness by increasing funding for research, surveillance, diagnosis, and treatment
2007	WIC food package revised	Designed to improve nutritional intake of WIC recipients by supporting and promoting long-term breastfeeding and adding fruits and vegetables, whole grains, soy-based foods, and a variety of culturally appropriate foods

TABLE 1.1 • Milestones in Federal Programs in Support of Children's Health

Date	Action	Impact
2008	Newborn Screening Saves Lives Act	Provided increased funding for newborn screening grants and provided more education and outreach, coordination of follow-up care after screening, and evaluation of newborn screening program effectiveness
2009	CHIP Reauthorization Act	Expanded the program to cover more children without insurance
2009	American Recovery and Reinvestment Act	Designated money to fund and expand programs such as Head Start, foster care, and the Supplemental Nutrition Assistance Program (food stamp program) as well as creating new jobs and improving services such as community health centers and unemployment benefits during the economic recession
2010	Affordable Care Act (Patient Protection and Affordable Care Act; Health Care and Education Reconciliation Act)	Increased coverage by expanding Medicaid; ending preexisting conditions exclusion for children; holding insurance companies accountable by ending lifetime coverage limits; requiring insurance companies to publicly justify premium increases; decreasing health care costs; increasing choice; and enhancing quality of care for all Americans by covering all preventive care
2014	Birth to Five: Watch Me Thrive	A federal initiative program that promotes developmental and behavioral screening for children with the goal of improving early diagnosis and treatment of children with developmental delays
2018	Helping Ensure Access for Little One, Toddlers, and Hopeful Youth by Keeping Insurance Delivery Stable (HEALTHY KIDS) Act	Extended funding for CHIP through 2027
2018	Maternal, Infant, and Early Childhood Home Visiting (MIECHV) program	The Bipartisan Budget Control Act extended funding for 5 years for the MIECHV program, which provides home visits to improve health and development outcomes for at-risk children.

National Conference of State Legislatures. (2020). *Children's Health Insurance Program Overview.* Retrieved September 1, 2022, from https://www.ncsl.org/research/health/childrens-health-insurance-program-overview.aspx; Yarrow, A. L. (2011). A history of federal child antipoverty and health policy in the United States since 1900. *Child Development Perspectives, 5*(1), 66–72; GovTrack. (2022). *H.R. 3921—115th Congress: HEALTHY KIDS Act.* Retrieved September 1, 2022, from https://www.govtrack.us/congress/bills/115/hr3921; Maternal and Child Health Bureau, Health Resources and Services Administration, & U.S. Department of Health and Human Services. (n.d.). *MCH timeline.* Retrieved August 10, 2022, from https://mchb.hrsa.gov/about/timeline/index.asp; HHS.gov/HealthCare. (2022). *About the Affordable Care Act.* Retrieved September 6, 2022, from https://www.hhs.gov/healthcare/about-the-aca/index.html

Referring back to the Romano family at the beginning of the chapter, what federal programs may be available to assist them?

Measurement of Children's Health Status

In 1979, the U.S. Surgeon General's Healthy People initiative presented an agenda for the nation that identified the most significant preventable threats to health. With the series of updates that followed, including the present one, Healthy People 2030, the United States has a comprehensive health promotion and disease prevention agenda with specific goals and objectives for improving the quantity and quality of life in the United States. Overarching goals are to attain healthy, thriving lives and eliminate preventable disease, disability, injury, and premature death; achieve health equity, eliminate disparities, and attain health literacy to improve the health of all groups; create physical, economic, and social environments that promote good health and well-being for all; promote healthy development and behaviors across every stage of life; and engage leadership, the public, and key constituents to take action and develop policies that will improve the health and well-being of all (U.S. Department of Health and Human Services, Office of Disease Prevention and Health Promotion, 2021a). The principle behind this report is that setting national objectives and monitoring their progress can motivate action and change. The report incorporates input from public health and prevention experts; federal, state, and local governments; over 2,000 organizations; and the public to develop health objectives.

There are specific health topic areas, including children's health topics, that serve as a method for evaluation of progress made in public health. These topic areas also serve as focal points to coordinate national health improvement efforts. For example, one objective under the physical activity topic is to increase the proportion of adolescents who meet current federal physical activity guidelines for aerobic physical activity and for muscle strengthening activity (U.S. Department of Health and

Human Services, Office of Disease Prevention and Health Promotion, 2021b). See the Healthy People 2030 features throughout the text for specific objectives, nursing implications, and guidance related to working toward achieving these objectives.

Measuring a child's health status is not always a simple process. For example, some children with chronic illnesses do not see themselves as "ill" if their disease is under control. A traditional method of measuring health is to examine mortality and morbidity data. This information is collected and analyzed to provide an objective description of a population's health.

Mortality Data

Mortality is the number of individuals who have died over a specific period. This statistic is generally presented as rates per 100,000 population and is calculated from a sample of death certificates. The National Center for Health Statistics, under the U.S. Department of Health and Human Services, collects, analyzes, and disseminates these data.

NEONATAL AND INFANT MORTALITY RATE

Neonatal mortality is the number of infant deaths occurring in the first 28 days of life per 1,000 live births. The infant mortality rate refers to the number of deaths occurring in the first 12 months of life. It is also documented as the number of deaths in relation to 1,000 live births. The infant mortality rate is used as an index of the general health of a country. Generally, this statistic is one of the most significant measures of children's health. In 2020, the infant mortality rate in the United States was 5.4 per 1,000 live births (CDC, 2022). See Figure 1.1.

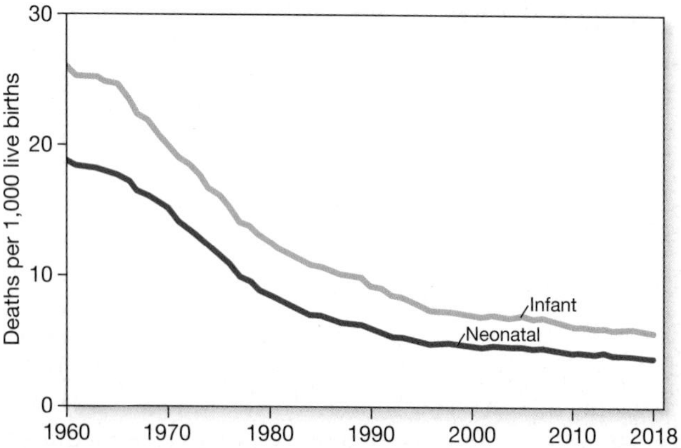

NOTE: Rates are infant (under 1 year) and neonatal (under 28 days) deaths per 1,000 live births in specified group.
SOURCE: NCHS, National Vital Statistics System, Mortality.

FIGURE 1.1 Infant and neonatal mortality from 1995 to 2020. (Data from Ely, D. M., & Driscoll, A. K. [2022]. Infant mortality in the United States, 2020: Data from the period linked birth/infant death file. *National Vital Statistics Reports, 71*[5], 1–17. https://doi.org/10.15620/cdc:120700.)

The infant mortality rate varies greatly from state to state as well as among ethnic groups. The United States has one of the highest gross national products in the world and is known for its technologic capabilities, but its infant mortality rate is much higher than—in some cases doubled—that of most other nations with similar resources (Central Intelligence Agency, 2022). The main causes of early infant death in the United States include congenital malformations, short gestation, low birth weight, sudden infant death syndrome, unintentional injuries, and maternal complications during pregnancy (Ely & Driscoll, 2022).

TAKE NOTE!

Non-Hispanic Black infants have consistently had higher infant mortality rates compared to other ethnic groups (CDC, 2022).

Preterm births and low birth weight are key risk factors for infant death; the lower the birth weight, the higher the risk of infant mortality. The percentage of infants born preterm in the United States hit a peak in 2006; thus, preterm-related causes of infant death increased during this time. From 2007 to 2014, preterm birth rates declined each year, but from 2015 until 2019, they began to rise again. In 2021, preterm birth rates hit an all-time high (Hamilton et al., 2022). This rising trend will need to be closely monitored to understand what is contributing to this increase and what can be done to help decrease the incidence of preterm birth.

CHILDHOOD MORTALITY RATE

Childhood mortality is defined as the number of deaths per 100,000 population in children between 1 and 14 years of age. The childhood mortality rate in the United States has decreased significantly since 1980, but disparities by sex, age, race, and ethnicity persist (America's Health Rankings, United Health Foundation, 2022). In 2020, the mortality rate for children between ages 1 and 4 years was 22.7 per 100,000, with the leading cause of death being unintentional injuries followed by congenital malformations, then homicide (CDC/NCHS, 2022c). The mortality rate for children aged 5 to 14 years was 13.7 per 100,000, with the leading cause being unintentional injuries followed by cancer, then congenital malformations (CDC/NCHS, 2022c). Other causes of childhood mortality include suicide, diseases of the heart, influenza, and pneumonia.

Even as research continues into the preventable nature of childhood injuries, unintentional injury, such as from motor vehicle collisions, fires, drowning, bicycle or pedestrian mishaps, poisoning, and falls, remains a leading cause of mortality and morbidity in children (Federal Interagency Forum on Child and Family Statistics, 2021). These injuries have far-reaching consequences for children, families, and society in general. Risk factors associated with childhood injuries include young age, male sex, low socioeconomic status, parents who are unmarried or single, low maternal education level, poor housing, parental drug or alcohol misuse, and low support within the family. These deaths can often be prevented through education about the value of using car seats and seat belts; the dangers of driving under the influence of alcohol and other substances; and the importance of pedestrian and bicycle safety, fire safety, water safety, and home safety.

TAKE NOTE!

In the United States, American Indian and Alaska Native children and Black children have the highest unintentional injury death rate (CDC, 2021).

Morbidity Data

Morbidity is the measure of prevalence of a specific illness in a population at a particular time. It is presented in rates per 1,000 population. Morbidity is often difficult to define and record because the definitions used vary widely. For example, morbidity may be defined as visits to the health care provider or diagnosis for hospital admission. Data may also be difficult to obtain. Morbidity statistics are revised less frequently because of the difficulty in defining or obtaining the information.

In general, however, as reported in a summary of health statistics for children, the vast majority of children are considered to be in excellent, very good, or good health, with only 2.1% reporting fair or poor health based on data collected via survey (CDC/NCHS, 2022a). Factors that may increase morbidity include homelessness, poverty, low birth weight, chronic health disorders, foreign-born adoption, attendance at day care centers, and barriers to health care. For example, 16.1% of children live in poverty and have a higher incidence of disease, limited coordination of health services, and limited access to health care, except for visits to the emergency department (Creamer et al., 2022). The overall poverty rate in 2021 was 11.6%, marking the second increase in the past 5 years (Shrider et al., 2021). However, the poverty rate among Black and Hispanic Americans is 19.5% and 17.1%, respectively; these children are particularly at increased risk for illness (Creamer et al., 2022).

The most important aspect of morbidity is the degree of disability it produces, which is identified in children as the number of days missed from school or confined to bed. In 2021, 4.4% of school-age children (ages 5 to 17) missed 11 or more days of school because of injury or illness (CDC/NCHS, 2022b).

Common health problems in children include respiratory disorders, gastrointestinal disturbances that lead to malnutrition and dehydration, and injuries. In 2018, acute bronchitis, asthma, pneumonia, epilepsy/convulsions, and depressive disorders were the major causes of hospitalization in children 1 to 17 years of age (McDermott & Roemer, 2021). Inpatient hospital stays due to depressive disorders were twice as high for females as for males (McDermott & Roemer, 2021).

As more immunizations become available, common childhood communicable diseases affect fewer children. The tracking of the leading topics from Healthy People provides some positive information related to improving children's health. Improvements have occurred in child health, but morbidity and disability from some conditions, such as asthma, diabetes, attention deficit disorders, and higher weight, have increased in recent decades. Also, disparities in health status among U.S. children reflect widening social inequalities.

One trend in the United States is the increasing number of children with mental health disorders and related emotional, social, or behavioral problems. It is estimated that one in five children in the United States have a mental, emotional, developmental, or behavioral disorder (Office of the Surgeon General, 2021). Recent research has found that depressive and anxiety symptoms increased during the COVID-19 pandemic (Office of the Surgeon General, 2021). These problems may limit the child's educational success and increase the risk for significant mental health problems later in life, emotional problems, possible use of firearms, reckless driving, risky sexual activity, and substance misuse during adolescence. Overall, these behavioral, social, and educational problems can interfere with children's social and academic development. Often, insurance may not reimburse for treating these problems, leading to additional concerns about access to treatment.

TAKE NOTE!

The U.S. Surgeon General issued an advisory to call the American people's attention to the increasing concerns regarding the mental health of our youth and the negative effects of social media on our youth's mental health (Office of the Surgeon General, 2023).

Environmental and psychosocial factors are an area of concern in children. They include academic difficulties, complex psychiatric disorders, self-harm and harm to others, use of firearms, hostility at school, substance misuse, human immunodeficiency virus (HIV)/acquired immunodeficiency syndrome (AIDS), and adverse effects of the media.

Referring back to Isabelle Romano and her family from the beginning of the chapter, what changes in child health in the United States may have affected them?

PEDIATRIC NURSING

Pediatric nursing is the practice of nursing involved in the health care of children from infancy through adolescence. In the United States, the number of children younger than age 18 years is approximately 72.8 million, accounting for almost 22% of the population (Federal Interagency Forum on Child and Family Statistics, 2021). The definition of nursing, "the protection, promotion, and optimization of health and abilities; prevention of illness and injury; facilitation of healing; alleviation of suffering through the diagnosis and treatment of human response; and advocacy in the care of individuals, families, groups, communities, and populations," also applies to the practice of pediatric nursing (American Nurses Association [ANA], n.d.). However, the overall goal of pediatric nursing practice is to promote and assist the child in maintaining optimal levels of health while recognizing the influence of the family on the child's well-being. This goal involves the practice of health promotion and disease prevention as well as assisting with care during disease or illness.

Evolution of Pediatric Nursing

In 1870, the first pediatric professorship for a health care provider was awarded in the United States to Abraham Jacobi, who is known as the founder of pediatrics. For the first time, the medical community realized there was a need to provide specialized training and education about children to health care providers. In the early 1900s, Lillian Wald established the Henry Street Settlement House in New York City; this was the start of public health nursing. This facility provided medical and other services to families with limited resources. These services included home nurse visits to teach families about health care.

During this time, health care personnel were trained to take care of children in hospitals, but parents of hospitalized children were discouraged from visiting to prevent the spread of infection. Restricting parents from being involved in their child's care was also thought to minimize emotional stress.

Nursing in public schools began in 1902 with the appointment of Lina Rogers as a full-time public school nurse in New York. A professional course in pediatric nursing was started in the early 1900s at the Teachers College of Columbia University.

In the 1960s, changes in the health care delivery system and shifts in the population's health status led to the development of the nurse practitioner role. Loretta Ford was the founder of the first nurse practitioner program. Cost-control systems from the federal government due to rapid escalation of health care expenditures were instituted in the 1970s. In addition, the considerable changes in the U.S. health care system in the 1980s affected pediatric nursing and child health care. The emphasis of care was on quality outcomes and cost containment. Some of these changes brought more advanced practice nurses into the field of pediatrics.

In the 1980s, the division of Maternal and Child Health Nursing Practice of the ANA developed maternal and child health standards to provide important guidelines for delivering nursing care.

In the 1990s, the Institute of Medicine published reports pointing out the need to improve quality and safety of the American health care system. This led to an increased focus on improving health care outcomes. As the health care environment continued to increase in complexity and hospitalized patients got sicker, programs were created for nurses to obtain a level of expertise and to validate mastery of their skills and knowledge by passing a national standardized examination. Registered nurses and nurse practitioners can be certified in different specialties, including pediatrics. These certifications show a commitment to lifelong learning and the ability to stay up to date in the rapidly changing health care environment. In recent years, pediatric nursing certifications have become increasingly specialized; for example, certifications are available in pediatric hematology/oncology nursing and pediatric emergency nursing.

Philosophy of Pediatric Nursing

Children need access to care that is continuous, comprehensive, coordinated, family centered, and compassionate. This care needs to focus on their changing physical, developmental, and emotional needs. Pediatric nurses provide this care by focusing on the family, providing atraumatic therapeutic care, and using evidence-based practice. These three concepts represent an overarching philosophy of pediatric nursing care and are integrated throughout the chapters of this book.

Parents and caregivers play a critical role in the health and well-being of children. Providing care through a family-centered approach leads not only to better outcomes but also to better consumer satisfaction. The family is the child's primary source of support and strength. The knowledge that the family has about a child's health or illness is vital. Family-centered care involves a mutually beneficial partnership among the child, the family, and the health care professionals (American Academy of Pediatrics, Committee on Hospital Care, Institute for Patient, and Family-Centered Care, 2012, reaffirmed 2018). It applies to the planning, delivery, and evaluation of health care for children of all ages in any setting (see Chapter 8).

Children may undergo a wide range of interventions, many of which can be traumatic, stressful, and painful. The various settings in which the child receives care can be scary and overwhelming to the child and the family, and interacting with health care personnel in various settings can cause anxiety. Thus, another major component of the pediatric nursing philosophy is providing atraumatic care. This is a philosophy of providing therapeutic care through interventions that minimize physical and psychological distress for children and their families (see Chapter 8).

Evidence-based practice involves the use of research findings in establishing a plan of care and implementing that care. It is a clinical decision-making approach involving the integration of the best scientific evidence, patient values and preferences, clinical circumstances, and clinical expertise to promote best outcomes (Melnyk & Fineout-Overholt, 2015). It is important that nurses develop the skills and knowledge necessary to ask pertinent clinical questions, search for current best evidence, analyze the evidence, integrate the evidence into practice when appropriate, and evaluate the outcomes. Evidence-based practice will lead to a decrease in variations in care while at the same time increasing quality and improving health care and patient outcomes.

Role of the Pediatric Nurse

The primary role of the pediatric nurse is to provide direct nursing care to children and their families, while being an educator and manager. As a child and family advocate, the nurse safeguards and advances the interests of children and their families by knowing their needs and resources, informing them of their rights and options, and assisting them in making informed decisions. In the role of educator, the nurse instructs and counsels children and their families about all aspects of health and illness. The pediatric nurse ensures that communication with the child and family is based on the child's age and developmental level. The pediatric nurse uses and integrates research findings to establish evidence-based practice, managing the delivery of care in a cost-effective manner to promote continuity of care and an optimal outcome for the child and family.

The pediatric nurse also serves as a collaborator, care coordinator, and consultant. Collaborating with the interdisciplinary health care team, the pediatric nurse integrates the child's and family's needs into a coordinated plan of care. In the role of consultant, the pediatric nurse ensures that the child's and family's needs are met through such activities as support group facilitation or working with the school nurse to plan the child's care.

The dimensions of pediatric health care are changing. We live in a global community in which distances have been minimized, enabling all of us to learn, share, and exchange information. The pediatric nurse needs to be alert to the wide-ranging developmental and mental health needs of children as well as to the traits and behaviors that may lead to serious health problems. The scope of pediatric health care practice is much broader today, and pediatric nurses must include quality evidence-based interventions when developing the plan of care. In addition, pediatric nurses must incorporate new information about genetics and neurobiology and must continue to keep up with the technology explosion.

Providing Culturally Focused Care

The United States is a society that includes various cultures and ethnicities, and each distinct individual brings a diversity and richness that enriches the country as a whole. Children do not fit into set categories or groups. Children and families vary by culture, family structure, socioeconomic status, background, and circumstances, so each child who enters the health care system should be considered a unique individual. Pediatric nurses must have greater sensitivity to the background of each child and must be able to provide care that addresses the child's uniqueness.

Providing Care Across the Health–Illness Continuum

As a result of improved diagnosis and treatment, the pediatric nurse now cares for children who have survived once-fatal situations, are living well beyond the usual life expectancy for a specific illness, or are functioning and attending school with chronic disabilities. While positive and exciting, these advances and trends pose new challenges for the health care community. For example, as care for premature newborns improves and survival rates have increased, so too has the incidence of long-term chronic conditions such as respiratory airway dysfunction or developmental delays. As a result, pediatric nurses care for children at all stages along the health–illness continuum, from well children to those who are occasionally ill to those with chronic, sometimes disabling conditions.

Providing Family-Centered Care

Due to the influence of managed care and the focus on prevention, better education, and technologic advances, people have taken increased responsibility for their own health. Families now want information about their child's illness, they want to participate in making decisions about treatment, and they want to accompany their children to all health care situations. As child advocates who value family-centered care, pediatric nurses can provide such empowerment and can address specific issues for children and families. Pediatric nurses must respect the family's views and concerns, address those issues and concerns, regard the parents and caregivers as important participants in their child's health, and always include the child and family in the decision-making process (see Chapter 8 for more information).

Providing Preventive Care

Efforts to reduce costs have also led to an increased emphasis on preventive care. Anticipatory guidance is vital during each health contact with children and their families. Education of the family includes everything from keeping the home safe to preventing illness. These are major points of emphasis for pediatric nurses as they deliver care to children and their families.

Providing a Continuum of Care

In an effort to become more cost-effective and to provide care more efficiently, the nursing care of children now encompasses a continuum of care that extends from acute care settings such as hospitals to outpatient settings such as ambulatory care clinics, primary care offices, rehabilitative units, community care settings, long-term facilities, homes, and schools. For example, after an acute hospital stay, a child may be able to complete therapy at home, school, or another community setting and can reenter the hospital for short periods for specific treatments or illness. Nurses play a primary role in providing better follow-up and smoother transitions from one setting to the next.

Providing Child and Family Teaching

The nurse's role in relation to child morbidity and mortality involves educating the family and community regarding the usual causes of deaths, the types of childhood illnesses, and the symptoms that require health care. The goal is to raise awareness and provide guidance and counseling to prevent unnecessary deaths and illnesses in children. The health of children is basic to their well-being and development, and the attention given to children's health in this country has slowly increased over the years. The pediatric nurse is in an excellent position to improve the future health of children.

Participating in Research

Pediatric nursing involves all the essential components of contemporary nursing practice. The pediatric nurse makes use of theories and research pertaining specifically to children as well as general nursing concepts and research. Nurses must know about current trends in child health so that they can provide appropriate anticipatory guidance, counseling, and teaching for children and families and can identify high-risk groups so that interventions can be initiated early, before illness or death occurs.

Implementing the Nursing Process

The pediatric nurse performs all of these tasks using the framework of the **nursing process**. The nursing process is used to care for the child and family during health promotion, maintenance, restoration, and rehabilitation. It is a problem-solving method based on the scientific method that allows nursing care to be planned and implemented in a thorough, organized manner to ensure quality and consistency of care. The nursing process is applicable to all health care settings and consists of five steps: assessment, nursing analysis, outcome identification and planning, implementation, and outcome evaluation.

1. Assessment: Assessment involves collecting data about the child and family and performing physical assessment during community-based health services, at admission to an acute care setting, at periodic times during the child's hospitalization or care, and during home care visits.
2. Nursing analysis: The nurse analyzes the data collected during assessment to make clinical judgments about the child's health and developmental status. The actual or potential health problems that result from this clinical judgment process describe health promotion and health patterns that pediatric nurses can manage.
3. Planning and expected outcomes: The next step in the process involves developing nursing care plans that incorporate goals or expected outcomes that improve the child's dysfunctional health patterns, promote appropriate health patterns, or provide for optimal developmental outcomes. The care plan includes the specific nursing actions that assist in obtaining these outcomes.
4. Implementation: The planned interventions are implemented, adapted to the child's developmental level and family status, and modified if the child's response indicates the need. The care plan incorporates the family in addition to the child.
5. Evaluation: The process is continually evaluated and updated during the partnership with the child and family.

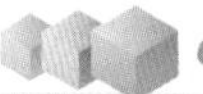
Concept Mastery Alert

Assessment

When prioritizing care for children who witnessed a traumatic incident, the nurse must remember that assessment is the first step in the nursing process.

Standardized care plans for specific patient problems and critical pathways for case management may be used in various pediatric settings. In general, care plans and critical pathways are becoming more evidence based, using a combination of research, group consensus, and past health care decisions to identify the most effective interventions for the child and family. Evidence-based care planning systems or tools can help bring evidence-based practices to the point of care. These templates can help improve the quality of patient care. The nurse is responsible for individualizing these standardized care plans based on the data collected during the assessment of the child and family and for evaluating the child's and family's response to the nursing interventions.

Nursing Practice Roles in Various Health Care Settings

The professional pediatric registered nurse provides care for children in a variety of settings. Acute care focuses on the diagnosis and treatment of illness and occurs in such settings as general pediatric hospital units, pediatric intensive care units, emergency departments, ambulatory clinics, surgical centers, and psychiatric centers. In the community, the focus is usually on health promotion and illness prevention. Various community settings include health clinics or offices, schools, homes, day care centers, and summer camps. Restorative, rehabilitative, or quality-of-life care generally takes place in rehabilitation centers or hospice programs or through service with a home health agency.

There are various practice roles for which the nurse's experience, competence, and educational level determine the nurse's position. For example, a clinical coordinator typically holds a baccalaureate degree and fills a leadership role in a variety of settings. The case manager, also usually a baccalaureate-prepared nurse, is responsible for integrating care from before admission to after discharge. The case manager coordinates the implementation of the interdisciplinary team in a collaborative manner to ensure continuity of care that is cost-effective, quality oriented, and outcome focused.

Various changes in the health care system continue to encourage the development of the advanced practice role for pediatric nursing. The advanced practice role is an expanded nursing role that requires additional education and skills in the assessment and care of children and their families. The pediatric nurse practitioner (PNP) has a master's degree and national certification in the specialty area. The PNP is an independent and autonomous practitioner. The PNP provides health maintenance care for children (such as well-child examinations and developmental screenings) and diagnoses and treats common childhood illnesses. The practitioner manages children's health in primary, acute, or intensive care settings or provides long-term care of the child with a chronic illness. The family nurse practitioner (FNP) and neonatal nurse practitioner (NNP) function in a similar manner to the PNP but provide care to individuals throughout the lifespan and to newborns, respectively. The clinical nurse specialist has a master's degree and provides expertise as an educator, clinician, or researcher, meeting the needs of staff, children, and families.

TAKE NOTE!

In 2004, the American Association of Colleges of Nursing (AACN) recommended that nurse practitioner education be moved from the master's to the doctoral level by the year 2015 due to the increasing complexity of the health care environment. Progress has been made in reaching this goal as doctoral nurse practitioner (DNP) programs offered have increased; all 50 states plus the District of Columbia have DNP programs available and there has also been a rise in enrollment in these programs (AACN, 2022).

Standards of Care and Performance in Today's Environment

In any role, the professional pediatric nurse is held accountable for nursing actions that adhere to standards of care. A **standard of care** is a minimally accepted action expected of an individual of a certain skill or knowledge level and reflects what a reasonable and prudent person would do in a similar situation. Professional standards from regulatory agencies, state or federal laws, nurse practice acts, and other specialty groups regulate nursing practice in general. The National Association of Pediatric Nurse Practitioners (NAPNAP), the Society of Pediatric Nurses (SPN), and the ANA have formulated specific standards of care and professional performance for pediatric clinical nursing practice (Table 1.2).

These standards are tools that determine if care constitutes adequate, effective, and acceptable nursing practice. They also serve as guides and legal measures for this special area of practice. These standards promote consistency in practice, provide important guidelines for care planning, assist with the development of outcome criteria, and ensure quality nursing care. The ANA–SPN standards specify what is adequate and effective for general pediatric nursing and promote consistency in practice.

Based on the Institute of Medicine's competencies for nursing, Quality and Safety Education for Nurses (QSEN) initiatives were developed to be integrated into nursing education. These quality and safety initiatives or competencies helped nurses improve the quality and safety of the health care system. Nurses need to understand these competencies and utilize them to continue to improve the quality and safety of their nursing practice.

TABLE 1.2 • National Association of Pediatric Nurse Practitioners, Society of Pediatric Nurses, and the American Nurses Association Scope and Standards of Pediatric Nursing Practice

	Standard: Description
Standards of practice	1. **Assessment:** The pediatric nurse collects comprehensive health data.
	2. **Diagnosis:** The pediatric nurse analyzes the assessment data in determining diagnosis.
	3. **Outcomes identification:** The pediatric nurse identifies expected outcomes individualized to the patient.
	4. **Planning:** The pediatric nurse develops a plan of care that prescribes interventions to attain expected outcomes.
	5. **Implementation:** The pediatric nurse implements the interventions identified in the plan of care, including coordination of care, health teaching, health promotion, and strategies to ensure a safe environment.
	6. **Evaluation:** The pediatric nurse evaluates the child's and family's progress toward attainment of outcomes.
Standards of professional performance	7. **Ethics:** The pediatric nurse's decisions and actions in all areas of practice are determined in an ethical manner.
	8. **Education:** The pediatric nurse acquires and maintains current knowledge and competency in pediatric nursing practice.
	9. **Evidence-based practice and research:** The pediatric nurse uses research findings in practice and participates in the generation of new knowledge.
	10. **Quality of practice:** The pediatric nurse systematically improves the quality and effectiveness of pediatric nursing practice.
	11. **Communication:** The pediatric nurse will communicate effectively in all areas of practice and in a variety of formats based on child, family, and colleague preferences.
	12. **Leadership:** The pediatric nurse demonstrates leadership in the practice setting and the profession.
	13. **Collaboration:** The pediatric nurse collaborates with the child, family, and other health care providers in providing patient care.
	14. **Professional practice evaluation:** The pediatric nurse evaluates their own nursing practice in relation to professional practice standards and relevant statutes and regulations.
	15. **Resource utilization:** The pediatric nurse considers factors related to safety, effectiveness, cost in planning and delivering care, and the impact on practice.
	16. **Environmental health:** The pediatric nurse practices and utilizes strategies that promote care in an environment that is safe and healthy.
	17. **Advocacy:** The pediatric nurse is an advocate for the patient and family.

From American Nurses Association, National Association of Pediatric Nurse Practitioners, & Society of Pediatric Nurses. (2015). *Pediatric Nursing: Scope and standards of practice* (2nd ed.). Nursebooks.org.

ETHICAL AND LEGAL ISSUES RELATED TO CARING FOR CHILDREN

Parents and guardians generally make choices about their child's health and services. As the legal custodians of minor children, they decide what is best for their children. Nurses caring for children and their families make the child's and family's needs a priority. Moral development (the ability to function in an ethical manner) and the legal requirements involved in working with children affect pediatric nurses on a daily basis. Pediatric nurses must function within ethical and legal boundaries related to care. They must understand their state's legal requirements for routine care, consent for treatment, hospitalization, and research.

TAKE NOTE!

As advocates for children, nurses support policies that protect children's rights and improve children's health care.

Ethical Issues Related to Working With Children and Their Families

Pediatric nurses must examine their own values so that they can provide nursing care in an ethical manner. Each situation must be evaluated individually. The nurse's relationship with the child and family is of prime importance. Every day, pediatric nurses encounter families from a wide variety of religious, cultural, and ethnic backgrounds, and it is critical to treat each family with respect. Family-centered care focuses on the needs of the child and family together and involves ethical treatment of the child.

Advances in science and technology have led to an increased number of ethical dilemmas in health care. Many facilities have formed institutional ethics committees. These committees not only provide case-by-case review and resolution of ethical dilemmas but also review existing institutional policies; develop new policies; and provide education to staff, health care providers, children, and families on ethical issues (Moon & Committee on Bioethics, 2019).

Practicing ethically begins with being sensitive to the sanctity and quality of human life. An ethical nurse is accountable and uses sound reasoning to resolve ethical challenges. Ethics includes the basic principles of autonomy, beneficence, nonmaleficence, justice, veracity, and fidelity. The nurse must understand these principles in order to analyze and respond to ethical dilemmas. Autonomy refers to the freedom to choose and self-determination in regard to making health care decisions. Generally, parents have the autonomy to make health care decisions for their children. In certain situations, however, older children have the autonomy to give assent to care (see the "Assent" section later in this chapter), and in special situations, adolescents are granted the autonomy to consent to health care procedures without their parents' knowledge. Beneficence refers to actions that will benefit others. In pediatric care, this means actions of kindness that will benefit the child rather than harming them. Nonmaleficence means avoiding causing harm, intentionally or unintentionally. Justice refers to acting fairly. Treatment decisions will not be based on factors such as age, sex, gender, religion, socioeconomic status, or ethnicity. Veracity is telling the truth, and fidelity is keeping promises and maintaining confidentiality and privacy. The pediatric nurse must balance these ethical components when dealing with families from a variety of backgrounds who are making health care decisions for their children. The process is as follows:

1. Identify the problem.
2. Gather information about the problem.
3. Weigh the risks against the benefits.
4. Choose a solution.
5. Implement the solution.
6. Evaluate the outcome of the situation.

Many pediatric institutions have adopted a "bill of rights" for children's health care. This bill might include the rights:

- To be called by name
- To receive compassionate health care in a careful, prompt, and courteous manner
- To know the names of all providers caring for the child
- To have basic needs met and usual schedules or routines honored
- To make choices whenever possible
- To be kept without food or drink when necessary for the shortest time possible
- To be unrestrained if able
- To have parents or other important people with the child
- To have an interpreter for the child and family when needed
- To object noisily if desired
- To be educated honestly about the child's health care
- To be respected as a person (not having people talk about the child within earshot unless the child knows what is happening)
- To have their confidentiality about their condition respected at all times by all health care providers (Society of Pediatric Nurses, 2021)

Legal Issues Related to Working With Children and Their Families

Minors (children younger than 18 years) generally require adult guardians to act on their behalf. Parents usually are the ultimate decision makers for their children. Biologic or adoptive parents are usually considered to be the child's legal guardian. When divorce occurs, one or both parents may be granted custody of the child. In certain cases (such as child abuse or neglect, or during foster care), a guardian ad litem may be appointed by the courts. This person generally serves to protect the child's best interests. States generally require parental or guardian consent for minors to receive medical treatment, but some exceptions exist (refer to the "Consent" section). Confidentiality of patient information should always be maintained within the context of the state law and the institution's policies.

Consent

Generally, only individuals over the age of majority (18 years of age) can legally provide consent for health care. Since children are minors, the process of consent involves obtaining written permission from a parent or legal guardian. In cases requiring a signature for consent, usually the parent gives consent for care for children younger than 18 years except in certain situations.

TAKE NOTE!

Never assume that the adult accompanying the child is the parent or legal guardian. Always clarify the relationship of the accompanying adult.

INFORMED CONSENT

Most care given in a health care setting is covered by the initial consent for treatment signed when the child becomes a patient at that office or clinic or by the consent to treatment signed upon admission to the hospital or other inpatient facility. Certain procedures, however, require a specific process of **informed consent**. Procedures that require informed consent include major and minor surgery; invasive procedures such as lumbar puncture or bone marrow aspiration; treatments placing the child at higher risk, such as chemotherapy or radiation therapy; procedures or treatments involving research; application of restraints; and photography involving children.

The informed consent process, which must be done before the procedure or specific care, addresses the legal and ethical requirement of informing the child and parent about the procedure. It originates from the right of the child and family to direct their care and the ethical responsibility of health care providers to involve the child and family in health care decisions. Nurses should involve children and adolescents in the decision-making process to the extent possible, though the parent is still ultimately responsible for giving consent. The health care provider or advanced practitioner providing or performing the treatment or procedure is responsible for informing the child and family about the procedure and obtaining consent by providing a detailed description of the procedure or treatment, the potential risks and benefits, and alternative methods available. The nurse's responsibility related to informed consent includes:

- Determining that the parents or legal guardians understand what they are signing by asking them pertinent questions
- Ensuring that the consent form is completed with signatures from the parents or legal guardians
- Serving as a witness to the signature process

Box 1.1 describes the key elements of informed consent, though laws vary from state to state.

Nurses must become familiar with state laws as well as the policies and procedures of the health care agency. Treating children without obtaining proper informed consent is a violation of the child's rights, and the health care provider or facility may be held liable for any damages (Olson & Middleman, 2022).

BOX 1.1 Key Elements of Informed Consent

- The decision maker must be of legal age in that state with full civil rights and be competent (have the ability to make the decision).
- Present information that is simple, concise, and appropriate to the level of education and language of the individual responsible for making the decision.
- The decision must be made voluntarily and without coercion, force, or influence of duress.
- Have a witness to the process of informed consent.
- Have the witness sign the consent form.

SPECIAL SITUATIONS TO INFORMED CONSENT

There are special situations related to informed consent. If the parent is not available, then the person in charge (relative, babysitter, or teacher) may give consent for emergency treatment if that person has a signed form from the parent or legal guardian allowing them to do so. During an emergency situation, verbal consent via telephone may be obtained. Two witnesses must be listening simultaneously and will sign the consent form, indicating that consent was received via telephone. Health care providers can provide emergency treatment to a child without consent if they have made reasonable attempts to contact the child's parent or legal guardian (American Academy of Pediatrics, Committee on Pediatric Emergency Medicine, & Committee on Bioethics, 2011, reaffirmed 2021). In urgent or emergent situations, appropriate medical care should never be delayed or withheld due to an inability to obtain consent (American Academy of Pediatrics, Committee on Pediatric Emergency Medicine, & Committee on Bioethics, 2011, reaffirmed 2021). Certain federal laws, such as the Emergency Medical Treatment and Labor Act (EMTALA), require that every child who presents at an emergency department is given a medical examination to determine if an emergency medical condition exists, regardless of informed consent or reimbursement ability (American Academy of Pediatrics, Committee on Pediatric Emergency Medicine, & Committee on Bioethics, 2011, reaffirmed 2021). Table 1.3 gives further information about other special situations.

EXCEPTIONS TO PARENTAL CONSENT REQUIREMENT

In some states, a **mature minor** may give consent to certain medical treatment. The health care provider must determine that the adolescent (usually older than 14 years) is sufficiently mature and intelligent to make the decision for treatment. The provider also considers the complexity of the treatment, its risks and benefits, and whether the treatment is necessary or elective before obtaining consent from a mature minor (American Academy of Pediatrics, Committee on Pediatric Emergency Medicine, & Committee on Bioethics, 2011, reaffirmed 2021).

State laws vary in relation to the definition of an **emancipated minor** and the types of treatment that may be obtained by an emancipated minor (without parental consent). The nurse must be familiar with their particular state's law. Emancipation may be considered in any of the following situations, depending on the state's laws:

- Membership in a branch of the armed services
- Marriage
- Court-determined emancipation
- Financial independence and living apart from parents
- Pregnancy
- Birthing parent younger than 18 years

The emancipated minor is considered to have the legal capacity of an adult and may make their own health

TABLE 1.3 • Special Considerations Related to Informed Consent

Issue	Definition	Nursing Considerations
Child not living with biologic or adoptive parents	Child living: • In foster care • With potential adoptive parent • With a relative	Legally appointed guardian must provide consent. Verify authority and include documentation of legally appointed guardian in the child's medical record.
Parent consent after divorce	Ability to give consent for health care rests with parent who has legal custody by divorce decree.	Determine if the parents have joint custody or if there is sole custody by one parent. Even the parent with only physical custody may give consent for emergency care. Court involvement may be needed if there is joint legal custody and parents disagree on care.
Consent for organ donation	For a minor to donate, the parents must be aware of the risks and benefits and must provide emotional support to the child, and there should be a close relationship between the donor and recipient if living-related donation is occurring.	Potential donors should be referred to local organ procurement organization. Educate the family about policies related to organ donation.The legal guardian or parent consents to organ donation.
Consent for medical experimentation	Requirements include consent of parents, assent of child, and perceived benefit to the child.	Comply with all federal regulations if federal funds are received. Refer to the "Assent" section.

American Academy of Pediatrics, Committee on Hospital Care, Section on Surgery, & Section on Critical Care. (2010, reaffirmed 2019). Pediatric organ donation and transplantation. *Pediatrics, 125*(4), 822–828. https://doi.org/10.1542/peds.2010-0081; Office for Human Research Protection. (2016). *Children: Information on special protections for children as research subjects.* Retrieved September 27, 2022, from https://www.hhs.gov/ohrp/regulations-and-policy/guidance/special-protections-for-children/index.html

care decisions (American Academy of Pediatrics, Committee on Pediatric Emergency Medicine, & Committee on Bioethics, 2011, reaffirmed 2021).

Many states do not require the consent or notification of parents or legal guardians when providing specific care to minors. Depending on the state law, health care may be provided to minors for certain conditions in a confidential manner without including the parents. These types of care may include pregnancy counseling, prenatal care, contraception, testing for and treatment of sexually transmitted infections and communicable diseases (including HIV), substance use disorder, and mental illness counseling and treatment (American Academy of Pediatrics, Committee on Pediatric Emergency Medicine, & Committee on Bioethics, 2011, reaffirmed 2021). These exceptions allow children to seek help in a confidential manner; they might otherwise avoid care if they were required to inform their parents or legal guardians. Again, laws vary by state, so the nurse must be knowledgeable about the laws in the state where they are licensed to practice.

PARENTAL REFUSAL OF MEDICAL TREATMENT

Parental autonomy (the right to decide for or against medical treatment) is a fundamental, constitutionally protected right but not an absolute one. The general assumption is that parents act in the best interest of their children. Ideally, medical care without informed consent should be given only when the child's life is in danger.

In some cases, parents may refuse medical treatment for their child. This refusal may arise when treatment conflicts with their religious or cultural beliefs, and the nurse should be aware of some of these common beliefs. Some religions, such as Christian Science, may prefer prayer or faith healing to allopathic medicine, and some Jehovah's Witnesses refuse blood product administration based on their religious beliefs. Muslims may refuse the use of any potentially addictive substances such as narcotics or medicines containing alcohol. Sometimes, common ground may be reached between the family's religious or cultural beliefs and the health care team's recommendations; adequate communication and education are the keys in this situation.

TAKE NOTE!

Do not assume what a family's beliefs are based on religious affiliation. Assess the views of each family and child on an individual basis.

In other cases, parents may refuse treatment if they perceive that their child's quality of life may be significantly impaired by the medical care that is offered. The health care team must appropriately educate the family and communicate with them, ensuring they can understand. The child and family should be informed of what to expect with certain tests or treatments. The health care team should make a clinical assessment of the child's and family's understanding of the situation and their reasons for refusing treatment. Active listening may allow the health care provider to address the concerns, fears, or reservations the family may have regarding their child's care.

Refusal of medical care may be considered a form of child neglect. If providing medical treatment may prevent substantial harm or suffering or save a child's life, providers and the judicial system strive to advocate for the child. The state has an overriding interest in the health and welfare of the child and can order that medical treatment proceed without signed informed consent; this is referred to as "parens patriae" (the state has a right and a duty to protect children). If the parents refuse treatment and the health care team feels the treatment is reasonable and warranted, the case should be referred to the institution's ethics committee. If the issue remains unresolved or the case is complex, the judicial system may become involved (Katz et al., 2016, reaffirmed 2023).

Assent

Assent means agreeing to something. In pediatric health care, the term **assent** refers to the child's participation in the decision-making process about health care (Katz et al., 2016, reaffirmed 2023). The age of assent depends on the child's developmental level, maturity, and psychological state. The American Academy of Pediatrics recommends that children and adolescents be involved in the discussions about their health care and kept informed in an age-appropriate manner (Katz et al., 2016, reaffirmed 2023). As a child gets older, assent or dissent should be given more serious consideration. The pediatric patient needs to be empowered by health care providers to the extent of their capabilities, and as children mature and develop over time, they should become the primary decision maker regarding their health care (Katz et al., 2016, reaffirmed 2023). The American Academy of Pediatrics recommends that if a provider asks the child's opinion about the direction of treatment or participation in research, then the child's view and desires should be seriously considered (Katz et al., 2016, reaffirmed 2023).

When obtaining assent, first help the child to understand their health condition as appropriate for the child's developmental level. Next, inform the child of the treatment planned and discuss what they should expect. Then determine what the child understands about the situation and make sure they are not being unduly influenced to make a decision one way or another. Lastly, ascertain the child's willingness to participate in treatment or research (Katz et al., 2016, reaffirmed 2023). Assent is a process and should continue throughout the course of the treatment or research protocol.

The converse of assent, which is dissent (disagreeing with the treatment plan), needs to be carefully considered and respected if it occurs. If the health care provider is not going to honor the child's dissent, the argument can be made that they should not ask for the child's assent. In some cases, such as cases of significant morbidity or mortality, dissent may need to be overridden. These cases need to be looked at on an individual basis. If the decision is made to move forward with treatment despite the child's dissent, then this decision must be explained to the child in developmentally appropriate terms.

There has been an increased emphasis on including children in research studies. Children are not little adults; however, less than 50% of medications have labeling with specific pediatric information (American Academy of Pediatrics, Committee on Drugs, 2014, reaffirmed 2021). In research studies, investigators and institutional review boards (IRBs) are responsible for ensuring that measures are taken to protect the children in the studies. The nurse caring for these children also has the responsibility to ensure protection at all stages of the research process. Nurses can become members of the IRB as well as become familiar with studies that have been approved in their work setting to help ensure that their pediatric patients are protected.

TAKE NOTE!

Whenever possible, assent for participation should be obtained from the child.

Advance Directives

The Patient Self-Determination Act of 1990 established the concept of advance directives. Advance directives determine the child's and family's wishes should life-sustaining care become necessary. Parents are generally the surrogate decision makers for children; however, the American Academy of Pediatrics encourages health care providers to take into consideration the views of the child when possible (Weise et al., 2017). If the child's interests are not served by prolonged survival, then the health care provider or advanced practitioner should educate the parents about the extent of the child's illness, diagnostic and therapeutic options, and potential for ongoing quality of life (Weise et al., 2017). After discussion with other family members, friends, and spiritual advisors, the parents may make the decision to forego life-sustaining medical treatment, either withdrawing treatment or deciding to withhold certain further treatment or opt not to resuscitate in the event of cardiopulmonary arrest (Weise et al., 2017).

Life-sustaining care may include antibiotics, chemotherapy, dialysis, ventilation, cardiopulmonary resuscitation (CPR), and artificial nutrition and hydration. Some families may choose to withdraw these treatments if they are already in place or not begin them should the need arise. **Do not attempt resuscitation (DNAR) orders** are in place for some children, particularly those who are terminally ill. Some institutions have started using the term "allow natural death" (AND). No matter what term is used, these orders should include specific instructions regarding the child's and family's wishes (e.g., some families may desire oxygen but not chest compressions or code medications). When the child is hospitalized, the DNAR order must be documented in the health care provider orders and updated according to the facility's policy. DNAR orders may also be in place in the home, but only a few states allow emergency medical services to honor a child's DNAR order in the home. Children with DNAR orders may also still be attending school. In that case, the health care professionals involved should meet with the school officials (the board of education and its legal counsel) to discuss how the DNAR request can be upheld in the school setting. The health care provider should help educate the school about the child's condition, potential complications, and health care goals (Weise et al., 2017). They should work with the school and family on developing an individualized health care plan that will include what to do instead of CPR, such as comfort measures (Weise et al., 2017).

The Baby Doe regulations, which are an amendment to the U.S. Child Abuse Protection and Treatment Act, provide specific guidelines on how to treat extremely ill, premature, terminally ill, or disabled infants regardless of the parents' wishes (National Child Abuse and Neglect Training and Publications Project, 2014). These cases encompass complex ethical issues and continue to be surrounded by legal uncertainty. Therefore, providers must continue to work with parents of extremely sick or premature infants to ensure that they are accurately informed about the condition of their child and the risks and benefits to treatment. Health care providers must also be aware of federal, state, and hospital policies regarding care of newborns who are very ill, premature, or disabled. The nurse must be knowledgeable about the laws related to health care of children in the state where they practice as well as the policies of their health care institution. The nurse must be sensitive to the various ethical situations that they may become involved in and should apply knowledge of laws as well as concepts of ethics to provide appropriate care.

Confidentiality Issues in Caring for Children

With the establishment of the Health Insurance Portability and Accountability Act (HIPAA) of 1996, confidentiality of health care information became required. The primary intent of the law is to maintain health insurance coverage for workers and their families when they change or lose jobs. Another aspect of the law requires the U.S. Department of Health and Human Services to establish national standards for electronic transactions for health information on individuals. Due to the increased use of electronic medical records (EMRs) and electronic billing, there is an increased possibility that personal health information might be inappropriately distributed. Patient confidentiality and privacy must be maintained as it is with paper documentation. Nurses can ensure that privacy is maintained when using computerized documentation and an EMR by doing the following:

- Always maintain the security of your personal log-in information; never share it with other nurses or other people.
- Always log off when leaving the computer.
- Do not leave patient information visible on a monitor screen when the computer or monitor is unattended.
- Use safeguards, such as encryption, when using alternative means of communication, such as e-mail.

HIPAA also addresses security and privacy issues involving health information about individuals. The HIPAA Security Rule establishes national standards to protect electronic personal health information. The HIPAA Privacy Rule ensures proper protection of personal health information while allowing for the flow of health information needed to provide and promote high-quality care (U.S. Department of Health and Human Services, 2022). As long as reasonable precautions have been taken to protect the child's privacy, the privacy rule allows certain disclosures that assist in patient care. State privacy laws and professional practice standards also exist to protect personal health information, and care providers must follow whichever guidelines are more stringent. In the pediatric area, information is shared only with the legal parents or guardians or individuals as established in writing by the parents. This law, along with professional obligation, promotes the security and privacy of children's health information.

Exceptions to Confidential Treatment in Children

There are exceptions to confidential treatment in children. For example, all states require reporting of suspicion of physical or sexual child abuse and injuries caused by a weapon or criminal act. Abuse cases are reported to the child welfare authorities and criminal acts to the police. If the minor is a threat to themselves, information may need to be disclosed to protect the child. The provider must also follow public health laws that require reporting certain infectious diseases to the local health department (e.g., tuberculosis, hepatitis, HIV, and other sexually transmitted infections). Finally, there is a duty to warn third parties when a specific threat is made to an identifiable person.

Providers must strike a balance between confidentiality and required disclosure. Even if disclosure is required, it is recommended that the provider discuss the issue with the child and, when possible, inform the minor of the limits to confidentiality and consent prior to the initiation of care (Middleman & Olson, 2021).

In the beginning of the chapter, you were introduced to the Romano family. How can you empower this family to help them provide the best care to Isabelle? What ethical and legal issues may arise?

KEY CONCEPTS

- In the past, health was defined simply as the absence of disease; health was measured by monitoring the mortality and morbidity of a group. Over the past century, however, the focus of health has shifted to disease prevention, health promotion, and wellness. The WHO (2022) defines health as "a state of complete physical, mental, and social well-being, and not merely the absence of disease or infirmity."
- In the 21st century, unintentional injuries continue to be the leading cause of death in children older than 1 year, but health concerns such as higher weight, environmental toxins, allergies, drug use, child abuse and neglect, and mental health illnesses impact children's health today (CDC/NCHS, 2022c).
- Healthy People provides a comprehensive health promotion and disease prevention agenda with specific goals and objectives that emphasize children's health and improving the health and well-being for all. One method to establish the aggregate health status of infants, children, and adolescents is by using statistics such as mortality and morbidity rates.
- The infant mortality rate is low in the United States, but it is still higher than in other countries with similar resources. This high rate may be the result of the number of preterm and low birth weight infants born in this country.
- The three general concepts that form the philosophy of pediatric nursing care are family-centered care, atraumatic care, and evidence-based care. Pediatric nurses use these three concepts to provide quality, cost-effective care that is continuous, comprehensive, and compassionate.
- The primary role of the pediatric nurse is to provide direct nursing care to children and their families as an advocate, educator, and care manager. The pediatric nurse also serves as a collaborator, care coordinator, and consultant.
- A standard of care is a minimally accepted action expected of an individual of a certain skill or knowledge level and reflects what a reasonable and prudent person would do in a similar situation. Professional standards from regulatory agencies, state or federal laws, nurse practice acts, and other specialty groups regulate nursing practice in general.
- The nursing process, a problem-solving method based on the scientific method, is used to care for the child and family during health promotion, maintenance, restoration, and rehabilitation. The nursing process is applicable in all health care settings and consists of five steps: assessment, nursing analysis, outcome identification and planning, implementation, and outcome evaluation.
- Ethical nursing care includes the basic principles of autonomy, beneficence, nonmaleficence, justice, veracity, and fidelity.
- Advances in science and technology have led to ethical dilemmas in health care; when parents refuse treatment or the child's desires conflict with the parents' decision, an ethical dilemma results.
- Children are entitled to a health care bill of rights just as adults are.
- Minor children (younger than age 18) must have their parents or legal guardians provide consent for health care in most cases.
- Nurses must be knowledgeable about the laws related to health care of children in the states where they practice as well as the policies of their health care institutions.
- Informed consent is required for major and minor surgery; invasive procedures such as lumbar puncture or bone marrow aspiration; treatments placing the child at higher risk, such as chemotherapy or radiation therapy; procedures or treatments involving research; application of restraints; and photography involving children.
- The nurse's responsibility related to informed consent includes determining that the parents or legal guardians understand what they are signing by asking them pertinent questions, ensuring that the consent form is completed with signatures from the parents or legal guardians, and serving as a witness to the signature process.
- In certain states, mature minors and emancipated minors may consent to their own health care.
- Depending on state law, certain health care may be provided to adolescents without parental notification, including pregnancy counseling, prenatal care, contraception, testing for and treatment of sexually transmitted infections and communicable diseases (including HIV), substance use disorder and mental illness counseling and treatment, and health care required as a result of a crime-related injury.

REFERENCES AND RECOMMENDED READINGS

American Academy of Pediatrics, Committee on Drugs. (2014, reaffirmed 2021). Policy statement: Off-label use of drugs in children. *Pediatrics, 133*(3), 563–567. https://doi.org/10.1542/peds.2013-4060

American Academy of Pediatrics, Committee on Hospital Care, Institute for Patient and Family-Centered Care. (2012, reaffirmed 2018). Policy statement: Patient and family-centered care and the pediatrician's role. *Pediatrics, 129*(2), 394–404. https://doi.org/10.1542/peds.2011-3084

American Academy of Pediatrics, Committee on Hospital Care, Section on Surgery, & Section on Critical Care. (2010, reaffirmed 2019). Pediatric organ donation and transplantation. *Pediatrics, 125*(4), 822–828. https://doi.org/10.1542/peds.2010-0081

American Academy of Pediatrics, Committee on Pediatric Emergency Medicine, & Committee on Bioethics. (2011, reaffirmed 2021). Consent for emergency medical services for children and adolescents. *Pediatrics, 128*(2), 427–433. https://doi.org/10.1542/peds.2011-1166

American Academy of Pediatrics, Council on Community Pediatrics. (2016, reaffirmed 2021). Poverty and child health in the United States. *Pediatrics, 137*(4), e20160339. https://doi.org/10.1542/peds.2016-0339

American Association of Colleges of Nursing. (2022). *DNP factsheet.* https://www.aacnnursing.org/News-Information/Fact-Sheets/DNP-Fact-Sheet

American Nurses Association. (n.d.). *Practice & policy: Scope of practice.* Retrieved September 22, 2022, from https://www.nursingworld.org/practice-policy/scope-of-practice/

American Nurses Association, National Association of Pediatric Nurse Practitioners, & Society of Pediatric Nurses. (2015). *Pediatric nursing: Scope and standards of practice* (2nd ed.). Nursesbooks.org.

America's Health Rankings, United Health Foundation. (2022). *Public health impact: Child mortality.* Retrieved September 12, 2022, from https://www.americashealthrankings.org/explore/health-of-women-and-children/measure/child_mortality_a/state/ALL

Centers for Disease Control and Prevention. (2021). *Injuries among children & teens.* Retrieved September 7, 2022, from https://www.cdc.gov/injury/features/child-injury/index.html

Centers for Disease Control and Prevention. (2022). *Reproductive health: Infant mortality.* Retrieved September 7, 2022, from https://www.cdc.gov/reproductivehealth/maternalinfanthealth/infantmortality.htm

Centers for Disease Control and Prevention/National Center for Health Statistics. (2022a). *Percentage of fair or poor health status for children under age 18 years, United States, 2019–2020.* National Health Interview Survey. Retrieved September 13, 2022, from https://wwwn.cdc.gov/NHISDataQueryTool/SHS_child/index.html

Centers for Disease Control and Prevention/National Center for Health Statistics. (2022b). *Percentage of missing 11 or more school days due to illness, injury, or disability in the past 12 months for children aged 5–17 years, United States, 2019–2020.* National Health Interview Survey. Retrieved September 19, 2022, from https://wwwn.cdc.gov/NHISDataQueryTool/SHS_child/index.html

Centers for Disease Control and Prevention/National Center for Health Statistics. (2022c). *Child health.* Retrieved September 1, 2022, from https://www.cdc.gov/nchs/fastats/child-health.htm

Central Intelligence Agency. (2022). *The World Factbook: Field listing—Infant mortality rate.* Retrieved September 7, 2022, from https://www.cia.gov/the-world-factbook/field/infant-mortality-rate

Creamer, J., Shrider, E. A., Burns, K., & Chen, F. (2022). *Poverty in the United States: 2021* (U.S. Census Bureau, current population reports, P60-277). U.S. Government Publishing Office. https://www.census.gov/library/publications/2022/demo/p60-277.html#:~:text=The%20official%20poverty%20rate%20in,and%20Table%20A%2D1

Ely, D. M., & Driscoll, A. K. (2022). Infant mortality in the United States, 2020: Data from the period linked birth/infant death file. *National Vital Statistics Reports, 71*(5), 1–17. https://doi.org/10.15620/cdc:120700

Federal Interagency Forum on Child and Family Statistics. (2021). *America's children: Key national indicators of well-being, 2021.* U.S. Government Printing Office.

GovTrack. (2022). *H.R. 3921—115th Congress: HEALTHY KIDS Act.* Retrieved September 1, 2022, from https://www.govtrack.us/congress/bills/115/hr3921

Guyer, B., Freedman, M. A., Strobino, D. M., & Sondik, E. J. (2000). Annual summary of vital statistics: Trends in the health of Americans during the 20th century. *Pediatrics, 106*(6), 1307–1317. https://doi.org/10.1542/peds.106.6.1307

Hamilton, B. E., Martin, J. A., & Osterman, M. J. K. (2022). Births: Provisional data for 2021. *Vital Statistics Rapid Release, 20.* National Center for Health Statistics. https://doi.org/10.15620/cdc:116027

HHS.gov/HealthCare. (2022). *About the Affordable Care Act.* Retrieved September 6, 2022, from https://www.hhs.gov/healthcare/about-the-aca/index.html

Katz, A. L., Webb, S. A., & AAP Committee on Bioethics. (2016, reaffirmed 2023). Informed consent in decision-making in pediatric practice. *Pediatrics, 138*(2), e20161485. https://doi.org/10.1542/peds.2016-1485

Mandy, G. T. (2022). Preterm birth: Definitions of prematurity, epidemiology, and risk factors for infant mortality. *UpToDate.* Retrieved July 24, 2023, from https://www.uptodate.com/contents/preterm-birth-definitions-of-prematurity-epidemiology-and-risk-factors-for-infant-mortality

Mandy, G. T. (2023). Overview of the long-term complications of preterm birth. *UpToDate.* Retrieved July 24, 2023, from https://www.uptodate.com/contents/overview-of-the-long-term-complications-of-preterm-birth

Maternal and Child Health Bureau, Health Resources and Services Administration, & U.S. Department of Health and Human Services. (n.d.). *MCH timeline.* Retrieved August 10, 2022, from https://mchb.hrsa.gov/about/timeline/index.asp

McDermott, K. W., & Roemer, M. (2021). *Most frequent principal diagnoses for inpatient stays in U.S. hospitals, 2018.* HCUP Statistical Brief #277. Agency for Healthcare Research and Quality. https://www.ncbi.nlm.nih.gov/books/NBK573113/pdf/Bookshelf_NBK573113.pdf

Melnyk, B. M., & Fineout-Overholt, E. (2015). *Evidence-based practice in nursing and health care: A guide to best practice* (3rd ed.). Wolters Kluwer Health.

Middleman, A. B., & Olson, K. A. (2021). Confidentiality in adolescent healthcare. *UpToDate.* Retrieved September 28, 2022, from https://www.uptodate.com/contents/confidentiality-in-adolescent-health-care

Moon, M., & AAP Committee on Bioethics. (2019). Institutional ethics committees. *Pediatrics, 143*(5), e20190659. https://doi.org/10.1542/peds.2019-0659

National Child Abuse and Neglect Training and Publications Project. (2014). *The Child Abuse Prevention and Treatment Act: 40 years of safeguarding America's children.* U.S. Department of Health and Human Services, Children's Bureau.

National Conference of State Legislatures. (2020). *Children's health insurance program overview.* Retrieved September 1, 2022, from https://www.ncsl.org/research/health/childrens-health-insurance-program-overview.aspx

Office for Human Research Protection. (2016). *Children: Information on special protections for children as research subjects.* Retrieved September 27, 2022, from https://www

.hhs.gov/ohrp/regulations-and-policy/guidance/special-protections-for-children/index.html

Office of the Surgeon General. (2021). *Protecting youth mental health: The U.S. Surgeon General's Advisory*. https://www.hhs.gov/sites/default/files/surgeon-general-youth-mental-health-advisory.pdf

Office of the Surgeon General. (2023). *Social media and youth mental health: The U.S. Surgeon General's Advisory*. https://www.hhs.gov/sites/default/files/sg-youth-mental-health-social-media-advisory.pdf

Olson, K. A., & Middleman, A. B. (2022). Consent in adolescent healthcare. *UpToDate*. Retrieved September 27, 2022, from https://www.uptodate.com/contents/consent-in-adolescent-health-care

Shrider, E. A., Kollar, M., Chen, F., & Semega, J. (2021). *Income and poverty in the United States: 2020* (U.S. Census Bureau, current population reports P60-273). U.S. Government Publishing Office. https://www.census.gov/content/dam/Census/library/publications/2021/demo/p60-273.pdf

Society of Pediatric Nurses. (2021). *SPN Informational Paper: Pediatric Bill of Rights*. https://www.pedsnurses.org/assets/docs/Informational-Papers/SPN%20Informational%20Paper-%20Pediatric%20Bill%20of%20Rights.pdf

U.S. Department of Health and Human Services. (2022). *Summary of the HIPPA privacy rule*. Retrieved September 28, 2022, from https://www.hhs.gov/hipaa/for-professionals/privacy/laws-regulations/index.html

U.S. Department of Health and Human Services, Office of Disease Prevention and Health Promotion. (2021a). *Healthy People 2030 framework*. Retrieved September 7, 2022, from https://health.gov/healthypeople/about/healthy-people-2030-framework

U.S. Department of Health and Human Services, Office of Disease Prevention and Health Promotion. (2021b). *Healthy People 2030 physical activity: Overview and objectives*. Retrieved September 7, 2022, from https://health.gov/healthypeople/objectives-and-data/browse-objectives/physical-activity

U.S. Department of Health and Human Services, Public Health Service. (1979). *Healthy People: The surgeon general's report on health promotion and disease prevention* (DHEW Publication No. PHS 79–5507). U.S. Government Printing Office.

U.S. Food and Drug Administration. (2019). *FDA approves innovative gene therapy to treat pediatric patients with spinal muscular atrophy, a rare disease and leading genetic cause of infant mortality*. https://www.fda.gov/news-events/press-announcements/fda-approves-innovative-gene-therapy-treat-pediatric-patients-spinal-muscular-atrophy-rare-disease#:~:text=The%20U.S.%20Food%20and%20Drug,genetic%20cause%20of%20infant%20mortality

U.S. National Library of Medicine, ClinicalTrials.gov. (2022). *Afrezza® INHALE-1 study in pediatrics (INHALE-1)*. https://clinicaltrials.gov/ct2/show/NCT04974528

Weise, K. L., Okun, A. L., Carter, B. S., & Christian, C. W.; Committee on Bioethics, Section on Hospice and Palliative Medicine, & Committee on Child Abuse and Neglect. (2017). Policy statement: Guidance on forgoing life-sustaining medical treatment. *Pediatrics*, *140*(3), e20171905. https://doi.org/10.1542/peds.2017-1905

World Health Organization. (2022). *Constitution*. Retrieved August 2, 2022, from https://www.who.int/about/governance/constitution

Yarrow, A. L. (2011). A history of federal child antipoverty and health policy in the United States since 1900. *Child Development Perspectives*, *5*(1), 66–72. https://doi.org/10.1111/j.1750-8606.2010.00157.x

DEVELOPING CLINICAL JUDGMENT

PRACTICING FOR NCLEX

1. The nurse is developing a community outreach program to help reduce childhood mortality. Which topic(s) would be essential to include? Select all that apply.
   a. HIV routes of transmission
   b. Treatment options for congenital anomalies
   c. Appropriate restraints in motor vehicles
   d. Low birth weight prevention strategies
   e. Proper bicycle helmet fit
   f. Water safety

2. The nurse is assessing the vital signs of a child who is being evaluated in an urgent care center. The child is to be seen by the PNP. The parent asks, "Why is my child seeing the PNP and not the doctor?" What is the best response by the nurse?
   a. "The PNP functions similar to the health care provider's assistant, so you should be perfectly at ease."
   b. "The child may be seen by the health care provider instead if you'd like."
   c. "Seeing the PNP is just one more step in having your child evaluated in this setting."
   d. "The PNP is an experienced RN with advanced education in the diagnosis and treatment of children."

3. When caring for an adolescent, in which case must the nurse share information with the parents no matter where care is provided?
   a. Pregnancy counseling
   b. Depression
   c. Contraception
   d. Tuberculosis

4. The school nurse is planning a screening program. What items should be included to address issues related to the "new morbidity?"
   a. Academic difficulties, violence, and other mental health issues
   b. The number of children with chronic illness at the school
   c. Statistics related to health insurance coverage of the children
   d. HIV infection, asthma, and respiratory allergy testing

CRITICAL THINKING EXERCISES

1. Detail how the nursing process fits into the framework of pediatric nursing.
2. Discuss how the role of the pediatric nurse differs from the role of the advanced practice pediatric nurse.
3. At your next staff meeting, you have been asked to present material to your nursing unit discussing special situations to informed consent related to children. Describe the topics that you should address.

STUDY ACTIVITIES

1. Research the IRB at the local hospital and become informed about which studies have been approved in your clinical setting.
2. Research a current policy, bill, or issue being debated on the community, state, or national level pertaining to child health or welfare. Summarize the major facts and supporting or opposing perspectives and present them in a class presentation or paper.
3. Obtain a standardized care plan from the hospital unit. Evaluate whether it is based on evidence-based practice. Develop an individualized plan of care for a child for whom you are caring. Compare and contrast the two types of care plans.

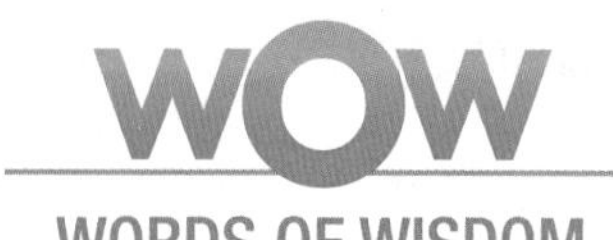

WORDS OF WISDOM

Learning rather than accomplishing should be the focus of raising children.

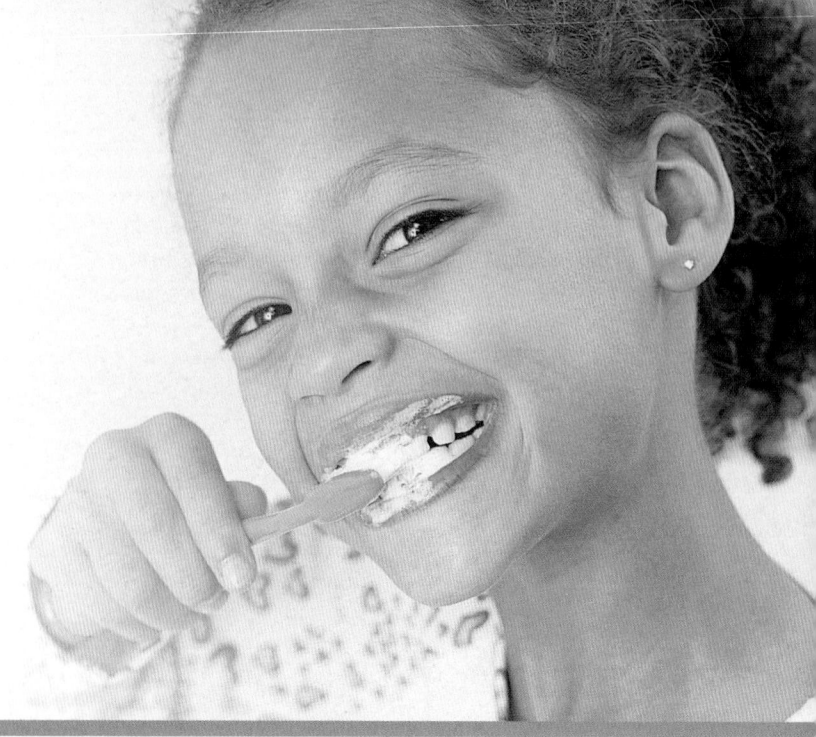

2

Factors Influencing Child Health

LEARNING OBJECTIVES

Upon completion of the chapter, you will be able to:

1. Discuss genetic influences on child health.
2. Compare and contrast the factors associated with health status and lifestyle that affect a child's health.
3. Discuss adverse childhood experiences (ACEs) and explain the concept of resiliency as it relates to children and their health status.
4. Examine access and barriers to health care and its effect on child health.
5. Delineate the structures, functions, and roles of families and the influence on children and their health.
6. Differentiate discipline from punishment.
7. Consider culture and ethnicity in relation to child health.
8. Discuss community and its effects on a child's health.
9. Examine the sources of violence and how exposure to violence affects children.
10. Describe the impact of social determinants of health on children.

KEY TERMS

discipline
enculturation (en-kŭl′chŭr-ā′shŭn)
family structure
foster care
genetics
heredity
punishment
resilience (rez-il′yŭns)
social determinants of health

Miguel Delgado is a 10-month-old who is admitted to the pediatric unit for treatment of pneumonia. He is accompanied by his parents and 3-year-old sister, Luisa. Miguel's parents speak Spanish and very little English. The family is Roman Catholic. As the nurse admitting Miguel, how will you facilitate communication? What steps can you take to help ensure ongoing communication with this family?

INTRODUCTION

When they come into the world, children are members of a family and have already been influenced by myriad factors such as genetics and the environment. As members of a family, they are also members of specific populations, cultures, communities, and societies. Children live, learn, and grow in environments that are affected by everchanging cultural, spiritual, community, and social factors. It is projected that over the next four decades, the United States will experience a dramatic increase in racial and ethnic diversity, and beginning around 2,030 immigration, will account for more than half of population growth (Vespa et al., 2018, revised 2020). The population that identifies with two or more races is expected to more than double, the Asian population is expected to double, the Hispanic population is expected to nearly double, and all other racial groups will see an increase with the exception of non-Hispanic White people, who are expected to decline in number (Vespa et al., 2018, revised 2020). Globalization has led to an international focus on the health of children. In addition, access to health care and the types of health care available for children have changed due to modifications in health care delivery and financing. Furthermore, the United States continues to grapple with issues such as violence, immigration, poverty, and homelessness. The interplay of all of these factors creates a situation unique to each child. These factors may affect the child positively, promoting healthy growth and development, or negatively, exposing the child to health risks.

Nursing care for children and their families involves astute assessment of all of the factors that may affect the health of children. Nurses play a key role in determining the impact of these factors on children and their families. Pediatric nurses need a sound knowledge base about the individual child, including genetics, race, temperament, and overall health status and lifestyle. Family, including the different structures, roles, and functions found in today's society, is also an important component of child health. Knowledge of various situations such as single-parent or adopted families is important to provide individualized care. The nurse should also assess the family's level of stress based on the demands they face and their ability to meet those demands. Do they have the coping behaviors, patterns, and strategies needed to have a positive impact on the child's health?

Other assessments need to focus on culture; ethnicity; spirituality; and the child's community and society, including social roles and social determinants of health (such as economic stability and homelessness). Information gathered from these assessments can help the nurse refer the family to community resources that may assist them with stability and health needs. Resources such as state and federal agencies and community agencies such as the United Way or Salvation Army may be of assistance to families.

Nurses work with children and their families in a variety of settings and need to be alert to subtle yet important indicators that may suggest a problem. For example, the child or family may give an inaccurate address or may provide the address of a shelter. Parents or children may be embarrassed or ashamed, feeling the stigma associated with poverty or homelessness. Other clues to problems may include a history of repeated infectious diseases, multiple health problems, or complaints that the child is always hungry. The key is to link children and their families with community resources that will assist with financial stability and with meeting the health needs of the children.

Due to changing demographics, patterns of immigration and the global nature of society, nurses must make sure that the care they provide is culturally sensitive. Nursing interventions need to incorporate the family's unique values, beliefs, and actions to ensure that their needs are met. To gain the knowledge and skills needed to plan effective care for children, pediatric nurses need to understand how all these factors affect the quality of nursing care and children's health outcomes. By doing so, nurses can create appropriate strategies and plan interventions for achieving the best possible outcomes for children and their families.

GENETIC INFLUENCES ON CHILD HEALTH

Genetics, the study of heredity and its variations, is a field that has applications to all stages of life and all types of diseases. **Heredity** is the process of transmitting genetic characteristics from parent to offspring. The child's sex and race; the child's biologic traits, including some behavioral traits or aspects of temperament; and certain diseases or illnesses are directly linked to genetic inheritance.

Sex

A child's sex is established when the sex chromosomes join. Sex can influence physical characteristics and personal attributes. In addition to the development of male or female genitalia, body development, and hair distribution, some diseases or illnesses can be sex-related; for example, scoliosis is more prevalent in those assigned female at birth, and color blindness is more common in those assigned male at birth. Survival rates of premature infants are correlated with sex; premature females have a higher survival rate than premature males (Mandy, 2022).

Race

Race indicates classification of a particular group of humans who have biologic physical characteristics that are transmitted by descent; they may share physical features such as skin color, bone structure, or blood type. Some of the physical variations may be common among those of a particular race but may be considered an identifying characteristic of a disorder if identified in those of other races. For example, epicanthal folds (the vertical folds of skin that partially or completely cover the inner canthi of the eye) are normal in children of Asian descent but may occur with genetic conditions such as Down syndrome. In addition, specific malformations and diseases have higher prevalences among people of specific races. For example, sickle cell anemia occurs more often in Black or African American children.

Temperament

Temperament is the manner in which a child interacts with the environment. The way a child experiences a particular event will be influenced by their temperament, and the child's temperament will influence the responses of others, including the parents, to the child. Early on, infants demonstrate differences in their behaviors in response to stimuli. These responses are an integral part of the infant's developing personality and individuality. Knowing a child's temperament can help parents and caregivers understand and accept the characteristics of the child without feeling responsible for having caused them.

It is important to recognize that there is a wide range of temperaments within normal development. If the definition of temperament is too narrow, certain behaviors may be mislabeled as development delays or concerns. Children's temperaments are commonly categorized into groups: even-tempered, challenging, and slow to warm up; various temperaments exist that are a combination of these groups (Bogues & Levine, 2023). Even-tempered children have regular biologic functions, predictable behavior, and positive attitudes toward new experiences. Challenging children have irregular biologic functions and are highly active and intense; they react to new experiences by withdrawing and are frustrated easily. Children in the slow-to-warm-up category are moody and less active and have more irregular reactions; they react to new experiences with mild but passive resistance and need extra time to adjust to new situations. Many children will have a mix of these temperament types.

A child's temperament may cause problems in the family if it conflicts with that of the parents (e.g., a challenging 2-year-old with slow-to-warm-up parents). If parents want and expect their child to be predictable but that is not the child's style, parents may perceive the child to have problems; this conflict may then affect the child's health. The key is not to label the child but to recognize the strengths and limitations of each group. Knowing a child's temperament can help parents understand a child's characteristics and behaviors and allow parents to adjust their parenting styles.

Genetically Linked Diseases

New technologies in molecular biology and biochemistry have led to a better understanding of the mechanisms involved in hereditary transmission, including those associated with genetic disorders. These advances are now leading to better diagnostic tests and management options.

Two major areas of study in genetics that are important to pediatrics are cytogenetics and the Human Genome Project. Cytogenetics is the study of genetics at the chromosome level. Chromosomal anomalies, such as trisomies 21, 18, and 13, occur in 0.6% of all live births and negatively affect fetal viability (Breilyn & Levy, 2023); anomalies are even more common among spontaneous abortions and stillbirths. The Human Genome Project is an international research effort involving the localization, isolation, and characterization of human genes and investigation of the function of the gene products and their interaction with one another. This research project will provide information about genetic diseases to aid in developing new ways to identify, treat, cure, or even prevent them. Chapter 27 offers a more detailed discussion of genetics.

HEALTH STATUS AND LIFESTYLE

Obviously, the general health status of a child and specific lifestyles can influence a child's health. Health status may be a factor soon after birth. Babies born prematurely or who suffered other in utero complications such as intrauterine growth restriction experience a higher rate of chronic health problems (Mandy, 2023). Children with chronic health conditions may also have developmental delays, especially in acquiring skills related to cognition, communication, adaptation, social functioning, and motor functioning. Thus, the beginning health status of a child may affect their long-term health and development. Lifestyle choices will also have an effect on a child's overall health status.

Development and Disease Distribution

The way a child develops is the result of genetics and the environment within the context of a variety of biopsychosocial forces. Biologic influences include genetics, in utero exposure to teratogens, postpartum illnesses, exposure to hazardous substances, and maturation. Chapters 3 through 7 discuss the forces affecting growth and development for each age group.

Developmental level has a major impact on the health status of children. In general, the distribution of diseases varies with age. For example, certain communicable diseases are more commonly associated with certain age groups. Roseola, which is a viral illness resulting in high fevers and rash, is most often seen in infants 7 to 13 months old, whereas scarlet fever, which is an infection from group A streptococci, is a disease that primarily affects children older than 3 (Centers for Disease Control and Prevention [CDC], 2022i; Tremblay & Brady, 2023). The physiologic immaturity of an infant's body system increases the risk of infection. Ingestion of toxic substances and risk of poisoning are major health concerns for toddlers as they become more mobile and inquisitive. Because preschool- and school-age children are generally very active, they are more prone to injuries. Adolescents are establishing their identity, which may lead them to separate from family values and traditions for a period of time and attempt to conform to their peers. This journey may lead to risk-taking behaviors, resulting in injuries or other situations that may impair their health.

Nutrition

Adequate nutrition is beneficial for the developing child; conversely, nutritional deprivation can seriously interfere with brain development and other functions. Nutritional requirements change over the child's life and have a great influence on the child's physical growth and intellectual development. Good nutrition provides the essentials required to maintain health and prevent illness (Fig. 2.1). Chapters 3 through 7 discuss the specific nutritional requirements and the impact of deficiencies for each developmental stage.

Nutritional deficiencies, such as iron-deficiency anemia, or excesses, such as that which can lead to higher weight in children, are still common problems in the United States. Some factors contributing to poor nutrition include inadequate food intake; nutritionally unsound social and cultural food practices; the easy accessibility of processed and nutritionally inadequate foods; lack of nutrition education in homes and schools; and the presence of illness that interferes with ingestion, digestion, and absorption of food. In a growing child, inadequate nutrition is associated with delayed development, increased susceptibility to childhood illnesses and infections, increased risk for morbidity and mortality, delayed development, and stunted physical growth (Buchanan & Marquez, 2023a). Higher weight in childhood places the child at a higher risk for higher weight in adulthood and for certain diseases, such as type 2 diabetes and cardiovascular disease, at an earlier age (Buchanan & Marquez, 2023b).

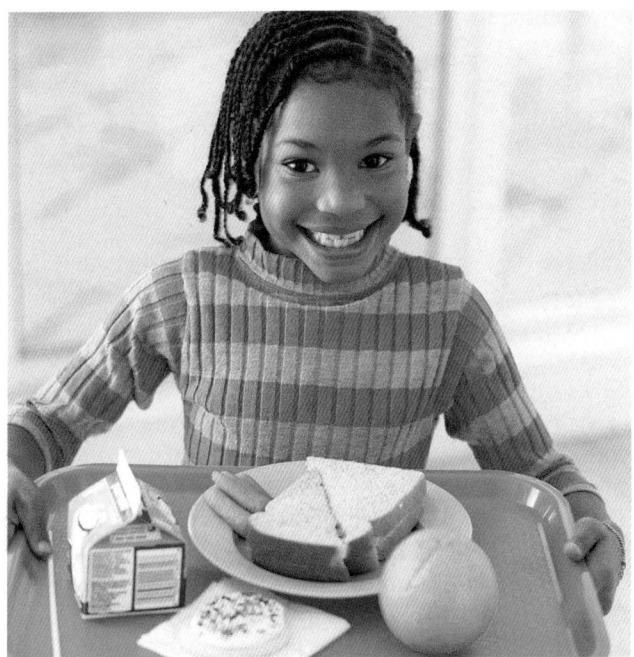

FIGURE 2.1 The dietary habits established early in life can have a long-lasting impact on the health of the child and their quality of life.

Lifestyle Choices

Lifestyle choices that can affect a child's health include patterns of eating; exercise; use of tobacco, drugs, or alcohol; and methods of coping with stress. For children, the lifestyle of the parents is basically the lifestyle of the child. Parents who are not as physically active and who have less healthy eating habits commonly have children with the same habits, which can contribute to diabetes, higher weight, and early heart disease. Once thought of as adult problems, these conditions are being diagnosed more frequently in children and adolescents today (Drozdz et al., 2021). Parents should first self-evaluate their own dietary and activity habits, make changes as necessary, and then strive to encourage healthy eating habits and an appropriate level of physical activity in the child's life through sports and hobbies, such as dancing, or family activities.

Gender and Sexual Identity

In addition to the specific biologic and physical traits related to the sex of the child, there are social factors related to the gender of the child. The child develops specific gender attitudes and behaviors that are aligned with their culture. Interactions with family members and peers as well as activities and societal values affect how children perceive themselves as a specific gender. A child is assigned a sex at birth, and in many cases this is congruent with their gender identity. In some cases, however, their sex and gender do not match, and the child may identify as transgender or gender diverse (Forcier & Olson-Kennedy, 2022).

Sexual identity can also have an impact on a child's overall health and development. People in the lesbian, gay, bisexual, transgender, queer, and more (LGBTQ+) population experience challenges in health care due to factors like discrimination, social pressure, and limited health care access (Bass & Nagy, 2022). Due to these challenges, LGBTQ+ individuals experience higher rates of depression, tobacco use, and sexually transmitted infections (Bass & Nagy, 2022). Health care providers need to learn and understand the special needs of this population and provide them with congruent, compassionate, comprehensive, and high-quality care. This will lead to improved health outcomes. Providers need to understand respectful terminology for this population; use gender-neutral language; and understand, assess, and treat them for the unique risks and challenges they may face, as appropriate. See Box 2.1 for commonly used terms related to gender identity. This list is not all-inclusive, and the exact terms a health care provider uses are secondary to the importance of being sensitive to and aware of an individual's unique psychosexual profile. One way to do this is to use the terms each individual patient prefers. Strong parental and social support are key to healthy development for LGBTQ+ children.

Environmental Exposure

Environmental exposure to dangerous substances can have a detrimental impact on the child. In utero, poor nutrition or exposure to the pregnant parent's use of alcohol, tobacco, or drugs or infections can affect the fetus. It is important for pregnant people to be aware of the risks associated with certain drugs, chemicals, and dietary agents as well as illnesses that may lead to problems for the child. These agents, known as teratogens, may be linked to birth defects in children. However, not all drugs or agents are associated with fetal effects, and research is ongoing to identify the correlations between teratogens and other variables.

The environment continues to affect a child's health after birth. Exposure to air pollution, tobacco, and water or food contaminants can impair a child's health status. Safety hazards in the home or community can contribute to falls, burns, drowning, or other injuries. Exposure to second-hand smoke and other pollutants, such as from radiation or chemicals, is a health hazard for children. Because children are smaller and still developing, environmental exposures can cause more health problems for them. For example, lead exposure is a common preventable poisoning in children, especially among children younger than 6 years (Sample, 2022). Due to young children's rapidly developing nervous systems, they are more sensitive to the effects of lead. Sources include lead paint, lead-contaminated dust, and lead contained in soil and water. Lead exposure can result in developmental and behavioral problems ranging from inattentiveness and hyperactivity to permanent brain damage and death, depending on the level of exposure.

BOX 2.1 Gender Identity Terms

- Binary: Identifying as a man or woman
- Nonbinary: Identifying one's gender identity as not fitting into the categories of man or woman
- Cisgender/cis: Describes a person whose gender identity aligns with their sex assigned at birth
- Transgender/trans: Describes a person whose gender identity is different than their sex assigned at birth
- Agender: Describes a person who does not identify as any gender
- Genderqueer: Describes a person whose gender identity is not binary
- Gender-expansive: Describes a more flexible gender identity beyond the binary
- Gender transition: The process of bringing oneself and one's body in alignment with one's gender identity
- Gender dysphoria: distress or discomfort experienced due to the lack of alignment between one's assigned sex at birth and one's gender identity
- Bigender: A gender identity that includes two genders or is moving between two genders
- Affirmed gender: Refers to a person's true gender, not just to their gender assigned at birth
- Genderfluid: Moving among genders and not adhering to one fixed gender

Adapted from Bass, B., & Nagy, H. (2022). Cultural competence in the care of LGBTQ patients. *StatPearls* [Internet]. StatPearls Publishing. https://www.ncbi.nlm.nih.gov/books/NBK563176/; PFLAG, (2023). *LGBTQ+Glossary*. Retrieved October 8, 2023, from https://pflag.org/glossary/

TAKE NOTE!

Third-hand smoke is residual tobacco smoke and carcinogens that remain after a cigarette is extinguished. These toxins cling to the hair and clothes of the person smoking and can be present on any surface in the house, such as carpet and cushions. Children are particularly susceptible to third-hand smoke since they breathe near, crawl on, touch, and may put their mouths on contaminated surfaces (Samet & Sockrider, 2022).

Stress, Coping, and Adverse Childhood Experiences

Children are exposed to various situations and events that can produce stress. These events can be associated with the common problems associated with growth and development, such as entering a new classroom, learning a new skill, or being teased by a classmate. However, they can also be associated with exposure to or experience with issues such as poverty, illness, divorce, violence, suicide, substance use, mental illness, or other traumas. These experiences are referred to as adverse childhood experiences (ACEs). Exposure to ACEs in childhood leads to an increased risk of chronic health problems, mental illness, and substance use in adulthood (CDC, 2022h). ACEs are preventable, and health care providers can help families and communities create safe, stable environments with nurturing healthy relationships for children.

TAKE NOTE!

People assigned female at birth and non-Hispanic American Indians or Alaska Natives had a higher risk of experiencing one or more ACEs (CDC, 2022h).

Some children can adapt and respond to the stress, while others have more difficulty. **Resilience** refers to the ability to adapt to and cope with significant adverse events or stresses and to recover and function successfully with positive outcomes.

Various internal and external protective factors promote resiliency. Internal factors include the person's ability to take control and be proactive; to be responsible for their own decisions; to understand and accept their own limits and abilities; and to be goal-directed, knowing when to continue or when to stop. External factors include caring relationships with a family member; a positive, safe learning environment at school (including memberships in clubs and social organizations); and positive influences in the community (see the discussion later in this chapter about protective factors and violence). Promoting the development of resiliency in children aids in the achievement of positive developmental and health outcomes (Gartland et al., 2019).

Access to Health Care

The health care system, including the delivery and financing of this system, continues to change and evolve. In the United States, changes in the health care system result from pressures from many directions. These changes reflect shifts in the social and economic realities and results of biomedical and technologic progress over the past several decades. The effects are felt by everyone who seeks health care in any form.

Access to health care is negatively affected by lack of health insurance. Families without insurance may delay care for their children and are less likely to have a usual place of care for their children (Federal Interagency Forum on Child and Family Statistics, 2021). The percentage of children without health insurance for 12 months has declined since 2010 and is currently at 5% (Federal Interagency Forum on Child and Family Statistics, 2022). This decrease is largely attributed to the expansion of Medicaid and the Child's Health Insurance Program (CHIP) (Mykyta et al., 2022). Medicaid is a joint federal and state program that provides health insurance to families with lower incomes. It is state-administered, and each state has its own set of guidelines. In 1997, the U.S. Congress passed legislation that led to the creation of the State Children's Health Insurance Program (SCHIP), now known as CHIP. The purpose of this program is to help insure children whose families are ineligible for Medicaid but cannot afford private health insurance. This program is also jointly funded by the federal and state governments but administered by individual states.

Medicaid or CHIP provides insurance coverage for 36% of children overall, while over 60% of children are covered by private insurance or employer-based health insurance (Mykyta et al., 2022). In recent years, Medicaid and CHIP have focused on increasing enrollment by increasing outreach, simplifying enrollment procedures, and retaining eligible enrollees. Legislation such as the Children's Health Insurance Program Reauthorization Act of 2009 (CHIPRA) and the Affordable Care Act have helped support this effort. Medicaid and CHIP provide a good base of coverage for children from families with lower incomes, but eligibility for parents is much more limited. These programs rely on adequate state and federal funding. Therefore, the continued success of these programs depends on future legislation. Changes in employer-based and private health insurance will continue to challenge the nation in ensuring adequate health care for all children.

Barriers to Health Care

Even with the federal and state programs available to assist children and families, barriers to appropriate, cost-effective, coordinated, and timely health care remain. Barriers can be financial, sociocultural, or part of the health care system itself.

Financial Barriers

In 2021, 29% of children were living in families with lower incomes, and 15.3% were living in poverty (Shrider & Creamer, 2023; Wildsmith & Alvira-Hammond, 2023). Many children and families do not have insurance, do not have enough insurance to cover services obtained, or cannot pay for services. Nurses need to assess for financial barriers to health care and be aware of resources available to help these families overcome these barriers.

Sociocultural Barriers

Lack of transportation and the need for both caregivers to work are examples of sociocultural barriers to seeking health care. Knowledge barriers (e.g., lack of understanding of the importance of prenatal care or preventive health care); language barriers (e.g., speaking a different language than the health care provider); and spiritual barriers (e.g., religious beliefs discouraging some forms of treatment) also exist.

Health Care Delivery System Barriers

The health care delivery system itself can create barriers, such as the cost containment movement. The majority of employed families with insurance are covered by some type of managed health care plan such as a health maintenance organization (HMO), a preferred provider organization (PPO), or a point-of-service (POS) plan. This prospective payment system, based on diagnosis-related groups (DRGs), limits the amount of health care the family may receive. This also includes Medicaid reimbursement. As a result, the trend is to discharge children as soon as possible and deliver care in the home or through community-based services. The overall plan may improve access to preventive services but may limit the access to specialty care, which has a major impact on children with chronic or long-term illnesses.

Health Disparities and Health Equity

Health equity is the concept that every person lives under different circumstances and has different life experiences, and some may need more resources, services, and support to achieve their optimal levels of health than others. Health disparities are preventable differences in the occurrence of disease, injury, violence, or optimal health often due to social or economic status, geographic location, and/or the surrounding environments (CDC, 2022f). Examples of people who may experience health disparities include people from underrepresented groups, people with disabilities, women, and people who are LGBTQ+. Examining and addressing social determinants of health can help us better understand how to improve health outcomes and work toward achieving health equity. Nurses need to develop and support policies, programs, and systems that improve health equity and address the needs of the community and society.

The COVID-19 Pandemic

The COVID-19 pandemic, caused by the severe acute respiratory syndrome coronavirus 2 (SARS-CoV-2) virus had a vast effect on child well-being and health beginning in 2019. The unprecedented pandemic and resultant lockdowns and quarantines affected many aspects of children's lives. It caused disruptions in school and learning, access to preventable health care, routines, food availability, and socialization and activity levels. Although children are less likely than adults to suffer serious illness from COVID-19, some children have been diagnosed with long COVID, which is continued or recurring symptoms such as fatigue, shortness of breath, headache, cognitive difficulties, loss of smell, sore throat, and sore eyes (Deville et al., 2022). Children with underlying conditions are at risk for severe illness, and a rare but serious complication seen in children is multisystem inflammatory syndrome (MIS-C; Deville et al., 2022; refer to Chapter 18 for more information about COVID-19 infection). Many studies are underway to learn more about the effects of COVID-19 infection and the pandemic on children. This research will help aid in decisions related to future interventions for COVID-19 (National Institutes of Health, 2021).

FAMILY THEORY

The family is considered the basic social unit. The U.S. Census Bureau (2021) defines a family as a group of two or more people related by birth, marriage, or adoption and living together. Traditional definitions of family emphasize the legal ties or genetic relationships of people living in the same household with specific roles. However, given the diversity of families in today's society, some believe that family should be defined as whatever the child says it is (Fig. 2.2) (Patterson, 1995).

The family into which a child is born greatly influences their development and health. Children learn health care activities, health beliefs, and health values from their families. The family's structure, the roles assumed by its members, and societal changes that affect the family's life can affect the child and their health. Children and families are unique: Each has different views and requires different methods for support.

Various theories and models have been generated to define a family, to understand its structure and function, and to assess a family's coping and adaptation (Table 2.1).

Family Structure

Family structure is the way the family is organized and the way the family members interact with one another on a regular, recurring basis in socially sanctioned ways. Family members can be gained or lost through divorce, marriage, birth, death, abandonment, and incarceration. With these events, the family structure changes, and roles are redefined or redistributed.

The nuclear family is no longer considered the dominant family structure in the United States. From 1960 to 2020, the percentage of children who were living with two parents decreased from 88% to 67% (Federal Interagency Forum on Child and Family Statistics, 2021; U.S. Census Bureau, 2016). Table 2.2 lists some of the family structures found in today's society. Nurses working with children need to understand the child's family structure and any changes that are occurring in it so they can help the family maintain or achieve optimal health and well-being.

Special Family Situations

Families face complex challenges as they try to nurture, develop, and socialize their children. When the family structure changes, the effects on children can be lifelong. Some situations may require astute assessment and proactive intervention to minimize the risk to the child and family.

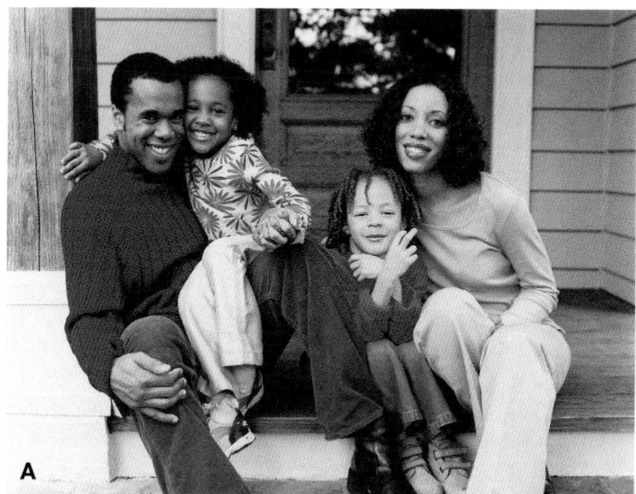

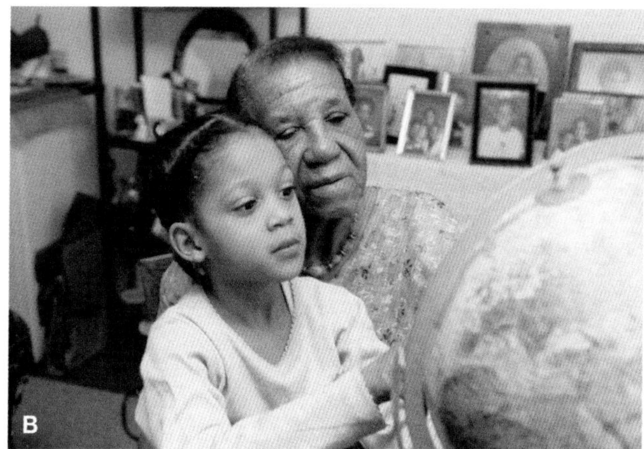

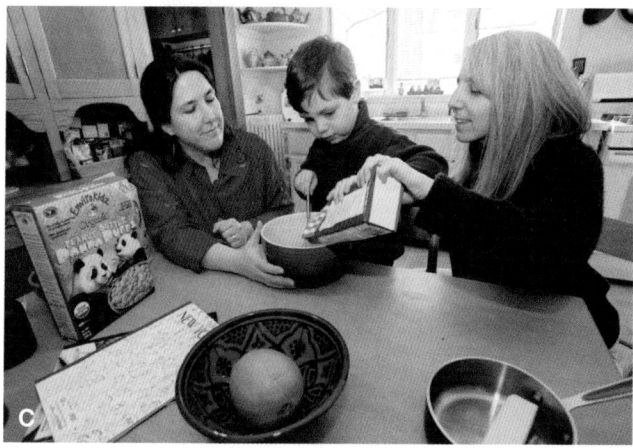

FIGURE 2.2 Nurses must recognize family dynamics when providing health care to children. There are many different family structures, and they influence child needs. **A.** The nuclear family is composed of two parents and their children. **B.** The extended family includes other family members, such as grandparents, aunts, uncles, and cousins. **C.** LGBTQ+ families may include two people of the same sex or same gender sharing a committed relationship with or without children.

TABLE 2.1 • Summary of Major Theories Related to Family

Theory	Description	Key Components
Friedman's structural functional theory (1998)	Emphasizes the social system of family, such as the organization or structure of the family and how the structure relates to the function	Identified five functions of families: 1. Affective function: meeting the love and belonging needs of each member 2. Socialization and social placement function: teaching children how to function and assume adult roles in society 3. Reproductive role: continuing the family and society in general 4. Economic function: ensuring the family has necessary resources with appropriate allocation 5. Health care function: involving the provision of physical care to keep family healthy
Duvall's developmental theory (1977)	Emphasizes the developmental stages that all families go through, beginning with marriage; the longitudinal career of the family is also known as the family life cycle	Described eight chronologic stages with specific predictable tasks that each family completes: 1. Marriage: beginning of family 2. Childbearing stage 3. Family with preschool children 4. Family with school-age children 5. Family with adolescents 6. Family with young adults 7. Middle-aged parents 8. Family in later years

(continued)

TABLE 2.1 • Summary of Major Theories Related to Family (*continued*)

Theory	Description	Key Components
Von Bertalanffy: general system theory applied to families (1968)	Emphasizes the family as a system with interdependent, interacting parts that endure over time to ensure the survival, continuity, and growth of its components; the family is not the sum of its parts but is characterized by wholeness and unity	Used to define how families interact with and are influenced by family and society and how to analyze the interrelationships of the members and the impact that change affecting one member will have on other members
Family stress theory	Addresses the way families respond to stress and how the family copes with the stress as a group as well as how each individual member copes	Described elements of stress as occurring internally within the family (e.g., values, beliefs, structure) that the family can control or change or externally from outside the family (e.g., culture of the surrounding community, genetics, the family's current time or place) over which the family has no control Described mobilization of family resources resulting in either a positive response of constructive coping or a negative response of a crisis Identified the main determinant of adequate coping based on the meaning of the stressful event to the family and its individual members
Resiliency model of family stress and family adjustment, and adaptation response model	Addresses the way families adapt to stress and can rebound from adversity	Identified the elements of risks and protective factors that aid a family in achieving positive outcomes

Adapted from Friedman, M. M. (1998). *Family nursing: Theory and practice* (4th ed.). Appleton & Lange; Duvall, E. (1977). *Marriage and family development* (5th ed.). J. B. Lippincott; Von Bertalanffy, L. (1968). *General systems theory.* Penguin Press; Boss, P. (2001). *Family stress management: A contextual approach* (2nd ed.). Sage Publications, Inc; Patterson, J. (2002). Integrating family resilience and family stress theory. *Journal of Marriage and Family, 64*(2), 349–360.

TABLE 2.2 • Types of Family Structures

Structure	Description	Specific Issues
Nuclear family	Husband, wife, and children living in same household	May include biologic or adopted children Once considered the traditional family structure; decreased due to trends in divorce rates and increases in alternative structures
Binuclear family	Child who is member of two families due to joint custody; parenting is considered a joint venture	Always better for the child when their interests are put above the parents' needs and desires
Single-parent family	One parent responsible for care of children	May encounter several challenges because of economic, social, and personal restraints; one person as household manager, caregiver, and financial provider
Commuter family	Adults in the family living and working apart for professional or financial reasons, often leaving the daily care of children to one parent	Similar to single-parent family
Blended family	Adults with children from previous marriages and/or from the new marriage	May lead to family conflict due to different expectations for the child and adults; may have different views and practices related to child care and health
Extended family	May include grandparents, cousins, aunts, and uncles	Need to determine decision maker as well as primary caregiver of the children Extended families may be more involved in child's life in some cultures than in others
LGBTQ+ family	May include adults of the same sex or same gender living together with or without children	May face prejudice and discrimination

TABLE 2.2 • Types of Family Structures

Structure	Description	Specific Issues
Communal family	Group of people living together to raise children and manage household, unrelated by blood or marriage	May face prejudice and discrimination Need to determine the decision maker and caregiver of children
Foster family	A temporary family for children who are placed away from their parents to ensure their emotional and physical well-being	May include foster family's children and other foster children in the home Foster children more likely to have unmet health needs and chronic health problems because they may have been living in a variety of settings
Grandparents-as-parents families	Grandparents raising their grandchildren if parents are unable to do so	May increase the risk of physical, financial, and emotional stress on older adults May lead to confusion and emotional stress for child if parents are in and out of the child's life
Adolescent families	Young parents still mastering the developmental tasks of their own childhoods	Greater risk for health problems during pregnancy and for delivery of premature infants, leading to risk of subsequent health and developmental problems Probably still need support from their families related to financial, emotional, and school issues

Divorced Families

Divorce is a common reason why the family structure changes. Today, just under 40% of marriages end in divorce, and many of these marriages include children (Fortin & Downes, 2023). Divorce can have a great impact on the child, sometimes with chronic and devastating results. Changes may have been occurring in the family for years, and children may have been exposed to turmoil, violence, or changes in structure before the actual divorce. Children may feel scared and confused by the threat divorce poses to their security. The initial response of children to divorce depends on their age as well as their developmental level, temperament, and the circumstances surrounding the divorce. Problems for children are often most apparent the first couple of years immediately following the divorce, and children may feel anger, anxiety, guilt, and depression and may exhibit nonadherence; however, most children show effective adjustment a few years after divorce (Fortin & Downes, 2023). Children in divorced families may experience long-term distress and require psychological help two to three times more than children whose parents remained married (Fortin & Downes, 2023).

Parents need to understand the impact divorce can have on their children so they can place the child's interest in the forefront. By appropriately supporting the child and utilizing the strengths of the child and family, children can be helped with constructively adjusting to divorce. Parents can use the suggestions in Box 2.2 to help reduce tension and conflict, thereby minimizing the impact of separation and divorce on their children. Health care providers can offer support, guidance, and resources to help make the strain of divorce easier on the entire family.

BOX 2.2 Recommendations for Divorcing Parents

1. Tell your children about the divorce and the reasons for the divorce in terms they can understand. Be sure you and your spouse are both present when telling the children; tell all the children at the same time.
2. Reassure your children that the divorce is not their fault. Repeat this as often as possible and as necessary.
3. Inform the children well in advance of anyone moving out of the house (except when abuse is present or there are concerns for immediate safety).
4. Clearly inform the children about the family structure after the divorce, such as who will live with whom and where; also discuss visitation clearly and honestly.
5. Do not expect your children to be or act like adults. Seek support from other adults in your life.
6. Do not discuss money or finances with your children.
7. Minimize unpredictable schedules and maintain routines, rules, and discipline, and be consistent in this area.
8. Never force or allow your children to take sides.
9. Avoid belittling your former spouse when the children can hear. However, do not lie to cover for irresponsible behavior by the other parent.
10. Never put your children in the middle between you and your ex-spouse.
11. Keep each parent involved in the child's life. Use letters, e-mails, phone calls, and text messages to continue communication. This shows the child they remain important to you even when they are with the other parent.
12. Communicate directly with the other parent. Avoid making the child your messenger.
13. Allow and assist the child to express their feelings about the divorce, and offer support.

Adapted from Kemp, G., Smith, M., & Segal, J. (2022). *Children and divorce.* https://www.helpguide.org/articles/parenting-family/children-and-divorce.htm; Fortin, K., & Downes, A. H. (2023). Section 5: Psychosocial Issues. In K. J. Marcdante, R. M. Kleigman, & A. M. Schuh (Eds.), *Nelson essentials of pediatrics* (9th ed., pp. 79–100). Elsevier.

Single-Parent Families

Divorce or separation, death of a partner, an unmarried person raising their own child, or adoption by a single caregiver are all circumstances that may result in single-parent families. Approximately 26% of children younger than 18 years live with one parent, with 21% living with the female parent only and 5% living with the male parent only (Federal Interagency Forum on Child and Family Statistics, 2021).

Single-parent families may face multiple factors that can affect the health of the children. Life in a single-parent household may include unique stressors for both the adult and the children. The single parent may feel overwhelmed if they have no one to share with the day-to-day responsibilities of care of the children, maintaining a job, and keeping up with the home and finances. These issues may be compounded by other pressures, such as custody problems, limited time to spend with children, continuing conflicts between parents who are separated or divorced, or changes in relationships with extended family members.

Communication and support are essential to the optimal functioning of the single-parent family. The parent and children need to be able to express their feelings and work through any problems together. Single parents must provide greater support for their children. Even though single parents may feel alone, they need to ensure they treat their children as children and not a substitute for a partner; they must receive support and comfort from sources who aren't their children. Community resources can be helpful. "Parents Without Partners," for instance, is an international organization that has over 200 chapters in the United States and Canada.

Blended Families

Creating a blended family (parents and their stepchildren), even though increasingly common, can be stressful for the parents and children alike. Although it can create new structure and stability and reduce some of the financial stress of single parenthood, making the transition to a blended family takes time. Children may feel jealous of a stepparent or feel disloyal toward the other biologic parent. There may be competition or rivalry among stepchildren. The child may fear that a stepparent is interfering with the child's relationship with their parent or taking away their source of love, affection, and attention.

Mutual respect and open, honest communication among all individuals involved are key, and this should include the child's biologic parents when possible. Responsibilities for parenting must be shared, including decisions about expectations, limits, and discipline. The continued role of both biologic parents and stepparents in the child's life is important to address.

Adoptive Families

Adoption is the process of a nonbiologic parent or parents creating a legal relationship with a child. Adoption can occur domestically (through an agency or intermediary such as an attorney in the family's own area or country), or the family may choose to adopt a child from another country. The child may be of a different culture, race, or ethnicity than the parents (Fig. 2.3). Most children in need of adoption in the United States and overseas are not infants (Schulte, 2022). Recent trends in adoption include an increase in transracial, same-sex parent, and single-parent adoptions along with increases in adoption of children with disabilities and increased openness in the adoption process (Schulte, 2022).

The amount of contact between the child and the birthing parent can vary greatly. In a closed adoption, there is no contact between the adoptive parents, the adopted child, and the birthing parent. In an open adoption, there is as much contact among the individuals as desired. Regardless of these decisions, adoptive families may be faced with unique issues. The children may have been exposed to poverty; neglect; infectious diseases; and lack of adequate food, clothing, shelter, and nurturing, placing them at risk for medical problems; physical growth and development delays or abnormalities; and behavioral, cognitive, and emotional problems. The adoptive parents may know about these problems, but in other situations, little, if any, history may be available.

Differences in culture, ethnicity, or race can further influence the adopted child's sense of identity (Jones & Schulte, 2012, reaffirmed 2017). Children in underrepresented groups may be subjected to racism or bigotry. Extended family members may not accept the child as part of the family. Parents need to emphasize that the

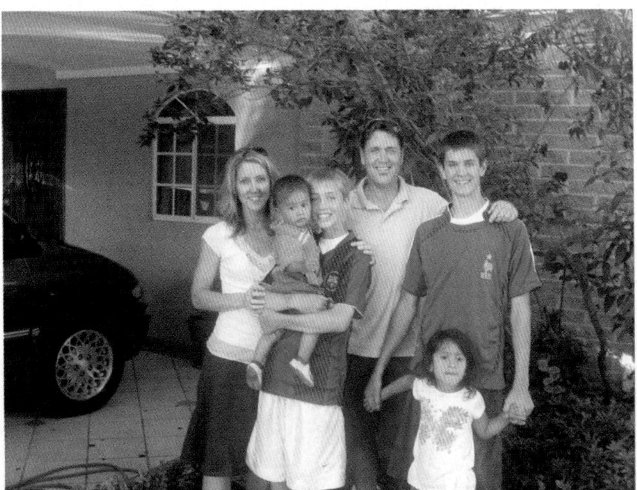

FIGURE 2.3 An adoptive family with children from a different culture.

adopted child is their child and is as much a part of the family as any other member. Parents need to openly recognize differences that exist between them and their child. They should encourage and assist the child in learning about the child's heritage, culture, and ethnic group (Jones & Schulte, 2012, reaffirmed 2017). Adopted adolescents and adults may feel a need to identify their biologic parents. Children adopted from other countries may travel to the country of their birth, and children adopted domestically may search for biologic relatives. Although this search is an indicator of healthy emotional growth, it can upset the adoptive parents, who may feel rejected.

TAKE NOTE!

Adolescents face vast challenges adjusting to adoption at this age because of the added complexity of identity issues facing this age group (Jones & Schulte, 2012, reaffirmed 2017).

Clear, open, honest communication and discussion are essential to promote a healthy, strong relationship. Support, guidance, and open communication are key for all parties involved. Open acknowledgment of the adoptive relationship helps nurture trust, security, and a child's self-esteem as they learn to understand what it means to be part of a family through adoption (Jones & Schulte, 2012, reaffirmed 2017).

The pediatric nurse needs to be sensitive, understanding, and supportive when interacting with adopted children and their families. "Positive" adoption language should be used. This includes saying "birth parent" when referring to biologic parents instead of "natural" or "real parent" and just "parents" when talking about adoptive parents (Jones & Schulte, 2012, reaffirmed 2017). Also, it is inappropriate to refer to the child as the "adopted child" or other children as "natural children" (Jones & Schulte, 2012, reaffirmed 2017). When discussing adoption, using terms such as "make an adoption plan" instead of "give away" or "give up for adoption" are preferred (Schulte, 2022). The nurse also needs to provide reassurance and understanding regarding missing health information and provide appropriate resources and referrals to resources that are knowledgeable about adoption and sensitive to the issues that may arise.

Foster Care Families

Foster care is a situation in which a child is cared for in an alternative living situation apart from their parents or legal guardians. The child may be placed in this living situation because of difficulties in the family situation, such as abuse, neglect, abandonment, or the parents' inability to meet the child's needs due to illness, substance use disorder, or death. The child may be sent to live with relatives (kinship care) or foster parents, who are strangers providing protection and shelter in a state-approved foster home.

There are about 407,493 children in the United States living in some form of foster care as of 2020 (U.S. Department of Health and Human Services, Administration for Children and Families, Administration on Children, Youth and Families, Children's Bureau, 2021). There has been a decline in the number of children in foster care over the past several years, and about 45% of children in foster care live in nonrelative homes (U.S. Department of Health and Human Services, Administration for Children and Families, Administration on Children, Youth and Families, Children's Bureau, 2021). In 2020, 48% of children who left foster care were reunified with their parents, 6% went to live with other relatives, and 25% were adopted (U.S. Department of Health and Human Services, Administration for Children and Families, Administration on Children, Youth and Families, Children's Bureau, 2021). The goal of foster care is to provide temporary services that protect the child's safety and health until the child can return home to their family or be adopted. However, children may remain in foster care for several years or longer and may be moved from one foster family to another.

Many children who are placed in foster care have been the victims of abuse or neglect. Children in foster care are more likely to exhibit a wide range of medical, emotional, behavioral, educational, or developmental problems (Fortin & Downes, 2023). They may experience certain issues, including the following:

- Unmet health care needs
- Significant mental health problems, such as depression, social problems, anxiety, and posttraumatic stress disorder due to trauma, loss, and unpredictability
- Behavioral problems such as substance use disorder, legal problems, and self-destructive behaviors
- Interruptions in developmental stages and developmental delays
- Educational obstacles due to frequent moves and gaps in education
- Self-blame and feelings of guilt
- Feelings of being unwanted
- Feelings of helplessness and powerlessness
- Insecurity about the future
- Ambivalent feelings related to foster parents and/or feelings of being disloyal to birth parents (Fortin & Downes, 2023)

Individual attention to the child in foster care is essential. A multidisciplinary approach to care that includes the birth parents, foster parents, child, health care professionals, and support services is important to meet the child's needs for growth and development. Nurses play a key role in advocating for the child.

Family Roles and Functions

The role of the family in caring for the child includes not only providing physical and emotional care but also imparting the rules and expected behaviors of society through teaching and discipline techniques. These expected behaviors depend on the culture, values, and beliefs of the family and the child's developmental stage and physical and cognitive abilities. Roles and functions are further defined by each family's own traditions and values and the family's set of standards for interaction within and outside the family. For instance, some families may value privacy more than others.

Caregiver–Child Interaction

The caregiver–child interaction is critical to the survival and healthy development of a young child (World Health Organization [WHO], 2012). Most often, the primary caregivers are the parents. Ideally, parents nurture their children and provide them with an environment in which they can become competent, productive, self-directed members of society. For young children, in particular, growth, health, and their personhood itself depend on the ability of the adults in their life to understand and respond to them.

Parental Roles

Parenting is an enormous responsibility and takes a lot of time and physical and mental energy. Parental roles are vast and numerous. Typical parental roles include nurturer/caregiver, financial provider, decision maker, schedule manager, financial manager, problem solver, counselor, teacher, behavior support manager, and health manager.

CHANGES IN PARENTAL ROLES OVER TIME

Parental roles evolve due to societal and economic changes as well as individual family changes. In the past in the United States, the role of provider was most often assigned to the parent. However, with increased numbers of women in the workplace and more households with two parents working, today, both parents are often the providers as well as the nurturers to the children. Technologic innovations have provided parents with opportunities to work at home, allowing some parents to maintain the provider role while simultaneously fulfilling the nurturer and health manager roles. Parents are taking on greater responsibilities related to household management and child care. Additionally, a significant number of children are being raised by their grandparents (Joshi & Lebrun-Harris, 2022). Moreover, as Baby Boomers age, Generation X and Millennial parents may find themselves caring for both their children and their own parents.

PARENTING STYLES

Research in the 1960s by Baumrind, a psychologist, and further research in the 1980s by Maccoby and Martin led to the conceptualization of four major parenting styles common in our society: authoritarian; authoritative; permissive; and uninvolved, rejecting, or neglecting (Baumrind, 1966; Cherry, 2022). The styles are defined by the amount of support and control exerted over the child during parenting. Many parents may use more than one parenting style and may fall somewhere in between styles instead of adhering strictly to just one. Also, some parents may change parenting styles as the child ages and matures. Nurses need to recognize different parenting styles and provide support to parents by discussing the effects of different parenting models and teaching parenting skills.

Authoritarian

The *authoritarian* parent expects obedience from the child and discourages the child from questioning the family's rules. The parent provides low support and high control over the child. The rules and standards set forth by the parents are strictly enforced and firm. The parents expect the child to accept the family's beliefs and values and demand respect for these beliefs. The parents are the ultimate authority and allow little, if any, participation by the child in making decisions. Behavior that does not adhere to the family's rules and standards is punished. This parenting style is associated with children who are obedient and proficient but who may also experience negative effects on self-esteem, happiness, and social skills as well as increased aggression and defiance (Cherry, 2022).

Authoritative

The *authoritative* or democratic parent shows some respect for the child's opinions. Although parents still have the ultimate authority and expect the child to adhere to the rules, authoritative parents allow children to be different and believe that each child is an individual. They exhibit warmth and consistently, fairly, and firmly enforce the family's rules and standards without emphasizing punishment. This type of parenting is associated with increased independence, happiness, and self-confidence, helping children become socially responsible individuals (Cherry, 2022).

Permissive

Permissive or laissez-faire parents have little control over the behavior of their children. Rules or standards may be inconsistent, unclear, or nonexistent. Permissive parents allow their children to determine their own standards and rules for behavior. Discipline can be lax, inconsistent, or absent. Parents can be warm, cool, or uninvolved. There are more negative than positive effects associated with this style of parenting. Negative effects include impulsivity, low happiness, poor school performance, problems with authority, and lack of responsibility and independence (Cherry, 2022).

Uninvolved, Rejecting, or Neglecting

Uninvolved parents are indifferent. They do not provide rules or standards. The child's basic needs are often met, but the parent is disconnected from the child's life. In some cases, the parents may neglect or reject the child. They can be cold and uninterested in meeting the child's needs. They minimize their interactions and time with the children. This type of parenting is associated with negative effects such as disinterest in school, disinterest in the future, and limited emotional and self-control (Cherry, 2022). This type of parenting may also lead to issues with trust, low self-esteem, and children having less competency than their peers (Cherry, 2022).

Discipline

Much of parenting involves increasing desirable behavior and decreasing or eliminating undesirable behavior, a process generally known as **discipline**. There are various opinions in U.S. society about the best or most effective method of discipline. Each child and family is unique. Discipline that works with one child or within one family may not work for another family. Discipline should focus on the development of the child while ensuring that their self-esteem and dignity are preserved. It should be based on age-appropriate expectations with clear, consistent guidelines while offering meaningful choices when possible. Discipline involves teaching and is ongoing, not something that is done only when the child misbehaves.

The American Academy of Pediatrics focuses on the importance of teaching good behavior rather than punishing bad behavior and teaching the child to manage or regulate their behavior (Sege et al., 2018). Effective discipline relies on understanding a child's normal growth and development, and nurses can assist families by educating them on their child's development along with effective discipline techniques. Teaching Guideline 2.1 provides some tips to help a child learn acceptable behavior as they grow.

TEACHING GUIDELINES 2.1 Teaching to Promote Effective Discipline

- Set clear, consistent, and developmentally appropriate expected behaviors; offer choices whenever possible.
- Maintain consistency in responding to behaviors; provide encouragement and affection.
- Role model appropriate behaviors.
- Provide an age-appropriate explanation of the consequence that will occur if the child demonstrates unacceptable behavior.
- Always administer the consequence soon after the unacceptable behavior.
- Keep the consequence appropriate to the age of the child and the situation.
- Stay calm but firm without showing anger when administering the consequence.
- Always praise the child for displaying appropriate behavior.
- Set up the environment to assist the child in accomplishing the appropriate behavior; remove temptations that may lead to inappropriate behavior.
- Reinforce that the child's behavior was bad, not that the child was bad.

POSITIVE REINFORCEMENT

Attention from parents is a powerful form of positive reinforcement and can help increase desirable behaviors. The key is to focus on the child's appropriate behaviors rather than emphasizing the inappropriate ones. Immediate, consistent, and frequent feedback is crucial. This feedback can be in the form of smiles, praise, special attention, or rewards such as extra privileges or a special token or activity. Providing the feedback immediately is important so that the child learns to associate the feedback with the appropriate behavior, thereby reinforcing the behavior.

EXTINCTION

Another form of discipline is extinction, which focuses on reducing or eliminating the positive reinforcement for inappropriate behavior. Examples are ignoring the temper tantrums of a toddler, withholding or removing privileges, and requiring a "time-out." Withholding or removing privileges such as TV, music, or computer or phone use is most effective for older children and adolescents. The adolescent may be grounded for a short time or not allowed to drive the car. To be effective, the privilege being withheld or removed must be something that the child values.

Time-out is an extinction discipline method that is most effective with toddlers, preschoolers, and early school-age children. It involves removing the child from the problem area and placing them in a neutral, nonthreatening, safe area where no interaction occurs between the child and parents or others for a specifically determined period (Fig. 2.4).

TAKE NOTE!

The amount of time a child spends in time-out is typically 1 minute per year of age; around the age of 3, the parent could allow the child to dictate their own time-out length, such as saying "Come back when you feel ready and calm." This allows the child to learn self-management skills (American Academy of Pediatrics [AAP], 2018).

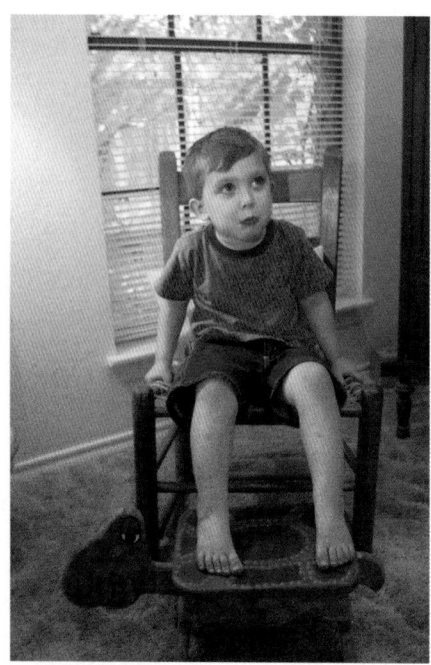

FIGURE 2.4 Although they might not like it, quiet solitude helps children develop inner control.

PUNISHMENT

Discipline is often confused with punishment, but **punishment** involves a negative or unpleasant experience or consequence for doing or not doing something. Punishment may be verbal or corporal. Verbal punishment commonly takes the form of reprimands or scolding (the use of disapproving statements). The statements are intended to change or eliminate the inappropriate behavior. Verbal reprimands can be effective in the short term if they are used sparingly and are focused on the child's specific behavior. If verbal reprimands are used frequently and indiscriminately, they lose their effectiveness, can provoke anxiety in the child, and encourage the child to ignore the parent.

Corporal punishment involves the use of physical pain as a means to decrease inappropriate behavior. The most common form of corporal punishment is spanking (the use of an open hand to the buttocks or an extremity with the intention of modifying behavior without causing injury) (Sege et al., 2018). Recent research shows that the use of corporal punishment is declining, with only 50% of parents reporting ever spanking their child (Sege et al., 2018).

Initially, spanking may be effective because of its sudden and shocking nature. However, over time it loses its effectiveness because its shock value declines. Spanking may stop the negative behavior, but it also increases the chance for physical injury, especially for infants and young children, and may lead to altered caregiver–child relationships (Sege et al., 2018). Because the effects of spanking diminish, the intensity of the spanking must be increased to achieve the same effects. Thus, it is important for parents to understand the consequences of its use.

Various studies have linked spanking in childhood with subsequent aggressive behavior in childhood and persistent anger in adulthood (Sege et al., 2018). Because of the negative consequences of spanking and because it has been shown to be no more effective than other methods for managing inappropriate behavior, the AAP recommends parents use methods other than spanking to respond to inappropriate behavior (Sege et al., 2018).

CULTURE

Culture (the view of the world and implementation of a set of traditions that are used by a specific social group in order to pass these traditions along to the next generation) plays a critical role in shaping a child, including their health and health practices. Culture is a complex phenomenon involving the integration of many components such as beliefs, values, language, time, and personal space that shape a person's actions and behavior. Children learn these patterns of cultural behaviors from their families and communities through a process called **enculturation**, which involves acquiring knowledge and internalizing values.

Culture influences every aspect of development and is reflected in childrearing beliefs and practices designed to promote healthy adaptation. Typically, a child begins to understand their culture at approximately 5 years of age (Andrews, 2020). The child's cultural background affects the way the child socializes, learns values, and experiences the world. The child's developing beliefs, customs, mode of communication, dress, and actions may all be shaped by their culture.

With today's changing demographic patterns, nurses must be able to incorporate cultural knowledge into their interventions so that they can care effectively for culturally diverse children. They must be aware of the wide range of cultural traditions, values, and ethics that exist in the United States today. All nurses must establish cultural knowledge about a child's culture so that health care interventions can be adapted to meet the needs of the child. The nurse should know about various culture-based health practices and how they may affect children, as well as the demographics of the local population.

The goal is for the nurse to view culture as a point of congruence rather than a potential source of conflict. The nurse needs to combine cultural respect with cultural humility. This is an ongoing process that includes self-reflection of one's own biases, a continued willingness to learn from others, and a desire to honor each individual's personal beliefs, customs, and values. By combining cultural respect and knowledge with cultural humility, the nurse will be able to provide more effective care to children and their families.

The relationship of culture to health care can become obscured by the use of broad group titles. In reality, there are many distinct cultural groups, and within a group there may be many subcultures. It is crucial that the nurse remembers that diversity exists within cultures, and this is as important as the diversity among different cultures. Every child is a unique individual with their own beliefs, values, and history. The nurse needs to assess each child and family and ask questions to understand their unique beliefs and values.

Cultural Health Practices

Health practices are often the result of health beliefs derived from a person's culture. For example, do the child and family view health and illness as the result of natural forces, supernatural forces, or the imbalance of forces? Many cultures have remedies that people may use or consider before they seek professional health care. Families may go to complementary or alternative medicine practitioners who they believe can cure certain illnesses.

If culturally influenced complementary and alternative care practices are compatible with the health regimen and support appropriate health practices, these practices do no harm; in fact, they can be beneficial to the child and family. However, these practices should not lead to a delay in beneficial treatment or create other problems.

TAKE NOTE!

Pediatric nurses can help to shape an individual's lifelong perceptions of health and health services. An understanding of how the child's and family's culture affects their health practices gives the nurse an opportunity to incorporate appropriate and beneficial health practices into the family's cultural milieu, providing sources of strength rather than areas of conflict.

Recall Miguel, the infant described at the beginning of the chapter. Propose appropriate nursing interventions that would assist in providing culturally competent care. How can you best determine the child's and family's cultural preferences?

Changing Cultural Demographics

Although the proportion of children is decreasing in relationship to the adult population, the racial, ethnic, and cultural diversity among children is significantly increasing in the United States (Federal Interagency Forum on Child and Family Statistics, 2021). Thus, the diversity among children entering the health care system in the United States is increasing. In 2022, approximately 49% of the population identified as White non-Hispanic, 26% as Hispanic; 14% as Black non-Hispanic; 6% as Asian; and 6% as non-Hispanic, all other races (Federal Interagency Forum on Child and Family Statistics, 2023). It is projected that by 2050, 31% of the U.S. population of children will identify as Hispanic; 39% as White non-Hispanic; 14% as Black non-Hispanic; 7% as Asian; and 9% as non-Hispanic, all other races (Federal Interagency Forum on Child and Family Statistics, 2023). In addition, the increasing number of relationships between individuals from different backgrounds is producing an increasing number of children whose heritage represents more than one cultural group.

Immigration

Employment and economic opportunities, expanded human rights, educational opportunities, and other types of freedoms and opportunities encourage many people from other countries to move to the United States. Approximately one in four children in the United States are immigrants or members of an immigrant family (Children's Defense Fund, 2023). This includes both children born outside the United States and those with at least one foreign-born parent. Some communities welcome newcomers, but others do not.

Immigration can affect the health, educational, and social services provided in the United States. It also is related to access to care and the types of care that need to be offered. Families who have immigrated face higher rates of poverty, lack of health insurance coverage, and low educational attainment than those who have not immigrated (Kaiser Family Foundation, 2022). Immigration can impose unique stresses on children and families, including:

- Depression, grief, or anxiety associated with leaving their country of origin and pressure for acculturation
- Separation from family and other support systems
- Language barriers
- Differences in social, professional, and economic status between their country of origin and the United States
- Traumatic events, such as war, that may have occurred in the countries they left (Linton et al., 2019)

Inability to speak English can hinder educational attainment, economic opportunities, and the ability to join the societal mainstream. Thirteen percent of children born in families who immigrated have difficulty speaking English, with 18% of children in such families living in a linguistically isolated home (i.e., no person 14 years or older speaks English "very well") (Kids Count Data Center, 2020a, 2020b). Parents who do not speak English may have trouble accessing health care and health insurance, enrolling their children in school, becoming involved in school activities, and accessing work or higher-paying jobs.

Children from other countries may arrive in the United States with significant health problems. They may present with diseases that are more common in their countries of origin and rarely seen in the United States, such as malaria. Their health status may be compromised due to the lack of at-birth and early childhood screenings, which may manifest in problems such as inborn errors of metabolism, lack of preventive care, no immunizations, and no dental care. Due to financial, language, cultural, and other types of barriers that immigrant families sometimes face, children may not receive the necessary preventive care or receive care for minor conditions until the conditions become more serious. Stressors, such as those associated with relocation, separation, and traumatic events, can also have a negative impact on psychological and physical health.

SPIRITUALITY AND RELIGION

Spirituality is a belief in something greater than oneself and a faith that affirms life positively. It is a major influence in many people's lives, providing a meaning or purpose to life and a foundation for and a source of love, relationships, and service. Spirituality is considered a universal human phenomenon with an assumption of the wholeness of individuals and their connectedness to a higher being. During life-changing events and crises, such as the birth of a child with a congenital defect or a serious or terminal illness, families often turn to spirituality for hope, comfort, and relief.

The word "religion" is often used interchangeably with spirituality in U.S. society. However, "spirituality" can be used to describe a more private and individual belief, while "religion" indicates an organized way of sharing beliefs and practicing worship. Eighty one percent of Americans report believing in God (Jones, 2022); therefore, spirituality and religion are an important focus when working with children and their families. A person's reaction to health and illness may be affected by these beliefs. Different religions may view illness as a punishment for sin or wrongdoing, a curse, or a test of strength (Andrews, 2020).

Children view spirituality and religion differently at different developmental stages. Typically, children imitate their parents' rituals when they are toddlers and then develop an increasingly sophisticated understanding of their parents' views during the years leading up to adolescence. (Refer to Chapters 3 through 7 for a discussion on how children of different ages and developmental levels view spirituality and religion.)

Families appreciate the recognition of and respect for their beliefs. Therefore, identifying the child's and family's religious beliefs and customs is important. Families may adhere to special dietary restrictions, rituals such as baptism or communion, use of amulets or icons, or practices related to dying that can be incorporated into the child's plan of care. Using open-ended questions and observing for the use of religious articles during assessment can provide clues to the family's beliefs and practices. Visits from spiritual leaders may also be noted.

Recall the Delgado family described at the beginning of the chapter. What, if any, influence might the family's culture and religious beliefs have on Miguel's care?

TAKE NOTE!

Never make assumptions about a family's religious or spiritual affiliation. Although they may belong to a particular religion, they may not adhere to all of the beliefs or participate in all aspects of the religion.

COMMUNITY

Community encompasses a broad range of concepts, from a person's particular neighborhood or group to an individual's nation of residence. The community surrounding a child affects many aspects of their health, development, and general welfare. The child's community consists of the family, school, neighborhood, youth organizations, and other peer groups.

The quality of life within the community has a great influence on a child's ability to achieve developmental tasks and become a functional member of society. The child's school, which is a community itself, and peer groups are important influences. School programs and community centers can also affect the child's overall health and well-being.

Children need to feel supported by, cared for, and valued by their community. They need to be surrounded by supportive, loving parents; safe schools and neighborhoods; adult mentors and role models; and caring teachers. They need to know what is expected of them and what behaviors are outside the boundaries of the community.

Schools and Other Community Centers

Children today start school at an earlier age, spend more time in child care settings, and are involved in various community centers and activities. By age 3 or 4, many children are in a preschool setting for several hours a day. Some children spend more awake time in school and child care settings than in their family homes. Thus, schools and child care settings have become major influences on children.

School also provides a means of socialization. School rules about attendance and authority relationships and the system of sanctions and rewards based on achievement help teach children behavioral expectations they will need for future employment and relationships in the adult world. Although the primary role of schools has always been academic education, today schools are performing more health-related functions. Schools play an important role in promoting healthy behaviors and educating children about proper exercise, nutrition, safety, sex, drugs, and mental health.

Academic success is linked to healthy behaviors. Academic success is a good indicator of child well-being and is a predictor of adult health outcomes (CDC, 2022a). Academic failure is linked to health risk behaviors such as substance use, unhealthy diets, and physical inactivity (CDC, 2022a). School health programs have positive impacts on health outcomes and health risk behaviors along with educational outcomes (CDC, 2022a).

Because in many families both parents need to work, many children are enrolled in child care and afterschool programs. Thus, the socialization process begins earlier and involves a larger percentage of the child's waking hours (Fig. 2.5).

Afterschool hours are a critical time during which children may participate in risky health behaviors if they are not provided with supervised, structured activity in which they can learn and grow. Community centers and afterschool programs can provide an opportunity for children to learn new skills, have new experiences, and develop relationships with caring adults in a safe and supportive environment.

Peer Groups

A child's friends can have a major influence on their growth and development. Peer group relationships often begin early and are a large part of the child's world, particularly with school-age children and adolescents. This influence starts in playgroups in preschool or elementary school. The child is confronted with a variety of values and belief systems from interactions with their friends. To be accepted, the child must conform to the specific values and beliefs of the group. When these values and beliefs differ from those of the adults in the child's world, conflicts can occur, possibly separating children from the adults and strengthening their sense of belonging to the peer group.

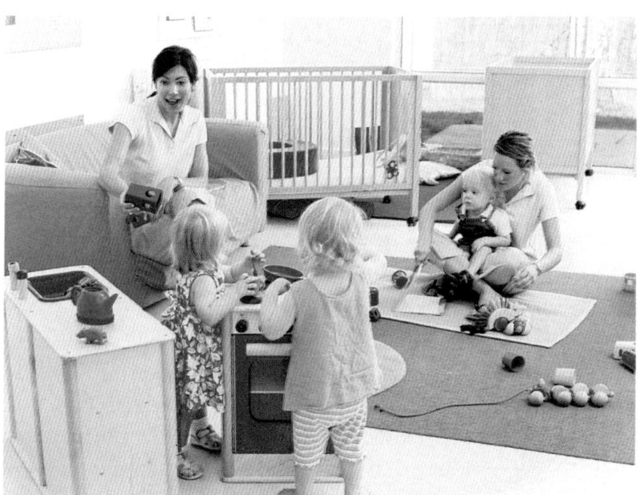

FIGURE 2.5 Day care centers can provide socialization and support for young children.

When the child's friends are successful in school or other activities, the growth and development of the child continues in a healthy and positive way. When these groups demonstrate healthy behaviors, the influence is positive; however, peer groups can also exert negative influences on the child. Thus, it is vital to identify the important peer groups in a child's life and the positive or negative behaviors connected with these groups.

Violence in the Community

Youth violence affects the community as well as the child and family. Studies have shown that youth violence is associated with a disruption in social services, negative impact on school attendance, an increase in health care costs, and a decline in property values (CDC, 2022b). Research continues to show that children exposed to violence suffer serious lifelong consequences, such as problems with development, behavior, and physical and mental health (CDC, 2022b).

Violent Crimes

Violent crimes include murder, rape, robbery, and aggravated assault. Statistics from the CDC (2022b) show that for people of ages 10 to 24 years:

- More than 1,000 individuals are treated each day in emergency departments for injuries due to physical violence.
- Homicide is the third leading cause of death for all people in this age group and is the leading cause of death for non-Hispanic Black or African American young people.

Suicide

Suicide is a serious public health problem affecting young people today. It is the third leading cause of death in people ages 10 to 17, with almost two thirds due to firearms (Kennebeck & Bonin, 2021). Of these reported suicides, males were more likely than females to die by suicide (Kennebeck & Bonin, 2021).

A nationwide survey of students in grades 9 to 12 in public and private schools found that one in five participants had reported seriously considering suicide. One in six made a plan for how they would carry out suicide, and one in 11 attempted suicide in the previous 12 months (Ivey-Stephenson et al., 2020).

TAKE NOTE!

Suicide rates vary among different demographic groups; non-Hispanic Native American/Alaskan Native and non-Hispanic White individuals have the highest rates of suicide in the United States (CDC, 2022c).

School Violence

In recent years, due to several high-profile cases of school shootings, much attention has been directed at school violence, and concern for student safety has increased. Statistically, however, less than 2% of homicides of school-age children occur on the way to or from school, at school events, or during school hours (CDC, 2021c). Although students are much less likely to be victims of crime at school, some schools continue to have violence problems, highlighting the importance of school violence prevention (CDC, 2021a). The CDC conducted a nationwide survey of high school students about high-risk behavior and found that in 2019, approximately 8% of the students reported that they had been involved in a physical altercation on school property, while 7% reported being injured or threatened by a weapon on school grounds (CDC, 2021a).

Much of school violence involves bullying, which is repeated negative actions that are clearly malicious and unwarranted by one or more people directed at a victim. It has been estimated that one in five students between ninth and 10th grades in the United States are a target of bullying (CDC, 2021b). Many cases of bullying go unreported; however, bullying can have long-lasting traumatic effects, such as depression, low self-esteem, anxiety, academic problems, sleep problems, and violence later in adolescence and adulthood (CDC, 2021b). School nurses need to be aware of bullying and offer support and guidance and intervention when necessary to students and staff.

Safe schools are essential for proper learning, growth and development, development of healthy relationships, and overall health of children. Violence in schools has a negative effect not only on students but also on the school and the entire community. The continued coordination among schools, law enforcement, social services, and mental health systems and the development of effective programs will help reduce these risk behaviors.

Violence in the Home

Violence that occurs in the home, known as domestic violence, affects the lives of many people in the United States, including children. Domestic violence includes intimate partner violence and violence between family members. Females between the age of 18 and 34 have the highest rate of being victims of intimate partner violence (Franchek-Roa, 2022) and are more likely than males to be victims of these types of crimes.

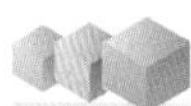 Concept Mastery Alert

Children who are exposed to frequent adverse events in the family often exhibit early initiation of smoking, sexual activity, and recreational drug use.

Children exposed to family violence are more likely to be a victim or perpetrator of violence in adulthood (Franchek-Roa, 2022). The Federal Child Abuse Prevention and Treatment Act (CAPTA) defines child abuse and neglect as any recent act or failure to act on the part of a parent or caregiver that results in death, serious physical or emotional harm, or sexual abuse or exploitation, or an act or failure to act that presents an imminent risk of serious harm to a child (U.S. Department of Health and Human Services, 2014). In 2020, approximately 618,000 cases of child maltreatment occurred in the United States (CDC, 2022). Of the number of children identified as being maltreated, 76.1% were victims of neglect, 16.5% were victims of physical abuse, and 9.4% were victims of sexual abuse (U.S. Department of Health and Human Services, Administration for Children and Families, Administration on Children, Youth and Families, Children's Bureau, 2022). Approximately 1,750 children died from abuse and neglect in 2020; 68% of those children were younger than 3 years (U.S. Department of Health and Human Services, Administration for Children and Families, Administration on Children, Youth and Families, Children's Bureau, 2022).

TAKE NOTE!

American Indian or Alaska Native and African American children experience higher rates of abuse and neglect, according to the U.S. Department of Health and Human Services, Administration for Children and Families, Administration on Children, Youth and Families, Children's Bureau (2022). The incidence of child abuse and neglect is five times higher for children from families with low socioeconomic status (CDC, 2022d).

Children who are exposed to stressors such as domestic violence or who are victims of childhood abuse or neglect are at high risk for short- and long-term problems. These problems manifest differently based on the child's age and developmental ability; the younger the child and the longer the exposure, the more serious the problems. Short-term problems may include sleep disturbances, headaches, stomachaches, depression, asthma, enuresis, aggressive behaviors such as increased peer aggression and bullying, decreased social competencies, withdrawal, avoidant attachment, developmental regression, fears, anxiety, and learning problems. Long-term problems may include poor school performance, truancy, absenteeism, and difficulty with adult relationships and tasks. There is a strong correlation between the number of exposures to ACEs and negative behaviors and health concerns such as early initiation of smoking, sexual activity, and illicit drug use; adolescent pregnancy; higher weight; depression; and suicide attempts (National Conference of State Legislators (NCSL), 2022).

TAKE NOTE!

Witnessing and being exposed to violence in childhood results in a higher tolerance and greater risk of use of violence as an adult (Franchek-Roa, 2022).

Due to the potential impact of violence on children and families, it is important to perform a thorough assessment to identify violence in the family (Box 2.3). Providing referrals to shelters and child advocacy centers and intervening to assist children in dealing with this issue are key.

Not all children who are exposed to violence suffer negative consequences. Studies have identified protective factors that can help buffer children from the effects of violence and reduce the risk that the child will develop violent behaviors in the future (CDC, 2022g). Examples of protective factors include:

- Feelings of connectedness or a secure attachment to a nonviolent parent or caregiver
- Strong commitment to school and academic performance
- Involvement in social activities
- Social and community support
- Positive sibling and peer relationships
- Ability to discuss problems with parents or a supportive adult
- Consistent presence of a parent at least once during the day, such as in the morning on awakening, when getting home from school, at dinnertime, or when going to bed
- Positive view of self
- Strong cultural and/or spiritual identity

Thus, interventions need to focus on reducing children's exposure to violence and fostering protective factors.

BOX 2.3 Assessing for Violence

Questions for the Parent

- Do you ever feel afraid in your home?
- What happens when you and (partner's name) argue?
- Do arguments ever become physical (hitting, kicking, pushing, throwing, or punching/breaking objects)?
- Have you ever been threatened with a weapon (e.g., gun, knife)?
- Have you ever felt trapped or like a prisoner in your own home? Does your partner ever lock you in/out of the house or take your car keys?
- Have your children ever seen or heard violence in the home?
- Have the police ever been involved due to violence in your home?
- Is the violence ever directed at the children? Does (partner's name) ever hit, kick, push, or yell at your child when they are angry?
- How do you and (partner's name) discipline the children?

Questions for the Child

- What happens when Mommy and Daddy (or appropriate partner names) argue or fight? Is there any hitting, pushing, and so forth?
- How do you feel when Mommy and Daddy (or appropriate partner names) fight?
- What happens to you when you get in trouble?
  - If hitting or other physical forms of discipline occur, ask:
- What are you hit with? Where on your body? Does it ever leave a mark or bruise?
- Who hits or kicks you? How often does it happen?

SOCIETY

Society has a major impact on the health of a child. Major societal factors that influence children and their health include social roles, social determinants of health, the media, and the expanding global nature of society. Each of these areas may influence children's self-concept, the communities they live in, their choice of lifestyle, and their health. Pediatric nurses need to assess these areas and their influence on the child and family so that individualized strategies can be designed and implemented to enhance any positive effects and minimize any negative effects on the child's and family's health.

Social Roles

Societal norms dictate that specific people behave in specific ways: certain behaviors are permitted, and others are prohibited. These patterns influence social roles and can be an important factor in the development of self-concept. A person's self-concept can strongly influence their health.

For children, social roles influence their ideas about themselves. Box 2.4 lists some typical roles children have

BOX 2.4 Examples of Social Roles for Children

- Child (daughter or son)
- Sibling
- Grandchild
- School or day care roles, such as first-grader, honor student
- Community member
- Organized religion roles (e.g., acolyte, altar server)
- Specialized roles such as developing musician, artist, or athlete

in our society. These social roles are generally carried out in groups, such as the family, school, peers, or religious or community organizations. At times, there may be a conflict in how the different groups expect a child to behave. There may also be conflict for parents related to childrearing practices. For example, the child's family may believe in creationism, while the school the child attends is teaching evolution. Thus, the child may feel confused as they try to reconcile the differences between the different groups.

Social Determinants of Health

Social determinants of health are conditions in the environment where people live, work, learn, and play that affect their health, well-being, and quality of life. Examples include education access and quality, economic stability, neighborhood and built environments, health care access and quality, and social and community context (Healthy People 2030, U.S. Department of Health and Human Services, Office of Disease Prevention and Health Promotion, n.d.).

Socioeconomic Status and Economic Stability

An important influence on children is the family's socioeconomic status (relative position in society), which takes into account the family's economic, occupational, and educational levels. Children are raised differently by parents with different educational levels, occupations, and incomes. Despite advances and improvements in quality and access to health care, discrepancies in health status among socioeconomic classes have continued (Agency for Healthcare Research and Quality, 2021). Income inequality is an important factor in explaining this variation. Parents with lower incomes may need to work longer hours to provide basic necessities and have little time or money to enrich the child's life with outside resources or make healthy lifestyle choices. However, these families may have stronger family relationships if they need to rely on the broader family network to meet some of their physical and emotional needs.

Low socioeconomic status can have an adverse influence on children's health. Some families may not be able to afford health insurance or health care. Meals may be unbalanced or irregular. The family's house or apartment may be overcrowded and may have poor sanitation or lead paint. These families may not understand the importance of preventive care or may not be able to afford it, and, as a result, the children may be inadequately immunized against communicable diseases or lack preventive care. Studies have documented that children from low socioeconomic backgrounds are more likely to suffer negative physical and mental health outcomes, such as depression, behavioral problems, substance misuse, and injuries (Bitsko et al., 2022). Basic financial stability enhances the general health and well-being of children; thus, an important negative influence on children's health is poverty. Children living in poverty are more likely to have poor health, complete fewer years of school, experience violent crimes, and become adults with lower incomes (Federal Interagency Forum on Child and Family Statistics, 2021).

The poverty threshold is based on the family's size and income and is used to determine whether a family is living in poverty (Table 2.3). According to the U.S. Census Bureau in 2020, the official poverty rate was 11.4%, the first increase after 5 consecutive years of decline (Shrider et al., 2021). Overall, 16.1% of children younger than 18 years were living in poverty (Shrider et al., 2021). According to the Children's Defense Fund (2023), 11.1 million American children live in poverty, with 5.5 million living in extreme poverty. The rate of poverty is closely tied to the overall health of the economy; therefore, in times of recession, a rise is usually seen.

Family structure is an important factor associated with poverty rates for children. The poverty rate for married-couple families is lower than that for families headed by a single parent. Of the families living below the poverty level, 38.1% were single-parent families with no spouse present; 17.8% were single-parent families with no spouse present; and 7.5% were married couples (Shrider et al., 2021). Educational level is another important factor; as education increases, unemployment declines and annual income rises. However, a chronic physical or emotional problem in any wage earner may lead to unemployment, and this can cause the family to experience economic declines.

The effects of poverty on children's health can be wide ranging. The family may be able to afford only

TABLE 2.3 • 2022 U.S. Poverty Guidelines

Size of Family Unit	48 Contiguous States and Washington, DC ($)	Alaska ($)	Hawaii ($)
1	13,590	16,990	15,630
2	18,310	22,890	21,060
3	23,030	28,790	26,490
4	27,750	34,690	31,920
5	32,470	40,590	37,350

Data from U.S. Department of Health and Human Services. (2022). *2022 poverty guidelines*. Retrieved October 14, 2022, from https://aspe.hhs.gov/topics/poverty-economic-mobility/poverty-guidelines

inadequate housing or a house or an apartment in a neighborhood with unsanitary conditions, toxins, or violence. These families may also experience homelessness.

Neighborhoods, Built Environments, and Homelessness

The neighborhood and environment where a child lives, plays, and learns is an important determinant of their health. Refer to the content discussed under the "Community" section earlier in the chapter. Housing is a critical social determinant of health in children. During the 2020–2021 school year, approximately 1.1 million children who were enrolled in school were not securely housed, this equates to 1 in 45 children enrolled in public school experiencing homelessness (Children's Defense Fund, 2023). It is impossible to measure homelessness with 100% accuracy. Therefore, looking at trends is important to demonstrate whether progress is being made. Recent data do suggest that homelessness among families is increasing (Children's Defense Fund, 2023).

Homelessness occurs across geographic regions. The principal causes of homelessness are poverty and lack of affordable housing. Other causes include cutbacks in public welfare programs; mental health issues; traumatic events such as unemployment, illness, or injuries; and personal crises such as divorce, domestic violence, and substance use disorder. Children may be forced out of their houses or choose to run away and become homeless because they have been abused or neglected, lived in foster homes, or were placed in residential treatment or juvenile detention centers.

The basic need for a stable shelter goes unmet for children experiencing homelessness. This is not conducive to appropriate growth and development in children. These children are more likely to suffer behavioral and emotional problems, be diagnosed with a mental illness, be victims of physical and sexual abuse, and suffer educational disabilities. They also have a higher incidence of acute and chronic health problems, such as increased rates of asthma; ear infections; gastrointestinal disorders such as diarrhea; speech problems; mental health problems, such as anxiety, depression, and withdrawal; violence and victimization; substance use disorder; pregnancy; and sexually transmitted diseases. They may be exposed to environmental hazards in homeless shelters or overcrowded housing, or they may experience exposure to the elements, lack of sanitary facilities, and an increased risk of injuries. An unbalanced diet may place children without homes at risk for nutritional deficits, which can lead to delayed growth and development. Adolescents without homes often engage in risky behaviors such as drug use or unprotected sex with multiple partners, so they are more likely to need emergency care, experience depression, contract sexually transmitted diseases, or become pregnant (AAP, 2013, reaffirmed 2022).

Children experiencing homelessness may have limited access to health care services, especially preventive care such as immunizations, dental care, and well-child services. Lack of immunizations can lead to delayed enrollment in school, and education is vital for these children to help break the cycle of homelessness. Families may need to use their money for food and shelter instead of health care. If they do seek health care, they may need to use an emergency department or a free clinic rather than a consistent family care provider, and such sporadic care is not conducive to the ongoing health needs of a growing child. The family may not be able to follow through with care because they cannot afford it, lack health insurance, or do not have transportation to the clinic or pharmacy.

Some children experiencing homelessness do not go to school or go to various schools because the family moves from place to place. The stress experienced by the family creates an environment that is not conducive to learning. As a result, children may present with learning problems, socialization issues, or other behavioral issues.

Media

Today's children are inundated with various forms of media via television, mobile phones and tablets, video and computer games, social media, the internet, movies, magazines, books, and newspapers (Fig. 2.6). Media can have both positive and negative effects on the development of children, and much depends on the content to which they are exposed (AAP, Council on Communications and Media, 2016b, reaffirmed 2022b; Chassiakos et al., 2016). Positive effects include exposure to early learning; new knowledge and information, including health promotion messages; increased awareness of current events and issues; and increased social contact and support (AAP, Council on Communications and Media, 2016b, reaffirmed 2022b; Chassiakos

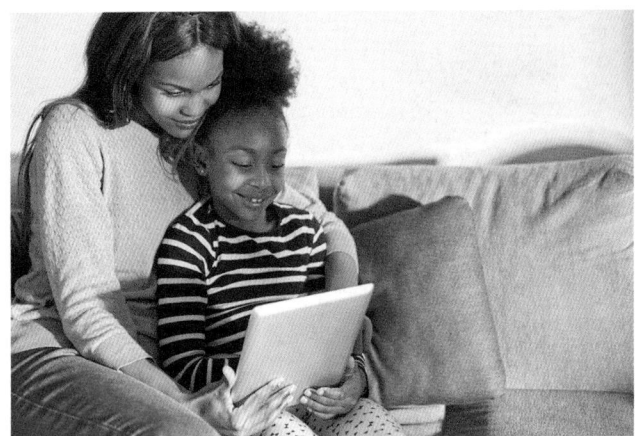

FIGURE 2.6 Technology can be fun and educational, but the child should be monitored while using the tablet or other forms of media to minimize negative effects.

et al., 2016). Negative effects include adverse health effects on sleep, attention, learning, activity, and mental health (AAP, Council on Communications and Media, 2016b, reaffirmed 2022b; Chassiakos et al., 2016). Increased support and connection from social media used in moderation has been found to be beneficial to a child's mental health (AAP, Council on Communications and Media, 2016b, reaffirmed 2022b). Increased risk of depression has been found with both high and low amounts of social media usage (AAP, Council on Communications and Media, 2016b, reaffirmed 2022b). Some of the images and information are not always in the best interests of children. Children may identify with and mimic characters who engage in risk-taking behaviors or lifestyles. Evidence is clear that media exposure can contribute to many different risks and health problems, such as excessive caloric intake, physical inactivity, smoking, early initiation of sexual behaviors, and underage drinking (AAP, Council on Communications and Media, 2016b, reaffirmed 2022b; Chassiakos et al., 2016). Research has established a strong link between media violence and violent, aggressive behavior (Chassiakos et al., 2016). If an image or type of behavior is portrayed as the norm, children may view this as acceptable behavior without examining the potential health risks or other long-term consequences. For example, when thinness is overvalued in the media, this can lead some children to develop unhealthy dieting or other behaviors in an attempt to attain that body type. For the child who has a body type that does not match the ones they see in media, depression or self-esteem issues may develop.

Overall, the images children view every day will affect their behavior and possibly their health, and pediatric nurses should take this into account when working with children and their families.

The media's influence does not only stem from content but also from total viewing time. For example, excessive TV viewing has been linked to higher weight, poor cognitive skills, and irregular sleep patterns. Overuse of computer or video games may lead to poor school performance. Media has become a major factor in children's lives, with TV remaining the dominant medium (AAP, Council on Communications and Media, 2016b, reaffirmed 2022b). The media can be a positive influence, such as when it offers educational programming or public service messages on the negative effects of substance use and misuse, smoking, or gang involvement. Public broadcasting networks often offer valuable programming.

A media history is helpful and important information to obtain. The nurse is encouraged to ask questions regarding media use, such as the amount of recreational screen time a child engages in and if the child has a television or internet-connected device in their bedroom (Chassiakos et al., 2016). The AAP recommends that families develop a family media plan. This allows a family to develop and individualize family rules and guidelines surrounding media use. The AAP Family Media Use Plan can be accessed at www.healthychildren.org/MediaUsePlan (AAP, Council on Communications and Media, 2016b, reaffirmed 2022b; Chassiakos et al., 2016). It is important for parents to set limits and know what their children are viewing, regardless of the device.

TAKE NOTE!

The AAP discourages the use of media, with the exception of video chatting, in children younger than 18 months. In children 18 to 24 months, media should be limited to educational programming with adult interaction during the media viewing and no more than 1 hour a day of media for children 2 to 5 years of age. For children older than 5 years, the recommendation includes 2 hours or less of sedentary screen time daily and no screens during meals or 1 hour before bed (AAP, Council on Communications and Media, 2016a, reaffirmed 2022a, 2016b, reaffirmed 2022b; Chassiakos et al., 2016).

Widespread access to the internet has fostered a connection to other areas of the world that would not have been possible in previous years. Children are no longer limited to their immediate surroundings, and they have access to a wealth of information. The internet can be a valuable resource for parents and children to access information, learn new things, and communicate with friends and family. However, online threats exist that can affect the child's health and safety, such as sexual predators, pornography, violence, and bigotry. Parents need to be alert to these hazards and set up safety guidelines (Teaching Guideline 2.2).

Global Society

The world is connected in many ways today; people travel from one nation to another easily, new products are distributed globally every day, people immigrate to new countries at increasing levels, and the internet makes worldwide communication simple. The United Nations Children's Fund (UNICEF) and the WHO lead the world in dealing with global children's issues. Every year, about 5.2 million children younger than 5 years and 500,000 children ages 5 to 9 die around the world (WHO, 2020). Thousands of children born in resource-limited countries are moving to resource-abundant nations such as the United States as refugees, immigrants, or international adoptees. These children become part of this nation.

TEACHING GUIDELINES 2.2 Teaching to Promote Safe Internet Use

- Develop a family media use plan.
- Determine a time limit that your child can spend on digital media each day or week, and maintain consistency in enforcing this time limit.
- Ensure that use of the internet does not replace or interfere with homework, sleep, physical activity, friends, or household or school activities.
- Tell your child *never* to share personal information with anyone online unless you know the person and the child has your permission to do so.
- Urge your child *never* to share their password with anyone, even friends.
- Review internet sites with your child, and explain which sites are appropriate. Use the safety and parental controls offered by your internet service provider.
- Avoid placing the computer or having digital media in the child's room. Rather, place the computer and encourage digital media use in a public area of your home, such as the den or kitchen, so that you can monitor your child's use.
- Discuss with your child the need for safety while using the internet. Explain potential hazards in terms the child can understand.
- Advise your child to immediately close any sites or stop any communication that makes them confused or uncomfortable. Tell your child *never* to arrange any face-to-face meetings with people they meet online. Urge your child to tell you if someone suggests such a situation.
- Teach the child *never* to open e-mail from any unknown senders.
- Be aware of digital media use policies in your child's school.

Pediatric nurses need to be aware of the impact of worldwide events, such as natural and human-made disasters, on children. Children can be displaced by events such as hurricanes or wars, placing them at increased risk for problems such as infectious diseases, malnutrition, and psychological trauma.

Young children bear the brunt of the global burden of disease, but progress has been made in reducing mortality in children younger than 5 years (WHO, 2020). UNICEF and the WHO have identified major problems affecting child growth and development and survival:

- Preterm birth complications and birth asphyxia
- Acute respiratory infections, such as pneumonia
- Malnutrition, including micronutrient deficiency
- Diarrhea related to lack of clean water and sanitation
- Vaccine-preventable diseases such as measles
- Malaria
- Poor health care of pregnant and nursing people (WHO, 2020)

These organizations work to propose ways to eradicate these conditions to improve the health of children around the world.

Today, society as a whole, families, and children have concerns over world threats and safety. Disasters such as terrorist attacks, school shootings, and extreme weather events can have significant impact on the well-being of children. The increase in these stressors puts children at risk for experiencing mental health difficulties. Children who have experienced these events are at risk for issues such as posttraumatic stress disorder, behavioral problems, depression, anxiety, sleep disturbances, restlessness, irritability, aggression, abnormal eating patterns, physiologic responses such as gastrointestinal symptoms, decline in academic performance, social isolation, and safety and security concerns (Fortin & Downes, 2023; UNICEF, 2022). Children's coping abilities may be reduced, and alterations in growth and development may be seen. Children's reactions depend on age and developmental level and are highly influenced by the emotional state of their caregivers. Pediatric nurses must be aware of the effects of world threats on children so that they can assess for alterations and intervene to promote security and stability.

KEY CONCEPTS

- The child's sex, race; biologic traits, including some behavioral traits or aspects of temperament; and certain diseases or illnesses are directly linked to genetic inheritance.
- The way a child experiences a particular event will be influenced by their temperament, and the child's temperament will influence the responses of others, including the caregivers, to the child.
- Developmental level has a major impact on the health status of children. Generally, the distribution of diseases varies with age.
- Adequate nutrition can support the developing child; conversely, nutritional deprivation can seriously interfere with brain development and other functions.
- Lifestyle choices that can affect a child's health include patterns of eating; exercise; use of tobacco, drugs, or alcohol; and methods of coping with stress. With advances in medicine, many chronic health problems today arise due to a person's lifestyle. In the case of children, the lifestyle of the caregivers is basically the lifestyle of the child.
- Environmental exposures can have a detrimental impact on the child.

- Resilience refers to the ability to adapt and cope with significant adverse events or stresses, recover, and function competently with positive outcomes.
- Internal factors that promote resiliency include the person's ability to take control and be proactive, to be responsible for their own decisions, to understand and accept their own limits and abilities, and to be goal-directed, knowing when to continue or when to stop.
- External factors that promote resiliency include caring relationships with a family member; a positive, safe learning environment at school (including clubs and social organizations); and positive influences in the community.
- Access to health care is negatively affected by lack of health insurance.
- Medicaid and CHIP are both public programs available to provide health insurance to families with limited resources.
- Despite the public programs available to assist children and families, barriers to appropriate, cost-effective, coordinated, and timely health care remain.
- The family is considered the basic social unit. The family into which a child is born will greatly influence their development and health. Children learn health care activities, health beliefs, and health values from their families.
- Typical parental roles include nurturer/caregiver, financial provider, decision maker, schedule manager, financial manager, problem solver, counselor, teacher, behavior support manager, and health manager.
- Major parenting styles can be categorized as authoritarian; authoritative; permissive; and uninvolved, rejecting, or neglecting. Each represents the amount of support and control exerted over the child by the parent.
- Discipline is a process that aims to increase desirable behavior and decrease or eliminate undesirable behavior. Punishment involves a negative or unpleasant experience or consequence for doing or not doing something.
- Culture plays a critical role in shaping a child, including their health and health practices.
- With today's changing demographic patterns, nurses must be able to incorporate cultural knowledge into their interventions so they can care effectively for culturally diverse children.
- Spirituality, a major influence for many individuals, provides a meaning and purpose to life and is a foundation for and a source of love, relationships, and service. Spiritual and religious beliefs and views can provide strength and support to children and families during times of stress and illness. Religion can also determine the way in which a family interprets and responds to illness; for example, some religions view illness as a punishment for wrongdoing or as a test of strength.
- The community surrounding a child affects many aspects of their health, development, and general welfare. The child's community consists of the family, school, neighborhood, youth organizations, and other peer groups.
- Some children spend more awake time in school and child care settings than in their family homes. Thus, schools and child care settings have become major influences on children.
- A child's friends can have a major influence on their growth and development.
- Suicide is a serious public health problem affecting young people today.
- Youth violence affects both the family and the community in terms of disrupted social services, increased health care costs, and decreased property values.
- Children may witness violent acts in the school, home, or community. They may also be victims of violence. However, not all children exposed to violence suffer negative consequences. In addition to resiliency, certain protective factors can help buffer them from the effects of violence, helping reduce the risk that they too will develop violent behaviors.
- Basic financial stability enhances the general health and well-being of children, and thus an important negative influence on children's health is poverty. Children experiencing poverty are more likely to have poor health, complete fewer years of school, experience violent crimes, and become adults with lower incomes (Federal Interagency Forum on Child and Family Statistics, 2023).
- Children who are experiencing homelessness are exposed to an environment that is not conducive to growth and development. They commonly experience physical health problems such as upper respiratory, ear, and skin infections; gastrointestinal disorders; and infestations.

REFERENCES AND RECOMMENDED READINGS

Agency for Healthcare Research and Quality. (2021). *2021 national healthcare quality and disparities report: Disparities in healthcare.* https://www.ncbi.nlm.nih.gov/books/NBK578532/

American Academy of Pediatrics. (2013, reaffirmed 2022). Policy statement. Providing care for children and adolescents facing homelessness and housing insecurity. *Pediatrics, 131*(6), 1206–1210. http://pediatrics.aappublications.org/content/early/2013/05/22/peds.2013-0645

American Academy of Pediatrics. (2018). What's the best way to discipline my child? *HealthyChildren.* http://www.healthychildren.org/english/family-life/family-dynamics/communication-discipline/pages/disciplining-your-child.aspx

American Academy of Pediatrics, Council on Communications and Media. (2016a, reaffirmed 2022a). Policy statement: Media and young minds. *Pediatrics, 138*(5). https://doi.org/10.1542/peds.2016-2591

American Academy of Pediatrics, Council on Communications and Media. (2016b, reaffirmed 2022b). Policy statement: Media use in school-aged children and adolescents. *Pediatrics, 138*(5). https://doi.org/10.1542/peds.2016-2592

Andrews, M. M. (2020). Transcultural perspectives in nursing care of children. In M. M. Andrews, J. S. Boyle, & J. W. Collins (Eds.), *Transcultural concepts in nursing care* (8th ed., pp. 172–208). Wolters Kluwer.

Bass, B., & Nagy, H. (2022). Cultural competence in the care of LGBTQ patients. In *StatPearls* [Internet]. StatPearls Publishing. https://www.ncbi.nlm.nih.gov/books/NBK563176/

Baumrind, D. (1966). Effects of authoritative parental control on child behavior, *Child Development, 37*(4), 887–907. https://doi.org/10.2307/1126611

Bitsko, R. H., Claussen, A. H., Lichstein, J., Black, L. I., Jones, S. E., Danielson, M. L., Jennifer, M. Hoenig, J. M., Jack, S. P. D., Brody, D. J., Gyawali, S., Maenner, M. J., Warner, M., Holland, K. M., Ruth Perou, R., Crosby, A. E., Blumberg, S. J., Shelli Avenevoli, S., Kaminski, J. W., & Ghandour, R. M. (2022). Mental health surveillance among children — United States, 2013–2019. *MMWR Suppl, 71*(Suppl 2), 1–42. https://doi.org/10.15585/mmwr.su7102a1

Bogues, L., & Levine, D. A. (2023). Section 2: Growth and development. Chapter 7: Normal development. In K. J. Marcdante, R. M. Kleigman, & A. M. Schuh (Eds.), *Nelson essentials of pediatrics* (9th ed., pp. 14–16). Elsevier.

Boss, P. (2001). *Family stress management: A contextual approach* (2nd ed.). Sage Publications, Inc.

Breilyn, M. S., & Levy, P. A. (2023). Section 9: Human genetics and dysmorphology. Chapter 49: Chromosomal disorders. In K. J. Marcdante, R. M. Kleigman, & A. M. Schuh (Eds.), *Nelson essentials of pediatrics* (9th ed., pp. 189–192). Elsevier.

Buchanan, A. O., & Marquez, M. L. (2023a). Section 6: Pediatric nutrition and nutritional disorders. Chapter 30: Pediatric undernutrition. In K. J. Marcdante, R. M. Kleigman, & A. M. Schuh (Eds.), *Nelson essentials of pediatrics* (9th ed., pp. 114–118). Elsevier.

Buchanan, A. O., & Marquez, M. L. (2023b). Section 6: Pediatric nutrition and nutritional disorders. Chapter 29: Obesity. In K. J. Marcdante, R. M. Kleigman, & A. M. Schuh (Eds.), *Nelson essentials of pediatrics* (9th ed., pp. 109–114). Elsevier

Centers for Disease Control and Prevention. (2021a, September 2). *Fast fact: Preventing school violence.* https://www.cdc.gov/violenceprevention/youthviolence/schoolviolence/fastfact.html

Centers for Disease Control and Prevention. (2021b). *Preventing bullying.* https://www.cdc.gov/violenceprevention/pdf/yv/Bullying-factsheet_508_1.pdf

Centers for Disease Control and Prevention. (2021c, September 2). *School-associated violent death study.* https://www.cdc.gov/violenceprevention/youthviolence/schoolviolence/SAVD.html

Centers for Disease Control and Prevention. (2022a, August 19). *Health & academics.* https://www.cdc.gov/healthyschools/health_and_academics/index.htm

Centers for Disease Control and Prevention. (2022b). *Preventing youth violence.* https://www.cdc.gov/violenceprevention/pdf/yv/YV-factsheet_2022.pdf

Centers for Disease Control and Prevention. (2022c, November 2). *Disparities in suicide.* https://www.cdc.gov/suicide/facts/disparities-in-suicide.html

Centers for Disease Control and Prevention. (2022d). *Preventing child abuse & neglect.* https://www.cdc.gov/violenceprevention/pdf/can/CAN-factsheet_2022.pdf

Centers for Disease Control and Prevention. (2022e, May 17). *Lead in foods, cosmetics, and medicines.* https://www.cdc.gov/nceh/lead/prevention/sources/foods-cosmetics-medicines.htm

Centers for Disease Control and Prevention. (2022f, July 1). *What is health equity?* https://www.cdc.gov/healthequity/whatis/index.html

Centers for Disease Control and Prevention. (2022g, April 6). *Child abuse and neglect: Risk and protective factors.* https://www.cdc.gov/violenceprevention/childabuseandneglect/riskprotectivefactors.html

Centers for Disease Control and Prevention. (2022h, April 6). *Fast facts: Preventing adverse childhood experiences.* https://www.cdc.gov/violenceprevention/aces/fastfact.html

Centers for Disease Control and Prevention. (2022i, June 27). *Scarlet fever.* https://www.cdc.gov/groupastrep/diseases-hcp/scarlet-fever.html#riskfactors

Chassiakos, Y. R., Radesky, J., Christakis, D., Moreno, M. A., Cross, C., & Council on Communications and Media. (2016). Technical report: Children and adolescents and digital media. *Pediatrics, 138*(5). https://doi.org/10.1542/peds.2016-2593

Cherry, K. (2022). *Why parenting styles matter when raising children.* https://www.verywellmind.com/parenting-styles-2795072

Children's Defense Fund. (2023). The state of America's children: 2023.HYPERLINK " https://ww" https://www.childrens-defense.org/the-state-of-americas-children/

Deville, J. G., Song, E., & Ouellette, C. P. (2022). COVID-19: Clinical manifestations and diagnosis in children. *UpToDate.* Retrieved October 17, 2022, from https://www.uptodate.com/contents/covid-19-clinical-manifestations-and-diagnosis-in-children

Drozdz, D., Alvarez-Pitti, J., Wójcik, M., Borghi, C., Gabbianelli, R., Mazur, A., Herceg-Čavrak, V., Lopez-Valcarcel, B. G., Brzeziński, M., Lurbe, E., & Wühl, E. (2021). Obesity and cardiometabolic risk factors: From childhood to adulthood. *Nutrients, 13*(11), 4176. https://doi.org/10.3390/nu13114176

Duvall, E. (1977). *Marriage and family development* (5th ed.). J. B. Lippincott.

Federal Interagency Forum on Child and Family Statistics. (2021). *America's children: Key national indicators of well-being, 2021.* U.S. Government Printing Office. https://www.childstats.gov/pdf/ac2021/ac_21.pdf

Federal Interagency Forum on Child and Family Statistics. (2022). *America's children in brief: Key national indicators of well-being, 2022.* U.S. Government Printing Office. https://www.childstats.gov/pdf/ac2022/ac_22.pdf

Federal Interagency Forum on Child and Family Statistics. (2023). *America's children: Key national indicators of well-being, 2023.* U.S. Government Printing Office. https://www.childstats.gov/pdf/ac2023/ac_23.pdf

Forcier, M., & Olson-Kennedy, J. (2022). Gender development and clinical presentation of gender diversity in children and adolescents. *UpToDate.* Retrieved January 12, 2023, from https://www.uptodate.com/contents/gender-development

-and-clinical-presentation-of-gender-diversity-in-children-and-adolescents

Fortin, K., & Downes, A. H. (2023). Section 5: Psychosocial issues. Chapter 26: Divorce, Separation, and Bereavement. In K. J. Marcdante, R. M. Kleigman, & A. M. Schuh (Eds.), *Nelson essentials of pediatrics* (9th ed., pp. 96–100). Elsevier.

Franchek-Roa, K. M. (2022). Intimate partner violence: Childhood exposure. *UpToDate*. Retrieved October 13, 2022, from https://www.uptodate.com/contents/intimate-partner-violence-childhood-exposure

Friedman, M. M. (1998). *Family nursing: Theory and practice* (4th ed.). Appleton & Lange.

Gartland, D., Riggs, E., Muyeen, S., Giallo, R., Afifi, T. O., MacMillan, H., Herrman, H., Bulford, E., & Brown, S. J. (2019). What factors are associated with resilient outcomes in children exposed to social adversity? A systematic review. *BMJ Open*, *9*(4). e024870. https://doi.org/10.1136/bmjopen-2018-024870

Healthy People 2030, U.S. Department of Health and Human Services, Office of Disease Prevention and Health Promotion. (n.d.). *Social determinants of health*. https://health.gov/healthypeople/objectives-and-data/social-determinants-health

Ivey-Stephenson, A. Z., Demissie, Z., Crosby, A. E., Stone, D. M., Gaylor, E., Wilkins, N., Lowry, R., & Brown, M. (2020). Suicidal ideation and behaviors among high school students—Youth Risk Behavior Survey, United States, 2019. *MMWR*, *69*(1), 47–55. https://doi.org/10.15585/mmwr.su6901a6

Jones, J. M. (2022). *Belief in God in U.S. Dips to 81%, a new low*. Retrieved October 13, 2022, from https://news.gallup.com/poll/393737/belief-god-dips-new-low.aspx

Jones, V. F., Schulte, E. E., & Committee on Early Childhood and Council on Foster Care, Adoption, and Kinship Care. (2012, reaffirmed 2017). The pediatrician's role in supporting adoptive families. *Pediatrics*, *130*(4), e1040–e1049. https://doi.org/10.1542/peds.2012–2261

Joshi, D. S., & Lebrun-Harris, L. A. (2022). Child health status and health care use in grandparent- versus parent-led households. *Pediatrics*, *150*(3), e2021055291. https://doi.org/10.1542/peds.2021-055291

Kaiser Family Foundation. (2022). *Health coverage of immigrants*. https://www.kff.org/racial-equity-and-health-policy/fact-sheet/health-coverage-of-immigrants/

Kemp, G., Smith, M., & Segal, J. (2022). *Children and divorce*. https://www.helpguide.org/articles/parenting-family/children-and-divorce.htm

Kennebeck, S., & Bonin, L. (2021). Suicidal behavior in children & adolescents: Epidemiology and risk factors. *UpToDate*. Retrieved October 13, 2022, from https://www.uptodate.com/contents/suicidal-behavior-in-children-and-adolescents-epidemiology-and-risk-factors

Kids Count Data Center. (2020a). *Children who have difficulty speaking English by family nativity*. Retrieved October 12, 2022, from https://datacenter.kidscount.org/data/tables/128-children-who-have-difficulty-speaking-english-by-family-nativity?loc=1#detailed/1/any/false/1729,870/78,79/470,471

Kids Count Data Center. (2020b). *Children living in linguistically isolated households by children in immigrant families*. Retrieved October 12, 2022, from https://datacenter.kidscount.org/data/tables/129-children-living-in-linguistically-isolated-households-by-family-nativity?loc=1&loct=2#detailed/1/any/false/1729,870,38,35/78,79/472,473

Linton, J. M., Green, A., & AAP Council on Community Pediatrics. (2019). Providing care for children in immigrant families. *Pediatrics*, *144*(3), e20192077. https://doi.org/10.1542/peds.2019-2077

Mandy, G. T. (2022). Preterm birth: Definitions of prematurity, epidemiology, and risk factors for infant mortality. *UpToDate*. Retrieved October 6, 2022, from https://www.uptodate.com/contents/preterm-birth-definitions-of-prematurity-epidemiology-and-risk-factors-for-infant-mortality

Mandy, G. T. (2023). Overview of the long-term complications of preterm birth. *UpToDate*. Retrieved September 25, 2023, from https://www.uptodate.com/contents/overview-of-the-long-term-complications-of-preterm-birth

Mykyta, L., Keisler-Starkey, K., & Bunch, L. (2022). More children were covered by Medicaid and CHIP in 2021. *United States Census Bureau*. https://www.census.gov/library/stories/2022/09/uninsured-rate-of-children-declines.html#:~:text=Medicaid%20and%20CHIP%20Drove%20Drop,change%20between%202020%20and%202021

National Conference of State Legislators (NCSL). (2022). Adverse Childhood Experiences. https://www.ncsl.org/health/adverse-childhood-experiences

National Institutes of Health. (2021). *News release: Long-term study of children with COVID-19 begins, NIH-supported research will track effects of COVID-19 infection on children over three years*. https://www.nih.gov/news-events/news-releases/long-term-study-children-covid-19-begins

Patterson, J. (1995). Promoting resilience in families experiencing stress. *Pediatric Clinics of North America*, *42*(1), 47–63. https://doi.org/10.1016/S0031-3955(16)38907-6

Patterson, J. (2002). Integrating family resilience and family stress theory. *Journal of Marriage and Family*, *64*(2), 349–360. https://doi.org/10.1111/j.1741-3737.2002.00349.x

PFLAG. (2023). *LGBTQ+Glossary*. Retrieved October 8, 2023, from https://pflag.org/glossary/

Samet, J. M., & Sockrider, M. (2022). Control of secondhand smoke exposure. In A. G. Hoppin (Ed.), *UpToDate*. Retrieved October 6, 2022, from https://www.uptodate.com/contents/control-of-secondhand-smoke-exposure

Sample, J. A. (2022). Childhood lead poisoning: Clinical manifestations and diagnosis. *UpToDate*. Retrieved September 26, 2023, from https://www.uptodate.com/contents/childhood-lead-poisoning-clinical-manifestations-and-diagnosis

Schulte, E. E. (2022). Adoption. *UpToDate*. Retrieved October 11, 2022, from https://www.uptodate.com/contents/adoption

Sege, R. D., Siegel, B. S., AAP Council on Child Abuse and Neglect & AAP Committee on Psychosocial Aspects of child and Family Health. (2018). Effective discipline to raise healthy children. *Pediatrics*, *142*(6), 20183112. https://doi.org/10.1542/peds.2018-3112

Shrider, E. A., & Creamer, J. (2023). *Poverty in the United States: 2022* (U.S. Census Bureau, Current Population Reports, P60-280). U.S. Government Publishing Office. https://www.census.gov/content/dam/Census/library/publications/2023/demo/p60-280.pdf

Shrider, E. A., Kollar, M., Chen, F., & Semega, J. (2021). *Income and poverty in the* United States: 2020 (U.S. Census Bureau, Current Population Reports, P60-273). U.S. Government Printing Office.

Tremblay, C., & Brady, M. T. (2023). Roseola infantum (exanthem subitum). *UpToDate*. Retrieved September 25, 2023, from https://www.uptodate.com/contents/roseola-infantum-exanthem-subitum

United Nations Children's Fund. (2022). *Mental health and psychosocial support in emergencies.* https://www.unicef.org/protection/mental-health-psychosocial-support-in-emergencies

U.S. Census Bureau. (2016). *The majority of children live with two parents, Census Bureau reports.* https://www.census.gov/newsroom/press-releases/2016/cb16-192.html

U.S. Census Bureau. (2021). *Subject definitions.* Retrieved October 11, 2022, from https://www.census.gov/programs-surveys/cps/technical-documentation/subject-definitions.html#family

U.S. Department of Health and Human Services. (2014). *What is child abuse or neglect? What is the definition of child abuse and neglect?* https://www.hhs.gov/answers/programs-for-families-and-children/what-is-child-abuse/index.html#:~:text=%C2%A7%205106g)%2C%20as%20amended%20by,sexual%20abuse%20or%20exploitation%22%3B%20or

U.S. Department of Health and Human Services. (2022). *2022 poverty guidelines.* Retrieved October 14, 2022, from https://aspe.hhs.gov/topics/poverty-economic-mobility/poverty-guidelines

U.S. Department of Health and Human Services, Administration for Children and Families, Administration on Children, Youth and Families, Children's Bureau. (2021). *The AFCARS report.* https://www.acf.hhs.gov/sites/default/files/documents/cb/afcarsreport28.pdf

U.S. Department of Health and Human Services, Administration for Children and Families, Administration on Children, Youth and Families, Children's Bureau. (2022). *Child maltreatment 2020.* https://www.acf.hhs.gov/cb/data-research/child-maltreatment

Vespa, J., Medina, L., & Armstrong, D. M. (2018, revised 2020). *Demographic turning points for the United States: Population projections for 2020 to 2060. Population estimates and projections current population reports.* https://www.census.gov/content/dam/Census/library/publications/2020/demo/p25-1144.pdf

Von Bertalanffy, L. (1968). *General systems theory.* Penguin Press.

Wildsmith, E., & Alvira-Hammond, M. (2023). Data on families with low incomes across America can inform two-generation approaches. *Child Trends.* https://doi.org/10.56417/1147h453i

World Health Organization. (2012). *Care for child development: Participant manual.* https://www.unicef.org/media/91176/file/3-CCD-Participant-Manual.pdf

World Health Organization. (2020). *Children: Improving survival and well-being.* https://www.who.int/en/news-room/fact-sheets/detail/children-reducing-mortality

DEVELOPING CLINICAL JUDGMENT

PRACTICING FOR NCLEX

1. A single parent asks the nurse for suggestions on disciplining their 2-year-old child. Which suggestion would be most appropriate?
   a. Encourage the parent to emphasize the inappropriate behavior.
   b. Wait an hour or so before enforcing the discipline.
   c. Have the child spend 2 minutes in time-out.
   d. Withhold a privilege from the toddler for a week.

2. The nurse is teaching a group of students about the possible effects of immigration on the health status of children. Which statement by a student would indicate the need for additional teaching?
   a. "The children of immigrants have better access to preventive care."
   b. "The children of immigrants may have limited involvement in activities due to language barriers."
   c. "The children of immigrants may lack adequate support systems."
   d. "The children of immigrants face increased stressors due to relocation."

3. The nurse is working with a group of adolescents who have been exposed to violence in their homes. Which examples would the nurse identify as protective factors that will help buffer the adolescents from the effects of violence? Select all that apply.
   a. Participating in a mentorship program
   b. Limiting involvement in social activities to help at home
   c. Limiting communication with parents
   d. Committing to school work
   e. Joining student government at school

4. In an effort to control health care costs for a family, what is the best recommendation by the nurse?
   a. "Shop around to find the most inexpensive health insurance plan."
   b. "Find a job that provides family health insurance at a minimal cost."
   c. "Focus on primary prevention, using the health care system for check-ups."
   d. "Avoid seeing a health care provider until your child becomes ill."

CRITICAL THINKING EXERCISES

1. A couple has adopted an 11-month-old infant from China and has brought her to the health care facility for a check-up. The couple had no contact with the infant's birth parents. The infant spent 7 months in an orphanage before being adopted. Describe the issues that may affect this family.
2. Vanessa Walters brings her 3-year-old son, Tyler, for a well-child visit. Vanessa states, "Tyler is a handful. He always seems to be misbehaving. I just don't know what to do." How should the nurse respond, and what suggestions might be helpful?
3. You have been asked by the local school district to speak to a group of middle school students about internet safety. Describe the topics that you should address.

STUDY ACTIVITIES

1. Discuss with fellow students the different types of family structures. Include information about your own family structure. Compare and contrast the roles assumed by each member in the different structures.
2. Create a culture diary or journal for use in clinical practice. Record observations made while caring for children and families of backgrounds different from your own. Address the preferences that the children and families had relating to food, health care, decision making for the family, view of children, and general health practices.
3. Perform a "spiritual inventory" on yourself. Identify your beliefs about higher authority, life after death, purpose in life, and the value of others who have different beliefs.
4. Search the internet for websites with information about violence and its impact on children's health.
5. The nurse is preparing a class for a group of students about children and families experiencing homelessness. Which factors contribute to homelessness? Select all that apply.
   a. Increase in family income
   b. Job loss
   c. Exposure to abuse or neglect
   d. Cutbacks in public welfare programs
   e. Development of community crisis centers

UNIT

II

Health Promotion of the Growing Child and Family

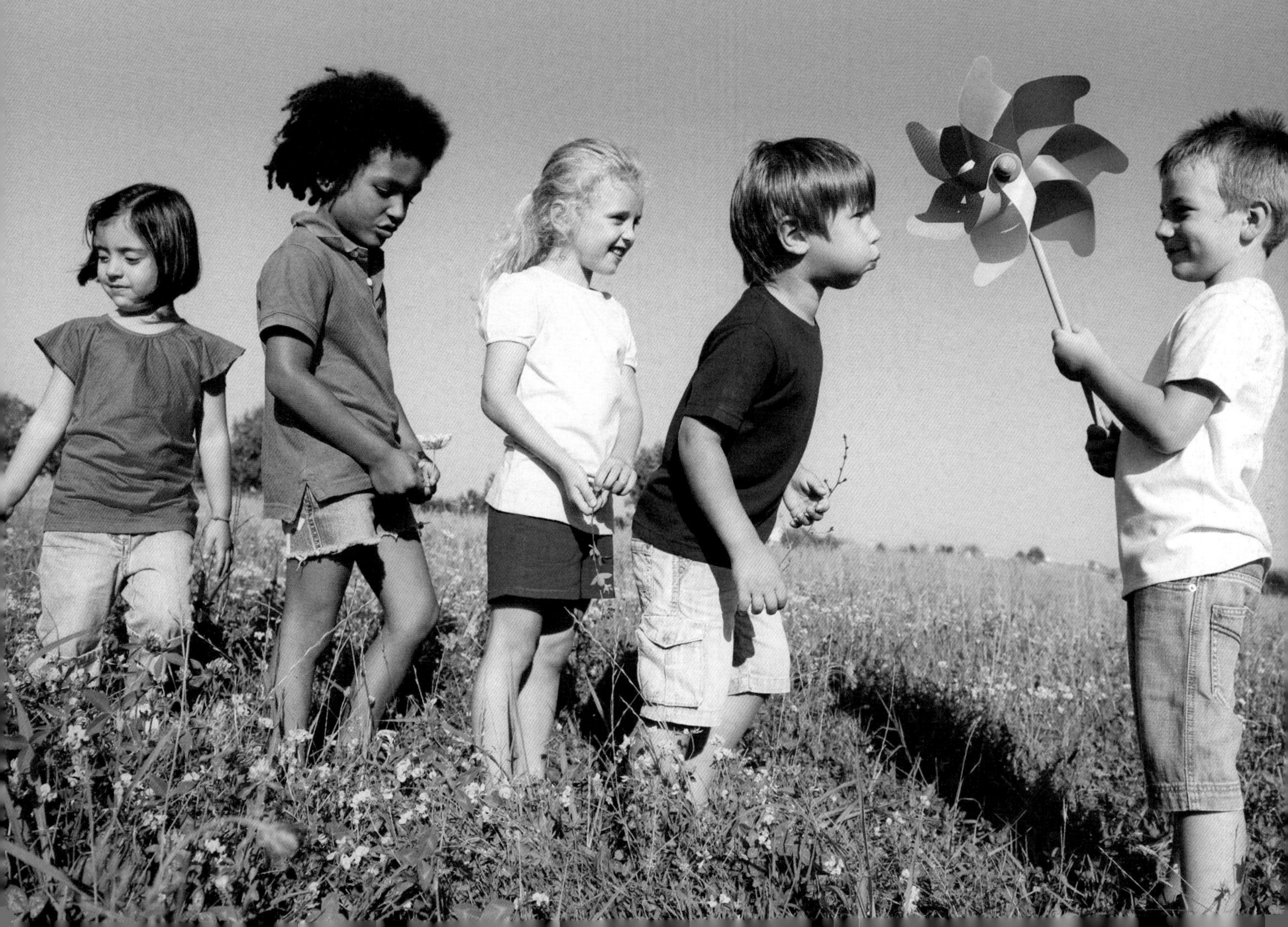

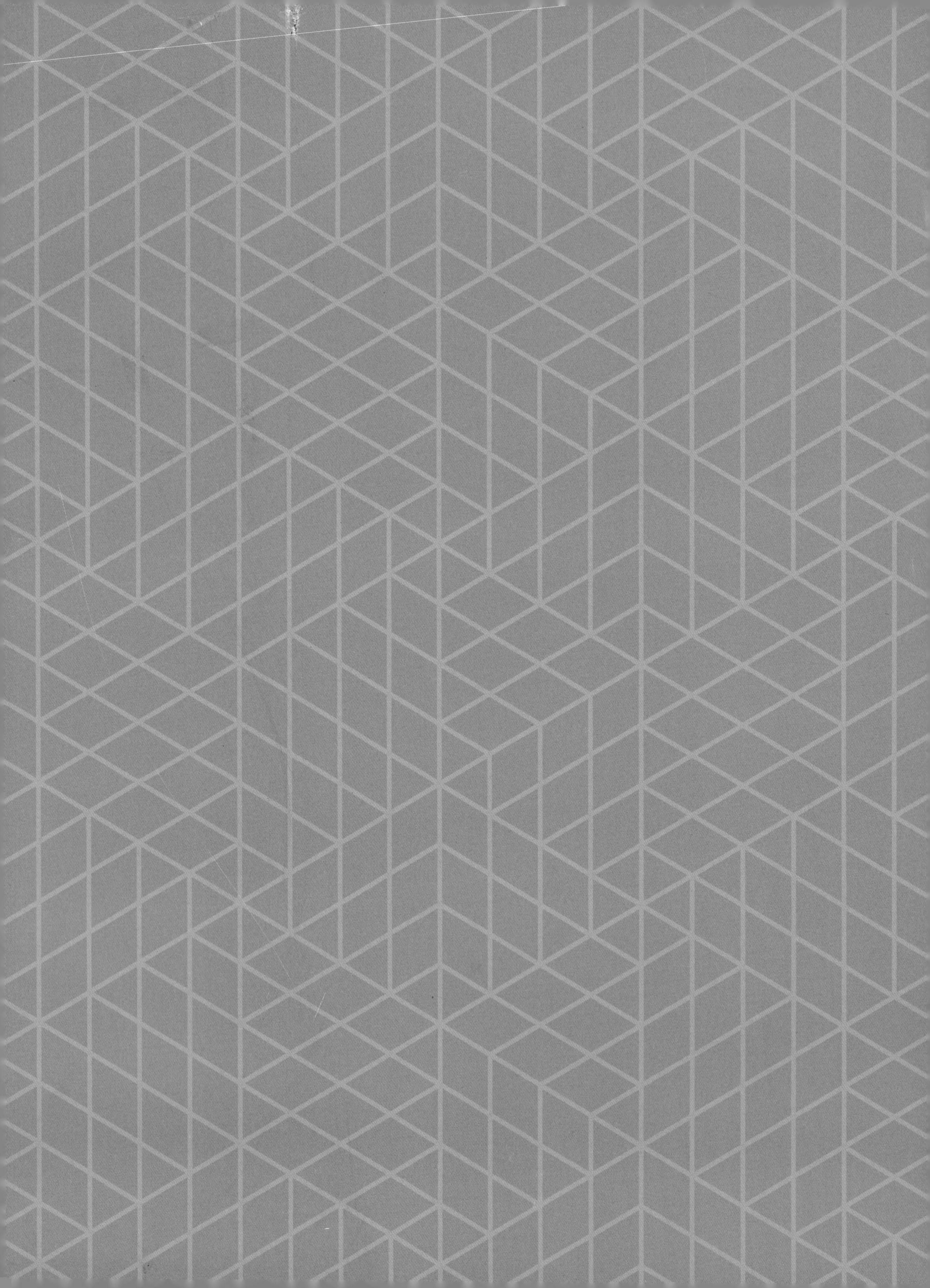

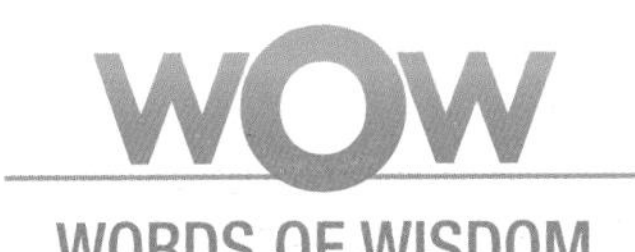

WORDS OF WISDOM

The miracle of a newborn infant... the commitment of raising a child... the nurse's presence helps guide this journey.

3

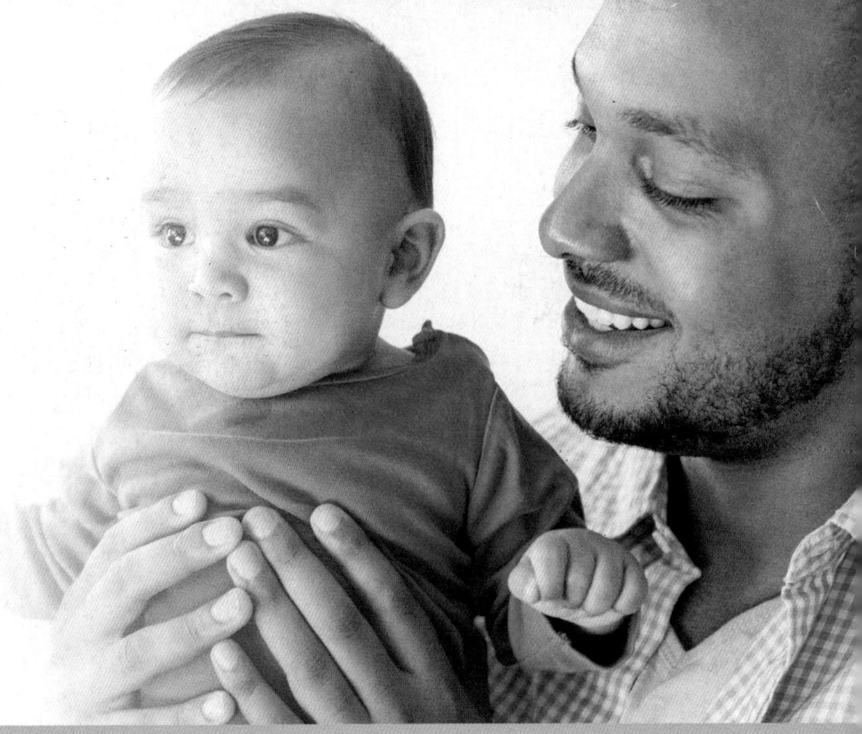

Growth and Development of the Newborn and Infant

KEY TERMS

anticipatory guidance
binocularity
cephalocaudal (sef´ă-lō-kaw´dăl)
colic
colostrum (kŏ-los´trŭm)
development
foremilk
growth
hindmilk
let-down reflex
maturation
object permanence
proximodistal (prok´si-mō-dis´tăl)
solitary play
stranger anxiety
temperament

LEARNING OBJECTIVES

Upon completion of the chapter, you will be able to:

1. Describe typical physical growth, physiologic changes, and sensory development in the newborn and infant.
2. Identify the gross and fine motor milestones of the newborn and infant.
3. Examine expected language development in the first year of life.
4. Implement a nursing care plan to address common issues related to growth and development in infancy.
5. Describe nutritional requirements of the newborn and infant.
6. Develop a nutritional plan for the first year of life.
7. Examine common issues related to growth and development in infancy.
8. Demonstrate knowledge of appropriate anticipatory guidance for common developmental issues.

Allison Johnson is a 6-month-old brought to the clinic by her parents for her 6-month check-up. As new parents, they have a list of questions and concerns. As the nurse caring for Allison, assess growth and development, and then teach the parents what changes to expect in Allison over the next few months.

INTRODUCTION

The newborn or neonatal period of infancy is defined as the period from birth until 28 days of age. Infancy is defined as the period from birth to 12 months of age. Growth and development are interrelated, ongoing processes in infancy and childhood. **Growth** refers to an increase in physical size. **Development** is the sequential process by which infants and children gain various skills and functions. Heredity influences growth and development by determining the child's potential, while environment contributes to the degree of achievement. **Maturation** refers to an increase in functionality of various body systems or developmental skills.

GROWTH AND DEVELOPMENT OVERVIEW

Growth and developmental changes in the first year of life are numerous and dramatic. Physical growth, maturation of body systems, and gross and fine motor skills progress in an orderly and sequential fashion. Although timing may vary from infant to infant, the order in which developmental skills are acquired is consistent. Infants also exhibit vast amounts of learning in the psychosocial and cognitive, language and communication, and social/emotional domains. Adequate growth and development are indicative of health in the infant or young child. Nurses must be familiar with normal developmental milestones so that they can accurately assess the infant's development as well as provide age-appropriate anticipatory guidance to the parents.

Achievement of developmental milestones may be assessed in a variety of ways. While obtaining the health history, the nurse may ask the parent or caregiver if the skill is present and when it was attained. The infant may also demonstrate the skill during the interview or examination, or the nurse may elicit the skill from the infant. A number of screening tools are also used to assess development, such as the Ages and Stages Questionnaire (ASQ), Infant–Toddler Checklist (ITC), Infant Development Inventory (IDI), and Parents' Evaluation of Developmental Status-Developmental Milestones (PEDS-DM).

Ill or premature infants may exhibit delayed acquisition of physical growth and developmental skills. When assessing the growth and development of a premature infant, use the infant's adjusted age to determine expected outcomes. To determine adjusted age, subtract the number of weeks that the infant was premature from the infant's chronologic age. Plot growth parameters and assess developmental milestones based on adjusted age. For example, a 6-month-old who was born at 28 weeks' gestation was born 12 weeks early (3 months), so subtract 3 months from their chronologic age of 6 months to obtain an adjusted age of 3 months. This infant would demonstrate healthy growth if they were the size of a 3-month-old, and they should be expected to achieve the developmental milestones of a 3-month-old rather than a 6-month-old.

PHYSICAL GROWTH

Ongoing assessments of growth are important so that too-rapid or inadequate growth can be identified early. With early identification, the cause can be diagnosed and the potential for further appropriate growth maximized. Infants grow rapidly over the first 12 months of life. Weight, length, and head and chest circumference are all indicators of physical growth in the newborn and infant.

Weight

The average newborn weighs 3.400 kg (7.5 lb) at birth, with males being slightly heavier than females. Newborns may lose 5% to 10% of their body weight over the first week of life. The average newborn then gains about 20 to 30 g per day and regains their birth weight by 7 to 10 days of age. Most infants double their birth weight by 4 to 5 months of age and triple their birth weight by the time they are 1 year old (Branchford & Levine, 2023).

Length

The average newborn is 50 cm (20 in) long at birth. The infant grows more quickly in length over the first 6 months than during the second 6 months. By 12 months of age, the infant's length has increased by 50% (Branchford & Levine, 2023).

Head Circumference

The average head circumference of the full-term newborn is 35 cm (13.5 in). Similarly to the weight and length, the head circumference increases rapidly during the first 6 months. Head circumference increases about 10 cm from birth to 1 year of age (Branchford & Levine, 2023).

Remember Allison Johnson, the 6-month-old introduced at the beginning of the chapter? Allison's weight is 7.26 kg (16 lb), her length is 65.41 cm (25.75 in), and her head circumference is 43.18 cm (17 in).

PHYSIOLOGIC CHANGES

The newborn's and infant's organ systems undergo significant changes as the infant grows. Systems that undergo significant change include the neurologic system, the cardiovascular system, the respiratory system, the gastrointestinal (digestive) system, the renal system, the hematopoietic system, the immunologic system, and the integumentary system.

Neurologic System

The infant experiences tremendous changes in the neurologic system over the first year of life. Critical brain growth and continued myelination of the spinal cord occur. Involuntary movement progresses to voluntary control, and immature vocalizations and crying progress to the ability to speak as a result of maturational changes of the neurologic system.

States of Consciousness

The typical newborn's ability to move sequentially through states of consciousness reassures parents and health care providers that the neurologic system, though immature, is intact. An average newborn will ordinarily move through six states of consciousness:

1. Deep sleep: Sleeping with eyes closed and no movement.
2. Light sleep: Sleeping with eyes closed; rapid eye movements and irregular movements may be noticed.
3. Drowsiness: Eyes may close or be half-lidded; the infant may be dozing.
4. Quiet alert state: The infant's eyes are wide open, and the body is calm.
5. Active alert state: The infant's eyes are open; body movements occur.
6. Crying: The infant cries or screams, and it is difficult to gain the infant's attention (Olsson, 2020).

Newborns usually progress through these states slowly, rather than going from deep sleep immediately into outright crying.

Brain Growth

The nervous system continues to mature throughout infancy, and the increase in head circumference is indicative of brain growth. The brain undergoes tremendous growth during the first 2 years of life. By 6 months of age, the infant's brain weighs half that of the adult brain. At age 12 months, the brain has grown considerably, weighing 2.5 times what it did at birth. Usually, the anterior fontanel remains open until 12 to 18 months of age to accommodate this rapid brain growth. However, the fontanel may close as early as 9 months of age, and this is not of concern in the infant with age-appropriate growth and development.

In general, the neurologic system matures a significant amount over the first year of life. Myelination of the spinal cord and nerves continues over the first 2 years. Maturation of the nervous system and continued myelination are necessary for the tremendous developmental skills that are achieved in the first 12 months. During the first few months of life, reflexive behavior is replaced with purposeful action.

Reflexes

Primitive reflexes are subcortical and involve a whole-body response. Selected primitive reflexes present at birth include Moro, root, suck, asymmetric tonic neck, plantar and palmar grasp, step, and Babinski. Except for the Babinski, which disappears around 1 year of age, these primitive reflexes diminish over the first few months of life, giving way to protective reflexes. Protective reflexes (also termed postural responses or reflexes) are gross motor responses related to maintenance of equilibrium. These responses are prerequisites for appropriate motor development and remain throughout life once they are established. The protective reflexes include the righting and parachute reactions. Appropriate presence and disappearance of primitive reflexes, as well as development of protective reflexes, are indicative of a healthy neurologic system. Persistence of primitive reflexes beyond the usual age of disappearance may indicate an abnormality of the neurologic system and should be investigated.

Table 3.1 gives descriptions and illustrations of several primitive and protective reflexes, as well as the timing of appearance and disappearance of these reflexes.

Respiratory System

The respiratory system continues to mature over the first year of life. The respiratory rate slows from an average of 30 to 60 breaths in the newborn to about 20 to 30 in the 12-month-old. The newborn breathes irregularly, with periodic pauses. As the infant matures, the respiratory pattern becomes more regular and rhythmic.

In comparison with the adult, in the infant:

- The nasal passages are narrower.
- The trachea and chest wall are more compliant.
- The bronchi and bronchioles are shorter and narrower.
- The larynx is more funnel shaped.
- The tongue is larger.
- There are significantly fewer alveoli.

These anatomic differences place the infant at higher risk for respiratory compromise. The respiratory system does not reach adult levels of maturity until about 7 years of age. The lack of immunoglobulin A (IgA) in the mucosal lining of the upper respiratory tract also contributes to the frequent infections that occur in infancy.

Cardiovascular System

The heart doubles in size over the first year of life. As the cardiovascular system matures, the average pulse rate decreases from 120 to 140 in the newborn to about 100 in the 1-year-old. Blood pressure steadily increases over the first 12 months of life, from an average of 60/40 in the newborn to 100/50 in the 12-month-old. The peripheral

TABLE 3.1 • Select Primitive and Protective Reflexes in Infancy

	Description	Age Reflex Appears	Age Reflex Disappears
Primitive Reflexes			
Root 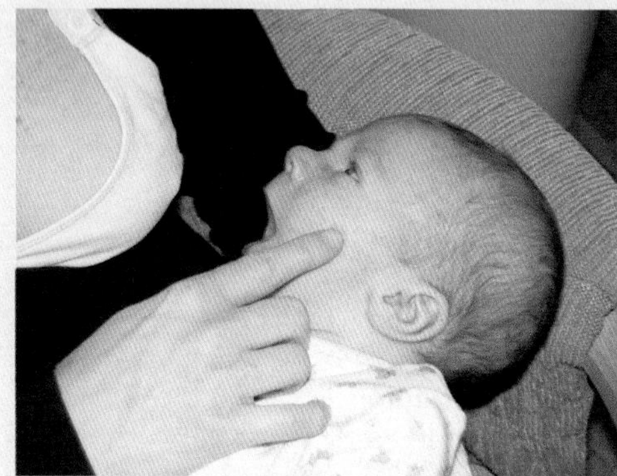	When infant's cheek is stroked, the infant turns to that side, searching with the mouth.	Birth	3 months
Suck 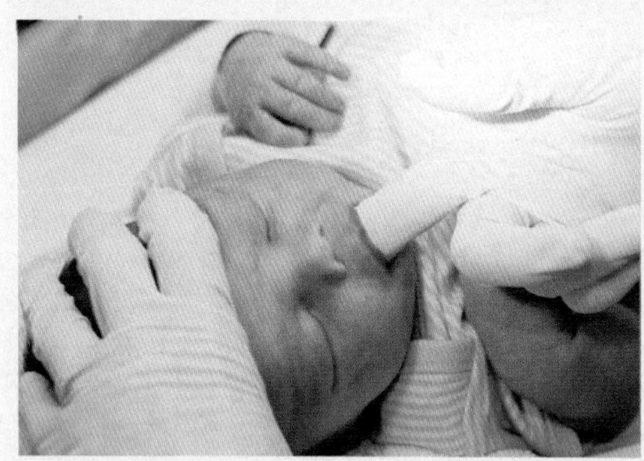	Reflexive sucking when the nipple or finger is placed in the infant's mouth	Birth	2–5 months
Moro 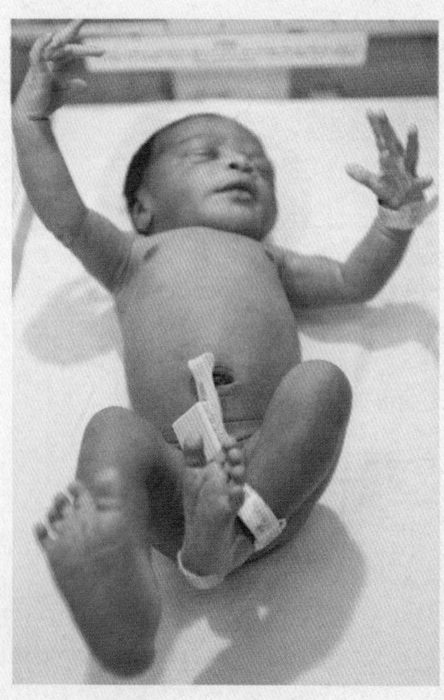	With sudden extension of the head, the arms abduct and move upward, and the hands form a "C."	Birth	4 months

TABLE 3.1 • Select Primitive and Protective Reflexes in Infancy

	Description	Age Reflex Appears	Age Reflex Disappears
Asymmetric tonic neck 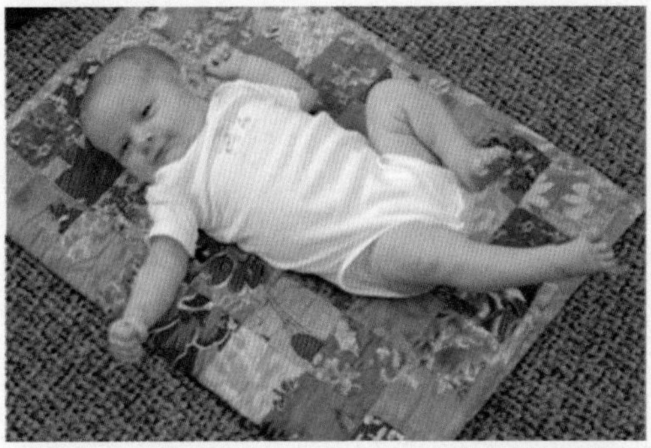	While lying supine, extremities are extended on the side of the body to which the head is turned, and opposite extremities are flexed (also called the "fencing" position).	Birth	4 months
Palmar grasp 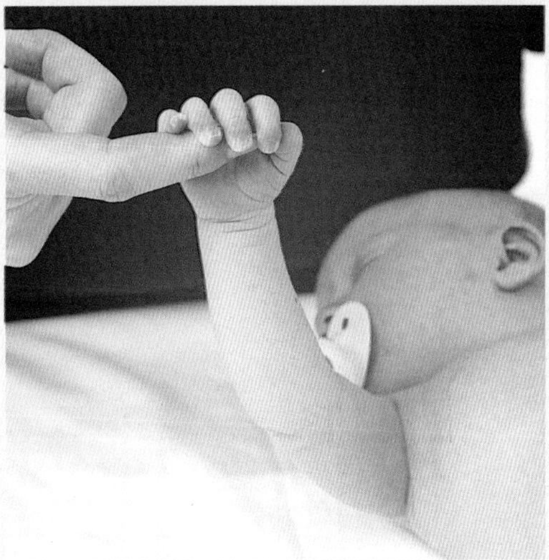	Infant reflexively grasps when the palm is touched.	Birth	4–6 months
Plantar grasp 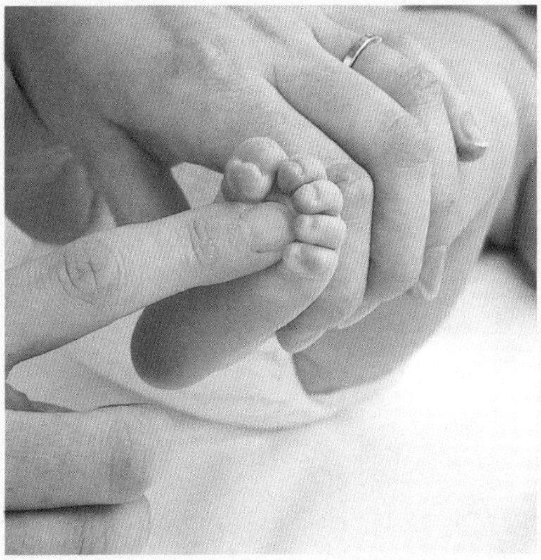	Infant reflexively grasps with the bottom of the foot when pressure is applied to the plantar surface.	Birth	9 months

(*continued*)

TABLE 3.1 • SelectPrimitive and Protective Reflexes in Infancy (*continued*)

	Description	Age Reflex Appears	Age Reflex Disappears
Babinski 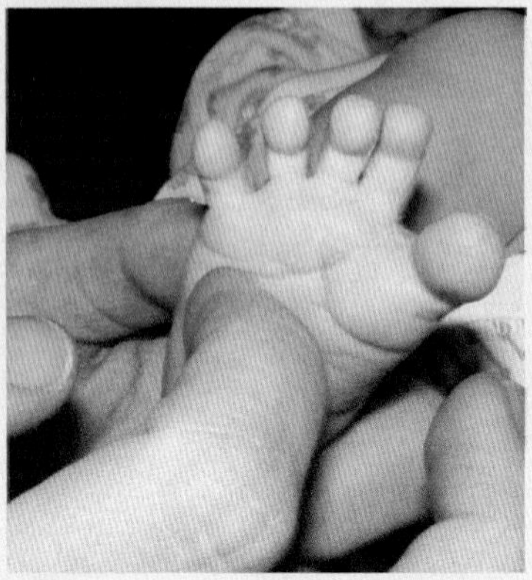	Stroking along the lateral aspect of the sole and across the plantar surface results in fanning and hyperextension of the toes.	Birth	12 months
Step 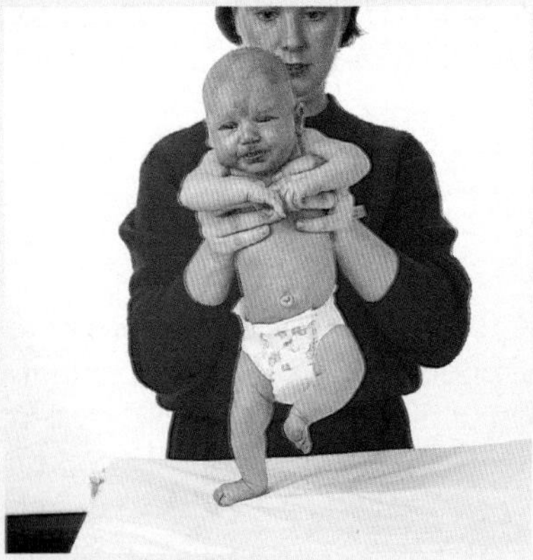	With one foot on a flat surface, the infant puts the other foot down as if to "step."	Birth	4–8 weeks
Protective Reflexes			
Neck righting	Neck keeps the head in an upright position when the body is tilted.	4–6 months	Persists
Parachute (sideways)	Protective extension with the arms when tilted to the side in a supported sitting position	6 months	Persists
Parachute (forward) 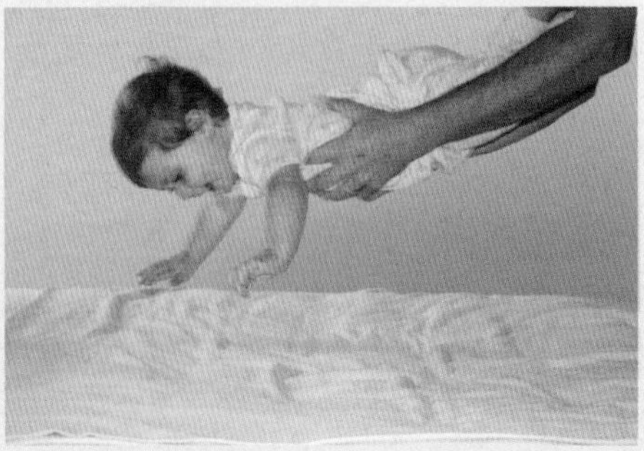	Protective extension with the arms when held up in the air and moved forward; the infant reflexively reaches forward to catch themselves.	6–7 months	Persists
Parachute (backward)	Protective extension with the arms when tilted backward	9–10 months	Persists

capillaries are closer to the surface of the skin, thus making the newborn and young infant more susceptible to heat loss. Over the first year of life, thermoregulation (the body's ability to stabilize body temperature) becomes more effective: The peripheral capillaries constrict in response to a cold environment and dilate in response to heat.

Gastrointestinal System

Teeth

The vast majority of newborns do not have teeth at birth, nor do they develop them in the first month of life. Occasionally, an infant is born with one or more teeth (termed natal teeth) or develops teeth in the first 28 days of life (termed neonatal teeth). The presence of natal or neonatal teeth may be associated with other birth anomalies. On average, the first primary teeth begin to erupt between the ages of 6 and 8 months. The primary teeth (also termed deciduous teeth) are lost later in childhood and will be replaced by the permanent teeth. The gums around the emerging tooth often swell. The lower central incisors are usually the first to appear, followed by the upper central incisors (Fig. 3.1). The average 12-month-old has four to eight teeth.

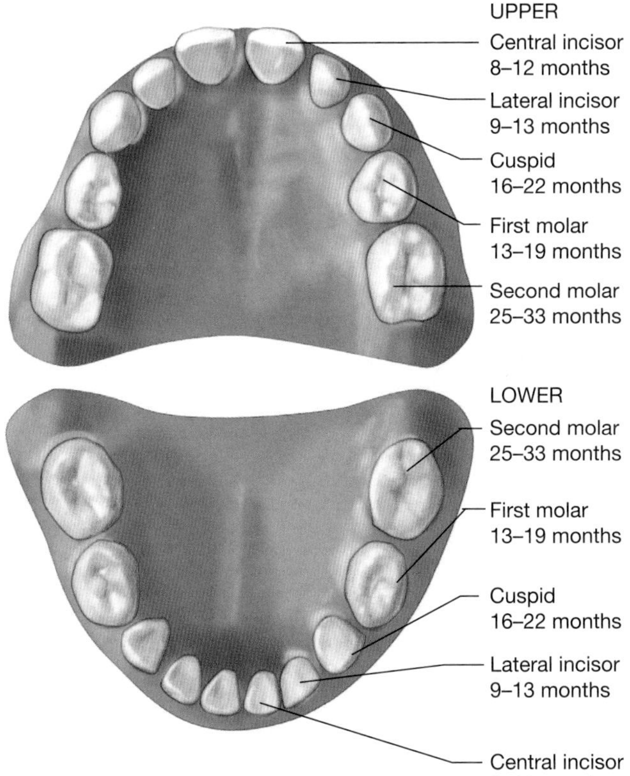

FIGURE 3.1 Sequence and average age of tooth eruption.

Digestion

The newborn's digestive system is not fully developed. Small amounts of saliva are present for the first 3 months of life, and ptyalin is present only in small amounts in the saliva. Gastric digestion occurs as a result of the presence of hydrochloric acid and rennin. The small intestine is about 270 cm (106.29 in) long and grows to the adult length by about 4 years of age (Maqbool & Liacouras, 2020). The stomach capacity is relatively small at birth, holding about 0.5 to 1 oz. However, by 1 year of age the stomach can accommodate three full meals and several snacks per day. In the duodenum, three enzymes, in particular, are important for digestion. Trypsin is available in sufficient quantities for protein digestion after birth. Amylase (needed for complex carbohydrate digestion) and lipase (essential for appropriate fat digestion) are both deficient in the infant and do not reach adult levels until about 5 months of age.

The liver is also immature at birth. The ability to conjugate bilirubin and secrete bile is present after about 2 weeks of age. Conjugation of medications may remain immature over the first year of life. Other functions of the liver, including gluconeogenesis, vitamin storage, and protein metabolism, remain immature during the first year of life.

Stools

The consistency and frequency of stools change over the first year of life. The newborn's first stools (meconium) are the result of digestion of amniotic fluid swallowed in utero. They are dark green to black and sticky (Fig. 3.2). In the first few days of life, the stools become yellowish or tan. Generally, the formula-fed infant has stools the consistency of peanut butter. Breastfed infants' stools are usually looser in texture and appear seedy. Newborns may have as many as eight to 10 stools per day or as few as one stool every day or two. After the newborn period, the number of stools may decrease, and some infants do not have a bowel movement for several days. Infrequent stooling is considered normal if the bowel movement remains soft. Due to the immaturity of the gastrointestinal system, newborns and young infants often grunt, strain, or cry while attempting to have a bowel movement. This is not of concern unless the stool is hard and dry. Stool color and texture may change depending on the foods that the infant is ingesting (Kaiser Permanente, n.d.).

TAKE NOTE!

Parents should call the primary care provider if the infant's stools are red, white, or black; mucus-like; frequent and watery; frothy or foul-smelling; or hard, dry, formed, or pellet-like; or if the baby is vomiting.

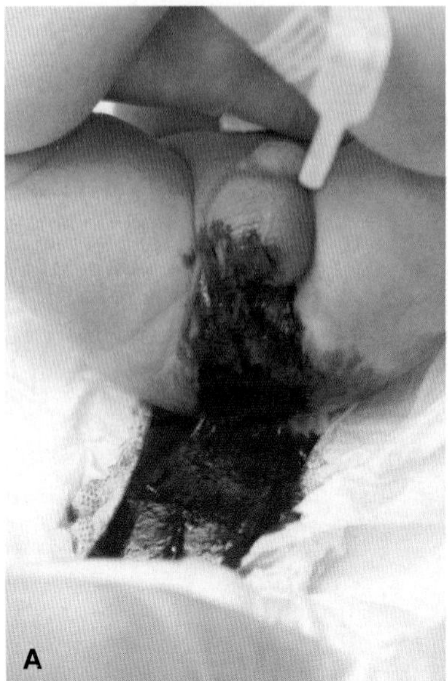

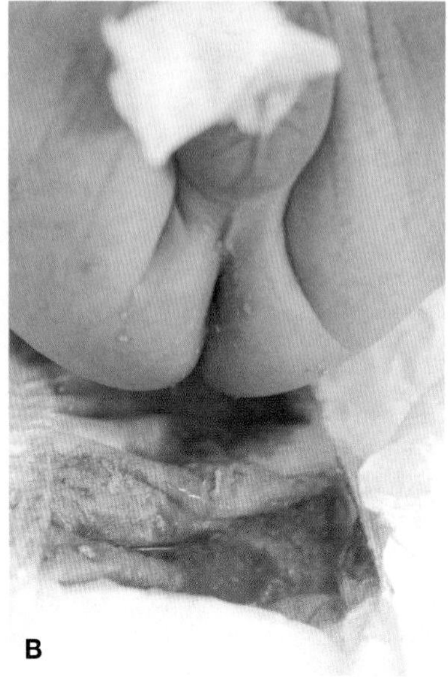

FIGURE 3.2 **A.** Meconium stool. **B.** Typical stool after the first few days. Note the yellowish, seedy stool of a breastfed infant.

Genitourinary System

In the infant, total body water is a greater percentage of weight than it is in the adult. Thus, the infant is more susceptible to dehydration. Over the first 12 months of life, extracellular fluid (lymph, interstitial fluid, and blood plasma) decreases, while the intracellular fluid volume increases, reaching the adult levels of 20% to 25% and 30% to 40%, respectively (Greenbaum & Londeree, 2023). Infants urinate frequently, and the urine has a relatively low specific gravity. The renal structures are immature and the glomerular filtration rate, tubular secretion, and reabsorption as well as renal perfusion are all reduced compared with those in the adult. The glomeruli reach full maturity by 2 years of age.

Integumentary System

In utero, the infant is covered with vernix caseosa, which protects the developing infant's skin. At birth, the infant may be covered with vernix (earlier gestational age), or vernix may be found in the folds of the skin, axilla, and groin areas (later gestational age). Production of vernix ceases at birth. Fine downy hair (lanugo) covers the body of many newborns. Often, this hair is lost over time and is not replaced. Darker-skinned neonates tend to have more lanugo present at birth than those with light skin.

Acrocyanosis (blueness of the hands and feet in light-skinned infants, noted on the soles and palms in darker-skinned infants) is normal in the newborn; it decreases over the first few days of life (Fig. 3.3). Newborns often experience mottling of the skin (a pink-and-white marbled appearance easily noted in light-skinned infants, more difficult to distinguish in darker-skinned infants) because of their immature circulatory system. Mottling decreases over the first few months of life (see Fig. 3.3). The newborn and young infant's skin is relatively thinner than that of the adult, with the peripheral capillaries being closer to the surface. This may cause increased absorption of topical medications.

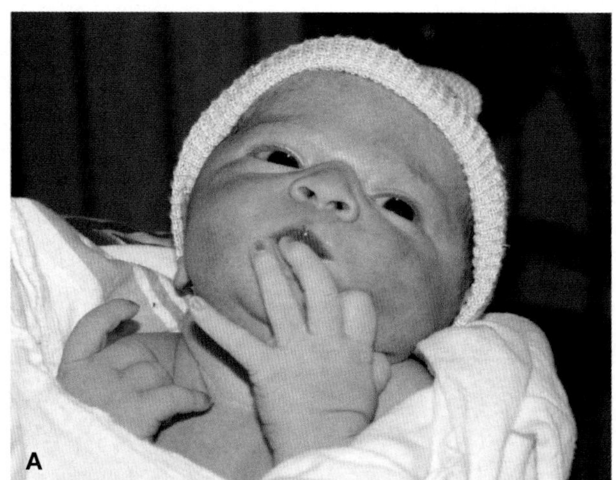

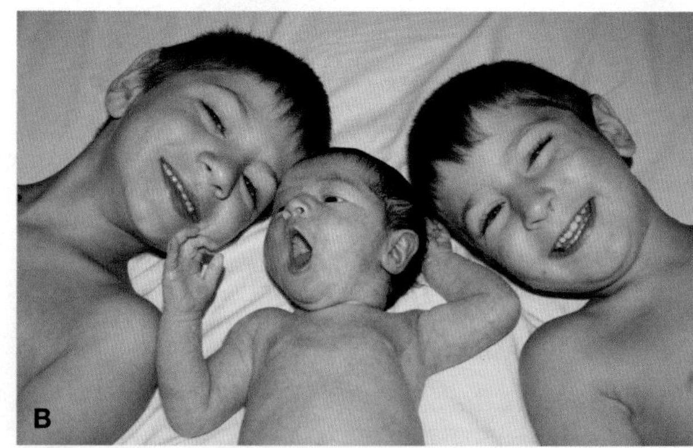

FIGURE 3.3 **A.** Acrocyanosis. Note blueness of the hands. **B.** Mottling of the skin in a young infant.

Hematopoietic System

Significant changes in the hematopoietic system occur over the first year of life. After birth, erythrocyte production decreases significantly, resulting in a relatively low hemoglobin and hematocrit around 2 to 3 months of age (physiologic anemia of infancy) (Nuss et al., 2022). During the last 3 months of gestation, maternal iron stores are transferred to the fetus. Healthy newborns typically have sufficient iron stores at birth. As the high hemoglobin concentration of the newborn decreases over the first 2 to 3 months, iron is reclaimed and stored. These stores may be sufficient for the first 6 to 9 months of life but will become depleted if iron intake is not sufficient (Powers, 2021).

TAKE NOTE!

Maternal iron stores are transferred to the fetus throughout the last trimester of pregnancy. Infants born prematurely miss all or at least a portion of this iron store transfer, placing them at increased risk for iron-deficiency anemia compared with term infants.

Immunologic System

Newborns receive large amounts of IgG through the placenta. This confers immunity during the first 3 to 6 months of life for antigens to which the birthing parent was previously exposed. Infants then synthesize their own IgG, reaching approximately 60% of adult levels at age 12 months (Cherry et al., 2019). IgM is produced in significant amounts after birth, reaching adult levels by 9 months of age. IgA, IgD, and IgE production increase very gradually, maturing in early childhood (Cherry et al., 2019).

PSYCHOSOCIAL DEVELOPMENT

Erik Erikson (1963) identifies the psychosocial crisis of infancy as trust versus mistrust. Development of a sense of trust is crucial in the first year, as it serves as the foundation for later psychosocial tasks. The parent or primary caregiver can have a significant impact on the infant's development of a sense of trust. When the infant's needs are consistently met, the infant develops this sense of trust. But if the parent or caregiver is inconsistent in meeting the infant's needs in a timely manner, then the infant develops a sense of mistrust. Table 3.2 lists activities that promote a sense of trust in infancy.

COGNITIVE DEVELOPMENT

The first stage of Jean Piaget's theory of cognitive development is referred to as the sensorimotor stage (birth to 2 years) (Piaget, 1969). Infants learn about themselves and the world through their developing sensory and motor capacities. Infants' development from birth to 1 year of age can be divided into four substages within the sensorimotor stage: reflexes, primary circular reactions, secondary circular reactions, and coordination of secondary schemes. Cause and effect guides most of the cognitive development seen in infancy (Table 3.2).

TABLE 3.2 • Developmental Theories

Theorist	Stage	Activities
Erikson	Trust vs. mistrust (birth to 1 year)	Caregivers respond to the infant's basic needs by feeding, changing diapers, cleaning, touching, holding, and talking to the infant. This creates a sense of trust in the infant. As the nervous system matures, infants realize they are separate beings from their caregivers. Over time, the infant learns to tolerate small amounts of frustration and trusts that although gratification may be delayed, it will eventually be provided.
Piaget	Sensorimotor (birth to 2 years)	Infant uses senses and motor skills to learn about the world.
	Substage 1: use of reflexes (birth to 1 month)	Reflexive sucking brings the pleasure of ingesting nutrition. Infant begins to gain control over reflexes and recognizes familiar objects, odors, and sounds.
	Substage 2: primary circular reactions (1–4 months)	Thumb sucking may occur by chance; then the infant repeats it on purpose to bring pleasure. Imitation begins. Object permanence begins. Infant shows affect.
	Substage 3: secondary circular reactions (4–8 months)	Infant repeats actions to achieve wanted results (e.g., shakes rattle to hear the noise it makes). The infant's actions are purposeful, but the infant does not always have an end goal in mind.
	Substage 4: coordination of secondary schemes (8–12 months)	Infants coordinate previously learned schemes with previously learned behaviors. They may grasp and shake a rattle intentionally or crawl across the room to reach a desired toy. Infant can anticipate events. Object permanence is fully present at about 8 months of age. The infant begins to associate symbols with events (e.g., waving goodbye means someone is leaving).
Freud	Oral stage (birth to 1 year)	Pleasure is focused on oral activities: feeding and sucking.

Adapted from Erikson, E. H. (1963). *Childhood and society* (2nd ed.). W. W. Norton and Company; Piaget, J. (1969). *The theory of stages in cognitive development*. McGraw-Hill; Reynolds, A., Angulo, A., Breheney, M., Green, J., & Goldson, E. (2022). Child development and behavior. In M. Bunik, W. W. Hay, M. J. Levin, & M. J. Abzug (Eds.), *Current diagnosis & treatment: Pediatrics* (26th ed.). McGraw-Hill Education.

The concept of **object permanence** begins to develop between 4 and 7 months of age and is solidified by about 8 months of age (Piaget, 1969). If an object is hidden from the infant's sight, the infant will search for it in the last place it was seen, knowing it still exists. This development of object permanence is essential for the development of self-image. By age 12 months, the infant knows they are separate from the parent or caregiver. Self-image is also promoted through the use of mirrors. By 12 months of age, infants can recognize themselves in the mirror. The 12-month-old will explore objects in different ways, such as throwing, banging, dropping, and shaking. The infant may imitate gestures and knows how to use certain objects correctly (e.g., puts phone to ear, turns up cup to drink, attempts to comb hair) (Piaget, 1969).

MOTOR SKILL DEVELOPMENT

Infants exhibit phenomenal increases in their gross and fine motor skills over the first 12 months of life.

Gross Motor Skills

The term "gross motor skills" refers to those that use the large muscles (e.g., head control, rolling, sitting, and walking). Gross motor skills develop in a **cephalocaudal** fashion (from the head to the tail) (Fig. 3.4). In other words, the baby learns to lift the head before learning to roll over and sit (Reynolds et al., 2022). At birth, babies have poor head control and need to have their necks supported when being held. They can lift their heads only slightly while in a prone position. Over the next several months, the infant's motor skills progress at a dramatic rate. First, the infant achieves head control, then the ability to roll over, sit, crawl, pull to stand, and, usually around 1 year of age, walk independently. Table 3.3 gives details on when the infant develops each specific gross motor skill. Progression of gross motor skills is illustrated in Figures 3.5 through 3.7.

> *TAKE NOTE!*
>
> Warning signs that may indicate problems with motor development include the following: arms and legs are stiff or floppy; child cannot support head at 3 to 4 months of age; child reaches with one hand only; child cannot sit with assistance at 6 months of age; child does not crawl by 12 months of age; child cannot stand supported by 12 months of age.

Fine Motor Skills

Fine motor development includes the maturation of hand and finger use. Fine motor skills develop in a **proximodistal** fashion (from the center to the periphery) (see Fig. 3.4). In other words, the infant first bats with the whole hand, eventually progressing to gross grasping, before being capable of fine fingertip grasping (Reynolds et al., 2022) (Fig. 3.8). The newborn's hand movements

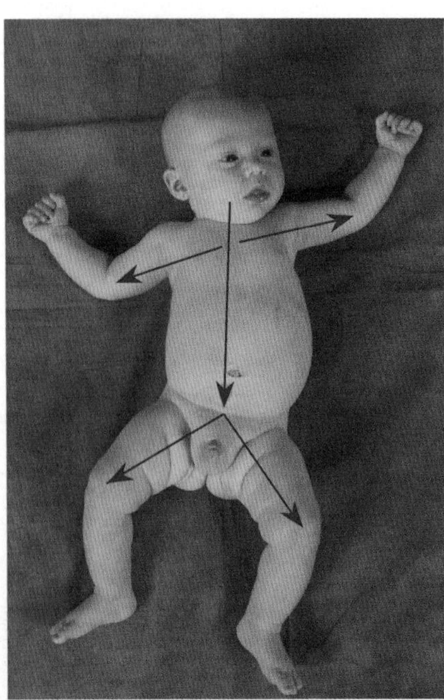

FIGURE 3.4 Gross motor skills develop in a cephalocaudal direction, fine motor skills in a proximodistal fashion.

TABLE 3.3 • Key Gross Motor Skills in Infancy

Age (months)	Gross Motor Skills
2	Holds head up when prone Moves all four extremities
4	Holds head steady without support When prone, pushes up on forearms/elbows
6	Rolls from prone to supine Tripod sits When prone, uses arms to push up straight
9	Sits unsupported Gets to sitting on own
12	Pulls to stand Cruises (walks holding onto furniture)

Adapted from Centers for Disease Control and Prevention. (2022b). *CDC's developmental milestones.* http://www.cdc.gov/ncbddd/actearly/milestones/index.html; Zubler, J. M., Wiggins, L. D., Macias, M. M., Whitaker, T. M., Shaw, J. S., Squires, J. K., Pajke, J. A., Wolf, R. B., Slaughter, K. S., Broughton, A. S., Gerndt, K. L., Mlodoch, B. J., & Lipkin, P. H. (2022). Evidence-informed milestones for developmental surveillance tools. *Pediatrics, 149*(3), e2021052138. https://doi.org/10.1542/peds.2021-052138

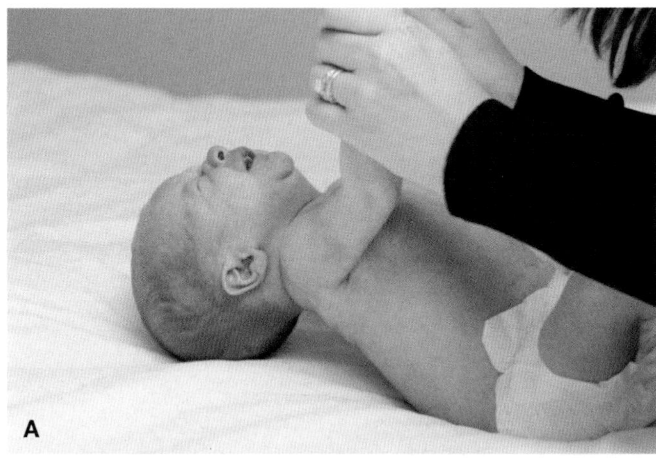

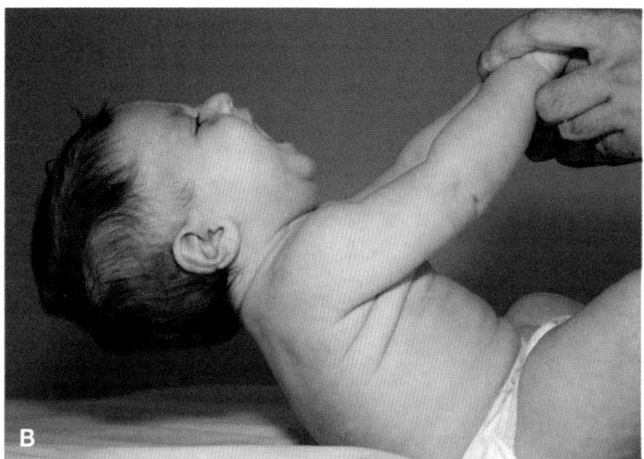

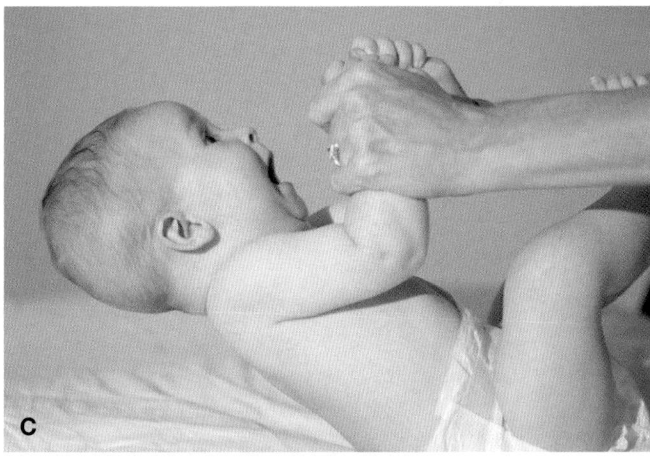

FIGURE 3.5 When pulled to sit, an infant shows significant head lag (newborn; 2 or 3 weeks old) (**A**), improving head control (2 months old) (**B**), and no head lag (4 months old) (**C**).

are involuntary in nature, whereas the 12-month-old is capable of feeding themselves with a cup and spoon. By 12 months of age, the infant should be able to eat with their fingers and assist with dressing (e.g., pushing an arm through the sleeve). Table 3.4 provides details on when the infant develops each specific fine motor skill.

SENSORY DEVELOPMENT

Although hearing should be fully developed at birth, the other senses continue to develop as the infant matures. Although they mature at different rates, sight, smell, taste, and touch all continue to develop after birth.

Sight

The newborn is nearsighted, preferring to view objects at a distance of 20 to 38 cm (8 to 15 in). Newborns prefer the human face to other objects and may even imitate the facial expressions made by those caring for them. In addition to human faces, newborns show a preference for certain objects, particularly those with contrasts such as black-and-white stripes. The newborn's eyes wander and occasionally cross. At 1 month of age, the infant can recognize by sight the people the infant knows best. The infant will study objects within their visual range closely. The ability to fuse two ocular images into one cerebral picture (**binocularity**) begins to develop at 6 weeks of age and is well established by 4 months of age. Full color vision develops by 7 months of age, as do distance vision and the ability to track objects.

Hearing

The newborn's hearing is intact at birth and as acute as that of an adult. Newborns prefer the sound of human voices to nonhuman sounds. By 1 month of age, the infant can recognize the sounds of people the infant knows best.

Smell and Taste

The sense of smell develops rapidly: The 7-day-old infant can differentiate the smell of their lactating parent's breast milk from that of another and will preferentially turn toward their parent's smell. Newborns prefer sweet tastes to all others. This persists for several months, and, eventually, the infant will accept nonsweet flavors.

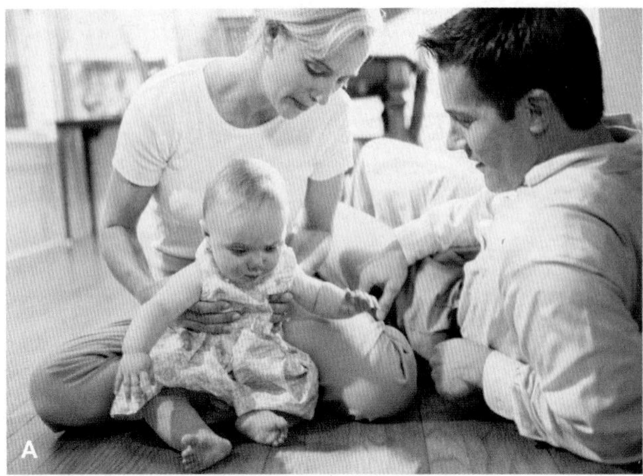

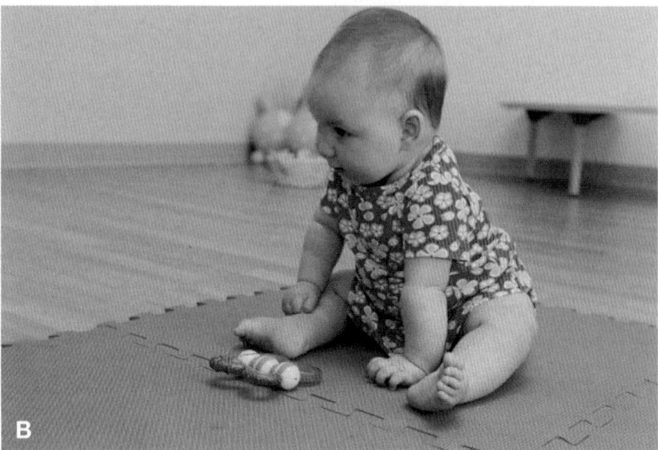

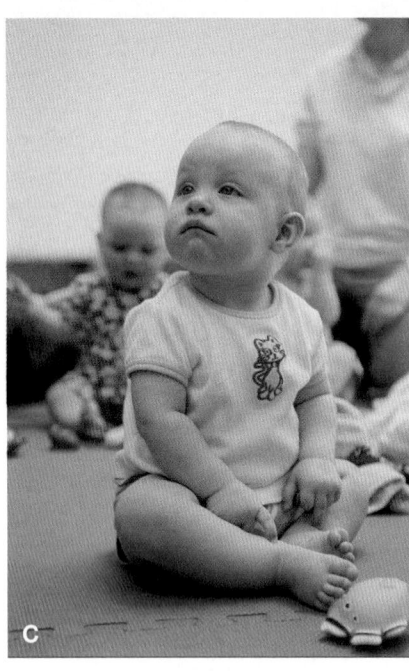

FIGURE 3.6 Development of sitting. **A.** At 4 months, the infant requires significant support. **B.** The 6-month-old infant sits in tripod fashion. **C.** The 8-month-old sits alone.

Touch

The sense of touch is perhaps the most important of all the senses for newborn communication. Even the most immature infant responds to soothing stroking. The infant prefers soft sensations to coarse sensations. The infant dislikes rough handling and may cry. Holding, stroking, rocking, or cuddling calms infants when they are upset and makes them more alert when they are drowsy. Infants learn to understand their caregiver's moods by the way they touch them.

TAKE NOTE!

Warning signs that may indicate problems with sensory development include the following: young infant does not respond to loud noises; child does not focus on a near object; infant does not start to make sounds or babble by 4 months of age; infant does not turn to locate sound at age 4 months; infant crosses eyes most of the time at age 6 months.

COMMUNICATION AND LANGUAGE DEVELOPMENT

For several months, crying is the only means of communication for the newborn and infant. The basic reason for crying is unmet needs. The 2-month-old baby reacts to loud sounds, coos, makes other vocalizations, and demonstrates differentiated crying. At 4 to 5 months of age, the infant makes simple vowel sounds, vocalizes in response to voices, and laughs aloud. The 6-month-old performs "raspberries," and squeals (in joy or displeasure). At age 9 months, babbling occurs in strings (e.g., mamama, dadada) without meaning, and the infant lifts their arms to be picked up. At 9 to 12 months of age, the infant begins to attach meaning to "mama" and "dada" and starts to imitate other speech sounds. The 12-month-old also babbles with inflection (this babbling has the rhythm and timing of spoken language, but few of the "words" make sense) (Reynolds et al., 2022; Zubler et al., 2022).

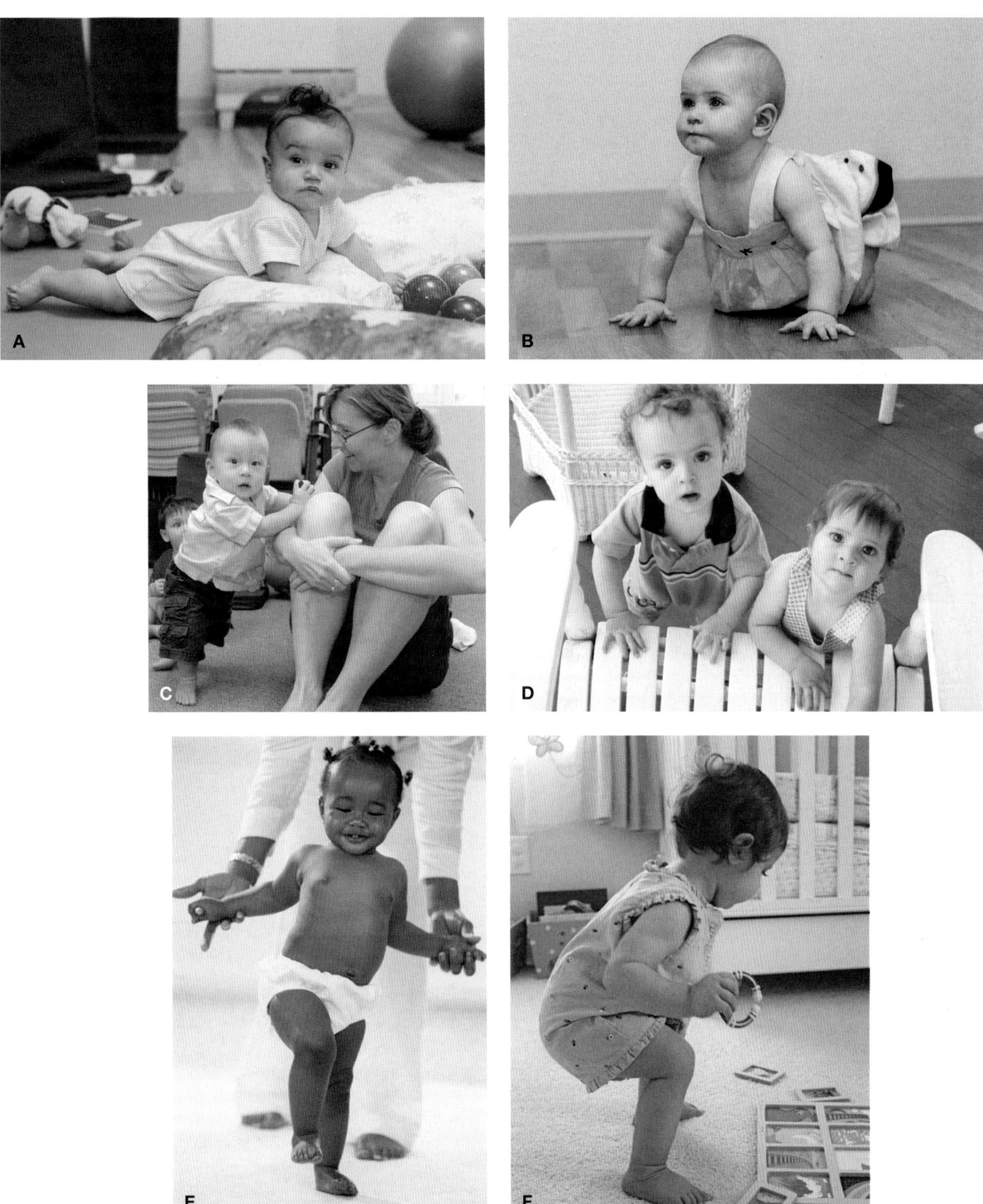

FIGURE 3.7 Development of locomotion. **A.** At 4 months, the infant pushes up from a prone position. **B.** At 8 months of age, the infant crawls with the abdomen off the floor. **C.** The infant pulls to stand by 10 months of age. **D.** The infant cruises along furniture or **(E)** takes steps with assistance at 10 to 11 months of age. **F.** The infant independently stands from a crouched position and walks around 12 months of age (+/− 3 months).

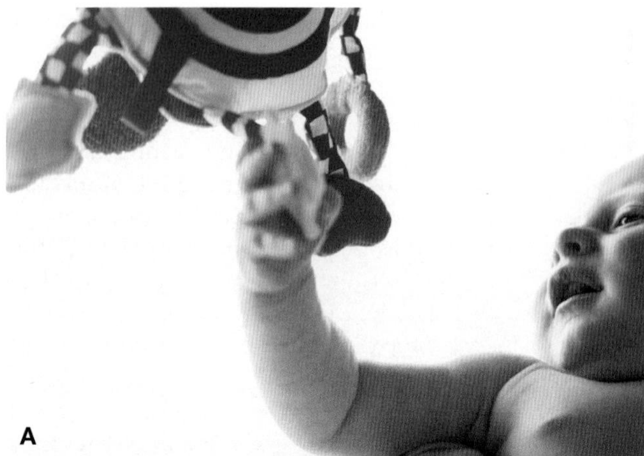

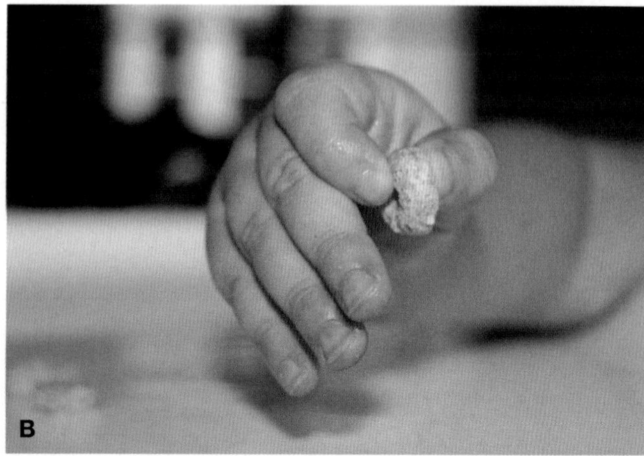

FIGURE 3.8 Development of the pincer grasp. Note the gross (whole-hand) approach to grasping a small object (**A**), compared with the fine (thumb-to-finger) ability (**B**).

It is very important for the parent or caregiver to talk to the infant in order for the infant to learn communication skills. Sometimes, regression in language development occurs briefly when the child is focusing energy on other skills, such as crawling or walking. As long as the infant's hearing is normal, language acquisition should continue to progress. Infants in bilingual families may "language mix" (uses some words from each language). This is considered to be a normal progression in language development for these children (Linguistic Society of America, 2023), but it makes it more difficult for the health care provider or nurse practitioner to determine delays in communication skills.

TABLE 3.4 • Key Fine Motor Skills in Infancy

Age (months)	Fine Motor Skills
2	Briefly opens hands
4	Bats at objects Holds toy when put in hand Brings hands to mouth
6	Reaches for desired item
9	Gross pincer grasp (rakes) Transfers objects from one hand to the other
12	Fine pincer grasp

Adapted from Centers for Disease Control and Prevention. (2022b). *CDC's developmental milestones.* http://www.cdc.gov/ncbddd/actearly/milestones/index.html; Zubler, J. M., Wiggins, L. D., Macias, M. M., Whitaker, T. M., Shaw, J. S., Squires, J. K., Pajke, J. A., Wolf, R. B., Slaughter, K. S., Broughton, A. S., Gerndt, K. L., Mlodoch, B. J., & Lipkin, P. H. (2022). Evidence-informed milestones for developmental surveillance tools. *Pediatrics, 149*(3), e2021052138. https://doi.org/10.1542/peds.2021-052138

TAKE NOTE!

Warning signs that may indicate problems in language development are as follows: infant does not make sounds at 4 months of age; infant does not laugh or squeal by 6 months of age; infant does not babble by 8 months of age; infant does not use single words with meaning at 12 months of age ("mama," "dada").

As you assess Allison (the 6-month-old introduced at the beginning of the chapter), what would you expect her gross motor, fine motor, and language skills to be at this age? How would this be different if Allison had been born 8 weeks premature?

SOCIAL AND EMOTIONAL DEVELOPMENT

The newborn spends much of the time sleeping, but by 2 months of age, the infant is ready to start socializing. The infant exhibits a first real smile at age 2 months and spends a great deal of time while awake watching and observing what is going on. By about 4 months of age, the infant will start an interaction with a caregiver by smiling widely and possibly gurgling. This prompts the caregiver to smile back and talk to the infant. The infant responds with more smiling, cooing, and gurgles as well as moving the arms and legs. The 4-month-old will also smile, chuckle, and move or vocalize to get the caregiver's attention. The baby may hesitate at first, but once the other person responds pleasantly to the infant, the infant engages and gets into the interaction. The infant may cry when the pleasant interaction stops. At 6 months of age, the infant knows familiar people, likes to look at themselves in the mirror, and laughs aloud (Zubler et al., 2022).

Stranger Anxiety

Around the age of 9 months, the infant may develop **stranger anxiety**. The previously happy and very friendly infant may become clingy and whiny when approached by strangers or people not well known. Stranger anxiety is an indicator that the infant is recognizing themselves as separate from others. As the infant becomes more aware of new people and new places, they may view an interaction with a stranger as threatening and may start crying, even if the parent is right there. Family members whom the child sees infrequently, as well as others the child does not spend a lot of time with, should approach the infant calmly and slowly, with the parent in sight. Sometimes, this will prevent a sudden crying spell (Branchford & Levine, 2023; Zubler et al., 2022).

Separation Anxiety

Separation anxiety may also start in the last few months of infancy. The infant becomes quite distressed when the parent leaves. The infant will eventually calm down and become engaged with the current caregiver. It is not until the infant is older that cognition and memory are sufficient for them to understand that the parent will come back (Reynolds et al., 2022).

TAKE NOTE!

Warning signs of possible problems with social/emotional development include: child does not smile at people at 3 months of age; child refuses to cuddle; child does not seem to enjoy people; child shows no interest in peek-a-boo at 8 months of age.

Temperament

Temperament is an individual's nature; it is the child's inborn traits that determine how they interact with the world (Child Development Institute [CDI], 2019). Temperament ranges from low or moderately active, regular, and predictable to highly active, more intense, and less adaptable. These are all considered normal along a continuum. An infant's innate temperament affects the way they respond to the environment. As parents take note of their infant's usual activity level, how intensely they react with others and the environment, and how stimulated they become with interactions, parents start to learn about their infant's temperament. The parent should note how adaptable and flexible the infant is as well as how predictable and persistent the baby is.

When parents are familiar with how the baby approaches life on a routine basis, they will be better able to recognize when the baby is not acting like themselves. Nurses can help parents interpret observations about their infant's temperament and recommend ways to support the infant's individual behavior. Some infants are slower to warm up than others; those infants should be approached slowly and calmly. Some infants exhibit increased levels of activity compared with quieter, more passive babies; those infants generally require more direct play with the parent or caregiver and will be the type of older infant who is in constant motion. Some infants are loud and some are not. The quiet infant may become overwhelmed with excessive stimulation, whereas the very active baby may need additional stimulation to be satisfied. Becoming familiar with the infant's temperament also helps the parents describe the best approach to the infant by others (e.g., child care workers or health care professionals) (CDI, 2019).

CULTURAL INFLUENCES ON GROWTH AND DEVELOPMENT

Many cultural differences have an impact on growth and development. For instance, certain groups tend to be shorter than others because of their genetic makeup (Sinha, 2021). These children will not grow to be as tall as those of another background that doesn't share the same genetic makeup. Cultural feeding practices in some cultures may lead to excess weight in some children. Some cultures and certain religions advocate for vegetarianism; those children need nutritional assessment to ensure they are getting enough protein intake for adequate growth.

Parenting styles and health promotion behaviors can also be significantly influenced by culture. Parents and extended family are the most significant influences in an infant's life in most cultures. Certain cultures place a high value on independence and may encourage their infants to develop quickly, while other cultures "baby" their infants for longer periods. Different cultures assign responsibility to major health-related decisions to different family members.

Health beliefs are often strongly influenced by an individual's religious or spiritual background. Sometimes, this creates conflict in the health care setting when the health providers have a different value system than that of the infant's family.

In some cultures, infants and children share a bed with their parents. When an infant or child is hospitalized and is accustomed to sleeping with the parents, it may be difficult and distressing for them to try to sleep alone.

The nurse should explore the family's cultural practices related to growth and development. Usually, these practices are not harmful and can be supported by the health care team, but safety must always be considered. The nurse should not make assumptions about a family's cultural practices based on their appearance or background; rather, the nurse should perform an adequate assessment for each individual and family (Centers for Disease Control and Prevention [CDC], 2021).

TAKE NOTE!

Many communities include people from a variety of cultures, so it is important for nurses to practice transcultural nursing (nursing care that is directed by cultural aspects and that respects the individual's differences). Many nurse researchers are exploring the cultural aspects of health care and the impact that cultural diversity has on health.

THE NURSE'S ROLE IN NEWBORN AND INFANT GROWTH AND DEVELOPMENT

Growth and development affect every aspect of the infant's life. As infants progress through various stages of development, they do so in a predictable fashion. Growth and development are sequential and orderly, although some children develop at faster rates than others. It is important for the nurse to understand growth and development. Health care visits through infancy often focus primarily on **anticipatory guidance** (educating parents and caregivers about what to expect in the next phase of development). The purpose of anticipatory guidance is to give parents the tools they need to support their infant's development in a safe fashion.

Clinical Judgment and the Nursing Process

After the infant's current growth and development status has been assessed, problems related to growth and development may be identified. The nurse may then identify one or more nursing diagnoses. The following nursing diagnoses with identified outcomes and interventions provide suggestions for nursing care planning or concept mapping. Care planning should be individualized based on the infant's and family's needs.

Nursing Analysis

Breastfeeding difficulty related to insufficient parental knowledge regarding breastfeeding techniques or the importance of breastfeeding, inadequate infant opportunity for breast suckling, inadequate milk supply, or parental ambivalence or anxiety as evidenced by insufficient infant weight gain or sustained weight loss, infant resistance to latching onto breast, or infant inability to correctly latch onto breast

Goal/Outcome

Lactating parent/infant dyad will experience successful breastfeeding: Infant will latch on, suck, and swallow at the breast; lactating parent will not experience sore nipples.

Promoting Effective Breastfeeding (interventions with *rationale*)

- Educate lactating parent on recognition of and response to infant hunger cues *to promote on-cue breastfeeding, which will establish milk supply.*
- Educate lactating parent on appropriate diet and fluid intake *to ensure ability to manufacture adequate supply of breast milk.*
- Demonstrate breastfeeding positions with infant at the breast (*appropriate positioning increases probability of successful latch*).
- Assess infant's latch technique, sucking motion, and audible swallowing (*an appropriately latched infant will take most of the areola in the mouth, suck in spurts, and demonstrate audible swallowing*).
- Assess infant voiding/stool patterns: *at least six voids per day and passage of stool ranging from one or more per day to one every several days is a normal pattern for breastfed infants.*
- Assess infant weight gain; *gain of 15 to 30 g per day after the second week of life indicates infant is receiving appropriate nutrition.*
- Assess lactating parent's nipples for redness or soreness; *if infant appropriately latches on, nipples will not become sore.*

Nursing Analysis

Desire for improved nutrition as evidenced by caregiver expression of readiness to enhance infant's nutrition.

Goal/Outcome

Infant will demonstrate adequate growth and appropriate feeding behaviors: steady increases in weight, length, and head circumference; infant feeds appropriately for age.

Promoting Enhanced Nutrition (interventions with *rationale*)

- Observe lactating parent/infant dyad breastfeeding or bottle-feeding *to determine need for further education or identify infant difficulties with feeding.*
- Educate parent about appropriate breastfeeding or bottle-feeding *so that they are aware of what to expect in normal feeding pattern.*

- When infant is old enough, provide education about addition of solid foods, spoon, and cup feeding: *after 6 months of age, breast milk or formula needs to be supplemented with a variety of foods.*
- Determine need for additional caloric intake if necessary (*premature infants and infants with chronic illnesses or metabolic disorders often need adjustments in caloric intake to demonstrate adequate or catch-up growth*).
- Obtain daily weights if hospitalized (weekly if outpatient) and weekly length and head circumference *to determine whether nutritional intake is sufficient to promote adequate growth.*

Nursing Analysis

Alteration in nutritional status related to insufficient dietary intake, as evidenced by failure to gain weight or by inadequate increases in weight, length, and head circumference over time.

Goal/Outcome

Infant will take in adequate nutrients using effective feeding pattern: Infant will demonstrate adequate weight gain (15 to 30 g/day) and steady increases in length and head circumference.

Promoting Adequate Nutritional Intake (interventions with *rationale*)

- Assess current feeding pattern and daily intake *to determine areas of concern.*
- Increase frequency of breastfeeding or volume of bottle-feeding *if needed to meet caloric needs.*
- Introduce solid foods on age-appropriate schedule: *introducing solids at the right time improves the chances that the child will learn to take solid foods.*
- Limit juice intake or discontinue altogether (*juice has little nutritive value and displaces nutrients from breast milk or formula*).
- Use human milk fortifier (if ordered) *to increase caloric density of breast milk.*
- Increase caloric density of formula (if ordered) by mixing to a more concentrated level or with additives (fats or carbohydrates) *to provide increased calories needed to support adequate growth.*
- If infant is taking solids already, choose higher-calorie foods *to maximize nutrient intake.*

Nursing Analysis

Altered attachment risk; risk factors include premature infant, disordered infant behavior and/or resulting parental conflict, or parental substance misuse.

Goal/Outcome

Parent and infant will demonstrate appropriate attachment via eye contact, parental response to infant cues, parental verbalization of caring for infant, and infant response to parent's caregiving behaviors.

Encouraging Appropriate Parent–Infant Attachment (interventions with *rationale*)

- Assess parent's response to infant cues *to determine degree of attachment and level of parent's knowledge about infant care.*
- Assess infant's response to parent's caregiving behaviors *to determine degree of attachment.*
- Determine infant's temperament *to counsel parent effectively about responses appropriate for that type of temperament.*
- Encourage en face positioning for holding or feeding the young infant *to encourage give-and-take response between infant and parent.*
- Encourage parent to meet infant's needs promptly and with affection *to promote sense of trust in the infant.*
- Reinforce parent's attempts at improving attachment with infant (*positive reinforcement naturally encourages appropriate behaviors*).

Nursing Analysis

Delayed growth and development risk; risk factors include prematurity, chronic illness, impaired attachment, or failure to thrive.

Goal/Outcome

Development will be maximized: Infant will make continued progress toward attainment of developmental milestones.

Maximizing Development (interventions with *rationale*)

- Perform developmental evaluation of the infant *to determine infant's current level of functioning.*
- Offer age-appropriate play, activities, and toys *to encourage further development.*
- Carry out interventions as prescribed by developmental specialist, physical therapist, occupational therapist, or speech therapist (*repeated exposure to the activities or exercises is needed to make developmental progress*).
- Provide support to parents of infants with developmental concerns, *as developmental progress can be slow and it is difficult for families to stay motivated and maintain hope.*

Nursing Analysis

Caregiver fatigue risk; risk factors include inexperience with caregiving, insufficient assistance, and not being developmentally ready for caregiving role.

Goal/Outcome

Parent will experience competence in role: will demonstrate appropriate caregiving behaviors and verbalize comfort in new role.

Preventing Caregiver Fatigue (interventions with *rationale*)

- Assess parent's knowledge of newborn/infant care and the issues that arise as a part of normal development *to determine parent's needs.*

- Provide education on normal newborn/infant care *so that parents have the knowledge they need to appropriately care for their new baby.*
- Provide anticipatory guidance related to normal infant development *to prepare parents for what to expect next and how to intervene.*
- Encourage respite for parents (*even a few hours away from the demands of an infant's care can rejuvenate the parents*).

Nursing Analysis

Injury risk; risk factors include extremes of age, infant curiosity, rapidly progressing motor abilities, or unsafe mode of transport.

Goal/Outcome

Infant safety will be maintained: Infant will remain free from injury.

Preventing Injury (interventions with *rationale*)

- Encourage car seat safety *to decrease risk of injury related to motor vehicles.*
- Childproof home; *as infant becomes more mobile, they will want to explore everything, increasing risk of injury.*
- Parents should have the Poison Control Center phone number available; *should an inadvertent ingestion occur, Poison Control can give parents the best advice for appropriate intervention.*
- Never leave an infant unattended in the sink, bathtub, or swimming pool *to prevent drowning.*
- Teach parents first aid measures and infant cardiopulmonary resuscitation (CPR) *to minimize consequences of injury should it occur.*
- Parents should watch the infant at all times (*no amount of childproofing can replace the watchful eye of a caring parent*).

PROMOTING HEALTHY GROWTH AND DEVELOPMENT

Adding a new person to the family produces both excitement and anxiety. Newborns are completely reliant on their parents or caregivers to fill every need. It is quite a burden and precious responsibility that new parents are taking on. Many parents read the latest books about caring for newborns, while others rely on information received from family and friends. Newborns and their parents spend only a short time in the hospital after delivery, so it is important that parents can care for their newborn and know when to call the primary care provider with concerns.

Periodic screening for adequate growth and development is recommended by the American Academy of Pediatrics (AAP) for all infants and children. The prevention of devastating disease is another priority for infants and children. The AAP and the Advisory Committee on Immunization Practices (ACIP) have made recommendations for immunization schedules. Immunizations are a very important part of the newborn's and infant's health visits. Nurses caring for newborns and infants should be familiar with the recommended infant/child periodic screenings (check-ups) as well as the current immunization schedule (see Chapter 9 for further information on immunizations).

Promoting Growth and Development Through Play

Experts in child development and behavior have said repeatedly that play is the work of children. Infants practice their gross and fine motor skills and language through play (Reynolds et al., 2022). Play is a natural way for infants and children to learn. Play is critical to infant development, as it gives infants the opportunity to explore their environment, practice new skills, and solve problems. The newborn prefers interacting with the parent to toys. Parents can talk to and sing to their newborns while participating in the daily activities that infants need, such as feeding, bathing, and changing diapers. Newborns and young infants love to watch people's faces and often appear to mimic the expressions they see.

As infants become older, toys may be geared toward the motor skills or language skills that the child is developing. Parents can promote fine motor development in infants by providing age-appropriate toys. For example, a rattle that a young infant can hold promotes reaching and attaining. The older infant builds fine motor skills by stacking cups or placing smaller toys inside of larger ones. Gross motor skills are reinforced and practiced over and over again when the infant wants to reach something they are interested in.

When playing with toys, the infant usually engages in **solitary play**; they do not share with other infants or directly play with other infants (Reynolds et al., 2022). A wide variety of toys are available for infants, but infants often enjoy the most basic ones, such as plastic containers of various shapes and sizes, soft balls, and wooden or plastic spoons. Books are also very important toys for infants. Reading to all ages of infants is appropriate, and the older infant develops fine motor skills by learning to turn book pages. Table 3.5 lists age-appropriate toys.

Promoting Early Learning

Research has shown that reading aloud and sharing books during early infancy are critical to the development of neural networks that are important in the later tasks of reading and word recognition. Reading books increases listening comprehension. Infants

TABLE 3.5 • Appropriate Toys for Newborns and Infants

Age	Appropriate Toys
Newborn to 1 month	Mobile with contrasting colors or patterns Unbreakable mirror Soft music Soft, brightly colored toys
1–4 months	Bright mobile Unbreakable mirror Rattles Singing by parent or caregiver, varied music High-contrast patterns in books or images
4–7 months	Fabric or board books Different types of music Easy-to-hold toys that do things or make noise (fancy rattles) Floating, squirting bath toys Soft dolls or animals
8–12 months	Plastic cups, bowls, buckets Unbreakable mirror Large building blocks Stacking toys Busy boxes (with buttons or knobs that make things happen) Balls Dolls Board books with large pictures Toy telephone Push–pull toys (older infants)

Adapted from National Association for the Education of Young Children. (n.d.). *Good toys for young children by age and stage.* http://www.naeyc.org/toys

demonstrate their excitement about picture books by kicking and waving their arms and babbling when looking at them. At 6 to 12 months, the infant reaches for books and brings them to the mouth. Over time, reading leads to acquisition of language skills. Reading picture books and simple stories to infants starts a good habit that should be continued throughout childhood (Lewis, 2019).

Promoting Safety

Hundreds of children younger than 1 year of age die each year as a result of injury (AAP, 2018a). As infants become more mobile, they risk injury from falls down stairs and off chairs, tables, and other structures. Curiosity leads the infant to explore potentially dangerous items, such as electrical outlets, hot stove or furnace vents, mop buckets, and toilets. Since infants explore so much with their mouths, small objects or hard foods pose a choking hazard. The infant will invariably pick up any accessible object and bring it to the mouth. With increasing dexterity, poisoning from medications, household cleaning products, or other substances also becomes a problem.

Safety in the Car

Motor vehicle crashes are one source of injury, particularly if the infant is improperly restrained. Infants should never be transported in a motor vehicle without proper restraint. Infant car seats should face the rear of the car throughout infancy (Smola et al., 2020). The car seat should be secured tightly in the center of the back seat. The infant should never be placed in a front seat that is equipped with an airbag.

Infants should never be left unattended in a motor vehicle. The temperature rises very quickly inside a closed vehicle, and an infant can suffocate from heat in a closed vehicle in the summer. Even during cooler weather, the heat generated within a closed vehicle can reach three to five times the exterior temperature. Kidnapping is also a concern if the baby is left unattended in a vehicle.

Safety in the Home

The baby's crib should have a firm mattress that fits snugly in the crib on a secure support. The distance between crib slats should be no wider than a soda can (6 cm [2.36 in] or less) to prevent injury (Safe Kids Worldwide, 2023). All crib edges should be smooth. Only well-fitting crib sheets should be used, not sheets intended for large beds. Crib side rails should always be raised when the parent is not right next to the crib.

Even before the infant can roll over, the baby wiggles and pushes with the feet. The infant can easily fall from a changing table, sofa, or crib with the side rails down, so the infant should never be left unattended on any surface. If infant seats, bouncy seats, or swings are used, the infant should always be restrained in the seat with the appropriate straps.

The AAP (2022) does not recommend the use of infant walkers, because the walker may tip over, and the baby may fall out of it or the infant may fall down the stairs in it. Walkers allow infants access to things they may not otherwise be capable of reaching until they are able to walk alone, such as hot stoves and items on the edge of the countertop.

As the infant becomes more mobile, learning to crawl and walk, new safety issues arise. Safety gates should be used at the tops and bottoms of stairways. Gates may also be used to block curious infants from rooms that may pose physical danger to them because of sharp-edged furniture or decorative objects. Electrical outlets should be covered with approved safety covers. Cabinets and drawers should be secured with child safety latches. Medications, household cleaning supplies, and other potentially hazardous substances should be stored completely out of reach of infants (AAP, 2018a).

Choking is a risk because infants immediately bring small items to the mouth for exploration. To avoid choking, recommend the following to parents:

- Use only toys recommended for children of 0 to 12 months of age.
- Avoid stuffed animals with eyes or buttons that can be dislodged by the persistent infant.
- Keep the floor free of small items (unintentionally dropped coins, paper clips, straight pins).
- Avoid feeding popcorn, nuts, carrot slices, grapes, and hot dog pieces to infants.

Suffocation is also a risk for infants. Cribs should not have pillows, comforters, stuffed animals, or other soft items in them. Keep plastic bags of any size away from infants. Avoid the risk of strangulation by keeping window blind and drapery cords out of the infant's reach (AAP, 2017, 2018a).

Although no safety measure is as effective as close supervision by a watchful parent or caregiver, the aforementioned safety measures can be critical to the infant's well-being.

Safety in the Water

Infants can drown in a small amount of water. Never leave an infant unattended in the sink, a baby bathtub or standard bathtub, a swimming or wading pool, or any other body of water, even if it is quite shallow. The bathroom door should be kept closed and the toilet lid down. Water should be emptied from tubs, pails, or buckets immediately after use. If the family has a swimming pool, a locked fence or locked screen enclosure should surround it. Exterior doors should be kept locked to prevent the older infant from wandering out to the pool (AAP, 2018a). The AAP recommends that parents use caution when enrolling their infant in an aquatic or swim program. Research has not sufficiently demonstrated that water survival skills taught to infants are effective (AAP, 2019). Completing an aquatic program does not decrease the risk of drowning; vigilant supervision is still always required.

Remember Allison Johnson, the infant described at the beginning of the chapter? What anticipatory guidance related to safety would you provide to Allison's parents?

Promoting Nutrition

Adequate nutrition is essential for growth and development. Breastfeeding and bottle-feeding of infant formula are both acceptable means of nutrition in the newborn and infant. Breast milk or formula supplies all of the infant's daily nutritional requirements until 6 months of age, at which time solid foods may be introduced (Buchanan & Marquez, 2023).

Cultural Factors

Many dietary practices are affected by culture, both in the types of food eaten and in the approach to progression of infant feeding. Some groups tend to be lactose intolerant (particularly Black, Native American, and Asian individuals); therefore, alternative sources of calcium must be offered. Explore the cultural practices of the family related to infant feeding so that you can support the family's cultural values.

Nutritional Needs

Newborns and infants are experiencing tremendous growth and need diets that support these rapid changes. Table 3.6 compares fluid and caloric needs in the newborn and infant.

Breastfeeding

The National Association of Pediatric Nurse Practitioners (NAPNAP), the AAP, the American College of Obstetrics and Gynecology, the American Dietetic Association, and the U.S. Breastfeeding Committee of the Department of Health and Human Services all recommend breastfeeding as the natural and preferred method of newborn and infant feeding (Busch et al., 2019). In their position statement on breastfeeding, NAPNAP recommends exclusive breastfeeding for the first 6 months as optimal since breast milk provides complete infant nutrition (Busch et al., 2019).

Breastfeeding or feeding of expressed human milk is recommended for all infants, including sick or premature newborns (with rare exceptions). The exceptions include infants with galactosemia, maternal use of illicit drugs and a few prescription medications, maternal untreated active tuberculosis, and maternal HIV infection

TABLE 3.6 • Nutritional Requirements

Nutritional Requirements	Newborn	Infant
Fluid	140–160 mL/kg/day	100 mL/kg/day for first 10 kg 50 mL/kg/day for next 10 kg
Calories	105–108 kcal/kg/day	1–6 months: 108 kcal/kg 6–12 months: 98 kcal/kg

Adapted from Kleinman, K., McDaniel, L., & Molloy, M. (Eds.). (2021). *The Harriet Lane handbook* (22nd ed.). Elsevier.

HEALTHY PEOPLE 2030

Objective	Nursing Significance
Increase the proportion of infants who are breastfed exclusively through 6 months. Increase the proportion of infants who are breastfed at 1 year.	• Encourage breastfeeding in all birthing parents beginning with the prenatal visit if applicable. • Provide accurate education related to breastfeeding. • Be available for questions or problems related to initiation and continuation of breastfeeding. Consult a lactation consultant as needed or available. • Encourage pumping of breast milk when birthing parent returns to work in order to continue breastfeeding. • Refer to local breastfeeding support groups such as La Leche League.

Healthy People Objectives retrieved from http://www.healthypeople.gov

in developed countries. Data from the CDC's *Breastfeeding Report Card* indicate that 83.2% of U.S. infants were ever breastfed, 55.6% of infants were breastfeeding at 6 months of age, and only 35.9% were receiving some breast milk at 1 year of age (2022a). Even partial breastfeeding is helpful and offers some of the health benefits of breastfeeding. Pediatric nurses in the community and the hospital are in an excellent position to promote and support breastfeeding, thereby contributing to the Healthy People 2030 goal of increasing the proportion of birthing parents who exclusively breastfeed their babies for the first 6 months (see Evidence-Based Practice 3.1).

BOX 3.1 Benefits of Breastfeeding

Infant

- Increased bonding with parent
- Immunologic protection
- Breast milk has anti-infective properties.
- Decreased incidence and severity of diarrhea
- Decreased incidence of asthma, otitis media, bacterial meningitis, botulism, urinary tract infection
- Possible enhancement of cognitive development
- Decreased incidence of higher weight in later childhood

Parental

- Increased bonding with infant
- Lessens birthing parent blood loss in the postpartum period
- Decreased risk of ovarian and premenopausal breast cancer
- Reduced incidence of pregnancy-induced, long-term higher weight
- Possible delay of return of ovulation in some
- Always ready; no mixing
- Economic advantage

Adapted from La Leche League International. (2023). *Breastfeeding info A to Z.* https://www.llli.org/breastfeeding-info/

BREAST MILK COMPOSITION

Breast milk includes lactose, lipids, polyunsaturated fatty acids, and amino acids. The ratio of whey to casein protein in breast milk makes it readily digestible. The high concentration of fats and the balance of amino acids are believed to contribute to proper myelination of the nervous system. The concentration of iron in breast milk is less than that of formula, but the iron has increased bioavailability and is sufficient to meet the infant's requirements for the first 4 to 6 months of life. In addition to complete nutrition, immunologic protection is transferred from lactating parent to infant via breast milk, and parental–infant bonding is promoted. The benefits of breastfeeding are listed in Box 3.1.

EVIDENCE-BASED PRACTICE 3.1

Milk Boosters for Breastfeeding Term Infants

STUDY

Earlier weaning from the breast and earlier formula supplementation often occur as a result of poor milk supply (as identified by the lactating parent). The authors performed a comprehensive review of research studies related to the use of galactagogues (milk boosters) by parents breastfeeding their term infants. The authors evaluated 41 eligible studies involving 3,005 parents and 3,006 infants from at least 17 countries. The studies evaluated increased milk production in relation to the use of medications, herbal supplements, and foods.

Findings

Upon analysis of the various research studies, the authors reached the conclusion that since the studies were so varied in their approach and report, it is difficult to conclude which (if any) galactagogue increases milk supply most effectively. Minor adverse effects may occur with medication as well as natural milk boosters. The authors were unable to make a recommendation as to the most effective milk booster to use, as well as if any galactagogue was effective.

Nursing Implications

Given the importance of breastfeeding and the Healthy People goal of increasing the proportion of infants exclusively breastfeeding for the first 6 months, it is important for parents to experience adequate milk production. According to current published research studies, neither medications, herbal, nor food galactagogues reigned superior at increasing milk production. Nurses should continue to provide appropriate education and support to breastfeeding parents and ensure they consult with their health care provider or advanced practice nurse if they decide to use galactagogues. Additional research is needed in this area, which nurses could initiate.

Adapted from Foong, S. C., Tan, M. L., Foong, W. C., Marasco, L. A., Ho, J. J., & Ong, J. H. (2020). Oral galactagogues (natural therapies or drugs) for increasing breast milk production in mothers of non-hospitalised term infants. *Cochrane Database of Systematic Reviews.* https://doi.org/10.1002/14651858.CD011505.pub2

BREAST MILK SUPPLY AND DEMAND

Frequent, on-demand breastfeeding of the newborn is necessary to establish an adequate milk supply. After delivery of the placenta, levels of progesterone drop dramatically, which stimulates the anterior pituitary to produce prolactin. Prolactin stimulates the production of milk in the acinar or alveolar cells of the breast. When the infant sucks at the breast, nervous impulses stimulate further production of breast milk.

The first "milk" to be produced by the breasts is termed **colostrum**. It is produced for the first 2 to 4 days after birth. Colostrum is a thin, watery, yellowish fluid that is easy to digest, as it is high in protein and low in sugar and fat. Colostrum is complete nutrition and all that is needed by the newborn for the first 2 to 4 days of life (La Leche League International [LLLI], 2023). Transitional breast milk replaces colostrum on days 2 to 4 after birth. By day 10 after birth, mature breast milk is produced. Mature breast milk has a slightly bluish color and appears thin.

The breastfeeding parent produces milk continually. Called **foremilk**, it collects in the lactiferous sinuses, which are small tubules serving as reservoirs for milk located behind the nipples. The **let-down reflex** is responsible for the release of milk from these reservoirs. When the baby sucks at the breast, oxytocin is released from the posterior pituitary, causing the lactiferous sinuses to contract. This allows milk to "let down" into the nipples, and the infant then sucks the milk. The let-down reflex is triggered not only by suckling at the breast but also by thinking of the baby or by the sound of a baby crying. After the foremilk is let down, new, fattier milk is formed. This **hindmilk** helps the breastfed infant to grow quickly (LLLI, 2023). Parents should be informed that the production of oxytocin during suckling may also cause uterine contractions and may cause afterpains during breastfeeding.

BREASTFEEDING TECHNIQUE

Breastfeeding parents may not have established adequate breastfeeding prior to leaving the hospital after birth of the newborn. The pediatric nurse may encounter an infant–parent dyad experiencing difficulty with breastfeeding for a variety of reasons. Thus, the pediatric nurse must be competent in counseling the breastfeeding parent.

Before each breastfeeding session, the breastfeeding parent should wash their hands. It is not necessary to wash the breast in most cases. The parent should be positioned comfortably. A number of positions are possible, and they should be varied throughout the day. The parent may hold the breast in a "C" position if that is helpful (Fig. 3.9). Stroke the nipple against the baby's cheek (Fig. 3.10). This should stimulate the infant to open the mouth widely. Bring the baby's wide-open mouth to the breast

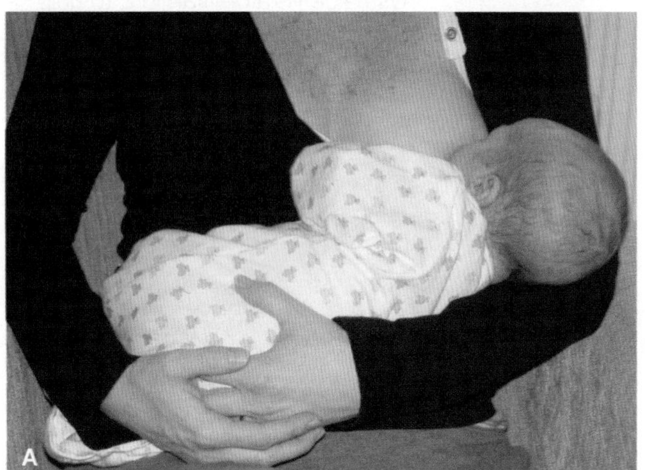

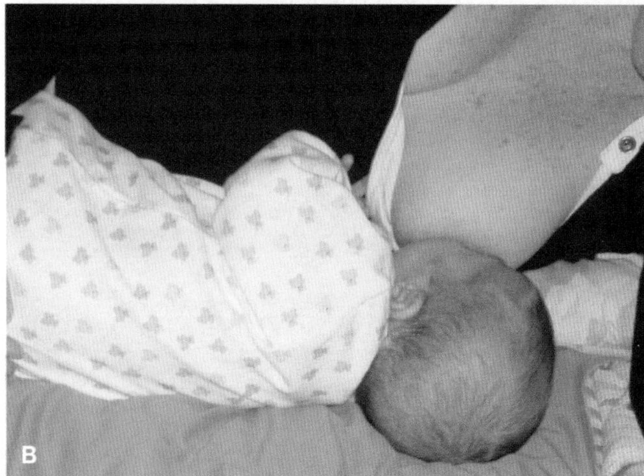

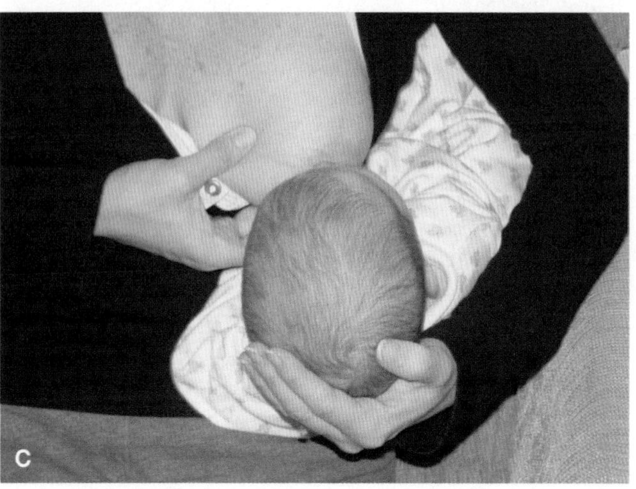

FIGURE 3.9 Various positions may be used during breastfeeding: cradle hold (**A**), side-lying (**B**), football hold (**C**). (Note the "C" position for holding the breast during latching on.)

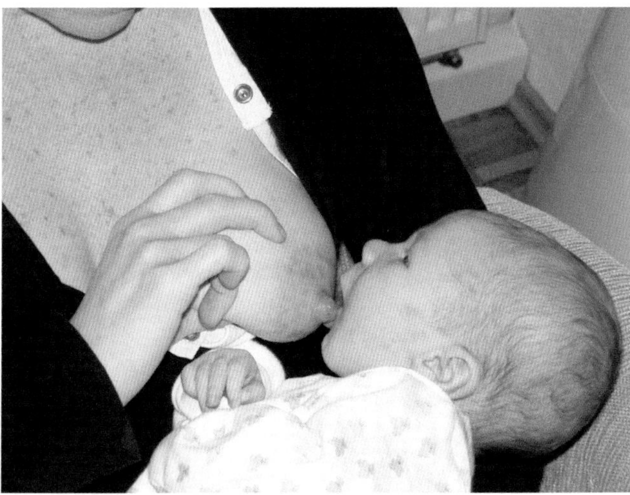

FIGURE 3.10 Stroking the infant's cheek with the nipple will elicit the rooting reflex.

to form a seal around all of the nipple and areola. When the infant is finished feeding, the parent can break the suction by inserting their finger into the baby's mouth, thus releasing the mouth from the nipple (Fig. 3.11). This technique may prevent the infant from pulling on the nipple, which can lead to soreness and cracking.

Watching and listening to the infant feed may help assess the adequacy of the baby's latch technique. The infant who is properly latched onto the breast will suck rhythmically, taking most or all of the areola into the mouth. Audible swallowing should be heard as milk is delivered into the infant's mouth. Assess the lactating parent for pain related to breastfeeding. They should not be in pain if the baby is latched on properly.

Establishment of breastfeeding is best achieved if the infant is allowed to feed on demand, whenever they are hungry. This may be as often as every 1.5 to 3 hours in the neonate. Infants may feed for 10 to 20 minutes on each breast at each feeding, or longer on just one breast, alternating the breast at each feeding. Both methods are acceptable.

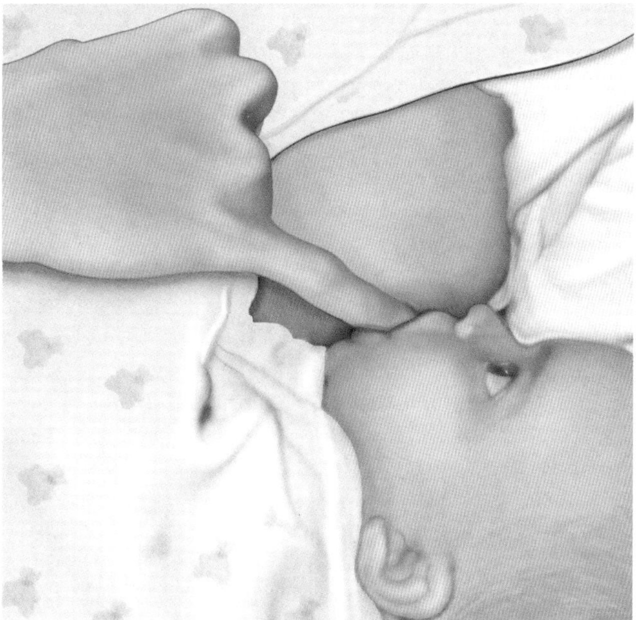

FIGURE 3.11 Inserting the little finger between the areola and the infant's mouth helps to break the suction.

The breastfeeding infant does not need supplementation with water or formula even in the first few days of life as long as the newborn continues to wet six to eight diapers per day. After several days of age, the lactating parent's milk supply should be well established. Adequate urine output and bowel movements, as well as continued weight gain in the infant, indicate the adequacy of breastfeeding. Working parents, in particular, may need additional support from the nurse in order to continue breastfeeding if they desire to do so. Common problems occurring with breastfeeding are addressed in Teaching Guidelines 3.1.

TEACHING GUIDELINES 3.1 Promoting Breastfeeding

Problem	Solutions
Sore nipples	Prevention: encourage appropriate latch-on from the beginning. Expose nipples to air between feedings. Allow breast milk to dry on nipples. Use aloe vera or vitamin E to help heal sore nipples. May use medical-grade lanolin or preservative-free lanolin
Engorgement	Apply warm compresses or encourage the lactating parent to take a warm shower prior to having the baby latch on (warmth encourages some of the milk to be released, allowing the breast to soften and making it easier for the infant to latch on).
Poor sucking	Feed on cue, not on a schedule. Encourage the sleepy infant by stroking the feet, undressing, and rubbing the head.
Inadequate milk supply	Decrease parental stress. Encourage adequate parental diet and fluid intake. Instruct working parents to pump in order to keep up milk supply when away from infant.
Other parent feels left out.	Encourage nonlactating parent to participate in other aspects of care.
Parent worries about adequacy of breast milk.	If infant is voiding six times per day and gaining weight, then the infant is receiving enough milk and appropriate nutrition.

BOTTLE-FEEDING

For the parent who does not desire to or cannot breastfeed, commercially prepared formulas are available for bottle-feeding. These formulas are designed to imitate human milk. Standard infant formulas based on cow's milk provide 20 kcal/oz and use lactose as a source for carbohydrates (Buchanan & Marquez, 2023). Vegetable oil is used as the source of fat; whey or casein provides protein. Newer cow's milk–based formulas contain long-chain polyunsaturated fatty acids that are thought to improve brain development. Ordinary cow's milk is not recommended for the first year of life.

> **TAKE NOTE!**
>
> Cow's milk does not provide an adequate balance of nutrients for the growing infant, especially iron. It may also overload the infant's renal system with inappropriate amounts of protein, sodium, and minerals.

Only formulas that are fortified with iron should be used. Iron stores that the infant received prenatally are depleted by 4 to 6 months of age. To prevent iron-deficiency anemia, poor growth patterns, and impaired development, iron-fortified formulas must be used. The AAP recommends that commercial formulas provide 10 to 12 mg of iron per liter (Buchanan & Marquez, 2023). Commercial formulas also provide an adequate blend of essential vitamins and minerals.

FEEDING PATTERNS

Infant feeding is an opportune time to establish good eating behaviors. The infant should always be held while being bottle-fed. Cradling in a semiupright position allows for additional bonding time, as the infant can see the caregiver's face while feeding (Fig. 3.12). Talking or singing during feeding time also increases bonding. As with breastfed infants, the bottle-fed infant should be fed on cue. Overfeeding with the bottle increases the incidence of spitting up and higher weight, so families need to learn their baby's cues to hunger and satiety (AAP, 2023).

It is important to feed the baby when the infant displays signs of hunger. Crying is a late sign of hunger; earlier signs include making sucking motions, sucking on hands, or putting the fist to the chin. The infant should be burped two or three times per feeding, when the infant slows feeding or stops sucking. Newborns may only take a half to 1 oz per feeding initially, working up to 2 to 3 oz in the first few days. They need to feed about six to 10 times per day. The infant will gradually be able to ingest more formula per feeding. By 6 months of age, babies feed four or five times per day and take 6 to 8 oz per feeding. Most infants will not require specific amounts per feeding; the infant should be fed until full. To prevent overfeeding, healthy bottle-fed infants should be allowed to self-regulate the amount of formula ingested per feeding. When the baby is satiated, they might fall asleep, spit out the nipple or formula, play with the nipple, or lie quietly, only sucking once in a while (AAP, 2023).

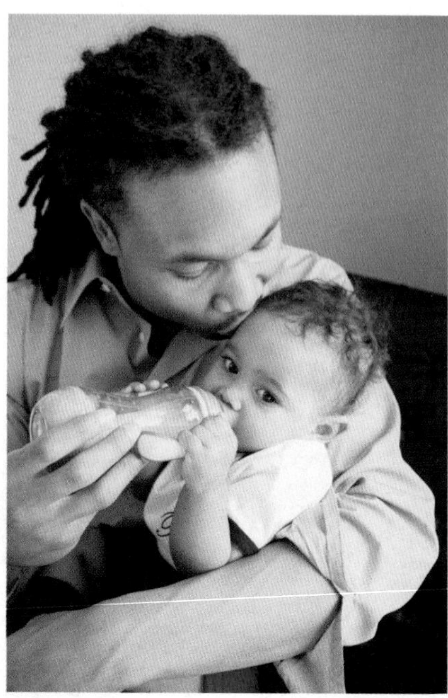

FIGURE 3.12 Technique for bottle-feeding the infant.

TYPES OF FORMULAS AND BOTTLES

Parents may choose to use commercial formulas that are ready to feed or available as a concentrate or as a powder. Parents should follow the instructions for mixing the concentrate or powder to avoid dehydration or fluid and electrolyte imbalances. Ready-to-feed formula should be used as is and never diluted (Buchanan & Marquez, 2023). A wide variety of baby bottle and nipple types are available for formula feeding, and the choice is purely individual. Few infants require special nipples or bottles. Box 3.2 gives guidelines on preparation and storage of formula and care of bottles.

SPECIAL FORMULAS

Special formulas may be needed for the infant who is allergic to a particular component of standard formula or has a renal, hepatic, metabolic, or intestinal disorder. For example, lactose-free cow's milk formulas are available for the lactose-intolerant child. Formulas using soy as the base ingredient instead of whey or casein are also available. Soy formulas are necessary for infants with a milk allergy, and they may be appealing to the vegetarian family.

These special formulas are designed to meet the nutritional needs of infants, depending on the disorder.

BOX **3.2** **Preparation and Storage of Bottles and Formula**

- Wash nipples and bottles in hot soapy water and rinse well OR run nipples and bottles through the dishwasher.
- Store the tightly covered ready-to-feed formula can after opening in refrigerator for up to 48 hours.
- After mixing concentrate or powdered formula, store tightly covered in refrigerator for up to 48 hours.
- Do not reheat and reuse partially used bottles. Throw away the unused portion after each feeding.
- Do not add cereal to the formula in the bottle.
- Do not sweeten formula with honey.
- Warm formula by placing bottle in a container of hot water.
- Do not microwave formula.

Adapted from American Academy of Pediatrics. (2023). *Formula feeding.* https://www.healthychildren.org/English/ages-stages/baby/formula-feeding/Pages/default.aspx

Infants who fail to gain weight may be placed on standard infant formula prepared to deliver a higher caloric density per ounce. Preterm infants (those born earlier than 36 weeks' gestation) need adequate nutrition to exhibit catch-up growth. Good catch-up growth (quadrupling or even quintupling the birth weight) in the first year or so of life is critical for adequate head growth and avoidance of neurodevelopmental consequences. Premature infant follow-up formulas are designed to provide additional calories, protein, and a particular calcium-to-phosphorus ratio as well as the vitamins and minerals needed for adequate catch-up growth.

Progressing to Solid Foods

After 6 months of age, infants usually require the nutrients available in solid foods in addition to their breast milk or formula. Progressing to feeding solid foods can be exciting and trying. Before solid foods are attempted, the infant should be assessed for readiness to progress. Parents need instruction in choosing appropriate solid foods and support in the progression process.

ASSESSING INFANT READINESS

Several factors contribute to the appropriate timing of solid food introduction. The tongue extrusion reflex is necessary for sucking to be an automatic reaction—that is, when a nipple or other item is placed in the mouth, the tongue extrudes and sucking begins. This reflex disappears at about 4 to 6 months of age (Duryea & Fleisher, 2022). Introducing solid food with a spoon prior to 4 to 6 months of age will result in extrusion of the tongue. The parent may think that the infant does not want the food and is spitting it out intentionally, but this is not the case; the infant simply must be mature enough to eat with a spoon (absence of extrusion reflex).

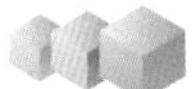
Concept Mastery Alert

Cow's milk should never be given to an infant because of its potential to cause an allergic reaction. Parents should avoid adding fruit juice to the infant's diet because the infant needs the protein and fat in breast milk or formula. Fruit juice would displace these important nutrients.

The ability to swallow solid food does not become completely functional until 4 to 6 months of age. Enzymes to appropriately digest food other than breast milk and formula are also not present in sufficient quantities until the age of 4 to 6 months.

Before the introduction of solid foods and the cup, the infant should be able to sit supported in a highchair. Solids should be fed with a spoon, with the infant in an upright position.

CHOOSING APPROPRIATE SOLID FOODS

Iron-fortified rice cereal mixed with a small amount of breast milk or formula is a good choice for the first solid food. The cereal is easily digested, and its taste is generally well accepted. The cereal should be quite thin at first; it can be mixed to a thicker consistency as the infant gets older. Once the feeding of cereal with a spoon is successful, other single foods may be introduced. The foods should be puréed to a smooth consistency, whether prepackaged "baby food" or puréed at home.

The introduction of one new food every 3 to 5 days is recommended (Buchanan & Marquez, 2023). This allows for identification of food allergies (Box 3.3). No salt, sugar, or other seasoning should be added to these first foods. Previously, avoidance of peanut-containing food until at least 12 months of age was recommended. Recent research recommends early introduction (around 6 months of age) of developmentally appropriate peanut food in skin prick-negative infants to decrease the incidence of developing peanut allergy (McCarthy, 2020).

Generally, by 8 months of age, the infant is ready for more texture in foods. Soft, smashed table food without large chunks is appropriate. Finger foods such as Cheerios, soft green bean pieces, or soft peas may also be offered. Avoid hard foods that the infant may choke on.

BOX **3.3** **Foods to Avoid in Infancy**

- Cow's milk
- Honey
- Excessive amounts of fruit juice
- Foods likely to cause choking
  - Popcorn
  - Other small hard foods (e.g., raw carrot chunks)
  - Grapes and hot dog slices (must be cut in smaller pieces)

Adapted from Schmitt, B. (2022a). *Solid foods (baby foods).* Schmitt Pediatric Guidelines LLC. https://doi.org/10.1542/ppe_schmitt_222

Strained, puréed, or mashed meats may be introduced at 10 to 12 months of age.

The cup should be introduced at 6 to 8 months of age. One ounce of breast milk or formula should be placed in the cup while the infant is learning. This will decrease the amount of mess should the cup be spilled. Old-fashioned sippy cups are generally acceptable for use, although older infants quickly learn to drink from an ordinary cup with assistance when they are thirsty. Older infants are also able to drink from a straw. Newer no-spill sippy cups are not recommended for general home use. They require sucking much like a bottle and do not really encourage the child to learn cup drinking. In addition, the no-spill sippy cup allows for juice or milk to be in constant contact with the baby's teeth, increasing the risk of dental caries (Hagan et al., 2017). Fruit juice is unnecessary and should not be introduced until 6 months of age. If juice is given, it should be limited to 2 to 4 oz per day. Fruit itself is much more nutritious than fruit juice. If infants are allowed to consume larger quantities of juice, it can displace important nutrients from breast milk or formula (Buchanan & Marquez, 2023).

PROMOTING HEALTHY EATING HABITS

Infants and children learn about food within a social context, so the family plays an important role in creating healthy eating habits. Families "model" eating behaviors; infants and children learn about eating through watching others. Lifelong eating patterns are often established in childhood, so it is important to emphasize healthy eating practices beginning in infancy. Parents should not let infants eat whatever they want (permissive feeding style); this will lead to fights over eating in the future. Infants may require as many as 20 exposures to a new food before it is accepted. On the other hand, infants should not be coerced into eating all that is provided (authoritarian feeding style). Forcing an infant to eat when they are full sets the child up for overeating in the future and may lead to more power struggles (Duryea & Fleisher, 2022). Parents need to find a balance between the permissive and authoritarian feeding styles to establish lifelong healthy eating patterns in their children. By providing education about appropriate diet and feeding behaviors, the nurse can help the family accomplish this goal.

Think back to Allison Johnson. What questions should you ask Allison's parents related to her nutritional intake? What anticipatory guidance related to nutrition would be appropriate?

Promoting Healthy Sleep and Rest

Newborns sleep about 10 to 19 hours a day, waking frequently to feed and quickly returning to sleep. By 3 months of age, most infants sleep 7 to 8 hours per night without waking. They will continue to take about three naps a day. By 6 months of age, the infant is more active and alert and may have more trouble going to sleep in the evening. Night waking may occur, but the infant should be capable of sleeping through the night and does not require a night feeding. By 12 months of age, infants sleep 9 to 12 hours per night and take one to two naps per day (Reynolds et al., 2022).

Discuss safe sleeping practices with parents of newborns and infants; the baby should sleep on a firm mattress without pillows or comforters. The baby's bed should be placed away from air conditioner vents, open windows, and open heaters. Sudden infant death syndrome (SIDS) has been associated with prone and side-lying positioning of newborns and infants, so the infant should be placed to sleep alone (no pillows, stuffed animals, fluffy blankets), on their back, and in their own crib (Moon et al., 2022). See the Healthy People 2030 box.

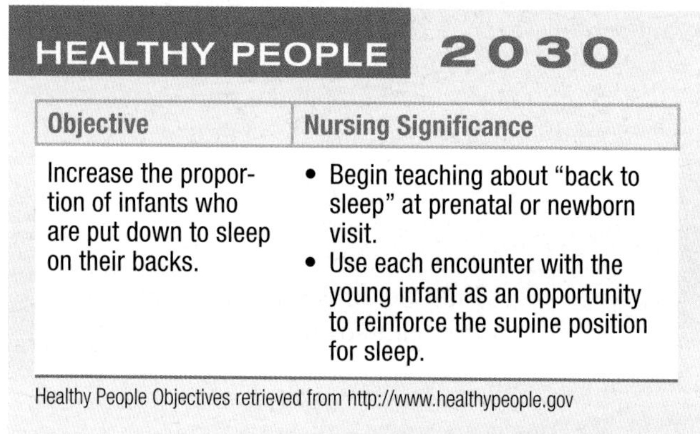

HEALTHY PEOPLE 2030

Objective	Nursing Significance
Increase the proportion of infants who are put down to sleep on their backs.	• Begin teaching about "back to sleep" at prenatal or newborn visit. • Use each encounter with the young infant as an opportunity to reinforce the supine position for sleep.

Healthy People Objectives retrieved from http://www.healthypeople.gov

TAKE NOTE!

The AAP has determined that side sleeping is not as safe as supine sleeping.

In the newborn period, the primary caregiver should try to sleep when the baby is sleeping. Since newborns need to be fed every 1.5 to 3 hours around the clock, parents may become exhausted quickly and are often eager for the infant to sleep through the night. Adding rice cereal to the evening bottle has not been proven to discourage night waking and is not recommended (CDC, 2022c). Provide support to parents of newborns and educate them on infant sleeping patterns.

It is important to establish a bedtime routine around 4 months of age due to the infant's increased alertness and activity level. The baby who is 4 months or older needs a time of calming and relaxation before going to sleep. A consistent bedtime routine should be established, perhaps a bath followed by rocking, singing, or reading. The infant should fall asleep in their own crib rather than being rocked to sleep or held until sleeping and then put in the crib. After 4 months of age, infants must learn to soothe themselves back to sleep following night waking. Older infants may exhibit head banging as a form of self-soothing and use it to fall asleep at night. Parents should minimize attention and stimulation provided during a night waking. Briefly checking on the infant to ascertain their safety, followed by placing the infant back in a lying position and telling them good night, is all that is needed. This may have to be repeated several times before the infant falls back to sleep. It is important to keep interactions brief during the night waking so that the infant learns to fall back to sleep on their own. Continued issues with night waking should be discussed with the infant's primary care provider.

Promoting Healthy Teeth and Gums

Healthy teeth and gums require proper oral hygiene and appropriate fluoride supplementation. Early childhood dental caries can result from pooling of milk or juice around teeth and gums. Before tooth eruption, parents should clean the child's gums after feeding with a damp washcloth. After teeth have erupted, parents can continue to use a soft cloth for tooth cleaning and then eventually use a small soft-bristled toothbrush. Toothpaste is unnecessary in infancy.

Infants should not be allowed to take milk or juice bottles to bed, as the high sugar content of the fluid in contact with the teeth all night leads to dental caries. Weaning from the bottle at age 12 to 15 months may help prevent dental caries. No-spill sippy cups have also been implicated in the development of dental caries and should be avoided. The American Academy of Pediatric Dentistry (AAPD) recommends that infants receive their first dental visit by the age of 1 year (2021). Children older than 6 months of age who are at risk for developing dental caries and whose drinking water source is not optimally fluoridated may require fluoride supplementation (AAPD, 2021). Excess fluoride ingestion may result in discoloration of the teeth (fluorosis), so ensure parents understand the dosage.

Promoting Appropriate Discipline

Parenting requires everchanging adaptations to the developing infant's needs. Unconditional love, patience, and compassion must be balanced with the parents' needs. Discipline refers to the molding of a child's behavior through instruction, practice, and consistency. Discipline helps build self-esteem in children as well as sets standards for social interactions. The primary goal of discipline is to teach an infant limits. Discipline should be used to help the infant solve problems. The infant's activities are based on the basic needs of food, security, warmth, love, and comfort. Misbehavior is the result of an unmet need, and the parents should respond accordingly.

As the infant is undergoing rapid changes in motor skills, safety needs increase. Nurses should encourage the parents to "childproof" their home so that the infant can develop physical skills without being at risk. In a childproof home, fewer restrictions need to be placed on the infant's behavior, and the infant can more readily explore.

Physical punishment or spanking should never be used in infancy. Infants are at increased risk for physical injury from spanking and cannot make the connection between the spanking and the undesirable behavior. Providing a safe environment, redirection away from undesirable behaviors, and saying "no" in appropriate instances are far more effective. For example, when the infant is in potential danger (e.g., inserting a key into an electrical outlet, attempting to ingest a poisonous substance, or reaching into the toilet), the parent must use a firm but calm and brisk approach. If the infant knows the parent is serious, adherence will usually come more quickly (AAP, 2018b).

Remaining calm, firm, and consistent is necessary. Immediacy is also an important component of appropriate discipline. The infant cannot make the connection between a subsequent punishment and discussion of behavior with the earlier event itself. Positive reinforcement should be used to support good behavior (AAP, 2018b).

Addressing Child Care Needs

Many parents work outside the home, there are many single-parent families, and many families live a distance away from relatives. In all of these circumstances, infants may need to be cared for outside the home, often in child care settings or home day care centers.

Parents contemplating child care must consider a number of factors. Do they want a sitter to come to their home? Will they use a traditional day care center or a home care situation with fewer children? How much can they afford? If families choose to use a freestanding day care center or a home-based day care center, they should make sure that the provider is appropriately licensed. Parents should feel comfortable with the caregiver-to-child ratio. Are the caregivers trained in infant CPR and first aid? Families may need to visit or interview several facilities before finding one that meets their requirements.

When an older infant is attending a child care situation for the first time, it may be helpful to visit the center once or twice beforehand so that the infant can get used to the caregivers from the comfort and security of the parent's lap. Warn parents that separation anxiety in late infancy can cause a disturbing crying episode when the parent leaves. Reassure parents that the infant will not suffer harm due to the separation.

ADDRESSING COMMON DEVELOPMENTAL CONCERNS

Parents commonly have multiple concerns during normal infant growth and development. Although most of these issues are not actual disease states or behavior problems, nurses must be aware of these issues to recognize them and to intervene appropriately.

Colic

Colic is defined as inconsolable crying that lasts 3 hours or longer per day and for which there is no physical cause. It may begin as early as 2 weeks of age, and healthy infants cry for a total of about 3 hours daily, 3 to 7 days per week. Crying and fussing are more prevalent in the evenings. Typically, colic resolves by 3 months of age, coinciding with the age at which infants are better able to soothe themselves (e.g., by finger sucking). The cause of colic is thought to be problems in the gastrointestinal or neurologic system (probably system immaturity), temperament, or parenting style. Some parents are overly anxious or overly attentive or, at the other extreme, may not give the infant the attention needed. Any of these may contribute to a baby's fussing and crying.

Prolonged crying leads to increased stress among caregivers. Failure to stop the crying leads to frustration, and crying that prevents the parents from sleeping contributes to the exhaustion they are already experiencing. Educate parents that normal crying increases by the time the infant is 6 weeks old and diminishes by about 12 weeks. When faced with a colicky baby, parents should develop a stepwise approach to checking that all of the infant's basic needs are met. When these needs are met, attempts at soothing the infant may be used. Reducing stimulation may decrease the length of crying. Carrying the infant more may also be helpful. Some infants respond to the motion of an infant swing or a car ride. Vibration, white noise, or swaddling may also help to decrease fussing in some infants. Pacifiers can be soothing to babies who need additional nonnutritive sucking. Parents should try one intervention at a time, taking care not to stimulate the infant excessively in the process of searching for solutions. Nurses should provide ongoing support to the parents of a colicky infant and reassure them that this is a temporary condition that will resolve in time (Reynolds et al., 2022).

Spitting Up

Spitting up (regurgitating small amounts of stomach contents) occurs in all infants, and a significant number of infants spit up excessively. Although spitting up after feeding is normal, it can be a cause of great concern to parents. Overfed babies who feed based on a parent-designed schedule and those who burp poorly are more likely to spit up. For some infants, the amount and frequency of spitting up are significant, and those babies should be evaluated by the health care provider or nurse practitioner (AAP, 2019).

Teach parents that feeding smaller amounts on a more frequent basis may help to decrease spitting-up episodes. Always burp the baby at least two or three times per feeding. Keep the baby upright for 30 minutes after feeding, and do not lay the infant prone after feeding. Avoid bouncing or excess activity immediately after feeding. Avoid compressing the stomach after meals with tummy time or positioning in an infant seat (AAP, 2019).

Reassure parents that if the infant is wetting at least six diapers per 24 hours and gaining weight, the spitting up is normal. If the infant vomits one third or more of most feedings, chokes when vomiting, or experiences forceful emesis, the primary care provider should be notified.

Thumb Sucking, Pacifiers, and Security Items

Infants demonstrate a clear need for nonnutritive sucking; even fetuses can be observed sucking their thumbs or fingers in utero. Thumb sucking is a healthy self-comforting activity. Infants who suck their thumbs or pacifiers often are better able to soothe themselves than those who do not. Studies have not shown that sucking either thumbs or pacifiers leads to the need for orthodontic braces unless the sucking continues well beyond the early school-age period. However, pacifier use has been associated with the increased incidence of otitis media (Reynolds et al., 2022). Hygiene is always a concern as pacifiers often fall on the floor. Infants may also become attached to a doll, stuffed animal, or blanket. Just like thumb sucking, the attachment item gives the infant the security to self-soothe when uncomfortable.

Families need to explore their feelings and cultural preferences about sucking habits and security items. Parents should not try to break the habit during a stressful time for the infant. When the infant is intensely trying to master a new skill such as sitting or walking, the infant may need the sucking or security item to self-soothe. Pacifiers and security items can be physically taken away at some point, but the thumb is attached. The infant who has become attached to thumb sucking should not have additional attention drawn to the issue, as that may prolong thumb sucking.

Families of infants who use pacifiers may want to wean the infant from the pacifier when the child approaches 1 year of age, as this is the time when the need for additional sucking naturally decreases. Otherwise, weaning from the pacifier should occur by 18 months of age in order to limit adverse effects upon dentition (AAPD, 2022). Attempts to wean the child from a security blanket or toy should probably be reserved for after infancy.

Teething

Discomfort is common as the tooth breaks through the periodontal membrane. Infants may drool, bite on hard objects, or increase finger sucking. Some infants may become very irritable, refuse to eat, and not sleep well. Fever, vomiting, and diarrhea are generally not considered a sign of teething but rather of illness.

Teething pain results from inflammation. Teach parents that gum massage or application of cold may be soothing to the gums. The parent should rub the inflamed gum with a clean finger for 2 minutes. The infant may chew on a chilled (not frozen) teething ring, or parents can rub an ice cube wrapped in a washcloth on the gums. Occasionally, oral acetaminophen or ibuprofen may be given to relieve pain (Schmitt, 2022b).

TAKE NOTE!

Advise against the use of over-the-counter topical anesthetics containing benzocaine (such as baby Orajel), as they can cause serious side effects, do not work very well, and are not approved for use by the Food and Drug Administration (Schmitt, 2022b).

Refer back to 6-month-old Allison Johnson. List some common developmental concerns of 6-month-old infants. What anticipatory guidance related to these concerns would you provide to her parents?

KEY CONCEPTS

- Infancy encompasses the period from birth to age 12 months.
- The infant exhibits tremendous growth, doubling the birth weight by 6 months of age and tripling it by 12 months of age.
- Most organ systems are immature at birth and develop and mature over the first year of life.
- Child development is orderly, sequential, and predictable, progressing in a cephalocaudal and proximodistal fashion.
- The infant is mastering the psychosocial task of trust versus mistrust.
- Cognitive development in infancy is sensorimotor; infants use their senses and progressing motor skills to master their environments.
- The 12-month-old babbles expressively and uses two or three words with meaning.
- Promotion of safety is of key importance throughout infancy.
- Breastfeeding is the natural and preferred method for infant feeding.
- Breastfed and bottle-fed infants should both be fed on cue rather than on a parent-designed schedule.
- Solid foods should be introduced at age 4 to 6 months. New foods should be introduced no more frequently than every 3 to 5 days.
- The cup may be introduced at 6 months of age. No-spill sippy cups are generally not recommended.
- Spitting up and colic are parts of normal development in the otherwise thriving infant and do not require medical intervention.

REFERENCES AND RECOMMENDED READINGS

American Academy of Pediatrics. (2017). *Safety for your child: Birth to 6 months*. http://www.healthychildren.org/English/tips-tools/Pages/Safety-for-Your-Child-Birth-to-6-Months.aspx

American Academy of Pediatrics. (2018a). *Safety for your child: 6 to 12 months*. http://www.healthychildren.org/English/tips-tools/Pages/Safety-for-Your-Child-6-to-12-Months.aspx

American Academy of Pediatrics. (2018b). *What's the best way to discipline my child?* http://www.healthychildren.org/English/family-life/family-dynamics/communication-discipline/Pages/Disciplining-Your-Child.aspx

American Academy of Pediatrics. (2019). *Swim lessons: When to start & what parents should know*. https://www.healthychildren.org/English/safety-prevention/at-play/Pages/swim-lessons.aspx

American Academy of Pediatrics. (2022). *Baby walkers: A dangerous choice*. https://www.healthychildren.org/English/safety-prevention/at-home/Pages/Baby-Walkers-A-Dangerous-Choice.aspx

American Academy of Pediatrics. (2023). *Formula feeding*. https://www.healthychildren.org/English/ages-stages/baby/formula-feeding/Pages/default.aspx

American Academy of Pediatric Dentistry. (2021). *Perinatal and infant oral health care: Latest revision*. https://www.aapd.org/media/Policies_Guidelines/BP_PerinatalOralHealthCare.pdf

American Academy of Pediatric Dentistry. (2022). *Policy on pacifiers*. https://www.aapd.org/globalassets/media/policies_guidelines/p_pacifiers.pdf

Branchford, B. R., & Levine, D. A. (2023). Section 2: Growth and development. In K. J. Marcdante, R. M. Kliegman, & A. M. Schuh (Eds.), *Nelson's essentials of pediatrics* (9th ed.). Elsevier.

Buchanan, A. O., & Marquez, M. L. (2023). Section 6: Pediatric nutrition and nutritional disorders. In K. J. Marcdante, R. M. Kliegman, & A. M. Schuh (Eds.), *Nelson's essentials of pediatrics* (9th ed.). Elsevier.

Busch, D. W., Silbert-Flagg, J., Ryngaert, M., & Scott, A. (2019). NAPNAP position statement on breastfeeding: National Association of Pediatric Nurse Practitioners, Breastfeeding Education Special Interest Group. *Journal of Pediatric Health Care, 33*(1), A11–A15. https://doi.org/10.1016/j.pedhc.2018.08.011

Centers for Disease Control and Prevention. (2021, September 10). *Cultural competence in health and human services*. https://npin.cdc.gov/pages/cultural-competence#what

Centers for Disease Control and Prevention. (2022a, August 31). *Breastfeeding report card*. https://www.cdc.gov/breastfeeding/data/reportcard.htm

Centers for Disease Control and Prevention. (2022b, December 29). *CDC's developmental milestones.* http://www.cdc.gov/ncbddd/actearly/milestones/index.html

Centers for Disease Control and Prevention. (2022c, May 17). *Infant and toddler nutrition, FAQs.* https://www.cdc.gov/nutrition/InfantandToddlerNutrition/faqs.html

Cherry, J., Harrison, G. J., Kaplan, S. L., Steinbach, W. J., & Hotez, P. (2019). *Feigin and Cherry's textbook of pediatric infectious diseases* (8th ed.). Elsevier.

Child Development Institute. (2019). *Temperament and your child's personality.* https://childdevelopmentinfo.com/uncategorized/temperament_and_your_child/

Duryea, T. K., & Fleisher, D. M. (2022). Patient education: Starting solid foods during infancy (beyond the basics). *UpToDate.* Retrieved September 22, 2022, from https://www.uptodate.com/contents/starting-solid-foods-during-infancy-beyond-the-basics

Erikson, E. H. (1963). *Childhood and society* (2nd ed.). W. W. Norton and Company.

Foong, S. C., Tan, M. L., Foong, W. C., Marasco, L. A., Ho, J. J., & Ong, J. H. (2020). Oral galactagogues (natural therapies or drugs) for increasing breast milk production in mothers of non-hospitalised term infants. *Cochrane Database of Systematic Reviews.* https://doi.org/10.1002/14651858.CD011505.pub2

Greenbaum, L. A., & Londeree, J. T. (2023). Maintenance fluid therapy. In K. J. Marcdante, R. M. Kliegman, & A. M. Schuh (Eds.), *Nelson's essentials of pediatrics* (9th ed.). Elsevier.

Hagan, J. F., Shaw, J. S., & Duncan, P. M. (2017). *Bright futures: Guidelines for health supervision of infants, children, and adolescents* (4th ed.). American Academy of Pediatrics.

Kaiser Permanente. (n.d.). *Bowel movements in babies.* https://healthy.kaiserpermanente.org/health-wellness/health-encyclopedia/he.bowel-movements-in-babies.abo3062

Kleinman, K., McDaniel, L., & Molloy, M. (Eds.). (2021). *The Harriet Lane handbook* (22nd ed.). Elsevier.

La Leche League International. (2023). *Breastfeeding info A to Z.* https://www.llli.org/breastfeeding-info/

Lewis, K. N. (2019). *Reading books to babies.* https://kidshealth.org/en/parents/reading-babies.html

Linguistic Society of America. (2023). *FAQ: Raising bilingual children.* https://www.linguisticsociety.org/resource/faq-raising-bilingual-children

Maqbool, A., & Liacouras, C. A. (2020). Normal development, structure, and function of the stomach and intestines. In R. M. Kliegman, J. W. St Geme, N. J. Blum, S. S. Shah, R. C. Tasker, & K. M. Wilson, *Nelson textbook of pediatrics* (21st ed.). Elsevier.

McCarthy, C. (2020). *Peanut allergies: What you should know about the latest research & guidelines.* https://www.healthychildren.org/English/health-issues/conditions/allergies-asthma/Pages/Peanut-Allergies-What-You-Should-Know-About-the-Latest-Research.aspx

Moon, R. Y., Carlin, R. F., Hand, I., & the Task Force on Sudden Infant Death Syndrome and the Committee on Fetus and Newborn. (2022). Sleep-related infant deaths: Updated 2022 recommendations for reducing infant deaths in the sleep environment. *Pediatrics, 150*(1), e2022057990. https://doi.org/10.1542/peds.2022-057990

National Association for the Education of Young Children. (n.d.). *Good toys for young children by age and stage.* http://www.naeyc.org/toys

Nuss, R., McKinney, C., & Wang, M. (2022). Hematologic disorders. In M. Bunik, W. W. Hay, M. J. Levin, & M. J. Abzug (Eds.), *Current diagnosis & treatment: Pediatrics* (26th ed.). McGraw-Hill.

Olsson, J. (2020). The newborn. In R. M. Kliegman, J. W. St Geme, N. J. Blum, S. S. Shah, R. C. Tasker, & K. M. Wilson (Eds.), *Nelson textbook of pediatrics* (21st ed.). Elsevier.

Piaget, J. (1969). *The theory of stages in cognitive development.* McGraw-Hill.

Powers, J. M. (2021). Iron deficiency in infants and children <12 years: Screening, prevention, clinical manifestations, and diagnosis. *UpToDate.* Retrieved September 21, 2022, from https://www.uptodate.com/contents/iron-deficiency-in-infants-and-children-less-than12-years-screening-prevention-clinical-manifestations-and-diagnosis

Reynolds, A., Angulo, A., Breheney, M., Green, J., & Goldson, E. (2022). Child development and behavior. In M. Bunik, W. W. Hay, M. J. Levin, & M. J. Abzug (Eds.), *Current diagnosis & treatment: Pediatrics* (26th ed.). McGraw-Hill Education.

Safe Kids Worldwide. (2023). *Baby sleep safety and suffocation prevention.* https://www.safekids.org/safetytips/field_age/babies-0–12-months/field_risks/sleep-safety

Schmitt, B. (2022a). Solid foods (baby foods). Schmitt Pediatric Guidelines LLC. https://doi.org/10.1542/ppe_schmitt_222

Schmitt, B. (2022b). Teething. Schmitt Pediatric Guidelines LLC. https://doi.org/10.1542/ppe_schmitt_235

Sinha, S. K. (2021). *Short stature.* http://emedicine.medscape.com/article/924411-overview

Smola, C., Sorrentino, A., Shah, N., Nichols, M., & Monroe, K. (2020). Child passenger safety education in the emergency department: Teen driving, car seats, booster seats, and more. *Injury Epidemiology, 7*(Suppl. 1), 26. https://doi.org/10.1186/s40621-020-00250-5

U.S. Department of Health and Human Services. (n.d.). *Healthy People 2030.* https://health.gov/healthypeople

Zubler, J. M., Wiggins, L. D., Macias, M. M., Whitaker, T. M., Shaw, J. S., Squires, J. K., Pajke, J. A., Wolf, R. B., Slaughter, K. S., Broughton, A. S., Gerndt, K. L., Mlodoch, B. J., & Lipkin, P. H. (2022). Evidence-informed milestones for developmental surveillance tools. *Pediatrics, 149*(3), e2021052138. https://doi.org/10.1542/peds.2021-052138

DEVELOPING CLINICAL JUDGMENT

PRACTICING FOR NCLEX

1. The parent of a 3-month-old infant asks the nurse about starting solid foods. What is the most appropriate response by the nurse?
  a. "It's okay to start puréed solids at this age if fed via the bottle."
  b. "Infants don't require solid food until 12 months of age."
  c. "Solid foods should be delayed until age 6 months, when the infant can handle a spoon on their own."
  d. "The tongue extrusion reflex disappears at age 4 to 6 months, making it a good time to start solid foods."

2. The parent of a 2-month-old infant is expressing concern that the infant may be getting spoiled. What is the nurse's best response?
  a. "The baby just needs love and attention. Don't worry; the baby's too young to spoil."
  b. "Consistently meeting the infant's needs helps promote a sense of trust."
  c. "Infants need to be fed and cleaned; if you are sure those needs are met, just let your baby cry."
  d. "Consistency in meeting needs is important, but you are right, holding the infant too much will spoil the baby."

3. Parents of an 8-month-old infant express concern that the infant cries when left with the babysitter. How does the nurse best explain this behavior?
  a. "Crying when left with the sitter may indicate difficulty with building trust."
  b. "Stranger anxiety should not occur until toddlerhood; this concern should be investigated."
  c. "Separation anxiety is normal at this age; the infant recognizes parents as separate beings."
  d. "Perhaps the sitter doesn't meet the infant's needs; choose a different sitter."

4. The nurse is providing anticipatory guidance to the parent of a 6-month-old infant. What is the best instruction by the nurse in relation to the infant's oral health?
  a. "Start brushing the teeth after all the baby teeth come in."
  b. "Use a washcloth with toothpaste to clean the mouth."
  c. "Clean your baby's gums, then new teeth, with a washcloth."
  d. "Rinse your baby's mouth with water after every feeding."

5. A 9-month-old infant's parent is questioning why cow's milk is not recommended in the first year of life as it is much cheaper than formula. What rationale does the nurse include in the response?
  a. It is permissible to substitute cow's milk for formula at this age as the infant is so close to 1 year old.
  b. Cow's milk is poor in iron and does not provide the proper balance of nutrients for the infant.
  c. As long as the parent provides whole milk, rather than skim, they can start cow's milk in infancy.
  d. If the parent cannot afford the infant formula, they should dilute it to make it last longer.

6. Parents report to the nurse that their young infant breastfeeds and sleeps well on their abdomen on a soft mattress, with a light blanket covering them. The nurse determines the infant is at risk for ____ related to _____ and ______.
  Blank 1:
  a. Shaken baby syndrome (SBS)
  b. Sudden infant death syndrome (SIDS)
  c. Gastroesophageal reflux disease (GERD)
  Blanks 2 and 3:
  a. Prone sleeping
  b. Supine sleeping
  c. Soft crib mattress
  d. Breastfeeding

7. A 12-month-old infant was born full-term without any difficulties. The infant weighed 8 lb at birth. Which assessment findings would the nurse expect for this infant? (Select four items.)
  a. Current weight is 24 lb.
  b. Anterior fontanel is closed.
  c. Posterior fontanel is slightly open.
  d. The infant is now walking.
  e. The infant tries to build a two-block tower.
  f. The infant says 10 words with meaning.

CRITICAL THINKING EXERCISES

1. The parent of an 11-month-old infant who was born at 24 weeks' gestation is concerned about the infant's size and motor skills. What information should the nurse provide?

2. An infant's parent thinks there may be something wrong because "he spits up so much." What further information should the nurse obtain?

3. If you determine that the infant in the preceding question is experiencing normal spitting up associated with his developmental age, develop a brief teaching plan to review with the parent.

STUDY ACTIVITIES

1. Parents bring their 9-month-old infant to the clinic for a well-child check-up. They have questions about feeding, speech, and walking. Develop a teaching plan of anticipatory guidance for the 9-month-old infant.
2. Develop a home and car safety plan for the 12-month-old infant.
3. In the clinical setting, observe two infants of the same age, one who is developing appropriately for their age and one who is experiencing delays. Note the similarities and differences between the two infants.

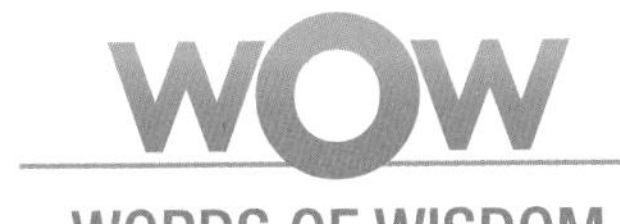

WORDS OF WISDOM

Toddlers will take risks and make many mistakes; nurses can help parents remember that both are an essential part of their growth.

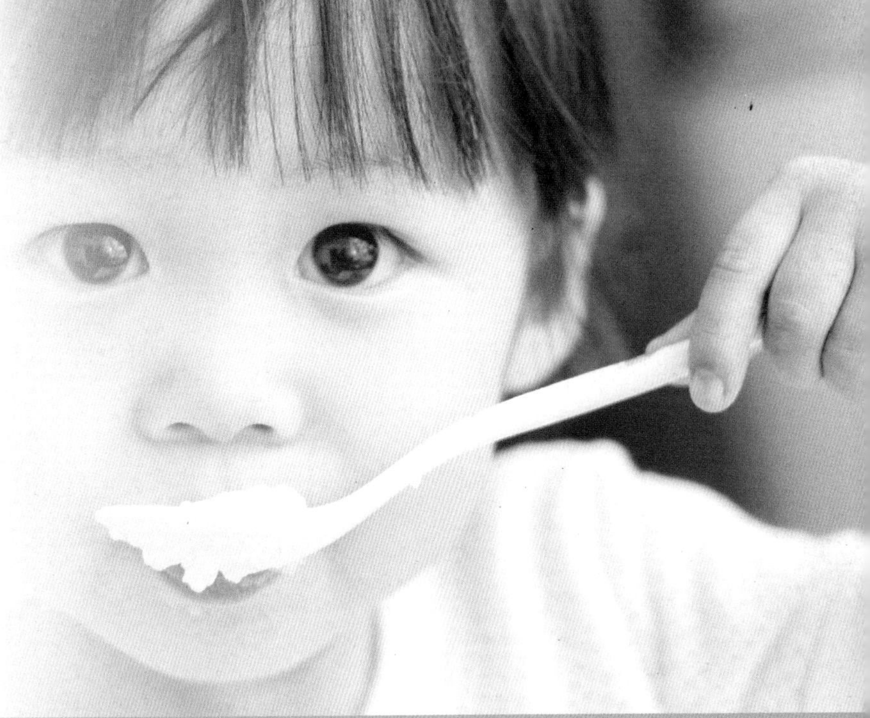

4

Growth and Development of the Toddler

KEY TERMS

animism (an´i-mizm)
echolalia (ek´ō-lā´lē-ă)
egocentrism (ē´gō-sen´trizm)
expressive language
food jag
individuation (in´di-vij´yū-ā´shŭn)
negativism
parallel play
physiologic anorexia (fiz´ē-ō-loj´ik an´ō-rek´sē-ă)
receptive language
regression
separation
separation anxiety
sibling rivalry
telegraphic speech

LEARNING OBJECTIVES

Upon completion of the chapter, you will be able to:

1. Describe normal physical growth, physiologic changes, and sensory development in the toddler.
2. Examine psychosocial, cognitive, social/emotional, and moral/spiritual development in the toddler.
3. Identify the gross and fine motor milestones of the toddler.
4. Explain normal language development in toddlerhood.
5. Implement a nursing care plan to address common issues or delays related to growth and development in toddlerhood.
6. Develop a teaching plan for safety promotion in the toddler period.
7. Examine common issues related to growth and development in toddlerhood.
8. Develop a nutritional plan for the toddler based on average nutritional requirements.
9. Consider appropriate methods of discipline for use during the toddler years.
10. Provide appropriate anticipatory guidance for common developmental issues that arise in the toddler period.

Jose Gonzales is a 2-year-old brought to the clinic by his parents for his 2-year-old check-up. As the nurse caring for him, assess Jose's growth and development, and then teach the parents what changes to expect in Jose over the next few months.

INTRODUCTION

The toddler period encompasses the second 2 years of life, from age 1 year to age 3 years. This period is a time of significant advancement in growth and development for the child. It can also be quite a challenging time for parents. The theme during the toddler years is one of holding on and letting go. Having learned that parents are predictable and reliable, the toddler is now learning that their behavior has a predictable, reliable effect on others. The challenge is to encourage independence and autonomy while keeping the curious toddler safe.

TAKE NOTE!

As more grandparents are assuming the primary caregiver role for their grandchildren, nurses should be alert to the possibility of increased stress that is placed upon the older caregiver, particularly during the active and sometimes trying years of toddlerhood (Smith & Segal, 2023).

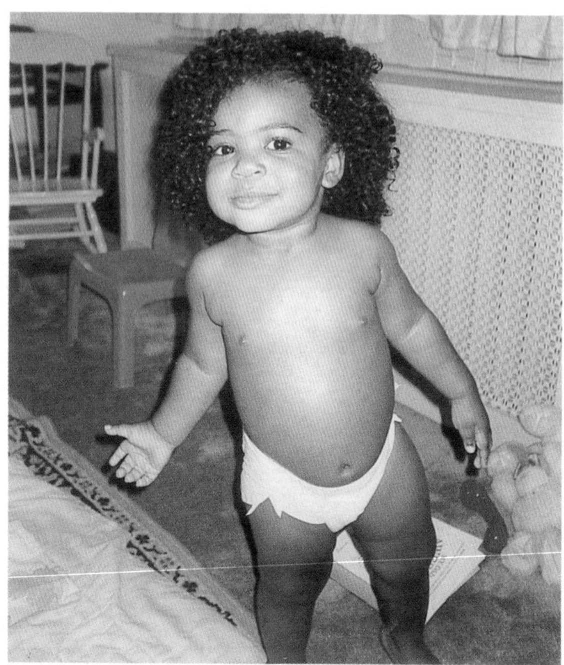

FIGURE 4.1 The typical toddler appearance is that of a rounded abdomen, a slight swayback, and a wide-based stance.

GROWTH AND DEVELOPMENT OVERVIEW

Infancy is a time of intense growth and development. Both physical growth and acquisition of new motor skills slow somewhat during the toddler years. Refinement of motor skills, continued cognitive growth, and acquisition of appropriate language skills are of prime importance during toddlerhood. The nurse uses the knowledge of normal toddler development as a roadmap for assessment of the 1- to 3-year-old child.

PHYSICAL GROWTH

The toddler's height and weight continue to increase steadily, although the increase occurs at a slower velocity compared to infancy. Toddler gains in height and weight tend to occur in spurts, rather than in a linear fashion (Fig. 4.1). The average toddler weight gain is 1.36 to 2.27 kg (3 to 5 lb) per year. Length/height increases by an average of 7.62 cm (3 in) per year. Toddlers generally reach about half of their adult height by 2 years of age. Head circumference increases about 2.54 cm (1 in) from age 1 to 2 years, then increases an average of 1.27 cm (0.5 in) per year until age 5. The anterior fontanel should be closed by the time the child is 18 months old. Head size becomes more proportional to the rest of the body near the age of 3 years (Carter & Feigelman, 2020a, 2020b; Reynolds et al., 2022).

Remember Jose Gonzales, introduced at the beginning of the chapter? During your assessment, you find that his weight is 13.6 kg (30 lb), height 83.82 cm (33 in), and head circumference 49.53 cm (19.5 in).

PHYSIOLOGIC CHANGES

Although not as pronounced as the changes occurring during infancy, the toddler's organ systems continue to grow and mature in their functioning. Significant functional changes occur within the neurologic, gastrointestinal, and genitourinary systems. The respiratory and cardiovascular systems undergo changes as well.

Neurologic System

Brain growth continues through toddlerhood, and head circumference (reflective of brain growth) reaches about 90% of its adult size by 2 years of age (Carter & Feigelman, 2020b). Myelination of the brain and spinal cord continues to progress and is complete around 24 months of age. Myelination results in improved coordination and equilibrium as well as the ability to exercise sphincter control, which is important for bowel and bladder mastery. Integration of the primitive reflexes occurs in infancy, allowing for the emergence of the protective reflexes near the end of infancy or early in toddlerhood. The forward or downward parachute reflex is particularly helpful when the child starts to toddle. Rapid increase in language skills is evidence of continued progression of cognitive development.

Respiratory System

The respiratory structures continue to grow and mature throughout toddlerhood. The alveoli continue to increase in number, not reaching the adult number until about

7 years of age. The trachea and lower airways continue to grow but remain small compared with the adult. The tongue is relatively large in comparison to the size of the mouth. Tonsils and adenoids are large, and the eustachian tubes are relatively short and straight.

Cardiovascular System

The heart rate decreases, and blood pressure increases in toddlerhood. Blood vessels are close to the skin surface and so are compressed easily when palpated.

Gastrointestinal System

The stomach continues to increase in size, allowing the toddler to consume three regular meals per day. Pepsin production matures by 2 years of age. The small intestine continues to grow in length, although it does not reach the maximum length of 2 to 3 m until adulthood. Stool passage decreases in frequency to one or more per day. The color of the stool may change (yellow, orange, brown, or green) depending on the toddler's diet. Since the toddler's intestines remain somewhat immature, the toddler often passes whole pieces of difficult-to-digest food such as corn kernels. Bowel control is generally achieved by the end of the toddler period.

Genitourinary System

Bladder and kidney function reach adult levels by 16 to 24 months of age. The bladder capacity increases, allowing the toddler to retain urine for longer periods. Urine output should be about 1 mL/kg/hour. The urethra remains short in both the male and the female toddler, making them more susceptible to urinary tract infections compared to adults.

Musculoskeletal System

During toddlerhood, the bones increase in length, and the muscles mature and become stronger. The abdominal musculature is weak in early toddlerhood, resulting in a pot-bellied appearance. The toddler appears to have a swayback along with the potbelly. Around 3 years of age, the musculature strengthens, and the abdomen is flatter in appearance.

PSYCHOSOCIAL DEVELOPMENT

Erikson defines the toddlerhood period as a time of autonomy versus shame and doubt. It is a time of asserting independence. Since the toddler developed a sense of trust in infancy, they are ready to give up dependence and to assert their sense of control and autonomy (Erikson, 1963). The toddler is struggling for self-mastery, to learn to do for themselves what others have been doing for them. Toddlers often experience ambivalence about the move from dependence to autonomy, resulting in emotional lability. The toddler may quickly change from happy and pleasant to crying and screaming. Assertion of independence also results in the toddler's favorite response, "no." The toddler will often answer "no" even when they really mean "yes." This **negativism**—always saying "no"—is a normal part of healthy development and is occurring as a result of the toddler's attempt to assert their independence. Table 4.1 gives further information related to developing a sense of autonomy.

COGNITIVE DEVELOPMENT

According to Jean Piaget (1969), toddlers move through the last two substages of the first stage of cognitive development, the sensorimotor stage, between 12 and 24 months of age. Young toddlers engage in tertiary circular reactions and progress to mental combinations. Rather than just repeating a behavior, the toddler is able to experiment with a behavior to see what happens. By 2 years of age, toddlers are capable of using symbols to allow for imitation. With increasing cognitive abilities, toddlers may now engage in delayed imitation. For example, they may imitate a household task that they observed a parent doing several days ago.

Piaget identified the second stage of cognitive development as the preoperational stage. It occurs in children between ages 2 and 7 years. During this stage, toddlers begin to become more sophisticated with symbolic thought. The thinking of the older toddler is far more advanced than that of the infant or young toddler, who views the world as a series of objects. During the preoperational stage, objects begin to have characteristics that make them unique from one another. Objects are considered large or small, having a particular color or shape, or having a unique texture. This moves beyond the connection of sensory information and physical action. Words and images allow the toddler to begin this process of developing symbolic thought by providing a label for the objects' characteristics (Piaget, 1969).

Toddlers also use symbols in dramatic play. First, they imitate life with appropriate toy objects, and then they are able to substitute objects in their play. A bowl may be used to pretend to eat from, but then later it can be used upside down on the head as a hat (Fig. 4.2). Human feelings and characteristics may also be attributed to objects (**animism**) (Martorell, 2022). See Table 4.1 for further explanation of cognitive development in toddlerhood.

TAKE NOTE!

Birthing parents who are depressed may not be as sensitive to their children as those who are not depressed. For this reason, maternal depression is a risk factor for poor cognitive development. Be alert to the mental status of a toddler's birthing parent so that appropriate referrals can be made if needed (Viguera, 2023).

TABLE 4.1 • Developmental Theories

Theorist	Stage	Activities
Erikson	Autonomy vs. shame and doubt Age: 1–3 years	Achieves autonomy and self-control Separates from parent/caregiver Withstands delayed gratification Negativism abounds. Imitates adults and playmates Spontaneously shows affection Is increasingly enthusiastic about playmates Cannot take turns in games until age 3 years
Piaget	Sensorimotor Substage 5: tertiary circular reactions Age: 12–18 months Substage 6: Mental combinations Age: 18–24 months Preoperational Age: 2–7 years	Differentiates self from objects Increased object permanence (knows that objects that are out of sight still exist [e.g., cookies in the cabinet]) Uses ALL senses to explore environment Places items in and out of containers Imitates domestic chores (domestic mimicry) Imitation is more symbolic. Starting to think before acting Understands requests and is capable of following simple directions Has a sense of ownership (my, mine) Time, space, and causality understanding is increasing. Uses mental trial and error rather than physical Makes mechanical toys work Plays make-believe with dolls, animals, and people Increased use of language for mental representation Understands concept of "two" Starting to make connections between an experience in the past and a new one that is currently occurring Sorts objects by shape and color Completes puzzles with four pieces Play becomes more complex.
Freud	Anal stage Age: 1–3 years	Focus is on achieving anal sphincter control. Satisfaction and/or frustration may occur as the toddler learns to withhold and expel stool.

Data from Erikson, E. H. (1963). *Childhood and society* (2nd ed.). W.W. Norton and Company; Reynolds, A., Angulo, A., Breheney, M., Green, J., & Goldson, E. (2022). Child development and behavior. In M. Bunik, W. W. Hay, M. J. Levin, & M. J. Abzug (Eds.), *Current diagnosis & treatment: Pediatrics* (26th ed.). McGraw-Hill Education; Piaget, J. (1969). *The theory of stages in cognitive development.* McGraw-Hill.

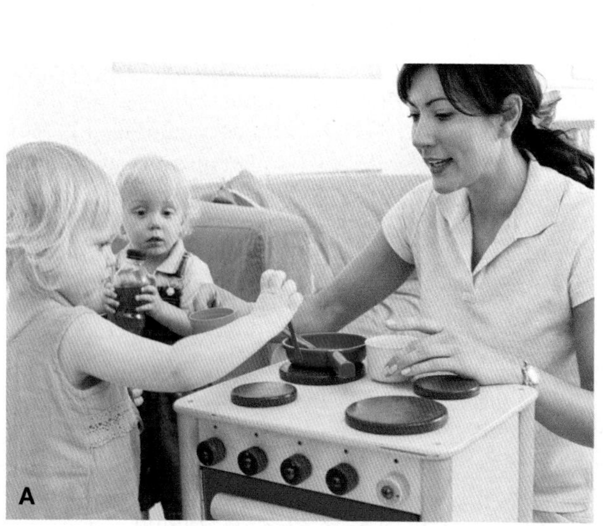

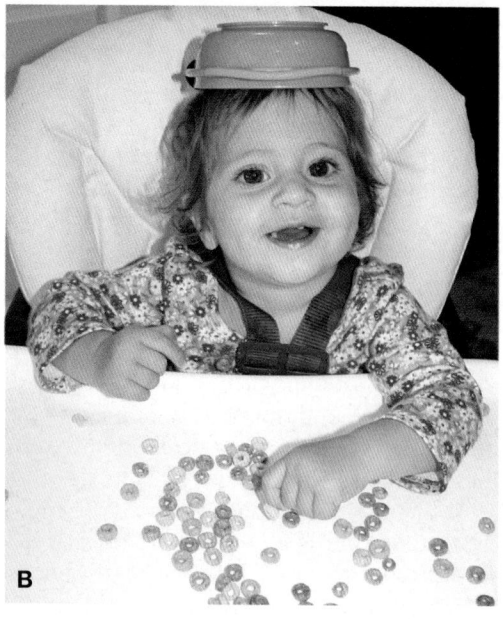

FIGURE 4.2 The toddler will pretend with items in the way they are intended to be used (**A**) as well as find other creative uses for them (**B**).

MOTOR SKILL DEVELOPMENT

Toddlers continue to gain new motor skills as well as refine others. Walking progresses to running, climbing, and jumping. Pushing or pulling a toy, throwing a ball, and pedaling a tricycle are accomplished in toddlerhood. Fine motor skills progress from holding and pinching to the ability to manage utensils, hold a crayon, string a bead, and use a computer. Development of eye–hand coordination is necessary for the refinement of fine motor skills. These increased abilities of mobility and manipulation help the curious toddler explore and learn more about their environment (Fig. 4.3). As the toddler masters a new task, they have confidence to conquer the next challenge. Thus, mastery in motor skill development contributes to the toddler's growing sense of self-esteem. The toddler who is eager to face challenges will likely develop more quickly than one who is reluctant. The senses of sight, hearing, and touch are useful in helping to coordinate gross and fine motor movement.

Gross Motor Skills

As gross motor skills are mastered and then used repeatedly, the large muscle groups in the toddler are strengthened. The "toddler gait" is characteristic of new walkers. The toddler does not walk smoothly and maturely. Instead, the legs are planted widely apart, toes are pointed forward, and the toddler seems to sway from side to side while moving forward (Fig. 4.4). Often, the toddler seems to speed along, be pitching forward, and may appear ready to topple over at any moment. The toddler may fall often but will use outstretched arms to catch themselves (parachute reflex). After about 6 months of practice walking, the toddler's gait is smoother, and the feet are closer together. By 3 years of age, the toddler walks in a heel-to-toe fashion similar to that of adults. Toddlers often use physical actions such as running, jumping, and hitting to express their emotions because they are only just learning to express their thoughts and feelings verbally. Table 4.2 lists motor skill expectations in relation to age.

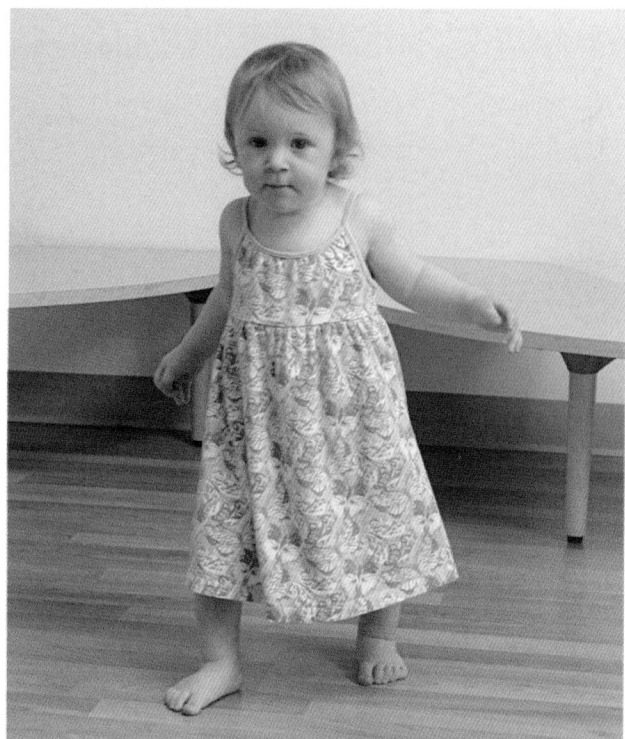

FIGURE 4.4 The young toddler (early walker) walks with a wide-based stance, feet pointing forward, and arms akimbo.

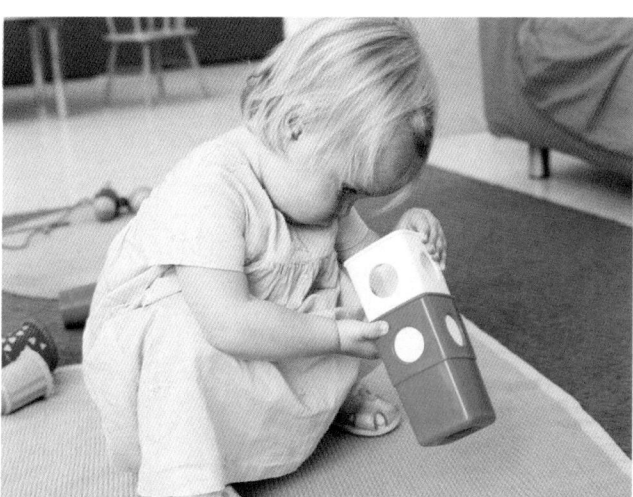

FIGURE 4.3 The toddler's curiosity about the world increases, as does their ability to explore it.

Fine Motor Skills

Fine motor skills in the toddler period are improved and perfected. Holding utensils requires some control and agility, but even more is needed for buttoning and zipping. Adequate vision is necessary for the refinement of fine motor skills because eye–hand coordination is crucial for directing the fingers, hand, and wrist to accomplish small muscle tasks such as fitting a puzzle piece or stringing a bead. See Table 4.2 for age expectations for various motor skills.

SENSORY DEVELOPMENT

Toddlers use all of their senses to explore the world around them. Toddlers examine new items by feeling them, looking at them, shaking them to hear what sound they make, smelling them, and placing them in their mouths. Toddler vision continues to progress and should be 20/50 to 20/40 in both eyes. Depth perception

TABLE 4.2 • Motor Skill Development

Age (months)	Expected Gross Motor Skill	Expected Fine Motor Skills
15	Takes few steps on own	Feeds self finger foods
18	Walks independently Climbs on/off furniture Climbs stairs with assistance Seats self in chair	Scribbles Tries to use a spoon Throws a ball Stacks three to four cubes
24	Runs Kicks ball Walks upstairs with assistance (not climbing) Kicks a ball	Eats with a spoon Stacks six to seven cubes Points to named pictures and objects Starting to turn knobs
30	Jumps with both feet	Turns knobs Turns book page one at a time Takes off some clothing items
36	Puts on some clothes by self	Strings items together Uses a fork Puts on some clothes by self Copies circle

Data from Carter, R. G., & Feigelman, S. (2020a). The preschool years. In R. M. Kliegman, J. W. St. Geme III, N. J. Blum, S. S. Shah, R. C. Tasker, K. M. Wilson, & R. E. Behrman (Eds.), *Nelson's textbook of pediatrics* (21st ed.). Elsevier; Carter, R. G., & Feigelman, S. (2020b). The second year. In R. M. Kliegman, J. W. St. Geme III, N. J. Blum, S. S. Shah, R. C. Tasker, K. M. Wilson, & R. E. Behrman (Eds.), *Nelson's textbook of pediatrics* (21st ed.). Elsevier; Reynolds, A., Angulo, A., Breheney, M., Green, J., & Goldson, E. (2022). Child development and behavior. In M. Bunik, W. W. Hay, M. J. Levin, & M. J. Abzug (Eds.), *Current diagnosis & treatment: Pediatrics* (26th ed.). McGraw-Hill Education; Zubler, J. M., Wiggins, L. D., Macias, M. M., Whitaker, T. M., Shaw, J. S., Squires, J. K., Pajke, J. A., Wolf, R. B., Slaughter, K. S., Broughton, A. S., Gerndt, K. L., Mlodoch, B. J., & Lipkin, P. H. (2022). Evidence-informed milestones for developmental surveillance tools. *Pediatrics, 149*(3), e2021052138. https://doi.org/10.1542/peds.2021-052138

also continues to mature. Hearing should be at the adult level, as infants are ordinarily born with hearing intact. The sense of smell continues to mature, and toddlers may comment if they do not care for the scent of something. Although taste discrimination is not completely developed, toddlers may exhibit preferences for certain flavors of foods. The toddler is more likely to try a new food if its appearance or smell is familiar. Lack of complete taste discrimination places the toddler at risk for inadvertent ingestion.

COMMUNICATION AND LANGUAGE DEVELOPMENT

Language development occurs rapidly during the toddler years. The acquisition of language is a dynamic and complex process. The child's age and social interactions and the types of language to which they have been exposed influence language development. **Receptive language** development (the ability to understand what is being said or asked) is typically far more advanced than **expressive language** development (the ability to communicate one's desires and feelings) (Carter & Feigelman, 2020b; Reynolds et al., 2022). In other words, the toddler understands language and is able to follow commands far sooner than they can actually use the words themselves. Language is a very important part of the toddler's ability to organize their world and actually make sense of it. Thoughtfully planned use of language can provide behavior guidance and contribute to the avoidance of power struggles. In regard to expressive language development, the young toddler begins to use short sentences and will progress to a vocabulary of 50 words by 2 years of age (Carter & Feigelman, 2020b; Reynolds et al., 2022). **Echolalia** (repetition of words and phrases without understanding) normally occurs in toddlers younger than 30 months of age. "Why" and "what" questions dominate the older toddler's language. Telegraphic speech is common in the 3-year-old. **Telegraphic speech** refers to speech that contains only the essential words to get the point across, much like a telegram. Rather than "I want a cookie and milk," the toddler might say, "Want cookie milk." In telegraphic speech, the nouns and verbs are present and are verbalized in the appropriate order (Carter & Feigelman, 2020b). Table 4.3 gives an overview of receptive and expressive language development in the toddler.

Early identification and referral of children with potential speech delays is critical. If a delay is identified, early intervention may increase the child's potential to acquire age-appropriate receptive and expressive language skills. Children with preexisting conditions

TABLE 4.3 • Language Development in Toddlers

Age (months)	Receptive Language	Expressive Language
12	Understands the word "no"	Imitates or uses gestures such as waving goodbye
15	Follows a command accompanied by a gesture	Uses a finger to point to things Looks for a familiar object when named Tries to say one to two words other than "dada" and "mama"
18	Follows a one-step command without gesture	Tries to say three or more words other than "dada" and "mama"
24	Points to named body parts Points to pictures in books	Sentences of two words ("me up," "want cookie") Uses gestures like blowing a kiss or nodding yes
30	Follows a series of two independent commands Names items when pointed to and asks, "what's this?"	Vocabulary of approximately 50 words Sentences of two words with an action word ("cat run")
36	Uses at least two back-and-forth exchanges when conversing Understands physical relationships (on, in, under)	Most outside the family understand speech. Asks "why," "where," and "what?" Verbalizes actions happening in a picture Says first name when asked

Data from Carter, R. G., & Feigelman, S. (2020a). The preschool years. In R. M. Kliegman, J. W. St. Geme III, N. J. Blum, S. S. Shah, R. C. Tasker, K. M. Wilson, & R. E. Behrman (Eds.), *Nelson's textbook of pediatrics* (21st ed.). Elsevier; Carter, R. G., & Feigelman, S. (2020b). The second year. In R. M. Kliegman, J. W. St. Geme III, N. J. Blum, S. S. Shah, R. C. Tasker, K. M. Wilson, & R. E. Behrman (Eds.), *Nelson's textbook of pediatrics* (21st ed.). Elsevier; Reynolds, A., Angulo, A., Breheney, M., Green, J., & Goldson, E. (2022). Child development and behavior. In M. Bunik, W. W. Hay, M. J. Levin, & M. J. Abzug (Eds.), *Current diagnosis & treatment: Pediatrics* (26th ed.). McGraw-Hill Education; Zubler, J. M., Wiggins, L. D., Macias, M. M., Whitaker, T. M., Shaw, J. S., Squires, J. K., Pajke, J. A., Wolf, R. B., Slaughter, K. S., Broughton, A. S., Gerndt, K. L., Mlodoch, B. J., & Lipkin, P. H. (2022). Evidence-informed milestones for developmental surveillance tools. *Pediatrics, 149*(3), e2021052138. https://doi.org/10.1542/peds.2021-052138.

such as genetic syndromes that are known to have an effect on language development should be referred to a speech–language pathologist as soon as the condition is recognized rather than waiting until the child exhibits a delay.

Of special concern in the toddler years is the development of speech and language in potentially bilingual children. At the age of 1 to 2 years, the potentially bilingual child may blend two languages—that is, parts of the word in both languages are blended into one word. At age 2 to 3 years, the potentially bilingual toddler may mix languages within a sentence. Thus, the assessment of adequate language development is more complicated in bilingual children. There are websites that may be helpful to parents of potentially bilingual children, where they can find support and resources.

TAKE NOTE!

Young children exposed to more than one language may experience simultaneous acquisition of both languages. The first word may be slightly delayed as compared with single language speakers, but still occurs within the normal range (Linguistic Society of America, 2023).

As you assess Jose (the 2-year-old introduced at the beginning of the chapter), what would you expect his gross motor, fine motor, and language skills to be at this age? How would this be different if Jose had been born 12 weeks premature?

EMOTIONAL AND SOCIAL DEVELOPMENT

Emotional development in the toddler years is focused on separation and individuation (Martorell, 2022). Seeing oneself as separate from the parent or primary caregiver (**separation**) is accompanied by forming a sense of self and learning to exert control over one's environment (**individuation**). As this need to feel in control of their world emerges, the toddler displays **egocentrism** (focus on self). This need for control results in emotional lability: happy and pleasant one moment, then overreacting to limit setting with a temper tantrum in the next moment (Lieberman, 2018). As toddlers identify the boundaries between themselves and the parent or primary caregiver, they learn to negotiate a balance between attachment and independence. Toddlers initially rely on the parents' communication and signals in order to initiate appropriate behavior or inhibit undesirable behavior. They have a difficult time choosing between sets of behaviors as

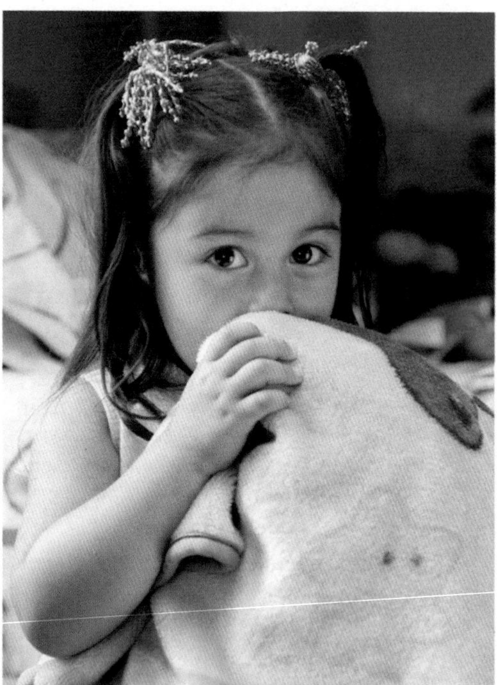

FIGURE 4.5 The toddler may be able to self-soothe and produce a sense of comfort during this stage of establishing autonomy by relying on a security item, such as a doll, bear, or blanket.

they occur in different situations. Power struggles often occur in this age group, and it is important for parents and caregivers to thoughtfully and intentionally develop the rituals and routines that will provide stability and security for the toddler (Carter & Feigelman, 2020b). Many toddlers rely on a security item (blanket, doll, or bear) to comfort themselves in stressful situations (Fig. 4.5). This ability to self-soothe is a function of autonomy and is viewed as a sign of a nurturing environment, rather than, as one might suspect, one of neglect.

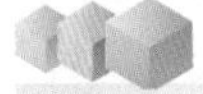 *Concept Mastery Alert*

When teaching parents interventions appropriate to the emotional development of their toddler, nurses can teach parents that they may offer a toddler limited choices (usually two are sufficient) to assist with control over their environment. Nurses should advise parents that aggressive behavior is normal in the toddler period, so parents should not blame toddlers for the behavior but should help toddlers understand the results of their behavior.

Children also begin to learn about sex and gender differences in the toddler years. They observe the differences between male and female body parts if they are exposed to them. Toddlers may question parents about these differences and may begin to explore their own genitals. Toddlers also begin to understand and mimic social gender differences. They make observations about gender-specific behavior dependent on what they are exposed to.

Aggressive behaviors are typically displayed during the toddler years. Toddlers may hit, bite, or push other children and grab toys. Adults can assist the toddler in building empathy by pointing out when someone is hurt and explaining what happened. Toddlers should not be blamed for their impulsive behavior; rather, they should be guided toward socially acceptable actions in order to foster development of appropriate social judgment. It is particularly important for the parent or caregiver to serve as a role model for appropriate behavior, rather than losing their own temper, in order for the toddler to be able to learn how to acceptably handle frustrations. Offering limited choices is one way of allowing toddlers some control over their environment and helping them to establish a sense of mastery. Since toddlers naturally have a short attention span, they tend to dawdle. As the toddlers become more self-aware, they start to develop emotions of self-consciousness such as embarrassment and shame.

Although toddlers are becoming more self-aware, they still do not have clear body boundaries. They do not clearly understand the body's functions, although they are beginning to make appropriate connections. Feces may be viewed as a part of the child, and the toddler may become upset at seeing it disappear in the toilet. The toddler will protect their body by resisting intrusive procedures such as temperature or blood pressure measurement.

Separation Anxiety

As toddlers become increasingly skilled at mobility, they realize that if they have the capability to leave, then so does the parent. As self-awareness develops and conflicts over closeness versus exploration occur, **separation anxiety** may reemerge in the 18- to 24-month period (Lieberman, 2018). Power struggles may escalate, and distress at separating from the parent may increase. Again, a predictable routine with appropriate limit setting may help toddlers to feel safer and more secure during this period. From the age of 24 to 36 months, separation anxiety again eases. The older toddler begins to have a concept of object constancy: they have an internal representation of the parent or caregiver and are better able to tolerate separation, knowing that a reunion will occur.

Temperament

Temperament is the biologic basis for personality. It is our emotional and motivational core, around which the personality develops over time (Child Development Institute, 2022). Temperament affects how the toddler interacts with the environment. The easygoing toddler may adapt more easily and not mind changes in routine as much as other toddlers. The easygoing toddler usually sleeps and eats well and has more predictable and regular behaviors. However, the toddler may still express frustration by having a temper tantrum. The challenging toddler is more likely to have intense reactions, negative or positive, with temper tantrums being more likely, more frequent, and more intense than in other toddlers. The structure and routine that toddlers need to feel secure are essential for this toddler; otherwise, the child feels insecure and, as a result, is more likely to behave inappropriately. The challenging toddler is also the most active of the three temperament types. The slow-to-warm-up toddler is more of a loner and may be very shy. They may experience more difficulty with separation anxiety. The behavior of the slow-to-warm-up toddler is more passive; the toddler may be watchful and withdrawn and may take longer to mature. Changes in routine usually do not result in as much upset, since the toddler's natural reaction is one of passivity (Lieberman, 2018).

Based on the toddler's temperament, make suggestions to the parents for interacting with the toddler in various situations. For example, to avoid temper tantrums in the challenging toddler, suggest that the parent should be especially diligent about maintaining structure and routine as well as avoiding tantrum triggers such as fatigue and hunger. Explain to parents that they may need to exercise additional patience with new activities to which the slow-to-warm-up toddler may need extra time becoming accustomed.

Fears

Common fears of toddlers include loss of parents (which contributes to separation anxiety) and fear of strangers. Some toddlers may be slow to warm up to people they do not know. The nurse caring for a toddler in the outpatient or hospital setting should take the time to establish a relationship with the toddler in order to allay the toddler's fears. Toddlers may be afraid of loud noises and large or unfamiliar animals. Going to sleep may be a scary time for toddlers as they may be afraid of the dark. A nightlight in the toddler's room may be helpful.

MORAL AND SPIRITUAL DEVELOPMENT

During the toddler years, children may feel comfort from the routine of praying, but they do not understand religious beliefs because of their limited cognitive abilities. Reading simple religious or moral allegories can lay a foundation for later related teachings. Kohlberg's (1984) description of moral development places the older toddler at the preconventional level. The toddler is only just beginning to learn right from wrong and does not understand the larger concept of morality. The toddler will base their actions on the avoidance of punishment and the attainment of pleasure. Older toddlers begin to feel empathy for others.

SOCIOCULTURAL INFLUENCES ON GROWTH AND DEVELOPMENT

Homelessness or poverty may directly influence the toddler's ability to grow adequately, as resources for the purchase and preparation of appropriate food may be lacking. Safe, appropriate toys may also not be available in those situations. Food customs continue to have an impact on the child's diet and ability to ingest appropriate nutrients. Individual families' value systems have an impact on the toddler's development as well. Some parents desire to keep their child a "baby" for a longer period, thus delaying weaning or continuing to feed the child baby food or puréed food for a longer period. Other families may highly value independence and encourage the toddler to walk everywhere on their own rather than carrying the child.

Culture may also affect emotional development. Some families start to discourage crying in male children. Ridicule for crying at this age may hurt the toddler's self-concept. Educating families about normal growth and development while continuing to value and support cultural practices is important (Martorell, 2022).

> Remember Jose Gonzales, whom you met at the beginning of the chapter? What developmental milestones would you expect him to have reached at his age?

THE NURSE'S ROLE IN TODDLER GROWTH AND DEVELOPMENT

The toddler's growth and development affect their everyday life as well as the family's. Although some toddlers may grow more quickly or reach developmental milestones sooner than others, growth and development remains orderly and sequential. Health care visits throughout toddlerhood continue to focus on growth and development. The nurse must have a good understanding of the changes that occur during the toddler years in order to provide appropriate anticipatory guidance and support to the family.

When the toddler is hospitalized, growth and development may be altered. The toddler's primary task is establishing autonomy, and the toddler's focus is mobility and language development. Hospitalization removes most opportunities for the toddler to learn through exploration of the environment. Isolation for contagious illness further constrains the toddler's ability to find some control over the environment. The nurse caring for the hospitalized toddler must use knowledge of normal growth and development to be successful in interactions with the toddler, promote continued development, and recognize delays (see Chapter 11) (Fig. 4.6).

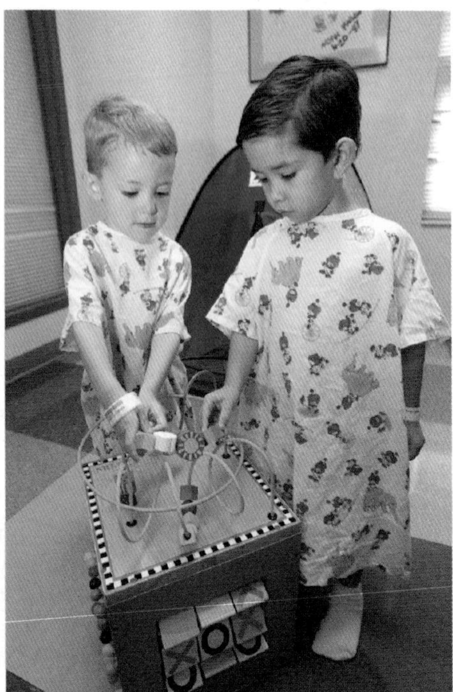

FIGURE 4.6 The hospitalized toddler continues to enjoy developmental tasks appropriate for their age, such as playing with manipulative toys.

Clinical Judgment and the Nursing Process

On completion of assessment of the toddler's current growth and development status, problems or issues related to growth and development may be identified. The nurse may then identify one or more nursing diagnoses. The following nursing diagnoses with identified outcomes and interventions provide suggestions for nursing care planning or concept mapping. Care planning should be individualized, based on the toddler's and family's needs.

Nursing Analysis

Injury risk due to extremes of age (e.g., curiosity, increased mobility, developmental immaturity) or unsafe mode of transport (e.g., lack of car seat and helmet use)

Goal/Outcome

Toddler safety will be maintained: Toddler will remain free from injury.

Preventing Injury (interventions with *rationale*)

- Teach and encourage appropriate use of rear-facing car seat until 2 years of age and forward-facing car seat after 2 years of age *to decrease risk of toddler injury related to motor vehicles.*
- Teach toddlers to stay away from the street and provide constant supervision *to prevent pedestrian injury.*
- Require bicycle helmet use while riding any wheeled toy *to prevent head injury and form habit of helmet use.*
- Childproof the home *to provide a developmentally safe environment for the curious and increasingly mobile toddler.*
- Post Poison Control Center phone number *in case of inadvertent ingestion.*
- Never leave a toddler unattended in a tub or pool or near any body of water *to prevent drowning.*
- Teach parents first-aid measures and child cardiopulmonary resuscitation (CPR) *to minimize consequences of injury should it occur.*
- Provide close observation and keep side rails up on crib/bed in hospital *because toddlers are at particularly high risk for falling or becoming entangled in tubing as they attempt mobility.*

Nursing Analysis

Alteration in nutritional status related to inappropriate nutritional intake to sustain growth needs (e.g., excess juice or milk intake, inadequate food variety intake), as evidenced by failure to attain adequate increases in length/height and weight over time.

Goal/Outcome

Toddler will consume adequate nutrients while using an appropriate feeding pattern: Toddler will demonstrate weight gain and increases in length/height.

Promoting Appropriate Nutrition (interventions with *rationale*)

- Assess current feeding schedule and usual intake, as well as methods used to feed, *to determine areas of adequacy versus inadequacy.*
- Determine toddler's ability to drink from cup, finger feed, swallow, and consume textures *to determine if additional exposure is needed or if further interventions such as speech or occupational therapy are required.*
- Weigh toddler daily on same scale if hospitalized, weekly on same scale if at home, and plot growth patterns weekly or monthly as appropriate on standardized growth charts *to determine if growth is improving.*
- Wean from bottle by 15 months of age *to discourage excess milk or juice intake in toddler who can carry bottle around.*
- Limit juice to 4 to 6 oz per day and milk to 16 to 24 oz per day *to discourage sense of fullness achieved with excess milk or juice intake, thereby increasing appetite for solid foods.*
- Provide three nutrient-dense meals and at least two healthy snacks per day *to encourage adequate nutrient consumption.*

- Feed toddler on a similar schedule daily without distractions and with the family; *toddlers respond well to routine and structure and may eat better in the social context of meals, and they become distracted easily (television should be off).*

Nursing Analysis

Delayed development risk; risk factors include inadequate nutrition, abuse, chronic illness, prematurity, technology dependence, behavioral disorder, or involvement with the foster care system.

Goal/Outcome

Development will be enhanced: Toddler will make continued progress toward realization of expected developmental milestones.

Enhancing Development (interventions with *rationale*)

- Screen for developmental capabilities *to determine toddler's current level of functio*ning.
- Offer age-appropriate toys, play, and activities (including gross motor) *to encourage further development.*
- Perform interventions as prescribed by physical, occupational, or speech therapist; *participation in those activities helps to promote function and accomplish acquisition of developmental skills.*
- Provide support to families of toddlers at risk for developmental delay *(progress in achieving developmental milestones can be slow and ongoing motivation is needed).*
- Reinforce positive attributes in the toddler *to maintain motivation.*
- Model age-appropriate communication skills *to illustrate suitable means for parenting the toddler.*

Nursing Analysis

Risk for body mass index (BMI) over 85th percentile for age 2+, or weight for length approaching 95th percentile for age (1 to 2 years of age); risk factors include portion sizes larger than recommended, excess milk or juice intake, late bottle weaning, and frequent snacking.

Goal/Outcome

Toddler will grow appropriately and not become overweight or obese: Toddler will achieve weight for length less than 85th percentile for age (less than 2 years old) or BMI less than 85th percentile (greater than 2 years old).

Promoting Proportionate Growth (interventions with rationale)

- Wean from bottle and discourage use of no-spill sippy cups by 15 months of age *(will keep mobile toddler from carrying around and continually drinking from cup or bottle).*
- Provide juice (4 to 6 oz per day) and milk (16 to 24 oz per day) from a cup at meal and snack time *to encourage appropriate cup drinking and limit intake of nutrient-poor, high-calorie fluids.*
- Provide only nutrient-rich foods without high sugar content for meals and snacks; *even if the toddler will not eat, it is inappropriate to provide high-calorie junk food just so the toddler eats something.*
- Ensure adequate physical activity *to stimulate development of motor skills and provide appropriate caloric expenditure. This also sets the stage for forming lifelong habit of appropriate physical activity.*

Nursing Analysis

Altered family functioning related to shift in family roles (toddler illness or hospitalization) as evidenced by change in family satisfaction/assigned tasks/communication pattern or decrease in available emotional support.

Goal/Outcome

Family will demonstrate adequate functioning: Family will display coping and psychosocial adjustment.

Enhancing Family Functioning (interventions with *rationale*)

- Assess the family's level of stress and ability to cope *to determine family's ability to cope with multiple stressors.*
- Engage in family-centered care *to provide a holistic approach to care of the toddler and family.*
- Encourage the family to verbalize feelings (*verbalization is one method of decreasing anxiety levels*) and acknowledge feelings and emotions.
- Encourage family visitation and provide for sleeping arrangements for a parent or caregiver to stay in the hospital with the toddler (*contributes to family's sense of control of situation*).
- Involve family members in toddler's care, *giving them a feeling of control and connectedness.*

Nursing Analysis

Desire for strengthened parenting related to parental expression of desire for enhanced skills.

Goal/Outcome

Parent will provide safe and nurturing environment for the toddler.

Increasing Parenting Skill Set (interventions with *rationale*)

- Use family-centered care *to provide holistic approach.*
- Educate parent about normal toddler development *to provide basis for understanding the parenting skills needed in this time period.*

- Acknowledge and encourage parent's verbalization of feelings related to chronic illness of child or difficulty with normal toddler behavior *to validate the normalcy of the parent's feelings.*
- Encourage positive parenting with respect to toddlers and their normal development *to help parents develop approaches to toddlers that can be used in place of anger and frustration.*
- Acknowledge and admire positive parenting skills already present *to contribute to parents' confidence in their abilities to parent.*
- Role model appropriate parenting behaviors related to communicating with and disciplining the toddler *to actually show rather than just tell the parent what to do.*

PROMOTING HEALTHY GROWTH AND DEVELOPMENT

Parents who give their toddler love and respect regardless of the child's sex, behavior, or capabilities are helping to lay the foundation for self-esteem. Self-esteem is also built through familiarity with the daily routine. Routine and ritual help toddlers develop a conscience. Making expectations known through everyday routines helps to avoid confrontations. If the toddler knows the routine, they know what to expect and how they are expected to act. When routine and limits are absent, the toddler develops feelings of uncertainty and anxiety. Limit setting (and remaining consistent with those limits) helps toddlers master their behavior, develop self-esteem, and become successful participants in the family. Children are then able to learn about cooperation throughout the predictable flow of daily life. Nurses need to be aware of normal developmental expectations in order to determine whether the toddler is progressing appropriately. Table 4.4 lists potential signs of developmental delay. Any toddler with one or more of these concerns should be referred for further developmental evaluation.

TABLE 4.4 • Signs of Developmental Delay

Age or Time Frame	Concern
After independent walking for several months	• Persistent tiptoe walking • Failure to develop a mature walking pattern
By 18 months	• Not walking • Not speaking 15 words • Does not understand function of common household items
By 2 years	• Does not use two-word sentences • Does not imitate actions • Does not follow basic instructions • Cannot push a toy with wheels
By 3 years	• Difficulty with stairs • Frequent falling • Cannot build tower of more than four blocks • Difficulty manipulating small objects • Extreme difficulty in separation from parent or caregiver • Cannot copy a circle • Does not engage in make-believe play • Cannot communicate in short phrases • Does not understand simple instructions • Little interest in other children • Unclear speech, persistent drooling

Promoting Growth and Development Through Play

Play is the major socializing medium for toddlers. Parents should limit television viewing and encourage creative and physical play instead. Toddlers typically play alongside another child (**parallel play**) rather than cooperatively (Fig. 4.7). The short attention span of the toddler will make them often change toys and types of play. It is important to provide a variety of safe toys to allow the toddler many different opportunities for exploring the environment. Toddlers do not need expensive toys; in fact, regular household items sometimes make the most enjoyable toys. Toddlers are egocentric, a normal part of their development (Piaget, 1969). This makes it difficult for them to share. As they are developing a sense of self (who they are as a person), they may see their toys as an extension of themselves. Learning to share occurs in later toddlerhood. Toddlers also like dramatic play and play that recreates familiar activities in the home. Toddlers like to listen to music of all kinds and will often dance to whatever they hear on the radio. Toddlers enjoy

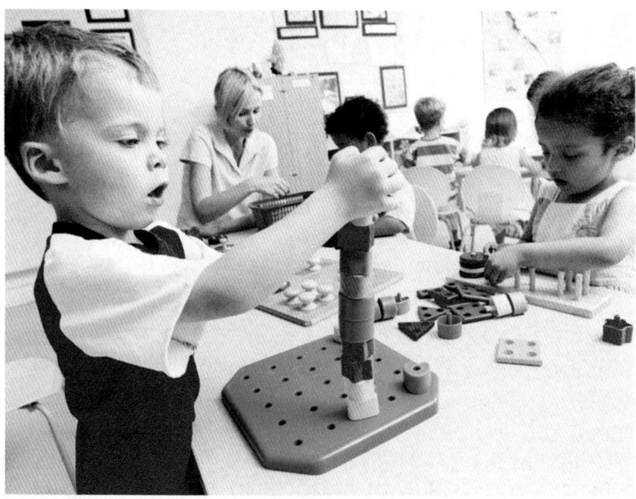

FIGURE 4.7 Parallel play. The toddler usually plays alongside another child rather than cooperatively.

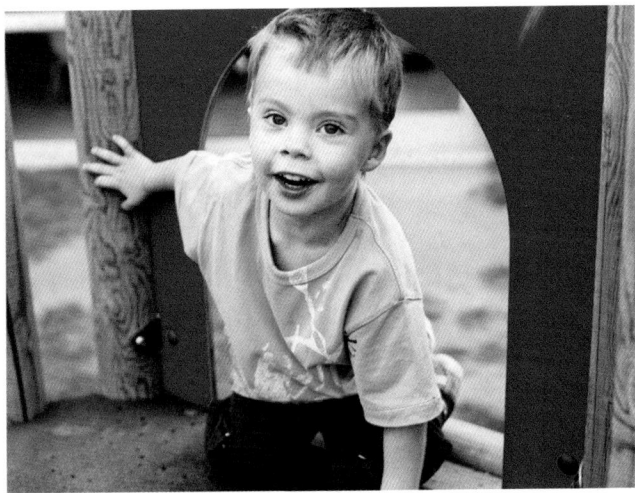

FIGURE 4.8 Toddlers love outdoor physical play, such as climbing on playground equipment. An adult should always supervise toddlers when they are playing outdoors.

BOX 4.1 Appropriate Toys for Toddlers

- Familiar household items such as plastic bowls and cups of various sizes, large plastic serving utensils, pots and pans, wooden spoons, cardboard boxes and tubes (from paper towel rolls), old magazines, baskets, purses, hats
- Child-size household item toys (kitchen, broom, vacuum cleaner, lawnmower, telephone, and so on)
- Blocks, cars and trucks, plastic animals, trains, plastic figures (family, community helpers), simple dolls, stuffed animals, balls, doll beds, and carriages
- Manipulative toys with knobs, wind-ups, and buttons that make things happen; putting large pegs or shapes into matching holes; stringing large beads on shoelaces; blocks and containers that stack; jigsaw puzzles with large pieces; toys that can be taken apart and put back together again
- Gross motor toys: play gym, push and pull toys, wagons, tricycle or other ride-on toys, tunnels
- Devices for playing music, various musical instruments
- Chalk, large crayons, finger paint, Play-Doh, washable markers
- Bucket, plastic shovel, and other containers for sand and water play
- Squeaking, floating, and squirting toys for the bath

Data from National Association for the Education of Young Children. (n.d.). *Good toys for young children by age and stage.* http://www.naeyc.org/toys

drums, xylophones, cymbals, and toy pianos. Musical instruments made at home are also enjoyed. A few pebbles or coins inside an empty water bottle with the top tightly secured is a great music maker; an empty butter tub with a lid and a pair of wooden spoons makes a nice drum.

Adequate physical activity is necessary for the development and refinement of movement skills. Toddlers need at least 60 minutes of structured physical activity and anywhere from 1 to several hours of unstructured physical activity per day (Hagan et al., 2017). Indoor and outdoor play areas should encourage play activities that use the large muscle groups. The activity must occur within a safe environment. Outdoor play structures should be positioned over surfaces that are soft enough to absorb a fall, such as sand, wood chips, or sawdust (Fig. 4.8). Box 4.1 lists recommended age-appropriate toys.

Promoting Early Learning

The parent–child relationship and the interactions between parent and child form the context for the toddler's early learning.

Promoting Language Development

Talking and singing to the toddler during routine activities such as feeding and dressing provide an environment that encourages conversation. Frequent, repetitive naming helps the toddler learn appropriate words for objects. The parent or caregiver should be attentive to what the toddler is saying as well as to their moods. Using clarification validates the toddler's emotions and ideas. Parents should listen to and answer the toddler's questions. They should sit down quietly with the toddler and gently repeat what the toddler is saying. Encouragement and elaboration convey confidence and interest to the toddler. The toddler needs time to complete their thoughts without being interrupted or rushed, because they are just starting to be able to make the connections necessary to transfer thoughts and feelings into language.

Parents should not overreact to the child's use of the word "no." They can give the toddler opportunities to use the word "no" appropriately by asking silly questions such as "Can a cat drive a car?" or "Is a banana purple?" When promoting language development, the parent or primary caregiver should teach the toddler appropriate words for body parts and objects and should help the toddler choose appropriate words to label feelings and emotions. Toddlers' receptive language and interpretation of body language and subtle signs far surpass their expressive language, especially at a younger age (Carter & Feigelman, 2020b; Reynolds et al., 2022).

Parents should avoid discussing scary or serious topics in the presence of the toddler, since the toddler is very adept at reading emotions. If the parents speak a foreign language in addition to English, both languages should be used in the home.

Encouraging Reading

Reading to the toddler every day is one of the best ways to promote language and cognitive development (Fig. 4.9). Toddlers particularly enjoy homemade or purchased books about feelings, family, friends, everyday life, animals and nature, and fun and fantasy. Board books have thick pages

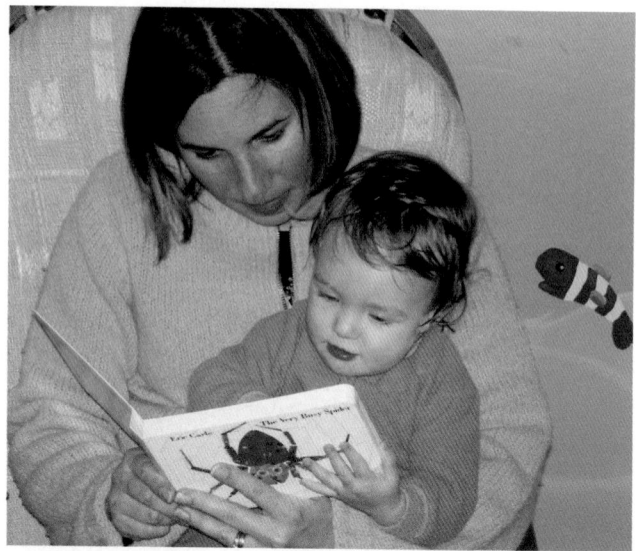

FIGURE 4.9 Reading to a toddler daily is one of the best ways to promote language development and school readiness.

that are easier for young toddlers to turn; older toddlers can turn paper pages one at a time. The toddler may also enjoy "reading" the story to the parent. Reach Out and Read, a program designed to promote early literacy, offers tips for reading with young children (see Teaching Guidelines 4.1).

Choosing a Preschool

The older toddler may benefit from the structure and socialization provided by attending preschool. Attending preschool will help the toddler become more mature and independent and give the toddler a different source for a sense of accomplishment. At this age, toddlers need supervised play with some direction that fosters their cognitive development. A strict curriculum is not necessary in this age group. When choosing a preschool, the parent or caregiver should look for an environment that has the following qualities:

- Goals and an overall philosophy with which the parents agree (promotion of independence and self-confidence through structured and free play)
- Teachers and assistants trained in early childhood development as well as child CPR
- Small class sizes and an adult-to-child ratio with which the parent feels comfortable
- Disciplinary procedures consistent with the parents' values
- Parents can visit at any time
- School is childproofed inside and out
- Appropriate hygiene procedures, including prohibiting sick children from attending

TEACHING GUIDELINES 4.1 Tips for Reading With Young Children

- Read often for a short time.
- Keep reading fun, short, and simple.
- Reading stories over and over, rhyming, and singing songs help the toddler learn.
- Be engaging: use voices for the story characters.
- Use body motions during the story (toddlers will too).
- Ask questions about the story and about the pictures.

Data from Reading Rockets. (2023). *Tips for parents of toddlers*. https://www.readingrockets.org/topics/activities/articles/reading-tips-parents-toddlers

Teach the parents how to ease the toddler's transition to attending preschool. Encourage parents to talk about going to preschool, and visit the school a couple of times. On the first day, parents should calmly and in a matter-of-fact tone tell the toddler that they will return to pick the child up. If the toddler expresses separation anxiety, the parent should remain calm and follow through with the plan for school attendance. After a few days of attendance, the toddler will be accustomed to the new routine, and crying when parting from the parent should be minimal.

Promoting Safety

Safety is of prime concern throughout the toddler period. Curiosity, mobility, and lack of impulse control all contribute to the incidence of unintentional injury in toddlerhood. Even the most watchful and caring parents have toddlers who run into the street, otherwise disappear from parents, and fall down the stairs. Toddlers require direct observation and cannot be trusted to be left alone. A childproof environment provides a safe place for the toddler to explore and learn. Motor vehicle crashes, drowning, choking, burns, falls, and poisoning are the most common injuries suffered by toddlers. Safety and injury prevention focus on these categories.

Safety in the Car

The safest place for the toddler to ride is in the back seat of the car. Parents should use the appropriate size and style of car seat for the child's weight and age as required by state law. At a minimum, toddlers should be in a rear-facing car seat with harness straps and a clip until 2 years of age (American Academy of Pediatrics [AAP], 2023b). After age 2 years, a forward-facing seat may be used if the toddler has reached the height and weight requirements. A toddler riding in a pickup truck should never ride in the cargo area or truck bed. A full rear seat in the truck is the preferred placement for the toddler car seat. If an appropriate rear seat is unavailable, the airbag should be disarmed, and the forward-facing car seat should be secured appropriately in the truck seat. The lower anchor and top tether are additionally required for all forward-facing car seats manufactured since 2002 and are accommodated by motor vehicles manufactured since that time (Fig. 4.10). In older vehicles or car seats,

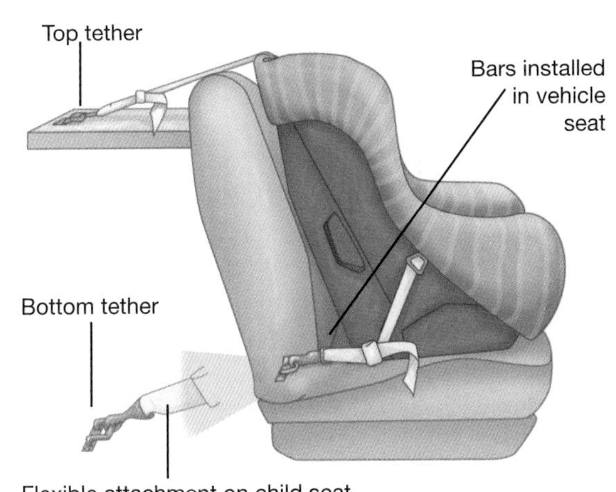

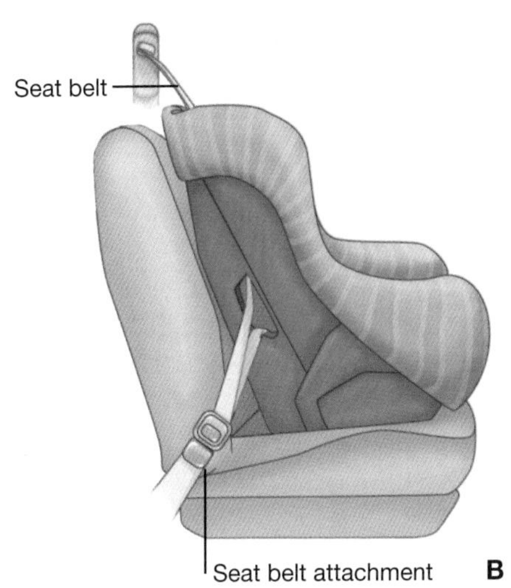

FIGURE 4.10 **A.** A lower anchor and top tether secure the forward-facing car seat. **B.** The shoulder safety strap may also be used to secure the toddler seat. (Adapted from US Department of Transportation, National Highway Traffic Safety Administration. [2011]. *LATCH makes child safety seat installation as easy as 1-2-3*. NHTSA. DOT HS publication 809 489.)

seat belts are utilized for installation. Drivers should avoid using the cell phone or attempting to intervene with the children while they are driving.

Safety in the Home

Key areas of concern for keeping toddlers safe in the home include avoiding exposure to tobacco smoke, preventing injury, and preventing poisoning.

AVOIDING EXPOSURE TO TOBACCO SMOKE

Environmental exposure to tobacco smoke has been associated with increased risk of respiratory disease and infection, decreased lung function, and increased incidence of middle ear effusion and recurrent otitis media (Samet & Sockrider, 2023). Parents should avoid cigarette smoking entirely to best protect their children. Even smoking outside of the home is suboptimal because smoke lingers on parents' clothing, and children who are often carried (such as younger toddlers) face more exposure. Counsel parents to stop smoking (optimal), but if they continue smoking never to smoke inside the home or car with children present.

PREVENTING INJURY

The toddler is able to open drawers and doors, unlock dead bolts, and climb anywhere they want to go. Toddlers have a limited concept of body boundaries and essentially no fear of danger. Toddlers may fall from any height to which they can climb (e.g., play structures, tables, counters). They may also fall from wheeled toys such as tricycles. As toddlers gain additional height and hand dexterity, they are able to reach potentially dangerous items on the counter or stove, leading to an inadvertent ingestion, burn, or cut.

The AAP advises against having guns in homes with children. If a gun is kept in the home, it should be stored unloaded and locked away (Schaechter, 2023).

To prevent injury in the home, stress the following to parents:

- Never leave a toddler unsupervised outdoors.
- Lock doors to dangerous rooms.
- Install safety gates at the top and bottom of staircases.
- Ensure that window locks are operable; if windows are left opened, then secure all window screens.
- Keep pot handles on the stove turned inward, out of an inquisitive toddler's reach.
- Teach the toddler to avoid the oven, stove, and iron.
- Keep electrical equipment, cords, and matches out of reach.
- Remove firearms from the home or keep them in a locked cabinet out of the toddler's reach.
- Always require the child to wear a helmet approved by the Consumer Products Safety Commission (CPSC) when riding a wheeled toy. This starts the habit of helmet wearing early, so it can be more easily carried over to the bicycle-riding years of the future.
- Begin teaching the toddler about watching for cars when crossing the street, but always carry or hold the hand of the toddler when crossing the street.
- Teach the toddler to avoid unknown animals (AAP, 2021b, 2022).

TAKE NOTE!

Bernie Burn, by Sarah Cruz, RN, is a book designed to educate parents and their toddlers about burn prevention while entertaining them. It is endorsed by the *American Journal of Nursing*.

PREVENTING POISONING

As toddlers become more mobile, they are increasingly able to explore their environment and more easily and efficiently gain access to materials that may be unsafe for them to handle. Their natural curiosity leads them into situations that may place them in danger. Poor taste discrimination in this age group allows for ingestion of chemicals or other materials that older children would find too unpleasant to swallow. Box 4.2 lists most potentially dangerous ingested poisons. Discuss poison prevention in the home at each well-child visit. The AAP (2021a) recommends that potentially poisonous substances (e.g., medications, cleaners, hair care products, car care products) be stored out of the toddler's reach, out of the toddler's sight, and in a childproof, locked cabinet.

Encourage all families to take the following safety measures:

- Store all substances in original containers only.
- Never store any liquid other than water or soda in beverage containers.
- Do not allow toddlers access to baby powder, lotion, cream, or other toddler hygiene products.
- Ensure all medications have child-safety caps.
- Do not leave within the toddler's reach medications such as lozenges or samples that are not packaged in safety bottles.
- Be very careful with medications that are provided in transdermal patch form.
- Do not refer to medicines as candy, as the toddler may mistake pills for candy and ingest them.
- Do not expose toddlers to hazardous vapors such as paints, cleaners, tobacco or cannabis smoke, and especially illicit drugs.
- Keep "button" batteries secured and away from a toddler's reach.
- Keep house plants off the floor, remove them from the home, or hang them or place them on a high shelf (AAP, 2021a; American Association of Poison Control Centers, n.d.).

TAKE NOTE!

The AAP (2021a) recommends that all families post the Poison Control Center number in a readily accessible place in the home: (800) 222-1222. Since 2003, the AAP has discouraged the use of syrup of ipecac in the home to induce vomiting after an unintentional ingestion. Instead, families should call the Poison Control Center right away.

Safety in the Water

Drowning is the leading cause of unintentional injury and death in U.S. children, with nearly half of drowning victims being 4 years old and younger (Safe Kids, 2023a). Drowning may occur in very small volumes of water such as a toilet, bucket, or bathtub, as well as the obvious sites such as swimming pools and other bodies of water. Toddlers' large heads in relation to their body size place them at risk for toppling over into a body of water that they are inquisitive about. Toddlers should be supervised at all times when in or around the water. In general, most children do not have the physical and cognitive capabilities necessary to truly learn how to swim until 4 years of age. Parents who want to enroll a toddler in a swimming class should be aware that a water safety skills class would be most appropriate. However, even toddlers who have completed a swimming program still need *constant* supervision in the water (Safe Kids, 2023a). Box 4.3 gives recommendations for the prevention of drowning.

Remember Jose Gonzales, the 2-year-old described at the beginning of the chapter? What anticipatory guidance related to safety should you provide to Jose's parents?

Promoting Nutrition

The toddler's ability to chew and swallow is improving, and they learn to use utensils effectively to feed themselves. The early years lay a foundation for the future, and

BOX 4.2 Most Dangerous Potential Poisons

- Medicines (especially iron)
- Cleaning products
- Antifreeze, windshield washer solution
- Alcohol
- Pesticides
- Gasoline, kerosene, lamp oil, furniture polish
- Wild mushrooms

Data from American Association of Poison Control Centers. (n.d.). *In the home safety tips.* https://aapcc.org/prevention/in-the-home

BOX 4.3 Preventing Drowning

- Pools should be fenced with locked gates or screened with locked doors.
- Interior doors should be kept locked.
- Young children should never be left unattended in or near water.
- Water wings or "floaties" are not a substitute for adult supervision or for personal flotation devices.
- U.S. Coast Guard–approved life preservers or personal flotation devices should be available when a young child is in or near a body of water.
- Parents and caregivers should be trained in child CPR.

Data from Safe Kids. (2023b). *Water safety tips at home.* https://www.safekids.org/tip/water-safety-home-tips

a great deal of parental and societal interest is focused on nutrition and eating. Forming healthy eating habits has its foundation early in life, and diet has a significant influence on the child's future health status. By establishing healthier food choice patterns early in life, the child is better able to continue these healthy choices later in life. The child younger than 2 years should not have their fat intake restricted, but unhealthy foods and sweets should not be eaten liberally. A diet high in nutrient-rich foods and low in nutrient-poor high-calorie foods such as sweets is appropriate for children of all ages. See the Healthy People 2030 box.

HEALTHY PEOPLE 2030

Objective	Nursing Significance
Reduce household food insecurity and in doing so reduce hunger.	• Counsel families about the appropriate toddler diet. • Refer eligible families to the special supplemental nutrition program for women, infants, and children (WIC).

Healthy People Objectives retrieved from http://www.healthypeople.gov

Weaning

The timing of weaning from breastfeeding or chestfeeding is influenced by a number of factors such as cultural beliefs, local and regional ethnic beliefs, the lactating parent's work schedule, desired child spacing, or societal feelings about the nature of the lactating parent–infant relationship. The AAP recommends breastfeeding for at least 6 months, then for as long as is mutually agreeable to the breastfeeding parent and child (AAP, 2023a). Extending breastfeeding or chestfeeding into toddlerhood is believed to be beneficial to the child. It provides nutritional, immunologic, and emotional benefits to the child. Contrary to popular belief, it is biologically possible to become pregnant while breastfeeding. Breastfeeding a newborn appropriately can occur while continuing to nurse the older sibling.

Weaning from breastfeeding or chestfeeding tends to occur earlier in the United States than in countries around the world, despite recommendations on length of breastfeeding by a number of organizations. Most professional organizations recommend breastfeeding for at least 1 year (National Association of Pediatric Nurse Practitioners [NAPNAP] et al., 2019). Weaning is a highly individualized decision. Educate parents about the benefits of extended breastfeeding, and support the decision to wean at a given time.

Weaning from the bottle should occur by 12 to 15 months of age. Prolonged bottle-feeding is associated with the development of dental caries. No-spill "sippy cups" contain a valve that requires sucking by the toddler in order to obtain fluid, thus functioning similarly to a baby bottle. Hence, no-spill sippy cups can also be associated with dental caries and are not recommended (Hagan et al., 2017). Cups with spouts that do not contain valves are acceptable. The 12- to 15-month-old is developmentally capable of consuming adequate fluid amounts using a cup.

Teaching About Nutritional Needs

Adequate calcium intake and appropriate exercise lay the foundation for proper bone mineralization. The toddler requires an average intake of 700 mg of calcium per day (Ben-Joseph, 2018). Dairy products are considered the primary sources of dietary calcium. One cup of low-fat or whole milk, 8 oz of low-fat yogurt, and 1½ oz of cheddar cheese each provide 300 mg of calcium. Broccoli, oranges, sweet potatoes, tofu, and dried beans or legumes are also good sources of calcium (35- to 120-mg calcium per serving).

Iron-deficiency anemia in the first 2 years of life may be associated with developmental and psychomotor delays (Powers, 2023). Although it is important for toddlers to consume adequate amounts of iron, they tend to have the lowest daily iron intake of any age group. When breastfeeding or formula-feeding ends (most often at 1 year of age), it is often replaced with iron-poor cow's milk. Limiting milk intake to 16 oz per day, as well as limiting juice intake, can be helpful. Encourage the parents to provide iron-fortified cereals and other foods rich in iron and vitamin C.

TAKE NOTE!

Toddlers who consume a strictly vegan diet (no food from animal sources) are at risk for deficiencies in vitamin D, vitamin B_{12}, and iron. Supplementation with these nutrients should occur to promote adequate nutrition and growth (Parks et al., 2020).

Fat or cholesterol intake should not be restricted in children younger than age 2 years. The first 2 years of life require high energy intake because they are a time of very rapid growth and development. Due to daily variations and the pickiness of the toddler, fat intake should be evaluated over a period of several days. Encourage parents to feed toddlers foods containing adequate amounts of fiber and limit processed foods. Generally, toddler serving sizes should be about two thirds of that of an older child. Box 4.4 lists common sources of several nutrients.

BOX 4.4 Key Nutrients Provided by Fruits and Vegetables

Dietary fiber: Apples, artichokes, berries, oranges, green peas, pears, prunes
Folate: Asparagus, Brussels sprouts, fruits, spinach, and dark greens
Vitamin A: Fruits, leafy green vegetables, orange and yellow vegetables, tomatoes
Vitamin C: Berries, broccoli, Brussels sprouts, cauliflower, cantaloupe, citrus fruits, kiwi, mango, papaya, green peas, pineapple, sweet and white potatoes, tomatoes, watermelon, winter squash

Data from Division of Agriculture. (2023). Fruits and vegetables: Important sources of nutrients and vitamins. *University of Arkansas*. https://www.uaex.uada.edu/counties/miller/news/fcs/fruits-veggies/fruits-and-vegetables-important-sources-of-nutrients-and-vitamins.aspx

Parents should encourage toddlers to drink water. Juice intake should be limited to 4 to 6 oz per day. Milk intake should be limited to no more than 24 oz per day. Juice and milk should be served along with meals or snacks. Water should be offered for between-meal drinking. Toddlers should drink from a cup.

Advancing Solid Foods

Parents should offer three full meals and two snacks daily. Portion sizes for toddlers are about one quarter of the size of adult portions. Large portions of a new or different food on the toddler's plate may intimidate the toddler. Normal toddler behaviors of mouthing, handling, tasting, extruding the food from the mouth, and then resampling the food often occur. These behaviors are distasteful to some parents but are a normal part of toddler development. Parents need to understand and tolerate these behaviors rather than scolding the toddler for them (Lieberman, 2018).

Toddlers are often afraid to try new things anyway, so the parent or caregiver should be flexible with the toddler's acceptance or rejection of new foods. If the toddler refuses healthy food choices at meal or snack time, parents should not substitute high-fat, high-sugar, processed food just to make sure that the child eats something (Parks et al., 2020). This sets the stage for future power struggles. The parent decides which foods will be served or offered. The toddler decides how much will be eaten. The toddler self-regulates the amount of food needed to sustain and allow further growth and development. The toddler may not eat well every day but, generally, over the course of several days, will consume the foods they need (Satter, 2023).

Foods should be served near room temperature. Some of the food on the plate should be soft and moist. Food should always be cut into bite-size pieces. Teaching Guidelines 4.2 gives recommendations on ways to prevent choking.

TEACHING GUIDELINES 4.2 Avoiding Choking

- Slowly add foods that are more difficult to chew as the toddler becomes more adept at chewing.
- Cut all foods into bite-sized pieces.
- Avoid foods that are hard to chew and that may become lodged in the airway, such as:
  - Nuts
  - Gumdrops or other chewy candies, hard candy
  - Raw carrots
  - Peanut butter (by itself)
  - Popcorn
- Cut hotdogs and grapes into quarters. Cook carrots until soft; if serving raw, then grate them.
- Always supervise the toddler while they are eating.

Adapted from Durani, Y. (2023). *Preventing choking*. https://kidshealth.org/en/parents/safety-choking.html

Promoting Self-Feeding

Toddlers most often eat with their fingers, but they do need to learn to use utensils properly. The following are suggestions for parents:

- Use a child-sized spoon and fork with dull tines.
- Seat the toddler in a highchair or at a comfortable height in a secure chair. The toddler should have their feet supported rather than dangling (Fig. 4.11).
- Never leave the toddler unattended while eating.
- Minimize distractions during mealtime. Serve food to the toddler along with the other members of the family (Satter, 2023).

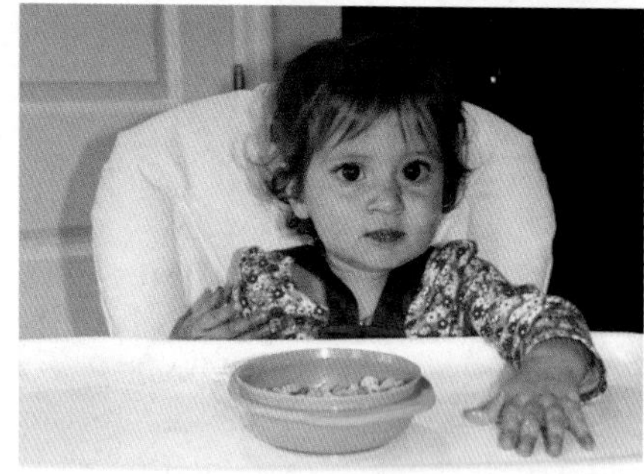

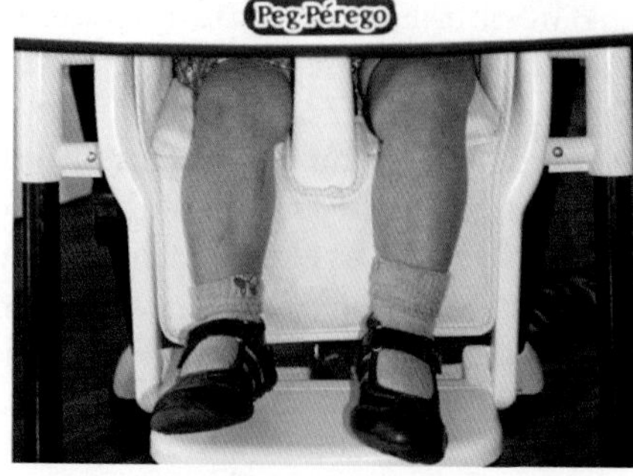

FIGURE 4.11 The toddler should be appropriately and safely seated in the highchair. The safety strap is secure, the toddler's feet are supported, and the tray table is locked in place.

Promoting Healthy Eating Habits

Since the toddler's rate of growth has slowed somewhat compared to that in infancy, the toddler requires less caloric intake for their size compared to the infant. This results in **physiologic anorexia**: toddlers simply do not require as much food intake for their size as they did in infancy. The toddler will also exhibit **food jags**. During a food jag, the toddler may prefer only one particular food for several days, then not want it for weeks. Again, it is important for the parent to continue to offer healthy food choices during a food jag and not give in by allowing the toddler to eat junk food (Satter, 2023).

The normal developmental issue of testing limits will also occur for the toddler at mealtime. Since toddlers still have limited ability to express their emotions with words, they use nonverbal behaviors to do so. While eating, the toddler may dislike the taste of a particular food or experience a feeling of fullness but will communicate that feeling by screaming or throwing food. When the child exhibits these behaviors, the parent must remain calm and remove the toddler from the situation. Meals should be eaten in a calm and pleasant environment. Parents should serve as role models for appropriate eating habits, but toddlers may also be willing to try more foods if they are exposed to other children who eat those foods. Praise the child for trying a new food, and never punish the toddler for refusing to try something new. A new food may need to be offered many times in a row before the toddler chooses to try it. Parents should be sure to include foods the child is familiar with and likes to eat at the same meal that the new food is being introduced (Satter, 2023). Teaching Guidelines 4.3 lists alternative foods that meet nutritional needs and a list of books for picky eating.

Preventing Overweight and Higher Weight

In children, the greatest risk factor for the development of overweight and higher weight is having a parent with a high BMI (Skelton & Klish, 2023). The nurse can screen for overweight and higher weight in the child older than 2 years of age by calculating the BMI and plotting the BMI on the standardized age- and sex-appropriate growth charts (see Appendix A for growth charts, and refer to Chapter 10 for BMI calculation instructions). Trends over time may be predictive of the development of overweight and higher weight. See the Healthy People 2030 box.

Another factor in the development of excess weight in young children is juice intake (Parks et al., 2020). Since most young children like the sweet taste of juice, they may drink excessive amounts of it. Toddlers who drink excess fruit juice and eat well may gain excess weight because of the high sugar content in the juice. On the other end of the spectrum, some children may feel

TEACHING GUIDELINES 4.3 Meeting Nutritional Needs for Picky Eating

Alternative Food Choices for Picky Eating

- Won't drink milk? Obtain calcium through yogurt (frozen or regular), cheese, pudding, and hot cocoa.
- Poor meat intake? Obtain iron through unsweetened iron-fortified cereals or breakfast bars, or raisins; cook with an iron skillet.
- Loves processed white bread? Encourage fiber intake with fresh fruits and vegetables, bran muffins, beans, or peas (can be in soup).
- Refuses vegetables? Encourage vitamin A intake with apricots, sweet potatoes, and vegetable juices.

Books for Picky Eating

- *Feeding with Love and Good Sense* by E. Satter. Kelcy Press, 2022.
- *First Foods* by M. Stoppard. Dorling-Kindersley Publishing, Inc., 2002.
- *Food Chaining: The Proven 6-Step Plan to Stop Picky Eating, Solve Feeding Problems, and Expand Your Child's Diet* by C. Fraker, M. Fishbein, S. Cox, & L. Walbert. Da Capo Lifelong Books, 2007.
- *Helping Your Child with Extreme Picky Eating: A Step-By-Step Guide for Overcoming Selective Eating, Food Aversion, and Feeding Disorders* by K. Rowell & J. McGlothlin. New Harbinger Publications, 2015.
- *Raising a Healthy, Happy Eater: A Parent's Handbook* by N. Fernando & M. Potock. The Experiment. 2022.
- *The No-Cry Picky Eater Solution: Gentle Ways to Encourage Your Child to Eat - and Eat Healthy* by E. Pantley. McGraw-Hill, 2011.
- *The Healthy Baby Meal Planner: Mom-Tested, Child-Approved Recipes for your Baby and Toddler* by A. Karmel. Fireside, 2005.

HEALTHY PEOPLE 2030

Objective	Nursing Significance
Reduce the proportion of children and adolescents aged 2–19 years who have higher weight.	• Counsel families about the appropriate toddler diet. • Educate families to decrease excess toddler intake of milk or juice and offer only nutrient-rich foods.

Healthy People Objectives retrieved from http://www.healthypeople.gov

full from juice consumption and decrease their intake of solid foods. These children are at risk for malnutrition. Fruit juice intake should be limited to 4 to 6 oz per day. See Evidence-Based Practice 4.1.

TAKE NOTE!

Young children should consume only pasteurized juice, as unpasteurized juice consumption places the toddler at increased risk of *Escherichia coli, Salmonella,* and *Cryptosporidium* infection.

Think back to Jose Gonzales. What questions should you ask Jose's parents related to his nutritional intake? What anticipatory guidance related to nutrition would be appropriate?

Promoting Healthy Sleep and Rest

The 18-month-old requires 13.5 hours of sleep per day, the 24-month-old 13 hours, and the 3-year-old 12 hours (Carter & Feigelman, 2020a, 2020b). A typical toddler should sleep through the night and take one daytime nap. Most children discontinue daytime napping at around 3 years of age. The toddler who slept in a crib as an infant will need to move to a youth or toddler bed or even a full-size bed usually sometime in the toddler period. When the crib becomes unsafe (i.e., when the toddler becomes physically capable of climbing over the rails), then they must make the transition to a bed.

Consistent bedtime rituals help the toddler prepare for sleep. Choose a bedtime and stick to it as much as possible. The nightly routine might include a bath followed by reading a story. The routine should be a calm period with minimal outside distractions. Toddlers often require a security item to help them get to sleep. Older toddlers may be afraid of the dark, so a nightlight is often helpful.

Night waking is a problem for some toddlers. This may occur as a result of change in routine or as a desire for nighttime attention. Attention during night waking should be minimized so that the toddler receives no reward for being awake at night. The book *No-Cry Sleep Solution,* by Elizabeth Pantley (2020) is an excellent resource for the family with a toddler who resists bedtime or is a persistent night waker. For some toddlers, night waking is caused by nightmares. As the imagination and capacity for make-believe grow, the toddler may not be able to distinguish between reality and pretend. The parent should hold and comfort the toddler after a nightmare. Limiting television viewing (especially shortly before bedtime) may be helpful in limiting nightmares.

Some families practice "co-sleeping" (when children sleep in the parents' bed). Although some professionals believe that co-sleeping may interfere with the toddler's struggle for independence, this theory has not been proven. The nurse should support the family's choice for sleep arrangements unless the co-sleeping is unsafe either physically or psychologically (SafeBedSharing.org, 2023). Refer to http://www.safebedsharing.org for bed-sharing safety guidelines.

What anticipatory guidance should you provide to Jose's parents in relation to sleep?

EVIDENCE-BASED PRACTICE 4.1
Higher Weight in Childhood Research Demonstration Projects

STUDY

Excess weight is a reliable predictor of poor health across the lifespan. While the four protective factors of healthy eating habits, self-regulation, parental responsive feeding practices, and parental sensitive scaffolding are known to be protective against higher weight development, they are less prevalent among families living in poverty (Nix et al., 2021). Few home-based interventions have been demonstrated to decrease the development of excess weight in toddlers living in poverty.

The researchers enrolled and retained 66 families of toddlers in Early Head Start, who were aged 18 to 36 months. Families were randomly assigned to an intervention or control group. Those in the intervention group received the Recipe 4 Success curriculum during a series of home visits.

Findings

A variety of measures were used to determine toddler healthy eating habits, toddler self-regulation, parental responsive feeding practices, and parental sensitive scaffolding. The study results revealed toddlers in the intervention (Recipe 4 Success) group were more likely to eat balanced meals and snacks rather than sweets and junk food. Additionally, these toddlers showed improved self-regulation (gratification delay in the presence of highly desired food). Parents in the intervention group were more likely to engage in responsive feeding practices and to demonstrate sensitive scaffolding (structuring task for engagement without overwhelming the toddler).

Nursing Implications

Overweight and higher weight in childhood places children at risk for negative cardiovascular events and excess weight continuing into adulthood. Nurses are in an ideal position to educate and support families in their decisions related to providing nutrition to their young children. Assisting parents in making healthy food decisions and appropriately involving their toddlers in the eating process may lead to decreased incidence of excess weight in toddlerhood.

Data from Nix, R. L., Francis, L. A., Feinberg, M. E., Gill, S., Jones, D. E., Hostetler, M. L., & Stifter, C. A. (2021). Improving toddlers' healthy eating habits and self-regulation: A randomized controlled trial. *Pediatrics, 147*(1), e20193326. https://doi.org/10.1542/peds.2019-3326

Promoting Healthy Teeth and Gums

By 30 months of age, the toddler should have a full set of primary ("baby") teeth. Parents may not be aware of the importance of preventing cavities in primary teeth since they will eventually be replaced by the permanent teeth. Poor oral hygiene, prolonged use of a bottle or no-spill sippy cup, lack of fluoride intake, and delayed or absent professional dental care may all contribute to the development of dental caries (Nowak & Warren, 2023). Cleaning of the toddler's teeth should progress from brushing with water alone to using a very small amount (pea-sized) of fluoridated toothpaste, with brushing beginning at 2 years of age (Fig. 4.12). Weaning from the bottle no later than 15 months of age and severely restricting use of a no-spill sippy cup (the kind that requires sucking for fluid delivery) is recommended.

By the age of 1 year, the toddler should have their first dentist visit to establish current health of the teeth and gums. Eating should be limited to meal and snack times, as "grazing" throughout the day exposes the teeth to food throughout the day. Carbohydrate-containing foods combined with oral bacteria create a decreased oral pH level that is optimal for the development of dental caries (cavities).

Public water fluoridation is a public health initiative that ensures that most children receive adequate fluoride intake to prevent dental caries. If the water supply contains adequate fluoride, no other supplementation is necessary other than brushing with a small amount of fluoride-containing toothpaste after age 2 years. Excess fluoride ingestion should be avoided, as it contributes to the development of fluorosis (mottling of the enamel). Risk factors for fluorosis development include:

- High fluoride levels in the local water supply
- Use of fluoride-containing toothpaste prior to age 2 years
- Excessive ingestion of fluoride either in toothpaste or foods
- Fluoride-containing foods: tea, ready-to-eat infant foods containing chicken, white or purple grape juice, and beverages, processed foods, and cereals that were manufactured with fluoride-containing water

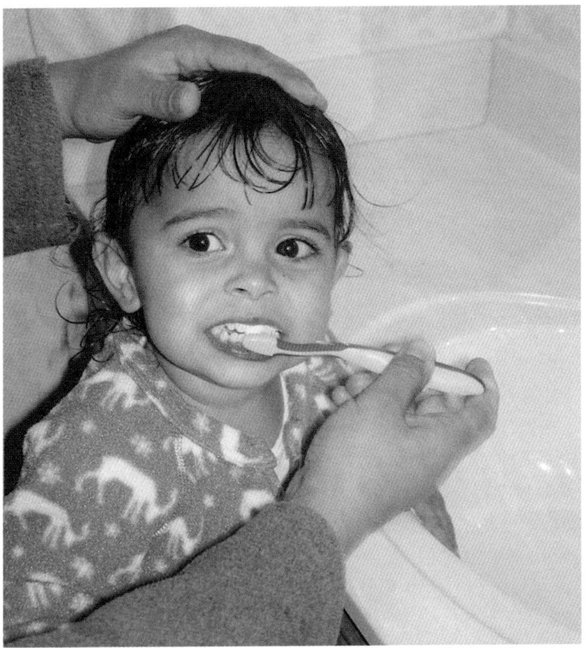

FIGURE 4.12 The parent should brush the toddler's teeth to ensure proper cleaning of the teeth, gums, and tongue. Use only water for brushing before 2 years of age and a pea-sized amount of fluoride-containing toothpaste after age 2 years.

Promoting Appropriate Discipline

Discipline is a common concern during toddlerhood. The toddler's intense personality and extreme emotional reactions can be difficult for parents to cope with and understand. The toddler needs firm, gentle guidance to learn what the expectations are and how to meet them. The parent's love and respect for the toddler teach the toddler to care about themselves and others. Affection is as important as the guidance aspect of discipline. Having realistic expectations of what the toddler is capable of learning and understanding can help the parent in the disciplinary process. The toddler's intense push for autonomy can often test a parent's limits. The easygoing infant usually becomes more challenging in toddlerhood. The toddler's continual quest for new experiences often places the toddler at risk, and their negativism often taxes the parent's patience.

In an effort to prevent the toddler from experiencing harm and in response to their continual testing of limits, parents often resort to spanking. Although commonly accepted, the AAP and the NAPNAP recommend against corporal or physical punishment (American Academy of Child and Adolescent Psychiatry, 2018; NAPNAP et al., 2022). Recent research points out the dangers inherent in the use of corporal punishment as well as the possibilities for negative effects on the child's future behavior (Box 4.5). Spanking or other forms of corporal punishment lead to a pro-violence attitude, create resentment and anger in some children, and contribute to the cycle of violence (NAPNAP et al., 2022).

TAKE NOTE!

Toddlers younger than 18 months should *never* be spanked, as there is an increased possibility of physical injury in this age group. Also, the infant/young toddler is not capable of linking the spanking with the undesired behavior (AAP, 2018).

BOX 4.5 Negative Impact of Physical Punishment

- Spanking is less effective than time-out or other disciplinary measures to reduce undesired behavior in children.
- The toddler younger than 18 months of age:
  - Is not capable of making the appropriate connections between spanking and the undesired behavior
  - Is at increased risk for physical injury from spanking than older children
- Physical punishment:
  - May lead to a pro-violence attitude
  - May create resentment in the toddler
  - Is a poor model for learning effective problem-solving
  - May be correlated with antisocial and criminal behavior later in life
  - Leads to increased aggression in preschoolers, school-age children, and adults
  - When used frequently, may weaken the parent–child relationship
- Childhood corporal punishment increases the probability of depression and substance use disorder in adulthood.
- Spanking may lead to more severe forms of punishment and to actual child abuse and maltreatment.
- The more frequently children are hit or spanked, the more likely they are to hit their own children and to be involved in spouse abuse as adults.

Data from Global Initiative to End All Corporal Punishment of Children. (2018). *Global initiative to end corporal punishment.* http://www.endcorporalpunishment.org/; National Association of Pediatric Nurse Practitioners, Child Maltreatment and Neglect Special Interest Group, VanGraafeiland, B., Hornor, G. A., Herendeen, P. A., Chiocca, E. M., Loyke, J. A., Dietzman, H., Boucher, N. L., Nielsen, A., & Record, S. C. (2022). NAPNAP position statement on using positive parenting to eliminate corporal punishment. *Journal of Pediatric Health Care, 36*, 202–204. https://doi.org/10.1016/j.pedhc.2021.09.001

Normal toddler development includes natural curiosity, which often results in dangerous or problematic activities for the toddler (Buckloh, 2023). Toddlers have a difficult time learning the rules and, in general, do not behave badly intentionally. Providing a childproof environment will allow the toddler to participate in safe exploration, which will meet their developmental needs and decrease the frequency of intervention needed on the part of the parents.

Discipline should focus on limit setting, negotiation, and techniques to assist the toddler to learn problem-solving. Parents should provide consistency and commit to the limits that are set. Offering realistic choices helps give the toddler a sense of mastery. Rules should be simple and limited in number. Maintaining the toddler's schedule of meals and rest/sleep will help to prevent conflicts that occur as a result of hunger or fatigue. Toddlers should not be made to share, as this is a concept they do not understand. Parents should encourage simple activities enjoyed by the children involved and avoid confrontation over toys. Parents should offer toddlers appropriate choices to help them develop autonomy but should not offer a choice when none exists.

Positive reinforcement should be used as much as possible. "Catching" a child being good helps to reinforce appropriate or desirable behaviors. When the toddler is displaying appropriate behavior, the parent should reward the child consistently with praise and physical affection.

"Time-out" can be used effectively at around 2.5 to 3 years of age (refer to Chapter 5 for details). "Extinction" is a particularly useful technique with 2- and 3-year-olds. Extinction involves systematically ignoring the undesired behavior. Parents sometimes unknowingly contribute to the occurrence of an unwanted behavior simply by the attention they give the toddler (even if it is negative in nature, it is still attention). Parents who want to extinguish an annoying (non-dangerous) behavior should resolve to ignore it every time it occurs. When the child withholds the behavior or performs the opposite (appropriate) behavior, parents should use compliments and praise. It may be difficult to ignore a difficult behavior, but the results are well worth the effort. Teaching Guidelines 4.4 provides tips on avoiding power struggles and offers appropriate guidance to toddlers.

TEACHING GUIDELINES 4.4 Providing Toddlers With Guidance

- When giving the toddler instructions, tell the child what to do, NOT what not to do. This allows for a positive focus. If you must say "no," "don't," or "stop," then follow with a direction of what to do instead.
- Offer limited choices, when a choice is truly available. Say, "Do you want to wear your blue hat or your red hat?" *not* "Do you want to put on your hat?" This gives the toddler some, but not all, control.
- Role model appropriate communication, but don't feel like you have to speak nicely all the time. If the situation warrants, use a firm and even tone to get the point across. Avoid yelling.
- Pay attention to the inflection in your voice. A statement or direction should not end in a questioning tone or with "Okay?" Be clear. Statements should sound like statements, and only questions should end in a questioning tone.
- When a toddler behaves aggressively, label the child's feelings calmly, but be firm and consistent with the expectation. For example, "I know you're mad at your friend, but it is not okay to hit."

Adapted from Buckloh, L. M. (2023). *Disciplining your toddler*. https://kidshealth.org/en/parents/toddler-tantrums.html#; Sears, W., & Sears, M. (2020b). *8 tools for toddler discipline*. http://www.askdrsears.com/topics/parenting/discipline-behavior/8-tools-toddler-discipline

ADDRESSING COMMON DEVELOPMENTAL CONCERNS

Common developmental concerns of the toddler period are toilet teaching, temper tantrums, thumb sucking or pacifier use, sibling rivalry, and regression. An understanding of the normalcy of negativism, temper tantrums, and sibling rivalry will help the family cope with these issues. Prepare parents for these developmental events by giving appropriate anticipatory guidance.

Toilet Teaching

When myelination of the spinal cord is achieved around age 2 years, the toddler is capable of exercising voluntary control over the sphincters. Female children may be ready for toilet teaching earlier than male children (Gavin, 2019). Toddlers are ready for toilet teaching when:

- Bowel movements occur on a fairly regular schedule.
- The toddler expresses knowledge of the need to defecate or urinate. This may be through verbalization, change in activity, or gestures such as:
  - Looks into or grabs diaper
  - Squats
  - Crosses legs
  - Grimaces and grunts
  - Hides behind a door or the couch when defecating
- The diaper is not always wet (this indicates the ability to hold the urine for a period of time).
- The toddler is willing to follow instructions.
- The toddler walks well alone and is able to pull down their pants.
- The toddler follows caregivers to the bathroom.
- The toddler climbs onto the potty chair or toilet (AAP, 2023c).

Parents should approach toilet teaching with a calm, positive, and nonthreatening manner. Initially it may be helpful to allow the toddler to observe a same-sex family member using the toilet. Start with the toddler fully clothed on the potty chair or toilet while the parent or caregiver talks about what the toilet is used for and when. The toddler will feel most comfortable with a toddler potty chair that sits on the floor (Fig. 4.13). If a potty chair is unavailable, facing toward the toilet tank may make the toddler feel more secure, as the buttocks remain on the front of the seat rather than sinking through the toilet seat opening. After a week or longer, remove a dirty diaper and place the contents in the toilet. Next, try having the toddler sit on the potty chair or toilet without pants or diaper on. The toddler may benefit from watching a caregiver or friend use the toilet. It may also be beneficial to demonstrate using the potty chair with a baby doll that wets.

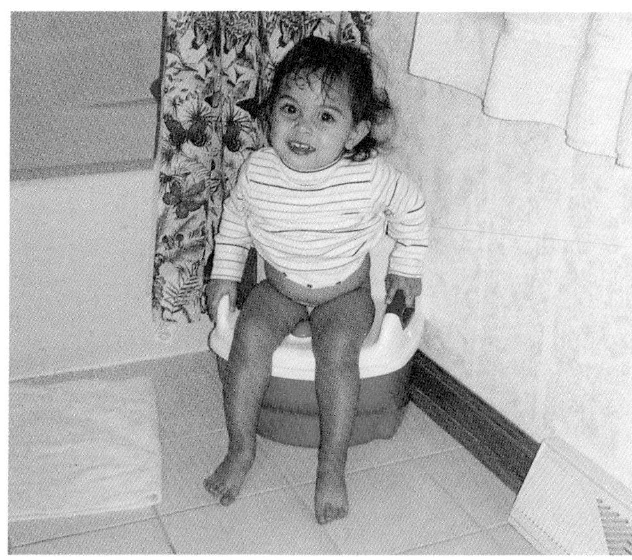

FIGURE 4.13 The toddler will feel most comfortable with a potty chair that sits on the floor.

Parents should always use gentle praise and no reproaches. Usually, the best time to achieve success with defecation on the toilet is following a meal. When the toddler has achieved success with bowel control, bladder control will come next. It may be many months before nighttime bladder control is achieved, and the toddler may still require a diaper at night. Parents should use appropriate words for body parts, urination, and defecation, then use those words consistently so the toddler understands what to say and do (AAP, 2023c).

After a couple of weeks of successful toileting, the toddler may start wearing training pants. When toddlers have an accident and do not make it to the toilet, gently remind them about toileting and let them help clean up. Toddlers should never be punished for bowel or bladder "accidents."

With so much attention focused on the genitalia during toilet teaching and the frequency of being without a diaper, it is natural for toddlers to become more focused on their own genitalia. Boys and girls both will explore their genitalia and discover the resulting pleasurable sensation. Masturbation in the toddler often causes a great deal of discomfort in the parent. The parent should not draw attention to the activity, as that may increase its frequency. The parent should calmly explain to the toddler that this is an activity that may only be done in private (Carter & Feigelman, 2020b). If the toddler is masturbating excessively or refuses to stop when in public, then there may be additional stressors in the toddler's life that should be explored.

Negativism

Negativism is common in the toddler period (Lieberman, 2018). As the toddler separates from the parent, recognizes their own individuality, and exerts autonomy, negativism abounds. Parents should understand that this negativism is a normal developmental occurrence and not necessarily deliberate defiance (although that also occurs). Avoid asking yes-or-no questions, as the toddler's usual response will be "no," whether they mean it or not. Offering the child simple choices will give the toddler a sense of control. The parent should not ask the toddler if they "want" to do something if there is actually no choice. "Do you want to use the red cup or the blue cup?" is more appropriate than "Do you want your milk now?" When it is time to go outside, don't ask, "Do you want to put your shoes on?" Instead, state in a matter-of-fact tone that shoes must be worn outside and give the toddler a choice of type of shoe or color of socks. If the child continues with negative answers, then the parent should remain calm and make the decision for the child.

Temper Tantrums

Even children who displayed an easygoing personality as infants may lose their temper frequently during the toddler years (Fig. 4.14). A toddler who was more intense as an infant may have more temper tantrums. Temper tantrums are a natural result of the frustration that toddlers experience. Toddlers are eager to explore new things, but their efforts are often thwarted (usually for safety reasons). Toddlers do not behave badly on purpose. They need time and maturity to learn the rules and regulations. Some of their frustration may come from lack of language skills to express themselves. Toddlers are just starting to learn how to verbalize feelings and to use alternative actions rather than just "pitching a fit."

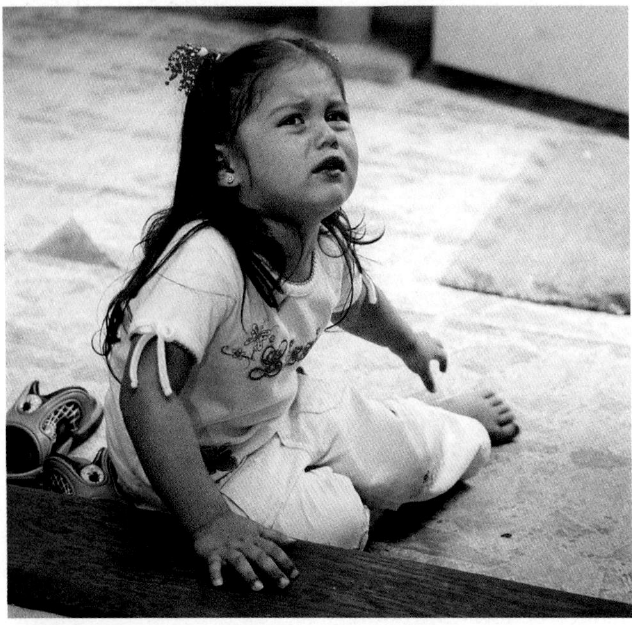

FIGURE 4.14 Tantrums are a normal component of toddler development.

The temper tantrum may be manifested as a screaming and crying fit or a full-blown episode in which the toddler throws themselves on the floor kicking, screaming, and pounding, perhaps even holding the breath. Fatigue or hunger may limit the toddler's coping abilities and promote negative behavior and temper tantrums (Buckloh, 2023).

Although tantrums are annoying to parents and caregivers, they are a normal part of the toddler's quest for independence. As toddlers mature, they become better able to express themselves and to understand their environment. Parents need to learn their toddler's behavioral cues in order to limit activity that is frustrating. When the parent notes the beginnings of frustration, a friendly warning might be given. Intervening early with an activity change might prevent a tantrum. Use distraction, refocusing, or removal from the situation.

When a temper tantrum does occur, the best course of action is to ignore the behavior and ensure that the child is safe during the tantrum. Physical punishment will probably just prolong the tantrum and, in fact, produce more intense negative behavior. If the tantrum occurs in public, it may be necessary for the parent to immobilize the child with a big bear hug and use a calm voice to soothe the toddler. It is important for parents to model self-control. Since toddlers' tantrums most often result from frustration, the role-modeled behavior of self-control helps to teach toddlers to control their temper when they can't get what they want (Buckloh, 2023).

Thumb Sucking and Pacifiers

Infants bring their hands to their mouths and begin thumb sucking as a form of self-soothing (Sears & Sears, 2020c). This habit may continue into the toddler years and beyond. The pacifier is used for the same reason. Toddlers may calm themselves in a stressful situation by thumb sucking or sucking on a pacifier. Opinions about thumb and finger sucking and pacifier use are significantly affected by family history and culture. For most children, there is no need to worry about a sucking habit until it is time for the permanent teeth to erupt. Prolonged and frequent sucking in the withdrawn child is more likely to yield changes to the tooth and jaw structure than sucking that is primarily used for self-soothing. Parents must sort through their own feelings about thumb sucking and pacifier use and then decide how they want to handle the habit.

To ensure safety with pacifier use:

- Use only one-piece pacifiers.
- Replace worn pacifiers with new ones.
- Never tie a pacifier around a toddler's neck.

Parents may want to limit thumb sucking and pacifier use to bedtime, in the car, and in stressful situations. The parent should calmly discuss these limits with the toddler and then remain consistent about enforcing them (Sears & Sears, 2020a, 2020c).

Sibling Rivalry

Many families have subsequent children when their first child is a toddler. The toddler has been accustomed to being the baby and receiving a great deal of attention, both at home and with the extended family. Since toddlers are normally egocentric, bringing a new baby into the home may be quite disruptive. To minimize issues with **sibling rivalry** (competition or jealousy between siblings), parents should attempt to keep the toddler's routine as close to normal as possible. Spend individual time with the toddler on a daily basis. Involve the toddler in the care of the baby. The toddler is capable of fetching a diaper or T-shirt, entertaining the baby with a toy, or helping sing a song to calm the baby (Schmitt, 2023). "Helping" the parent care for the baby gives the toddler a sense of importance (Fig. 4.15). The toddler will need significant support while holding the baby.

Regression

Some toddlers experience regression during a stressful event (e.g., the birth of a sibling, hospitalization). Stress in a toddler's life affects their ability to master new developmental tasks. During **regression**, the toddler may want to go back to an earlier stage. They may desire a bottle or pacifier forgotten long ago. The toddler may stop displaying previously achieved language or motor skills. A significant stress in the toddler's life may also disrupt the toilet teaching process (toilet teaching may not be achieved near the time a sibling is born). When regression occurs, parents should ignore the regressive behavior and offer praise for age-appropriate behavior or attainment of skills (AAP, 2021c).

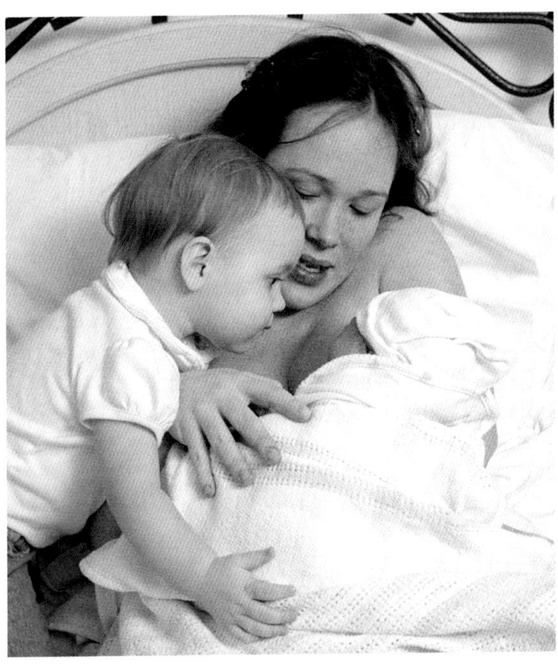

FIGURE 4.15 The toddler may be more likely to accept the new baby in a positive manner if they feel that this is "our baby," not just "Mommy's baby." This toddler is meeting their new sibling for the first time.

Refer to Jose Gonzales, the 2-year-old. List common developmental concerns of the toddler. What anticipatory guidance related to these concerns would you provide to Jose's parents?

Unfolding Patient Stories: Jackson Webber • Part 1

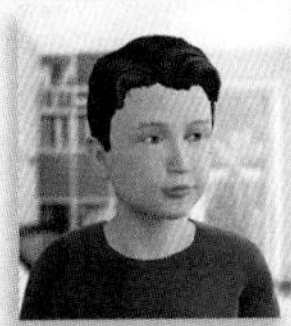

Jackson Webber, age 3, is diagnosed with generalized seizures and started on phenobarbital. His parent is single and employed full time. She is concerned about his recent developmental regression and how it will affect his return to child care. What education can the nurse provide on normal growth and development for a 3-year-old and the relationship between developmental milestones and the new onset of an illness? What questions can the nurse ask to evaluate the adequacy and safety of the child care center that Jackson attends when considering his new diagnosis of seizures? (Jackson Webber's story continues in Chapter 16.)

Care for Jackson and other patients in a realistic virtual environment: ***vSim** for Nursing* (thepoint.lww.com/vSimPediatric). Practice documenting these patients' care in DocuCare (thepoint.lww.com/DocuCareEHR).

KEY CONCEPTS

- The toddler's organ systems are continuing to mature, and growth slows during this period as compared with infancy.
- The psychosocial task of the toddler years is to attain a sense of autonomy and to experience separation and individuation.
- Cognitive development in toddlerhood progresses from sensorimotor in nature to preoperational.
- The toddler refines gross motor skills after learning to walk and builds fine motor skills through the use of utensils and various manipulative toys.
- The toddler progresses from limited expressive language capabilities to a vocabulary of 900 words by age 3 years.
- Toddlers use all of their senses to explore and learn about their environment.
- Visual acuity progresses to at least 20/50 in the toddler period.
- Negativism abounds in toddlers as they attempt to assert their independence.

- Very ritualistic, toddlers feel safer and more secure when clear limits are enforced and a structured routine is followed.
- The toddler is starting to learn right from wrong and bases actions on punishment avoidance.
- Toddler development may be promoted through active gross motor play, books, music, and block building.
- Safety is a primary concern in the toddler years as the child is more mobile, very curious, and experimenting with autonomy.
- Poisoning in the toddler period may be prevented through proper storage of medications and other potentially poisonous substances and appropriate supervision.
- Consistent bedtime rituals help ease the toddler's transition to sleep.
- All primary teeth are erupted by 30 months of age and may be kept healthy with appropriate tooth brushing and fluoride supplementation.
- The toddler may experience a decrease in appetite as growth slows, yet they still need appropriate nutritional intake for continued development.
- Toilet teaching can be achieved after myelination of the spinal cord is complete, usually around 2 years of age.
- Thumb sucking, pacifier use, security items, and temper tantrums are expected issues in the toddler years.
- Toddler discipline should focus on clear limits and consistency. It should not involve spanking. It should be balanced with a caring and nurturing environment along with frequent praise for appropriate behavior.
- Parental role modeling of appropriate behavior, especially related to dealing with frustration, is beneficial to toddlers.
- Parents play an important role in toddler development, not only by providing a loving environment but also by role modeling appropriate behavior in most areas of daily life.

REFERENCES AND RECOMMENDED READINGS

American Academy of Child and Adolescent Psychiatry. (2018). *Physical punishment.* https://www.aacap.org/aacap/families_and_youth/facts_for_families/fff-guide/Physical-Punishment-105.aspx

American Academy of Pediatrics. (2018). *Where we stand: Spanking.* https://www.healthychildren.org/English/family-life/family-dynamics/communication-discipline/Pages/Where-We-Stand-Spanking.aspx

American Academy of Pediatrics. (2021a). *Poison prevention & treatment tips for parents.* https://www.healthychildren.org/English/safety-prevention/all-around/Pages/Poison-Prevention.aspx

American Academy of Pediatrics. (2021b). *TIPP—2 to 4 years: Safety for your child.* https://doi.org/10.1542/peo_document303

American Academy of Pediatrics. (2021c). *Welcoming a new sibling: How to help your child adjust.* https://doi.org/10.1542/peo_document133

American Academy of Pediatrics. (2022). *Safety for your child: 1 to 2 years.* https://www.healthychildren.org/English/ages-stages/toddler/Pages/Safety-for-Your-Child-1-to-2-Years.aspx

American Academy of Pediatrics. (2023a). *Breastfeeding.* https://www.healthychildren.org/English/ages-stages/baby/breastfeeding/Pages/default.aspx

American Academy of Pediatrics. (2023b). *Car seats: Information for families.* https://www.healthychildren.org/English/safety-prevention/on-the-go/Pages/Car-Safety-Seats-Information-for-Families.aspx

American Academy of Pediatrics. (2023c). *Potty training.* https://www.healthychildren.org/English/ages-stages/toddler/toilet-training/Pages/default.aspx

American Association of Poison Control Centers. (n.d.). *In the home safety tips.* https://aapcc.org/prevention/in-the-home

Ben-Joseph, E. P. (2018). *Nutrition guide for toddlers.* https://kidshealth.org/en/parents/toddler-food.html

Buckloh, L. M. (2023). *Disciplining your toddler.* https://kidshealth.org/en/parents/toddler-tantrums.html#

Carter, R. G., & Feigelman, S. (2020a). The preschool years. In R. M. Kliegman, J. W. St. Geme III, N. J. Blum, S. S. Shah, R. C. Tasker, K. M. Wilson, & R. E. Behrman (Eds.), *Nelson's textbook of pediatrics* (21st ed.). Elsevier.

Carter, R. G., & Feigelman, S. (2020b). The second year. In R. M. Kliegman, J. W. St. Geme III, N. J. Blum, S. S. Shah, R. C. Tasker, K. M. Wilson, & R. E. Behrman (Eds.), *Nelson's textbook of pediatrics* (21st ed.). Elsevier.

Child Development Institute. (2022). *Temperament and your child's personality.* https://childdevelopmentinfo.com/uncategorized/temperament_and_your_child/

Division of Agriculture. (2023). Fruits and vegetables—Important sources of nutrients and vitamins. *University of Arkansas.* https://www.uaex.uada.edu/counties/miller/news/fcs/fruits-veggies/fruits-and-vegetables-important-sources-of-nutrients-and-vitamins.aspx

Durani, Y. (2023). *Preventing choking.* https://kidshealth.org/en/parents/safety-choking.html

Erikson, E. H. (1963). *Childhood and society* (2nd ed.). W. W. Norton and Company.

Gavin, M. L. (2019). *Toilet training.* https://kidshealth.org/en/parents/toilet-teaching.html

Global Initiative to End All Corporal Punishment of Children. (2018). *Global initiative to end corporal punishment.* https://endcorporalpunishment.org

Hagan, J. F., Shaw, J. S., & Duncan, P. M. (2017). *Bright futures: Guidelines for health supervision of infants, children, and adolescents* (4th ed.). American Academy of Pediatrics.

Kohlberg, L. (1984). *Moral development.* Harper & Row.

Lieberman, A. (2018). *The emotional life of a toddler.* Simon & Schuster.

Linguistic Society of America. (2023). *FAQ: Raising bilingual children.* https://www.linguisticsociety.org/resource/faq-raising-bilingual-children

Martorell, G. (2022). *Life: The essentials of human development* (2nd ed.). McGraw-Hill Publishing.

National Association for the Education of Young Children. (n.d.). *Good toys for young children by age and stage.* http://www.naeyc.org/toys

National Association of Pediatric Nurse Practitioners, Breastfeeding Education Special Interest Group, Busch, D. W., Silbert-Flagg, J., Ryngaert, M., & Scott, A. (2019). NAPNAP position statement on breastfeeding. *Journal of Pediatric Health Care, 33*(1), A11–A15. https://doi.org/10.1016/j.pedhc.2018.08.011

National Association of Pediatric Nurse Practitioners, Child Maltreatment and Neglect Special Interest Group, VanGraafeiland, B., Hornor, G. A., Herendeen, P. A., Chiocca, E. M., Loyke, J. A., Dietzman, H., Boucher, N. L., Nielsen, A., & Record, S. C. (2022). NAPNAP position statement on using positive parenting to eliminate corporal punishment. *Journal of Pediatric Health Care, 36*, 202–204. https://doi.org/10.1016/j.pedhc.2021.09.001

Nix, R. L., Francis, L. A., Feinberg, M. E., Gill, S., Jones, D. E., Hostetler, M. L., & Stifter, C. A. (2021). Improving toddlers' healthy eating habits and self-regulation: A randomized controlled trial. *Pediatrics, 147*(1), e20193326. https://doi.org/10.1542/peds.2019-3326

Nowak, A. J., & Warren, J. J. (2023). Preventive dental care and counseling for infants and young children. *UpToDate.* Retrieved September 23, 2023, from https://www.uptodate.com/contents/preventive-dental-care-and-counseling-for-infants-and-young-children

Pantley, E. (2020). The *no-cry sleep solution* (2nd ed.). McGraw Hill.

Parks, E. P., Shaikhkhalil, A., Sainath, N. N., Mitchell, J. A., Brownell, J. N., & Stallings, V. A. (2020). Feeding healthy infants, children, and adolescents. In R. M. Kliegman, J. W. St. Geme III, N. J. Blum, S. S. Shah, R. C. Tasker, K. M. Wilson, & R. E. Behrman (Eds.), *Nelson's textbook of pediatrics* (21st ed.). Elsevier.

Piaget, J. (1969). *The theory of stages in cognitive development.* McGraw-Hill.

Powers, J. M. (2023). Iron deficiency in infants and children <12 years: Screening, prevention, clinical manifestations, and diagnosis. *UpToDate.* Retrieved September 23, 2023, from https://www.uptodate.com/contents/iron-deficiency-in-infants-and-children-less-than12-years-screening-prevention-clinical-manifestations-and-diagnosis

Reading Rockets. (2023). *Reading tips for parents of toddlers.* https://www.readingrockets.org/topics/activities/articles/reading-tips-parents-toddlers

Reynolds, A., Angulo, A., Breheney, M., Green, J., & Goldson, E. (2022). Child development and behavior. In M. Bunik, W. W. Hay, M. J. Levin, & M. J. Abzug (Eds.), *Current diagnosis & treatment: Pediatrics* (26th ed.). McGraw-Hill Education.

SafeBedSharing.org. (2023). *Bed sharing or co-sleeping.* http://www.safebedsharing.org/safetyguidelines.html

Safe Kids. (2023a). *Swimming.* https://www.safekids.org/poolsafety

Safe Kids. (2023b). *Water safety tips at home.* https://www.safekids.org/tip/water-safety-home-tips

Samet, J. M., & Sockrider, M. (2023). Secondhand smoke exposure: Effects in children. *UpToDate.* Retrieved September 23, 2023, from https://www.uptodate.com/contents/secondhand-smoke-exposure-effects-in-children

Satter, E. (2023). *Child feeding ages and stages.* https://www.ellynsatterinstitute.org/how-to-feed/child-feeding-ages-and-stages/

Schaechter, J. (2023). *Guns in the home: How to keep kids safe.* https://www.healthychildren.org/English/safety-prevention/at-home/Pages/Handguns-in-the-Home.aspx

Schmitt, B. (2023). *Sibling rivalry toward a newborn.* https://doi.org/10.1542/ppe_schmitt_205

Sears, W., & Sears, M. (2020a). *Choosing & using a safe pacifier.* http://www.askdrsears.com/topics/parenting/child-rearing-and-development/bringing-baby-home/pacifiers-in-or-out/choosing-using

Sears, W., & Sears, M. (2020b). *8 tools for toddler discipline.* http://www.askdrsears.com/topics/parenting/discipline-behavior/8-tools-toddler-discipline

Sears, W., & Sears, M. (2020c). *Thumbsucking: Harmful or helpful?* http://www.askdrsears.com/topics/parenting/discipline-behavior/bothersome-behaviors/thumbsucking

Skelton, J. A., & Klish, W. J. (2023). Definition, epidemiology, and etiology of obesity in children and adolescents. *UpToDate.* Retrieved September 23, 2023, from https://www.uptodate.com/contents/definition-epidemiology-and-etiology-of-obesity-in-children-and-adolescents

Smith, M. A., & Segal, J. (2023). *Grandparents raising grandchildren: The rewards & challenges of parenting the second time around.* https://www.helpguide.org/articles/parenting-family/grandparents-raising-grandchildren.htm?pdf=13581

U.S. Department of Health and Human Services. (n.d.). *Healthy People 2030.* https://health.gov/healthypeople

Viguera, A. (2023). Postpartum depression: Adverse consequences in mothers and their children. *UpToDate.* Retrieved September 23, 2023, from https://www.uptodate.com/contents/postpartum-depression-adverse-consequences-in-mothers-and-their-children

Zubler, J. M., Wiggins, L. D., Macias, M. M., Whitaker, T. M., Shaw, J. S., Squires, J. K., Pajke, J. A., Wolf, R. B., Slaughter, K. S., Broughton, A. S., Gerndt, K. L., Mlodoch, B. J., & Lipkin, P. H. (2022). Evidence-informed milestones for developmental surveillance tools. *Pediatrics, 149*(3), e2021052138. https://doi.org/10.1542/peds.2021-052138

DEVELOPING CLINICAL JUDGMENT

PRACTICING FOR NCLEX

1. The nurse is caring for a hospitalized 30-month-old who is resistant to care, is angry, and yells "no" all the time. The nurse identifies this toddler's behavior as
   a. problematic, as it interferes with needed nursing care.
   b. normal for this stage of growth and development.
   c. normal because the child is hospitalized and out of his routine.

2. The parent of a 15-month-old is concerned about a speech delay. They describe the toddler as being able to understand what is said, sometimes following commands, but using only one or two words with any consistency. What is the nurse's best response to this information?
   a. The toddler should have a developmental evaluation as soon as possible.
   b. If the parent would read to the child, then speech would develop faster.
   c. Receptive language normally develops earlier than expressive language.
   d. The parent should ask the child's health care provider for a speech therapy evaluation.

3. A 2-year-old is having a temper tantrum. What advice should the nurse give the parent?
   a. For safety reasons, the toddler should be restrained during the tantrum.
   b. Punishment should be initiated, as tantrums should be controlled.
   c. The parent should promise the toddler a reward if the tantrum stops.
   d. The tantrum should be ignored as long as the toddler is safe.

4. What is the best advice about nutrition for the toddler?
   a. Encourage cup drinking and give water between meals and snacks.
   b. Encourage unlimited milk intake, because toddlers need the protein for growth.
   c. Avoid sugar-sweetened fruit drinks and allow as much natural fruit juice as desired.
   d. Allow the toddler unlimited access to the sippy cup to ensure adequate hydration.

5. To gain cooperation from a toddler, what is the best approach by the nurse?
   a. Immediately pick the toddler up from the parent's lap.
   b. Kneel in front of the toddler while they are on the parent's lap.
   c. Do the nursing tasks quickly so the toddler can play.
   d. Ask the toddler if it is okay if you begin the needed task.

6. The nurse is teaching the parents of a 2-year-old about toilet training. Which statements by the nurse are correct? Select all that apply.
   a. "Bowel training is usually accomplished before bladder training."
   b. "Wanting to please the parents helps motivate the child to use the toilet."
   c. "Watching older siblings use the toilet can provide role modeling for the child."
   d. "Children must be forced to sit on the toilet when first learning."
   e. "Children should never be scolded if they have an accident during toilet training."
   f. "Once toilet training is established, children never regress."

7. The nursing instructor has taught a group of nursing students about toddler physical growth and development. The nursing students verbalize the toddler is at increased risk for ___ related to ___ and ___.

   Blank 1:
   a. respiratory distress
   b. diarrhea
   c. infection

   Blanks 2 and 3:
   a. slower pulse and respiratory rate than in infancy
   b. less efficient defense mechanisms than in infancy
   c. abdominal respirations
   d. large lymphatic tissues
   e. immature intestinal functions
   f. short, straight eustachian tube

CRITICAL THINKING EXERCISES

1. Develop a teaching plan about safety to present to a toddler-age preschool class.
2. Construct a 3-day menu that is realistic and that will provide the nutrients needed for a 2-year-old.
3. Develop a plan for educating the parent of a 34-month-old who has been resistant to toilet teaching. Include assessments the nurse will make as well as the plan for teaching.

STUDY ACTIVITIES

1. Visit a preschool that provides care for toddlers with special needs as well as typical toddlers. Perform a developmental assessment on a typical toddler and one with special needs (both the same age). Compare and contrast your findings.
2. Care for two average 2-year-olds in the clinical setting. Describe each toddler's behavior, response to the parent, and response to the nurse, and list strategies used to gain adherence and minimize stress to the toddler.
3. Observe in the toddler classroom of a typical preschool. Choose two toddlers the same age with different temperaments. Record the toddlers' differences and similarities in response to structure and authority, interactions with classmates, attention levels, and language and activity levels.

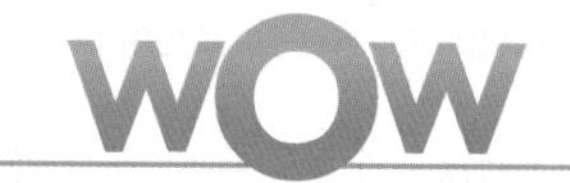

WORDS OF WISDOM

Preschoolers have been called the "little scientists" for their bold and inquisitive natures.

5

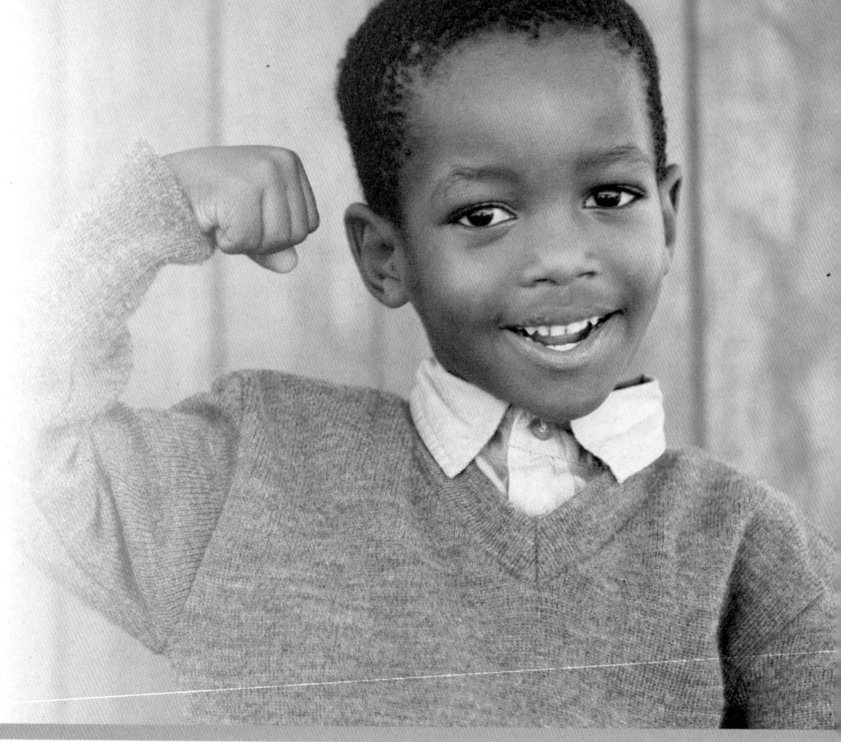

Growth and Development of the Preschooler

LEARNING OBJECTIVES

Upon completion of the chapter, you will be able to:

1. Describe expected physical growth, physiologic changes, and sensory development in the preschooler.
2. Examine psychosocial, cognitive, and moral/spiritual development in the preschooler.
3. Identify the gross and fine motor skills milestones of the preschooler.
4. Explain expected language and social/emotional development, and cultural influences on development in the preschool years.
5. Implement a nursing care plan that addresses common concerns or delays in the preschooler's development.
6. Develop a nutrition plan for the preschool-age child.
7. Provide appropriate anticipatory guidance for common developmental issues that arise in the preschool period.

KEY TERMS

animism (an′i-mizm)
empathy
imaginary friend
magical thinking
preoperational thought
school readiness
transduction

Nila Patel is a 4-year-old brought to the clinic by her parents for her school check-up. As the nurse caring for her, assess Nila's growth and development and then teach the parents what changes to expect in Nila over the next few months.

INTRODUCTION

The preschool period is the period between 3 and 6 years of age. This is a time of continued growth and development. Physical growth continues more slowly than in earlier years. Gains in cognitive, language, and psychosocial development are substantial throughout the preschool period. Many tasks that began during the toddler years are mastered and perfected during the preschool years. The child has learned to tolerate separation from parents, has a longer attention span, and continues to learn skills that will lead to later success in the school-age period. Preparation for success in school continues during the preschool period because most children enter elementary school by the end of the preschool period.

GROWTH AND DEVELOPMENT OVERVIEW

The healthy preschooler is slender and agile with an upright posture. The formerly clumsy toddler becomes more graceful, demonstrating the ability to run more smoothly. Athletic abilities may begin to develop. Major development occurs in the area of fine motor coordination. Psychosocial development is focused on the accomplishment of initiative. Preconceptual thought and intuitiveness dominate cognitive development. The preschooler is an inquisitive learner and absorbs new concepts like a sponge absorbs water.

PHYSICAL GROWTH

The average preschool-age child will grow 6.35 to 7.62 cm (2.5 to 3 in) per year. The average 3-year-old is 94 cm (37 in) tall, the average 4-year-old is 102.9 cm (40.5 in) tall, and the average 5-year-old is 109.2 cm (43 in) tall. Average weight gain during this time period is about 1.8 to 2.3 kg (4 to 5 lb) per year (Carter & Feigelman, 2020). The average weight of a 3-year-old is 14.5 kg (32 lb), increasing to an average weight of 18.6 kg (41 lb) by age 5. The loss of baby fat and the growth of muscle during the preschool years give the child a stronger, more mature appearance (Fig. 5.1). The length of the skull also increases slightly, with the lower jaw becoming more pronounced. The upper jaw widens through the preschool years in preparation for the emergence of permanent teeth, usually starting around age 6.

During your assessment of Nila (the 4-year-old introduced at the beginning of the chapter), you measure her weight to be 20 kg (44 lb) and her height to be 101.6 cm (40 in).

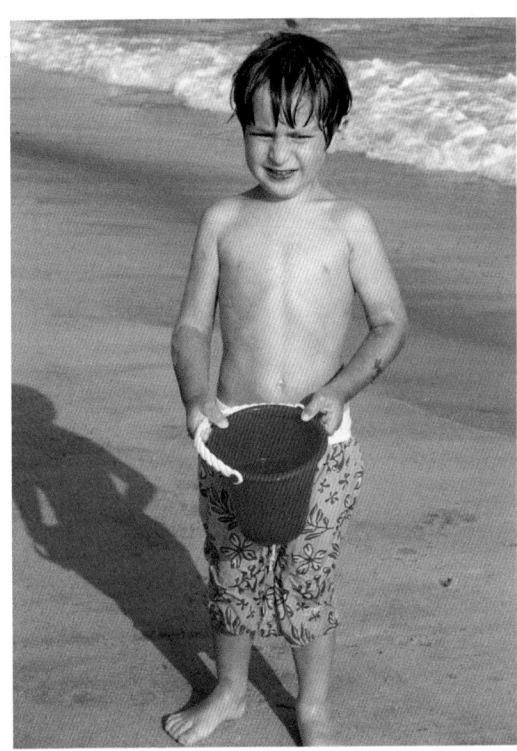

FIGURE 5.1 The preschool child has a slenderer appearance and erect posture than the toddler.

PHYSIOLOGIC CHANGES

Most of the body systems have matured by the preschool years. Myelination of the spinal cord allows for bowel and bladder control to be complete in most children by age 3 years. The respiratory structures are continuing to grow in size, and the number of alveoli continues to increase, reaching the adult number at about 7 years of age. The eustachian tubes remain relatively short and straight. Heart rate decreases and blood pressure increases slightly during the preschool years. An innocent heart murmur may be heard upon auscultation, and splitting of the second heart sound may become evident. The preschooler should have 20 deciduous teeth present.

The small intestine is continuing to grow in length. Stool passage usually occurs once or twice per day in the average preschooler. The 4-year-old generally has adequate bowel control. The urethra remains short, making preschoolers more susceptible to urinary tract infections than adults. Bladder control is usually present in 4- and 5-year-old children, but an occasional injury may occur, particularly in stressful situations or when the child is absorbed in an interesting activity.

The bones continue to increase in length, and the muscles continue to strengthen and mature. However, the musculoskeletal system is still not fully mature, making the preschooler susceptible to injury, particularly with overexertion or excess activity.

SENSORY DEVELOPMENT

Hearing is intact at birth and should remain so throughout the preschool years. The senses of smell and touch continue to develop throughout the preschool years. The young preschooler may have a less discriminating sense of taste than the older child, putting them at increased risk for inadvertent ingestion. Visual acuity continues to progress and should be equal bilaterally. The typical 5-year-old has visual acuity of 20/40 or 20/30. Color vision is intact at this age.

PSYCHOSOCIAL DEVELOPMENT

According to Erik Erikson (1963), the psychosocial task of the preschool years is establishing a sense of initiative versus guilt. The preschooler is an inquisitive learner, enthusiastic about learning new things. Preschoolers feel a sense of accomplishment when succeeding in activities (Fig. 5.2), and feeling pride in one's accomplishment helps the child to use initiative. However, when the child extends themselves further than current capabilities allow, they may feel a sense of guilt. The superego or conscience development is completed during the preschool period, and this is the basis for moral development (understanding right and wrong). Table 5.1 gives examples illustrating the stage of initiative versus guilt.

COGNITIVE DEVELOPMENT

According to Jean Piaget's theory (1969), the preschool-age child continues in the preoperational stage. **Preoperational thought** dominates during this stage and is based on a self-centered understanding of the world. In the preconceptual phase of preoperational thought, the child remains egocentric and is able to approach a problem from a single point of view only. The young preschooler may understand the concept of counting and begins to engage in fantasy play.

Magical thinking is a normal part of preschool development. In magical thinking, the preschooler believes that their thoughts are all-powerful. The fantasy experienced through magical thinking allows the preschooler to make room in their world for the actual or the real. Through make-believe and magical thinking, preschool-age children satisfy their curiosity about differences in the world around them.

The preschooler often has an **imaginary friend** as well (Reynolds et al., 2022). The imaginary friend is not real and exists only in the child's imagination. This friend serves as a creative way for the preschooler to sample different activities and behaviors and practice conversational skills. Despite this imaginative practice, the preschooler is able to switch easily between fantasy and reality throughout the day.

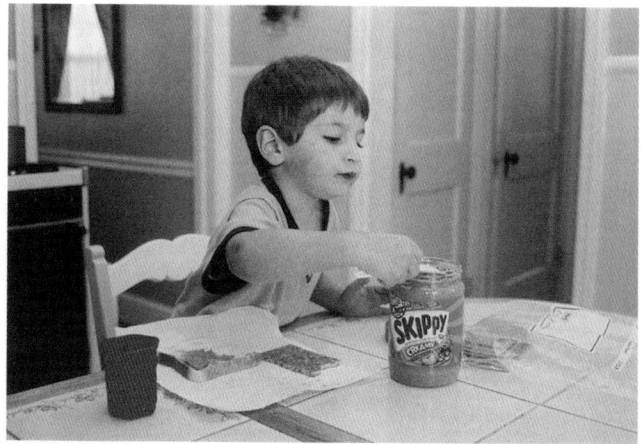

FIGURE 5.2 Allowing the preschooler to assist with simple household tasks, such as preparing a sandwich, encourages the development of initiative.

The child in the intuitive phase can count 10 or more objects, correctly name at least four colors, and better understand the concept of time. They know about things that are used in everyday life, such as appliances, money, and food. The preschooler uses **transduction** when reasoning; they extrapolate from a particular situation to another, even though the events may be unrelated. The preschooler also attributes life-like qualities to inanimate objects (**animism**). Table 5.1 gives further examples illustrating this developmental stage.

The acquisition of language skills in the toddler period is enhanced in the preschool period. The expansion of vocabulary enables the preschooler to progress further with symbolic thought. At this age, children do not completely understand the concept of death or its permanence: They may ask when their grandparent or pet who died is returning.

MORAL AND SPIRITUAL DEVELOPMENT

The preschool-age child can understand the concepts of right and wrong and is developing a conscience. That inner voice that warns or threatens is developing in the preschool years. Kohlberg (1984) identified this stage (between 2 and 7 years) as the preconventional stage, which is characterized by a punishment-and-obedience orientation. Preschool children see morality as external to themselves; they defer to power (that of the adult). The child's moral standards are those of their parents or other adults who influence them, not necessarily their own. Preschoolers adhere to those standards to gain rewards or avoid punishment. Since the preschool-age child is facing the psychosocial task of initiative versus guilt, it is natural for the child to experience guilt when something goes wrong.

TABLE 5.1 • Developmental Theories

Theorist	Stage	Activities
Erikson	Initiative vs. guilt Age: 3–6 years	Likes to please parents Begins to plan activities, make up games Initiates activities with others Acts out the roles of other people (real and imaginary) Develops sexual identity Develops conscience May take frustrations out on siblings Likes exploring new things Enjoys sports, shopping, cooking, working Feels remorse when making the wrong choice or behaving badly Cooperates with other children Negotiates solutions to conflicts
Piaget	Preoperational substage: preconceptual phase Age: 2–4 years	Exhibits egocentric thinking, which lessens as the child approaches age 4 Has a short attention span Learns through observing and imitating Displays animism Forms concepts that are not as complete or as logical as the adult's Is able to make simple classifications By age 4 understands the concept of opposites (hot/cold, soft/hard) Reasoning is that of specific to specific. Has an active imagination
	Preoperational substage: intuitive phase Age: 4–7 years	Is able to classify and relate objects Has intuitive thought processes; knows if something is right or wrong, though cannot state why Tolerates others' differences but does not understand them Is curious about facts Knows acceptable cultural rules Uses words appropriately but often without true understanding of their meaning Has a more realistic sense of causality May begin to question parents' values
Kohlberg	Punishment–obedience orientation Age: 2–7 years (preconventional morality)	Determines good vs. bad depending on associated punishment Children may learn inappropriate behavior at this stage if parental intervention does not occur (if the child hits, bites, or is verbally disrespectful but is not punished for these activities, the child will view those behaviors as good and continue to participate in them).

Data from Erikson, E. H. (1963). *Childhood and society* (2nd ed.). W. W. Norton and Company; Carter, R. G., & Feigelman, S. (2020). The preschool years. In R. M. Kliegman, J. W. St. Geme III, N. J. Blum, S. S. Shah, R. C. Tasker, K. M. Wilson, & R. E. Behrman (Eds.), *Nelson's textbook of pediatrics* (21st ed.). Elsevier; Kohlberg, L. (1984). *Moral development.* Harper & Row; Piaget, J. (1969). *The theory of stages in cognitive development.* McGraw-Hill.

As the child's moral development progresses, they learn how to deal with angry feelings. Sometimes the way the child chooses to deal with those feelings may be inappropriate, such as fighting and biting. Lying begins to occur in the preschool period. Younger preschoolers have difficulty differentiating between reality and their imagination and fantasies, whereas older preschoolers are more aware of right and wrong. Preschoolers also use their limited life experiences to make sense of and help them cope with crises. They need to learn the socially acceptable limits of behavior and are also learning the rewards of manners. The preschool-age child begins to help out in the family and begins to understand the concept of give-and-take in relationships.

During the preoperational phase of cognitive development, the preschooler's concept of faith is intuitive and projective in nature (Chromey, 2021). The preschool-age child's imagination allows for anything to be possible, so they do not have a logical view of the world as adults do. Preschool-age children have limited life experiences, so they may project a feeling onto a new person or situation. They may use this projection to help them understand what is going on around them. Preschoolers may project their parents' or caregivers' feelings or characteristics onto "God;" if Mommy gets angry, then God is probably also angry.

The family's religious beliefs may affect the child's diet, the mode of discipline that parents use, and even how the parents view their children. Knowing about a family's practices of prayer or meditation is helpful to the pediatric nurse, who can help continue the ritual when the child is ill or hospitalized (Fig. 5.3).

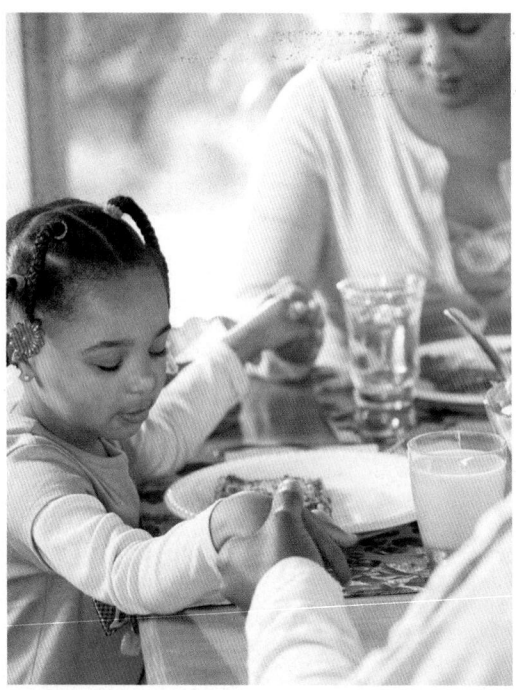

FIGURE 5.3 The preschool child may participate in religious rituals without having full understanding of their meaning.

MOTOR SKILL DEVELOPMENT

As the preschooler's musculoskeletal system continues to mature, existing motor skills become refined and new ones develop. The preschooler has more voluntary control over their movements and is less clumsy than the toddler. Significant refinement in fine motor skills occurs during the preschool period (Table 5.2).

Gross Motor Skills

The preschooler is agile while standing, walking, running, and jumping (Fig. 5.4). They can go up and down stairs and walk forward and backward easily. Standing on tiptoes or on one foot still requires extra concentration. The preschooler seems to be in constant motion. They also use the body to understand new concepts (such as using the arms in a "chug-chug" motion when describing how the train wheels work).

Fine Motor Skills

The 3-year-old can move each finger independently and is capable of grasping utensils and crayons in adult fashion, with the thumb on one side and the fingers on the other. They can also scribble freely, copy a circle, trace a square, and feed themselves without spilling much. These skills become refined over the next 2 years, and by 5 years of age, the child can write letters, cut with scissors more accurately, and tie shoelaces (Fig. 5.5).

COMMUNICATION AND LANGUAGE DEVELOPMENT

The acquisition of language allows the preschool-age child to express thoughts and creativity. The preschool years are a time of refinement of language skills. The

TABLE 5.2 • Motor Skill Development

Age	Expected Gross Motor Skills	Expected Fine Motor Skills
3 years	• Climbs well • Pedals tricycle • Runs easily • Walks up and down stairs with alternate feet • Bends over easily without falling	• Undresses self, puts on loose clothing items independently • Uses a fork • Builds a tower of 9 or 10 cubes • Strings beads or macaroni • Screws/unscrews lids, nuts, bolts • Copies circle
4 years	• Throws ball overhand • Kicks ball forward • Catches bounced ball • Stands on one foot for up to 5 seconds • Alternates feet going up and down steps • Moves backward and forward with agility	• Uses scissors successfully • Copies capital letters • Draws circles and squares • Traces a cross or diamond • Draws a person with two to four body parts • Laces shoes
5 years	• Hops on one foot • Stands on one foot for 10 seconds or longer • Swings and climbs well • May skip • Somersaults • May learn to skate and swim	• Prints some letters • Draws a person with a body and at least six parts • Fastens some buttons • Dresses/undresses without assistance • Can learn to tie laces • Uses fork, spoon, and knife (supervised) well • Copies triangle and other geometric patterns • Mostly cares for own toileting needs

Data from Carter, R. G., & Feigelman, S. (2020). The preschool years. In R. M. Kliegman, J. W. St. Geme III, N. J. Blum, S. S. Shah, R. C. Tasker, K. M. Wilson, & R. E. Behrman (Eds.), *Nelson's textbook of pediatrics* (21st ed.). Elsevier; Reynolds, A., Angulo, A., Breheney, M., Green, J., & Goldson, E. (2022). Child development and behavior. In M. Bunik, W. W. Hay, M. J. Levin, & M. J. Abzug (Eds.), *Current diagnosis & treatment: Pediatrics* (26th ed.). McGraw-Hill Education; Zubler, J. M., Wiggins, L. D., Macias, M. M., Whitaker, T. M., Shaw, J. S., Squires, J. K., Pajke, J. A., Wolf, R. B., Slaughter, K. S., Broughton, A. S., Gerndt, K. L., Mlodoch, B. J., & Lipkin, P. H. (2022). Evidence-informed milestones for developmental surveillance tools. *Pediatrics, 149*(3), e2021052138. https://doi.org/10.1542/peds.2021-052138

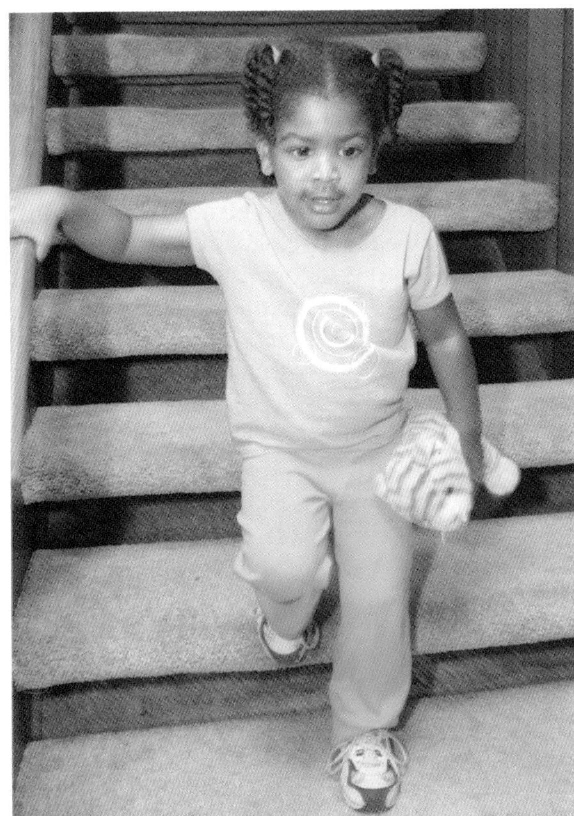

FIGURE 5.4 The preschooler runs well, navigates stairs, and can balance on one foot.

3-year-old exhibits telegraphic speech, using short sentences that contain only the essential information. Language development in the preschool years is extensive. At 2 years of age, a child uses 50 to 100 words and by 5 years of age uses about 2,000 words (Carter & Feigelman, 2020). By the end of the preschool period, the child is using sentences that are adult-like in structure (Table 5.3).

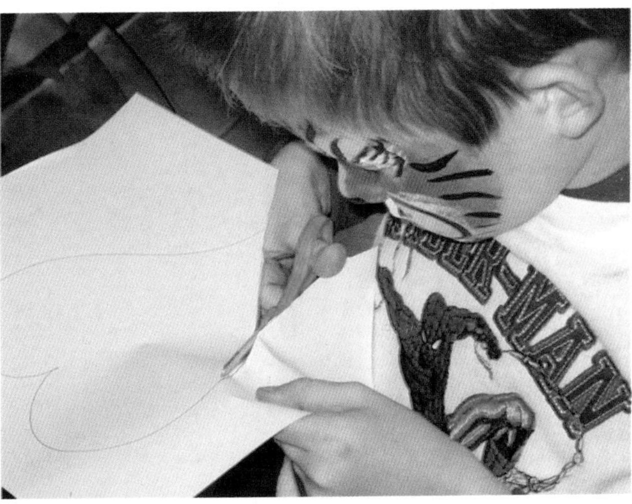

FIGURE 5.5 The 5-year-old has the fine motor dexterity to cut well with scissors.

TABLE 5.3 • Communication Skills in the Preschool Child

Age	Communication Abilities
4 years	• Speaks in complete sentences (four or more words) using adult-like grammar • Tells a story that is easy to follow • 75% of speech understood by others outside of family • Asks questions with "who," "how," and "how many" • Stays on topic in a conversation • Understands the concepts of "same" and "different" • Asks many questions • Knows names of familiar animals • Names common objects in books and magazines • Knows at least one color • Uses language to engage in make-believe • Follows a three-part command • Can count a few numbers • Vocabulary of 1,500 words
5 years	• People outside of the family can understand most of the child's speech. • Explains how an item is used • Participates in long, detailed conversations • Tells stories • Talks about past, future, and imaginary events • Answers questions that use "why" and "when" • Uses and recognizes simple rhymes • Can count to 10 • Recalls part of a story • Speech should be completely intelligible, even if the child has articulation difficulties. • Speech is generally grammatically correct. • Vocabulary of 2,100 words • Says name and address

Data from Centers for Disease Control and Prevention. (2023). *CDC's developmental milestones.* http://www.cdc.gov/ncbddd/actearly/milestones/index.html; Carter, R. G., & Feigelman, S. (2020). The preschool years. In R. M. Kliegman, J. W. St. Geme III, N. J. Blum, S. S. Shah, R. C. Tasker, K. M. Wilson, & R. E. Behrman (Eds.), *Nelson's textbook of pediatrics* (21st ed.). Elsevier; Zubler, J. M., Wiggins, L. D., Macias, M. M., Whitaker, T. M., Shaw, J. S., Squires, J. K., Pajke, J. A., Wolf, R. B., Slaughter, K. S., Broughton, A. S., Gerndt, K. L., Mlodoch, B. J., & Lipkin, P. H. (2022). Evidence-informed milestones for developmental surveillance tools. *Pediatrics, 149*(3), e2021052138. https://doi.org/10.1542/peds.2021-052138

The 3- to 6-year-old is starting to develop fluency (the ability to smoothly link sounds, syllables, and words when speaking). Initially, the child may exhibit disfluency or stuttering. Speech may sound choppy, or the child may say repeated consonants or "um." Stuttering usually has its onset in the preschool years and will resolve in 80% of children by age 8 years (Carter & Feigelman, 2020). Parents should slow down their speech and should give the child time to speak without rushing or interrupting. Some sounds remain difficult for the preschooler to enunciate properly: "f," "v," "s," and "z" sounds are usually mastered by age 5 years, but some children do not master the sounds of "sh," "l," "th," and "r" until age 6 or later. The potentially bilingual child may lag slightly behind the single-language speaker but will be able to differentiate and use both languages by the end of the preschool period (Linguistic Society of America, 2023).

Communication in preschool children is concrete in nature, as they are not yet capable of abstract thought. Despite its concrete nature, the preschooler's communication can be quite elaborate and involved; they may talk about dreams and fantasies. In addition to acquiring vocabulary and learning the correct use of grammar, the preschool child's receptive language skills are also becoming refined.

The preschooler is in tune with the parents' moods and easily picks up on negative emotions in conversations. If the preschooler hears parents discussing things that are frightening to the child, the preschooler's imagination may fuel the development of fears and lead to misinterpretation of what the child has heard.

As you assess Nila, the 4-year-old introduced at the beginning of the chapter, what would you expect her gross motor, fine motor, and language skills to be at this age?

EMOTIONAL AND SOCIAL DEVELOPMENT

By the time a child enters kindergarten, they should have developed a useful set of social skills that will help them have successful experiences in the school setting as well as in life in general. These skills include cooperation, sharing (of things and feelings), kindness, generosity, affection display, conversation, expression of feelings, helping others, and making friends.

Preschoolers tend to have strong emotions. They can be excited, happy, and giddy in one moment, then extremely disappointed in the next. The preschool-age child has a vivid imagination, and fears are very real to preschoolers. Most children this age have learned to control their behaviors. They should be able to name the feelings they are having rather than acting on them. Strong feelings may be expressed through outlets such as clay or Play-Doh, water play, drawing or painting, or dramatic play such as with puppets.

Preschoolers are developing a sense of identity. They may identify as boys or girls. They know that they belong to a particular family, community, or culture. They take pride in using self-control rather than giving in to their impulses. The preschool-age child is capable of helping others and being involved in routines and transitions.

Parents can encourage and assist preschool-age children with developing the social and emotional skills that will be needed when the child enters school. Preschool-age children thrive on one-to-one communication with a parent. During interactive communication, children learn to express their feelings and ideas. Interactive communication fosters not only emotional and moral development but also self-esteem and cognitive development. Asking the preschool child questions requires the child to think through their own intention or motivation and encourages vocabulary development. Parents may use individual communication as a time to explore right and wrong, thus further contributing to moral development. Being listened to while answering parents' questions gives preschoolers a sense that they are valued, that what they think and have to say matters.

Establishing a few simple rules and then enforcing them consistently gives preschoolers the structure and security they need while promoting moral development. Parents or caregivers can help the child give a name to the emotion that is being experienced. Fears are very real to preschoolers because of their active imaginations and may result in a variety of emotions. Parents should validate the feeling or emotion and then discuss with the child alternatives for dealing with the emotion.

Preschoolers are developing their senses of identity, and parents should encourage preschoolers to do simple things for themselves, like dressing and washing their hands and faces (Fig. 5.6). Parents should give the child the time needed to complete the task. This helps to establish a sense of accomplishment.

At this age, the child may begin to show an interest in basic sexuality. The preschooler may want to know why male and female bodies are different, how the reproductive organs function, and where babies come from. The parent should answer the child honestly and directly, using the correct anatomic terms. Long explanations are not necessary, just simple answers. This curiosity is a normal function of the preschool years, and the curiosity may also involve playing with the genitals (see the "Masturbation" section later in this chapter).

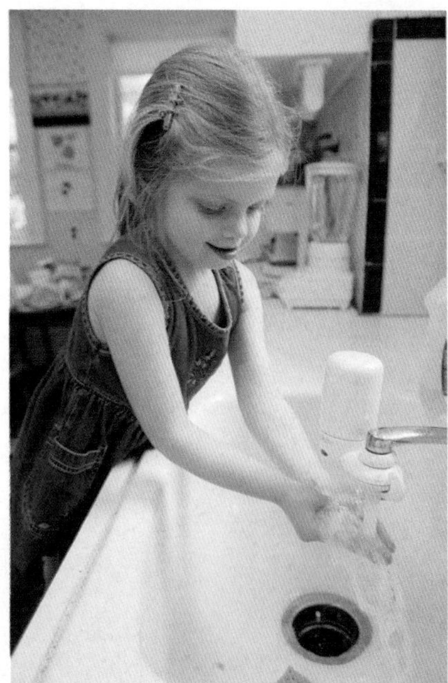

FIGURE 5.6 Encouraging the preschooler to complete simple tasks by themselves helps build self-esteem.

Friendships

Preschoolers need interactions with friends as well. Learning how to make and keep a friend is an important part of social development. Friends may be other children in the neighborhood or those at preschool or day care. A special friend is someone the preschooler can care about, talk to, and play with (Fig. 5.7). The preschooler is more likely to agree to rules and wants to please friends and be like them. The preschooler loves to sing, dance, and act and will enjoy these activities with friends. Disagreements may occur, but the parent can encourage the children to express their views, discuss and resolve conflicts, and continue being friends.

Temperament

By the time children are 3 years old, they recognize that what they do matters. It is helpful for the parent to view the child as an active participant in the parent–child relationship. The child's temperament has become a reliable indicator of how a parent might expect the child to react in a certain situation. When the parent is in tune with the preschooler's temperament, it is easier to find ways to ease transitions and changes for that child. In the area of task orientation, temperament may range from the highly attentive and persistent to the more distractible and active (Child Development Institute, 2022).

A child's social flexibility is also evident by this age. A child who is adaptable will handle stimuli from the outside world in an approaching rather than a withdrawing manner. Temperament also determines the extent of reactivity (the child's sensory threshold of responsiveness). This determines the quality of the child's mood and the intensity of reactions to stimuli, change, or situations. When the parents are familiar with the child's task orientation, social flexibility, and reactivity, they can better structure activities and situations for the child.

The 4-year-old is better at learning self-control and can use setbacks in appropriate behavior as opportunities for growth. Temper tantrums should ease by this age, as the child's language skills are more capable of keeping up with complex ideas. The 4-year-old is able to see the rewards of growing up. However, this awareness of self-power may lead to additional fears. The 5-year-old, who has a more vulnerable as opposed to a confident temperament, may be more apt to experience fears.

Fears

With their vivid imaginations, preschoolers experience a variety of fears. Preschoolers may be scared of loud noises such as fire engine sirens or barking dogs. Imaginary monsters may scare the child. Preschoolers are often afraid of people they do not know and of strange people (Santa Claus or people who look or dress differently from what they are accustomed to). Many preschoolers are afraid of the dark. Preschoolers may also fear insects as well as animals they are not familiar with. The preschooler's memory is long enough that they may fear returning to the doctor's office when a painful procedure occurred during the prior visit.

Parents should acknowledge fears rather than minimizing them. They can then collaborate with the child on strategies for dealing with the fear.

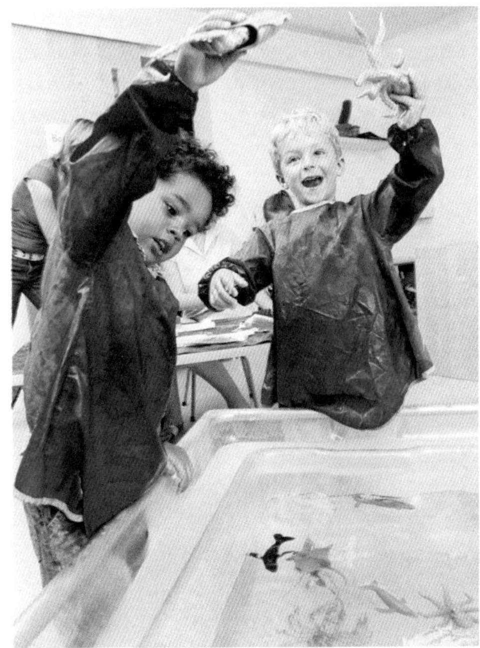

FIGURE 5.7 The preschool child begins to develop friendships.

CULTURAL INFLUENCES ON GROWTH AND DEVELOPMENT

Children may learn prejudice or bias at home before entering school or day care. The ways families view people of other races or cultures may be subtly or overtly demonstrated in routine daily activities. The preschool-age child is developing a conscience, so attitudes of tolerance or bias may influence the child's values. As in the toddler period, the value that the family places on independence will affect the child's development of a healthy self-concept.

Some families value reading and education more than others. If reading is not valued in the home, the preschool-age child's first experience with books may not occur until they are in school. Food served in the home is often specific to the family's cultural background. As the preschool-age child is exposed to people of other cultures in school, they may or may not like the food that is served. Exploring customs or cultural practices that the family participates in is important so that these practices may be safely incorporated into the child's plan of care.

THE NURSE'S ROLE IN THE GROWTH AND DEVELOPMENT OF PRESCHOOL-AGE CHILDREN

Growth and development in the preschool-age child remains orderly and sequential. Some preschoolers grow faster than others or reach various developmental milestones sooner than others. Nurses must be aware of the usual growth and development patterns for this age group so that they can assess preschool-age children appropriately and provide guidance to their families. The changes that the preschool-age child is experiencing affect not only the child but also the family. Health care visits throughout the preschool period continue to focus on expected growth and development and anticipatory guidance. An additional concern is the preparation for school entry (**school readiness**).

If the preschooler is hospitalized, growth and development may be altered. Hospitalization hinders the preschool-age child's ability to explore the environment and engage in make-believe play, thus presenting a challenge for the curious and inquisitive child. If the child must be isolated for a contagious illness, the opportunities for exploration and experimentation are further restricted. In addition, a sick preschooler may feel a sense of guilt, worrying that they may have caused the illness with negative thoughts or behaviors.

When caring for the hospitalized preschooler, the nurse must use knowledge of expected growth and development to recognize potential delays, promote continued appropriate growth and development, and interact successfully with the preschooler.

Clinical Judgment and the Nursing Process

After recognizing and analyzing cues from a thorough assessment of the preschool-age child's growth and development status, the nurse might identify several hypotheses, including:

- Injury risk
- Alteration in nutritional status
- Delayed growth and development risk
- Risk for body mass index (BMI) beyond 85th percentile for age
- Altered family functioning
- Desire for improved parenting skills

The above hypotheses provide suggestions for nursing care planning or concept mapping. The nurse will then generate solutions by planning interventions (suggested with rationales). Care planning should be individualized based on the preschooler's and family's needs.

Nursing Analysis

Injury risk; risk factors include extremes of age (e.g., curiosity, increased mobility, developmental immaturity) and unsafe mode of transport (e.g., lack of car seat and helmet use).

Goal/Outcome

Preschooler safety will be maintained: Preschooler will remain free from injury.

Preventing Injury (interventions with *rationale*)

- Teach and encourage appropriate use of forward-facing car seat or booster seat *to decrease risk of injury related to motor vehicles.*
- Teach preschoolers to stay away from the street and to cross the street only when holding the hand of an adult *to prevent pedestrian injury.*
- Require bicycle helmet use while riding any wheeled toy *to prevent head injury and form a habit of helmet use.*
- Teach the preschooler appropriate safety rules in the home (e.g., avoiding electric outlets); *the preschooler is able to follow simple directions and carry out directives. Limits help them organize the environment.*
- Post Poison Control Center phone number *in case of accidental ingestion; the preschool child is curious.*
- Never leave a preschool child unattended in a tub or pool or near any body of water *to prevent drowning.*
- Provide swimming lessons for children of ages 4 or 5 *to encourage water safety but not as a replacement for adult supervision.*
- Teach parents first aid measures and child cardiopulmonary resuscitation (CPR) *to minimize consequences of injury should it occur.*
- Provide close observation and keep side rails up on the bed in the hospital *because the preschool child continues to be at risk for falling or injuring themselves on equipment or tubing due to curiosity.*

Nursing Analysis

Alteration in nutritional status related to insufficient dietary intake (excess juice or milk intake, inadequate variety of food intake) as evidenced by failure to attain adequate increases in height and weight over time.

Goal/Outcome

Child will consume adequate nutrients: Child will demonstrate weight gain and increases in height.

Promoting Appropriate Nutrition (interventions with *rationale*)

- Assess current feeding schedule and usual intake as well as methods used to feed *to determine areas of adequacy versus inadequacy.*
- Determine if the preschooler is unable to drink from a cup or does not finger feed or use utensils properly or if

the child has difficulty swallowing or tolerating certain textures of foods *to determine if further interventions such as speech or occupational therapy are required.*

- Weigh child daily on the same scale if hospitalized, weekly on the same scale if at home, and plot growth patterns weekly or monthly as appropriate on standardized growth charts *to determine if growth is improving.*
- Limit juice to 4 to 6 oz per day and milk to 16 to 24 oz per day *to discourage the sense of fullness achieved with excess milk or juice intake, thereby increasing appetite for appropriate solid foods.*
- Provide three nutrient-dense meals and at least two healthy snacks per day *to encourage adequate nutrient consumption.*
- Feed the child on a similar schedule daily without distractions and with the family; *preschool children continue to respond well to routine and structure. They are more interested in the social context of meals and are still apt to become distracted easily, so the television should be off at mealtimes.*

Nursing Analysis

Delayed growth and development risk; risk factors include inadequate nutrition, abuse, chronic illness, prematurity, technology dependence, behavioral disorders, or involvement with the foster care system.

Goal/Outcome

Development will be enhanced: The child will make continued progress toward realization of expected developmental milestones.

Enhancing Development (interventions with *rationale*)

- Screen for developmental capabilities *to determine the child's current level of functioning.*
- Offer age-appropriate toys, play, and activities (including those using gross motor skills) *to encourage further development.*
- Perform interventions as prescribed by a physical, occupational, or speech therapist; *participation in those activities helps promote function and accomplish acquisition of developmental skills.*
- Provide support to families of preschoolers with developmental delay (*progress in achieving developmental milestones can be slow, and ongoing motivation is needed*).
- Reinforce positive attributes in the child *to maintain motivation.*
- Model age-appropriate communication skills *to illustrate suitable means for parenting the preschooler.*

Nursing Analysis

Risk for BMI beyond 85th percentile for age; risk factors include portion sizes larger than recommended, excess milk or juice intake, and excess snacking.

Goal/Outcome

Child will grow appropriately and achieve BMI within the fifth to 85th percentiles for age on standardized growth charts.

Promoting Appropriate Growth (interventions with *rationale*)

- Discourage use of no-spill sippy cups *which contribute to dental caries and allow unlimited access to fluids, possibly decreasing appetite for appropriate solid foods.*
- Provide juice (4 to 6 oz per day) and milk (16 to 24 oz per day) from a cup at meal and snack time and water in between *to avoid the child drinking excessive juice or milk.*
- Provide only nutrient-rich foods without high sugar content for meals and snacks; *even if the preschooler is a picky eater, it is inappropriate to provide high-calorie junk food just to get the child to eat something.*
- Teach parents to role model appropriate eating (nutrient-rich, varied diet) *to encourage the child to try and accept new foods as well as to become familiar with a variety of foods.*
- Severely limit the intake of fast foods and foods with high sugar and fat content *to decrease intake of nutrient-poor, high-calorie foods.*
- Ensure adequate physical activity *to stimulate development of motor skills and provide appropriate caloric expenditure. This also sets the stage for forming a lifelong habit of appropriate physical activity.*
- Teach parents to limit entertainment screen time to 1 hour per day *to encourage participation in physical activities.*

Nursing Analysis

Altered family functioning related to a shift in family roles (preschooler illness or hospitalization) as evidenced by a change in family satisfaction/assigned tasks/communication pattern or decrease in available emotional support.

Goal/Outcome

Family will demonstrate adequate functioning: Family will display coping and psychosocial adjustment.

Enhancing Family Functioning (interventions with *rationale*)

- Assess the family's level of stress and ability to cope *to determine family's ability to cope with multiple stressors.*
- Engage in family-centered care *to provide a holistic approach to care of the preschooler and family.*
- Encourage the family to verbalize feelings (*verbalization is one method of decreasing anxiety levels*) and acknowledge feelings and emotions.
- Use puppets or dramatic play with the child *to elicit the preschooler's feelings about the current situation.*

- Encourage family visitation and provide for sleeping arrangements for a parent or caregiver to stay in the hospital with the preschooler; *this contributes to the family's sense of control in a situation.*
- Involve family members in the preschooler's care, *giving them a feeling of control and connectedness.*

Nursing Analysis

Desire for improved parenting skills related to parental expression of readiness for enhanced skills.

Goal/Outcome

Parents will provide a safe and nurturing environment for the preschool child: Parents will verbalize new skills they will employ in the family.

Increasing Parenting Skill Set (interventions with *rationale*)

- Use family-centered care *to provide a holistic approach.*
- Educate the parent about normal preschool development *to provide a basis of understanding for parenting skills needed in this time period.*
- Acknowledge and encourage parents' verbalization of feelings related to chronic illness of the child or difficulty with normal preschool behavior; *this validates the normalcy of parents' feelings.*
- Encourage positive parenting and respect for the preschooler and their normal development *to help parents develop approaches to preschoolers that can be used in place of anger and frustration.*
- Role model appropriate parenting behaviors related to communicating with and disciplining the child; *role modeling demonstrates rather than just verbalizes what the parent should strive for.*

PROMOTING HEALTHY GROWTH AND DEVELOPMENT

The building of self-esteem continues throughout the preschool period. It is of particular importance during these years, as the preschooler's developmental task is focused on the development of initiative rather than guilt. A sense of guilt will contribute to low self-esteem, while a child who is rewarded for their initiative will have increased self-confidence. The parent who provides a loving and nurturing environment for the preschooler builds upon the earlier foundation.

Routine and ritual continue to be important throughout the preschool years, as they help the child develop a sense of time as well as provide the structure for the child to feel safe and secure. Daily routine continues to assist with the development of conscience in the preschooler. As in toddlerhood, making expectations known through everyday routines helps avoid confrontations. The preschooler is developing the maturity to know how to behave in various situations and is capable of learning manners.

Setting limits (and remaining consistent with those limits) continues to be important in the preschool period. Consistent limits provide the preschooler with expectation and guidance. As the preschooler increasingly participates in fantasy and imagination, the limits of routine and structure help guide their behavior and ability to distinguish reality.

Nurses caring for preschoolers should have knowledge of typical developmental expectations, so they can determine whether the preschool child is progressing appropriately. Table 5.4 lists potential signs of developmental delay. A preschool child with one or more of these concerns should be referred for further developmental evaluation.

Promoting Growth and Development Through Play

Providing sincere encouragement for the preschool child's efforts and accomplishments helps them develop a sense of initiative. Giving children opportunities to

TABLE 5.4 • Signs of Developmental Delay

Age	Concern
4 years	• Cannot jump in place or ride a tricycle • Cannot stack four blocks • Cannot throw ball overhand • Does not grasp crayon with thumb and fingers • Has difficulty with scribbling • Cannot copy a circle • Does not use sentences with three or more words • Cannot use the words "me" and "you" appropriately • Ignores other children or does not show interest in interactive games • Will not respond to people outside the family; still clings or cries if parents leave • Resists using the toilet, dressing, sleeping • Does not engage in fantasy play
5 years	• Is often unhappy or sad • Has little interest in playing with other children • Is unable to separate from parent without major protest • Is extremely aggressive • Is extremely fearful or timid, or unusually passive • Cannot build a tower of six to eight blocks • Is easily distracted; cannot concentrate on a single activity for 5 minutes • Rarely engages in fantasy play • Has trouble with eating, sleeping, or using the toilet • Cannot use plurals or past tense • Cannot brush teeth, wash and dry hands, or undress efficiently

decide how and with whom they want to play also helps them develop initiative. Preschool children like to write, color, draw, paint with a brush or their fingers, and trace or copy patterns (Fig. 5.8). They may start small collections that may be sorted. They like using toys for their intended purposes as well as for whatever invented purpose they can imagine.

Preschoolers begin to play cooperatively with one another. Play may be focused on a distinct theme. They define roles, make up rules, and assign jobs. They are able to work together toward a common goal such as building a house or fort with discarded boxes. Cooperative play encourages the preschool child to learn to share, take turns and compromise, listen to others' opinions, consider the feelings of others, use self-control, and overcome fears.

Preschoolers have incredible imaginations and love to play "make-believe" (Fig. 5.9). Encouraging pretend play and providing props for dress-up stimulate curiosity and creativity. Fantasy play is usually cooperative in nature. It encourages the preschooler to develop social skills such as taking turns, communication, paying attention, and responding to one another's words and actions. Fantasy play also allows preschoolers to explore complex social ideas such as power, compassion, and cruelty. Through role-play, children begin to develop their sexual identity as well.

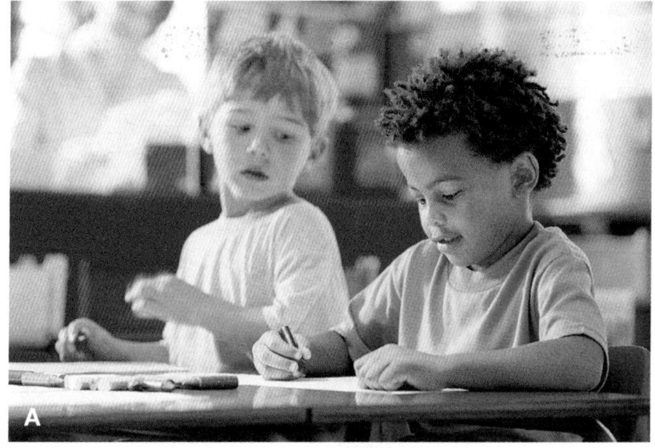

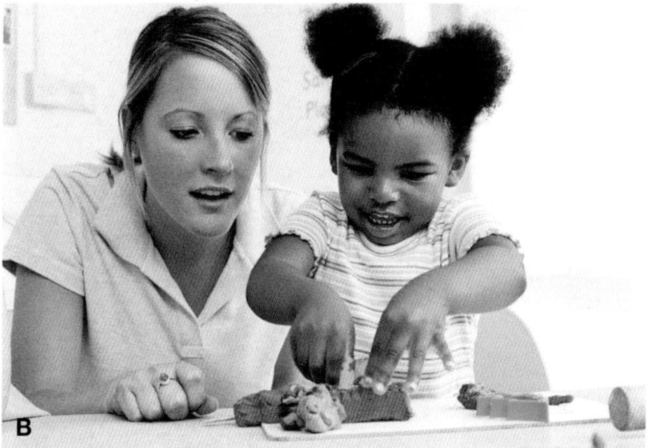

FIGURE 5.8 The preschool child loves to create things, so coloring (**A**) and molding clay (**B**) are ideal activities for children at this age.

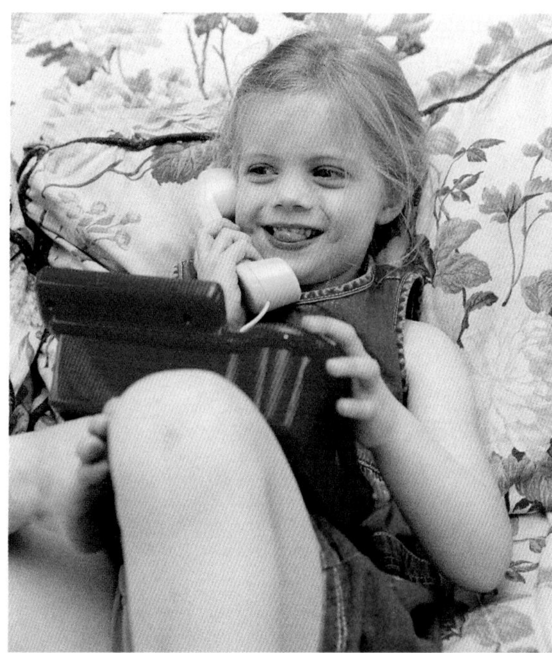

FIGURE 5.9 Preschool children enjoy imitative play.

Since preschool children have vivid imaginations, it is important to be careful about what television they watch. The preschooler should be limited to no more than 1 hour per day of quality television or other digital media programming (American Academy of Child and Adolescent Psychiatry [AACAP], 2020). The violence in some television programs may scare the preschool child or inspire them to act out the violent behavior.

Most preschoolers also engage in dramatic play, fueled by their innate curiosity and vivid imaginations. Three-year-olds may not realize that they are pretending. They run from scary creatures, make plans, and pack their backpacks (never intending to actually leave). Four-year-olds are more sophisticated with dramatic or pretend play; they know they are pretending, and they use dress-up clothes and props to act out more complex roles and scenarios (Fig. 5.10). Five-year-olds are capable of quite complex scenarios. They pretend they are real or fantasy characters. They often use dramatic play to express anxiety, try out negative feelings, or conquer their fears. For example, a child who is afraid of getting a shot at the doctor's office may work through that feeling with pretend play.

Parents should encourage physical activity in the preschool child. Regular physical activity improves gross motor skills, may enhance the child's self-confidence, and allows the child to expend excess energy. Establishing the habit of daily physical activity in the early years is important in the long-term goal of avoiding excess weight. The main goal of organized sports at this age should be

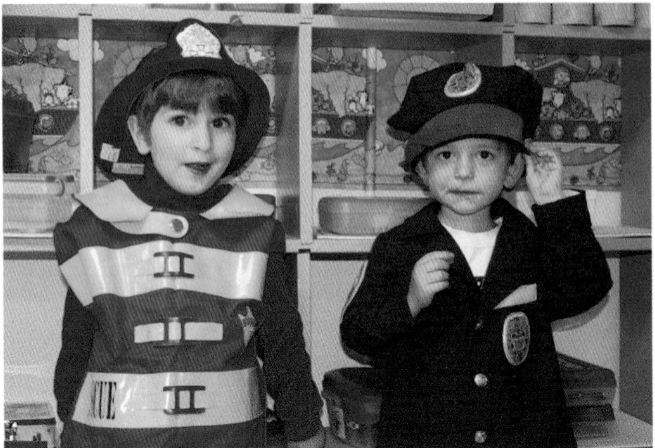

FIGURE 5.10 Preschool children love to dress up and pretend.

fun and enjoyment, though safety must remain a priority. Expensive toys that claim to teach the young child are not necessary. Toys that require interactive rather than passive play and that may include the involvement of the parent are recommended (National Association for the Education of Young Children, n.d.). Box 5.1 lists appropriate playthings for the preschool child.

Promoting Early Learning

The family is the foundation for the child's early growth and development. Parents serve as role models for behavior related to education and learning, as well as instilling values in their children. School readiness is a topic that has received a significant amount of national attention in recent years. To succeed in school, children need safe, responsive home environments that allow them to learn and explore as well as structure and limits that allow them to learn the socially acceptable behaviors that they will need in school. Language development is critical to the ability to succeed in school and can be encouraged through books and reading. Each of these components is important in readying the child for education in a more formal setting (Williams et al., 2019). Promoting language development, choosing a preschool, and making the transition to kindergarten are discussed in more detail in the sections that follow.

Promoting Language Development

The parent serves as the child's first teacher. The interactions between parent and child in relation to books and other play activities model the types of interactions that the child will later have in school. Asking open-ended questions stimulates the development of thinking as well as language in the preschool child. The preschooler is a great imitator, so the parent should serve as a role model for appropriate language. Parents should avoid swearing, as the child is sure to repeat "bad words" even if they do not understand what they mean. Allowing children to pursue interests at their own pace will help them to develop the literacy and numeric skills that will enable them to later focus on academic skills.

Preschoolers enjoy books with pictures that tell stories (Fig. 5.11). Stories with repeated phrases help keep the child's attention. Children like stories that describe experiences similar to their own. The preschool child

BOX 5.1 Appropriate Toys for Preschoolers

- Blocks, simple jigsaw puzzles (four to six large pieces), pegboards, wooden bead with string
- Supplies for creativity: chalk, large crayons, finger paint, Play-Doh or clay, washable markers, paper, paint and paintbrush, scissors, paste, or glue
- Puppets, dress-up clothes, and props for dramatic play
- Bucket, plastic shovel, and other containers for sand and water play
- Play kitchen with accessories and pretend food (Empty food boxes can be recycled for kitchen play.)
- Squeaking, floating, and squirting toys for the bath
- Sandbox with a shovel and various toys for building
- Dolls that can be dressed and undressed (large buttons, zippers, and snaps), doll care accessories (diapers, bottles, carriage, crib)
- Gross motor toys: tricycle or big wheel (with helmet), jungle gym or swing set (with supervision), Hula-Hoop, tunnel, wagon
- Blocks, Legos, cars and trucks, plastic animals, trains, plastic figures (family, community helpers), stuffed animals, balls, sewing cards
- Tape/CD/record players or streaming devices for music, various musical instruments
- Simple card and board games (older preschoolers)
- Dollhouse with furniture and accessories, people, and animals

Data from National Association for the Education of Young Children. (n.d.). *Good toys for young children by age and stage.* http://www.naeyc.org/toys

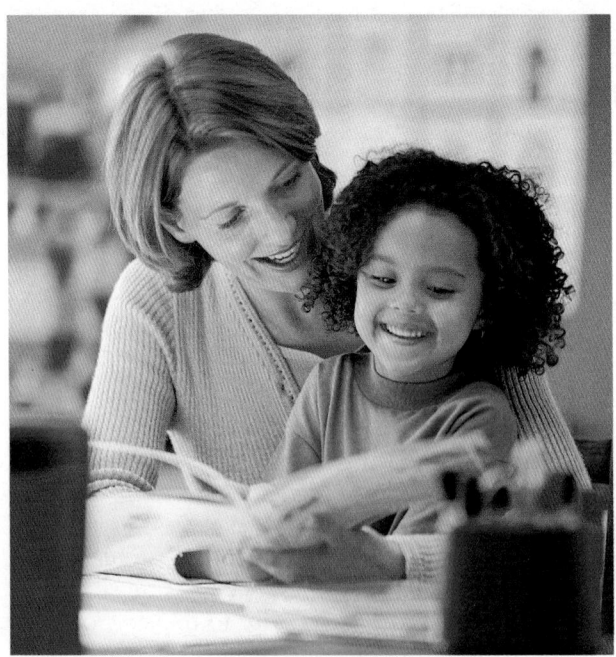

FIGURE 5.11 Preschool children enjoy being read to and looking at the pictures that go along with the story.

demonstrates early literacy skills by reciting stories or portions of books. They may also retell the story from the book, pretend to read books, and ask questions about the story. The preschool child has enough focus and expanded attention to notice when a page is skipped during reading and will call it to the parent's attention.

Choosing a Preschool and Starting Kindergarten

Many parents choose to enroll their child in preschool. Preschool should be used primarily as an opportunity to foster the child's social skills and accustom them to the group environment. When selecting a preschool, the parent may want to consider the accreditation of the school, the teachers' qualifications, and recommendations of other parents. The focus of the school environment is also important: What is the daily schedule of activities? Is the school very structured, or does it have a looser environment? The parents must decide how focused on curriculum they want the school to be. The parent should observe the classroom, evaluating the environment, noise level, and sanitary practices as well as how the children interact with each other and how the teachers interact with the children.

The type of discipline used in the school is also an important factor. Parents should not choose a preschool that uses corporal punishment. The American Academy of Pediatrics (AAP) discourages the use of corporal punishment in the school setting (Sege, 2018). Recent research demonstrates that corporal punishment may hurt a child's self-esteem, result in adverse behavioral outcomes, and result in harmful brain changes leading to cognitive differences affecting the child's ability to succeed in school (Cuartas et al., 2021). It may also lead to disruptive and violent behavior in the classroom (Sege, 2018). As preschool is the foundation for later education, the child should have the opportunity to build self-esteem and the skills needed for the more formal setting of elementary school.

Kindergarten will be the next big step. Kindergarten hours may be longer than preschool hours, and kindergarten is usually held 5 days per week. This may be a significant change for some children. For most children, the setting and personnel in kindergarten will be new. Rules and expectations are often different as well. When discussing starting kindergarten with the preschool child, parents should do so in an enthusiastic fashion, keeping the conversation light and positive. Parents should meet with the child's teacher prior to the start of school, if possible, to discuss any particular needs or concerns. Parents may want to schedule a tour of the school for the preschooler or attend the school's open house with the child to ease the transition. Practicing the new daily routine prior to the start of school will also be helpful.

Most states require up-to-date immunizations and a health screening of the child before they enter kindergarten, so advise parents to plan ahead and schedule these in a timely fashion so that school entrance is not delayed (Public Health Law Program, 2022).

TAKE NOTE!

Risk factors for lack of social and emotional readiness for school include insecure attachment in the early years, parental depression, parental substance use disorder, and low socioeconomic status. Nurses should screen for these factors and make referrals if appropriate.

Promoting Safety

In the United States, unintentional injury remains the leading cause of death for children between the ages of 1 and 14 years (National Center for Injury Prevention and Control, 2020). Preschoolers are at an ideal age to be taught about safety and safe behaviors. They are cognitively able to absorb concrete information and they desire to master the situations they are in, but they continue to display poor judgment related to safety issues. Their engagement in fantasy is so strong that it makes it difficult for them to master complicated cause-and-effect relationships. The preschool child is capable of learning safe behaviors but may not always be able to transfer those behaviors to a different situation. Parents must continue to closely supervise preschool children to avoid accidental injury during this period.

Safety in the Car

The preschooler up until 4 years of age, whose height meets the car seat size requirement, should use a forward-facing car seat with harness and top tether. All preschoolers after reaching the car seat height restriction should ride in a booster seat that uses both the lap and shoulder belts (Fig. 5.12). It is recommended that

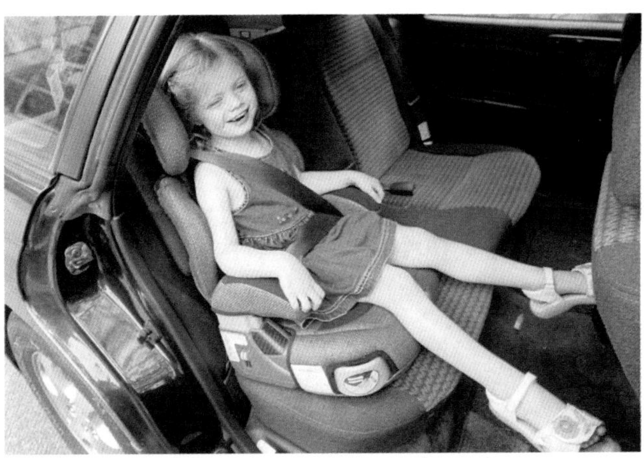

FIGURE 5.12 The older preschool child should be appropriately secured in an approved booster seat.

the booster seat continue to be used until a height of 145 cm (4 ft 9 in) and age of 8 to 12 years are reached (AAP, 2023a). The back seat of the car is always the safest place for a child to ride. If a child younger than 12 years must sit in the front seat because there are not enough rear seats available, then the front passenger seat air bag should be deactivated. Young children should never ride in the cargo area of a pickup truck as their risk for dying in the event of a crash is increased 10-fold as compared with riding appropriately restrained inside a motor vehicle (Stanford Medicine, 2023). See the Healthy People 2030 box.

HEALTHY PEOPLE 2030

Objective	Nursing Significance
Reduce the proportion of passenger vehicle occupant deaths that weren't buckled in.	Encourage car seat and booster seat use until the child is of the appropriate size and age to progress to seat belts.

Healthy People Objectives retrieved from http://www.healthypeople.gov

TAKE NOTE!

Although motor vehicle crashes remain a major cause of injury and death in the preschool-age group, many families do not use appropriate car seat/seat belt safety with their children. Child passenger safety technicians are available to provide proper installation of car seats. To find one in your area, visit http://cert.safekids.org/ or http://www.seatcheck.org. The National Highway Traffic Safety Administration (NHTSA) Auto Safety Hotline may be reached at (888) 327-4236.

Safety in the Home

Handguns, matches, bodies of water, bicycle riding, and poisons continue to be sources of potential injury during the preschool years. Falls account for the highest percentage of nonfatal injuries among preschoolers. In this age group, drowning is responsible for the most fatal injuries followed by motor vehicle crashes. A significant number of injuries also occur in or around the home, including burns and poisoning (National Safety Council, 2023).

PREVENTING EXPOSURE TO TOBACCO SMOKE

Parents should protect their preschoolers from second-hand tobacco smoke. Exposure to tobacco smoke is associated with an increased incidence of otitis media and respiratory infections, as well as increased symptoms and medication use in children with asthma. Other effects include decreased lung function and behavioral difficulties (World Health Organization, n.d.). The preschool child should never be in an enclosed space, such as a car, where tobacco smoke is present.

PREVENTING INJURY

The preschool child who runs out into the street is at risk for being struck by a car. Teach preschoolers to stop at the curb and never go into the street without a grown-up. The preschooler may learn to ride a bicycle (with or without training wheels). The child must wear an approved bicycle helmet any time they ride the bicycle, even if it is just in the driveway. Requiring helmet use in the early years may lead to the habit of helmet use as the child gets older. Allowing the preschooler to choose their own helmet may encourage the child to use the helmet.

Bicycles should be safe for this age group. The size must be correct; the balls of the feet should reach both pedals while the child is sitting on the seat and has both hands on the handlebars. Children younger than 5 years have difficulty learning to use hand-operated brakes, so traditional pedal-back brakes are recommended in this age group. Preschoolers are not mature enough to ride a bicycle in the street even if they are riding with adults, so they should always ride on the sidewalk (AAP, 2022c).

It is important to make the inside of the home safe for the preschool child. Parents should install and maintain smoke alarms as well as carbon monoxide detectors in the home. Increased physical dexterity and refinement of motor skills enable the preschooler to strike matches or use a lighter and start a fire. The preschool child is capable of washing their hands independently, so the water heater should be set at 49°C (120°F) or below to prevent scalding (AAP, 2022b).

The preschooler's active imagination and desire to play make-believe may result in a firearm injury. The average preschooler is physically capable of handling and firing a gun, particularly a handgun, which is smaller and lighter. If present in the home, firearms should be kept in a locked cabinet with the ammunition stored elsewhere (AAP, 2022a).

PREVENTING POISONING

Though it is continuing to develop, preschoolers still have unrefined taste discrimination, placing them at risk for accidental ingestion. Parents should never try to coax a child to take a vitamin supplement, tablet, or pill by calling it "candy." Dangerous fluids should be stored in their original containers and should be kept out of reach of preschoolers; they should not be poured into containers that look like ordinary drinking glasses or cups. Potentially dangerous cleaning or personal health and beauty products, gardening and pool chemicals, and automotive materials should be kept out of reach of preschoolers and in a locked cabinet if possible.

Medications should have childproof caps and should be kept in a locked cabinet. The Poison Control Center telephone number should be posted on or near the home phone (1-800-222-1222) (American Association of Poison Control Centers, n.d.).

Safety in the Water

Children 4 years of age are able to voluntarily hold their breath, making this age an appropriate time for a child to learn to swim (AAP, 2023b). Children at this age are physically capable of this activity and have the cognitive maturity to accomplish the task of swimming and basic water safety. If developmentally appropriate, water survival skills may be started at age 1 year and can help decrease the risk of drowning (AAP, 2023b). Swimming programs should focus on appropriate swim techniques as well as safety measures. Parents and caregivers should be trained in infant/child CPR. Homes with swimming pools should have lifesaving devices readily accessible. Preschoolers should be taught never to dive into water until an adult has verified its depth. Preschoolers are still too young to be left unattended around any body of water, even if they know how to swim. Preschoolers should never be allowed to swim in a canal or any fast-moving water. Preschoolers who are riding in boats or fishing off riverbanks should wear a personal flotation device. Parents should also be cautioned about close supervision of young children walking, skating, or riding near thin or weak ice.

TAKE NOTE!

All swimming pools should be secured by a fence that is at least 5 ft in height with a self-latching gate to protect young children from entering a pool area unattended (SafeKids, 2023).

Recall Nila Patel, the 4-year-old presented at the beginning of the chapter. What anticipatory guidance related to safety should you provide to her parents?

Promoting Nutrition

The preschool child has a full set of primary teeth, is able to chew and swallow competently, and has learned to use utensils fairly effectively to feed themselves (Fig. 5.13). As in the toddler years, it is important for the preschool child to continue to learn and build upon healthy eating habits. These habits will last throughout the child's life. A diet high in nutrient-rich foods such as whole grains, vegetables, fruits, appropriate dairy foods, and lean meats is appropriate for the preschooler. Nutrient-poor, high-calorie foods such as sweets and typical fast foods should be offered only in limited amounts.

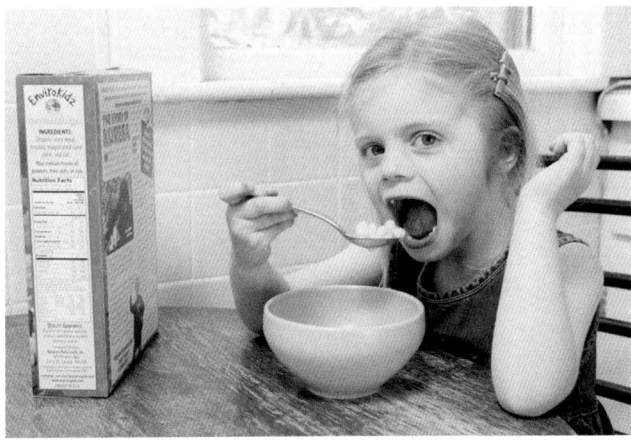

FIGURE 5.13 The preschool child has the manual dexterity to handle utensils appropriately and feed themselves independently.

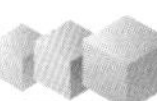

Concept Mastery Alert

Preschoolers are erratic eaters and may eat well one day and then eat little the next day. Food jags are not common in preschoolers but are common in toddlers.

Nutritional Needs

The 3- to 5-year-old requires 700 to 1,000 mg of calcium (Gavin, 2021) and 7 to 10 mg of iron daily (Powers, 2023). Box 5.2 lists calcium and iron sources. For dietary fiber, 3-year-olds should consume 8 g daily, 4-year-olds should eat 9 g, and 5-year-olds should eat 10 g (Diab et al., 2022).

BOX 5.2 Daily Calcium and Iron Recommendations for Preschool Children

Calcium: 700 mg (3-year-old), 1,000 mg (4- to 8-year-old)

Calcium in Foods

- 8 oz low-fat or whole milk: 275–300 mg
- 8 oz low-fat yogurt: 313–415 mg
- 1½ oz cheddar cheese: 307 mg
- 1 oz dried white beans (cooked): 75 mg
- ¼ c tofu: 138–253 mg
- ½ c raw broccoli: 21 mg

Iron: 7 mg (3-year-old), 10 mg (4- to 8-year-old)

Iron in Foods

- ¾ c 100% fortified prepared cereal: 18 mg
- 3 oz beef: 3 mg
- 3 oz chicken (dark meat): 1.1 mg
- ½ c cooked lentils: 3 mg
- 3 oz chicken (white meat): 0.9 mg
- 15.2-cm (6-in) slice watermelon: 0.7 mg
- ¼ c fresh cooked spinach: 1.6 mg
- ¼ c tofu: 1.7 mg
- ¼ c raisins: 1 mg
- 1 slice enriched bread: 0.8–0.9 mg
- ¼ c frozen spinach, cooked: 0.85 mg

Data from National Institutes of Health. (2023). *Iron dietary supplement fact sheet.* http://ods.od.nih.gov/factsheets/Iron-HealthProfessional/#h4; National Institutes of Health. (2022). *Calcium dietary supplement fact sheet.* http://ods.od.nih.gov/factsheets/Calcium-HealthProfessional/#h3

The typical preschooler requires about 85 kcal/kg of body weight. Saturated fats should account for less than 10% of total calories. Preschool children's diets should include a daily total fat intake of not less than 10% and not more than 35% of total calories to promote and maintain healthy cholesterol levels (Diab et al., 2022).

TAKE NOTE!

Drinking excess amounts of milk may lead to iron deficiency, as the calcium in milk blocks iron absorption.

Promoting Healthy Eating Habits

Preschool children may be selective eaters. They may eat a limited variety of foods or foods prepared in certain ways and may not be willing to try new things. The 3- or 4-year-old may exhibit "food fads," eating only certain foods over a several-day period. As the child gets older, pickiness lessens. By 5 years of age, the child is more focused on the social context of eating—table conversation and manners. The 5-year-old is generally more willing to at least try new foods and may like to help with meal preparation and clean-up as appropriate.

If the preschooler is growing well, then the pickiness is not a cause for concern. A larger concern may be the negative relationship that can develop between the parent and child relating to mealtime. The more the parent coaxes, cajoles, bribes, and threatens, the less likely the child is to try new foods or even eat the ones they like. The parent must maintain a positive and patient demeanor at mealtime.

The child should be offered a healthy diet with foods from all groups over the course of the day as recommended by the U.S. Department of Agriculture (USDA, n.d.). Parents may visit the USDA's website at https://www.myplate.gov/myplate-plan to develop a personalized daily food plan for their child based on age and activity level.

The parent should maintain a matter-of-fact approach, offer the meal or snack, and then allow the child to decide how much of the food, if any, they are going to eat. High-fat, nutrient-poor snacks should not be substituted for healthy foods just to coax the child to "eat something." See the Healthy People 2030 box.

HEALTHY PEOPLE 2030

Objective	Nursing Significance
Increase consumption of calcium in the population aged 2 years and older.	• Screen preschoolers for appropriate dietary intake of calcium. • Educate families about calcium content in foods. • Assist families with choosing a diet that meets calcium needs and is appealing to the young child.

Healthy People Objectives retrieved from http://www.healthypeople.gov

Maintaining Healthy Body Weight

Worldwide, over 22 million children younger than 5 years have BMIs classified as obese. In the past 30 years, the number of U.S. children and adolescents with overweight BMIs has doubled. According to the National Health and Nutrition Examination Survey, 13.9% of 2- to 5-year-olds have BMIs classified as obese (Centers for Disease Control and Prevention, 2022). Children are now developing traditionally adult onset-associated diseases related to higher weight such as type 2 diabetes mellitus, dyslipidemia, and nonalcoholic fatty liver disease (Cunningham et al., 2022). This risk is increased if one or both parents have overweight BMIs (Fan & Zhang, 2022).

Parents are in an opportune position to exert a positive influence on their preschooler's nutritional intake and activity level. The habits learned in early childhood will likely carry over into the school-age, adolescent, and adult years. Children whose parents take an authoritarian approach to mealtime may learn to overeat, as they are encouraged to finish the entire meal ("Clean your plate!"). If they are offered appropriate, healthy food choices and access to high-calorie, nutrient-poor food is limited, preschoolers will learn to self-regulate (eat only until full). Food should not be used as either reward or punishment.

Parents should remain positive and patient at mealtime. Mealtimes should continue to be structured. Unstructured meals lead to an increase in fat and calorie consumption. Nutrient-dense (increasingly plant-based) foods and beverages with lower fat and sugar content are recommended to decrease the incidence of developing excess weight (Fisher et al., 2022). To limit the chance that overeating will occur, preschoolers should be offered a variety of healthy foods at each meal. This may include one each of a protein source, grain, vegetable, and fruit. The preschool child's serving size is usually one third to one half of the recommended size of an adult serving. The preschool child may imitate the other eaters at the table. Parents have a prime chance to be good role models, setting an example by eating vegetables and fruits.

As with toddlers, fruit juice should be limited to 4 to 6 oz per day, as excess consumption can lead to excess weight gain. Preschoolers should be encouraged to drink water.

Limiting television viewing time and encouraging physical activity are also important strategies for maintaining a healthy weight. See Evidence-Based Practice 5.1.

Refer back to Nila Patel, the 4-year-old introduced at the beginning of the chapter. What questions should you ask Nila's parents related to nutritional intake? What anticipatory guidance related to nutrition would be appropriate? Nila's parent expresses concern regarding higher weight. How would you address these?

EVIDENCE-BASED PRACTICE **5.1**

Preventing Higher Weight in Preschoolers

STUDY

One of the most pressing public health issues is the continued rise in excess weight gain during childhood. Early childhood higher weight is associated with immediate health consequences as well as long-term issues such as adult higher weight and early-onset metabolic syndrome. Early childhood is a prime time for establishing healthy eating and activity habits that may persist into adulthood.

The authors of this study conducted a meta-analysis of existing literature on interventions for the prevention of higher weight in children.

Findings

The authors noted that during early childhood, providing a healthy diet and ensuring physical activity for children until age 5 years helps reduce BMI. Neither diet nor activity alone affects BMI as significantly as the two interventions together. The authors therefore recommend utilizing both interventions.

Nursing Implications

Nurses are in a unique position to provide ongoing, repeated education about the importance of maintaining healthy weight in preschoolers to families wherever they encounter them. Nurses should encourage families to:

- Provide meals seated with the family and in a positive atmosphere.
- Ensure the preschooler receives a varied diet with plenty of plant-based foods.
- Encourage water as the beverage of choice.
- Instruct families to avoid high-sugar foods and beverages.
- Encourage daily physical activity: structured, at least 60 minutes daily; and unstructured, 60 minutes to several hours daily.
- Teach families to limit media consumption to 30 minutes daily and to not put a television in the child's bedroom.

Data from Brown, T., Moore, T. H. M., Hooper, L., Gao, Y., Zayegh, A., Ijaz, S., Elwenspoek, M., Foxen, S. C., Magee, L., O'Malley, C., Waters, E., & Summerbell, C. D. (2019). Interventions for preventing obesity in children. *Cochrane Database of Systematic Reviews.* https://doi.org/10.1002/14651858.CD001871.pub4

Promoting Healthy Sleep and Rest

The preschool child needs about 10 to 13 hours of sleep each day, including naps if taken (AAP, 2020). Unless very tired, many preschool children will resist going to bed from time to time. Bedtime rituals continue to be reassuring to children, and it is important to continue them in the preschool years. Having a time of relaxation with a decrease in stimulation will allow the child to fall asleep more easily. Some children continue to need a security item at bedtime or naptime. A nightlight in the bedroom may be necessary, as many children this age are afraid of the dark. Teaching Guidelines 5.1 gives information about assisting parents to establish a bedtime routine.

Nightmares often occur in preschool children as a result of the child's struggle to distinguish what is real from what is not. When a child awakens from a nightmare, they are often crying and may be able to recount what the dream was about. Parents should validate the child's fear rather than discount it (Reynolds et al., 2022). Saying, "Yes, I agree, monsters are scary; it's a good thing they aren't real" is more appropriate than, "Don't be silly; monsters aren't real." Sometimes children benefit from reading stories about dreams. Recommended books include:

- *Bedtime for Frances* by Russell Hoban
- *Ben's Dream* by Chris Van Allsburg
- *In the Night Kitchen* by Maurice Sendak
- *There's a Nightmare in My Closet* by Mercer Mayer

Nightmares should not be confused with night terrors. After a nightmare, the child is aroused and interactive, but night terrors are different: A short time after falling asleep, the child partially awakens and is screaming. The child usually does not respond much to the parent's soothing, but they eventually stop screaming and go back to sleep. Night terrors are often frightening for parents because the child does not seem to be responding to them. One technique that may help to decrease the incidence of night terrors is to wake the child about 30 to 45 minutes into the sleep cycle. If continued nightly for about a week, the cycle of night terrors may be broken (Morse & Kotagal, 2021). See Comparison Chart 5.1.

TEACHING GUIDELINES **5.1** Bedtime Routines

- Establish a bedtime as well as morning wake-up time.
- Avoid sugar or caffeine consumption in the evening.
- Avoid stimulating activities such as roughhousing before bedtime.
- Do not allow television watching in bed.
- Make the child's bedroom an inviting and comfortable area of the home.
- Provide a nightlight in the child's bedroom if they are afraid of the dark.
- Conform to a nightly routine:
  - Television off at a certain time
  - Bath
  - Quiet game or story reading/telling
  - Bedtime prayer or song
- Maintain quiet in the bedroom and nearby to increase the child's ability to fall asleep.

Data from American Academy of Pediatrics. (2020). *Healthy sleep habits: How many hours does your child need?* https://www.healthychildren.org/English/healthy-living/sleep/Pages/Healthy-Sleep-Habits-How-Many-Hours-Does-Your-Child-Need.aspx; Reynolds, A., Angulo, A., Breheney, M., Green, J., & Goldson, E. (2022). Child development and behavior. In M. Bunik, W. W. Hay, M. J. Levin, & M. J. Abzug (Eds.), *Current diagnosis & treatment: Pediatrics* (26th ed.). McGraw-Hill Education.

COMPARISON CHART 5.1 Nightmares Versus Night Terrors

	Nightmare	Night Terror
Definition	Scary or bad dream followed by awakening	Partial arousal from deep sleep
When parents become aware	The child awakens the parent after episode is over.	Screaming and thrashing during the episode awakens the parent.
Timing	Usually in the second half of the night	Usually about an hour after falling asleep
Behavior	Crying, may be scared after awakening	Sits up, thrashes, cries, screams, talks, looks wild-eyed. Sweats, may have racing heartbeat
Responsiveness	Responsive to parents' soothing and reassurances	Child unaware of parents' presence, may scream and thrash more if restrained
Return to sleep	Difficulty going back to sleep if afraid	Rapidly returns to sleep without full awakening
Memory of occurrence	May remember the dream and talk about it later	No memory of the event

Data from Morse, A. M., & Kotagal, S. (2021). Sleepwalking and other parasomnias in children. *UpToDate*. Retrieved October 13, 2022, from https://www.uptodate.com/contents/sleepwalking-and-other-parasomnias-in-children#H27172832

Think back to Nila Patel. What anticipatory guidance would you provide to her parents in relation to sleep during the preschool years?

Promoting Healthy Teeth and Gums

Prevention of dental caries continues to be important for the preschool child and can be achieved through daily brushing and flossing. Parents should use only a pea-sized amount of toothpaste to prevent excess fluoride consumption, which can contribute to fluorosis (Nowak & Warren, 2023). The preschooler may brush their own teeth, but the parent must continue to supervise to ensure adequate brushing. Parents must perform flossing because the preschool child cannot perform this task adequately. Cariogenic foods should be avoided. If sugary foods are consumed, the mouth should be rinsed with water if it is not possible to brush the teeth immediately (Nowak & Warren, 2023). The preschool child should visit the dentist every 6 months.

TAKE NOTE!

Prevention of dental caries is important in the primary teeth, because loss of these teeth to caries may affect the proper formation of permanent teeth as well as the width of the dental arch.

Promoting Appropriate Discipline

Successful discipline results from a loving and nurturing environment in which the preschooler's self-esteem is fostered and limits are well chosen and enforced consistently. Spanking (striking with the open hand) is the least effective discipline practice and is discouraged by the AACAP (2018) and the National Association of Pediatric Nurse Practitioners (2022). Belts, switches, paddles, or other items should never be used to strike a child. The use of physical punishment has been associated with a number of additional problems in adulthood, such as antisocial and criminal behaviors (AACAP, 2018; see Chapter 4).

If parents are consistent with discipline while encouraging the preschooler's normal growth and development of imagination and make-believe, the child will learn to accept that certain things are not allowed. The sense of initiative can be preserved and guilt avoided if the rules are clear and enforced consistently (Sears & Sears, 2020a).

TAKE NOTE!

Corporal punishment not only causes physical and emotional pain, it also decreases learning capacity (AACAP, 2018).

Minimize the occurrence of misbehavior by anticipating conditions likely to lead to the undesired or risky action. When the situation becomes difficult, parents should use distraction to change the preschooler's focus. When discussing the misbehavior, be certain to label the behavior and not the child. This helps preserve the preschooler's self-esteem. When teaching preschoolers about undesired behavior, be sure they also understand the reason why it is wrong or unacceptable to do it. This helps encourage the child to use internal controls over behavior. Parents should serve as role models for self-control, including choice of words, the tone they are delivered in, and the actions that accompany them.

Children work harder to obtain praise than to receive punishment, so always reward positive behaviors. Preschool children are becoming capable of understanding the concept of right and wrong. They start to understand each other's feelings (**empathy**) and are cognitively capable of remembering basic rules.

Time-out or time away from the situation can be effective in this age group. This punishment should be used only for intentional misbehavior (knowing something is forbidden but doing it anyway). It is particularly helpful with dangerous or destructive behavior. The preschooler is given a warning that time-out will occur if the behavior does not stop. The preschooler is removed from the situation and must stay in time-out for a specified period of time. A particular time-out area is helpful; a boring corner of the room without distractions available is a good location. The generally recommended period of time is to require 1 minute of time-out per year of age; thus, a 4-year-old would be in time-out for 4 minutes (Sears & Sears, 2020b). Set the timer so the child will know when the time-out is over. If the child gets up before the prescribed time, replace the child in time-out and restart the timer. Time-out works best if used each and every time the undesirable behavior occurs. It is also important to praise the child when they follow the rules and behave appropriately.

A simple and clear explanation of the misbehavior should be given to the child; parents should also talk about acceptable alternative strategies that the child can use in the future instead of the undesired behavior. Removal of a privilege such as playing with a favorite toy can be as effective as time-out. Books and other media that are available to help educate parents about appropriate discipline and to help the child learn self-control are listed in Box 5.3.

BOX 5.3 Selected Resources for Parents and Preschoolers

Books for Parents (About Discipline)

- *How to Talk so Kids Will Listen and Listen so Kids Will Talk* by A. Faber & E. Mazlish (Harper Resource)
- *Kids Are Worth It: Giving Your Children the Gift of Inner Discipline* by B. Colorosos (Harper Collins Publishers)
- *Positive Discipline A to Z: 1001 Solutions to Everyday Parenting Problems* by J. Nelson, L. Lott, & S. G. Glenn (Three Rivers Press)
- *Setting Limits With Your Strong-Willed Child: Eliminating Conflict by Establishing Clear, Firm and Respectful Boundaries* by R. MacKenzie (Three Rivers Press)
- *The Case Against Spanking: How to Discipline Children Without Hitting* by I. A. Hyman (Jossey-Bass)
- *The Nurturing Parent: How to Raise Creative, Loving, Responsible Children* by J. S. Dacey & A. J. Packer (Fireside)
- *Without Spanking or Spoiling: A Practical Approach to Toddler and Preschool Guidance* by E. Crary (Parenting Press)

Books for Preschoolers (About Dealing With Feelings and Learning How to Behave)

- *Hands Are Not for Hitting* by M. Agassi (Free Spirit Publishing)
- *I Can't Wait* by E. Crary (Parenting Press)
- *I Want It* by E. Crary (Parenting Press)
- *I Want to Play* by E. Crary (Parenting Press)
- *I Was so Mad* by M. Mayer (Golden Books)
- *I Was so Mad* by N. Simon & D. Leder (Albert Whitman & Company)
- *I'm Excited* by E. Crary (Parenting Press)
- *I'm Frustrated* by E. Crary (Parenting Press)
- *I'm Mad* by E. Crary (Parenting Press)
- *I'm Scared* by E. Crary (Parenting Press)
- *Feet Are Not for Kicking* by E. Verdick (Free Spirit Publishing)
- *Teeth Are Not for Biting* by E. Verdick (Free Spirit Publishing)
- *When Sophie Gets Angry … Really, Really Angry* by M. Bang (Blue Sky Press)
- *Words Are Not for Hurting* by E. Verdick (Free Spirit Publishing)

ADDRESSING COMMON DEVELOPMENTAL CONCERNS

Common developmental concerns of the preschool period include lying, how to address sex education, and masturbation. Parents often express difficulty in dealing with these issues with their preschool children. Offering appropriate anticipatory guidance may give the parents the support and confidence they need to deal with these issues.

Lying

Lying is common in preschool children. It may occur because the child fears punishment, has gotten carried away with imagination, or is imitating what they see the parent do. The parent should ascertain the reason for the lie before punishing the child. If the child has broken a rule and fears punishment, then the parent must determine the truth. The child needs to learn that lying is usually worse than the misbehavior itself. The punishment for the misbehavior should be lessened if the child admits the truth. The parent should remain calm and serve as a role model of an even temper. The next time the misbehavior occurs, the child will be more apt to simply tell the truth.

If the child's lying is their imagination getting carried away, then the parent should guide the child in distinguishing between myth and reality (Sears & Sears, 2020c). The preschooler's imagination is vivid, and the child needs direction in the use of that faculty. Parents should serve as role models of appropriate behavior for their children to learn it. Children who lie because they hear their parents lying must not see or hear their parents do it.

Sex Education

Preschoolers are keen observers but are still not able to interpret all that they see correctly. The child may recognize but not understand sexual activity. Preschoolers are inquisitive and want to learn about everything around them; therefore, they are likely to ask questions about sex and where babies come from. Before attempting to answer questions, parents should try to find out first exactly what the child is asking and what the child already thinks about that subject. Then they should provide a simple, direct, and honest answer. The child needs only the information that they are requesting. Additional questions will occur in the future and should be addressed as they arise.

Masturbation

The normal curiosity of the preschool years often leads children to explore their own genitals (Carter & Feigelman, 2020). This behavior may be upsetting to some parents, but masturbation is a healthy and natural part of normal preschool development if it occurs in moderation. If the parent overreacts to this behavior, then it may occur more frequently. Masturbation should be treated in a matter-of-fact way by the parent. The child needs to learn certain rules about this activity; nudity and masturbation are not acceptable in public. The child should also be taught safety; no other person can touch the child's private parts unless it is the parent, doctor, or nurse checking to see when something is wrong.

Think back to Nila Patel. What are some developmental concerns that are common during the preschool years? What anticipatory guidance related to these concerns would you provide to Nila's parents?

Unfolding Patient Stories: Sabina Vasquez • Part 1

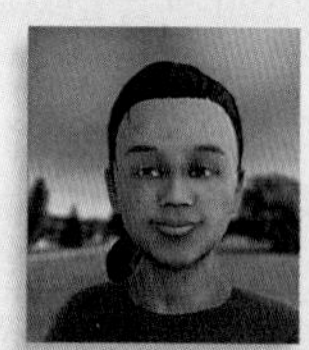

Sabina Vasquez, age 8, was diagnosed with asthma at age 4. At her first visit to the primary care provider's office with asthma symptoms as a 4-year-old, what appropriate age-related strategies would have been used in planning asthma education for this patient and her family? How would patient education strategies differ when explaining asthma to an 8-year-old compared with a 4-year-old? (Sabina Vasquez's story continues in Chapter 18.)

Care for Sabina and other patients in a realistic virtual environment: ***vSim** for Nursing* (thepoint.lww.com/vSimPediatric). Practice documenting these patients' care in DocuCare (thePoint.lww.com/DocuCareEHR).

KEY CONCEPTS

- The preschool child grows at a slower rate and takes on a more slender and upright appearance than the toddler.
- The primary psychosocial task of the preschool period is developing a sense of initiative.
- Cognitive development moves from an egocentric approach to the world toward a more empathetic understanding of what happens outside of the self.
- The preschooler gains additional motor skills and displays significant refinement of fine motor abilities.
- Cognitive and language skills that develop in the preschool years help prepare the child for success in school.
- Disfluency or hesitancy in speech is a normal finding in the preschool period and occurs as a result of the fast pace with which the preschooler is gaining language skills and vocabulary.
- The vocabulary of a preschooler increases to about 2,100 words, and the child speaks in full sentences with appropriate use of tense and prepositions.
- Appropriate growth and development should be maintained in the child who is ill or hospitalized.
- Recognizing concerns or delays in growth and development is essential so that the appropriate referrals may be made and intervention can begin.
- The preschool child requires a well-balanced diet with fat content between 20% and 30% of calories consumed.
- Adequate physical activity and provision of a nutrient-dense diet (rather than foods high in fat and sugar) are the foundation for maintaining healthy weight in the preschool child.
- Adequate dental care is important for the health of the primary teeth.
- Preschoolers need about 12 hours of sleep per day and benefit from a structured bedtime routine.
- Due to the active imagination of the preschooler, nightmares and night terrors may begin during this period.
- Safety and injury prevention remain a focus in the preschool years.
- Structure, appropriate limit setting, and consistency are the keys for effective discipline in the preschool period.
- Time-out is an effective disciplinary measure for preschoolers.
- Masturbation may occur as the preschooler discovers their body. If not excessive, it is considered a normal part of growth and development.

REFERENCES AND RECOMMENDED READINGS

American Academy of Child and Adolescent Psychiatry. (2018). *Physical punishment.* https://www.aacap.org/aacap/families_and_youth/facts_for_families/fff-guide/Physical-Punishment-105.aspx

American Academy of Child and Adolescent Psychiatry. (2020). *Screen time and children.* https://www.aacap.org/AACAP/Families_and_Youth/Facts_for_Families/FFF-Guide/Children-And-Watching-TV-054.aspx

American Academy of Pediatrics. (2020). *Healthy sleep habits: How many hours does your child need?* https://www.healthychildren.org/English/healthy-living/sleep/Pages/Healthy-Sleep-Habits-How-Many-Hours-Does-Your-Child-Need.aspx

American Academy of Pediatrics. (2022a). *Gun safety: Where we stand.* https://www.healthychildren.org/English/safety-prevention/all-around/Pages/where-we-stand-gun-safety.aspx

American Academy of Pediatrics. (2022b). *Safety for your child: 2 to 4 years*. https://www.healthychildren.org/English/ages-stages/toddler/Pages/Safety-for-Your-Child-2-to-4-Years.aspx

American Academy of Pediatrics. (2022c). *Your child's first tricycle or bike: Important safety rules*. https://www.healthychildren.org/English/safety-prevention/at-play/Pages/your-childs-first-tricycle-or-bike-teaching-them-to-ride-safely.aspx

American Academy of Pediatrics. (2023a). *Car seats: Information for families*. https://www.healthychildren.org/English/safety-prevention/on-the-go/Pages/Car-Safety-Seats-Information-for-Families.aspx

American Academy of Pediatrics. (2023b). *Swim lessons: When to start & what parents should know*. https://www.healthychildren.org/English/safety-prevention/at-play/Pages/Swim-Lessons.aspx

American Association of Poison Control Centers. (n.d.). *Prevention*. https://poisoncenters.org/prevention

Brown, T., Moore, T. H. M., Hooper, L., Gao, Y., Zayegh, A., Ijaz, S., Elwenspoek, M., Foxen, S. C., Magee, L., O'Malley, C., Waters, E., & Summerbell, C. D. (2019). Interventions for preventing obesity in children. *Cochrane Database of Systematic Reviews*. https://doi.org/10.1002/14651858.CD001871.pub4

Carter, R. G., & Feigelman, S. (2020). The preschool years. In R. M. Kliegman, J. W. St. Geme III, N. J. Blum, S. S. Shah, R. C. Tasker, K. M. Wilson, & R. E. Behrman (Eds.), *Nelson's textbook of pediatrics* (21st ed.). Elsevier.

Centers for Disease Control and Prevention. (2022, May 17). *Childhood obesity facts*. https://www.cdc.gov/obesity/data/childhood.html

Centers for Disease Control and Prevention. (2023, June 6). *CDC's developmental milestones*. http://www.cdc.gov/ncbddd/actearly/milestones/index.html

Child Development Institute. (2022). *Temperament and your child's personality*. https://childdevelopmentinfo.com/uncategorized/temperament_and_your_child/

Chromey, R. (2021). *Do you know the ABCs of spiritual growth in children?* https://childrensministry.com/abcs-spiritual-growth/

Cuartas, J., Weissman, D. G., Sheridan, M. A., Lengua, L., & McLaughlin, K. A. (2021). Corporal punishment and elevated neural response to threat in children. *Child Development, 92*(3), 831–832. https://doi.org/10.1111/cdev.13565

Cunningham, S. A., Hardy, S. T., Jones, R., Ng, C., Kramer, M. R., & Narayan, K. M. V. (2022). Changes in the incidence of childhood obesity. *Pediatrics, 150*(2), e2021053708. https://doi.org/10.1542/peds.2021-053708

Diab, L. K., Haemer, M., Primark, L. E., & Krebs, N. R. (2022). Normal childhood nutrition and its disorders. In M. Bunik, W. W. Hay, M. J. Levin, & M. J. Abzug (Eds.), *Current diagnosis & treatment: Pediatrics* (26th ed.). McGraw-Hill Education.

Erikson, E. H. (1963). *Childhood and society* (2nd ed.). W. W. Norton and Company.

Fan, H., & Zhang, X. (2022). Influence of parental weight change on the incidence of overweight and obesity in offspring. *BMC Pediatrics, 22*, 330. https://doi.org/10.1186/s12887-022-03399-8

Fisher, E. F., Lemus, T. P., Reichert, A., Alsopp, M., & Harvey, T. S. (2022). *Reframing childhood obesity: Cultural insights on nutrition, weight, and food systems*. Vanderbilt Cultural Contexts of Health Initiative. https://www.vanderbilt.edu/cultural-contexts-health/wp-content/uploads/sites/350/2022/06/Reframing-Childhood-Obesity-CCH-Report.pdf

Gavin, M. L. (2021). *Calcium*. https://kidshealth.org/en/parents/calcium.html?WT.ac=p-ra

Kohlberg, L. (1984). *Moral development*. Harper & Row.

Linguistic Society of America. (2023). *FAQ: Raising bilingual children*. https://www.linguisticsociety.org/resource/faq-raising-bilingual-children

Morse, A. M., & Kotagal, S. (2021). Sleepwalking and other parasomnias in children. *UpToDate*. Retrieved September 29, 2023, from https://www.uptodate.com/contents/sleepwalking-and-other-parasomnias-in-children#H27172832

National Association for the Education of Young Children. (n.d.). *Good toys for young children by age and stage*. https://www.naeyc.org/resources/topics/play/toys

National Association of Pediatric Nurse Practitioners, Child Maltreatment and Neglect Special Interest Group, VanGraafeiland, B., Hornor, G. A., Herendeen, P. A., Chiocca, E. M., Loyke, J. A., Dietzman, H., Boucher, N. L., Nielsen, A., & Record, S. C. (2022). NAPNAP position statement on using positive parenting to eliminate corporal punishment. *Journal of Pediatric Health Care, 36*, 202–204. https://doi.org/10.1016/j.pedhc.2021.09.001

National Center for Injury Prevention and Control. (2020). *10 leading causes of death by age group, United States 2020, all races, both sexes*. https://www.cdc.gov/injury/wisqars/pdf/leading_causes_of_death_by_age_group_2020-508.pdf

National Institutes of Health. (2022). *Calcium dietary supplement fact sheet*. https://ods.od.nih.gov/factsheets/Calcium-HealthProfessional/#h3

National Institutes of Health. (2023). *Iron dietary supplement fact sheet*. https://ods.od.nih.gov/factsheets/Iron-HealthProfessional/#h4

National Safety Council. (2023). *Top 10 preventable injuries*. https://injuryfacts.nsc.org/all-injuries/deaths-by-demographics/top-10-preventable-injuries/data-details/

Nowak, A. J., & Warren, J. J. (2023). Preventive dental care and counseling for infants and young children. *UpToDate*. Retrieved September 29, 2023, from https://www.uptodate.com/contents/preventive-dental-care-and-counseling-for-infants-and-young-children

Piaget, J. (1969). *The theory of stages in cognitive development*. McGraw-Hill.

Powers, J. M. (2023). Iron deficiency in infants and children <12 years: Screening, prevention, clinical manifestations, and diagnosis. *UpToDate*. Retrieved September 29, 2023, from https://www.uptodate.com/contents/iron-deficiency-in-infants-and-children-less-than12-years-screening-prevention-clinical-manifestations-and-diagnosis

Public Health Law Program. (2022). *State school immunization requirements and vaccine exemption laws*. Centers for Disease Control and Prevention. https://www.cdc.gov/phlp/docs/school-vaccinations.pdf

Reynolds, A., Angulo, A., Breheney, M., Green, J., & Goldson, E. (2022). Child development and behavior. In M. Bunik, W. W. Hay, M. J. Levin, & M. J. Abzug (Eds.), *Current diagnosis & treatment: Pediatrics* (26th ed.). McGraw-Hill Education.

SafeKids. (2023). *Swimming*. https://www.safekids.org/poolsafety

Sears, W., & Sears, M. (2020a). *Shape children's behavior*. https://www.askdrsears.com/topics/parenting/discipline-behavior/shape-childrens-behavior

Sears, W., & Sears, M. (2020b). *10 time-out for children techniques*. https://www.askdrsears.com/topics/parenting/discipline-behavior/10-time-out-techniques

Sears, W., & Sears, M. (2020c). *Why do kids lie?* https://www.askdrsears.com/topics/parenting/discipline-behavior/morals-manners/why-do-kids-lie

Sege, R. D. (2018). *AAP policy opposes corporal punishment, draws on recent evidence.* https://www.aappublications.org/news/2018/11/05/discipline110518

Stanford Medicine. (2023). *Motor vehicle safety for children.* https://www.stanfordchildrens.org/en/topic/default?id=motor-vehicle-safety-for-children-85-P01038

U.S. Department of Agriculture. (n.d.). *MyPlate plan.* https://www.myplate.gov/myplate-plan

Williams, P. G., Lerner, M. A., Council on Early Childhood; Council on School Health, Sells, J., Alderman, S. L., Hashikawa, A., Mendelsohn, A., McFadden, T., Navsaria, D., Peacock, G., Scholer, S., Takagishi, J., Vanderbilt, D., De Pinto, C. L., Attisha, E., Beers, N., Gibson, E., Gorski, P., … Weiss-Harrison, A. (2019). School readiness. *Pediatrics, 144*(2), e20191766. https://doi.org/10.1542/peds.2019-1766

World Health Organization. (n.d.). *Passive smoking.* http://www.who.int/tobacco/en/atlas10.pdf

Zubler, J. M., Wiggins, L. D., Macias, M. M., Whitaker, T. M., Shaw, J. S., Squires, J. K., Pajke, J. A., Wolf, R. B., Slaughter, K. S., Broughton, A. S., Gerndt, K. L., Mlodoch, B. J., & Lipkin, P. H. (2022). Evidence-informed milestones for developmental surveillance tools. *Pediatrics, 149*(3), e2021052138. https://doi.org/10.1542/peds.2021-052138

DEVELOPING CLINICAL JUDGMENT

PRACTICING FOR NCLEX

1. The nurse is caring for a 4-year-old who is hospitalized and insists on having the nurse perform every assessment and intervention on their imaginary friend first. The child then agrees to have the assessment or intervention done to themselves. The nurse identifies this preschooler's behavior as:
   a. problematic; the child is old enough to begin to have a basis in reality.
   b. normal, because the child is hospitalized and out of their routine.
   c. normal for this stage of growth and development.
   d. problematic, as it interferes with needed nursing care.
2. The parent of a 3-year-old is concerned about their child's speech. They describe the preschooler as hesitating at the beginning of sentences and repeating consonant sounds. What is the nurse's best response?
   a. "Hesitancy and disfluency are normal during this period of development."
   b. "Reading to the child will help model appropriate speech."
   c. "Expressive language concerns warrant a developmental evaluation."
   d. "You should ask your child's health care provider for a speech therapy evaluation."
3. The parent of a 4-year-old asks for advice on using time-out for discipline with their child. What advice should the nurse give the parent?
   a. If spanking is not working, then time-out is not likely to be helpful either.
   b. Place the child in time-out for 4 minutes.
   c. Use time-out only if removing privileges is unsuccessful.
   d. The child should stay in time-out until crying ceases.
4. A 5-year-old child is not gaining weight appropriately. Organic problems have been ruled out. What is the priority action by the nurse?
   a. Allow the child unlimited access to the sippy cup to ensure adequate hydration.
   b. Encourage sweets for the extra caloric content.
   c. Teach the parent about nutritional needs of the preschooler.
   d. Assess the child's usual intake pattern at home.
5. The nurse is providing teaching about accidental poisoning to the family of a 3-year-old. The nurse understands that a child of this age is at increased risk of accidental ingestion due to which sensory alteration?
   a. A lack of fully developed hearing
   b. A less discriminating sense of touch
   c. Visual acuity that has not fully developed
   d. A less discriminating sense of taste
6. The nurse is caring for a 4-year-old. Which behaviors does the nurse expect to observe in this child, indicating Piaget's stage of preoperational thought? Select all that apply.
   a. Egocentrism
   b. Temper tantrums
   c. Magical thinking
   d. Trust issues
   e. Having an imaginary friend
   f. Initiative
7. The nursing instructor has taught a group of nursing students about preschooler physical growth and development. The nursing students state that the 3-year-old should have been able to achieve control over ___ and ___ as a result of ____.

   Blanks 1 and 2:
   a. bowel elimination
   b. emotions
   c. urinary elimination
   d. utensil use
   e. social skills
   f. writing skills

   Blank 3:
   a. increased psychosocial maturity
   b. complete myelination of the spinal cord
   c. improved fine motor control
   d. skillful toilet teaching

DOSAGE CALCULATION QUESTIONS

1. A child who weighs 33 lb has an order for acetaminophen 10 mg/kg/dose, every 4 hours as needed for pain or fever.
   a. How many milligrams will the child receive per dose?
   b. Acetaminophen elixir is provided as 160 mg/5 mL. How many milliliters will the nurse administer per dose?

CRITICAL THINKING EXERCISES

1. Teach a preschool class about bicycle and street safety. Be certain to design the content at an appropriate developmental level.
2. Construct a 3-day menu for a 4-year-old who is selective about eating. Include three daily meals and two snacks. Follow the nutritional guidelines recommended by the USDA.
3. Color or draw with a preschool child. Analyze the drawings and interactions or discussions you have with the child, relating them to psychosocial and cognitive development expected at this age.

STUDY ACTIVITIES

1. Care for two average 3-, 4-, or 5-year-old children in the clinical setting (make sure both are of the same age). Describe each child's development level, response to hospitalization, and family dynamics.

2. Visit a preschool that provides care for children with developmental delays as well as children exhibiting expected development. Perform a developmental assessment on a child with expected development and one with developmental delays (both of the same age). Compare and contrast your findings.

3. Observe a 3-, 4-, or 5-year-old's classroom of a typical preschool. Choose two children who are of the same age with different temperaments. Record the differences and similarities in their response to structure and authority, interactions with classmates, attention levels, and language and activity levels.

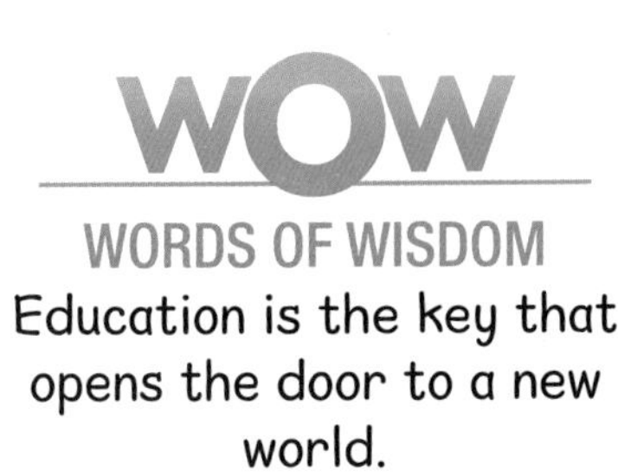

WORDS OF WISDOM

Education is the key that opens the door to a new world.

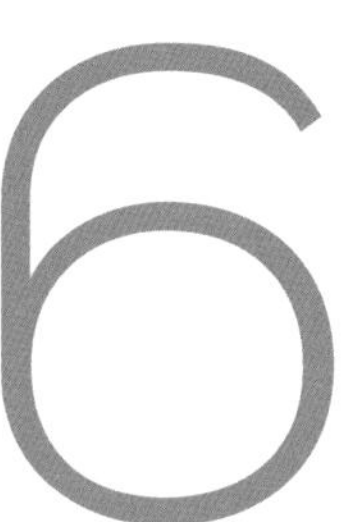

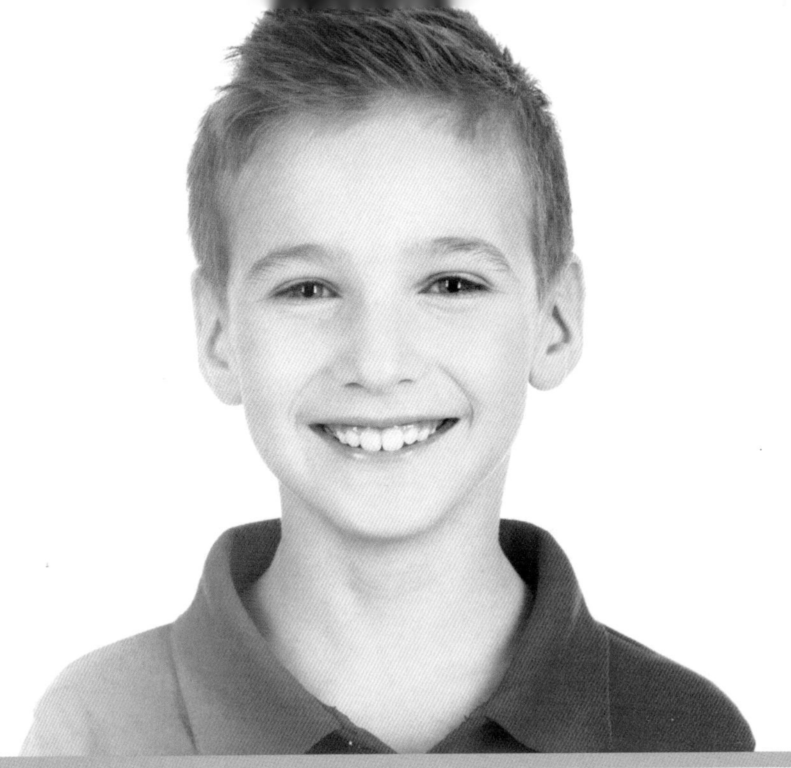

Growth and Development of the School-Age Child

LEARNING OBJECTIVES

Upon completion of the chapter, you will be able to:

1. Identify normal physiologic, cognitive, and moral changes occurring in the school-age child.
2. Describe the role of peers and schools in the development and socialization of the school-age child.
3. Identify the developmental milestones of the school-age child.
4. Describe the role of the nurse in promoting safety for the school-age child.
5. Demonstrate knowledge of the nutritional requirements of the school-age child.
6. Identify common developmental concerns in the school-age child.
7. Demonstrate knowledge of the appropriate nursing guidance for common developmental concerns.

KEY TERMS

bruxism (brŭk´sizm)
caries
industry
inferiority
malocclusion (mal´ō-klū´zhŭn)
prepubescence (prē´pyū-bes´ĕnt)
principle of conservation
school-age child
school refusal
self-esteem

Lawrence Jones is a 10-year-old brought to the clinic by his parent for his annual school check-up. As the nurse caring for him, assess Lawrence's growth and development, and then provide appropriate anticipatory guidance to his parent.

INTRODUCTION

School-age children, between the ages of 6 and 12 years, are experiencing a time of slow progressive physical growth, while their social and developmental growth accelerate and increase in complexity. The focus of their world expands from family to teachers, peers, and other outside influences (e.g., coaches, media). The child at this stage becomes increasingly more independent while participating in activities outside the home.

GROWTH AND DEVELOPMENT OVERVIEW

The school-age years are a time of continued maturation of the child's physical, social, and psychological characteristics. It is during this time that children move toward abstract thinking and seek approval of peers, teachers, and parents. Their eye–hand–muscle coordination allows them to participate in organized sports in school or the community. The **school-age child** typically values school attendance and school activities. The nurse uses knowledge of normal growth and development of the school-age child to assist the child in coping with disruptions and changes during this period.

PHYSICAL GROWTH

From 6 to 12 years of age, children grow an average of 6 to 7 cm (2 to 2.5 in) per year, increasing their height by at least 1 ft (CHOC, 2021). An increase of 2 to 3 kg (4 to 7 lb) per year in weight is expected (CHOC, 2021). In the early school-age years, female and male children are similar in height and weight and appear thinner and more graceful than in previous years (Cincinnati Children's, 2023). In later school-age years, most female children begin to surpass males in both height and weight (Biro & Chan, 2023; Cincinnati Children's, 2023; see Appendix A for growth charts).

Preadolescent children generally do not want to be different from peers, although there are biologic sex-based differences in physical and physiologic growth during the school-age years. These differences, especially secondary sexual characteristics, may be concerning to children and are often a source of embarrassment.

Sex-based differences are more apparent at the end of the middle school years and may become extreme and a source of emotional problems. These differences in height and weight relationships, and changes in growth patterns, should be explained to parents and children (Fig. 6.1). Physical maturity is not necessarily associated with emotional and social maturity. An 8-year-old who is the size of an 11-year-old will think and act like an 8-year-old. Many times, the expectations placed on these children are unrealistic and can impact their self-esteem and competence. This can work in reverse, to similar effect, for an 11-year-old who is the size of an 8-year-old and is therefore treated as such.

Remember Lawrence Jones, the 10-year-old introduced at the beginning of the chapter? Lawrence's weight is 28.1 kg (62 lb) and his height is 137.2 cm (54 in). Plot Lawrence's measurements on the appropriate growth chart.

PHYSIOLOGIC CHANGES

Maturation of organs may differ with age or sex. Maturation of organs remains fairly consistent until late school age. In the late school-age years (10- to 12-year-olds),

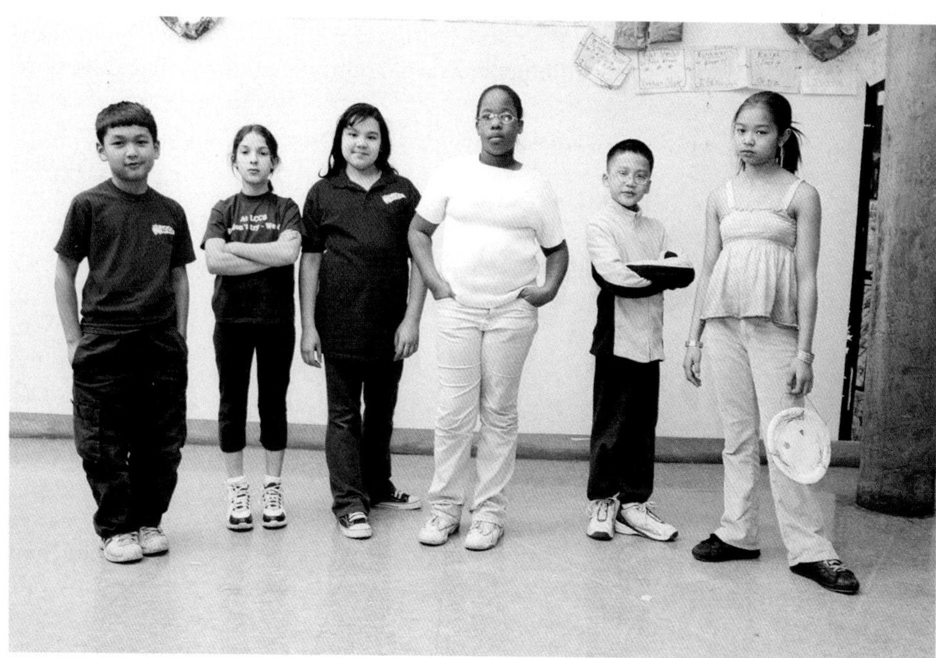

FIGURE 6.1 The different growth rates of school-age children are depicted by these same-age school-age children.

male children experience a slowed growth in height and increased weight gain, which may lead to excess weight. During this time, female children may begin to have changes in the body that soften body lines. Preadolescence is a period of rapid growth, especially for female children.

Neurologic System

The brain and skull grow slowly during the school-age years. Brain growth is complete by the time the child is 10 years of age. The shape of the head is longer, and the growth of the facial bones changes facial proportions.

Respiratory System

The respiratory system continues to mature with the development of the lungs and alveoli, resulting in fewer respiratory infections. Respiratory rates decrease, abdominal breathing disappears, and respirations become diaphragmatic in nature. The frontal sinuses are developed by 7 years of age. Tonsils decrease in size from the preschool years, but they remain larger than those of adolescents. The adenoids and tonsils may appear large normally, even in the absence of infection.

Cardiovascular System

The school-age child's blood pressure increases, and the pulse rate decreases. The heart grows more slowly during the middle years and is smaller in size in relation to the rest of the body than at any other development stage.

Gastrointestinal System

During the school-age years, all 20 primary deciduous teeth are lost and replaced by 28 of 32 permanent teeth, with the exception of the third molars (commonly known as wisdom teeth). The school-age child experiences fewer gastrointestinal upsets compared with earlier years. Stomach capacity increases, which permits retention of food for longer periods. In addition, the caloric needs of the school-age child are lower than in the earlier years.

Genitourinary System

Bladder capacity increases, but this varies among individual children. Female children generally have a greater bladder capacity than male children. Urination patterns vary with the amount of fluids ingested, the time they were ingested, and the stress level of the child. The formula for bladder capacity is age in years plus 2 oz. Therefore, the bladder capacity of the 7-year-old would be 9 oz. The larger capacity of the bladder allows for the child to experience longer periods between voiding.

Prepubescence

The late school-age years are also referred to as *preadolescence* (the time between middle childhood and the 13th birthday). During preadolescence, **prepubescence** occurs. Prepubescence typically occurs in the 2 years before the beginning of puberty and is characterized by the development of secondary sexual characteristics, a period of rapid growth for female children, and a period of continued growth for male children. There is approximately 2 years' difference in the onset of prepubescence between males and females. Sexual development, especially if there is a mismatch between timing of puberty and chronologic age, can have an effect on psychosocial functioning (Biro & Chan, 2023). Early development in female children can lead to concern over physical appearance and lower self-esteem (Biro & Chan, 2023). Delayed development in male children can lead to psychological and social issues such as depression and anxiety (Biro & Chan, 2023). It is important for the nurse and parents to educate the late school-age child about body changes to help minimize psychosocial issues such as anxiety, depression, and low self-esteem and promote comfort with these body changes.

Musculoskeletal System

Musculoskeletal growth leads to greater coordination and strength, yet the muscles are still immature and can be injured easily. Bones continue to ossify throughout childhood, but mineralization is not complete until maturity.

Immune System

Lymphatic tissues continue to grow until the child is 9 years old; immunoglobulins A and G (IgA and IgG) reach adult levels at around 10 years of age. Due to the lymphatic system becoming more competent in localizing infections and producing antibody–antigen responses, school-age children may have fewer infections. They may experience more infections during the first 1 to 2 years of school due to exposure to other children who may have infections.

PSYCHOSOCIAL DEVELOPMENT

Erikson (1963) describes the task of the school-age years to be a sense of **industry** versus **inferiority**. During this time, the child is developing their sense of self-worth by becoming involved in multiple activities at home, at school, and in the community, which develops their cognitive and social skills. The child is interested in learning how things are made and work. The school-age child's satisfaction from achieving success in developing new skills leads them to an increased sense of self-worth and level of competence. It is the role of the parents, teachers, coaches, and nurses of the school-age child to identify areas of competency and to build on the child's successful experiences to promote mastery, success, and self-esteem. If the expectations of adults are set too high, the child will develop a sense of inferiority and incompetence that can affect all aspects of their life. See Table 6.1 for a further explanation of psychosocial development in school-age children.

COGNITIVE DEVELOPMENT

Piaget's stage of cognitive development for the 7- to 11-year-old is the period of concrete operational thoughts (Piaget, 1969). In developing concrete operations, the child is able to assimilate and coordinate information about their world from different dimensions. The child is able to see things from another person's point of view and think through an action, anticipating its consequences and the possibility of having to rethink the action. They are able to use stored memories of past experiences to evaluate and interpret present situations. The school-age child also develops the ability to classify or divide things into different sets and to identify their relationships to each other. The school-age child is able to classify members of four generations on a family tree vertically and horizontally and at the same time see that one person can be a father, son, uncle, and grandson. It is at this time that the school-age child develops an interest in collecting objects. The child starts out collecting multiple objects and becomes more selective as they get older. Also, during concrete operational thinking, the school-age child develops an understanding of the **principle of conservation**—that matter does not change when its form changes. For example, if the child pours a half cup of water into a short, wide glass and into a tall, thin glass, they still only have a half cup of water even though it looks like the tall, thin glass has more (Fig. 6.2). The child learns about conserving matter in a sequence ranging from the simplest to the more complex. See Table 6.1 for further information about cognitive development of school-age children.

TABLE 6.1 • Developmental Theories

Theorist	Stage	Activities
Erikson	Industry vs. inferiority	Interested in how things are made and run Success in personal and social tasks Increased activities outside home—clubs, sports Increased interactions with peers Increased interest in knowledge Needs support and encouragement from important people in child's life Needs support when child is not successful Inferiority occurs with repeated failures with little support or trust from those who are important to the child.
Piaget	Concrete operational	Learns by manipulating concrete objects Lacks ability to think abstractly Learns that certain characteristics of objects remain constant Understands concepts of time Engages in serial ordering, addition, subtraction Classifies or groups objects by their common elements Understands relationships among objects Starts collections of items Can reverse thought process
Kohlberg	Conventional Stage 3: interpersonal conforming, "good child, bad child," age 7–10 years Stage 4: "law and order," age 10–12 years	An act is wrong because it brings punishment. Behavior is completely wrong or right. Does not understand the reason behind rules If child and adult differ in opinions, the adult is right. Can put self in another person's position Begins to exercise the "golden rule" Acts are judged in terms of intention, not just punishment.
Freud	Latency	A time of tranquility between the Oedipal phase of early childhood and adolescence—focuses on activities that develop social and cognitive skills Develops social skills in relating to same-sex friends through joining clubs like Brownies, Girl Scouts, Boy Scouts

Data from Erikson, E. (1963). *Childhood and society* (2nd ed.). Norton; Kohlberg, L. (1984). *Moral development.* Harper & Row; Piaget, J. (1969). *The theory of stages in cognitive development.* McGraw-Hill; Feigelman, S. (2020). Developmental & behavioral theories. In R. M. Kleigman, J. W. St. Geme III, N. J. Blum, S. S. Shah, R. C. Tasker, K. M. Wislon, & R. E. Behrman (Eds.), *Nelson textbook of pediatrics* (21st ed., pp. 1233–1257). Elsevier.

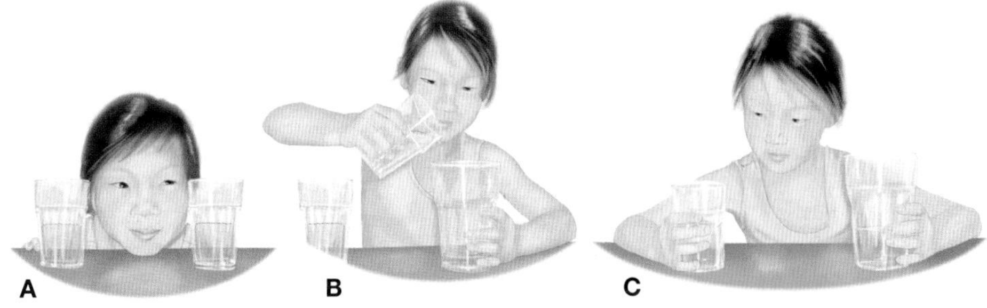

FIGURE 6.2 School-age children understand the theory of conservation (**A**). If you pour an equal amount of liquid into two glasses of unequal shape (**B**), the amount of water you have remains the same despite the unequal appearance in the two glasses (**C**).

MORAL AND SPIRITUAL DEVELOPMENT

During the school-age years, the child's sense of morality is constantly being developed. According to Kohlberg (1984), the school-age child is at the conventional stage of moral development. The 7- to 10-year-old usually follows rules out of a sense of being a "good" person. They want to be a good person to parents, friends, and teachers and to themselves. The adult is viewed as being right. This is stage 3: interpersonal conformity (good child, bad child), according to Kohlberg. The 10- to 12-year-olds progress to stage 4: the "law and order" stage. At this stage, the child can determine if an action is good or bad based on the reason for the action, not just on the possible consequences of the action. The older school-age child's behavior is guided by their desire to cooperate and by their respect for others. This leads to the school-age child's ability to understand and incorporate into their behavior the concept of the "golden rule," to treat others how you would like to be treated (Finkelstein & Feigelman, 2020). See Table 6.1 for additional information about the moral development of school-age children.

During school age, children are still concrete thinkers and are guided by their family's religious and cultural beliefs. They may be comforted by the rituals of their religion, but they are just beginning to understand the differences between natural and supernatural. Incorporating spiritual or religious practices in their lives can assist school-age children in coping with different stressors.

MOTOR SKILL DEVELOPMENT

Gross and fine motor skills continue to mature throughout the school-age years. Refinement of motor skills occurs, and speed and accuracy increase. To assess the motor skills of school-age children, ask questions about participation in sports and afterschool activities, band membership, constructing models, and writing skills.

Gross Motor Skills

During the school-age years, coordination, balance, and rhythm improve, facilitating the opportunity to ride a two-wheel bike, jump rope, dance, and participate in a variety of other sports (Fig. 6.3). Older school-age children may become awkward because their bodies grow faster than their ability to compensate.

School-age children between the ages of 6 and 8 enjoy gross motor activities such as bicycling, skating, and swimming. They are enthralled with the world and are in constant motion. Sometimes, fear is limited due to the strong impulses of exploration. Children between 8 and 10 years of age are less restless, but their energy level continues to be high, with activities more subdued and directed. These children exhibit greater rhythm and gracefulness of muscular movements, allowing them to participate in physical activities that require longer and more concentrated attention and effort, such as baseball or soccer.

Between the ages of 10 and 12 years (the pubescent years for female children), energy levels remain high but are more controlled and focused. Physical skills in this

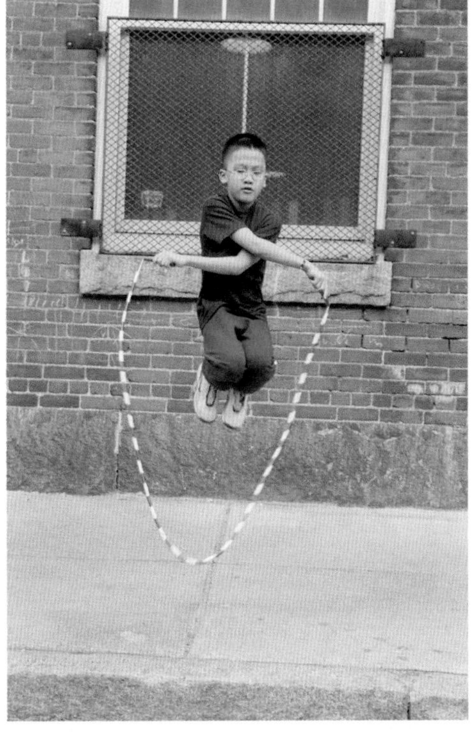

FIGURE 6.3 Jumping rope is an example of the increased development of gross motor skills of the school-age child.

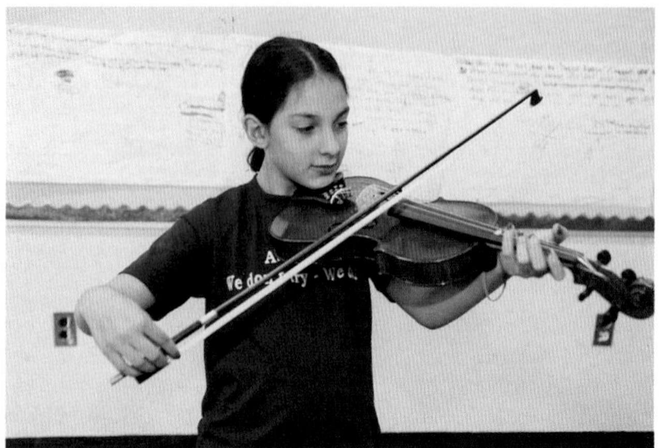

FIGURE 6.4 School-age children improve their fine motor skills so they can play musical instruments well.

age group are similar to those of adults, with strength and endurance increasing during adolescence.

All school-age children should be encouraged to engage in physical activities and learn physical skills that contribute to their health for the rest of their lives. Cardiovascular fitness, weight control, emotional tension release, and development of leadership and following skills are enhanced through physical activity and team sports.

Fine Motor Skills

Myelinization of the central nervous system is reflected by refinement of fine motor skills. Eye–hand coordination and balance improve with maturity and practice. Hand usage improves, becoming steadier and independent and granting an ease and precision that allows these children to write, print words, sew, or build models or other crafts. The child between 10 and 12 years of age begins to exhibit manipulative skills comparable to adults. School-age children take pride in activities that require dexterity and fine motor skills such as playing musical instruments (Fig. 6.4). Talent and practice become the keys to proficiency.

SENSORY DEVELOPMENT

All senses are mature early in the school-age years. Good vision is essential to the physical development and educational progression of school-age children. Vision screening programs conducted by school nurses identify problems with vision and result in appropriate referrals when warranted. Some problems frequently identified include amblyopia (lazy eye), uncorrected refractive errors or other eye defects, and malalignment of the eyes (called *strabismus*). Amblyopia is reduced vision in an eye that has not been adequately used during early development. Inadequate use can result from conditions such as strabismus, one eye being more nearsighted, farsighted, or astigmatic than the other eye. If untreated in childhood, it can persist into adulthood and cause permanent visual impairments (American Association for Pediatric Ophthalmology and Strabismus [AAPOS], 2021). This condition is correctable with glasses or patching, which forces the child to use the weaker eye. A recent study by the National Institutes for Health confirmed that older children (up to 14 years of age) can achieve some improvement in vision, but success remains higher when started at a younger age (AAPOS, 2021). Proper screening and referral, as well as notification to parents of the existing condition, are essential to the education and socialization of the school-age child.

Hearing deficits that are severe are usually diagnosed in infancy, but the less severe may not be diagnosed until the child enters school and has difficulty learning or with speech. It is important to screen children for hearing deficits to ensure proper educational and social progression.

The sense of smell is mature and can be tested in the school-age child by using scents that children are familiar with, such as chocolate or other familiar odors. In addition, the school-age child may be tested for the sense of touch with objects to discriminate cold from hot, soft from hard, and blunt from sharp.

COMMUNICATION AND LANGUAGE DEVELOPMENT

Language skills continue to accelerate during the school-age years and vocabulary expands. Culturally specific words are used, with bilingual children speaking English in school and a second language at home. The school-age child learns to read, and reading efficiency improves language skills. Reading skills are improved with increased reading exposure. School-age children begin to use more complex grammatical forms such as plurals and pronouns. Also, they develop metalinguistic awareness—an ability to think about language and comment on its properties. This enables them to enjoy jokes and riddles due to their understanding of double meanings and play on words and sounds. They are also beginning to understand metaphors such as "a stitch in time saves nine." School-age children may experiment with profanity and dirty jokes if exposed. This age group tends to imitate parents, family members, or others. Therefore, role modeling is important.

Refer back to Lawrence Jones, who was introduced at the beginning of this chapter. What developmental milestones would you expect him to have reached by this age? What would you expect his gross motor, fine motor, and language skills to be at this age?

EMOTIONAL AND SOCIAL DEVELOPMENT

Patterns of temperamental traits identified in infancy may continue to influence behavior in the school-age child. Analyzing past situations may provide clues to the way a child may react to new or different situations. Children may react differently over time due to their experiences and abilities. **Self-esteem** is the child's view of their individual worth. This view is impacted by feedback from family, teachers, and other authority figures.

Temperament

Temperament has been described as the way individuals behave. Three commonly grouped temperaments in children are *even-tempered and adaptable, slow to warm up, and challenging and easily frustrated* (Bogues & Levine, 2023). Variations and combinations of these categories are seen. Not every child can be placed into one of these groups. Understanding a child's temperament can help care providers and parents to understand the child's behavior, actions, and how they relate to the world.

The child who is even-tempered may adapt to school entry and other experiences smoothly and with little or no stress. The slow-to-warm child may be slow to adapt to changes. The slow-to-warm school-age child may exhibit discomfort when placed in different or new situations such as school. This child may need time to adjust to the new place or situation and may demonstrate frustration with tears or somatic complaints. The slow-to-warm child should be allowed time to adjust to new situations and people (such as teachers) within their own time frame. All of these factors may impact the younger school-age child upon entering the school environment, with changes in authority and the introduction of many peers. The challenging or easily distracted child may benefit from an introduction to the new experience and people by role-playing, by visiting the site and being introduced to the teachers, and by hearing stories or participating in conversations about the upcoming school experience. These children require patience, firmness, and understanding to make the transition into a new situation or experience such as school.

Assessment of temperament by a professional would include a combination of interview, observation, and a standardized questionnaire. Better understanding a child's temperament can assist parents with adjusting their parenting style to better fit their child and may help limit emotional and behavioral problems that occur when these areas are in conflict.

Self-Esteem Development

Self-esteem mirrors the child's individual self-worth and consists of both positive and negative qualities. Children strive to achieve internalized goals of attainment, although they continually receive feedback from individuals they perceive as authorities (parent or teacher). By the school-age years, children have received feedback related to their performance or tasks. The direction of this feedback influences the child's opinion of self-worth, which influences self-esteem and self-evaluation.

Children face the process of self-evaluation from a framework of either self-confidence or self-doubt. Children who have mastered the earlier developmental task of autonomy and initiative face the world with feelings of pride rather than shame (Erikson, 1963).

If school-age children regard themselves as worthwhile, they have a positive self-concept and high self-esteem. Significant adults in school-age children's lives can manipulate the environment to facilitate success. This success impacts the self-esteem of the child.

Body Image

Body image is how the school-ager perceives their body. School-age children are knowledgeable about the human body but may have different perceptions about body parts. School-age children are very interested in peers' views and acceptance of their body, body changes, and clothing. This age group may model themselves after parents, peers, and people in movies or on television. It is important for late school-agers to feel accepted by peers. If they feel different and are teased, there may be lifelong effects.

School-Age Fears

The school-age child's fears shift away from pretend things, like monsters, to things that could happen to them in real life, such as natural disasters, others hurting them, and the death of a loved one (Radcliff, 2023). School-age children are less fearful of harm to their body than in their preschool years but fear being kidnapped or undergoing surgery. They may continue to fear the dark but are less fearful of animals, such as dogs and noises. The school-age child needs reassurance that their fears are normal for this developmental age. Parents, teachers, and other caregivers should listen to the child's fears with sympathy and support. Recognize the child's fears, but do not cater to them. Help the child face their fears, and teach the child coping strategies, for instance, using positive self-statements such as "I can do this" and relaxation techniques such as deep breathing and visualization (Radcliff, 2023).

Peer Relationships

The school-age child's concept of self is shaped not only by their parents but also by relationships with others. Peer relationships influence children's independence from parents. Peers play an important role in the approval and critiquing of skills of school-age children. Previously, only adults such as parents and teachers have been authorities; now, peers influence school-age children's perceptions of themselves. Peer relationships help to support the school-age child by providing enough security to risk the parental conflict brought about when establishing independence. School-age children associate with peers of the same sex or same gender most of the time. Although games and other activities are shared by all children, the child's concept of the appropriate gender role is influenced by their relationship with peers.

Continuous peer relationships provide the most important social interaction for school-age children. Valuable lessons are learned from interactions with children of their own age. Children learn to respect differing points of view that are represented in their groups. Peer groups establish norms and standards that signify acceptance or rejection. Children may modify behavior to gain acceptance. A characteristic of school-age children is their formation of groups with rules and values.

Teacher and School Influences

School serves as a means to transmit values of society and to establish peer relationships. Secondary only to the family, school exerts a profound influence on the social development of the child. Often, school requires changes for the child and parent. The child enters an environment that requires conforming to group activities that are structured and directed by an adult other than the parent. The parent's attitude and support influence the child's transition into the school setting. Parents who are positive and supportive promote a smooth entry into school. Parents who encourage clinging behaviors may delay a successful transition into school.

To facilitate the transition from home to school, the teacher must have the personality and knowledge of development that will allow them to meet the needs of young children. Even though the teacher's responsibilities are primarily to stimulate and guide intellectual development, they must share in shaping the child's attitudes and values. The system of awards and punishment administered by teachers affects the self-concept of children and influences their response to school. Teachers and school are important in shaping the socialization, self-concept, and intellectual development of children.

Family Influences

The school-age years are a time for peer relationships, questioning of parents, and the potential for parental conflict but continued respect for family values. School-age years are the beginning of the time of peer-group influence, with testing of parental and family values. Although the peer group is influential, the family's values usually predominate when parental and peer-group values come into conflict. Even though the school-age child may question the parents' values, the child will usually incorporate the values from parents into their values.

Often, in the late school age and preadolescent period, the child may prefer to be in the company of peers and show a decreased interest in family functions. This may require an adjustment for parents. Parents' awareness of this developmental trend and their continuing support for the child are important while they continue to enforce restrictions and control of behaviors. The school-ager is beginning to strive for independence, but parental authority and controls continue to impact choices and values.

TAKE NOTE!

School-age children continue to need parenting. They do not need parents as friends.

CULTURAL INFLUENCES ON GROWTH AND DEVELOPMENT

Culture influences habits, beliefs, language, and values. School-age children thrive on learning the music, language, traditions, holidays, games, values, gender roles, and other aspects of culture. Nurses must be aware of the effects on children of various groups' family structures and traditional values. The school-age child's cultural and ethnic backgrounds must be considered when assessing growth and development. Cultural implications must be considered for all children and families in order to provide appropriate care.

THE NURSE'S ROLE IN SCHOOL-AGE GROWTH AND DEVELOPMENT

Growth and development in the school-age child occurs in irregular spurts, with a wide variation of sizes, shapes, and abilities seen. Nurses must be aware of the usual growth and development patterns for this age group so that they can assess school-age children appropriately and provide guidance to the child and their family. This is a time when children compare themselves to peers, and self-esteem is a central issue. The school-age child is separating from their parents and seeks acceptance from peers and adults outside of their family. Health care visits throughout the school-age period continue to focus on expected growth and development and anticipatory guidance. Visits are more infrequent during the school-age years; therefore, the nurse needs to assess the child's functioning not only at home but also at school and within the community.

If the school-age child is hospitalized, growth and development may be altered. The school-age child is able to understand the reason for hospitalization and what will happen. They are often worried about pain or changes that may occur to their body. It is important for health care providers and family members to be honest and open with the school-age child. The school-age child may miss school and the interactions with their peers. The school-age child may regress and exhibit behaviors of a younger child, such as needing special comfort toys or demanding attention from their parents. Hospitalization for the school-age child can bring with it a loss of control. The school-age child is used to controlling their self-care and making choices about their meals and activities.

When caring for the hospitalized school-age child, the nurse must use knowledge of normal growth and development to recognize potential delays, promote continued appropriate growth and development, and interact successfully with the school-age child. Provide opportunities for the school-age child to maintain independence, gain control, and increase self-esteem.

Clinical Judgment and the Nursing Process

On completion of assessment of the school-age child's current growth and development status, problems or issues related to growth and development may be identified. The nurse may then identify one or more nursing diagnoses. The following nursing diagnoses with identified outcomes and interventions provide suggestions for nursing care planning or concept mapping. Care planning should be individualized.

Nursing Analysis

Risk for excess weight; risk factors include average daily physical activity being less than recommended for sex and age, consumption of sugar-sweetened beverages, frequent snacking, high frequency of restaurant or fried food, insufficient knowledge of modifiable factors, sedentary behavior occurring for more than 2 hours a day, portion sizes larger than recommended, body mass index (BMI) approaching 85th percentile, and parental excess weight.

Goal/Outcome

The school-age child will maintain a healthy weight for age, BMI of less than the 85th percentile; lose weight at an appropriate rate: Increase the amount of exercise; make appropriate eating choices; and decrease caloric intake to an appropriate amount for age and sex.

Promoting Healthy Weight (interventions with *rationale*)

- Assess knowledge of parents and child about nutritional needs of school-age children *to determine deficits in knowledge.*
- Plot out height, weight, and BMI *to detect weight loss or weight gain.*
- Have child keep food and exercise diary for 1 week *to determine current patterns of eating and exercise.*
- Interview parents in relation to their eating habits and exercise habits *to determine where adjustments might need to be made.*
- Analyze preceding data, and base recommendations for changes on these data, *to best develop a further plan.*
- Educate primary caregiver about appropriate serving sizes and foods *so that primary caregiver is aware of what to expect for school-age children.*
- Discuss ways to decrease temptation to overeat and to make good meal choices *to assist the child with developing healthy eating habits* (see Teaching Guidelines 6.2).
- Have child assist in meal planning and grocery shopping *to allow them some sense of control in process.*
- Incorporate increase in daily exercise, which will stress sense of self-improvement, *to increase caloric expenditure and self-esteem.*
- Decrease television/computer/device time *to increase caloric expenditure.*
- Develop reward system *to increase self-esteem.*
- Investigate joining weight-loss program for school-age children *to increase self-esteem and to increase awareness that other children have the same problem.*

Nursing Analysis

Delayed growth and development risk; risk factors include inadequate nutrition, presence of abuse, substance misuse, technology dependence, behavioral disorder, low socioeconomic status involvement with the foster care system, prematurity, chronic illness, genetic disorder.

Goal/Outcome

Growth and development will be maximized: School-age child will make continued progress toward attainment of expected standards of school performance.

Promoting Development (interventions with *rationale*)

- Perform developmental evaluation of the school-age child *to determine current functioning.*
- Develop realistic multidisciplinary plan *to ensure maximizing resources.*
- Carry out interventions as prescribed by developmental specialist, physical therapist, occupational

therapist, or speech therapist at home and at school *to maximize benefit of interventions.*
- Have scheduled evaluation meetings *to be able to adapt interventions as soon as possible.*

Nursing Analysis

Injury risk due to exposure to toxic chemicals, insufficient knowledge of modifiable factors, unsafe mode of transport, extremes of age (e.g., developmental stage including high level of curiosity and increasing cognitive skills and motor abilities).

Goal/Outcome

School-age child's safety will be maintained: They will remain free from injury.

Preventing Injury (interventions with *rationale*)

- Discuss safety measures needed for the following: bikes, scooters, guns, skateboards, cars, water, and playground *to decrease risk of injury related to those areas.*
- Discuss and develop a fire safety plan *to decrease risk of injury related to fire.*
- Discuss appropriate safety equipment needed for each sport *to decrease risk of injury.*
- Discuss appropriate sports to participate in depending on age and maturity of child *to prevent possible injury* and *to promote child's self-esteem.*
- Instruct parents to post the Poison Control Center phone number (*in the event of accidental ingestion, Poison Control can give parents the best advice for appropriate intervention*).
- Teach parents and child first-aid measures and child cardiopulmonary resuscitation (CPR) *to minimize consequences of injury should it occur.*
- Discuss influence of peers on actions of school-age children *to prevent possible injury due to mimicking behavior.*

Nursing Analysis

Caregiver role strain risk; risk factors include dependency, discharged home with significant needs, problematic behavior, caregiver substance misuse, unstable health condition, insufficient knowledge about community resources, social isolation.

Goal/Outcome

Parent will experience competence in role: They will demonstrate appropriate caregiving behaviors and verbalize comfort in caring for a school-age child.

Preventing Caregiver Role Strain (interventions with *rationale*)

- Assess parents' knowledge of school-age children and the issues that arise as a part of normal development *to determine parents' needs.*
- Provide education on normal issues of school-age children *so that parents have the knowledge they need to appropriately care for their school-age child.*
- Provide anticipatory guidance related to upcoming expected issues related to school-age development *to prepare parents for what to expect next and how to intervene.*

PROMOTING HEALTHY GROWTH AND DEVELOPMENT

The family plays a critical role in promoting healthy growth and development of the school-age child. Respectful interchange of communication between the parent and child will foster self-esteem and self-confidence. This respect will give the child confidence in achieving personal, educational, and social goals appropriate for their age. The nurse should study interactions between parents and school-age children to observe for this respect or lack of respect ("putting the child down"). The nurse can model appropriate behaviors by listening to the child and making appropriate responses. The nurse can be a resource for parents and an advocate for the child in promoting healthy growth and development.

Promoting Growth and Development Through Play

Cooperative play is exhibited by the school-age child. Play for the school-age child includes both organized cooperative activities (such as team sports) and solitary activities. School-age children have the coordination and intellect to participate with other children of their age in sports such as soccer, baseball, football, and tennis. The school-age child comprehends that their cooperation with others will lead to a unified whole for the team. In addition, the child learns rules and the value of playing by the rules.

School-age children also enjoy solitary activities, including board, card, video, and computer games, and dollhouse and other small-figure play (Fig. 6.5). Many school-agers start collections of stamps, cars, or other valuable or not-so-valuable items. During the school-age years, children may also begin a scrapbook or keep a diary. They may participate in activities, such as dance or karate, and join clubs or special interest groups (Fig. 6.6).

Active play has decreased in recent years as television viewing, multimedia device use, and video games have increased (Oh et al., 2022). This trend has resulted in health risks such as excess weight, type 2 diabetes, and cardiovascular problems (CDC, 2022b).

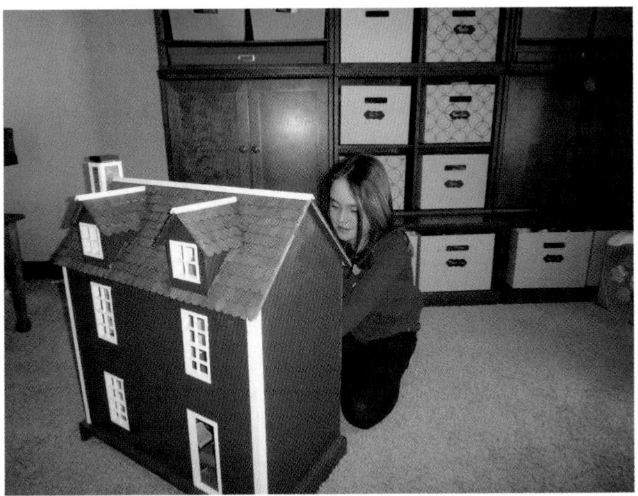

FIGURE 6.5 This school-age child enjoys solitary play with their dollhouse and dolls.

Promoting Learning

School attendance and learning are important to the school-age child. Parent–child, child–teacher, and child–peer relationships and activities influence the school-age child's learning.

Formal Education

Most children are excited about starting school and making new friends. They like the notion of getting books, having book bags, and having homework assignments. The reality of the work involved with school and homework may decrease the enthusiasm about school.

Peers are important within this age group. Both peers and teachers influence children. Attending school may be their first experience interacting with a large number of children of their own age. Through this interaction, children learn cooperation, competition, and the importance of following the rules. Peer approval and influences grow as the child matures. Teachers have significant influences on children. They help to guide the child's intellectual development by rewarding successes and helping the child deal with failures. The student–teacher relationship is a key to success. Teachers play a role in fostering feelings of industry and preventing feelings of inferiority (Fig. 6.7). School-age children also learn skills, rules, values, and other ways to work with peers and other authority figures.

Parental support is important for school adjustment and achievement. Parents must collaborate with teachers and school personnel to ensure that the child is fulfilling the expectations and requirements for this age group in school. Parents must monitor the child's homework assignments and friends and observe for any changes in behavior that would indicate school or behavioral problems.

Reading

Encouraging reading is an excellent way to promote learning in the school-age child. Trips to the library and purchasing books help to promote a love of reading. School-age children enjoy being read to as well as reading on their own. Younger school-age children (6 to 8 years) enjoy books that are simple to read, with few words on a page, such as the Dr. Seuss books. They enjoy books about animals and trains and simple mysteries. Children 8 to 10 years of age have more advanced reading skills and enjoy those books from early childhood, as well as more classic novels and adventures such as the *Harry Potter* series. Older children enjoy horror stories, mysteries, romances, and adventure stories as well as classic novels. School-age children of all ages benefit from books on topics related to things they may be experiencing, such as a visit to the hospital for a surgical procedure. See Box 6.1 for ideas for parents to promote reading in the school-age child.

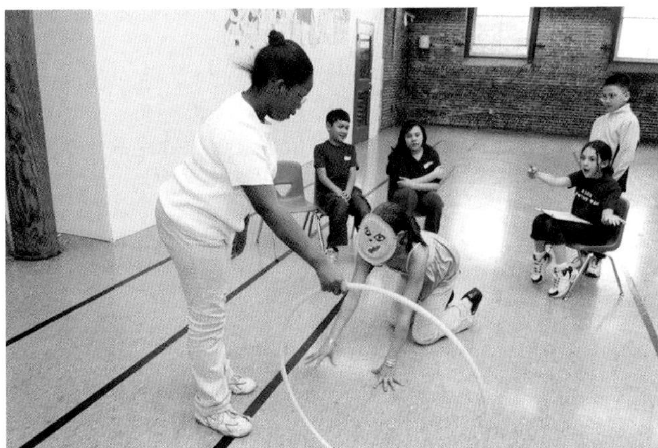

FIGURE 6.6 School-age children like to join clubs. These children, in the acting club at school, are rehearsing for a play.

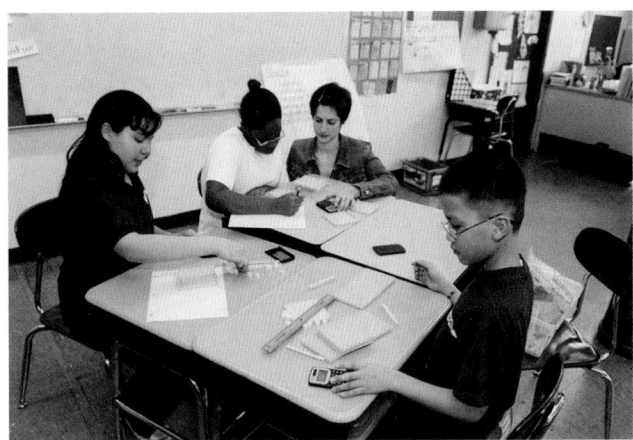

FIGURE 6.7 School is important to the school-age child.

BOX 6.1 Promotion of Reading in School-Age Children

- Parents, read to and with your children.
- Ask teachers and librarians for advice on books appropriate for your child.
- Choose stories that the child can relate to if the child has difficulty reading.
- Choose books with movement if the child has a short attention span.
- Take advantage of all reading opportunities (cereal boxes, road signs).
- Provide choices for the child to select a book of interest.
- Talk about the text and ask questions to improve understanding.
- Keep a record of what the child is reading.
- Visit a library, get a library card, and check out books.
- Parents, demonstrate role modeling through reading books.

Promoting Safety

School-age children become more independent with age. This independence leads to an increased self-confidence and decreased fears, which may contribute to accidents and injuries. School age is a time that the child may walk to school with peers who may influence their behavior. Increased independence may also increase exposure to dangerous situations such as the approach of strangers or unsafe streets. Promotion of safe habits during the school-age years is important for parents and nurses. See Teaching Guidelines 6.1 for additional information on safety education for nurses and parents.

TEACHING GUIDELINES 6.1 Safety Issues and Interventions of the School-Age Child

Safety Issue	Interventions
Car safety	• A seat belt or age- and weight-appropriate booster seat should be used at all times. The lap belt should lie low and flat on the hips, and the shoulder belt should lie on the shoulder, not the neck or face (proper fitting of adult shoulder and lap belts without a booster seat usually occurs when the child is about 144.8 cm [57 in] tall). • Seat belts should be fastened before car is started. • Children under 13 years must sit in the back seat. • Childproof locks should be used in the back seat. • Rules of conduct for car rides must be established.
Pedestrian safety	• The child should be instructed to stop at the curb and look right, left, then right again before crossing the street and to cross only at safe crossings. • Older children and adults should provide supervision of younger children. • Walking should only be done on sidewalks. • Phones, headphones, and devices should be put away when crossing the street. • In parking lots, children should know to watch for cars backing up and not dart out between parked cars. • If children are playing outside, drivers should be aware of their presence before backing up.
Bike safety: general	• The child should know to wear a properly fitted, Consumer Product Safety Commission (CPSC) or Snell-approved helmet every time they ride a bike. • A properly fitting helmet should sit level, not tilted, and firmly and comfortably on the head; have strong wide Y-shaped straps and when you open your mouth should pull down a bit; not move with sudden pulling or twisting; never be worn over anything else (hat, scarf, etc.). • Bikes should be well maintained and appropriately sized. • The child should be oriented to the bike and demonstrate ability to ride the bike safely before being allowed to ride on street. • Safe areas for bike riding should be established, as should routes to and from the area of activities. • Riding a bike barefoot, with someone else on the bike, or with clothing that might get entangled in the bike should be prohibited. • The child should know to wear sturdy, well-fitting shoes. • The bike should be inspected often to ensure it is in proper working order. • A basket should be used to carry heavy objects.
Bike safety in traffic	• All traffic signs and signals must be observed. • Avoid riding at night; if riding at night occurs, the bike should have lights and reflectors, and the rider should wear light-colored clothes. • The child should know to ride on the side of the road traveling with traffic and keep close to the side of the road in single file.

TEACHING GUIDELINES **6.1** Safety Issues and Interventions of the School-Age Child

Safety Issue	Interventions
	• The child should learn to watch and listen for cars and to stop and check for traffic in both directions when leaving driveways, alleys, or curbs. • Headphones should not be used while riding a bike. • Never hitch a ride on any vehicle.
Sports safety	• Sports should be matched to child's ability and desire. • The sports program should have a warm-up procedure. • Coaches should be trained in CPR and first aid. • Appropriate protection devices should be used for individual sports.
Skateboarding and inline skating safety	• The child should wear a helmet and protective padding on knees, elbows, and wrists. • The child should know not to skate in traffic or on streets or highways. • Homemade ramps should be assessed for hazards before skating.
All-terrain vehicle safety	• The child should be at least 16 years of age to operate vehicle. • Take a hands-on safety course before riding. • Helmets designed for motorcycles must be worn in addition to protective coverings. • No nighttime riding • No double riding • Use should be avoided on public roads. • Never stand up in the vehicle or ride in a person's lap.
Fire safety	• All homes should have working smoke detectors and fire extinguishers. Change the batteries at least twice a year. • Have a fire-escape plan. • Practice the fire-escape plan routinely. • Nobody should smoke in the home, especially in bed. • Teach what to do in case of a fire: use a fire extinguisher, call 911, and know how to put out clothing fire. • Use the stove and other cooking facilities under adult supervision. • All flammable materials and liquids should be stored safely. • Fireplaces should have protective gratings. • Teach children to avoid touching wires they might encounter while playing.
Water safety	• Teach children how to swim and to never play around or in water without adult supervision. • If swimming skill is limited, the child must wear a life preserver at all times. • The child should know never to swim alone—if at all possible, they should swim only where there is a life guard. • Understand basic CPR. • Teach the child to never run or fool around at the edge of the pool. • Drains in pool should be covered with appropriate cover. • Life jackets should be worn when on a boat. • Make sure the water is deep enough to support diving.
Firearm safety	• Teach the child never to touch guns and to tell an adult when they encounter a gun. • If there are guns in household, secure them in a safe place, use gun safety locks, and store bullets in a separate place. • Never point a gun at a person.
Toxin safety	• Teach the child the hazards of accepting recreational drugs, alcohol, or dangerous drugs. • Store potentially dangerous material in a safe place.

Data from American Academy of Pediatrics, HealthyChildren. (2021). *Booster seats for school-age children*. https://www.healthychildren.org/English/safety-prevention/on-the-go/Pages/Booster-Seats-for-School-Age-Children.aspx; Jennissen, C. (2022). *ATVs are not safe for children: AAP policy explained.* https://www.healthychildren.org/English/safety-prevention/at-play/Pages/ATV-Safety-Rules.aspx; Gill, A. C. (2022). Bicycle injuries in children: Prevention. *UpToDate*. Retrieved October 17, 2022, from https://www.uptodate.com/contents/bicycle-injuries-in-children-prevention

Unintentional injuries are the leading cause of death in children older than 1 year of age (Gill & Kelly, 2022). In 2020, more than 6 million children sought medical attention at a hospital emergency room for nonfatal unintentional injuries (Gill & Kelly, 2022). School-age children are very active at home, in the community, and at school. This increased mobility, activity, and time away from parents increase the risk of unintentional injuries. School-age children continue to need supervision and guidance. They need information and rules about car safety, pedestrian safety, bicycle and other sport safety, fire safety, and water safety.

Car Safety

Motor vehicle crashes are a common cause of injury in the school-age child. While traveling in the car, school-age children should always sit in the rear seat. The front seat is dangerous because of passenger-side airbags in most new-model cars. A school-age child over 18.1 kg (40 lb; generally 4 to 8 years of age) should use a belt-positioning, forward-facing booster seat using both lap and shoulder belts (American Academy of Pediatrics [AAP], HealthyChildren, 2021). School-age children who outgrow the convertible restraint can sit in a booster seat until the vehicle seat belt restraint fits properly over the hips and shoulder, typically when they are 144.8 cm (4 ft 9 in) or taller, usually between 8 and 12 years of age (AAP, HealthyChildren, 2021). The seat belt needs to lie low and flat over the hip bones and across the shoulder, not the neck or face. Children younger than 13 years of age should not ride in the front seat of a vehicle with an airbag (AAP, HealthyChildren, 2021).

Pedestrian Safety

In 2021, about 9,250 children were injured as pedestrians, with 385 suffering fatal injuries (Safe Kids Worldwide, 2023). The highest risk age group is 12 to 19 years (Safe Kids Worldwide, 2023). Children younger than 10 years should not be unsupervised pedestrians. Young school-age children, therefore, should walk to school or the bus with an older friend, sibling, or parent. Darting out into the street without looking both ways or from between cars is a common occurrence in the school-age years. Teach children safe street and pedestrian practices.

Bicycle and Sport Safety

Bicycling, riding scooters, skateboarding, and inline skating or roller skating are common activities of school-age children. Laws in some states require helmets for riding bicycles and scooters. In addition, when skating or skateboarding, school-age children should wear a helmet, kneepads, and elbow pads.

Research has shown that brain injuries due to bicycle crashes have been reduced by wearing a well-fitting helmet (Gill, 2022; see Healthy People 2030). It is important for children to wear helmets that fit and that do not obstruct their vision or hearing. Because school-age children have completed most of their skull growth, a helmet can be worn into adolescence. It is important for the child to have a bicycle that is appropriate for their size and age. The child should be able to plant both feet on the ground when sitting on the seat of the bike (Fig. 6.8). It is important to stress to parents the importance of appropriate size and not to get a bike for the child to "grow into." If older school-agers are using the bike for transportation on busy streets, they should be taught to use bike lanes and to give appropriate hand signals for turning. Nonmotorized and motorized scooters also place children at risk for injury, so counsel families about the use of protective gear, including helmets, elbow pads, and kneepads.

Fire Safety

School-age children are eager to help parents with cooking and ironing. They are curious about fire and are drawn to play with fire, matches, and fireworks. Serious burns can occur from any exposure to fire. Educate children about the hazards of fire. In addition, teach children proper behavior around fires at home and outdoors.

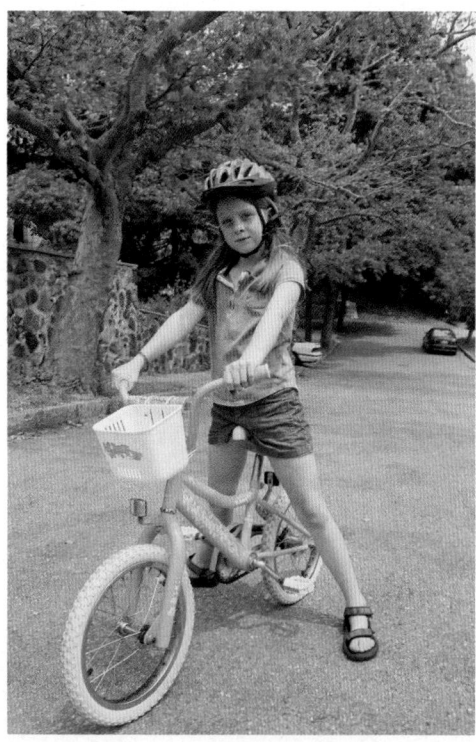

FIGURE 6.8 Wearing the appropriate safety equipment and having an appropriately sized bicycle are important to prevent injuries in school-age children.

HEALTHY PEOPLE 2030

Objective	Nursing Significance
Reduce fatal traumatic brain injuries.	• Provide education to children and their parents about avoiding head injury through helmet use. • Encourage child to choose a helmet that appeals to them (one that looks "cool").

Healthy People Objectives retrieved from http://www.healthypeople.gov

Always supervise children in the use of matches. In the home setting, parents should develop a fire safety plan with their children, teach children what to do if their clothes catch fire, and practice evacuating the house in the event of a fire. In the school setting, children should be aware of the appropriate response to fire drills, and fire drills should be conducted on a regular basis.

Water Safety

Teach school-age children swimming and water safety. An adult should always supervise children when they are swimming to prevent water-related accidents.

Remember Lawrence Jones, the 10-year-old presented in the case study? What anticipatory guidance related to safety should you provide to his parent?

Child Abuse

Child abuse, including physical abuse and sexual abuse, is a common crime of violence against children. An estimated 2.1 million reports of child abuse are made annually to child protective services in the United States (U.S. Department of Health and Human Services, Administration for Children and Families, Administration on Children, Youth and Families, Children's Bureau, 2022). Nationally, 618,000 cases were substantiated in 2020; in 76.1% the children were victims of neglect in, 16.5% they were victims of physical abuse, in 9.4% they were victims of sexual abuse, and in 6% they were victims of other abuse, such as drug or alcohol use disorder, emotional or psychological abuse (U.S. Department of Health and Human Services, Administration for Children and Families, Administration on Children, Youth and Families, Children's Bureau, 2022). The perpetrators may be family, friends, and strangers. It is important for parents to teach children the concept of "good touch" versus "bad touch" prior to school-age years. Whenever the school-age child's behavior yields suspicion of physical or sexual abuse, the nurse should report to the appropriate authorities in their state. These topics will be discussed in more depth in Chapter 28.

Promoting Nutrition

Growth, body composition, and body shape remain constant during late school-age years. Needed calories decrease while the appetite increases. In preparation for adolescence, the body fat composition of school-age children increases. This tendency toward increased body fat occurs earlier in female children than in male children, with the amount of increase greater in females. Males tend to have more lean body mass per inch of height than females.

Diet preferences established in the preschool years continue during the school-age period. As the child grows older, influences of family, media, and peers can impact the eating habits of this age group. Some of these influences are parents' work schedule, outside activities, and exercise level of the child. Decreased exercise levels and poor nutritional choices lead to the higher weight more frequently seen in this age group. See Box 6.2 for appropriate questions to ask the child and parent regarding nutritional status. Healthy People 2030 provides objectives and actions to improve the nutritional health of children.

Nutritional Needs

The school-age child's calorie needs vary based on age, sex, and activity level. Children 4 to 8 years old who are moderately active will need about 1,400 to 1,600 calories a day (U.S. Department of Agriculture [USDA] & U.S. Department of Health and Human Services [HHS],

BOX 6.2 Dietary Questions

Questions for the Child

- How often do you eat together as a family?
- What are the usual mealtimes?
- How often does the family eat out?
- Do you eat breakfast regularly?
- Where do you eat lunch?
- What do you drink/how much?
- What foods do you eat most often?
- What is your favorite food?
- How often do you eat fast foods?
- What type of exercise do you do?

Questions for the Parents

- How would you describe your child's usual appetite?
- Do you have any special cultural/religious practices regarding food?
- Has your child gained or lost weight recently?
- Do you have any concerns about their eating behaviors?
- How does your child exercise? Your family?
- Is there a family history of cancer, hypertension, diabetes, higher weight, or heart disease?

HEALTHY PEOPLE 2030

Objective	Nursing Significance
Increase fruit consumption by people aged 2 years and older. Increase vegetable consumption by people aged 2 years and older. Increase consumption of dark green vegetables, red and orange vegetables, and beans and peas by people aged 2 years and older. Increase whole grain consumption by people aged 2 years and older. Reduce consumption of added sugars by people aged 2 years and older. Reduce consumption of saturated fat by people aged 2 years and older. Reduce consumption of sodium by people aged 2 years and older. Increase calcium consumption by people aged 2 years and older. Increase potassium consumption by people aged 2 years and older.	• Educate families about the importance of whole grains, fruits, and vegetables in the diet. • Encourage the child to choose fruits and vegetables that appeal to them. • Provide creative suggestions for vegetable preparation to make them more appealing to children. • Educate families about saturated fat–containing foods. • Offer suggestions for alternative sources of proteins and fats (chicken or fish, olive oil).

Healthy People Objectives retrieved from http://www.healthypeople.gov

2020). Males 9 to 13 years old who are moderately active need about 1,800 to 2,200 calories a day, while females of this age who are moderately active need about 1,600 to 2,000 calories a day (USDA & HHS, 2020). Of these calories, 45% to 65% should come from carbohydrates, 10% to 30% from protein, and 25% to 35% from fat (USDA & HHS, 2020). The 4- to 8-year-old child needs 1,000 mg of calcium, while the 9- to 13-year-old needs 1,300 mg of calcium for maintenance of growth and good nutrition (USDA & HHS, 2020). Calcium is needed for the development of strong bones and teeth. Milk, yogurt, and cheese provide protein, vitamins, and minerals and are an excellent source of calcium. Meats, poultry, fish, and eggs provide protein, vitamins, and minerals.

Promoting Healthy Eating Habits

School-age children should choose culturally appropriate foods and snacks from the USDA's MyPlate. MyPlate illustrates the five food groups and encourages children to make half of their plate fruits and vegetables, to make half of their grains whole grains, and to choose lean proteins and calcium-rich foods. The website https://www.choosemyplate.gov/kids offers many tools for the child to use, including development of personalized goals and menus, online diet and physical activity assessment tools, games, activities, and tips for parents. School-age children need to limit intake of fat and processed sugars. A prudent diet limits the use of fatty meats, high-fat dairy products, and hydrogenated shortenings and promotes the consumption of fish and the substitution of polyunsaturated vegetable oils and margarines.

Maintaining a Healthy Body Weight

Maintenance of a healthy body weight weight remains a serious health concern for children in the United States, with 20.7% of school-age children having a BMI greater than 95% (CDC, 2022a). According to the CDC (2022a), overweight is classified as a BMI greater than 85%, and obese is classified as a BMI greater than 95% (see Healthy People 2030 objectives).

Some factors linked to higher weight include family role modeling, lack of exercise, unstructured meals, consumption of sugar-sweetened beverages, large portion sizes, lack of sleep, recreational media use such as television viewing and video gaming as well as genetic, environmental, and socioeconomic factors (Skelton & Klish, 2023). Some factors that influence lack of exercise include the decreased number of days that school systems offer physical education programs and recess. Some children live in neighborhoods or communities that lack sidewalks or parks and have no safe place to play outside; therefore, they spend time doing sedentary activities such as watching TV or playing video or computer games. Children with higher weight are at higher risk for cardiovascular diseases such as high cholesterol and hypertension; type 2 (non–insulin-dependent) diabetes; respiratory complications such as obstructive sleep apnea; mental health issues such as depression, anxiety

HEALTHY PEOPLE 2030

Objective	Nursing Significance
Reduce the proportion of children and adolescents with higher weight	• Screen all children for the development of overweight, as indicated by an increasing BMI for their age. • Provide accurate diet counseling. • Encourage daily physical activity. • Counsel parents to limit television/computer time daily.

Healthy People Objectives retrieved from http://www.healthypeople.gov

and eating disorders; and orthopedic problems (USDA & HHS, 2020). When parents do not have knowledge of nutrition, do not monitor snacks or meals, and have unstructured meals, habits are established that contribute to higher weight.

Maintaining healthy body weight in childhood is important because childhood higher weight often carries over into adolescence and adulthood and contributes to disease (Skelton & Klish, 2023). Due to the risk of higher weight, encourage parents to never use food as a reward. To achieve a healthy weight, caregivers should establish regular mealtimes and offer healthy foods and snacks. Encourage parents to praise their child's good food choices and to role model appropriate eating and exercise.

Think back to Lawrence Jones; what questions should you ask Lawrence's parent related to nutritional intake? What anticipatory guidance related to nutrition would be appropriate?

Promoting Healthy Sleep and Rest

The number of hours of sleep required for growth and development decreases with age. Children between the ages of 6 and 8 years require about 12 hours of sleep per night, children between 8 and 10 years of age require 10 to 12 hours of sleep per night, and children between 10 and 12 years of age need 9 to 10 hours of sleep per night. Young school-age children may need an occasional brief nap for an energy boost after being in school for most of the day. Bedtime rituals and consistent schedules continue to be important throughout the school-age years. Parents must facilitate a bedtime schedule and quiet time before bed. Bedtime is a special time for parents and children. They can spend time together reading, listening to soothing music, and discussing the day's events. This time continues to be important during the school-age years as the child gains independence from their parents. Children should have bedtime expectations as well as wake-up times and methods for waking up (alarm, calling by parent, and so forth). Night terrors or sleepwalking may occur in young children but typically resolve as the child gets older (Morse & Kotagal, 2021).

What anticipatory guidance should you provide to Lawrence Jones's parent in relation to proper sleep for their 10-year-old?

Promoting Healthy Teeth and Gums

Dental **caries** remain a leading chronic disease in children even though the incidence has declined since the 1970s, mostly due to the introduction of fluoride (Nowak & Warren, 2022). Recent statistics show that 45.8% of children have treated or untreated dental caries (Nowak & Warren, 2022). Dental caries disproportionately affect children living below 100% of the poverty level and non-Hispanic Black and Hispanic children. (Clark et al., 2020).

Dental care with emphasis on prevention of caries is important in this age group. School-age children need to brush their teeth two to three times per day for 2 to 3 minutes each time with fluorinated toothpaste (Fig. 6.9). Parents should replace the toothbrush (soft) every 3 to 4 months. Flossing the teeth at least once daily is recommended along with limiting the intake of sugar to aid in the prevention of cavities and improved oral health. Parents must monitor toothbrushing, observe for abnormal alignment of their child's teeth, and schedule regular dental examinations every 6 months to ensure good dental health and prevent dental problems. Children will need help with brushing teeth until they are between 7 and 10 years of age.

Dental sealants are an easy way to protect a child's primary or permanent teeth. The sealant is a plastic coating applied to biting surfaces to seal out tooth decay on back teeth and sometimes to cover deep pits or grooves. In addition, parents should give a fluoride supplement (as directed by the dentist) to their children if fluoride is not in the town's water supply (Clark et al., 2020). The school-age child should have an established dental home; if not, provide appropriate resources to establish one. See Healthy People 2030.

Proper alignment of teeth is important to tooth formation, speech development, and physical appearance. Many school-age children need braces or other orthodontic devices to correct **malocclusion**, a condition in which the teeth are crowded, crooked, or misaligned. **Bruxism** or teeth grinding while asleep may continue in the school-age years. Bruxism may result in grinding away of tooth enamel. Teeth grinding may be due to malalignment. A dental evaluation should be scheduled if consistent teeth grinding occurs.

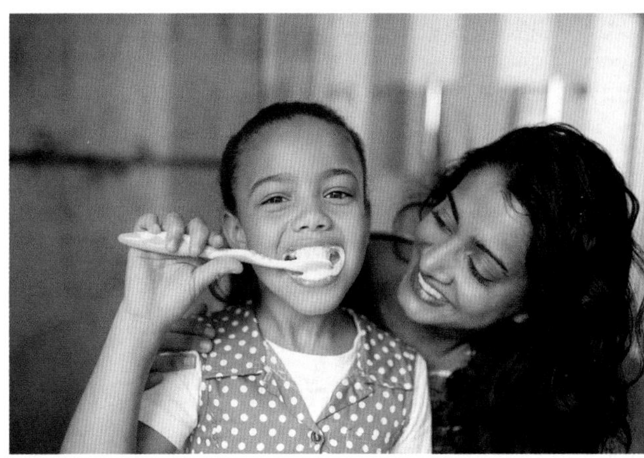

FIGURE 6.9 Using correct technique to brush the teeth is important in the prevention of cavities.

HEALTHY PEOPLE 2030

Objective	Nursing Significance
Reduce the proportion of children and adolescents with lifetime tooth decay. Reduce the proportion of children and adolescents with active and untreated tooth decay. Increase the proportion of children and adolescents who have dental sealants on one or more molars. Increase the proportion of children from families with low income who have a preventive dental visit.	• Encourage appropriate toothbrushing and flossing. • Educate child and family about fluoride use. • Refer school-age children to dentist for regular check-ups and interventions such as molar sealants. • Assist families lacking dental insurance to find resources for the provision of dental care.

Healthy People Objectives retrieved from http://www.healthypeople.gov

Children wearing braces are more prone to cavities; encourage them to brush their teeth after meals and snacks. School nurses can assist these children with brushing after lunch. In addition, the school nurse should promote dental health through education on dental care and gum problems that result from lack of proper dental care. Diet can play a part in dental health. Limiting sticky, high-sugar, and high-carbohydrate foods will decrease the possibility of cavities.

Promoting Appropriate Discipline

Because of the increasing ability of the school-age child to view situations from different angles, the school-age child should be able to see how their actions affect others. The school-age child is aware of the cause and effect of their behaviors and realizes that their behaviors have consequences. School-age children should be able to express emotions without using violence. Discipline techniques with consequences have both *natural* and *logical* consequences. Natural consequences allow the child to learn the results of their actions. For example, if the child throws a toy out of the window, they cannot play with the toy anymore. In logical consequences, if the child does not put away their bike, they do not get to ride the bike for the rest of the day.

In disciplining children, parents should teach children the rules established by the family, values, and social rules of conduct. Rules should provide the school-age child with guidelines about behavior that is acceptable and unacceptable. School-age children look to their parents for guidance and as role models. Parents should role model appropriate expressions of feelings and emotions and allow the child to express emotions and feelings. Discuss the effects of the child's temperament on their behavior, as well as what constitutes age-appropriate behavior. Include how the parents' temperament can influence the child's temperament.

Effective guidance and discipline focus on the development of the child. They can preserve the child's self-esteem and dignity. Discuss with parents guidelines regarding discipline. Explain to parents that they should never belittle the child. Children may view parents and caregivers negatively if they are consistently belittled or insulted. These negative actions can inhibit learning and teach the child to react unkindly to others. Instead, parents should discipline with praise. Positive acknowledgments of appropriate behavior and setting consistent appropriate limits are likely to encourage healthy development and appropriate behavior (Sege et al., 2018). Discuss with parents how to be realistic when planning activities so as not to overwhelm the child, resulting in misbehavior. Encourage parents to say "no" only when they mean it, to avoid a negative atmosphere in the home, and to avoid inconsistency.

When misbehaviors occur, the type and amount of discipline are based on different factors:

- Developmental level of both the child and the parents
- Severity of the misbehavior
- Established rules of the family
- Temperament of the child
- Response of the child to rewards

Keep in mind that school-age children should participate in developing a plan of action for their misbehavior. Whatever methods of discipline are chosen, it is important that parents are consistent in providing discipline in a nurturing environment.

ADDRESSING COMMON DEVELOPMENTAL CONCERNS

According to Erikson (1963), the developmental task of the school-age child is industry. The school-age child is busy learning, achieving, and exploring. As the school-age child becomes more independent, forces other than the family such as television, video games, and peers influence them. Some of these influences are positive and others are negative. Some of the common developmental concerns for the school-age child are discussed in the following sections. Guidelines to assist the parents and nurses when encountering these concerns are included in Teaching Guidelines 6.2.

TEACHING GUIDELINES 6.2 Addressing Common Developmental Concerns

Television, Video Games, and the Internet

- Establish a consistent time limit for any media use and develop a family media plan.
- Establish media-free times, such as mealtimes and car rides.
- Monitor television programs and internet activity.
- Prohibit television or video games with violence.
- Do not put television, video games, or internet-connected devices in children's bedrooms.
- Place computers in an open area that allows easy monitoring by an adult.
- Co-view television, video games, and internet content with the child.
- Encourage sports, interactive play, and reading.
- Teach your child internet safety, such as never to share personal information or meet a friend they have only met online without parental permission, never to share passwords, never to respond to a message that hurts their feelings or makes them uncomfortable, and never to send mean messages over the internet.
- Teach proper social media use.
- Be a good role model.

Maintaining Healthy Weight

- Provide healthy meals and snacks.
- Schedule and encourage daily exercise.
- Encourage involvement in sports and activities.
- Restrict TV, digital media, and video game use.
- Limit the amount of fast food intake.
- Provide education about healthy nutrition.
- Never use food as a reward.
- Be a good role model.

School Refusal

- Return the child to school.
- Investigate the cause of the fear.
- Support the child.
- Collaborate with teachers.
- Praise success in school attendance.

Children Who Are Home Alone

- Provide rules to follow and expectations, such as:
  - Not answering the door or phone
  - No friends in the house when parents are not home
  - No playing with fire
- Teach the child to call a trusted neighbor when help is needed and 911 in the event of emergency.
- Post all resource numbers (even numbers you think your child may have memorized), including afterschool help lines, if available, in a clearly viewable spot. Include the pediatrician's number and preferred hospital.
- Enroll the child in an afterschool program, if available.
- Discuss limitations of outside play.
- Discuss limitations of television viewing and video game use.
- Make sure the child knows how to contact the parent.
- Set clear homework expectations.
- *Do not* keep guns in the home.
- Teach the child where first-aid supplies are located.
- Teach the child household emergency procedures including for circuit breakers and water shut-off valves.
- Practice with your child. Have a trial run by leaving for a short time but staying close and role-playing situations that may occur.
- Always check in with your child while you are away.

Stealing

- Educate parents about the possibility of stealing.
- Discuss ways to teach the concepts of ownership and property rights.
- Handle the situation openly.
- Assist the child in developing and enacting a plan to return what was stolen.
- Make sure the punishment is appropriate for the action.

Lying

- Help parents in understanding why the child is lying.
- When the child lies, calmly confront the child and explain why the behavior is not acceptable.
- Educate parents that their behavior should reflect what they teach and expect from their child.
- Educate parents that too rigid or severe punishments can decrease the child's sense of worth.
- Seek professional help if lying persists in the older school-age child, to rule out underlying problems.

Cheating

- Educate parents that the child must be mature enough to understand the concept of rules.
- Handle cheating situations openly.
- Help parents to understand why their child is cheating and to modify the trigger.
- Develop an appropriate punishment; inappropriate punishment could undermine the child.
- Educate parents that their behavior should reflect what they expect from their child.
- Seek professional help if cheating persists in the older school-age child, to rule out underlying problems.

(*continued*)

TEACHING GUIDELINES **6.2** Addressing Common Developmental Concerns (*continued*)

Bullying

The Bullied Child

- Educate parents whose children are at risk for being bullied, such as:
  - Children who appear different from the majority
  - Children who act different from the majority
  - Children who have low self-esteem
  - Children with a mental or psychological problem
- Teach parents to role play different scenarios the child may face at school; show the child different ways to react to being bullied.
- Impress upon the child that they did not cause the bullying.
- Develop ways to increase the child's self-esteem at home.
- Discuss the situation with the teacher and develop a plan of care.

The Bullying Child

- Educate parents on reasons why it is important to correct the behavior.
- Discuss ways the child can appropriately show their anger and feelings.
- Have parents help the child to see how it feels to be bullied.
- Do not allow fighting at home.
- Reward settling of conflicts without violence.

Tobacco and Alcohol Education

- Inquire about tobacco and alcohol use.
- Discuss the physical and social dangers of tobacco and alcohol use.
- Urge parents to be good role models.
- Limit reading and media materials about alcohol and tobacco use.
- Discuss the influences of tobacco and alcohol use by peers.
- Educate the child on chewing tobacco. Let them know it is just as dangerous as smoking tobacco.
- Educate the child on e-cigarettes and the dangers associated with them.
- Advocate for a smoke-free environment in the home and other places frequented.
- Avoid having tobacco and alcohol products readily available in the home.

Television, Video Games, and the Internet

The influence of television, video games, digital media, and the internet on the school-age child is a growing concern for parents and child specialists. In today's world, the child is surrounded by digital media. School-age children use digital media for education, communication, and entertainment. They have access to thousands of apps, live streaming, streaming movies and TV shows, videos, games, and social media, all on multiple devices, from TVs and computers to smartphones and tablets. By the age of 18, a child will have seen 200,000 violent acts (Ben-Joseph, 2022). Although a school-age child can determine what is real from what is fantasy, research has shown that too much time in front of a screen—watching it or playing video games—can lead to aggressive behavior, less physical activity, and excess weight (Ben-Joseph, 2022; see Healthy People 2030).

Some television shows, video games, and internet activity can have positive influences on children, but parents should be taught guidelines on the use of TV, video games, digital media, and the internet. Parents should set limits on how much screen time the child can have. The AAP recommends that parents place consistent limits on media time and type and that there should be designated media-free times (American Academy of Pediatrics [AAP], Council on Communications and Media, 2016, reaffirmed 2022).

HEALTHY PEOPLE 2030

Objective	Nursing Significance
Increase the proportion of parents who follow AAP recommendations on limiting screen time for children aged 6 to 17 years.	• Encourage the family to develop a family media plan. • Assist families to identify activities other than television or video games for the child to participate in. • Praise craft, music, and sports participation.

Healthy People Objectives retrieved from http://www.healthypeople.gov

Television watching, internet activity, or video gaming should not be used as a reward. The parents should be aware of what the child is watching and doing online. This can be accomplished by parents and children watching programs together and parents using that opportunity to discuss the subject matter with the child. There should be no TV during dinner and no TV or internet-connected devices in the child's room. The parents need to set an example for the child by reading instead of using digital media or by doing a physical activity together as a family. If the TV or digital media causes fights or arguments, it should be turned off for a period of time.

TAKE NOTE!

According to the AAP age-based guidelines, school-age children need supervision and monitoring when using the internet to ensure they are not exposed to inappropriate material or content (AAP, Council on Communications and Media, 2016, reaffirmed 2022). Encourage parents of children in this age group to utilize internet safety tools that limit access to content and websites and that provide information on internet activities.

School Refusal

School refusal (also called *school phobia* or *school avoidance*) has been defined as a refusal to attend school or difficulty remaining in school for an entire day. Behaviors include frequent absences, skipping classes, being chronically late for school, severe misbehavior before school, or attending school with great fear. School phobia needs to be defined both symptomatically and operationally as the cause for the anxiety.

Some of the fears expressed by school-refusing children include separating from parents, riding the bus, tests, bullying, teacher reprimands, anxieties over toileting in a public bathroom, physical harm, or undressing in the locker room. Due to the emotional distress caused in these children when attending school, they are frequently classified as having school phobia. Young children may complain of stomachache or headache, and older children may complain of palpitations or feeling faint.

It is important to investigate specific causes of school refusal/school phobia and take appropriate actions. Often, school phobia is a symptom of deeper problems. The health care provider or nurse practitioner should conduct a physical examination of the child to rule out any physical illness. After these measures are taken, the parent, teacher, school counselor, and school administrator may devise a plan to assist the student to overcome a specific fear. In uncomplicated cases, parents must return the child to school as soon as possible. There may be altered schedules (partial days or decreased hours) to help promote a successful transition back to school. Another idea to help desensitize the child may be to have them spend part of the day in the counselor's or school nurse's office.

Children Who Are Home Alone

With the increasing incidence of both parents in the workforce and many children living with just one parent, children often return home alone without adult supervision for a number of hours. Most young children are not capable of handling stress or making decisions on their own before 11 or 12 years of age. However, some school-age children are more mature and can be left alone by 8 to 10 years of age; maturity is the key, not the age. Parents not only need to consider their child's maturity and readiness to be home alone but must also comply with legal requirements if present. Many states offer guidelines concerning when it is okay to leave a child alone at home, and a few states have laws with a minimum age, but these vary by state; therefore, the nurse needs to be familiar with the state and local laws in order to assist parents in making decisions about when it is appropriate for their child to be home alone (Child Welfare Information Gateway, 2018). However, the AAP continues to recommend that a school-age child come home to a parent or other responsible adult (AAP, 2022).

If children come home to no supervision, they should know the names, addresses, and phone numbers of parents and a neighbor, as well as emergency numbers. They should be given rules about answering the door and the phone. They should not answer the door and should tell anyone who calls that a parent is home but busy at this time. Directions as to the handling of the house key and fire safety should be taught and demonstrated (see Teaching Guidelines 6.2).

Stealing, Lying, and Cheating

Stealing, lying, and cheating are inappropriate behaviors that may occur during the school-age years. In most cases, these behaviors will result in a good lesson learned, and the child will outgrow them. In some cases, they may indicate a more severe psychological or behavioral problem. Parents are usually disturbed by these behaviors. In turn, they have difficulty in addressing these issues and need help providing appropriate interventions.

Children between 6 and 8 years old do not fully understand the concepts of ownership and property rights. These children may steal things because they like the look of the item. By the age of 9, the child should respect others' possessions and property and understand that stealing is wrong. The school-age child may steal because they desire the item, because they feel peer pressure and are trying to impress their peers, or because they have a sense of low self-esteem. Stealing becomes a concern if the child steals and does not have remorse or steals continuously or if stealing is accompanied by other behavioral problems (Johns Hopkins Medicine, n.d.).

Stealing and lying are both more common in boys and in children between 5 and 8 years old (Johns Hopkins Medicine, n.d.). It is acceptable for these children to tell tall tales, but they should know what truth is and what make-believe is. These younger children typically lie to avoid punishment. However, they do not like others to lie and will tell on them if they lie. Children between 8 and 12 years old typically lie because they are unable to meet expectations of family and peers, they are testing the rules and limits placed on them, or they are unable to explain bad behavior (Johns Hopkins Medicine, n.d.). If lying persists in older school-age children, if it is accompanied by other behavioral problems, or if the child does not show remorse with lying, parents should discuss the matter with a health care provider because the lying may be evidence of underlying problems.

The concept of cheating is not well understood until the child is about 6 to 7 years old. Before this age, the desire to "win" is most important, and rigid rules are hard to understand. In children between 8 and 12 years old, the concept of cheating is fully understood, and following of rules becomes more important (Johns Hopkins Medicine, n.d.). If cheating persists in older school-age children, parents should discuss the matter with a health care provider because the behavior may indicate underlying problems.

In dealing with children who exhibit stealing, lying, or cheating behaviors, parents must first realize the importance of their own behaviors in those areas. Parents are role models to the school-age child. Therefore, when the child sees or hears that parents lie, steal, or cheat (e.g., parents bragging about cheating on their taxes), they think it is all right to mimic those behaviors. Secondly, parents must directly confront any stealing, lying, or cheating behaviors and discuss (and follow through consistently with) the consequences of such behaviors (see Teaching Guideline 6.2).

Bullying

Bullying, which is inflicting unwanted, repeated verbal, emotional, or physical aggression on others and involves a power imbalance, is widespread and negatively impacts all parties involved (CDC, 2021). Utilizing e-mail, text messages, social media, and instant messaging, often referred to as cyberbullying, is a growing concern. Bullies often look for victims who appear shy, weak, and defenseless.

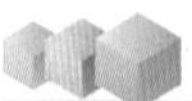

Concept Mastery Alert

Most often, children who bully have low self-esteem, poor grades, and poor interpersonal skills. Both male and female children are bullied, but male children tend to bully other male children and more often show force when bullying.

Being bullied can have negative results on children throughout life. These children often have increased episodes of headaches, stomachaches, sleep problems, anxiety, loneliness, depression, substance use, lower academic achievement, and suicidal tendencies (Moreno & Englander, 2020). After the problem of either being bullied or being the bully has been identified, parents must work with the child, the school, and the health care provider or nurse practitioner to solve the problem (see Teaching Guidelines 6.2 and Evidence-Based Practice 6.1).

Tobacco and Alcohol Education

School-age children are eager to grow up and be independent. Peers and acceptance are very important at this time. School-age children may be exposed to messages that are in conflict with their parents' values regarding smoking and alcohol. Peers often exert pressure for children to experiment with tobacco and alcohol.

School-age children are ready to absorb information that deals with drugs and alcohol. Information from parents or other adults who are major influences in the child's life is essential at this time to set clear rules and

EVIDENCE-BASED PRACTICE **6.1**

Meta-Analysis of the Effectiveness of School-Based Programs to Reduce Bullying Perpetration and Victimization

STUDY

Bullying perpetration and victimization continue to pose a problem in elementary schools. In addition to the behavioral disruption that occurs as a result of bullying perpetration and victimization, prior research has demonstrated that child bullies and victims are at increased risk for mental health problems, such as depression, anxiety, low self-esteem, suicidal ideation, and low social competence. Adverse consequences from bullying have led to prevention programs to decrease peer victimization. This systematic review and meta-analysis summarized 100 studies to evaluate the effectiveness of face-to-face school-based antibullying programs.

Findings

The results of this analysis found that school-based antibullying programs are effective in reducing bully perpetration by approximately 18% to 19% and bully victimization by approximately 15% to 16%. Variations in the effectiveness of intervention programs were found and demonstrate a need for further research to explore these variations.

Nursing Implications

Nurses should continue to educate parents and teachers about bullying. Become actively involved in the local elementary school bullying-prevention program, and encourage a whole school comprehensive approach. Further research is needed to determine which programs are most effective.

Data from Gaffney, H., Ttofi, M. M., & Farrington, D. P. (2021). Effectiveness of school-based programs to reduce bullying perpetration and victimization: An updated systematic review and meta-analysis. *Campbell Systematic Reviews*, *17*(2), e1143. https://doi.org/10.1002/cl2.1143

model behaviors for children to embrace. Discussions with children need to be based on facts and focused on the present. Some topics for discussion include:

- What alcohol and drugs are like and how they harm you
- Differences in medical use versus illegal use of drugs
- How to think critically to interpret messages seen in advertising, media, and sports and from entertainment personalities

Recall Lawrence Jones, the 10-year-old presented at the beginning of the chapter. List potential developmental problems he may experience. What anticipatory guidance related to these concerns should you provide to his parent?

Unfolding Patient Stories: Charlie Snow • Part 1

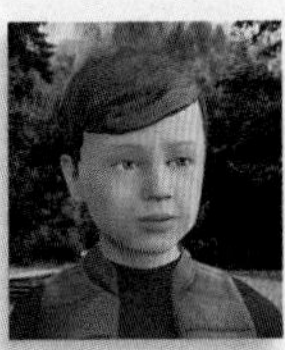

Charlie Snow, a 6-year-old with a known hypersensitivity to perfumes and dyes and an allergy to peanuts, comes for a routine clinic visit accompanied by his aunt. He is living with his aunt and uncle while his parents are serving in the military. The nurse discovers a rash in multiple areas underneath his clothing. What questions should the nurse ask to determine the cause of the rash? What education should the nurse provide for his aunt, who has limited knowledge of allergies and child care experience? (Charlie Snow's story continues in Chapter 25.)

Care for Charlie and other patients in a realistic virtual environment: ***vSim** for Nursing* (thepoint.lww.com/vSimPediatric). Practice documenting these patients' care in DocuCare (thePoint.lww.com/DocuCareEHR).

KEY CONCEPTS

- Physical growth is slow and steady, with social and cognitive development progressing rapidly, during the school-age years of 6 to 12. Height increases approximately 6 to 7 cm (2.5 in) per year, and weight gain is 3 to 3.5 kg (7 lb) per year. Males are generally taller and heavier than females during this period.
- With entrance into the school system, school-age children have the influences of peers and teachers.
- With the development of gross motor skills and involvement in sports at school and in the community, safety education and practices are required. Also, with participation in cooperative sports, injuries occur.
- Increased independence leads to increased exposure to safety hazards.
- The school-age child develops the cognitive ability to classify objects and to identify relationships among objects.
- Dental care is very important to prevent dental caries, malocclusion, and other problems. In early school age, the first primary teeth will be lost.
- The onset of puberty may occur by the later school-aged years.
- Erikson's (1963) developmental task for the age group is the development of a sense of industry.
- Peers are important, especially peers of the same gender. School-age children usually have a best friend and belong to clubs. They have collections of nonvaluable items such as rocks, clips, and so forth.
- School-age children are capable of concrete operations, solving problems, and making decisions. They continue to need guidance, rules, and direction from parents.
- The school-age child develops a conscience and knows cultural and social values. They can understand and obey rules.
- The school-age child incorporates spiritual or religious practices into their life, which may be a source of comfort during stressful times.
- The nurse's role includes educating parents and school-age children in promoting health and safety.
- Nurses should inform the school-age child about expected developmental changes in the body to promote self-esteem and self-confidence.

REFERENCES AND RECOMMENDED READINGS

American Academy of Pediatrics. (2022). *Back-to-school tips for families.* https://www.healthychildren.org/English/ages-stages/gradeschool/school/Pages/Back-to-School-Tips.aspx

American Academy of Pediatrics, Council on Communications and Media. (2016, reaffirmed 2022). Policy statement: Media use in school-aged children and adolescents. *Pediatrics, 138*(5), e20162592. https://doi.org/10.1542/peds.2016-2592

American Academy of Pediatrics, HealthyChildren. (2021). *Booster seats for school-aged children.* https://www.healthychildren.org/English/safety-prevention/on-the-go/Pages/Booster-Seats-for-School-Aged-Children.aspx

American Association for Pediatric Ophthalmology and Strabismus. (2021). *Amblyopia.* https://aapos.org/glossary/amblyopia

Ben-Joseph, E. P. (2022). *How media use can affects kids.* https://kidshealth.org/en/parents/tv-affects-child.html#catsafe-play

Biro, F. M., & Chan, Y.-M. (2023). Normal puberty. UpToDate. Retrieved October 10, 2023, from https://www.uptodate.com/contents/normal-puberty

Bogues, L., & Levine, D. A. (2023). Section 2: Growth and development. Chapter 7: Normal development. In K. J. Marcdante, R. M. Kleigman, & A. M. Schuh (Eds.), *Nelson essentials of pediatrics* (9th ed., pp. 14–16). Elsevier.

Centers for Disease Control and Prevention. (2021). *Preventing bullying.* https://www.cdc.gov/violenceprevention/pdf/yv/Bullying-factsheet_508_1.pdf

Centers for Disease Control and Prevention. (2022a). *Childhood obesity facts.* https://www.cdc.gov/obesity/data/childhood.html

Centers for Disease Control and Prevention. (2022b). *Physical activity facts*. https://www.cdc.gov/healthyschools/physicalactivity/facts.htm

Child Welfare Information Gateway. (2018). *Leaving your child home alone*. U.S. Department of Health and Human Services, Children's Bureau. https://www.childwelfare.gov/pubPDFs/homealone.pdf

CHOC. (2021). *Growth & development: 6 to 12 years (school age)*. https://www.choc.org/primary-care/ages-stages/6-to-12-years/

Cincinnati Children's. (2023). *Growth, range of height and weight*. https://www.cincinnatichildrens.org/health/g/normal-growth

Clark, M. B., Keels, M. A., Slayton, R. L., & AAP Section on Oral Health. (2020). Fluoride use in caries prevention in the primary care setting. *Pediatrics, 146*(6), Article e2020034637. https://doi.org/10.1542/peds.2020-034637

Erikson, E. (1963). *Childhood and society* (2nd ed.). Norton.

Feigelman, S. (2020). Developmental & behavioral theories. In R. M. Kleigman, J. W. St. Geme, III, N. J. Blum, S. S. Shah, R. C. Tasker, K. M. Wislon, & R. E. Behrman (Eds.), *Nelson textbook of pediatrics* (21st ed., pp. 1233–1257). Elsevier.

Finkelstein, L. H., & Feigelman, S. (2020). Middle childhood. In R. M. Kleigman, J. W. St. Geme, III, N. J. Blum, S. S. Shah, R. C. Tasker, K. M. Wislon, & R. E. Behrman (Eds.), *Nelson textbook of pediatrics* (21st ed., pp. 1358–1373). Elsevier.

Gaffney, H., Ttofi, M. M., & Farrington, D. P. (2021). Effectiveness of school-based programs to reduce bullying perpetration and victimization: An updated systematic review and meta-analysis. *Campbell Systematic Reviews, 17*(2), e1143. https://doi.org/10.1002/cl2.1143

Gill, A. C. (2022). Bicycle injuries in children: Prevention. *UpToDate*. Retrieved October 17, 2022, from https://www.uptodate.com/contents/bicycle-injuries-in-children-prevention

Gill, A. C., & Kelly, N. R. (2022). Pediatric injury prevention: Epidemiology, history, and application. *UpToDate*. Retrieved October 19, 2022, from https://www.uptodate.com/contents/pediatric-injury-prevention-epidemiology-history-and-application

Jennissen, C. (2022). *ATVs are not safe for children: AAP policy explained*. https://www.healthychildren.org/English/safety-prevention/at-play/Pages/ATV-Safety-Rules.aspx

Johns Hopkins Medicine. (n.d.). *Lying and stealing. Health Library*. Retrieved October 22, 2022, from https://www.hopkinsmedicine.org/healthlibrary/conditions/pediatrics/lying_and_stealing_90,P02241

Kohlberg, L. (1984). *Moral development*. Harper & Row.

Moreno, M. A., & Englander, E. (2020). Bullying, cyberbullying, and school violence. In R. M. Kleigman, J. W. St. Geme, III, N. J. Blum, S. S. Shah, R. C. Tasker, K. M. Wislon, & R. E. Behrman (Eds.), *Nelson textbook of pediatrics* (21st ed., pp. 1083–1087). Elsevier.

Morse, A. M., & Kotagal, S. (2021). Parasomnias of childhood, including sleepwalking. *UpToDate*. Retrieved October 13, 2023, from https://www.uptodate.com/contents/parasomnias-of-childhood-including-sleepwalking

Nowak, A. J., & Warren, J. J. (2022). Preventive dental care and counseling for infants and young children. *UpToDate*. Retrieved October 17, 2022, from https://www.uptodate.com/contents/preventive-dental-care-and-counseling-for-infants-and-young-children

Oh, C., Carducci, B., Vaivada, T., & Bhutta, Z. A. (2022). Interventions to promote physical activity and healthy digital media use in children and adolescents: A systematic review. *Pediatrics, 149*(Suppl. 6), e2021053852I. https://doi.org/10.1542/peds.2021-053852I

Piaget, J. (1969). *The theory of stages in cognitive development*. McGraw-Hill.

Radcliff, Z. (2023). Childhood Fears and Worries. https://kidshealth.org/en/parents/anxiety.html

Safe Kids Worldwide. (2023). *FAST facts pedestrian injuries among children in 2021*. https://www.safekids.org/sites/default/files/documents/fast_facts_-_2021_-_pedestrian_injuries.pdf

Sege, R. D., Siegel, B. S., AAP Council on Child Abuse and Neglect, & AAP Committee on Psychosocial Aspects of Child and Family Health. (2018). Effective discipline to raise healthy children. *Pediatrics, 142*(6), Article 20183112. https://doi.org/10.1542/peds.2018-3112

Skelton, J. A., & Klish, W. J. (2023). Definition, epidemiology, and etiology of obesity in children and adolescents. *UpToDate*. Retrieved October 12, 2023, from https://www.uptodate.com/contents/definition-epidemiology-and-etiology-of-obesity-in-children-and-adolescents

U.S. Department of Agriculture, & U.S. Department of Health and Human Services. (2020). *Dietary guidelines for Americans, 2020–2025*. (9th ed.) https://www.dietaryguidelines.gov/sites/default/files/2021-03/Dietary_Guidelines_for_Americans-2020-2025.pdf

U.S. Department of Health and Human Services. (n.d.). *Healthy People 2030*. https://health.gov/healthypeople

U.S. Department of Health and Human Services, Administration for Children and Families, Administration on Children, Youth and Families, Children's Bureau. (2022). *Child maltreatment 2020*. https://www.acf.hhs.gov/cb/data-research/child-maltreatment

DEVELOPING CLINICAL JUDGMENT

PRACTICING FOR NCLEX

1. The successful resolution of developmental tasks for the school-age child, according to Erikson, would be identified by:
   a. learning from repeating tasks.
   b. developing a sense of worth and competence.
   c. using fantasy and magical thinking to cope with problems.
   d. developing a sense of trust.
2. Which of the following are reasons that school-age children steal? Select all that apply.
   a. To escape punishment
   b. High self-esteem
   c. Low expectations of family/peers
   d. Lack of sense of property
   e. Strong desire to own something
3. Which activities will promote weight loss in a school-age child with higher body weight? Select all that apply.
   a. Unlimited computer and TV time
   b. Role modeling by family
   c. Becoming active in sports
   d. Eating unstructured meals
   e. Involving the child in meal planning and grocery shopping
   f. Drinking seven to eight glasses of water per day
4. Samantha, a 10-year-old, is brought into your clinic for a well-child examination. The parent states, "Samantha's friend group seems to be so much more important to them these days." As the nurse caring for the child, how would you explain the role of peers in the school-age child?
   a. This allows them the opportunity to learn conflict management.
   b. This helps them to shape their concept of self and provides security as they gain independence from their parents.
   c. This will encourage them to remain dependent on their teachers and family.
   d. This will help them to work through their fears of body safety.
5. The parent of two children, ages 6 and 9, states the children want to play on the same baseball team. As the school nurse, what advice would you give their parent?
   a. Having the children on the same team will make it more convenient for the family.
   b. Levels of coordination and concentration differ, so the children need to be on different teams.
   c. Put the children on the same team because they are both school-age children.
   d. It is best to avoid putting the children on the same team to prevent sibling rivalry.
6. The nursing student is caring for a 9-year-old child. According to Piaget's cognitive development theory, the nurse can expect the child to understand the principle of __________ and have a concept of __________ as the school-age child is in the __________ stage.

   Blanks 1 and 2:
   a. Spatial reasoning
   b. Space
   c. Conservation
   d. Elasticity
   e. Time
   f. Representation

   Blank 3:
   a. Preoperational
   b. Sensorimotor
   c. Formal operational
   d. Concrete operational

CRITICAL THINKING EXERCISES

1. Ms. Sams brings her 8-year-old, Frank, to the health care provider's office for his annual examination. She states that she is concerned about his recent behavior. He went to the grocery store with his friend and his friend's parent, and he came home with a Matchbox car. The friend's parent stated she had not purchased the car.
   a. What would be your response to Ms. Sams?
   b. Ms. Sams said she still has the car. What would you advise Ms. Sams to do to make Frank aware of the consequences of his actions?
2. Sally's parent is asking the nurse for advice about purchasing a two-wheeled bike for her 7-year-old. What guidance should the nurse offer this parent?
3. Ms. Shaw brings in her 11-year-old daughter for a well-child check-up. The school-ager says to the nurse, "I look different from my friends. I do not wear bras, and my friends are already wearing bras." What would be an appropriate response to this school-ager?
4. Johnny is a 9-year-old whose parents both work during the day. He returns home alone after school. How should the parents prepare Johnny for this experience? What safety rules would be included in the education for Johnny?

STUDY ACTIVITIES

1. Attend a sporting event (such as soccer or baseball) with school-age teams. Describe the coordination and gross motor functioning of this group.
2. Attend a first-grade class. Observe the behaviors exhibited by the school-age children in this class. How do these behaviors compare with expected values for this age group?

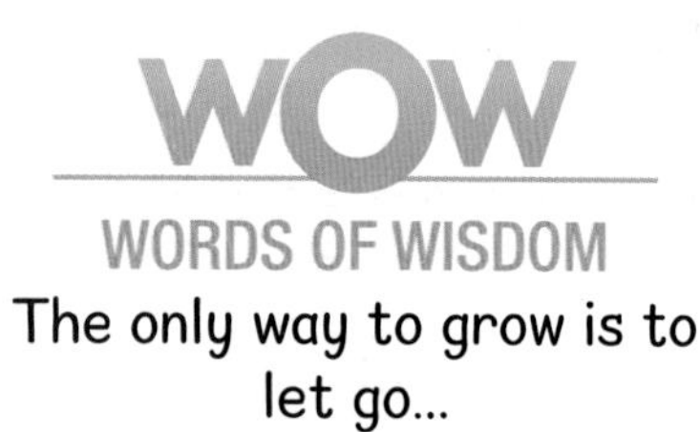

The only way to grow is to let go...

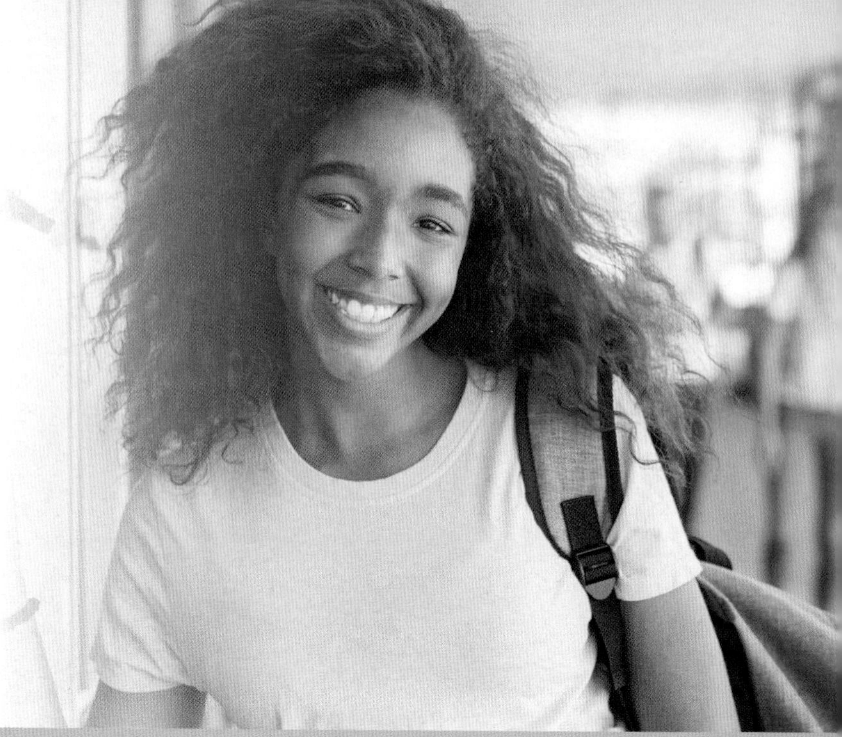

7

Growth and Development of the Adolescent

LEARNING OBJECTIVES

Upon completion of the chapter, you will be able to:

1. Identify normal physiologic changes, including puberty, occurring in the adolescent.
2. Discuss psychosocial, cognitive, social, and moral changes occurring in the adolescent.
3. Identify changes in relationships with peers, family, teachers, and community during adolescence.
4. Describe interventions to promote safety during adolescence.
5. Demonstrate knowledge of the nutritional requirements of the adolescent.
6. Demonstrate knowledge of the development of sexuality and its influence on dating during adolescence.
7. Identify common developmental concerns of the adolescent.
8. Demonstrate knowledge of the appropriate nursing guidance for common developmental concerns.

KEY TERMS

adolescence
menarche (men-ahr′kē)
peer groups
puberty
risk-taking behaviors
sexuality
thelarche (thē-lahr′kē)

Cho Chung is a 15-year-old brought to the clinic by her parent for her annual school check-up. As the nurse caring for her, assess Cho's growth and development, and then provide appropriate anticipatory guidance to her parent.

INTRODUCTION

Adolescence spans the years of transition from childhood to adulthood, which is usually between the ages of 11 and 20 years. There is some overlap between late school age and adolescence. The adolescent experiences drastic changes in the physical, cognitive, psychosocial, and psychosexual areas. With this rapid growth during adolescence, the development of secondary sexual characteristics, and amorous interest in peers, the adolescent needs the support and guidance of parents and nurses to facilitate a healthy lifestyle and to reduce **risk-taking behaviors** such as drinking, drug use, unsafe sexual activity, and participating in reckless behavior or dangerous activities. Not all adolescents will align with the sex they are assigned at birth; in this chapter, the term "male" will be used to refer to those born with male internal and external genitalia, and "female" will be used to refer to those born with female internal and external genitalia.

GROWTH AND DEVELOPMENT OVERVIEW

Adolescence is a time of rapid growth with dramatic changes in body size and proportions. The magnitude of these changes is second only to the growth in infancy. During this time, sexual characteristics develop, and reproductive maturity is achieved. The age of onset and the duration of the physiologic changes vary from individual to individual. Generally, females enter puberty earlier (at 9 to 10 years of age) than males (at 10 to 11 years; Table 7.1). Adolescents will represent varying levels of identity formation and will offer unique challenges to the nurse.

PHYSIOLOGIC CHANGES ASSOCIATED WITH PUBERTY

The secretion of estrogen in females and testosterone in males stimulates the development of breast tissue in females, pubic hair in both sexes, and changes in male genitalia. These biologic changes that occur during adolescence are known as **puberty**. Puberty is the result of triggers from the environment, the central nervous system, the hypothalamus, the pituitary gland, the gonads, and the adrenal glands. Gonadotropin-releasing hormone (GnRH), produced by the hypothalamus, travels to the anterior pituitary gland to stimulate the production and secretion of follicle-stimulating hormone (FSH) and luteinizing hormone (LH). The increased levels of FSH and LH stimulate the gonadal response. LH stimulates ovulation in females and acts on testicular Leydig cells in males, prompting maturation of the testicles and testosterone production. FSH with LH stimulates sperm production. Estrogen, progesterone, and testosterone and other androgens are released from the gonads and affect biologic changes and changes in various organs, including alterations in muscles, bones, skin, and hair follicles.

Females reach physical maturity before males, and **menarche**, the first menstrual period, usually begins between the ages of 9 and 15 years (average 12.8 years). Breast budding (**thelarche**) occurs at approximately age 9 to 11 years and is followed by the growth of pubic hair.

TABLE 7.1 • Physiologic Changes of Adolescence

Stage of Adolescence	Changes in Females	Changes in Males
Early adolescence (10–13 years)	Pubic hair begins to curl and spread over mons pubis; genitalia pigmentation increases. Breast bud and areola continue to enlarge; no separation of breasts. First menstrual period (average 12 years, normal range 9–16 years)	Pubic hair spreads laterally, begins to curl; pigmentation increases. Growth and enlargement of testes in scrotum (scrotum reddish in color) and continued lengthening of penis Leggy look due to extremities growing faster than the trunk
Middle adolescence (15–17 years)	Pubic hair becomes coarse in texture and continues to curl; amount of hair increases. Areola and papilla separate from the contour of the breast to form a secondary mound.	Pubic hair becomes coarser in texture and takes on adult distribution. Testes and scrotum continue to grow; scrotal skin darkens; penis grows in width, and glans penis develops. May experience breast enlargement Voice changes; more masculine due to rapid enlargement of the larynx and pharynx as well as lung changes
Late adolescence (18–21 years)	Mature pubic hair distribution and coarseness	Mature pubic hair distribution and coarseness Breast enlargement disappears Adult size and shape of testes, scrotum, and penis; scrotal skin darkening

Data from Holland-Hall, C. (2020). Adolescent physical and social development. In R. M. Kleigman, J. W. St. Geme, III, N. J. Blum, S. S. Shah, R. C. Tasker, K. M. Wilson, & R. E. Behrman (Eds.), *Nelson textbook of pediatrics* (21st ed., pp. 5550–5576). Elsevier.

TAKE NOTE!

Black females, on average, reach menarche slightly earlier than White females (Blake & Van Eyk, 2023a).

The first sign of pubertal changes in males is testicular enlargement in response to testosterone secretion, usually occurring in Tanner stage 2. As testosterone levels increase, the penis and scrotum enlarge, hair distribution increases, and scrotal skin texture changes. During late puberty, males will typically experience their first ejaculation, which may occur while they are sleeping (nocturnal emissions). Nurses should provide anticipatory guidance to adolescent males regarding involuntary nocturnal emissions (wet dreams) to assure them that this is an expected occurrence.

Tanner stages 3 to 5 usually occur during adolescence. Refer to Figures 10.28, 10.36, and 10.34 for an illustration of the increase in breast tissue and pubic hair distribution in females and scrotal and penile changes as well as hair distribution changes in males. The nurse should provide guidance to adolescents about the normalcy of the sexual feelings and evolving body changes that occur during puberty.

PHYSICAL GROWTH

Diet, exercise, and hereditary factors influence the height, weight, and body build of the adolescent. Over the past three decades, adolescents have become taller and heavier than their ancestors, and the beginning of puberty is earlier. During the early adolescent period, there is an increase in the percentage of body fat, and the head, neck, and hands reach adult proportions.

The rapid growth during adolescence is secondary only to that of the infant years and is a direct result of the hormonal changes of puberty. Adolescents experience changes in appearance and size. Height in females increases rapidly before menarche and usually ceases 2 to 2½ years after menarche. The growth spurt in males occurs later than in females and usually begins between the ages of 10½ and 16 years and ends sometime between the ages of 13½ and 17½ years. Muscle mass increases in males, and fat deposits increase in females (Fig. 7.1).

During early adolescence, growth is rapid, but it decreases in middle and late adolescence. Height for adolescent males who are between the 50th and 95th percentile ranges from 132 cm (52½ in) to 176.8 cm (69½ in). Weight of males in these percentiles ranges from 35.3 kg (77¼ lb) to 95.76 kg (211 lb). On average, males will gain 10 to 30 cm (4 to 12 in) in height and 7 to 30 kg (15 to 65 lb) in weight.

Height for females who are between the 50th and 95th percentile ranges from 144.8 cm (57 in) to 173.6 cm (68½ in), with weight ranging from 27.24 kg (60 lb) to 82.47 kg (181 lb). On average, females will gain 5 to 20 cm (2 to 8 in) in height and 7 to 25 kg (15 to 55 lb) in weight during adolescence. See Appendix A for growth charts for this age group. Refer to Chapter 10, Box 10.1, for instructions for calculating body mass index (BMI).

Remember Cho Chung, the 15-year-old introduced at the beginning of the chapter. During your assessment, you measure Cho's weight at 49.89 kg (110 lb) and her height at 152.4 cm (60 in). Plot Cho's measurements on the appropriate growth chart.

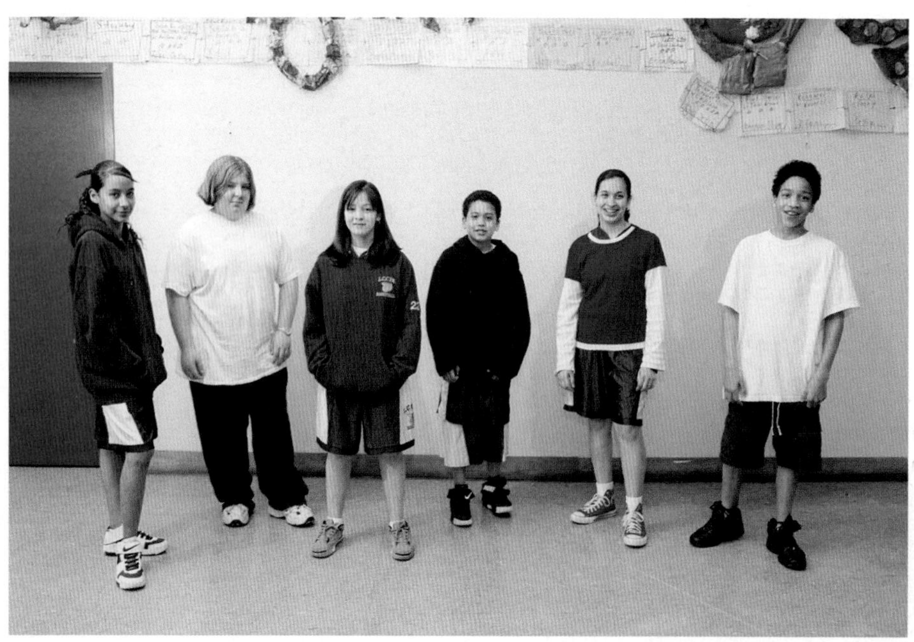

FIGURE 7.1 These adolescents reflect the differences in sizes and shapes seen in adolescents of the same age.

PHYSIOLOGIC CHANGES

Adolescence is a time of metabolic slowing and of increasing size of some organs. The basal metabolic rate (BMR) reaches the adult level during late adolescence.

Neurologic System

During adolescence, there is continued brain growth, although the size of the brain does not increase significantly. Neurons do not increase in number, but growth of the myelin sheath enables faster neural processing.

Respiratory System

The adolescent years see an increase in diameter and length of the lungs. Respiratory rate decreases and reaches the adult rate of 15 to 20 breaths/min. Respiratory volume and vital capacity increase. Volume and capacity are greater in males than females, which may be associated with increased chest and shoulder size in males. The growth of the laryngeal cartilage, larynx, pharynx, vocal cords, and lungs produces the voice changes experienced in adolescence. These changes in the quality of the child's voice are often preceded by some voice instability, where voice cracking is heard. Deepening of both male and female voices occurs but is more pronounced in males.

Cardiovascular System

There is an increase in size and strength of the heart. Systolic blood pressure increases and heart rate decreases. Blood volume reaches higher levels in males, which may be due to their greater muscle mass.

Gastrointestinal System

The adolescent has a full set of permanent teeth with the exception of the last four molars (wisdom teeth), which may erupt between the ages of 17 and 20 years. The liver, spleen, kidneys, and digestive tract enlarge during the growth spurt in early adolescence, but do not change in function. These systems are mature in early school age.

Musculoskeletal System

The ossification of the skeletal system is incomplete until late adolescence in males. Ossification is more advanced in females and occurs at an earlier age. During the growth spurt, muscle mass and strength increase. At similar stages of development, muscle development is generally greater in males. Estrogen, progesterone, and testosterone (sex steroids) and other androgens are released from the gonads and affect changes in the muscles and bones. Low estrogen levels tend to stimulate skeletal growth, while higher levels inhibit growth. During middle adolescence, shoulder, chest, and hip breadth increase.

Integumentary System

During adolescence, the skin becomes thick and tough. Under the influence of androgens, the sebaceous glands become more active, particularly on the face, back, and genitals. Due to the increased levels of testosterone during Tanner stages 4 and 5, adolescents may have increased sebum production, which may lead to the development of acne and oily hair.

The exocrine and apocrine sweat glands function at adult levels during adolescence. The exocrine glands are all over the body, and they produce sweat, which helps to eliminate body heat through evaporation. The apocrine glands are found in the axillae, genital, and anal areas and around the breasts. The apocrine sweat glands produce sweat in response to hair follicles. This sweat is produced continuously and is stored and released in response to emotional stimuli.

PSYCHOSOCIAL DEVELOPMENT

According to Erikson, it is during adolescence that individuals achieve a sense of identity (Erikson, 1963). As the adolescent is trying out many different roles in regard to their relationships with peers, family, community, and society, they are developing their own individual sense of self. If the adolescent is not successful in forming their own sense of self, they develop a sense of role confusion or diffusion. The adolescent culture becomes important to the individual. It is through their involvement with adolescent groups that the individual finds support and help with developing their own identity.

Erikson (1963) believed that during the task of developing their own sense of identity, the adolescent revisits each of the previous stages of development. The sense of trust is encountered as the adolescent strives to find out in whom and in what ideals they can have faith. In revisiting the stage of autonomy, the adolescent is seeking out ways to express their individuality in an effective manner. The adolescent would avoid behaviors that would "shame" or ridicule them in front of their peers. The sense of initiative is revisited as the adolescent develops their vision for what they might become. And the sense of industry is again encountered as the adolescent makes their choice to participate in different activities at school, in the community, at church, and in the workforce.

The ability of the adolescent to successfully form a sense of self is dependent on how well the adolescent successfully completed the former stages of development.

TABLE 7.2 • Developmental Theories

Theories	Stages	Activities
Erikson (psychosocial)	Identity vs. role confusion or diffusion Early (10–13 years)	Focuses on bodily changes Experiences frequent mood changes Importance placed on conformity to peer norms and peer acceptance Strives to master skills within peer groups Defining boundaries with parents and authority figures Early stage of emancipation—struggles to separate from parents while still desiring dependence on them Identifies with same-sex peers Takes more responsibility for own behaviors
	Middle (14–16 years)	Continues to adjust to changed body image Tries out different roles within peer groups Need for acceptance by peer group at the highest level Interested in being romantically attractive to peers Time of greatest conflict with parents/authority figures
	Late (17–20 years)	Able to understand implications of behavior and decisions Roles within peer groups established Feels secure with body image Has matured sexual identity Has idealistic career goals Importance of individual friendships emerges Process of emancipation from family almost complete
Piaget (cognitive)	Formal operations Early (10–13 years)	Limited abstract thought process Egocentrical thinking Eager to apply limited abstract process to different situations and to peer groups
	Middle (14–17 years)	Increased ability to think abstractly or in more idealistic terms Able to solve verbal and mental problems using scientific methods Thinks they are invincible—risky behaviors increase Likes making independent decisions Becomes involved/concerned with society, politics
	Late (17–20 years)	Abstract thinking establishes Develops critical thinking skills—tests different solutions to problems Less risky behaviors Develops realistic goals and career plans
Kohlberg	Postconventional level III	Morals based on peer, family, church, and societal morals
	Early (10–13 years)	Asks broad, usually unanswerable questions about life
	Middle (14–17 years)	Developing own set of morals—evaluates individual morals in relation to peer, family, and societal morals
	Late (17–20 years)	Internalizes own morals and values Continues to compare own morals and values with those of society Evaluates morals of others

Data from Erikson, E. (1963). *Childhood and society* (2nd ed.). Norton; Kohlberg, L. (1984). *Moral development.* Harper & Row; and Piaget, J. (1969). *The theory of stages in cognitive development.* McGraw-Hill.

Erikson (1963) believed that if the adolescent has been successful, they can develop resources during adolescence to overcome any gaps in previous developmental stages. If the adolescent believes that they cannot express themselves in any manner due to societal restrictions, they will develop role confusion. See Table 7.2 for additional information.

COGNITIVE DEVELOPMENT

According to Piaget, the adolescent progresses from a concrete framework of thinking to an abstract one (Piaget, 1969). During this formal operational period, the adolescent develops the ability to think outside of the present; that is, they can incorporate into thinking concepts that do exist as well as concepts that might exist. The adolescent's thinking becomes logical, organized, and consistent. They are able to think about a problem from all points of view, ranking the possible solutions while solving the problem. Not all adolescents achieve formal operational reasoning at the same time.

In the early stages of formal operational reasoning, the adolescent's thinking is egocentric, thinking they are at the center of everyone's attention. The adolescent is idealistic, constantly challenging the way things are and wondering why things cannot change. These activities lead to the adolescent's feeling of being omnipotent. The adolescent must undergo this way of thinking, even though it can frustrate adults, in their quest to reach formal operational reasoning. As the individual progresses toward middle adolescence, their thinking becomes introspective. They assume others are just as interested in what interests them, which leads them to feel unique, special, and exceptional. That feeling of "being exceptional" leads to the risk-taking behaviors for which adolescents are well known. Also, the adolescent feels very committed to their viewpoints. They try very hard to convince others of their viewpoints and strongly embrace those causes that support their opinions. This idealism can cause the adolescent to reject their family, culture, religion, and community beliefs, which can cause conflict. See Table 7.2 for additional information.

MORAL AND SPIRITUAL DEVELOPMENT

It is during the adolescent years that individuals develop their own set of values and morals. According to Kohlberg, adolescents are experiencing the postconventional stage of moral development (Kohlberg, 1984). It is only because adolescents are developing their formal operational way of thinking that they can experience the postconventional stage of moral development. At the beginning of this stage, adolescents begin to question the status quo. The majority of their choices are based on emotions while they are questioning societal standards. As they progress to developing their own set of morals, adolescents realize that moral decisions are based on rights, values, and principles that are agreeable to a given society. They also realize that those rights, values, and principles can be in conflict with the laws of the given society, but they are able to reconcile the differences. Because adolescents undergo the process of developing their own set of morals at different rates, they might find that their friends view a situation differently. This difference can lead to conflicts and the forming of different friendships. See Table 7.2 for additional information.

Adolescents may also begin to question their formal religious practices or in some cases cling to them (Ford, 2007). As they progress through adolescence, individuals may become more interested in the spiritualism of their religion than in the actual practices of their religion. Adolescents are searching for ideals and may exhibit intense emotions along with introspection (Ford, 2007). Increased spirituality and religious activities are related to increased healthy behaviors and decreased high-risk behaviors (Ford, 2007).

Referring back to Cho Chung, identify the stage of psychosocial development that she should be in according to Erikson. What approaches for assessment and teaching would be most effective based on the stage you identified?

MOTOR SKILL DEVELOPMENT

During adolescence, the individual refines and continues to develop their gross and fine motor skills. Because of this period of rapid growth spurts, adolescents may experience times of decreased coordination and have a diminished ability to perform previously learned skills, which can be worrisome for the adolescent.

Gross Motor Skills

It is usually during early adolescence that individuals begin to develop endurance. Their concentration has increased, so they can follow complicated instructions. Coordination can be a problem because of the uneven growth spurts. During middle adolescence, speed and accuracy increase while coordination also improves. Adolescents become more competitive with each other (Fig. 7.2). During late adolescence, the individual usually narrows their areas of interest and concentrates on the needed relevant skills.

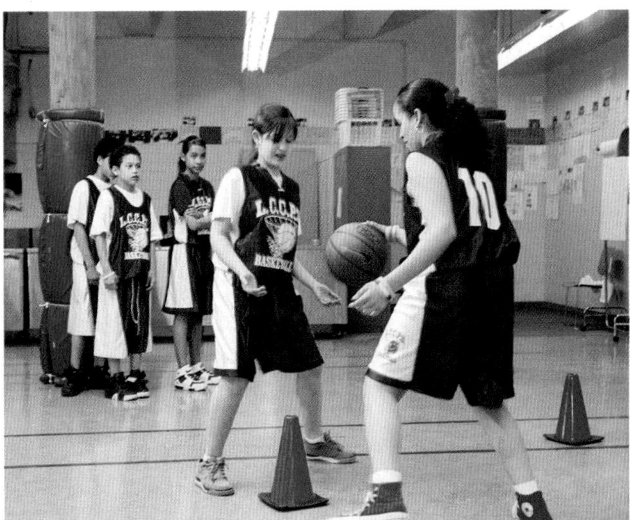

FIGURE 7.2 Adolescents become involved in competitive sports, which draw upon their gross motor skills.

Fine Motor Skills

In the early adolescent years, the individual increases their ability to manipulate objects. The adolescent's handwriting is neater, and they have increased finger dexterity. The middle adolescent years see the individual refining their dexterity skills. By late adolescence, the individual has developed precise eye–hand coordination and finger dexterity.

COMMUNICATION AND LANGUAGE DEVELOPMENT

Language skills continue to develop and be refined during adolescence. Adolescents have improved communication skills, using correct grammar and parts of speech. Vocabulary and communication skills continue to develop during middle adolescence. However, the usage of colloquial speech (slang) increases, causing communication with people other than peers to be difficult at times. By late adolescence, language skills are comparable to those of adults.

As you assess Cho (the 15-year-old introduced at the beginning of the chapter), what would you expect her gross motor, fine motor, and language skills to be at this age?

EMOTIONAL AND SOCIAL DEVELOPMENT

Adolescents undergo a great deal of change in the areas of emotional and social development as they grow and mature into adults. Areas that are affected include the adolescent's relationship with parents; self-concept and body image; importance of peers; and sexuality and dating.

Relationship With Parents

Families and parents of adolescents experience changes and conflict that require adjustments and the understanding of adolescent development. The adolescent is striving for self-identity and increased independence. They spend more time with peers and less time with family and attending family functions. Parents sense that they have less influence on the adolescent as the adolescent questions family values and becomes more mobile. This may lead to a family crisis, and the parents may respond by setting stricter limits or asking questions about the adolescent's activities and friends. Other parents may drop all rules and assume that the adolescent can manage themselves. Both of these responses increase tension in the family.

With the adolescent attempting to establish some level of independence—and the family learning to let go while focusing on aging parents, their marriage, and other children—a state of disequilibrium occurs. The family may experience more stress than at any other time.

Some families have better outcomes with their adolescents than others. Families who listen to and continue to demonstrate affection for and acceptance of their adolescent have a more positive outcome. This does not mean that the family accepts all of the adolescent's ideas or actions, but they are willing to listen and attempt to negotiate some limits. For tips to improve communication with adolescents, see Box 7.1.

Siblings experience changes in the relationship with the adolescent; the older sibling may attempt to parent, and the younger sibling may regress in an attempt to avoid the family conflict. Understanding the status of the adolescent–family relationship is essential for the nurse.

Self-Concept and Body Image

Self-concept and self-esteem are often tied to body image. Adolescents who perceive their body as being different than their peers' bodies or as less than ideal may view themselves negatively.

Sexual characteristics are important to the adolescent's self-concept and body image. Adolescents are concerned about the size of their penis or breasts, facial hair, and the onset of menstruation. Larger breasts are often considered more feminine, and menstruation is considered a rite of passage into adulthood. All of these body changes are important to the adolescent's self-concept.

Importance of Peers

Peer groups play an essential role in the identity of the adolescent (Holland-Hall, 2020). Adolescent peer relationships are important in providing opportunities to learn about negotiating differences; for recreation, companionship, and someone to share problems with; for learning peer loyalty; and for creating stability during transitions or times of stress. Learning to work out differences with peers is a skill that is important throughout life. Peers serve as someone safe to discuss family issues with, as the adolescent emotionally moves away from the

BOX **7.1** **Ways to Improve Communication With Adolescents**

- Set aside an appropriate amount of time to discuss subject matter without interruptions.
- Talk face-to-face. Be aware of body language.
- Ask questions to see why they feel the way they do.
- Ask them to be patient as you tell your thoughts.
- Choose words carefully so they understand you.
- Tell them exactly what you mean.
- Give praise and approval to your adolescent often.
- Speak to your adolescent as an equal—don't talk down to them.
- Be aware of your tone of voice and body language.
- Don't pretend you know all the answers.
- Admit that you do make mistakes.
- Set rules and limits fairly.

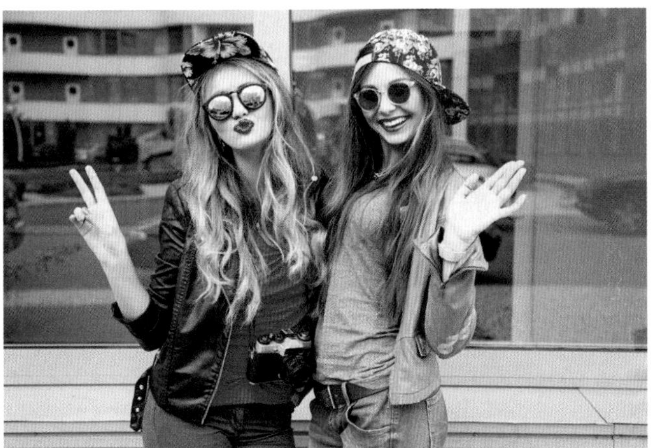

FIGURE 7.3 Peers play an important role in shaping the adolescent's identity.

family while trying to find their identity. Due to changes that have taken place within family systems in society, peer groups play a significant role in the socialization of adolescents (Fig. 7.3).

Peers serve as credible sources of information, role model social behaviors, and act as sources of social reinforcement. Friends provide an opportunity for fun and excitement. Peers impact each other's appearance, dress, social behavior, and language. Peers can also have positive influences on each other, such as promoting college attendance, or negative influences, such as involvement with alcohol, drugs, or gangs. Early and middle adolescence are periods when adolescents may consider joining gangs. Peer role modeling and peer acceptance may lead to the formation of a gang that provides a collective identity and gives a sense of belonging. Peer pressure, companionship, and protection are the most frequent reasons given for joining gangs, particularly those associated with criminal activity.

Parents must know their adolescent's friends and continue to be aware of potential problems while allowing the adolescent the independence to become their own person. Nurses must remind parents of the importance of peers and the impact they have on the adolescent's decisions and life choices. The transition to greater peer involvement requires guidance and support. Adolescents who do not have parental or adult supervision and opportunities for conversation with adults may be more susceptible to peer influences and at higher risk for poor peer selections.

Sexuality

Adolescence is a critical time in the development of sexuality. **Sexuality** includes the thoughts, feelings, and behaviors related to the adolescent's sexual identity. Adolescence is a time when individuals may begin experimentation related to their sexual identity, orientation, and behavior. This experimentation is part of the process of sorting through their sexuality and does not always define their sexual identity or orientation.

Adolescents who identify as lesbian, gay, bisexual, transgender, queer, intersex, asexual, and identities that defy discrete labels (LGBTQ+) face the same health concerns as other adolescents, but additional challenges may include questioning of their sexual identity, the complexity of coming out, and possible societal discrimination (Forcier & Olson-Kennedy, 2020). The majority of LGBTQ+ adolescents are healthy and well, but some are at an increased risk for adverse outcomes such as depression, suicide, substance use disorder, homelessness, sexually transmitted infections (STIs), unplanned pregnancy, and victimization (Forcier & Olson-Kennedy, 2020). See Evidence-Based Practice 7.1. Personal, societal, and family acceptance are crucial and lead to decreased adverse outcomes.

EVIDENCE-BASED PRACTICE 7.1

Reducing Behavioral Health Symptoms by Addressing Minority Stressors in LGBTQ+ Adolescents: A Randomized Controlled Trial of Proud & Empowered

STUDY

LGBTQ+ adolescents have an increased incidence of depression, anxiety, self-harm, suicidal attempts and ideation, and substance use. Discrimination, violence, and victimization place the LGBTQ+ adolescent at higher risk for mental health conditions. Previous studies have shown evidence that improving adolescents' ability to cope with stress improves mental health outcomes. This study was a randomized control trial (RCT) of a program called Proud & Empowered, to be delivered in school settings. It is a small group program for LGBTQ+ adolescents, consisting of 10 sessions lasting about 45 minutes each.

Nursing Implications

Nurses should support school-based programs. School staff and school officials should be educated on the increased mental health risks for LGBTQ+ youth and programs that have demonstrated effectiveness at decreasing mental health symptoms and reducing stress. Further research is needed to evaluate the effectiveness of school-based programs, utilizing larger sample sizes. Nurses should work with a multidisciplinary team that includes medical and mental health professionals, school and educational professionals, and adolescents and their families to incorporate appropriate interventions into their local schools.

Data from Goldbach, J. T., Rhoades, H., Mamey, M. R., Senese, J., Karys, P., & Marsiglia, F. F. (2021). Reducing behavioral health symptoms by addressing minority stressors in LGBTQ adolescents: A randomized controlled trial of Proud & Empowered. *BMC Public Health*, *21*, 2315. https://doi.org/10.1186/s12889-021-12357-5

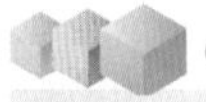

Concept Mastery Alert

When providing care to an adolescent who shares information about their sexual identity, the nurse must remember that assessment is the first step in the nursing process.

Dating

An interest in romantic partnerships occurs during adolescence (Fig. 7.4). Some of the reasons cited for this developing interest are physical development and body changes, peer-group pressure, and curiosity. During the past couple of decades, dating has become less common (Eickmeyer et al., 2020). The percentage of adolescents who date frequently increases with age. As of 2020, 51% of high school seniors reported dating, a decrease from 78% 20 years before (Eickmeyer et al., 2020). Adolescent dating can range from group dating to single dating to serious relationships.

During early adolescence, individuals tend to date for fun and recreation.

Middle and late adolescents have group and single dates. Romantic relationships become more central to the social life of this age group. Dating or spending time with a potential romantic partner is viewed as a major developmental marker for adolescents and is one of the most challenging adjustments. Both positive and negative developmental outcomes can result depending on the quality of the relationship that forms. Some adolescents who date may report slightly higher levels of self-esteem, self-worth and social support (Emerson et al., 2023; Kansky & Allen, 2018). However, other types of dating relationships may result in an adolescent having lower academic success and motivation, higher depression rates, increased anxiety, and increased risk of substance use (Emerson et al., 2023; Kansky & Allen, 2018). Trends in dating are everchanging, but dating remains a developmental milestone for the adolescent.

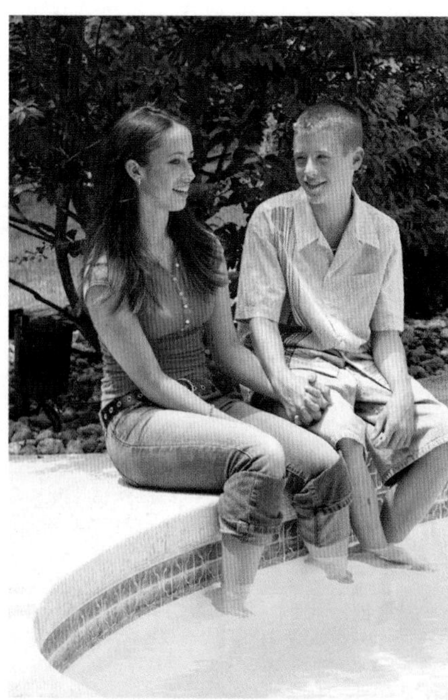

FIGURE 7.4 Dating becomes an important aspect of the adolescent's life.

Healthy romantic relationships can assist the adolescent in developing a strong sense of self-identity, self-regulation; self-expression; emotional autonomy from their family; and interpersonal skills, such as empathy; and are related to increased quality of adult relationships (Emerson et al., 2023; Kansky & Allen, 2018). The emotional ups and downs that accompany dating can help develop emotional resilience and coping skills. Romantic relationships at this stage are a great source of emotional support. Risks of being involved in unhealthy romantic relationships include dating violence and risky sexual activity such as STIs and pregnancy. Adolescents do not automatically know what makes for a healthy relationship. They need to be educated on the right and wrong behaviors of dating and what behaviors make up a healthy relationship, such as open communication, honesty, and trust. They need to know the signs of an unhealthy relationship and how to seek help if needed.

Refer back to Cho, the 15-year-old from the beginning of the chapter. Cho's parent states they are concerned about the changes that have occurred in their relationship over the past year. Cho seems much more self-centered, always wants to be with her friends, is critical of her parents, and seems to be constantly in conflict with them. Based on what you know about this stage of development, what guidance, including approaches and techniques, can you discuss with Cho's parent to address these concerns?

CULTURAL INFLUENCES ON GROWTH AND DEVELOPMENT

Although the adolescent's culture continues to influence them, the desire to be in harmony with peers becomes paramount. That desire can cause conflict with the adolescent's family and culture. Today's adolescents live in a rapidly changing, increasingly culturally diverse world. They may be exposed to people from many different cultures and ethnic groups.

Attitudes regarding adolescence vary among cultures. Certain cultures may have more permissive attitudes toward issues facing adolescents, while others are more conservative (e.g., toward sexuality). Experiencing a rite-of-passage ceremony to signal the adolescent's movement to adult status varies among cultures. American culture does not have a universal rite of passage for adolescents. Some religious and social groups do have ceremonies that signal a movement toward the maturity of adulthood (e.g., the Jewish bar or bat mitzvah, the Catholic confirmation, and social debuts). In many parts of the world, separate "youth cultures" have developed in an attempt to blend traditional and modern worlds for the adolescent.

It is important for the nurse to recognize the background of each adolescent. Research has shown that certain demographic groups are at higher risk for certain diseases. For example, Black and Hispanic adolescents are at higher risk for developing hypertension (Mattoo, 2021). But the major influence on the adolescent's health and successful achievement of the tasks of adolescence is socioeconomic status. Adolescents at a lower socioeconomic level are at higher risk for developing physical and psychological health care problems and risk-taking behaviors; this may be in part due to lack of access to health care and necessary services (American Psychological Association, 2019). In caring for adolescents, recognize the influence of their unique backgrounds on their health.

THE NURSE'S ROLE IN ADOLESCENT GROWTH AND DEVELOPMENT

Growth and development in the adolescent is rapid. Nurses must be aware of the expected growth and development patterns for this age group so that they can assess the adolescent appropriately and provide guidance to the adolescent and their family.

During adolescence, the individual faces many challenges. Their fluctuating relationships with parents and other adult figures may limit the adolescent from seeking assistance in dealing with the common issues of adolescence. In dealing with adolescents, be aware that they may behave unpredictably, may be inconsistent with their need for independence, may have sensitive feelings, may interpret situations differently from what they are, may think friends are extremely important, and may have a strong desire to belong. During health care visits, the adolescent or parent may have concerns that they are hesitant or uncomfortable talking about in front of each other. Try to provide an opportunity for them to have private time with a health care provider to discuss issues. The adolescent may greatly appreciate the opportunity for time to discuss concerns with a nonjudgmental informed adult.

If the adolescent is hospitalized, growth and development may be altered. The adolescent may be concerned about how the illness or injury will affect their body and body image. They may fear pain and loss of privacy. The adolescent may experience anxiety about separation from friends and loss of control.

When caring for the hospitalized adolescent, the nurse must use knowledge of expected growth and development to recognize potential delays, promote continued appropriate growth and development, and interact successfully with the patient. Provide opportunities for them to maintain independence, participate in decisions, and encourage socialization with friends through phone, e-mail, and visits when possible.

Clinical Judgment and the Nursing Process

On completion of assessment of the adolescent's current growth and development status, problems or issues related to growth and development may be identified. The nurse may then identify one or more nursing diagnoses. The following nursing diagnoses with identified outcomes and interventions provide suggestions for nursing care planning or concept mapping, which should be individualized, based on the adolescent's and family's needs.

Nursing Analysis

Alteration in nutritional status related to anxiety, depression, eating disorders, excessive family mealtime control, stressful mealtimes, inadequate choice of food, media influence on eating behaviors of high-calorie unhealthy foods, irregular mealtimes, changes to self-esteem on entering puberty, as evidenced by avoiding participation in regular mealtimes, frequently eating from fast-food restaurants, poor quality or overprocessed foods, overeating, or undereating.

Goal/Outcome

Adolescents will demonstrate adequate growth: appropriate weight gain and increase in height for age and sex; BMI between 5th and 85th percentiles

Promoting Appropriate Eating Dynamics (interventions with *rationale*)

- Assess parents' and adolescent's knowledge of nutritional needs of adolescents and family eating patterns *to determine need for further education.*
- Educate parents and adolescent about appropriate serving sizes and foods *so that they are aware of what to expect for adolescents.*
- Determine need for additional caloric intake if necessary (*if* adolescent is *very active in sports or has a chronic illness, caloric intake needs to meet body's demands*).
- Plot out height, weight, and BMI *to detect possible pattern.*
- Assess for risk factors for developing an eating disorder *to identify need for early intervention.*

Nursing Analysis

Excess weight risk; risk factors include average daily physical activity being less than recommended for sex and age, consumption of sugar-sweetened beverages, frequent snacking, high frequency of restaurant or fried food, insufficient knowledge of modifiable factors, portion sizes being larger than recommended, sedentary behavior occurring for more than 2 hours/day, BMI approaching 85th percentile, parental excess weight.

Goal/Outcome

Adolescent will maintain a healthy weight for age, BMI less than 85th percentile, and lose weight at an appropriate rate: increase amount of exercise, make appropriate eating choices, decrease caloric intake to appropriate amount for age and sex.

Promoting Healthy Weight (interventions with *rationale*)

- Assess knowledge of parents and adolescent about nutritional needs of adolescents *to determine deficits in knowledge.*
- Have adolescent keep a detailed food and exercise diary for 1 week *to determine current patterns of eating and exercise.*
- Interview family in relation to their eating habits and exercise habits *to determine where adjustments might need to be made.*
- Discuss changes in a positive manner—talk about developing healthy eating habits instead of dieting *to promote adherence.*
- Analyze preceding data, and base recommendations for changes on these data *to promote adherence and to prioritize recommendations.*
- Discuss ways to decrease temptation to overeat, for example, eat slowly, put down the fork between bites, serve food on smaller plates, and count mouthfuls, *to allow time to realize that they are full.*
- Have adolescent create meal plans and grocery shop *to allow them some sense of control and decision making.*
- Incorporate increase in daily exercise, which will stress sense of self-improvement *to increase caloric expenditure and self-esteem.*
- Decrease screen time *to increase caloric expenditure.*
- Encourage peer exercise activities *to increase peer interactions and to help adolescent to realize that others are like them.*
- Develop reward system *to increase self-esteem.*
- Investigate weight loss programs for adolescents *to increase self-esteem and encourage weight loss.*

Nursing Analysis

Delayed growth and development risk; risk factors include inadequate nutrition, presence of abuse, substance misuse, technology dependence, behavioral disorder, economic disadvantage, involvement with the foster care system, prematurity, chronic illness, and genetic disorders.

Goal/Outcome

Growth and development will be maximized: Adolescent will make continued progress toward attainment of expected school performance.

Promoting Development (interventions with *rationale*)

- Perform scheduled evaluation of the adolescent by school and health care provider *to determine current functioning.*
- Develop realistic multidisciplinary plan *to ensure maximizing resources.*
- Carry out interventions as prescribed by developmental specialist, physical therapist, occupational therapist, or speech therapist at home and at school *to maximize benefit of interventions.*
- Have scheduled evaluation meetings *to be able to adapt interventions as soon as possible.*

Nursing Analysis

Injury risk; risk factors include exposure to toxic chemicals, insufficient knowledge of modifiable factors, unsafe mode of transport, extremes of age (developmental stage including increased motor and cognitive skills and feeling of invincibility).

Goal/Outcome

Adolescent's safety will be maintained: will remain free from injury.

Preventing Injury (interventions with *rationale*)

- Discuss safety measures needed for the following: bikes, scooters, guns, skateboards, cars, and water *to decrease risk of injury related to those areas.*
- Discuss and develop a fire safety plan *to decrease risk of injury related to fire.*
- Discuss appropriate safety equipment needed for each sport *to decrease risk of injury.*
- Discuss appropriate sports to participate in depending on age, sex, and maturity of adolescent *to prevent possible injury.*
- Teach parents and adolescent first-aid measures and cardiopulmonary resuscitation (CPR) *to minimize consequences of injury should it occur.*
- Discuss influence of peers on actions of adolescents *to prevent possible injury due to mimicking behavior.*
- Educate adolescents about the risk of overdose with substance use *to prevent injury or death due to substance use.*

Nursing Analysis

Ineffective coping related to inability to conserve adaptive energies, inadequate confidence in ability to deal with a situation, inadequate opportunity to prepare for stressors, inadequate resources, insufficient social support as evidenced by alteration in sleep pattern, destructive behavior toward others or self, frequent illness, inability to meet basic needs, insufficient coping strategies, risk-taking behavior, substance misuse.

Goal/Outcome

Adolescent will demonstrate adequate coping abilities as evidenced by management of stress of adolescence and no evidence of participating in risk-taking behaviors.

Ineffective Coping (interventions with *rationale*)

- Assess adolescent's knowledge of normal stress facing adolescents *to determine current knowledge.*
- Assess adolescent's present coping skills *to determine areas for improvement/support.*
- Encourage parents to accept adolescent as a unique individual *to improve self-esteem.*
- Discuss with parents and adolescent normal developmental issues facing adolescents *to give them knowledge needed to cope.*
- Provide different situations the adolescent might be faced with, and encourage adolescent to develop different solutions *to assist adolescent in developing problem-solving strategies.*
- Allow for increasing independence and opportunities to solve own problems *to improve coping skills.*
- Encourage parents to provide unconditional love *to improve self-esteem.*
- Assess for any evidence of any risk-taking behaviors (drugs, smoking, self-harm) *to identify need for early interventions.*

Nursing Analysis

Caregiver role strain risk; risk factors include dependency, discharge home with significant needs, substance misuse, unstable health condition, insufficient knowledge about community resources, and social isolation.

Goal/Outcome

Parent will experience competence in role: will demonstrate appropriate caregiving behaviors and verbalize comfort in caring for an adolescent.

Preventing Caregiver Role Strain (interventions with *rationale*)

- Assess parents' knowledge of adolescents and the issues that arise as a part of expected development *to determine parents' needs.*
- Provide education on normal issues of adolescence *so that parents are prepared with the knowledge they need to appropriately care for their adolescents.*
- Provide anticipatory guidance related to upcoming expected issues related to adolescent development *to prepare parents for what to expect next and how to intervene in an appropriate manner.*

PROMOTING HEALTHY GROWTH AND DEVELOPMENT

It takes multiple groups who address multiple issues to promote healthy growth and development in the adolescent. Some of these groups include sports teams in the school or the community, peers, teachers, band and choir members, and so forth. Also, the family's support and love will influence growth and development.

Promoting Growth and Development Through Sports and Physical Fitness

Many adolescents are involved in team sports that provide avenues for exercise. High levels of physical activity may reduce cardiovascular disease risk factors and provide disease prevention against cancer, higher weight, osteoporosis, diabetes, and depression (Centers for Disease Control and Prevention [CDC], 2022a). Adolescents probably spend more time and energy participating in sports than any other age group. Participation in sports contributes to the adolescent's development, educational process, and better health. Sports and games provide an opportunity to interact with peers while enjoying socially accepted stimulation and conflict. Competition in sports activities helps the adolescent in processing self-appraisal and in developing self-respect and concern for others.

Every sport has some potential for injury. Rapidly growing bones, muscles, joints, and tendons are more vulnerable to unusual strains and fractures. Incidence of concussions (which is considered a mild traumatic brain injury) is a growing concern in all adolescent athletes. To help prevent injury, parents and coaches need to be aware of early warning signs of fatigue, dehydration, and injury. See Chapter 22 for a discussion of sports injuries.

In relation to youth sports, the role of the nurse is to educate to prevent injuries (Fig. 7.5). This education

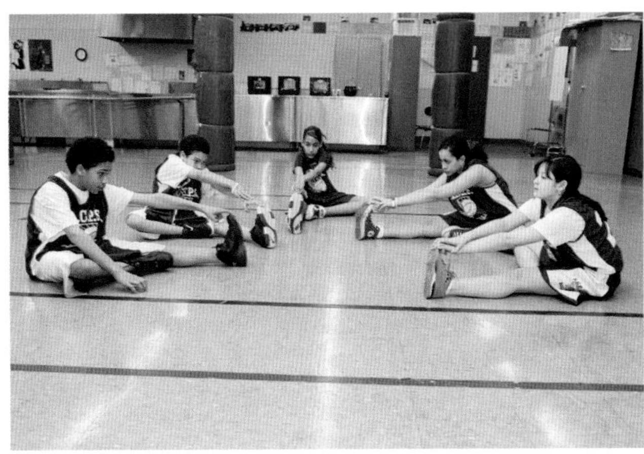

FIGURE 7.5 Stretching before exercise is an important part of exercise.

should include discouraging participation when the adolescent is tired or has an existing injury, encouraging the use of proper well-fitting protective gear, and ensuring the adolescent learns how to play a sport before participating in it.

In addition, adolescence is a good time to develop an exercise program. The U.S. Department of Health and Human Services (HHS) recommends that adolescents participate in 60 minutes of moderate to vigorous physical activity each day (CDC, 2022a). Nurses should encourage all adolescents to be physically active daily.

Promoting Learning

School, teachers, family, and peers influence education and learning for the adolescent. Also, activities such as athletics and club membership enhance learning through interactions with peers, coaches, club leaders, and others.

School

School plays an essential part in preparing adolescents for the future. Completing school prepares the adolescent for college or employment to make an adequate income. Schools in the United States may not meet the developmental needs of all adolescents. Students from historically marginalized communities may not be at the appropriate grade level, and the dropout rate may be higher than in students from communities that have not been historically marginalized. Dropout rates have declined since the 1970s but still remain a concern. Dropout rates are highest among Hispanic students (National Center for Education Statistics, 2022). Those who drop out of school may lack skills needed to function in today's society. They are more likely to be unemployed, have higher rates of incarceration, and have lower income levels and occupational status than those with a high school diploma (American Public Health Association [APHA], 2018; National Center for Education Statistics, n.d.; see Healthy People 2030).

HEALTHY PEOPLE 2030

Objective	Nursing Significance
Increase the proportion of high school students who graduate in 4 years.	• Encourage school attendance and completion when encountering adolescents for well-child or sick visits. • Refer children who have difficulty concentrating or learning for further evaluation. • Praise school accomplishments.

Healthy People Objectives retrieved from http://www.healthypeople.gov

There is evidence that the transition from elementary school to middle school, at age 12 or 13, and then the transition to high school, both of which occur at the time of physical changes, may have a negative effect on adolescents. It is important to observe for transition problems into middle or high school, which may be exhibited by failing grades or behavior problems. Also, students who experience difficulties in school, resulting in negative evaluations and failing grades, may feel alienated from school. Students with poor grades and low academic achievement exhibit more unhealthy behaviors such as physical inactivity and poor diet and are more likely to engage in risky behaviors such as early sexual initiation and substance use (CDC, 2022b). Schools that support peer-group relationships, promote health and fitness, encourage parental involvement, and strengthen community relationships have better student outcomes. Parents, teachers, and health care providers should provide guidance and support.

Other Activities

Adolescents are involved in many other activities that influence learning. Some of these activities include (1) school activities such as band, choir, or clubs; (2) athletic activities in the school and community and sometimes in the state or region; (3) art, sewing, and building classes; and (4) work activities when the late adolescent has a part-time job. These activities all contribute to the growth, development, and education of the adolescent.

Promoting Safety

Unintentional injury is the leading cause of death in adolescents (CDC, 2021a). Motor vehicle crashes are the leading cause of unintentional injury death, followed by poisoning, primarily due to drug overdose from opioids, and drowning (CDC, 2021a). Males are more likely than females to die of any type of injury (CDC, 2021a).

Influencing factors related to the prevalence of adolescent injuries include increased physical growth, insufficient psychomotor coordination for the task, abundance of energy, impulsivity, peer pressure, and inexperience. Impulsivity, inexperience, and peer pressure may place the adolescent in a vulnerable situation between knowing what is right and wanting to impress peers. On the other hand, adolescents have a feeling of invulnerability, which may contribute to negative outcomes. Alcohol and other drugs are contributing factors in automobile crashes and unintentional firearm injuries among adolescents. Most of the serious or fatal injuries in adolescents are preventable (Fig. 7.6). Nurses must educate parents and adolescents on car, gun, and water safety to prevent unintentional injuries. See Teaching Guidelines 7.1 for information on promoting safety.

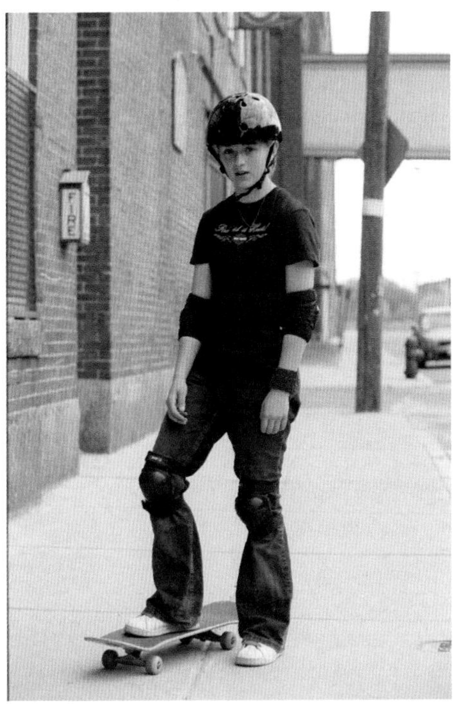

FIGURE 7.6 Wearing appropriate safety equipment can prevent injuries.

TAKE NOTE!

A sharp increase in firearm-related deaths in children 0 to 19 years of age was seen from 2019 to 2020, along with drug overdose and poisonings (CDC/National Center for Health Statistics, 2022; Goldstick et al., 2022). Nurses need to follow this trend to ensure we are providing interventions to help protect our youth from these preventable causes of death.

Motor Vehicle Safety

The largest numbers of adolescent injuries are due to motor vehicle crashes. When the adolescent passes their driving test, they are able to drive legally. However, driving is complex and requires judgments that the adolescent is often incapable of making. Also, the typical adolescent is opposed to authority and is interested in showing peers and others their independence. It is also normal for adolescents to take risks. These factors, coupled with inexperience with driving, may lead to underestimating hazardous and dangerous situations. Adolescents and young adults are the least likely age group to wear a seat belt (CDC, 2021b). Crashes involving

TEACHING GUIDELINES 7.1 Promoting Safety

Safety Issue	Activity
Motor vehicle	• Wear a seat belt at all times. • Do not drive impaired or drive with someone who is impaired. • Take a driver-education course. • Parents should drive with the adolescent for 30–50 hours prior to obtaining license, at different times of the day, in different heavy and light traffic and during different weather conditions. • Restrict nighttime driving. • Establish driving rules between parent and adolescent prior to the adolescent getting license. • Have all passengers wear seat belts. • Do not use cell phone or text while driving, drink and drive, or drive when tired. • Maintain the car's good condition. • Drive with adult supervision for a period of time after receiving a license. • Encourage a limit on the number of adolescent passengers.
Bike: General	• Have a well-maintained and appropriate-size bike for adolescent. • Adolescent should demonstrate their ability to ride the bike safely before being allowed to ride on the street. • Safe areas for bike riding should be established as well as routes to and from area of activities. • Do not ride bike barefoot, with someone else on bike, or with clothing that might get entangled in the bike. • Wear sturdy, well-fitting shoes and Consumer Product Safety Commission (CPSC) or Snell-approved helmets. • A properly fitting helmet should: sit level, not tilted, and firmly and comfortably on the head; have strong wide Y-shaped straps and when you open your mouth should pull down a bit; not move with sudden pulling or twisting; never be worn over anything else (hat, scarf, etc.). • The bike should be inspected often to ensure it is in proper working order. • A basket should be used to carry heavy objects.

(continued)

TEACHING GUIDELINES 7.1 Promoting Safety (*continued*)

Safety Issue	Activity
Bike: In traffic	• All traffic signs and signals must be observed. • If the adolescent is riding at night, the bike should have lights and reflectors, and the rider should wear light-colored clothes. • Ride on the side of the road traveling with traffic and keep close to the side of the road in single file. • Watch and listen for cars and never hitch a ride on any vehicle. • Do not wear headphones while riding a bike.
All-terrain vehicles	• The vehicle not be operated by an adolescent younger than 16 years of age. • Take a hands-on safety course before riding. • Helmet and protective coverings are required. • No nighttime or double riding • Not for use on public roads or if the adolescent has been drinking or using drugs • Do not stand up in the vehicle or ride in a person's lap.
Skateboards/skates	• Wear a helmet, and protective padding on knees, elbows, and wrists. • Do not skate in traffic or on streets or highways. • Skating on homemade ramps could be dangerous—assess ramps for any hazards before skating.
Water safety	• Learn how to swim; if swimming skill is limited, wear a life preserver at all times. • Never swim alone; if at all possible, swim only where there is a life guard. • Learn basic cardiopulmonary resuscitation (CPR). • Do not run or fool around at the edge of the pool. • Drains in the pool should be covered with appropriate cover. • Wear a life jacket when on a boat. • Make sure there is enough water to support diving. • Do not swim if drinking alcohol or using drugs.
Firearms	• If guns are in the household, take a firearm safety class, secure guns in a safe place, use gun safety locks, and store bullets in a separate place. • Never point a gun at a person.
Fire safety	• All homes should have working smoke detectors and fire extinguishers. Change the batteries at least twice a year. • Have a fire-escape plan and practice the plan routinely. • No smoking in bed • Teach what to do in case of a fire—use a fire extinguisher, call 911, and know how to put out clothing fire. • All flammable materials and liquids should be stored safely. • Fireplaces should have protective gratings. • Avoid touching any downed power lines.
Machinery	• Use safety devices. • Receive training on how to use equipment. • Do not use machinery when alone.
Sports	• Match the sport to the adolescent's ability and desire. • Sports programs should have a warm-up procedure and hydration policy. • Undergo a sports physical before start of activity. • Coaches should be trained in CPR and first aid. • Wear appropriate protection devices for the individual sport.
Sun	• Use sunscreen with both ultraviolet A (UVA) and ultraviolet B (UVB) protection. • Apply sunscreen prior to going out, and reapply sunscreen often. • Limit sun exposure, especially between 10 a.m. and 2 p.m. • Wear protective clothing and a hat and sunglasses while outside. • Do not suntan, and avoid using tanning beds.

TEACHING GUIDELINES 7.1 Promoting Safety

Safety Issue	Activity
Personal safety	• Never go with a stranger. • Do not enter a car when the driver has been drinking. • Notify an adult about where you are when out after dark. • Keep your cell phone fully charged. • Never give out personal information over the internet. • Say "no" to drugs, alcohol, smoking, and to being touched when you do not want to be touched.
Toxins	• Teach the hazards of accepting illegal drugs, alcohol, and dangerous drugs. • Store potentially dangerous material in a safe place.

Data from American Academy of Pediatrics. (2010, reaffirmed 2016). The teen driver. *Pediatrics*, *118*(6), 2570–2581. http://pediatrics.aappublications.org/content/118/6/2570.full; Centers for Disease Control and Prevention. (2021c). *Keep teen drivers safe*. https://www.cdc.gov/injury/features/teen-drivers/index.html; American Academy of Pediatrics, Council on Environmental Health and Section on Dermatology. (2011, reaffirmed 2017). Policy statement—Ultraviolet radiation: A hazard to children and adolescents. *Pediatrics*, *127*(3), 588–597. https://doi.org/10.1542/peds.2016-4205; American Academy of Pediatrics, HealthyChildren. (2022). *ATVs are not for children: AAP urges these safety rules*. https://www.healthychildren.org/English/safety-prevention/at-play/Pages/ATV-Safety-Rules.aspx; Centers for Disease Control and Prevention. (2022c). *Drowning facts*. http://www.cdc.gov/HomeandRecreationalSafety/Water-Safety/waterinjuries-factsheet.html; Gill, A. C. (2022). Bicycle injuries in children: Prevention. *UpToDate*. Retrieved October 17, 2022, from https://www.uptodate.com/contents/bicycle-injuries-in-children-prevention

adolescents are more likely to involve speeding, driving too fast for conditions, or following too close to the car in front of them (CDC, 2021b). More crashes occur when passengers, mostly other adolescents, are present in the car; during driving at night; or when driving under the influence of alcohol or drugs (American Academy of Pediatrics, 2010, reaffirmed 2016; CDC, 2021b).

It is essential to promote driver education, to teach about the importance of wearing seat belts, and to explain laws about adolescent driving and curfews (Fig. 7.7). See Teaching Guidelines 7.1 for additional information.

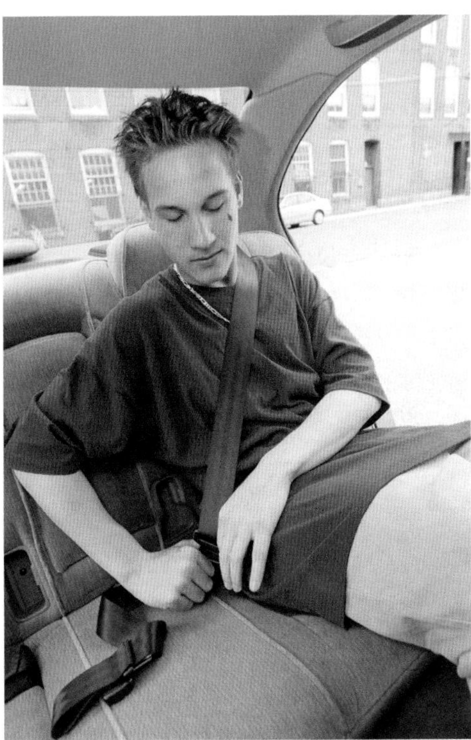

FIGURE 7.7 The use of seat belts has led to fewer fatal injuries in car crashes.

TAKE NOTE!

All states, although varied, have enacted a Graduated Driving License (GDL) program, which allows adolescents to gain driving experience and limits risky circumstances (such as nighttime driving and driving with passengers) by providing a license in three stages (learner's permit, provisional license, and full license; CDC, 2021b). Studies have shown this program to be highly effective in reducing adolescent driver crashes (CDC, 2021b).

Firearm Safety

The risk of dying from a firearm injury among 15- to 19-year-olds has been rising. In 2019, firearms became the leading cause of death in children 0 to 19 years of age, exceeding motor vehicle crashes (Naik-Mathuria & Gill, 2022). Seventy-four percent of homicides involved firearms, and 45% of suicides in children and adolescents involved firearms (Naik-Mathuria & Gill, 2022). Homicides in adolescent males account for the majority of pediatric firearm deaths (Naik-Mathuria & Gill, 2022). Provide education about gun safety. Emphasize that an absence of guns in the home is the most effective way to prevent firearm injuries. If there are guns in the home, they must be kept locked in a safe location, with ammunition kept separately. Parents must teach adolescents about the dangers of playing with firearms. See Teaching Guidelines 7.1 for additional information on gun safety.

Water Safety

Drowning is a needless cause of death in adolescents. Many drownings are a result of risk-taking behaviors. With the independence of the adolescent, adult supervision is often not prevalent, and the adolescent takes a risk that results in drowning. Provide water safety education and proper supervision to decrease the incidence of risk taking. Teach about swimming lessons for nonswimmers. See Teaching Guidelines 7.1 for additional information.

Remember Cho Chung, the 15-year-old presented at the beginning of the chapter? What anticipatory guidance related to safety should you provide to Cho and her parent?

Promoting Nutrition

Nutritional needs are increased during adolescence due to accelerated growth and sexual maturation. Adolescents may appear to be constantly hungry and need regular meals and snacks with adequate nutrients to meet the body's needs. Multiple factors influence the adolescent's diet and eating habits (Box 7.2).

According to CDC data, since the 1970s, the obesity rate in adolescents has more than tripled (CDC, 2022d). Poor diet and physical inactivity have contributed to higher weight in this age group. Excess weight in adolescence is associated with excess weight in adulthood, along with numerous adverse health conditions such as diabetes, heart disease, certain types of cancer, osteoarthritis, and overall poorer physical and mental health (CDC, 2022e).

Nutritional Needs

Adolescents have a need for increased calories, zinc, calcium, and iron for growth. However, the number of calories needed during adolescence depends on the individual's age and activity level as well as growth patterns. Female adolescents who are moderately active require about 2,000 calories per day (U.S. Department of Agriculture [USDA] & Health and Human Services [HHS], 2020). Male adolescents who are moderately active require between 2,200 and 2,800 calories per day (USDA & HHS, 2020). Of these calories, 45% to 65% should come from carbohydrates, 10% to 30% from protein, and 25% to 35% from fat (USDA & HHS, 2020). Adolescents require about 1,300 mg of calcium each day (USDA & HHS, 2020). Adolescents should be made aware of foods high in calcium, including fortified ready-to-eat cereals, cheese, yogurt, almond milk, white beans, and broccoli. Adolescent males require 11 mg of iron each day, and females require 15 mg each day (USDA & HHS, 2020). Advise adolescents about foods high in iron (Box 7.3; see Healthy People 2030).

BOX 7.2 Factors Influencing the Adolescent's Diet

- Peer pressure
- Busy schedules
- Concern about weight control
- Convenience of fast food

BOX 7.3 Foods High in Iron

- Beef, chicken, seafood, liver
- Tofu
- Nuts and seeds
- Lentils and legumes
- Eggs
- Dark leafy vegetables such as spinach
- Iron-fortified cereals, whole-grain breads, and pastas

Protein requirements for adolescent females, 14 to 18 years of age, are 46 g/day, and for adolescent males, 14 to 18 years of age, 52 g/day (USDA & HHS, 2020). Some foods high in protein are meats, fish, poultry, beans, and dairy products.

HEALTHY PEOPLE 2030

Objective	Nursing Significance
Reduce iron deficiency in females aged 12–49 years. Increase calcium consumption by people aged 2 years and older. Increase vitamin D consumption by people aged 2 years and older. Increase consumption of potassium in the population aged 2 years and older. Reduce consumption of sodium in the population aged 2 years and older.	• Educate parents and adolescents about iron, calcium, vitamin D, and potassium-containing foods. • Encourage adolescent females to consume a diet high in iron-rich foods. • Educate adolescents on vitamin D–fortified foods and vitamin D supplements. • Educate the parent and adolescent about sodium reduction and high sodium-containing foods.

Healthy People Objectives retrieved from http://www.healthypeople.gov

Promoting Healthy Eating Habits

The nurse must understand expected growth and development of the adolescent in order to provide guidance that fits the quest for independence and the need for adolescents to make their own choices. Assess the eating habits and diet preferences of the adolescent. The assessment should include an evaluation of foods from the different food groups that the adolescent eats each day. Also, assess the number of times that fast foods, unhealthy snacks, and other junk food are eaten per week. This assessment will help the nurse to guide the adolescent in making better food choices at home and in fast-food establishments. Many fast-food restaurants offer baked chicken sandwiches and salads with fewer calories and less fat. Adolescents may be guided in alternating hamburgers and fries with more nutritious choices. Remember that planning should always include the adolescent.

The USDA provides a personalized food plan called MyPlatePlan based on an individual's age, sex, weight, height, and amount of physical activity. Refer to Figure 7.8

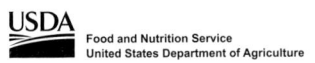

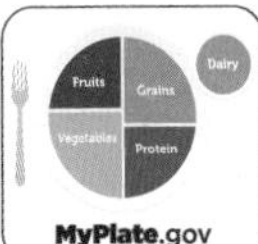

Start *simple* with **MyPlate** Plan

The benefits of healthy eating add up over time, bite by bite. Small changes matter. Start Simple with MyPlate.

A healthy eating routine is important at every stage of life and can have positive effects that add up over time. It's important to eat a variety of fruits, vegetables, grains, protein foods, and dairy or fortified soy alternatives. When deciding what to eat or drink, choose options that are full of nutrients. Make every bite count.

Food Group Amounts for 2,800 Calories a Day for Ages 14+ Years

 Fruits	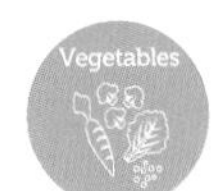 Vegetables	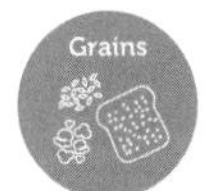 Grains	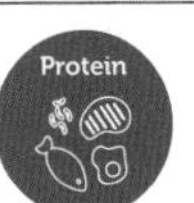 Protein	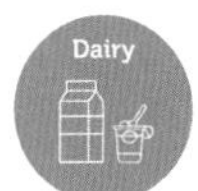 Dairy
2½ cups	**3½ cups**	**10 ounces**	**7 ounces**	**3 cups**
Focus on whole fruits	Vary your veggies	Make half your grains whole grains	Vary your protein routine	Move to low-fat or fat-free dairy milk or yogurt (or lactose-free dairy or fortified soy versions)
Focus on whole fruits that are fresh, frozen, canned, or dried.	Choose a variety of colorful fresh, frozen, and canned vegetables—make sure to include dark green, red, and orange choices.	Find whole-grain foods by reading the Nutrition Facts label and ingredients list.	Mix up your protein foods to include seafood; beans, peas, and lentils; unsalted nuts and seeds; soy products; eggs; and lean meats and poultry.	Look for ways to include dairy or fortified soy alternatives at meals and snacks throughout the day.

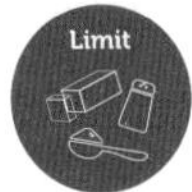

Choose foods and beverages with less added sugars, saturated fat, and sodium.
Limit:
- Added sugars to <**70 grams** a day.
- Saturated fat to <**31 grams** a day.
- Sodium to <**2,300 milligrams** a day.

Be active your way:
Children 6 to 17 years old should move **60 minutes** every day. Adults should be physically active at least 2½ **hours** per week.

MyPlate Plan

Write down the foods you ate today and track your small changes, bite by bite.

Food group targets for a 2,800-calorie* pattern are:	Write down your food choices for each food group.	Did you reach your target?
Fruits — **2½ cups** 1 cup of fruits counts as • 1 cup raw or cooked fruit; or • ½ cup dried fruit; or • 1 cup 100% fruit juice.		Y N
Vegetables — **3½ cups** 1 cup of vegetables counts as • 1 cup raw or cooked vegetables; or • 2 cups leafy salad greens; or • 1 cup 100% vegetable juice.		Y N
Grains — **10-ounce equivalents** 1 ounce of grains counts as • 1 slice bread; or • 1 ounce ready-to-eat cereal; or • ½ cup cooked rice, pasta, or cereal.		Y N
Protein — **7-ounce equivalents** 1 ounce of protein foods counts as • 1 ounce seafood, lean meats, or poultry; or • 1 egg; or • 1 Tbsp peanut butter; or • ¼ cup cooked beans, peas, or lentils; or • ½ ounce unsalted nuts or seeds.		Y N
Dairy — **3 cups** 1 cup of dairy counts as • 1 cup dairy milk or yogurt; or • 1 cup lactose-free dairy milk or yogurt; or • 1 cup fortified soy milk or yogurt; or • 1½ ounces hard cheese.		Y N

Limit:
- Added sugars to <**70 grams** a day.
- Saturated fat to <**31 grams** a day.
- Sodium to <**2,300 milligrams** a day.

Y N

Be active your way:
Children 6 to 17 years old should move **60 minutes** every day. Adults should be physically active at least 2½ **hours** per week.

Y N

* This 2,800-calorie pattern is only an estimate of your needs. Monitor your body weight and adjust your calories if needed.

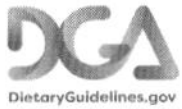

FNS-904-29
July 2021
USDA is an equal opportunity provider, employer, and lender.

FIGURE 7.8 MyPlatePlan for a 15-year-old male 63.5 kg (140 lb), 162.56 cm (5 ft 4 in), 30 to 60 minutes of exercise daily. (USDA. [2021, July]. *Start simple with MyPlate Plan*. FNS-904-29. Retrieved November 4, 2022, from https://myplate-prod.azureedge.us/sites/default/files/2021-08/2020MyPlatePlan_2800cals_Age14%2B.pdf)

for an example. At https://www.myplate.gov/life-stages/teens, the adolescent can create their customized food plan. Nurses may use the information in MyPlatePlan to help adolescents plan a healthy diet for themselves. See Healthy People 2030.

HEALTHY PEOPLE 2030

Objective	Nursing Significance
Increase whole-grain consumption by people aged 2 years and older. Increase fruit consumption by people aged 2 years and older. Increase vegetable consumption by people aged 2 years and older. Increase consumption of dark green vegetables, red and orange vegetables, and beans and peas by people aged 2 years and older. Reduce consumption of added sugars by people aged 2 years and older. Reduce consumption of saturated fat by people aged 2 years and older.	• Educate adolescents and families about the importance of whole grains, fruits, and vegetables in the diet. • Encourage the adolescent to choose fruits and vegetables that appeal to them. • Educate adolescents and families about saturated fat–containing foods and ways to reduce them in their diet. • Educate adolescents and families about foods with added sugar and how to avoid them. • Offer suggestions for alternative sources of proteins and fats (chicken or fish, olive oil).

Healthy People Objectives retrieved from http://www.healthypeople.gov

Maintaining Healthy Body Weight

The prevalence of BMIs classified as obese in children aged 12 to 19 years old is 19.7% (CDC, 2022f). Although excess weight has increased in all segments of the U.S. population, there are differences specific to race, ethnicity, and socioeconomic status. The prevalence of BMIs classified as obese is highest in Hispanic and non-Hispanic Black children and adolescents (CDC, 2022f).

This increase in excess weight in adolescents has led to increases in hypertension, heart disease, and type 2 diabetes. Influential factors causing excess weight include poor food choices, unhealthy eating practices, and lack of exercise. Around 15% of youths reported drinking sugary beverages at least once a day, and 25.9% reported attending physical education classes in school (Merlo et al., 2020). Overall, measures of how well Americans' food choices follow the dietary guidelines have remained low (USDA & HHS, 2020). Adolescents are busy and eat on the run, with many meals from fast-food facilities. In addition, many schools have decreased or discontinued physical education, which has resulted in a more sedentary lifestyle, leading to weight gain (APHA, 2021). Interest in computer games, smartphones, and television watching at home has decreased physical activity and exercise and further contributed to weight gain and higher weight (Woessner, 2021; see Healthy People 2030).

HEALTHY PEOPLE 2030

Objective	Nursing Significance
Reduce the proportion of children and adolescents with obesity. Increase the proportion of adolescents who do enough aerobic physical activity. Increase the proportion of adolescents who do enough muscle strengthening activity. Increase the proportion of children and adolescents who play sports.	• Screen all children for the development of excess weight, as indicated by an increasing body mass index (BMI) for their age. • Provide accurate diet counseling. • Encourage daily physical activity. • Counsel adolescents and parents to limit television screen time daily. • Educate the adolescent on the health risks associated with excess weight. • For the nonexercising adolescent, advise them to start slowly by walking. • Work with the adolescent to identify physical activities that interest them. • Praise efforts to participate in a routine exercise plan. • Identify an athletic individual that the adolescent identifies with, and encourage similar activities in the adolescent. • Encourage involvement in organized sports through school or local programs.

Healthy People Objectives retrieved from http://www.healthypeople.gov

Nurses must make parents and adolescents aware of factors leading to excess weight. Nurses should recommend:

- Proper nutrition and healthy food choices
- Good eating habits, including eating a healthy breakfast daily
- Decreased fast-food intake
- Physical activity for at least 60 minutes daily
- Parents/adolescents exercising more at home
- Parents living a healthy lifestyle
- Decreasing nonactive screen viewing and use

Think back to Cho Chung. What questions should you ask Cho and her parent related to nutritional intake? What anticipatory guidance related to nutrition would be appropriate?

Promoting Healthy Sleep and Rest

The average number of hours of sleep that adolescents require per night is 9 hours (Paul & Wallace, 2023). The adolescent often experiences a change in sleep patterns that leads to feeling more awake at night and the desire to sleep later in the morning (Paul & Wallace, 2023). Also, in this independence-seeking phase of adolescence, the adolescent may stay up later to do homework, to complete projects, or to participate in activities and may have difficulty awakening in the morning. Surveys show that 72.7% of high schoolers and 57.8% of middle schoolers do not get enough sleep on school nights (CDC, 2020). Inadequate sleep leads to an increased risk of certain health and cognitive problems such as higher weight, diabetes, poor mental health, problems with attention, and negative effects on mood and motivation (CDC, 2020). Early school start times contribute to this pattern of not getting enough sleep for adolescents (see Healthy People 2030). Adolescents will often try to make up for needed sleep by sleeping longer hours on weekends. Rapid growth and increased activities may produce fatigue and the need for more rest. Parents may report that the adolescent sleeps all the time and never has the time or energy to help with household chores. Explain to parents the need to discourage late hours on school nights because they may affect school performance. Encourage the adolescent to go to bed at the same time each night and awaken at the same time in the morning, even on weekends (CDC, 2020). Provide advice to adolescents and parents about having realistic expectations; encourage them to agree on a level of normalcy and adequate rest for the adolescent so that they can still fulfill responsibilities in the home.

HEALTHY PEOPLE 2030

Objective	Nursing Significance
Increase the proportion of high school students who get enough sleep. Increase proportion of secondary schools with a start time of 8:30 a.m. or later.	• Encourage consistent bedtimes. • Encourage adolescent to make bedroom dark, relaxing, and quiet. • Encourage no electronic devices in bedroom, and limit light exposure and technology use in the evening hours. • Encourage regular exercise. • Limit caffeine and tobacco. • Educate and encourage local school officials to adopt later start schedule for adolescents.

Healthy People Objectives retrieved from http://www.healthypeople.gov

What anticipatory guidance to Cho Chung and her parent in relation to sleep during the adolescent years should you provide?

Promoting Healthy Teeth and Gums

Most permanent teeth have erupted with the possible exception of the third molars (wisdom teeth). These molars may be impacted and require surgical removal. The rate of cavities decreases, but the need for routine dental visits every 6 months and brushing two to three times per day are important. Some of the conditions that occur during adolescence include malocclusion, gingivitis, and tooth avulsion. Malocclusion (a poor bite) occurs from facial and mandibular bone growth that results in misalignment of the top teeth with the bottom teeth. It is the most common reason for referral to an orthodontist. The treatment includes braces and other dental devices. Teach the adolescent to brush the teeth more frequently if they have braces or other dental devices. Gingivitis is inflammation of the gums and breakdown of gingival epithelium due to diet and hormonal changes. The use of dental devices/braces makes cleaning more difficult and contributes to gingivitis. Tooth avulsion (knocked-out teeth) may occur during sports and other activities such as falls. The avulsed tooth should be reimplanted as soon as possible. The nurse may see the adolescent first, so it is important that nurses know the proper procedure, which is to reinsert the tooth into its socket, if possible, or to store it in cool milk or normal saline for transport to the dentist.

Promoting Personal Care

Promotion of personal care during adolescence is an important topic to cover with the adolescent and their parents. Topics to discuss include general hygiene tips, caring for body piercings and tattoos, preventing sun-tanning, and promoting a healthy sexual identity.

General Hygiene Tips

Adolescents find that frequent baths and deodorant use are important due to apocrine sweat gland secretory activity. Also, to decrease oily skin, teach the adolescent to wash their face two to three times per day with plain unscented soap. Vigorous scrubbing should be discouraged because it could irritate the skin and lead to follicular rupture. The hair should be shampooed daily or every other day to remove excess oil from the hair and scalp. Many over-the-counter medications are available for beginning acne or acne with a few lesions. These preparations may cause drying or redness. Discourage adolescents from squeezing acne lesions to prevent further irritation and permanent scarring. If the adolescent has severe acne, encourage them to ask a parent to make an appointment with a dermatologist.

Caring for Body Piercings and Tattoos

It is not uncommon for an adolescent to experiment with body piercing (Fig. 7.9). Generally, body piercing is safe, but nurses should caution adolescents about obtaining these procedures under nonsterile conditions and should educate them about potential complications. Qualified personnel using sterile needles should perform the procedure. Teach the adolescent to cleanse the pierced area twice a day and more often at some sites.

Infections from body piercing usually result from unclean tools of the trade. Some infections that may occur as a result of unclean tools include hepatitis, tetanus, tuberculosis, and human immunodeficiency virus (HIV). Also, keloid formation and allergies to metal may occur. The navel is an area prone to infection because it is a moist area that endures friction from clothing. Naval piercings, particularly after a navel infection occurs, may take up to a year to heal (Desai, 2023). Pierced ear cartilage also heals slowly and is prone to infection (Desai, 2023). Potential concerns with tongue piercing include tooth damage from biting on the jewelry or partial paralysis if the jewelry pierces a nerve.

Tattoos are continuing to grow in popularity among adolescents and are more commonplace among both adolescents and adults than in the past (Desai, 2021). Tattoos serve to define one's identity and are a form of self-expression (see Fig. 7.9). Because of the invasiveness of the tattooing procedure, it should be considered a health risk situation. Like piercings, tattoos begin as open wounds predisposing to infection.

Nurses should educate adolescents about the risk of tattooing under unsafe conditions, including bloodborne infections, such as hepatitis B and C, skin infections, scarring, bleeding, and allergic reactions to dyes used in the tattoo process (Desai, 2021). They need to encourage the adolescent to go to a licensed facility with licensed tattoo artists and to double check that all equipment used is disposable and sterilized (Desai, 2021). Teach adolescents to cleanse tattoos with an antibacterial soap and water several times a day and to keep the area moist with an ointment to prevent scab formation while it is healing. Refer to Box 7.4 for additional information about tattoos.

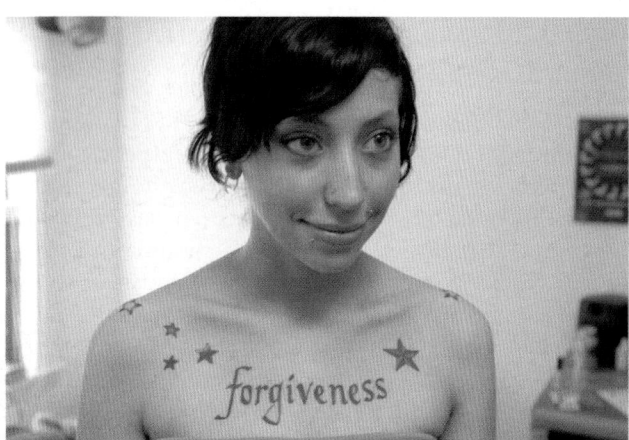

FIGURE 7.9 Having multiple piercings and tattoos can lead to certain health risks.

Preventing Sun-Tanning

Sun-tanning is popular among some adolescents and is influenced by the American media, which promotes a link between tan skin and beauty in light-skinned individuals. There is no such thing as a good tan. Most exposure to ultraviolet rays occurs during childhood and adolescence, thereby putting people at risk for the development of skin cancer. However, it can be difficult to convince adolescents that tanning is harmful to their skin and puts them at risk for skin cancer later in life (see Healthy People 2030).

HEALTHY PEOPLE 2030

Objective	Nursing Significance
Reduce the proportion of students in grades 9 through 12 who report sunburn.	• Remind adolescents to use sunscreen during outdoor organized-sports practice. • Encourage adolescents to use sunscreen-containing makeup. • Educate adolescents and families about the risks associated with sun exposure. • Educate adolescents and their families to avoid the sun between 10 a.m. and 4 p.m., wear sun-protective clothing when exposed to sunlight, use sunscreen with a sun protection factor (SPF) of 15 or higher, and avoid artificial sources of UV light.

Healthy People Objectives retrieved from http://www.healthypeople.gov

BOX 7.4 What Adolescents Need to Know About Tattooing

- Infections occur as a result of nonsterile equipment used in the procedure.
- New tattoos are open wounds predisposed to infection; sites require proper care. Keep bandaged for the first 24 hours, then wash with soap and warm water several times per day, and apply antibiotic ointment or fragrance-free lotion three times a day for the first week.
- Do not let the tattoo dry out. Do not expose it to direct sunlight until fully healed, and then keep it protected from the sun with sunscreen.
- Avoid pools, hot tubs, or long baths/showers until healed.
- For most people, a tattoo is permanent; new procedures for removal can be painful and expensive.

Educate adolescents about the benefits and effects of different sun protection products. Explain that sun damage and skin cancers can be prevented if sunscreens are used as directed on a regular basis. Encourage sunscreen or sunblock use for water sports, beach activities, and participation in outdoor sports. Also, make adolescents aware of allergies to some sunscreen products. See Teaching Guidelines 7.1 for additional information.

Promoting a Healthy Sexual Identity

Encourage parents and adolescents to have discussions about sexuality. In addition, nurses should ensure that adolescents have the knowledge, skills, and opportunities that enable them to make responsible decisions regarding sexual behaviors. Education for the adolescent should include a discussion about media influences and the use of sexuality to promote products. This discussion should make the adolescent aware of the motives of the media and the need to be an individual and not be influenced by television, magazines, and other forms of advertisement. Encourage parents to be aware of whom their adolescents are dating and where they go on their dates. Refer to Teaching Guidelines 7.2 for information on counseling related to adolescent sexuality.

Promoting Appropriate Discipline

Adolescents naturally misbehave or do not follow the rules of the house, and parents must determine how to respond. Adolescents need to know the rules and expectations. After rules are established, parents must explain to the adolescent the consequences of breaking the rules.

Offer guidance to parents related to disciplining adolescents. The parent and the adolescent should collaborate on what the consequences will be if the rules are broken. Parents must acknowledge and offer reinforcement and support when the adolescent follows the rules. Consistency and predictability are the cornerstones of discipline, and praise is the most powerful reinforcer of learning.

TEACHING GUIDELINES 7.2 Adolescent Sexuality

- It should be your choice to engage in sexual relations. Do not be influenced by peers. When you say "no," be firm and clear about your position. If someone says "no" to you, you must respect their choice.
- Pregnancy, sexually transmitted infections (STIs), and human immunodeficiency virus (HIV) infection can occur with any sexual encounter without the use of barrier methods of contraception. Use appropriate contraception if you are sexually active. Discuss abstinence as a contraceptive method.
- Sexual activity in a mature relationship should be pleasurable to both parties. If your sexual partner is not interested in your pleasure, you need to reconsider the relationship.

Promoting Proper Media Use

Television, the internet, social media, and other forms of media, are a large force in the lives of adolescents today. Adolescents are immersed daily in a variety of different media. Of adolescents, 95% report owning a smartphone, and 35% report using the top five social media platforms (i.e., YouTube, TikTok, Instagram, Snapchat, and Facebook) almost constantly (Pew Research Center, 2022). With greater technology and media access come benefits such as enhancing communication skills, increasing social connections, and improving technical skills, but risks also exist, such as cyberbullying, exposure to inappropriate content, privacy issues, internet addiction, and sleep deprivation. Health care providers need to assess media use and advise parents on ways to decrease media risks. Parents should be advised to evaluate websites their adolescent wants to participate in and verify they are age-appropriate. Parents should talk to their adolescent children daily about online use and activity and help them to balance online and offline activity. They need to discuss the dangers of sharing too much information and posting images or photographs. Parents should emphasize that once something is online, it is available for others to see and share and may be difficult to remove. Parents need to be educated on the technology their children are using and encourage the development of a family media use plan that involves establishing consistent, reasonable rules about use of cell phones, texting, the internet and social media. Such rules could include no media during meals and regular checking of privacy settings and online profiles for inappropriate content (American Academy of Pediatrics, Council on Communications and Media, 2016, reaffirmed 2022).

ADDRESSING COMMON DEVELOPMENTAL CONCERNS

Adolescence is a time of rapid growth and development with maturation of sexuality. The adolescent period begins with a child and ends with the expectation of adulthood. Many developmental concerns are present during this period, including violence, suicide, homicide, and substance misuse. The following is an overview of some of these concerns.

Violence

The CDC's Injury Center defines youth violence as occurring when young people between the ages of 10 and 24 years intentionally use physical force or power to threaten or harm others (CDC, 2022g). More than 1,000 youth are

BOX 7.5 Factors Contributing to Adolescent Violence

- Crowded conditions/housing
- Low socioeconomic status
- Limited parental supervision/involvement
- Single-parent families/both parents in workforce
- History of violent victimization
- Poor family functioning
- Access to guns or cars
- Drug or alcohol use
- Low self-esteem
- Racism
- Peer or gang pressure
- Aggression

treated in an emergency department as a result of injuries from physical violence every day (CDC, 2022g). The issue of youth violence is a growing concern in America's communities. The health and well-being of adolescents and society are threatened by this violence. See Box 7.5 for factors contributing to adolescent violence. Health care providers need to provide education on the effects and ways to prevent youth violence along with supporting programs developed to curb youth violence.

Suicide

Suicide is the third leading cause of death in people 10 to 19 years old (Kennebeck & Bonin, 2021). Certain factors can put adolescents at risk for suicide, but having these risk factors does not mean suicide will occur. Refer to Box 7.6 for risk factors for suicide in adolescents (see Healthy People 2030). Most people are not comfortable discussing the topic of suicide and therefore do not communicate openly about it. It is important that health care providers address this significant health problem and work to prevent suicide. The National Center for Injury Prevention and Control (NCIPC) is working to create awareness of suicide as a serious public health problem and is developing strategies to reduce injuries and deaths due to suicide.

BOX 7.6 Risk Factors for Suicide in Adolescents

- Depression or other mental illness
- Mental health changes
- Family history of suicide or mood disorders
- History of previous suicide attempt
- Poor school performance
- Family disorganization
- Substance misuse
- Marginalization for identifying as LGBTQ+
- Access to means to attempt suicide
- Social isolation
- History of physical or sexual abuse
- Exposure to violence or bullying
- Incarceration

Homicide

Homicide is the second leading cause of death in children between 10 and 24 years old, with the majority of victims being male and killed by firearms (CDC, 2022g; Naik-Mathuria & Gill, 2022). It is the leading cause of death for non-Hispanic Black or African American individuals 10 to 24 years old (CDC, 2022g). Refer to Box 7.5 for factors that contribute to violence among adolescents. In a nationwide survey conducted in 2019, 13% of participants reported carrying a weapon (e.g., gun, club, knife) on one or more days within the past 30 days (Sege, 2022; see Healthy People 2030).

HEALTHY PEOPLE 2030

Objective	Nursing Significance
Reduce physical fighting among adolescents. Reduce gun carrying among adolescents. Reduce suicide attempts by adolescents. Reduce suicidal thoughts in lesbian, gay, or bisexual high school students. Reduce suicidal thoughts in transgender students.	• Screen adolescents at all encounters for indications of violent behaviors. • Provide education related to decreasing school violence at middle and high schools. • Encourage alternative, appropriate methods for dispelling anger. • Screen adolescents at all encounters for indications of depression. • Assist schools to implement school-based initiatives that foster supportive, inclusive, antidiscriminatory environments.

Healthy People Objectives retrieved from http://www.healthypeople.gov

Dating Violence

Violent behavior that takes place in a context of dating is not a rare event and can have serious short-term and lifelong effects. In a recent survey, approximately 1 in 12 high school students reported physical violence, and one in 12 reported sexual violence from a dating partner in the past 12 months (CDC, 2022h). Dating violence in the adolescent years is a risk factor for continued violence exposure in adulthood. Risk factors for dating violence include inadequate parental supervision, substance misuse, history of physical or sexual abuse in childhood, early-onset puberty, early onset of sexual activity, identifying as LGBTQ+, low socioeconomic status, and risky sexual practices (Miller & Wiemann, 2020). Nurses need to assess for and provide interventions to those adolescents experiencing dating violence or those at risk for being a victim or perpetrator. Education on development of healthy relationships is important. See Healthy People 2030.

HEALTHY PEOPLE 2030

Objective	Nursing Significance
Reduce sexual or physical adolescent dating violence.	• Screen adolescents at all encounters for indications of dating violence. • Teach safe and healthy relationship skills. • Discuss with the adolescent good relationship role models in their life.

Healthy People Objectives retrieved from http://www.healthypeople.gov

Gangs

Much of youth violence is a result of the behavior of adolescent gangs. The risk factors for gang involvement are similar to those for aggressive or delinquent behavior. See Box 7.7 for risk factors for adolescent gang involvement. Gang membership occurs in cities and in suburban areas but may differ in composition. All socioeconomic groups are represented in gang membership. Gang membership may aid in the formation of identity by providing status and a sense of belonging. However, adolescents who are gang members are more likely to commit serious and violent crimes. Identifying those at risk and providing early intervention is important. Research has shown that increasing parental monitoring, increasing involvement in extracurricular activities, improving coping skills to deal with conflict, and educating about the negative consequences of gang membership may be beneficial in preventing gang membership (American Academy of Child and Adolescent Psychiatry, 2017).

Nursing Interventions to Decrease Youth Violence

Nurses working with adolescents should include violence prevention in anticipatory guidance. Violence is a learned behavior. It is often reinforced by the media, television, music, and personal example. Explain to parents, teachers, and peers the importance of being good role models. Parents should monitor video games, music, television, and other media to decrease exposure to violence. Parents need to know who their adolescent's friends are and monitor for negative behaviors and actions. Pediatric nurses play a key role in identifying at-risk youth and developing, planning, implementing, and evaluating interventions to prevent youth violence.

BOX 7.7 Risk Factors for Gang Involvement

- Delinquency involvement, especially at a young age
- History of or victim of physical violence or aggression
- Alcohol and drug use; drug dealing
- Association with violent or aggressive peers
- Low socioeconomic status
- Family with criminal history, drug or alcohol problems, violence in the home
- Poor parental supervision/involvement
- Poor academic performance
- Living in a community with a high rate of crime among adolescents and access to firearms and drugs

Substance Use

Agents commonly misused by children and adolescents include alcohol; nicotine; cannabis; prescribed medications such as Ritalin and OxyContin; hallucinogens; sedatives; analgesics; anxiolytics; steroids; inhalants (inhaling fumes of common household products); stimulants; opiates; and various club drugs such as ecstasy, gamma-hydroxybutyrate (GHB), and lysergic acid diethylamide (LSD). The substance misused is related to its availability and cost. Overall, the use of illicit drugs showed a decline in 2021 (Johnston et al., 2022). The occurrence of substance use varies by age, sex, race, ethnicity, and sociodemographic factors. Two common substances that are more accessible and have the highest incidence of use are alcohol and nicotine. Drug use often progresses from beer or wine to nicotine or hard liquor and then to cannabis, followed by illicit drugs.

Some of the long-term effects and consequences of drug and alcohol use include the possibility of overdose and death, unintentional injuries, irrational behaviors, inability to think clearly, unsafe driving and legal consequences, problems with relationships with family and friends, sexual activity and STIs, and health problems such as liver problems (hepatitis) and cardiac problems (sudden death with cocaine). Refer to Table 7.3 for commonly misused drugs and behaviors exhibited.

Tobacco/Nicotine

Smoking remains the leading preventable cause of death in the United States (CDC, 2023). Long-term consequences of adolescent smoking are reinforced by the fact that most young people who smoke regularly continue to smoke throughout adulthood. Each day in the United States, approximately 21,600 children younger than 18 years try their first cigarette, with 200 becoming regular smokers; nine out of 10 adult people who smoke started smoking before age 18 (CDC, 2022i). One in 13 Americans will die early from the effects of smoking (CDC, 2022i). The overall rate of use of any tobacco product has been declining, with the latest estimates at 4% of middle schoolers and 13.4% of high schoolers reporting use of any form of tobacco in the past 30 days (CDC, 2022i). There are many forms of tobacco use, such as e-cigarettes, flavored cigars, smokeless tobacco, hookahs, pipes, nicotine pouches, heated tobacco products,

TABLE 7.3 • Drugs Commonly Misused

Drug	Manifestations	Considerations
Cannabis	Red eyes; dry mouth; euphoria; relaxation; decreased motivation; difficulty with coordination, thinking, and problem solving; loss of inhibition; appetite stimulation	Considered a gateway drug
Synthetic cannabis	Laboratory-synthesized liquid chemicals mimic the effect of tetrahydrocannabinol (THC), the psychoactive ingredient in the naturally grown cannabis plant; relaxed feeling, mild changes in perception, extreme paranoia, anxiety, hallucinations	Unpredictable effect; not clear what chemicals are used and how they can harm the body; symptoms reported include increased heart rate, vomiting, agitation, confusion, hallucinations; has been associated with heart attacks
Cocaine and crack	Powerful stimulant; weight loss, euphoria, elation, agitation, increased motor activity, pressured speech, dilated pupils, tachycardia, hypertension, anorexia, insomnia	Psychotic behavior with large doses; if combined with other drugs can be fatal
Heroin	Elation, euphoria, detachment, drowsiness, constricted pupils, slurred speech, impaired judgment	Tolerance, dependence, and highly addictive; self-neglect with malnutrition and dehydration; criminal behaviors to get drugs; infections at injection sites; at risk for acquiring human immunodeficiency virus (HIV)/acquired immunodeficiency syndrome (AIDS) and hepatitis; highly addictive; can lead to coma or death
Prescription opiate drugs: • Oxycodone • Hydrocodone • Diphenoxylate • Morphine • Codeine • Fentanyl • Propoxyphene • Hydromorphone • Meperidine • Methadone	Feelings of relaxation and euphoria	Can lead to addiction and drug-seeking behaviors; high doses can lead to breathing complications and death
Methamphetamine	Euphoria, increased energy and alertness, agitation, weight loss, insomnia, tachycardia, hypertension	Increased risk of human immunodeficiency virus (HIV)/acquired immunodeficiency syndrome (AIDS) or hepatitis; risk for dysrhythmia and hyperthermia; repeated use can cause violent behavior and psychosis; possible paradoxical effect of depression in children
MDMA (3,4-methylenedioxymethamphetamine) and other club drugs (lysergic acid diethylamide [LSD], ketamine, phencyclidine [PCP])	Hallucinations, illusions, euphoria, hyperalertness, depersonalization, heightened sensual awareness, dilated pupils, hypertension, increased salivation, distorted perceptions. agitation, violence, antisocial behaviors, loss of sense of time, forceful clenching of the teeth	Panic flashbacks long after use of drugs; psychotic behaviors; can lead to hyperthermia as it interferes with the body's ability to regulate temperature; memory loss with long-term use; high blood levels lead to increased risk of seizures and dysrhythmia
Inhalants	Similar effects as alcohol but high only lasts a few minutes, slurred speech, lack of coordination, euphoria, dizziness	Long-term use can break down myelin and damage brain cells.
Bath salts	Similar effect as stimulants such as methamphetamines and MDMA; hallucinatory effects	Much is still unknown about how these substances affect the brain; linked to a high number of emergency room and Poison Control Center visits
Prescription stimulants such as dextroamphetamine and methylphenidate	Increased alertness, attention, and energy; feelings of exhilaration; increased heart rate and blood pressure	High doses increase risk for dysrhythmia, hyperthermia, heart failure, and seizures. If mixed with antidepressants or over-the-counter cold medicines can lead to dangerously high blood pressure and dysrhythmia.

TABLE 7.3 • Drugs Commonly Misused

Drug	Manifestations	Considerations
Prescription central nervous system depressants: • Mephobarbital; sodium pentobarbital • Diazepam • Alprazolam • Lorazepam • Estazolam • Zolpidem • Zaleplon Eszopiclone	Euphoria followed by depression or hostility, decreased anxiety, drowsiness, impaired judgment, decreased inhibitions, slurred speech, incoordination	Often used with stimulants; may have a paradoxical effect of hyperactivity in children
Dextromethorphan	Taken in very large amounts; effects similar to phencyclidine (PCP) and ketamine; feelings of being detached from oneself and the environment	Found in over-the-counter cold medicines; can lead to impaired motor function, numbness, nausea, vomiting, increased heart rate and blood pressure; risk of hypoxic brain damage

Data from Breuner, C. C. (2020). Substance abuse. In R. M. Kleigman, J. W. St. Geme, III, N. J. Blum, S. S. Shah, R. C. Tasker, K. M. Wilson, & R. E. Behrman (Eds.), *Nelson textbook of pediatrics* (21st ed., pp. 5678–5765). Elsevier; Blake, K., & Van Eyk, N. (2023b). Section 12: Adolescent medicine. Substance abuse. In K. J. Marcdante, R. M. Kleigman, & A. M. Schuh (Eds.), *Nelson essentials of pediatrics* (9th ed., pp. 297–300). Elsevier.

and bidis. Electronic nicotine delivery systems (ENDSs), such as vaporizers, vapes, and e-cigarettes, may look like conventional cigarettes or resemble things such as pens and USB flash drives. There was an upward trend in the use of ENDSs in middle and high school students from 2013 to 2019, but it has since declined (Rigotti & Reddy, 2022). Adolescents need to be aware that e-cigarettes are not a safe alternative to smoking. Nicotine, which is highly addictive, and other harmful chemicals are absorbed through the lungs and into the body with the use of e-cigarettes. Nicotine is harmful to the developing brain and can have lasting effects.

TAKE NOTE!

In 2016, the U.S. Food and Drug Administration extended their regulation on all tobacco and nicotine products and has a comprehensive plan to help better protect our youth and decrease the number of adolescents using Electronic Nicotine Delivery Systems (ENDSs). Most states have enacted minimum legal age for sales of ENDSs ranging from 18 to 21 years old.

Adolescents who smoke are more likely than those who don't to use alcohol and illegal drugs (American Cancer Society, 2020). Smoking is associated with other risky behaviors, including fighting, carrying weapons, mental health problems such as depression, attempting suicide, and engaging in unprotected sex (American Cancer Society, 2020). Studies have found that the use of e-cigarettes (or vaping) in youth is strongly linked to the use of regular cigarettes and other tobacco products in adulthood (American Cancer Society, 2022). The short-term health effects of smoking include damage to the respiratory system, addiction to nicotine, and the associated risk of other drug use. Smoking negatively impacts physical fitness and lung growth and increases the potential for addiction in adolescents. Smokeless tobacco may also cause many problems. It can lead to bleeding gums and sores in the mouth that never heal. Smokeless tobacco use leads to discoloration of the teeth and may eventually lead to cancer.

HEALTHY PEOPLE 2030

Objective	Nursing Significance
Reduce current use of tobacco products among adolescents. Reduce current use of e-cigarettes among adolescents. Reduce current use of cigarettes among adolescents. Reduce current use of cigars among adolescents. Reduce current use of flavored tobacco products among adolescent tobacco users. Reduce current use of cigarettes among adolescents. Reduce current use of smokeless tobacco products among adolescents.	• Provide education in the office, hospital, or school related to adverse effects of tobacco/nicotine. • Emphasize the dangers of tobacco/nicotine. • Praise adolescents for abstaining from the use of tobacco/nicotine products and rising above peer pressure.

Healthy People Objectives retrieved from http://www.healthypeople.gov

Alcohol

Although alcohol remains the most widely used and misused drug among youths in the United States, its use among adolescents has continued a downward trend (Johnston, 2022). A national survey on drug use found that 26% of eighth graders and 61.5% of 12th graders reported ever trying alcohol, while 7% of eighth graders, 13% of 10th graders, and 26% of 12th graders reported drinking alcohol in the past 30 days (Johnston, 2022). The incidence of alcohol use increases throughout adolescence, and adolescents who begin drinking before the age of 15 are 5.6 times more likely to develop alcohol dependence later in life (NIH/National Institute on Alcohol Abuse and Alcoholism, 2022). Alcohol use in adolescence can lead to prevailing alcohol use in adulthood; contributes to physical health problems, school problems, and legal problems; leads to increased injuries; impairs judgment; increases the risk of sexual and physical assault; and interferes with brain development (NIH/National Institute on Alcohol Abuse and Alcoholism, 2022). It may also precede other drug misuse.

HEALTHY PEOPLE 2030

Objective	Nursing Significance
Reduce the proportion of adolescents reporting use of alcohol during the past 30 days. Reduce the proportion of adolescents reporting use of any illicit drugs during the past 30 days. Reduce the proportion of adolescents reporting use of cannabis in the past 30 days. Reduce the proportion of persons under 21 engaging in binge drinking of alcoholic beverages. Reduce the proportion of motor vehicle crash deaths involving an alcohol-impaired driver with a blood alcohol concentration (BAC) of 0.08 g/dL or higher. Increase the proportion of adolescents who perceive great risk associated with substance misuse.	• Provide education in the office, hospital, or school related to adverse effects of alcohol and illicit substance use. • Emphasize the dangers of substance use and driving, and educate the adolescent to never get in a car with someone who is under the influence of alcohol or drugs. • Praise adolescents for abstaining from the above substances and rising above peer pressure.

Healthy People Objectives retrieved from http://www.healthypeople.gov

TAKE NOTE!

Research shows adolescents who have parents who are actively involved in their lives are less likely to drink alcohol (NIH/National Institute on Alcohol Abuse and Alcoholism, 2022).

Illicit Drugs

Adolescents may also experiment with or misuse illicit drugs. Substance misuse remains a widespread problem among American adolescents, even though prevalence is trending downward. Cannabis remains the most widely used illicit drug (Johnston et al., 2022). A national survey on drug use showed the annual prevalence rate for illicit drugs remaining stable at the lowest levels in over 20 years, with a significant decline seen in 2021 (Johnston et al., 2022). During this time, the COVID-19 pandemic led to changes in adolescent lives and decreased social and school activities (Johnston et al., 2022). The trends in adolescent drug use need continued monitoring to assess if the decline will persist over time.

Factors that primarily affect drug use include the psychoactive potential and benefits reported, how risky the drug is to use, how acceptable it is to peer groups, and the accessibility and availability of the drug. The riskier or less accepted a drug is by peers, the less likely the adolescent will use it.

Nursing Interventions to Decrease Substance Misuse Among Adolescents

Adolescents' brains are still developing, leaving them particularly vulnerable to the damaging effects of drugs. Substance misuse in adolescence is related to poorer health outcomes; therefore, it is important that nurses be aware of interventions to decrease these behaviors. Adolescent drug misuse is related to social factors, including times of life transitions and stress, such as changing schools, moving, or divorce, as well as peer factors such as peer pressure. Therefore, nurses need to target assessments and programs at these critical times. Based on reviews of programs and interventions, it has been found that certain methods work. Programs that reach children and adolescents through a variety of sources such as school, family, community, and media campaigns are more successful. Programs that are culturally competent and address all forms of drug use (alcohol, tobacco, and illicit drugs) tend to work well. Programs that focus on increasing awareness of the risks and health consequences of substance use are important. Certain factors have been found to help adolescents remain drug-free. These include strong connections to parents, family, school, and religion; presence of parents in the home at key times of the day; and limited access to substances such as alcohol, tobacco, and cannabis (NIH/National Institute on Alcohol Abuse and Alcoholism, 2022). Programs that focus on decreasing risk factors and increasing protective factors such as enhancing self-esteem, social and parental support, and stress-specific coping skills are beneficial. Topics that should be discussed include:

- Short- and long-term effects of alcohol, tobacco, and drugs on health
- Risk factors and implications for unintentional injuries and sexual activity

- Short- and long-term effects of alcohol, tobacco, and drugs on relationships and school performance and progression
- The how and why of chemical dependency
- Impact of substance abuse on society
- Importance of maintaining a healthy lifestyle
- Importance of resisting peer pressure to use drugs and alcohol
- Importance of having confidence in one's own judgment

Refer back to 15-year-old Cho. List some common developmental concerns of the adolescent. What anticipatory guidance related to these concerns would you provide?

KEY CONCEPTS

- Adolescence is a period of rapid and variable growth in the areas of physical, psychosocial, cognitive, and moral development.
- The adolescent is developing their own identity, becoming an abstract thinker, and developing their own set of morals and values. Inability to successfully develop an individual identity leads to poor preparation for the challenges of adulthood.
- Relationships with parents fluctuate widely during adolescence. The adolescent eventually gains independence from their parents.
- Peers become most important—guiding mainly the early and middle adolescent in their decisions—while the late adolescent can usually formulate their own decisions.
- Adolescence is a critical time in the development of sexuality. Sexuality includes the thoughts, feelings, and behaviors surrounding the adolescent's sexual identity.
- The egocentric and invincible thought processes of the adolescent can lead to injuries. Health care providers must emphasize safety regarding cars, bikes, water, firearms, and fire.
- Unintentional injury is the leading cause of death in adolescents (CDC, 2021a). Motor vehicle crashes are the leading cause of unintentional injury death followed by poisoning, primarily due to drug overdose from opioids, and drowning (CDC, 2021a).
- Nutritional habits of the adolescent lead to deficiency in vitamins and minerals needed for the rapid growth during this period.
- Excess weight in adolescents is a growing health concern. Health care providers are facing increased numbers of adolescents with hypertension, type 2 diabetes, and hyperlipidemia.
- Substance misuse and experimentation is common during adolescence; it is associated with other risk-taking behaviors such as injuries and sexual activity.
- Health care providers must work collaboratively with the adolescent in the development of interventions to promote health.

REFERENCES AND RECOMMENDED READINGS

American Academy of Child and Adolescent Psychiatry. (2017). *Gangs and children.* https://www.aacap.org/AACAP/Families_and_Youth/Facts_for_Families/FFF-Guide/Children-and-Gangs-098.aspx

American Academy of Pediatrics. (2010, reaffirmed 2016). The teen driver. *Pediatrics, 118*(6), 2570–2581. http://pediatrics.aappublications.org/content/118/6/2570.full

American Academy of Pediatrics, Council on Communications and Media. (2016, reaffirmed 2022). Policy statement: Media use in school-aged children and adolescents. *Pediatrics, 138*(5), Article e20162592. https://doi.org/10.1542/peds.2016-2592

American Academy of Pediatrics, Council on Environmental Health and Section on Dermatology. (2011, reaffirmed 2017). Policy statement—Ultraviolet radiation: A hazard to children and adolescents. *Pediatrics, 127*(3), e791–e817. https://doi.org/10.1542/peds.2010-3502

American Academy of Pediatrics, HealthyChildren. (2022). *ATVs are not safe for children: AAP policy explained.* https://www.healthychildren.org/English/safety-prevention/at-play/Pages/ATV-Safety-Rules.aspx

American Cancer Society. (2020). *Health risks of smoking tobacco.* https://www.cancer.org/content/dam/CRC/PDF/Public/8345.00.pdf

American Cancer Society. (2022). *What do we know about e-cigarettes?* https://www.cancer.org/content/dam/CRC/PDF/Public/9309.00.pdf

American Psychological Association. (2019). *Children, youth, families and socioeconomic status.* Retrieved January 21, 2019, from https://www.apa.org/pi/ses/resources/publications/children-families.aspx

American Public Health Association. (2018). *The dropout crisis: A public health problem and the role of school-based health care.* https://www.apha.org/-/media/Files/PDF/SBHC/Dropout_Crisis.ashx

American Public Health Association. (2021). *Supporting physical education in schools for all youth.* https://apha.org/Policies-and-Advocacy/Public-Health-Policy-Statements/Policy-Database/2022/01/07/Supporting-Physical-Education-in-Schools-for-All-Youth

Blake, K., & Van Eyk, N. (2023a). Adolescent medicine: Overview and assessment of adolescents. In K. J. Marcdante, R. M. Kleigman, & A. M. Schuh (Eds.), *Nelson essentials of pediatrics* (9th ed., pp. 281–287). Elsevier.

Blake, K., & Van Eyk, N. (2023b). Adolescent medicine: Substance abuse. In K. J. Marcdante, R. M. Kleigman, & A. M. Schuh (Eds.), *Nelson essentials of pediatrics* (9th ed., pp. 297–300). Elsevier.

Breuner, C. C. (2020). Substance abuse. In R. M. Kleigman, J. W. St. Geme, III, N. J. Blum, S. S. Shah, R. C. Tasker, K. M. Wilson, & R. E. Behrman (Eds.), *Nelson textbook of pediatrics* (21st ed., pp. 5678–5765). Elsevier.

Centers for Disease Control and Prevention. (2020). *Sleep in middle and high school students.* https://www.cdc.gov/healthyschools/features/students-sleep.htm

Centers for Disease Control and Prevention. (2021a). *Injuries among children and teens.* https://www.cdc.gov/injury/features/child-injury/index.html#:~:text=That%20is%20about%2020%20deaths,Child%20injury%20is%20often%20preventable

Centers for Disease Control and Prevention. (2021b). *Teen drivers: Get the facts.* https://cdctransportation.org/www.cdc.gov/transportationsafety/teen_drivers/teendrivers_factsheet.html

Centers for Disease Control and Prevention. (2021c). *Keep teen drivers safe.* https://www.cdc.gov/injury/features/teen-drivers/index.html

Centers for Disease Control and Prevention. (2022a). *CDC healthy schools: Physical activity facts.* https://www.cdc.gov/healthyschools/physicalactivity/facts.htm

Centers for Disease Control and Prevention. (2022b). *CDC healthy schools: Health & academics.* https://www.cdc.gov/healthyschools/health_and_academics/index.htm

Centers for Disease Control and Prevention. (2022c). *Drowning facts.* Replace with this link please https://www.cdc.gov/drowning/facts/index.html

Centers for Disease Control and Prevention. (2022d). *Obesity.* https://www.cdc.gov/healthyschools/obesity/facts.htm

Centers for Disease Control and Prevention. (2022e). *Consequences of obesity.* https://www.cdc.gov/obesity/basics/consequences.html

Centers for Disease Control and Prevention. (2022f). *Overweight and obesity: Childhood obesity facts.* https://www.cdc.gov/obesity/data/childhood.html#:~:text=Prevalence%20of%20Childhood%20Obesity%20in%20the%20United%20States&text=The%20prevalence%20of%20obesity%20was,to%2019%2Dyear%2Dolds

Centers for Disease Control and Prevention. (2022g). *Preventing youth violence.* https://www.cdc.gov/violenceprevention/youthviolence/fastfact.html?CDC_AA_refVal=https%3A%2F%2Fwww.cdc.gov%2Fviolenceprevention%2Fyouthviolence%2Fdefinitions.html

Centers for Disease Control and Prevention. (2022h). *Preventing teen dating violence.* https://www.cdc.gov/violenceprevention/pdf/ipv/TDV-factsheet_2022.pdf

Centers for Disease Control and Prevention. (2022i). *Smoking & tobacco use: Youth and tobacco use.* https://www.cdc.gov/tobacco/data_statistics/fact_sheets/youth_data/tobacco_use/index.htm

Centers for Disease Control and Prevention. (2023). *Smoking and tobacco use: Fast facts and fact sheets.* https://www.cdc.gov/tobacco/data_statistics/fact_sheets/fast_facts/index.htm

Centers for Disease Control and Prevention, & National Center for Health Statistics. (2022). *All injuries.* https://www.cdc.gov/nchs/fastats/injury.htm

Desai, N. (2021). Tattooing in adolescents and young adults. *UpToDate.* Retrieved November 2, 2022, from https://www.uptodate.com/contents/tattooing-in-adolescents-and-young-adults

Desai, N. (2023). *Body piercing in adolescents and young adults. UpToDate.* Retrieved October 15, 2023, from https://www.uptodate.com/contents/body-piercing-in-adolescents-and-young-adults

Eickmeyer, K., Hemez, P., Manning, W. D., Brown, S. L., & Guzzo, K. B. (2020). *Trends in relationship formation and stability in the United States dating, cohabitation, marriage, and divorce.* http://mastresearchcenter.org/wp-content/uploads/2020/05/MAST-PA1-Trends-Brief_May-2020_final.pdf

Emerson, A., Pickett, M., Moore, S., & Kelly, P. J. (2023). A scoping review of digital health interventions to promote healthy romantic relationships in adolescents. *Prevention Science, 24*(4), 625–639. https://doi.org/10.1007/s11121-022-01421-0

Erikson, E. (1963). *Childhood and society* (2nd ed.). Norton.

Forcier, M., & Olson-Kennedy, J. (2020). Lesbian, gay, bisexual, and other sexual minoritized youth: Epidemiology and health concerns. *UpToDate.* Retrieved October 23, 2022, from https://www.uptodate.com/contents/lesbian-gay-bisexual-and-other-sexual-minoritized-youth-epidemiology-and-health-concerns

Ford, G. S. (2007). Hospitalized kids: Spiritual care at their level. *Journal of Christian Nursing, 24*(3), 135–140. https://doi.org/10.1097/01.cnj.0000279357.48047.a3

Gill, A. C. (2022). Bicycle injuries in children: Prevention. *UpToDate.* Retrieved October 17, 2022, from https://www.uptodate.com/contents/bicycle-injuries-in-children-prevention

Goldbach, J. T., Rhoades, H., Mamey, M. R., Senese, J., Karys, P., & Marsiglia. F. F. (2021). Reducing behavioral health symptoms by addressing minority stressors in LGBTQ adolescents: A randomized controlled trial of proud & empowered. *BMC Public Health, 21*, 2315. https://doi.org/10.1186/s12889-021-12357-5

Goldstick, J. E., Cunningham, R. M., & Carter, P. M. (2022). Current causes of death in children and adolescents in the United States [Editorial]. *New England Journal of Medicine, 386*(20), 1955–1956. https://doi.org/10.1056/NEJMc2201761

Holland-Hall, C. (2020). Adolescent physical and social development. In R. M. Kleigman, J. W. St. Geme, III, N. J. Blum, S. S. Shah, R. C. Tasker, K. M. Wilson, & R. E. Behrman (Eds.), *Nelson textbook of pediatrics* (21st ed., pp. 5550–5576). Elsevier.

Johnston, L. D., Miech, R. A., O'Malley, P. M., Bachman, J. G., Schulenberg, J. E., & Patrick, M. E. (2022). *Monitoring the future national survey results on drug use 1975–2021: Overview, key findings on adolescent drug use.* Institute for Social Research, University of Michigan. https://monitoringthefuture.org/wp-content/uploads/2022/08/mtf-overview2021.pdf

Kansky, J., & Allen, J. P. (2018). Long-term risks and possible benefits associated with late adolescent romantic relationship quality. *Journal of Youth and Adolescents, 47*(7), 1531–1544. https://doi.org/10.1007%2Fs10964-018-0813-x

Kennebeck, S., & Bonin, L. (2021). Suicidal behavior in children and adolescents: Epidemiology and risk factors. *UpToDate.* Retrieved November 3, 2022, from https://www.uptodate.com/contents/suicidal-behavior-in-children-and-adolescents-epidemiology-and-risk-factors

Kohlberg, L. (1984). *Essays on moral development.* Harper & Row.

Mattoo, T. K. (2021). Epidemiology, risk factors, and etiology of hypertension in children and adolescents. *UpToDate.* Retrieved October 23, 2022, from https://www.uptodate.com/contents/epidemiology-risk-factors-and-etiology-of-hypertension-in-children-and-adolescents

Merlo, C. L., Jones, S. E., Michael, S. L., Chen, T. J., Sliwa, S. A., Lee, S. H, Brener, N. D., Lee, S. M., & Parket, S. (2020). Dietary and physical activity behaviors among high school students—

Youth Risk Behavior Survey, United States, 2019. *MMWR Supplements, 69*(Suppl. 1), 64–76. http://doi.org/10.15585/mmwr.su6901a8

Miller, E., & Wiemann, C. M. (2020). Adolescent relationship abuse including physical and sexual teen dating violence. *UpToDate*. Retrieved November 3, 2022, from https://www.uptodate.com/contents/adolescent-relationship-abuse-including-physical-and-sexual-teen-dating-violence

Naik-Mathuria, B., & Gill, A. C. (2022). Firearm injuries in children: Prevention. *UpToDate*. Retrieved October 31, 2022, from https://www.uptodate.com/contents/firearm-injuries-in-children-prevention

National Center for Education Statistics. (n.d.). Trends in high school dropout and completion rates in the United States. https://nces.ed.gov/programs/dropout/intro.asp

National Center for Education Statistics. (2022). *Condition of education: Status dropout rates*. U.S. Department of Education, Institute of Education Sciences. https://nces.ed.gov/programs/coe/indicator/coj

NIH/National Institute on Alcohol Abuse and Alcoholism. (2022). *Underage drinking*. https://www.niaaa.nih.gov/sites/default/files/publications/NIAAA_Underage_Drinking_1.pdf

Paul, C. R., & Wallace, C. M. (2023). Behavioral disorders: Normal sleep and pediatric sleep disorders. In K. J. Marcdante, R. M. Kleigman, & A. M. Schuh (Eds.), *Nelson essentials of pediatrics* (9th ed., pp. 54–58). Elsevier.

Pew Research Center. (2022). *Teens, social media and technology 2022*. https://www.pewresearch.org/internet/2022/08/10/teens-social-media-and-technology-2022/

Piaget, J. (1969). *The theory of stages in cognitive development*. McGraw-Hill.

Rigotti, N. A., & Reddy, K. P. (2022). Vaping and e-cigarettes. *UpToDate*. Retrieved November 3, 2022, from https://www.uptodate.com/contents/vaping-and-e-cigarettes

Sege, R. D. (2022). Peer violence and violence prevention. *UpToDate*. Retrieved November 3, 2022, from https://www.uptodate.com/contents/peer-violence-and-violence-prevention

U.S. Department of Agriculture, & U.S. Department of Health and Human Services. (2020). *Dietary guidelines for Americans, 2020–2025* (9th ed.). https://www.dietaryguidelines.gov/sites/default/files/2021-03/Dietary_Guidelines_for_Americans-2020-2025.pdf

U.S. Department of Health and Human Services. (n.d.). *Healthy people 2030*. https://health.gov/healthypeople

Woessner, M. N., Tacey, A., Levinger-Limor, A., Parker, A. G., Levinger, P., & Levinger, I. (2021). The evolution of technology and physical inactivity: The good, the bad, and the way forward. *Frontiers in Public Health, 9*, 655491. https://doi.org/10.3389/fpubh.2021.655491

DEVELOPING CLINICAL JUDGMENT

PRACTICING FOR NCLEX

1. When giving parents guidance for the adolescent years, which would the nurse advise the parents to do? Select all that apply.

a. Accept the adolescent as a unique individual.
b. Provide strict, inflexible rules.
c. Listen and try to be open to the adolescent's views.
d. Screen all of their friends.
e. Respect the adolescent's privacy.
f. Provide unconditional love.

2. In developing a weight loss plan for an adolescent, which would the nurse include? Select all that apply.

a. Have parents make all of the meal plans.
b. Eat slowly and place the fork down between each bite.
c. Have the family exercise together.
d. Refer to an adolescent weight loss program.
e. Keep a food and exercise diary.

3. Which is associated with the period of early adolescence? Select all that apply.

a. Uses scientific reasoning to solve problems
b. At times, still wants to be dependent on parents
c. Incorporates own set of morals and values
d. Is influenced by peers and values memberships in cliques

4. What has the most influence in deterring an adolescent from beginning to drink alcohol?

a. Drinking habits of parents
b. Drinking habits of peers
c. Drinking philosophy of adolescent's culture
d. Drinking philosophy of adolescent's religion

5. The nurse is teaching a parent about adolescent growth and development. After the teaching session, the parent should be able to verbalize that adolescence is a time of __________growth and the adolescent needs ____________ and __________.

Blank 1:
a. rapid
b. slow
c. continual
d. gradual

Blanks 2 and 3:
a. more than 8 hours of sleep
b. increased calories
c. a low-calcium diet
d. decreased calories
e. fewer than 8 hours of sleep
f. a low protein diet

6. The nurse is caring for an 11-year-old female. What changes in puberty should the nurse expect to find on assessment? Select all that apply.

a. Hip girth widening
b. Pubic hair beginning to curl
c. Breasts beginning to separate
d. Breast buds enlarging
e. Genital pigmentation increasing

CRITICAL THINKING EXERCISES

1. During a sports physical examination, Susan, a 16-year-old, tells her health care provider that she is overweight. What additional information would the nurse obtain?

2. The parents of Joe, a 14-year-old, talk to the school nurse about Joe's behavior at home. He is moody, fights with his younger siblings, only wants to be on his computer, and does not want to go on the family vacation. What advice would the nurse give the parents?

3. Jane tells the school nurse that she thinks she might be a lesbian. What additional information would the nurse obtain?

4. Alicia's parents are worried because all of Alicia's friends wear heavy makeup and have multiple piercings and hair colors. What advice would the nurse give Alicia's parents?

STUDY ACTIVITIES

1. Talk to an early, middle, and late adolescent. Compare and contrast their interactions with you. Identify what psychosocial, cognitive, and moral stage they are in, using examples from their conversations with you.

2. Have an adolescent keep a food and exercise diary for 1 week. Analyze the information. Develop with the adolescent any interventions needed to promote healthy eating and exercise habits.

3. Plan a class on the dangers of smoking and electronic nicotine delivery systems (ENDSs) for 15-year-olds.

4. Plan a class for parents on how to keep the lines of communication open for adolescents.

5. Go to https://www.myplate.gov/myplate-plan and create and compare a customized meal plan for an adolescent at a healthy weight versus an adolescent with excess weight.

UNIT

III

Working With Children and Families

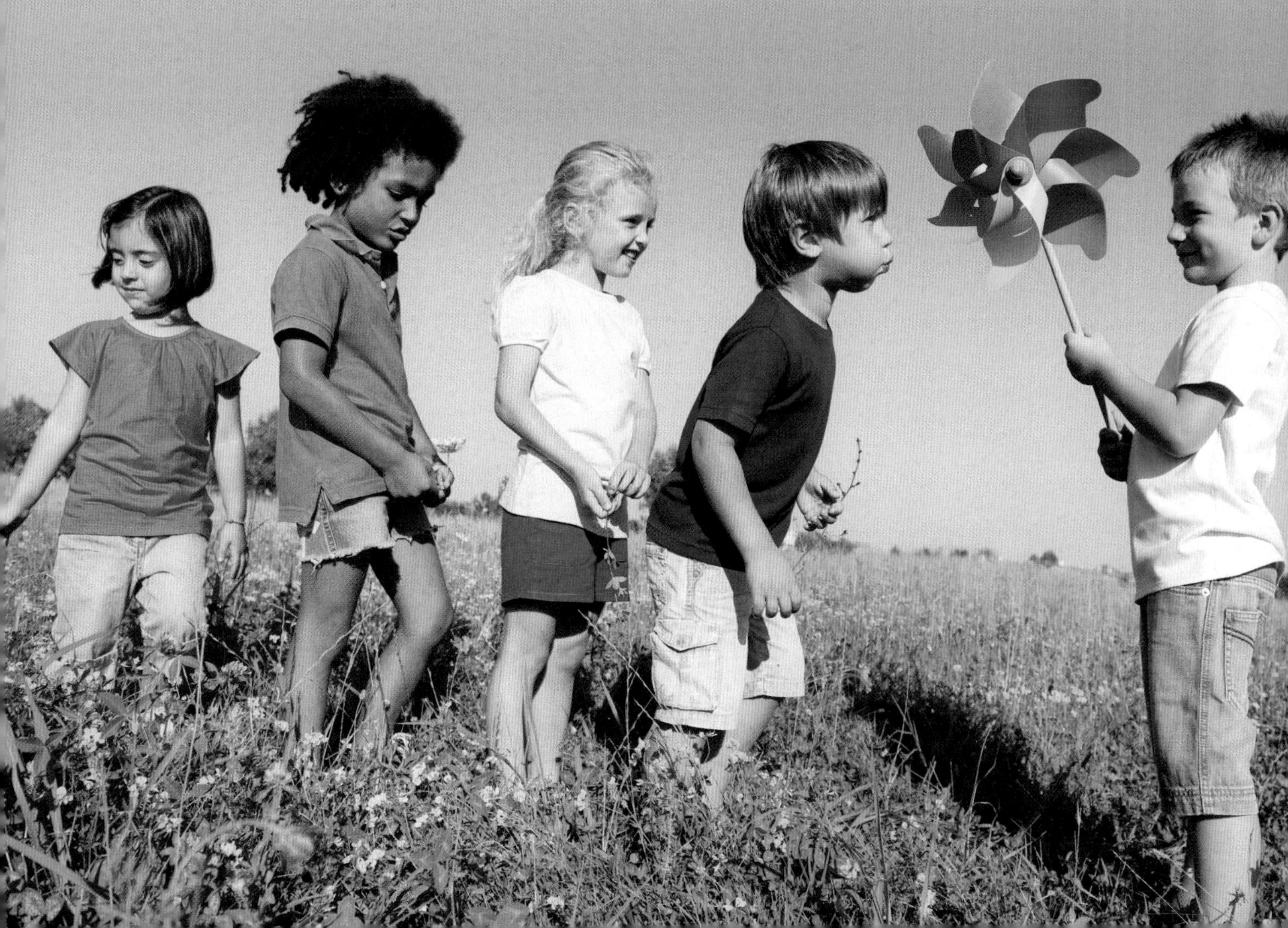

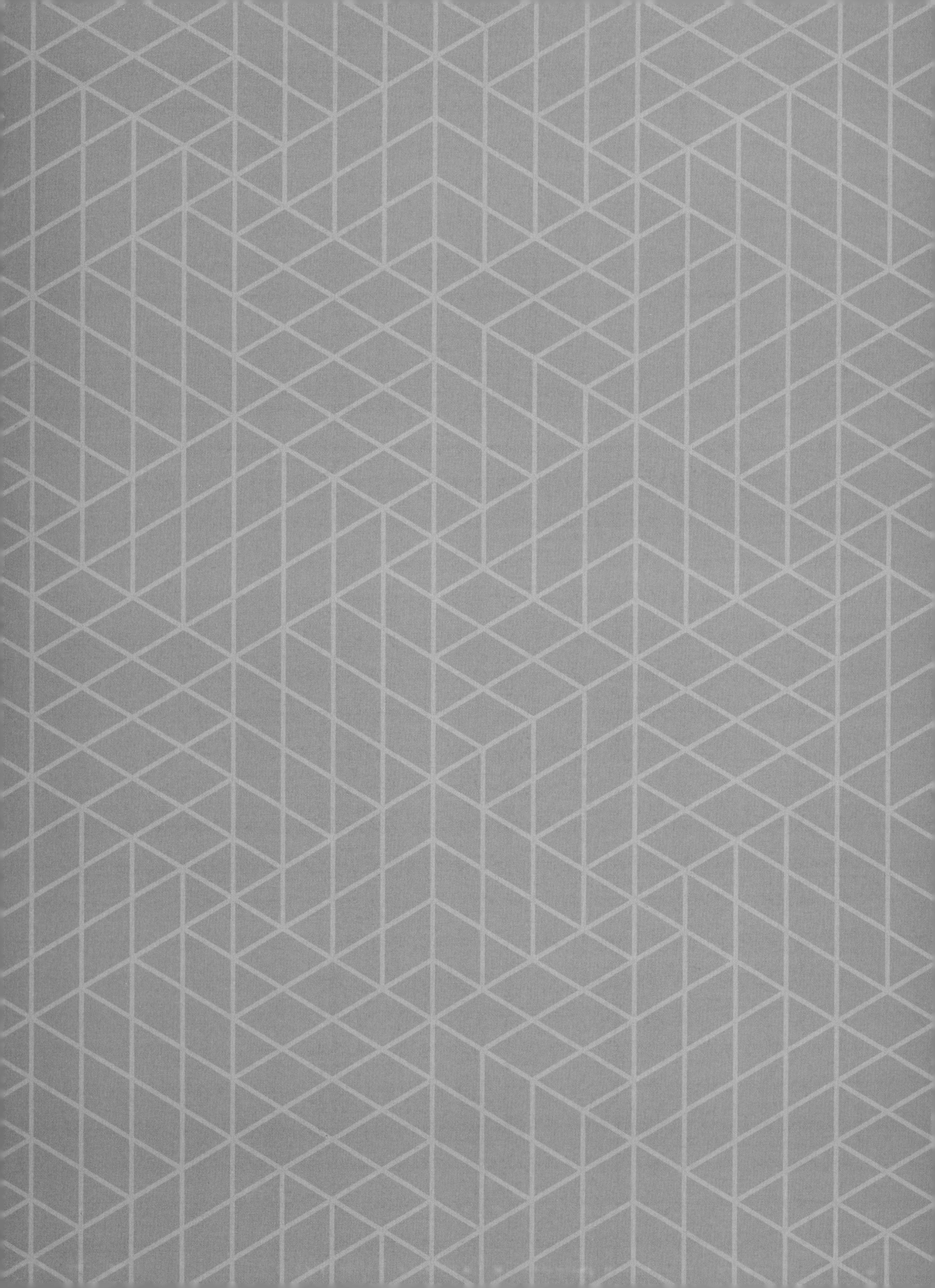

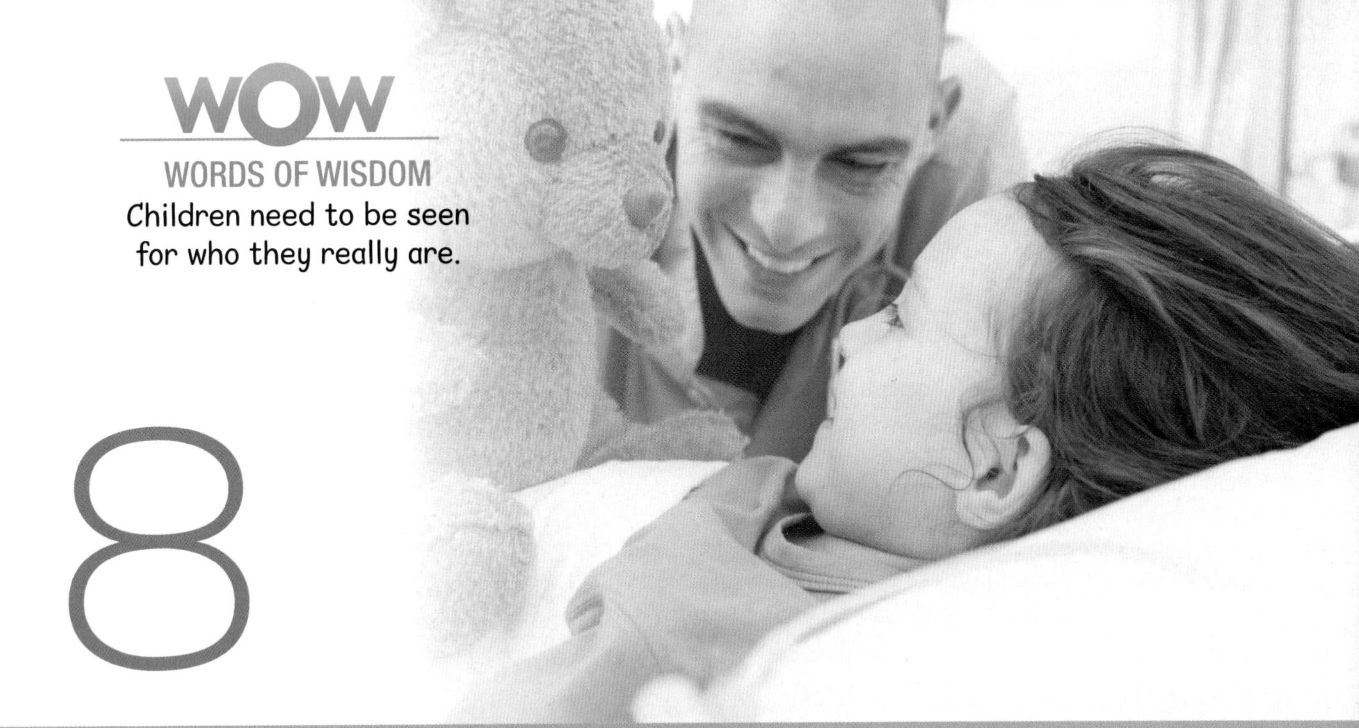
WOW
WORDS OF WISDOM
Children need to be seen
for who they really are.
8

Atraumatic Care of Children and Families

LEARNING OBJECTIVES

Upon completion of the chapter, you will be able to:

1. Describe the major principles and concepts of atraumatic care.
2. Describe interventions to incorporate atraumatic care to prevent and minimize physical stress for children and families.
3. Explain the major components and concepts of family-centered care.
4. Discuss appropriate therapeutic communication skills when interacting with children and their families.
5. Understand the concept of culturally respectful communication when working with children and their families.
6. Describe the process of health teaching as it relates to children and their families.

Emma Moore, 4 years old, is admitted to the pediatric unit with a suspected head injury from a fall. She was playing at a playground with a babysitter and fell from the top of the slide.

KEY TERMS

atraumatic care
child life specialist
family-centered care
personal health literacy
therapeutic hugging

INTRODUCTION

Atraumatic care is defined as therapeutic care that minimizes or eliminates the psychological and physical distress experienced by children and their families in the health care system (Wong, 1995). This concept is based on the underlying premise of "do no harm." Box 8.1 highlights the major principles of atraumatic care.

Pediatric nurses must be vigilant for any situation that may cause distress and must be able to identify potential stressors. It is important to provide nursing care that decreases the child's exposure to stressful situations and prevents or minimizes pain and bodily injury; take steps to minimize separation of the child from the family; and utilize techniques of communication and provide teaching that promotes a sense of control. Atraumatic care involves guiding children and their families through the health care experience using a family-centered approach by promoting family roles, fostering family support of the child, and providing appropriate information. Help children cope with this experience by using age-appropriate and child-specific interventions. Preparation can help children and their families adjust to illness and hospitalization. Use appropriate techniques for therapeutic communication (goal-directed, focused, purposeful communication); therapeutic play (type of play that provides an emotional outlet or improves the child's ability to cope with the stress of illness and hospitalization); and education to help the child and family understand the reason for the hospitalization and the necessary tests and procedures. In addition, help the family and other health care personnel obtain the resources and relationships they need for optimal care.

The best pediatric nursing care encompasses the concepts of atraumatic care. Minimizing physical stressors during procedures, providing family-centered care, and utilizing excellent communication skills on the part of the nurse enhance the health care experience for the child and family. Having an informed and educated family is the best way to provide optimal health care for children.

Table 8.1 gives suggestions for incorporating the principles of atraumatic care into nursing care for the child and family. Look for tips on atraumatic care as it relates to specific topics throughout the text.

BOX 8.1 Principles of Atraumatic Care

- Prevent or minimize physical stressors, including pain, discomfort, immobility, sleep deprivation, inability to eat or drink, and changes in elimination.
  - Avoid or reduce intrusive and painful procedures, such as injections, multiple punctures, and urethral catheterization.
  - Avoid or reduce other kinds of physical distress, such as noise, smells, shivering, nausea and vomiting, sleeplessness, restraints, and skin trauma.
  - Control pain via frequent assessments and use of pharmacologic and nonpharmacologic interventions.
- Prevent or minimize parent–child separation.
  - Promote family-centered care, treating the family as the patient.
  - Use core primary nursing.
  - Consider research findings related to preferences of parents and children and whether to be together.
- Promote a sense of control.
  - Elicit the family's knowledge about the child and their health condition, promoting partnerships, empowerment, and enabling.
  - Reduce fear of the unknown through education, familiar articles, and decreasing the threat of the environment.
  - Provide opportunities for control, such as participating in care, attempting to normalize a daily schedule, and providing direct suggestions.

Adapted from Wong, D. (1995). *Whaley & Wong's nursing care of infants and children* (5th ed.). Mosby.

PREVENTING AND MINIMIZING PHYSICAL STRESSORS

The health care facility or hospital is an unfamiliar environment for children and parents and may upset or intimidate them. They may feel anxiety, fear, helplessness, anger, or loss of control. Even health care procedures performed in the home or school may be perceived as threatening to children. To prevent and minimize the physical stress experienced by children and their families in relation to health care, pediatric nurses, child life specialists (CLSs), and other health care professionals recommend the use of atraumatic care.

Utilizing the Child Life Specialist

The **child life specialist** (CLS) is an individual specially trained in the developmental impact of illness, injury, and trauma and who provides programs that prepare children for hospitalization, surgery, and other procedures that could be painful or distressing (Association of Child Life Professionals, 2022). The CLS is a member of the multidisciplinary team and works in conjunction with the health care provider and parents to foster an atmosphere that promotes the child's well-being. Services provided by a CLS include:

- Nonmedical preparation for hospitalization, clinic visits, tests, surgeries, and other medical procedures
- Support during medical procedures
- Therapeutic play
- Activities to support normal growth and development
- Education for the child and family about health conditions
- Teaching and support with coping and pain management strategies
- Sibling support
- Advocacy for the child and family
- Grief and bereavement support
- Emergency room interventions for children and families

TABLE 8.1 • Suggestions for Atraumatic Care

Principle	Suggestions for Nursing Care
Preventing or minimizing physical stressors	• For painful injections, blood draws, or IV insertion, use numbing techniques (see Chapter 14). • During painful or invasive procedures, avoid traditional restraint or "holding down" of the child. Use alternative positioning such as "therapeutic hugging." • If the aforementioned positions are not an option, have the parent stand near the child's head to provide comfort. • Insert a saline lock if the child requires multiple doses of parenteral medications. • Advocate for minimal laboratory blood draws. • Minimize intramuscular or subcutaneous injections. • Provide appropriate pain management (refer to Chapter 14).
Preventing or minimizing child and family separation	• Promote family-centered care. • In the hospital, provide comfortable accommodations for the parent. • Allow the family the choice about whether to stay for an invasive procedure, and support them in their decision.
Promoting a sense of control	• Maintain the child's home routine related to activities of daily living. • In the hospital, use primary nursing. • Encourage the child to have a security item present if desired. • Involve the child and family in planning care from the moment of the first encounter. • Empower the family and child by providing knowledge. • Allow the child and family choices when they are available. • Make the environment more inviting and less intimidating.

- Hospital preadmission tours and information programs
- Outpatient consultation with families (Romito et al., 2021).

The goal of the CLS is to decrease the child's anxiety and fear while improving and encouraging the child's understanding and cooperation. The CLS considers the needs of siblings or other children who may be affected by the child's illness or trauma. The CLS provides engaging and uplifting events by coordinating special entertainment and activities. The CLS is an excellent resource and provides education to health care providers and families. The American Academy of Pediatrics (AAP) recommends child life services because they are "a quality benchmark of an integrated patient- and family-centered health care system, a recommended component of medical education, and an indicator of excellence in pediatric care" (Romito et al., 2021, p. 5).

Minimizing Physical Stress During Procedures

Children undergo numerous diagnostic and therapeutic procedures in a wide range of settings during their development. These procedures may be performed in the community or outpatient setting or in a care facility. Regardless of the procedure and the setting, children, like adults, need thorough preparation before the procedure and support during and after the procedure to promote the best outcome and to ensure atraumatic care.

Using positions that are comforting to the child during painful procedures is an important aspect of atraumatic care (Fig. 8.1). **Therapeutic hugging** (a holding position that promotes close physical contact between the child and a parent or caregiver) may be used for certain procedures or treatments where the child must remain still. For example, the parent can hold the child in their lap snugly to prevent the child from moving during an injection or venipuncture. When using this technique, make sure the parent understands their role and knows which body parts to hold still in a safe manner. Alternatively, distraction or stimulation (such as with a toy) can help to gain the child's cooperation. Refer to Box 8.2 for distraction methods (Fig. 8.2).

Before the Procedure

Appropriate preparation for procedures helps decrease the child's and family's anxiety level; promote the child's cooperation; support the child's and family's coping skills; improve recovery; and increase trust between the child, their family, and the health care team (Romito et al., 2021). Adequate preparation and explanation also help encourage long-term coping and build trust and rapport that will positively impact future medical situations (Romito et al., 2021).

Preparation may include preparing the child psychologically (including explanation and education) as well as physically. It is important to employ the concepts of atraumatic care when preparing children for a procedure. General guidelines for preparation include:

- Provide a description of and the reason for the procedure using age-appropriate language ("The doctor will look at your blood to see why you are sick").

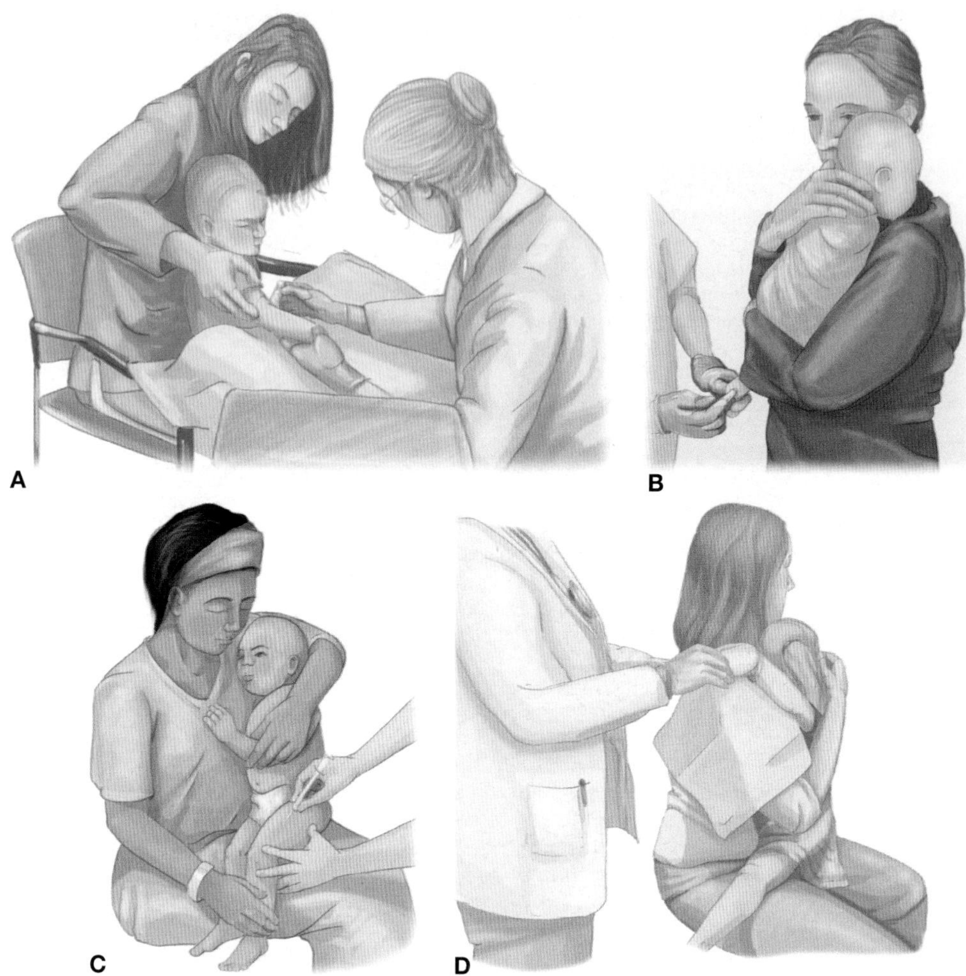

FIGURE 8.1 Positioning a child for comfort during a painful procedure. **A.** Sitting on the parent's lap while undergoing allergy testing provides this toddler with a sense of comfort. **B.** Position the infant cuddled over the parent's or the nurse's shoulder when obtaining a heel stick. The parent is preferable to the nurse. **C.** Use "therapeutic hugging" to maintain a child's position when the child is receiving an intramuscular injection. **D.** Use "therapeutic hugging" to position a child while the child is having an IV line inserted.

- Describe where the procedure will occur ("The x-ray department has big machines that won't hurt you; it's a little cold there too").
- Introduce strange equipment the child may see ("You will lie on a special bed that moves in the big machine, but you can still see out").
- Describe how long the procedure will last ("You will be in the x-ray department until lunchtime").

BOX 8.2 Distraction Methods

- Have the child point toes inward and wiggle them.
- Ask the child to squeeze your hand.
- Encourage the child to count aloud.
- Sing a song and have the child sing along.
- Point out the pictures on the ceiling.
- Have the child blow bubbles.
- Play music appealing to the child.

- Identify unusual sensations that may occur during the procedure ("You may smell something different" or "The machine makes loud noises").
- Inform the child if any pain is involved.
- Tell the child it is okay to cry or yell.
- Identify any special care required after the procedure ("You will need to lie quietly for 15 minutes afterward").
- Discuss ways that may help the child stay calm, such as using distraction methods or relaxation techniques ("During the procedure, you may want to count from 1 to 100 or sing your favorite song").

TAKE NOTE!

In the hospital, perform all invasive procedures in the treatment room or a room other than the child's room. The child's room should remain a safe and secure area (Ernst & AAP Committee on Hospital Care, 2020).

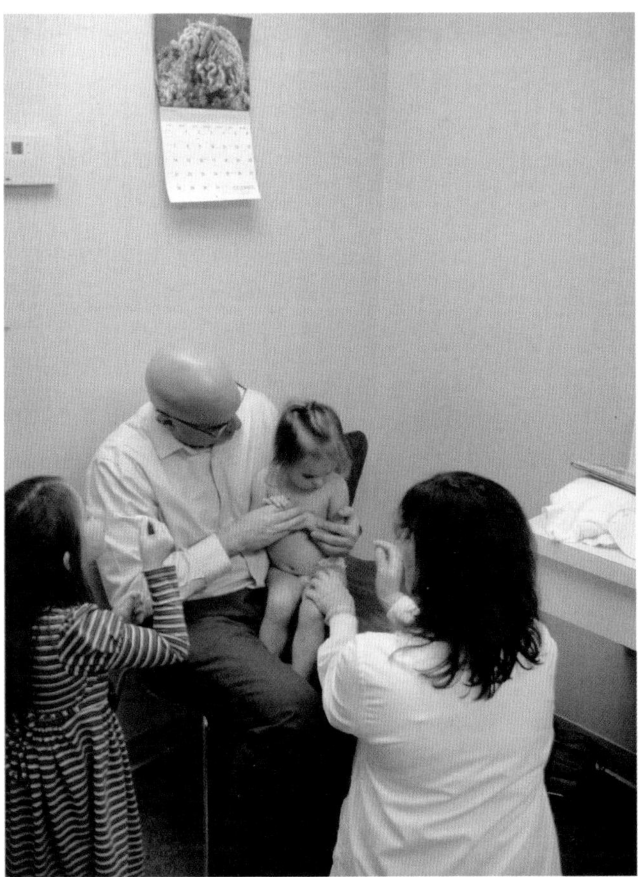

FIGURE 8.2 When possible, allow the caregiver to assist with providing positions of comfort and involve a sibling to assist with distraction techniques such as blowing bubbles, singing, or reading to the child during procedures.

A major aspect of preparation involves play. Toys and dolls provide an excellent way to demonstrate procedures that will occur. Consider the child's temperament, coping strategies, and previous experiences as well as developmental needs and cognitive abilities. First, gain trust and provide support. Include the child's parents, because parents are usually the greatest source of comfort for the child. Be short, simple, and appropriate in explaining situations at the child's level of development. Explain what is to be done and what is expected of the child. Avoid terms that have double meanings or that might be confusing. Table 8.2 lists alternative words or phrases to use for terms that may be confusing or misunderstood. Allow the child time to play with a toy or dolls and medical equipment as appropriate. Watch for signs of anxiety or fears.

During the Procedure

Use a firm, positive, confident approach that provides the child with a sense of security. Encourage cooperation by involving the child in decision making and allowing the child to select from a list or group of appropriate choices. Allow the child to express feelings of anger, anxiety, fear, frustration, or any other emotions. Often, this is how a child communicates and copes with the situation. Remind the child that it is okay to scream or cry but that it is important to hold still. Use distraction methods such as those listed in Box 8.2.

Toddlers and preschoolers often resist procedures despite preparation for them. Being held down or restrained is often more traumatizing to the young child than the procedure itself. Use alternative methods (positions that provide comfort for the child) to keep the child still during the procedure (see Fig. 8.1). The older child can be held while using a book or story for distraction.

After the Procedure

After the procedure, hold and comfort the child. Cuddle and soothe infants. Encourage children to express their feelings through play, such as dramatic play, or use of puppets. Gross motor activities such as pounding or throwing are also helpful for children to discharge pent-up feelings and energy. School-age children and adolescents may not outwardly demonstrate behavior indicating the need for comforting; however, provide them with opportunities to express their feelings and be comforted. Remember to praise children for appropriate behavior during the procedure and after all interventions are completed.

TAKE NOTE!

Remember to utilize CLSs when available.

Remember Emma Moore, the 4-year-old introduced at the beginning of the chapter? The health care provider's orders for Emma include starting intravenous (IV) fluids and obtaining blood work upon arrival at the unit. As the admitting nurse, how will you provide atraumatic care?

PREVENTING OR MINIMIZING CHILD AND FAMILY SEPARATION: PROVIDING CHILD- AND FAMILY-CENTERED CARE

Family-centered care involves a partnership between the child, family, and health care providers in planning, providing, and evaluating care (American Academy of Pediatrics, Committee on Hospital Care, Institute for Patient and Family-Centered Care, 2012, reaffirmed 2018; Kuo & Turchi, 2023). It works well for children of any age and in all arenas of health care, from preventive care of the healthy child to long-term care of the child with a chronic or terminal illness. Family-centered

TABLE 8.2 • Alternatives for Confusing or Misunderstood Terms

Term to Avoid	How Children Might Interpret It	Use These Terms Instead
Catheter	Too technical	Tube
Deaden	Kill	Make sleepy
Dye	Die	Special medicine to help the doctor see (part of the body) better
Electrodes	Too technical	Stickers, ticklers, snaps
ICU	I see you.	Special room with your own nurse
Incision, cut open, make a hole	Too explicit	Special or small opening
Monitor	Too technical	Screen
Dressing change	To change clothes	Clean bandage/Band-Aid
Pain	May be too explicit	Child's word for hurt; "boo-boo"
Put to sleep, anesthesia	May confuse with putting a pet to sleep	Special kind of sleep
Shot	Children are scared of shots.	Medication under the skin
Stool	Like you sit on	"Poop" or child's word for it
Stretcher or gurney	"Stretch her"	Rolling bed or special bed on wheels
Take your temperature/blood pressure	Where are you going to "take" them?	See how warm you are/hug your arm.
Test	Like at school (the child will need to perform)	See how your heart is working.
Tourniquet	Too technical	Special kind of rubber band
Urine	"You're in"	"Pee" or child's word for it
X-ray	Don't understand	Picture or big camera to take pictures of the inside of your body

Based on Gaynard, L., Wolfer, J., Goldberger, J., Redbum, L., Laidley, L., & Thompson, R. (1998). *Psychosocial care of children in hospitals: Clinical practice manual from the ACCH Child Life Research Project* (1st ed.). Child Life Council.

care enhances parents' and caregivers' confidence in their own skills and also prepares children and young adults for assuming responsibility for their own health care needs. It is based on the concept that the family is the constant in the child's life and the primary source of strength and support for the child (American Academy of Pediatrics, Committee on Hospital Care, Institute for Patient and Family-Centered Care, 2012, reaffirmed 2018; Kuo & Turchi, 2023).

According to the American Academy of Pediatrics, Committee on Hospital Care, Institute for Patient and Family-Centered Care (2012, reaffirmed 2018), family-centered care focuses on several core principles:

- Respect for the child and family
- Recognition of the effects of cultural, racial, ethnic, and socioeconomic factors on the family's health care experience
- Identification of and expansion of the family's strengths
- Support of the family's choices related to the child's health care
- Maintenance of flexibility
- Provision of honest, unbiased information in an affirming and useful approach
- Assistance with the emotional and other support the child and family require
- Collaboration with families
- Empowerment of families

When children's health care is provided through a family-centered approach, many positive outcomes are possible, including:

- Anxiety is decreased.
- Children are calmer and pain management is enhanced.
- Recovery times are shortened.
- Families' confidence and problem-solving skills are improved.

- Communication between the health care team and the family is also improved, leading to greater satisfaction for both health care providers and health care consumers (families).
- A decrease in health care costs is seen and health care resources are used more effectively (American Academy of Pediatrics, Committee on Hospital Care, Institute for Patient and Family-Centered Care, 2012, reaffirmed 2018).

Ways to increase collaboration between the family and the health care team may include a family advisory board, a newsletter, conferences, or parent resource notebooks. Methods for increasing communication between the health care team and the family may include the use of mailboxes or dry-erase boards for updating the daily plan of care, including the parents' participation in rounds or through a daily assessment of health status by the child or family.

Vigilant parents are committed to the child's care, and most want to be present for all aspects of their child's care. They want to be part of the decision-making process regarding their child's care; they want to be heard and develop a rapport with the health care professionals caring for their child. They demonstrate resilience in their ability to make it through the emotional upheaval associated with an illness. It is important to be sensitive to the inconveniences that a child's illness may impose on the family. Address the family's emotional and spiritual needs, attend to their concerns, and provide the best accommodations possible when the child is hospitalized (Fig. 8.3). Practicing true family-centered care may empower the family, strengthen family resources, and help the child and family feel more secure and supported throughout the process.

TAKE NOTE!

Some parents will not know how to advocate or speak up for their child; as a nurse, you must help open this door for them.

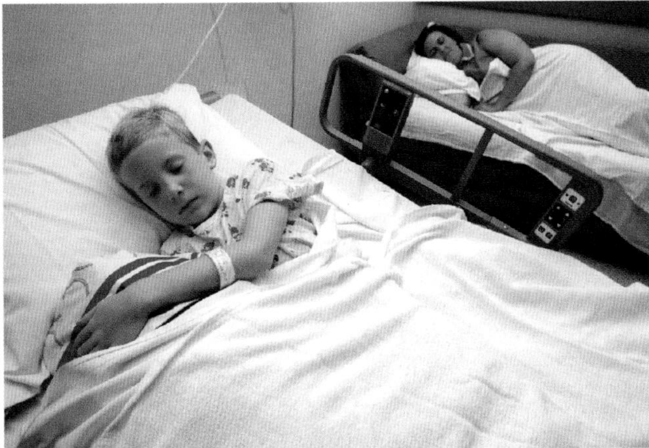

FIGURE 8.3 Providing a comfortable area for the parent to rest is an important component of family-centered care.

PROMOTING A SENSE OF CONTROL

During times of illness, hospitalization, or health-related interventions, the child and family can experience an extreme sense of loss of control. Providing effective communication and teaching can help foster feelings of control and improve the child's and family's ability to cope. Assisting the family with obtaining necessary information, resources, and relationships contributes to optimal health care for the child and family. Communication and teaching are skills that are used continuously in pediatric nursing, no matter what the setting or the child's state of health.

Enhancing Communication

Effective communication with children and their parents is critical to providing atraumatic quality nursing care. Child- and parent-centered communication enhances child outcomes and child and family satisfaction with nursing care. Effective communication is the foundation of the therapeutic relationship and leads to increased knowledge and health care behaviors on the part of the child and family (Betancourt et al., 2021; Levetown & American Academy of Pediatrics Committee on Bioethics, 2008, reaffirmed 2017). Nurses are in an ideal position to improve communication in the health care environment. They need to ensure inclusion of the child and family in health conversations and to clarify misconceptions following medical encounters.

Children are often socialized to be passive participants in health care, doing as they are told with or without protests. "As pediatric nurses, we have an obligation to listen, to hear, and to feel the voices of the children in our care" (McPherson & Thorne, 2000, p. 28). Children can inform nurses of their experiences in an accurate fashion, and nurses need to be able to discern this information from communication with the child. Children want to be respected, listened to, and understood.

Communication patterns can vary greatly from one child to the next. Some children are talkative, while others are quiet. Children may be more apt to communicate if they are engaged in another activity. Children often use fewer words than adults and may rely more on nonverbal communication and silence. Communicating in the pediatric setting can be complicated and more difficult than in the adult setting, but it remains crucial. The pediatric nurse needs to consider the age of the child and the child's cognitive and developmental level as well as communicating at an appropriate level with the parents.

Verbal Communication

Communicating through the use of words, either written or spoken, is termed verbal communication. Nurses use verbal communication throughout the day when interacting with children. Good verbal communication skills are necessary when performing nursing assessments and providing child and family teaching. General guidelines for appropriate verbal communication include:

- Use open-ended questions that do not restrict the child's or parent's answers.
- Redirect the conversation to maintain focus.
- Use reflection to clarify the parent's feelings.
- Paraphrase the child's or parent's feelings to demonstrate empathy.
- Acknowledge emotions.
- Demonstrate active listening by using the child's or family's own words.

Remember that most parents are laypeople, so avoid using medical jargon. The abbreviations and shortened terms that health care providers use, sometimes without thinking, may sound scary or foreign to children and parents. When medical terminology is necessary, provide a definition using developmentally appropriate language.

Nonverbal Communication

Nonverbal communication is also referred to as body language. It includes attending to others and active listening. The nurse should listen to the other person's verbal communication from the beginning of the interaction. When children and parents feel they are being heard, trust and rapport are established. Guidelines for appropriate nonverbal communication include:

- Relax; maintain an open posture, with the arms uncrossed.
- Sit opposite the family and lean forward slightly.
- Maintain eye contact.
- Nod your head to demonstrate interest.
- Note the child's or parent's posture, eye contact, and facial expressions.

Active listening is critical to the communication process. Listening may uncover fears or concerns that the nurse may not have discovered through questioning. Paying attention while children and parents talk is a powerful communication tool. By not listening, the nurse may miss critical information, and the family may be reluctant to share further. When interacting with the child and family, determine whether the messages sent by the child's or parent's verbal and nonverbal communication are congruent.

Developmental Techniques for Communicating With Children

Effective communication with children involves a variety of age-appropriate methods. If the child is shy, talk to the parents first to give the child time to warm up to you. Use specific and clear phrases in an unhurried, quiet, yet confident manner. Communicate at the child's eye level (Fig. 8.4A). Spending time and incorporating play with younger children, even just a few moments, may help them feel more at ease with you and help open the door to communication. Instead of direct questioning, use dolls, puppets, or stuffed animals with younger children (Fig. 8.4B). The use of metaphors (e.g., referring to white blood cells as "bad guy fighters") and stories can help illustrate health concepts to young and school-age children.

Older children need privacy. Provide the child or adolescent with honest answers at a developmentally appropriate level. Allow children to express their thoughts and feelings. Offer the child choices when possible but only when they truly exist. Encourage children to write and draw about their experiences. This may increase their understanding and also draw attention to any misconceptions or fears. Box 8.3 lists requirements for communication with children and adolescents.

Children feel empowered when health care professionals communicate directly with them. Include children in discussions and avoid talking about them in their presence. Children may also desire advice about their health care and reassurance about their health status. To be effective when communicating with children of

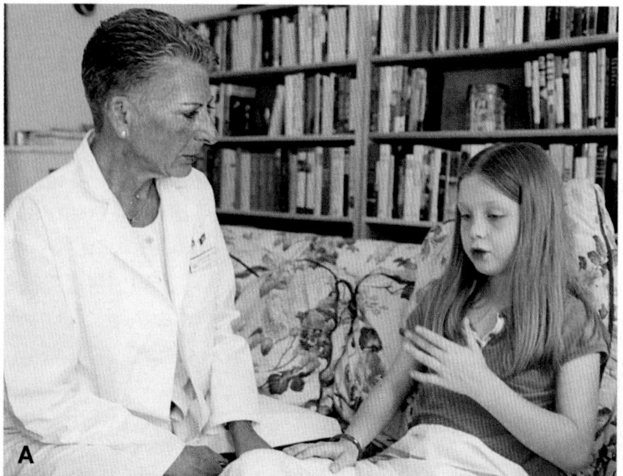

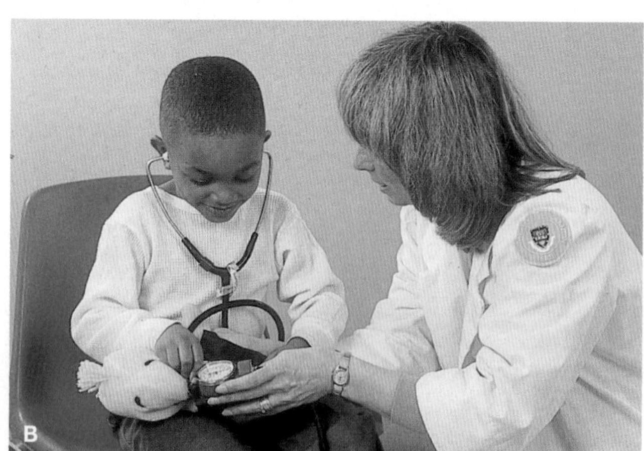

FIGURE 8.4 A. Sitting at the child's level and allowing the child time for self-expression are steps that improve therapeutic communication. **B.** Communication or teaching with dolls may be useful with younger children.

BOX 8.3 Basics for Communicating With Children

- Introduce yourself and explain your role.
- Position yourself at the child's level.
- Allow the child to remain near the parent if needed so the child can remain comfortable and relaxed.
- Smile and make eye contact with the child if culturally appropriate.
- Direct your questions and explanations to the child.
- Listen attentively and pause to allow time for the child to formulate their thoughts.
- Use the child's or family's terms for body parts and medical care when possible.
- Speak in a calm, quiet, confident, and unhurried voice.
- Use positive rather than negative statements and directions.
- Encourage the child to express their feelings and ask questions.
- Observe for nonverbal cues.
- Ask for permission if you need to approach the child to avoid appearing threatening.

different developmental stages, the nurse must become familiar with how children of different ages communicate and then use age-appropriate techniques for effective communication.

- Infants communicate primarily through touch, sight, and hearing. Communication with the infant can occur by cuddling, holding, rocking, and singing to the infant.
- When working with toddlers and preschoolers, allow them time to complete their thoughts. Although language acquisition at this age is exponential, it often takes longer for the young child to find the right words, particularly in response to a question.
- School-age children are interested in learning and appreciate simple but honest and straightforward responses. When addressed first and allowed to respond, the school-age child may be eager to communicate. The school-age child is beginning to utilize more sophisticated language and developing problem-solving and critical thinking skills.
- Adolescents may experience strong feelings and emotions and perceive situations in extreme terms. Building a trusting, respectful rapport is essential.

For communication tips related to the child's age, see Table 8.3.

TABLE 8.3 • Communicating Effectively With Children

Age	Techniques
Infants	• Respond to crying in a timely fashion. • Allow the infant time to warm up to you. • Use a soothing and calming tone when speaking to the infant. • Talk to the infant directly. • Communication through play may be helpful with older infants. • Watch for signs of overstimulation such as closing eyes, turning away, yawning, and irritability.
Toddlers	• Approach toddlers carefully; they are often not only fearful but also can be resistant. • Use the toddler's preferred words for objects or actions so they are better able to understand. • Toddlers enjoy stories, dolls, and books. • Participate in parallel play to help start communication. • Prepare toddlers for procedures just before they are about to occur.
Preschoolers	• Use play, puppets, or storytelling via a third-party approach. • Speak honestly. • Use simple, concrete terms. • Ask specific questions. • Allow the child to have choices as appropriate. • Participate in imaginative play to help open communication. • Prepare preschoolers about 1 hour prior to a procedure.
School-age children	• Use diagrams, illustrations, books, and videos. • Allow the child to honestly express feelings. • Use third-party stories to elicit desired information (such as "some children feel anxious about…"). • Allow the child to ask questions related to care and treatment. Give the child adequate time for all of the questions to be answered. • Prepare the child a few days in advance for a procedure.
Adolescents	• Always respect the adolescent's need for privacy. • Ensure confidentiality. • Remain nonjudgmental. • Listen attentively and speak respectfully. • Use appropriate medical terminology, defining words as necessary. • Use creativity and humor. • Do not force the adolescent to talk as this may shut down communication. • Prepare the adolescent up to 1 week prior to a procedure.

Tips for Communicating With Parents

When communicating with parents, be honest. Parents want to feel valued and should be equal partners with the health care team. Allow the parent to express concerns and ask questions. Explain equipment and procedures thoroughly. Help the parents understand the long-term as well as short-term effects of the treatment. Teach the parents what the child will feel like and how they will look during a procedure. Teach and encourage the parent to perform as much of the child's care as is reasonable and permitted. Ask the parent about their perception of the child's progress. Allowing the parents to be involved in the care of their child gives them a sense of control and lets them know they are valued by the health care team. Provide parents with positive reinforcement, reassurance, guidance, and support.

Communicating Across Cultures

Understanding and respecting the child's culture helps foster good communication and improves child and family education about health care. Culture is shaped by religion, spirituality, race, ethnicity, geography, income, education, sexual orientation, and gender identity or expressions (Betancourt et al., 2021). These factors are intertwined and affect the child's and family's communication styles, health status, and health beliefs. It is important to be aware of the family's background, lifestyle, and health care practices to meet their information needs.

Learning about the practices of various cultures is just the beginning; the nurse must assess each family's individual beliefs and practices rather than generalizing. The best way to assess the family's cultural practices is to ask and then listen. Determine the language spoken at home, and observe the use of eye contact and other physical contact. Demonstrate a caring, nonjudgmental attitude and sensitivity to the child's and family's unique background.

WORKING WITH AN INTERPRETER

Attempting to communicate with a family who does not speak the nurse's language can be frustrating. In this situation, trained interpreters are an invaluable aid and an essential component of child and family education. Whether working with an interpreter in person or over the phone/computer, it is important to coordinate efforts so that both the family and the interpreter understand the information to be communicated. Working as a team, the nurse questions or informs, and the interpreter conveys the information to the child and family completely and accurately. Well-trained translators can also help prevent cultural missteps and can help guide the health care provider to provide information in a more culturally accepted manner; therefore, the use of untrained translators, such as family members, is not appropriate (American Academy of Pediatrics, 2021; Betancourt et al., 2021). Box 8.4 presents tips on working with an interpreter to maximize teaching efforts.

COMMUNICATING WITH CHILDREN WHO ARE DEAF OR HARD OF HEARING AND THEIR FAMILIES

For children who are deaf or hard of hearing and their families, determine the method of communication they use (e.g., lip reading, American Sign Language [ASL], another method, or a combination). If the nurse is not proficient in ASL and the child or family uses it, then an ASL interpreter must be available. According to the

BOX 8.4 Tips on Working With an Interpreter

- **Help the interpreter prepare and understand what needs to be done ahead of time.** A few minutes of preparation may save a lot of time and help communication flow more smoothly in the long run.
- **The interpreter is the "communication bridge," not the "content expert."** The nurse's presence at teaching sessions is vital.
- **Ensure enough time is allotted.** It may take longer to say in some languages what has already been said in English; therefore, plan for more time than you normally would.
- **Speak slowly and clearly.** Avoid jargon. Use short sentences and be concise. Avoid interrupting the interpreter.
- **Pause every few sentences so the interpreter can translate your information.** After 30 seconds of speaking, stop and let the interpreter express the information.
- **Talk directly to the child and family, not the interpreter.** This demonstrates that the information is coming from you and facilitates communication between you and the child and family. This also helps to limit side conversations that may occur between the interpreter and the child and family.
- **Give the family and the interpreter a break.** Keep sessions short; sessions that last longer than 20 or 30 minutes are too long for attention spans and concentration.
- **Express the information in two or three different ways if needed.** There may be cultural barriers as well as language and dialect differences that interfere with understanding. Interpreters may know the correct communication protocols for the family.
- **Use an interpreter to help ensure the family can read and understand translated written materials.** The interpreter can also help answer questions and evaluate learning.
- **Avoid side conversations during sessions.** These can be uncomfortable for the family and jeopardize child and family–provider relationships and trust.
- **Just because someone speaks another language doesn't mean they will make an effective interpreter.** An interpreter who has no medical background or training may not understand or interpret correctly, no matter how fluent they are.
- **Children should not be used as interpreters.** Doing so can affect family relationships, proper understanding, and adherence to health care.

Based on Levetown, M., & American Academy of Pediatrics Committee on Bioethics. (2008, reaffirmed 2017). Communicating with children and families: From everyday interactions to skill in conveying distressing information. *Pediatrics*, 121(5), e1441–e1460. https://doi.org/10.1542/peds.2008-0565; Betancourt, J. R., Green, A. R., & Carillo, J. E. (2021). The patient's culture and effective communication. *UpToDate*. Retrieved November 9, 2022, from https://medilib.ir/uptodate/show/2753

Americans with Disabilities Act, children and family members who are deaf or hard of hearing must be provided with the ability to communicate effectively with health care providers (National Association of the Deaf, 2022).

At the beginning of the chapter, you were introduced to Emma Moore, a 4-year-old with a suspected head injury. Discuss ways to facilitate communication with Emma and her family.

Teaching Children and Families

Regardless of the type of practice or health care setting, nurses are in a unique position to help families manage the health care needs of their child. Indeed, the family has a right and a responsibility to participate fully in making decisions about health care processes for their child. This is true whether the child is hospitalized with a long-term, devastating illness or needs only health maintenance activities. To accomplish this, families need to be knowledgeable about their child's condition, the health care management plan, and when and how to contact health care providers. With the limited time available in all health care arenas and shortened stays in inpatient facilities, the pediatric nurse must focus on teaching goals and begin teaching at the earliest opportunity.

TAKE NOTE!

"There is no prescription more valuable than knowledge."
–C. Everett Koop, MD, former Surgeon General of the United States

Patient education occurs when nurses share information, knowledge, and skills with families, thus empowering them to take responsibility for their child's health care. Through patient education, families can overcome feelings of powerlessness and helplessness and gain the confidence and ability to step to the forefront of the health care team. Nurses spend innumerable hours teaching children and families; in fact, on some days in the hospital, more teaching than nursing care is provided. Given the importance of and the amount of time spent on child and family education, each nurse should become an expert at basic patient education principles. See the Healthy People 2030 box.

HEALTHY PEOPLE 2030

Objective	Nursing Significance
Increase the proportion of people who report their health care provider always asked them to describe how they will follow instructions. Reduce the proportion of people who report poor patient/provider communication (e.g., listening, explanations, disrespect, time). Increase the proportion of adults with limited English proficiency who say their providers explain things clearly. Increase the health literacy of the population.	• Assess health learning needs of children and their families. • Plan health care education in collaboration with children and their families. • Provide health education at each patient encounter and evaluate for effective learning. • Practice universal literacy precautions. • Focus on providing easy-to-understand information during every patient encounter.

Healthy People Objectives retrieved from http://www.healthypeople.gov

Goals of Child and Family Education

The goals of child and family education are to:

- Improve the child's and family's health literacy
- Encourage communication with health care providers
- Improve health outcomes and promote healthy lifestyles
- Encourage involvement of the child and family in care and decision making about care
- Improve adherence to the care and treatment plan
- Promote a sense of autonomy and control

Overall goals for the child and family include the ability of children and families to make informed decisions, perform basic health care skills, recognize when the child has a problem and know how to respond to the problem, and know how to get answers when questions arise.

TAKE NOTE!

Today, health care consumers have information available at their fingertips. It is important to steer children and their families to reliable and credible health care resources.

Steps of Child and Family Education

The steps of child and family education are similar to the steps of the nursing process. The nurse must assess, plan, implement, evaluate, and document education. Once the nurse reaches a level of comfort and experience with each of these steps, they all blend together into one harmonious whole that becomes an everyday part of nursing practice. Child and family education begins with the first encounter and proceeds through discharge and beyond. Reassessment after each step or change in the process is critical to success.

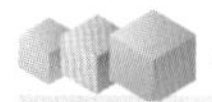
Concept Mastery Alert

When given a diagnosis that will have a significant impact on a family's life, it is important for the nurse to allow the parents time to take in the information about the disorder. The nurse should give parents only small amounts of information at a time to allow them time to absorb it.

ASSESSING TEACHING AND LEARNING NEEDS

Excellent nursing care begins with a thorough assessment of the child. In the same way, child and family education begins with a learning needs assessment that includes the child's and family's learning needs, learning styles and preferences, and potential barriers to learning. Based on the results of the assessment, an individualized plan can be developed to reduce the time and effort required for teaching while maximizing learning for the child and family. Although actual nursing care in pediatrics is given to the child, the educational process is targeted toward both the child (when developmentally appropriate) and the adult members of the family. Therefore, it is advisable to conduct a learning needs assessment on both the adult caregivers and the child when appropriate. Box 8.5 describes the components of a learning needs assessment. This is also a good time to establish rapport with the family, demonstrating your interest in them and your confidence in their ability to learn.

In addition to determining the language spoken in the home and use of eye and physical contact, investigate the following during the assessment:

- Who is the person caring for the child at home?
- Who is the authority figure in the family?
- What is the social support structure?
- Are there any special dietary needs and concerns?
- Are any alternative and complementary health practices used?
- Are any special clothes or other items used to help maintain health?
- What religious beliefs, ceremonies, and spiritual practices are important?

BOX 8.5 Learning Needs Assessment

Assess:

- Learner characteristics: Find out more about the child's and family's life and how the child's illness has affected it. Learn more about the child's and family's social, cultural, and spiritual values.
- Learner needs and readiness: This includes what the child and family want and need to know and what they know already; their readiness and willingness to learn; their motivation to learn and emotional concerns; and their capacity to learn, such as physical or cognitive abilities, including the ability to read and developmental level.
- Learning style: Determine how the child and family learn best, as well as preferred learning methods and modalities, such as audio, video, written, or modeling.
- Learning barriers: Identify cultural or language barriers, cognitive or physical disabilities, presence of pain, and lack of a support network.

This information will help the nurse direct their teaching and adapt their teaching style to meet the learning needs for each individual family. Learning needs can then be negotiated with the family and met based on the assessment. Pediatric issues encountered when teaching families of various backgrounds might include confusion regarding the use of the imperial versus the metric scale; preparing formulas and medicines using a "handful" or "pinch" of ingredients, rather than specific measurements such as a measuring cup or syringe; access to refrigeration for liquid antibiotics; and breastfeeding practices.

Share the assessment with all members of the interdisciplinary team so that the entire team can support the child's and family's learning. Although assessment generally takes place during the first or second meeting with the child and family, it should also occur with each encounter to check for any changes that may occur.

Malcolm Knowles outlined core learning principles to consider when teaching adults (Knowles et al., 2015). He found that instruction for adults needs to focus more on the process than on the content. Box 8.6 lists adult learner–centered principles.

LITERACY ISSUES

Adequate literacy skills are essential for child and family education, yet many people in America have marginal reading capabilities. In the United States, more than 54%

BOX 8.6 Specific Learning Principles Related to Adults

- **Adults are self-directed.** Adults value independence and want to learn on their own terms. Teaching strategies that include such concepts as role playing, demonstration, and self-evaluation are most helpful. Using this model, nurses can partner with families to ensure that education is interactive and adopt the role of facilitator, rather than lecturer.
- **Adults are problem-focused and task-oriented.** Adults learn best when they perceive there is a gap in their knowledge base and want information and skills to fill the gap. Providing a reason to learn can motivate families that appear slow to adhere to their child's care and education.
- **Adults are goal-oriented.** Adults learn best at a time when learning meets an immediate need. Presenting information in an organized, sequential, and timely fashion can often help families understand the importance of learning a particular piece of information or task.
- **Adults value past experiences and beliefs.** Adults bring an accumulated wealth of experiences to each health care encounter; this provides a rich base for new learning. Education should take into account a wide range of backgrounds. Appreciating and using individual differences during teaching encounters can help improve compliance and reduce resistance to educational goals.

Based on Knowles, M. S., Holton, E. F., 3rd, & Swanson, R. A. (2015). *The adult learner: The definitive classic in adult education and human resource development* (8th ed.). Routledge.

of adults ages 16 to 74 read at a level of the average sixth grader or below (Rothwell, 2020).

Even people with adequate literacy skills may have difficulty reading, understanding, and applying information to health care situations (Fig. 8.5). **Personal health literacy** is the ability to obtain, read, process, understand, and use health care information and services to make appropriate health care decisions (Centers for Disease Control and Prevention [CDC], 2022a). It is not simply the ability to read and understand health care information but also includes listening, oral, analytical, and decision-making skills. Applying these skills to health care situations allows the child and family to use the information to make well-informed health care decisions. The inability to comprehend health care information is an enormous problem for many Americans today, with 45% of all American adults having low health literacy (Betancourt et al., 2021).

Organizational health literacy refers to the ability of an organization to equitably empower an individual to find, read, process, understand, and use health care information and services to make appropriate health care decisions (CDC, 2022a). Practices that improve personal and organizational health literacy have the potential to decrease health disparities and improve health equity. Research has shown that health literacy leads to improved health outcomes, increased patient satisfaction, increased use of preventive health care, fewer dosing errors, decreased unneeded emergency room visits, and decreased hospital readmissions (Health Resources & Service Administration [HRSA], 2022). See the previous Healthy People 2030 box.

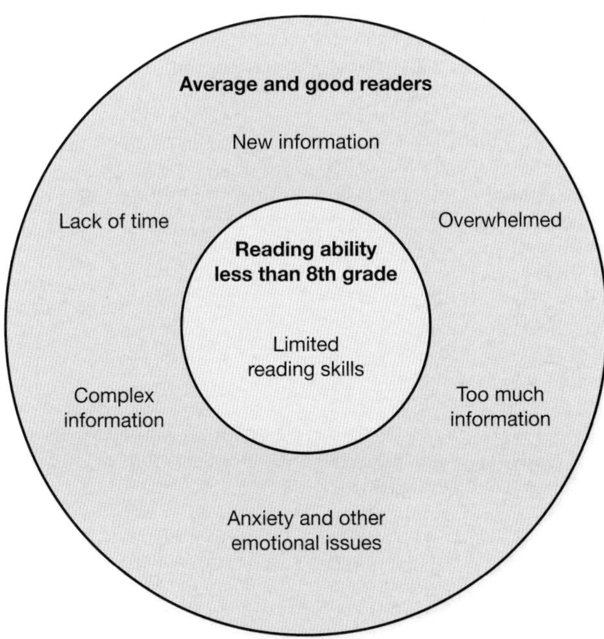

FIGURE 8.5 Factors contributing to poor health literacy.

TAKE NOTE!

Health literacy is a central focus of Healthy People 2030. One of the overarching goals is to "eliminate health disparities, achieve health equity, and attain health literacy to improve the health and well-being of all" (U.S. Department of Health and Human Services, n.d.).

Medical information is becoming increasingly complex, while the amount of time nurses have to spend with children is decreasing. Also, when unfamiliar information is introduced or when emotional distress is present, reading ability and understanding are further reduced. Therefore, all health care providers should use universal literacy precautions and focus on providing easy-to-understand information during every patient encounter.

TAKE NOTE!

Federal programs, such as the Affordable Care Act of 2010, the Department of Health and Human Services' National Action Plan to Improve Health Literacy, and the Plain Writing Act of 2010 have been developed to improve health literacy (CDC, 2022b; Koh et al., 2012).

Poor literacy and health literacy skills are difficult to recognize; appearance, verbal ability, employment status, and educational level cannot reliably indicate a person's literacy or health literacy abilities. Many people who do not read well go to great lengths to hide this. Poor health literacy affects all segments of the population, but certain groups such older adults, people with limited resources, people from underrepresented groups, people who are medically underserved, and people who speak English as a second language are at a higher risk (Hickey et al., 2018).

Potential indications of poor literacy skills include (Center for Health Care Strategies, 2024):

- Difficulty filling out registration forms, questionnaires, and consent forms; forms are incomplete, incorrect, or inaccurate
- Frequently missed appointments
- Nonadherence and lack of follow-up with treatment regimens
- History of medication errors
- Responses such as "I forgot my glasses" or "I'll read this when I get home"
- Inability to answer common questions about their treatment or medications
- Avoiding asking questions for fear of looking "stupid"

PLANNING EDUCATION

Once the assessment is completed, plan mutually agreed-upon, achievable, individualized learning goals and objectives. It is important that both the teacher and the learner believe the goals can be accomplished. Finding common ground and building a bridge between the child's and family's concerns and what the health care team believes they need to know is a critical part of an education plan. This is also an excellent time to consider which child education materials and resources can be used to maximize learning and retention. No single teaching method will suit every child and family; individualize educational methods to meet the learning needs and abilities of the audience.

Research has shown that 40% to 80% of verbal information given during an office visit is forgotten immediately and that almost half of what is retained is incorrect (Brega et al., 2015; Krontoft, 2021). Verbal instruction continues to be an important component of patient education, but it is not always effective and should be used along with other teaching methods. Using multiple teaching strategies, such as using videos, dolls, play therapy, or computer-based instruction along with written material at an appropriate reading level for the general population for future reference is beneficial. Visual aids, such as pictures and illustrations, are helpful and can assist those with low literacy. Planning child and family education should involve input from the entire interdisciplinary team when appropriate. Through good communication and collaboration, team members can work together to empower the child and family to become knowledgeable and skillful caregivers. Leaving behind the traditional path of teacher-centered education and providing family-centered education instead requires thought and skill.

PRACTICAL INTERVENTIONS TO ENHANCE LEARNING

The assessed needs and planned learning objectives lead to good teaching interventions. Evaluate these interventions frequently to ensure that the child and family are learning and meeting agreed-upon goals. Table 8.4 presents techniques that can help improve learning.

Experts, including the American Medical Association and the Agency for Healthcare Research and Quality (AHRQ), recommend practicing universal literacy precautions, which means delivering care as if everyone has low health literacy (AHRQ, 2010, reviewed 2020).

Nurses are in an excellent position to create a "blame-free" environment and offer help. It is entirely appropriate to say to the child or family member, "Many people have a problem reading and remembering the

TABLE 8.4 • Techniques to Improve Learning

Technique	Explanation
Slow down and repeat information often.	Since most of the education in a health care setting is done verbally, repeat important information at least four or five times.
Speak in conversational style using plain, nonmedical language.	When writing directions, write only several words, bullet points, or phrases. Use common, "living room-type" language containing one or two syllables whenever possible.
Group information and teach it in small amounts using logical steps.	This is especially important when there are large amounts of complex information for the family to learn. Teach for 10–15 minutes, give the learner a break, and return later to teach again.
Prioritize information and teach "survival skills" first.	Due to time constraints and multiple demands on the part of staff coupled with the rapid turnaround times of health care encounters for children, there rarely seems to be enough time to teach. Nurses must provide the child and family with the necessary information to meet their immediate needs. This may include information about: • The child's medical condition • Treatment information • Why the information is important • Possible problems, adverse effects, or concerns • What to do if problems arise • Whom to contact for further help, information, or supplies
Use visuals such as pictures, videos, and models.	Use visual resources to enhance and reinforce learning when available. Drawing simple pictures and charts or using alternative methods such as color coding often allows learning to occur for families who are having difficulty grasping information or concepts.
Teach using an interactive, "hands-on" approach.	When the learner uses hands-on practice or participates in care, learning occurs more quickly and easily. Learning first on a doll or model can ease anxiety and bolster self-confidence before care or procedures on the child are actually performed.
Teach using demonstration, return demonstration, and teach-back, tell-back.	Show the learner how to do something, have them show you what they learned to do, have the learner state in their own words what they know or have learned to do.

information on this teaching sheet (booklet, manual). Is this ever a problem for you?"

The nurse can take several steps to enhance learning, such as:

- Draw pictures or use medical illustrations.
- Use videos.
- Color-code medications or the steps of a procedure.
- Record audio.
- Repeat verbal information often and group it into small amounts.
- Teach a "back-up" family member.

TEACHING CHILDREN AND ADOLESCENTS

Teaching children and adolescents is a vital part of pediatric nursing practice. Children and adolescents have a great need for information about their illness as they attempt to master their anxiety and restore feelings of competency, self-confidence, and hope. As with adults, they learn best when their input is valued, and they are actively involved in the learning process. The age and developmental level of the child will determine the amount, format, and timing of the information given. Before beginning to teach a child, it is important to establish rapport and lay the foundation for good communication. Refer to the "Developmental Techniques for Communicating With Children" section and Table 8.3 for additional information related to communicating well with children and adolescents.

Teaching Preschool Children

When teaching young children, the nurse or family assumes part or all of the responsibility for what is learned, how it is learned, and when it is learned. Because they have vivid imaginations, young children often attempt to invent pieces of information, or they pick up bits and pieces of misinformation that can lead to false assumptions. Skillfully delivered and timed information can promote trust, calmness, and control in an otherwise apprehensive and uncooperative preschooler. Table 8.5 presents some general guidelines for teaching young children.

Teaching School-Age Children

Unless they are quite ill, school-age children often want to participate in their care. They have a need to cooperate and achieve. When teaching, speak directly to them and include them in the education plan. Teach the school-age child and parent together, as parents can often learn by observing the care being given and taught to their child. Table 8.6 provides some general guidelines to keep in mind when teaching school-age children.

Teaching Adolescents

Adolescents are particularly sensitive about maintaining body image and feelings of control and autonomy. This is especially important with health care processes and decisions that affect them. Table 8.7 gives guidelines to use when teaching adolescents.

TABLE 8.5 • General Teaching Tips for Young Children

Teaching Tips	Practical Application
Offer simple, concise, concrete explanations based on the assessed needs, questions, and developmental level of the child.	Use a child's senses and relate what a procedure will look, sound, smell, taste, or feel like ("The machine will sound very loud, like a big train").
Be honest, even when the information you need to convey is not positive. This helps the child form a bond of trust and confidence with caregivers.	Use the family's words that the child understands; use "soft words" ("This will feel warm" instead of "This will burn").
Time explanations to decrease anxiety and excess worry before the event. Avoid telling unpleasant news close to bedtime.	As a general rule, give toddlers information about procedures, medicines, and other interventions immediately beforehand; give 4–7-year-olds information 1 or 2 days in advance.
Parents know their child best. Eliciting information from them about their child's past behaviors and coping skills can often mean the difference between a positive and negative experience for their child.	Teach parents how to coach their child with pain management, visualization, or other methods of distraction when appropriate ("Remember when we went to the beach...").
Provide an active role for the child. This helps foster a child's sense of self-confidence and control over the situation.	Allow the child to help with simple self-care activities such as holding a dressing or piece of tape. Provide props and dolls to touch and feel as much as possible ("Your job is to keep your hands still").
Children's wishes must be respected when they verbalize or demonstrate that they do not want more information.	Keep explanations short and simple; know when to stop teaching.
Praise the child and let them know how much you appreciate their help and cooperation.	Use "please" and "thank you" often ("Thank you. I like the way you held still for me").

TABLE 8.6 • General Guidelines When Teaching School-Age Children

Teaching Tips	Practical Application
Allow the child some control and involvement in the decision-making process.	Offer choices whenever possible (taking the medicine with juice or milk), but don't offer choices when there are no alternatives (taking the medicine or not).
Children can relate present-day happenings to past experiences.	Use examples and past experiences that are familiar to the child ("Remember when you were first learning to swim…").
Achievement and accomplishment are important to children at this age, so anything they can be actively involved in will help them adjust and learn.	Provide an active role and allow the child to do as much of their care as possible. Use props, dolls, games, and computers to enhance learning.
At this age, most children are able to sequence, understand cause and effect, and make sense of time.	Teach children the steps involved and how long it will take ("Today I'm going to teach you how to change your dressing. This will help keep your cut clean. First, wash your hands …").
Gaining control over the situation and preparing mentally are important for the child's self-confidence.	Provide information 3–7 days in advance, depending on the child's age and developmental level.
Praise the child and let them know how much you appreciate their help and cooperation.	Use "please" and "thank you" often ("Thanks! You did a great job using your inhaler").

Remember Emma Moore, the 4-year-old described at the beginning of the chapter? What teaching methods would be appropriate to facilitate learning?

EVALUATING LEARNING

Teaching, even when done well, does not necessarily mean learning has occurred. Evaluation of learning is critical to ensure that the child and family have actually learned what was taught. In a health care setting, perform an evaluation with each educational encounter and adjust goals and interventions accordingly. The nurse, along with the rest of the interdisciplinary team, is responsible for child and family learning. Help ensure understanding by asking for feedback and offering an opportunity for questions. Also, assessing for signs of confusion, such as increased anxiety, can help evaluate learning. If the child or family has not learned the information, the health care team ensures that teaching strategies are adjusted so that the child or family does learn it.

The ultimate goal of education is a change in behavior on the part of the child and family; this change can occur in their level of knowledge, skill, or both. Evaluation can occur in several different ways, depending on the topic and the method of teaching. The child or family may:

- Demonstrate a skill, often referred to as return demonstration. Learning can quickly and easily be identified using this method.
- Repeat back or teach back the information using their own words.

TABLE 8.7 • General Guidelines When Teaching Adolescents

Teaching Tips	Practical Application
Allow adolescents to be in control and involved in the decision-making process.	Speak directly to adolescents; consider their input in all decisions about their care and education.
Adolescents can process abstract information and understand how their actions affect long-term outcomes.	Provide reasons why something is important, and discuss how their lives will be affected by their decision to take care of their health needs ("If you take your asthma medicine, you'll be better able to play tennis").
Adolescents are concerned about how they look and how they fit in with peers.	Collaborate with the adolescent to develop acceptable solutions and strategies for dealing with health issues that affect personal appearance and peer acceptance (e.g., wigs or head scarves for hair loss from chemotherapy).
Adolescents strive for independence and have personal values and ideologies that may conflict with those of parents and the medical community.	Expect some potential lack of adherence to the care plan, despite best educational efforts. Work together to achieve win–win outcomes of educational goals.

- Answer open-ended questions. Open-ended questions provide an opportunity to assess for missing or incorrect information. Open-ended questions are those that cannot be answered with a simple "yes" or "no."

Another option to evaluate learning is to provide a "pretend" scenario for the family, mentally placing them in their own home. Have them verbalize all the steps needed to care for their child, from routine care to handling an emergency situation. They will need to convey information accurately and completely as they walk through the steps necessary to provide care for their child independently at home.

DOCUMENTING EDUCATION FOR THE CHILD AND FAMILY

Documenting child care and education on the medical record is part of every nurse's professional practice and serves four main purposes. First and foremost, the child's medical record serves as a communication tool that the entire interdisciplinary team can use to keep track of what the child and family have learned already and what learning still needs to occur. Next, it serves to testify to the education the family has received if and when legal matters arise. Third, it verifies standards set by The Joint Commission, Centers for Medicare & Medicaid Services (CMS), and other accrediting bodies that hold health care providers accountable for child and family education activities. And last, it informs third-party payers of goods and services provided for reimbursement purposes.

Documentation of child and family education is imperative. It is the only way to ensure that the family's educational plan and objectives have been completed and that the family is ready for discharge. Documentation of child and family education should include such topics as follows:

- The learning needs assessment
- Information on the child's medical condition and plan of care
- Goals of child education and the dates goals are met
- Teaching method used and how it is received by child and family
- Medications, including drug–drug and drug–food interactions
- Modified diets and nutritional needs
- Safe use of medical equipment
- Follow-up care and community resources

CONSIDER THIS!

Elsa is a 5-year-old on your unit who was recently diagnosed with diabetes. She is getting ready to be discharged home at the end of the week. Her grandparents are her primary caregivers.

- What concerns regarding learning would you take into consideration during your assessment?
- Describe different teaching strategies you would utilize with Elsa and her family.
- How would you evaluate learning with Elsa and her family?

KEY CONCEPTS

- Atraumatic care focuses on minimizing stressors and separation from the family and promoting a sense of control for the child and family.
- Children and families need appropriate explanation and education before a procedure is performed. Preparation may include explaining the procedure as well as physically preparing the child. Appropriate preparation helps decrease the child's and family's anxiety, promote the child's cooperation, and support the child's and family's coping skills.
- A major aspect of preparation involves play.
- Include the child's parents in preparation because parents are usually the greatest source of comfort for the child.
- Be short, simple, and appropriate in explaining situations at the child's level of development. Explain what is to be done and what is expected of the child.
- Utilize a CLS when available.
- Family-centered care involves a beneficial partnership among the patient, family, and health care providers in planning, providing, and evaluating care.
- Family-centered care is based on the concept that the family is the primary source of strength and support for the child.
- Family-centered care includes respect for the child and family, recognition of cultural diversity, identification of the family's strengths, assistance with emotional and other support of the family, providing honest and unbiased information, and collaborating and empowering families.
- Maintain open and honest lines of communication with children and their families.
- Therapeutic communication involves the use of open-ended questions, reflection, paraphrasing, acknowledgment of emotions, and active listening.
- To communicate effectively with children, provide information and support on the child's developmental level and utilize age-appropriate methods.
- When communicating with parents, be honest. Parents want to feel valued and should be equal partners in the health care team.
- It is vital for the family to have knowledge about their child's health.
- The nurse should assess the family's culture and language before planning teaching. An interpreter may be needed if the family does not speak English. The nurse must assess each family's individual beliefs and practices rather than generalizing.
- The steps of health education are assessment of learning needs and styles, collaborative establishment of the goals and plan of education, implementation, evaluation, and documentation of education.

- Patient education begins with the first patient encounter and proceeds through discharge and beyond. Reassessment after each step or change in the process is critical to success.

REFERENCES AND RECOMMENDED READINGS

Agency for Healthcare Research and Quality. (2010, reviewed 2020). *AHRQ health literacy universal precautions toolkit.* https://www.ahrq.gov/health-literacy/improve/precautions/index.html

American Academy of Pediatrics. (2021). *Addressing low health literacy and limited English proficiency.* https://www.aap.org/en/practice-management/providing-patient--and-family-centered-care/addressing-low-health-literacy-and-limited-english-proficiency/

American Academy of Pediatrics, Committee on Hospital Care, Institute for Patient and Family-Centered Care. (2012, reaffirmed 2018). Policy statement: Patient and family-centered care and the pediatrician's role. *Pediatrics, 129*(2), 394–404. https://doi.org/10.1542/peds.2011-3084

Association of Child Life Professionals. (2022). *The child life profession: What is a certified child life specialist?* https://www.childlife.org/the-child-life-profession

Betancourt, J. R., Green, A. R., & Carillo, J. E. (2021). The patient's culture and effective communication. *UpToDate.* Retrieved November 9, 2022, from https://www.uptodate.com/contents/the-patients-culture-and-effective-communication

Brega, A. G., Barnard, J., Mabachi, N. M., Weiss, B. D., DeWalt, D. A., Brach, C., Cifuentes, M., Albright, K., & West, D. R. (2015). *AHRQ health literacy universal precautions toolkit* (2nd ed.). Agency for Healthcare Research and Quality. https://www.ahrq.gov/sites/default/files/publications/files/healthlittoolkit2_4.pdf

Centers for Disease Control and Prevention. (2022a). *What is health literacy.* https://www.cdc.gov/healthliteracy/learn/index.html

Centers for Disease Control and Prevention. (2022b). *CDC's health literacy action plan.* https://www.cdc.gov/healthliteracy/planact/cdcplan.html

Center for Health Care Strategies. (2024). *Health literacy fact sheets: Identifying limited health literacy.* https://www.chcs.org/media/2-Identifying-Limited-Health-Literacy_2024.pdf

Ernst, K. D., & AAP Committee on Hospital Care. (2020). Recommended for the care of pediatric patients in hospitals. *Pediatrics, 145*(4), e20200204. https://doi.org/10.1542/peds.2020-0204

Gaynard, L., Wolfer, J., Goldberger, J., Redbum, L., Laidley, L., & Thompson, R. (1998). *Psychosocial care of children in hospitals: Clinical practice manual from the ACCH Child Life Research Project* (1st ed.). Child Life Council.

Health Resources & Services Administration. (2022). *Health literacy.* https://www.hrsa.gov/about/organization/bureaus/ohe/health-literacy/index.html

Hickey, K. T., Masterson Creber, R. M., Reading, M., Sciacca, R. R., Riga, T. C., Frulla, A. P., & Casida, J. M. (2018). Low health literacy: Implications for managing cardiac patients in practice. *The Nurse Practitioner, 43*(8), 49–55. https://doi.org/10.1097/01.NPR.0000541468.54290.49

Knowles, M. S., Holton, E. F., 3rd, & Swanson, R. A. (2015). *The adult learner: The definitive classic in adult education and human resource development* (8th ed.). Routledge.

Koh, H. K., Berwick, D. M., Clancy, C. M., Baur, C., Brach, C., Harris, L. M., & Zerhusen, E. G. (2012). New federal policy initiatives to boost health literacy can help the nation move beyond the cycle of costly "crisis care". *Health Affairs, 31*(2), 434–443. https://doi.org/10.1377/hlthaff.2011.1169

Krontoft, A. (2021). How do patients prefer to receive patient education material about treatment, diagnosis and procedures?—A survey study of patients preferences regarding forms of patient education materials; leaflets, podcasts, and video. *Open Journal of Nursing, 11,* 809–827. https://doi.org/10.4236/ojn.2021.1110068

Kuo, D. Z., & Turchi, R. M. (2023). Children and youth with special health care needs. *UpToDate.* Retrieved October 17, 2023, from https://www.uptodate.com/contents/children-and-youth-with-special-health-care-needs

Levetown, M., & American Academy of Pediatrics Committee on Bioethics. (2008, reaffirmed 2017). Communicating with children and families: From everyday interactions to skill in conveying distressing information. *Pediatrics, 121*(5), e1441–e1460. https://doi.org/10.1542/peds.2008-0565

McPherson, G., & Thorne, S. (2000). Children's voices: Can we hear them? *Journal of Pediatric Nursing, 15*(1), 22–29. https://doi.org/10.1016/S0882-5963(00)80020-2

National Association of the Deaf. (2022). *Questions and answers for healthcare providers.* http://www.nad.org/issues/health-care/providers/questions-and-answers

Romito, B., Jewell, J., Jackson, M., & AAP Committee on Hospital Care; Association of Child Life Professionals. (2021). Child life services. *Pediatrics, 147*(1), e2020040261. https://doi.org/10.1542/peds.2020-040261

Rothwell, J. (2020). Assessing the economic gains of eradicating illiteracy nationally and regionally in the United States. *Gallup.* https://www.barbarabush.org/wp-content/uploads/2020/09/BBFoundation_GainsFromEradicatingIlliteracy_9_8.pdf

U.S. Department of Health and Human Services. (n.d.). *Healthy People 2030.* https://health.gov/healthypeople

Wong, D. (1995). *Whaley & Wong's nursing care of infants and children* (5th ed). Mosby.

DEVELOPING CLINICAL JUDGMENT

PRACTICING FOR NCLEX

1. When providing atraumatic care to a child, which action would be the most appropriate?
   a. Applying restraints for any procedure that would be uncomfortable
   b. Keeping the lights on in the child's room throughout the day and night
   c. Limiting the use of topical anesthetics for painful injections
   d. Allowing parents and children an informed choice about being together
2. When caring for children, how does the nurse best incorporate the concept of family-centered care?
   a. Encourages the family to allow the health care provider to make health care decisions for the child
   b. Uses the concepts of respect, family strengths, diversity, and collaboration with the family
   c. Advises the family to choose a pediatric provider who is on the child's insurance plan
   d. Recognizes that families undergoing stress related to the child's illness cannot make good decisions
3. When working with children and families, which are strategies for promoting therapeutic communication? Select all that apply.
   a. Detailed explanations
   b. Attentive listening
   c. Comforting touch
   d. Closed-ended questions
   e. Demonstrating empathy
   f. Acknowledging the child's emotions
4. The nurse is caring for a 2-year-old in the hospital, and the parent expresses concern that the toddler will be scared. Which response by the nurse would be most appropriate?
   a. "Don't worry; we practice family-centered and atraumatic care here."
   b. "We will do our best to minimize the stress your child experiences."
   c. "It will probably be upsetting for you as well, so you should stay home."
   d. "Our practice of atraumatic care will eliminate all pain and stress for your child."
5. When planning education for a child and their parents, what is the first step the nurse should take?
   a. Decide what procedures and medications the child will be discharged with.
   b. Determine the child's and family's learning needs and styles.
   c. Ask the family if they have ever performed this type of procedure.
   d. Tell the child and family what the goals of the teaching session are.
6. Which statement indicates the novice nurse has a good understanding of health literacy? Select all that apply.
   a. "Health literacy includes actions and skills created to help the educator."
   b. "Health literacy is not necessary for children."
   c. "Health care providers should practice universal health literacy."
   d. "Health literacy leads to improved health outcomes and may decrease health inequities."
   e. "Health literacy allows children and their families to use health information, not to just understand it."

CRITICAL THINKING EXERCISES

1. A 5-year-old is being admitted to your unit. The health care provider has ordered IV fluids along with laboratory work including a complete blood count, electrolytes, and a urine culture. As the nurse, how will you prepare the child and family before the procedure and support them during and after the procedure to promote the best outcomes and to ensure atraumatic care?
2. A 3-year-old from another country has become seriously ill while visiting the United States and will require a lengthy hospital stay. Describe the steps the nurse should take to communicate effectively with and provide extensive health care teaching to this child's family.

STUDY ACTIVITIES

1. Develop a teaching plan for one of the families you care for in the clinical setting. Be sure to follow the appropriate steps for providing education.
2. Interview a CLS about the effects that the traditional (not atraumatic) approach to restraining a child for procedures might have on a child of various ages.
3. Research the availability of language interpreters and translators in your local community, compiling a list of the available resources.

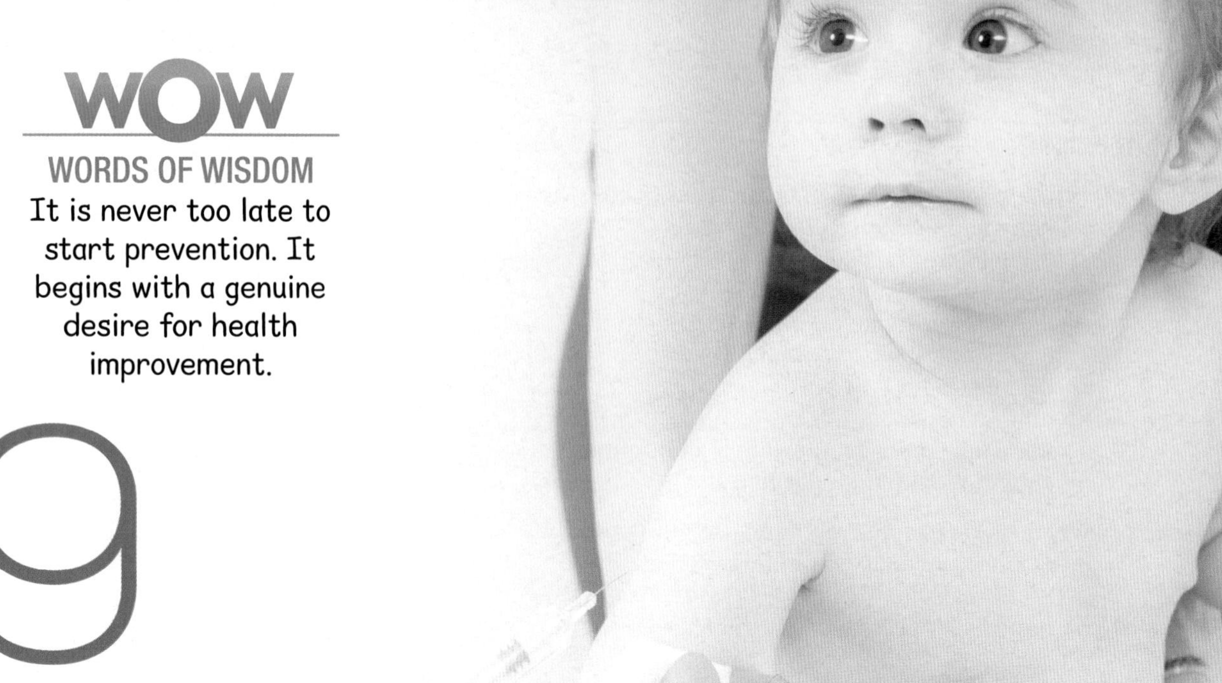

WOW

WORDS OF WISDOM

It is never too late to start prevention. It begins with a genuine desire for health improvement.

9

Health Supervision

LEARNING OBJECTIVES

Upon completion of the chapter, you will be able to:

1. Describe the principles of health supervision.
2. Identify challenges to health supervision for children with chronic illnesses.
3. List the three components of a health supervision visit.
4. Discuss developmental surveillance and developmental screening of children.
5. Demonstrate knowledge of the principles of immunization.
6. Identify barriers to immunization.
7. Explain key components of health promotion.
8. Describe the role of anticipatory guidance in health promotion.

KEY TERMS

active immunity
developmental screenings
developmental surveillance
immunity
medical home
passive immunity
risk assessment
screening tests
selective screening
universal screening

Three-year-old **Maya Randall** and 9-month-old **Evan Randall** are brought to the clinic by their parent. Maya was last seen in the clinic when she was 1 year old, and Evan has never been seen. The parent says that both children have been healthy, so they did not need to come to the clinic before this. Maya is complaining of a sore throat, which is what prompted today's visit.

PRINCIPLES OF HEALTH SUPERVISION

Health supervision involves providing services proactively with the goal of optimizing the child's level of functioning. It ensures the child is growing and developing appropriately, and it promotes the best possible health of the child by teaching parents and children about preventing injury and illness (e.g., proper immunizations and anticipatory guidance). This chapter is organized around the three components of health supervision: developmental surveillance and screening; injury and disease prevention; and health promotion. Health supervision of the child begins at birth and continues through adolescence. It is vital to every child and is most effective when the child has a centralized source of health care. Any place publicly accessible by children and families can be an appropriate setting for health supervision services—private health care providers' offices, community health departments, sliding-scale clinics, homeless shelters, day care centers, and schools. The framework for the health supervision visit is developed from national guidelines available through the U.S. Department of Health and Human Services (USDHHS), the American Medical Association (AMA), and the American Academy of Pediatrics (AAP). These organizations also provide guidelines for children with chronic illness and services and information regarding unique situations such as the internationally adopted child.

Wellness

The focus of pediatric health supervision is wellness. The health supervision visit provides an opportunity to maximize health promotion for the child, family, and community. Nurses have the ability to promote optimal health during these encounters. Health supervision visits must be viewed as part of a continuum of care, not as the accomplishment of isolated tasks.

Medical Home

A **medical home** is an approach to care that builds a long-term and comprehensive relationship with the family. This continuing relationship promotes trust between the pediatric care team and the family and leads to comprehensive, continuous, coordinated, and cost-effective care. The medical home is the setting that allows the highest level of health supervision. To be effective, the medical home must be accessible, family-centered, culturally effective, and community based. It must be integrated into the child's world, not adjacent to it. Characteristics of a medical home are displayed in Box 9.1.

BOX 9.1 Characteristics of a Medical Home

- Care accessible and in the child's community
- All insurance, including Medicaid, accepted
- Family-centered care provided
- Child or family able to speak directly to the health care provider when needed
- Partnership based on mutual trust and respect between the family and pediatric care team
- Preventive care activities provided
- Ambulatory and inpatient care are accessible.
- Continuity of care from infancy through adolescence
- Coordinated care with other care providers
- Comprehensive care where all health care needs can be met: well care, sick care, and behavioral care
- Availability of subspecialty consultation and referrals
- Work with family to meet the nonmedical and medical needs of the child and family.
- Interactive relationships with school and community agencies
- A centralized database containing all pertinent information
- Concern and compassion for the well-being of the child and family expressed
- Respect for family's cultural and religious beliefs.

Adapted from American Academy of Pediatrics, National Resource Center for Patient and Family Centered Medical Home. (2022). What is medical home. https://www.aap.org/en/practice-management/medical-home/medical-home-overview/what-is-medical-home/

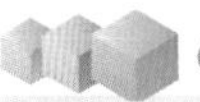
Concept Mastery Alert

Medical Home

A pediatric medical home provides continuity of care from infancy through adolescence. A medical home contains a centralized database that contains all information about a child that pertains to their health status.

Partnerships

The child is the focus of the health supervision visit. However, the child's health is linked to the needs and resources of their family and community. For instance, if the family is in turmoil because of divorce, drug misuse, or parental health problems, the child is less likely to receive the attention and energy that they need to thrive. Likewise, a community with high federal poverty levels, poor infrastructure, and lack of resources will not be able to provide the support services needed to allow children to reach their full potential. To be effective, the nurse must offer commitment and develop an ongoing partnership with the child, family, and community. These partnerships allow for mutual goal setting, marshaling of resources, and development of optimal health practices.

The partnership between the child and the health supervision team develops over time. In infancy, the family is the surrogate for the child in the partnership. The child's participation in the partnership increases at a rate that is developmentally appropriate. The child's increasing influence in the partnership allows the nurse to tailor health supervision to the child's needs. The partnership allows the child to take increasing responsibility for their personal health and optimizes health promotion.

Nurses must validate and enhance the role of family members as they influence and inform the child's concept of wellness. The health care community must involve the family to have a significant impact on a child's health. The family wants the best possible outcome for their child, and health care decisions are based on the knowledge they possess. The nurse can greatly facilitate trust by acknowledging that the family has unique insights to offer on their child's health. Nurses can also strengthen the partnership between the family and the health care community by recognizing the family's healthy practices, addressing their health issues, and strengthening their skills. By contributing to the partnership, both the nurse and the family enhance the chance of success for health care plans, but families are the ones who must implement any health care strategy and know what expected outcomes are reasonable. Their feedback is invaluable to formulating an effective long-term health supervision plan that optimizes their child's wellness.

TAKE NOTE!

Observe the parent–child interaction during the health supervision visit. The nurse can learn much about the family dynamic by observing the family for behavioral clues:

- Does the parent make eye contact with the infant?
- Does the parent anticipate and respond to the infant's needs?
- Are parents effective when dealing with a toddler's temper tantrum?
- Do the parents' comments increase the school-age child's sense of self-worth?

Behavioral observations are crucial to the proper assessment of the family's needs and issues.

Partnerships between the community and the health promotion team benefit the community as well as individual children. When nurses develop partnerships with community agencies such as schools, places of worship, and ancillary health facilities, barriers to care can be overcome. The nurse becomes aware of available resources in the community that can benefit an individual family. With input from community partners, the nurse can perform an assessment of the community's needs. The assessment then provides the foundation for the development of community-based health promotion programs. These programs expand the resources of the community, which in turn enhances the health of its members.

Special Issues in Health Supervision

Special issues in health supervision include cultural influences, community influences, health supervision and the child with a chronic illness, and health supervision and the child who was internationally adopted.

Cultural Influences on Health Supervision

A person's definition of health is influenced by their culture. Successful interactions result when the nurse is aware of the beliefs and interactive styles that are often present in members of a specific culture. If the goals of the health care plan are not consistent with the health belief system of the family, the plan has little chance of success. Optimal wellness for the child requires the nurse and the family to partner to establish a mutually acceptable plan of care. A plan must balance the cultural beliefs and practices of the family with those of the health care establishment. The nurse must possess cultural respect, humility, and sensitivity for the partnership to be successful.

Most health promotion and disease prevention strategies in the United States have a future-based orientation and view the child as an active and controlling agent in their own health. This may reflect many families in the United States, but the nurse must be prepared to develop strategies that are meaningful to children whose cultures do not align with this orientation. Significant numbers of children belong to cultures with a present-based orientation. These cultures are more concerned about what is going on now. For these children and families, health promotion activities need shorter-term goals and outcomes to be useful. Families with a fatalistic worldview will see any actions on their part as ineffective. They may feel that a higher power controls their fate and that health is a gift to be appreciated, not a goal to be pursued. Certain cultures believe health is the result of being in harmony within oneself and the larger universe. From this viewpoint, taking a medication or receiving a treatment may not be perceived as an effective way to restore health because it does not address the problem of being "out of harmony." It is important to remember that each individual does not necessarily subscribe to all of the beliefs and practices of their cultural group. The nurse should explore each child's and family's specific beliefs during the health interview.

Community Influences on Health Supervision

The child is a member of a community as well as a family and a culture. Each community has unique strengths, weaknesses, and values. A community can be a contributor to a child's health or the cause of their illnesses. The child's health cannot be totally separated from the health of the surrounding community.

Ideally, the child's medical home is within the family's community. If home and access to medical care are close, barriers such as lack of transportation, expense of travel, and time away from the parents' workplace are reduced. Having the medical home within the community facilitates bonds between the health team and schools, places of worship, and support services and agencies. Community support and resources are necessary for children with significant problems. A close working relationship between the child's health care provider and community agencies is an enormous benefit to the child (see the "Partnerships" section).

The community assessment may reveal problems that are causing or contributing to the child's health problems. A deteriorating infrastructure can contribute to decreased access to care and increased risk of injury or illness. Poverty has been linked to low birth weight and can lead to food insecurity and hunger or higher weight, among other health problems (Carlson & Neuberger, 2021). Housing is an important social determinant of health. Substandard housing can be directly related to lead poisoning and asthma, for example (Bryant-Stephens et al., 2021; National Center for Healthy Housing, 2022). A thorough knowledge of the family's community is needed before a health surveillance program can be effective.

Health Supervision and the Child With Chronic Illness

Effective health supervision must be responsive to the individual child's situation. The child with a chronic illness needs to be assessed repeatedly to determine their health maintenance needs. These assessments determine the frequency of visits and types of interventions needed. The impact of the illness on the child's functional health patterns determines whether standard health supervision visits need to be augmented.

An effective partnership among the child's medical home, family, and community is vital for a child with a chronic illness. Coordination of specialty care, community agencies, and family support networks enhances the quality of life and health of these children. Access to care and services minimizes the risk of injury from the illness. Support groups and community-based resources optimize the family's adaptation to the stressors of chronic illness.

Comprehensive health supervision includes frequent psychosocial assessments. Issues to be covered include:

- Health insurance coverage
- Transportation to health care facilities
- Financial stressors
- Family coping
- School's response to the chronic illness

These are often stressful and emotionally charged issues. The nurse with a trusting and ongoing relationship with the child and family is in the best position to help with these issues. The nurse can assist the family to find financial and medical assistance programs, take advantage of community resources, and participate in support groups. The nurse can also educate school personnel about the child's illness and assist them in maximizing the child's potential for academic success.

Health Supervision and the Child Adopted Internationally

In 2021, approximately 1,785 children were adopted from countries outside the United States, many from areas with a high prevalence of infectious diseases (Intercountry Adoption, Bureau of Consular Affairs, U.S. Department of State, 2022). International adoptions have been decreasing over the past 10 years, and many countries ceased adoptions during the COVID-19 pandemic. In 2021, Colombia supplied nearly half of all international adoptees, followed by India, Ukraine, and South Korea (Intercountry Adoption, Bureau of Consular Affairs, U.S. Department of State, 2022).

Health supervision of the child who is internationally adopted must include comprehensive screening for infectious diseases and disorders of growth and development, along with dental, vision, hearing, and any further testing based on diseases common in their country of origin (Schulte, 2020). A complete blood cell count and blood lead level screening in young infants is also recommended (Schulte, 2020). A thorough review of immunization records should be performed. Intestinal parasites are a common problem, and infected children are frequently symptom-free, so a thorough history and physical examination along with universal screening is recommended (Schulte, 2020).

Universal screening for hepatitis B, C, and A; varicella virus; HIV; syphilis; and tuberculosis infections is recommended (Schulte, 2020). Due to lack of resources in the home country, screening and treatment for these diseases are sporadic and ineffective. If testing is documented, it is likely to be unreliable. Testing supplies may have been outdated or improperly stored. Also, the test may have been performed before the child's seroconversion occurred.

Proper screening is important not only to the child's health but also to the adopting family and the larger community. Screening is recommended within the first few weeks of the child's arrival in the United States.

COMPONENTS OF HEALTH SUPERVISION

Developmental surveillance and screening, injury and disease prevention, and health promotion are the critical components of health supervision for children. Health supervision visits for children without health problems and with appropriate growth and development are recommended at birth, within the first week of life, by 1 month, then at 2 months, 4 months, 6 months, 9 months, 12 months, 15 months, 18 months, 24 months, 30 months, and then yearly until age 21 (Bright Futures/ American Academy of Pediatrics [AAP], 2022). Children with disabilities or concerns will have more frequent and intensive visits. Health supervision visits include assessment of physical health along with intellectual and social development and parent–child interaction.

Each health supervision visit will include:

- A history and physical assessment, including head circumference (until 2 years of age), height, and weight
- Developmental surveillance or screening and behavioral–social–emotional screening
- Sensory screening (vision and hearing)
- Appropriate at-risk screening (such as lead screening, anemia screening, tuberculin test, hypertension screening, cholesterol screening)
- Immunizations
- Health promotion/anticipatory guidance (injury prevention, violence prevention, nutrition counseling) (Bright Futures/AAP, 2022)

Disease prevention and health promotion are concepts well established in adult health supervision. Injury prevention and developmental surveillance/screening are additional components of pediatric health supervision visits that help every child achieve their optimal state of wellness.

Developmental Surveillance and Screening

Developmental surveillance is an ongoing collection of skilled observations made over time during health care visits. Components include:

- Noting and addressing parental concerns
- Obtaining a developmental history
- Making accurate observations
- Consulting with relevant professionals

Developmental screenings are brief assessment procedures that identify children who warrant more intensive assessment and testing. Developmental screening assessments may be observational or by caregiver report (Fig. 9.1).

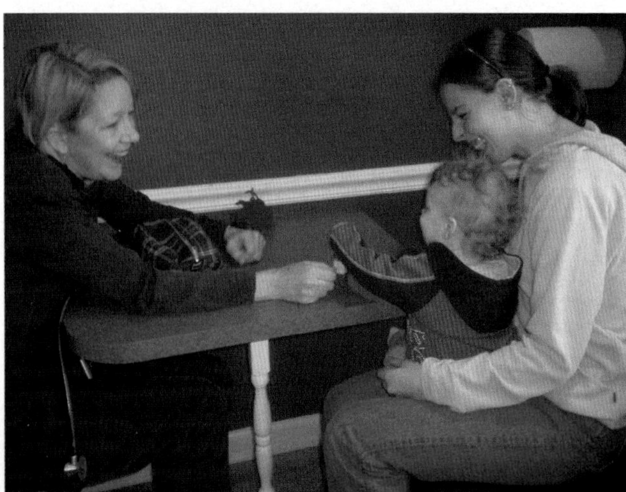

FIGURE 9.1 Developmental screening provides the opportunity for the nurse to identify problems in the child's development.

Development, or the emergence of the child's abilities, is a longitudinal process. Within the trust and security of the medical home, family and health care providers can share observations and concerns. In collaboration, the family and the health care provider observe the child's accomplishments or milestones over time. Data collection for developmental surveillance of infants and young children is performed through developmental questionnaires, health care provider observations, and a thorough physical examination. School records and test results can provide academic performance data for the older child. Input from teachers, coaches, and other adults involved with the child can give insight into the child's emotional and social development. Early identification of developmental delays leads to improved outcomes (Zubler et al., 2022).

When developmental delay is suspected, frequent developmental surveillance is warranted. Reemphasizing parental roles and responsibilities fosters cooperation and adherence. It is therefore crucial that parents understand the need for frequent assessments. A pattern of developmental delays warrants a formal evaluation.

The pediatric nurse must understand expected growth and development and become proficient at screening for problems related to development. The historical information obtained from the parent or primary caregiver about developmental milestones may identify risks for developmental delay. To access the most recent developmental milestone checklists, go to the Developmental Milestones website of the Centers for Disease Control and Prevention (CDC). Special attention to developmental surveillance is recommended at 4 to 5 years of age before a child enters school (Lipkin et al., 2020). If at any time there is a concern about development or a developmental delay is suspected, developmental screening should occur.

TAKE NOTE!

In 2022, the CDC's Learn the Signs. Act Early. program provided funding for the AAP to revise its developmental surveillance checklists. The goal was to provide milestone checklists when most children (at least 75%) would be expected to attain a milestone. In the past, the checklist incorporated milestones that 50% of children met, and this may have led to delays in diagnosis and a "wait-and-see" approach. Additional goals included aligning the developmental checklist with the recommended AAP health supervision visits by adding 15-and 30-month checklists and clarifying milestones, eliminating repetition of milestones across ages, and eliminating warning signs to minimize confusion (Zubler et al., 2022).

Factors placing the infant or toddler at risk for developmental problems include:

- Birth weight less than 1.5 kg
- Gestational age less than 33 weeks
- Central nervous system abnormality
- Hypoxic ischemic encephalopathy
- Alcohol or drug misuse by the pregnant parent
- Hypertonia
- Hypotonia
- Hyperbilirubinemia requiring exchange transfusion
- Kernicterus
- Congenital malformations
- Symmetric intrauterine growth deficiency
- Perinatal or congenital infection
- Suspected sensory impairment
- Chronic (more than 3 months) otitis media with effusion
- Inborn error of metabolism
- HIV infection
- Lead level above 5 mg/dL
- Inappropriate parental concern about developmental issues (e.g., not allowing a developmentally appropriate 3-year-old to feed themselves)
- Parent with less than high school education
- Single parent
- Sibling with developmental problems
- Parent with developmental disability or mental illness

Infants or children with any of these risk factors should be screened carefully for developmental delays. This screening should occur in a prospective manner, with screenings occurring at frequent intervals to identify concerns early.

TAKE NOTE!

Any child who "loses" a developmental milestone—for example, the child able to sit without support who now cannot—needs an immediate full evaluation, since this may indicate a significant neurologic problem.

A number of developmental screening tools are available to guide the nurse in assessing development. Screening tools can be general and covering all developmental domains or targeted and focusing on one area of development. Table 9.1 provides a few examples of

TABLE 9.1 • Common Developmental Screening Tools Used in Primary Care

Age	Screening Tool	Definition	Nursing Implications
Birth–66 months	Survey of Well-Being of Young Children	Simple questions to screen for social–emotional, developmental milestones, as well as autism and family risk (including parent mental health concerns, substance use, food insecurity, and family violence)	A parental-report tool, requires scoring manually or electronically after completion to determine risk level or presence of delays; written at sixth-grade reading level; takes about 10 minutes to complete and 5 minutes to score; available in several languages
Birth–66 months	Ages and Stages Questionnaire (ASQ), 3rd edition	Assesses communication, gross motor, fine motor, personal–social, and problem-solving skills	A parental-report screening tool, scored by the nurse after completion to determine child's progress in each of the developmental areas; written at a fourth- to sixth-grade reading level; takes 10–15 minutes to complete, 2–3 minutes to score; many languages available
Birth–7 years, 11 months	Parents' Evaluation of Developmental Status (PEDS)	Screens for a wide range of developmental, behavioral, social–emotional/mental health, self-help, early academic, and family issues	A short 10-question parental-report screening tool that can also be used in nurse interview format. Effective regardless of parents' level of education, income, race, marital status, or child's age or birth order; written at a fourth- to fifth-grade reading level; 5 minutes to complete, 2 minutes to score; available in Spanish
Birth–7 years, 11 months	Parents' Evaluation of Developmental Status -Developmental Milestones (PEDS-DM)	Screens for fine motor, gross motor, expressive and receptive language, self-help, social–emotional issues and reading and math issues for older children	A short six- to eight-question parental-report screening tool that can also be used in nurse interview format Includes an assessment level version for use in neonatal intensive care unit and early childhood intervention programs; written at a second- to fourth-grade reading level; 5 minutes to complete, 1 minute to score; available in Spanish

Adapted from Aites, J., & Schonwald, A. (2022). Developmental-behavioral surveillance and screening in primary care. *UpToDate*. Retrieved December 12, 2022, from https://www.uptodate.com/contents/developmental-behavioral-surveillance-and-screening-in-primary-care

common developmental screening tools. The AAP provides an online screening tool finder in their Screening Technical Assistance and Resource (STAR) Center, which can be found on their website. Many screening methods assist the nurse in identifying infants and children who may have developmental delays, thus allowing for prompt identification and referral for evaluation. Additional data can be used to determine a school-age child's developmental level, including handwriting samples, ability to draw, school performance, and social skills.

In addition to developmental and behavioral surveillance at every visit, the AAP recommends performing the following additional screening tests. Perform a developmental screening at 9, 18, and 30 months and a screening test for autism spectrum disorder (ASD) with a standardized developmental tool at 18 and 24 months or at any point that concerns about ASD are raised (Lipkin et al., 2020). Also, perform a risk assessment for tobacco, alcohol, and drug use at every visit from 11 to 21 years of age, as well as a depression screening at every visit from 12 to 21 years of age. For the latest recommendations for preventive pediatric health care and links to recommended screening tools, visit the AAP website for the preventive care/periodicity schedule.

Injury and Disease Prevention

Disease prevention is defined as interventions performed to protect children from a disease or to identify it at an early stage and lessen its consequences. These interventions are determined by the results of the nurse's assessment, nationally accepted practice guidelines, and the family's goals. Components of disease prevention include screening tests and immunizations.

Injury prevention is accomplished primarily through education, anticipatory guidance, and physical changes in the environment. Injuries can be unintentional (poisoning, falls, or drowning) or intentional (child abuse, homicide, or suicide). The types of injuries a child is most likely to encounter vary greatly among age groups. Although aggressive public health initiatives have decreased mortality rates of childhood unintentional injuries significantly in the past 50 years, injury is still the leading cause of death in children and adolescents, and rates remain higher in some populations. Therefore, continued vigilance and public health action remain necessary (CDC, 2021a). The nurse, in partnership with the family and the community, can have an enormous impact on child safety. Specific interventions are discussed in Chapters 3 to 7.

Screening Tests

Screening tests are procedures or laboratory analyses used to identify children with a certain condition. These tests are done to ensure that no child with the disorder is missed. They have a high sensitivity (a high false-positive rate) and a low specificity (a low false-negative rate). If a screening test is positive, follow-up tests with higher specificity are performed. A **risk assessment** is performed by the health care provider or nurse practitioner in conjunction with the child and includes objective as well as subjective data to determine the likelihood that the child will develop a condition.

In **universal screening**, an entire population is screened regardless of the child's individual risk. This type of screening is performed when a reliable risk assessment procedure is not available. In contrast, **selective screening** is done when a risk assessment indicates the child has one or more risk factors for the disorder.

TAKE NOTE!

To increase cooperation from young children during screenings, set up a reward system. Easy-to-do rewards include:

- Stamping the back of the child's hand with a "smiley face"
- Making an eye cover by placing two stickers back to back over a tongue blade and letting the child keep the cover after the screening
- Copying a design onto a sheet of paper and letting the child take it home to color
- Letting the child play with a simple device such as a penlight or stethoscope

NEWBORN SCREENING

Newborn screening is performed on every newborn at birth for health disorders that would not have been found otherwise. These disorders, if left untreated, would lead to significant morbidity or death. State law determines which metabolic screening tests are mandatory in that state. The March of Dimes would like to see all states provide newborn screening for 35 health conditions (March of Dimes, 2020). Go online to Baby's First Test to see a list of conditions tested for by state. To decrease variability across states, the United States Secretary of the USDHHS has established the Recommended Uniform Screening Panel (RUSP) (Kemper, 2021). For the latest RUSP, visit the Health Resources & Services Administration website at www.hrsa.gov. These disorders include:

- Amino acid metabolism disorders (these newborns cannot process amino acids) such as classic phenylketonuria, maple syrup urine disease, and homocystinuria
- Organic acid metabolism disorders (these newborns cannot metabolize food correctly) such as isovaleric acidemia, glutaric acidemia, and propionic acidemia
- Fatty acid oxidation disorders (these newborns cannot change fat to energy) such as medium-chain acyl-CoA

dehydrogenase deficiency, trifunctional protein deficiency, and carnitine uptake defect

- Hemoglobinopathies (these newborns have problems with their red blood cells) such as sickle cell anemia and hemoglobin S/beta-thalassemia
- Lysosomal storage disorders (these newborns cannot break down certain types of complex sugars) such as mucopolysaccharidosis type-1 (MPS 1) and Pompe disease
- Endocrine disorders (these newborns have problems with certain glands that help the body make hormones) such as congenital adrenal hyperplasia (CAH) and congenital hypothyroidism
- Others such as biotinidase deficiency, classical galactosemia, cystic fibrosis, critical congenital heart defect, severe combined immunodeficiency (SCID), spinal muscular atrophy, and hearing loss

During the initial health supervision visit, the nurse should confirm that newborn screening was performed prior to discharge from the birthing unit. If the test was not performed or was performed before 48 hours of age, the screening should be performed at that visit. The metabolic screening results need to be noted in the child's permanent record at the medical home.

HEARING SCREENING

The AAP recommends hearing screening of all infants. Hearing loss is a common condition in newborns, and even mild hearing loss can cause serious delays in social and emotional development, language acquisition, and cognitive function (Vohr, 2022). Identification of hearing loss by 6 months of age is crucial to reduce the impact on the child's development (Delaney, 2022). Refer to Healthy People 2030 box. Targeted screening based on risk factors will identify only 50% to 75% of infants with hearing loss, and with reliable screening tests available, universal screening has been implemented (Vohr, 2022). Screening should be done before discharge from the birthing unit; if not, the newborn needs to be screened before 1 month of age. Behavioral observations of the infant's response to sounds, such as a ringing bell or clapping hands, are not sensitive enough to preclude mild to moderate hearing loss (Delaney, 2022). Accepted methodologies for screening newborn hearing are displayed in Table 9.2.

TABLE 9.2 • Hearing Screening Methods

Test Name	Age Group	Characteristics	Nursing Implications
Automated auditory brain stem response (AABR)	Newborn–6 months	Measures electroencephalographic waves; electrodes placed on forehead, mastoid, and nape of neck Click stimulus delivered via earphones. Test results may be affected by ear debris.	Infant must be quiet (sedation may be needed). Can be conducted in presence of background noise
Otoacoustic emissions (OAEs)	Newborn–6 months or developmentally delayed children at the infant's level of functioning	The machine produces clicks that stimulate cilia in the cochlea and measures the response.	Infant must be quiet. Test results may be inaccurate in first 24 hours of life. Not sufficient to detect neural hearing loss
Visual reinforcement audiometry (VRA)	6 months–2 years	Visual reward is linked to a tone signal. Child looks to the visual reward in response to the tone. Reward is activated, reinforcing the response.	Child must be alert and happy for best results. Schedule for after sleep/rest period.
Tympanometry	Over 7 months	Measures tympanic membrane mobility and determines middle ear pressure	The probe must form a seal with the canal. The child must remain still to obtain a valid result.
Conditioned play audiometry (CPA)	2–4 years	Similar to VRA except uses "listening games" Child does listening game at the tone and receives social reward. May be used when developmental age is 2 years	See Nursing Implications for VRA.

(continued)

TABLE 9.2 • Hearing Screening Methods (*continued*)

Test Name	Age Group	Characteristics	Nursing Implications
Pure-tone (conventional) audiometry	4 years and older	Measures hearing acuity through a range of frequencies and intensities Child must wear earphones. Performed in a soundproof room if possible	Teach the child the desired motor response before screening. Administer conditioning trials. Offer two presentations of stimulus to ensure reliability. At a minimum, screen 1,000-, 2,000-, and 4,000-Hz levels at 20 dB
Whisper test	4 years and older	One ear is occluded. Examiner stands behind the child and whispers a word. The child must accurately repeat the whispered word.	The child must be in a quiet room and away from distractions. The child should be alert and well rested for accurate results. Consider a reward system to increase adherence.
Weber test	6 years and older	Place a vibrating tuning fork in the middle of the top of the head. Ask if the sound is in one ear or both ears. The sound should be heard in both ears.	The child must understand the instructions and be able to cooperate.
Rinne test	6 years and older	Place a vibrating tuning fork on the mastoid process to assess bone conduction. The child signals when the sound is gone. Next, place a vibrating tuning fork outside the ear to test air conduction. The child signals when the sound is gone. For a passing test, air conduction time should be twice as long as bone conduction time.	The child must understand the instructions and be able to cooperate.

HEALTHY PEOPLE 2030

Objective	Nursing Significance
Increase the proportion of newborns who are screened for hearing loss by no later than age 1 month. Increase the proportion of infants who did not pass the hearing screening test that receive diagnostic audiologic evaluation for hearing loss no later than age 3 months. Increase the proportion of infants with confirmed hearing loss who are enrolled for intervention services no later than age 6 months.	• Determine results of newborn hearing screening at first newborn check-up. • Refer any infant with possible hearing deficit for further evaluation. • Ensure infants with hearing loss receive appropriate augmentation (hearing aids). • Ensure all children and adolescents receive hearing screenings with well-child check-ups as appropriate.

Healthy People Objectives retrieved from http://www.healthypeople.gov

Screening for hearing loss in older children begins with a history from the primary caregivers. If any problems are noted, audiometry should be performed. When the child is capable of following simple commands reliably, the nurse can perform some basic procedures to screen for hearing loss. The whisper test is easy to perform but in order to be valid requires a quiet room that is away from distractions. The Weber and Rinne tests are typically performed together and can be used to screen for sensorineural or conductive hearing loss. Refer to Table 9.2, for hearing screening methods.

Universal hearing screening with objective testing is recommended at ages 4, 5, 6, 8, and 10 (Bright Futures/AAP, 2022). Screening with audiometry should occur once between the ages of 11 and 14, once between 15 and 17, and again between 18 and 21 (Bright Futures/AAP, 2022). See Box 9.2 for examples of risk assessment. More frequent screening is recommended if there is any behavior that indicates the child's hearing may be impaired. Repeated hearing screenings are recommended if a child has risk factors for acquired hearing loss such as those listed in Box 9.3.

BOX 9.2 Hearing Risk Assessment

Ages 3 Months–4 Years

- Auditory skill monitoring
- Developmental surveillance
- Assessment of parental concerns

Age 4 Years

- Difficulty hearing on the telephone
- Difficulty hearing people in a noisy background
- Frequent asking of others to repeat themselves
- Turning the television up too loudly

BOX 9.3 Risk Factors for Hearing Impairment

- Family history of hearing loss
- Prenatal or neonatal infection
- Anomalies of the head, face, or ears (craniofacial anomalies)
- Low birth weight (<1.5 kg)
- Hyperbilirubinemia requiring exchange transfusion
- Ototoxic medications
- Low Apgar scores: 4 or less at 1 minute or 6 or less at 5 minutes
- Mechanical ventilation or extracorporeal membrane oxygenation (ECMO)
- Neonatal intensive care unit admission lasting 5 days
- Syndrome associated with hearing loss
- Head trauma
- Bacterial meningitis
- Neurodegenerative disorders
- Persistent pulmonary hypertension
- Otitis media with effusion for 3 months

Adapted from Delaney, A. M. (2022). Newborn hearing screening. *eMedicine.* https://emedicine.medscape.com/article/836646-overview?form=fpf; Vohr, B. R. (2022). Screening the newborn for hearing loss. *UpToDate.* Retrieved December 13, 2022, from https://www.uptodate.com/contents/screening-the-newborn-for-hearing-loss

VISION SCREENING

Newborns with ocular structural abnormalities are at high risk for vision impairment. Vision screening with objective testing is recommended at ages 3, 4, 5, 6, 8, 10, 12, and 15 years, with risk assessment being performed at all other health supervision visits (Bright Futures/AAP, 2022). The screening procedures for children younger than 3 years of age or for nonverbal children involve evaluating the child's ability to fixate on and follow objects. The neonate should be able to fixate on an object approximately 25 to 30 cm (10 to 12 in) from the face. After fixation, the infant should be able to follow the object to the midline. By 2 months of age, the infant should be able to follow the object 180 degrees. The technique of photoscreening can help identify problems such as ocular malalignment, refractive error, and lens and retinal problems.

TAKE NOTE!

Use objects with black-and-white patterns when performing vision screening on an infant younger than 6 months. The infant's vision at this age is more attuned to high-contrast patterns than to colors. Try checkerboard patterns or concentric circles. Animal figures like pandas and Dalmatians also work well.

After the age of 3 years, a variety of standardized age-appropriate vision screening charts are available. These charts include the "tumbling E" and Allen figures (Fig. 9.2A, B). These charts allow for a more precise vision assessment and aid the nurse in identifying preschool

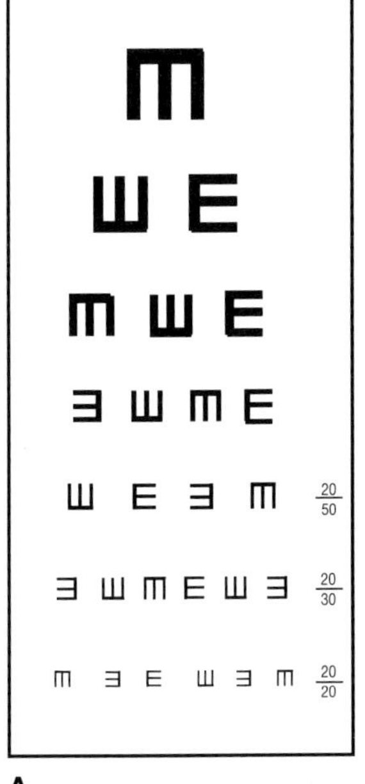

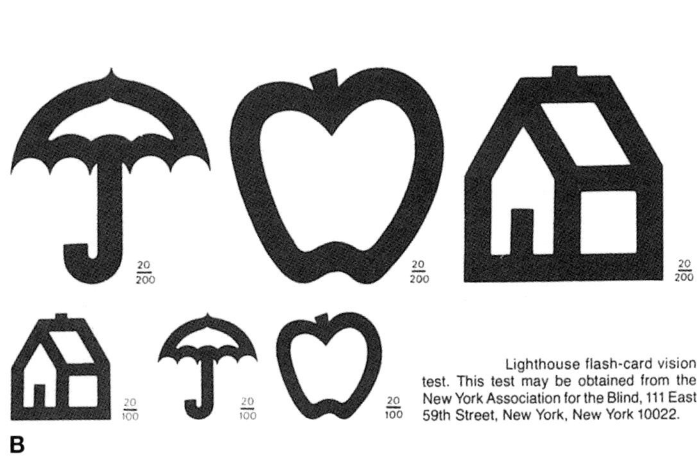

E
H N
D F N
P T X Z
U Z D T F
D T F P D H
P H U N T D Z
C

FIGURE 9.2 **A.** The "tumbling E" chart is appropriate for children who do not yet know the alphabet but who can follow instructions to indicate the direction in which the arms of the "E" are pointing. **B.** A picture chart similar to the Allen object recognition chart is appropriate for vision screening in the preschool-age child. **C.** The Snellen eye chart may be used for children 6 years or older who know the alphabet. The test can be obtained at www.preventblindness.org/children or by calling 1-800-331-2020.

TABLE 9.3 • Vision Screening Tools

Screening Tool	Age	Nursing Implications
Snellen letters or numbers	School-age	The child must know their letters or numbers for the test to be valid.
"Tumbling E"	Preschool	The child points in the direction that the "E" is facing.
LEA symbols or Allen figures	Preschool	The child should first identify the pictures with both eyes at a comfortable distance prior to monocular testing to ensure validity of the test.
Ishihara	School-age	Screens for color discrimination (numbers composed of dots, hidden within other dots)
Color Vision Testing Made Easy (CVTME)	Preschool	Uses dot pictures like the Ishihara, but instead of numbers has easily identified shapes embedded in the dots

children with visual acuity problems. By age 5 or 6, most children know the alphabet well enough to use the traditional Snellen chart for vision screening (Fig. 9.2C). Refer to the Healthy People 2030 box. Table 9.3 gives further information about vision screening tools.

Screenings should be performed when children are alert, as fatigue and lack of interest can mimic poor vision. When using any vision screening chart, several simple steps need to be followed:

- Place the chart at the child's eye level.
- Make sure there is sufficient lighting.
- Place a mark on the floor approximately 300 to 600 cm (10 to 20 ft) from the chart (distance depends on what the tool is calibrated for).
- Align the child's heels on the mark.
- Have the child read each line, first, with one eye covered and then with the other eye covered. Explain to the child to keep the eye covered but open (Fig. 9.3).
- Have the child read each line with both eyes.

In addition to visual acuity screening, children should also be screened for color discrimination. Any child who has eye abnormalities or who has failed visual screening needs to be evaluated by a specialist appropriately trained to treat children.

HEALTHY PEOPLE 2030

Objective	Nursing Significance
Increase the proportion of preschool children aged 3–5 years who receive vision screening.	• Use a preschool-appropriate vision screening tool to assess vision. • Ensure screening begins at age 3 years.

Healthy People Objectives retrieved from http://www.healthypeople.gov

IRON-DEFICIENCY ANEMIA SCREENING

Iron deficiency is the leading nutritional deficiency in children (Powers, 2021). Iron deficiency can cause cognitive and motor deficits resulting in developmental delays and behavioral disturbances. The increased incidence of iron-deficiency anemia is directly associated with periods of diminished iron stores, rapid growth, and high metabolic demands. At 6 months of age, the in utero iron stores of a full-term infant are almost depleted (Powers, 2021). The adolescent growth spurt warrants constant iron replacement. Pregnant adolescents are at even higher risk for iron deficiency due to the demands of the adolescent's growth spurt and the needs of the developing fetus.

The AAP recommends assessing for risk factors related to iron-deficiency anemia at 4, 15, 18, 24, and 30 months and then annually and performing a hematocrit or hemoglobin at 12 months (Bright Futures/AAP, 2022). Refer to Box 9.4 for risk factors for iron-deficiency anemia.

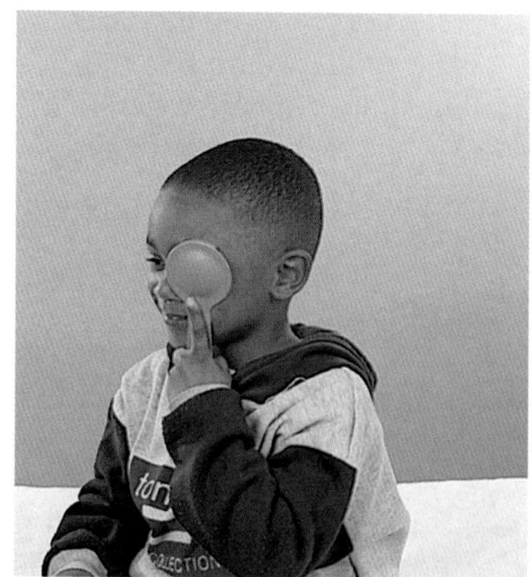

FIGURE 9.3 One eye must be covered while the other is tested in order to detect discrepancies in visual acuity between the two eyes and identify amblyopia early.

BOX 9.4 Risk Factors for Iron-Deficiency Anemia

- Periods of rapid growth
- Low-birth-weight or preterm infants
- Low dietary intake of meat, fish, poultry, and ascorbic acid
- Higher weight
- Inappropriate consumption of cow's milk
- Use of infant formula not fortified with iron
- Exclusive breastfeeding after age 4 months without iron-fortified supplemental foods
- Meal skipping, frequent dieting
- Exposure to lead
- Feeding problems
- Pregnancy or recent pregnancy
- Intensive physical training
- Recent blood loss, heavy/lengthy menstrual periods
- Chronic use of aspirin or nonsteroidal antiinflammatory drugs
- Parasitic infections

Children at High Risk for Iron-Deficiency Anemia

- Families with low income
- Those eligible for the Special Supplemental Nutrition Program for Women, Infants, and Children (WIC)
- Hispanic/Latin American and Asian American children
- Migrants or recently arrived refugees

Data from Powers, J. M. (2021). Iron deficiency in infants and children <12: Screening, prevention, clinical manifestations, and diagnosis. *UpToDate.* Retrieved December 14, 2022, from https://medilib.ir/uptodate/show/5925

LEAD SCREENING

Elevated blood lead levels (3.5 mcg/dL or higher) remain a preventable environmental health threat. Approximately half a million children have blood levels greater than 3.5 mcg/dL, which can lead to a wide variety of symptoms and problems, such as headaches, stomach pain, inattentiveness, irritability, hyperactivity, decreased bone and muscle growth, poor muscle coordination, problems with language and speech, cognitive impairments, hearing problems, and seizures (CDC, 2022a; Gavin, 2021). Although the prevalence of elevated lead levels has declined significantly over the past two decades, mainly due to the banning of lead-based paint in 1978, the elimination of lead from motor vehicle gasoline, banning the use of lead pipes for plumbing, and the removal of lead for solder in food cans, certain communities still possess a high level of lead exposure (Sample, 2022; United States Environmental Protection Agency, 2018). Lead poisoning is a problem that affects children younger than 6 years the most because children of this age are crawling on the ground and putting things in their mouths, and their developing neurologic system is more sensitive to the effects of lead. It has also been found that even low blood lead levels can harm children and result in IQ deficits, attention-related behavior problems, and poor academic achievement (Sample, 2022). Therefore, the AAP and CDC state that there is no safe blood lead level in children and that a shift to primary prevention is the key (Sample, 2022). Ensuring that no children spend time or live in homes, buildings, or environments where they are exposed to lead hazards is the key. Educate parents on lead hazards, and encourage them to avoid exposure of their children. Lead-based paint continues to be the highest hazard and most dangerous source of lead exposure in children (Gavin, 2021). Lead hazards include homes or buildings built before 1978, contaminated soil and dust, water that flows through old lead pipes or faucets, foods stored in containers that are painted with lead paint (such as lead-glazed pottery or lead crystal) or canned food that is sealed with lead (such as those imported from other countries), toys or toy jewelry that may be painted with lead paint or have lead components, and folk remedies that contain lead, such as greta and azarcon (Sample, 2022).

TAKE NOTE!

A healthy diet that includes calcium, iron, and vitamin C can also help decrease the way the body absorbs lead (Gavin, 2021).

The AAP Bright Future guidelines recommends performing a risk assessment and, if positive, screening at 6, 9, 12, 18, and 24 months and at 3, 4, 5, and 6 years (Bright Futures/AAP, 2022). At-risk children should have a blood lead level drawn at ages 12 and 24 months (Bright Futures/AAP, 2022). Refer to the Healthy People 2030 box.

HEALTHY PEOPLE 2030

Objective	Nursing Significance
Reduce blood lead level in children aged 1–5 years.	• Screen for lead exposure. • Ensure that high risk children have blood lead levels measured.

Healthy People Objectives retrieved from http://www.healthypeople.gov

TAKE NOTE!

Many cases of elevated blood lead levels have been reported in children who are recent immigrants, refugees, or international adoptees. In addition to blood lead testing for all children between ages 6 months and 6 years, it is also recommended for these children on entering the United States and again 3 to 6 months after placement in a permanent residence (Sample, 2022).

HYPERTENSION SCREENING

Higher weight and resulting hypertension have been on the rise in children and can lead to adult cardiovascular disease. Universal hypertension screening for children beginning at 3 years of age is recommended (Bright Futures/AAP, 2022). If the child has risk factors for systemic hypertension, such as preterm birth, very low birth weight, kidney disease, organ transplant, congenital heart defect, or other illnesses associated with hypertension, then screening begins when the risk factor becomes apparent (Bright Futures/AAP, 2022).

The guidelines for determining hypertension in children and adolescents utilize body size in order to be more precise. Sex and age are used to determine specific systolic and diastolic blood pressure percentiles. Refer to Appendix B for Blood Pressure Charts for Children and Adolescents. Auscultation is the preferred method of measuring blood pressure in children, and an elevated blood pressure must be confirmed on repeated visits before a diagnosis of hypertension is given. Refer to Box 9.5 for hypertension guidelines. Anticipatory guidance on activity is appropriate for any child with the inclusion of weight management for children with elevated blood pressure, stage 1 or 2 hypertension (Flynn et al., 2017). Refer to Chapter 19 for additional information on hypertension.

BOX 9.5 Childhood Hypertension Guidelines

	Children 1 to <13 Years Old	Children >13 Years Old
Optimal/normal	<90th percentile for sex, age, and height	BP <120/<80 mm Hg
Elevated blood pressure	BP 120/80 mm Hg to <95th percentile for sex, age, and height (whichever is lower) or BP ≥90th percentile to ≤95th percentile for sex, age, and height	BP 120/<80–129/<80 mm Hg
Stage 1 hypertension	≥95th percentile to <95th percentile + 12 mm Hg for sex, age, and height, or 130/80 to 139/89 mm Hg (whichever is lower) on at least three separate occasions	130/80–139/89 mm Hg
Stage 2 hypertension	≥95th percentile + 12 mm Hg for sex, age, and height or ≥140/90 mm Hg (whichever is lower) on at least three separate occasions	≥140/90 mm Hg

Data from Flynn, J. T., Kaelber, D. C., Baker-Smith, C. M., Blowey, D., Carroll, A. E., Daniels, S. R., de Ferranti, S. D., Dionne, J. M., Falkner, B., Flinn, S. K., Gidding, S. S., Goodwin, C., Leu, M. G., Powers, M. E., Rea, C., Samuels, J., Simasek, M., Thaker, V. V., Urbina, E. M., & Subcommittee on Screening and Management of High Blood Pressure in Children. (2017). Clinical practice guideline for screening and management of high blood pressure in children and adolescents. *Pediatrics, 140*(3), e20171904. https://doi.org/10.1542/peds.2017-1904

HYPERLIPIDEMIA SCREENING

Atherosclerosis has been documented in children, and a link exists between high lipid levels and the development of these lesions. Bright Futures Guidelines recommends universal screening for dyslipidemia once between 9 and 11 years of age and again between 17 and 21 years of age (Bright Futures/AAP, 2022). Performing a risk assessment screening at 24 months and 4, 6, 8, and 12 through 17 years of age is also recommended. Refer to Box 9.6 for details regarding screening for hyperlipidemia.

Remember Maya and Evan, the children introduced at the beginning of the chapter? How would you assess their growth and development? Which screening tests are warranted for them, and why? What further information would you need to determine which tests should be performed?

Immunizations

Immunization is the key disease prevention activity during childhood health supervision visits. The development of effective vaccines, beginning in the 1940s, revolutionized children's health care. Immunization allowed the focus to shift from disease treatment to disease prevention. The nurse needs to understand the principles of immunizations, the proper use of vaccines, and barriers to immunization. Armed with this knowledge, the nurse can partner with families to provide the highest level of disease protection to children (Fig. 9.4). Refer to the Healthy People 2030 box. For information on vaccine-preventable communicable diseases, refer to Chapter 15.

BOX 9.6 Hyperlipidemia Screening

Screen if parents, grandparents, aunts/uncles, siblings have/had documented:
- Coronary atherosclerosis
- Myocardial infarction
- Angina pectoris
- Peripheral vascular disease
- Cerebrovascular disease/stroke
- Coronary artery bypass graft/stent/angioplasty at <55 years in males, <65 years in females
- Sudden cardiac death

Screen if a parent's blood cholesterol level is 240 mg/dL or higher.
Screen at health care provider's discretion:
- Parental history is unobtainable.
- Child has diabetes or hypertension.
- Child has lifestyle risk factors:
  - Cigarette smoking
  - Higher weight
  - Sedentary lifestyle
  - High-fat dietary intake

Data from National Heart, Lung, and Blood Institute. (2012). *Expert panel on integrated guidelines for cardiovascular health and risk reduction in children and adolescents.* Summary Report (NIH Publication No. 12-7486). U.S. Department of Health and Human Services. http://www.nhlbi.nih.gov/guidelines/cvd_ped/peds_guidelines_sum.pdf

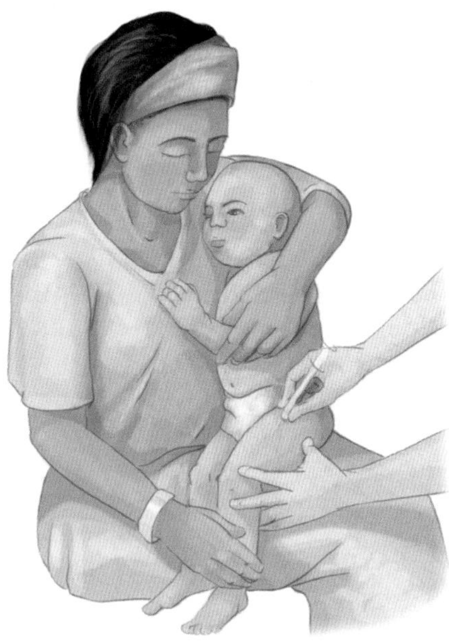

FIGURE 9.4 Nurse administering intramuscular injection into the vastus lateralis of an infant.

PRINCIPLES OF IMMUNIZATION

The immune system has the ability to recognize materials present in the body as "self" or "nonself." Foreign materials (nonself) are called antigens. When an antigen is recognized by the immune system, the immune system responds by producing antibodies (immunoglobulins) or directing special cells to destroy and remove the antigen.

HEALTHY PEOPLE 2030

Objective	Nursing Significance
Increase the vaccination coverage level of 4 doses of the diphtheria–tetanus–acellular pertussis (DTaP) vaccine among children by age 2 years. Maintain the vaccination coverage level of 2 doses of measles–mumps–rubella (MMR) vaccine for children in kindergarten. Maintain the vaccination coverage level of 1 dose of MMR among children by age 2 years. Reduce the proportion of children in the United States who receive 0 doses of recommended vaccines by age 2 years. Increase the percentage of adolescents who receive recommended doses of human papillomavirus (HPV) vaccine. Increase the proportion of people who are vaccinated annually against seasonal influenza.	• Immunize at every opportunity. If a child is due or past due for vaccinations, provide them at a sick visit if not contraindicated. • Educate families about the benefits and risks of immunization.

Healthy People Objectives retrieved from http://www.healthypeople.gov

Immunity is the ability to destroy and remove a specific antigen from the body. The acquisition of immunity can be active or passive. **Passive immunity** is produced when the immunoglobulins of one person are transferred to another. This immunity lasts only weeks or months. Passive immunity can be obtained by injection of exogenous immunoglobulins. It can also be transferred from birthing parents to infants via colostrum or the placenta. **Active immunity** is acquired when a person's own immune system generates the immune response. Active immunity lasts for many years or for a lifetime. This long-term protection is the result of immunologic memory. After the initial immune response, specialized cells for that antigen continue to exist. When an antigen returns, these memory cells rapidly produce a fresh supply of antibodies to reestablish protection. This immunity can occur after exposure to natural pathogens or after exposure to vaccines. Vaccines mimic the characteristics of the natural antigen. The immune system mounts a response and establishes an immunologic memory as it would for an infection.

The classification of vaccines is based on the characteristics of the antigen present. The antigen may be viral or bacterial. It may be live attenuated (weakened) or killed. It may be the whole antigen or a portion of it (fractional).

- Live attenuated vaccines are modified living organisms that are weakened. The organism can produce an immune response but does not produce the complications of the illness.
- Inactivated vaccines contain whole dead organisms; they are incapable of reproducing but are capable of producing an immune response.
- Toxoid vaccines contain protein products produced by bacteria called toxins. The toxin is heat-treated to weaken its effect, but it retains its ability to produce an immune response.
- Conjugate vaccines are the result of chemically linking the bacterial cell wall polysaccharide (sugar-based) portions with proteins. This dramatically increases the immune response compared to presenting the polysaccharide portion alone.
- Recombinant vaccines use genetically engineered organisms. For example, the hepatitis B vaccine (HepB) is produced by splicing a gene portion of the virus into a gene of a yeast cell. The yeast cell is then able to produce hepatitis B surface antigen to use for vaccine production.
  - Messenger RNA (mRNA) vaccines make a specific type of protein to trigger an immune response. This technology was used to make some of the COVID-19 vaccines.
  - Viral vector vaccines use a modified harmless version of a different virus as a vector to deliver protection. This type of technology was used to make some of the COVID-19 vaccines.

The safety and efficacy of existing vaccines are constantly being reviewed, and research to improve vaccines is ongoing. The goal is to refine vaccines so that a maximum immune response is produced with the least amount of risk for the child.

IMMUNIZATION MANAGEMENT

The Advisory Committee on Immunization Practices (ACIP), a branch of the CDC, reviews the recommended immunization schedules at least yearly and updates the schedule to ensure that it reflects current best practices. In addition to the recommended schedule, the ACIP publishes a "catch-up" schedule for children who have not been adequately immunized. The child's immunization record must be compared with the latest edition of these schedules when assessing the need for immunization. For the latest immunization schedule, visit the CDC immunization schedules website.

TAKE NOTE!

When obtaining an immunization history from the parent, ask, "When and where did your child receive their last immunization?" The answer will provide more information than simply asking, "Are your child's immunizations up to date?" The nurse can compare this information with that on the immunization record, discover in what settings the child is getting health care, and use the information as a starting point in a discussion of any reactions to previous immunizations.

Vaccine storage and administration affect the efficacy of a vaccine. Improperly stored or reconstituted vaccines can be ineffective (CDC, 2022b). The vaccine must be given by the correct route; not all vaccines are given intramuscularly (Fig. 9.5). The manufacturer's package insert is the best reference source for any vaccine.

TAKE NOTE!

Proper vaccine storage is critical to vaccine efficacy. If you suspect that a vaccine was not maintained at the proper storage temperature, do not use it! An ineffective vaccine is of no use in preventing disease.

Any vaccine can have side effects, and the most common ones are mild, such as redness, tenderness, and swelling at the site; low-grade fever; and fussiness. These symptoms usually resolve within a few days. The National Childhood Vaccine Injury Act (NCVIA) requires that Vaccine Information Statements (VISs) (Fig. 9.6) be provided to parents before an immunization is given (CDC, 2021b). These inform about the benefits and risks and discuss specific side effects that may be seen for each immunization. In accordance with the concept of partnership with the parents, allow ample time for them to read the VIS and to discuss their concerns. If the parents do not understand the information presented, they should feel comfortable asking questions. If the parents do not have reading literacy, present the information orally and verify that the parents understand it. If the information in the VIS is not in the parent's native language, have a translator present the information.

At this time, ask the parents about the child's reactions to previous immunizations, and screen for precautions and contraindications for each vaccine to be administered. Before the vaccine is given, the parents must sign consent forms.

Any clinically significant adverse event that occurs after an immunization should be reported to the Vaccine Adverse Event Reporting System (VAERS), which is a cosponsored surveillance program by the CDC and the U.S. Food and Drug Administration (FDA) (VAERS, n.d.). For assistance in obtaining and completing a VAERS form, call 800-822-7967 or visit www.vaers.hhs.gov.

Documentation in the child's permanent record includes the following:

- Date the vaccine was administered
- Name of vaccine (commonly used abbreviation is acceptable)
- Lot number and expiration date of vaccine
- Manufacturer's name
- Site and route by which vaccine was administered (e.g., left deltoid, intramuscularly)
- Edition date of VIS given to the parents
- Name and address of the facility administering the vaccine (where the permanent record will be kept)
- Name of the person administering the immunization

Families should be provided with a copy of the child's immunizations. This reinforces the importance of the procedure and reminds the parents to keep the child's immunizations up to date.

Figure 9.7 shows a typical vaccine administration record.

VACCINE DESCRIPTIONS

This section reviews the most commonly used vaccines. These immunizations are recommended by the ACIP and the AAP. Each state has laws that determine which immunizations are required for school admittance. These requirements can be waived if a contraindication or precaution to the vaccine exists. *Contraindications* are conditions that justify withholding an immunization either permanently or temporarily. The majority of contraindications are temporary, and the vaccine can be administered at a later date when the contraindication has resolved. The only permanent contraindication to all vaccines is an anaphylactic or systemic allergic reaction to a vaccine component. If severe allergic reaction occurs, this is a contraindication for any subsequent doses of that specific vaccine (Kroger et al., 2022). Children who are severely immunocompromised or people who are pregnant should not receive live vaccines (such as MMR and varicella) (see further on). With pertussis immunization (DTP, DTaP, or Tdap) (see the following section), encephalopathy without an identified cause within 7 days of the immunization permanently contraindicates further immunization with pertussis-containing vaccine. Children with SCID disease or a history of intussusception are both contraindications to the immunization

Administering Vaccines: Dose, Route, Site, and Needle Size

Vaccine	Dose	Route
COVID-19 *For product and dosage information for COVID-19 vaccine primary series and booster doses for both immunocompetent and immunocompromised adults, see CDC's "COVID-19 Vaccine Interim COVID-19 Immunization Schedule for Persons 6 Months of Age and Older."**		IM
Dengue (DENV4CYD)	0.5 mL	Subcut
Diphtheria, Tetanus, Pertussis (DTaP, DT, Tdap, Td)	0.5 mL	IM
***Haemophilus influenzae* type b** (Hib)	0.5 mL	IM
Hepatitis A (HepA)	≤18 yrs: 0.5 mL ≥19 yrs: 1.0 mL	IM
Hepatitis B (HepB) *People 11–15 yrs may be given Recombivax HB(Merck) 1.0 mL adult formulation on a 2-dose schedule.*	Engerix-B; Recombivax HB ≤19 yrs: 0.5 mL ≥20 yrs: 1.0 mL Heplisav-B ≥18 yrs: 0.5 mL PreHevbrio ≥18 yrs: 1.0 mL	IM
Human papillomavirus (HPV)	0.5 mL	IM
Influenza, live attenuated (LAIV4)	0.2 mL (0.1 mL in each nostril)	Intranasal spray
Influenza, inactivated (IIV4); 6 thru 35 mos • Egg-based IIV4: Afluria, Fluzone, Fluarix, FluLaval • Cell-culture based (ccIIV4): Flucelvax	Afluria: 0.25 mL Fluzone: 0.25 or 0.5 mL Fluarix, Flucelvax, FluLaval: 0.5 mL	IM
Influenza, inactivated (IIV4) and • Cell-culture based (ccIIV4), 3+ yrs; • Recombinant (RIV4, Flublok), 18+ yrs; • Adjuvanted (aIIV4, Fluad) 65+ yrs	0.5 mL	IM
Influenza, high-dose (IIV4-HD) 65+ yrs	0.7 mL	IM
Measles, Mumps, Rubella (MMR)	0.5 mL — MMR II (Merck)	IM or Subcut
	0.5 mL — Priorix (GSK)	Subcut
Meningococcal serogroups A, C, W, Y (MenACWY)	0.5 mL	IM
Meningococcal serogroup B (MenB)	0.5 mL	IM
Mpox (Jynneos)	0.5 mL	Subcut†
Pneumococcal conjugate (PCV)	0.5 mL	IM
Pneumococcal polysaccharide (PPSV23)	0.5 mL	IM or Subcut
Polio, inactivated (IPV)	0.5 mL	IM or Subcut
Respiratory Syncytial Virus (RSV) vaccine	0.5 mL	IM
RSV preventive antibody (RSV-mAb)	0.5 mL, 1 mL, or 2 mL based on weight and/or age	IM
Rotavirus (RV)	Rotarix: 1.0 mL Rotateq: 2.0 mL	Oral
Varicella (VAR)	0.5 mL	IM or Subcut
Zoster (Zos)	Shingrix: 0.5‡ mL	IM
Combination Vaccines		
DTaP-HepB-IPV (Pediarix) DTaP-IPV/Hib (Pentacel) DTaP-IPV (Kinrix; Quadracel) DTaP-IPV-Hib-HepB (Vaxelis)	0.5 mL	IM
MMRV (ProQuad)	0.5 mL	IM or Subcut
HepA-HepB (Twinrix)	1.0 mL	IM

*www.cdc.gov/vaccines/covid-19/downloads/COVID-19-immunization-schedule-ages-6months-older.pdf

†Administer mpox vaccine (Jynneos) 0.5 mL Subcut or, in adults, 0.1 mL intradermally. Subcut is the route indicated on the package insert. Intradermal administration to adults is permitted under FDA emergency use authorization (see www.fda.gov/media/160774/download).

‡The Shingrix (RZV) vial may contain more than 0.5 mL. Do not administer more than 0.5 mL.

Injection Site and Needle Size

Subcutaneous (Subcut) injection

Use a 23–25 gauge needle. Choose the injection site that is appropriate to the person's age and body mass.

AGE	NEEDLE LENGTH	INJECTION SITE
Infants (1–12 mos)	⅝"	Fatty tissue over anterolateral thigh muscle
Children 12 mos or older, adolescents, and adults	⅝"	Fatty tissue over anterolateral thigh muscle or fatty tissue over triceps

Intramuscular (IM) injection

Use a 22–25 gauge needle. Choose the injection site and needle length that is appropriate to the person's age and body mass.

AGE	NEEDLE LENGTH	INJECTION SITE
Newborns (1st 28 days)	⅝"[1]	Anterolateral thigh muscle
Infants (1–12 mos)	1"	Anterolateral thigh muscle
Toddlers (1–2 yrs)	1–1¼"	Anterolateral thigh muscle[3]
	⅝[2]–1"	Deltoid muscle of arm
Children (3–10 yrs)	⅝[2]–1"	Deltoid muscle of arm[3]
	1–1¼"	Anterolateral thigh muscle
Adolescents and teens (11–18 yrs)	⅝[2]–1"	Deltoid muscle of arm[3]
	1–1½"	Anterolateral thigh muscle
Biological sex and weight of patient 19 yrs or older		
Female or male <130 lbs	⅝[2]–1"	Deltoid muscle of arm
Female or male 130–152 lbs	1"	Deltoid muscle of arm
Female 153–200 lbs Male 153–260 lbs	1–1½"	Deltoid muscle of arm
Female more than 200 lbs Male more than 260 lbs	1½"	Deltoid muscle of arm
Female or male, any weight	1[2]–1½"	Anterolateral thigh muscle

1 If skin is stretched tightly and subcutaneous tissues are not bunched.

2 Alternate needle lengths may be used if the skin is stretched tightly and subcutaneous tissues are not bunched, as follows: a) a ⅝" needle in toddlers, children, and patients weighing less than 130 lbs (less than 60 kg) for IM injection in the deltoid muscle only, or b) a 1" needle for administration in the thigh muscle for adults of any weight.

3 Preferred site

NOTE: Always refer to the package insert included with each biologic for complete vaccine administration information. CDC's Advisory Committee on Immunization Practices (ACIP) recommendations for the particular vaccine should be reviewed as well. Access the ACIP recommendations at www.immunize.org/acip.

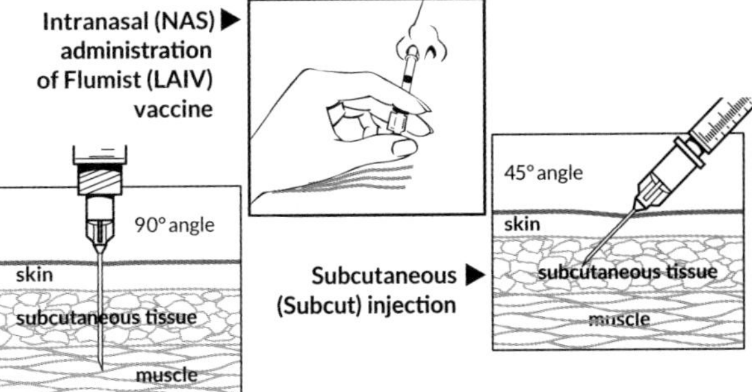

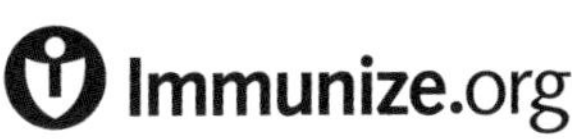

FOR PROFESSIONALS www.immunize.org / FOR THE PUBLIC www.vaccineinformation.org

www.immunize.org/catg.d/p3085.pdf
Item #P3085 (2/19/2024)

Scan for PDF

FIGURE 9.5 Administering vaccines: Dose, route, site, and needle size. (Reprinted from Immunize.org. (2024). *Administering vaccines: Dose, route, site, and needle size*. https://www.immunize.org/wp-content/uploads/catg.d/p3085.pdf.)

VACCINE INFORMATION STATEMENT

DTaP (Diphtheria, Tetanus, Pertussis) Vaccine: *What You Need to Know*

Many vaccine information statements are available in Spanish and other languages. See www.immunize.org/vis

Hojas de información sobre vacunas están disponibles en español y en muchos otros idiomas. Visite www.immunize.org/vis

1. Why get vaccinated?

DTaP vaccine can prevent **diphtheria, tetanus,** and **pertussis.**

Diphtheria and pertussis spread from person to person. Tetanus enters the body through cuts or wounds.

- **DIPHTHERIA (D)** can lead to difficulty breathing, heart failure, paralysis, or death.
- **TETANUS (T)** causes painful stiffening of the muscles. Tetanus can lead to serious health problems, including being unable to open the mouth, having trouble swallowing and breathing, or death.
- **PERTUSSIS (aP),** also known as "whooping cough," can cause uncontrollable, violent coughing that makes it hard to breathe, eat, or drink. Pertussis can be extremely serious especially in babies and young children, causing pneumonia, convulsions, traumatic brain injury, or death. In adolescents and adults, it can cause weight loss, loss of bladder control, passing out, and rib fractures from severe coughing.

2. DTaP vaccine

DTaP is only for children younger than 7 years old. Different vaccines against tetanus, diphtheria, and pertussis (Tdap and Td) are available for older children, adolescents, and adults.

It is recommended that children receive 5 doses of DTaP, usually at the following ages:

- 2 months
- 4 months
- 6 months
- 15–18 months
- 4–6 years

DTaP may be given as a stand-alone vaccine, or as part of a combination vaccine (a type of vaccine that combines more than one vaccine together into one shot).

DTaP may be given at the same time as other vaccines.

3. Talk with your health care provider

Tell your vaccination provider if the person getting the vaccine:

- Has had an **allergic reaction after a previous dose of any vaccine that protects against tetanus, diphtheria, or pertussis**, or has any **severe, life-threatening allergies**
- Has had **a coma, decreased level of consciousness, or prolonged seizures within 7 days after a previous dose of any pertussis vaccine (DTP or DTaP)**
- Has **seizures or another nervous system problem**
- Has ever had **Guillain-Barré Syndrome** (also called "GBS")
- Has had **severe pain or swelling after a previous dose of any vaccine that protects against tetanus or diphtheria**

In some cases, your child's health care provider may decide to postpone DTaP vaccination until a future visit.

Children with minor illnesses, such as a cold, may be vaccinated. Children who are moderately or severely ill should usually wait until they recover before getting DTaP vaccine.

Your child's health care provider can give you more information.

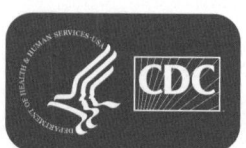

U.S. Department of Health and Human Services
Centers for Disease Control and Prevention

FIGURE 9.6 Federal law mandates the use of Vaccine Information Statements (VISs). These should be given to the parent or primary caregiver for each vaccine the child receives. (Reprinted from Centers for Disease Control and Prevention. [2021c]. *DTaP (Diphtheria, Tetanus, Pertussis) vaccine:* What you need to know. https://www.cdc.gov/vaccines/hcp/vis/vis-statements/dtap.pdf)

4. Risks of a vaccine reaction

- Soreness or swelling where the shot was given, fever, fussiness, feeling tired, loss of appetite, and vomiting sometimes happen after DTaP vaccination.
- More serious reactions, such as seizures, nonstop crying for 3 hours or more, or high fever (over 105°F) after DTaP vaccination happen much less often. Rarely, vaccination is followed by swelling of the entire arm or leg, especially in older children when they receive their fourth or fifth dose.

As with any medicine, there is a very remote chance of a vaccine causing a severe allergic reaction, other serious injury, or death.

5. What if there is a serious problem?

An allergic reaction could occur after the vaccinated person leaves the clinic. If you see signs of a severe allergic reaction (hives, swelling of the face and throat, difficulty breathing, a fast heartbeat, dizziness, or weakness), call **9-1-1** and get the person to the nearest hospital.

For other signs that concern you, call your health care provider.

Adverse reactions should be reported to the Vaccine Adverse Event Reporting System (VAERS). Your health care provider will usually file this report, or you can do it yourself. Visit the VAERS website at www.vaers.hhs.gov or call **1-800-822-7967**. *VAERS is only for reporting reactions, and VAERS staff members do not give medical advice.*

6. The National Vaccine Injury Compensation Program

The National Vaccine Injury Compensation Program (VICP) is a federal program that was created to compensate people who may have been injured by certain vaccines. Claims regarding alleged injury or death due to vaccination have a time limit for filing, which may be as short as two years. Visit the VICP website at www.hrsa.gov/vaccinecompensation or call **1-800-338-2382** to learn about the program and about filing a claim.

7. How can I learn more?

- Ask your health care provider.
- Call your local or state health department.
- Visit the website of the Food and Drug Administration (FDA) for vaccine package inserts and additional information at www.fda.gov/vaccines-blood-biologics/vaccines.
- Contact the Centers for Disease Control and Prevention (CDC):
  - Call **1-800-232-4636** (**1-800-CDC-INFO**) or
  - Visit CDC's website at www.cdc.gov/vaccines.

Vaccine Information Statement
DTaP (Diphtheria, Tetanus, Pertussis) Vaccine

42 U.S.C. § 300aa-26
8/6/2021

OFFICE USE ONLY

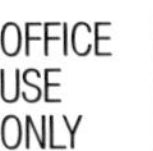

FIGURE 9.6 *(continued)*

Vaccine Administration Record for Children and Teens

Patient name ______________________

Birthdate______________ Chart number ____________

PRACTICE NAME AND ADDRESS

Before administering any vaccines, give copies of all pertinent Vaccine Information Statements (VISs) to the child's parent or legal representative and make sure they understand the risks and benefits of the vaccine(s). Always provide or update the patient's personal record card.

Vaccine	Type of Vaccine[1]	Date vaccine given (mo/day/yr)	Funding Source (F,S,P)[2]	Site[3]	Vaccine		Vaccine Information Statement (VIS)		Vaccinator[5] (signature or initials and title)
					Lot #	Mfr.	Date on VIS[4]	Date given[4]	
Hepatitis B[6] (e.g., HepB, DTaP-HepB-IPV, DTaP-IPV-Hib-HepB) Give IM.[7]									
RSV-mAb[8] Give IM.[7]									
Diphtheria, Tetanus, Pertussis[6] (e.g., DTaP, DTaP-HepB-IPV, DTaP-IPV-Hib-HepB, DTaP-IPV/Hib, DTaP-IPV, Tdap, Td) Give IM.[7]									
***Haemophilus influenzae* type b**[6] (e.g., Hib, Hib-DTaP-IPV/Hib, DTaP-IPV-Hib-HepB) Give IM.[7]									
Polio[6] (e.g., IPV, DTaP-HepB-IPV, DTaP-IPV/Hib, DTaP-IPV, DTaP-IPV-Hib-HepB) Give IPV Subcut or IM.[7] Give all others IM.[7]									
Pneumococcal (e.g., PCV13, PCV15, PCV20; PPSV23) Give PCV IM.[7] Give PPSV23 Subcut or IM.[7]									
Rotavirus (RV1, RV5) Give orally (po).									

Abbreviation	Trade Name and Manufacturer
DTaP	Daptacel (Sanofi); Infanrix (GSK); Tripedia (Sanofi)
DTaP-HepB-IPV	Pediarix (GSK)
DTaP-IPV/Hib	Pentacel (Sanofi)
DTaP-IPV	Kinrix (GSK); Quadracel (Sanofi)
DTaP-IPV-Hib-HepB	Vaxelis (MCM Vaccine)
Tdap	Adacel (Sanofi); Boostrix (GSK)
Td	Tenivac (Sanofi); Tdvax (MA Biological Labs)
HepB (see note #1)	Engerix-B (GSK), Recombivax HB (Merck); Heplisav-B (Dynavax); PreHevbrio (VBI Vaccines) for 18 yrs & older
HepA-HepB	Twinrix (GSK) for teens age 18 yrs & older
Hib	ActHIB (Sanofi), Hiberix (GSK), PedvaxHIB (Merck)
IPV	IPOL (Sanofi)
RSV-mAb	Beyfortus (Sanofi & AstraZeneca)
PCV13; PCV15: PCV20	PCV13: Prevnar 13 (Pfizer); PCV15: Vaxneuvance (Merck); PCV20: Prevnar 20 (Pfizer)
PPSV23	Pneumovax 23 (Merck)
RV1; RV5	RV1: Rotarix (GSK); RV5: RotaTeq (Merck)

CONTINUED ON THE BACK ▶

How to Complete this Record

1. Record the standard abbreviation (e.g., Tdap) or the trade name for each vaccine (see table at right). Use trade name for HepB if vaccinating an older teen (schedule varies by brand).
2. Record the funding source of the vaccine given as either F (federal), S (state), or P (private).
3. Record the site where vaccine was administered as either RA (right arm), LA (left arm), RT (right thigh), LT (left thigh), or NAS (intranasal).
4. Record the publication date of each VIS as well as the date the VIS is given to the patient.
5. To meet the space constraints of this form and federal requirements for documentation, a healthcare setting should keep a reference list of vaccinators that includes their initials and titles.
6. For combination vaccines, fill in a row for each antigen in the combination.
7. IM is the abbreviation for intramuscular; Subcut is the abbreviation for subcutaneous.
8. RSV monoclonal antibody (mAb) is a passive immunization product, not a vaccine, routinely recommended for seasonal prevention of RSV disease in infants. Record administration in an equivalent manner.

www.immunize.org/catg.d/p2022.pdf
Item #P2022 (9/18/2023)

Scan for PDF

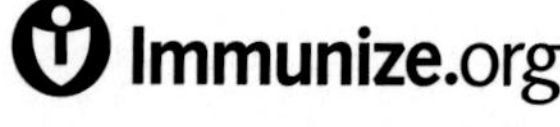

FOR PROFESSIONALS www.immunize.org / FOR THE PUBLIC www.vaccineinformation.org

FIGURE 9.7 Sample of a vaccine administration record. (Reprinted from Immunize.org. [2023]. *Vaccine administration record for children and teens*. http://www.immunize.org/catg.d/p2022.pdf)

Vaccine Administration Record for Children and Teens (continued)

Patient name ____________

Birthdate ____________ Chart number ____________

Before administering any vaccines, give copies of all pertinent Vaccine Information Statements (VISs) to the child's parent or legal representative and make sure they understand the risks and benefits of the vaccine(s). Always provide or update the patient's personal record card.

PRACTICE NAME AND ADDRESS

Vaccine	Type of Vaccine[1]	Date vaccine given (mo/day/yr)	Funding Source (F,S,P)[2]	Site[3]	Vaccine		Vaccine Information Statement (VIS)		Vaccinator[5] (signature or initials and title)
					Lot #	Mfr.	Date on VIS[4]	Date given[4]	
Measles, Mumps, Rubella (e.g., MMR, MMRV) Give MMRII and MMRV Subcut or IM; give Priorix Subcut.[6]									
Varicella (e.g., VAR, MMRV) Give Subcut or IM.[6]									
Hepatitis A (HepA) Give IM.[6]									
Meningococcal ACWY (MenACWY) Give IM.[6]									
Meningococcal B (MenB-4C, MenB-FHbp) Give IM.[6]									
Human papillomavirus (HPV) Give IM.[6]									
Influenza (IIV, ccIIV, RIV, LAIV) Give IIV, ccIIV, and RIV IM.[6] Give LAIV NAS.[6]									
COVID-19 (e.g., COV-mRNA; COV-aPS) Give IM.[6]									
Other (e.g., dengue)									

Abbreviation	Trade Name and Manufacturer
MMR	MMR II (Merck); Priorix (GSK)
VAR	Varivax (Merck)
MMRV	ProQuad (Merck)
HepA	Havrix (GSK); Vaqta (Merck)
HepA-HepB	Twinrix (GSK) for teens age 18 and older
MenACWY	MenQuadfi (Sanofi); Menveo (GSK)
MenB-4C (see note #1)	Bexsero (GSK)
MenB-FHbp (see note #1)	Trumenba (Pfizer)
HPV	Gardasil 9 (Merck)
ccIIV (cell culture-based IIV)	Flucelvax (Seqirus) for teens 18 and older
IIV (inactivated influenza vaccine)	Fluarix, FluLaval (GSK); Afluria (Seqirus); Flubok (Sanofi)
LAIV (live attenuated influenza vaccine)	FluMist (AstraZeneca)
RIV (recombinant influenza vaccine)	RIV: Flublok (Sanofi) for teens 18 and older
COV-mRNA (see note #1)	Comirnaty (Pfizer-BioNTech); Spikevax (Moderna)
COV-aPS (see note #1)	Novavax (Novavax)
Other (e.g., dengue)	Dengue vaccine: Dengvaxia (Sanofi)

How to Complete this Record

1. For meningococcal B and COVID-19 vaccines, record the trade name (see table at right); for all other vaccines, record the standard abbreviation (e.g., HPV) or trade name for each vaccine (see table at right).
2. Record the funding source of the vaccine given as either F (federal), S (state), or P (private).
3. Record the site where vaccine was administered as either RA (right arm), LA (left arm), RT (right thigh), LT (left thigh), or NAS (intranasal).
4. Record the publication date of each VIS as well as the date the VIS is given to the patient.
5. To meet the space constraints of this form and federal requirements for documentation, a healthcare setting should keep a reference list of vaccinators that includes their initials and titles.
6. IM is the abbreviation for intramuscular; Subcut is the abbreviation for subcutaneous; NAS is the abbreviation for intranasal.
7. For combination vaccines, fill in a row for each antigen in the combination.

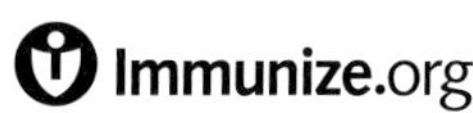

www.immunize.org/catg.d/p2022.pdf / Item #P2022 (9/18/2023)

FIGURE 9.7 *(continued)*

of rotavirus vaccines (Kroger et al., 2022). Current, recent, or upcoming anesthesia, surgery, or hospitalization is not a contraindication for vaccination, and hospitalization can be used as an opportunity to provide recommended immunizations (Kroger et al., 2022).

Precautions are conditions that increase the risk of an adverse reaction, may cause diagnostic confusion, or may impair the child's ability to acquire immunity from the vaccine (Kroger et al., 2022). The presence of a moderate to severe acute illness with or without fever is a precaution for all vaccines (Kroger et al., 2022). However, with minor illness the safety and efficacy of immunizations has been documented (Kroger et al., 2022). In general, immunizations should be postponed when a precaution is present; however, on an individualized basis, providers must weigh the benefits of immunization against the likelihood of an adverse event (Kroger et al., 2022).

Diphtheria, Tetanus, and Pertussis Vaccines

Immunization against diphtheria, tetanus, and pertussis diseases is given via a combination vaccine. The vaccine currently used for children younger than 7 years is diphtheria, tetanus, acellular pertussis (DTaP). It contains diphtheria and tetanus toxoids and pertussis cell wall proteins. The older version of this vaccine—diphtheria, tetanus, pertussis (DPT)—contained killed whole cells of pertussis bacteria and caused more frequent and severe adverse reactions than DTaP. Diphtheria and tetanus (DT) vaccine is used for children younger than 7 years who have contraindications to pertussis immunization. Full-strength diphtheria toxoid causes significant adverse reactions in people older than 7 years. For this group, the Tdap adolescent preparation vaccine is used: it contains tetanus toxoid, reduced diphtheria toxoid, and acellular pertussis vaccine. The lowercase "d" is used to designate the lower dose of diphtheria toxoid. The ACIP recommends that Tdap be used for all tetanus boosters in older children (11 to 12 years) and adolescents because Tdap provides a boost to diphtheria and pertussis immunization.

Haemophilus Influenzae Type B Vaccines

Haemophilus influenzae type B is a bacterium that causes several life-threatening illnesses in children younger than 5 years. These infections include meningitis, epiglottitis, and septic arthritis. *H. influenzae* type B conjugate vaccines (Hib) have been extremely effective in cutting the rates of these diseases in children. There are several different types of Hib conjugate vaccines. Two or three doses are needed for the primary infant series depending on the vaccine product used (e.g., PedvaxHIB requires two doses, while ActHIB, Hiberix, Vaxelis, and Pentacel require three doses) (CDC, 2022c). A booster vaccine is needed at 12 to 15 months. These vaccine products are interchangeable, but if different brands are administered to a child, then a total of three doses is necessary to complete the primary series in infants. Hib vaccine is not routinely given to children aged 5 years or older and is contraindicated in children younger than 6 weeks (CDC, 2021d).

Polio Vaccine

Wild polio has been eliminated in the United States, and since 2000, inactivated polio vaccine (IPV) is the only polio vaccine currently recommended (ACIP, 2000; CDC, 2021e, 2022g). It is a killed virus vaccine that poses no risk of vaccine-acquired disease. The CDC recommends four doses of IPV. IPV is available in combination vaccines, which has several vaccines in one injection; this may result in a child getting five doses of IPV. This has been determined to be safe in children. Children who will be traveling to an area outside of the United States where polio is prevalent should complete the series before leaving, and an accelerated schedule is encouraged to accomplish this if necessary (CDC, 2022c).

Measles, Mumps, and Rubella Vaccines

MMR is a live attenuated virus combination vaccine. It is the one most commonly used in childhood immunizations. MMR can be given the same day as other live attenuated virus vaccines such as varicella vaccine (Var). However, if not given on the same day, the immunizations should be spaced at least 28 days apart (Kroger et al., 2022). Anaphylactic reactions are believed to be associated with the neomycin or gelatin components of the vaccine rather than the egg component. The vaccine is not prepared from the allergenic albumen portion of the egg, so egg allergy is no longer a contraindication for measles vaccine (Kroger et al., 2022). Pregnancy in a child's parent is not a contraindication to the vaccination of the child (Kroger et al., 2022).

> **TAKE NOTE!**
>
> During mumps outbreaks, children in the area who are identified as high risk, such as those living in close, prolonged contact at universities, schools, or close-knit communities, should receive a third dose of a mumps-containing vaccine (CDC, 2021f).

Hepatitis A Vaccine

Hepatitis A vaccine (HepA) is an inactivated whole virus vaccine. Hepatitis A is spread through close physical contact and by eating or drinking contaminated food or water. It is one of the most frequently reported vaccine-preventable diseases in the United States. Young children are particularly susceptible to hepatitis A because of their close contact with other children, inadequate hygiene practices, and tendency to place everything in their mouths. HepA is recommended to be given to all children at age 12 months, followed by a repeat dose with a minimum interval of 6 to 18 months (CDC, 2022c).

Hepatitis B Vaccine

The hepatitis B vaccine (HepB) is a recombinant vaccine. Hepatitis B virus can result in a serious infection that affects the liver. It is spread through contact with blood and body fluids and can be spread from an infected gestational parent to a newborn at birth. Hepatitis B vaccination is recommended at birth, preferably within the first 12 hours, then at 1 to 2 months and 6 to 18 months (CDC, 2022c). A total of four doses is acceptable when a combination vaccine with hepatitis B is used after birth (CDC, 2022c). Because hepatitis B is a sexually transmitted infection, it is important to verify the immunization status of all adolescents.

Varicella Vaccine

Varicella vaccine is a live attenuated virus vaccine. All children aged 12 to 15 months who have not had varicella (chickenpox) should be immunized. A second dose is recommended at age 4 to 6 years. The vaccine provides effective postexposure prophylaxis if administered within 3 to 5 days after exposure. The ACIP does recommend vaccination even if exposure is greater than 5 days in children without evidence of immunity and eligible for the vaccination (not recommended for children younger than 12 months of age) (Immunization Action Coalition, 2022b). Varicella may be given the same day as other live attenuated virus vaccines. However, if not given on the same day, the immunizations should be spaced at least 28 days apart (Kroger et al., 2022). Pregnancy in a child's parent is not a contraindication to the vaccination of the child (Kroger et al., 2022).

Pneumococcal Vaccines

Streptococcus pneumoniae (pneumococcus) is a common cause of pneumonia, sepsis, meningitis, and otitis media in young children (CDC, 2022d). In 2022, the ACIP recommended PCV15 or PCV13 for use in routine vaccination for children (Kobayashi et al., 2022). It stimulates an immune response in infants and is given at 2, 4, 6, and 12 to 15 months of age as part of the initial immunization series (CDC, 2022d). PPSV contains 23 strains of *S. pneumoniae*. It does not provoke an immune response in children under 2 years of age (Kobayashi et al., 2022). PPSV is given to children over 2 years of age who are at high risk for pneumococcal sepsis. This group includes children with anatomic/functional asplenia; sickle cell disease; chronic cardiac, pulmonary, or kidney disease; diabetes mellitus; cerebrospinal fluid leak or HIV infection; children getting or who have cochlear implants; and children with immunosuppression (Kobayashi et al., 2022).

Influenza Vaccines

Influenza immunization is recommended yearly for all people 6 months of age or older. All children 6 months to 8 years of age who have not received at least two doses of the influenza vaccine will require two doses separated by 4 weeks (CDC, 2022c). The ACIP provides yearly recommendations for the use of the influenza vaccine. Ensure you are aware of the most up-to-date recommendations available.

There are three influenza vaccines available: the inactivated influenza vaccine (IIV), recombinant influenza vaccine (RIV), and live attenuated influenza vaccine (LAIV). These vaccines are available as trivalent or quadrivalent, depending on the number of virus strains they vaccinate against. Quadrivalent seasonal influenza vaccine protects against two B virus strains and provides broader protection against influenza. LAIV is given intranasally and should not be given to anyone who is immunocompromised or who will be in close contact with an immunosuppressed person. It is also contraindicated in children 2 to 4 years old diagnosed with asthma or with a history of wheezing or medically attended wheezing in the past 12 months, children who have received influenza antiviral therapy in the past 48 hours, or children who are taking aspirin or other salicylates (Grohskopf et al., 2022). The ACIP provides no preference of which type of age-appropriate, licensed influenza vaccine is administered (Grohskopf et al., 2022).

Rotavirus Vaccine

Prior to the availability of the rotavirus vaccine, rotavirus was the most common cause of severe gastroenteritis among young children (CDC, 2021g). The virus is shed in the stool and easily spreads via the fecal–oral route. Severe, watery, crampy diarrhea quickly leads to dehydration in the infected child. The rotavirus vaccine is a live vaccine targeting five strains of rotavirus and is given via the oral route to infants. Two vaccine products are currently available. Rotarix requires two doses (at 2 and 4 months) and RotaTeq requires three doses (at 2, 4, and 6 months) (CDC, 2022c). If RotaTeq was used for any doses or the vaccine product is unknown, a total of three doses should be administered (CDC, 2022c). Administration of rotavirus vaccine is contraindicated in children with SCID or a history of intussusception (Kroger et al., 2022).

Human Papillomavirus Vaccine

Human papillomavirus (HPV) is a DNA tumor virus transmitted through direct skin-to-skin contact. HPV is contracted most often during vaginal or anal penetrative sexual acts. HPV infection is the most common sexually transmitted infection in the United States (CDC, 2022e). HPV causes genital warts and is responsible for the development of cancer. For these reasons, the ACIP and AAP have recommended that HPV vaccination occur in all preadolescent children (CDC, 2022c). Children 11 to 12 years old, and as young as 9 years old, should receive two shots 6 to 12 months apart. If the child is 15 years or older, they will need to receive the three-dose series (CDC, 2022c).

Meningococcal Vaccine

Meningococcal disease may manifest as meningitis, a deadly blood infection (meningococcemia), or bacteremic pneumonia. It is caused by the bacterium *Neisseria meningitidis*, which is spread through direct contact or by air droplets. It develops quickly, usually in healthy children and adolescents, and results in high rates of morbidity and mortality. For these reasons, the meningococcal conjugate vaccine is recommended for all previously unvaccinated children at age 11 to 12 years with a booster dose at the age of 16 years (CDC, 2022c). Routine vaccination is also recommended for children 2 months to 10 years old who are at an increased risk for the disease due to certain medical conditions such as anatomic or functional asplenia (including sickle cell disease); taking a medicine called Soliris; complement component deficiency; HIV infection; part of a community where there is an outbreak of serogroup A, C, W, or Y meningococcal disease; or traveling to a country where meningococcal disease is common (CDC, 2021h). Vaccination with serogroup B meningococcal vaccine is recommended in adolescents and preadolescents who are at an increased risk for the disease due to certain medical conditions such as anatomic or functional asplenia (including sickle cell disease), taking a medicine called a complement inhibitor such as Soliris, complement component deficiency, or part of a community where there is an outbreak of serogroup B meningococcal disease (CDC, 2021h). Specific populations such as military recruits and first-year college students living in residence halls who are unvaccinated or incompletely vaccinated need the immunization (CDC, 2023a).

TAKE NOTE!

In October 2023, the CDC recommended that if meningococcal groups A,C,Y & W-135 (MenACWY) and serogroup B meningococcal (MenB) are both indicated at the same visit, a new vaccine pentavalent meningococcal (MenABCWY) may be given (CDC, 2023b).

Respiratory Syncytial Virus Vaccine

Respiratory syncytial virus (RSV) is a common respiratory virus that causes mild, cold like symptoms in people of all ages. In some infants and young children, it can be dangerous and lead to difficulty breathing, low oxygen levels, dehydration, and severe lung complications. RSV is the most common cause of bronchiolitis and hospitalization among infants in the United States (CDC, 2023c). It is easily spread through contact with infected respiratory secretions or objects contaminated with the virus. Seasonal outbreaks occur (refer to Chapter 18 for further information regarding bronchiolitis and RSV).

The RSV preventive antibody (nirsevimab) can help prevent severe illness in infants and young children. The ACIP released new recommendations in August 2023 (CDC, 2023b). All infants younger than 8 months and born shortly before or during the RSV season should receive one dose of nirsevimab within 1 week of birth (in most infants, if the parent received the RSV vaccine during pregnancy, they do not need to receive nirsevimab). Those not born during the RSV season should receive one dose of nirsevimab shortly before the start of their first RSV season (CDC, 2023b, 2023c). Infants aged 8 to 19 months who are at increased risk for severe RSV disease should receive nirsevimab before the start of their second RSV season (CDC, 2023b).

TAKE NOTE!

The ACIP recommends COVID-19 vaccination for everyone 6 months or older. It is safe to administer the COVID-19 vaccine on the same day as other vaccines. Refer to the CDC website for updated COVID-19 vaccine information.

Recall the Randall children, introduced at the beginning of the chapter. What immunizations would be appropriate for them to receive? Explain how you would administer the injections, and discuss any contraindications or precautions.

BARRIERS TO IMMUNIZATION

A fully immunized child is protected from the discomforts and complications of many infectious diseases. Disease prevention spares the family the emotional and financial burdens that serious illnesses can cause. Immunization programs prevent devastating epidemics in a community. Health care dollars not spent treating preventable diseases can be used for other urgent issues. Immunization rates for routine, recommended pediatric vaccines remain above 90%, with the exception of the influenza and HPV vaccines (USDHHS, 2021). Despite the numerous advantages of immunization and these high immunization rates, gaps among children receiving vaccines still exist. Disparities in immunization rates by race, sex geography, ethnicity, and social determinants of health, such as employment, income, housing, education, and transportation, reflect health inequities in the United States (USDHHS, 2021).

Many factors lead to children not being fully immunized. Parental concerns about vaccine safety and side effects are a significant cause of inadequate immunization (Boom & Healy, 2020). Other parental objections include "vaccines do not work," "my child is not at risk," "the disease prevented by the vaccine is not dangerous," and "natural immunity is better" (Boom & Healy, 2020). Parents may also have a lack of trust in governmental and health organizations, as well as pharmaceutical companies (Boom & Healy, 2020). See Evidence-Based Practice 9.1. Parents may want to postpone some of the scheduled immunizations because they are concerned about the effects of multiple injections on their child. Postponing a portion of the immunizations puts the child at risk for contracting disease. Disrupting the optimal spacing of the immunizations can decrease the efficacy of vaccine, putting the child at further risk.

Misconceptions of what constitutes a contraindication to vaccination and having more than one health care provider are major contributors to inadequate immunization

EVIDENCE-BASED PRACTICE 9.1

COVID-19 Vaccine Hesitancy Among Racially Diverse Parents

STUDY

As of October 2021, 1.9 million cases of COVID-19 were diagnosed in children 5 to 11 years of age in the United States. Underrepresented groups have borne the greatest burden of COVID-19 infections and hospitalization in the United States. Non-Hispanic Black children experienced higher rates of hospitalization and higher incidence of the COVID-19–associated complication, multisystem inflammatory syndrome. The COVID-19 pandemic seems to have worsened and magnified the already existing health disparities in the United States. Early research in the general population has shown a high rate of vaccine hesitancy. This study was an online survey of 400 English-speaking racially diverse female guardians of children 5 to 10 years of age. The aim of the study was to understand how race/ethnicity influenced the decision of a parent to vaccinate their child against the COVID-19 infection.

Findings

Overall, 34.5% of parents surveyed would not vaccinate their child against COVID-19, while 40.85% would vaccinate and 24.75% were unsure. In parents who did not plan to vaccinate their child, the study found significantly higher levels of COVID-19 misconceptions, including the perception that children are less susceptible to infection, the belief that symptoms were less severe, a general mistrust of vaccines, a lower confidence in the safety and efficacy of the COVID-19 vaccine, less community support for the vaccine, and a lower likelihood of being influenced by the FDA or doctor recommendation for the vaccine. Analysis of the findings found that race/ethnicity, parental vaccine status, education, financial security, perceived childhood COVID-19 susceptibility and severity, vaccine safety and efficacy concerns, community support, and FDA and health care provider recommendations accounted for 70.3% of the differences for vaccine hesitancy. The study found 62% of non-Hispanic Asian parents, 45% of Hispanic parents, 31% of non-Hispanic Black parents, and 25% of non-Hispanic White parents planned to vaccinate their child. A higher number of non-Hispanic Asian parents were vaccinated themselves compared to other racial/ethnic groups. A significantly higher number of non-Hispanic Asian parents intended to vaccinate their child, while more non-Hispanic Black parents were unsure, and a higher proportion of non-Hispanic White parents did not plan to vaccinate their child.

Nursing Implications

Parents often have concerns regarding immunizations. The findings of this study emphasize the importance of understanding and addressing racial and ethnic differences when designing public health strategies regarding immunizations. Nurses are in a unique position to educate families and the community about current research findings. Even though the number of routine immunizations has increased dramatically over the past two decades, the total number of antigens the child is exposed to is actually less. This is due to the fact that newer vaccines are less crude and less antigenic than before.

Data from Fisher, C. B., Gray, A., & Sheck, I. (2021). COVID-19 pediatric vaccine hesitancy among racially diverse parents in the United States. *Vaccines, 10*(1), 31. https://doi.org/10.3390/vaccines10010031

status. The more children there are in a family, the less likely the children are to be fully vaccinated. The costs of vaccines or lack of access to health services can also deter families from obtaining immunizations.

OVERCOMING BARRIERS TO IMMUNIZATION

The use of a manufacturer-produced combination vaccine is encouraged when appropriate, particularly whenever it will reduce the number of injections at a visit (CDC, 2022c). These combination vaccines have been studied and approved by the FDA. The nurse should never mix separate vaccines in the same syringe unless expressly permitted in the product insert for all vaccines involved. Examples of combination vaccines are:

- ProQuad: measles, mumps, rubella, varicella
- Kinrix/Quadracel: DTaP–IPV
- Pediarix: DTaP–HepB–IPV
- Pentacel: DTaP–IPV/Hib
- Vaxelis: DTaP–IPV–Hib–HepB (CDC, 2022c)

Vaccines for Children (VFC) is a federally funded program that was implemented in 1994 in response to the 1989–1991 measles epidemic (CDC, 2016). Prior to this program, free vaccines were available only through public health agencies. The goal of this program is to improve immunization rates by providing free vaccines to families with low income and uninsured through private health care providers who are registered VFC providers. Additional information on the VFC program is available at http://www.cdc.gov/vaccines/programs/vfc/. The Affordable Care Act of 2010 requires new health plans to cover preventive services, including ACIP-approved immunizations, without charging a deductible, copayment, or coinsurance (USDHHS, 2022). The goal of these programs is to increase access to vaccines.

Establishing a medical home for every child will alleviate many of the factors associated with lack of immunization. Parents who have a long-term, trusting relationship with a health care provider are more likely to have their concerns about vaccine safety discussed and removed. Missed opportunities for immunizations can be reduced by:

- Maintaining a centralized immunization record
- Verifying immunization status at every visit, not just health supervision visits
- Verifying the status of siblings accompanying the child to the appointment
- Providing parents with up-to-date information on vaccines geared to their concerns and needs

Two excellent resources for vaccination recommendations in the United States are the CDC's Vaccines and Immunizations website (https://www.cdc.gov/vaccines/) and the CDC Hotline (800-232-4636 or 800-CDC-INFO).

What are some potential barriers to the Randall children being fully immunized? As a nurse, how can you help overcome these barriers?

Health Promotion

Health promotion focuses on maintaining or enhancing the physical and mental health of children. The principal components of health promotion are identifying risk factors for a disease, facilitating lifestyle changes to eliminate or reduce those risk factors, and empowering children at the individual and community level to develop resources to optimize their health. The nurse implements health promotion through education and anticipatory guidance.

Partnership development is the key strategy for success when implementing a health promotion activity. Identifying key stakeholders from the community allows problems to be solved and provides additional venues for disseminating information. Health promotion messages can be reinforced at schools, dayHealthy People Objectives retrieved from http://www.healthypeople.govcare centers, community agencies, and places of worship. If families have difficulty getting to health care facilities, the community arenas may be the primary source of health promotion.

Providing Anticipatory Guidance

Anticipatory guidance is primary prevention. The nurse partners with the parents to create a "road map" to optimal health for the child. The Healthy People 2030 box provides a framework for determining health promotion goals. *Bright Futures: Guidelines for Health Supervision of Infants, Children, and Adolescents* (Hagan et al., 2017) is another valuable resource.

The "skeleton" of the guidance provided involves common childhood health problems. The nurse fleshes out that information using the results of risk assessments and screening tests, health concerns unique to the child, and the interests and concerns of the parents. Age-related anticipatory guidance information is provided in Chapters 3 to 7.

> Provide appropriate anticipatory guidance for 3-year-old Maya and 9-month-old Evan.

Promoting Oral Health Care

Effective oral health practices are essential to the overall health of children and adolescents. Dental caries are one of the most common chronic illnesses seen in children (Nowak & Warren, 2022). Poor oral health can have significant negative effects on systemic health. Children who suffer from untreated dental caries have an increased incidence of pain and infections and may have problems with eating and playing, difficulty at school, and sleep pattern disturbances (CDC, 2022f). Refer to the Healthy People 2030 box.

Optimal oral health is not limited to the prevention and treatment of dental caries. It includes anticipatory guidance about nonnutritive sucking habits, injury

HEALTHY PEOPLE 2030

Objective	Nursing Significance
Reduce the proportion of children and adolescents with lifetime tooth decay experience in their primary or permanent teeth. Reduce the proportion of children and adolescents with active and currently untreated tooth decay in their primary or permanent teeth. Increase the proportion of youth from families with low income who have a preventive dental visit.	• Teach children and adolescents appropriate tooth brushing and flossing techniques. • Encourage use of fluoride-containing toothpastes. • Encourage routine dental visits.

Healthy People Objectives retrieved from http://www.healthypeople.gov

prevention, oral cancer prevention, and tongue and lip piercing. Preventing and treating malocclusion can have a significant benefit for children. Comprehensive health care is not possible if oral health is not a priority in the health delivery system.

Optimizing oral health can benefit the community as well as the individual child. The cost of pediatric oral health care can be reduced by 50% with the proper use of fluoride treatments coupled with other preventive measures (AAPD, 2018a). These health care dollar savings will enhance community resources.

Having a dental home enhances the likelihood that the child will obtain appropriate preventive and routine care. The AAPD adopted the policy of the dental home in 2001 (AAPD, 2018b). It is modeled on the AAP medical home policy. The dental home provides the same benefits to the child as the medical home. Characteristics of a dental home are listed in Box 9.7. The AAPD (2018b) recommends that the dental home be established by the infant's first birthday.

Promoting Healthy Weight

Higher weight in children is an important public health issue. The number of children with higher weight has continued to rise over the past 20 years. The principal causes

BOX 9.7 Characteristics of the Dental Home

- Preventive health program based on risk assessment
- Anticipatory guidance on oral health developmental issues, including dietary counseling related to oral health
- Plans for emergency dental trauma, management of oral pain and infection
- Anticipatory guidance on oral hygiene
- Comprehensive, evidence-based dental care (acute and preventive services)
- Comprehensive assessment for oral diseases
- Referral to specialists for care not available at the dental home

Based on American Academy of Pediatric Dentistry. (2018b). *Policy on the dental home*. http://www.aapd.org/media/Policies_Guidelines/P_DentalHome.pdf

of this increase are unhealthy eating habits and decreased physical activity. Weight is best managed by balancing calories with a combination of diet and exercise. Nurses can have the maximum effect in promoting healthy weight in children by encouraging activities that address both healthy eating patterns and physical fitness. Children, parents, and communities are all targets for healthy weight promotion by nurses. Refer to the Healthy People 2030 box.

HEALTHY PEOPLE 2030

Objective	Nursing Significance
Reduce the proportion of children and adolescents with higher weight	• Screen all children for the development of overweight as indicated by an increasing body mass index (BMI) for their age. • Provide accurate diet counseling. • Encourage daily physical activity. • Counsel parents to limit television/computer time daily.

Healthy People Objectives retrieved from http://www.healthypeople.gov

The focus of healthy weight promotion should be health centered, not weight centered. Linking success to numbers on a scale increases the possibility of developing eating disorders, nutritional deficiencies, and body hatred. Instead, emphasizing the benefits of health through an active lifestyle and nutritious eating creates a nurturing environment for the child. This allows the child to maintain their self-esteem. In addition, a health-centered orientation also allows the family to develop a lifestyle that incorporates its cultural food patterns and traditions.

Parents who have a healthy eating pattern are likely to maintain and encourage those patterns in their children. The nurse provides parents with anticipatory guidance about age-related eating patterns during each health supervision visit. Parents with toddlers and preschoolers may need training in ways to cope with the child's growing autonomy while providing a variety of nutritious options.

The nurse can begin directly advising the young child on healthy foods. Information and teaching modalities need to be age appropriate. With colorful posters and games, the nurse can teach the preschool child the difference between healthy and unhealthy food choices. As children enter school, group and peer-led activities can be effective. The nurse must gear material toward the adolescent's growing autonomy in making self-care decisions.

Before providing education to school-age and adolescent children, it is important to obtain nutritional histories directly from them because increasingly they are eating meals away from the family table. As they spend more time away from their parents, they need to develop the ability to make nutritious choices. The goal is to help older children develop strategies for making healthy choices as part of their increasingly independent lifestyle. Detailed anticipatory guidance is provided in Teaching Guidelines 9.1 and in Chapters 3 to 7.

TEACHING GUIDELINES 9.1 Healthy Eating

Breakfast

1. Don't skip breakfast. You will not have enough energy to play well later in the day. Skipping breakfast can also lower your grades in school.
2. Avoid eating high-sugar foods at breakfast. They will make you sleepy during the day.
3. Start your breakfast with some fruit. A small glass of juice, berries on your cereal, or a banana is a good choice.
4. Protein is important at breakfast. Milk, either in a glass or on cereal, is a good source of protein; so is yogurt or peanut butter.

Lunch

1. Check the quality of school-provided lunches. If they are high in fat or sugar, bring your lunch. Many schools publish their daily menus in advance. Check online or ask the school for a copy.
2. Add a variety of healthy alternatives to your lunches.
   a. Try different types of breads. Pitas, wraps, bagels, and taco shells can be a good change of pace in the sandwich routine.
   b. Freeze fruits before putting them in the lunch box. This will keep the lunch items cool and the fruit fresh tasting. Canned pineapple and grapes freeze well; so do bananas.
   c. Try alternatives to high-fat chips. Dried fruits, baked pretzels, and animal crackers are a few examples of tasty, healthy treats.
   d. Low-fat chocolate milk is more nutritious than prepackaged juice boxes, which have high sugar concentrations.

Snacks

1. Limit snacks to afterschool and bedtime. Light snacks such as yogurt or fruit provide good hunger management. A very hungry child will tend to overeat at meals.
2. Children need to learn to eat only when they are hungry. Children often eat out of boredom. Discourage nonstop grazing by planning activities to occupy the child.
3. A small bedtime snack is okay if the child is hungry but should not become a habit. A light carbohydrate such as graham crackers or a piece of fruit works well.

(continued)

(*continued*)

Dinner

1. Plan your menu a week ahead. Planning ahead reduces the likelihood of eating out or getting take-out food. Restaurant foods are more likely to be high in fats and refined carbohydrates.
2. Prepare homemade healthy versions of take-out favorites. Top prepared pizza crust with cooked chicken, vegetables, mushrooms, and cheese. Serve the pizza with a salad for a complete and healthy meal. "Make your own tacos" nights, using lean hamburger and low-fat sour cream, can be a lot of fun for children.
3. Don't turn dinner into a battle zone. Forcing children to eat foods they do not like will only deepen their dislike of them. Give them the healthy foods they do enjoy, and eventually they will explore more options.
4. Lead by example. Children eventually adopt the eating patterns of their parents. If they see their parents eat vegetables, they will eventually try them.

Promoting Healthy Activity

Healthy physical activity can take many forms. During the preschool years, encourage parents to provide a wide variety of physical activities. This exposure to multiple types of exercise allows the child to find the one that is most enjoyable and increases the chances that they will maintain an active lifestyle. The focus should be on noncompetitive, fun activities. When the child enters school, the lure of television and computers can significantly diminish the amount of time spent in physical activity. Parents can encourage their children to stay physically active in several ways. They can limit the amount of time spent in sedentary activities and actively encourage the child to pursue any exercise that they enjoy. In addition to verbal encouragement, parents can promote exercise by participating in exercise with the child. A simple family walk can increase physical fitness while providing time for interaction between parent and child. Refer to the Healthy People 2030 box. Teaching Guidelines 9.2 gives additional suggestions for promoting physical activity.

TEACHING GUIDELINES 9.2 Healthy Activity

1. Plan physical activities that your family can do as a group.
2. Write exercise activities on your family's daily schedule.
3. Look for activities that appeal to your child's interest, such as dance, team sports, or swimming.
4. Place value on noncompetitive as well as competitive activities.
5. Show your child you believe exercise is important. Exercise daily yourself.
6. Encourage the community to develop safe areas for spontaneous games and activities.

TAKE NOTE!

The USDHHS recommends all children 6 to 17 years of age participate in at least 60 minutes of physical activity every day (U.S. Department of Agriculture & USDHHS, 2020).

HEALTHY PEOPLE 2030

Objective	Nursing Significance
Increase the proportion of children and adolescents who meet the current aerobic physical activity guideline. Increase the proportion of adolescents who meet the current muscle strengthening activity guideline. Increase the proportion of adolescents who walk or use a bicycle to get to and from places. Increase the proportion of children and adolescents who participate on a sports team or take sports lessons afterschool or on weekends.	• For the adolescent who does not exercise, advise them to start slowly by walking. • Work with the adolescent to identify physical activities that interest them. • Praise efforts to participate in a routine exercise plan. • Identify an athletic individual with whom the adolescent identifies, and encourage similar activities in the adolescent.

Healthy People Objectives retrieved from http://www.healthypeople.gov

Promoting Personal Hygiene

Handwashing is the first personal hygiene topic that needs to be introduced to children. Handwashing prevents disease by limiting a child's exposure to pathogens. The nurse can introduce the topic to preschool children using cartoons and games. Have the child sing "Twinkle, Twinkle Little Star" while washing their hands; this encourages adequate cleansing time. Use soap containers and towels with colorful characters to make the experience more fun. The school-age child can understand the concepts of germs and disease. Slogans such as "Let's drown a germ" can serve as a reminder of the importance of handwashing. The Glo Germ program (n.d.) is effective in this age group. A nontoxic substance that shines under a black light is placed on the children's hands. The children can follow how germs travel from object to object. After washing their hands, the children can see if they did a good job (Glo Germ, n.d.).

In response to peer pressure, adolescents are usually stringent about personal hygiene. Younger adolescents may need guidance in dealing with pubescent body changes such as body odor, fungal infections such as tinea pedis (athlete's foot), and acne.

Promoting Safe-Sun Exposure

Skin cancer is a significant health problem in the United States. Blistering sunburns in children substantially increase the risk of melanoma and other skin cancers (American Academy of Dermatology, 2022). People with fair skin are at highest risk for skin cancers, but anyone can become sunburned and develop skin cancer. When teaching children about safe-sun exposure, remind them that harmful ultraviolet (UV) rays can reflect off water, snow, sand, and concrete, so being in the shade or under an awning does not guarantee protection. Adequate sun protection requires using sunscreen, avoiding peak sun hours, and wearing proper clothing. Teaching Guidelines 9.3 gives more detailed instructions. Refer to the Healthy People 2030 box.

TEACHING GUIDELINES 9.3 Safe-Sun Exposure

Sunscreen

1. Use sunscreen lotions every day. Harmful UV rays penetrate clouds and cause damaging sunburns.
2. Use sunscreens with a sun protection factor (SPF) of 30 or higher and with UVA and UVB protection. An adequate amount for an average-sized child is half an ounce.
3. Apply sunscreens half an hour before sun exposure.
4. Reapply every hour if the child is perspiring heavily.
5. Reapply immediately after swimming.
6. Infants 6 months old or younger should not use sunscreens. Take steps to avoid sun exposure completely with this age group.

Clothing

1. Wear hats. The brim of the hat should be 10.16 cm (4 in) or more and should shade the ears. Straw hats need to have a sunproof liner to be effective. Children introduced to hats as infants usually accept hats as part of the "outfit."
2. Wear UV-blocking sunglasses. The eye is the second most common site for melanoma.
3. Wear long, loose, and lightweight clothing for maximum sun protection.

Lifestyle

1. Avoid sun exposure between 10 a.m. and 4 p.m. This is when UV rays are the strongest.
2. Ask your health care provider if your medication will increase your sensitivity to UV rays. If the answer is yes, take extra precautions to reduce sun exposure.
3. Avoid tanning beds. The devices emit UV rays just like the sun and can cause damage.
4. Check the UV index before going out. The higher the index, the more precautions you should take. UV index figures are available online and in TV and radio weather reports.
5. Advocate for safe-sun scheduling of recreational activities. Talk to others about scheduling outdoor activities before 10 a.m., after 4 p.m., or in the shade.
6. Consider UV-blocking plastic film for your house and car windows.

HEALTHY PEOPLE 2030

Objective	Nursing Significance
Reduce the proportion of students in grades 9–12 who report sunburn.	• Educate families to start skin protection from the sun in childhood to reduce the risk of skin cancer as an adult. • Teach parents to use PABA-free sunscreen (formulated specifically for children) after age 6 months with an SPF of 15 or greater and to reapply sunscreen frequently while the child is out of doors. • Advocate for schools to encourage a sun-safe environment.

Healthy People Objectives retrieved from http://www.healthypeople.gov

TAKE NOTE!

Give children the following physical reference when doing health promotion on safe-sun exposure. Tell the child, "Play outside only when your shadow is taller than you are." The child's shadow will be "taller" before 10 a.m. and after 2 p.m. The nurse can demonstrate this concept by placing a ruler on end and shining a bright light over it. As the nurse moves the light, the child will see the ruler's shadow lengthen.

KEY CONCEPTS

- Health supervision for children is a dynamic process. Optimal wellness for the child can occur only if the nurse forms meaningful partnerships with the child, the family, and the community. These partnerships allow for free exchange of information and the establishment of mutually agreed upon goals. The medical home exists when there is a single primary care provider for the child. The medical home establishes a trusting long-term relationship with the child and family. This relationship leads to comprehensive, coordinated, and cost-effective care for the child.
- Children with chronic illnesses have a critical need for comprehensive and coordinated health supervision. Children with chronic illnesses require more frequent health supervision assessments. These children must have a medical home. The location of that medical home may be with a knowledgeable primary health care provider or at a multidisciplinary specialty facility. The location is determined by the child's needs and the family's preferences.
- The nurse incorporates frequent assessments of the many psychosocial stressors faced by families of children with chronic illnesses when establishing health care plans for them.

- Health supervision has three components: developmental surveillance and screening; injury and disease prevention; and health promotion.
- Developmental surveillance is an ongoing process requiring a skilled observer and interviewer. To be effective, the nurse must understand normal growth and development expectations and be proficient at developmental screening procedures and techniques. Caregivers are most likely to reveal risk factors for developmental delay when the nurse has a long-term and trusting relationship with the family.
- Screening tests are part of injury and disease prevention. They are modalities that identify treatable disease in an early or asymptomatic state and allow for cure or lessening of the disease's injury.
- Vision and hearing screening are functional testing modalities that the nurse must be proficient in administering in order for the child's results to be valid.
- Immunizations are a cornerstone of pediatric disease prevention. The nurse increases the effectiveness of immunization by understanding the principles of immunization and applying them to the child's individual circumstances. Adhering to good immunization management practices, as outlined by the ACIP and the AAP, enhances the benefits and reduces the risks of immunization.
- Barriers to full immunization include fragmentation of health care, concerns about vaccine safety, financial constraints, and lack of knowledge. The nurse can be pivotal in ensuring that children and adolescents are fully immunized by serving as child educator and advocate.
- The principal components of health promotion are identifying risk factors for a disease, facilitating lifestyle changes to eliminate or reduce those risk factors, and empowering children at the individual and community level to develop resources to optimize their health.
- The nurse implements health promotion through education and anticipatory guidance.
- Anticipatory guidance provided involves common childhood health problems and seeks to prevent or improve the health of children.
- The nurse uses the results of risk assessments and screening tests, health concerns unique to the child, and the interests and concerns of the parents to develop appropriate anticipatory guidance for each child and family.

REFERENCES AND RECOMMENDED READINGS

Advisory Committee on Immunization Practices. (2000). Recommendations and reports: Poliomyelitis prevention in the United States: Updated recommendations of the Advisory Committee on Immunization Practices (ACIP). *Morbidity and Mortality Weekly Report (MMWR), 49*(RR05), 1–22. http://www.cdc.gov/mmwr/preview/mmwrhtml/rr4905a1.htm

Aites, J., & Schonwald, A. (2022). Developmental-behavioral surveillance and screening in primary care. *UpToDate*. Retrieved December 12, 2022, from https://www.uptodate.com/contents/developmental-behavioral-surveillance-and-screening-in-primary-care

American Academy of Dermatology. (2022). *Skin cancer*. https://www.aad.org/media/stats/conditions/skin-cancer

American Academy of Pediatric Dentistry. (2018a). *Policy on use of fluoride*. http://www.aapd.org/media/Policies_Guidelines/P_FluorideUse.pdf

American Academy of Pediatric Dentistry. (2018b). *Policy on the dental home*. http://www.aapd.org/media/Policies_Guidelines/P_DentalHome.pdf

American Academy of Pediatrics, National Resource Center for Patient and Family Centered Medical Home. (2022). *What is medical home*. https://www.aap.org/en/practice-management/medical-home/medical-home-overview/what-is-medical-home/

Boom, J. A., & Healy, C. M. (2020). Standard childhood vaccines: Caregiver hesitancy or refusal. *UpToDate*. Retrieved December 20, 2022, from https://www.uptodate.com/contents/standard-childhood-vaccines-parental-hesitancy-or-refusal

Bright Futures/American Academy of Pediatrics. (2022). *Recommendations for preventive pediatric health care*. https://downloads.aap.org/AAP/PDF/periodicity_schedule.pdf?_ga=2.17675389.55149517.1670352585-1010168752.1655126485&_gac=1.21185481.1667484109.CjwKCAjwzY2bBhB6EiwAPpUpZvGVWommkXC3nD4TQGqyFG8j5TGVRbeF_LzRU01f-VGezeqJ-uf2ExoCRJEQAvD_BwE

Bryant-Stephens, T. C., Strane, D., Robinson, E. K., Bhambhani, S., & Kenyon, C. C. (2021). Housing and asthma disparities. *The Journal of Allergy and Clinical Immunology, 148*(5), 1121–1129. https://doi.org/10.1016/j.jaci.2021.09.023

Carlson, S., & Neuberger, Z. (2021). *WIC works: Addressing the nutrition and health needs of low-income families for more than four decades*. https://www.cbpp.org/research/food-assistance/wic-works-addressing-the-nutrition-and-health-needs-of-low-income-families

Centers for Disease Control and Prevention. (2016). *Vaccines for children program (VFC)*. http://www.cdc.gov/vaccines/programs/vfc/about/index.html

Centers for Disease Control and Prevention. (2021a). *Injuries among children and teens*. https://www.cdc.gov/injury/features/child-injury/index.html

Centers for Disease Control and Prevention. (2021b). *Vaccine information statements (VIS): Facts about VISs*. http://www.cdc.gov/vaccines/hcp/vis/about/facts-vis.html

Centers for Disease Control and Prevention. (2021c). *DTaP (diphtheria, tetanus, pertussis) vaccine: What you need to know*. https://www.cdc.gov/vaccines/hcp/vis/vis-statements/dtap.pdf

Centers for Disease Control and Prevention. (2021d). *Vaccines and preventable diseases: Hib vaccination: Information for healthcare professionals*. https://www.cdc.gov/vaccines/vpd/hib/hcp/index.html

Centers for Disease Control and Prevention. (2021e). *Vaccines and preventable diseases: Polio vaccination*. https://www.cdc.gov/vaccines/vpd/polio/index.html

Centers for Disease Control and Prevention. (2021f). *Vaccines and preventable diseases: Mumps vaccination*. https://www.cdc.gov/vaccines/vpd/mumps/index.html

Centers for Disease Control and Prevention. (2021g). *Rotavirus in the U.S.* https://www.cdc.gov/rotavirus/surveillance.html

Centers for Disease Control and Prevention. (2021h). *Vaccines and preventable diseases: Meningococcal vaccination: What everyone should know.* https://www.cdc.gov/vaccines/vpd/mening/public/index.html

Centers for Disease Control and Prevention. (2022a). *Overview of childhood lead poisoning prevention.* https://www.cdc.gov/nceh/lead/overview.html

Centers for Disease Control and Prevention. (2022b). *Vaccine storage and handling tool kit.* https://www.cdc.gov/vaccines/hcp/admin/storage/toolkit/storage-handling-toolkit.pdf

Centers for Disease Control and Prevention. (2022c). *Recommended child and adolescent immunization schedule, United States.* https://www.cdc.gov/vaccines/schedules/hcp/imz/child-adolescent.html

Centers for Disease Control and Prevention. (2022d). *Pneumococcal vaccination: Information for health professional.* https://www.cdc.gov/vaccines/vpd/pneumo/hcp/index.html

Centers for Disease Control and Prevention. (2022e). *Human papillomavirus (HPV): Genital HPV infection—Basic fact sheet.* http://www.cdc.gov/std/HPV/STDFact-HPV.htm

Centers for Disease Control and Prevention. (2022f). *Oral health: Children's oral health.* https://www.cdc.gov/oralhealth/basics/childrens-oral-health/index.html

Centers for Disease Control and Prevention. (2022g). *Polio in the United States.* https://www.cdc.gov/polio/us/index.html

Centers for Disease Control and Prevention. (2023a). *Meningococcal disease: Risk factors.* https://www.cdc.gov/meningococcal/about/risk-factors.html

Centers for Disease Control and Prevention. (2023b). *Addendum—Child and adolescent recommended immunization schedule for ages 18 years or younger, United States, 2023.* https://www.cdc.gov/vaccines/schedules/hcp/imz/child-adolescent.html#addendum-child

Centers for Disease Control and Prevention. (2023c). *Respiratory syncytial virus (RSV) preventive antibody: Immunization information statement (IIS): What you need to know.* https://www.cdc.gov/vaccines/vpd/rsv/immunization-information-statement.html

Delaney, A. M. (2022). Newborn hearing screening. *eMedicine.* https://emedicine.medscape.com/article/836646-overview#a1

Fisher, C. B., Gray, A., & Sheck, I. (2021). COVID-19 pediatric vaccine hesitancy among racially diverse parents in the United States. *Vaccines, 10*(1), 31. https://doi.org/10.3390/vaccines10010031

Flynn, J. T., Kaelber, D. C., Baker-Smith, C. M., Blowey, D., Carroll, A. E., Daniels, S. R., de Ferranti, S. D., Dionne, J. M., Falkner, B., Flinn, S. K., Gidding, S. S., Goodwin, C., Leu, M. G., Powers, M. E., Rea, C., Samuels, J., Simasek, M., Thaker, V. V., Urbina, E. M., & Subcommittee on Screening and Management of High Blood Pressure in Children. (2017). Clinical practice guideline for screening and management of high blood pressure in children and adolescents. *Pediatrics, 140*(3), e20171904. https://doi.org/10.1542/peds.2017-1904

Gavin, M. L. (2021). *Lead poisoning.* http://kidshealth.org/parent/medical/brain/lead_poisoning.html#

Glo Germ. (n.d.). *Glo Germ.* http://www.glogerm.com

Grohskopf, L. A., Blanton, L. H., Ferdinands, J. M., Chung, J. R., Broder, K. R., Talbot, H. K., Morgan, R. L., & Fry, A. M. (2022). Prevention and control of seasonal influenza with vaccines: Recommendations of the advisory committee on immunization practices—United States, 2022–23 Influenza Season. *Morbidity and Mortality Weekly Report (MMWR), 71*(RR-1), 1–28. http://doi.org/10.15585/mmwr.rr7101a1

Hagan, J. F., Shaw, J. S., & Duncan, P. M. (Eds.). (2017). *Bright futures: Guidelines for health supervision of infants, children, and adolescents* (4th ed.). American Academy of Pediatrics. https://brightfutures.aap.org/materials-and-tools/guidelines-and-pocket-guide/Pages/default.aspx

Immunization Action Coalition. (2022a). *Administering vaccines: Dose, route, site, and needle size.* http://www.immunize.org/catg.d/p3085.pdf

Immunization Action Coalition. (2022b). *Ask the experts: Varicella (chickenpox).* http://www.immunize.org/askexperts/experts_var.asp

Immunization Action Coalition. (2023). *Vaccine administration record for children and teens.* http://www.immunize.org/catg.d/p2022.pdf

Intercountry Adoption, Bureau of Consular Affairs, U.S. Department of State. (2022). *Annual report on intercountry adoption—FY 2021.* https://travel.state.gov/content/dam/NEWadoptionassets/pdfs/FY21%20Annual%20Report%20on%20Intercountry%20Adoption.pdf

Kemper, A. R. (2021). Newborn screening. *UpToDate.* Retrieved December 13, 2022, from https://www.uptodate.com/contents/newborn-screening

Kobayashi, M., Farrar, J. L., Gierke, R., Leidner, A. J., Campos-Outcalt, D., Morgan, R. L., Long, S. S., Poehling, K. A., Cohen, A. L., ACIP Pneumococcal Vaccines Work Group, & CDC Contributors. (2022). Use of 15-Valent pneumococcal conjugate vaccine among U.S. children: Updated recommendations of the advisory committee on immunization practices—United States. *Morbidity and Mortality Weekly Report (MMWR), 71*(37), 1174–1181. http://doi.org/10.15585/mmwr.mm7137a3

Kroger A, Bahta L, & Hunter P. (2022). *General best practice guidelines for immunization. Best practices guidance of the Advisory Committee on Immunization Practices (ACIP).* www.cdc.gov/vaccines/hcp/acip-recs/general-recs/downloads/general-recs.pdf

Lipkin, P. H., Macias, M. M., Norwood, K. W., Brei, T. J., Davidson, L. F., Davis, B. E., Ellerbeck, K. A., Houtrow, A. J., Hyman, S. L., Kuo, D. Z., Noritz, G. H., Yin, L., Murphy, N. A., Levy, S. E., Weitzman, C. C., Bauer, N. S., Childers D. O. Jr., Levine, J. M., Peralta-Carcelen, A. M., & AAP Council on Children with Disabilities, Section on Developmental and Behavioral Pediatrics. (2020). Promoting optimal development: Identifying infants and young children with developmental disorders through developmental surveillance and screening. *Pediatrics, 145*(1), e20193449. https://doi.org/10.1542/peds.2019-3449

March of Dimes. (2020). *Newborn screening tests for your baby.* https://www.marchofdimes.org/baby/newborn-screening-tests-for-your-baby.aspx

National Center for Healthy Housing. (2022). *Lead.* https://nchh.org/information-and-evidence/learn-about-healthy-housing/health-hazards-prevention-and-solutions/lead/

National Heart, Lung, and Blood Institute. (2012). *Expert panel on integrated guidelines for cardiovascular health and risk reduction in children and adolescents.* Summary report (NIH Publication No. 12-7486). U.S. Department of Health and Human Services. http://www.nhlbi.nih.gov/guidelines/cvd_ped/peds_guidelines_sum.pdf

Nowak, A. J., & Warren, J. J. (2022). Preventive dental care and counselling for infants and young children. *UpToDate.*

Retrieved December 21, 2022, from https://www.uptodate.com/contents/preventive-dental-care-and-counseling-for-infants-and-young-children

Powers, J. M. (2021). Iron deficiency in infants and children <12: Screening, prevention, clinical manifestations, and diagnosis. *UpToDate*. Retrieved December 14, 2022, from https://www.uptodate.com/contents/iron-deficiency-in-infants-and-children-less-than12-years-screening-prevention-clinical-manifestations-and-diagnosis

Sample, J. A. (2022). Childhood lead poisoning: Clinical manifestations and diagnosis. *UpToDate*. Retrieved December 14, 2022, from https://www.uptodate.com/contents/childhood-lead-poisoning-clinical-manifestations-and-diagnosis

Schulte, E. E. (2020). Domestic and international adoption. In R. M. Kleigman, J. W. St. Geme III, N. J. Blum, S. S. Shah, R. C. Tasker, K. M. Wilson, & R. E. Behrman (Eds.), *Nelson textbook of pediatrics* (21st ed., pp. 960–976). Elsevier.

U.S. Department of Agriculture, & U.S. Department of Health and Human Services. (2020). *Dietary guidelines for Americans, 2020–2025* (9th ed.). DietaryGuidelines.gov

U.S. Department of Health and Human Services. (2021). *Vaccines National Strategic Plan 2021–2025*. https://www.hhs.gov/sites/default/files/HHS-Vaccines-Report.pdf

U.S. Department of Health and Human Services. (2022). *About ACA: Preventative care*. https://www.hhs.gov/healthcare/about-the-aca/preventive-care/index.html

U.S. Department of Health and Human Services. (n.d.). *Healthy People 2030*. https://health.gov/healthypeople

United States Environmental Protection Agency. (2018). *Protecting children from lead exposures*. https://www.epa.gov/sites/production/files/2018-10/documents/leadpreventionbooklet2018-v11_web.pdf

Vaccine Adverse Event Reporting System. (n.d.). *About the VAERS program*. https://vaers.hhs.gov/index.html

Vohr, B. R. (2022). Screening the newborn for hearing loss. *UpToDate*. Retrieved December 13, 2022, from https://www.uptodate.com/contents/screening-the-newborn-for-hearing-loss

Zubler, J. M., Wiggins, L. D., Macias, M. M., Whitaker, T. M., Shaw, J. S., Squires, J. K., Pajek, J. A., Wolf, R. B., Slaughter, K. S., Broughton, A. S., Gerndt, K. L., Mlodoch, B. J., & Lipkin, P. H. (2022). Evidence-informed milestones for developmental surveillance tools. *Pediatrics, 149*(3), e2021052138. https://doi.org/10.1542/peds.2021-052138

DEVELOPING CLINICAL JUDGMENT

PRACTICING FOR NCLEX

1. During the health interview, the parent of a 4-month-old says, "I'm not sure my baby is doing what they should be." What is the nurse's best response?
   a. "I'll be able to tell you more after I do the physical."
   b. "Fill out this developmental screening questionnaire and then I can let you know."
   c. "Tell me more about your concerns."
   d. "All parents worry about their babies. I'm sure they're doing well."
2. An infant is at your facility for their initial health supervision visit. They are 2 weeks old and respond to a bell during the examination. You review all the birth records and find no documentation that a newborn hearing screening was performed. What is the best action by the nurse?
   a. Do nothing; responding to the bell proves the infant does not have a hearing deficit.
   b. Schedule the infant immediately for newborn hearing screening.
   c. Ask the parent to observe for signs that the infant is not hearing well.
   d. Screen again with the bell at the infant's 2-month health supervision visit.
3. A 15-month-old is having their first health supervision visit at your facility. Their parent has not brought a copy of the child's immunization record but believes the child is fully immunized: "They had immunizations 3 months ago at the local health department." Which would be the best action by the nurse?
   a. Ask the parent to bring the records to the 18-month health supervision visit.
   b. Start the "catch-up" schedule because there are no immunization records.
   c. Keep the child at the facility while the parent returns home for the records.
   d. Call the local health department and verify the child's immunization status.
4. A 4-year-old child is having a vision screening performed. Which screening chart would be best for determining the child's visual acuity?
   a. Snellen
   b. Ishihara
   c. Allen figures
   d. CVTME
5. Which facility fulfills the characteristics of a medical home?
   a. Urgent care center
   b. Primary care pediatric practice
   c. Mobile outreach immunization program
   d. Dermatology practice
6. The nurse understands that a live attenuated vaccine is contraindicated in which children? Select all that apply.
   a. A child currently being treated with antibiotics due to an ear infection
   b. A child who received the rotavirus vaccine last week
   c. A pregnant adolescent
   d. A child currently receiving chemotherapy
   e. A child who is scheduled for surgery next week

CRITICAL THINKING EXERCISES

1. During a health supervision visit for a 5-year-old, the parent tells you they are worried about the child's hearing. Your facility has been his medical home since birth. The child was the product of a normal pregnancy and delivery. They have had frequent ear infections since the age of 8 months. Six months ago, the child had a ruptured appendix and was treated with an aminoglycoside. The child has been fully recovered for 4 months.
   a. During the health interview, what information should the nurse elicit from the parent?
   b. What information should the nurse verify from the permanent medical record?
   c. What risk factors for hearing loss does this child have?
   d. What is the best course of action at this time?
2. The nurse is examining a 4-year-old to determine their readiness for school. Describe the developmental, vision, and hearing screening tools that will help the nurse to identify any problems.

STUDY ACTIVITIES

1. Develop an immunization plan for the following well children: a 2-month-old, an 18-month-old who has never been immunized, and a 5-year-old who was current with all immunizations at age 2.
2. This is the first health supervision visit for a 3-year-old adoptee from Russia since arriving in this country 1 week ago. Develop a plan for this visit.
3. Develop a healthy weight program for the following: a preschool class, a family in which the parents and the two school-age children have mildly overweight BMIs, and an adolescent girl who is of healthy weight but fears "getting fat."

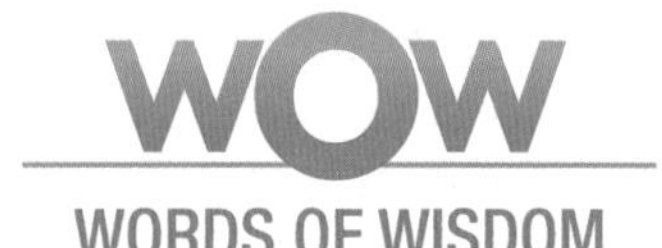

WORDS OF WISDOM

Astute nursing assessment of the child provides a snapshot of the child's overall health, growth, and development.

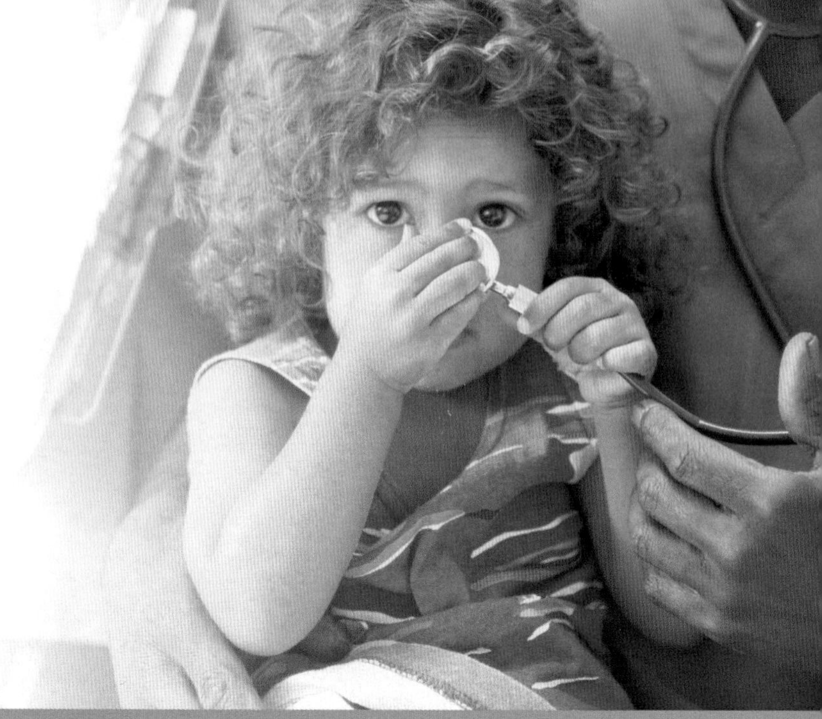

10 Health Assessment of Children

KEY TERMS

accommodation
acrocyanosis (ak′rō-sī-ă-nō′sis)
body mass index (BMI)
chief complaint
fontanels
lanugo
obligate nose breather
PERRLA
point of maximum intensity (PMI)
stadiometer
Tanner stages
tympanometer

LEARNING OBJECTIVES

Upon completion of the chapter, you will be able to:

1. Demonstrate an understanding of the appropriate health history to obtain from the child and the parent or primary caregiver.
2. Individualize elements of the health history depending on the age of the child.
3. Discuss important concepts related to health assessment in children.
4. Identify health assessment approaches that relate to the age and developmental stage of the child.
5. Describe the appropriate sequence of the physical examination in the context of the child's developmental stage.
6. Distinguish normal variations in the physical examination from differences that may indicate serious alterations in health status.
7. Determine sexual maturity based on evaluation of the secondary sex characteristics.

Elliot Simmons, 3 years old, is brought to the clinic for his annual examination. His parent states that he is very fearful and anxious about this visit.

INTRODUCTION

Assessment of the child's health status involves many components: the health interview and history; observation of the parent–child interaction; assessment of the child's emotional, physiologic, cognitive, and social development; and physical examination. The nurse's skills are vital to the success of the assessment process. The nurse must:

- Establish rapport and trust.
- Demonstrate respect for the child and the parent or caregiver.
- Communicate effectively by listening actively, demonstrating empathy, and providing feedback.
- Observe systematically (especially while the child is quiet).
- Obtain accurate data.
- Validate and interpret data accurately (Treitz et al., 2022).

The focus of the assessment process depends on the purpose of the visit and the needs of the child. Assessment is an ongoing process and is repeated to varying degrees at every encounter. The expert nurse is constantly evaluating the children in their care, whether directly or indirectly as part of conversation and play. Indeed, some of the most subtle developmental signs may express themselves only during relaxed and casual interaction with a child (Brazelton & Sparrow, n.d.). The nurse may observe gait while watching a child run down the hall, assess fine motor skills and social adaptation while the child is playing a board game, or observe balance and coordination while the child is bouncing a ball. Play activities can give the nurse feedback related to upper body strength, such as when the child pushes the nurse's arms away when tickled. The nurse must also learn to perform a comprehensive and thorough examination of a child in an efficient manner.

A thorough and thoughtful assessment of a child is the foundation on which the nurse determines the needs of the child. A comprehensive history, a thorough examination, and developmental or cognitive testing as appropriate will provide practical information about the health of a child and guide the nurse's plan of care (developmental testing is covered in Chapter 9). The history and physical examination also provide a time for health education, teaching about expected growth and development, and discussing healthy lifestyle choices. The nurse uses critical thinking skills to analyze the data and establish priorities for nursing intervention or follow-up care (Chiocca, 2020).

The health assessment may be documented using a number of formats such as a written narrative, a written flow sheet, or an electronic health record. The information should be easily retrievable and available to all members of the child's health care team.

HEALTH HISTORY

The health history provides the nurse with an overall picture of what the child has experienced, highlighting areas of concern such as recurrent upper respiratory infections or headaches. This not only helps the nurse to assess those specific areas more comprehensively but also provides the opportunity to ask focused questions and identify areas where education may be needed. The time used to obtain the health history also gives the nurse an opportunity to interact with the child in a nonthreatening manner while the child watches the interactions between the nurse and the primary caregiver (Drutz & White-Satcher, 2023; Miller, n.d.).

Preparing for the Health History

Appropriate materials and a suitable environment are needed when performing a thorough health history. Take into account family roles and values. Consider the age and developmental stage of the child in order to approach the child appropriately and possibly involve them in the health history. Observe the child–parent interaction. Determine the extent of the health history that is needed in a given situation. Being well organized and staying flexible will help ensure success (Chiocca, 2020).

Gathering Materials

Before beginning, make sure the following are available: materials to record the history data (either a computer or chart paper and a pen), a private space with adequate lighting, chairs for adults and the nurse, and a bed or examination table for the child. The space should be safe for the child's developmental stage. Sit down for as much of the history taking as possible to demonstrate a relaxed and welcoming manner.

Approaching the Parent or Caregiver

Greet the parent or caregiver by name. While interviewing the parent, provide toys or books to occupy the child, allowing the parent to concentrate on the questions. Use open-ended questions and avoid making judgmental comments. Show respect by remaining approachable. Remember that the structure of the family and its roles and dynamics will affect how the family communicates and how they make decisions about health care. Demonstrate patience and help the parent stay on track when there are several children in the family. Throughout the interview, refer to the child by name and use the preferred gender when referring to the child, demonstrating interest and competence.

TAKE NOTE!

Illness can cause great stress in families and individuals, so nurses must remember to protect themselves from potentially threatening behavior on the part of the family. Sit close to the door, and if uncomfortable with a family member, ask for assistance. The nurse may need to alert security personnel in certain cases (Mento et al., 2020).

Approaching the Child

Show a professional demeanor while still being warm and friendly to the caregivers and child. To have a positive impact on the interaction, wear a child-friendly lab coat, uniform, or character pins, or use a colorful stethoscope cover. These may allow the child to see the nurse as friendly or nonthreatening (Drutz & White-Satcher, 2023). Make eye contact if possible and address the child by name. Use slow deliberate gestures rather than very quick or grand ones, which may be frightening to shy children.

Some young children will warm up when given time to be invisible in the room, such as hiding behind a parent before they tentatively appear. Make physical contact with the child in a nonthreatening way at first. Briefly cuddling a newborn before returning them to the caregiver, laying a hand on the head or arm of toddlers and preschoolers, and warmly shaking the hand of older children and adolescents will convey a gentle demeanor. A joke, a puppet, a silly story, or even a simple magic trick may coax the child into warming up. Being at the same eye level as the child can also be more reassuring than standing over the child (Miller, n.d.). This may require having extra seating for the nurse at the same level as the child and parent or caregiver. Aim to be seen as a trustworthy adult who is the child's partner in feeling better and staying healthy.

Elicit the child's cooperation by allowing them control over the pace and order of the health history, or anything else that the child can control while still allowing the nurse to obtain the information needed. All of this establishes a personal relationship with the child and helps gain their cooperation (Miller, n.d.).

Communicating With the Child During the Health History

Give the child opportunities to actively participate in the health history and assessment process. For young children, such as toddlers and preschoolers, ask them to point to where it hurts and allow them to answer questions. Validation of the information by the parent or caregiver is essential because of the limited comprehension and language use of children at these ages. The school-age child can answer more accurately because of their increased language skills and maturity level.

Initially, address the child and obtain as much information from them as possible. School-age children should be able to answer questions about interactions with friends and siblings and school and activities they enjoy or in which they are involved. Ask the parent or caregiver if any additional information or observations should be included.

Adolescents may not feel comfortable addressing health issues, answering questions, or being examined in the presence of the parent or caregiver. The nurse must establish a trusting relationship with the adolescent to provide them with optimal health care. Ask adolescents whether they would be more comfortable answering questions alone in the examination area or whether they prefer their parents to be present. Either way, the parent or caregiver will have an opportunity to talk with the nurse after the health history and assessment are completed (Sass & Richards, 2022).

Demonstrate an interest in the adolescent by asking questions about school, work, hobbies or activities, and friendships. Begin with these topics to make the adolescent feel comfortable in communicating with the nurse. Communicate honestly with the adolescent and explain the rationale for various aspects of the health history. Adolescents can be sensitive to nonverbal communication, so be aware of gestures and expressions (Sass & Richards, 2022). Once a rapport has been established, move on to more emotionally charged questions that relate to sexuality, substance use, depression, and suicide.

Always assure the adolescent that complete confidentiality will be maintained to the extent possible. Current state law will determine the types of information that may be withheld from parents. If the information that the nurse receives indicates that the adolescent may be in danger, then the nurse must inform the adolescent that the information will be shared with other providers and the parents (Sass & Richards, 2022).

TAKE NOTE!

Do not try to become the adolescent's peer. Remain in the role of the nurse while demonstrating respect and acceptance toward the adolescent. Clarify the meaning of jargon or slang that the adolescent uses, but do not use these words yourself; the adolescent will simply not accept the nurse as a peer.

Observing the Parent–Child Interaction

Observation of the parent–child interaction begins during the focused conversation of the health interview and continues throughout the physical examination. Explore the family dynamics, not only through questions but also by observing the family for behavioral clues. Does the parent make eye contact with the infant? Does the parent anticipate and respond to the infant's needs? Are the parents ineffective when dealing with a toddler's temper tantrum? The plan of care may need to be adjusted to teach appropriate responses to the infant's needs or toddler's behavior. Do the parents' comments increase the school-age child's sense of self-worth? Behavioral observations are crucial to proper assessment of the family's needs (Columbia University, College of Physicians and Surgeons, n.d.; Drutz & White-Satcher, 2023).

Further observe the parent–child interaction to determine if the parent appears to be overwhelmed and if their behavior seems appropriate. Monitor the child's behavioral cues. Does the child look at the parent or caregiver before answering? Does the child seem relaxed and happy with the parent or caregiver, or is the child tense? The infant will appear calm and relaxed if their needs are generally met. Crying may occur when the baby is ill or frightened but may also indicate discomfort with the parent or caregiver. Use a calm and comforting voice with the infant. Infants respond well to higher-pitched and soothing voices.

When observing the relationship between the adolescent and the parent or caregiver, does the parent or caregiver allow the adolescent to speak, or do they frequently interrupt? Does the parent or caregiver contradict what is being said? Observe the body language of the adolescent: does the adolescent seem relaxed or tense? Since adolescents are between childhood and adulthood, they have unique needs. They are experiencing a time of multiple physical and emotional changes, many of which they cannot control. They need to know that the nurse is interested in what they have to say (Sass & Richards, 2022). The use of open-ended questions allows the adolescent to talk. "Tell me about your …" or "What have you noticed about …?" are comfortable phrases to use to elicit the information needed. Be aware of your own reactions to the adolescent's questions or behaviors, such as nonverbal and facial expressions. Talk with the adolescent using accurate language that is developmentally and age appropriate.

Determining the Type of History Needed

The purpose of the examination will determine how comprehensive the history must be. If the health care provider or nurse practitioner rarely sees the child or if the child is critically ill, a complete and detailed history is in order, no matter what the setting. The child who has received routine health care and presents with a mild illness may need only a problem-focused history. In critical situations, some of the history taking must be delayed until after the child's condition is stabilized. Evaluate the situation to determine the best timing and the extent of the history (Quinlin & Gawlik, 2021). Also, be sensitive to repetitive interviews in hospital situations, and collaborate with health care providers or other members of the health care team to ensure that a family already under stress does not need to undergo prolonged or repetitive questioning.

CLINICAL REASONING ALERT!

Immediately report absence of the red reflex in one or both eyes, as this may indicate the presence of cataracts (Chiocca, 2020).

Performing a Health History

The health interview is the foundation of an accurate health assessment. Careful conversation and interview with the child or the caregiver will provide important information about the child's health. Depending on the intent of the health assessment, many of the questions will be direct, and many will require the caregiver or child to answer simply "yes" or "no." In other than emergency situations, though, asking open-ended questions offers an excellent opportunity to learn more about the patient's life. For example, "Are you happy at school?" may elicit a brief nod of the head, whereas "Tell me what it's like on your school playground" may result in a story about the child's friends, the kind of activities the child enjoys, any bullying that goes on, and so forth. These stories will provide the nurse with clues to the child's stage of physical, emotional, and moral development as well as their functional status (Columbia University, College of Physicians and Surgeons, n.d.; Drutz & White-Satcher, 2023).

Establish a therapeutic relationship with the child and family. Without the trust that comes from this therapeutic relationship, the family may not reveal vital information due to fear, embarrassment, or mistrust (Treitz et al., 2022). Use therapeutic communication techniques such as active listening, open-ended questions, and eliminating barriers to communication. Establishing a "medical home" where ongoing health supervision occurs encourages trust through continuity of care and the family's continuing relationships with primary care providers (see Chapter 9).

The structure of the health interview is determined by the nature of the visit. At an initial visit, large amounts of historical data are collected. Having the family fill out a questionnaire can save time, but a questionnaire is not a substitute for the health interview. The questionnaire may serve as a springboard to begin structured conversations between the family and the nurse. At subsequent visits, the health interview can focus on the pertinent issues of that visit as well as any health issues that are being monitored.

The health history includes demographics, chief complaint and history of present illness, past health history, review of systems, family health history, developmental history, functional history, and family composition, resources, and home environment.

TAKE NOTE!

Any questionnaires used in the health care setting should be written at a fourth- to sixth-grade reading level and be in the primary language of the person completing them (National Institutes of Health, 2021).

Demographics

Initially, questions should be simple and nonintrusive; once a rapport between the nurse and the patient has started, sensitive questions can be asked. First, obtain data such as the child's name, nickname, birth date, and sex and gender. Determine the child's race or ethnicity, the language the child understands, and the language the child speaks. Record the child's address and home telephone number and the parent's or caregiver's work telephone number. Identify who the historian is (the child or the parent or caregiver) and note how reliable this source of information is considered to be. Do not assume that an adult with the child is the child's parent. Establish the relationship of the adult to the child, and ask who cares for the child if that person does not. Determine the composition of the household, including other children and other family members or other people who live there.

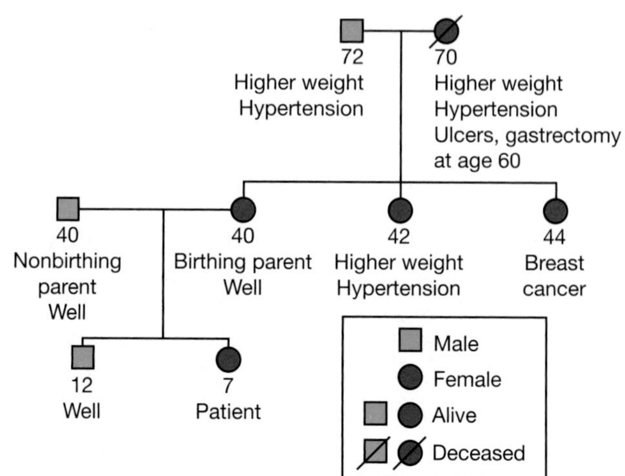

FIGURE 10.1 Genogram.

Chief Complaint and History of Present Illness

Next, ask about the **chief complaint** (reason for the visit). The reason may not always be apparent to you. A question such as "What can I help you with today?" or "What did you notice in your baby or child that you wanted to have checked today?" is welcoming. The response from the child or parent may be a functional problem, a developmental concern, or a disease. Record the chief complaint in the child's or parent's own words.

Next, address the history related to the present illness. For each concern, determine its onset, duration, characteristics, and course (location, signs, symptoms, exposures, and so on), previous episodes in the patient or the family, previous testing or therapies, what makes it better or worse, and what the concern means to the child and the family. Inquire about any exposure to infectious agents.

Past Health History

Ask about the prenatal history (any problems with pregnancy), perinatal history (any problems with labor and delivery), past illnesses, or any other health or developmental problems. Document the child's prior history of illnesses (recurrent, chronic, or serious) and any accidents or injuries in the past. Inquire about any operations or hospitalizations the child has had. Document the child's diet. Note the child's allergies to foods, medications, animals, environmental or contact agents, or latex products. Determine the child's reaction to the allergen as well as its severity. Determine the child's immunization status (refer to Chapter 9 for further information on immunizations). Record any medications the child is taking, the dosage and schedule, as well as when the last dose was given. Determine menstrual history as appropriate.

Family Health History

Obtaining information about the family's health is a key part of a health interview. Perform a three-generation family health history. This information may be documented in a genogram (Fig. 10.1). Asking about the age and health status of parents, siblings, and other family members helps to identify trends and specific health issues (Bryant & Speck, 2022). For example, do the grandparents have early-onset coronary artery disease? If they do, the child may benefit from additional health screening. Siblings may exhibit a genetic disease or carry a trait for the disease. This family health information helps to guide future health planning.

Review of Systems

Inquire about current or past history of problems related to:

- Growth and development
- Skin
- Head and neck
- Eyes and vision
- Ears and hearing
- Mouth, teeth, and throat
- Respiratory system and breasts
- Cardiovascular system
- Gastrointestinal system
- Genitourinary system
- Musculoskeletal system
- Neurologic system
- Endocrine system
- Hematologic system

Table 10.1 provides specific questions related to each of these systems.

Developmental History

Determine the age when landmarks in gross motor control were achieved, such as sitting, standing, walking, pedaling, and so on. Ask whether the child has attained

TABLE 10.1 • Questions for the Review of Systems

Systems	Has the Child Experienced
Growth and development	Weight loss or gain; appropriate energy and activity levels; fatigue; behavioral changes such as irritability, nervousness, anger, or increased crying
Skin	Easy bruising or bleeding, rash, lesion, skin disease, pruritus, birthmarks, or change in mole, pigment, hair, or nails
Head and neck	Head injury, headache, dizziness, syncope
Eyes and vision	Pain, redness, discharge, diplopia, strabismus, cataracts, vision changes, reading difficulties, need to sit close to the board at school or close to the TV at home
Ears and hearing	Earache, recurrent ear infection, tubes in eardrums, discharge, difficulty hearing, ringing, excess cerumen
Mouth, teeth, and throat	Swollen gums, pain with teething, caries, tooth loss, toothache, sores, difficulty with chewing or swallowing, hoarseness, sore throat, mouth breathing, change in voice
Respiratory system and breasts	Nasal congestion or discharge, cough, wheeze, noisy breathing, snoring, shortness of breath or other difficulty breathing, problems with or changes in breasts
Cardiovascular system	Murmur, color change (cyanosis), exertional dyspnea, activity intolerance, palpitations, extremity coldness, high blood pressure, high cholesterol
Gastrointestinal system	Nausea, vomiting, abdominal pain, cramping, diarrhea, constipation, stool holding, anal pain or itching
Genitourinary system	Dysuria; polyuria; oliguria; narrow urine stream; dark, cloudy, or discolored urine; difficulty with toilet training; bedwetting Undescended testicles, pain in penis or scrotum, sores or lesions, discharge, scrotal swelling when crying, changes in scrotum or penis size, addition of pubic hair Vaginal discharge, itching rash, problems with menstruation or menstrual cycle, development of pubic hair
Musculoskeletal system	Joint or bone pain, stiffness, swelling, injury (e.g., broken bones or sprains), movement limitation, decreased strength, altered gait, changes in coordination, back pain, posture changes or spinal curvature
Neurologic system	Numbness, tingling, difficulty learning, altered mood or ability to stay alert, tremors, tics, seizures
Endocrine system	Increased thirst, excessive appetite, delayed or early pubertal changes, problems with growth
Hematologic system	Swelling of lymph nodes, pale color, excessive bruising

Data from Bryant, P., & Speck, P. M. (2022). Health assessment. In T. Kyle (Ed.), *Primary care pediatrics for the nurse practitioner.* Springer; Jarvis, C., & Eckhardt, A. (2020). *Physical examination and health assessment* (8th ed.). Elsevier.

fine motor skills such as grasping, releasing, pincer grasp, crayon or utensil use, and handwriting skills. Note the child's age and extent of language acquisition. Document speech problems such as a lisp or stuttering. The rate of developmental skill acquisition may vary from child to child, but the sequence of skill attainment should remain the same. Inquire about self-care ability (e.g., tying shoes, dressing, brushing teeth) and, in the younger child, how toilet training is progressing. Question the parents about the child's feeding skills, including how well the child drinks from a cup and uses utensils or whether the child has any special requirements. Inquire about social skills and comfort articles (e.g., blankets, stuffed animals). Note whether the child has a habit of thumb or finger sucking or using a pacifier. Document day care attendance and preschool or school adjustment and achievements.

Functional History

The functional history should contain information about the child's daily routine. Inquire about:

- Safety measures (e.g., car seats and their placement, use of seat belts, smoke detectors, bike helmets)
- Routine health care and dental care (including dates of dental care and what was done)
- Nutrition, including a 24-hour dietary recall or week-long food diary, use of supplements and vitamins, feeding pattern and satisfaction with diet, amount of "junk food" consumed, food likes and dislikes, and the parent's perception of the child's nutrition (refer to Chapters 3 to 7 for nutritional needs at various ages)
- Physical activity, recreation, play, and organized sports
- Television and computer habits
- Sleep behavior and bedtime

- Elimination patterns and any concerns
- Hearing or vision problems (dates of last screenings and results)
- Relationships with other family members and friends, coping and temperament, discipline strategies, attention or school behavior problems
- Religious involvement and other spiritual practices
- Use of adaptive and assistive devices such as eyeglasses or contact lenses, hearing aids, walker, braces, wheelchair
- Sexual practices (Bryant & Speck, 2022)

Family Composition, Resources, and Home Environment

Determine the marital status of the parents. Does the child live with the parents, a stepparent, or other family member? Is the child adopted or in foster care? Are the parents the primary caregivers for the child? If not, the primary caregiver should be included in the interview process if possible. Parents may not know some of the child's routines if the child spends much of the time being cared for by someone else. Working parents may learn about a health or behavior issue only after being alerted by the child's day care center or babysitter. It may be helpful to expand the family history to include the grandparents and their interaction with the child.

Determine the employment status of the parents and their occupations, as this can affect the child's overall well-being; for example, the parents' work schedule may not allow them to spend much time with the child. Assess family income and financial resources, including health insurance and Supplemental Nutrition Assistance Program (SNAP); Special Supplemental Nutrition Program for Women, Infants, and Children (WIC); or other governmental supplemental income. Major family changes can also affect how the parents and child interact, so evaluate for relationship problems or changes.

Ask about the family's home and its age and environment. Is there a safe outdoor play area? If there is a pool, are safety features in place? Determine whether the home has electricity and an indoor water supply. Also determine whether the home has heating, air conditioning, and refrigeration. What pets does the family have? How are they housed? Are there infestations of insects or rodents in the home?

TAKE NOTE!

Homes or apartments built prior to 1978 may contain lead-based paint, and children who live there are at an increased risk for the development of lead poisoning (Centers for Disease Control and Prevention [CDC], 2023).

PHYSICAL EXAMINATION

The next step after the health history is the physical examination. It should focus on the chief complaint or any of the systems that engaged the nurse's critical thinking while obtaining the history. The examination will reflect the nurse's general practice style, the developmental stage and age of the child, the temperament of the child and caregiver, and the health status of the child. For example, a very ill child will not waste energy protesting the examination, so the nurse can move quickly in that situation. A healthy child, however, will express their expected developmental stage and will show varying degrees of resistance to the examination (Columbia University, College of Physicians and Surgeons, n.d.; Miller, n.d.).

Preparing for the Physical Examination

When performing the physical examination, being prepared and organized ensures that the needed information will be obtained efficiently. The appropriate methods to use and ways to approach the child depend on the child's developmental stage.

Gathering Materials

The examination area should include an examination table or the child's hospital crib or bed. Appropriate lighting is necessary for adequate observation and inspection. Gather the equipment necessary for the examination such as clean gloves, stethoscope, thermometer, sphygmomanometer, tape measure, reflex hammer, penlight, otoscope/ophthalmoscope, tongue depressor, and cotton ball. An infant or adult scale is needed, as well as a stadiometer for children capable of standing independently. Young children may be frightened by seeing a large amount of equipment, so take out one piece of equipment at a time. Some children can be very resistant to what they see as a threat or an invasion of their privacy, so it may help to have washable toys in the examination area to use as distractions during the assessment (Drutz & White-Satcher, 2023; Miller, n.d.).

Children and their parents may be able to sense any frustration or anxiety on the part of the examiner, so display a confident and matter-of-fact approach. If the child is not cooperative, do not become discouraged; more time and explanation will usually do the trick.

Regardless of the child's age, if the examination room is cold, the child will be uncomfortable and possibly less cooperative. Provide appropriate covers to ensure the child's comfort, or have the child remain dressed until the time of the examination (Miller, n.d.).

Approaching the Child

Approach the child according to their developmental age and stage. Table 10.2 outlines a general approach to

TABLE **10.2** • Developmental Considerations for Examination

	Newborn	Infant	Toddler	Preschool	School-Age	Early Adolescent	Late Adolescent
Place to perform examination	May lie on examination table or in caregiver's lap	In caregiver's lap or on examination table with caregiver right beside infant	Allow some freedom of movement when possible; child may stand between seated caregiver's legs or sit on the lap.	Some may be willing to sit on examination table with caregiver standing close by with hand on the leg.	Sitting on examination table where they still have eye contact with caregiver	Some may be willing to have their caregiver wait outside the examination room.	Explain to the caregiver that the adolescent needs privacy and that they should wait outside the examination room.
Examination direction	Keep up a running dialogue with the caregiver, explaining each step as you do it.	Continue to explain each step to the caregiver; address child by name. Perform most invasive parts last.	Introduce yourself to caregiver and child; explain most steps to the child and all steps to caregiver; allow child to handle instruments. Perform most invasive parts last.	Allow child to decide the order of the examination; explain what the instruments do and let the child try them; speak to the caregiver before and after the examination.	Include the child in all parts of the examination; use head-to-toe approach with genital examination last. Speak to the caregiver before and after the examination.	Speak to the child using mature language; appeal to their desire for self-care. Use a head-to-toe approach, with genital examination last.	Explain confidentiality to caregiver and adolescent; allow time talking with them together and separately. Use a head-to-toe approach, with genital examination last.

Data from Chiocca, E. M. (2020). *Advanced pediatric assessment* (3rd ed.). Springer Publishing Company; Miller, S. (n.d.). *Pediatric physical exam video* [Video]. http://www.columbia.edu/itc/hs/medical/clerkships/peds/Student_Information/Reference_Materials/PE_Video.html; Columbia University, College of Physicians and Surgeons. (n.d.). *Points on the pediatric physical exam.* http://www.columbia.edu/itc/hs/medical/clerkships/peds/Student_Information/Reference_Materials/Pediatric_PE.html

the physical examination in each broad developmental category.

If several children are to be seen at the same time, begin with the child who will be most cooperative. If the other children do not see anything scary and realize that their sibling was examined without a problem, it sets the stage for better cooperation from the younger ones.

NEWBORNS AND INFANTS

If the infant is asleep, auscultate the heart, lungs, and abdomen first while the baby is quiet. Count the heart rate and respiratory rate before undressing the baby. Completely undress newborns and infants down to their diaper, removing it just at the end to examine the genitalia, anus, spine, and hips. It is best to examine the infant 1 to 2 hours before a feeding. Having the parent or caregiver hold the child during the examination can help to alleviate fears and anxieties (Fig. 10.2). Allow the parent or caregiver to be a nurturer rather than assisting with painful procedures, unless there are no other choices available (Miller, n.d.).

Perform the assessment in a head-to-toe manner, leaving the most traumatic procedures, such as examination of the ears, nose, mouth, and throat, until the end (Bryant & Speck, 2022; Miller, n.d.). Also delay eliciting the Moro reflex until the end of the examination, as the startling sensation may make the infant cry. Use firm, gentle handling while examining the infant. Make sure your hands and the stethoscope are warm. Perform the assessment as quickly and completely as possible. Use a soft and crooning voice, smile, and engage the infant in eye contact. In addition, use brightly colored objects to help distract them. If the baby is crying, a pacifier may be useful.

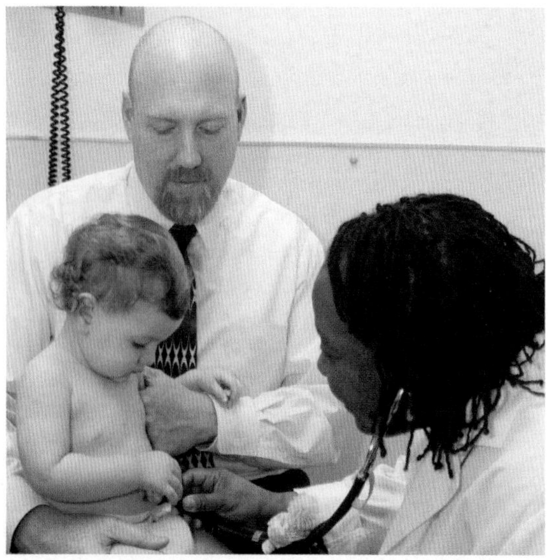

FIGURE 10.2 The infant or toddler may feel more comfortable and secure being examined while sitting in the parent or caregiver's lap.

TAKE NOTE!

Many older infants demonstrate stranger anxiety as a normal part of development. If the parent is not holding the infant, make sure the parent is within the infant's view; this will increase the baby's comfort and cooperation (Miller, n.d.).

TODDLERS

Toddlers usually prefer to remove their clothing one item at a time as needed for the examination. After one area is examined, the child may feel more comfortable replacing that item of clothing before removing another one (Treitz et al., 2022). An examination gown is usually not necessary before school age. Again, make certain the room temperature is comfortable.

When the nurse enters the room, a child of this age is often sitting or standing by the parent. Incorporate play as appropriate during the health assessment. Remember your own facial expressions and tone. Use little touch at the beginning of the encounter with the child and the caregiver.

Introduce the equipment to be used slowly, explaining briefly what is going to happen. Let the child touch and hold the equipment whenever possible, even taking a parent's temperature or putting the blood pressure cuff on a teddy bear (Fig. 10.3). The toddler will prefer to sit on the caregiver's lap. When the toddler must be supine for the abdominal examination, sit in your chair knee-to-knee with the caregiver so the toddler may lie back on the caregiver's and your laps. Praise the child for being cooperative during the examination. "You did such a good job holding still while I listened to your chest" and similar phrases give positive feedback to the child.

If the child is uncooperative, assess as thoroughly as possible and move on to the next area to be assessed. The caregiver may need to place an arm around the toddler's body to provide restraint for invasive procedures. Use

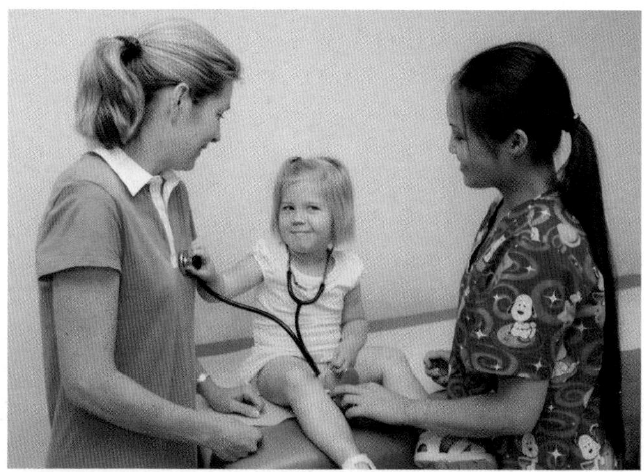

FIGURE 10.3 The preschooler enjoys listening to the parent's heart first.

short phrases to tell the toddler what you are going to do, rather than asking if it is okay (Chiocca, 2020; Miller, n.d.).

TAKE NOTE!

Toddlers are egocentric. Telling a toddler how well another child behaved probably will not be helpful in gaining the young child's cooperation.

PRESCHOOLER

The preschooler may fear body invasion and mutilation and will withdraw from any procedure or assessment that is viewed as intrusive. Otherwise, the sense of initiative often leads the preschooler to be cooperative. Use simple explanations to inform the child about each step of the examination, offering reassurance as appropriate. Allow them to "help" by holding the stethoscope or penlight. If choices are available, offer them to the child. Again, always compliment the child on their cooperation.

TAKE NOTE!

Preschoolers like to play games. To encourage deep breathing during lung auscultation, hold up a finger or a lit penlight and instruct the child to "blow it out" (Miller, n.d.).

SCHOOL-AGE CHILDREN

The school-age child's thinking is still very concrete, but they can be objective and realistic. Avoid using medical jargon and words that may have a double meaning to a young child. Instead of "take your temperature," "take your blood pressure," "hit your knee," or "test," say, "Let's see how warm you are," "I want to listen to you breathe," and other phrases that describe, in words the child can understand, what you are preparing to do. The school-age child may be interested in how things work and why certain things need to be done and will be responsive to truthful and simple explanations. Instruments that are colorful or look like toys are helpful throughout early childhood and the early school-age period (Drutz & White-Satcher, 2023; Miller, n.d.).

Always respect a child's desire to avoid pain and insult. Allow children to wear their underpants under the examination gown to provide a sense of security until the genitalia need to be examined. Allow the child to replace their clothing as soon as possible. Privacy and respect for the child's feelings are important to children of this age (Treitz et al., 2022).

TAKE NOTE!

Describing and commenting on your findings during the physical examination is interesting to the school-age child, as children of this age like to learn about how the body works (Miller, n.d.).

ADOLESCENTS

Provide privacy while the adolescent is undressing and putting on a gown. Demonstrate an attitude of respect. Perform the assessment in a head-to-toe manner, exposing only the area to be examined. Provide information about physical changes in a matter-of-fact way, such as "The hair on your legs is what is expected at this time." This provides information related to sensitive areas that the adolescent may be reluctant to ask about. It also provides the adolescent with information about the sexual development that is normal and expected. Allow opportunities for the adolescent to ask questions without the caregiver being present. Assure the adolescent that there are no "dumb questions" about the changes being experienced. The nurse should ask adolescents to remove their bras so that the nurse can perform a breast examination, teach breast self-examination, and check for scoliosis. During the breast and genital examination, it is appropriate to have a staff member present whose gender the adolescent is comfortable with, such as having a female staff member present when a male nurse examines a female patient (Sass & Richards, 2022).

Steps of the Physical Examination

The physical examination of children, just as for adults, begins with a systematic inspection: checking color, warmth, characteristics, and texture visually and smelling for any odor. Palpation follows inspection to validate your observations. Percussion is a useful tool for determining the location, size, and density of organs or masses. Tapping with the reflex hammer elicits deep tendon reflexes. The stethoscope is used to auscultate the heart, lungs, and abdomen.

Performing a Physical Examination

A complete examination includes assessment of the general appearance, vital signs, body measurements, and pain, as well as examination of the head, neck, eyes, ears, nose, mouth and throat, skin, thorax and lungs, breasts, heart and peripheral perfusion, abdomen, genitalia and rectum, musculoskeletal system, and neurologic system. The nurse in most settings will not be assessing the breasts, genitalia, eyes, or ears in detail. Be aware of the role of the nurse in different settings and how the nurse can facilitate the assessment process.

General Appearance

Never discount first impressions. Does the child give an impression of being ill or well? What is the child's expression and energy level? Note lethargy, listlessness, excessive activity, or inappropriate attention span for the child's age. Observe the child's state of alertness and whether they are responding appropriately to the stress of the situation. Note the child's posture and positioning:

- The newborn's posture is flexed, with arms and legs tucked in.
- The older infant should have improving head and then trunk control.
- The toddler demonstrates lordosis (swayback) and bowlegs, with a relatively large head and protuberant belly.
- The preschooler is slenderer and upright in appearance.
- The school-age child and adolescent should demonstrate an upright, straight, and well-balanced posture.

Note whether the child's development appears appropriate. Observing the child initially may yield a wealth of information about the child's development. Is the child active, moving about the room? Does the child's speech seem appropriate for their age? Notice whether the family interacts appropriately with one another and the child. Does the child appear clean and well cared for? Does the child appear well nourished or small for age, or is higher weight a concern? Note the scent of tobacco smoke or alcohol on family members. Notice if the baby bottle or pacifier is nearby and whether the child has a toy or transitional object. Assess whether the siblings appear equally well cared for. Observe for tension in the room between adults and children or adolescents. This initial quick assessment of general appearance will serve the nurse well if it is objective; delay interpretation of this assessment until additional data are gathered.

Measurement of Vital Signs

Measure, document, and interpret the vital signs of children using age-appropriate equipment and approaches. The child's age and size, as well as knowledge of underlying health conditions, will affect analysis of the vital signs. Vital signs are the temperature, pulse rate, respiratory rate, and blood pressure. These measurements fluctuate normally in children; assessing vital signs while the child is quiet is most appropriate. Comforting an infant or distracting a young child may be necessary while obtaining vital signs. If the child is crying or otherwise active during the assessment, document that fact. Many acute care settings require continuous measurement of vital signs using specific monitoring equipment. Also assess the child's pain level when assessing the vital signs.

TEMPERATURE

Temperature is measured as it is in adults. Thermometers are available in electronic and digital types. Use the same type of equipment consistently to allow reliable comparisons to be made and to permit tracking of temperatures during the course of illness. No matter which type of thermometer is used, ensure accuracy by carefully following the manufacturer's instructions.

The routes for taking the child's temperature are tympanic, temporal, oral, axillary, and rectal. Numerous research studies have been undertaken to determine the best method for temperature assessment in children. Take the child's temperature using the least invasive method that is best accepted by the child, parent, and health care provider or nurse practitioner.

> **TAKE NOTE!**
>
> Although they may continue to be available in some instances, glass thermometers are not recommended for use due to the mercury they contain (Vorvick et al., 2022).

Choosing a method of measuring temperature depends on what is available at the facility and the child's age and physical condition. Tympanic temperature reflects the pulmonary artery temperature and can be measured with the tympanic thermometer within seconds. The accuracy of a tympanic temperature reading depends on the user's technique and can be safely and effectively used in children 6 months of age and older (American Academy of Pediatrics [AAP], 2021). Refer to Nursing Procedure 10.1.

Temporal scanning uses infrared scanning on the skin over the temporal artery combined with a

NURSING PROCEDURE 10.1 Measuring Tympanic Temperature

1. Note age of child. If younger than 3 years, pull the earlobe back and down.
2. Insert the tympanic thermometer gently into the ear canal with the infrared sensor beam directed toward the center of the tympanic membrane rather than the sides of the ear canal.
3. Push the button to take the temperature and hold until a reading is obtained. The length of time required for the temperature to register varies per manufacturer but is only a few seconds at most.

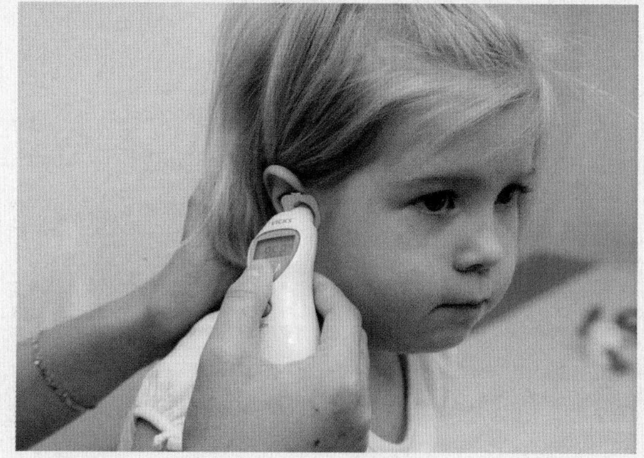

mathematical computation to determine the child's arterial temperature. Temporal artery thermometry may be used with any child over the age of 3 months (AAP, 2021). Measure temperature on the exposed side of the head (not the side that has been lying on a pillow or covered by a hat). Depress the sensor button and slide the sensor tip externally in a horizontal line across the child's forehead, midway between the eyebrows and hairline and ending at the lateral hairline (Fig. 10.4). Continuing to depress the button, lift the sensor from the forehead and then place it on the soft spot behind the ear lobe. Hold it there until the device registers the temperature reading, which usually requires 1 second. Accuracy may be affected by excessive sweating (Exergen Corporation, n.d.).

Oral temperature is highly reliable if the child can cooperate. By 5 years of age, the child can hold an electronic oral thermometer in the mouth well enough to obtain a reading. Place the probe under the tongue, and ensure the child's mouth remains closed until the device registers the temperature. Oral intake, oxygen administration, and nebulized medications or treatments may affect oral temperature.

The axillary method may be used for children who have difficulty cooperating, neurologic impairment, immunosuppression, or injuries or recent surgery to the oral cavity. Place the tip of the electronic or digital thermometer in the axilla to obtain the reading. Make sure the tip is indeed in the axilla and not just between the arm and the child's side. Hold the thermometer parallel rather than perpendicular to the child's side to obtain the most accurate reading. Keep the child's arm pressed down to the side until the thermometer registers, which will be as little as 10 seconds with certain electronic models but 2 or 3 minutes with digital models commonly used at home.

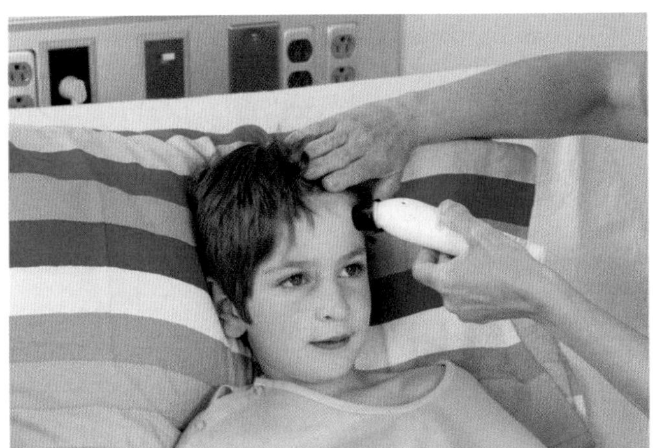

FIGURE 10.4 Temporal artery thermometers are noninvasive and well tolerated by young children. For an accurate reading, move hair to expose forehead and hairline.

Although long considered to reflect core temperature, the rectal route is invasive, not well accepted by some children, and probably unnecessary with the modern alternative methods now available (Chiocca, 2020). To take the rectal temperature, position the young infant supine with legs flexed. The older infant or child should be prone or side-lying. Small children may lie across the parent's lap for additional comfort. Apply a water-soluble jelly to the covered probe, insert the thermometer past the anal sphincter no more than 2.5 cm (1 in), and hold it there until the temperature registers (as little as 15 seconds with certain electronic models but longer with digital models).

TAKE NOTE!

Avoid the rectal route of temperature measurement in the child with immunosuppression or neutropenia, as well as the child who has diarrhea, a bleeding disorder, or a history of rectal surgery (Perry et al., 2022).

PULSE

Assess the heart rate while the child is resting or sleeping. The heart rate in infants is much faster than in adults. It also varies in infants and children who are anxious, fearful, or crying. As the child grows, the heart rate slows, and the range of normal values narrows. Table 10.3 lists heart rate ranges according to the child's age. The radial pulse is difficult to palpate accurately in children younger than 2 years of age because the blood vessels lie close to the skin surface and are easily obliterated (Bryant & Speck, 2022). For children younger than 10 years of age, auscultate the apical pulse with the stethoscope for a full minute (Jarvis & Eckhardt, 2020). In older children, palpate the radial pulse for a full minute (Fig. 10.5).

TABLE 10.3 • Heart Rate and Respiratory Rate Ranges by Age Group

	Infant	Toddler	Preschooler	School-Age	Adolescent
Heart rate	80–150	70–120	65–110	60–100	55–95
Respiratory rate	25–55	20–30	20–25	14–26	12–20

Data from Kleinman, K., McDaniel, L., & Molloy, M. (2021). *The Harriet Lane handbook: A manual for pediatric house officers* (22nd ed.). Elsevier; Chiocca, E. M. (2020). *Advanced pediatric assessment* (3rd ed.). Springer Publishing Company.

Note any irregularities in strength or rhythm. Finally, document the method used to obtain pulse measurement as well as any activity of the child during the assessment and any action taken.

TAKE NOTE!

In the infant and young child, the heart rate is often quite elevated due to fear or anxiety when the stethoscope is placed on the chest initially. For an accurate heart rate, wait several seconds until the rate slows, and then count for 1 full minute.

RESPIRATORY RATE

Assess respirations when the child is resting or sitting quietly, since respiratory rate often changes when infants or young children cry, feed, or become more active. They also tend to breathe faster when they are anxious or scared. The most accurate respiratory rate is obtained before disturbing the infant or child. This can often be done easily when the parent or caregiver is holding the child before any clothing is removed. Count the respiratory rate for a full minute to ensure accuracy. Infants' respirations are primarily diaphragmatic, so count the abdominal movements. After 1 year of age, count the thoracic movements. Table 10.3 lists ranges of respiratory rate according to the child's age. Document the rate, activity of the child, any deviations from normal, and any action taken.

TAKE NOTE!

Infants normally display an uneven or irregular breathing pattern, with short pauses between some breaths. This may be accentuated when they are ill (Kyle, 2022).

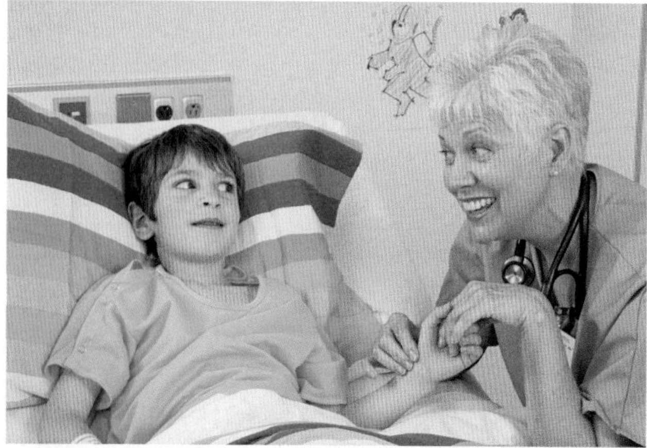

FIGURE 10.5 Assessing the radial pulse of a young child.

MEASURING OXYGEN SATURATION

Since the incidence of respiratory dysfunction is high in children during an illness, pulse oximetry is often routinely included in the vital signs assessment. This method is reliable and noninvasive. Pulse oximetry determines the oxygen saturation (SaO_2) in blood by using a sensor that measures the absorption of light waves as they pass through highly perfused areas of the body. The pulse rate on the oximeter should coincide with the apical pulse rate to ensure that the oxygen saturation reading is accurate. Nursing Procedure 10.2 details how to use the pulse oximeter. Identify whether pulse oximetry monitoring will be continuous or intermittent (as with vital signs).

A few guidelines to follow when using pulse oximetry are as follows:

- The probe may be placed on the finger, toe, ear, foot, or forehead. Avoid placing the probe on the same extremity with a blood pressure cuff or an intravenous or other type of line.
- Use the health care provider's or nurse practitioner's orders or health care agency guidelines to set parameters for high and low pulse rate as well as high and low oxygen saturation. Never turn off the alarm settings.
- Ensure that the probe is not applied too tightly, as this will prevent venous flow and cause inaccurate readings.
- It is helpful to use the provided cover over the sensor to prevent disruption from ambient light.

Potential sources of errors in pulse oximeter readings include abnormal hemoglobin value, poor perfusion, ambient light interference, motion artifact, and skin breakdown. Falsely low readings may be associated with a nonsecure connection (movement of child's foot or hand), and poor perfusion. Falsely normal readings may be associated with carbon monoxide poisoning and severe anemia (Mechem, 2022).

BLOOD PRESSURE

The AAP recommends that children older than 3 years have their blood pressure measured at least once during every health care episode (Flynn et al., 2017). Children younger than 3 years old should have blood pressure measured if they have one of the following risk factors:

- History of prematurity, very low birth weight, or other neonatal intensive care complication
- Congenital heart defect
- Recurrent urinary tract infections, hematuria, proteinuria, known kidney disease or urologic malformations, family history of congenital kidney disease
- Malignancy, bone marrow transplant, or solid organ transplant
- Treatment with medications that raise blood pressure
- Systemic illnesses associated with hypertension such as neurofibromatosis and tuberous sclerosis
- Increased intracranial pressure (Flynn et al., 2017)

NURSING PROCEDURE 10.2 Pulse Oximetry Monitoring

1. Explain the procedure to the child and family (use a penlight to show how the sensor "looks through the skin").
2. Attach the probe to the child and connect to the monitor.
3. Set the parameters for the alarm if monitoring pulse oximetry continuously.
4. Observe and record pulse rate and oxygen saturation.
5. Record the activity level of the child and the percentage of oxygen in use.
6. Check skin condition and rotate sensor position every few hours if adhesive type used.

Types of Sensors

a. Nonadhesive for infants (continuous use)

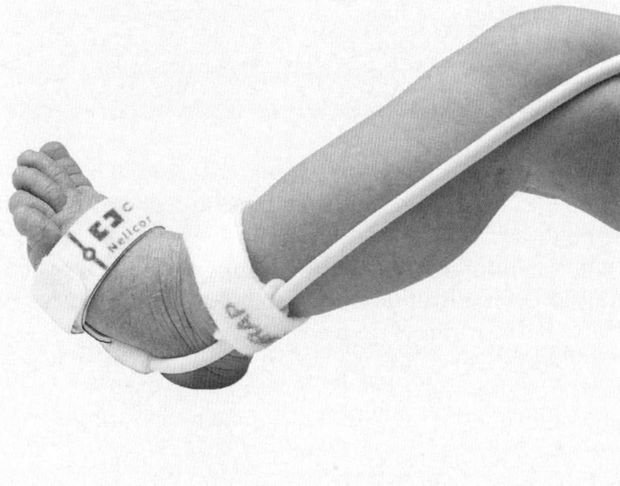

b. Finger adhesive (continuous use)

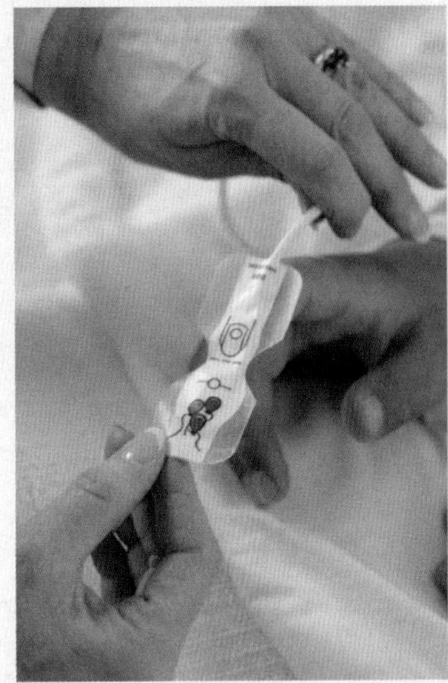

c. Finger reusable (intermittent use)

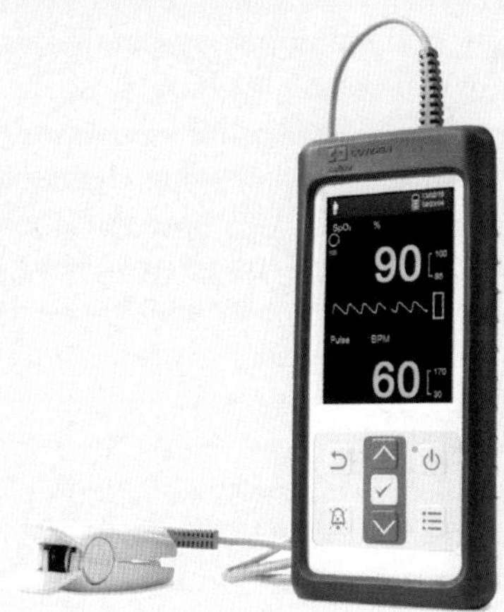

In the hospital or outpatient setting when a child is ill or undergoing surgery or a procedure, the frequency of blood pressure measurement will depend on the child's physical status. Measurement of blood pressure can be frightening to a young child, so include an age-appropriate explanation and perform the procedure after obtaining the pulse rate and respirations (Fig. 10.6). Accuracy of blood pressure measurement depends on the cuff size, as well as the operator's skill and accurate calibration of an electronic device. The cuff bladder width should be at least 40% of the circumference of the upper arm at its midpoint, and the cuff bladder length should cover 80% to 100% of the circumference of the upper arm (Flynn et al., 2017). Various pediatric and infant cuffs are available, as well as larger thigh cuffs that may be used on an arm in an adolescent with higher weight.

TAKE NOTE!

Using an accurate cuff size is important: a wider cuff yields a lower reading, and a narrower cuff yields a higher reading.

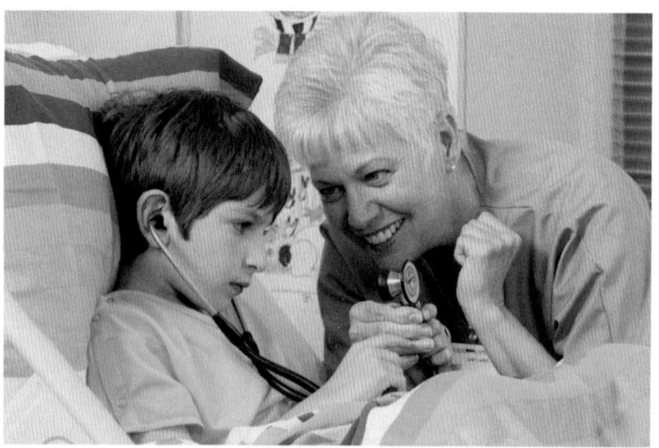

FIGURE 10.6 Allowing children to handle the equipment gives them some control over the situation.

Measure blood pressure in the upper arm, lower arm, thigh, or calf/ankle. The size of the cuff should match the extremity used. The measurement should be taken in the same limb, at the same place, and in the same position with each subsequent measurement to ensure consistency in tracking the blood pressure. To measure blood pressure using the upper arm, place the limb at the level of the heart, place the cuff around the upper arm, and auscultate at the brachial artery. When obtaining blood pressure in the lower arm, again, position the limb at the level of the heart, place the cuff above the wrist, and auscultate the radial artery. For measurement in the thigh, place the cuff above the knee and auscultate the popliteal artery. To obtain blood pressure on the calf or ankle, place the cuff above the malleolus or at the midcalf and auscultate the posterior tibial or dorsal pedal artery. Figure 10.7 shows appropriate cuff placement and auscultation points for the various sites.

When using auscultation to obtain blood pressure readings in children, note systolic pressure at the moment the first Korotkoff sound is heard as the manometer pressure is lowered (Fig. 10.8). The point at which the sound disappears is the diastolic pressure. The systolic blood pressure can sometimes be heard to a measurement of zero, so document the reading as systolic pressure over "P" for pulse.

Alternative methods for obtaining blood pressure measurements in children include the use of Doppler or oscillometric devices. The Doppler ultrasound method uses high-frequency sound waves that bounce off body parts to obtain blood pressure. Apply the gel to the Doppler end, and listen with the Doppler device where Korotkoff sounds would normally be auscultated.

With either the Doppler method or auscultation, inflate the cuff 20 mm Hg past the point where the distal pulse disappears. Oscillometric equipment measures the mean arterial pulse and then calculates the systolic and diastolic readings. The accuracy of this method depends heavily on ongoing validation and calibration. Also, the cuff inflates to a preset value often far higher than the infant or child's blood pressure, resulting in a tight, uncomfortable cuff being in place for a longer period of time.

TAKE NOTE!

If the oscillometric device yields a blood pressure greater than the 90th percentile for sex and height, repeat the reading using auscultation.

In children older than 1 year, the systolic pressure in the thigh tends to be 10 to 40 mm Hg higher than in the arm; the diastolic pressure remains the same. Refer to Appendix B for the National Heart, Lung, and Blood Institute (NHLBI) blood pressure levels based on sex and height. Systolic blood pressure increases if the child is crying or anxious, so measure the blood pressure with the child quiet and relaxed. If the reading is lower in the leg than in the arm, always consider coarctation of the aorta or interference with circulation to the lower extremities.

Pain Assessment

Pain is considered to be the fifth vital sign. Use the Face, Legs, Activity, Cry, Consolability (FLACC) pain scale to measure pain in children who are too young to verbally or conceptually quantify their pain or when there is a

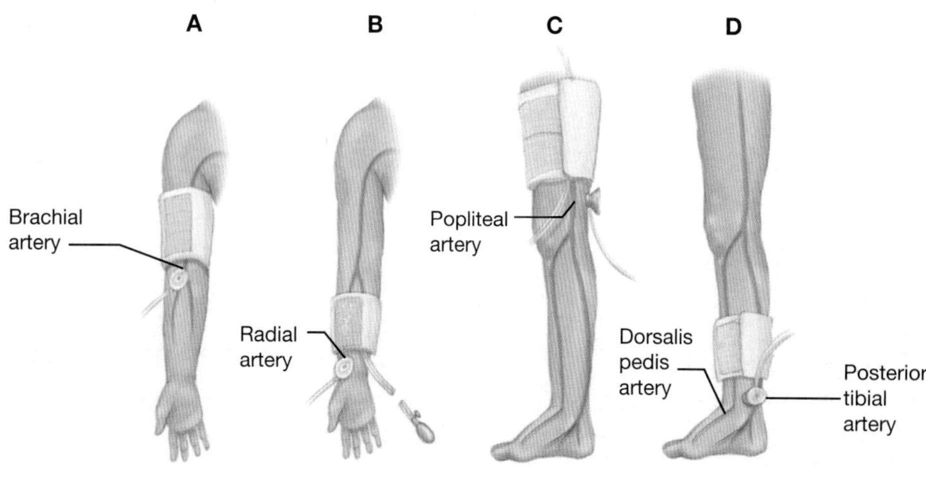

FIGURE 10.7 Various positions of cuff placement and auscultation area for obtaining blood pressure. **A.** Upper arm. **B.** Lower arm. **C.** Thigh. **D.** Calf/ankle.

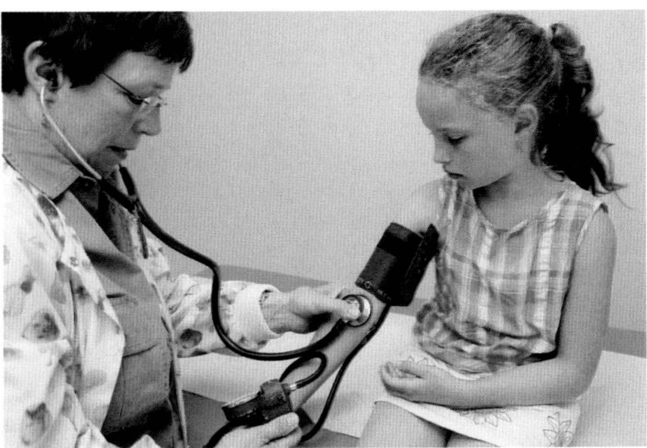

FIGURE 10.8 Auscultation is the preferred method for measuring blood pressure in children.

language barrier (Choueiry et al., 2020). The FLACC pain scale consists of a possible 10 points, with 0, 1, or 2 points given for each of five clinical signs (see Table 14.7).

Children who are older and can express that pain is worsening or improving should use the Pain Faces Scale (see Fig. 14.3). Explain that each face represents a person who is happy or sad, depending on how much or how little pain they have: 0 is for a person who is "very happy because they don't hurt at all;" 1 means "it hurts just a little bit;" 2, "it hurts a little more;" 3, "it hurts even more;" 4, "it hurts a whole lot;" and 5, "it hurts as much as you can imagine—but you don't have to be crying to feel this bad." Then ask the child to point to the face that best describes the amount of pain being felt (Wong & Baker, 1988).

For additional information related to pain assessment, refer to Chapter 14.

Body Measurements

Appropriate growth in children is usually an indicator of good health. A child who is not growing well may be in poor health, have inappropriate or inadequate dietary intake, or have a chronic disease. Accurate assessment of growth is a critical skill for the pediatric nurse.

Determine the child's height or length, weight, and weight for length or **body mass index (BMI)**. BMI is a reflection of weight in relation to height. Measure the head circumference for healthy children younger than age 2. Plot these measurements on a graph so they can be compared with earlier measurements and those of the child's peers' measurements. Additional anthropometric measurements used in children may include the chest circumference, midupper arm circumference, and skinfold measurement at the triceps, abdomen, or subscapular regions, but these are not performed routinely and are usually used only when a nutritionist consultation is necessary.

The growth chart is a screening tool for nutritional problems as well as a useful screen for chronic illness. Record each measurement in ink with a small dot at the correct location for the child's age and the date of the measurement written above it. Then use a plastic straightedge to connect the previous measurement to the most current one. Children grow at variable rates; in infancy and prepuberty, the growth velocity is normally more rapid. The growth chart allows the nurse to compare the child to other children of the same age and sex while allowing for normal genetic variation. When measurements fall close to the same percentiles over time, growth is normal for that child. Measurements falling within the following percentiles for age are generally considered the expected growth range:

- World Health Organization (WHO) growth charts (age birth to 2 years)—2nd to 98th percentile
- CDC growth charts (age 2 to 20 years)—5th to 85th percentile (CDC, 2022)

Sudden or sustained changes in percentile may indicate a chronic disorder, emotional difficulty, or nutritional intake problem. These findings require further assessment of the physical status of the child as well as other types of evaluations such as dietary intake or serum laboratory measurements. Appendix A provides growth charts for ages birth to 24 months and 2 to 20 years. The AAP and CDC recommend the use of these growth charts with all children, although special growth charts are also available for children with specific conditions (CDC, 2017). Look for a trend over time of healthy growth that is neither too fast nor too slow.

LENGTH OR HEIGHT

Calculate the length of the infant and toddler in a lying position until the age of 24 months. Use a measuring board (Fig. 10.9) or a cloth or paper measuring tape. Stretch out the legs to get a full extension of the body. Marking the examination paper at the child's head and extended foot is an option. Make sure that the growth chart where the measurement is plotted is marked for length and not height, as the two measurements differ. Document the length in centimeters and inches.

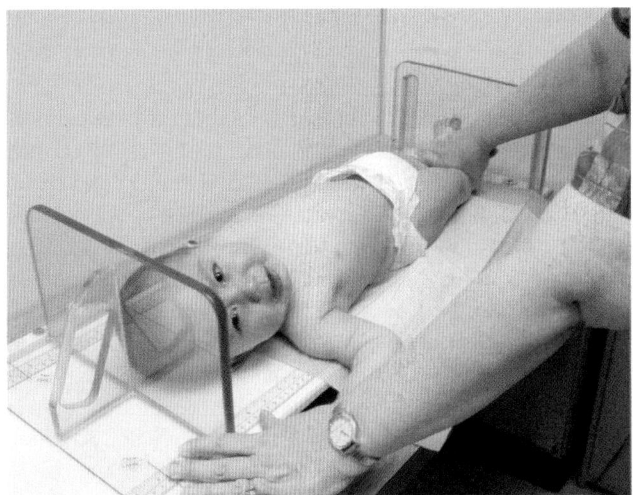

FIGURE 10.9 The recumbent measuring board is the most accurate method for obtaining a length measurement in infants and very young children.

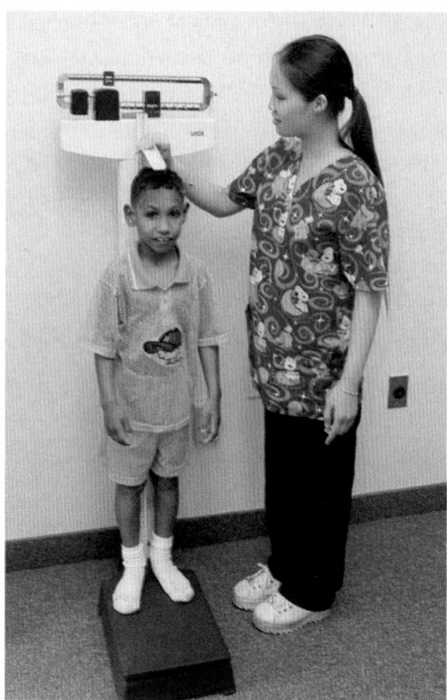

FIGURE 10.10 Standing height is most accurately measured with the stadiometer.

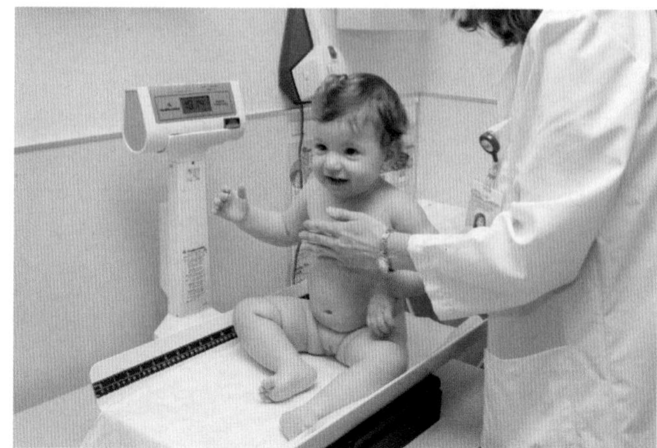

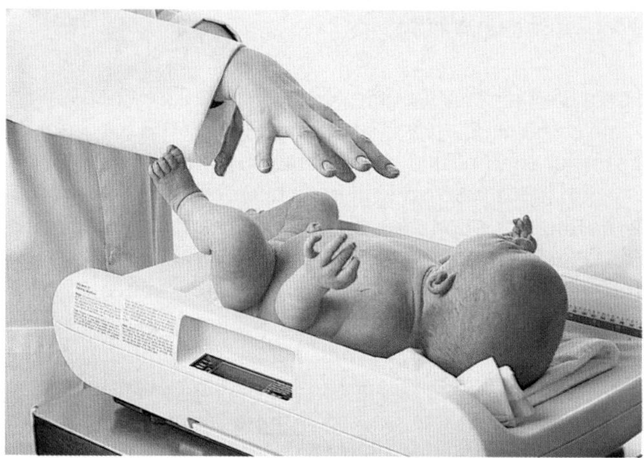

FIGURE 10.11 A nurse or caregiver should remain nearby while weighing the infant or toddler.

Once the child can cooperate and stand independently, begin measuring the standing height. Using a **stadiometer** is best (Fig. 10.10), but a cloth or paper tape can be used. Ask the child to remove their shoes and check that the back, shoulders, buttocks, and heels are against the wall, with the pelvis tucked as much as possible to correct for lordosis. The chin should be parallel to the floor. Plot this measurement on a growth chart marked for height rather than length. Record the height in centimeters as well as feet and inches.

TAKE NOTE!

Cloth and paper measuring tapes may stretch over time. Periodically replace or recalibrate all measuring tools.

WEIGHT

Measure weight on a scale that is calibrated between every measurement. Just before placing the child on the electronic scale, press the "zero" or "tare" button and make sure the reading is 0. Calibrate the balance-type scale by setting the weight at zero, observing the beam balance, and making adjustments as necessary. Infants and toddlers should be weighed on a platform-type electronic or balance scale, with an examination paper placed between the child and the scale surface. Calibrate the scale with the examination paper in place. Remove the infant's diaper immediately before placing them on the scale. Toddlers may sit on the scale with the nurse or caregiver nearby to avoid falls (Fig. 10.11). Weigh older children and adolescents on a standing scale (Fig. 10.12). They may keep their underpants on and wear a lightweight examination gown.

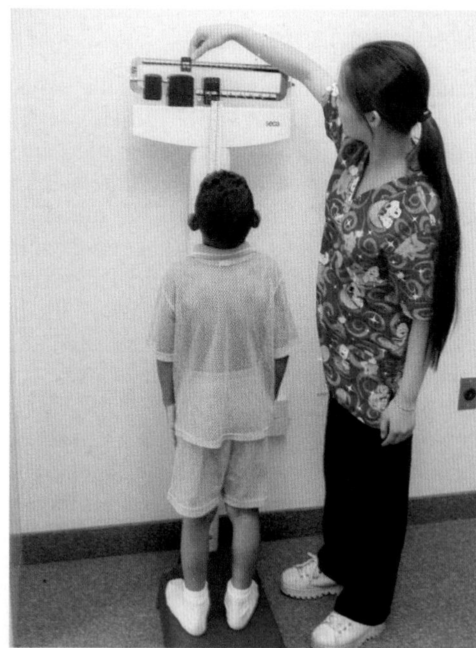

FIGURE 10.12 Children who can stand independently can be weighed on a regular standing balance scale.

An alternate method for obtaining weight, although much less accurate, is to weigh the caregiver initially and then weigh the caregiver holding the child. The difference between the two weights is the child's weight. Regardless of the method used, weigh the infant to the nearest 10 g (or half-ounce) and the toddler and older child to the nearest 100 g (or quarter pound). Record the weight in kilograms and in pounds.

WEIGHT FOR LENGTH

For children between the ages of newborn and 24 months, plot weight on the growth chart in comparison to the child's length. This allows the nurse to determine whether the child is a healthy weight for how long they are. Children placing less than the fifth percentile on the weight-for-length chart are considered lower weight. Those placing greater than the 95th percentile are considered to be overweight.

BODY MASS INDEX

BMI is determined by comparing the child's height and weight. Calculate the BMI using the child's weight and height by either the English or the metric method. Box 10.1 provides BMI calculation formulas. BMI is included on the charts for children ages 2 to 20 years. Plot the BMI on the growth chart according to the child's age. A child whose BMI for age plots at less than the fifth percentile is considered to be lower weight. BMI for age between the 85th and 95th percentiles indicates risk of overweight. BMI for age greater than the 95th percentile indicates the child is higher weight (CDC, 2022).

The growth chart can indicate when a child is not growing adequately and can also be used to predict the development of overweight and higher weight. Refer to the Healthy People 2030 box.

HEAD CIRCUMFERENCE

Measure head circumference at well-child visits and upon hospital admission until the third birthday. Then measure it at the annual well-child visit until 6 years old if there are problems such as microcephaly or macrocephaly present at age 3. Measure the largest point across the skull, not including the ears, with a nonstretching cloth or paper tape. Begin at the forehead just above the eyebrows and bring the tape around the head in a taut circle just above the occipital prominence at the back of the head (Fig. 10.13). Plot this measurement in relation to the child's age on the appropriate standardized growth chart (usual growth charts include head circumference only up to age 2 years).

BOX 10.1 Calculation of Body Mass Index (BMI)

English Formula

$$\frac{\text{weight in pounds}}{(\text{height in inches}) \times (\text{height in inches})} \times 703$$

Metric Formula

$$\frac{\text{weight in kilograms}}{(\text{height in meters}) \times (\text{height in meters})} \times 10{,}000$$

HEALTHY PEOPLE 2030

Objective	Nursing Significance
Reduce the proportion of children and adolescents with higher weight.	• Screen for overweight in all children by plotting weight for length of children younger than 24 months and body mass index for age for children aged 2–20 years. • Assess dietary intake and activity level in all children at risk for or overweight. • Provide diet and activity recommendations to attain a healthy weight or BMI. • Refer children with significant higher weight to a pediatric endocrinologist.

Healthy People Objectives retrieved from http://www.healthypeople.gov

Monitoring Equipment

Sometimes, children in acute care settings require continuous monitoring of vital signs. This monitoring could be via an apnea monitor or a cardiopulmonary monitor. The apnea monitor measures abnormal or irregular breathing in infants. The cardiopulmonary monitor generally measures heart rate and respiratory rate. Additional equipment on this monitor also allows for blood pressure and temperature monitoring. Set high and low alarm limits according to the health care facility's policies. Figure 10.14 indicates the placement of electrodes for the apnea and cardiopulmonary

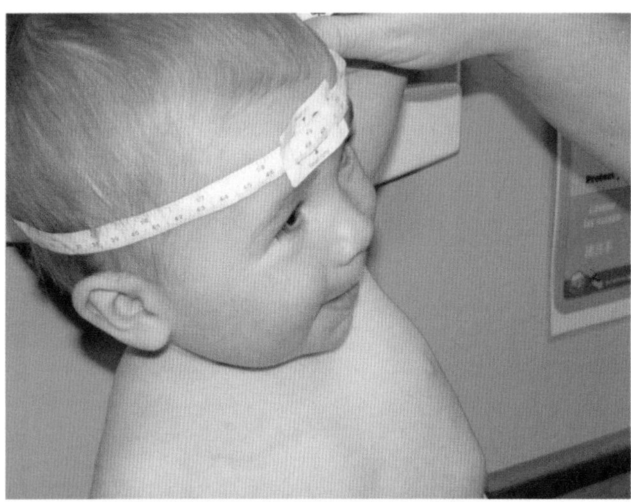

FIGURE 10.13 Measure occipitofrontal head circumference at the largest point.

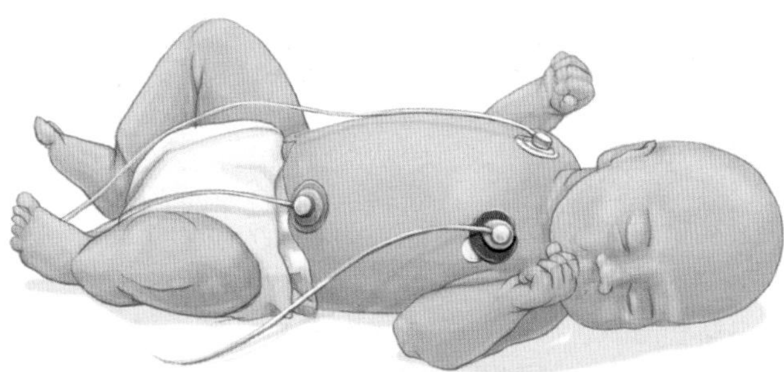

FIGURE 10.14 Placement of cardiac apnea monitor leads: white on the right upper chest, black on the left upper chest, green or red on the abdomen (not over bone).

monitors. Assess the skin where the electrodes are placed to ensure there is no skin breakdown. If the alarm sounds, immediately check the child to ensure the leads are not disconnected or the child is not in distress.

Skin

The skin is the body's largest organ and reveals information about a child's nutrition, respiratory, cardiac, endocrine, and hydration status at a glance. A careful skin examination provides an invaluable understanding of a child's health (Chiocca, 2020).

INSPECTION

Inspect the color of the skin. The color should be appropriate to the child's racial or ethnic background, with the nail beds, conjunctivae, soles of the feet, and palms of the hands appearing pink. Normal variations include the following:

- Blueness of the hands and feet, known as **acrocyanosis**, is normal in babies up to several days of age and results from an immature circulatory system completing the switch from fetal to extrauterine life (see Fig. 3.3A).
- Cooling or warming the newborn and young infant may produce a vasomotor response that causes a mottling of the skin over the trunk and extremities (see Fig. 3.3B).
- Babies of darkly pigmented parents will be paler than their parents for many months until the melanocytes in the epidermis begin production.
- Dark-skinned infants commonly have hyperpigmented areolas, genitals, and linea nigra.

Other variations related to skin color are discussed in Box 10.2.

Inspect the skin for the presence of lanugo. All infants display some degree of **lanugo** (soft, downy hair on the body, particularly the face and back). Lanugo is more abundant in infants of Hispanic descent and in premature infants and recedes over the first few weeks of life.

Inspect the entire body for nevi and vascular and other lesions. Note their location, size, distribution, characteristics, and color. Pigmented nevi (also termed "birthmarks") are indicated by a darker patch of skin and generally do not fade over time. Note the presence of hyperpigmented nevi (formerly called Mongolian spots), which appear as blue or gray, variably and irregularly shaped macules (Fig. 10.15). These are a common finding in dark-skinned infants. These nevi fade over months to years as the child's skin pigment darkens. Do not mistake hyperpigmented nevi for bruises. Inspect the skin for vascular lesions. Table 10.4 describes vascular lesions and their significance.

Rashes are common in children and are often associated with communicable diseases. Describe the rash in detail, noting types of lesions, distribution, drying, scabbing, scaling, and any drainage. The newborn and young infant may display milia (small white papules) on the forehead, chin, nose, and cheeks. These recede spontaneously. In adolescents, the skin examination may reveal open or closed comedones (pimples or blackheads) across the face, chest, and back. Adolescents may sport

BOX 10.2 Variations in Skin Color and Their Causes

- **Pallor** (defined as decreased pinkness in light-skinned patients, ashy-gray in dark-skinned) is caused by anemia, shock, fever, or syncope.
- **Central cyanosis** (blueness of the lips, tongue, oral mucosa, trunk) is caused by hypoxia or circulatory collapse.
- Overall yellow color (**jaundice**) may be physiologic in the newborn or related to liver or hematopoietic disease in any age child.
- **Yellowing** of nose, palms, and soles may result from excess intake of yellow vegetables.
- **Redness** of the skin results from blushing, exposure to cold, hyperthermia, inflammation (localized), or alcohol ingestion.
- **Lack of color** in skin, hair, and eyes is related to albinism

Data from Chiocca, E. M. (2020). *Advanced pediatric assessment* (3rd ed.). Springer Publishing Company; Jarvis, C., & Eckhardt, A. (2020). *Physical examination and health assessment* (8th ed.). Elsevier.

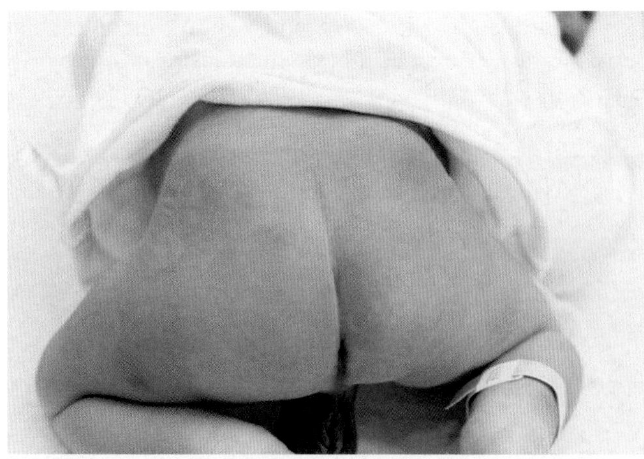

FIGURE 10.15 Transient hyperpigmentation most often occurs in darker-skinned infants.

TABLE 10.4 • Vascular Lesions and Their Significance

Description	Significance
Salmon nevi: light pink macule usually on eyelids, nasal bridge, back of neck ("stork bite")	Usually fade over time but may never go away completely. No complications
Strawberry nevus: raised reddish papule made of blood vessels (hemangiomas)	Present at or develop after birth; recede over time, usually by the age of 9 years. Usually no complications
Nevus flammeus: dark purple-red flat patch, grows with the child ("port-wine stain")	May be associated with Sturge–Weber syndrome. May be disfiguring; may be removed with laser therapy
Ecchymosis: purplish discoloration, changing to blue, brown, black (bruise)	Common on lower extremities in young children. Should correlate with the injury
Petechiae: pinpoint reddish-purple macules that do not blanch when pressed	Broken tiny blood vessels; occur with coughing, bleeding disorders, meningococcemia
Purpura: larger purple macules that do not blanch when pressed	Bleeding under the skin; occur with bleeding disorders, meningococcemia

Data from Chiocca, E. M. (2020). *Advanced pediatric assessment* (3rd ed.). Springer Publishing Company; Jarvis, C., & Eckhardt, A. (2020). *Physical examination and health assessment* (8th ed.). Elsevier.

tattoos, brandings, or various body piercings; inspect these areas for signs of infection such as erythema or drainage (Fig. 10.16).

Document the presence of any lacerations, abrasions, or burns. Note the distribution of the injury and whether it seems consistent with the mechanism described in the health history. Be alert to the possibility of child abuse if the type or number of burns, lacerations, or bruises seems unusual for the situation.

TAKE NOTE!

Petechiae or ecchymosis may be found over areas traumatized by the birth process; these may take a few weeks to resolve. Certain cultures use "cupping" or "coining" when a child is ill, and these practices may yield bruises or mild burns (Boos, 2022).

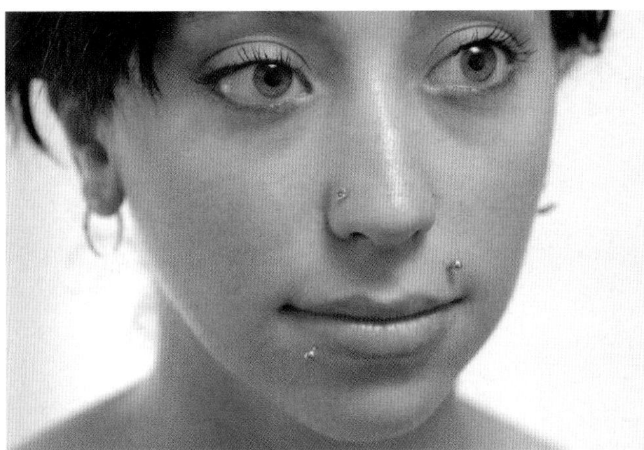

FIGURE 10.16 Adolescent with multiple piercings.

PALPATION

Palpate the skin for temperature, moisture, texture, turgor, and edema. Use the back of your hand to assess the skin's temperature, comparing the right side of the body to the left and the upper body to the lower. The skin should feel uniformly warm. Cool extremities are associated with environmentally cool temperatures as well as impending circulatory collapse and shock. Warm skin may be associated with fever or sunburn, or locally a burn or infectious process. The skin should feel fairly dry, occasionally moister in the creases. Dry, flaking skin may occur in the young infant, particularly if born postmaturely. Overall skin dryness in the well-hydrated child may occur with excess sun exposure, poor nutrition, or overbathing. Moist skin occurs with perspiration, fever resolution, and shock. The infant's and young child's skin is ordinarily soft. Older children should continue to have a smooth and even skin texture. The preadolescent and adolescent may have oily-feeling skin on the face, shoulders, or back.

Assess skin turgor by elevating the skin on the abdomen in the infant or on the back of the hand in the older child or adolescent. The "pinched-up" skin should quickly return to place. Skin that remains tented is strongly suggestive of moderate to severe dehydration. When edema is present, palpate the edematous area to determine its extent. Palpate any lumps or protrusions to determine firmness or tenderness. Palpate lesions or rashes with a gloved hand to document the size and extent of the lesions.

Hair and Nails

Inspect the hair and scalp, noting distribution of hair as well as color, texture, amount, and quality. The young infant's hair may be entirely absent or quite thick; it will be replaced by hair that is of a texture and color closer to what the child will have throughout childhood. Coarse, dry hair at any age may indicate a thyroid disorder or nutritional deficiency. Inspect the scalp thoroughly; it should be free from lesions and infestations. Note the presence of a greasy, scaly plaque on the scalp of infants; termed "seborrheic dermatitis" or "cradle cap," it is benign and easily treated.

Inspect the nails for color, shape, and condition. Full-term infants may have long, papery fingernails that can scratch their skin if not trimmed. Children should have healthy nails. Dry, brittle nails may indicate a nutritional deficiency. Inspect the skin around the nails to ensure that it is intact and without signs of infection. Many children (especially school-age children) have a nervous habit of nail biting or hangnail biting or pulling.

Inspect the school-age child's or adolescent's toenails to ensure they are trimmed in a horizontal fashion. Self-trimming of toenails either too low or in a curved fashion places the child at risk for the development of ingrown nails. Clubbing of the nails indicates chronic hypoxemia related to respiratory or cardiac disease. Nails that curve inward or outward may be hereditary or linked with injury, infection, or iron-deficiency anemia.

Head

Examining the head is critical in the newborn and infant periods but should not be overlooked in older children as an opportunity to check for diseases of the scalp and functional and developmental problems that are reflected in poor hygiene of the head and scalp. Note hair distribution and any bald or thinning areas. Use of gloves may be indicated, depending on the overall scalp cleanliness and chance of infestation by head lice (seen as small grayish specks near the base of hair shafts).

INSPECTION

Examine the head and face for shape and symmetry. In newborns, the head may be temporarily misshapen from uterine positioning or a lengthy vaginal delivery. Some infants have a slight flattening of the back of the head since the recommended sleeping position is supine. Note any irregularities or asymmetry. Observe the infant's head shape by looking down on it from above. Observe whether the head appears centered on the neck or tilts to one side. After 4 months of age, the infant should have achieved enough head control to hold the head erect and in midline when placed in a vertical position. Pull the infant from the supine position into sitting to determine the extent of head lag. To determine the extent of head control in older infants and children, ask the child to turn the head in different directions, either by simple commands or by following a colorful object.

Observe the infant's face when crying, smiling, or babbling for symmetry of muscle movement. In children who are old enough to follow directions, a game of "Simon Says" is a playful way to determine facial symmetry and strength; ask them to puff out their cheeks, make kisses, look surprised, stick out their tongue, and so on (effectively testing function of cranial nerve VII [facial]) (Chiocca, 2020).

> **TAKE NOTE!**
>
> When you note a flattened occiput in an infant, encourage the parent or caregiver to allow the infant "tummy time" while awake and observed and to change the infant's head position frequently when upright in an infant seat (Fahrenkopf et al., 2020).

PALPATION

Gently palpate the anterior and posterior fontanels (Fig. 10.17). The **fontanels** are the soft areas on the skull that remain open in infancy to allow for rapid brain growth in the first few months of life. Note the size of the fontanels. The anterior fontanel's size is 1 to 4 cm in either direction until it can no longer be felt when it is closed by the age of 9 to 18 months (Chiocca, 2020). The posterior fontanel is much smaller and may close any time between shortly after birth and approximately 2 months of age. The fontanels should not be depressed or taut and bulging, although it is not uncommon to see them pulsate or briefly bulge if the baby cries. In an acutely ill infant, assess the fontanels while obtaining the vital signs. Dehydration can cause the fontanels to be sunken; increased intracranial pressure and overhydration can cause them to bulge. Palpate the skull for asymmetry, overriding or open sutures, and lumps or other deformities. Palpate the jaw joints as the child bites down to assess cranial nerve V (trigeminal). Use the fingertips to palpate for occipital, postauricular, preauricular, submental, and submandibular lymph nodes, noting their size, mobility, and consistency (Fig. 10.18).

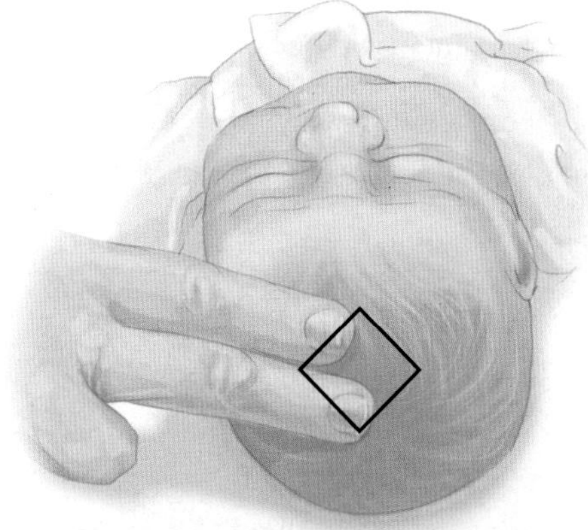

FIGURE 10.17 Note location and size of the fontanels. The anterior fontanel is diamond shaped and closes between the ages of 9 and 18 months.

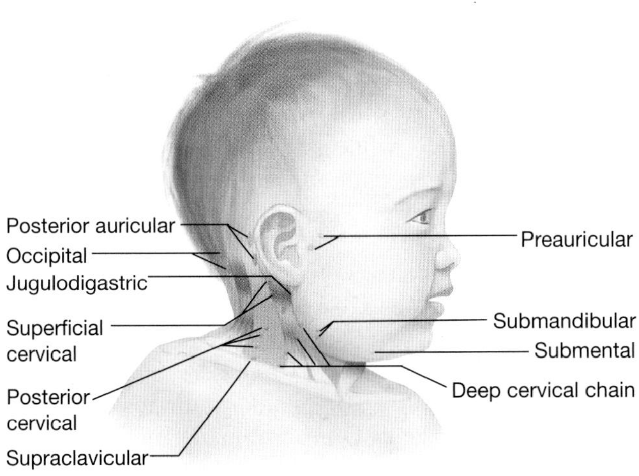

FIGURE 10.18 Location of lymph nodes.

> *TAKE NOTE!*
>
> A large fontanel may be associated with congenital hypothyroidism. Sagittal fontanel presence may occur with Down syndrome. A fontanel that becomes larger over time rather than smaller may indicate the development of hydrocephalus, especially if accompanied by an accelerated increase in head circumference (Chiocca, 2020).

Neck

Inspect the neck for symmetry. The infant's neck is short, but by 4 years of age the child's neck should be similar in appearance to the adult's. Webbing or excessive neck skinfolds may be associated with Turner syndrome, and lax neck skin may occur with Down syndrome. Assess the flexibility of the neck through a full range of motion. Take younger children through a passive range of motion. Older children will be able to look in all directions on command and stretch their chins to their chests themselves. Test cranial nerve XI (accessory) in the older child by having the child attempt to turn the head against resistance. Assessment of neck mobility is particularly important when infections of the central nervous system are suspected. Pain or resistance to range of motion may indicate meningeal irritation. Do not assess neck mobility in the trauma victim.

> *TAKE NOTE!*
>
> The infant or child who has experienced trauma should have the cervical spine maintained completely immobile until a radiologist has determined that the spinal cord is not damaged.

Palpate the neck for masses and lymph nodes. Palpate the cervical and clavicular lymph nodes with the distal part of the fingers using gentle but firm pressure in a circular motion. Tilt the child's head upward slightly to allow better access. Assess the lymph nodes for swelling, mobility, temperature, and tenderness. In healthy infants and adolescents, the cervical lymph nodes are usually not palpable; in healthy children between 1 and 11 years, the cervical nodes are often found to be small, nontender, and mobile (see Fig. 10.18 for locations of lymph nodes). Enlarged cervical lymph nodes frequently occur in association with upper respiratory infections and otitis media. Report significant enlargement to the health care provider or nurse practitioner. Palpate the trachea; the thyroid is usually palpable only in older children.

Eyes

Assessment of the eyes includes evaluation of the external and internal structures as well as screening for visual acuity. Any nurse caring for a child should be adept at examining the external structures. Assessment of the internal structures will also be covered later but is usually performed only by the advanced nurse practitioner. Refer to Chapter 9 for information on vision screening. Determination of visual acuity tests the function of cranial nerve II (optic).

EXTERNAL STRUCTURES

Observe the eyes for symmetry and spacing, even distribution of eyelashes and eyelids, and presence of epicanthal folds. Note the child's ability to blink and report an inability to do so. The eyes should look symmetric, and both should be facing forward in the midline when the child is looking directly ahead. The iris should be perfectly round, and the sclerae should be clear. The cornea should be uniformly transparent. Inspect the corners of the eye (medial and lateral canthus) and the conjunctiva (lining of the eyelids). They should be free of discharge, inflammation, or swelling. Epicanthal folds may be present in children of Asian descent, children with genetic abnormalities, or those with fetal alcohol spectrum disorder. Using a small penlight or ophthalmoscope, inspect the function and clarity of the pupil by putting your nondominant hand on the child's forehead and moving the light toward and away from each eye. This will elicit the blink reflex. Next, observe whether the pupil contracts with the light and expands when the light is removed. Make the same motion with a small toy or object, and direct the child to look at it. The eyes demonstrate **accommodation**, or focusing at different distances, if the pupil constricts as the object moves closer. If normal findings are present, report **PERRLA** (pupils are equal, round, reactive to light and accommodation) (Fig. 10.19). This is a particularly important assessment in head and eye injuries, as well as when other neurologic concerns are present.

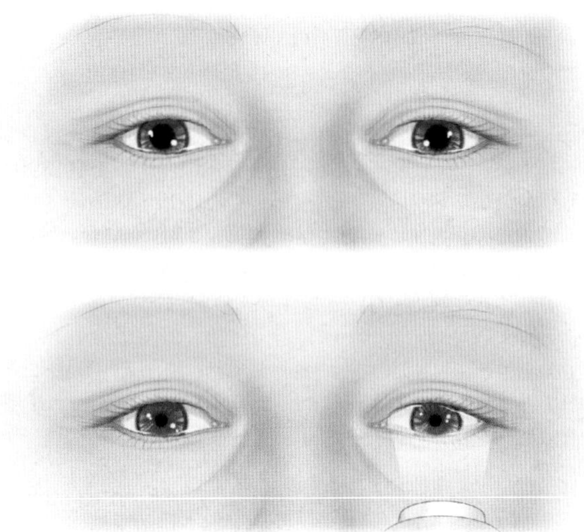

FIGURE 10.19 The pupils should be equal, round, and reactive to light and accommodation (PERRLA).

TAKE NOTE!

The infant may exhibit intermittent strabismus (crossing of the eyes) until about 4 months of age. However, persistent strabismus at any age or intermittent strabismus after 4 months of age should be evaluated by a pediatric ophthalmologist (Andre & Rockwell, 2022).

Check extraocular muscle motility and function of cranial nerves III and IV (oculomotor and abducens) by instructing the child to follow the light through the six cardinal positions of gaze. Infants and very young children will follow an interesting object. Instruct the older child to look downward and inward (testing cranial nerve IV [trochlear]). Assess eye muscle strength using two tests. Using the Hirschberg test, bring the penlight to the middle of your face and direct the child to look at it. The small dot of reflected light seen in the iris should be placed symmetrically in each eye (Fig. 10.20). The cover test also assesses eye muscle strength. Cover one of the child's eyes and instruct the child to focus on an interesting object. The eye should not waver. While the child is still focusing with the first eye, remove the cover from the second. Observe the uncovered eye for movement. Report any movement or drift.

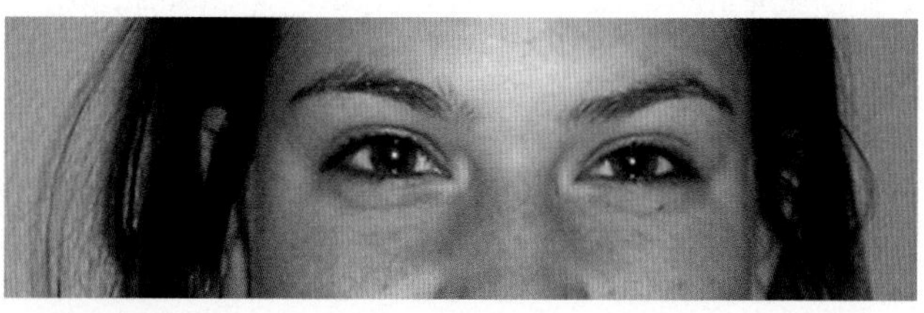

FIGURE 10.20 Note reflected light falling symmetrically on each pupil with the Hirschberg test.

To test peripheral vision, have the child focus on a specific point or object directly in front. Bring a finger or a small object from beyond the range of vision into the area of the peripheral vision. When the child sees the object from the side, while still focusing on the object or point in front, the child should say "stop." This also tests cranial nerve II (optic).

INTERNAL STRUCTURES

An advanced nurse practitioner with experience in this type of assessment best accomplishes assessment of the internal structures of the eye. An adequate assessment requires that the child cooperate. Restraint for eye examination does not usually prove fruitful, as movement and tearing of the eyes interfere with the accuracy of the examination. Use the ophthalmoscope to inspect the internal eye structures. Observe the glow of the pupil, which appears red (creamy colored in children with very dark eye color). Inspect the optic disc, macula, fovea, and blood vessels. Refer any child with blurring or bulging of the optic disc or hemorrhage of vessels to a pediatric ophthalmologist for further evaluation.

CLINICAL REASONING ALERT!

A child in an emergent situation should have a health history that is focused on the child's most immediate need. On the other hand, a comprehensive health history is appropriate for the child who is having his first visit at a pediatrician's office, for example.

Remember Elliot, the 3-year-old being seen for his annual examination? When you enter the room, he is hiding behind his parent's legs.

Ears

Assessment of the ears includes evaluation of the external and internal structures as well as screening for hearing. Any nurse caring for a child should be adept at examining the external structures. Assessment of the internal structures will also be covered further on but is usually performed only by the advanced nurse practitioner. Refer to Chapter 9 for information on hearing screening. Testing of hearing also tests the function of cranial nerve VIII (acoustic).

EXTERNAL STRUCTURES

Assess the placement of the external ears on the head. They should be symmetric and placed no lower than the eyes. The pinna should deviate no more than 10 degrees from an imaginary line that is perpendicular to a line drawn between the outer canthus of the eye and the top of the ear. Low-set ears may be associated with genetic abnormalities or syndromes (Fig. 10.21). Note protrusion or flattening of the ears, which may be normal for that child or may indicate inflammation (protrusion) or persistent side-lying

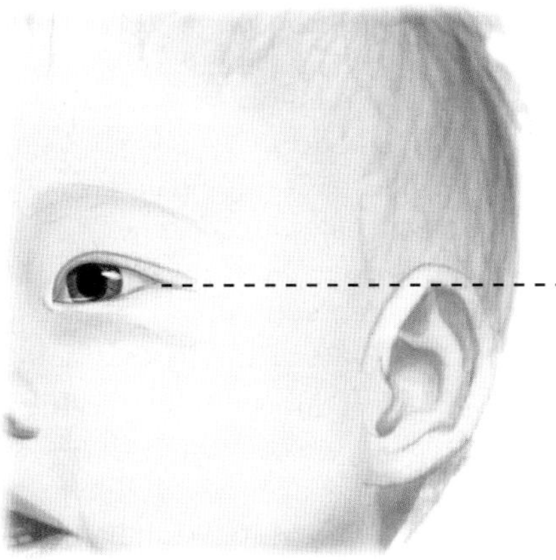

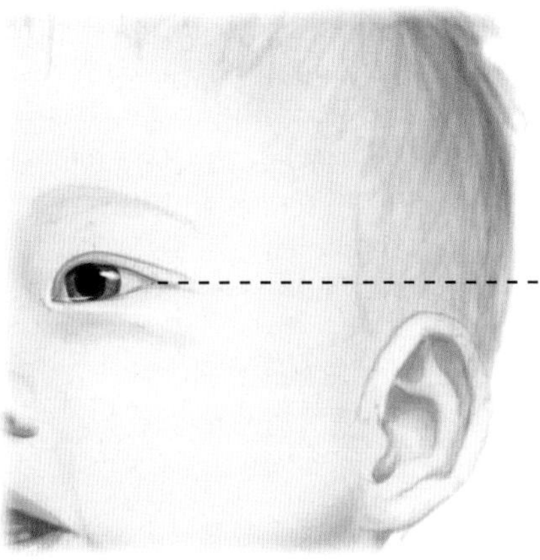

FIGURE 10.21 Low-set ears may be associated with chromosomal or other genetic anomalies.

(flattening). Note the presence of pits or skin tags in the preauricular area. Observe the exterior ear canal. A waxy cerumen that is soft and an orangish-brown color is normally found lubricating and protecting the external ear canal and should be left in place or washed gently away when bathing. Note drainage from the ear canal, which is always considered abnormal. Pull on the auricle and palpate the mastoid process, neither of which should result in pain in the healthy child.

TAKE NOTE!

Impacted and dry cerumen can be softened with a few drops of peanut, olive, or almond oil and then gently irrigated from the canal with an ear syringe and warm water (Sevy et al., 2023).

INTERNAL STRUCTURES

Use a **tympanometer** to assess the mobility of the eardrum (tympanic membrane). Gently pull down on the earlobe of infants and toddlers and up on the outer edge of the pinna in older children to straighten the ear canal, and press the tip of the tympanometer over the external canal. A reading of air pressure is recorded by the instrument, and this is useful to assess middle ear disease. Many tympanometers record a wave pattern that may be printed to include in the child's chart.

A nurse practitioner or health care provider generally performs inspection of the ear canal and tympanic membrane with an otoscope (Fig. 10.22). The otoscopic examination is usually performed near the end of the physical assessment for infants and young children, as they are often quite resistant to this intrusive procedure. The infant or toddler may require restraint in the parent's lap for the otoscopic evaluation. The preschooler may cooperate if the nurse uses a game such as looking for pretend puppies or potatoes in the child's ear. As with the tympanometer, gently pull down on the earlobe of the infant or toddler and up on the outer edge of the pinna in older children to straighten the ear canal. Use an otoscopic speculum appropriate to the size of the child's ear canal. Insert the speculum into the ear canal to visualize the canal and the tympanic membrane. The canal should be pink, should have tiny hairs, and should be free from scratches, drainage, foreign bodies, and edema. The tympanic membrane should appear pearly pink or gray and should be translucent, allowing visualization of the bony landmarks. It may be red if the child has been crying recently. Compress the pneumatic insufflator bulb to provide a puff of air; this causes motion of the tympanic membrane when the middle ear is healthy. Note abnormalities such as a fluid level; bubble or pus behind the tympanic membrane; tympanic membrane immobility; holes or perforations in the tympanic membrane; and the presence of tympanostomy tubes, scarring, or vesicles.

TAKE NOTE!

Never attempt to flush a foreign object out with water until it has been identified, because small pieces of sponge, clay, or vegetative material like peas or beans swell with water, further obstructing the ear canal (Yoon et al., 2022).

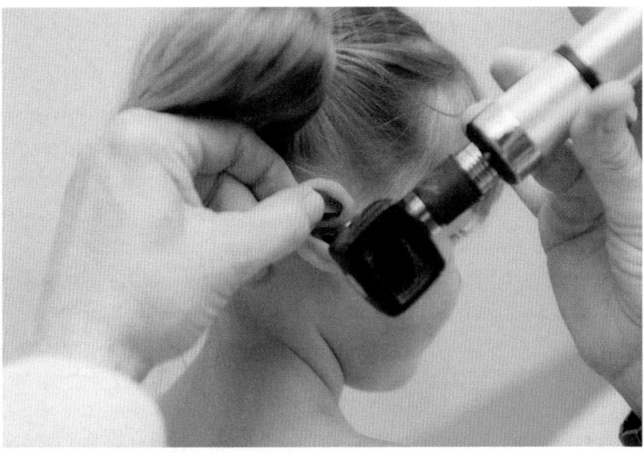

FIGURE 10.22 Otoscopic examination allows visualization of the internal structures of the ear.

Nose and Sinuses

The nose, as with all facial features in a child, should be symmetric, but it can be displaced temporarily by birth trauma in newborns. Ensure the nares provide unobstructed airflow by alternately occluding one nostril at a time and observing for air movement through the other nostril. If the child is breathing comfortably, there should be little nostril movement visible. Adolescents may have pierced their nose or nasal septum; ensure that the site is free from infection or loose jewelry that could migrate into the sinuses. Ideally, the nose should not be draining, although clear mucus may be present if the child has been crying. Assess the amount, color, thickness, and presence of any odor if drainage is present. Inspect the interior of the nose by tilting the child's head backward and pushing the tip of the nose upward. Direct the beam of a penlight in the nostril. The nasal mucosa should be uniformly firm, pink, and free from edema, excoriation, or masses. Test the older child's sense of smell by having the child close the eyes and identify a familiar scent such as peppermint or coffee (cranial nerve I [olfactory]). Palpate the sinuses for tenderness.

TAKE NOTE!

Infants younger than 1 month of age are **obligate nose breathers**, which allows for swallowing without aspiration during breast or artificial nipple feeding (Smith, 2022).

Mouth and Throat

Wear a powder-free glove to examine the mouth, teeth, and throat. Inspection of the exterior of the mouth may be done at any point in the examination. Infants and young children may find assessment of the mouth and particularly the pharynx and uvula to be quite intrusive, so delay that part of the assessment until the end of the examination, after otoscopic evaluation. Assess the character and quality of the child's voice and the infant's cry. It should be neither too hoarse nor too shrill.

INSPECTION OF THE MOUTH

Observe the lips for color, symmetry, and absence of inflammation or edema. Salivation in infants begins at about 3 months of age; drooling occurs because the infant does not learn to swallow saliva until several months later. Next, inspect the interior of the mouth. The mouth is the first part of the digestive system, and a pink, moist, healthy mucosal lining is indicative of a healthy gastrointestinal tract. In infants, the tongue should lie within the mouth at rest and should be capable of extending over the lower gum line to help the baby feed. The tongue extrusion reflex is normal in infants until the age of 6 months and allows the infant to suckle easily from birth. Observe movement of the tongue when the infant or young child babbles or cries. Ask the older child to touch the tongue to the roof of the mouth and then stick out the tongue and move it from side to side (testing cranial nerve XII [hypoglossal]). Full movement should be present, and the tongue should be free from lesions or exudate. Visualize the hard and soft palate (which should be intact) or palpate with the gloved finger.

Most infants have no teeth before the fifth to sixth month. When the teeth begin to erupt, they usually erupt symmetrically at the rate of about one a month, until toddlers have 20 teeth by 30 months of age. The infant may drool for several months before teething. During teething, the gums will be swollen at the location of the impending tooth. In older children, the secondary teeth replace the primary teeth much more slowly and with little discomfort from ages 5 to 20. Figure 10.23 shows the usual permanent tooth eruption pattern.

Look for dental caries or alignment problems, and inspect the gums for signs of infection. Test cranial nerve IX (glossopharyngeal) by having the child identify taste with the posterior portion of the tongue.

TAKE NOTE!

Natal (present at birth) or neonatal (erupting by 30 days of age) teeth should be evaluated by a pediatric dentist for potential extraction, as they may pose an aspiration risk (Smith, 2022).

INSPECTION OF THE THROAT

Inspect the tonsils, uvula, and oropharynx. Assess the infant's throat during a yawn or cry, as any forcible attempt to depress the tongue with a tongue depressor produces a strong reflex elevation of the base of the tongue that completely blocks the view of the pharynx. The young child will require restraint so that the nurse can depress the tongue and visualize the back of the mouth without injuring the child (Fig. 10.24). Asking the older child to open wide, stick out the tongue, and say "aaaah" simultaneously will allow for a quick look at the tonsils and pharynx without the need to use a tongue depressor, but the nurse must be quick because the tongue rises rapidly after those maneuvers are performed.

Tonsils usually cannot be seen in the infant. As the child becomes a toddler, the tonsils become dramatically larger and then begin to decrease in size again by age 9. The tonsils should be pink and often have crypts on their surfaces, which are sometimes filled with debris. Ensure that the uvula is midline and rises if the gag reflex is elicited (cranial nerve X [vagus]). Inspect the oropharynx, which should be pink and free from exudate.

Thorax and Lungs

Assessment of the thorax and lungs begins by observing the shape and contour of the thorax and determining the

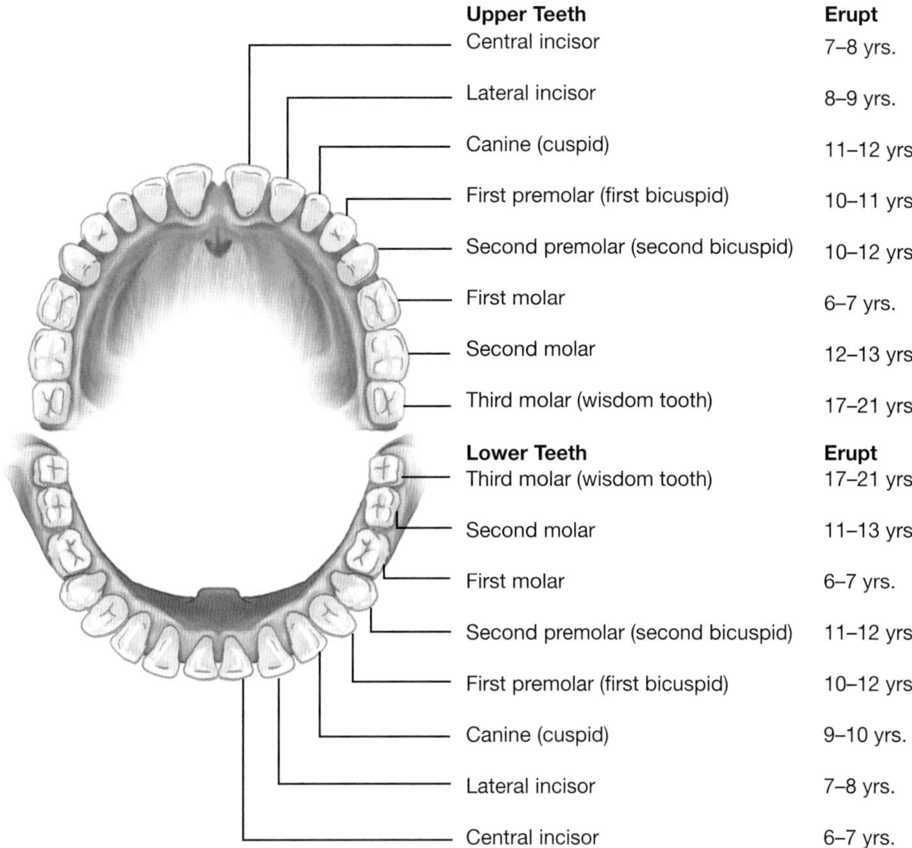

FIGURE 10.23 Usual sequence of permanent tooth eruption.

work of breathing. Accurate auscultation of the lungs is essential since children often have respiratory infections and disorders and may exhibit alterations in respiratory effort and breath sounds. Note the child's color, which should be pink; cyanosis indicates hypoxia. Listen for audible stridor (inspiratory high-pitched sound), expiratory grunting or snoring, audible wheezing (heard with the naked ear), or cough. Document type and extent of cough. Observe the nail beds for clubbing, which occurs with diseases inducing chronic hypoxic states.

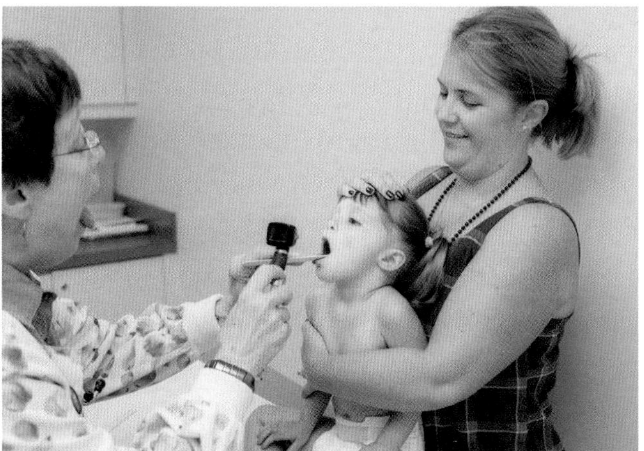

FIGURE 10.24 The young child may need to be restrained so that the throat examination can be done safely.

THORAX

Examine the chest with the head in a midline position to determine size and shape as well as symmetry, movement, and bony landmarks. The newborn's chest should be smooth and round, with the transverse diameter nearly equal to the anterior–posterior diameter. The shape of the chest progresses to that of the adult by the age of 5 to 6 years. At that time, the anterior–posterior diameter is about half the transverse diameter (Fig. 10.25). At the point where the xiphoid process and the right and left costal margins meet, the costal angle should measure 90 degrees or less. Inspect for structural deformity such as pectus excavatum (depressed sternum) or pectus carinatum (protuberant sternum) (Fig. 10.26). Note symmetric movement of the chest wall with respiration. Infants and younger children are primarily diaphragmatic breathers, so the abdomen and chest will rise and fall together. Older children, particularly adolescent females, demonstrate thoracic breathing, yet the abdomen and chest should continue to rise and fall together. Asymmetry of chest wall movement is an abnormal finding.

Observe the depth and regularity of respirations, noting the length of the inspiratory and expiratory phases

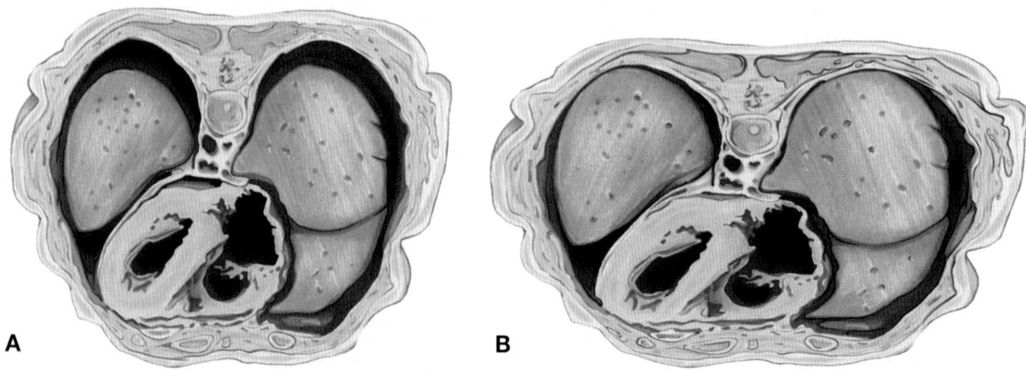

FIGURE 10.25 **A.** The newborn's chest is round. **B.** The adult chest has an anterior–posterior diameter about half the transverse diameter.

in relation to each other. The newborn and young infant demonstrate an irregular respiratory pattern. Older infants and children should have a more regular respiratory pattern.

Assess the child's respiratory effort by first observing for nasal flaring, which indicates labored breathing. Observe the chest wall and shoulders for accessory muscle use, which normally is not present. If retractions are present, note their location and severity. Typical locations for retraction include the intercostal, subcostal, substernal, suprasternal, and clavicular regions (Fig. 10.27). Pay attention to the position the child naturally assumes to breathe comfortably; children in respiratory distress often sit forward and are uncomfortable lying down or talking (Jarvis & Eckhardt, 2020).

LUNGS

Experienced examiners may palpate and percuss the lungs before using auscultation to evaluate the breath sounds.

Palpation and Percussion

Palpate for symmetric respiratory excursion by placing the thumbs and fingers together along the costal margin on the chest or back. Movement should be symmetric with each breath. Palpate for the normal presence of tactile fremitus with the palms or fingertips while the infant is crying or while the older child says "99." Indirectly percuss the lungs of older children, noting resonance over lung fields. Hyperresonance may be present in conditions resulting in hyperaeration of the lungs, such as asthma.

Auscultation

Use the bell of the stethoscope or switch to a small diaphragm to auscultate lung sounds in the infant or child. The adult-sized diaphragm may be used for the adolescent. Auscultate the lung fields with the infant or child in a sitting position, even if that requires propping the infant in a parent's lap. Infants and young children have loud breath sounds because of their thin chest walls. Breath sounds should be clear with adequate aeration throughout all lung fields. Listen to a full inspiration and expiration at the apices of the lungs as well as symmetrically across the entire lung field, systematically comparing the right to the left side. Listen on the anterior chest, on the posterior chest, and in the axillary regions.

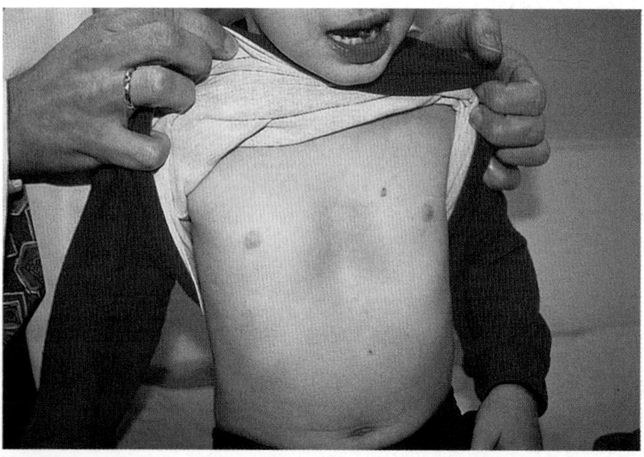

FIGURE 10.26 Pectus excavatum: note depression in xiphoid area.

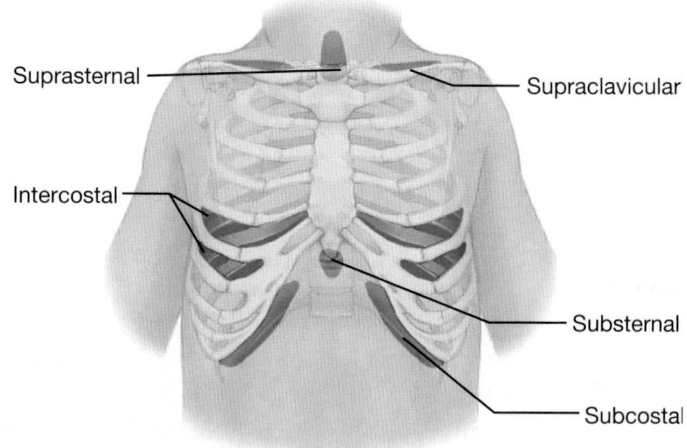

FIGURE 10.27 Location of retractions.

Playing games may encourage younger children to cooperate with deep breathing during lung assessment. The child can blow a cotton ball up in the air, blow a pinwheel, or "blow out" the light of the penlight (Miller, n.d.). Older children are capable of deep breathing when instructed to do so.

The child who has a respiratory disorder or who is experiencing respiratory distress may exhibit diminished breath sounds, most often in the lung bases. Diminished breath sounds are softer and quieter than lung sounds demonstrating adequate aeration. In the healthy infant or child, no adventitious sounds should be heard. If noisy breath sounds are heard in the infant or young child, particularly over all lung fields, compare the sound to the noises heard over the trachea or below the nares. Infants and young children with secretions in the nasopharyngeal area may have those sounds transmitted over the lung fields. These sounds usually clear with coughing or airway suctioning; they are not true adventitious sounds. Note adventitious breath sounds such as wheezes or crackles, documenting their location and whether they are present on inspiration, expiration, or both. It is most important to describe the abnormal breath sounds being heard rather than attempting to classify the sounds. Adventitious lung sounds are associated with a variety of disorders, and extensive experience is required to appropriately classify lung sounds. Adventitious breath sounds should be reported for further evaluation.

Breasts

Assess the breasts of children of all ages and sexes. Note the size of the breasts in relation to the age of the child. Palpate the axillary lymph nodes during the breast assessment.

INSPECTION

Observe the breasts for position, shape, size, symmetry, and color. Newborns of any sex may have swollen nipples from the influence of maternal estrogen, but by several weeks of age, the nipples should be flat and should continue to be so in all prepubertal children. In children, the nipples are located lateral to the midclavicular line, usually between the fourth and fifth ribs. The areola becomes darker in color as the child approaches puberty. Children with higher weight may appear to have enlarged breasts due to adipose tissue. Note the location of additional (supernumerary) nipples if present (usually located along the mammary ridge); they may appear as darkly pigmented, elevated, or nipple like spots. These are usually of no concern as they do not change over time, but they may be associated with kidney disorders.

Inspect the breasts for the current stage of development: widening of the areola, elevation of the nipple, and increase in breast size. Female breast development may begin as early as age 8 but usually starts by age 13. Breast development then continues in a characteristic, but usually asymmetric, pattern, with one breast larger than the other throughout the lifespan. The sexual maturity rating scale developed by Tanner in 1962 is used to describe breast development (**Tanner stages**) (Fig. 10.28). Adolescent males may develop gynecomastia (enlargement of the breast tissue) due to hormonal pubertal changes. When the hormone levels stabilize, male adolescents then have flat nipples. Occasionally, gynecomastia is caused by cannabis use, H_2 blockers, phenytoin, or hormonal dysfunction (Gilmore & Hay, 2021).

PALPATION

Palpate the breasts in a systematic fashion. A tender nodule palpated just under the nipple confirms pubertal changes. This change may be difficult to assess in patients with excessive adipose tissue. Normal breast tissue should feel smooth, firm, and elastic. Note masses or nodules if present. Palpate for axillary lymph nodes with the child's arms relaxed at the side but slightly abducted. Note size and texture of nodes if present.

Heart and Peripheral Perfusion

The examination of the heart in children is identical to that of adults except for the focus of the examiner's attention. Congenital heart defects are the most common cause of heart problems in children, and children with these defects present differently than adults with heart disease.

TAKE NOTE!

The younger the child, the more responsive the heart rate is to activity changes. It increases with fever, fear, crying, or anxiety and decreases with sleep, sedation, or vagal stimulation (Jarvis & Eckhardt, 2020).

INSPECTION

Observe the child's posture. Note the presence of pallor, cyanosis, mottling, or edema, which may indicate a cardiovascular problem. Inspect the anterior chest from the side or at an angle, noting symmetry in shape as well as movement. Observe for the apical impulse, which is visible in about half of children. It occurs at the **point of maximum intensity (PMI)**, which is located at the third to fourth intercostal space just medial of the child's left midclavicular line until the age of 4 years, at the fourth intercostal space at the left midclavicular line in children ages 4 to 6 years, and then lateral to the left midclavicular line at the fifth intercostal space in children ages 7 years and older (Fig. 10.29). Note clubbing of the fingertips or distention of neck veins, both of which may be associated with congenital heart defect.

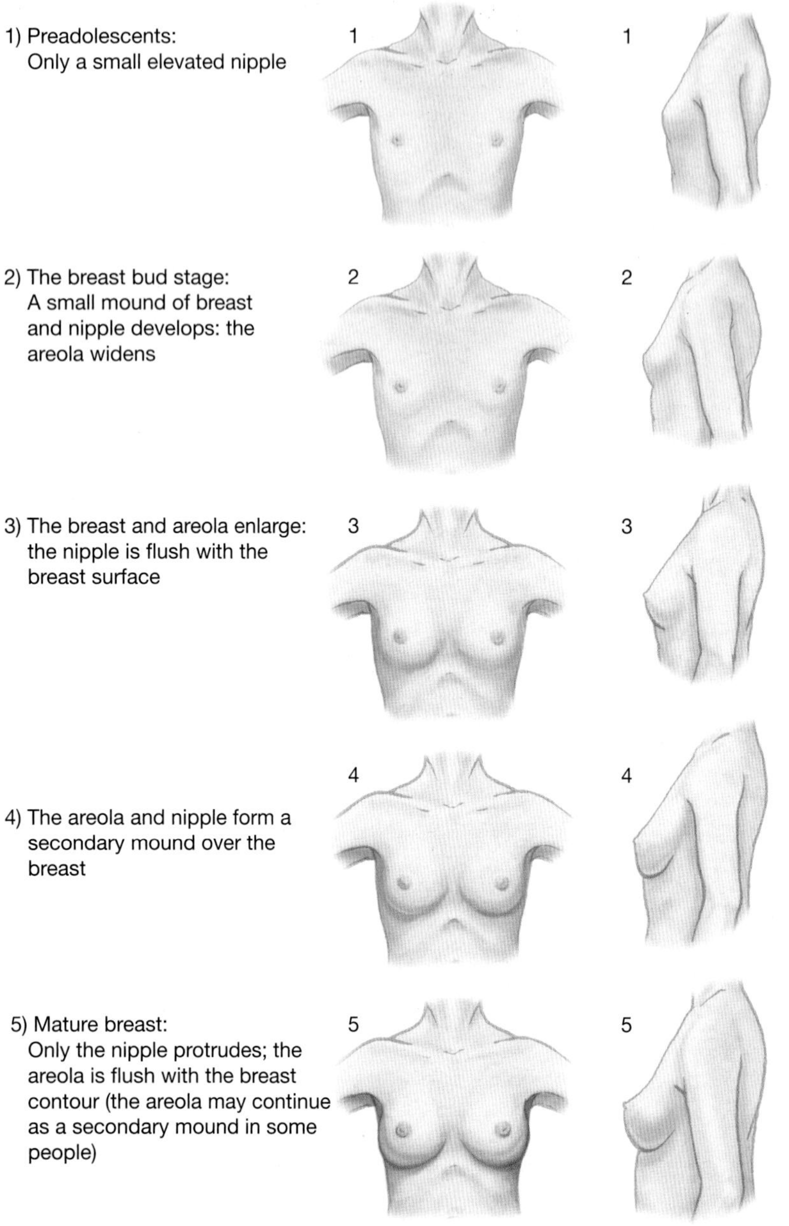

1) Preadolescents:
Only a small elevated nipple
1
1
2) The breast bud stage:
A small mound of breast and nipple develops: the areola widens
2
2
3) The breast and areola enlarge:
the nipple is flush with the breast surface
3
3
4) The areola and nipple form a secondary mound over the breast
4
4
5) Mature breast:
Only the nipple protrudes; the areola is flush with the breast contour (the areola may continue as a secondary mound in some people)
5
5

FIGURE 10.28 Tanner sexual maturity rating for breast development. (Adapted from Tanner, J. M. [1962]. *Growth at adolescence*. Blackwell Scientific Publications.)

Left Midclavicular line
Birth to 4 years
Ages 4 to 6 years
7 years and older

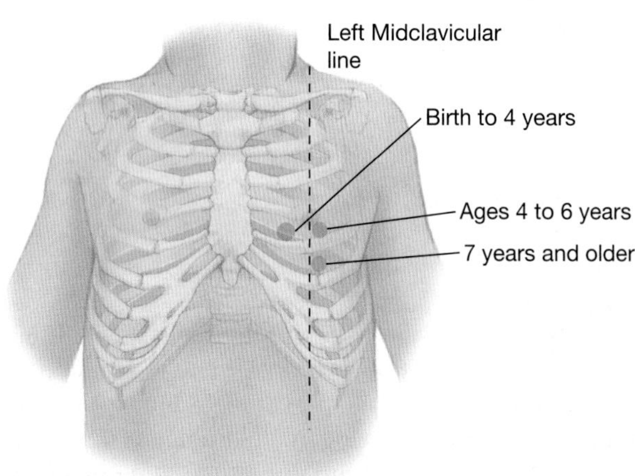

FIGURE 10.29 The point of maximum intensity (PMI) or apical impulse.

PALPATION

Using the fingertips, palpate the chest for lifts and heaves or thrills, which are not normal. Palpate the apical pulse in the area of the PMI (see Fig. 10.29). Check the pulses and compare the upper body to the lower body pulses, as well as left versus right, noting strength and quality (Fig. 10.30). The pedal, brachial, and femoral pulses are usually easily palpated. The radial pulse is very difficult to palpate in children younger than 2 years. Note the warmth of the distal extremities. To assess capillary refill time, place slight pressure on the nail beds and quickly release it. Observe the length of time required for refill and return to original color. Compare capillary refill time of the fingers to the toes. A capillary refill time of less than 3 seconds indicates adequacy of perfusion.

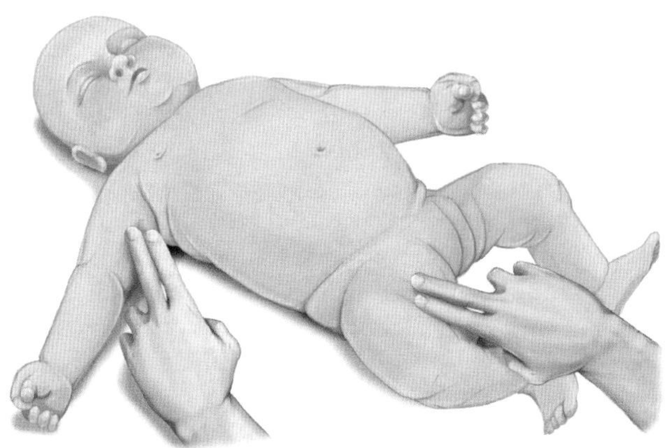

FIGURE 10.30 It is important to assess brachial and femoral pulses simultaneously to determine equality or differences in strength and intensity.

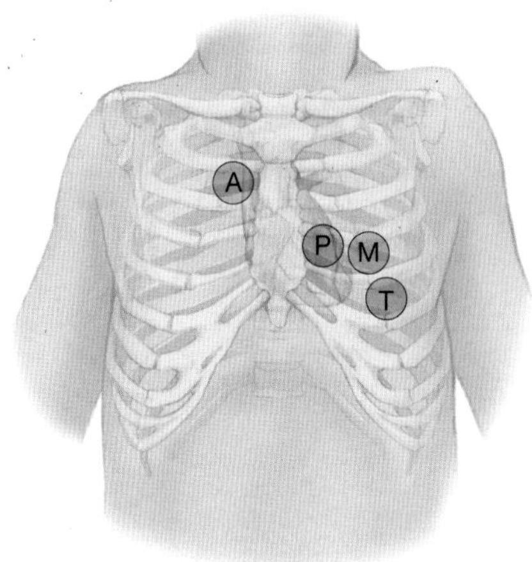

FIGURE 10.32 Areas where the sounds of heart valves radiate. A, Aortic valve—second intercostal space, just right of sternum; P, Pulmonic valve—second intercostal space, just left of sternum; T, Tricuspid valve—fourth intercostal space, just left of sternum; M, Mitral valve—fourth intercostal space at left midclavicular line.

AUSCULTATION

Perform auscultation of the heart with the child in two different positions, upright and reclined (Fig. 10.31). Auscultate the heart rate in the area of the PMI as this is the point on the chest wall where the heartbeat is heard most distinctly (see Fig. 10.29). As you begin auscultation, listen first for respirations and note their timing so as not to confuse the heart sounds with the lung sounds. A crying infant may help by briefly holding their breath between cries. Once you are confident that you are listening to the heart, be sure to listen for 1 full minute because of the irregularity of rhythms in some children. Count the heart rate, which should be consistent with the palpated pulse (either radial or brachial, depending on the child's age).

Develop a systematic approach to auscultation of the heart. Listen over all four valvular areas anteriorly (Fig. 10.32). In the infant or younger child, also auscultate the heart in the axillary region and posteriorly (certain murmurs radiate to these areas). Note S_1, S_2, extra heart sounds, or murmurs. S_1 is usually loudest at the mitral and tricuspid areas and increases in intensity with fever, exercise, and anemia. S_2 is usually most intense at the aortic and pulmonic areas. A split S_2 heard at the apex occurs in many infants and young children. S_3 may be heard in many healthy children and is considered normal, although the child with a chronic cardiac condition may develop an S_3 when congestive heart failure is present. S_4 is usually considered abnormal, most often occurring with cardiac disease.

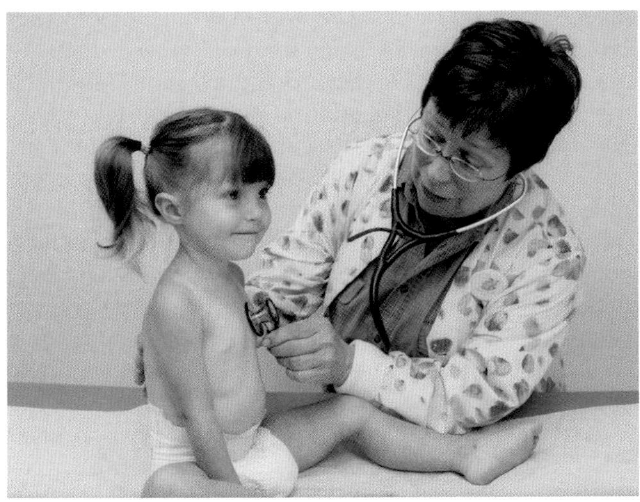

FIGURE 10.31 Auscultating the child's heart.

Sinus arrhythmia is a common and normal finding in children and adolescents. It results in an irregular heart rhythm: the heart rate increases with inhalation and decreases with exhalation. If the child holds their breath, the rhythm becomes regular.

Auscultate for murmurs. Note the location (where it is heard best or loudest) and timing of the murmur. A systolic murmur occurs in association with S_1 (closure of the atrioventricular valves), a diastolic murmur in association with S_2 (closure of the semilunar valves). Also note the duration of murmur. Does it occur early or late in diastole or systole? Does it occur all the way across systole (holosystolic)? Note the intensity of the murmur. Table 10.5 discusses grading of murmur intensity.

Innocent murmurs occur in about 40% to 50% of children at some point throughout childhood. A Still murmur is most common, usually occurring between 2 and 7 years of age. It occurs in early systole, is best heard between the apex and left lower sternal border, and is usually medium pitched and musical. A venous hum that is heard in the infraclavicular area and possibly radiating down the chest is considered an innocent murmur. Often an innocent murmur disappears when the child changes position. Refer any child with a murmur to an experienced practitioner for further evaluation (Jone et al., 2022).

TABLE 10.5 • Grading Heart Murmurs in Children

Grade	Sound
1	Barely audible; sometimes heard, sometimes not. Usually heard only with intense concentration
2	Quiet, soft; heard each time the chest is auscultated
3	Audible, intermediate intensity
4	Audible, with a palpable thrill
5	Loud, audible with edge of the stethoscope lifted off the chest
6	Very loud, audible with the stethoscope placed near but not touching the chest

Data from Jone, P.-N., Kim, J. S., Burkett, D., Jacobson, R., & Von Alvensleben, J. (2022). Cardiovascular diseases. In M. Bunik, W. W. Hay, M. J. Levin, & M. J. Abzug (Eds.), *Current diagnosis & treatment: Pediatrics* (26th ed.). McGraw-Hill.

Abdomen

The abdomen contains organs related to the genitourinary and lymphatic systems, in addition to the gastrointestinal system. These structures lie within the abdomen in approximately the same location as they do in adults. Dividing the abdomen into quadrants simplifies the description of normal organ location and the reporting of abnormalities. Draw an imaginary vertical line from the xiphoid process to the symphysis pubis. Cross this with an imaginary perpendicular line through the umbilicus. The sequence of physical examination is altered for the abdominal assessment: auscultation is done before percussion and palpation because manipulation of the lower abdomen may affect the bowel sounds (Chiocca, 2020).

INSPECTION

Inspect the abdomen for size, shape, and symmetry. The abdomen in the infant and toddler is rounded and protuberant until the abdominal musculature becomes well developed. Although rounded, the abdomen should not be distended (at any age). By adolescence, the stature is more erect, and the abdomen begins to appear flat when standing and concave when supine. The thin skin of a young child may allow the visualization of superficial venous circulation across the abdomen. Inspect the abdomen for movement. At eye level with the abdomen, note abdomen and thorax movement occurring simultaneously. Visible peristaltic waves are abnormal and should be reported immediately.

Inspect the newborn's umbilicus for color, bleeding, odor, and drainage. The umbilical stump should slowly dry, become black and hard, and fall away from the cutaneous navel by the end of the second week of life. Note drainage or granulation at the umbilical site, indicating delayed drying of the umbilical stump. Inspect the umbilicus in older infants and young children for the presence of umbilical hernia. Because the umbilicus divides the rectus abdominis muscle, it is not uncommon to see an umbilical hernia protrude through and become larger when the infant or toddler strains or cries. This is a benign finding and will usually disappear as the abdomen becomes stronger. Adolescents may have jewelry piercing the umbilicus.

AUSCULTATION

Auscultate the abdomen using the diaphragm or the bell of the stethoscope pressed firmly against the abdomen. Count the bowel sounds in each of the four quadrants for a full minute. Bowel sounds should be present by a few hours after birth and should remain active throughout life. Note whether bowel sounds are normally active, hyperactive, hypoactive, or absent. Normal bowel sounds can be described as growls, gurgles, and clicking sounds. Hypoactive bowel sounds may occur postoperatively. Hyperactive bowels sounds are common with diarrhea. Classify bowel sounds as absent after listening for 5 full minutes in each area. Absent bowel sounds may indicate ileus or peritonitis.

PERCUSSION

Indirectly percuss all areas of the abdomen. Normal findings include dullness along the costal margins and tympany over the remainder of the abdomen. A full bladder may yield dullness to percussion.

PALPATION

Palpate the abdomen with the child in a supine position. If the child's legs are small enough, the knees may be brought up with the nondominant hand to flex the hips and relax the abdomen. Palpate all four quadrants of the abdomen in a systematic fashion, first lightly and then deeply. Apply light pressure with the fingertips to perform light palpation, assessing for tenderness and muscle tone (Fig. 10.33). Note skin turgor by gently elevating a piece of skin and allowing it to fall back into place. Perform deep palpation to assess the organs and any masses. Place one hand on top of the other and palpate from the lower quadrants to the upper (see Fig. 10.33). The edge of the liver may be felt at the right costal margin, and the tip of the spleen can be felt at the left costal margin. The descending colon may be felt in the left lower quadrant as a small column and the bladder as a soft balloon below the umbilicus. The kidneys are rarely palpable. The abdomen should be soft and nontender to palpation. Report firmness, tenderness, or masses. Palpate the inguinal area for the presence of hernia or enlarged lymph nodes.

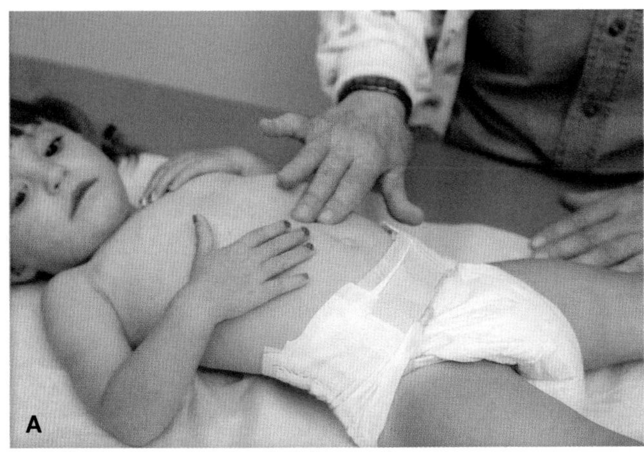

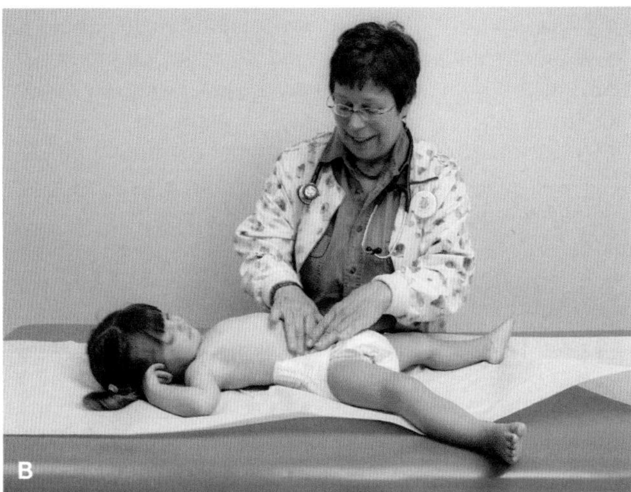

FIGURE 10.33 (**A**) Light and (**B**) deep palpation of the abdomen.

TAKE NOTE!

To decrease ticklishness with abdominal palpation, place a flat, warm, still hand on the abdomen while distracting the child before palpation begins. An alternate technique is to first palpate with the child's hand over the examiner's hand.

Genitalia and Anus

Examination of the genitals should immediately follow the abdominal assessment in the younger child and should be reserved for the end of the assessment in the adolescent. Although the anus is part of the gastrointestinal tract, it is best assessed during the genital examination. The AAP recommends that a parent chaperone the genitalia and anus examination of the infant and the child. In the case of the adolescent, a medical provider chaperone is recommended (Dev & Cruz, 2017).

Ensure privacy for the older child and adolescent. Keep the child covered as much as possible. Use a casual, matter-of-fact approach to place the child or adolescent at ease. During the genital examination, teach the child or adolescent about normal variations and changes with puberty, as well as issues related to health promotion.

MALE

Inspect the penis and scrotum for size, color, skin integrity, and obvious masses. With higher weight, the penis may appear small because of additional skinfolds. Penis size should correlate with pubertal stage (Fig. 10.34). The penis may have a foreskin that covers the glans, protecting and lubricating it. If present, do not forcibly retract the foreskin. In circumcised penises, the urinary meatus is

From top to bottom:

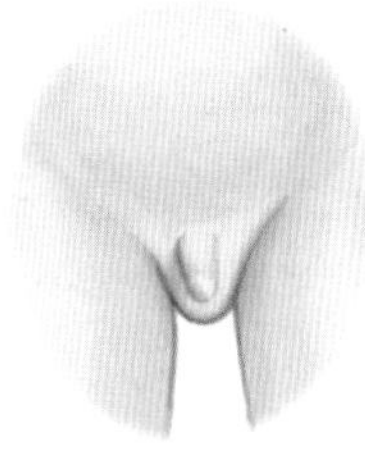

1) No pubic hair and scrotum size and proportion the same as during childhood

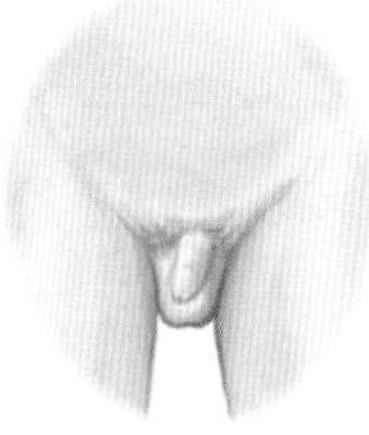

2) Few straight hairs at base of penis, little or no penis enlargement, testes/scrotum begin to enlarge

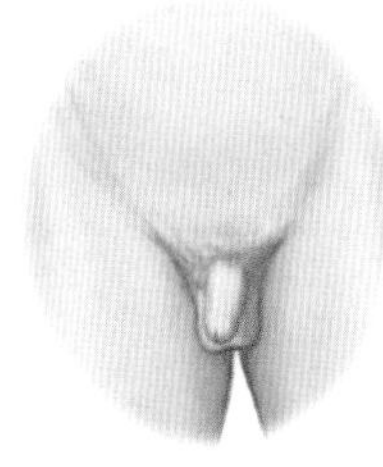

3) Sparse pubic hair growth over entire pubis, penis begins to lengthen, scrotum continues to enlarge

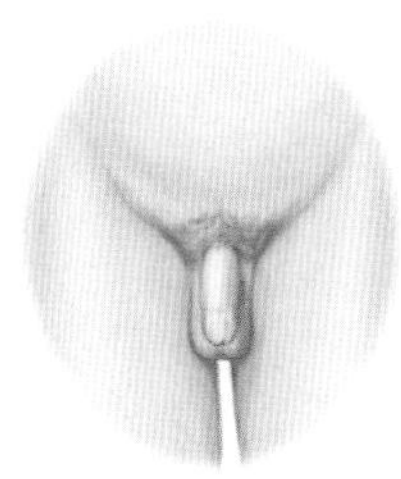

4) Thick pubic hair growth but not on thighs, penis grows in length and diameter, testes almost full grown

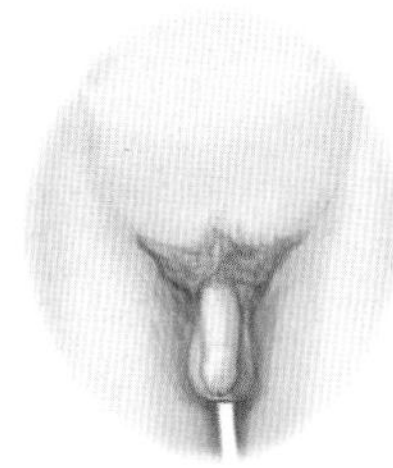

5) Pubic hair growth spread over medial thighs, penis and scrotum are adult size and shape

FIGURE 10.34 Tanner male sexual maturity rating for genitalia and pubic hair. (Adapted from Tanner, J. M. [1962]. *Growth at adolescence*. Blackwell Scientific Publications.)

exposed and should be at the tip of the glans. Assess the meatus for absence of discharge. If possible, observe the stream of urine for strength of flow and patency of the urethral orifice. Skin lesions may indicate sexually transmitted infection. A foreskin that cannot be retracted in a person older than 3 years may indicate phimosis. Report abnormal findings.

TAKE NOTE!

When you first remove a male infant's diaper, this is the ideal time to assess the force of the urine stream and the erection reflex, as the cool air may make the infant void and briefly experience an erection.

Assess the presence and distribution of pubic hair. Inspect the scrotum for size, slight asymmetry, color, and absence of edema. The scrotum may initially be swollen from birth trauma or maternal hormones, but this swelling should decrease in the first few days of life. The scrotum is ordinarily more deeply pigmented than the rest of the skin. Figure 10.34 illustrates scrotal changes that occur with puberty. Assess the testicles by placing one finger over the inguinal canal and palpating the scrotum with the other. This prevents the retractile testes in a young child from slipping back up the inguinal canal. The testicles should be smooth, of similar sizes, and freely movable. The infant's testicles may be palpated in the scrotum or in the inguinal canal, where they can be easily moved into the scrotum with gentle pressure from the examiner's nondominant hand (Fig. 10.35). Beyond infancy, allow the child to sit cross-legged to reduce the cremasteric reflex that retracts the testicles during palpation. An adolescent may need to stand for the nurse to fully palpate the scrotum. Document the presence of both testicles in the scrotal sac, if they are retractile, or if they are absent. Report undescended testicle or other abnormal findings.

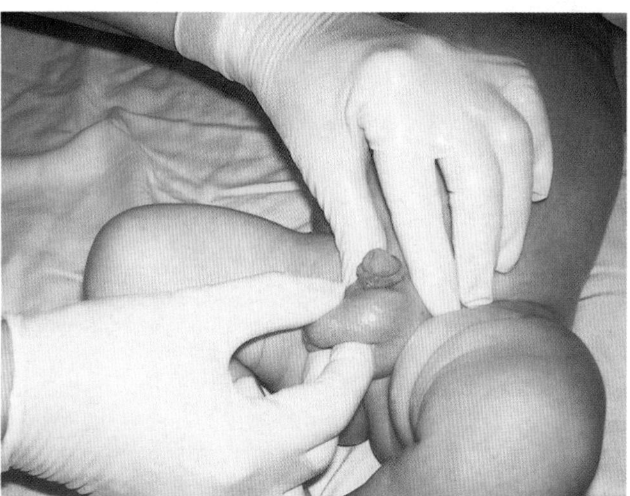

FIGURE 10.35 Placing a digit over the inguinal canal during testicular palpation prevents retraction of the testis into the canal.

FEMALE

In most cases, the female genitalia examination is limited to assessment of the external genitalia. Internal examination is not routinely performed before maturity unless the adolescent anticipates becoming or is sexually active or requests birth control, or if pathology is suspected. If an internal examination is needed, refer the child or adolescent to the appropriate advanced nurse practitioner or health care provider.

Position the infant in the parent's lap or on the examination table or crib. The toddler or preschooler should be examined in the parent's lap, in a frog-legged position. The school-age or adolescent female should lie on the examination table or bed. Provide for privacy by keeping the genital area covered until it is time for the examination.

Perform the assessment of the external genitalia in a systematic fashion. First, determine the presence and distribution of pubic hair. Infants and young females may have a small amount of downy pubic hair. Otherwise, the appearance of pubic hair indicates the onset of pubertal changes, sometimes prior to breast changes. Pubic hair generally begins to appear by age 11 years, with age 13 being the latest. Figure 10.36 illustrates the development of pubic hair on the vulva through puberty.

Inspect the labia majora and minora for size, color, and skin integrity. The newborn's labia minora are swollen from the effects of maternal estrogen but will decrease in size and be hidden by the labia majora within the first few weeks of life. Redness or swelling of the labia may occur with infection, sexual abuse, or masturbation. Lesions on the external genitalia may indicate sexually transmitted infection. Gently spread the labia to inspect the clitoris, urethral meatus, and vaginal opening. Some children may prefer to spread the labia themselves. The urinary meatus and vaginal orifice should be visible and not occluded by the hymen. It is not uncommon to see a hymenal tag. Note clitoral size. Inspect the urinary meatus and vaginal opening for edema or redness, which should not be present. Observe for any vaginal discharge. A small amount of blood-tinged or mucoid discharge may be noted in the first few weeks of life as a result of maternal hormone exposure. A small amount of clear mucous like discharge is normal in all females. If present, document labial adhesion or other abnormal findings.

ANUS

Inspect the anal area for fissures, rash, hemorrhoids, prolapse, or skin tags. Examine the infant's anal area while examining the genitalia. The younger child may lie back in the parent's lap and flex the knees to the chest. The

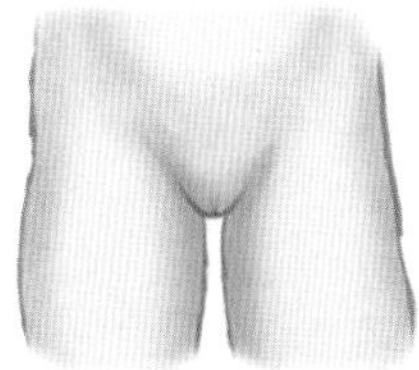

Stage 1 Preadolescents.
No pubic hair. Mons and labia covered with fine vellus hair as on abdomen.

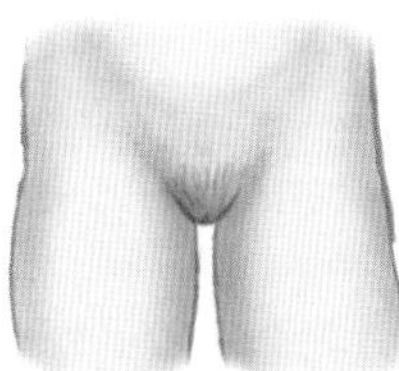

Stage 2 Growth sparse and mostly on labia. Long, downy hair, slightly pigmented, straight or only slightly curly.

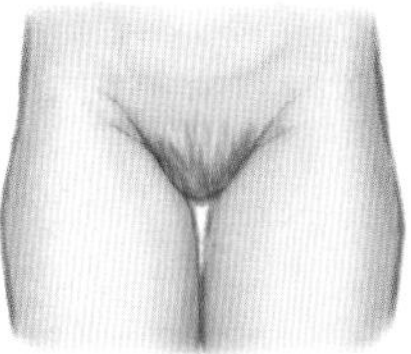

Stage 3 Growth sparse and spreading over mons pubis. Hair darker, coarser, curlier.

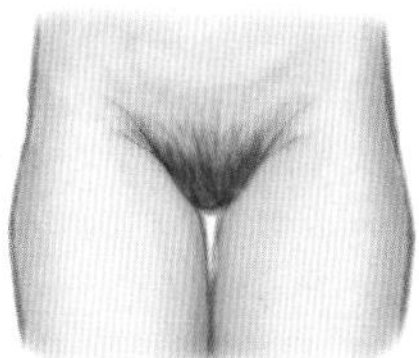

Stage 4 Hair is adult in type but over smaller area; none on medial thigh.

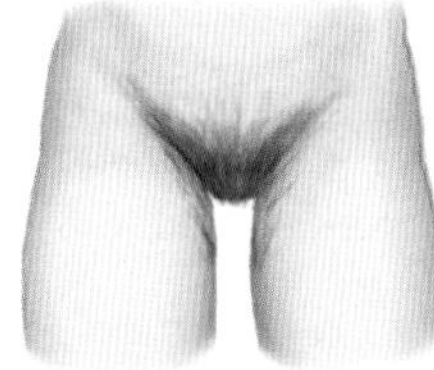

Stage 5 Adult in type and pattern; inverse triangle. Also on medial thigh surface.

FIGURE 10.36 Tanner female sexual maturity rating for pubic hair. (Adapted from Tanner, J. M. [1962]. *Growth at adolescence.* Blackwell Scientific Publications.)

older child or adolescent may be prone or in a side-lying position. If the adolescent is already standing for the scrotal assessment, have them bend forward so that you can assess the anal area. The anus should appear moist and hairless. Gently stroke the anal area to elicit the anal reflex (quick contraction). If indicated, inspect anal sphincter tone by inserting a gloved finger lubricated with water-soluble jelly just inside the anal sphincter.

Musculoskeletal

Assessment of the musculoskeletal system includes examination of the clavicles and shoulders, spine, extremities, joints, and hips. Determining the child's ability to move all extremities through the full range of motion is also important.

CLAVICLES AND SHOULDERS

Palpate the clavicles. In the newborn, tenderness or crepitus reveals a fracture sustained at birth. In the older infant or child, a bump indicates callus formation with clavicle fracture. Test shoulder strength and the function of cranial nerve XI in the older child by requesting that the child shrug the shoulders while you apply downward pressure.

SPINE

Observe the child's resting posture and alignment of the trunk. The newborn's position will look like the position the baby preferred in utero and is one of general flexion. The older infant moves more and can sit unassisted in the second half of the first year. Toddlers stand with a wide-based gait, a slightly swayed back, and the abdomen slightly protruding. The posture straightens in the preschool and school-age years. Adolescents often demonstrate kyphosis as the skeleton and muscles are both growing rapidly (Fig. 10.37).

Inspect the child's spine. The newborn's spine has a single C-shaped curve and remains rounded for the first 3 months of life. The cervical curve begins to develop around 3 to 4 months of age as the baby gains head control. By 12 to 18 months of age, the lumbar curve develops, which corresponds to the onset of walking. The S-shaped spine in older children and adolescents is similar to that of the adult. The spine should be flexible, with good muscle tone and no rigidity. Assess the back, and hip and shoulder heights for symmetry.

Examine the preadolescent and adolescent for the development of scoliosis. Refer to Chapter 22 for information about scoliosis screening. Scoliosis screening is

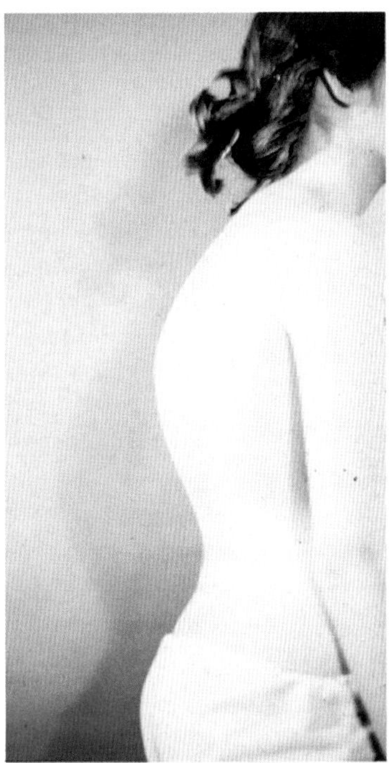

FIGURE 10.37 The adolescent's posture often demonstrates kyphosis.

generally performed during well-child examinations by the health care provider or nurse practitioner or by the middle or high school nurse on a particular day of the school year.

Note mobility of the vertebral column by having the child bend forward and side to side. Flex the neck and move it from side to side. No resistance or pain should occur. Inspect the back for discoloration, tufts of hair, or dimples. A normal pilonidal dimple is sometimes seen at the base of the spine, but there should be no tuft of hair or nevi along the spine. Document and report unexpected findings.

EXTREMITIES

All children, even newborns, should be able to move all extremities spontaneously. Screen the infant younger than 6 months for developmental dysplasia of the hip by performing the Ortolani and Barlow maneuvers (refer to Chapter 22 for additional information). These maneuvers are usually best performed by a proficient examiner. Inspect and palpate the child's upper and lower extremities. Assess for symmetry in size, contour, movement, warmth, and color of the extremities. The infant's feet and legs appear bowed secondary to in utero positioning but can be straightened through passive range of motion. Observe the child in a standing position. Bowing of the lower legs (internal tibial torsion) lessens as the toddler begins to bear weight and usually resolves in the second or third year of life as the strength of the muscles and bones increases. When it persists past that time, it is termed "genu varum" (bow legs). Genu valgum (knock knee) is usually present until the child is 7 years old. Observe the child walking, noting any difficulty with leg position or balance. If the child is reluctant to walk, use play as a way to elicit the behavior. The school-age child should have gait and leg appearance similar to that of the adult.

Note the normal flat foot in the toddler and young child. The arch develops as the child grows, and the muscles become less lax, although some children may continue with flexible flat feet; this is considered a normal variation.

Perform passive range of motion of the young infant's extremities. Inability to straighten the foot to midline may indicate clubfoot. Count the fingers and toes, noting abnormalities such as polydactyly (increased number of digits) or syndactyly (webbing of the digits). Palpate the joints for warmth or tenderness. Check the mobility of the joints of the upper and lower extremities by performing range of motion. Determine lower extremity muscle strength by having the child push against the examiner's hands with the soles of the forefoot. Assess upper extremity strength by having the child squeeze the examiner's crossed fingers or push up or down against the examiner's outstretched hands.

TAKE NOTE!

Slight tremors may be noticed in the infant's extremities in the first month of life.

Neurologic

The neurologic examination should include level of consciousness, balance and coordination, sensory function, reflexes, and a developmental screening. Motor function is assessed within the musculoskeletal section. Cranial nerve function is generally tested within other portions of the physical assessment as it applies to that section.

LEVEL OF CONSCIOUSNESS

Note the state of alertness and attentiveness to parents and the environment in the newborn and infant. Older infants become interactive with other people, as do toddlers and preschoolers. Younger children demonstrate orientation by positive interaction with family members and by crying or fussing when they feel threatened. By school age, the child should be oriented to name and place and a few years later should be able to state the date as well (even if only the day of the week).

BALANCE AND COORDINATION

The cerebellum controls balance and coordination. Observe the child's gait to assess balance and coordination. Observe toddlers and older children rising and walking from a seated and supine position. They should be able to stand and balance without straining or holding on to objects. Continue to test cerebellar function by having the younger child skip or hop and requesting that the older child or adolescent walk heel to toe. Further tests of cerebellar function responsible for balance and coordination are discussed in Box 10.3. Demonstrate each test and make sure the child understands your instructions.

BOX 10.3 Cerebellar Function Testing

- **Romberg:** Ask the school-age or older child to stand still with eyes closed and arms down by the sides. Observe the child for leaning (stand close in case this does occur). This is considered a positive Romberg test, indicating cerebellar dysfunction.
- For the following tests, the child should demonstrate accuracy and smoothness:
- **Heel-to-shin:** Have the child lie in a supine position, place one heel on the opposite knee, and run it down the shin.
- **Rapid alternating movements:** The child pats the thighs with the hands, lifts them, turns them over, pats the thighs with the back of the hands, and repeats the process multiple times. An alternate test is for the child to touch the thumb to each finger of the same hand, starting at the index finger, then reverse the direction and repeat.
- **Finger-to-finger:** The child's eyes are open. The child touches the examiner's outstretched finger with the index finger, then touches their own nose. The examiner moves the finger to a different spot, and the child repeats this process several times.
- **Finger-to-nose:** The child's eyes are closed. The child stretches the arm with the index finger extended, then touches their nose with that finger, keeping the eyes closed.

Data from Chiocca, E. M. (2020). *Advanced pediatric assessment* (3rd ed.). Springer Publishing Company; Jarvis, C., & Eckhardt, A. (2020). *Physical examination and health assessment* (8th ed.). Elsevier.

SENSORY TESTING

Portions of sensory testing related to most of the cranial nerves, vision, hearing, taste, and smell have already been incorporated into other sections as appropriate within the physical assessment. Test cranial nerve V (trigeminal) by lightly touching the child's cheek with a cotton ball. The young infant will root toward the side that is touched. With the child's eyes closed, ask the child to identify other locations where they are lightly touched (several different ones) to assess sensation. Ask the child to tell you when they are touched. Make a game of this activity to encourage cooperation in younger children. In the older child who knows the definition of sharp and dull, test for these sensations with the child's eyes closed. Use the rounded end of a tongue blade for dull and the broken edge of a tongue blade for the sharp sensation. The child should be able to discriminate the sensations of sharp and dull.

REFLEXES

Assess the infant's primitive and protective reflexes. The primitive reflexes involve a whole-body response and are subcortical in nature. Selected primitive reflexes present at birth include Moro, root, suck, asymmetric tonic neck, plantar and palmar grasp, step, and Babinski. Most of the primitive reflexes diminish over the first few months of life, giving way to protective or postural reflexes. Protective reflexes are motor responses related to maintenance of equilibrium. They are necessary for appropriate motor development and remain throughout life once they are established. The protective reflexes include the righting and parachute reactions.

Place one finger in each of the infant's hands to elicit the palmar grasp reflex (usually disappears by the age of 3 to 4 months). Touch the thumb to the ball of the infant's foot to elicit the plantar grasp reflex. The infant's toes will curl down (this reflex disappears by the age of 8 to 10 months). Refer to Table 3.1 for illustrations and additional explanation of the other reflexes. Appropriate presence and disappearance of primitive reflexes, as well as development of protective reflexes, is indicative of a healthy neurologic system. Primitive reflexes that persist beyond the usual age of disappearance may indicate an abnormality of the neurologic system and should be further investigated (Kotagal & Morse, 2022).

Assess deep tendon reflexes in all infants and children. Appropriate responses indicate that the reflex arc is intact. Use the reflex hammer in all ages or the curved tips of the two first fingers to elicit the responses in infants. The limb must be relaxed and the muscle partly stretched. Use a snapping motion of the wrist to tap with the fingertips or the reflex hammer. Test the biceps, triceps, patellar, and Achilles reflexes as you would in the adult. It may help to place a finger under the infant's knee to encourage relaxation. Young children who tense up when their reflexes are being tested may relax the area if you have them focus on another area, so have the child clasp the hands while testing the Achilles and patellar reflexes. As the child focuses on the hands, the lower extremities relax (Jarvis & Eckhardt, 2020). Distraction may also be helpful.

Grade the strength of the response using the standard scale from 0 to 4+:

- 0: no response
- 1+: diminished or sluggish
- 2+: average
- 3+: brisker than average
- 4+: very brisk, may involve clonus

The newborn's deep tendon reflexes are normally brisk (3+). They decrease to average (2+) usually by 4 months of age. Healthy children should have reflexes of 2+ if the reflex has been elicited properly. Absent, sluggish, or hyperreactive responses usually indicate disease (Bryant & Speck, 2022).

DEVELOPMENTAL SCREENING

An important component of the neurologic assessment and a comprehensive child health assessment is developmental screening. Developmental screening may be used to identify children whose developmental status may warrant additional evaluation. Become comfortable with the developmental screening tools used and what the results of the screening mean. On completion of the screening, discuss the child's abilities with the parent or caregiver. Developmental screening is often performed separately from the physical examination and is discussed in further detail in Chapter 9.

Refer back to Elliot, the 3-year-old from the beginning of the chapter. What are some important considerations when performing his physical examination?

Unfolding Patient Stories: Eva Madison • Part 1

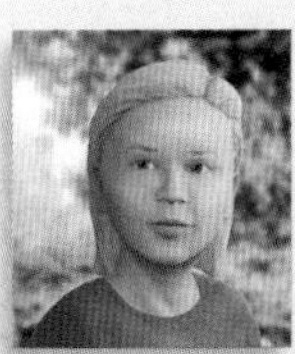

Eva Madison, a 5-year-old, is at the clinic with their parent for a routine check-up. How can the nurse create an environment that is conducive to obtaining health information? How can the nurse prepare the child and the parent for the physical examination? What key areas of the health history and physical assessment should the nurse evaluate in this 5-year-old? (Eva Madison's story continues in Chapter 20.)

Care for Eva and other patients in a realistic virtual environment: ***vSim** for Nursing* (thepoint.lww.com/vSimPediatric). Practice documenting these patients' care in DocuCare (thePoint.lww.com/DocuCareEHR).

KEY CONCEPTS

- The health history in children includes more than just the chief complaint, history of present illness, and past medical history; it is important to include the perinatal history and developmental milestones.
- Allow the chief complaint to determine which parts of the history require more in-depth investigation.
- The developmental history will warrant more attention in the younger child, while school performance and adjustment will be more important in the school-age child and adolescent.
- Although the parent will provide most of the health history for the infant and the young child, allow the young verbal child to answer questions during the health history as appropriate.
- Direct health history questions to the school-age child and adolescent, seeking clarification from the parents as needed.
- Provide confidentiality and privacy for the adolescent during the health history.
- Weight and length or height should be assessed at each well-child visit to determine adequacy of growth.
- Measure head circumference until age 3 years to monitor brain growth.
- Perform hearing and vision screenings for children of all ages.
- BMI can be used to identify children who are overweight or at risk for being overweight.
- The normal range of vital signs varies based on the child's age.
- The sequence of the physical examination in children should be based on the child's developmental age, their level of cooperation, and the severity of the illness.
- Obtain heart rate and respiratory rate, and auscultate the heart and lungs while the infant or young child is quiet.
- Perform intrusive procedures such as examination of the ears, mouth, and throat last in the infant or young child.
- Perform the health assessment in a head-to-toe fashion in the school-age child or adolescent, reserving the genitalia and anus examination for last.
- Plan the health assessment in such a way as to minimize trauma to the child or adolescent.
- Use age-appropriate measurement tools to assess pain in children.
- Allow the infant or young child to remain in the parent's lap for as much of the assessment as possible so that the child feels secure.
- Use age-appropriate games during the health assessment to gain cooperation in the younger child.
- Having the young child sit cross-legged for a testicular examination may reduce the cremasteric reflex.
- The newborn may exhibit a wide variety of normal skin variations.
- The infant's fontanels should be soft and flat; report a bulging fontanel immediately.
- Jaundice (outside of the newborn period), pallor, cyanosis, and poor skin turgor indicate illness and may need immediate intervention.
- Heart murmurs should be assessed for intensity, location, and duration. They may be innocent or may indicate a congenital heart defect.
- The infant's chest wall is relatively thin, allowing upper airway sounds to be transmitted throughout the lung fields.
- Substernal or xiphoid retractions indicate that the child is laboring to breathe, whereas a fixed, depressed sternum (pectus excavatum) is a structural abnormality.
- The Tanner stages of sexual maturity provide a basis for assessing pubertal development. Use the breast and pubic hair charts for females and the pubic hair and penis and scrotum size chart for males.

REFERENCES AND RECOMMENDED READINGS

American Academy of Pediatrics. (2021). *Fever and your child*. https://publications.aap.org/patiented/article/doi/10.1542/peo_document040/80029/Fever-and-Your-Child

Andre, J. H., & Rockwell, M. (2022). Management of eye disorders. In T. Kyle (Ed.), *Primary care pediatrics for the nurse practitioner* (pp. 269–285). Springer.

Boos, S. (2022). Differential diagnosis of suspected child physical abuse. *UpToDate*. Retrieved November 3, 2023, from https://www.uptodate.com/contents/differential-diagnosis-of-suspected-child-physical-abuse

Brazelton, T. B., & Sparrow, J. (n.d.). *The Touchpoints model of development*. https://www.brazeltontouchpoints.org/wp-content/uploads/2011/09/Touchpoints-Model-of-Development-April-2015.pdf

Bryant, P., & Speck, P. M. (2022). Health assessment. In T. Kyle (Ed.), *Primary care pediatrics for the nurse practitioner* (pp. 25–47). Springer.

Centers for Disease Control and Prevention. (2017, June 16). *Clinical growth charts*. https://www.cdc.gov/growthcharts/clinical_charts.htm

Centers for Disease Control and Prevention. (2022, September 24). *About child & teen BMI*. https://www.cdc.gov/healthyweight/assessing/bmi/childrens_bmi/about_childrens_bmi.html

Centers for Disease Control and Prevention. (2023, January 10). *Childhood lead poisoning prevention program*. http://www.cdc.gov/nceh/lead/

Chiocca, E. M. (2020). *Advanced pediatric assessment* (3rd ed.). Springer Publishing Company.

Choueiry, J., Reszel, J., Hamid, J. S., Wilding, J., Martelli, B., & Harrison, D. (2020). Development and pilot evaluation of an educational tool for the FLACC pain scale. *Pain Management Nursing*, *21*(6), 523–529. https://doi.org/10.1016/j.pmn.2020.06.002

Columbia University, College of Physicians and Surgeons. (n.d.). *Points on the pediatric physical exam.* http://www.columbia.edu/itc/hs/medical/clerkships/peds/Student_Information/Reference_Materials/Pediatric_PE.html#PhysicalExam

Dev, L. S., & Cruz, M. (2017). Healthy sexual development and sexuality. In T. K. McInerny, H. M. Adam, D. E. Campbell, J. M. Foy, & D. M. Kamat (Eds.), *American Academy of Pediatrics textbook of pediatric care* (2nd ed.). American Academy of Pediatrics.

Drutz, J. E., & White-Satcher, D. (2023). The pediatric physical examination: General principles and standard measurements. *UpToDate.* Retrieved November 3, 2023, from https://www.uptodate.com/contents/the-pediatric-physical-examination-general-principles-and-standard-measurements

Exergen Corporation. (n.d.). *Nurse's center.* https://medical.exergen.com/nurses-center/

Fahrenkopf, M. P., Adams, N. S., Mann, R. J., & Girotto, J. A. (2020). Deformational plagiocephaly. In R. M. Kliegman, J. W. St Geme, N. J. Blum, S. S. Shah, R. C. Tasker, & K. M. Wilson (Eds.), *Nelson textbook of pediatrics* (21st ed.). Elsevier.

Flynn, J. T., Kaelber, D. C., Baker-Smith, C. M., Blowey, D., Carrol, A. E., Daniels, S. R., de Ferranti, S. D., Dionne, J. M., Leu, M. G., Powers, M. E., Rea, C., Samuels, J., Simasek, M., Thaker, V. V., Urbina, E. M., & The Subcommittee on Screening and Management of High Blood Pressure in Children. (2017). Clinical practice guideline for screening and management of high blood pressure in children and adolescents. *Pediatrics, 140*(3), e20171904. https://doi.org/10.1542/peds.2017-1904

Gilmore, B. M., & Hay, B. B. (2021). Evidence-based assessment of the breasts and axillae. In K. S. Gawlik, B. M. Melnyk, & A. M. Teall (Eds.), *Evidence-based physical examination: Best practices for health and well-being assessment* (pp. 483–501). Springer.

Jarvis, C., & Eckhardt, A. (2020). *Physical examination and health assessment* (8th ed.). Elsevier.

Jone, P.-N., Kim, J. S., Burkett, D., Jacobson, R., & Von Alvensleben, J. (2022). Cardiovascular diseases. In M. Bunik, W. W. Hay, M. J. Levin, & M. J. Abzug (Eds.), *Current diagnosis & treatment: Pediatrics* (26th ed.). McGraw-Hill.

Kleinman, K., McDaniel, L., & Molloy, M. (2021). *The Harriet Lane handbook: A manual for pediatric house officers* (22nd ed.). Elsevier.

Kotagal, S., & Morse, A. M. (2022). Detailed neurologic assessment of infants and children. *UpToDate.* Retrieved November 3, 2023, from https://www.uptodate.com/contents/detailed-neurologic-assessment-of-infants-and-children

Kyle, T. (2022). Well-child visits during infancy. In T. Kyle (Ed.), *Primary care pediatrics for the nurse practitioner* (pp. 161-169). Springer.

Mechem, C. C. (2022). Pulse oximetry. *UpToDate.* Retrieved November 3, 2023, from https://www.uptodate.com/contents/pulse-oximetry

Medtronic. (2023). *Pulse oximetry.* https://www.medtronic.com/covidien/en-us/products/pulse-oximetry.html

Mento, C., Silvestri, M. C., Bruno, A., Muscatello, M. R. A., Cedro, C., Pandolfo, G., & Zoccali, R. A. (2020). Workplace violence against healthcare professionals: A systematic review. *Aggression and Violent Behavior, 51,* 101381. https://doi.org/10.1016/j.avb.2020.101381

Miller, S. (n.d.). *Pediatric physical exam video* [Video]. http://www.columbia.edu/itc/hs/medical/clerkships/peds/Student_Information/Reference_Materials/PE_Video.html

National Institutes of Health. (2021). *Clear & simple.* https://www.nih.gov/institutes-nih/nih-office-director/office-communications-public-liaison/clear-communication/clear-simple

Perry, A. G., Potter, P. A., Ostendorf, W. R., & Laplante, N. (2022). Chapter 5: Vital signs. In A. G. Perry, P. A. Potter, W. R. Ostendorf, & N. Laplante (Eds.), *Clinical nursing skills and tecchniques* (10th ed., pp. 68-107). Elsevier.

Quinlin, L., & Gawlik, K. (2021). Evidence-base history-taking approach for wellness exams, episodic visits and chronic care management. In K. S. Gawlik, B. M. Melnyk, & A. M. Teall (Eds.), *Evidence-based physical examination: Best practices for health and well-being assessment* (pp. 17-42). Springer.

Sass, A. E., & Richards, M. J. (2022). Adolescence. In M. Bunik, W. W. Hay, M. J. Levin, & M. J. Abzug (Eds.), *Current diagnosis & treatment: Pediatrics* (26th ed.). McGraw-Hill.

Sevy, J. O., Hohman, M. H., & Singh, A. (2023). Cerumen impaction removal. *StatPearls.* StatPearls Publishing. Retrieved November 3, 2023, from https://www.ncbi.nlm.nih.gov/books/NBK448155/

Smith, D. (2022). The newborn infant. In M. Bunik, W. W. Hay, M. J. Levin, & M. J. Abzug (Eds.), *Current diagnosis & treatment: Pediatrics* (26th ed.). McGraw-Hill.

Tanner, J. M. (1962). *Growth at adolescence.* Blackwell Scientific Publications.

Treitz, M., Nicklas, D., & Fox, D. (2022). Ambulatory & office pediatrics. In M. Bunik, W. W. Hay, M. J. Levin, & M. J. Abzug (Eds.), *Current diagnosis & treatment: Pediatrics* (26th ed.). McGraw-Hill.

U.S. Department of Health and Human Services. (n.d.). *Healthy People 2030.* https://health.gov/healthypeople

Vorvick, L. J., Zieve, D., Conaway, B., & the A.D.A.M. Editorial Team. (2022). *Temperature measurement.* https://medlineplus.gov/ency/article/003400.htm

Wong, D. L., & Baker, C. M. (1988). Pain in children: Comparison of assessment scales. *Pediatric Nursing, 14*(1), 9–17. https://pubmed.ncbi.nlm.nih.gov/3344163/

Yoon, P. J., Scholes, M. A., & Herrmann, B. W. (2022). Chapter 18: Ear, nose, & throat. In M. Bunik, W. W. Hay, M. J. Levin, & M. J. Abzug (Eds.), *Current diagnosis & treatment: Pediatrics* (26th ed.). McGraw-Hill.

DEVELOPING CLINICAL JUDGMENT

PRACTICING FOR NCLEX

1. A 5-year-old visits the pediatric office with an upper respiratory infection. Which approach would give the nurse the most information about the child's developmental level?
   a. Playing a game with the child
   b. Talking with the child about the teddy bear next to them
   c. Using a screening tool during a follow-up office visit
   d. Asking the 10-year-old sibling about the child
2. Which statement indicates the best sequence for the nurse to conduct an assessment in a nonemergency situation?
   a. Introduce yourself, ask about any problems, take a history, and do the physical examination.
   b. Perform the physical examination and then ask the family if there are any problems in the child's life.
   c. Do the physical examination while at the same time asking about the child's previous illnesses; then talk about the family's concerns.
   d. Get a complete history of the family's health beliefs and practices, and then assess the child.
3. What approach by the nurse would most likely encourage a child to cooperate with an assessment of physical and developmental health?
   a. Explain to the child what's going to happen when the child asks questions.
   b. Explain what is going to happen in words the child can understand.
   c. Force the child to cooperate by having a parent hold them down.
   d. Give the child a sticker before beginning the examination.
4. A sleeping 5-month-old is being held by the parent when the nurse comes in to do a physical examination. What assessment should be done initially?
   a. Listening to the bowel sounds
   b. Counting the heart rate
   c. Checking the temperature
   d. Looking in the ears
5. Which assessment finding is considered normal in children?
   a. Irregular respiratory rate and rhythm
   b. Split S_2 and sinus arrhythmia
   c. Decreased heart rate with crying
   d. Genu varum past the age of 5 years
6. A child's weight is 35 lb, 7 oz. Convert the weight to kilograms.
7. A child's height is 41 in. Convert the height to centimeters.

CRITICAL THINKING EXERCISES

1. A soft and muffled heart murmur is heard in a 4-year-old patient. The parent states that they have never been told that the child has a murmur. What should the nurse do?
2. A nurse is helping a new parent breastfeed their 4-day-old baby. The parent notices that the baby has a bluish cast to the skin on their hands and that sometimes the infant has a tremor. They ask the nurse if the baby is cold, although the baby is swaddled and comfortably resting against the parent's skin. How might the nurse help teach this parent?
3. Devise a plan for encouraging cooperation of the toddler or preschooler during various parts of the physical examination.

STUDY ACTIVITIES

1. In the clinical setting, obtain a health history on an infant, child, or adolescent.
2. In the clinical setting, compare the approach you use for the physical examination of a toddler versus a school-age child or adolescent.
3. No matter how thoughtfully and appropriately you plan your assessment, odds are good that you will have difficulty assessing a 2-year-old. Discuss with your classmates the strategies that you have used for success, and brainstorm with them about their ideas for assessing a crying or resistant young child.

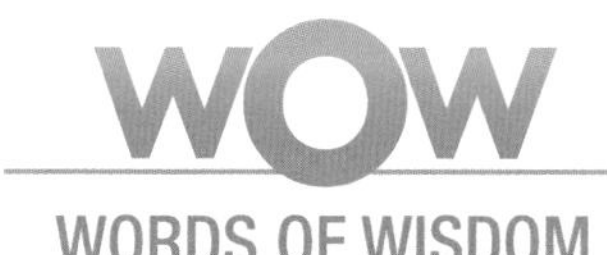

WORDS OF WISDOM

Nurses should leave their "comfort zone" of practice and reach out to children on their turf to make a difference.

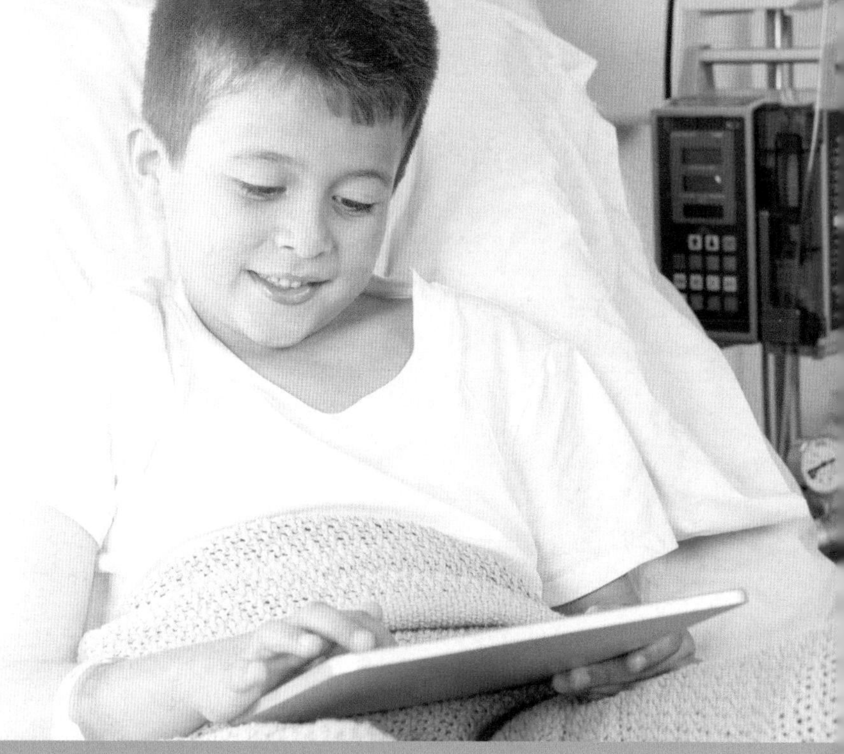

11

Caring for Children in Diverse Settings

LEARNING OBJECTIVES

Upon completion of the chapter, you will be able to:

1. Discuss the variety of settings in which nursing care occurs.
2. Describe the various roles of the nurse, including hospital and community settings and home care nurses.
3. Examine the nurse's role in home health care.
4. Explain the major stressors of illness and hospitalization for children.
5. Identify the reactions and responses of children and their families during illness and hospitalization.
6. Describe the nursing care that minimizes stressors for children who are ill or hospitalized.
7. Delineate the major components of admission for children to the hospital.
8. Discuss appropriate safety measures to use with hospitalized children.
9. Identify nursing responsibilities related to patients discharged from the hospital.

KEY TERMS

child with medical complexity
community
individualized health plan
therapeutic play

Jake Jorgenson, 8 years old, was brought to the clinic with a history of headaches, vomiting not related to feeding, and changes in his gait. Initial testing leads to a suspected brain tumor. Jake is to be admitted to the neurologic service at a pediatric hospital for further testing and treatment. Up to this point, he has been a healthy child with no previous hospitalizations. He lives at home with his parents and two siblings, Jenny, age 11, and Joshua, age 5.

INTRODUCTION

Nursing care of the child occurs in a variety of settings, from acute care in a hospital to well and ill care in community settings, such as health care providers' offices, schools, churches, health departments, community centers, and even within the child's own home. Within each setting, the nurse incorporates basic nursing care with specific strategies to help promote positive outcomes for the child, family, and community as a whole.

Children receive most of their health care, well and ill care, in the community setting. Nurses play an important role in the health and wellness of a community. They not only meet the health care needs of individuals but also go beyond to create interventions that affect the community. Community health nursing refers to nursing care that strives to improve the health of a specific community as a whole. For example, community health nurses working in the Department of Health and Human Services would strive to make sure that all children in their particular community were up-to-date on immunizations. Community-based nursing focuses more on providing care to the individual or family (which, of course, impacts the community) in settings outside of acute care. For example, a community-based nurse would work in the local public school to care for students' health needs. Nurses practicing in the community promote the health of individuals, families, groups, communities, and populations and promote an environment that supports health.

COMMUNITY HEALTH NURSING

Nursing in the community is aimed at disease prevention and improvement of the health of populations and communities. "Population" refers to all of the people occupying an area who may not necessarily interact, such as the population of the United States, or to all of those who share one or more characteristics, for example, the pediatric population (Rector, 2022). **Community** can be defined as a "collection of people who interact with one another and whose common interests or characteristics form the basis for a sense of unity or belonging" (Rector, 2022, p. 5). Community health nurses work in geographically and culturally diverse settings. They address current and potential health needs of the population or community. They promote and preserve the health of a population and are not limited to particular age groups or diagnoses. Public health nursing is a specialized area of community health nursing.

Epidemiology can help determine the health and health needs of a population and assist in planning health services. Community health nurses perform epidemiologic investigations to help analyze and develop health policy and community health initiatives. Community health initiatives can be focused on the community as a whole or a specific target population with specific needs. Healthy People 2030 is an example of national health initiatives developed using the epidemiologic process (U.S. Department of Health and Human Services, n.d.). Healthy People 2030 ensures that health care professionals look at the individual as well as the community. It addresses the link between the individual's health and the health of the community. Nurses play a key role in the health of a community and the individuals who reside in it.

Healthy People 2030 is the fifth edition of national health goals, which were launched in 1979. Healthy People 2030 is a comprehensive health initiatives plan. Nurses can help the nation meet these objectives by educating those in the community on appropriate prevention strategies, such as proper immunization and smoking cessation (see individual chapters for relevant Healthy People objectives and nursing implications). Healthy People 2030 is available online at https://www.healthypeople.gov. Refer to Chapter 1 for more information.

COMMUNITY-BASED NURSING

In the past, the major role of the nurse in the community was that of the community health nurse or public health nurse. Today, nurses practice in a variety of settings within a community, such as clinics and health care providers' offices, schools, camps, shelters, places of worship, health departments, community health centers, and homes.

Shifting Responsibilities From Hospital-Based to Community-Based Nursing Care

Over the past century, changes in health care such as strained health care funding, shorter hospital stays, and cost containment, have led to a shift in responsibilities of care for children from the hospital to homes and communities. Community care, especially home care, is a rapidly growing service in the United States. Community-based care has been shown to be a cost-effective way to provide care. It emphasizes wellness and prevention. Increases in disposable income and the longevity of children with chronic and debilitating health conditions have also contributed to the continued shift of health care to the community and home setting. Advances in technology have allowed for improved monitoring of children in community settings and at home, as well as allowing complicated procedures, such as intravenous administration of antibiotics, to be done at home.

Another major reason for the increase in community care of children, especially home care, is the understanding that an acute care setting is not an ideal environment for children's development. Caring for children at home and within their community not only improves their physical health but also allows for adequate growth and development while keeping them within their family. When they are in a familiar environment with the comfort and support of family, there is a better opportunity for improved care and quality of life.

Role of the Community-Based Nurse

With the shift in responsibilities from hospital care to community care have come changes in nursing care. More opportunities exist for nurses to provide direct care to children in the community setting, especially the home. Community-based nursing care differs from nursing care in the acute setting. In the community or home care setting, the nurse provides direct care for the child but spends more time in the role of educator, communicator, and manager than the nurse in the acute care setting. In home care, the nurse spends a significant amount of time in the supervision or management role. Community-based nursing focuses on the practice of nursing that provides personal care to individuals and families in the community. Community-based nurses focus on promoting and preserving health as well as preventing disease or injury. They are educators, managers of care, and advocates along with being direct providers of care.

Communication and Education

The community-based nurse must use the principles and techniques of interpersonal communication. The nurse must be able to assess the child's and family's learning needs and their readiness to learn. As hospital stays become shorter and admissions to the hospital become less frequent, teaching now begins wherever the child or family enters the health care system. Often, initial teaching occurs in the community setting, especially the home. In the community-based setting, teaching is often focused on assisting the child and family to achieve independence.

Discharge Planning and Care Coordination

Due to the short lengths of stay in acute settings and the shift to community settings for children with complex health needs, discharge planning and care coordination have become important nursing roles. Discharge planning involves the development and implementation of a comprehensive plan for the safe discharge of a child from a health care facility and for continuing safe and effective care in the community and at home. Successful discharge planning begins upon the child's admission to the facility.

Modern pediatric health care focuses on an interdisciplinary plan of care designed to meet the child's physical, developmental, educational, spiritual, and psychosocial needs. Nurses provide care coordination through the implementation of this interdisciplinary plan in a collaborative manner to ensure continuity of care that is cost-effective, quality oriented, and outcome focused.

Advocacy and Resource Management

Another important role of the community-based nurse is to advocate for the child and family to ensure that their needs are being met and that they have available resources and appropriate health care services. Working in a child's and family's home can lead a nurse to become overly involved or attached. To best serve the child and family, the community-based nurse must be an advocate and educator but avoid becoming a personal friend by maintaining professional boundaries and a therapeutic nurse–patient relationship (National Council of State Boards of Nursing [NCSBN], 2018).

Nurses must have a basic understanding of community, state, and federal resources to ensure they are providing families with the resources they may need. One such resource important in the community-based care of children with complex medical needs is Medicaid. Medicaid is a national program providing medical assistance for children and families with low incomes. It is jointly run by the federal and state governments but is administered at the state level; therefore, provisions vary widely. Additionally, medical model waivers are state-run programs that use federal and state funds to pay for health care for people with certain medical conditions. These waivers will refrain from enforcing one or more Medicaid rules to extend eligibility or services to children who qualify. Home- and community-based waiver programs, such as the Katie Beckett waiver (also known as the Deeming waiver), allow children and young adults with complex medical needs to be cared for at home and make them eligible for Medicaid based on their own income and assets, regardless of their parents' income (Kids' Waivers, 2022). Without medical waiver programs, many children with special needs would either go without health care or would be institutionalized in order to qualify for Medicaid.

Physical Care

The community-based nurse performs less direct physical care than the nurse in the acute care setting. Many times, the nurse observes the child or caregiver performing physical care tasks. Excellent assessment skills are especially important in the community care setting. The nurse often functions in a more autonomous role; after data collection, the community-based nurse will often decide whether to initiate, continue, alter, or end physical nursing care. Assessment will go beyond physical assessment of the child to include the environment and the community.

ILLNESS AND HOSPITALIZATION IN CHILDHOOD

In today's health care environment, children receive much of their care for illnesses in community health settings, as discussed previously. As a result of this trend, fewer children may actually be admitted to a hospital unit, and those who are hospitalized are generally acutely ill. In addition, hospital stays are often shorter due to economic trends in the health care environment, such as the delivery system of managed care and other factors that attempt to control costs. In all of the varied settings where health care is administered, nurses provide well care, episodic ill care, and chronic care. They work to promote, preserve, and improve the health of children and families in all these settings.

General Inpatient Unit

With inpatient unit stays for children that are shorter and that involve more acute conditions, there is little time for admission preparation. Often, the admission procedure and treatment actually occur simultaneously. Sometimes, the stay is in a special 23-hour observation unit, so the child is in the setting for less than 24 hours. General hospital stays may be in a pediatric hospital, a pediatric unit in a general hospital, or a general unit that occasionally admits children. General units often lack child-oriented services, such as play areas, child-size equipment, and staff familiar with caring for children.

Emergency Departments

A major cause of illness and hospitalization in children is injuries from accidents; the top seven nonfatal injuries are all unintentional (National Center for Injury Prevention and Control, Centers for Disease Control and Prevention [CDC], 2020). Many times, a family's first experience with the acute care setting is the emergency department. Due to the situation, the child and family may experience increased anxiety, and it may become overwhelming as uncertainties develop and critical decisions must be made. The family may be frightened, insecure, and in a state of shock.

Procedures and tests are performed quickly, with minimal time for preparation. The family is often ill-prepared for the visit, having little money or clothing with them. Siblings may be present if the parents did not have time to arrange other child care.

Due to the fast pace of the emergency department, the family may be hesitant to ask questions; hence, it is important for the nurse to keep the family and child well informed. Allow the family to stay with the child, provide support, and allow the family, and when appropriate the child, to participate in decisions.

Families may have a strong fear of the unknown and may be terrified that the child will die or be permanently disabled. Help the family to identify their concerns and their support systems. Prepare them for what they will experience. Provide comfort such as holding, touching, talking softly, and other appropriate interventions according to age, developmental level, and culture.

Pediatric Intensive Care Units

The pediatric intensive care unit (PICU) specializes in caring for children in crisis. The same principles and concepts of general care of children apply to this setting, but everything is intensified. Families will be faced with an unfamiliar, high-tech environment and interaction with a large team of care providers.

Families must deal with the critical situation that brought them to the PICU. The child will likely experience pain, unusual noises, and increased stimulation and will probably undergo uncomfortable procedures. Parents may face the possibility of losing their child. Sometimes, the child cannot talk, eat, or display other appropriate developmental behaviors. Sensory overload (increased stimulation) or sensory deprivation (lack of stimulation) can affect both child and family.

The nurse should welcome families (if institutional policy permits) and encourage them to stay with the child and participate in care. Explain everything to the parents and, when appropriate, to the child. Frequently touch the child and encourage the parents to comfort them. Listen for clues about what the child and family need during the PICU stay.

Rehabilitation Units/Facilities

The rehabilitation unit/facility provides care for children beyond the initial period of illness or injury. The care involves an interdisciplinary approach that assists the child to reach their potential and achieve developmental skills. For example, rehabilitation units help children regain abilities lost due to neurologic injuries or serious burns. The facilities often resemble a home environment, with special services to help children to relearn activities of daily living and to help them deal with the physical or mental challenges associated with the original illness or injury. Typically, families are encouraged to participate and are given support for their child's eventual return home. There is a balance of nurturing and firm discipline while the child reclaims independence.

Outpatient Facilities

Outpatient care is health care provided to individuals who do not require care in an acute setting. Due to advances in medical technology, more medical procedures (such as diagnostic tests, treatments, and surgeries) can be administered on an outpatient basis and do not require children to be hospitalized. Outpatient care delivers convenient and cost-effective health care to children and their families, often right within their own community. These settings allow for increased independence and permit children to return to their normal routine as quickly as possible. More and more outpatient care centers are opening, sponsored by health maintenance organizations (HMOs), health care providers' groups, community agencies and public health departments, and hospitals.

Outpatient units are used to keep hospital stays short and decrease the cost of hospitalization. Outpatient units may be a part of the hospital or a freestanding facility. The child and family arrive in the morning; the child undergoes the procedure, test, or surgery and then goes home in the evening. Examples of surgeries and procedures performed in outpatient settings include tympanostomy tube placement, hernia repair, tonsillectomy, cystoscopy, bronchoscopy, blood transfusions, dialysis, and chemotherapy. The advantages of this environment include minimal separation of the child from the family, minimal disruption of the family pattern, decreased risk of infection, and decreased cost. Disadvantages include lack of equipment for overnight stays, so if there are complications, the child will need to be transported to the hospital.

Many centers offer preoperative health assessment and teaching sessions. These allow the parent and child to ask questions and resolve them before the procedure. On the day of the procedure, parents should be allowed to be with their child until the procedure begins. Parents should also be allowed to be with their child in the postanesthesia recovery unit as quickly as possible. This provides reassurance and comfort to the child while meeting their physical and emotional needs.

The role of the nurse in the outpatient or ambulatory setting includes admission and assessment, preoperative teaching and preparation, patient assessment and support, postoperative monitoring, case management, discharge planning, and teaching. Before the procedure, the nurse reviews with the family the routine to be followed and any special instructions (such as NPO orders) and familiarizes the child with the setting to help alleviate fears. This may occur during the preoperative health assessment.

TAKE NOTE!

Encourage the parent to bring one of the child's favorite toys, blankets, or games to make the child feel more comfortable.

The nurse performs any surgical preparation and discusses intraoperative procedures as necessary. The nurse provides postoperative care and assessment of the child. Once the child's condition is stable and they meet the discharge criteria of the facility, the nurse reviews with the parent postoperative instructions, including pain management; care of the incision if appropriate; diet; activity, including return to school; necessary follow-up; and when to call the health care provider or nurse practitioner.

Health Care Provider's Office or Clinic, Health Departments, and Urgent Care Centers

Health care providers' offices, clinics, health departments, and urgent care centers are used by children and their families for well care, episodic ill care, acute care, and care of chronic conditions. For well care and illness or injury, children are often seen by their primary care health care provider. They may visit a health care provider's office or clinic or the health department. In more acute situations or for after-hours issues that cannot wait until clinic operating hours, a child may be seen in an urgent care center or may be referred to the emergency department. The American Academy of Pediatrics discourages children and families from using urgent care centers or the emergency department for routine care, since it is difficult to provide coordinated, comprehensive family-centered care consistent with a "medical home" concept (see "Medical Homes" section on Chapter 9) (Conners et al., 2017).

The nurse's role in these settings includes preparing patients, collecting pertinent health information, performing assessments, assisting the health care provider with diagnostic testing and procedures, administering injections and medications, changing wound dressings, assisting with minor surgery, helping to maintain records, and educating the child and family about home care and when to call the health care provider or nurse practitioner or return to be seen.

An essential component of primary care practice is telephone or virtual triage. Pediatric office nurses often fill this role. When parents feel comfortable with the providers in their child's medical home office, they often call or message for advice to treat their child at home. A triage nurse needs excellent assessment and critical thinking skills along with solid training and education. The triage nurse needs to assess the child's entire situation, including current signs and symptoms, history, and home treatment.

Protocols, standardized policies and procedures, and professional judgment guide the triage nurse in the decision-making process. Pediatric telephone protocols are available for purchase through the American Academy of Pediatrics (http://www.aap.org/). The triage nurse needs to determine whether the child requires emergency care, an office visit, or home management. Good listening and the ability to maintain a calm voice when talking to parents are skills necessary for successful telephone triage. The triage nurse should not discourage parents from bringing the child into the office to be seen; triage is not meant to keep children out of the office, and if a parent is concerned, that is reason enough to be seen.

TAKE NOTE!

Parents can often pick up on subtle problems in their children. They may not be able to accurately describe signs and symptoms, but they know that their child "isn't acting right." Nurses must listen to parents and act on their concerns.

Medical Care Centers

The **child with medical complexity** (CMC) is defined as a child with "substantial health care needs, one or more chronic conditions, functional limitations often associated with technology assistance, and health care use" (Elias et al., 2012, reaffirmed 2022, p. 997). The number of children with medical complexity accounts for less than 1% of the children in the United States, but they make up more than a third of the total pediatric health care costs (Murphy et al., 2020). The number of children with medical complexity is growing. Reasons include improvements in the treatment and care of complex medical conditions and increased sophistication of medical technology, which has led to infants and children surviving and thriving with previously fatal conditions (Gallo et al., 2021). For many years, these children lived in hospitals their entire lives. Due to concerns about the high cost of long-term hospitalization and the diminished quality of life for these children, alternative care settings in the community, such as medical day care centers, have been developed.

Medical day care centers are specifically designed to meet the needs of these children. Most centers accept children who have complicated medical needs or who are dependent on technology. Examples include children with multiple congenital anomalies, children who are ventilator dependent, children with respiratory conditions, children with cardiac conditions, and children with cancer. Some centers accept children with less complicated needs, such as cardiorespiratory monitoring or asthma, and some enroll children without health care needs to promote peer relationships and acceptance. Just as at a regular day care center, the parents or caregivers can drop the child off in the morning and pick the child up in the afternoon. Some centers offer afterschool, weekend, or respite services. The centers usually provide needed therapies and have indoor and outdoor play areas, educational activities, and arts and crafts.

Health professionals are present at these centers to provide for the children's medical, emotional, and developmental needs. Nurses trained in pediatric and neonatal care, physical therapists, occupational therapists, speech therapists, child-life specialists (CLSs), and social workers staff the centers; some centers have respiratory therapists on site. Children are able to receive all of their prescribed therapies while at the center. Nursing care includes direct care such as administering medication and changing dressings, assessing and evaluating the child's overall condition, identifying potential medical emergencies, determining the need for changes in care or treatment and monitoring, and providing frequent treatments or interventions to maintain life and health.

Most centers are located in the community to help ease transportation issues. Some centers provide transportation to and from home or school. Centers are licensed by the state day care licensing authorities or, in some states, prescribed pediatric extended care (PPEC) agencies. Families may be able to obtain financial assistance from their private insurance or Medicaid.

Schools

School nursing is a specialized practice of professional nursing and focuses on improving students' health, development, and safety to improve their achievement and success. School nurses work to remove or minimize health barriers to learning to provide students with the best opportunity for academic success. School nurses help bridge the gap between health care and education (National Association of School Nurses [NASN], 2023).

School nurses provide direct health care to students along with screening and referrals for health conditions. They provide leadership for health services, such as identifying health and safety concerns in the school environment and planning and training for emergencies and disasters. School nurses promote a healthy school environment by supporting healthy food services and promoting proper physical education and sports policies and practices. They promote health education through health counseling and education of students and staff. School nurses coordinate school health programs and link health service programs within the school and community. School nurses carry out a variety of roles in providing health care to children (Fig. 11.1). Box 11.1 lists some of the activities of the school nurse.

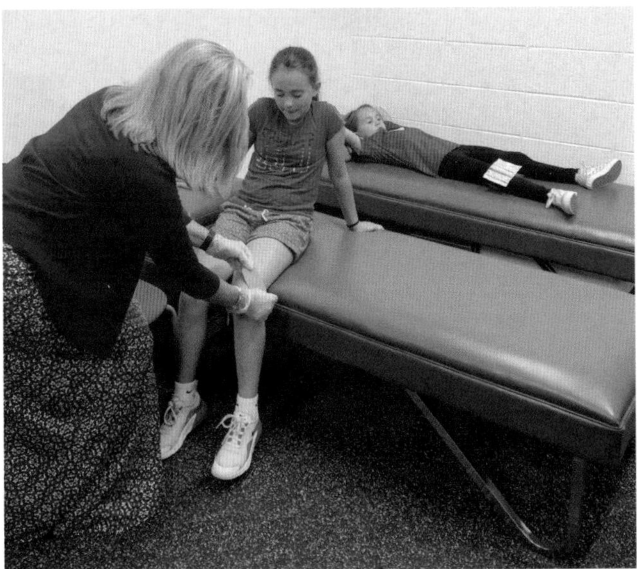

FIGURE 11.1 The school nurse provides nursing assessment as well as health education to students in the school setting.

The population of students has changed over the years. Access to public schools for children with disabilities is mandated. Due to improvements in technology, children with chronic conditions or special needs live longer and enter school. There has been an increase in the number of children with psychiatric conditions such as depression, attention-deficit/hyperactivity disorder, and more serious conditions such as bipolar disorder. All have contributed to an increase in the number of children with diverse and sometimes complex health needs in the school system. The essential role of the school nurse has not changed, but the responsibilities and expectations have. School nurses are challenged to meet the growing needs of the changing school population.

BOX **11.1 Examples of Activities of the School Nurse**

- Conduct health screenings (such as vision, hearing, and scoliosis).
- Assess growth and development.
- Provide emergency first aid, care for acute and chronic illnesses, such as medication administration and diabetes monitoring.
- Train and educate staff on cardiopulmonary resuscitation (CPR), first aid, and health issues.
- Assess, monitor, and refer students with communicable diseases.
- Educate on health promotion and disease prevention (such as immunizations; bike and car safety; decreasing high-risk behaviors, such as smoking, drinking, drug use, and sexual activity).
- Serve as a resource for health issues and education.
- Act as a liaison between health care provider and school.
- Reinforce patient and family health education (such as discharge instructions, self-care measures).
- Monitor long-term illness in students.
- Network with community agencies and make necessary referrals.

Nurses in the school setting develop **individualized health plans** (IHPs). It is the position of the National Association of School Nurses that school nurses develop an IHP to formalize the plan of support for a student with complex health care needs (NASN, 2020). It is a written agreement developed as part of an interdisciplinary collaboration of school staff along with the student, the student's family, and the student's health care provider. The plan describes the student's needs and how the school plans to meet these needs. The nurse plays a critical role in developing these plans. The nurse will use the nursing process and then, based on the nursing assessment and analysis, will develop goals and interventions to ensure that the child's needs are being met. Examples of students who may need an IHP are students with asthma, serious allergies, chronic conditions such as type 1 diabetes, physical disabilities, attention-deficit/hyperactivity disorder, and medication needs.

TAKE NOTE!

The IHP needs to include directions for care while the child is at school and must also take into account circumstances that may affect the student's health care needs, such as variations in school routine, absence of staff, special outings such as field trips and extracurricular activities, and a plan in case of emergency.

Home Health Care

Home care provides short- or long-term services for children and their families in the home. It is also used for medically needy and technology-dependent children, such as ventilator-dependent children. Among those who often benefit from home care are children with acute illness, such as a child with osteomyelitis requiring intravenous antibiotics, or chronic health care issues, such as a child with bronchopulmonary dysplasia, who may have required traditional in-hospital care.

It is important that the nurse practices family-centered home care that focuses on increasing support for the emotional and developmental needs of the child. This type of care encourages families to care for their children at home while health care professionals provide the support, empowerment, education, and expertise in caring for the child that they need. In family-centered home care, the family and health care professionals build a partnership of trust to meet the needs of the child. The nurse must value the role of the family and regard family members as the ultimate experts in caring for their child. In home care, the family is extensively involved in the child's care, and the home care nurse is there to facilitate.

Any illness, especially a chronic illness, affects the entire family and can disrupt family structure. There is a change in the role of the parent when they must care for an ill child. These role changes can result in stress for the family members and can affect their participation in the child's care. It is important for home care nurses to seek a partnership role with the family regarding care of the child. This can be difficult for both parties. Often, nurses set limits on parental involvement and do not consider the parents' perspective. Many nurses are concerned that the parents may not be able to care for the child safely. It is important for nurses to use self-awareness and reflective practice to help them understand and empower families as well as to develop a partnership for care. A communication framework, developed by Berlin and Fowkes (1983), that can assist nurses in the home care setting is the LEARN framework, which can help create cross-cultural collaboration and communication between nurses and families (Box 11.2).

Home care is geared toward the needs of the child and family. Private-duty nursing care is used when more extensive care is needed; it may be delivered hourly (several hours per day) or on a full-time, live-in basis. Periodic visiting nurse care is used when the child needs intermittent interventions such as intravenous antibiotic administration, follow-up with child and family teaching, and periodic monitoring, such as bilirubin monitoring. The goals of nursing care in the home setting include promoting, restoring, and maintaining the health of the child. Home care focuses on minimizing the effects of the illness or disability, along with providing the child or family with the means to care for the illness or disability at home. Nurses in the home care setting are direct providers of care, child and family educators, child and family advocates, and case managers.

There are some disadvantages to home care. The presence of health care professionals in the home can be an intrusion on family privacy. Also, caring for children with complex medical needs can be overwhelming for some families. Financial issues can become a large burden: families may have higher out-of-pocket costs if their insurance does not reimburse for home care. Having one parent at home full time and not earning an income can contribute to increased financial strain, not to mention social isolation of that parent. All of these factors can lead to increased stress on family members. The advantages of home care usually outweigh the disadvantages, but nurses need to be aware of these potential disadvantages and provide support and resources as necessary.

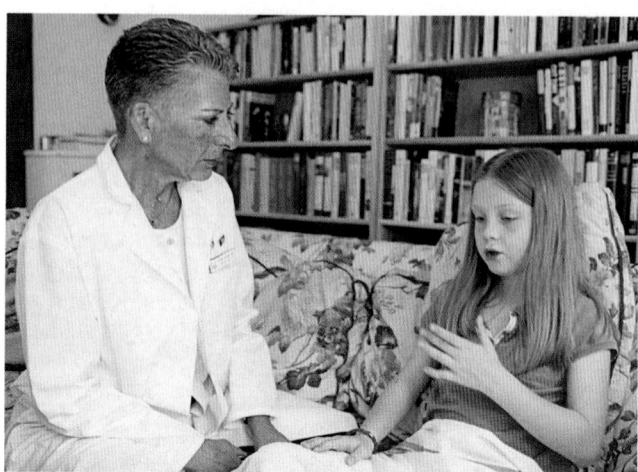

FIGURE 11.2 Listening to the child helps to develop a trusting relationship between the home care nurse and the child and her family.

The Nurse's Role in Home Care

Early discharge planning, teaching, and case management are keys to promoting a successful transition from the hospital setting to home. The environment differs greatly between the acute setting and home setting. In the acute setting, the nurse is in control of the environment; in the home setting, the nurse is a guest in the home. It is important for the nurse to establish a trusting relationship with both the child and the family (Fig. 11.2). A trusting therapeutic relationship will make all aspects of care more effective. Box 11.3 gives hints on building this relationship.

NURSING ASSESSMENT IN THE HOME SETTING

Nursing in the home care setting can be challenging. The focus is on meeting the child's physical and psychological needs while involving the family. In this role, the nurse uses the nursing process. Assessment in the home is similar to that in the acute care setting but also involves obtaining first-hand data about the family and the way

BOX 11.2 LEARN Framework

- L: Listen empathetically and with understanding to the family's perception of the situation.
- E: Explain your perception of the situation.
- A: Acknowledge and discuss the similarities as well as differences between the two perceptions.
- R: Recommend interventions.
- N: Negotiate and agree on the interventions.

Adapted from Berlin, E. A., & Fowkes, W. C., Jr. (1983). A teaching framework for cross-cultural health care—Application to practice. *The Western Journal of Medicine, 139*(6), 934–938.

BOX 11.3 Hints to Establishing a Trusting Relationship in Home Care

- Include the child in the conversation and make them feel a part of the interaction.
- Address caregivers formally unless otherwise instructed.
- Be friendly. Use a soft, calm voice.
- Be interested in the child's activities.
- Have the primary caregiver present at the initial visit.
- Listen to and show respect to the child and the family.

it functions. Assess the child's growth and development, and thoroughly assess the home environment (refer to Chapters 3 to 7 and 9 for additional information). Ensure that the home offers a safe and nurturing environment for the child. The U.S. Environmental Protection Agency (EPA) provides online training and resources for health care providers, including nurses (U.S. Environmental Protection Agency, 2022). These resources can be accessed on the EPA website under "Resources for Healthcare Providers about Children's Environmental Health."

Assess resources available to the family. This includes necessary equipment such as a hospital bed and oxygen, suitable physical and emotional surroundings (are the family members able to deal with the stress of the situation?), ability to contact emergency services, power backup if needed, and ease of evacuation of the child in case of a fire. Determine whether electricity, sanitary conditions, heat, air conditioning, and telephone access are present. If there is no phone in the home, the family needs to have plans for accessing a phone in case of emergency (perhaps a neighbor's phone). Identify areas of priority and provide appropriate referrals to resources.

During the assessment phase, the nurse identifies the person who is the primary caregiver; this may be a parent, grandparent, or older sibling. It is essential to include this person when developing the plan of care, as they are the expert on the child and family. The primary caregiver can provide insight into direct care and which strategies will be most effective with this child, taking into account the physical layout of the home, the financial ability of the family, and the way the family functions. The home care nurse must also assess the family's teaching and learning needs.

After the assessment is complete, develop appropriate nursing diagnoses, outcomes, and goals. This will include the frequency and duration of the home visits. Consider the individual needs of each patient in conjunction with state, federal, and agency policies, certification standards, and payer guidelines from private insurance and/or Medicaid regulations to assist in the development of the plan. The nurse may be the provider of direct care to the child, or the care may be indirect, in which case the nurse plans and supervises the care that is given by others, such as unlicensed personnel and parents.

NURSING MANAGEMENT IN THE HOME SETTING

Nursing care in the home requires excellent critical thinking skills. The nurse has a great deal of independence since there are no other nurses, supervisors, or health care providers on site. When complex care is provided in the home, the nurse may need to adjust procedures to fit the setting. For example, feeding schedules may be adjusted to fit a child's school schedule, or equipment may be adjusted to allow a child to receive feedings continuously while at school (Fig. 11.3).

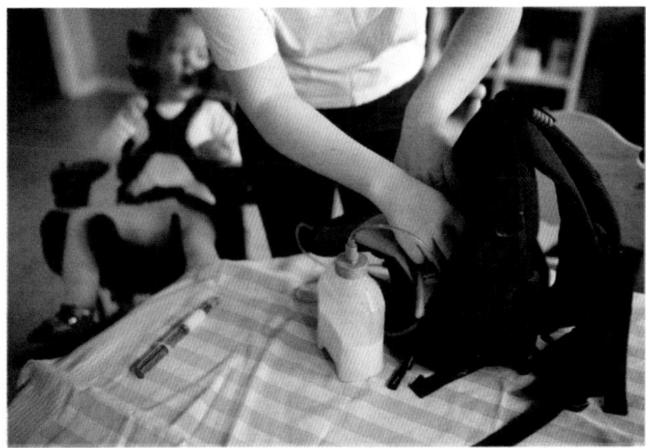

FIGURE 11.3 The home care nurse may have to adjust procedures and equipment use to fit the home setting. Placing a feeding pump in a backpack allows this child to receive feedings continuously while at school. (Shutterstock/Johner Images.)

Educating the Child and Family

An important role of the home care nurse is empowering children and their families through education (refer to Chapter 8 for further information related to teaching). Encourage the family to participate in the child's care. In many situations, parents or caregivers must learn caregiving procedures immediately so the child can be cared for at home, such as a child who needs dressing changes four times a day or a child who is ventilator dependent. A child newly diagnosed with diabetes will have some immediate teaching needs, but as the child grows and their condition changes, additional care will need to be taught.

As with any nursing care, the effectiveness of nursing interventions along with changes in the child's or family's status needs to be continuously evaluated and the plan of care altered as needed.

Other Community Settings

The primary focus of nursing in other community settings continues to be on promoting health, preventing disease and injury, and ensuring a safe environment. Nurses play important roles in child care centers, camps, health department clinics, and shelters. In child care centers, nurses help address infection control issues and assess for a safe environment. They provide education and training to staff members. A camp nurse ensures a safe environment for all campers and provides first-aid and acute illness care as needed. Camps for children with special needs exist, staffed by specially trained nurses. These camps cater to children with complex health care needs, such as diabetes, cancer, head injuries, and physical disabilities, and allow the children the opportunity to experience camp life while providing a safe environment and necessary medical care. Health department and shelter nurses focus on health supervision services and connecting patients to needed community resources.

TAKE NOTE!

Nurses have a unique opportunity to give back to their community by volunteering their services in various settings, such as shelters and clinics in medically underserved areas.

CHILDREN'S REACTIONS TO ILLNESS AND HOSPITALIZATION

In general, children are more vulnerable to the effects of illness and hospitalization because this is a change from their usual state of health and routine. They also have limited understanding and coping mechanisms to assist them in resolving the stressors that might occur during this time. Hospitalization and illness create a series of traumatic and stressful events in a climate of uncertainty for children and their families, whether it is an elective procedure that is planned in advance or an emergency situation resulting from trauma. The stressors that children experience in relation to hospitalization and illness may result in various reactions. Children react to the stresses of hospitalization before admission, during hospitalization, and after discharge.

Besides the physiologic effects of the health problem, the psychological effects of illness and hospitalization on a child include anxiety and fear related to the overall process and the potential for bodily injury, physical harm, and pain. In addition, children are separated from their homes, families, and friends and what is familiar to them, which may result in separation anxiety (distress related to removal from family and familiar surroundings). There is a general loss of control over their lives and sometimes their emotions and behaviors. The result may be feelings of anger and guilt, regression (return to a previous stage of development), acting out, and other types of defense mechanisms to cope with these effects. Children's typical coping strategies are tested during this experience.

Anxiety and Fear

For many children, entering a health care setting is like entering a foreign world. The result is anxiety and fear. Anxiety often stems from the rapid onset of the illness or injury, particularly when the child has limited experiences with disease or injury. Normal fears of childhood include the fear of separation from their parents and family or guardians, loss of control, and bodily injury, mutilation, or harm. Children's fears are similar to adult fears of the unknown, including fear of unfamiliar environments and losing control.

Therefore, when the child is in the hospital, they become distressed about the unfamiliar environment; health care procedures, especially the use of needles or associated pain that may occur; and situations such as the strange words being used, ominous-looking equipment, strangers in unusual attire (e.g., surgical caps, masks, gowns), unfamiliar and frightening noises and smells, or the sounds of other children crying. This exposure to people, situations, and procedures that may be new to them and that cause them pain leads to increased anxiety and fear (Fig. 11.4). Overall, illness and hospitalization are a difficult experience for children.

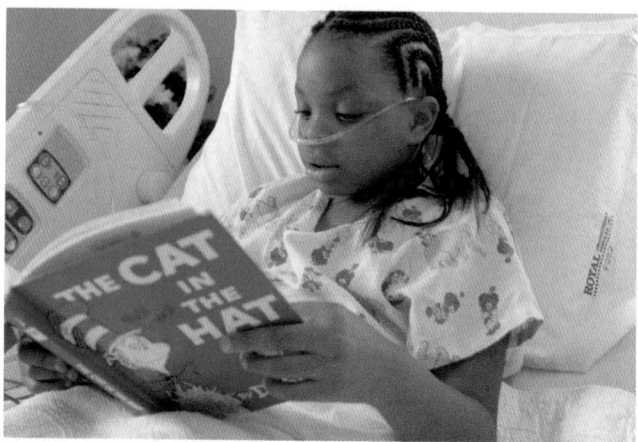

FIGURE 11.4 The presence of familiar objects and home routines normalizes the environment and helps the child cope with hospitalization. Reading a favorite bedtime story can be comforting.

Separation Anxiety

Separation anxiety is a major stressor for children of certain ages. Timing of separation anxiety varies among children. It typically begins once a child has developed object permanence (an understanding that things exist even when they are out of sight), which is usually around 4 to 8 months (Piaget, 1969).

James Robertson and John Bowlby described three stages that the infant and child goes through during separation anxiety—protest, despair, and detachment (Robertson & Bowlby, 1952). The first phase, protest, occurs when the child is separated from the parents or primary caregiver. This phase may last from a few hours to several days. The child reacts aggressively to this separation and exhibits great distress by crying, expressing agitation, and rejecting others who attempt to offer comfort. The child may also display anger and inconsolable grief.

If the parents do not return within a short time, the child exhibits the second phase, despair. The child displays hopelessness by withdrawing from others; becoming quiet without crying; and exhibiting apathy, depression, lack of interest in play and food, and overall feelings of sadness.

Detachment (also known as denial) is the third and final phase of separation anxiety. During this phase, the child forms coping mechanisms to protect against further emotional pain. This occurs more often in long-term separations. During this stage, the child shows interest in the environment, starts to play again, and forms superficial relationships with the nurses and other children. If the parents return, the child ignores them. A child in this phase of separation anxiety exhibits resignation, not contentment. It is more difficult to reverse this stage, and developmental delays may occur.

Today, health care providers primarily observe the first and second stages because of the shorter hospital stays and the more common use of a family-centered approach to care.

Loss of Control

When ill or hospitalized, children experience a significant loss of control. This loss of control increases the perception of threat and affects their coping skills. They lose control over routine self-care and their usual tasks and play as well as decisions related to the care of their own bodies. In the hospital, the child's usual routine is disrupted. They cannot choose what to do and at what time. The child can no longer accomplish simple tasks independently as they do at home or school. Confinement to the bed or crib worsens this loss of control. For example, if connected to tubes or intravenous lines, the child may not even be able to visit the bathroom alone.

Hospitalization also affects the child's control over decisions related to their own body. Many of the procedures and treatments that occur in the hospital are invasive or are at least disturbing to children, and much of the time they do not have the option to refuse to undergo them. Adults are presumed to be competent to make health care decisions, but, generally, children are not. Although the parents and nurses of hospitalized children have the children's best interest in mind, children often feel powerless when in the hospital, not having their feelings and wishes respected and having minimal control over events.

TAKE NOTE!

When advocating for a child, make sure to include the child's voice. Do not assume what their wishes may be; ask about them directly.

FACTORS AFFECTING CHILDREN'S REACTION TO ILLNESS AND HOSPITALIZATION

Various factors have a great impact on the ability of children to handle illness and hospitalization. These factors may increase or diminish the fears of the child who is ill and hospitalized. Each child responds differently and will perceive the hospital experience differently. Box 11.4 lists the various factors affecting a child's response to illness and hospitalization.

BOX 11.4 Factors Affecting a Child's Response to Illness and Hospitalization

- Amount of separation from parent/caregiver
- Age
- Developmental level
- Cognitive level
- Previous experience with illness and hospitalization
- Recent life stresses and changes
- Type and amount of preparation
- Temperament
- Innate and acquired coping skills
- Seriousness of the diagnosis/onset of illness or injury (e.g., acute or chronic)
- Support systems available, including the family and health care professionals
- Cultural background
- Parents' reaction to illness and hospitalization

Developmental Level

The child's age, cognitive level, and developmental level will affect their perceptions of actual events, and this in turn will affect their reaction to illness and hospitalization. Children's responses to the stressors of fear, separation anxiety, and loss of control vary depending on their age and developmental level. Younger children, with their limited life experience and immature intellectual capacities, have a more difficult time comprehending what is happening to them. This can be particularly true for toddlers and preschoolers, who perceive the intactness of their bodies to be exposed during physical intrusions. In addition, they frequently interpret illness as punishment for wrongdoing or hospital procedures as hostile, mutilating acts. Although children are increasingly able to adapt as they grow older, lack of understanding about the need for hospitalization and threatened sense of control can make adaptation difficult.

Infants

Newborns and infants are adapting to life outside the womb with rapid growth and development and establishment of a healthy attachment to parents or primary caregivers. They are dependent on others for nurturance and protection. They gain a sense of trust in the world through rhythmic and reciprocal patterns of contact and feeding, resulting in bonding to the primary caregiver. They need a secure pattern of restful sleep, satisfaction of oral and nutritional needs, relaxation of body systems, and spontaneous response to communication and gentle stimuli. The caregiver–infant attachment is critical for psychological health, especially during periods of illness and hospitalization.

Unfortunately, during illness and hospitalization, these critical patterns of feeding, contact, comfort, sleeping, elimination, and stimulation are disrupted, resulting in fear, separation anxiety, and loss of control. By 5 to 6 months of age, infants have developed an awareness of self as separate from the birthing parent. As a result, infants of this age are acutely aware of the absence of their primary caregiver and become fearful of unfamiliar people. Infants may be separated from their parents when hospitalized if the parents cannot room-in because of hospital policy or if they must work or care for other children. This results in separation anxiety.

The infant's oral needs, the basic source of infant satisfaction, are often not met in the hospital due to the condition of the child or the procedures that must be performed. The infant is accustomed to having their basic needs met by the parent when they cry or gesture. The constraints of hospitalization result in loss of control over the environment, leading to additional anxiety in the infant.

Toddlers

Toddlers are more aware of self and can communicate their desires. Because their autonomy is developing, toddlers need to master accomplishments to minimize the development of shame and doubt. Control becomes an issue for toddlers. Toddlers also need opportunities to explore, and they need consistent routines. In addition, toddlers are aware of the need for care and protection from others, so they need familiarity and closeness to the primary caregiver. When the toddler is ill or hospitalized, disruption occurs in this development of autonomy.

Toddlers are often fearful of strangers and can recall traumatic events. Simply walking toward the room where a traumatic procedure previously occurred may upset the toddler. Ordinarily, a resurgence in separation anxiety occurs during the toddler years. When the toddler is separated from their parents or caregivers in an unfamiliar environment, separation anxiety is compounded. In response to this anxiety, toddlers may demonstrate behaviors such as pleading for the parents to stay, physically trying to go after the parents, throwing temper tantrums, and refusing to comply with usual routines. Restrictions related to mobility and new skill acquisition result in loss of control. Disruption in usual routines also contributes to loss of control, and the toddler feels insecure. As a result, regression in toilet training and refusal to eat are common reactions in toddlers.

Preschoolers

The preschooler has better verbal and developmental skills to adapt to various situations, but illness and hospitalization can still be stressful. Preschoolers may understand that they are in the hospital because they are sick, but they may not understand the cause of their illness. Preschoolers fear mutilation and are afraid of intrusive procedures since they do not understand the body's integrity. They interpret words literally and have an active imagination. Therefore, when the nurse says, "I need to take some blood," preschoolers' fantasies may run wild. They may not understand the concept of blood and may think everything will come out of their body. They may think that blood is "taken" the same way a child picks up a toy to take it out of the room. Preschoolers' thinking is egocentric; they believe that some personal deed or thought caused their illness, which can lead to guilt and shame. These feelings may be internalized. Overall, preschoolers' concrete, egocentric, and magical thinking (type of thinking that allows for fantasies and creativity) limits their ability to understand, so communication and interventions must be on their level.

Separation anxiety may not be as much of an issue as it is for toddlers since preschoolers may already be spending time away from parents in preschool. They are, however, still acutely aware of the comfort and security that their family provides for them, so disruptions in these relationships lead to challenges. The preschooler may constantly ask for their parents or ask to call the parents. They may quietly cry, refuse to eat or take medication, or generally be uncooperative.

In addition, the ill or hospitalized preschooler loses control over the environment. The preschooler is naturally curious about their surroundings and learns best by observing and working with objects. This might be limited during illness or hospitalization. Because the preschooler cannot participate in typical activities and explore the environment as usual, the child's normal creative, curious nature may give rise to a variety of fantasies that may present challenges.

School-Age

School-age children, generally, are hospitalized because of long-term illnesses or trauma. The general task of their development stage, to develop confidence through a sense of industry, can be disrupted during illness or hospitalization. Even at this time, they generally want to continue to learn and maintain their skills and abilities. The stress of illness or anxiety related to diagnostic tests and therapeutic interventions may lead to inward or outward expressions of distress. If they have learned various coping skills, this distress may be minimized. After 11 years of age, there is an increased awareness of physiologic, psychological, and behavioral causes of illness and injury. Typically, the school-age child has a more realistic understanding of the reasons for the illness and can better comprehend explanations. School-age children are concerned about disability and death, and they fear injury and pain. They want to know why procedures and tests are being performed. They can understand cause and effect and how it relates to their illness. They are uncomfortable with any type of genital examination.

Separation anxiety is not as much of an issue for school-age children. They are accustomed to periods of separation and may already be experiencing some separation anxiety related to being in school. At the same time, they may be missing school and friends as they try to adjust to the unfamiliar environment. They may feel that friends will forget them if they remain ill or in the hospital for a long time. Some school-age children may regress and become needy, demanding their parents' attention or playing with special "comfort toys" they used at a younger age.

Since school-age children are accustomed to controlling self-care and are typically highly social, they like being involved. They are used to making choices about meals and activities. Illness or hospitalization presents loss of control by limiting their activities, making them feel helpless and dependent. This may result in feelings of loneliness, boredom, isolation, and depression. The key is to give them opportunities to maintain independence, retain a sense of control, enhance self-esteem, and continue to work toward achieving a sense of industry.

Adolescents

Adolescents fear injury and pain. Since appearance is important to them, they are concerned with how the illness or injury will affect their body image. Anything that changes their perceptions of themselves has a major impact on their response. Typically, adolescents do not like to be different; they like "being cool," which means being in control and not showing how afraid they really are. They may also feel ambivalent about wanting their parents. Adolescents typically do not experience separation anxiety from being away from their parents; instead, their anxiety comes from being separated from friends.

Loss of control is a key factor affecting the behavior of adolescents who are ill or hospitalized. Anger, withdrawal, or general lack of cooperation may occur due to the feelings of loss of control. In addition, their desire to appear confident may lead them to question everything that is being done or that they are asked to do. Their feelings of invincibility may cause them to take risks and be noncompliant with treatment. Overall, adolescents strive for independence, self-assertion, and liberation while developing their identity.

Previous Experiences

In general, children's lack of understanding and experience of illness, hospitalization, and hospital procedures contributes to their anxiety level. However, previous experience with hospitalization and other health-related experiences can either facilitate preparation or impair it if the experiences were perceived as negative. For example, the child who associates the hospital with the birth of a sibling may view this experience as positive. However, the child who associates the hospital with the serious illness or death of a relative or close friend will probably view the experience as negative.

The type of experience may contribute to increased anxiety and fear if the child must be admitted to the hospital. If children have had previous experiences, how the experience unfolded and their response to it will determine many of their reactions to illness or hospitalization. Older children may cling to their parents, kick, or create a scene because of their previous experience.

Recent Stresses and Changes and Individual Coping Skills

The effects of illness hospitalization on children are influenced by the nature and severity of the health problem, the condition of the child, and the degree to which activities and routines differ from those of everyday life. A lack of sensory stimulation in the hospital environment can lead to listlessness, indifference, unhappiness, and even appetite changes. When the child's motor activity is restricted, anger and hyperactivity may result. Play, recreation, and educational opportunities can provide an outlet to distract the child from the illness, provide pleasant experiences, and help the child understand their condition.

The child's ability to work through a situation will also affect their responses to illness and hospitalization. This ability depends on the age of the child, their perceptions of the event, previous encounters with health care personnel, and support from significant others. Box 11.5 lists various coping skills used by children and suggestions for promoting positive coping.

Parents' Response to Child's Illness and Hospitalization

Parents who do not tell children the truth or who do not answer their questions confuse and frighten them and may weaken the child's trust in the parents. Children take in their parents' anxiety and concern. Even whispers can set off children's imaginations. For example, preschoolers may invent elaborate stories to explain what is

BOX 11.5 Children and Coping

Behavior/Methods for Coping	Suggestions to Promote Coping
Ignore or negate the problem.	Breathing techniques such as blowing bubbles, pinwheels, or party noise makers
Stoicism, passive acceptance	Distraction with books or games
Acting out—yelling, kicking, screaming, crying	Imagery with tapes or scenarios
Anger, withdrawal, rejection	Music
Intellectualizing	Teaching before events or procedures

happening to them. It is important for children to believe that someone is in control and that the person can be trusted. Some parents, however, have their own fears and insecurities. Thus, a child's reaction is often related to the parents' reaction to the illness and hospitalization.

The relationship between the family and the health care staff may either add to or ease the child's stress. This relationship can contribute significantly to the quality of the environment. Health care personnel must assume responsibility for the care of ill or hospitalized children by maintaining good partnerships with families.

FAMILY'S REACTIONS TO THE CHILD'S ILLNESS AND HOSPITALIZATION

Whether planned or unplanned, hospitalization increases the family's stress and anxiety level. The illness or serious injury of one family member affects all members of the family because the process disrupts the family's usual routines and may alter family roles. Parents and siblings have their own reactions to this experience.

Reactions of Parents

Watching a child in pain is difficult, especially when the parent is assisting with the procedure by holding the child. The parent may feel guilty for not seeking care sooner. Parents may also exhibit other feelings such as denial, anger, depression, and confusion. Parents may deny that the child is ill. They may express anger, especially directed at the nursing staff, another family member, or a higher power, because of their loss of control in caring for the child. Depression may occur because of exhaustion and the psychological and physical requirements of spending long hours in a hospital caring for a child. Confusion may develop because of dealing with an unfamiliar environment or the loss of a parental role. Finally, the parents' relationship may be strained because of dual roles, long separation, and increased stress.

Reactions of Siblings

Siblings of children who are hospitalized may experience jealousy, insecurity, resentment, confusion, and anxiety. They may have difficulty understanding why their sibling is ill or getting all the attention, leaving little for them. They may wonder if their sibling is going to die or ever return home. They may worry that their sibling's illness is going to happen to them. Certain age groups, such as preschoolers, may feel that they caused the illness. Little information or understanding about what is happening, combined with their magical and egocentric thinking, contributes to their fears that they may have caused the illness or injury by their thoughts, wishes, or behaviors. If the family roles or routines change significantly, the siblings may feel insecure or anxious. They may develop changes in behavior or in school performance. See Evidence-Based Practice 11.1.

EVIDENCE-BASED PRACTICE **11.1**

What Personal Challenges Do Caregivers Face During Pediatric Hospitalization?

The stressors of an ill child in the hospital can affect all family members. Strong parent–provider partnerships can improve patient- and family-centered care and patient outcomes. Limited data are available describing challenges caregivers face in general pediatric hospitalization regardless of illness or diagnosis. Unaddressed caregiver needs may influence understanding and perceptions of the plan of care, caregiver decision-making skills, and caregiver engagement in care. Addressing caregiver needs optimizes family-centered care.

STUDY

A small qualitative study was performed. Caregivers at a children's hospital were interviewed to learn about their hospital experience and the personal challenges they faced and to obtain feedback on possible interventions to minimize their challenges.

Findings

The study found caregiver difficulties with their child's hospitalization were connected to physiologic challenges, including lack of sleep and inability to eat and tend to personal care; psychosocial challenges, including isolation, stress, and juggling multiple roles; and communication challenges between the family and medical team.

Nursing Considerations

Recognize that caregivers of a hospitalized child often experience personal challenges. Nurses are in the unique position to help caregivers overcome these challenges. Helping address caregivers' physiologic, psychosocial, and communication needs may be critical to improving the experience of hospitalization. Meeting caregiver's basic needs is crucial to assisting them to function as an advocate for their child. This study also sought out interventions that caregivers felt the hospital could implement to help address these challenges. Examples of interventions nurses could implement include clustering care and posting signs alerting staff to when the child or caregiver is sleeping. The nurse can offer personal hygiene items and improve access to food by educating the caregiver on food options available to them. Nurses can help uncover and address transportation issues and improve communication by using white boards in patient rooms to share key information, help caregivers sign up for the patient portal, thoroughly review all discharge paperwork with the caregiver, and answer all questions the caregiver or patient may have. Further research is warranted and needs to be focused on developing evidence-based interventions that address the challenges faced by caregivers of hospitalized children.

Based on Vaz, L. E., Jungbauer, R. M., Jenisch, C., Austin, J. P., Wagner, D. V., Everist, S. J., Libak, A. J., Harris, M. A., & Zuckerman; K. E. (2022). Caregiver experiences in pediatric hospitalizations: Challenges and opportunities for improvement. *Hospital Pediatrics, 12*(12), 1073–1080. https://doi.org/10.1542/hpeds.2022-006645

Factors Influencing Family Reactions

The parenting style and the family–child relationship can influence the hospital experience as well as the family members' coping skills. Cultural, ethnic, and religious variations, values, and practices related to illness; general response to stress; and attitudes about the care of a sick child have a significant influence on the family's response. For example, religious beliefs can increase problems or can be a source of strength to the family and child. Families already in crisis or without support systems have a more difficult time dealing with the added stress of hospitalization. Chapter 2 gives further explanations of some of these influences on children and their families.

Remember Jake, the 8-year-old with a suspected brain tumor introduced at the beginning of the chapter? What reactions to illness and hospitalization might you see from him and his family?

Clinical Judgment and the Nursing Process

In most instances, the nurse is the primary person involved in the care of a hospitalized or ill child. The nurse is probably the first one to see the child and family and will spend more time with them than other health care personnel. Nurses are part of a medical community that makes decisions in the child's best interest, but the nurse needs to bear in mind the child's rights and must try to minimize the child's distress so that the hospital stay will be as pleasant an experience as possible. When establishing strategies to care for children, nurses should examine the general effects of hospitalization and illness on children in each developmental stage and should strive to understand both the reactions of the child and family to illness and hospitalization and the factors affecting these reactions.

Nursing Analysis

After recognizing and analyzing cues from a thorough assessment, the nurse may identify several hypotheses, including:

- Anxiety
- Risk for powerlessness
- Decreased diversional activity engagement
- Interrupted family processes
- Bathing/dressing/feeding self-care deficit
- Risk for delayed development
- Deficient knowledge
- Risk for caregiver role strain

These hypotheses provide suggestions for nursing care planning or concept mapping. The nurse will then generate solutions by planning interventions (suggested along with rationales further on). The plan of care should be individualized, based on the child's and family's needs.

Nursing Analysis

Anxiety related to stressors (from hospital situation or illness, fear of injury or bodily mutilation, separation from family or friends, changes in routine, painful procedures and treatments, and unfamiliar events and surroundings) as evidenced by crying, fussing, withdrawal, or resistance

Goal/Outcome

Child and family will exhibit a decrease in anxiety level as evidenced by positive coping strategies, verbalization or playing out of feelings, appropriate behaviors, positive interactions with staff, child and parent cooperation and participation, and absence of signs and symptoms of increasing anxiety and fear.

Minimizing Anxiety (interventions with *rationale*)

- Orient child and family to the unit and the child's room *to familiarize them with the facility.*
- Assess for signs and symptoms of anxiety and fear *to establish a baseline and assess effectiveness of interventions.*
- Place the child in a room with another child of a similar age, developmental level, and condition severity *to promote sharing.*
- Provide atraumatic care *to minimize exposure to distress, which would increase anxiety.*
- Explain all events, treatments, procedures, and activities to the parents and child (at a level the child can understand) in a calm, relaxed manner *to help the child prepare for what is to come and decrease fear of the unknown. A calm, relaxed manner helps to establish rapport and instill trust.*
- Enlist the aid of a CLS *to assist in age-appropriate preparation for all events, treatments, and procedures.*
- Encourage parents to room-in if possible *to provide the child with support;* if parents cannot stay, encourage them to call *to reduce the child's fear of being alone.*
- Urge parents to inform the child when they will be leaving and when they are expected to return *to help the child cope with their absence and promote trust.*
- Assess child's usual routine at home and attempt to incorporate aspects of usual routine into hospital routine *to ease the transition to the hospital and promote the child's participation in routine.*
- Offer comfort measures such as holding, stroking, and rocking *to relieve distress.*
- Encourage the child to play (unstructured and therapeutic play as necessary) *to allow for expression of feelings and fears and promote energy expenditure.*

- Suggest that parents bring in a special toy or object from home *to promote feelings of security.*
- Provide positive reinforcement for participation in care activities *to foster self-esteem.*
- Assess for regression behaviors and inform parents that such behaviors are common *to alleviate their concerns about this behavior.*
- Provide consistency with care measures *to facilitate trust and acceptance.*

Nursing Analysis

Risk for powerlessness; risk factors include insufficient knowledge to manage a situation, ineffective coping strategies, pain, anxiety (lack of control over procedures, treatments, and care, changes in usual routine, continual hospital readmissions)

Goal/Outcome

Child and family will demonstrate an increase in control over the situation as evidenced by participation in care activities, identification of needs and choices, and incorporation of appropriate aspects of child's usual routine with that of the hospital routine.

Promoting Control (interventions with *rationale*)

- Encourage child and parents to identify areas of concern *to help determine priority needs.*
- Encourage parent and child to participate in care activities *to promote feelings of control.*
- Incorporate aspects of child's routine at home and use terms similar to those used at home *to foster a sense of normalcy.*
- Offer child choices as much as possible, such as options for foods, drinks, hygiene, activities, or clothing (if appropriate) *to promote feelings of individuality and control.*
- Allow child opportunities for being out of bed or room within limitations as appropriate *to foster independence.*
- Work with child, as age and development allow, and family to set up a schedule *to promote structure and routine.*

Nursing Analysis

Decreased diversional activity engagement related to the current setting/situation not allowing engagement in activity (confinement in bed or health care facility, lack of appropriate stimulation from toys or peers), impaired mobility (activity restrictions or equipment such as IV pump), insufficient energy, insufficient motivation, or physical discomfort as evidenced by verbalization of boredom or lack of participation in play, reading, or school work.

Goal/Outcome

Child will participate in diversional activities as evidenced by engagement in unstructured and therapeutic play that is developmentally appropriate and by interaction with family, staff, and other children.

Promoting Adequate Diversional Activities (interventions with *rationale*)

- Question child and family about favorite types of activities *to establish a baseline for developing appropriate choices during hospitalization.*
- Assist with planning activities within the limits of the child's condition *to maintain muscle tone and strength without overexerting the child.*
- Spend time with the child *to provide stimulation and foster trust.*
- Enlist the aid of a CLS *to provide suggestions for appropriate activities.*
- Encourage interaction with other children *to promote sharing and avoid loneliness.*
- Provide developmentally appropriate opportunities for unstructured and therapeutic play *to facilitate expression of feelings.*
- Encourage short trips to the playroom or activity room *to provide a change of scenery and sensory stimulation.*
- Integrate play activities with nursing care *to achieve therapeutic effect.*

Nursing Analysis

Interrupted family processes related to power shift among family members and shift in family roles (separation from child due to hospitalization, increased demands of caring for an ill child, changes in role function and routine, and effect of hospitalization on other family members such as siblings), as evidenced by parental verbalization of issues, parental presence in hospital, or child's hospitalization requiring parent to miss work.

Goal/Outcome

Family will demonstrate positive coping strategies and mutual support for one another as evidenced by visiting frequently and staying with the child as necessary, sharing of family responsibilities, obtaining assistance for relief or respite, and visiting by other members of the child's family and friends.

Maximizing Family Functioning (interventions with *rationale*)

- Encourage parents and family members to verbalize concerns about child's illness, diagnosis, and prognosis *to promote family-centered care and identify areas where intervention may be needed.*
- Explain therapies, procedures, child's behaviors, and plan of care to parents *to promote understanding of the child's status and plan of care, which helps to decrease anxiety.*
- Encourage parental involvement in care *to promote feelings of the parents being needed and valued,*

providing them with a sense of control over their child's health.
- Identify support system for family and child *to identify resources available for coping.*
- Educate family and child on additional resources available *to promote a wider base of support to deal with the situation.*
- Suggest ways that parents can divide time between child and other siblings *to prevent feelings of guilt.*
- Provide support and positive reinforcement *to promote family coping and foster family strength.*
- Encourage frequent visits by family members, including siblings as appropriate, *to promote ongoing family functioning.*
- Stress the need for adequate rest, sleep, exercise, and nutrition for family members *to promote family health and minimize stress of hospitalization on family.*
- Assist with referrals for resources and help from additional family members and friends as necessary *to allow for respite or relief of care responsibilities.*
- Encourage family to maintain usual routine as much as possible *to minimize the effects of hospitalization on family functioning.*
- Enlist the aid of a CLS to work with any siblings *to provide support and education and to address the needs of a sibling of a hospitalized child.*

Nursing Analysis

Bathing/dressing/feeding self-care deficit related to anxiety, decrease in motivation (regression), discomfort, environmental barrier (such as activity restrictions, immobility or use of equipment, devices, or prescribed treatments), fatigue, pain, or weakness as evidenced by inability to feed, bathe, or dress self or accomplish other activities of daily living.

Goal/Outcome

Child will participate in self-care within limitations of condition as evidenced by assisting with bathing and hygiene, feeding, toileting, and dressing and grooming.

Promoting Self-Care (interventions with *rationale*)

- Assess child's usual routine for self-care and self-care abilities *to provide a baseline for individualizing interventions.*
- Provide child-sized equipment and devices *to promote child's ability to complete the self-care task.*
- Encourage parents and child to do as much self-care as possible, within limitations of the child's condition and developmental level, *to promote feelings of independence and foster growth and development.*
- Offer praise and encouragement for activities performed *to foster self-esteem, confidence, and competence.*
- Ensure adequate rest periods *to minimize energy expenditure associated with self-care activities.*

Nursing Analysis

Risk for delayed development; risk factors include chronic illness and treatment regimen (resultant stressors associated with hospitalization, current condition or illness, separation from family, and sensory overload or sensory deprivation).

Goal/Outcome

Child will demonstrate developmentally appropriate milestones as evidenced by age-appropriate behaviors and activities.

Promoting Growth and Development (interventions with *rationale*)

- Assess child's developmental stage *to establish a baseline and determine appropriate strategies.*
- Use unstructured and therapeutic play and adaptive toys *to promote developmental functioning.*
- Provide stimulating environment when possible *to maximize potential for growth and development.*
- Praise accomplishments and emphasize child's abilities *to foster self-esteem and encourage feelings of confidence and competence.*
- Include parents in techniques to foster growth and development *to promote feelings of control in their child's care.*

Nursing Analysis

Deficient knowledge related to insufficient knowledge (regarding hospitalization, surgery, treatments, procedures, required care, and follow-up) as evidenced by questioning and verbalization, lack of prior exposure.

Goal/Outcome

Child and family will demonstrate understanding of all aspects of child's current situation as evidenced by identification of child's and family's needs, verbal statements of understanding and/or need for additional information, return demonstration of procedures and treatments, and verbalization of instructions for follow-up and continued care.

Providing Child and Family Teaching (interventions with *rationale*)

- Assess child's and family's willingness to learn *to ensure effective teaching.*
- Provide family with time to adjust to diagnosis *to facilitate their ability to learn and participate in the child's care.*
- Repeat information *to promote multiple opportunities for child and family to learn.*
- Teach in short sessions *to prevent overloading the child and parents with information.*

- Gear teaching to appropriate level of understanding for the child and the family (depends on age of child, physical condition, memory) *to promote learning.*
- Provide reinforcement and rewards *to facilitate the teaching/learning process.*
- Use multiple modes of learning, such as written information, verbal instruction, demonstrations, and media, when possible *to facilitate learning and retention of information.*
- Provide the child and family with written step-by-step instructions for procedures or care *to provide a reference, if needed, at a later date.*
- Have child and family provide return demonstrations of care procedures *to ensure effectiveness of teaching.*
- Arrange for trial home care during hospitalization and after discharge as appropriate *to ensure understanding and provide opportunities for additional teaching and learning.*

Nursing Analysis

Risk for caregiver role strain; risk factors include child's increased care needs, unstable health condition, competing role commitments, inexperience with caregiving, stressors, change in nature or complexity of care activities.

Goal/Outcome

Caregiver will exhibit emotional health: *verbalizes concerns calmly, participates in child's care, and demonstrates knowledge of resources.*

Easing Caregiver Role Strain (interventions with *rationale*)

- Assess parental behavior *to identify role strain.*
- Provide emotional support and encourage talking about feelings, fears, and concerns *to promote trust in nurse as a source of emotional support.*
- Arrange for and/or encourage respite care for child: *provides parent with time away from continual care.*
- Consult social services *to identify community resources available for caregiver support (home health, support group, etc.).*
- Encourage parent to meet own needs and find personal time *to increase energy level and self-esteem, ultimately enhancing the quality of care given.*

PREPARING THE CHILD AND FAMILY FOR SURGERY

If the child is to undergo a surgical procedure, whether in the hospital or an outpatient setting, special interventions are necessary. Preparation provides reassurance and comfort to the child and allows them to know what will happen and what is expected of them. The parents should be allowed to stay with the child until surgery begins. Parents should also be allowed to be with the child when they wake up in the postanesthesia recovery area.

Preoperative care for the child who is to undergo surgery is similar to that for an adult. The major difference is that the preparation and teaching must be geared to the child's age and developmental level. Many facilities offer special programs to help prepare children and families for the surgical experience. Preoperative preparation programs allow children and their families to experience a "trial run" in a supportive environment to help reduce anxiety, increase knowledge, increase comfort level, and enhance coping skills (Romito et al., 2021). The American Society of Anesthesiologists has prepared a coloring and activity book entitled *My Surgery Journey* (American Society of Anesthesiologists, n.d.). This book is designed to alleviate some of the fears that younger children may have related to the hospital experience. It describes the process from admission (whether it be to the hospital or the ambulatory surgery center) through discharge.

Many facilities have coloring or activity books specific to the facility and procedures that allow children to prepare and learn about their surgical and hospital experience through interactive activities like word searches, mazes, and matching games. These activities help the child and family prepare for what to expect and can provide a place to express thoughts, feelings, and questions through interactive and fun activities.

Providing Preoperative Teaching

Teaching the child and family is essential. Table 11.1 discusses strategies for preoperative teaching. Like any intervention, adapt the teaching to the child's developmental level. For example, when teaching a toddler or preschooler about breathing exercises, have the child blow a pinwheel or cotton balls across the table through a straw. The child will enjoy the activity while also reaping the respiratory benefits of the activity.

In preparation for surgery, use items such as stuffed animals or dolls to help children understand what is going to happen to them (Fig. 11.5). Allow

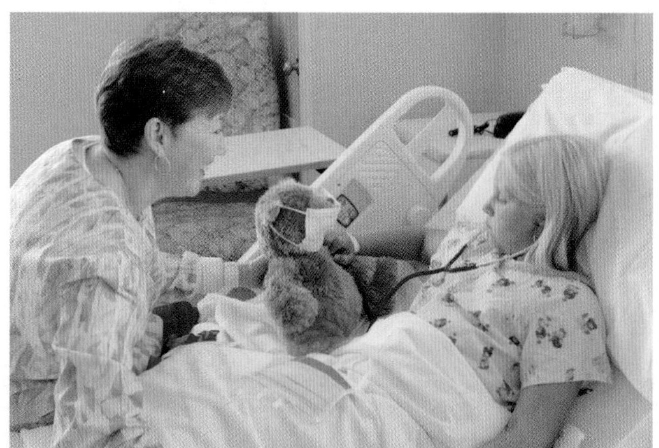

FIGURE 11.5 Using a stuffed animal to explain a surgical procedure to the child.

TABLE 11.1 • Strategies for Preoperative Teaching

Developmental Level	Implications for Teaching
Infants and toddlers	Encourage parents to use a soft tone of voice and stroking and secure, comfortable holding positions to promote calm. Remind parents to use positive facial expressions. Encourage the parent or caregiver to stay with the child as much as possible. Use terms that the child and parents can understand. For toddlers, provide information as close to the day of surgery as possible to prevent undue anxiety.
Preschoolers and school-age children	Provide factual explanations using terms the child and parents can understand. Incorporate pictures and other visual aids in explanation. Tailor the timing of education to meet the child's learning needs, allowing enough time for the child to ask questions. For preschoolers, provide information 1–2 days before surgery. For school-age children, provide information 3–5 days before surgery.
Adolescents	Provide detailed explanations of the procedure at least 7–10 days beforehand. Answer questions honestly, ensuring privacy at all times. Remain available for questions or concerns arising before or after surgery.

the child to role-play various experiences with dolls. Dolls designed to simulate surgical experiences have been developed. For example, Shadow Buddies are custom-made dolls that have the same illness or surgery as the child; the doll may have an ostomy, a scar, or a catheter (Shadow Buddies Foundation, n.d.). The dolls were developed to help children cope with their illness or disease and send the message that it is okay to be different. These dolls also provide the child with a companion to talk to.

SAFETY DURING HOSPITALIZATION OR PROCEDURES

Safety is a critical aspect of care of the child. Due to their age and developmental level, children are vulnerable to harm.

Maintaining the Child's Safety

Ensure the child has an identification band in place at all times. Sometimes, in implementing interventions, an armband is removed, so make sure it is attached to another extremity. Monitor children closely to avoid accidents such as a child pushing the wrong knob, picking up a piece of equipment or supplies left in the bed or room, or climbing out of bed (Fig. 11.6). Table 11.2 highlights nursing goals for ensuring safe, developmentally appropriate care for the hospitalized child.

Use of Restraints

When caring for children, some type of restriction may be necessary. The restriction, often referred to as a restraint, may be needed to ensure the child's safety, allow a therapeutic or diagnostic procedure to be done, immobilize a body part or limit movement, or prevent disruption of prescribed therapy. However, restraints can be overused and are not without risks to the child's safety and should be used as a last resort (Centers for Medicare & Medicaid Services [CMS], 2020). As a result, each facility will have specific procedures and policies in place related to the use of restraints based on standards developed by The Joint Commission, regulations developed by the CMS, state law, and facility requirements. These procedures and policies are designed to safeguard children's physical safety and psychological well-being.

TAKE NOTE!

Always refer to your institution's policy regarding restraint use.

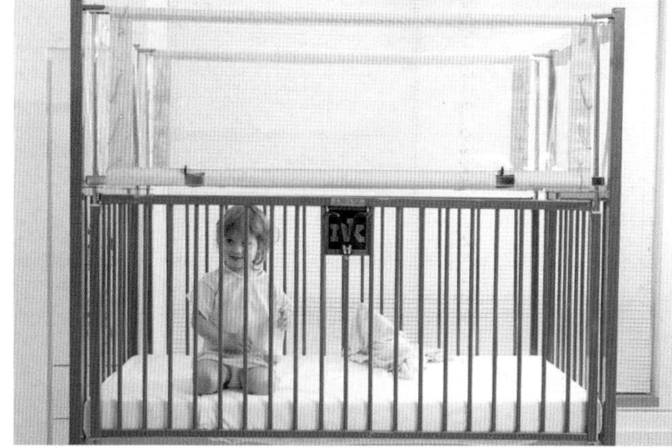

FIGURE 11.6 Safety is an essential aspect of pediatric nursing. A clear plastic cover over the crib prevents the older infant or toddler from climbing out and falling.

TABLE 11.2 • Nursing Considerations for Providing Safe, Developmentally Appropriate Care

	Ensuring Safety	Promoting Healthy Growth and Development
Infants	• Maintain close supervision of the infant. • Keep one hand on the infant when crib sides are down. • Keep crib rails up all the way when the infant is in the crib. • Avoid leaving small objects that are harmful or that can be swallowed in the crib. • Provide safe and appropriate toys for the infant. • Place infants in rooms close to the nurses' station. • Encourage a family member to stay with the infant at all times.	• Use the en face position when holding newborns. • Smile and talk to the infant during bathing, feeding, and other interactions. • Minimize the number of painful or uncomfortable procedures. • Provide comfort during and after procedures by holding or talking, using soothing tones and movements. • When handling the infant, use smooth, continuous movements. • Use gentle stroking and holding, which may reduce stress. • Serve as a role model for first-time parents. • Encourage the family to maintain home routines while in the hospital, planning nursing care around the usual feeding and sleep times. • Use the pacifier between feedings to satisfy nonnutritive sucking needs.
Toddlers	• Keep crib side rails up with overhead crib protection intact when the toddler is in the crib. • Never leave a toddler alone in the room unless secured in the crib. • Use a bed only for the older toddler who has an adult present in the room at all times. • Avoid leaving small objects that can be swallowed or are harmful in the crib or bed. • Place crib out of reach of cords, equipment, and electrical outlets. • Provide safe and appropriate toys for the toddler. • Place toddlers in rooms close to the nurses' station. • Always have someone with the toddler when ambulating.	• Encourage the parent to stay with the toddler to decrease separation anxiety. • To promote autonomy, allow the toddler to make appropriate choices, such as which juice to take the medicine with. • Encourage active play in the playroom or with push/pull toys in the hallway (accompanied by an adult). • Expect and plan for regression in areas of toilet training, eating, and other behaviors. • Expect increased temper tantrums, in general, and intense reactions to intrusive procedures. • Maintain home routine while in the hospital, planning nursing care around the usual feeding and sleep times. • Give simple directions with choices appropriate to the hospital situation. • Provide close supervision while encouraging independence.
Preschoolers	• Keep bed in low position with the side rails up when the preschooler is in the bed. • Instruct the child to call the nurse or caregiver for help getting out of bed. • Keep harmful objects out of reach of the child.	• Encourage parents to stay with the preschooler in the room as well as other areas of the hospital. • Encourage the preschooler to be involved in care by providing choices and opportunities for the child to help. • Use play as an opportunity to work through the preschooler's fears. • Explain activities in simple, concrete terms, being cautious with the words you use because of the preschooler's fantasies and magical thinking. • Expect reactions to pain and bodily injury to be verbally aggressive and specific. • Try to maintain home routines while the child is in the hospital, working them into the plan of care when possible.
School-Age Children	• Keep the bed in the low position with the side rails up while the child is in the bed, explaining that this is a hospital rule, not a punishment.	• Provide opportunities for the child to be involved in care. • Allow children to select their meals, assist with treatments, and keep their rooms neat. • Allow visits with other children if the condition allows. • Encourage parents to tell the child when they will return. • Plan care around the child's usual home routines (meals, sleep). • Encourage the child to do school work.
Adolescents	• Be aware of the adolescent's whereabouts. The adolescent may not wish to stay in the room but may become confused about where the room or unit is located in the hospital.	• Allow adolescents to interact with others. • Alter hospital routines as possible to allow the adolescent to sleep in or stay up later at night. • Provide others close to their age as roommates. • Encourage visits from friends. • Provide emotional support for feelings of being alone or away from friends; be alert for regression, which may result in the adolescent becoming emotional. • Answer questions honestly and with appropriate information. • Give the adolescent a sense of control by allowing choices. • Be sensitive to concerns about being "different."

Restraints can promote physical distress in a child and be stressful for the parents as well. Children may also view restraints as punishment. Before a restraint is used, other measures need to be considered and alternative attempts or rationales for not using alternatives need to be documented (CMS, 2020).

Restraining Children to Maintain Safety

When deciding whether it is necessary to restrain a child, consider the child's age, developmental level, mental status, and threat to others and self. If it is determined that a restraint is needed, select the most appropriate, least restrictive type of restraint (CMS, 2020). For example, if the child has an intravenous catheter in the antecubital space that stops flowing when the child bends the arm, an elbow restraint or arm board, rather than a soft wrist restraint or four-point extremity restraint, would be appropriate. Table 11.3 lists the types of restraints and the major issues associated with the use of restraints in children.

Explain why the child should not touch the intravenous site or should maintain a certain position so that they have a basic understanding of what is necessary. This may be all that is necessary for an older child. One-to-one supervision and behavior modification techniques may be other alternatives to the use of restraints.

ATRAUMATIC CARE

Therapeutic hugging should be used for procedures and treatments such as intravenous line insertion for which the child needs to remain still. Refer to Chapter 8 for further information.

TAKE NOTE!

When selecting a restraint, the nurse must choose the least restrictive type and apply it for the shortest time necessary (CMS, 2020).

TABLE 11.3 • Types of Restraints and Associated Safety Concerns

Type of Restraint	Purpose	Safety Concerns
Soft limb restraint	Wrist or ankle restraint to prevent range of motion of extremities	Check wrist or ankle for any sign of circulatory, integumentary, or neurologic compromise.
Elbow restraint 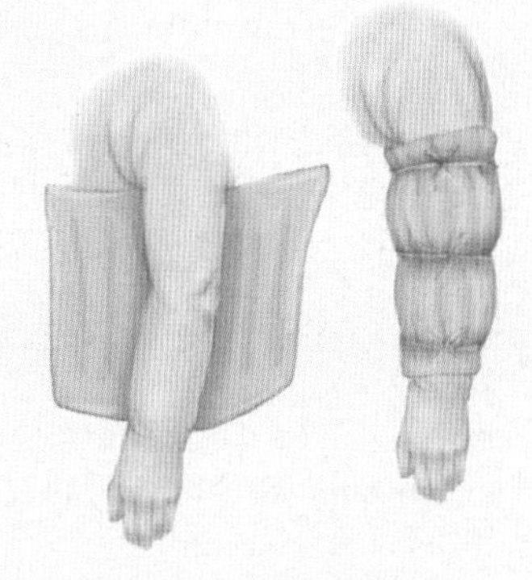	Prevents child from flexing and reaching face, head, IV, and other tubes 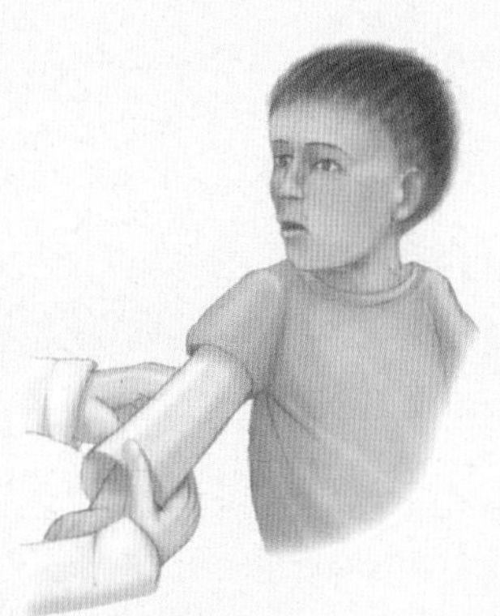	Position the restraint so that it does not rub against axilla. Check pulse, temperature, and capillary refill of the extremity.

(continued)

TABLE 11.3 • Types of Restraints and Associated Safety Concerns (*continued*)

Type of Restraint	Purpose	Safety Concerns
Mummy restraint	Body restraint using a sheet/blanket folded in a square appropriate to size of infant or young child to secure the whole body of the child or every extremity except for one	Ensure that all extremities are secured within the sheet. Ensure face is not covered or airway restricted.
Jacket (vest) restraint	Jacket worn by child with ties attached to the child's back and to side of bed. Used to keep children flat in bed, such as after surgery, or safe in chair	Ensure the child can turn head to side and that the head of the bed is elevated, if possible. Place ties in back so child cannot manipulate them. Ensure attached to nonmovable part of bed frame.

Before applying a restraint, explain the reason for the restraint to the child and the parents. Emphasize that the rationale is to maintain the child's safety; the restraint is not punishment. Having the child and parents state the reason for the restraint demonstrates their understanding.

In addition, the nurse must do the following:

- Ensure that the restraint fits properly.
- Secure the restraints with ties to the bed or crib frame, not the side rails.
- Use a clove-hitch type of knot to secure the restraints with ties (this allows for quick, easy access and release of the restraint).
- Check restraints 15 minutes following initial placement and then every hour for proper placement.
- Assess the temperature of the affected extremities, pulses, and capillary refill, initially after 15 minutes and then every hour after placement.
- Remove the restraint every 2 hours to allow for range of motion and repositioning, with documentation of this process and any findings.
- Encourage parent participation, providing continuous explanations about the reasons for the restraints and tentative time frame for use.
- Offer positive reinforcement to the child and parents.
- Review the criteria for removing the restraints; document removal and continued assessment.

It is important that the nurse is familiar with federal standards and regulations and state laws, and they should always follow facility policy and procedures.

TAKE NOTE!

Appropriate safety interventions that are age and developmentally appropriate and that would be used outside of the health care setting to protect an infant, toddler, or preschool child such as stroller, swing, highchair safety belts, and crib rails, crib covers, and enclosed or domed cribs, and raised padded side rails used for seizure precautions are not considered restraints (CMS, 2020).

Transport of the Child

Children may need to be transported to other units for diagnostic tests or surgery; to different areas in the same unit, such as the playroom or treatment room; or for discharge. When the child is transported to other areas, specific guidelines need to address safety issues, the age and developmental level of the child, the child's physical condition, and the destination. These factors need to be considered before transport so that the appropriate method can be used with the least amount of risk for the child. Various methods to transport children include carrying the infant and using strollers, wagons, or rolling beds (Fig. 11.7). If possible, the parents should accompany the child to offer support and comfort.

Providing Safe Transportation Within the Hospital

When carrying an infant, good support of the back and head is vital. Rails should be up on all beds and wagons. Use safety belts with strollers and wheelchairs.

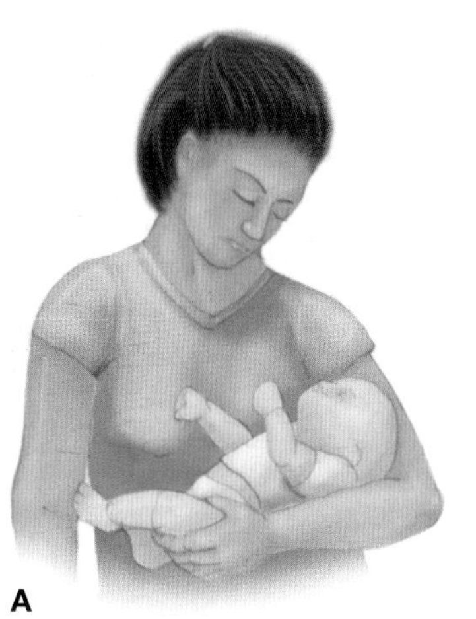
A

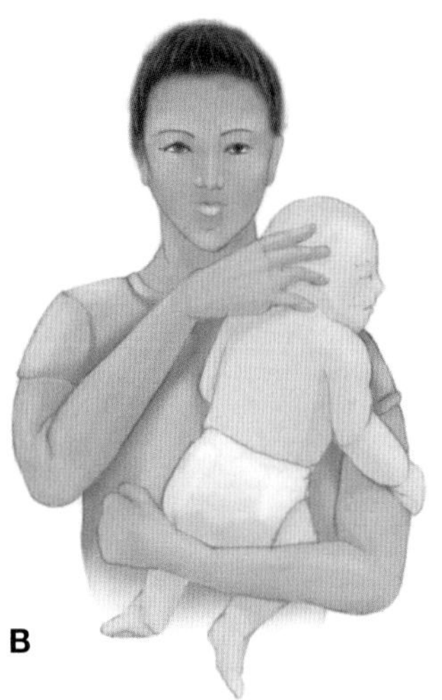
B

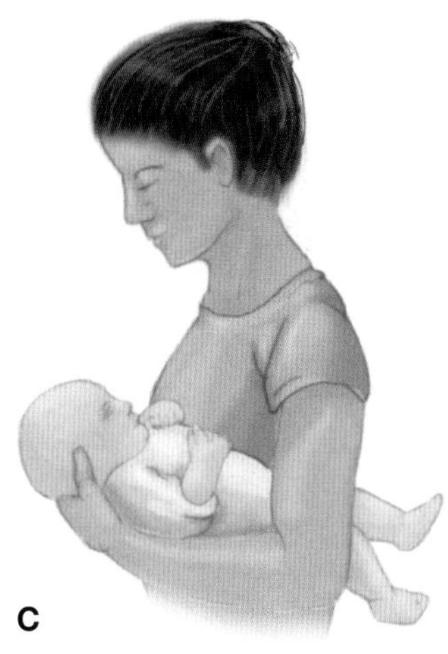
C

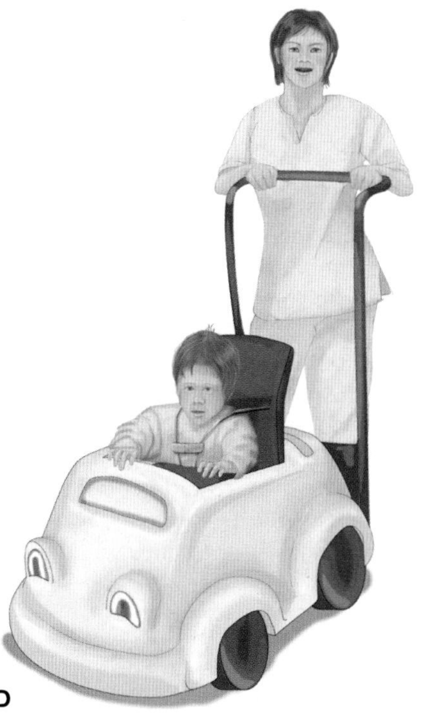
D

FIGURE 11.7 Methods for transporting the infant or child. **A.** Cradle method for carrying infants up to 3 months of age. One hand grasps the infant's thighs; the other arm supports the infant's head and back. **B.** The "over-the-shoulder" method for carrying infants up to 7 months of age. Support the head if the infant does not have head control. **C.** Football method for carrying infants up to 2 months of age. The forearm and hand support the body and head of the infant. **D.** A wagon with rails and padding is used to transport small children.

TAKE NOTE!

Never leave a child unattended during transport. Keep the child visible at all times during the transport.

THINKING ABOUT DEVELOPMENT

Discuss ways to maintain safety for an 8-year-old child in the hospital. How would this differ if the child was 3 years old?

HOSPITALIZATION IN CHILDHOOD

Hospitalization is often confusing, complex, and overwhelming for children and their families. Reactions and responses to illness and hospitalization depend on a number of factors, including the child's developmental stage. Nursing strategies are needed to prepare children and their families for this experience while minimizing negative effects. These strategies include identifying the needs of children and families through astute assessment of nonverbal and verbal behaviors, then validating the information with accurate interpretation and providing appropriate responses and interventions.

Although the nurse implements these strategies throughout the interaction with the child and family, a critical time to ensure the best outcome for the child and family is during the admission process. The nurse assesses the learning needs and abilities of the child and family. For the interventions to be successful, the nurse must communicate and teach in the most effective method for the individual child and family. The nurse also evaluates the child's and family's competence in performing specific activities prior to discharge.

In a study of hospitalized children, Crole and Smith (2002) found that the nursing care for a hospitalized child occurred in four phases: introduction, building a trusting relationship, decision-making phase, and providing comfort and reassurance. These phases remain relevant today. All of these phases are interconnected. For example, if trust is not established, it becomes difficult to move to the next phase.

The introduction phase involves the initial contact with children and their families, and it establishes the foundation for a trusting relationship. Use favorite toys and common television shows to establish rapport. Allow the child to participate in the conversation without the pressure of having to comply with requests or undergo any procedures. Next, a trusting relationship can be built by using appropriate language, games, and play such as singing a song during a procedure, preparing the child adequately for procedures, and providing explanations and encouragement. Get down to the child's level and play on their terms.

In the decision-making phase, the nurse gives some control over to the child by allowing them to participate in making certain decisions. This phase is critical to maintaining the trust the child has developed. For example, it is imperative to decide how much control the child will have during treatment, how much information to share with the child about upcoming events, and whether parents should participate. Reinforce the child's use of coping strategies that lead to healthy outcomes by providing options whenever it is safe to do so. Finally, the comfort and reassurance phase uses techniques such as praising the child and providing opportunities to cuddle with a favorite toy. This phase helps the nurse re-establish trust and provide comfort to the child to increase positive outcomes.

Preparing Children and Families for Hospitalization

When preparing children for hospitalization, be aware of the situations that may create distress in a child and try to minimize or eliminate them. Even the most minor situations may be frightening to young children. Remember, new experiences, unfamiliar sights and sounds, disruption of sleep patterns, and pain associated with procedures and treatments are major causes of stress for the hospitalized child and family.

Table 11.4 presents some hospital activities that may seem scary or stressful to a child and gives suggestions for preparing the child and family. Thoughtful preparation for these situations may help relieve stress. Educate children about what to expect so they can cope with their imagination and distinguish reality from fantasy. Describe the intervention and the sequence of steps that will occur, and include sensory information such as how the child will feel.

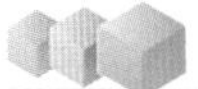 *Concept Mastery Alert*

Preparing the Child for Hospitalization

To help ease the stress of hospitalization in a child, encourage the parents and child to work with a child-life specialist at the hospital who can give the child a comprehensive preparation for the hospitalization.

Reduce the child's fears and increase their ability to cope with the hospital experience through good preparation. Preparation should include exploring the child's perceptions, reviewing previous experiences, and identifying coping strategies. The goal should be to decrease fear and anxiety by allowing the child to better understand what is happening. Useful techniques include the following:

- Perform nursing care on stuffed animals or dolls and allow the child to do the same.
- Avoid the use of medical terms.

TABLE 11.4 • Strategies to Reduce Fear of Common Hospitalization Situations

Situation	Strategies to Reduce Fear
Procedure involving intrusion into the body or use of equipment or technology	Describe the procedure and equipment in terms the child can understand. Review the steps of the procedure or steps involved with the use of the equipment. Explain what the child's role will be and what is or isn't allowed. If appropriate, have the child rehearse with the equipment or role-play.
Darkness, such as with radiologic examinations or at night	Keep a light on in the examination area. Use a nightlight in the child's room. If possible, allow the child to hold the caregiver's or nurse's hand or a favorite toy.
Transport to other areas of the hospital	Allow caregiver to accompany child, if possible. Inform the child of where they are going, about how long they will be there, and approximately when they will return. Introduce the child to the person who will be transporting the child.
Numerous personnel in and out of child's room	Identify all staff members working with the child (each shift and each day). Place a small board in the child's room with the name of the nurse caring for the child that shift or day. Inform the child how long the nurse will be caring for the child (adapt this information according to the child's cognitive level; for example, instead of saying that you'll be there for 8 hours, say, "I'll be your nurse until just before dinnertime" or "I'll be your nurse until you go for your test"). Say goodbye to the child when leaving for the day; tell the child about their new nurse; inform the child of when you will return.

- Allow the child to handle some equipment.
- Teach the child the steps of the procedure or inform them exactly what will happen during the hospital stay.
- Show the child the room where they will be staying.
- Introduce the child to the health care personnel with whom they will come in contact.
- Explain the sounds the child may hear.
- Let the child sample the food that will be served.

All techniques used to prepare the child for hospitalization should emphasize the philosophy of atraumatic care. Adapt all information to the cognitive and developmental level of the child. Identify what role the child will play in the situation: it is always helpful for children to have something to do, since it shows them that they are included. A rehearsal of what will occur in the hospital allows the child to become comfortable with the situation. If time permits, provide pamphlets that describe the procedure, and suggest preparation activities for the child at home before admission.

The child and family may be able to take a tour of the hospital unit or the surgical facility. Videos, photographs, and books on hospitalization and surgery can serve as resources for the family and child. Many institutions offer programs to familiarize children and families with the hospital experience with a guided tour. During the tour, opportunities are provided for role-playing, and during stops along the way the child can see, touch, and feel the equipment that may be used (Fig. 11.8). If the tour guide notes a child or family member is really scared or concerned about something, the pediatric staff can be alerted and therefore address this issue, leading to improved family-centered care.

Several children's books are available that focus on hospital stays and procedures, such as the coloring and activity book by Johns Hopkins Children's Center (2023), *My Trip to the Hospital* in the Little Critter Series by Mercer Mayer, and *Clifford Visits the Hospital* by Norman Bridwell. A list may be available at the hospital from the child-life department. Be familiar with these resources at your particular setting.

Parents are instrumental in preparing children by reviewing the materials that are given, answering questions,

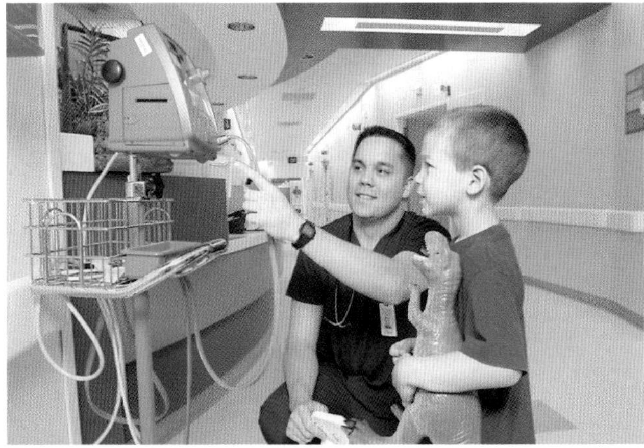

FIGURE 11.8 A child is being prepared for hospitalization by becoming familiar with some of the equipment that might be used.

TEACHING GUIDELINES 11.1 Preparing Your Child for Hospitalization

- Read stories about experiences with hospitals or surgery.
- Talk about going to the hospital and what it will be like coming home.
- Be honest and encourage the child to ask questions.
- Visit the hospital and go through the preadmission tour if time permits.
- Provide support to the child via your presence, phone or video calls, and special items brought from home.
- Encourage the child to draw pictures to express how they are feeling.
- Include siblings in the preparation.

and being truthful and supportive. Teaching Guidelines 11.1 provides suggestions for parents in preparing their child for hospitalization.

Remember Jake, the 8-year-old introduced at the beginning of the chapter? How can you help prepare Jake and his family for hospitalization?

Admitting the Child to the Facility

Admitting the child to the facility involves preparing them for admission and introducing the child to the unit where they will be staying. Use the appropriate hospital forms. Chapter 8 gives general information about communicating with and teaching children and families.

In today's health care environment, the admission process occurs quickly, with little time for extensive preparation; this is why preparation before admission is so important. Of course, the urgency of the child's medical condition may also limit the amount of preparation that can be done in advance.

TAKE NOTE!

When a child is admitted to a general unit, take extra time to orient and explain the routines and procedures to the child and family. Emphasize that the parents can stay with the child (if institutional policy permits). If possible, place the child in a room close to the nurses' station, and order food appropriate for the child's age and developmental level.

Types of Admissions and Nursing Care

The hospital units to which a child may be admitted include:

- General inpatient unit
- Emergency and urgent care department
- PICU
- Outpatient or special procedures unit
- Rehabilitation unit or hospital

ADMISSION ASSESSMENT

Obtain information about the child's history, routines, and reason for admission. Determine baseline vital signs and height and weight, and perform a physical assessment. Follow the facility's admission policy or procedure. Recognize the needs of the family and child during this process. If some of this information already exists, do not ask for it again, except to confirm vital information such as allergies, medications taken at home, and history of the illness. Typically, the information is collected immediately if the child's condition is urgent; otherwise, the information is collected within 8 hours, except for the information that is required for safe care.

COMMUNICATING WITH THE CHILD AND FAMILY

Regardless of the site of care, nursing care must begin by establishing a trusting, caring relationship with the child and family. Smile, introduce yourself, and give your title. Let the child and family know what will happen and what is expected of them. Ask the family and child what names they prefer to be called by. Maintain eye contact at the appropriate level. With a younger child, start with the family first so the child can see that the family trusts you. Communicate with children at age-appropriate levels. Orient the child and family to the hospital unit. Briefly explain policies and routines and the personnel who will be involved in the care of the child.

Isolation Rooms

Isolation rooms are used for situations involving the risk for infection. When a child is admitted with an infectious disease, or to rule out an infectious disease, or if the child has impaired immune function, isolation will be instituted. Children in this setting may experience sensory deprivation due to the limited contact with others and the use of personal protective equipment such as gloves, masks, and gowns.

CARING FOR THE CHILD IN ISOLATION

Encourage the family to visit often, and help them understand the reason for the isolation and any special procedures that are required. Introduce yourself before entering the room, and allow the child to view your face before applying a mask if possible. Continue to have contact with the child, and hold or touch the child often, especially if the parents are not present.

Addressing the Effects of Hospitalization Developmentally

When addressing the fears, separation anxiety, and loss of control that occur in hospitalized children, the nurse should consider the child's age and cognitive or developmental level. Interventions are then based on how the child experiences these stressors at that age or developmental level. The content, timing, setting, and method of preparation are also based on the child's age and cognitive or developmental level. General guidelines for addressing fear and anxiety, separation anxiety, and loss of control are provided in Box 11.6.

Caring for Newborns and Infants Who Are Hospitalized

Assess the developmental stage of the infant, and assess the baby's attachment to the parents or primary caregivers. Assess the infant's facial expression as it is the most consistent indicator of pain or bodily injury. Avoid separation from the primary caregiver, if possible, in order to decrease fear and minimize separation anxiety; this will also promote healthy attachment. Arrange for volunteers to provide consistent comfort to the baby if the parent or primary caregiver cannot stay with the infant. Maintain the infant's home routine related to sleep and feeding to help decrease feelings of loss of control. Weigh the infant daily, at the same time, on the same scale. Monitor intake and output closely. Be alert to signs of discomfort other than crying, such as a furrowed brow or tense body posture. Additional nursing considerations related to ensuring safety and promoting growth and development of the infant are presented in Table 11.2.

BOX 11.6 Guidelines to Address the General Effects of Hospitalization

Minimizing Fear and Anxiety

- Prepare the child and family for hospitalization and procedures.
- Explain everything to the child and their families before it occurs (see Chapter 8).
- Use age-appropriate communication techniques. Include the family in this process so they can help the child cope with fears.
- Allow time for children to play out their fears and concerns.
- Talk to the child and parents using a soft, friendly, comforting tone of voice.
- Have a calm, empathetic approach when caring for the child.

Addressing/Minimizing Separation Anxiety

- Know the stages of separation anxiety and be able to recognize them.
- Remember that behaviors demonstrated during the first stage do not indicate that the child is "bad."
- Encourage the family to stay with the child, and always use a family-centered approach to care.
- Help the child cope, and intervene before the behaviors of detachment occur.

Addressing Loss of Control

- Minimize physical restrictions, altered routines and rituals, and dependency issues, because they produce loss of control.
- Allow as much independence as possible within the constraints of the diagnosis.
- Allow the child to participate in care and decisions regarding care whenever possible.

Caring for Hospitalized Toddlers

Key nursing concerns when caring for toddlers are separation anxiety, growth and development, and autonomy. Establish a trusting relationship with the toddler through nonthreatening play to decrease the amount of fear the toddler feels. Be alert to subtle, nonverbal indicators of grief or discontent.

Encourage the parent or primary caregiver to stay with the toddler in the hospital to decrease separation anxiety. Maintain the home routine related to meals and sleep or a nap to provide structure, and help decrease the toddler's feelings of loss of control. If indicated, weigh the toddler daily. Closely monitor intake and output. Refer to Table 11.2 for additional nursing considerations related to ensuring safety and promoting growth and development in the hospitalized toddler.

Caring for Preschoolers Who Are Hospitalized

Nursing care for preschoolers who are hospitalized focuses on their special needs, fears, and fantasies. When working with preschoolers, remember that they use magical thinking and fantasy. Be honest and specific, providing information just prior to the intervention to allay the child's fears. As with toddlers, encourage parental involvement to decrease the amount of separation anxiety the preschooler experiences while in the hospital. Allow the preschooler to make simple decisions such as which color bandage to use or whether to take medicine from a cup or syringe. This will help the child to feel some sense of control. Table 11.2 gives specific nursing considerations related to ensuring safety and promoting growth and development for the preschooler in the hospital.

Caring for School-Age Children Who Are Hospitalized

Provide honest information using concrete, meaningful words to the school-age child to minimize fear of the unknown. Encourage parental involvement or rooming-in to decrease separation anxiety as school-age children are still very attached to their parents. Involve the child in making simple decisions and planning the schedule as appropriate to give them a sense of control. Table 11.2 provides additional nursing considerations when caring for hospitalized school-age children that include ensuring safety and promoting growth and development.

Caring for Adolescents Who Are Hospitalized

The adolescent may or may not express fears. Educate the adolescent honestly; younger adolescents require more concrete explanations, while older adolescents can process more abstract concepts. Respect the adolescent's need for privacy. Encourage visits from the adolescent's friends to minimize anxiety related to separation. Prepare a mutually agreeable schedule with the adolescent, as appropriate, that includes their preferences while incorporating the required nursing care. Collaborating with the adolescent will provide them with increased control. Refer to Table 11.2 for additional nursing considerations related to care of the adolescent in the hospital.

Providing Basic Care for the Child Who Is Hospitalized

Basic care involves general hygiene measures, including bathing, hair care, oral care, and nutritional care. Young children are dependent on an adult for most, if not all, of their self-care needs. If parents are present, allow them to provide care for the child to decrease the child's stress. Older children may perform hygiene measures themselves but may need some assistance from the nurse.

General Hygiene Measures

General hygiene measures help to maintain healthy skin, hair, and teeth. Skin is a complex structure; its primary function is to protect the tissues that it encloses and to protect itself. Injury to the child's skin may occur when inserting and maintaining an intravenous line, removing a dressing, positioning a child in bed, changing a diaper, using and removing electrode patches, and maintaining restraints. Risk factors for problems include impaired mobility, protein malnutrition, edema, incontinence, sensory loss, anemia, and infection. A good time to assess the skin is during bath time.

BATHING

Bathing infants and children is a common daily hygiene measure in the health care environment. Although a parent or primary caregiver often does this in today's family-centered environment, the nurse is still responsible for ensuring that bathing is done safely and hygienically. Adhere to safety principles to prevent falls, burns, and aspiration of water. Never leave a child alone in a bathtub. Use a gentle, pH-balanced soap with moisturizer if there is a need to rehydrate the skin. Note any condition that might require special considerations or further assessment, such as paralysis, loss of sensation, surgical incisions, skin traction/cast, external lines (intravenous lines, urinary catheters, or feeding tubes), or other alterations in skin integrity. Pay close attention to the ears, between skin folds, the neck, the back, and the genital area for alterations in skin integrity. Table 11.5 highlights specific developmental considerations for bathing.

Before bathing and performing other hygiene measures, assess the family's preferences and home practices for the child, such as time of day, rituals, special equipment, and allergies to products. This is a good time to assess the amount of assistance that might be required by the parents and to address learning needs related to hygiene. Follow general guidelines in bathing any patient with regard to equipment, room temperature, privacy, and use of products such as deodorant and lotion.

PROVIDING HAIR CARE

Lying in bed can make the hair matted and tangled. Avoid pulling on the child's hair when combing or brushing it. If necessary, use commercial detangling solutions to ease combing.

If the hair requires washing, this is often done during the daily bath for infants. Typically, shampooing once or twice a week is sufficient for younger children. Adolescents may need more frequent shampooing due to the increase in sebaceous gland secretion. The frequency of shampooing also varies based on the child's condition; for example, if the child has experienced diaphoresis, more frequent shampooing may be indicated.

Shampooing may be done at the bedside with specially adapted equipment, at a readily accessible sink while the child is sitting in a chair or lying on a stretcher, or in a tub or shower. Commercial no-rinse shampoos may be available for use. With these products, the shampoo is applied to the hair and then brushed or combed out.

If the child uses a tub or shower for hair care, monitor the child's safety throughout to ensure that the child does not slip and fall due to the slippery surface or is burned because of improper water temperature.

TABLE 11.5 • Developmental Considerations for Bathing

Age of Child	Special Considerations
Infants	Use a sponge bath or tub bath to bathe young infants who cannot sit unaided. Support the infant's body at all times. Ensure appropriate water temperature. Avoid use of talcum powder.
Toddlers	Bathe older infants and toddlers at the bedside or in a regular bathtub, depending on their health condition.
School-age children and adolescents	Older children may prefer a shower, if available and acceptable for their health condition. Assess whether a shower would be safe. Provide privacy.

The child's ethnicity may require special measures for hair care. For example, a child of African descent may use a broad-toothed comb for hair care. Ask the child's parents to bring one from home if one is not available. Also ask the child and parents about any products used on the hair that the child prefers; the parents can bring some from home. Encourage the parents to help with braiding or plaiting of the hair if desired.

PROVIDING ORAL HYGIENE

Oral hygiene is an important part of basic care. Wipe the infant's gums with a wet cloth after each feeding. Assist children in brushing and flossing their teeth after each feeding or meal and before bedtime. Provide special attention to oral hygiene of the immunosuppressed, such as using soft toothbrushes and moistened gauze sponges to prevent bleeding, and carefully inspect the oral cavity for areas of breakdown.

Nutrition

Adequate nutrition is necessary for growth and development and tissue repair, so it is an essential component of care for the ill or hospitalized child. Frequently, the ill or hospitalized child experiences a loss of appetite, which can affect the child's nutritional status. This may be compounded by other problems such as nausea and vomiting and nothing by mouth (NPO) restrictions for testing or surgery. The hospitalized child may adopt feeding habits that do not fit their age or stage of development, such as use of a bottle in an older infant/child or a child capable of self-feeding wanting to be fed. Readoption of these feeding habits should be accommodated when possible.

CLINICAL REASONING ALERT!

Relieve pain and nausea before meals are served.

PROVIDING NUTRITIONAL CARE

If possible, schedule procedures or treatments away from mealtimes. In younger children, refusing to eat may be related to the child's feeling of separation; in others, refusing to eat may reflect the child's attempt to control the situation. Encourage parents to use gentle persuasion instead of force to assist with intake. The use of force can lead to an aversion for food that carries beyond the hospital stay into the home environment. Give the child choices about what to eat; this reinforces the child's sense of control. Remind parents that the child's appetite will probably improve as their condition improves. Teaching Guidelines 11.2 provides tips for promoting nutrition in the hospitalized child. Although geared to parents, nurses can also incorporate these guidelines into the child's plan of care.

TEACHING GUIDELINES 11.2 Promoting Nutrition for Your Hospitalized Child

- Check with the nurse about any restrictions related to your child's diet. Find out if intake and output are being monitored.
- Encourage your child to eat their favorite foods.
- Assist your child with eating or drinking as necessary; be present at mealtimes to promote socialization.
- Frequently offer small cups of fluid and finger foods; avoid giving large quantities at one time.
- Try offering fluids at different temperatures at different times for variety.
- Remember that children can ingest greater amounts of thin liquids (e.g., gelatin or carbonated drinks) than thicker liquids (e.g., cream soups or milkshakes).
- Include ice chips as fluid intake. Ice is approximately equivalent to half the same amount of water (e.g., 1 cup of ice equals a half-cup of water).
- Use straws (unless not allowed) and brightly colored utensils, cups, or dishes to provide contrast and stimulation.
- Offer the child choices; allow the child to choose what they want from the menu.
- Talk with the dietitian to see if any special preferences can be addressed.
- Offer praise to your child for what they eat or drink.
- Never punish the child for not eating or drinking.
- Encourage the older child to help keep track of what they eat and drink.

Providing Play, Activities, and Recreation for the Child Who Is Hospitalized

Play is an important component in the child's plan of care. Today, many health care settings providing care for children have playrooms with age-appropriate toys, equipment, and other creative activities (Fig. 11.9). If the facility is large enough, there may even be a separate area for adolescents where they can listen to music, play video games, and visit with peers.

TAKE NOTE!

Avoid using the term "playroom" when caring for older school-age children and adolescents. Instead, call it the "activity room" or "social room." Doing so promotes a greater feeling of maturity and makes it more likely that they will use the area.

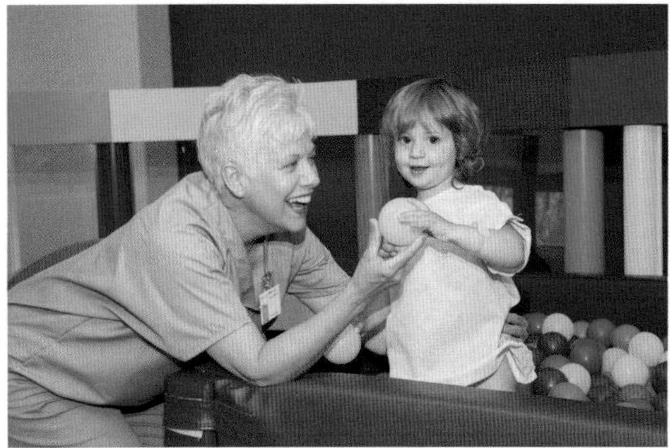

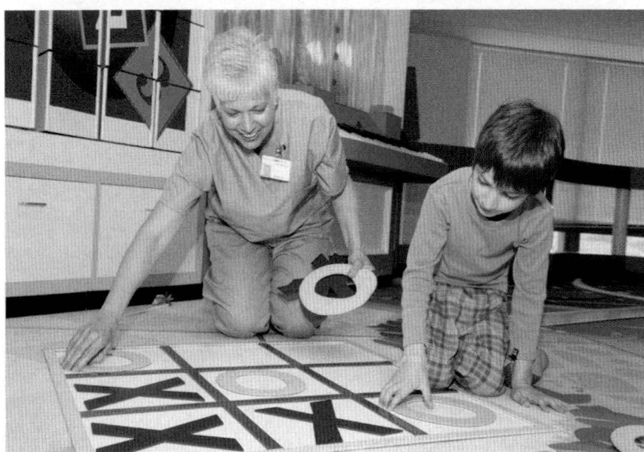

FIGURE 11.9 Children occupied in a hospital playroom. It is important to provide age-appropriate activities for younger and older children alike.

Obviously, some children will not be able to use these facilities if their activity level is restricted or if isolation is necessary. Children may also play in their rooms. Ensure that opportunities for unstructured play are provided to all children who can engage in play. Therapeutic play may be used to teach children about their health status or to allow them to work through issues in their lives.

TAKE NOTE!

Keep the bed or crib and playroom as "safe" places. Perform invasive procedures such as venipunctures in the treatment room, if possible. Never perform any nursing interventions in the playroom, no matter how nonthreatening they may appear to the nurse.

The nurse's greatest ally in the hospital in relation to atraumatic care is the CLS. They not only prepare the child for procedures but also provide activities and events to encourage play and normal growth and development.

Providing Unstructured Play

Encourage unstructured play as it allows children to control events, ideas, and relationships. Encourage parents to bring small toys and favorite stuffed animals from home to make the child feel more comfortable in the strange environment of the hospital. Children also enjoy receiving small new toys as surprises when they are hospitalized. Many children enjoy diversional activities such as playing board games or electronic games, reading books, and watching TV or videos. Quiet activities appropriate to the child's developmental level provide the opportunity for play and encourage the use and development of fine motor skills even if the child is confined to bed. Infants and toddlers enjoy manipulating blocks and playing with stacking toys. The preschooler may enjoy coloring, dollhouses, or playing with plastic building blocks such as Legos. School-age children and adolescents may enjoy playing video games, putting together a puzzle, or building a model geared toward their developmental level.

Play as Part of Nursing Care

Play is also an important part of nursing care. Use play as appropriate while providing routine nursing care to the child. An example of the use of play in nursing care involves the school-age child's love of competition and games. To increase range of motion in a school-age child who is hospitalized for traction due to a fracture, have the child throw a soft sponge ball or beanbag ball into a hoop, and compete against the child. To increase deep breathing, encourage the child to blow bubbles or blow a whistle. To increase intake of fluids, help the child create a graph to chart the number of glasses of fluids they drink over a period of time. Award the child a sticker, baseball card, special pencil, or other small item if they reach a certain level.

When using play as part of nursing care, it is important to evaluate the outcome of play. Play used in the manner described previously should enhance the child's outcome. For example, for the child blowing bubbles, determine whether this activity enhanced coughing and deep breathing.

Therapeutic Play

Another important aspect of play is **therapeutic play**. Therapeutic play is nondirected and focuses on helping the child cope with feelings and fears. Health care professionals use therapeutic play to help the child deal with the physical and psychological challenges of illness and hospitalization. Supervised play with medical equipment in the hospital environment can help children work through their feelings about what has happened to them (Fig. 11.10). In a large hospital or a children's hospital, the CLS typically coordinates these activities. Goals include maintaining normal living patterns, minimizing psychological trauma, and promoting optimal development of the child. If a CLS is not

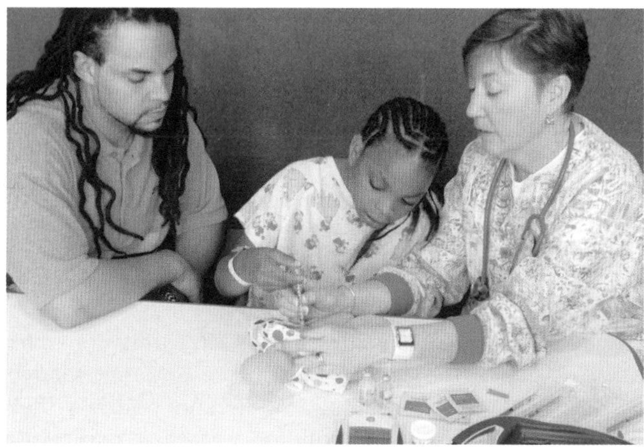

FIGURE 11.10 The nurse supervises play with medical equipment to help the child work through her feelings about being hospitalized.

available, the nurse provides this type of activity. There is a greater emphasis on the developmental and psychosocial implications of illness and hospitalization and validation of the child's voice.

In emotional outlet play or traumatic play, the child acts out or dramatizes real-life stressors. For example, using a wooden hammer and pegs, a soft sponge ball, or boxing gloves can allow the child to express anger over separation from family and friends. Commercial toys such as anatomically correct dolls and puppets have removable parts so children can see various organs of the body. Sometimes, younger children "talk" to puppets and dolls, allowing them to express their feelings to a nonthreatening "person" about a specific situation or what they want from the health care provider. For example, the Shadow Buddies dolls mentioned earlier in the chapter provide a way of coping with a specific condition. The company creates an ostomy buddy who has a stoma, a cancer buddy with thinning hair and a chest catheter for chemotherapy treatments, and a heart buddy who has a chest incision and a repaired heart (Shadow Buddies Foundation, n.d.).

Other types of therapeutic play include drawing and supervised "needle play." Drawing is a way for the child to express their thoughts and feelings. Supervised "needle play" assists children who must undergo frequent blood work, injections, or intravenous procedures. A doll can receive an injection as the child works out their anger and anxiety. Keep in mind safety and the child's growth and development level before planning this type of directed play; an adult must always be present.

Promoting School Work and Education During Hospitalization

Promote school work while the child is in the hospital. Determine the amount of school work that can be done by assessing the child's condition, the availability of teachers, and the family situation. Many children's hospitals have teachers at the hospitals; there may be classrooms too. These teachers work closely with the child's school to continue school work as the child's condition permits. Hospitals without an educational staff will rely on parents to coordinate with the child's school. Parents may bring in schoolbooks and the child's homework for completion while in the hospital. This connection to the child's school helps maintain normalcy for the child and minimizes the disruption of everyday life. Nurses and other health care providers, such as social workers, should help facilitate this process.

> Think back to Jake, the 8-year-old, from the beginning of the chapter. What nursing care could you provide that will help minimize stressors?

Family Members' Needs

Many factors may influence the family's reaction to the child's hospitalization. Parents or caregivers and siblings experience many emotions when a child is hospitalized, including disbelief, anger, guilt, fear, anxiety, frustration, and depression. Visiting restrictions, unexpected changes in the child's health status, lack of information or understanding of their child's health condition, changes in their routine and roles, financial stress, and feelings of being undervalued in the care of their child all contribute to the parents' or caregivers' feelings.

Family-centered care recognizes the need to treat the child in the context of the family, including siblings. Important questions that will affect how siblings deal with the hospitalization of the child include:

- Was the admission an emergency?
- Were there previous admissions, and how did the siblings perceive those hospitalizations?
- How serious is the illness or trauma?
- Is the prognosis known?

Addressing Parents' Needs

Assess the factors that may influence the family's reaction to the child's hospitalization and plan the care of the child to accommodate some of these issues. Encourage families to have support systems in place before, during, and after hospitalization. Help parents and caregivers to work through their feelings in order to decrease anxiety, thus decreasing the child's anxiety level. The philosophy of family-centered care places the family at the core of care; the family is the primary and continuing provider of care for the child. Practice family-centered care, which addresses the child's and family's needs and preferences and increases the child's and parents' satisfaction with the health care setting (American Academy of Pediatrics, Committee on Hospital Care, Institute for Patient and Family-Centered Care, 2012, reaffirmed 2018).

Encourage parents to room-in with the child throughout the hospital stay, if possible. Facilities can be designed to welcome family participation. For example, having charging ports, internet, and printers or scanners available and providing extra meals and beds for the parents can encourage parents to participate in care. View the parents as vital members of the health care team and partners in the care of the child who is ill.

Addressing Siblings' Needs

Address the siblings' possible feelings of guilt. Use educational materials, allow time for visits, send photographs back and forth between siblings, and allow siblings to talk on the phone.

Child and Family Teaching

Not all experiences with hospitalization are negative; in fact, the experience may enhance the child's and family's coping skills, bolster self-esteem, and provide new socialization experiences. It may allow the child to master self-care skills and provides an opportunity for the child and family to learn new information. Parents may learn more about their child's growth and development skills as well as additional parenting or caregiving skills, resulting in improved parenting abilities. In addition, the child's overall health may be improved because of the hospital stay if the child receives current immunizations and the parents learn more about health care practices.

The overall goals of child and family teaching are to minimize the child's and family's stress, educate them about treatment and nursing care in the hospital, and ensure the family can provide appropriate care at home on discharge. Providing support before, during, and after hospitalization may minimize stress. Preadmission programs can introduce the child and family to the setting. During the hospital stay, forming partnerships with the child and family, using strategies to promote coping, and providing appropriate preparation for procedures, tests, and surgery serve to decrease stress.

Educating the Child and Family

Assess the child's and family's knowledge of the illness and hospital experience. This provides a baseline for teaching. Include hospital rules in child and family teaching. Behavioral changes in hospitalized children often disturb parents or caregivers. Determine the child's usual patterns of behavior and explain to the parents about the child's reaction to hospitalization. Encourage the family to maintain consistent discipline even while in the hospital to provide structure for the child as well as to prevent discipline issues after discharge. Also discuss how siblings may react to the hospitalization, and provide appropriate teaching to the siblings. Every interaction the nurse has with the child or family provides an opportunity for teaching. Explain the purpose of even simple procedures such as vital signs assessment to the child and family. Provide ongoing information about the child's illness or trauma, treatment plan, and expected outcomes. Chapter 8 provides general principles related to teaching children and their families.

Preparing the Child and Family for Discharge

Discharge planning actually begins on admission. The nurse assesses the family's resources and knowledge level to determine what education and referrals they may need. On discharge, children and their parents or caregivers receive written instructions about home care, and a copy is retained in the medical record. These instructions are individualized for the child. Generally, discharge instructions should include:

- Follow-up appointment information
- Guidelines about when to contact the health care provider or nurse practitioner (e.g., new or worsening symptoms or indications that the child is not improving)
- Diet
- Activity level allowed
- Medications, including dose, times to be given, route, adverse effects, and special instructions; any prescriptions should be included
- Information on additional treatments the child requires at home
- Specific dates for when the child may return to school or day care
- Names and phone numbers of agencies the family has been referred to, such as durable medical equipment providers

Provide and review educational booklets that give basic health information or general care for a child with a particular disease (Fig. 11.11). Media such as videos may also be used, if available. The ability to watch a

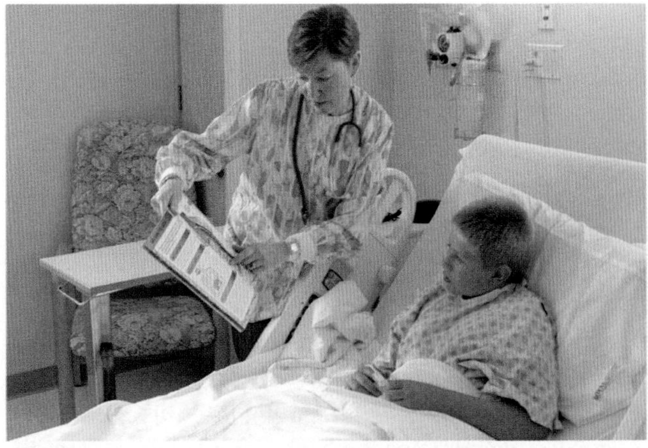

FIGURE 11.11 The nurse uses charts with pictures to perform patient teaching before the child goes home.

procedure over and over is helpful to some families. Explain, demonstrate, and request a return demonstration of any treatments or procedures to be done at home. Provide a written schedule if the child is to receive multiple medications, tube feedings, or other medical treatments. For complicated cases, a written teaching plan may be used to provide continuity of child/family education between various nurses. As the family attempts to perform each task, document whether the caregiver continues to require assistance or prompting with the task or whether they can perform the task independently.

Parents of children with multiple medical needs may benefit from a trial period of home care. This occurs while the child is still in the hospital, but the parents or caregivers provide all of the care that the child requires. Support the family and praise their accomplishments during this trial period.

KEY CONCEPTS

- Nursing care of the child occurs in a variety of settings, from acute care in a hospital to well and ill care in community settings, such as health care providers' offices, schools, places of worship, health departments, community centers, and even within the child's own home. Within each setting, the nurse incorporates basic nursing care with specific strategies to help promote positive outcomes for the child, family, and community as a whole.
- Advantages of community-based care, especially home care, include shorter hospital stays and decreased health care costs, but the major advantage of home care is the comfort and family support it provides, promoting an improved quality of life for these children. Caring for children at home not only improves their physical health but also allows for adequate growth and development while keeping them within their family.
- Community-based nurses focus on the practice of nursing that provides personal care to children and families in the community. These nurses focus on promoting and preserving health as well as preventing disease or injury. They help children and their families cope with illness and disease. They are direct providers of care as well as advocates and educators working to minimize and remove barriers to allow the child to develop to their full potential.
- Due to the short lengths of stay in acute settings and the shift to home care for children with complex health needs, discharge planning and care coordination have become important nursing roles. Discharge planning provides a comprehensive plan for the safe discharge of a child from a health care facility and for continuing safe and effective care at home. Care coordination focuses on coordinating health care services while balancing quality and cost outcomes. Both contribute to improved transitions from hospital to home for children, their families, and the health care team.
- In all of the varied settings where health care is administered, nurses provide well care, episodic ill care, and chronic care. They work to promote, preserve, and improve the health of children and families in these settings.
- Goals of the nurse in the home care setting include promoting, restoring, and maintaining the health of the child. Home care focuses on minimizing the effects of the illness or disability and providing the child or family with the means to care for the illness or disability at home. Nurses in the home care setting are direct providers of care, child and family educators, child and family advocates, and case managers.
- Disadvantages to home care include intrusion on family privacy. Caring for children with complex medical needs can be overwhelming for some families, and financial issues related to home care can become a large burden to families.
- Nursing in the home care setting can be challenging. The focus is on meeting the child's physical and psychological needs while involving the family. Health care professionals provide the support, empowerment, education, and expertise in caring for the child that families need.
- Stressors associated with hospitalization and illness include separation from family and routines; fear of an unknown environment; potential for pain, bodily injury, or mutilation; and loss of control.
- Responses of children to the general stressors of hospitalization include anxiety, fear, anger, guilt, and regression.
- The responses of children and families to illness and hospitalization can be influenced by the age and developmental level of the child, their perceptions of the situation, previous experiences, separation from family and peers, coping skills, and the preparation and support provided by the family, facility, and health care providers.
- Family-centered care and atraumatic care are philosophies that pay special attention to the concerns of the family and child during hospitalization.
- Providing support to children who are hospitalized and their families is critical for minimizing stress.
- Whatever the reason for admission, preparation for admission is vital.
- Upon admission to the hospital or outpatient unit, orient the child and family to the unit, discuss unit policies and routines and the personnel who will be involved in the care of the child, and begin child/family teaching.
- Establish a trusting, caring relationship with the child and family. Let the child and family know what will happen and what is expected of them. Obtain information about the child's history, routines, and reason for admission. Obtain baseline vital signs and height and weight, and perform a physical assessment. Each health care setting has its own policies and procedures for this.
- Due to their age and developmental level, children may be vulnerable to harm, and the nurse must use

appropriate safety measures in caring for children (e.g., identification of children, use of restraints and transportation, basic hygiene measures). These measures need to address developmental risks, such as that the infants, toddlers, and preschoolers require close supervision, and the nurse must avoid leaving small objects within reach.

- Play, including therapeutic play, is an important strategy to prepare children for hospitalization and to help them adapt to the effects of illness and hospitalization. It provides an emotional outlet, opportunities for teaching and learning, and the ability to become familiar with a situation and improve physiologic abilities. A CLS is a specially trained individual who is a member of the child's multidisciplinary team. They work in conjunction with the child's health care providers and parents to foster an atmosphere that promotes the child's well-being.
- Parents may experience anger or guilt related to the hospitalization of their child.
- Discharge planning begins on admission. Each interaction with the family is an opportunity for child and family teaching.
- Provide and review discharge instructions with the child and primary caregiver. Use educational booklets or media such as videos that give basic health information or general care for a child with a particular disease.
- Explain, demonstrate, and request a return demonstration of any treatments or procedures to be done at home. Provide a written schedule if the child is to receive multiple medications, tube feedings, or other medical treatments.

REFERENCES AND RECOMMENDED READINGS

American Academy of Pediatrics, Committee on Hospital Care, Institute for Patient and Family-Centered Care. (2012, reaffirmed 2018). Policy statement: Patient and family-centered care and the pediatrician's role. *Pediatrics, 129*(2), 394–404. https://doi.org/10.1542/peds.2011-3084

American Society of Anesthesiologists. (n.d.). My Surgery Journal. https://www.asahq.org/madeforthismoment/wp-content/uploads/2020/10/ASA-239-MFTM-Coloring-Book_BOY.pdf

Berlin, E. A., & Fowkes, W. C., Jr. (1983). A teaching framework for cross-cultural health care. Application in family practice. *The Western Journal of Medicine, 139*(6), 934–938. https://www.ncbi.nlm.nih.gov/pmc/articles/PMC1011028/pdf/westjmed00196-0164.pdf

Centers for Medicare & Medicaid Services. (2020). *State Operations Manual Appendix A—Survey protocol, regulations and interpretive guidelines for hospitals.* https://www.cms.gov/Regulations-and-Guidance/Guidance/Manuals/downloads/som107ap_a_hospitals.pdf

Conners, G. P., Kressly, S. J., Perrin, J. M., Richerson, J. E., Usha, M., Sankrithi, U. M., Committee on Practice and Ambulatory Medicine, Committee On Pediatric Emergency Medicine, Section On Telehealth Care, Section On Emergency Medicine, Subcommittee On Urgent Care, & Task Force On Pediatric Practice Change. (2017). Nonemergency acute care: When it's not the medical home. *Pediatrics, 139*(5), e20170629. https://doi.org/10.1542/peds.2017-0629

Crole, N., & Smith, L. (2002). Examining the phases of nursing care of the hospitalized child. *Australian Nursing Journal, 9*(8), 30–31.

Elias, E. R., Murphy, N. A., & the Council on Children with Disabilities. (2012, reaffirmed 2022). Clinical report: Home care of children and youth with complex health care needs and technology dependencies. *Pediatrics, 129*(5), 996–1005. https://doi.org/10.1542/peds.2012-0606

Gallo, M., Agostiniani, R., Pintus, R., & Fanos, V. (2021). The child with medical complexity. *Italian Journal of Pediatrics, 47*(1), 1. https://doi.org/10.1186/s13052-020-00935-z

John Hopkins Children Center. (2023). *Hopkins children's guide to surgery coloring book.* https://www.hopkinsmedicine.org/johns-hopkins-childrens-center/patients-and-families/your-visit/abcs-surgery/surgery-coloring-book.html

Kids' Waivers. (2022). *Full list.* http://www.kidswaivers.org/full-list/

Murphy, N. A., Alvey, J., Valentine, K. J., Mann, K., Wilkes, J., & Clark, E. B. (2020). Children with medical complexity: The 10-year experience of a single center. *Hospital Pediatrics, 10*(8), 702–708. https://doi.org/10.1542/hpeds.2020-0085

National Association of School Nurses. (2020). *Individualized healthcare plans: The role of the school nurse (Position Statement).* Author.

National Association of School Nurses. (2023). *About NASN: Definition of school nursing.* https://www.nasn.org/about-nasn/about

National Center for Injury Prevention and Control, Centers for Disease Control and Prevention. (2020). *WISQARS leading causes of nonfatal injury.* https://wisqars.cdc.gov/lcnf/

National Council of State Boards of Nursing. (2018). *A nurse's guide to professional boundaries.* https://www.ncsbn.org/public-files/ProfessionalBoundaries_Complete.pdf

Piaget, J. (1969). *The theory of stages in cognitive development.* McGraw-Hill.

Rector, C. (2022). The journey begins: Introduction. In C. Rector & M. J. Stanley (Eds.), *Community and public health nursing. Promoting the public's health* (10th ed., pp. xxiv–22). Wolters Kluwer Health.

Robertson, J., & Bowlby, J. (1952). Responses of young children to separation from their mothers II: Observations of the sequences of response of children aged 18 to 24 months during the course of separation. *Courrier du Centre International de l'Enfance, 2,* 131–142.

Romito, B., Jewell, J., Jackson, M., & AAP Committee on Hospital Care; Association of Child Life Professionals. (2021). Child life services. *Pediatrics, 147*(1), e2020040261. https://doi.org/10.1542/peds.2020-040261

Shadow Buddies Foundation. (n.d.). *Shadow buddies foundation.* http://www.shadowbuddies.org/

U.S. Department of Health and Human Services. (n.d.). *Healthy People 2030.* https://health.gov/healthypeople

United States Environmental Protection Agency. (2022). *Resources for healthcare providers about children's environmental health.* https://www.epa.gov/children/resources-healthcare-providers-about-childrens-environmental-health

Vaz, L. E., Jungbauer, R. M., Jenisch, C., Austin, J. P., Wagner, D. V., Everist, S. J., Libak, A. J., Harris, M. A., & Zuckerman, K. E. (2022). Caregiver experiences in pediatric hospitalizations: Challenges and opportunities for improvement. *Hospital Pediatrics, 12*(12), 1073–1080. https://doi.org/10.1542/hpeds.2022-006645

DEVELOPING CLINICAL JUDGMENT

PRACTICING FOR NCLEX

1. The nurse is preparing a 5-year-old for surgery on their lower leg. The parent is helping them into the hospital gown, and the child fights removal of their underwear. What is the most appropriate nursing action?
   a. Allow the parent to remove the underwear.
   b. Tell the child they are acting childishly.
   c. Notify the operating room that the underwear is on.
   d. Allow the child to keep their underwear on.
2. A 6-month-old infant requires restraint to prevent removal of a nasogastric tube. What is the priority nursing intervention?
   a. Tie the restraint loosely to prevent skin breakdown.
   b. Leave the baby unrestrained when directly observed.
   c. Position the restrained infant prone to prevent aspiration.
   d. Place the infant in a room near the nurses' station.
3. A 10-year-old child on a regular diet refuses to eat the food on the meal tray. They request chicken nuggets, French fries, and ice cream. What is the best nursing action?
   a. Ask that the child's desired foods be sent up from the kitchen.
   b. Negotiate with the child to eat at least part of the food on the tray.
   c. Remove a privilege.
   d. Offer the child cereal and milk from stock on the nursing unit.
4. The nurse providing home care to a 2-year-old listens to the child's parents talk about how the child and family are adjusting to the child's current illness. Which role is the nurse providing?
   a. Case management
   b. Child and family advocacy
   c. Direct nursing care
   d. Child and family education
5. A child is to undergo a tympanostomy tube placement in a freestanding outpatient surgery center. What are the major advantages associated with this location? Select all that apply.
   a. Decreased risk for infection
   b. Decreased health care costs
   c. Ability to be transferred if overnight stay is required
   d. Decreased disruption of family functioning
   e. Decreased risk of complications
   f. Ability to return to normal routine for the child quickly

CRITICAL THINKING EXERCISES

1. Becky, an 8-year-old, is admitted to the pediatric unit for an emergency surgery. She is in third grade and very active in afterschool programs. Her parent is with her during the admission process but will have to return to work shortly after Becky returns from surgery to the pediatric unit. Would the nurse expect Becky to show separation anxiety? What are the three top nursing concerns for Becky relating to the effects of hospitalization?
2. A 6-year-old is admitted to the general pediatric unit after spending several hours in the emergency department with an acute asthma attack. A parent and two younger siblings are present, but the parent plans to leave shortly to take the siblings home. The other parent will visit in about 2 hours, after work. What is the overall goal for this child's care? What could the nurse say to promote coping in this child? What would be the best answer if the parent asks if they should stay rather than take the siblings home?
3. A child with cerebral palsy is discharged from the hospital, where they have been receiving treatment for pneumonia. Home health care nurses, through a local agency, are to help the family administer intravenous antibiotic therapy and to monitor the child's health status.
   a. As the home health nurse assigned to this child, what should your nursing assessment include?
   b. In this situation, what are some nursing interventions that will help ensure family-centered care?
   c. When this child is stable and can go back to school, what will be the role of the school nurse in caring for this child?

STUDY ACTIVITIES

1. Follow a child and family during the admission process, from preadmission to initial time on the unit, to identify the procedures and tasks involved. Examine the response of the child and family and how the nursing staff responds to their needs.
2. Develop a teaching plan to orient a toddler or preschooler and their family to a nursing unit. Include the resources, personnel, and techniques to include in the teaching plan.
3. Shadow a nurse working in a community setting, such as a camp, school, shelter, or health department. Identify the role the nurse plays in the health of the children and families in the setting and the community.

4. Spend a day in a medical day care setting. Identify the needs of one child and their family, how they may differ from those of a child in a traditional day care setting, and the role of the nurse in meeting those needs.

5. Develop an IHP for a child with diabetes.

6. Shadow a nurse working in a home health care setting. Identify ways they help the family to promote the child's growth and development and to ensure that the child has as normal a childhood as possible. Identify interventions that embody the key concepts of family-centered care.

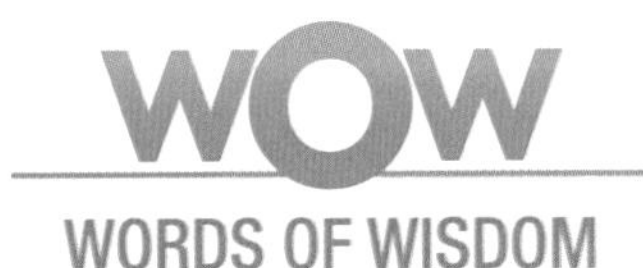

WORDS OF WISDOM

The touch of a parent's hand and the sound of their voice bring comfort to the child with special health care needs, and when the nurse brings comfort, you strengthen both of them.

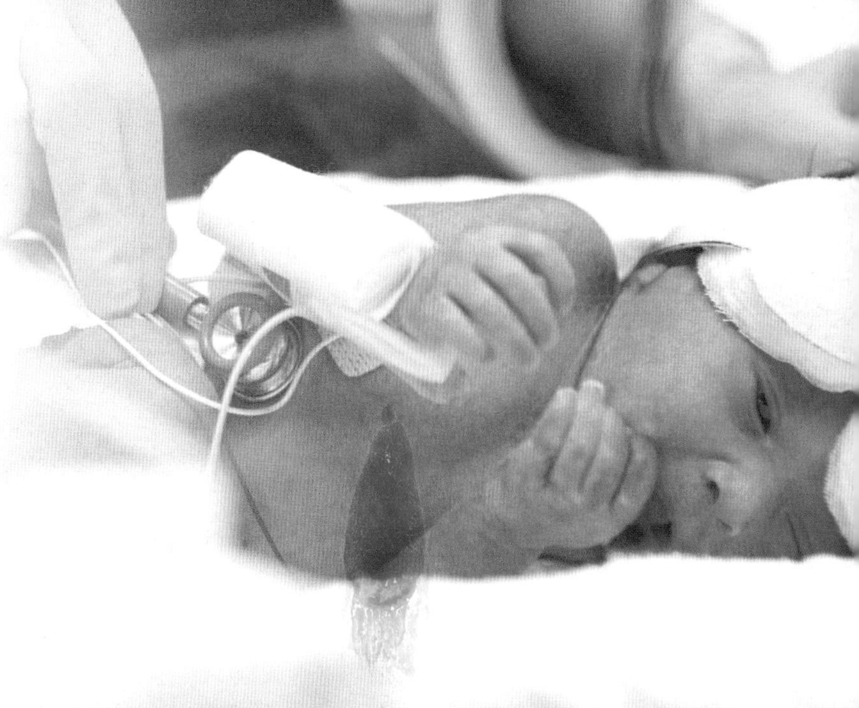

12

Caring for the Child With Special Health Care Needs

KEY TERMS

chronic illness

developmental delay

developmental disability

palliative care (pal´ē-ā-tiv kār)

respite care (res´pit kār)

terminal illness

LEARNING OBJECTIVES

Upon completion of the chapter, you will be able to:

1. Analyze the impact that special health care needs has on the child and family.
2. Identify anticipated times when the child and family will require additional support.
3. Describe ways that nurses assist children with special health care needs and their families to obtain optimal functioning.
4. Discuss early intervention and public school education for the child with special health care needs.
5. Plan for transition of the child with special health care needs from the inpatient facility to the home and from pediatric to adult medical care.
6. Discuss key elements related to pediatric end-of-life care.
7. Differentiate developmental responses to death and appropriate interventions.

Preet Singh, an 18-month-old who was born at 28 weeks' gestation, is seen in your clinic for the first time. He has a history of hydrocephalus and developmental delay. During the examination, his parent states, "I'm concerned about finding a good, affordable preschool for Preet. His older brother attends public school, but I can't imagine Preet going there."

INTRODUCTION

The Maternal Child Health Bureau (MCHB) defines children with special health care needs as "those who have or are at risk for chronic physical, developmental, behavioral, or emotional conditions" and who "also require health and related services of a type or amount beyond that required by children generally" (MCHB, 2023, para. 4). Children who have a terminal illness or are otherwise dying also require additional care. Nurses are in a unique position, in both the inpatient and the outpatient setting, to have a significant and positive influence on the lives of these children and their families. In addition to providing direct care, the nurse fills the critical role of child and family advocate and case manager. When a child is dying, nurses not only provide physical care to the child but also strive to meet the emotional needs of the child and family.

THE CHILD WITH SPECIAL HEALTH CARE NEEDS

The numbers of children with **chronic illnesses** (long-lasting or recurrent illnesses) are increasing. Children with special health care needs make up about 19% of the population of children in the United States, and nearly one in five families has a child with a special health care need (MCHB, 2023). Increasing numbers of children are being diagnosed with physical and mental disorders (Abdi et al., 2020), and larger numbers of children are living with the assistance of high-tech treatments and equipment (Brenner et al., 2021).

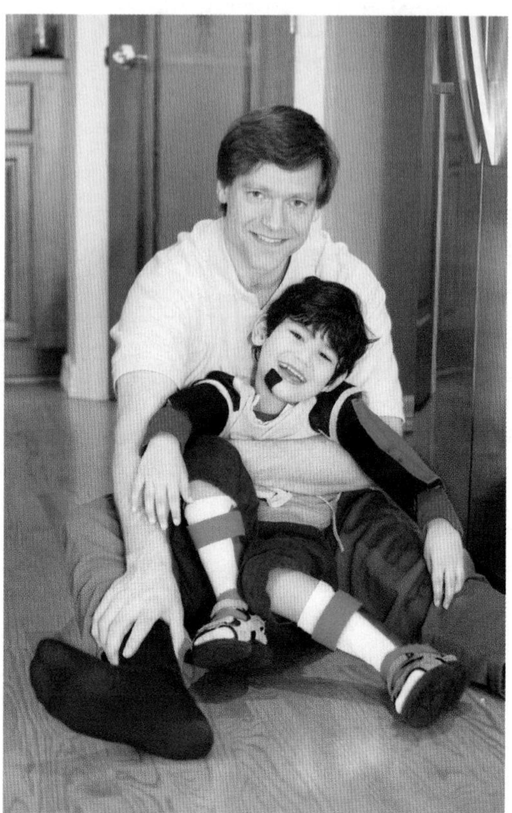

FIGURE 12.1 The child with special health care needs often requires a significant amount of care at home throughout life.

Impact of the Problem

Children with chronic physical, developmental, behavioral, or emotional conditions may use or need prescription medication, medical care, mental health services, or education services more than other children of the same age. They may need physical, occupational, or speech therapy (Fig. 12.1). Alternatively, they may require ongoing treatment for emotional, developmental, or behavioral problems (MCHB, 2023). These children and their families may be inadequately insured, have financial needs and unmet family support needs, or have difficulty obtaining the specialty care that the child requires (Kuo & Turchi, 2023). It can be challenging for the family of a child with these needs to navigate the system and obtain all of the services the child requires.

When an infant is born very prematurely, when a child is injured and requires long-term rehabilitation and special care, or when a child is diagnosed with a complex chronic health condition, the parents are often initially devastated. The parents may feel they must adapt to the risk and protect their child. They are interested in preserving their family while compensating for the past, and they cautiously look to the future and become hopeful again. While the infant or child is in the hospital, nurses can help families build on their strengths, empowering them to care for their medically fragile infant or special needs child. Education is paramount and should begin as early in hospitalization as possible (Cincinnati Children's Hospital Medical Center [CCHMC], 2023). In many situations, particular discharge needs are known early in the course of the hospitalization. Nurses should provide anticipatory guidance about the course of treatment and the expected outcome.

Most children with chronic illnesses or those who require technology progress through stages of growth and development just as typical children do, although sometimes at a slower pace. The exception is the child with significant psychomotor delays, although some developmental progression may occur. Children with developmental or functional needs desire to be treated as normal, and they want to experience the same events that other children do.

Remember Preet, the 18-month-old former 28-week premature neonate introduced at the beginning of the chapter? What would you expect his gross motor, fine motor, and language skills to be at this age?

Effects of Special Health Care Needs on the Child

When a child has a chronic physical, developmental, behavioral, or emotional condition, the child's coping ability is affected. In addition, the child's ability to cope is significantly affected by the family's response to stressors, which can be numerous for these families. Children experience differing effects of the chronic illness or disability based on their developmental level, which naturally changes over time for most children. These differences in their health and needs may lead to alterations in social–emotional development (Population Reference Bureau [PRB], 2023).

Infants may fail to develop a sense of trust, while the toddler may experience difficulty developing autonomy. The preschooler may experience limited opportunities for socialization. The school-age child may have limited opportunities to achieve a sense of industry because of school absence and inability to participate in activities or competitive events. Many school-age children who have medically complex conditions may often be absent from school, affecting their academic achievement (PRB, 2023).

Adolescents may feel as though they are different from their peers because of their different skills, abilities, or appearance. This may hinder the adolescent's ability to form a sense of personal identity. Since the adolescent may require significant amounts of support from the family, it may be difficult for the adolescent to achieve independence. If the earlier stages of cognitive development have been delayed, then reaching the level of abstract thinking may be blocked (American Academy of Child and Adolescent Psychiatry [AACAP], 2023).

The child with special health care needs may be able to focus on the positive experiences in their life as a method of coping, leading to as much independence as possible. Other children may always feel different from their peers in a negative sense and withdraw. Irritability and acting out may also occur. Some children may be compliant and seek support for themselves. The child's coping pattern may change over time or with certain situations, such as relapse or worsening of the condition. Children with more protective parents may display marked dependence and may be fearful (Schmitz, 2019). Children whose parents have been more indulgent may be more independent and defiant. The nurse must assess the child's individual response to the current health care status and intervene as appropriate.

Effects on the Family

Each member of the family experiences effects related to the child's situation. Family members' experiences and their responses influence each other directly (Fig. 12.2).

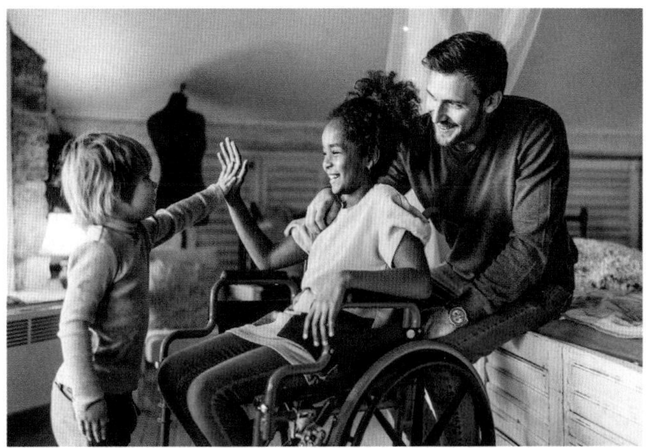

FIGURE 12.2 A child with special health care needs with their family. (Shutterstock/NDAB Creativity.)

Effects on Parents

Raising a child with special health care needs is generally not what parents expected. Some parents may adapt over time and accept the child's illness or disability. Others may adapt but do not find acceptance and experience the continual fading and reemergence of chronic sorrow. Denial of problems may prevent parents from progressing through grief, but it also gives them a sense of hope (Bally et al., 2018).

Caring for the child at home rather than in a facility may decrease the parents' feelings of anxiety and helplessness. As with healthy children, parents enjoy witnessing the emotional and social growth of the child. Parents of children with special health care needs experience a multitude of emotions and changes in their lives. They worry about the child's and family's well-being and, as experts in their child's care, often feel burdened with the demands of continual care. They may feel helpless and overwhelmed when their child is discharged from the hospital. Although willing to carry out the responsibility for care, they may experience fear, anger, sadness, guilt, frustration, or resentment. Many parents experience grief as a result of losing the child they expected (Bally et al., 2018).

STRESSORS OF DAILY LIVING

Families with children who have special health care needs experience life differently from other families. They may have to change their housing situations to accommodate the child's functional needs. Sleep may be affected. Constant supervision of a child who requests technologic assistive devices makes it difficult to carry out other basic household activities. In addition to basic child care and running of the household, medical and technical care must be incorporated into daily life. The family's identity and the parents' employment may be radically altered. Holidays and vacations may be affected, as it can be difficult to plan activities. Nursing and other health care professional visits can be disruptive to family life.

The extended caregiving responsibilities can also have adverse health effects on caregivers; often, families report emotional and physical burdens of their own (Blanco et al., 2021). In addition, these parents are at increased risk for the development of depression (Blanco et al., 2021). Parents may experience role conflicts, financial burdens, and difficulty balancing the independence of providing care with the isolation associated with it. It can be difficult to enjoy spontaneous events outside the home since extra planning is necessary.

The degree of independence can be influenced by mobility issues, education, and assistive technology. Although education for all children is federally mandated, parents have anxiety about educational decisions and may find it difficult to obtain the support and educational services the child needs.

Additional stress is associated with transition times in the care of a child with special health care needs. These transition times include:

- Initial diagnosis or change in prognosis
- Increased symptoms
- When the child moves to a new setting (hospital, school)
- During a parent's absence
- During periods of developmental change

VULNERABLE CHILD SYNDROME

Vulnerable child syndrome is a clinical state in which the parents' reactions to a serious illness or event in the child's past continue to have long-term psychologically harmful effects on the child and parents for many years (Schmitz, 2019). The parents view the child as being at higher risk for medical, developmental, or behavioral problems than the child may actually be. Parents exhibit excessive unwarranted concerns and seek health care for their child frequently. Risk factors for the development of vulnerable child syndrome include pregnancy-related problems (e.g., illness, history of miscarriage, infertility), preterm birth, low birth weight, and an illness or threat to life while the child is quite young (Verbeek et al., 2021). Parental fears result in extreme concern and overprotection, inability to trust another caregiver with their children, and lack of setting age-appropriate boundaries, thereby threatening the child's development (Verbeek et al., 2021). The child may also develop difficult behaviors such as aggression, conduct issues, or hyperactivity, or they may develop a disease role and have sleep issues, anxiety, and chronic physical complaints (Verbeek et al., 2021).

Effects on Siblings

The siblings of children with special health care needs may also be dramatically affected. Their relationship with their parents is different from what it would have been if their sibling had been healthy. Parents often need to spend more time with the child with special health care needs and have less time with the siblings (Sewell-Roberts, 2021). Children exhibit emotional and psychological responses to a sibling's long-term needs (Lummer-Aikey & Goldstein, 2021). The sibling's knowledge about the illness, their attitude toward and adjustment to it, their own self-esteem, how socially supported they are, and the parents' awareness of their feelings are all related to how well the sibling adjusts.

Nursing Management of the Child With Special Health Care Needs and Their Family

Family-centered care provides the optimal framework for caring for all children and their families. Family-centered care can also minimize the impact of chronic illness and maximize the child's developmental potential. To provide the best nursing care for children with special health care needs and their families, the nurse must first develop a trusting relationship with the family.

To ensure optimal functioning, children with special health care needs require comprehensive and coordinated services from multiple professionals. These professionals should work collaboratively to address the child's health, educational, psychological, and social service needs. In addition to case management and advocacy, nursing management focuses on screening and ongoing assessment of the child, provision of home care, care of the child with technology needs, education and support of the child and family, and referral for resources.

Developing a Therapeutic Relationship

Raising children always has the potential to be challenging, but a child's additional health care needs can completely overwhelm a parent. The parents' needs change continuously, so it is best if the family has a stable, long-term relationship with a primary health care provider. This promotes trust and a more efficient two-way flow of information.

Respect the parents' range of emotions and work with them as a team to manage the child's care. Nurses should recognize when parents are successful in adhering to the treatment plan or when other small gains are made. Empowering the family strengthens them and gives them self-confidence. Feeling supported and invigorated gives parents and caregivers strength, energy, and hope. Box 12.1 lists principles related to family involvement.

Screening and Ongoing Assessment

Nurses should perform screening to identify children with unmet health care needs. Children with special health care needs may attain developmental milestones

BOX 12.1 Principles Related to Family Involvement

Families:
- Are the constant in a child's life
- Need to have access to information and training
- Deserve to receive culturally respectful care
- Know their strengths, limitations, and fears
- Merit mutual respect and responsibility for outcomes

Adapted from de Leon Siantz, M. L., Kilanowski, J. F., & Thomas, T. L. (2018). Cultural values, beliefs, and preference are integral to family-centered care. In C. L. Betz, M. J. Krajicek, & M. Craft-Rosenberg (Eds.), *Guidelines for nursing excellence in the care of children, youth, and families* (2nd ed.). Springer Publishing Company.

more slowly than other children. If a developmental screening tool is used for ongoing developmental surveillance of the young child, then the results should be compared visit to visit to determine progress rather than using it as a screening tool. Assess these families for vulnerable child syndrome.

Promoting Home Care

Home is the most developmentally appropriate environment for all children, even those who have technology needs. The child's home can be an emotionally nurturing and socially stimulating environment. Receiving care in the home allows children with technology needs to display improved physical, emotional, psychological, and social status (Mitchell et al., 2022).

Technology needs for children may include supplemental oxygen, assisted ventilation, tracheostomy care, assisted enteral or parenteral feeding, or parenteral medication administration. With advances in technology, children with extensive medical and developmental needs may be cared for at home, and the decision for home care should be undertaken seriously by the health care team and family (Blanco et al., 2021). Early discharge planning is important, and parents will need detailed instructions and support in caring for children using these devices at home (CCHMC, 2022).

EARLY DISCHARGE PLANNING

Early discharge planning and ongoing inclusion and education of the family facilitates continuity of care. Box 12.2 provides information about preparing the child with special health care needs for discharge.

BOX 12.2 Preparing for Home Care Before Discharge

- Promote liaison with community resources. Develop communication between various services. Plan appointments. Set up home nursing care (either private duty or visits).
- Teach skills, encouraging active caregiving in the hospital setting to increase the caregivers' self-confidence.
- Discuss psychological and emotional issues with parents.
- Obtain and organize equipment and supplies (running out of supplies may cause significant stress on families).
- Refer the family for necessary financial resources.
- Ensure the family's home environment is adequate (e.g., enough room for equipment, electricity on, air conditioner for warm weather, heater for cold weather, refrigeration for food).
- For the baby being discharged from the neonatal intensive care unit (NICU):
  - Teach the parents about the infant's cues and behaviors and the different sleep–wake patterns.
  - Encourage kangaroo care and infant massage while in the NICU (as the infant's condition allows).
  - Educate the parents about possible effects on short- and long-term neurodevelopment.
  - Refer to a local early intervention program.
  - Assist the family with finding a primary care provider who is experienced in the ongoing follow-up of high-risk infants.

Adapted from Smith, V. C., & Stewart, J. (2023). Discharge planning for high-risk newborns. UpToDate. Retrieved on November 5, 2023, from https://www.uptodate.com/contents/discharge-planning-for-high-risk-newborns

CARING FOR THE CHILD WITH TECHNOLOGY NEEDS AT HOME

Home care nurses are often involved in the care of children with technology needs. Caring for a child who requires these devices at home can be a complex process, but children thrive in the home care setting with appropriate intervention and care. Improved collaboration between parents and home care nurses may decrease the parents' stress and maximize opportunities for appropriate growth and development in the child with technology needs. Thus, a strong relationship, good communication, and effective negotiation skills are assets to the family and child.

Help the family incorporate the medical regimen into daily life to minimize the child's potential perception of being different from other children. Teach families about the technical processes related to home and travel oxygen therapy, use of the ventilator, suctioning, chest percussion and postural drainage, tube feedings and care of the feeding tube, and medications. Assist parents with the planning and management of routine care, respiratory treatments, nutritional support, and developmental interventions. Reinforce exercises and techniques as prescribed by developmental therapists. Refer to Chapter 11 for additional information about home care nursing.

Providing Care Coordination

Once a child with special health care needs has been discharged to the home setting, the nurse plays a vital role in care coordination. Any child with special health care needs benefits from a medical home for their primary care, as it provides continuous, accessible, comprehensive services (National Resource Center for Patient/Family-Centered Medical Home, 2020). See the Healthy People 2030 box.

HEALTHY PEOPLE 2030

Objective	Nursing Significance
Increase the proportion of children with special health care needs who have a system of care that is family-centered, comprehensive, and coordinated.	Refer the child and family with special needs to an integrated health program that provides interdisciplinary, collaborative care for children requiring complex, coordinated care.

Healthy People Objectives retrieved from http://www.healthypeople.gov

The nurse in the medical home is a critical team member, providing ongoing care coordination and follow-up. The nurse can best benefit the family by being available to the family as needed and providing the support they need as they learn how to deal with the child's care needs at home. Refer to Box 12.3 for nursing interventions for families of children with special health care needs.

Providing Ongoing Follow-Up of the Former Premature Infant

Many former premature infants experience medical and developmental problems throughout infancy, early childhood, and beyond. Upon or following discharge, many former premature infants display one or more of the following medical or developmental problems:

- Chronic lung disease (bronchopulmonary dysplasia)
- Cardiac changes such as right ventricular hypertrophy and pulmonary artery hypertension
- Growth delays, poor feeding, anemia of prematurity, other nutrient deficiencies
- Apnea of prematurity, gastroesophageal reflux disease, bradycardia
- Sudden unexplained infant death (SUID)
- Osteopenia (rickets) of prematurity
- Hydrocephalus, ventriculomegaly, abnormal head magnetic resonance imaging results, ventriculoperitoneal shunt
- Inguinal or umbilical hernias
- Retinopathy of prematurity, strabismus, decreased visual acuity
- Hearing deficits
- Delayed dentition
- Gross motor skills, fine motor skills, and language development delay; sensory integration issues (Stewart, 2023)

BOX 12.3 Nursing Interventions for Families of Children With Special Health Care Needs

- Develop written health plans.
- Provide care coordination and collaboration with specialists in other disciplines, early intervention, schools, and public agencies.
- Address needs for prior authorization for treatments, medications, or specialist referrals; retain copies in the child's chart of authorization forms and approvals.
- Modify office routines to promote family and child comfort.
- Assist parents with child care decisions.
- Know community resources available to children with special health care needs.
- When the child is hospitalized, encourage high levels of parental participation.
- Provide care coordination across multiple health settings.
- Educate child care providers on child health needs.
- Help parents get involved with parent support networks.

Adapted from Cincinnati Children's Hospital Medical Center. (2023). *Ongoing support resources. https://www.cincinnatichildrens.org/patients/child/special-needs*; Kuo, D. Z., & Turchi, R. M. (2023). Children and youth with special health care needs. UpToDate. Retrieved on November 5, 2023, from https://www.uptodate.com/contents/children-and-youth-with-special-health-care-needs

Over the long term, former premature infants are at higher risk than full-term infants of developing cognitive delay, cerebral palsy, attention-deficit/hyperactivity disorder, learning disabilities, difficulties with socialization, and vulnerable child syndrome (Mandy, 2023; Stewart, 2023). In addition, many former premature infants display alterations in muscle tone at or shortly after discharge from the neonatal intensive care unit (NICU) that require physical therapy intervention.

For these reasons, former premature infants require special attention and thorough, appropriate assessment to discern subtle changes that may affect their long-term physical, cognitive, emotional, and social outcome. The pediatric nurse should have an understanding of the special concerns that former premature infants and children as well as their families may face (Fig. 12.3).

From the beginning, encourage families to keep all of the infant's pertinent check-up, insurance, and medical and developmental information; this will serve as a resource for the parents, and they will be able to supply complete information when visiting various providers.

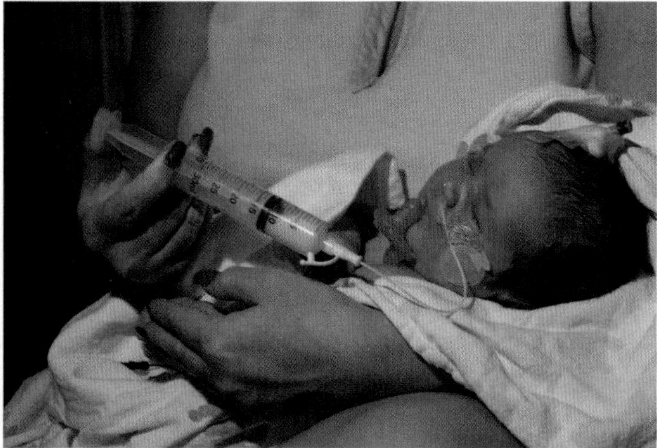

FIGURE 12.3 Parents of an infant discharged from the neonatal intensive care unit (NICU) may need to administer special care, such as feeding.

PROVIDING ROUTINE WELL-CHILD CARE TO THE FORMER PREMATURE INFANT

Former premature infants require similar well-child care as full-term infants do, with additional visits for management of any complex medical issues and developmental screenings or interventions. Teach families routine newborn care, including bathing, dressing, and avoidance of cigarette smoke. All visits for primary care follow-up will be scheduled based on the infant's chronologic age.

Prior to discharge from the NICU, the infant will be tested for oxygen desaturation while seated in the car seat (Smith & Stewart, 2023). Clearance will be obtained prior to the infant's discharge. Former premature infants require car seat use just as other infants do. Help the parents find methods of padding the car seat or adding an additional semifirm cushion inside the seat for the infant to ride in the car safely. Some infants may need to continue cardiac/apnea monitoring while in the car seat. Since the former premature infant is at increased risk for SUID compared to the general population, it is critical to teach parents to put the infant on their back to sleep (Stewart, 2023).

Give immunizations according to the current immunization schedule recommended by the Centers for Disease Control and Prevention (CDC) based on the infant's chronologic age. All former premature infants should receive the flu vaccine as recommended after 6 months' chronologic age. Respiratory syncytial virus (RSV) prophylaxis is critical for certain groups of premature infants (Stewart, 2023). Therefore, administer the palivizumab (Synagis) vaccine according to the recommended schedule (refer to Chapter 18 for additional information about RSV prophylaxis).

ASSESSING GROWTH AND DEVELOPMENT OF THE FORMER PREMATURE INFANT

When assessing growth and development of the infant or child who was born prematurely, determine the child's adjusted or corrected age so that you can perform an accurate assessment. The corrected or adjusted age should be used for evaluating progression in growth as well as development. For example, if a 6-month-old infant was born at 28 weeks' gestation (12 weeks, or 3 months early), their growth and development expectations are those of a 3-month-old (corrected age). Continue to correct age for growth and development until the child is 3 years old.

Although breast milk is the preferred form of nutrition for former premature infants, many require special diets to foster catch-up growth (Stewart, 2023). Extra calories are necessary for increased growth needs. Additional calcium and phosphorus are required for bone mineralization. For these reasons, former premature infants should be fed breast milk fortified with additional nutrients or a commercially prepared formula specifically for premature infants. When former premature infants demonstrate consistent adequate growth (usually by 6 months corrected age), they may be switched to a "term infant formula" such as Similac or Enfamil, concentrated to a higher caloric density if needed. Assess the infant's ability to suck efficiently and refer them to occupational or speech therapy if the infant is a slow feeder or has difficulty feeding.

All anticipatory guidance related to nutrition is based on the child's corrected age (The Warren Center, 2023). In other words, begin solid foods at 6 months' corrected age, not chronologic age, and delay the addition of whole milk until 12 months' corrected age, rather than chronologic age. Signs that the former premature infant may be ready to attempt spoon-feeding include interest in feeding, decrease in tongue thrust, and adequate head control.

Early screening and intervention for issues related to development are critical to the attainment of optimal development in the former premature infant. The comorbidities that they exhibit in the form of prior and current medical problems place these infants at high risk for **developmental delay** (lag in meeting developmental milestones). Even mild developmental delays warrant evaluation and intervention. Developmental screening tools may be used to screen for developmental concerns in the former premature infant, although they do not always identify children at risk. Parent-report questionnaires demonstrate fairly accurate estimations of developmental problems and are simple to use. Most importantly, assess the child's development based on corrected age until the child is 3 years old. Refer infants and children early if developmental concerns are suspected.

Identifying and Managing Undernutrition and Feeding Disorders in Children With Special Health Care Needs

Undernutrition can cause inadequate growth in infants and children. The child fails to demonstrate appropriate weight gain over a prolonged period of time. Length or height velocity and head circumference growth may also be affected. Risk factors for undernutrition include malignancy, developmental disability, and chronic illness, among others (Bamberger et al., 2022). Adequate nutrition is critical for appropriate brain growth in the first 3 years of life and for growth in general throughout childhood and adolescence (Seymour, 2021).

Undernutrition can be a multifactorial problem. **Developmental disability** (mental or physical or combination impairment resulting in lifelong disability) may contribute to undernutrition, as the child's ability to consume adequate nutrition is impaired because of sensory or motor delays, such as with cerebral palsy. Other organic causes of undernutrition include inability to suck or swallow correctly, malabsorption, diarrhea, vomiting, or alterations in metabolism and caloric/nutrient needs associated with a variety of chronic illnesses. Infants and children with cardiac or metabolic disease, chronic lung disease (bronchopulmonary dysplasia), cleft palate, or gastroesophageal reflux disease are at particular risk. Feeding disorders or food refusal may occur in infants or children who have required prolonged mechanical ventilation, long-term enteral tube feedings, or an unpleasant event such as a choking episode. Additional causes of undernutrition include family income below the poverty threshold, neglect, abuse, behavioral problems, lack of appropriate parental interaction, poor feeding techniques, lack of parental knowledge, or parental mental illness (Bamberger et al., 2022).

Screen all children for undernutrition to identify it early. In addition to poor growth, the infant or child with undernutrition may present with a history of developmental delay or loss of acquired milestones. Infants or children with feeding problems may display nipple, spoon, or food refusal; difficulty sucking; disinterest in feeding; or difficulty progressing from liquid to puréed to textured food. Perform a detailed dietary history, and instruct the parents to complete a 3-day food diary to identify what the child actually eats and drinks. Assess the parent–child interaction, with particular attention to the parent's ability to read and respond to the infant's or child's cues. Observe feeding, noting the child's oral interest or aversion, oral–motor coordination, and swallowing ability, as well as parent–child interactions before, during, and after the feeding (Bamberger et al., 2022).

Significant undernutrition may require hospitalization for evaluation and management. Sometimes, enteral tube feedings are necessary in order for children with undernutrition or feeding disorders to demonstrate adequate growth (Duryea, 2023). Box 12.4 lists nursing interventions for the hospitalized child with undernutrition.

TAKE NOTE!

Infants and children who have experienced neglect may not interact appropriately with their environment or caregiver (lack of eye contact) (Duryea, 2023).

BOX 12.4 Nursing Interventions During Hospitalization for Undernutrition

- Observe parent–child interactions, especially during feedings.
- Develop an appropriate feeding schedule.
- Provide feedings as prescribed (usually, 120 kcal/kg/day is needed to demonstrate proper weight gain).
- Weigh the child daily and maintain strict records of intake and output.
- Educate parents about proper feeding techniques and volumes.
- Provide extensive support to alleviate parental anxiety related to the child's inability to gain weight.

Adapted from Duryea, T. K. (2023). Poor weight gain in children younger than two years in resource-abundant countries: Management. *UpToDate.* Retrieved on November 5, 2023, from https://www.uptodate.com/contents/poor-weight-gain-in-children-younger-than-two-years-in-resource-abundant-countries-management

Promoting Growth and Development

When caring for the infant with special health care needs in the hospital, provide consistent caregivers to encourage the infant to develop a sense of trust. Allow and encourage the parent to stay with the infant, providing a comfortable place for the parent to sleep. To promote attachment, emphasize the baby's positive qualities. Encourage developmentally appropriate skills, and allow the infant to have pleasurable experiences through all of the senses.

For the toddler, begin developmentally appropriate limit setting and discipline. Encourage independence as the toddler is able. Modify gross motor and sensory activities to accommodate the toddler's limitations. To encourage a sense of control, offer the toddler simple choices.

As the preschooler develops, encourage mastery of self-help skills as the child is able. Encourage socialization with same-age peers to develop a sense of friendship. Reinforce to the child that an illness or disability is not a punishment for wrongdoing or the child's fault in any way.

Encourage the school-age child to attend school and make up work that must be missed for medical treatments or appointments. Provide education to the school staff and other students about the child's special needs. Promote involvement in appropriate sports activities; music, drama, or art activities; and clubs such as Boy Scouts or Girl Scouts. Educate the child about the illness or disability and the course of treatment.

Inform parents of adolescents that those with chronic illnesses often participate in the same activities as those without, such as risk taking, rebelling, and trying out different identities. Assist the adolescent with coping and interpersonal skills. Promote involvement in activities with other adolescents with special health care needs as well as those without. Ensure that the adolescent participates in rites of passage as able, such as attending the prom or obtaining a driver's license. Discuss future plans with the adolescent, such as college or vocation, as well as transition to a non-pediatric health care provider (Blanco et al., 2021).

Providing Resources to the Child and Family

Nurses should be familiar with community resources available to children with special health care needs. Educational opportunities for children with special health care needs include early intervention programs and programs offered through the public school system. Financial resources, respite care, and complementary therapies are other areas with which the nurse should become familiar.

EDUCATIONAL OPPORTUNITIES FOR THE CHILD WITH SPECIAL HEALTH CARE NEEDS

The foundation for health and development in children is laid during the first few years of life. Children with special health care needs often require multiple developmental interventions and special education in the early years in order to reach their developmental potential later in childhood. Children learn best when they are at the stage of maximal readiness, and the early years must not be missed as an opportunity for development. See the Healthy People 2030 box.

HEALTHY PEOPLE 2030

Objective	Nursing Significance
Increase the proportion of children and youth with disabilities who are usually in regular education programs.	• Ensure that children younger than 3 years who may qualify are referred to the local early intervention program. • Encourage families to advocate for their child's needs on the individualized education plan.

Healthy People Objectives retrieved from http://www.healthypeople.gov

Early intervention programs are intended to enhance the development of infants and toddlers with or at risk for disabilities, thereby minimizing educational costs and special education. Early intervention is also directed toward enhancing the capacity of families to meet their children's needs as well as to maximize the likelihood of independent living (CDC, 2022).

The Individuals with Disabilities Education Improvement Act of 2004 (formerly called Public Law 99–457) mandates government-funded care coordination and special education for children up to 3 years of age. This early intervention program is administered through each state. Federal law allows each state to define developmental disability differently, but, in general, qualified personnel perform an evaluation of the child's physical, language, emotional, and social capabilities to determine eligibility (U.S. Department of Education [USDE], n.d.). The law guarantees that eligible children will obtain access to services that will enhance their development. Children who qualify for services receive care coordination, and an individualized family service plan is developed by the service coordinator in conjunction with the family. The service coordinator manages the developmental services and special education that the child requires.

The intent of the program is that the child receives services in a nonmedical environment, so most services occur in the home or day care center. Home visits by the service coordinator and maintenance of regular contact with the family ensure the success of the program.

Refer children who may have developmental delay to the local early intervention program. For children receiving these services, collaborate with the service coordinator on an ongoing basis with particular involvement at hospital discharge and when transition of services occurs at age 3 years.

> Think back to Preet, the 2-year-old boy with a history of hydrocephalus and developmental delay, from the beginning of the chapter. After further discussion with Preet's parent, you realize he has not been involved in an early intervention program. Discuss with his parent the educational opportunities that are available for Preet and why they are important.

Schools may have a profound impact on the child's overall health and development. Some children with special needs do not require additional services to succeed in school. For these children, the nurse's role is to assess for school success or failure and determine the effect of the school environment on the child's health. The Individuals with Disabilities Education Act, reauthorized in 2004, provides for the education of children with special needs through the public school system, from ages 3 to 21 years. These services are provided within the public school system.

According to the law, each student with special health care needs is entitled to an individualized education program (IEP), which is a written plan designed to meet the preschool, primary, or secondary school student's individual needs. A committee consisting of the child's parent, a regular teacher, a special education teacher, and various other specialists develops the IEP. Nurses may be called to serve on this committee. The IEP must include measurable short- and long-term goals. Parents are informed of the student's progress routinely, and the IEP is reviewed at least annually (USDE, n.d.).

Preschool special education through the local public school system is provided from ages 3 to 5 years; access to the curriculum is ensured for all children. A child is eligible for special education preschool when a significant delay is present in the cognitive, language, adaptive, social–emotional, or motor development domains to the extent that it adversely affects the child's learning ability. In the school setting, the child receives developmental therapy as needed to augment their ability to participate in the education process. The least restrictive environment is preferred, with children with special health care needs participating in classes containing age-appropriate peers without special health care needs whenever possible (USDE, n.d.). Special education preschool services are often offered in the elementary school setting.

FINANCIAL AND INSURANCE RESOURCES

Many children with special health care needs whose families demonstrate financial need may be eligible for Supplemental Security Income (SSI). This program was created in 1972 through Public Law 92–603. SSI is a cash assistance program, and monthly benefits vary per individual. SSI qualification usually makes the child eligible for state-administered Medicaid (Social Security Administration [SSA], n.d.-a). Medicaid benefits vary slightly from state to state, but generally cover medical visits, medication, hospitalization, and limited adjuvant therapies. The Children's Health Insurance Program (CHIP) provides low-cost health insurance to eligible children. Eligibility and the extent of benefits provided by CHIP vary by state (Centers for Medicare and Medicaid Services, n.d.). Title V programs under the MCHB block grant program provide funds to the individual states for administration of services. State Title V programs provide community-based, comprehensive service coordination for children with special health care needs (SSA, n.d.-b). Online directories providing a wealth of links to resources for children with special health care needs include Children's Disabilities Information and Special Child.

RESPITE CARE

Primary caregivers of children with special health care needs must be dedicated, skillful, vigilant, and knowledgeable. Constant care can be a stress on the primary caregiver, who needs temporary relief from the daily caregiving demands. **Respite care** provides an opportunity for families to take a break from the daily intensive caregiving responsibilities. Respite care should meet the child's health care needs and offer the child developmental opportunities. Finding and using respite care that the family is comfortable with and trusts may decrease the family's stress and lead to an enhanced quality of life for these families. Nurses can facilitate access to respite care, educate respite providers, and ensure quality respite care practices through involvement in community agencies.

COMPLEMENTARY THERAPIES

Families of children with special health care needs often use adjuvant therapies. These may include homeopathic and herbal medicine, pet therapy, hippotherapy, music, and massage, among others. Many families may want to blend complementary and alternative therapies with mainstream medicine in search of palliation or a cure. When obtaining the health history, ask specifically about homeopathy or herbal medications the child may be taking.

TAKE NOTE!

Become familiar with the risks and benefits of homeopathic and herbal medications as well as any contraindications, as many families use these treatments in an effort to improve their child's quality of life or outcome.

Hippotherapy is the use of equine movement for the engagement of the sensory, neuromuscular, and cognitive systems resulting in achievement of functional outcomes. Occupational and physical therapists as well as speech-language pathologists utilize evidence-based practice and clinical reasoning to provide purposeful movement of the horse with the child riding. Hippotherapy should not be confused with therapeutic horseback riding or adaptive horseback riding. In hippotherapy, the pathologist or therapist chooses specific horse movements for therapeutic exercise, neuromuscular re-education, therapeutic activities, or treatment of speech, language, voice, communication, and auditory processing disorder. Additional information may be obtained through the American Hippotherapy Association (2022) at www.americanhippotherapyassociation.org.

Pet therapy may be used to decrease stress or as a component of psychotherapy. Music may be used to induce positive behavioral changes, reduce pain or stress, or induce various other positive effects (American Music Therapy Association, 2023). Massage therapy may be beneficial to a wide variety of children. It may be used to reduce pain, promote relaxation, decrease fear, and demonstrate a specific positive effect related to the child's particular medical condition (Genik et al., 2020).

Providing Support and Education

At the time of initial diagnosis, allow and encourage the family to express their feelings. Parents of children with special health care needs require emotional, practical, economic, and social support. Encourage parents to obtain help with daily routines. Encourage stress reduction for the parents through exercise and allowing time for themselves. Be a supportive and encouraging listener, and be sure to nurture the whole child, rather than just treating their condition. Refer to Evidence-Based Practice Box 12.1.

Parents may value peer support groups, sometimes feeling that only other parents in similar situations could understand the emotions they experience (Foster et al., 2022). Pediatric nurses should be proactive in helping families find support systems.

Each parent may react differently. It is important for nurses to involve each parent in the child's care. Teach skills to each parent, and actively involve both parents by asking about their observations and opinions.

Parents become the experts on their child's needs and care, and they should be recognized as such. Parents want to be taken seriously and do not like being ignored. They should be viewed as having reliable and valuable information about their children. By being an active and reflective listener, the nurse can demonstrate to the parents that their opinion is valued, in addition to finding out what the child really needs. Some parents may hesitate to volunteer information, unsure about what information the nurse needs. Show respect for the parents' knowledge of their child's needs by seeking advice on the child's daily care, medical and physical needs, and current developmental level, no matter what the site of care is (Foster et al., 2022).

Families may need additional support from the nurse at times of transition. As the equipment or treatment needs change, adjust the teaching plan. Educate the child and family about the use of adaptive equipment.

EVIDENCE-BASED PRACTICE 12.1

Caring for Children With Technology Needs at Home

STUDY

Caring for a child who has technology needs at home can be an overwhelming task for parents. A qualitative descriptive study examined parents' perceptions of what was most helpful versus what wasn't in providing this care. A convenience sample of 103 participants was utilized.

Findings

Items identified as helpful included emotional support from partners, other family members, and nurses; positive thoughts; hope; self-care; respite care; and work flexibility.

NURSING IMPLICATIONS

Provide emotional support to families caring for children with technology needs at home. Encourage parents to incorporate positivity and self-care into their daily routines. Assist families with obtaining resources for respite care.

Data from Toly, V. B., Blanchette, J. E., & Musil, C. M. (2019). Mothers caring for technology-dependent children at home: What is most helpful and least helpful? *Applied Nursing Research*, *46*, 24–27. https://doi.org/10.1016/j.apnr.2019.02.001

Ensure families understand how specific activities must be modified to accommodate the child's needs. Provide anticipatory guidance related to expected developmental changes, including resources and laws related to education. Act as a liaison between the family and the day care center or school. As the child grows and matures, encourage parents to relinquish caregiving tasks to the child as appropriate to encourage independence and promote self-esteem.

Assisting the Adolescent With Special Health Care Needs Making the Transition to Adulthood

Adolescence is a time of physical changes, psychosocial challenges, and initiation of independence from parents. The adolescent with a chronic illness or one who has technology needs may experience this period differently from others. Puberty can be affected by chronic illness, either delaying it or expediting it. Chronic illness may lead to isolation from peers at a time when peer interaction is the core of psychosocial development. Adolescents may struggle to fit in with their peers by hiding their illness or health care needs, not adhering well to treatment regimens, or participating in risky behaviors. At a time when the child should be developing independence from the parents, they may be experiencing significant dependence related to their health condition. For these reasons, the adolescent with special health care needs may require increased amounts of support from the nurse.

Making the transition to adult care for a child with special health care needs can be difficult, and advance planning leads to a smoother transition. Transition planning involves multidisciplinary care coordination; acknowledgment of the changing roles among the adolescent, family, and health care professionals; and fostering of the adolescent's self-determination skills. A written plan for transition to adult care should be initiated in midadolescence. Have ongoing conversations with the adolescent about this transition. Issues to be resolved prior to the transition include financial resources for medical care, college or vocational school attendance, living arrangements, and caregiving arrangements (Ellison et al., 2022).

Recommendations for successful transition include:

- At age 12 to 14 years, ensure that the adolescent is aware of the facility's transition policy, and continue to reinforce at visits.
- Track the adolescent's transition progress via a registry.
- Plan for transition services with the adolescent and family, including health care goals, emergency planning, and legal changes.
- With the adolescent and family, identify an adult provider.
- Complete a full transition plan/packet (Ellison et al., 2022).

Before moving to adult care with an adult medical provider, ensure that the adolescent understands the treatment rationale, symptoms of worsening condition, and especially danger signs. Teach the adolescent about when to seek help from a health professional. Introduce the adolescent to the medical insurance process. At transition, coordinate a seamless transfer by providing a detailed written plan to the care coordinator or advanced practice nurse after verbal collaboration. After the transition, serve as a consultant to the adult office in relation to the adolescent's needs. Consult with a transition services coordinator or other service agency as available in the local community. See the Healthy People 2030 box.

HEALTHY PEOPLE 2030

Objective	Nursing Significance
Increase the proportion of youth (ages 12–17) with or without special health care needs, who receive services to support their transition to adult health care.	• In the primary care setting, assist families with planning for transition beginning in early adolescence. • If available, refer families to multidisciplinary programs for children with medically complex needs.

Healthy People Objectives retrieved from http://www.healthypeople.gov

THE CHILD WHO IS DYING

Each year, the death rate for children 1 to 14 years of age is 17.2 per 100,000 children (Kaiser Family Foundation [KFF], 2023a). The death rate for infants is much higher, at 5.4 per 1,000 live births (KFF, 2023b). A child's chronic illness may progress to the point of becoming a **terminal illness**, one deemed to be noncurable, ultimately leading to death. Despite the increased survival rates for children with cancer as a result of improved treatment options and protocols, cancer remains the leading cause of death from disease in all children older than 1 year (CDC, n.d.). Less frequently, other diseases also lead to terminal illness in children, such as congenital defects and cardiovascular and neurologic disorders (Adistie et al., 2020). Pediatric nurses will inevitably encounter situations in which a child dies. These situations are extremely difficult for all people involved, and the nurse plays a key role in caring for the dying child and their family. Caring for the child who is dying is a family-centered, multidisciplinary process. Nurses must respond to the child's and family's physiologic, emotional, and spiritual needs during this difficult time. Children display differing responses to the dying process and impending death, depending on their developmental level. Children and their families need significant amounts of support throughout the process of dying.

End-of-Life Decision Making

Parents are obligated not only to protect their children from harm but also to do as much good for them as possible, from both an ethical and a legal standpoint. When the time comes for end-of-life decision making, parents are often torn about the "right" course of action. Parents may be asked to make decisions about stopping treatment, withdrawing treatment, providing palliative care, or consenting to "do not resuscitate" (DNR) orders. Children, parents, and health care providers are generally in agreement that continued suffering is not desired for any child with a terminal illness. When all possible curative attempts have been made, then survival is no longer possible (Shaw et al., 2021).

Nurses involved in this process must examine their own values related to dying and consider the American Nurses Association's *Code of Ethics for Nurses* (2015) as well. The family's feelings must also be acknowledged. During the process of end-of-life decision making, health care providers must assure families that the focus of care is changing and that the child is not being abandoned. Emphasize to parents that no matter what their decision is, the health care team is dedicated to the comfort and expert care of their child (Stokes, 2021).

Ensure communication is family-centered. Quality of life must be taken into consideration when making decisions to continue or withhold treatment. Provide parents facing end-of-life decisions with honest information and education from the time of the diagnosis and prognosis forward. Anticipate that parents may vacillate in the decision-making process. Clarify information for them and allow them private time to discuss the options. Do not make judgments about or question the parents' decision. Be sensitive to any ethnic, spiritual, or cultural preferences during the terminal stage of the illness. Encourage parents to interact with other parents who have a child with a terminal illness (Cacciatore et al., 2019).

Allowing Natural Death

The decision to institute a DNR order is one of the most difficult decisions a family may make. DNR refers to withholding cardiopulmonary resuscitation should the child's heart stop beating. Parents may initially feel like this means they are giving up on their child. Nurses must educate families that resuscitation may be inappropriate and lead to more suffering than if death were allowed to occur naturally. The parents need to understand that when a **palliative care** (specialized care for a serious or terminal illness) route is chosen, rather than continuing a curative or treatment route, the focus of the child's care is changing, but the child and family are not being abandoned. Families may wish to specify a certain extent of resuscitation that they feel more comfortable with (e.g., allowing supplemental oxygen but not providing chest compressions). Some institutions are now replacing the DNR terminology with "allow natural death" (AND), which may be more acceptable to families facing the decision to withhold resuscitation.

Involving the Child Who Is Dying in the Decision-Making Process

End-of-life decision making often involves ethical dilemmas for the child, family, and health care team. This is particularly true when the parents' wishes conflict with the child's or adolescent's desires. Children should be involved in decision making to the extent that they are able. Discuss intervention within the context of the child's condition and wishes. Children of sufficient maturity may assent to the continuation or withdrawal of treatment (National Association of Pediatric Nurse Practitioners et al., 2020). Be available to the older child or adolescent to provide support and information if they desire. Talk with the child or adolescent with the parents present, as well as in private. Maintain the child's comfort and dignity. Encourage the child to spend time with other children with a terminal illness. Assure the child that everything will be done to make them comfortable. Consult parents about the timing and depth of end-of-life discussions. Just as parents do, the child with a terminal illness may vacillate in the decision-making process. Remain sensitive and respect the child's decisions.

Organ or Tissue Donation

With large numbers of organ transplant candidates on waiting lists and the shortage of viable organs, pediatric organ and tissue donation is a priority (Vyas & Nakagawa, 2023). For many families, knowing that a child's organs or tissues may save another child's life provides a way to help others despite their own loss. A healthy child who dies unexpectedly is a good candidate for organ donation. Many chronic illnesses in children preclude the option of organ or tissue donation, although individual determinations of eligibility should be made.

The discussion of organ donation should be separated from the discussion of impending death or brain death notification. Written consent is necessary for organ donation, so the family must be appropriately informed and educated. Many families who never thought about it before may consider the option of donation if adequately educated about the process. All expenses for organ procurement are borne by the recipient's family, not the donor's. Ask whether the child who is dying ever expressed a wish to donate organs and whether the parents have considered it.

Families need to know that procurement of the organs does not mar the child's appearance, so an open casket at the child's funeral is still possible if the family desires. The donating child will not suffer further because of organ donation. The organs or tissues will be harvested in a timely fashion after the declaration of death, so the family need not worry about delay of end-of-life rituals. The family's cultural and religious beliefs must be considered, and the team discussing organ donation with the family must do so in a sensitive and ethical manner (Vyas & Nakagawa, 2023).

Palliative Care of the Child Who Is Dying

Appropriate palliative care is essential for any child with a life-threatening or progressive incurable condition (Hauer, 2023). Whether palliative care is provided in the home, hospital, or hospice setting, the goal is to provide the best quality of life possible at the end of life while alleviating physical, psychological, emotional, and spiritual suffering (Hauer, 2023). Palliative care of children should be based on the following principles:

- Respect for the child's goals, preferences, and choices
- Acknowledgment and addressing of caregiver's concerns
- Provision of a comprehensive, interdisciplinary continuum of care in the community
- Competent and ethical care

Hospice Care

Hospice allows for family-centered care in the child's home or a hospice facility. As with adult hospice care, the comfort of the entire family is important. The goal of pediatric hospice care is enhancement of quality of life for the child and family through an individualized plan of care. The recommended standards for pediatric hospice care allow for palliative care to be given concurrently with potentially curative treatments, and thus hope is not lessened (Hauer, 2023). Parents are educated on ways to comfort and interact with their dying child, such as massage, movement, or singing. Spiritual support is available through a chaplain, a social worker, or the family's minister. The nurse not only educates the family about the dying process but also assists them with providing basic care and pain management. The decision to withhold nutrition or hydration may be made in certain instances. Anticipating and preventing symptoms, including pain, while managing them if they do occur is of the utmost importance (Hauer, 2023). Ongoing bereavement care is also provided to the family by the hospice after the child's death.

Nursing Management of the Child Who Is Dying

Although interdisciplinary care is essential for quality care at the end of life, it is the nurse who plays the key role of child/family advocate and who is usually the constant presence throughout the dying process. Nursing management of the child who is dying focuses on managing pain and discomfort, providing nutrition, providing emotional support to the child and family, and assisting the family through the grief process. Throughout the process, it is important to focus on the family as the unit of care.

Managing Pain and Discomfort

Pain management is an essential component of care for the child with a terminal illness. Adequately managing pain may enhance the child's quality of life and minimize suffering. Assess pain using a developmentally appropriate tool (see Chapter 14 for further information). Provide pain medication around the clock rather than on an as-needed basis to prevent recurrence or escalation of pain. Determine the child's preferred comfort measures and use them to provide additional relief. Change the child's position frequently but gently to minimize discomfort. Limit nursing care to comfort measures that ease the child's discomfort. Maintain a calm environment, minimizing noise and light. Include integrative care interventions such as massage or healing touch as requested and tolerated.

Providing Nutrition

Since the body naturally requires less nutrition as the child is dying, do not excessively coax the child to eat or drink. Offer frequent small meals or snacks of the child's choosing. Soups and shakes require less energy to eat and so may be desirable. If the child desires a different food, provide that one. Keep strong odors away from the child to decrease nausea. Administer antiemetics as needed. Provide mouth care and keep the lips lubricated to keep the mouth feeling clean and prevent the discomfort associated with chapped lips. Make sure the environment is a pleasant one for eating.

Providing Emotional Support to the Child and Family

Be attuned to the entire family's needs and emotions in order to foster a holistic connection with the child and family. Nurses provide physical care through specific tasks and interventions for the child who is dying, but they also need to be fully present emotionally with the child and family. Many people are uncomfortable with the concept of a dying child. Nurses should work through their own feelings about the situation in order to stay fully present with the child and family, attending to their individualized needs. Families and children who are dying benefit from the presence of the nurse, not just the interventions they perform.

Ask yourself what you need to do in order to be fully present with the child and family. Listen to the child and family; be still and silent for a time to accomplish this. Foster respect for the whole child by attending to them as such (Broden et al., 2020).

Respect the parents by helping them honor the commitments they have made to their child. Acknowledge that parents have diverse needs for information and participation in decision making. Allow and encourage family customs or rituals in relation to death and dying. Families may want a faith leader to be present when the child's death is imminent. Certain rituals may be desired, depending on the family's religious or spiritual background. Ensure that these important events occur, and alter nursing care routines as needed to accommodate them. Respect the family's need to participate in these rituals and customs (Hauer, 2023).

Work collaboratively with the family and health care team to provide for the needs of the child and family. Resources for these families are listed in Box 12.5. The Make-a-Wish Foundation works to grant the wishes of children who are terminally ill, giving the child and family an experience of hope, strength, and love.

BOX 12.5 Resources for Families of a Dying Child

Websites

- Project Joy and Hope: www.joyandhope.org
- Children's Hospice International: www.chionline.org
- Compassionate Friends: www.compassionatefriends.org

Books

- *Gentle Willow: A Story for Children About Dying* by Joyce Mills
- *35 Ways to Help a Grieving Child* by the Dougy Center for Grieving Children
- *Sad Isn't Bad* by Michaeline Mundy
- *A Child Asks … What Does Dying Mean?* by Lake Pylant Monhollon
- *Talking with Children and Young People About Death and Dying: A Workbook* by Mary Turner
- *The Worst Loss: How Families Heal from the Death of a Child* by Barbara Rosof
- *I Have No Intention of Saying Goodbye: Parents Share Their Stories of Hope and Healing After a Child's Death* by Sandy Fox
- *Stars in the Deepest Night: After the Death of a Child* by Genesse Gentry
- *The Bereaved Parent* by Harriet Schiff
- *You Are Special* by Max Lucado

EASING ANXIETY OR FEARS

Parents may be afraid about the child dying alone or not know what to expect in the death process. This fear may contribute to increased anxiety, which the child may sense. Younger children may fear separation from their parents, and older children may not want to die alone or experience pain or discomfort associated with dying. Each child and family is individual; discuss their particular fears and anxieties in order to determine the child's and family's needs for education and support (Hauer, 2023).

Involve the parents and other family members in all phases of the child's care. Explain all aspects of care to the child to minimize anxiety related to nursing interventions. Answer the child's questions honestly. Involve the child in decision making whenever possible. Limit interventions to those related to palliation, rather than treatment, advocating for the child as needed. Remain with the child when a parent or family member is not in the room, so the child will not fear dying alone.

MEETING THE CHILD'S NEEDS ACCORDING TO DEVELOPMENTAL STAGE

It is important to provide the type of support and education that the child who is dying needs according to their developmental stage. For the infant, unconditional love and trust are of utmost importance. Ensure that the infant's family is available to the child. The toddler, 1 to 3 years old, thrives on familiarity and routine. Maximize the toddler's time with parents, be consistent, provide favorite toys, and ensure physical comfort. Spirituality in the preschool years focuses on the concept of right versus wrong. The 3- to 5-year-old may see death as punishment for wrongdoing; correct this misunderstanding. Use honest and precise language (Hauer, 2023). Help the parents teach the child that although the family will miss the child, it will continue to function without them.

The school-age child has a concrete understanding of death. Children who are 5 to 10 years old need specific, honest details as desired. Encourage the child to help make decisions and help the child establish a sense of control (Hauer, 2023). The young adolescent (10 to 14 years old) will benefit from reinforcement of self-esteem, self-respect, and a sense of worth. Respect the child's need for privacy and time alone as well as time requested with peers. Support the need for independence and encourage the child to participate in decision making. The older adolescent (14 to 18 years of age) has a more adult-like understanding of death and will need further support through honest, detailed explanations and will want to feel truly involved and listened to. They may also benefit from group activities away from family and unrelated to their medical diagnosis (Hauer, 2023).

Assisting the Family Through the Grief Process

The family may experience anticipatory grief when the diagnosis of a terminal illness is made. Family members may deny the prognosis, become angry at the health care system or a higher power, or experience depression. Acute grief is an intense process that occurs around the time of the actual death. Family members may feel short of breath or as though the throat is tight. They may verbalize that the situation is unreal to them or search for reasons why death was not prevented. Families may also display hostility or restlessness. Each individual will express grief in their own manner. Mourning the death of a loved one takes a long time, and families should be supported throughout the process (Broden et al., 2020). Local and national resources are available for grieving parents. Refer parents to bereavement resources as appropriate.

KEY CONCEPTS

- Children with special health care needs are those who have or who are at risk for a chronic physical, developmental, behavioral, or emotional condition that generally requires more intensive and diverse health services, as well as coordination of those services, than do other children.
- Most children with chronic illnesses or who are dependent on technology progress through stages of growth and development just as healthy children do, although possibly at a slower pace.
- Parents of children with special needs experience a multitude of emotions and changes in their lives, often carrying a heavy caregiving burden. They become the experts on their child's care and should be empowered and supported in their efforts.
- The child with special health care needs and their family may require additional support during times of transition, such as at initial diagnosis or change in prognosis, when symptoms increase, when the child moves to a new setting (hospital, school), during periods of developmental change, or during a parent's absence.
- Children with special health care needs and their families are at increased risk for the development of vulnerable child syndrome, which may have psychologically harmful effects on the child and family for many years.
- Home is the most developmentally appropriate environment for children with special health care needs. Children display an improved physical, emotional, psychological, and social status when they are cared for at home.
- Family-centered care provides the optimal framework for caring for children with special health care needs and their families. Empowering the family strengthens them. A medical home or a permanent relationship with the health care provider or nurse practitioner benefits the family as care coordination and advocacy are provided.
- Use adjusted or corrected age when assessing growth and development of the infant or child who was born prematurely. Provide early screening and intervention for issues related to development to maximize the former premature infant's potential for growth and development.
- Become familiar with the risks and benefits of adjuvant therapies used by some families of children with special health care needs.
- Screen children with special health care needs for undernutrition or a feeding disorder.
- Screening helps identify children with unmet health needs so that intervention may begin.
- Early intervention provides care coordination (developmental services and special education), as well as an individualized family service plan for qualifying children and their families.
- Each student with special health care needs is entitled to an IEP, which is a written plan that is designed to meet the preschool, primary, or secondary school student's needs.
- Early discharge planning and ongoing inclusion and education of the family facilitate continuity of care. During midadolescence, initiate a written plan to help the child make the transition to adult care.
- Support the child who is dying and their family throughout the end-of-life decision-making process, providing facts as desired about palliative care, hospice, and organ donation.
- Younger children who are dying generally need their families to be close and to trust their needs will be provided for. Older children require honest explanations given at a level appropriate for the child's age or developmental stage.

REFERENCES AND RECOMMENDED READINGS

Abdi, F. M., Seok, D., & Murphey, D. (2020). *Children with special health care needs face challenges accessing information, support, and services.* Child Trends. https://cms.childtrends.org/wp-content/uploads/2020/02/CYSHCN-Brief_ChildTrends_February2020.pdf

Adistie, F., Lumbantobing, V. B. M., & Maryam, N. N. A. (2020). The needs of children with terminal illness: A qualitative study. *Child Care in Practice, 26*(3), 257–271. https://doi.org/10.1080/13575279.2018.1555136

American Academy of Child and Adolescent Psychiatry. (2023). *Chronic illness and children.* https://www.aacap.org/AACAP/Families_and_Youth/Facts_for_Families/FFF-Guide/The-Child-With-A-Long-Term-Illness-019.aspx

American Hippotherapy Association. (2022). *FAQs for families.* https://www.americanhippotherapyassociation.org/frequently-asked-questions

American Music Therapy Association. (2023). *What is music therapy?* https://www.musictherapy.org/about/musictherapy/

American Nurses Association. (2015). *Code of ethics for nurses with interpretive statements (view only for members and non-members).* https://www.nursingworld.org/practice-policy/nursing-excellence/ethics/code-of-ethics-for-nurses/coe-view-only/

Bally, J., Smith, N., Holtslander, L., Duncan, V., Hodgson-Viden, H., Mpofu, C., & Zimmer, M. (2018). A metasynthesis: Uncovering what is known about the experiences of families with children who have life-limiting and life-threatening illnesses. *Journal of Pediatric Nursing, 38,* 88–98. https://doi.org/10.1016/j.pedn.2017.11.004

Bamberger, J. M., Nelson, C. S., & Westry, M. F. G. (2022). Management of nutritional disorders. In T. Kyle (Ed.), *Primary care pediatrics for the nursing practitioner* (p. 419-456). Springer.

Blanco, M. A., Lilly, C. M., Bavinger, B. C., Garcia, S., & Hojnicki, M. P. (2021). Caring for medically complex children in the outpatient setting. *Advances in Pediatrics, 68,* 89–102. https://doi.org/10.1016/j.yapd.2021.05.012

Brenner, M., Alexander, D., Quirke, M. B., Eustace-Cook, J., Leroy, P., Berry, J., Healy, M., Doyle, C., & Masterson, K. (2021). A systematic concept analysis of ‘technology dependent’: Challenging the terminology. *European Journal of Pediatrics, 180*(1), 1–12. https://doi.org/10.1007/s00431-020-03737-x

Broden, E. G., Deatrick, J., Ulrich, C., & Curley, M. A. Q. (2020). Defining a “good death” in the pediatric intensive care unit. *American Journal of Critical Care, 29*(2), 111–121. https://doi.org/10.4037/ajcc2020466

Cacciatore, J., Thieleman, K., Lieber, A. S., Blood, C., & Goldman, R. (2019). The long road to farewell: The needs of families with dying children. *Omega: Journal of Death & Dying, 78*(4), 404–420. https://doi.org/10.1177/0030222817697418

Centers for Disease Control and Prevention. (n.d.). *WISQARS leading causes of death visualization tool.* https://wisqars.cdc.gov/data/lcd/home

Centers for Disease Control and Prevention. (2022). *What is “early intervention”?* https://www.cdc.gov/ncbddd/actearly/parents/states.html

Centers for Medicare and Medicaid Services. (n.d.). *Children’s health insurance program (CHIP).* https://www.medicaid.gov/chip/index.html

Cincinnati Children’s Hospital Medical Center. (2023). *Ongoing support resources.* https://www.cincinnatichildrens.org/patients/child/special-needs

de Leon Siantz, M. L., Kilanowski, J. F., & Thomas, T. L. (2018). Cultural values, beliefs, and preference are integral to family-centered care. In C. L. Betz, M. J. Krajicek, & M. Craft-Rosenberg (Eds.), *Guidelines for nursing excellence in the care of children, youth, and families* (2nd ed., pp. 57-75). Springer Publishing Company.

Duryea, T. K. (2023). Poor weight gain in children younger than two years in resource-abundant settings: Management. *UpToDate.* Retrieved on November 5, 2023, from https://www.uptodate.com/contents/poor-weight-gain-in-children-younger-than-two-years-in-resource-abundant-countries-management

Ellison, J. L., Brown, R. E., & Ameringer, S. (2022). Parents’ experiences with health care transition of their adolescents and young adults with medically complex conditions: A scoping review. *Journal of Pediatric Nursing, 66,* 70–78. https://doi.org/10.1016/j.pedn.2022.04.018

Foster, C. C., Shaunfield, S., Black, L. E., Labellarte, P. Z., & Davis, M. M. (2022). Improving support for care at home: Parental needs and preferences when caring for children with medical complexity. *Journal of Pediatric Health Care, 36*(2), 154–164. https://doi.org/10.1016/j.pedhc.2020.08.005

Genik, L. M., McMurty, M., Marshall, S., Rapoport, A., & Stinson, J. (2020). Massage therapy for symptom reduction and improved quality of life in children with cancer in palliative care: A pilot study. *Complementary Therapies in Medicine, 48,* 102263. https://doi.org/10.1016/j.ctim.2019.102263

Hauer, J. (2023). Pediatric palliative care. *UpToDate.* Retrieved on November 5, 2023, from https://www.uptodate.com/contents/pediatric-palliative-care

Kaiser Family Foundation. (2023a). *Rate of child deaths (1-14) per 100,000 children.* https://www.kff.org/other/state-indicator/child-death-rate/?currentTimeframe=0&sortModel=%7B%22colId%22:%22Location%22,%22sort%22:%22asc%22%7D

Kaiser Family Foundation. (2023b). *Total infant deaths.* https://www.kff.org/other/state-indicator/infant-death-rate/?dataView=1¤tTimeframe=0&sortModel=%7B%22colId%22:%22Location%22,%22sort%22:%22asc%22%7D

Kuo, D. Z., & Turchi, R. M. (2023). Children and youth with special health care needs. *UpToDate.* Retrieved on November 5, 2023, from https://www.uptodate.com/contents/children-and-youth-with-special-health-care-needs

Lummer-Aikey, S., & Goldstein, S. (2021). Sibling adjustment to childhood chronic illness: An integrative review. *Journal of Family Nursing, 27*(2), 136–153. https://doi.org/10.1177/1074840720977177

Mandy, G. T. (2023). Overview of the long-term complications of preterm birth. *UpToDate.* Retrieved on December 29, 2023, from https://www.uptodate.com/contents/overview-of-the-long-term-complications-of-preterm-birth

Maternal and Child Health Bureau. (2023). *Children with special health care needs.* Health Resources and Services Administration. https://mchb.hrsa.gov/maternal-child-health-topics/children-and-youth-special-health-needs

Mitchell, T. K., Bray, L., Blake, L., Dickinson, A., & Carter, B. (2022). ‘I feel like my house was taken away from me’: Parents’ experiences of having home adaptations for their medically complex, technology-dependent child. *Health and Social Care in the Community, 30*(6), e4639–e4651. https://doi.org/10.1111/hsc.13870

National Association of Pediatric Nurse Practitioners, Research Committee, Ordway, M. R., Bahorski, J., Spratling, R., Sonney, J. T., & Danford, C. A. (2020). NAPNAP position statement on protection of children involved in research studies. *Journal of Pediatric Health Care, 34*(5), 510–513. https://doi.org/10.1016/j.pedhc.2020.04.012

National Resource Center for Patient/Family-Centered Medical Home. (2020). *Implementing medical homes for children and youth with special health care needs (CYSHCN) within Medicaid managed care.* National Academy for State Health Policy. https://downloads.aap.org/MedHome/pdf/Medical%20Home%20CYSHCN%20Fact%20Sheet5.pdf

Population Reference Bureau. (2023). *Summary: Impacts of special health care needs on children and families.* https://www.kidsdata.org/topic/15/impacts-of-special-health-care-needs-on-children-and-families/summary

Schmitz, K. (2019). Vulnerable child syndrome. *Pediatrics in Review, 40*(6), 313–315. https://doi.org/10.1542/pir.2017-0243

Sewell-Roberts, C. (2021). *Caring for siblings of kids with disabilities.* https://kidshealth.org/en/parents/siblings-special-needs.html

Seymour, K. (2021). *Supporting healthy brain development in children through nutrition.* https://ks.childcareaware.org/supporting-healthy-brain-development-in-children-through-nutrition/

Shaw, T., Winegard, B., & Timmons, Z. (2021). Determining futility—One free-standing children's hospital's experience with a policy. *Pediatrics, 147*(3_MeetingAbstract), 525–527. https://doi.org/10.1542/peds.147.3MA5.525

Smith, V. C., & Stewart, J. (2023). Discharge planning for high-risk newborns. *UpToDate.* Retrieved on November 5, 2023, from https://www.uptodate.com/contents/discharge-planning-for-high-risk-newborns

Social Security Administration. (n.d.-a). *Supplemental security income (SSI) for children.* https://www.ssa.gov/ssi/text-child-ussi.htm

Social Security Administration. (n.d.-b). *Title V—Maternal and child health services block grant.* https://www.ssa.gov/OP_Home/ssact/title05/0500.htm

Stewart, J. (2023). Care of the neonatal intensive care unit graduate. *UpToDate.* Retrieved on November 5, 2023, from https://www.uptodate.com/contents/care-of-the-neonatal-intensive-care-unit-graduate

Stokes, L. (2021). ANA position statement: Nursing care and do-not-resuscitate (DNR) decisions. *The Online Journal of Issues in Nursing, 26*(1). https://doi.org/10.3912/OJIN.Vol26No01PoSCol02

The Warren Center. (2023). *Corrected (adjusted) age for preemies.* https://thewarrencenter.org/help-information/premature-birth/corrected-adjusted-age-for-preemies/

Toly, V. B., Blanchette, J. E., & Musil, C. M. (2019). Mothers caring for technology-dependent children at home: What is most helpful and least helpful? *Applied Nursing Research, 46,* 24–27. https://doi.org/10.1016/j.apnr.2019.02.001

U.S. Department of Education. (n.d.). *IDEA.* https://sites.ed.gov/idea/

U.S. Department of Health and Human Services. (n.d.). *Healthy people 2030.* https://health.gov/healthypeople

Verbeek, I. N. E., van Onzenoort-Bokken, L., Hermanus, S., & Zegers, J. (2021). Vulnerable child syndrome in everyday paediatric practice: A condition deserving attention and new perspective. *Acta Paediatrica, 110*(2), 397–399. https://doi.org./10.1111/apa.15505

Vyas, H., & Nakagawa, T. A. (2023). Management of the potential pediatric organ donor following neurologic death. *UpToDate.* Retrieved on November 5, 2023, from https://www.uptodate.com/contents/management-of-the-potential-pediatric-organ-donor

DEVELOPING CLINICAL JUDGMENT

PRACTICING FOR NCLEX

1. The parents of a 5-year-old with special health care needs talk to the parents of a 10-year-old with a similar condition for quite a while each day. What is the nurse's interpretation of this behavior?
- **a.** The nurse has not provided enough emotional support for the parents.
- **b.** This relationship between the two families is potentially unhealthy.
- **c.** Support between families of children with special health care needs is extremely valuable.
- **d.** Confidentiality is a pressing issue in this particular situation.

2. The nurse is caring for a child who has received all possible medical care for cancer yet continues to experience relapse and metastasis. It is time to make the transition from curative care attempts to palliative care. What is the most important nursing consideration at this time?
- **a.** The health care professionals should make the decision about the child's care.
- **b.** The family may lose a sense of hope, so cancer treatments should continue.
- **c.** Involve the family in the decision-making process about the shift to palliative care.
- **d.** Palliative care can take place only at home, so the child should be discharged.

3. The nurse is caring for a 3-year-old with a gastrostomy tube and tracheostomy who is on supplemental oxygen and multiple medications. The parent is rooming in during this hospitalization. What is the priority nursing action?
- **a.** Incorporate the parent's assistance in care when convenient.
- **b.** Recognize the parent as the expert on the child's needs and care.
- **c.** Recommend that the parent go home to get some rest.
- **d.** Provide family-centered care since the parent is there.

4. The nurse is caring for a child with a developmental disability who is starting kindergarten this year. The parent is tearful and doesn't want the child to go to school. What is the best response by the nurse?
- **a.** "Do you need some time alone to collect yourself?"
- **b.** "You've known for a while this time would come."
- **c.** "Can I call your partner or a friend for you?"
- **d.** "It is normal to feel stressed or sad at this time."

5. The parents of a child with a developmental disability ask the nurse for advice about disciplining their child. What is the best response by the nurse?
- **a.** "You should choose methods that are most congruent with your values about discipline."
- **b.** "Children like this really can't follow directions, so they may be hard to discipline."
- **c.** "Punish your child only for socially unacceptable or offending behaviors."
- **d.** "Spanking works well for this type of child, as they really don't like pain."

CRITICAL THINKING EXERCISES

1. A 15-year-old is dying of cancer after all medical care options have been exhausted. Describe the plan of care for this child and family. What strategies should the nurse use to support the child and family through this difficult process?

2. A 5-month-old infant who was born at 24 weeks' gestation is ready to be discharged from the NICU. The infant will be going home on oxygen, gastrostomy tube feedings, and eight medications. Develop a teaching plan for the family.

STUDY ACTIVITIES

1. In the clinical setting, care for a child with a terminal illness. Reflect in your clinical journal about the feelings you had during the care of the child as well as the feelings and behaviors that you noticed in the child, siblings, parents, and nursing staff.

2. Visit a preschool that provides care for both children who have developmental delays and children developing as expected. Choose two same-age children, one with a disability and the other without. Perform a developmental screening on each of the two children. Compare your findings.

3. Spend the day with a home care nurse providing care for a child with technology needs. What obstacles has the family overcome to have this child at home? What adjustments does the nurse make to provide family-centered care in the home (as compared to the hospital setting)?

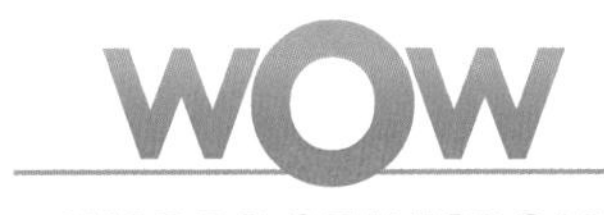

WORDS OF WISDOM

Quality technical skills delivered by a caring hand are a vital part of good nursing care.

13

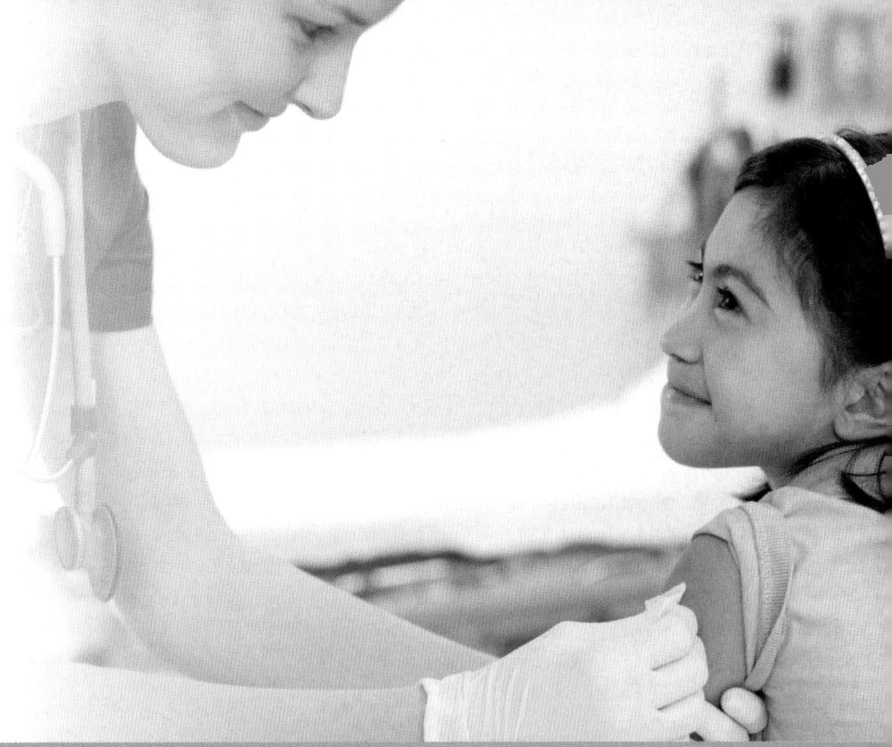

Key Pediatric Nursing Interventions

KEY TERMS

bolus feeding

enteral nutrition (en´tĕr-ăl nū-trish´ŭn)

gastric residual

gastrostomy (gas-tros´tŏ-mē)

gavage feedings (gă-vahzh´ fēd´ingz)

infiltration

parenteral nutrition (pă-ren´tĕr-ăl nū-trish´ŭn)

pharmacodynamics (fahr´mă-kō-dī-nam´iks)

pharmacokinetics (fahr´mă-kō-ki-net´iks)

total parenteral nutrition

LEARNING OBJECTIVES

Upon completion of the chapter, you will be able to:

1. Describe the "rights" of pediatric medication administration.
2. Explain the physiologic differences in children affecting a medication's pharmacodynamic and pharmacokinetic properties.
3. Accurately determine recommended pediatric medication doses.
4. Explain the proper technique for administering medication to children via the oral, rectal, ophthalmic, otic, intravenous, intramuscular, and subcutaneous routes.
5. Discuss atraumatic approaches to care in medication administration in children.
6. Identify the preferred sites for peripheral and central intravenous medication administration.
7. Describe nursing management related to maintenance of intravenous infusions and prevention of complications in children.
8. Explain nursing care related to enteral tube feedings.
9. Describe nursing management of the child receiving total parenteral nutrition.

Lily Kline, a 9-month-old, is admitted to your unit for malnutrition. The health care provider has ordered insertion of a nasogastric tube to begin gavage feedings. The parents are nervous and upset about this. They ask, "What will this tube do for Lily? It sounds uncomfortable. What do you have to do to insert it? Will it have to stay in all the time? Won't it move?" How would you address their concerns?

INTRODUCTION

The ill child often requires medications, intravenous (IV) therapy, or enteral nutrition to restore health. These interventions occur most often in the inpatient setting, but with today's advanced technology, many children may receive treatment in the home, day care center, school, health care provider's office, or other community setting.

This chapter will discuss the key elements of, and guidelines for, care related to medication administration, IV therapy, and nutritional support in children. Child and parent education is emphasized. The chapter will focus on adapting and modifying medication administration and nursing procedures based on the child's growth and development and providing these treatments using a family-centered, atraumatic approach. Refer back to Chapter 8 for an overview of the important aspects of caring for a child who is to undergo a procedure.

MEDICATION ADMINISTRATION

At one time or another, every child will need to receive medication. As with adults, pediatric medication administration is a critical component of safe and effective nursing care. The pediatric nurse must adapt administration principles and techniques to meet the child's needs. Medication administration, regardless of the route, requires a solid knowledge base about the drug and its action. As with medication administration to any person, the nurse must adhere to the "rights" of medication administration (Box 13.1). These rights were developed to ensure patient safety by decreasing the occurrence of medication errors. Some experts have added additional rights, such as right documentation, right to be educated, right to refuse, right approach, and right form. These additional rights are important to consider to increase patient safety and satisfaction.

BOX 13.1 Rights of Pediatric Medication Administration

Right Patient
- Confirm child identity by two ways. Children may deny their identity in an attempt to avoid an unpleasant situation, play in another child's bed, or remove ID bracelet.
- Confirm identity each time medication is given.
- Verify child's name with caregiver to provide additional verification.
- Use technology when available (i.e., bar code systems).

Right Medication
- Check order and expiration dates.
- Know action of medication and potential side effects (use pharmacy, drug formulary).
- Ensure that the medication provided is the medication that is ordered.

Right Route of Administration
- Check ordered route and ensure this is the most effective and safest route for this child; clarify any order that is confusing or unclear.
- Give the medication by the route ordered. If there is a need to change route, always check with prescriber (e.g., if a child is vomiting and has an order for an oral medication, the medication may need to be given via the IV or rectal route).

Right Time
- Give within 20 to 30 minutes of the ordered time.
- For a medication given on an as-needed (PRN) basis, know when it was last given and how much was given during the past 24 hours.

Right Dose
- Calculate the recommended dose according to child's weight, and double-check your calculations.
- Always question the pharmacist and/or prescriber if the ordered dose falls outside the recommended dose range.
- Unusually large or small volumes or dosages should always be verified.

Differences in Pharmacodynamics and Pharmacokinetics

Although a drug's mechanism of action is the same in any individual, the physiologic immaturity of some body systems in a child can affect a drug's **pharmacodynamics** (behavior of the medication at the cellular level). As a result, the body may not respond to the drug as intended. The intended effect may be enhanced or diminished, necessitating a change in the dosage to ensure optimal effectiveness without increasing the child's risk for toxicity.

The child's age, weight, body surface area (BSA), and body composition can also affect the drug's **pharmacokinetics** (movement of drugs throughout the body via absorption, distribution, metabolism, and excretion). Drugs are administered to children via many of the same routes that are used for adults. However, this similarity ends once the drug is administered. During the absorption process, drugs move from the administration site into the bloodstream. In infants and young children, the absorption of orally administered medications is affected by slower gastric emptying, increased intestinal motility, a proportionately larger small intestine surface area, higher gastric pH, and decreased lipase and amylase secretion compared with adults. Intramuscular (IM) absorption in infants and young children is affected by the amount of muscle mass, muscle tone and perfusion, and vasomotor instability. Similarly, decreased perfusion alters subcutaneous (SQ) absorption. Absorption by these routes is erratic and may be decreased. In contrast, topical absorption of medications is increased in infants and young children, which can result in adverse effects not seen in adults. Infants and young children have a greater BSA, leading to increased absorption of topical medications. Absorption in infants is also increased due to greater permeability of the infant's skin.

The distribution (movement of a drug from the blood to interstitial spaces and then into cells) of medications is also altered in infants and young children. Medication distribution in children is affected by the following:

- Higher percentage of body water than adults
- More rapid extracellular fluid exchange
- Decreased body fat
- Liver immaturity, altering first-pass elimination
- Decreased amounts of plasma proteins available for drug binding
- Immature blood–brain barrier, especially in neonates, allowing permeation by certain medications

Metabolism of medications in children is altered because of differences in hepatic enzyme production and the child's increased metabolic rate. Biotransformation (the alteration of chemical structures from their original form, which allows for the eventual excretion of the substance) is affected by the same variations affecting distribution in children. In addition, the immaturity of the kidneys until the age of 1 to 2 years affects renal blood flow, glomerular filtration, and active tubular secretion. This results in a longer half-life and increases the potential for toxicity of drugs primarily excreted by the kidneys.

Developmental Issues and Concerns

Children are constantly growing and developing. The specific psychosocial, cognitive, physical, and motor developmental levels of children are important. Nurses need a solid understanding of growth and development to ensure safe administration of medications to children. Table 13.1 details some growth and development issues related to administering medications to children. Always give developmentally appropriate, truthful explanations before administering medications to children, including:

- Why the drug is needed
- What the child will experience
- What is expected of the child
- How the parents can participate and support their child

Refer to Chapters 3 to 7 for further information about growth and developmental issues.

The child's past experiences with taking medications and the approaches that may have been used will often affect how the child reacts. Always approach children positively; let your manner convey the belief that they can accomplish this needed behavior. Never label the child as "bad" if they did not fully cooperate in taking medication. When medications must be administered with a needle (intramuscularly or subcutaneously), assure the child that this method is not a consequence of the child's behavior. Help parents to work through the feelings of frustration that may result from the child's

TABLE 13.1 • Growth and Development Issues Related to Pediatric Medication Administration

Stage of Development	Issue/Concern	Nursing Interventions
Infant	Development of trust, which is fostered by consistent care; development of stranger anxiety later in infancy	Involve parents in medication administration to reduce stress for infant. Ensure that parents hold and comfort infant during intervention.
Toddler	Development of autonomy with displays of negativism; rituals, routines, and choices necessary to maintain some sense of control	Follow routines and rituals from home in giving medications if these are safe and positive approaches. Involve parents in medication administration. Offer simple choices (e.g., "Do you want Mom or me to give you your medicine?"). Allow child to touch or handle equipment as appropriate.
Preschooler	Development of initiative, which is fostered when they sense they are helping	Provide an opportunity to play with the equipment and respond positively to explanations and comforting. Provide choices that are possible, and keep them simple (e.g., "Do you want juice or water with your medication?" or "Which medication do you want to take first?"). Do not ask, "Will you take your medicine now?" Involve parents in medication administration. Be aware that giving suppositories is particularly upsetting to this age group because of their fears of bodily intrusion and mutilation.
School-age child	Development of industry, benefiting from being a part of their care; generally cooperative	Explain to child in simple terms the purpose of the medication. Seek their assistance, such as putting pills in cup or opening the packet, and allow a broader range of choices. Establish a reward system to enhance their cooperation, if necessary.
Adolescent	Development of identity, benefiting from much more control over their care	Approach in same manner as adults, with respect and sensitivity to their needs. Maintain the adolescent's privacy as much as possible.

refusal to cooperate with medication administration. Provide parents with facts about growth and developmental issues and children's fears and anxiety related to medication administration. Model alternative ways for the parents to deal with undesirable behavior.

TAKE NOTE!

Always administer medications promptly, assist the child in holding still using a comforting position for the child, and reward positive behavior.

Determination of Correct Dose

Administering the correct dose is a key component of medication administration. Children are more vulnerable to medication errors due to the individual dosing necessary for proper medication administration. Improper dosing is a more common medication error reported in the pediatric population than the adult population (The Joint Commission, 2021). Many drug references list recommended pediatric dosages, and nurses are responsible for checking doses to ensure that they are appropriate for the child. Two common methods for determining pediatric doses are based on the unit of drug per kilogram of body weight or BSA.

Dose Determination by Body Weight

The most common method for calculating pediatric medication doses is based on body weight. The recommended dosage is usually expressed as the amount of drug to be given over a 24-hour period (mg/kg/day) or as a single dose (mg/kg/dose). It is important to differentiate between the 24-hour dosage and the single dose. Use these guidelines to determine the correct dose by body weight:

1. Weigh the child.
2. If the child's weight is in pounds, convert it to kilograms (divide the child's weight in pounds by 2.2).
3. Check a drug reference for the safe dose range (e.g., 10 to 20 mg/kg of body weight).
4. Calculate the low safe dose (Box 13.2).
5. Calculate the high safe dose (Box 13.2).
6. Determine if the dose ordered is within this range.

TAKE NOTE!

Pay close attention to ensure if the safe range dose is for 24 hours (mg/day) or a single dose period (mg/dose).

The pediatric dosage should not exceed the minimum recommended adult dosage. With many medications, once a child or adolescent weighs 40 to 50 kg or greater, the adult dose is frequently prescribed. However, it remains important to always verify that the dose does not exceed the recommended adult dose.

BOX 13.2 Dosage Calculation Using Body Weight

After converting the child's weight in pounds to kilograms and checking the safe dose range:

- Calculate the low safe dose range (e.g., 10 to 20 mg/kg, and the child weighs 30 kg):
  - Set up a proportion using the low safe dose range

  $10 \text{ mg}/1 \text{ kg} = x \text{ mg}/30 \text{ kg}$

  Solve for x by cross-multiplying:

  $1 \times x = 10 \times 30$

  $x = 300 \text{ mg}$
- Calculate the high safe dose range:
  - Set up a proportion using the high safe dose range

  $20 \text{ mg}/1 \text{ kg} = x \text{ mg}/30 \text{ kg}$

  Solve for x by cross-multiplying:

  $1 \times x = 20 \times 30$

  $x = 600 \text{ mg}$
- Compare the safe dose range (for this, e.g., 300 to 600 mg) with the ordered dose. If the dose falls within the range, the dose is safe. If the dose falls outside the range, notify the prescriber.

Dose Determination by BSA

Calculating the dosage based on BSA takes into account the child's metabolic rate and growth. It is commonly used for chemotherapeutic agents. Some recommended medication doses may read "mg/BSA/dose." To determine the dose using BSA, you will need to know the child's height and weight, which will be plotted on a nomogram (Fig. 13.1). A nomogram is a graph divided into three columns: height (left column), surface area (middle column), and weight (right column).

Use these guidelines to determine BSA:

1. Measure the child's height.
2. Determine the child's weight.
3. Using the nomogram, draw a line to connect the height measurement in the left column and the weight measurement in the right column.
4. Determine the point where this line intersects the line in the surface area column. This is the BSA, expressed in meters squared (m^2).

Once you have determined the BSA, use the recommended dosage range to calculate the safe dosage.

TAKE NOTE!

Prior to administration of any medication, wash hands and don gloves if necessary. Adhere to the rights of medication administration.

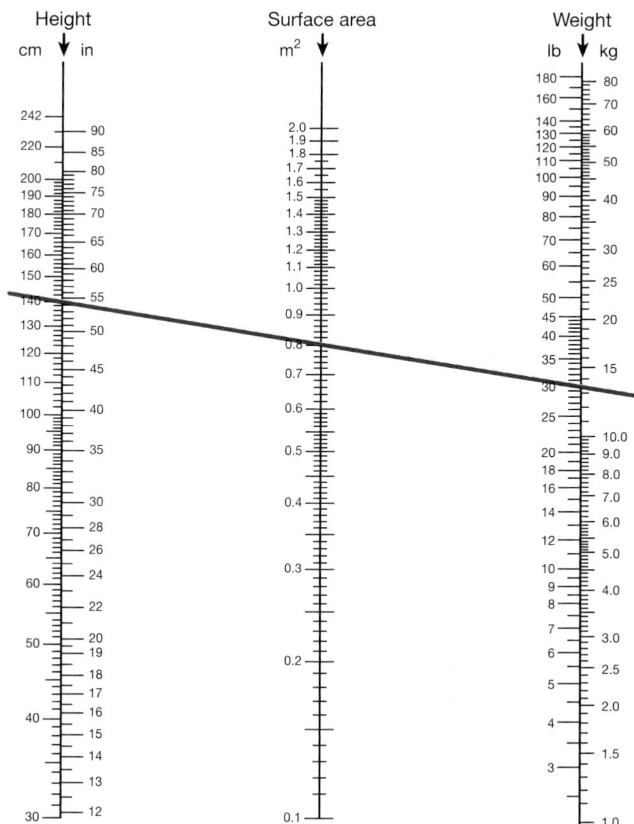

FIGURE 13.1 A nomogram to determine body surface area.

Oral Administration

Medications to be given via the oral route are supplied in many forms, including liquids (elixirs, syrups, or suspensions), powders, tablets, and capsules. Generally, children younger than 5 to 6 years are at risk for aspiration because they have difficulty swallowing tablets or capsules. Therefore, if a tablet or capsule is the only oral form available, it needs to be crushed or opened and mixed with a pleasant-tasting liquid or a small amount (generally no more than a tablespoon) of a nonessential food such as applesauce. However, never crush or open an enteric-coated or time-release tablet or capsule. The crushed tablet or inside of a capsule may taste bitter, so never mix it with formula or other essential foods. Otherwise, the child may associate the bitter taste with the food and later refuse to eat it.

CLINICAL REASONING ALERT!

Certain drug formulations should not be crushed. Before crushing a pill or opening a capsule, always check that this will not alter the intended effects of the drug. Crushing a time-release medication allows immediate absorption of the entire dose of the medication and can have lethal consequences.

Liquid medications, primarily suspensions, may be less concentrated at the top of the bottle than at the bottom of the bottle. Always shake the liquid to ensure even drug distribution. The key to administering liquid forms of oral medications is to use calibrated equipment such as a medicine cup, spoon, plastic oral syringe, or dropper (Fig. 13.2).

TAKE NOTE!

Use the medicine cup or syringe with proper calibration instead of household cups or measuring spoons, since they are not calibrated and may deliver an incorrect dose of medication.

If a dropper is packaged with a certain medication, never use it to administer another medication, since the drop size may vary from one dropper to another. If using a syringe for oral administration, only use the type intended for oral medications, not the one designed for parenteral administration. When using a dropper or oral syringe (without a needle) for infants or young children, direct the liquid toward the posterior side of the mouth. Give the drug slowly in small amounts (0.2 to 0.5 mL), and allow the child to swallow before more medication is placed in the mouth (Fig. 13.3). A nipple without the bottle attached is sometimes used to administer medication to infants. Place the medication directly in the nipple, and keep the nipple filled with medication as the infant sucks so no air is taken in while the infant takes the medication. Always place the infant or young child upright (at least a 45-degree angle) to avoid aspiration. The toddler or young preschooler may enjoy using the oral syringe to squirt the medicine into their own mouth. Older children can take oral medication from a medicine cup or measured medicine spoon.

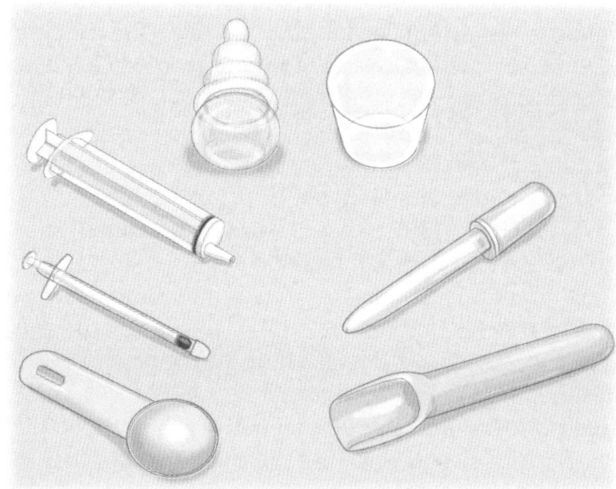

FIGURE 13.2 Devices used to administer oral medications to children.

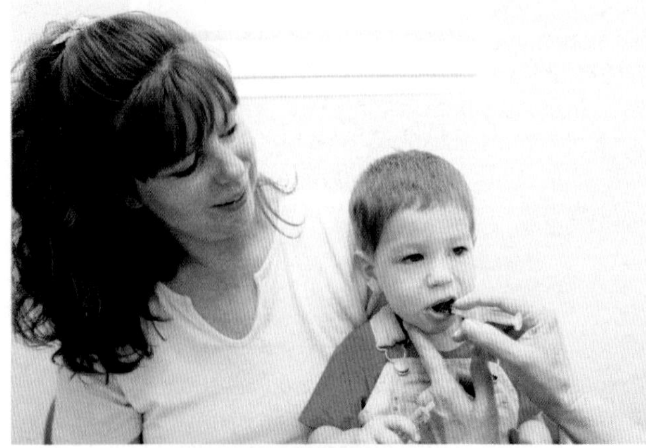

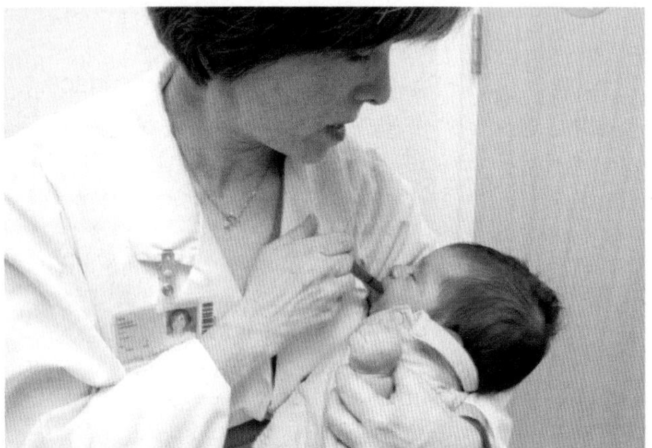

FIGURE 13.3 Position the infant or young child with head elevated for safe medication administration. Holding the child or having a parent hold the child is preferred unless contraindicated.

TAKE NOTE!

Never force an oral medication into a child's mouth or pinch the child's nose. Doing so increases the risk of aspiration and interferes with the development of a trusting relationship.

As children adapt to swallowing tablets or capsules, administration is similar to that of adults. When helping the younger child learn how to swallow medication, the tablet or capsule can be placed at the back of the tongue or in a small amount of food such as ice cream or applesauce. Always tell children if there is medicine in the food; otherwise, they may not trust you.

When the child has a nasogastric, orogastric, nasojejunal, nasoduodenal, **gastrostomy** (opening into the stomach), or jejunostomy tube, oral medications may be given via these devices. The tube allows for the medication to be placed directly into the stomach or small intestine area. Be aware that not all medications can be placed directly into the duodenum or jejunum. Medication for administration via a tube must be supplied in a liquid form, or a crushed tablet or opened capsule can be mixed with a liquid (Box 13.3). Always check tube placement before administering the medication. After administration, flush the tube to maintain patency.

BOX 13.3 Guidelines for Administering Medications via Gastrostomy or Jejunostomy Tubes

Verify correct placement (refer to Box 13.4).

- Give liquid medications directly into the medication port. Draw appropriate amount into syringe and clear air.
- Mix powdered medications well with warm water first.
- If medication is in pill or capsule form, verify it is okay to crush or open. Then, crush tablets or open capsules and mix with warm water to prevent tube occlusion.
- Label each syringe appropriately.
- Give medications one at a time. Flush the tube with water after administering each medication unless contraindicated to ensure that the entire amount of medication has been given and to prevent tube occlusion.

Adapted from Cincinnati Children's Hospital Medical Center. (2022). *Gastrostomy tube (G-tube) home care.* https://www.cincinnatichildrens.org/health/g/g-tube-care

TAKE NOTE!

Parental involvement in medication administration when possible helps decrease stress on the child and provides an opportunity for teaching and evaluating parental techniques.

Rectal Administration

Rectal medications are typically supplied in the form of suppositories. The rectal route is not a preferred route for medication administration in children because the drug's absorption may be erratic and unpredictable, and the method is invasive. The rectal route can be extremely upsetting to the toddler and preschooler because of age-related fears and may be embarrassing to the school-age child or adolescent. However, the rectal route may be used when the child is vomiting or receiving nothing by mouth (NPO). Use age-appropriate explanations and reassurance. Helping the child to maintain the correct position may be necessary to ensure proper insertion and safety of rectal suppositories.

Lubricate the suppository well with a water-soluble lubricant. With the child in the side-lying position, insert the suppository into the rectum quickly but gently. Use a gloved finger or a finger cot to insert the suppository. Insert the suppository above the anal sphincter. For an infant or child younger than 3 years, use the fifth finger for insertion. For an older child, use the index finger. To prevent expulsion of the suppository, hold the buttocks together for several minutes or until the child loses the urge to defecate. If the child has a bowel movement within 10 to 30 minutes after administration of the medication, examine the stool for the presence of the suppository. If it is observed, notify the health care provider or nurse practitioner to determine if the drug needs to be administered again.

Ophthalmic Administration

Ophthalmic medications are typically supplied in the form of drops or ointment. Many children have a fear of having anything placed in their eyes. Therefore, provide an age-appropriate explanation to gain their cooperation. Also, have the child keep their eyes closed until you are ready to administer the medication. Ensure that the medication is at room temperature, as chilled medication may be uncomfortable to the child. Proper positioning of the child is necessary to control the child's head, keep the child's hands from interfering, and prevent injury to the eye. Attempt to administer the medication when the child is not crying to ensure that the medication reaches its intended target area.

Place the child in the supine position, slightly hyperextending the neck with the head lower than the body so the medication will be dispersed over the cornea. Rest the heel of your hand on the child's forehead to stabilize it. Retract the lower eyelid, and place the medication in the conjunctival sac; maintain sterile technique by being careful not to touch the tip of the tube or dropper to the sac. For eye drops, place the prescribed number of drops into the lower conjunctival sac (Fig. 13.4). For ointment, apply the medication in a thin ribbon from the inner canthus outward without touching the eye or eyelashes. If the child is old enough to cooperate, instruct the child to gently close the eyes to allow the medication to be dispersed.

If a child is uncooperative, they may need to be immobilized in order to administer the eye drops. Alternatively, one or two drops on the inner canthus of the closed eye can be administered while the child is lying supine. Then instruct the child to open their eyes, and the drops will enter the eye. Wipe any excess medication from the skin. Punctal occlusion after application is also important to slow systemic absorption and ensure that the medicine stays in the eye.

Children often require ophthalmic medications at home. Parents or caregivers need instruction about how to administer this type of medication. Teaching Guidelines 13.1 provides information on administering eye drops and eye ointments.

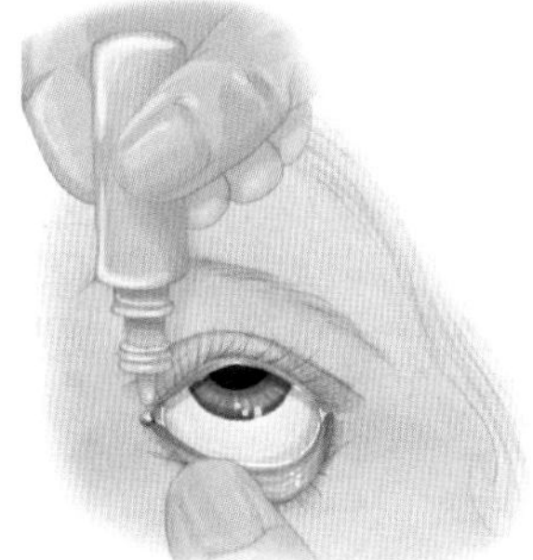

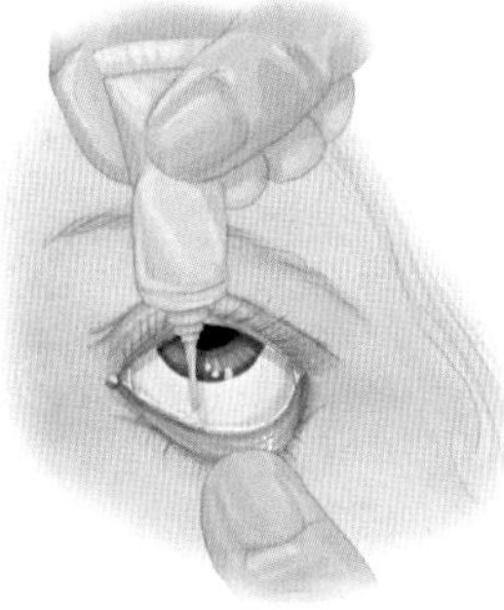

FIGURE 13.4 Administering eye medication: gently press the lower lid down, and have the child look up as the medication is instilled into the lower conjunctival sac.

TEACHING GUIDELINES 13.1 Applying Eye Medications

- Wash your hands with soap and water. Dry them thoroughly using a clean cloth.
- Cleanse the eye. Move from the nose side of the eye outward. Use a clean area of the cloth each time you wipe and a separate cloth for each eye. Use warm water to help clear crusty eye drainage. Wash your hands again.
- Allow the eye drops or ointment to come to room temperature (if the medication was stored in the refrigerator). If necessary, warm the eye drops or ointment tube in the palm of your hand. Keep the cap on to avoid any spillage. Make sure medication is well mixed if needed.
- Remove the cap, placing it on a dry, clean surface.
- For young children (3 years or younger), obtain assistance from an additional adult to keep their arms and fingers away during the procedure. If doing this procedure alone, wrap the child in a towel or blanket, keeping the arms inside.
- Have the child look up and to the other side. The eye drops should flow away from the child's nose.
- Place the wrist of the hand you will be using to give the drops against the child's forehead. With the other hand, gently pull down the lower eyelid. Have the medication about 2.54 cm (1 in) away from the eye.
- Gently squeeze the eye drop bottle, dispensing the proper number of drops away from the tear ducts that are in the inner corner of the eye, or gently squeeze the ointment tube, dispensing a small trail (about 2 cm) of ointment into the gap between the lower portion of the eye and the bottom eyelid. Twist or rotate the tube when you reach the outer eye to help disconnect the ointment from the tube.
- Make sure the tip of the bottle or tube does not make contact with the eye or any other surface.
- For eye drops, gently press your finger against the inside corner where the eye meets the nose for about 1 to 3 minutes, blocking the tears and medication from exiting through the tear duct. This will help the eye retain more of the medication. If the child is old enough, they may be able to do this unassisted.
- For ointment, have the child close their eye and not rub the area.
- Ask the child to close their eyes gently and not to blink or squeeze the eye shut more than normal, as this may wash away the medication prematurely.
- Gently dab away any tears or excess medication on the face with a clean tissue.
- Wash your hands again and dry them thoroughly.

Adapted from Lippincott Williams & Wilkins. (2023). *Lippincott nursing procedures* (9th ed.). Wolters Kluwer.

Otic Administration

Medications for otic administration are typically in the form of ear drops. This route of administration can be upsetting to the child because they cannot see what is happening. The child often receives otic drugs for an earache, and they may fear that the ear drops will increase the pain. Explain the procedure to the younger child in terms that they can understand to help allay these fears. Gain the older child's cooperation by explaining the purpose of the medication and the procedure for administration.

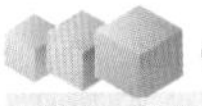

Concept Mastery Alert

Administering Pediatric Ear Drops

When administering pediatric ear drops, pulling the pinna down and back is correct if the child is under 3 years of age. To administer ear drops to a child who is 4 years old, the nurse should pull the pinna up and back.

Reinforce the need for the child to keep the head still. Younger children may require assistance to do so. Be sure that the ear drops are at room temperature. If necessary, roll the container between the palms of your hands to help warm the drops. Using cold ear drops can cause pain and possibly vertigo when they reach the eardrum (Cleveland Clinic, 2023).

Place the child in a supine or side-lying position with the affected ear exposed (Fig. 13.5). Pull the pinna downward and back in children under age 3 and upward and back in older children. Instill the prescribed amount of medication using a dropper, being careful not to contaminate the tip of the dropper. Then, have the child remain in the same position for several minutes to ensure that the medication stays in the ear canal. Soothe, comfort, and distract the child to allow the medication to instill. Massage the area anterior to the affected ear to promote passage of the medication into the ear canal. If necessary, place a piece of cotton or a cotton ball loosely in the ear canal to prevent the medication from leaking.

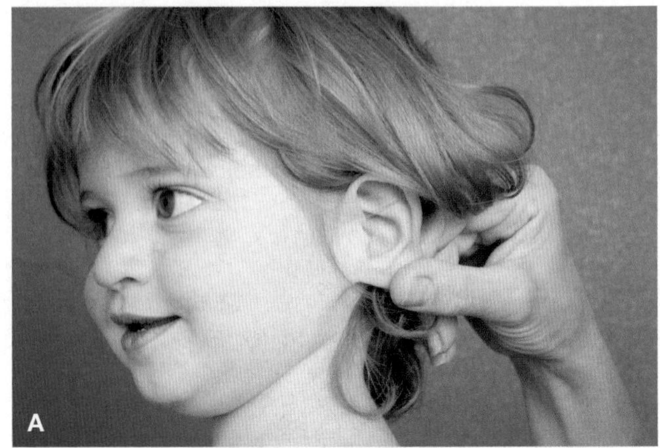

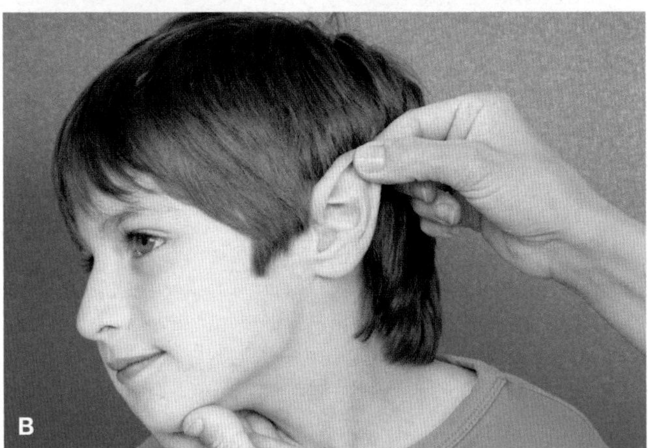

FIGURE 13.5 Administering ear drops. **A.** For the child younger than 3 years, the nurse pulls the pinna of the ear down and back. **B.** For a child older than 3 years, the nurse pulls the pinna of the affected ear up and back.

Nasal Administration

Nasally administered medications are typically drops and sprays. Administering nose drops to infants and young children may be difficult, and additional help may be needed to help maintain the child's position. Ensure medication is at room temperature. Have the child blow their nose or use a bulb syringe to clear nasal passage of secretions. For nose drops, position the child supine with the head hyperextended to ensure that the drops will flow back into the nares. A pillow or folded towel can be used to facilitate this hyperextension. Place the tip of the dropper just at or inside the nasal opening, taking care not to touch the nares with the dropper (Fig. 13.6). Doing so might stimulate the child to sneeze. Although the nasal membranes are not sterile, the drop solution is, and sneezing would contaminate the dropper, leading to contamination of the drop solution when the dropper is returned to the bottle. Once the drops are instilled, maintain the child's head in hyperextension for at least 1 minute to ensure that the drops have come in contact with the nasal membranes.

For nasal sprays, position the child upright with head tilted slightly back, and place the tip of the spray bottle just inside the nasal opening and tilted toward the back. Hold one nostril closed (or have the child do this if appropriate) and instruct the child to take a deep breath through the nostril while the medication is being administered. Squeeze the container, providing just enough force for the spray to be expelled from the container. Using too great a force can push the spray solution and secretions into the sinuses or eustachian tube.

TAKE NOTE!

In young infants, instill the medication in one naris at a time, since they are obligate nose breathers.

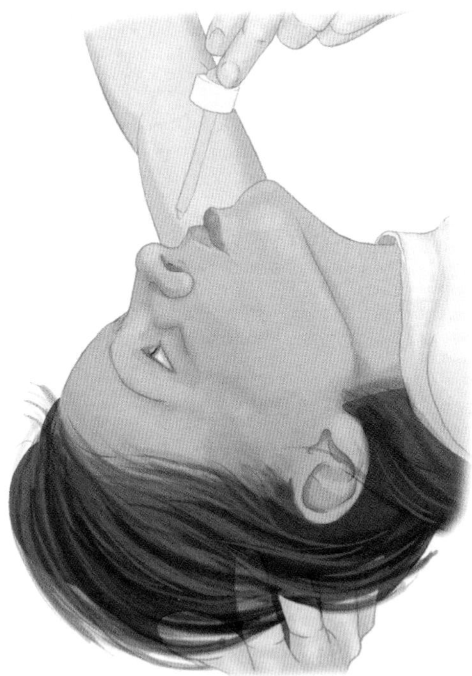

FIGURE 13.6 Administering nose drops. Tilt the head down and back to instill nose drops.

Intramuscular Administration

IM administration delivers medication to the muscle. In children, this method of medication administration is used as infrequently as possible because it is painful, and children often lack adequate muscle mass for medication absorption. However, IM administration is used to administer certain medications, such as many immunizations.

Muscle development and the amount of fluid to be injected determine IM injection sites in children. Needle size (gauge and length) is determined by the size of the muscle and the viscosity of the medication. For example, more viscous medications often require a larger-gauge needle. In addition, the needle must be long enough to ensure that the medication reaches the muscle.

The preferred injection site for infants 12 months or less is the vastus lateralis or anterolateral thigh muscle; in certain circumstances (such as physical obstruction of the anterolateral thigh), the gluteal muscle can be considered (Immunization Action Coalition, 2022; Kroger et al., 2023). In infants and children greater than 12 months, the vastus lateralis or anterolateral thigh muscle remains the preferred site, but the deltoid can be considered if sufficient mass is present (Immunization Action Coalition, 2022; Kroger et al., 2023).

TAKE NOTE!

Many experts no longer recommend use of the dorsogluteal site at any age due to the risk of damaging nerves and vasculature and the possibility of a suboptimal immune response (Drutz, 2023).

The deltoid muscle is used as an IM injection site in children older than 3 years and may be used in toddlers if the muscle mass is sufficient (Immunization Action Coalition, 2022; Kroger et al., 2023). Figure 13.7 illustrates IM injection sites.

Select the needle size and gauge based on the size of the child's muscle. The goal is to use the smallest length and gauge that will deposit the medication in the muscle. Table 13.2 provides general guidelines for solution amount, needle size, and needle gauge when administering IM medications.

Insert the needle into the skin at a 90-degree angle. Aspirating and, if no blood was present, injecting the medication was the traditional procedure. However, recent research has shown decreased discomfort and no associated complications with rapid injection of IM immunizations without aspiration (Centers for Disease Control and Prevention [CDC], 2021). In addition, there are no large blood vessels present in the currently recommended injection sites, the vastus lateralis and deltoid muscles (CDC, 2021). Therefore, the CDC and the Advisory Committee on Immunization Practices (ACIP) no longer recommend aspiration before injection of vaccines (CDC, 2021; Kroger et al., 2023).

Subcutaneous and Intradermal Administration

SQ administration distributes medication into the fatty layers of the body. It is used primarily for insulin administration, heparin, and certain immunizations, such as Measles, Mumps, Rubella (MMR). The amount of SQ tissue differs among individuals. Therefore, when selecting a site and needle size, choose the most appropriate based on adequacy and condition of the SQ tissue and the frequency and duration of the therapy. The preferred sites for SQ administration include the anterior thigh for infants younger than 12 months and the lateral upper triceps area (Kroger et al., 2023). Use a 3/8- or 5/8-in, 23- to 25-gauge needle. With the nondominant hand, pinch up the skin to isolate the tissue from the muscle or pull it taut depending on the amount of adipose tissue present and the length of needle. Insert the needle at a 45- to 90-degree angle, release the skin if pinched, and inject the medication. Remove the needle at the same angle it was inserted.

Intradermal (ID) administration deposits medication just under the epidermis. The forearm is the usual site for administration. ID administration is used primarily for tuberculosis screening and allergy testing. A 1-mL syringe with a 5/8-in, 25- or 27-gauge needle is commonly used to administer the medication. Insert the needle, with the bevel up, beneath the skin at a 5- to 15-degree angle. Keep the fingers and thumb resting on the sides of the syringe to ensure the proper angle.

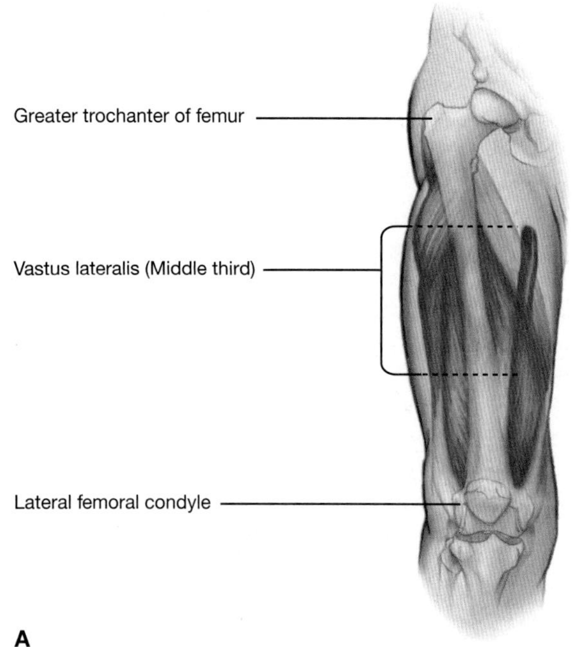

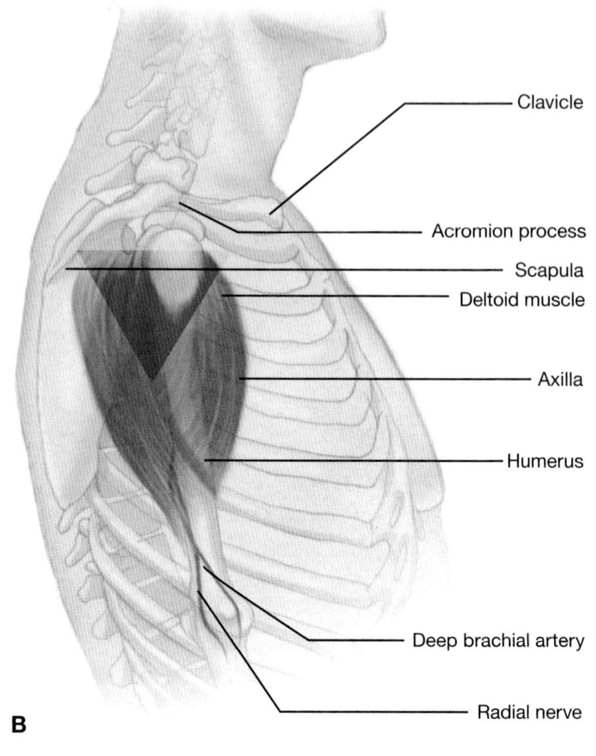

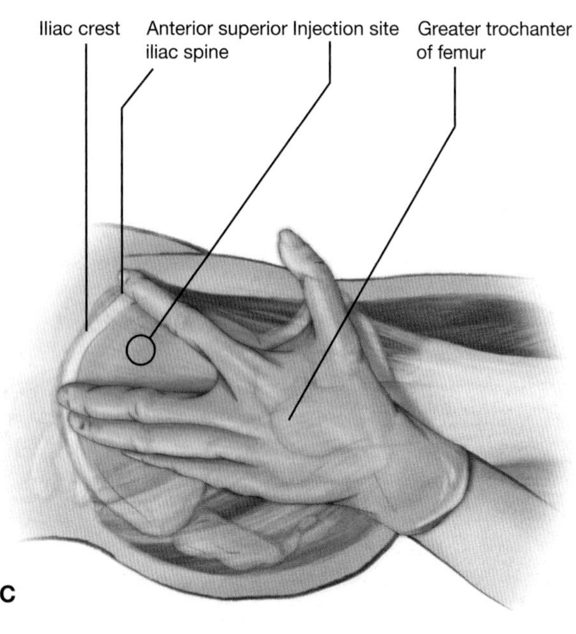

FIGURE 13.7 Locating intramuscular injection sites. **A.** Vastus lateralis: identify the greater trochanter and the lateral femoral condyle; inject in middle third and anterior lateral aspect. **B.** Deltoid: locate the lateral side of the humerus, one to two finger widths below the acromion process. Inject into upper third of muscle. **C.** Ventrogluteal: place palm of left hand on right greater trochanter so index finger points toward anterosuperior iliac spine, spread middle finger to form a V, and inject in the middle of the V.

Intravenous Administration

IV medication administration is commonly used with children, especially when a rapid response to a drug is desired or when absorption via other routes is difficult due to the child's illness or condition. In some cases, the IV route is the only effective method for administering a medication. Use of the IV route requires that the child have an IV device inserted, peripherally or centrally. Although insertion of this device is invasive and traumatic for the child, IV medication administration is considered to be less traumatic when compared to the trauma associated with multiple injections. Unfortunately, the veins of a child are small and easily irritated.

Most medications given by the IV route must be given at a specified rate and diluted properly to prevent overdose or toxicity due to the rapid onset of action that occurs with this route. Therefore, when administering medications via the IV route, knowledge of the drug, the amount of drug to be administered, the minimum dilution of the drug, the type of solution for dilution or infusion, the compatibility of various solutions and medications, the length of time for infusion, and the rate of infusion is required. Careful maintenance of the IV site is required to prevent complications.

TABLE 13.2 • Guidelines for Solution Amount, Needle Length, and Needle Gauge for Intramuscular Injections

	Solution Amount				
	Vastus Lateralis (Anterolateral)	Deltoid	Ventrogluteal	Length	Gauge
Infant <12 months old	0.5 mL	Not recommended	Not recommended until 7 months; then 0.5 mL	5/8 to 1 in	22–25
Toddler 12 months to 2 years	0.5–1 mL (preferred site)	0.5 mL	1 mL	5/8 to 1 in	22–25
Preschooler 3–5 years old	1 mL	0.5 mL (preferred site)	1.5 mL	5/8 to 1 in	22–25
School age 6–10 years old	1.5–2 mL	0.5–1 mL (preferred site)	1.5–2 mL	5/8 to 1.25 in	22–25
Late school-age/adolescent (11–18 years old)	Up to 3 mL	1–2 mL (preferred site)	1–5 mL	5/8 to 1.5 in	22–25

Needle size and site need to be individualized based on the size of the muscle, amount of adipose tissue, and amount of solution to be administered.

Data from Kroger, A., Bahta, L., Long, S., & Sanchez, P. (2023). *General best practice guidelines for immunization*. www.cdc.gov/vaccines/hcp/acip-recs/general-recs/downloads/general-recs.pdf; Schneider, M. (2022). *Clinical guidelines (Nursing): Intramuscular injections*. https://www.rch.org.au/rchcpg/hospital_clinical_guideline_index/Intramuscular_Injections/#:~:text=The%20anterolateral%20aspect%20of%20the,anaphylaxis%20management%20in%20all%20ages

The primary method for IV medication administration is a syringe pump. This method provides a highly precise rate of infusion. Nursing Procedure 13.1 outlines the steps for administering medication via a syringe pump.

If a pump is unavailable, the medication may be administered via a volume control device. The medication is added to the device with a specified amount of compatible fluid and then infused at the ordered rate.

Direct IV push medication is typically reserved for emergency situations and when therapeutic blood levels must be reached quickly to achieve the desired effect. Direct IV push administration requires that the drug be diluted appropriately and given at a specified rate, such as over 2 to 3 minutes. Care must be taken to prevent fluid overload, which may occur due to flushing needed to maintain IV patency and prevent drug incompatibilities, and from the administration of multiple drug therapies.

TAKE NOTE!

The use of clinical judgment is necessary when selecting injection or intravenous sites, needle length and gauge, and appropriate infusion devices.

NURSING PROCEDURE 13.1 Administering Medication via a Syringe Pump

Purpose: To provide accurate and safe administration of IV medication

1. Verify the medication order.
2. Gather the medication and necessary equipment and supplies.
3. Wash hands and put on gloves.
4. Attach the syringe pump tubing to the medication syringe, and purge air from the tubing by gently filling the tubing with medication from the syringe.
5. Insert the syringe into the pump according to the manufacturer's directions.
6. Clean the appropriate port on the child's IV access device or tubing, flush the device or tubing if appropriate (e.g., an intermittent infusion device [saline lock or heparin lock]), and attach the syringe tubing to the IV tubing or device.
7. Set the infusion rate on the pump as ordered.
8. When the medication infusion is completed, flush the syringe pump tubing to deliver any medication remaining in the tubing, according to institution protocol.
9. Document the procedure and the child's response to it.

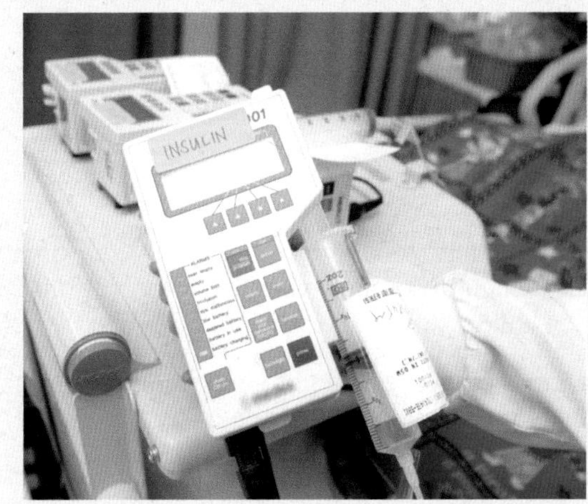

Providing Atraumatic Care

When administering any medication, including oral medications, use the principles of atraumatic care (see Chapter 8 for more information). Children can experience stress and fear or upset when they must take medications. The child may become upset or stressed when they must be secured snugly or positioned to minimize movement. The child may experience further discomfort if the medication has an unpleasant taste or results in pain, such as with an injection.

• • • ATRAUMATIC CARE • • •

Encourage the child to participate in care, and provide the child with developmentally appropriate options, such as which fluid to drink with the medication or which flavor of ice pop to suck on before or after the administration (see Table 13.1).

To decrease discomfort and pain for the child who is to receive an injection, apply a topical anesthetic such as a eutectic mixture of local anesthetic (EMLA) cream or vapocoolant spray to the site before injection when possible (Kroger et al., 2023), and inject the most painful medication last (see Chapter 14 for additional information). Also, utilize developmentally appropriate distraction techniques, such as music, books, blowing bubbles or a pinwheel, and deep breathing exercises (see Chapter 8 for additional information).

Ensuring that the child doesn't move is essential to prevent injury when administering an injection. When administering an injection to a young child, at least two adults should hold the child; this may also be necessary to help an older child to remain still.

TAKE NOTE!

According to research, children experience less pain and decreased fear if they are sitting versus lying down when receiving an injection (CDC, 2021).

• • • ATRAUMATIC CARE • • •

Use positions that are comforting to the child, such as therapeutic hugging, during injections. Have the child sit on the caregiver's lap, with the caregiver holding the child's arms and legs to their body. Refer to Chapter 8, Figure 8.1. After administration, encourage the parents or caregivers to hold and cuddle the child and offer praise.

Educating the Child and Parents

Teaching the child and parents or caregivers about medication administration is key. Many medications are given in the home, making the parents or caregivers responsible for administration. They need to know what medications they are giving and why, how to give them, and what to expect from the drug, including adverse effects. Caregivers and parents often make medication errors at home, such as incorrectly dosing over-the-counter medications and prescription medications or failing to follow or understand medication instructions given, for example, not completing the full course of the medication or missing doses (Lopez-Pineda et al., 2021). Therefore, ensure thorough instruction, including frequency of administration, when the next dose is due, and length of time the medication is to be given. Emphasize the importance of completing the prescribed dose. Demonstrate use with an actual syringe if possible, encourage return demonstration of medication administration, advise against the use of home-measuring devices (such as a spoon), and emphasize the importance of always using the calibrated dispensing device that was given with the medication. If the medication is to be given via injection, parents and caregivers need to learn how to administer the injection properly. Encourage questions or concerns from parents or caregivers.

Parents and caregivers commonly need suggestions about the best ways to administer the medication to their child. Provide them with tips for administration, such as mixing unpleasant-tasting medications with applesauce or yogurt or offering a favorite liquid as a chaser. Also teach the parents how to properly measure the amount of drug to be given. Teaching Guidelines 13.2 gives pointers about oral medication administration. Refer to Chapter 8 for further information on teaching children and families about medication administration.

Preventing Medication Errors

Experts agree that the incidence of potentially harmful medication errors is higher in the pediatric population compared to adults (The Joint Commission, 2021). This can be related to weight-based dosing calculations, fractional dosing, and the need for the use of decimal points. Children are also more susceptible because many drugs used in pediatrics are formulated and packaged for adults and lack U.S. Food and Drug Administration (FDA) approval and dosing guidelines for children. Recent legislative changes have led to a dramatic increase in pediatric drug studies and improvement in accurate pediatric dosing and labeling (FDA, 2023).

The need for safety takes on even greater importance due to the physiologic, psychological, and cognitive differences inherent in children. Children are more vulnerable to medication errors as they vary in weight,

TEACHING GUIDELINES 13.2 Administering Oral Medications

- Be firm when telling your child that it is time for their medication. State, "It's time for your medicine" instead of asking, "Will you take your medicine?" or "Can you take your medicine for me?"
- Allow your child to choose an appropriate liquid to help swallow the medication or drink after taking it. Limit the choices to two or three.
- Never bribe or threaten your child to take their medication.
- Never refer to the medication as "candy."
- Be honest about the taste of the medication. If necessary, mix it with another food such as applesauce, yogurt, or syrup to help mask the taste.
- Do not mix the medication with formula or baby food.
- Always check with your health care provider or nurse practitioner and pharmacy about opening capsules or crushing tablets and mixing them with food. Some medications should not be opened or crushed.
- If you are giving a liquid using an oral syringe or dropper, place the medication slowly along the inside of the cheek. Never squirt the medication forcibly to the back of the child's throat. It may cause the child to gag and spit out the medication or aspirate it into their lungs.
- Always praise the child after taking the medication and provide comfort and cuddling.

BSA, and organ maturity, which affect their ability to metabolize and excrete medications; they depend on others for medication administration; they are often unable to communicate if an adverse reaction is occurring; and they need special compound medication formulations (The Joint Commission, 2023). Confirming the child's identity and double-checking the dosage before administration of any medication are two critical safeguards that play a major role in preventing medication errors. Other ways to prevent medication errors include the following:

- Confirm that the children's weight is accurate.
- Always weigh children in kilograms.
- Double-check medication calculations; utilize another health care provider when possible, especially for high-risk medications.
- If a dose seems unusually small or large, verify the order.
- Utilize medication ordering and dispensing systems, if available.
- Always report medication errors or near-miss errors to help prevent future mistakes.
- Utilize The Joint Commission's official "Do Not Use" list. (The up-to-date list can be found on The Joint Commission's website.)

TAKE NOTE!

If a parent, caregiver, or child questions whether a medication should be given, listen attentively, answer their questions, and double-check the order.

INTRAVENOUS THERAPY

IV access provides a route for the administration of medications and fluids. It is commonly used for children because it is the quickest, and often the most effective, method of administration. As with adults, numerous sites and various devices and equipment may be used to provide IV therapy over a short or long period of time. When administering IV therapy, safety is crucial. The nurse must have a solid knowledge base about the fluids or medications to be given as well as a thorough understanding of the child's physical and emotional development. Venipuncture can be a terrifying and painful experience for children and their families. Nurses play a crucial role in providing support and education to the child and family before, during, and after the procedure (refer to Chapter 8 for additional information related to provision of atraumatic care with procedures).

Sites

IV therapy may be administered via a peripheral vein or a central vein. Peripheral IV therapy sites commonly include the hands, feet, and forearms (Fig. 13.8). In

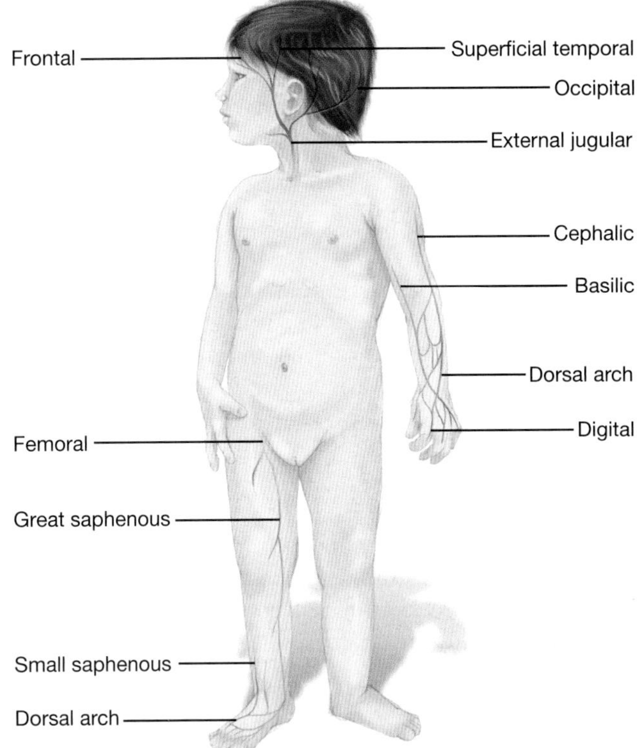

FIGURE 13.8 Preferred peripheral sites for IV insertion.

neonates and young infants, the scalp veins may be used (Doyle et al., 2022). The scalp veins are easily visualized, being covered only by a thin layer of SQ tissue. These veins do not have valves, so the device may be inserted in either direction, although the preference would be in the direction of blood flow. However, use of a scalp vein requires that that area of the infant's head be cleared of hair to enhance visualization. In addition, use of the scalp veins can be frightening to parents, who may think the fluid is infusing into the infant's brain. Thus, scalp veins are usually used only if other sites are assessed to be inferior or attempts at other sites have been unsuccessful (Doyle et al., 2022). When used, ensure appropriate education of the parents prior to insertion, and, if shaving the child's hair is needed, inquire if parents would like to keep the child's hair.

TAKE NOTE!

When selecting an IV site in an extremity, always choose the most distal site. Doing so prevents injury to the veins superior to the site and allows additional access sites should complications develop in the most distal site.

Central IV therapy is usually administered through a large vein, such as the subclavian, femoral, or jugular vein or the vena cava. The tip of the device lies in the superior vena cava just at the entrance to the right atrium. The device is inserted surgically or percutaneously and exits the body typically in the chest area, just below the clavicle. A device can be inserted via a peripheral vein, such as the median, cephalic, or basilic vein, and then threaded into the superior vena cava.

Equipment

The choice of equipment is determined by the solution or medication to be administered, the duration of the therapy, the age and developmental level of the child, the child's status, and the condition of their veins. Various types of IV devices are commercially available. In addition, different types of tubing and infusion control devices may be necessary.

Peripheral Access Devices

Devices used for peripheral venous access in a child include over-the-needle catheters or winged-infusion sets, commonly referred to as "butterflies" or scalp vein needles. These devices are inserted into the vein and then connected to the IV solution via tubing to provide a continuous infusion of fluid. These devices can also be inserted for intermittent use if the child does not require a continuous fluid infusion. Typically, the hub of the device is capped or plugged to allow intermittent access, such as for administering medications or obtaining blood specimens. When used in this manner, these devices are termed peripheral intermittent infusion devices or saline or heparin locks.

Needle size on the device also varies. Typically, the needle ranges from 21- to 25-gauge, depending on the child's size. Use the smallest-gauge catheter with the shortest length possible to prevent traumatizing the child's fragile veins. Typically, peripheral IV devices are used for short-term therapy, usually averaging 3 to 5 days. Midline catheters or peripherally inserted central catheters (PICCs) are also available and recommended for use if therapy is to exceed 7 days (Paterson et al., 2020).

Central Access Devices

Numerous devices for central venous access are available. The type chosen depends on several factors, including the duration of the therapy, the child's diagnosis, the risks to the child from insertion, and the ability of the child and family to care for the device. The device may have one or multiple lumens. Although central venous access devices can be used short term, the majority are used for moderate- to long-term therapy.

Central venous access devices are indicated when the child lacks suitable peripheral access, requires IV fluid or medication for a prolonged period of time, or is to receive specific treatments, such as the administration of highly concentrated solutions or irritating drugs like chemotherapeutic agents, parenteral nutrition, or blood and blood products. Child preference is also a consideration. Central venous access is advantageous because it provides vascular access without the need for multiple IV starts, thus decreasing discomfort and fear. However, central venous access devices are associated with complications such as infection at the site, sepsis due to the direct access to the central circulation, and thrombosis due to partial occlusion of the vessel. Typically, a chest radiograph is performed after a central venous access device is inserted to verify proper placement. No fluids are administered until correct placement is confirmed. Table 13.3 describes the major types of central venous access devices.

Infusion Control Devices

Infants and young children are at increased risk for fluid volume overload compared with adults. Also, malfunction at the IV insertion site, such as infiltration, may result in much greater injury than a similar incident would cause in an adult. Therefore, IV fluids must be carefully administered and monitored. To ensure accurate fluid administration, infusion control devices such as infusion

TABLE 13.3 • Types of Central Venous Access Devices

Device	Description
Peripherally inserted central catheter (PICC)	Short- to moderate-term therapy (few weeks to a few months) Insertion via a peripheral vein such as basilic, cephalic, or brachial vein Catheter typically threaded into superior vena cava; distal tip terminates in the superior vena cava, inferior vena cava, or proximal right atrium Insertion via saphenous vein with tip terminating in inferior vena cava above the diaphragm for infants Single or multiple lumens Can be inserted at the bedside; requires additional training and advanced skill Blood sampling is possible; child can be sent home with the line in place
Nontunneled central venous catheter (CVC)	Usually used short term (1–2 weeks) One or more lumens Percutaneous insertion most commonly via the subclavian, internal jugular, or femoral vein with the tip of the catheter at the top of the superior vena cava just above the right atrium Useful for emergency situations Catheter sutured in place at the exit site Increased rate of central line–associated bloodstream infection than tunneled CVC
Tunneled central venous catheter (e.g., Groshong, Hickman/Broviac)	Usually for long-term use (1–6 months) Catheter inserted by a health care provider via small incision in jugular or subclavian vein and tunneled in the subcutaneous tissue under the skin Initially sutured in place to stabilize position; sutures removed after approximately 1–2 weeks when cuff on catheter attaches to subcutaneous tissue Single or multiple lumens Some have valves that prevent backflow of blood and air entrance Radiologic confirmation of placement needed Blood sampling is possible; child can be sent home with the line in place Requires surgical removal
Implanted ports (e.g., Port-a-Cath, Infuse-a-Port, Mediport)	Long-term use (>3 months to years) Surgically inserted by a health care provider Stainless steel port with a polyurethane or silicone catheter attached Catheter tip lying in subclavian or jugular vein; port implanted under skin in a subcutaneous pocket, usually on the upper chest wall Port covered completely by skin and visible only as a slight bulging on the chest; possibly more appealing to the older child and adolescent because there are no visible parts or dressings Access to port via a specially angled, noncoring needle (Huber needle) Site preparation and pain relief measures necessary before accessing the port Lowest risk for central line–associated bloodstream infection Blood sampling is possible; child can be sent home with the line in place Surgical removal is required

Adapted from Naik, V. M., Mantha, S. S. P., & Rayani, B. K. (2019). Vascular access in children. *Indian Journal of Anaesthesia*, *63*(9), 737–745. https://doi.org/10.4103/ija.IJA_489_19

pumps, syringe pumps, and volume control sets may be used.

Infusion pumps used for children are similar to those used for adults. In addition, syringe pumps are often used to deliver fluid and medications to children. These pumps can be programmed to deliver minute amounts of fluid over controlled periods of time (syringe pumps are discussed further in the next section).

An IV solution bag may be attached to a calibrated volume control set that has been filled with a specified amount of IV solution (Fig. 13.9). The fluid chamber holds a maximum of 100 to 150 mL of fluid that can be infused over a specified period of time as ordered. Usually, a maximum of a 2-hour infusion amount in the chamber avoids accidental fluid overload in the pediatric population. This chamber can be filled every 1 to 2 hours so only small amounts of ordered quantities of fluid can infuse and the child is protected from receiving too much fluid volume. Due to the advances in pump technology and the introduction of "smart pumps," which include dose error reduction systems such as hospital-defined drug libraries (drug lists) with standard drug concentrations, and dose limits to potentially improve the safety of IV medication administration, the use of volume control devices has been reduced or eliminated in many facilities. Concerns include inability to identify the

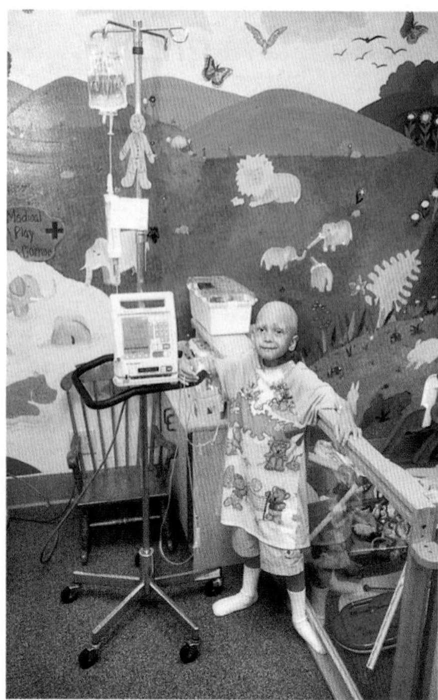

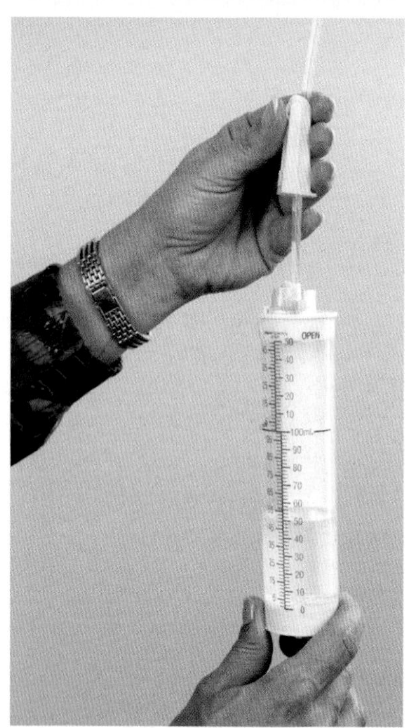

FIGURE 13.9 Volume control infusion device.

medication in the volume control device and the potential for interaction or precipitation that may occur when multiple medications are administered using the same volume control device. However, they are still available as a safety device for controlling the volume of fluid administered to children; therefore, nurses should be familiar with how to use them. Be familiar with your facility's policies and procedures. When using a volume control device, label the chamber when medications are added, and check for incompatibilities and potential interactions when multiple medications are given.

Inserting Peripheral IV Access Devices

Peripheral IV devices are used for most IV therapies. Prior to insertion, review the child's diagnosis and medical history for information that may affect therapy, such as site selection or insertion. For example, a child who has a history of chronic illness may have heightened fears and anxieties related to insertion due to previous experiences or difficulty in accessing IV sites. Typically, the nondominant extremity should be used for insertion, but this may not be possible in certain situations, such as if a right-handed child has a cast on their left arm.

Check the orders for the prescribed therapy. Determine the purpose and length of the IV therapy and the type of fluid or medication that is to be administered. This information aids in selecting the best device and insertion site. For example, the device needs to be of an adequate gauge to allow the solution or medication to infuse into the vein while at the same time allowing enough blood flow around the device to promote dilution of the infusion.

Establish rapport with the child and parents. Inform them about IV therapy and what to expect. Be honest with the child. Explain that the venipuncture will hurt but only for a short time. Provide the child with a time frame that they can understand, such as the time it takes to brush their teeth or eat a snack.

• • • ATRAUMATIC CARE • • •

Use therapeutic play to assist the child in preparing and coping for the procedure (see Chapter 11 for more information).

Insertion of an IV therapy device is traumatic. Follow the principles of atraumatic care, including the following:

- Gather all equipment needed before approaching the child.
- If possible, select a site using hand veins rather than wrist or upper arm veins to reduce the risk of phlebitis. Avoid sites where excessive movement may occur, such as the lower extremity veins and areas of joint flexion, if possible, because these are associated with an increased risk of thrombophlebitis and other complications (Lippincott Williams & Wilkins, 2023).
- Ensure adequate pain relief using pharmacologic and nonpharmacologic methods prior to insertion of the device (see Chapter 14 for more information about management of pain related to procedures).
- Allow the antiseptic used to prepare the site to dry completely before attempting insertion.
- Use a barrier such as gauze or a washcloth or the sleeve of the child's gown under the tourniquet to avoid pinching or damaging the skin.
- If the child's veins are difficult to locate, use a device to transilluminate the vein (utilizes a bright light, which illuminates the vein's size and direction of travel).

- Make only two attempts to gain access; if you are unsuccessful after two attempts, allow another individual two attempts to access a site. If still unsuccessful, evaluate the need for insertion of another device.
- Encourage parental participation as appropriate in helping to position the child or to provide comfort positioning, such as therapeutic hugging.
- Coordinate care with other departments such as the laboratory for blood specimen collection to minimize the number of venipunctures for the child.
- Secure the IV line using a minimal amount of tape or transparent dressing.
- Protect the site from bumping by using a security device such as the IV house dressing (Fig. 13.10).

TAKE NOTE!

Some facilities have policies in place allowing only one stick per nurse, with a maximum of two sticks; then the doctor needs to be notified unless the situation is an emergency.

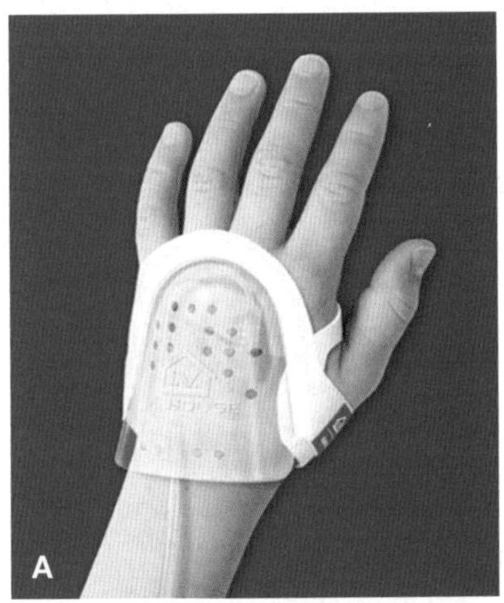

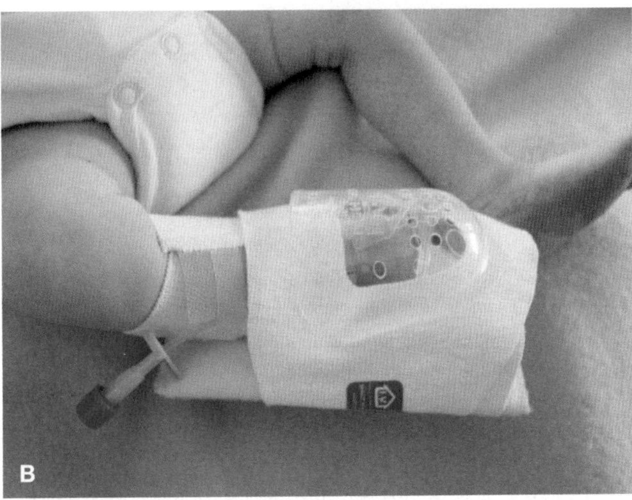

FIGURE 13.10 A. IV house over the IV site on a child's hand. **B.** IV house over the site on an infant's foot.

IV Fluid Administration

Administering IV fluids to an infant or child requires close attention to the child's fluid status. Typically, the amount of fluid to be administered in a day (24 hours) is determined by the child's weight (in kilograms) using the following approach:

- 100 mL/kg of body weight for the first 10 kg
- 50 mL/kg of body weight for the next 10 kg
- 20 mL/kg of body weight for the remainder of body weight in kilograms

Table 13.4 gives examples of calculating a child's fluid requirements using body weight. Once the 24-hour total fluid requirement is determined, this amount is divided by 24 hours to arrive at the correct hourly rate of infusion.

Maintaining IV Fluid Therapy

Throughout the course of therapy, monitor the fluid infusion rate and volume closely, as often as every hour. If a volume control set is used to administer the IV infusion, fill the device with the allotted amount of fluid that the child is to receive in 1 hour. Doing so prevents inadvertent administration of too much fluid. Never assume that just because an infusion pump is in use, the infusion is being administered without problems. Pumps can malfunction. The tubing can become blocked, or the IV device can move out of the vein lumen. Not enough fluid, fluid overload, or infiltration of the solution into the tissues can occur.

In addition to monitoring the fluid infusion, closely monitor the child's output. Expected urine output for children and adolescents is 1 to 2 mL/kg/hour.

TAKE NOTE!

When measuring the output of an infant or child who is not toilet trained or who is incontinent, weigh the diaper to determine the output. Remember that 1 g of weight is equal to 1 mL of fluid.

Flushing the IV line when the device is used intermittently may be necessary to maintain patency, such as before and/or after medication is administered and after obtaining blood specimens. However, there is much debate as to how often flushing should be done and the best flush solution to use, heparin or saline. Saline has been found to be more compatible with the numerous solutions and medications administered intravenously and is less expensive and less irritating to the vein. In addition, using saline lessens the incidence of pain and phlebitis. Heparin is expensive and incompatible with numerous medications and solutions, and it can affect clotting time, depending on the concentration of the flush solution used. However, it has also been found to increase catheter patency and decrease infusion failures. Evidence appears to support the effectiveness of both heparin and normal saline for maintaining

TABLE 13.4 • Intravenous Maintenance Fluid Calculations by Body Weight

<10 kg in weight	100 mL/kg of weight = # mL for 24 hours Example: A child weighs 7.4 kg 7.4 × 100 = 740 mL (daily requirement) 740/24 = 30.8 or 31 mL/hour
11–20 kg in weight	100 mL/kg of weight for the first 10 kg + 50 mL/kg for the next 10 kg = # mL for 24 hours Example: A child weighs 16 kg (10 × 100 = 1,000) plus (6 × 50 = 300) Total = 1,300 mL (daily requirement) 1,300/24 = 54 mL/hour
>20 kg in weight	100 mL/kg for the first 10 kg + 50 mL/kg for the next 10 kg + 20 mL/kg for each kg >20 kg = # mL for 24 hours Example: A child weighs 30 kg (10 × 100 = 1,000) plus (10 × 50 = 500) plus (10 × 20 = 200) Total = 1,700 mL (daily requirement) 1,700/24 = 70.8 or 71 mL/hour

patency of peripheral IV catheters, and which fluid is used will depend on provider and agency preference. The most effective flushing solution may depend on individual factors, such as catheter type, patient condition, and medications being infused. Additional research is needed to determine the best solution, volume and concentration of the flush solution, and interval for flushing. Flushing solutions and procedure will vary; therefore, it is important to always follow your agency's policy or provider order for flushing IV lines. See Evidence-Based Practice 13.1

If the child is receiving IV therapy via a central venous access device, provide site care using sterile technique and flush the device according to agency policy. Note the exit site for the device, and inspect it frequently for signs of infection. If the device has multiple lumens, label each lumen with its use (i.e., blood specimen, medication, or fluid). Always check the compatibilities of solutions and medications being given simultaneously.

TAKE NOTE!

When flushing or administering medications through a PICC line, follow the manufacturer's recommended syringe size, because PICC lines are fragile. Using a larger-volume syringe (i.e., 10 mL or larger) exerts less pressure on the PICC, thereby reducing the risk of rupture (Lippincott Williams & Wilkins, 2023).

Preventing Complications

IV therapy is an invasive procedure that is associated with numerous complications. Strict aseptic technique is necessary when inserting the device and caring for the site.

EVIDENCE-BASED PRACTICE 13.1

Which Is More Effective—Normal Saline or Heparin for Maintaining Patency and Avoiding Complications in Peripheral Intravenous Catheters (PIVC)?

The debate on flushing with heparin or saline has been investigated in a number of research studies for many years, with controversial results. Many differences in the maintenance of PIVCs exist even within the same facilities.

STUDY

A systematic review of research studies involving hospitalized patients with PIVC was performed to evaluate the efficacy of normal saline versus heparin in maintaining patency and preventing complications of peripheral venous catheters.

Findings

The review found that it is not fully documented if normal saline is superior to heparin in maintaining patency and preventing complications. Researchers tend to support the use of normal saline over heparin as it is safer, more compatible with other medications, more efficient, easier to use, and cost effective.

Nursing Implications

The use of normal saline (NS) seems to have more advantages over the use of heparin. These findings cannot be generalized due to the small number of studies. Therefore, further research is warranted. Nurses must be aware of and follow their agency policy and procedures. Nursing care needs to be based on current scientific evidence. Nurses need to continuously question their care practices and review current research and perform research on topics they feel need it.

Data from Sotnikova, C., Fasoi, G., Efstathiou, F., Kaba, E., Bourazani, M., & Kelesi, M. (2020). The efficacy of normal saline (N/S 0.9%) versus heparin solution in maintaining patency of peripheral venous catheter and avoiding complications: A systematic review. *Materia Socio-Medica*, *32*(1), 29–34. https://doi.org/10.5455/msm.2020.32.29-34

Adherence to standard precautions is key. Inspect the insertion site every 1 to 2 hours for inflammation or **infiltration** (inadvertent infusion of a nonirritant solution or medication into the surrounding tissue). Note signs of inflammation such as warmth, redness, induration, or tender skin. Check closely for signs of infiltration such as cool, blanched, or puffy skin. Use of a transparent dressing or IV house dressing provides easy access for assessing the IV insertion site. These types of dressings also help to prevent movement of the catheter hub, thus minimizing the risk of mechanical irritation, dislodgement, and complications such as phlebitis or infection (see Fig. 13.10).

Typically, in adults, an IV site is changed every 72 to 96 hours and at any time when the integrity of the system has been compromised or contamination is suspected (CDC, 2017). Recent clinical trials have suggested that routine replacement of a PIVC does not decrease the risk of infection (Ullman & Chopra, 2022). Current recommendations include replacement in children only when clinically indicated (CDC, 2017; Ullman & Chopra, 2022). Follow the agency's policies and procedures related to site changes. Consider an alternative route for fluid and medication administration or the insertion of an alternative IV device, such as a PICC line. Catheter-related bloodstream infections can often occur with the use of central venous lines. These infections result in increased morbidity, mortality, and health care costs (Haddadin et al., 2022). Prevention is paramount. Nurses need to practice proper hand hygiene, use maximal barrier protection during insertion, assess the site frequently, provide proper site care using strict sterile technique, and ensure that the child's central venous catheter is removed as soon as it is no longer needed. In children, it is also important to prevent the child from touching and playing with the central venous line site or dressing. The CDC and Healthcare Infection Control Practices Advisory Committee (HICPAC) currently recommends changing administration sets that are continuously used no more frequently than every 96 hours but at least every 7 days, except if fluids that increase microbial growth, such as blood, blood products, or parenteral nutrition, have been administered (CDC, 2017; Ullman & Chopra, 2022). In these cases, changing the administration sets every 24 hours is recommended (CDC, 2017; Ullman & Chopra, 2022). Replace administration sets per agency policy. Ensure proper disinfecting of all catheter hubs, needleless connectors, and injection ports before accessing them to minimize contamination.

TAKE NOTE!

Chlorhexidine-impregnated sponge (Biopatch) dressings may be used to help prevent infection in children over 2 months old (Ullman & Chopra, 2022). Always follow agency or institution policy and procedures regarding site care.

Discontinuing the IV Device

Prepare the child for removal of the IV device in much the same manner as for insertion. Many children may fear the removal of the device to the same extent that they feared its insertion. Explain what is to occur, and enlist the child's help in the removal.

• • • ATRAUMATIC CARE • • •

If appropriate, allow the child to assist in removing the tape or dressing. This gives the child a sense of control over the situation and also encourages their cooperation.

In addition, practice atraumatic care by doing the following:

- Use water or adhesive remover to help loosen the tape.
- If a transparent dressing is in place, gently lift off the dressing by pulling up opposite corners using a motion parallel to the skin surface.
- Avoid using scissors to cut the tape, but if cutting the tape is necessary, be sure that the child's fingers are clear of the tape and scissors.
- Turn off the infusion solution and pump.
- Once all tape and dressings are removed, gently slide the IV device out using a motion opposite to that used for the insertion.
- Apply pressure to the site with a dry gauze dressing, and then cover with a small adhesive bandage. If possible, allow the child to choose the bandage.

TAKE NOTE!

If the IV site was in the arm at or near the antecubital space, apply pressure until the bleeding stops. Do not have the child bend their arm after removal of the device as this is not sufficient pressure to prevent hematoma formation.

PROVIDING NUTRITIONAL SUPPORT

Adequate nutrition is important for all individuals but especially for children. During the growing years, the quality of a child's nutrition affects their overall health and development. The presence of a chronic illness, disease, or trauma can increase the child's nutritional demands; if the child cannot meet these even with oral supplementation, other measures may be necessary to provide nutritional support. Such measures may include **enteral nutrition** (delivery of nutrition into the gastrointestinal tract via a tube) and **parenteral nutrition** (IV delivery of nutritional substances). The nutritional plan is determined by the child's age, developmental level, and health status.

Enteral Nutrition

Enteral nutrition, commonly called tube feedings, involves the insertion of a tube so that feedings can be delivered directly into the child's gastrointestinal tract. The tube may be inserted via the nose or mouth or through an opening in the abdominal area, with the tube ending in the stomach or small intestine. Nasogastric or orogastric tube feedings, a tube from the nose to the stomach or from the mouth to the stomach, respectively, are commonly referred to as **gavage feedings**. Nasoduodenal or nasojejunal feedings involve a tube that is inserted through the nose and ends in either the duodenum or the jejunum. Gastrostomy feedings involve the insertion of a gastrostomy tube through an opening in the abdominal wall and into the stomach. Jejunostomy feedings are similar to gastrostomy feedings except that the tube lies in the jejunum.

Enteral nutrition is indicated for children who have a functioning gastrointestinal tract but cannot ingest enough nutrients orally. The child may be unconscious or have a severely debilitating condition that interferes with their ability to consume adequate food and fluids. Other conditions that may warrant the use of enteral nutrition include the following:

- Failure to thrive
- Inability to suck or tiring easily during sucking
- Abnormalities of the throat or esophagus
- Swallowing difficulties or risk of aspiration
- Respiratory distress
- Metabolic conditions
- Severe gastroesophageal reflux disease (GERD)
- Surgery
- Severe trauma

Enteral feedings may be given via nasogastric, orogastric, nasojejunal, nasoduodenal, gastrostomy, or jejunostomy tubes (Fig. 13.11). Table 13.5 provides additional information about these types of feeding tubes. Enteral feedings cost less, are associated with fewer complications, and are considered safer than parenteral feedings. However, tube misplacement is a serious complication.

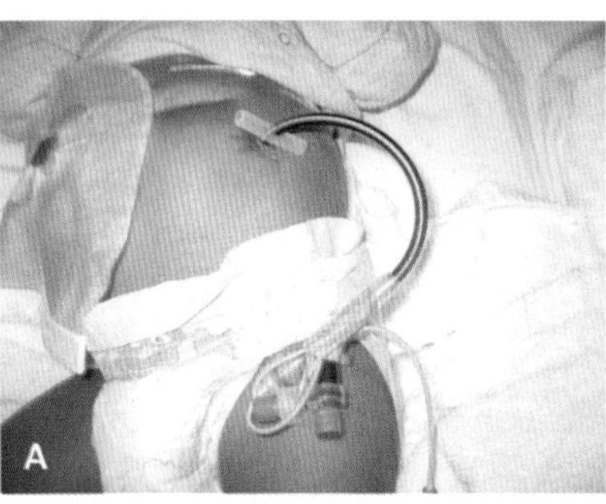

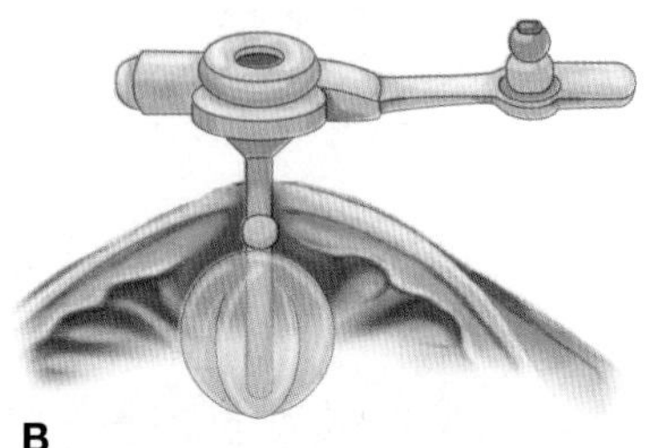

FIGURE 13.11 **A.** Gastrostomy tube. **B.** Low-profile (button) gastrostomy tube. The filled balloon keeps the tube in place inside the stomach.

Inserting a Nasogastric or Orogastric Feeding Tube

Tubes for gavage feeding can be inserted via the nose or mouth. For infants, who are obligate nose breathers, insertion via the mouth may be appropriate. Oral insertion also promotes sucking in the infant. For the older child, nasal insertion is usually the preferred method. If the tube is to remain in place, the nose is also considered to be more comfortable. Nursing Procedure 13.2 gives the steps for inserting a gavage feeding tube.

DETERMINING TUBING LENGTH FOR INSERTION

Several methods exist for determining proper tube length, and significant variation in clinical practice is common. Therefore, it is imperative to know your institution's policy and procedures and be up-to-date on current evidence-based practice guidelines. Traditionally, morphologic methods, measuring from the nose to ear to mid-xiphoid to umbilicus (NEMU) or just nose to ear to mid-xiphoid (NEX), have been used to determine tube length for insertion. Research supports the use of the NEMU method over the NEX method, as it demonstrates consistent placement into the body of the stomach (Irving et al., 2018).

Improving the accuracy of predicting tube length will lead to an increase in successful nasogastric tube placements and, therefore, improved outcomes and decreased health care costs.

Determining tubing length for insertion of a nasogastric tube has also been done by using age-related height-based (ARHB) methods. Recent research has shown this method may be more accurate for measuring tube length (Manzo et al., 2023). Refer to Table 13.7 for ARHB equations. Continued research is warranted, and nurses need to ensure they are following best evidence-based practices.

CHECKING TUBE PLACEMENT

Once the gavage feeding tube is inserted, checking for placement is essential. Tube placement must be confirmed each time the tube is inserted and before each use. Radiologic confirmation of tube placement is considered the most accurate method, but the risks associated with repeated radiation exposure, high costs, and the impractical nature of obtaining a radiograph before feeding tube use make it unrealistic (Irving et al., 2018). Several methods have been proposed as reliable for checking tube placement, but no single method has

TABLE 13.5 • Types of Enteral Feeding Tubes

Type of Tube	Indication	Nursing Implications
Nasogastric (inserted via the nose into the stomach) Orogastric (inserted via the mouth into the stomach)	Short-term enteral feeding Orogastric usually limited to young infants only	• Long-term use or repeated insertion causes irritation and discomfort. • Silicone and polyurethane tubes are very flexible and more comfortable; they require a stylet or guidewire for insertion. • Length of long-term use varies according to the type of tube used and the institution protocol. Periodically, a nasogastric tube is removed and reinserted via the opposite nostril to prevent pressure on the nasal mucosa. • Maintaining orogastric placement between feedings can be difficult due to oral secretions.
Nasoduodenal (inserted via the nose to the duodenum) or nasojejunal (inserted via the nose to the jejunum)	Short-term enteral feeding. Indicated if child has trouble digesting food, cannot use their gastrointestinal tract secondary to congenital anomalies or surgery, or is at risk for or has a history of severe reflux or aspiration	• Silicone and polyurethane tubes with weighted tip allow tube to pass from pylorus into small intestines. • Agency may require special training in order to place at bedside; may also be performed in radiology • Length of use same as nasogastric or orogastric tubes
Gastrostomy (surgically inserted through the abdominal wall into the stomach) Jejunostomy (surgically inserted through the abdominal wall into the jejunum)	Long-term enteral feeding or when esophageal atresia or stricture is present Jejunostomy tubes are indicated when gastric feeding is not tolerated.	• The inner section of the tube is below the skin surface, with the tip located in the stomach or jejunum (may be balloon, winged, or mushroom shaped). The outer section appears above the skin surface at the insertion site and has an opening or feeding port to which the feeding solution is attached. • Low-profile gastrostomy device (gastrostomy button) is flush with the abdominal surface. The flip-top opening is anchored by a dome that fits against the stomach wall. Less conspicuous, it allows the child to be more active and mobile. • After initial insertion, the tube length is measured from the insertion site to the far end of the tube and recorded. This measurement is checked at least daily to ensure that the tube has not moved. • There are many different devices available. For any gastrostomy or jejunostomy tube, the type and size of tube inserted as well as the amount required to fill the balloon, if present, should be known.

been shown to be consistently accurate for continually assessing tube placement.

Research has suggested alternative methods such as using measurements of bilirubin, trypsin, and pepsin levels, CO_2 monitoring, transillumination, and magnetic detection to enhance assessment of tube placement, but insufficient evidence is available to support these methods. Also, these methods have other limitations such as the cost, the availability of equipment, and the limited availability for bedside testing of these levels.

Refer to Box 13.4 for methods to verify feeding tube placement. However, keep in mind that even with these methods, tube malpositioning can occur. Therefore, nurses need to be vigilant in checking for tube placement using the recommended methods and be cautious and proactive if there is any suspicion that the tube may be misplaced.

TAKE NOTE!

Radiologic verification is recommended if bedside methods are conflicting, the nasogastric tube (NGT) was difficult to place, or the child is at high risk, such as children with swallowing problems, children with altered levels of consciousness, or children in the intensive care unit (Irving et al., 2018).

If the gavage feeding tube is to remain in place, secure it to the child's cheek. Do not tape the tube to the child's forehead, because this could lead to irritation and pressure on, and possible breakdown of, the nasal mucosa. Also, measure the length of the tube extending from the nose or mouth to the end, and record this information. Double-check this measurement before administering each intermittent tube feeding to verify that

NURSING PROCEDURE 13.2 Inserting a Gavage Feeding Tube

Purpose: To provide a means for delivering nutrition to the child's functioning gastrointestinal tract

1. Verify the order for gavage feeding, confirm identity, and review child's medical history for any contraindications to placing a feeding tube.
2. Explain the procedure to the child and parents using appropriate language geared to the child's development level.
3. Gather the necessary equipment; remove formula for feeding from refrigerator if appropriate, and allow it to come to room temperature.
4. Wash hands and put on gloves.
5. Inspect the child's nose and mouth for deformities that may interfere with the passage of the tube.
6. Position the infant supine with the head slightly elevated and with the neck slightly hyperextended so that the nose is pointed upward. If necessary, place a rolled towel or blanket under the neck to help in maintaining this position. Assist the older child to a sitting position, if appropriate. Alternatively, have the parent or another person hold the child to promote comfort and reassurance. Enlist the aid of additional people, such as a parent or other health care team member, to assist in maintaining the child's position.
7. Determine the proper tube circumference or French. This will depend on the indication for use of the tube (suction or nutrition), the expected duration the tube will be in place, and the size and age of the child. Use clinical judgment to determine the correct tube type and size. Refer to Table 13.6.
8. Determine the tubing length for insertion: Use morphologic measurement from the tip of the nose to the earlobe to the middle of the area between the xiphoid process and umbilicus or age-related height-based (ARHB) method, ensuring accurate height and calculations (Table 13.7). Mark this measurement on the tube with an indelible pen or with a piece of tape.
9. Lubricate the tube with a generous amount of sterile water (many small-bore feeding tubes have a water-activated lubricant) or water-soluble lubricant to promote passage of the tube and minimize trauma to the child's mucosa.
10. Insert the tube into one of the nares or the mouth. Direct a nasally inserted tube straight back toward the occiput; direct an orally inserted tube toward the back of the throat.
11. Advance the tube slowly to the designated length; encourage the child (if capable) to swallow frequently to assist with advancing the tube. If not contraindicated, the child can sip on water through a straw to help facilitate swallowing and advancement of the tube.
12. Watch for signs of distress, such as gasping, coughing, or cyanosis, indicating that the tube is in the airway. If these signs develop, withdraw the tube and allow the child to rest before attempting reinsertion.
13. Temporarily secure tube, remove stylet if applicable, and check for proper placement of the tube. Refer to Box 13.4.
14. Document the type of tube inserted; length of tubing inserted; measurement of external tubing length, from nares to end of tube, after insertion; and confirmation of placement.

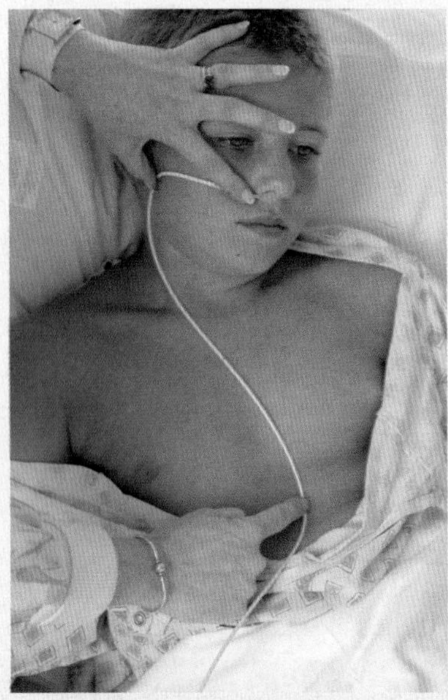

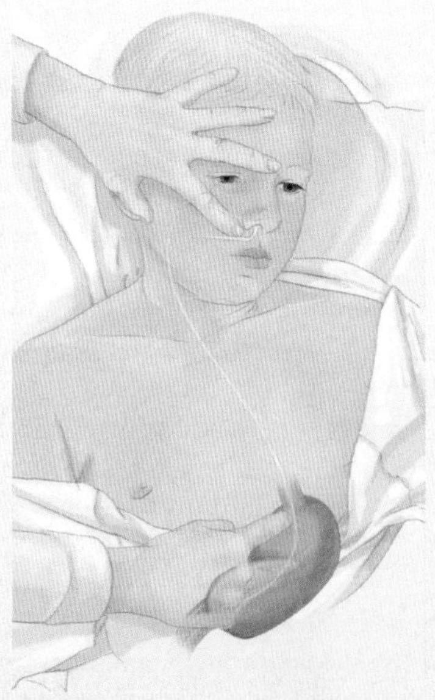

Adapted from Lippincott Williams & Wilkins. (2023). *Lippincott nursing procedures* (9th ed.). Wolters Kluwer.

TABLE 13.6 • General Gavage Feeding Tube Size Based on Age

Age	Size of Tube (Fr)
Newborn	6–8
0–5 years	6–10
6–12 years	8–12
>12 years	10–14

A larger tube will be utilized if tube is used for suction.

the feeding tube is in the proper position. Once the position of the gavage feeding tube is confirmed, the feeding solution or medication can be administered.

> Remember Lily, the 9-month-old infant diagnosed with malnutrition who is to receive gavage feedings with a nasogastric tube? What equipment will be needed, and what steps will you take to complete the procedure?

Administering Enteral Feedings

Enteral feedings can be given continuously or intermittently, regardless of the type of tube used. Intermittent feedings are commonly called bolus feedings. With a **bolus feeding**, a specified amount of feeding solution is given at specific intervals, usually over a short period of time such as 15 to 30 minutes. Given via a syringe, feeding bag, or infusion pump, bolus feedings most closely resemble regular meals. Continuous feedings are given at a slower rate over a longer period of time. In some cases, the feeding may be given during the night so that the child can be free to move about and participate in activities during the day. For continuous feedings, an enteral feeding pump is used to administer the solution at a prescribed rate.

Checking for tube placement is a priority before administering any intermittent tube feeding and periodically during continuous tube feedings, regardless of the type of tube being used. (Refer to Box 13.4.) For gastrostomy and jejunostomy tubes, ensure that the calibration, if present, has not changed. Measure the length of the tube daily from the exit site on the stomach to the end of the tube. Assess the abdomen for distension and bowel sounds. Also, measure the **gastric residual** (the amount remaining in the stomach, which indicates gastric emptying time) by aspirating the gastric contents with a syringe, measuring it, and then replacing the contents. Check the residuals periodically, according to the facility's policy, such as every 4 to 6 hours, and before each intermittent feeding. If the residual volume exceeds the amount specified by the health care provider's order, hold the feeding and notify the health care provider or nurse practitioner.

Begin the feeding by placing the child in a supine position with the head and shoulders elevated approximately 30 degrees so that the feeding will remain in the stomach area. Flush the tube with a small amount of water to clear it and prevent occlusion. This is not necessary for a gavage feeding if the tube is being inserted each time a feeding is given. Ensure that the feeding solution is at room temperature. Administer the feeding per the facility's policy.

Feeding solutions may be placed into the barrel of a syringe or into a feeding bag attached to the feeding tube and allowed to flow by gravity. The rate of flow for gravity-assisted feedings can be increased or decreased by raising or lowering the feeding solution container,

TABLE 13.7 • Age-Related Height-Based Equations for Predicting Orogastric/Nasogastric Tube Insertion Lengths

Route	Age Group	Predicted Internal Distance to the Body of the Stomach Determined by:
Oral	Age ≤28 months	16.6 + 0.183 (height, cm)
	Between ages 28 months and 100 months (8 years 4 months)	20.1 + 0.183 (height, cm)
	Between ages 100 months (8 years 4 months) and 121 months (~10 years)	17 + 0.218 (height, cm)
	Greater than 121 months (~10 years)	18.5 + 0.218 (height, cm)
Nasal	Age <28 months	17.6 + 0.197 (height, cm)
	Between ages 28 months and 100 months (8 years 4 months)	21.1 + 0.197 (height, cm)
	Between ages 100 months (8 years 4 months) and 121 months (~10 years)	18.7 + 0.218 (height, cm)
	Greater than 121 months (~10 years)	21.2 + 0.218 (height, cm)

Data from Cincinnati Children's Hospital Medical Center. (2011). *Best Evidence Statement (BESt). Confirmation of nasogastric/orogastric tube (NGT/OGT) placement.* Cincinnati Children's Hospital Medical Center. https://rightbiometrics.com/wp-content/uploads/2023/02/Confirmation-of-Nasogastric-Tube-NGT-Placement.pdf

BOX 13.4 Methods for Verification of Feeding Tube Placement

- Obtain radiographic confirmation of proper tube placement in children who are considered high risk for aspiration, such as children with neurologic impairment, children obtunded, sedated, unconscious, critically ill, having reduced gag reflex or static encephalopathy, or when nonradiologic methods are not feasible or bedside results are conflicting.
- Nonradiologic verification is used in children who are not considered high risk for aspiration; document pH of aspirate; document insertion distance and external length of tube in the chart. Mark and document the tube's exit site from the nose or mouth.
- Use bedside techniques at regular intervals to determine proper tube positioning.
  - Measuring pH: Gastric secretions have a pH less than 5. Small intestine secretions will usually have a pH greater than 6, but this does not reliably predict proper tube placement. A pH greater than 6 can occur with respiratory or esophageal placement, with proper tube placement (gastric or intestinal) when feedings are given continuously, or if the child is receiving acid-inhibiting medications. Therefore, if the pH is greater than 5, additional assessment is warranted.
  - Observing appearance of fluid aspirated from tube (can be used in conjunction with pH testing but is not a reliable single verification method)
    - Gastric secretions are usually grassy green or clear and colorless and can have off-white or tan mucous shreds. It may also be brown tinged if blood is present.
    - Intestinal secretions are often bile stained, light golden yellow to brownish green. They tend to be thicker and more translucent than gastric secretions.
    - Respiratory secretions can be white, yellow, straw colored, or clear.
  - Instill air into the tube, and then auscultate for the sound (gastric auscultation) (can be used in conjunction with other assessment methods).
  - Check external markings on tube and external tube length (tube remaining from nares to end of tube) to determine if the tube seems to have migrated or been misplaced.
- Continually assess for signs indicative of feeding tube misplacement, such as unexplained gagging, vomiting, or coughing; signs and symptoms of respiratory distress; and decreased oxygen saturations.
- If bedside techniques reveal conflicting results or the child is at high risk, radiologic confirmation is recommended.
- Review routine chest and abdominal radiographs (if obtained) to double-check correct tube position. Always follow agencies' policy and procedures.

Adapted from Irving, S. Y., Rempel, G., Lyman, B., Sevilla, W. M., Northington, L., Guenter, P., & The American Society for Parenteral and Enteral Nutrition. (2018). Pediatric nasogastric tube placement and verification: Best practice recommendations from the NOVEL Project. *Nutrition in Clinical Practice, 33*(6), 921–927; Lippincott Williams & Wilkins (2023). *Lippincott nursing procedures* (9th ed.). Wolters Kluwer.

respectively. Typically, intermittent feedings last from 15 to 30 minutes. A feeding bag may also be attached to a pump to control the rate of flow. Monitor the child's tolerance to the feeding.

Once the feeding is complete, but before the formula completely empties from the container, flush the tube with water. As the water leaves the syringe or tubing, clamp the tube to prevent air from entering the stomach. Then disconnect the syringe or tube-feeding bag from the tube.

CLINICAL REASONING ALERT!

If the child vomits during the feeding, stop the feeding immediately and turn the child onto their side or sit them up.

If the child has a gastrostomy button, open the cap and connect an adaptor or insert extension tubing through the one-way valve. This allows access to the gastric conduit. The feeding solution container is connected to the extension tubing or adaptor, and the feeding is given as described previously. After the feeding is completed, the extension tubing or adaptor is flushed with water and the flip-top opening is closed.

Burp the infant during and after any type of tube feeding in the same manner as for an infant who is bottle- or breast-fed. Also, position the child on their right side with the head slightly elevated, approximately 30 degrees, for about 1 hour after the feeding to facilitate gastric emptying and reduce the risk of aspiration and regurgitation. Some children have a difficult time with gas and burping on their own after tube placement. Venting, which helps relieve gas, may be ordered by the health care provider or nurse practitioner. It removes excess air and can be helpful if the child is bloated or the abdomen is distended. Use a catheter-tip syringe with the plunger removed and attach to the end of the tube. Hold the syringe above the child's stomach for a few minutes. Once the air or gas is removed, allow any stomach contents or formula to flow back into the stomach.

Weigh the child daily throughout enteral nutrition therapy to determine the effectiveness of the therapy.

Providing Skin and Insertion Site Care

Skin around the gastrostomy or jejunostomy insertion site may become irritated from movement of the tube, moisture, leakage of stomach or intestinal contents, or the adhesive device holding the tube in place. Keeping the skin clean and dry is important and will help prevent most of these problems.

The skin around a gastrostomy or jejunostomy tube requires cleaning at least once a day. Routine site care includes, for newly placed tubes, gentle cleansing with sterile water or saline or, for established tubes, soap and water, followed by rinsing or cleaning with water alone. To clean under an external disk or bumper, a cotton-tipped applicator may be used. During insertion site care, rotate the gastrostomy tube or button a quarter-turn to prevent skin adherence and irritation. Always follow agency or institution policies and procedures.

TAKE NOTE!

Do not rotate a jejunal or gastrojejunal tube because it can cause kinking.

Assess the insertion site and condition of the surrounding skin for signs and symptoms of infection, such as erythema, induration, foul drainage, or pain. A small amount of clear or tan drainage is normal. If any drainage is present, a dressing can be placed. Use a presplit 2 × 2 gauze, and place it loosely around the site. Change this dressing when it is soiled. If no drainage is present, do not place a dressing as it can cause undue pressure and trap moisture, leading to skin irritation.

Preventing movement of the tube also helps reduce skin irritation. Check the volume of the balloon with a balloon-tipped device about once or twice a week, and reinflate the balloon to the initial volume if needed. The tube should be able to move slightly in and out of the child's stomach. The plastic disk should be snug against the skin but not tight enough to cause pressure. Tube stabilization methods help prevent the tube from moving around and sliding further into the stomach or jejunum. Stabilize the tube by pulling gently on the tubing and sliding the stabilizer bar or disk snugly against the abdomen.

TAKE NOTE!

Rotate sites where the tube is secured to the abdomen to prevent tension on the stoma or skin breakdown.

Measure and record the length of the tube from the exit site of the abdominal wall to the end of the tube. All future measurements should be the same unless the tube length is changed. For tubes without a stabilizer bar or disk or for additional stabilization needs, several other methods may be used, including cut baby bottle nipples, taping methods, and commercially available stabilizers (Fig. 13.12). It is always important to follow agency policy.

TAKE NOTE!

When using the nipple method, make sure to cut several holes in the base of the nipple to allow air circulation and site assessment.

Promoting Growth and Development

Some children receive all of their nutritional needs through tube feedings, whereas other children use tube feedings as a supplement to eating by mouth. Feeding time is a special time for infants and children. Occasionally, babies who are fed solely through an enteral feeding tube may forget or lose the desire to eat by mouth. Use a pacifier to help avoid this, allowing the infant to associate the pacifier in their mouth with a feeding. The sucking motion will also exercise the jaw and promote the flow of the feedings. The saliva produced during sucking aids in digestion. Combined with holding the infant and cuddling, rocking, and talking to them, this promotes a more normal feeding time.

Talking with children, playing music, or reading a story promotes an active feeding time. At home, encourage parents to include the feeding as a part of regular family mealtime together to provide socialization for the child. Allow the child to participate in the feedings by gathering supplies and administering the actual feeding so that the child may experience independence and adaptation. If the child also eats food by mouth, feed them by mouth first and then administer the tube feeding. Children with feeding tubes should be allowed as normal a routine as possible. For example, they can crawl, walk, and jump just like children of the same age and developmental level. However, in some cases, contact sports such as football, hockey, and wrestling should be avoided because of

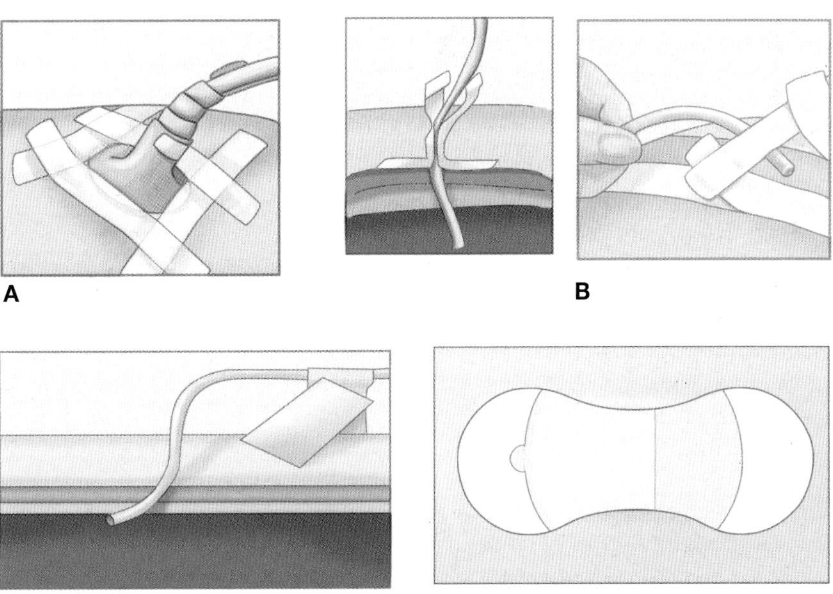

FIGURE 13.12 Methods to stabilize a gastrostomy tube include (**A**) the nipple method, (**B**) taping methods, (**C**) the tension loop method, and (**D**) commercially available stabilizing devices (GripLok; pictured here).

the higher risk of injury. Securing the tubing under the child's clothing will prevent it from becoming accidentally dislodged and prevent the child from pulling and playing with it. Using one-piece outfits, an Ace wrap, or stretchy gauze to cover the tube can help protect it.

Educating the Child and Family

Educate children receiving enteral feedings and their parents thoroughly about this method of nutritional support. Reinforce the reason for the therapy, and provide the child and parents with opportunities to verbalize their concerns and ask questions. Ensure that the parents understand the risks and benefits of the therapy and the expected duration.

Provide the child, if developmentally appropriate, and parents with opportunities to participate in the feeding sessions. This helps allay some of their fears and anxieties and promotes a sense of control over the situation. They will also gain valuable practice in learning the skill should the feedings be required at home. Teaching Guidelines 13.3 identifies important topics to include in the teaching plan for a child receiving enteral nutrition at home. Troubleshooting problems at home is an important topic to cover. Refer to Teaching Guidelines 13.4. Education also involves helping the family develop appropriate coping strategies to adapt, solve problems, and access the support and services they will need after discharge.

TEACHING GUIDELINES 13.3 Topics to be Covered for Home Enteral Nutrition

- Type and size of tube
- Type of nutritional support
- Rationale for therapy
- Expected results from therapy
- Duration of therapy
- Frequency of feedings
- Feeding solution and equipment
- Tube insertion technique (if appropriate)
- Methods to check for correct placement
- Steps for administering the feeding (and medication, if ordered)
- Procedure for flushing tube
- Procedure for venting the tube, if appropriate
- Frequency of weighing the child
- Signs and symptoms of complications and when to notify health care provider or nurse practitioner
- Troubleshooting problems, such as clogging of the tube or dislodgement (see Teaching Guidelines 13.4)
- Daily tube care (e.g., cleaning the site, rotating tube)
- Site assessment
- Technique for reinsertion/replacement of tube as appropriate
- Equipment suppliers
- Resources for support
- Follow-up visits and referrals

Remember Lily from the beginning of the chapter? She is to be discharged home after having a gastrostomy tube inserted to continue feedings at home. What teaching is needed for her family prior to discharge?

TEACHING GUIDELINES 13.4 Troubleshooting Complications at Home

- If a tube becomes clogged, instruct caregivers to slowly push warm water into the tube. Amount and size of syringe will vary based on child's size and facility policy. Repeat if necessary. Instruct caregivers to never use an object or put anything into the tube. They should call the doctor or nurse if they are unable to unclog the tube. Declogging medications may be prescribed.
- If a tube is inadvertently removed, instruct the caregiver to try to replace the tube into the opening 1 to 2 in, tape the tube to the child's abdomen, and do not use the tube. If unable to do this, cover the site with a small clean dressing tape. They should then call the health care provider or nurse immediately; the tube needs to be replaced as soon as possible (within 1 to 4 hours), or the tract will close. Some institutions may instruct the family on how to replace the tube once the tube is more than 6 weeks old and has formed an established G-tube tract.
- If the site is red or irritated, instruct caregivers to continue with routine cleaning, keep the area clean and dry, and call the health care provider. An antibiotic or skin barrier cream may be ordered. Assess for leakage and try to minimize, if possible. Check the tube's position, and ensure tube is stabilized and secure and not dangling.
- If the tube is leaking, the caregiver needs to keep the dressing clean and dry. Assess tube position and secure the tube to avoid dangling. Assess if leaking is from stoma area or tube valve, if applicable. More frequent venting may help, and the health care provider should be notified.

Always teach following the instructions per agency policy and procedure regarding home care.

Adapted from Cincinnati Children's Hospital Medical Center. (2022). *Gastrostomy tube (G-tube) home care*. https://www.cincinnatichildrens.org/health/g/g-tube-care

Parenteral Nutrition

Nutritional support can be administered IV through a peripheral or central venous catheter. The concentration and components of the solution determine the type of parenteral nutrition. Parenteral nutrition given via a central venous access device is termed **total parenteral nutrition** (TPN). Comparison Chart 13.1 gives information about peripheral and central parenteral nutrition.

Administering TPN

Typically, the health care provider or nurse practitioner determines the concentration and components of the TPN solution based on a thorough assessment of the child's status, including the results of laboratory testing. This information is used as a baseline for evaluating the effectiveness of therapy.

The solution is prepared under sterile conditions in the pharmacy. For TPN, a central venous access device is inserted and secured, if one is not already in place. Use specialized tubing with an in-line filter (to prevent small microparticles from entering the circulation).

TPN solutions may be refrigerated until they are to be used. Once started, a single solution of TPN should hang for no longer than 24 hours (Lippincott Williams & Wilkins, 2023). The infusion of the solution is initiated at a slow rate that is gradually increased as ordered based on how the child tolerates the therapy. TPN solutions are highly concentrated glucose solutions that can cause hyperglycemia if given too rapidly. Use of an infusion pump is essential to control the rate of infusion. Fat emulsions are administered periodically to meet the child's need for essential fatty acids. These solutions are given as a piggyback solution into the TPN line but below the in-line filter.

Throughout TPN therapy, be vigilant in monitoring the infusion rate, and report any changes in the infusion rate to the health care provider or nurse practitioner immediately. Gradual adjustments may be made to the rate, but only as ordered by the health care provider or nurse practitioner.

Initially, check blood glucose levels frequently, such as every 4 to 6 hours, to evaluate for hyperglycemia. These levels can be obtained with a bedside glucose meter. Minimize the trauma and discomfort associated with frequent invasive procedures by using the principles of atraumatic care. If blood glucose levels are elevated, SQ administration of insulin may be needed. Once the child's glucose levels stabilize, the frequency of blood glucose level testing decreases, such as every 8 to 12 hours, based on the facility's policy.

CLINICAL REASONING ALERT!

If for any reason the TPN infusion is interrupted or stops, be prepared to begin an infusion of a 5% to 10% dextrose solution at the same infusion rate as the TPN (Lippincott Williams & Wilkins, 2023). This helps to prevent rebound hypoglycemia that may occur due to the increased insulin secretion by the child's body in response to the use of the highly concentrated TPN solution.

Perform catheter site care, tubing and filter changes, and dressing changes according to the facility's policy. Inspect the insertion site closely for signs of infection.

COMPARISON CHART 13.1 Peripheral Parenteral Nutrition Versus Total Parenteral Nutrition

	Peripheral Parenteral Nutrition	Total Parenteral Nutrition
Indications/use	Primarily supplemental Short-term use to supply additional calories and nutrients (2 weeks or less)	Provides all nutrients to meet child's needs Enough calories supplied to restore nitrogen balance[a] Longer-term use (2 weeks or more)
Route	Peripheral vein	Central venous access to allow rapid dilution of hypertonic solution
Child's status	Nutritional status usually within acceptable parameters Oral intake decreased or absent	Child with a nonfunctioning gastrointestinal (GI) tract, such as a congenital or acquired GI disorder Severe failure to thrive Multisystem trauma or organ involvement Preterm newborns
Components	Less concentrated mixture of fluid, electrolytes, carbohydrates (dextrose), amino acids, vitamins, and minerals Carbohydrate concentration usually limited to 10% or less and osmolarity of <600 mOsm[a]	Highly concentrated solution of carbohydrates, electrolytes, vitamins, and minerals Lipid emulsion to supply need for essential fatty acids Total nutrient admixture (TNA) with components of TPN plus lipids and other additives in one container

[a]Lippincott Williams & Wilkins. (2023). *Lippincott nursing procedures* (9th ed.). Wolters Kluwer; Baker, R. D., Baker, S. S. & Bojczuk, G. (2022). Parenteral nutrition in infants and children. *UpToDate*. Retrieved March 1, 2023, from https://www.uptodate.com/contents/parenteral-nutrition-in-infants-and-children

Also, monitor the child's vital signs, daily weights, and intake and output closely for changes. In addition, review laboratory test results, which can aid in early detection of problems, such as infection or electrolyte excesses or deficits.

TPN can be administered continuously over a 24-hour period, or after initiation it may be given on a cyclic basis, such as over a 12-hour period during the night. When administering cycled TPN, the solution is infused at half the prescribed rate for the first and last hour to prevent hyper- and hypoglycemia.

Preventing Complications

Nurses play a key role in minimizing the risk for complications related to use of central venous access devices and TPN. Box 13.5 describes these complications. Key measures to reduce the risk of complications include the following:

- Monitor the child's vital signs closely for changes.
- Adhere to strict aseptic technique when caring for the catheter and administering TPN.
- Ensure that the system remains a closed system at all times. Secure all connections, and clamp the catheter or have the child perform the Valsalva maneuver during tubing and cap changes.
- Use occlusive dressings. Chlorhexidine-impregnated sponge (Biopatch) dressings may be used to help prevent infection. Always follow agency or institution policy and procedures.

BOX 13.5 Complications That Can Occur With Central Venous Access Devices and Total Parenteral Nutrition (TPN)

- Air embolism from inadvertent entry of air into the system during tubing or cap changes or accidental disconnection
- Cardiac tamponade due to catheter advancement with movement of the arm, neck, or shoulder
- Catheter occlusion from the development of a fibrin sheath or thrombus at the catheter tip, malpositioning or kinking, or the deposition of precipitates or a blood clot
- Venous thrombosis from injury to the vessel wall during insertion or movement of the catheter after insertion or from chemical irritation due to administration of concentrated solutions, vesicants, and other medications through the catheter
- Hyperglycemia, typically with too rapid an infusion of TPN
- Hypoglycemia, which may occur with rapid cessation
- Dehydration as the child's body attempts to rid itself of excess glucose through renal excretion
- Electrolyte imbalance (particularly potassium, sodium, calcium, magnesium, and phosphorus)
- Infection at the skin insertion site, along the catheter pathway, or in the bloodstream. Organisms can arise from the skin, hands of caregivers, or other areas such as wound drainage, droplets from the lungs, or urine. For example, connection sites can be contaminated during tubing or dressing changes.

- Adhere to agency policy for flushing of the catheter and maintaining catheter patency.
- Assess intake and output frequently.
- Monitor blood glucose levels and obtain laboratory tests as ordered to evaluate for changes in fluid and electrolytes.

Promoting Growth and Development

Meals are a time for meeting nutritional needs as well as a time for love, comfort, support, and socialization. TPN meets the child's nutritional needs, but the child's need for love and support also must be met. Implement measures similar to those for children receiving enteral nutrition (see discussion earlier in this chapter). Also provide opportunities for holding and cuddling the child. Allow the older child to participate in activities that can help to occupy the time associated with meals. When administering cyclic TPN, run the TPN over the nighttime hours, whenever possible, to allow the child to participate in developmentally appropriate activities during the day. Encourage the child and parents to participate in the care to promote a sense of independence as well as a sense of control over the situation.

Educating the Child and Family

Children who require long-term TPN therapy may receive TPN in the home. Administering TPN at home requires thorough education of the child and parents. This teaching can occur in the health care agency or in the child's home. The amount of information to be taught can be overwhelming, so ensure that ample time is available. Allow time for questions and concerns. Offer emotional support and guidance whenever necessary.

Provide written and verbal instructions about the care involved. Have the child (if appropriate) and parents demonstrate the care needed, including care of the central venous access device. Review with them the measures for obtaining, storing, and handling the solutions and supplies. Develop plans for troubleshooting problems with devices and equipment, and give instructions on how to recognize and treat complications. Also teach them about danger signs and symptoms that require immediate notification. Be sure they have the name and number of a contact person in case of emergency situations.

Initiate the appropriate referrals for support. Specialized home care infusion services are available for follow-up in the home. In addition, social services can be helpful in providing assistance with finances, health insurance reimbursement, scheduling, transportation, emotional support, and community resources.

Unfolding Patient Stories: Brittany Long • Part 1

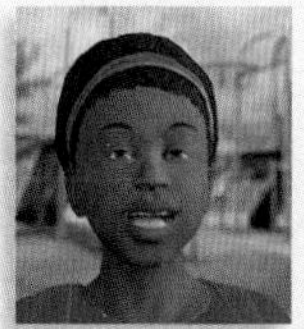

Brittany Long, a 5-year-old child diagnosed with sickle cell anemia, is having an acute pain crisis, and her parent brings her to the emergency department (ED). Her last visit to the ED was 1 year ago, when she was hospitalized for a vaso-occlusive crisis episode. How would the nurse prepare Brittany for insertion of an IV line and administration of IV fluids? How would the explanation differ for her parent? What nursing interventions safeguard the IV line and administration of fluids? (Brittany Long's story continues in Chapter 24.)

Care for Brittany and other patients in a realistic virtual environment: ***vSim** for Nursing* (thepoint.lww.com/vSimPediatric). Practice documenting these patients' care in DocuCare (thePoint.lww.com/DocuCareEHR).

KEY CONCEPTS

- The "rights" of pediatric medication administration are the right drug, right dose, right route, right time, and right patient. Some experts have added additional rights, such as right documentation, right to be educated, right to refuse, right form, and right approach. These additional rights are important to consider to increase patient safety and satisfaction.
- The physiologic immaturity of some body systems in children can affect a drug's pharmacodynamics, leading to differences in the body's response to the drug and thus enhancing or diminishing the drug's effects. The child's age, weight, BSA, and body composition can affect the drug's pharmacokinetics.
- The two most common methods for determining pediatric drug doses involve the use of the child's body weight and BSA.
- Children younger than 5 to 6 years are at risk for aspiration when receiving tablets or capsules because they have difficulty swallowing them; liquids may be more appropriate. When administering oral medications to children, always tell them whether a medication is being mixed with food.
- Medication administration via the rectal route is not preferred because the drug's absorption may be erratic and unpredictable, and children find this route extremely upsetting or embarrassing.
- When administering otic medications, pull the pinna downward and back if the child is under age 3, and up and back for older children.
- IM administration is used infrequently in children because it is painful and children often lack the adequate muscle mass. When used with infants up to 12 months old, the preferred site is the vastus lateralis muscle or anterolateral thigh muscle. In infants and children older than 12 months, the vastus lateralis or anterolateral thigh muscle remains the preferred site, but the deltoid can be considered if sufficient mass is present.
- Administration of medication via the IV route is common with children, especially when a rapid response to the drug is desired or when absorption via other routes is difficult or impossible. The primary method for IV medication administration is via a syringe pump.
- Preferred sites for peripheral IV therapy include the veins of the hands, feet, and forearms. The scalp vein may be used in infants but only if attempts at other sites have been unsuccessful. The general guideline for insertion of any peripheral devices is to use the smallest-gauge catheter for the shortest length of time possible to prevent trauma to the child's fragile veins.
- Central venous therapy is usually administered through a large vein, such as the subclavian, femoral, or jugular vein or vena cava. The tip of the device lies in the superior vena cava just at the entrance to the right atrium. Devices include single- or multiple-lumen short- and long-term catheters, PICCs, tunneled catheters, and vascular access ports.
- Monitoring intake and output is important when a child is receiving IV therapy. Site inspection, proper care of the site, and proper dressing changes are key to preventing complications.
- Nutritional support can be administered enterally via a nasogastric or orogastric tube (gavage feeding) or via a gastrostomy or jejunostomy device or administered parenterally through a peripheral or central venous access device.
- Enteral nutrition is indicated for children who have a functioning gastrointestinal tract but cannot consume adequate amounts of nutrients orally.
- Prior to any enteral feeding, placement of the feeding tube must be confirmed. The gold standard for confirming placement is with a radiograph. At the bedside, nonradiologic methods are used to confirm placement, including checking the color and pH of the aspirate, checking external markings on the tube and verifying external tube length, continually assessing for signs indicative of feeding tube misplacement, such as unexplained gagging, vomiting, or coughing; signs and symptoms of respiratory distress; and decreased oxygen saturations.
- Children receiving TPN require close monitoring of the infusion rate and volume, intake and output, vital signs, and blood glucose levels. Strict aseptic technique is necessary when caring for the central venous access site and TPN infusion.

REFERENCES AND RECOMMENDED READINGS

Baker, R. D., Baker, S. S. & Bojczuk, G. (2022). Parenteral nutrition in infants and children. *UpToDate*. Retrieved March 1, 2023, from https://www.uptodate.com/contents/parenteral-nutrition-in-infants-and-children

Centers for Disease Control and Prevention. (2017). *Guidelines for the prevention of intravascular catheter-related infections (2011)*. (Edit [February 2017]). https://www.cdc.gov/infectioncontrol/guidelines/bsi/recommendations.html#rec2

Centers for Disease Control and Prevention. (2021). *Epidemiology and prevention of vaccine-preventable diseases* (14th ed). In E. Hall, A. P. Wodi, J. Hamborsky, V. Morelli, & S. Schillies (Eds.). Public Health Foundation.

Cincinnati Children's Hospital Medical Center. (2011). *Best Evidence Statement (BESt). Confirmation of nasogastric/orogastric tube (NGT/OGT) placement.* Cincinnati Children's Hospital Medical Center. https://rightbiometrics.com/wp-content/uploads/2023/02/Confirmation-of-Nasogastric-Tube-NGT-Placement.pdf

Cincinnati Children's Hospital Medical Center. (2022). *Gastrostomy tube (G-tube) home care.* https://www.cincinnatichildrens.org/health/g/g-tube-care

Cleveland Clinic. (2023). *Ear drops.* https://my.clevelandclinic.org/health/treatments/24654-ear-drops

Doyle, T. D., Anand, S., & Edens, M. A. (2022). Scalp catheterization. *StatPearls* [Internet]. StatPearls Publishing. https://www.ncbi.nlm.nih.gov/books/NBK507856/

Drutz, J. E. (2023). Standard immunizations for children and adolescents: Overview. *UpToDate.* Retrieved February 22, 2023, from https://www.uptodate.com/contents/standard-immunizations-for-children-and-adolescents-overview

Haddadin, Y., Annamaraju, P., & Regunath, H. (2022). Central line associated blood stream infections. *StatPearls* [Internet]. StatPearls Publishing. https://www.ncbi.nlm.nih.gov/books/NBK430891/

Immunization Action Coalition. (2022). *How to administer intramuscular (IM) and how to administer subcutaneous (SC) injections.* http://www.immunize.org/catg.d/p2020.pdf

Irving, S. Y., Rempel, G., Lyman, B., Sevilla, W. M., Northington, L., Guenter, P., & The American Society for Parenteral and Enteral Nutrition. (2018). Pediatric nasogastric tube placement and verification: Best practice recommendations from the NOVEL project. *Nutrition in Clinical Practice, 33*(6), 921–927. https://doi.org/10.1002/ncp.10189

Kroger, A., Bahta, L., Long, S., & Sanchez, P. (2023). *General best practice guidelines for immunization.* https://www.cdc.gov/vaccines/hcp/acip-recs/general-recs/index.html

Lippincott Williams & Wilkins. (2023). *Lippincott nursing procedures* (9th ed.). Wolters Kluwer.

Lopez-Pineda, A., Gonzalez de Dios, J., Guilabert, M., Mira-Perceval Juan, G., & Joaquín Mira Solves, J. (2021). A systematic review on pediatric medication errors by parents or caregivers at home, *Expert Opinion on Drug Safety, 21*(1), 95–105. https://doi.org/10.1080/14740338.2021.1950138

Manzo, B. F., Marcatto, J. O., Ferreira, B., Galvão Diniz, C., & Parker, L. A. (2023). Comparison of 3 methods for measuring gastric tube length in newborns: A randomized clinical trial. *Advances in Neonatal Care, 23*(3), E79–E86. https://doi.org/10.1097/ANC.0000000000001065

Naik, V. M., Mantha, S. S. P., & Rayani, B. K. (2019). Vascular access in children. *Indian Journal of Anaesthesia, 63*(9), 737–745. https://doi.org/10.4103/ija.IJA_489_19

Paterson, R. S., Chopra, V., Brown, E., Kleidon, T. M., Cooke, M., Rickard, C. M., Bernstein, S. J., & Ullman, A. J. (2020). Selection and insertion of vascular access devices in pediatrics: A systematic review. *Pediatrics, 145*(Suppl. 3), S243–S268. https://doi.org/10.1542/peds.2019-3474H

Schneider, M. (2022). *Clinical guidelines (Nursing): Intramuscular injections.* https://www.rch.org.au/rchcpg/hospital_clinical_guideline_index/Intramuscular_Injections/#:~:text=The%20anterolateral%20aspect%20of%20the,anaphylaxis%20management%20in%20all%20ages

The Joint Commission. (2021). Preventing pediatric medication errors. *Sentinel Event Alert,* Issue 39. https://www.jointcommission.org/-/media/tjc/documents/resources/patient-safety-topics/sentinel-event/sea-39-ped-med-errors-rev-final-4-14-21.pdf

The Joint Commission. (2023). *Facts about the official "do not use" list.* https://www.jointcommission.org/resources/news-and-multimedia/fact-sheets/facts-about-do-not-use-list/

Ullman, A. J., & Chopra, V. (2022). Routine care and maintenance of intravenous devices. *UpToDate.* Retrieved February 28, 2023, from https://www.uptodate.com/contents/routine-care-and-maintenance-of-intravenous-devices

U.S. Food and Drug Administration. (2023). *Pediatric labeling changes.* https://www.fda.gov/science-research/pediatrics/pediatric-labeling-changes

DEVELOPING CLINICAL JUDGMENT

PRACTICING FOR NCLEX

1. A 3-year-old child is to receive a medication that is supplied as an enteric-coated tablet. What is the best nursing action?
   a. Crush the tablet and mix it with applesauce.
   b. Dissolve the medication in the child's milk.
   c. Place a pill in the posterior part of the pharynx, and tell the child to swallow.
   d. Check with the prescriber to see if an alternative form can be used.
2. The nurse is caring for an infant who weighs 8.2 kg and is NPO and receiving IV fluid therapy. What rate does the nurse calculate as meeting the child's daily fluid requirements?
   a. 82 mL per hour
   b. 41 mL per hour
   c. 34 mL per hour
   d. 22 mL per hour
3. When administering ear drops to a 2-year-old, which action would be most appropriate?
   a. Tell the child that the drops are to treat their infection.
   b. Pull the pinna of the child's ear down and back.
   c. Have the child turn their head to the opposite side after giving the drops.
   d. Massage the child's forehead to facilitate absorption of the medication.
4. An infant is to receive intermittent gavage feedings via a nasogastric tube every 6 hours. The feeding tube was inserted with a previous feeding and remains in place. The nurse is preparing to administer the next scheduled feeding. Place the events in the proper sequence.
   a. Check the placement of the feeding tube.
   b. Position the infant on their right side with the head of the bed slightly elevated.
   c. Allow the feeding to come to room temperature.
   d. Flush the tube with water.
   e. Clamp the tube to prevent air from entering the stomach.
   f. Pour the solution into the barrel of the syringe.
5. Which statements are appropriate when administering medication to children? Select all that apply.
   a. Prior to administering a liquid medication, always shake the bottle.
   b. If the child is upset or crying, administer oral liquid medication into the posterior side of the child's mouth, and pinch their nose to assist them to swallow.
   c. When administering a crushable medicine to an infant, place the medication in the infant's bottle before their next feeding.
   d. When administering liquid medication to a toddler, make sure the child is sitting at a 45-degree angle.
   e. When administering a medication using a dropper, ensure that the dropper is the one that was packaged with the medication.
   f. The nurse must administer all medications to ensure that the parents do not make an error.

CRITICAL THINKING EXERCISES

1. When reviewing the medical record of a child, the nurse notes that the ordered dose of medication is different from the recommended dose. How should the nurse proceed?
2. While caring for a 5-year-old child who is receiving IV fluid therapy at a rate of 100 mL per hour, the nurse notes that the infusion is running slowly. The insertion site appears slightly reddened and swollen. What should the nurse do next?
3. A school-age child is to be discharged, continuing TPN therapy at home. The child lives with their parents and two younger siblings. How would the nurse prepare this child and family for discharge? How could the nurse promote growth and development for this child during TPN therapy?

STUDY ACTIVITIES

1. Review the medical records of several children who are on a pediatric unit in your agency. Note the type of medication, route ordered, and what specific interventions are needed for each child related to the medication administration and developmental age of the child, including atraumatic care interventions. Compile a list of the most commonly used routes.
2. Interview several parents about their experiences in giving medications to their children. From these interviews, develop a teaching sheet that provides tips to facilitate oral medication administration to children.
3. Create a chart that compares the SQ, IM, and IV methods of medication administration. Include examples of medications given via these routes, onset of action, appropriate sites, and necessary safety measures for each.

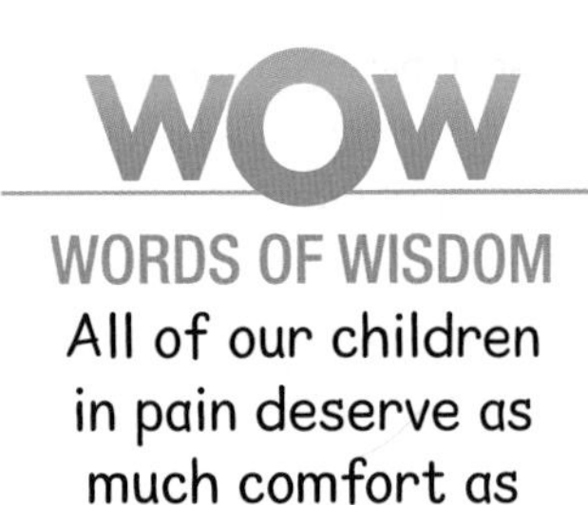

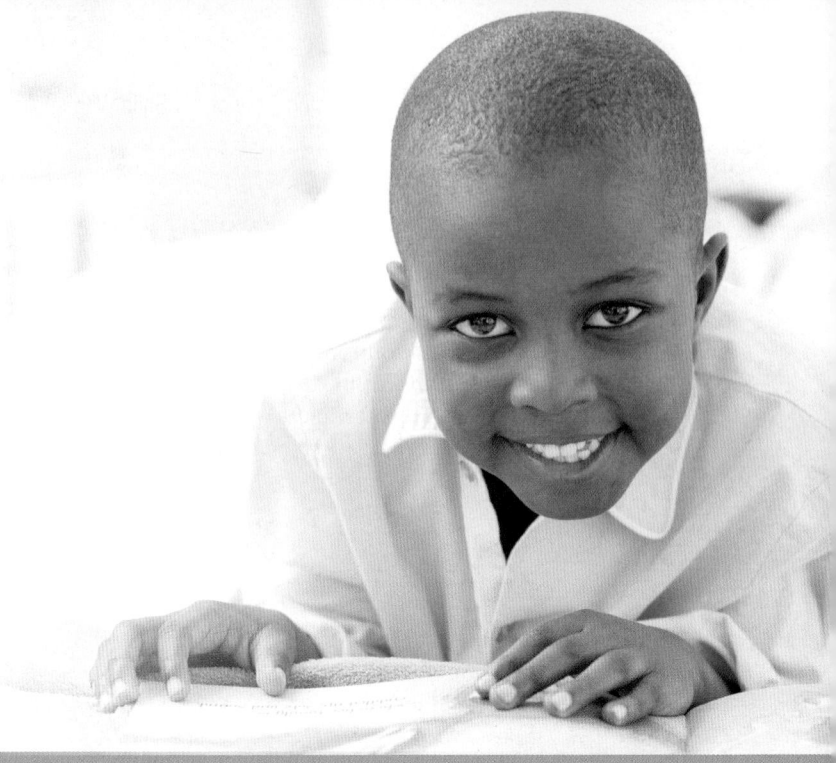

All of our children in pain deserve as much comfort as we can give.

14 Nursing Care of the Child With an Alteration in Comfort–Pain Assessment and Management

KEY TERMS

acute pain
chronic pain
drug tolerance
epidural analgesia (ep′i-dūr′ăl an′ăl-jē′zē-ă)
moderate sedation
neuromodulators (nŭr′ō-mod′yū-lā′tōrz)
neuropathic pain (nŭr′ō-path′ik pān)
nociceptive pain (nō′si-sep′tiv pān)
nociceptors (nō′si-sep′tŏrz)
pain
pain threshold
patient-controlled analgesia (PCA)
physical dependence
somatic pain (sō-mat′ik pān)
transduction
visceral pain (vis′ĕr-ăl pān)

LEARNING OBJECTIVES

Upon completion of the chapter, you will be able to:

1. Identify the major physiologic events associated with the perception of pain.
2. Distinguish different types of pain based on duration, etiology, and source or location.
3. Discuss the factors that influence the pain response.
4. Identify the developmental considerations for the effects and management of pain.
5. Explain the principles of pain assessment as they relate to children.
6. Understand the use of the various pain rating scales and physiologic monitoring for children.
7. Establish a nursing plan of care for children related to management of pain, including pharmacologic and nonpharmacologic techniques and strategies.

Aiden Russell is a 6-year-old on the pediatric unit admitted for a wound infection. He requires twice-daily (BID) dressing changes. In report, you are told that Aiden cries and fights during the dressing change but otherwise seems to be playing and not experiencing much pain.

INTRODUCTION

A child's comfort is affected by many factors such as hunger, sleep, temperature, presence of caregivers and family, presence of strangers, and the presence of pain. Alteration in comfort in children incorporates all of these factors. A major issue affecting a child's comfort is pain, and nurses have an integral role in helping children and families deal with pain. Therefore, in this chapter, the main focus will be pain assessment and pain management in children.

Pain is a highly individualized, subjective experience that can affect any person of any age. It is a complex phenomenon that involves multiple components and is influenced by myriad factors. **Pain** is defined by the International Association for the Study of Pain (2011) as "an unpleasant sensory and emotional experience associated with, or resembling that associated with, actual or potential tissue damage" (Hauer & Jones, 2021). Another definition of pain that is commonly used is as follows: It is whatever the person experiencing it says it is, existing whenever the person says it does (McCaffery, 1968). The person experiencing the pain is the only one who can identify pain and know what the pain is like.

Pain is a universal experience. Pain affects adults and children of all ages, even preterm infants. Pain can result from numerous causes, including disease processes, injuries, procedures, and surgical interventions. In 1995, the American Pain Society (1995) labeled it "the fifth vital sign." The American Pain Society's goal was to encourage health care professionals to assess pain every time temperature, pulse, respirations, and blood pressure were assessed and to institute measures to manage it.

Unlike adults, however, children may lack the verbal capacity to describe their pain effectively. In addition, many caregivers and health care providers have misconceptions about pain in children, it is difficult to assess the complex nature of the pain experience, and limited resources and research are available related to pain relief strategies for children. Therefore, pain is a major source of distress for children and their families as well as for health care providers.

If left unmanaged, pain in children can lead to serious physical and emotional consequences, such as increased oxygen consumption and alterations in blood glucose metabolism. In addition, the experience of untreated pain early in life may lead to long-term physiologic and psychological consequences for the child (Roué, 2023). For example, inadequately controlled pain can have long-lasting negative outcomes, such as increased distress during later procedures, nonadherence to treatment regimens, inactivity, prolonged bed rest, and the development of chronic pain. Detrimental effects on the course of a disease itself may also be seen with untreated pain. Preterm infants are at a greater risk due to long hospitalizations and numerous painful and invasive procedures (Roué, 2023).

All these factors make pain management a critical element in the plan of care for children. Pain management in children has improved, but underestimation and inadequate management still remain a problem (American Academy of Pediatrics [AAP] et al., 2016, reaffirmed 2020). Various national health associations have issued position papers and guidelines related to the need to treat pain and suffering in children. Effective pain management involves initial pain assessment, therapeutic interventions, and reassessment for all children in any health care setting.

This chapter describes the pain experience in children, including the types of pain, factors influencing pain, and common fallacies and myths associated with pain in children. The nursing process is applied to provide an overview of the care for a child in pain. Various pain management strategies are described, including nonpharmacologic and pharmacologic interventions and measures to address procedure-related and chronic pain.

PHYSIOLOGY OF PAIN

The sensation of pain is a complex phenomenon that involves a sequence of physiologic events in the nervous system. These events are transduction, transmission, perception, and modulation.

Transduction

Peripheral nerve fibers extend from the spinal cord to various locations in and throughout the body's tissues, such as the skin, joints, bones, and membranes covering the internal organs. At the end of these fibers are specialized receptors, called **nociceptors**, which become activated when they are exposed to noxious stimuli. The noxious stimuli can be mechanical, chemical, or thermal. Mechanical stimuli may include intense pressure to an area, a strong muscular contraction, or extensive pressure due to muscular overstretching. Chemical stimulation may involve the release of mediators, such as histamine, prostaglandins, leukotrienes, or bradykinin, as a response to tissue trauma, ischemia, or inflammation. Thermal stimuli typically involve extremes of heat and cold. This process of nociceptor activation is called **transduction**.

Transmission

When nociceptors are activated by noxious stimuli, the stimuli are converted to electrical impulses that are relayed along the peripheral nerves to the spinal cord and brain. Specialized afferent nerve fibers are responsible for moving the electrical impulse along. Myelinated A-delta fibers are large fibers that conduct the impulse at very rapid rates. The pain transmitted by these fibers is often referred to as "fast pain," most commonly associated with mechanical or thermal stimuli (Nath, 2023). Pain is also transmitted by unmyelinated small C fibers. These fibers transmit the impulse slowly and are often activated by chemical stimuli or continued mechanical or thermal stimuli (Nath, 2023). These fibers carry the impulse to the spinal cord via the dorsal horn. Neurotransmitters are released to facilitate the transmission process to the brain.

Several theories have been proposed in an attempt to explain the process of pain transmission. The best known of these is gate control theory. According to this theory, the dorsal horn of the spinal cord contains interneuronal or interconnecting fibers. Large-diameter, faster fibers carry nonnociceptive, tactile information, while smaller nerve fibers carry nociceptive or pain signals. Large fibers, when stimulated, close the gate or pathway to the brain, thereby inhibiting or blocking the transmission of the pain impulse. Subsequently, the impulse does not reach the brain, where it would be interpreted as pain. It is now known that pain modulation is a more complex process, but this theory helps explain why some nonpharmacologic therapies, such as massage and pressure, are effective in reducing pain (Nath, 2023).

Perception

Once in the dorsal horn of the spinal cord, the nerve fibers divide and then cross to the opposite side and rise upward to the thalamus. The thalamus responds quickly and sends a message to the somatosensory cortex of the brain, where the impulse is interpreted as the physical sensation of pain. The impulses carried by the fast A-delta fibers lead to the perception of sharp, stabbing localized pain that also commonly involves a reflex response to withdraw from the stimulus. The impulses carried by the slow C fibers lead to the perception of diffuse, dull, burning, or aching pain. The point at which the person first feels the lowest intensity of the painful stimulus is termed the **pain threshold**. In addition to sending a message to the cerebral cortex, the thalamus also sends a message to the limbic system, where the sensation is interpreted emotionally, and to the brain stem centers, where autonomic nervous system responses begin.

Modulation

Research has identified substances called **neuromodulators** that appear to modify the pain sensation. These substances have been found to change a person's perception of pain. Examples of these neuromodulators include serotonin, endorphins, enkephalins, and dynorphins.

Pain perception can be modified peripherally or centrally. In the peripheral nerve fibers, chemical substances are released that either stimulate the nerve fibers or sensitize them. Peripheral sensitization allows the nerve fibers to react to a stimulus that is of lower intensity than would be needed to cause pain. As a result, the person perceives more pain. Actions that block or inhibit the release of these substances can lead to a decrease in pain perception.

Modification of pain perception can occur centrally in the spinal cord at the dorsal horn. Substances released by the excited interneurons can potentiate the pain sensation. Other neurochemicals, through their binding to specific receptors, can inhibit the perception of pain. Figure 14.1 illustrates the physiology of pain.

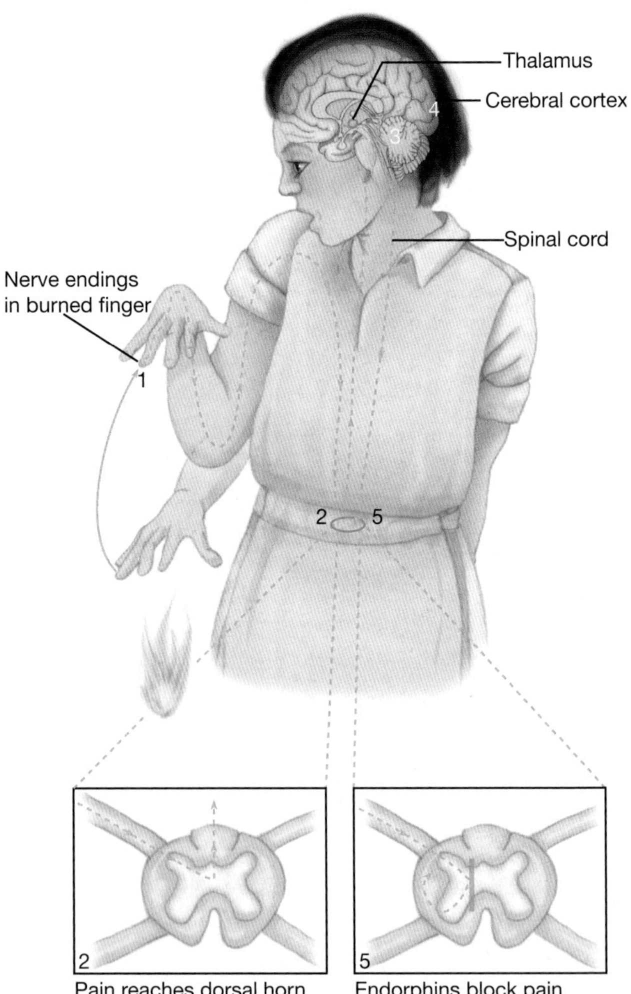

FIGURE 14.1 Physiology of pain. (*1*) Exposure to thermal noxious stimuli results in activation of nociception (transduction). (*2*) Impulses are relayed along the peripheral nerves to the spinal cord through the dorsal horn (transmission). (*3, 4*) This results in the individual feeling the sensation of pain (perception). (*5*) Neurons in the brain stem send signals back down to the dorsal horn, and these fibers release substances such as endorphins, which can inhibit painful impulses in the dorsal horn (modulation). These neurotransmitters are taken back by the body, therefore limiting the analgesic value.

TYPES OF PAIN

Many different systems can be used to classify pain. Most commonly, pain is classified based on its duration, etiology, or source or location.

Classification by Duration

Pain is classified by duration as either acute or chronic.

Acute Pain

Acute pain is defined as pain that is associated with a rapid onset of varying intensity. It usually indicates tissue damage and resolves with healing of the injury. Acute pain reflects stimulation of nociceptors and serves a protective function (i.e., alerting the person to a problem). Examples of causes of acute pain include trauma, invasive procedures, acute illnesses such as sore throat or appendicitis, and surgery. This type of pain generally lasts a few days.

TAKE NOTE!

Children often experience pain associated with various procedures done in health care settings. This type of pain is usually short in duration. Preparation of the child and family will help decrease fears or anxiety. Depending on the type of procedure and the child's age, cognitive level, and temperament, various techniques and methods can be used. Advocating for atraumatic care and adhering to its guidelines will help minimize procedure-related pain.

Chronic Pain

Chronic pain is defined as pain that continues past the expected point of healing for injured tissue. It provides no protective function. It may be continuous or intermittent, with and without periods of exacerbation or remission. It often interferes with sleep and performance of activities of daily living. It can result in loss of appetite and depression. Thus, chronic pain impairs a person's ability to function. In contrast to acute pain, environmental and psychological factors influence behaviors associated with chronic pain. In children, chronic, recurrent pain is most commonly associated with abdominal pain, nonspecific headache, limb pain, or chest pain. Some conditions, such as sickle cell disease and migraines, have characteristics of both acute and chronic pain. Children with chronic pain may not exhibit the same physical or emotional responses as seen with acute pain. As pain becomes prolonged and continuous, the autonomic nervous system response tends to diminish.

Classification by Etiology

Pain can be classified by etiology as nociceptive or neuropathic.

Nociceptive Pain

Nociceptive pain reflects pain due to noxious stimuli that damage normal tissues or have the potential to do so if the pain is prolonged. The pain perceived often correlates closely with the degree or intensity of the stimulus and the extent of real or possible tissue damage. With nociceptive pain, nervous system functioning is intact. Reports of nociceptive pain vary depending on the location of the nociceptors being stimulated. Nociceptive pain ranges from sharp or burning, to dull, aching, or cramping, and to deep aching or sharp stabbing. Examples of conditions that result in nociceptive pain include chemical burns, sunburn, cuts, appendicitis, and bladder distention.

Neuropathic Pain

Neuropathic pain is pain due to malfunctioning of the peripheral or central nervous system. It may be continuous or intermittent and is commonly described as burning, tingling, shooting, squeezing, or spasm-like pain. Examples of neuropathic pain include posttraumatic and postsurgical peripheral nerve injuries, pain after spinal cord injury, metabolic neuropathies, phantom limb pain after amputation, and poststroke pain.

Classification by Source or Location

Pain may also be classified by the source or location of the area involved. It can be somatic pain (superficial and deep) or visceral pain. These classifications typically indicate nociceptive pain.

Somatic Pain

Somatic pain refers to pain that develops in the tissues. It can be further divided into two groups—superficial and deep. Superficial somatic pain, often called cutaneous pain, involves stimulation of nociceptors in the skin, subcutaneous tissue, or mucous membranes. Typically, the pain is well localized and described as a sharp, pricking, or burning sensation. Superficial somatic pain may be due to external mechanical, chemical, or thermal injury or skin disorders. Tenderness is commonly present.

Deep somatic pain typically involves the muscles, tendons, joints, fasciae, and bones. It can be localized or diffuse and is usually described as dull, aching, or cramping. Deep somatic pain may be due to strain from overuse or direct injury, ischemia, and inflammation. Tenderness and reflex spasm may be present. In addition, the person may exhibit sympathetic nervous system activation such as tachycardia, hypertension, tachypnea, diaphoresis, pallor, and pupillary dilation.

Visceral Pain

Visceral pain is pain that develops within organs such as the heart, lungs, gastrointestinal (GI) tract, pancreas, liver, gallbladder, kidneys, or bladder. It is often produced by disease. It is usually diffuse and poorly localized and is described as a deep ache or sharp stabbing sensation that may be referred to other areas. Visceral pain may be due to distention of the organ, organ muscular spasm, contraction, pulling, ischemia, or inflammation. Tenderness, nausea, vomiting, and diaphoresis may be present.

FACTORS INFLUENCING PAIN

Children, like adults, experience neurologic events that result in the perception of pain. However, research has found that environmental and psychological factors may exert a greater influence on the child's perception of pain (McGrath, 2005). Certain factors such as age, sex, cognitive level, temperament, previous pain experiences, and family and cultural backgrounds cannot be changed. However, situational factors involving behavioral, cognitive, and emotional aspects can be modified.

Age and Sex

Research has demonstrated that the nervous system structures needed for pain impulse transmission and perception are present before birth (Roué, 2023). Therefore, children of any age, including preterm newborns, are capable of experiencing pain. Early on, children can interpret pain as an unpleasant sensation, but this interpretation is based on their comparison with other sensations. As they get older, they learn to use words to describe their pain more fully.

Gender and sex may also play a role in a child's perception of pain. It has been suggested that males and females differ in how they perceive, experience, express, and cope with pain and respond to analgesics (Osborne & Davis, 2022). This may be influenced by various factors, including genetics, hormones, family, and culture. Further research is warranted in this area to facilitate more focused care in pain management.

Cognitive Level

Cognitive level is a key factor affecting a child's pain perception and response and usually goes hand in hand with the child's age. Cognitive level typically increases with age, thereby influencing the child's understanding of the pain and its impact and their choices for coping strategies. In addition, as the child's cognitive level increases, their ability to communicate information about pain increases. However, this increased understanding and ability to communicate with advancing age may not apply to the child experiencing developmental delays. For example, a school-age child or adolescent with developmental delays may have the same cognitive level as a toddler or preschooler. Health care providers need to be cognizant of these differences when caring for the child in pain.

Temperament

Literature suggests that temperament plays a role in predicting distress and pain levels in a child during painful events (Favaretto et al., 2022; Horton et al., 2015). For example, a child with a challenging temperament is more likely to have an increased distress response to pain. Nurses can personalize interventions in the clinical environment and during the pain experience to better fit the child's temperament and other personality traits of the child and family.

Previous Pain Experiences

A child identifies pain based on their experiences with pain in the past. The number of episodes of pain, the type of pain, the severity or intensity of the previous pain experience, the effectiveness of treatment of pain, and how the child responded all affect how the child will perceive and respond to the current experience. Research suggests that severe pain experiences in the neonate or young infant can lead to increased pain sensitivity and chronic pain syndrome later in life (Roué, 2023). Previous pain experiences with inadequate pain control may lead to increased distress during future painful procedures. For example, research studies have demonstrated that neonates who had undergone painful procedures such as circumcision and heel lancing showed a stronger negative response to routine immunizations and venipuncture weeks to months later (Roué, 2023).

Family and Culture

The child's cultural and family background will influence how they will express and manage pain. Some cultures transmit the standard of accepting pain stoically; others encourage outward expression. Parents have a strong influence on the child's ability to cope. For example, if a parent reacts to the child's pain in a positive manner and offers comfort measures, the child may have an easier time coping. If the parent shows anger or disapproval, the pain experience may be intensified for the child.

Situational Factors

Situational factors involve factors or elements that interact with the child and their current situation involving the experience of pain. These factors are highly variable and dependent on the specific situation. Situational factors result from the context in which the child is experiencing pain and include cognitive factors, or what the child understands and believes about the pain experience; behavioral factors, or how the child and family react and what they do about the pain experience; and emotional factors, or how the child and family feel about the pain experience (McGrath, 2005). Due to children's limited experience with pain, situational factors may affect them more than adults (McGrath, 2005). A thorough pain assessment must include assessment for situational factors that may exacerbate pain. Examples of situational factors include:

- Child's lack of understanding of the source of pain
- Child's lack of ability to use coping mechanisms or pain-relieving strategies to decrease pain
- Stress and anxiety in anticipation of pain
- Child's lack of control of cause of pain
- Child's lack of ability to understand what to expect from potentially painful experiences
- Increased anxiety exhibited by the family
- Overly protective behaviors exhibited by the family
- Presence of emotions such as fear, anxiety, frustration, distress, underlying anxiety, and depression (McGrath, 2005).

DEVELOPMENTAL CONSIDERATIONS

Since children of various developmental ages respond differently to pain and perceive pain in different ways, it is important to review developmental considerations. Refer to Chapters 3 through 7 for a more complete understanding of childhood development. Nurses must understand how children of various ages respond to painful stimuli and what behaviors may be expected on the basis of their developmental level. By understanding these developmental considerations, the nurse can appropriately assess the child's pain and provide effective interventions.

Infants

Research has demonstrated that infants, including preterm infants, experience pain and can distinguish pain from other tactile experiences (Roué, 2023). Much of this research focuses on pain related to invasive procedures, such as heel sticks and intravenous catheter insertion. Research suggests that neonates actually have a lower pain threshold and pain tolerance and experience pain at a greater intensity than older-age children and adults (Luo et al., 2023).

Concept Mastery Alert

Levels of Pain

When obtaining a blood sample with a heel stick, the nurse should remember that neonates, and, in particular, preterm infants, feel pain and feel it with greater intensity than do older infants.

In preterm and term newborns, behavioral and physiologic indicators are used for determining pain. Behavioral indicators include facial expression, such as brow contracting and chin quivering; body movements; and crying (Roué, 2023). Physiologic signs include changes in heart rate, respiratory rate, blood pressure, oxygen saturation levels, breathing pattern, skin color, pupillary size, intracranial pressure, vagal tone, and palmar sweating (Roué, 2023).

In the younger infant, facial expression is the most common response to pain (Fig. 14.2). The brows may be lowered and drawn together, with the eyes tightly closed. The mouth is open, often forming a square. The body may be stiff, and thrashing may be seen. When the area is stimulated, the infant may demonstrate a generalized reflex withdrawal. The infant may exhibit a high-pitched, shrill cry.

The older infant often displays similar behavioral manifestations of pain. The older infant may display an angry facial expression, but the eyes are open. They often demonstrate a definite withdrawal response when

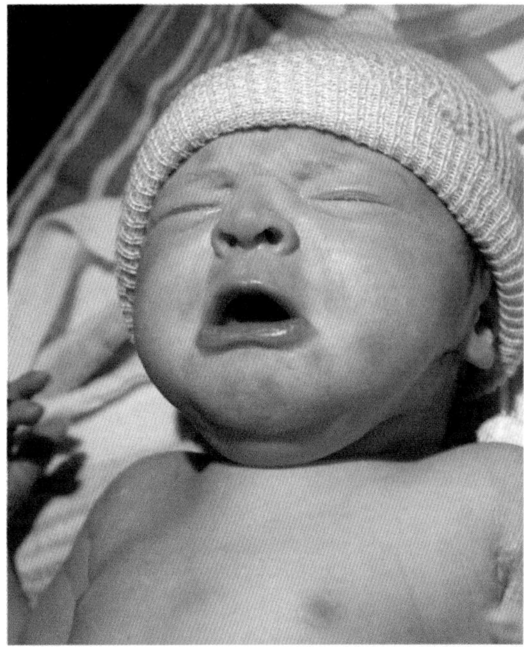

FIGURE 14.2 In the younger infant, facial expression is the most common response to pain.

the area is stimulated. The older infant cries loudly and tries to push away the stimulus that is causing the pain. Other manifestations include irritability, restless sleeping, and poor feeding.

TAKE NOTE!

Remember that anything that causes pain in an adult or older child will cause pain in a neonate or infant regardless of whether the neonate or infant exhibits typical behaviors indicating pain (Roué, 2023). The response to pain is highly variable.

Infants also demonstrate physiologic responses to pain. These may include:

- Increased heart rate, usually averaging approximately 10 bpm; possibly bradycardia in preterm newborns
- Decreased vagal tone
- Decreased oxygen saturation
- Palmar or plantar sweating (as measured by skin conductivity testing); not reliable in infants before 37 weeks' gestation

Toddlers

Toddlers can react to painless procedures as intensely as painful ones, with intense emotional upset and physical resistance or aggression. They may bite, hit, scream, or kick. Other behaviors may include being quiet, pointing to where it hurts, or saying such words as "ow." Facial grimacing and teeth clenching may be noted. They may also react with fear and try to hide or leave the room. They often have limited vocabularies, so it may be difficult for them to express pain. It is important to ask about and encourage the child to verbalize their pain. Ensure the use of words the toddler understands, such as "owie" or "boo-boo." Toddlers may demonstrate regressive behaviors, such as clinging to the parent or crying loudly.

TAKE NOTE!

Young children express pain by using simple words such as "hurt" or "ouchie" or by pointing to the area that hurts. By the age of 3 to 7 years, they can express the presence of pain, and they can usually describe it and its intensity, location, and quality (Zeltzer et al., 2020).

Preschoolers

Preschoolers may become quiet or try to withdraw and hide in response to actual or perceived pain. For example, the child may say they need to go to the bathroom or to get something from another room. Because of their magical thinking, preschoolers may believe pain is a punishment for misbehaving or having bad thoughts. Preschoolers may not verbally report their pain, thinking that pain is something to be expected or that the adults are aware of their pain. They can tell someone where it hurts and can use various tools to describe the severity of pain. However, because they may have limited experience with pain, they may have difficulty distinguishing among types of pain (e.g., sharp or dull), describing the intensity of the pain, and determining whether the pain is worse or better.

School-Age Children

School-age children can usually communicate the type, location, and severity of pain. Children older than the age of 8 can use specific words, such as "sharp as a knife," "burning," or "pulling" to describe their pain. However, they may deny pain in an attempt to appear brave or to avoid further pain related to a procedure or intervention. They may be more concerned with their fear about the illness and its effects rather than the pain. They may also fear being embarrassed by acting out behaviors in response to pain, such as screaming or thrashing. Thus, a typical response might be to withdraw by staring at the television. Other behaviors that may indicate pain in a school-age child include muscular rigidity, such as clenching the fists, stiffening the body, closing the eyes, wrinkling the forehead, or gritting the teeth.

Adolescents

Adolescents may be concerned primarily about body image and fear losing control over their behavior. This may result in denial or refusal of medications. Their mood and what they think is expected of them will also affect their response to pain. Adolescents often ask numerous questions and pay close attention to how others respond to them. Fearing that their behavior may be viewed as juvenile, they may attempt to remain stoic and not exhibit any emotion. Subtle changes such as increased muscle tension with clenched fists and teeth, rapid breathing, and guarding the affected body part may occur. They may also show lack of interest in everyday activities or a decreased ability to concentrate.

Common Fallacies and Myths About Pain in Children

In general, children respond to pain based on the type of pain, the extent of pain, and their age and developmental level. Table 14.1 highlights some common myths and misconceptions related to pain in children. Because of these myths, children have historically been medicated less than adults with similar diagnoses, leading to inadequate pain management (Gai et al., 2020; Roué, 2023).

TABLE 14.1 • Myths and Misconceptions About Children and Pain

Myth or Misconception	Fact
Newborns do not feel pain.	Newborns, including preterm newborns, do feel pain. The neurologic and hormonal systems needed for the transmission of painful stimuli are sufficiently developed.
Exposure to pain at an early age has little to no effect on the child.	Prolonged or severe pain can lead to increased newborn morbidity. Infants who have experienced pain during the neonatal period respond differently to subsequent painful events.[a]
Infants and small children have little memory of pain.	Repeated exposure to painful procedures and events can have long-term consequences. Memories of pain may be stored in the child's nervous system, influencing later reactions to painful stimuli.[a]
The intensity of a child's behavioral reaction indicates the intensity of the child's pain.	Numerous factors affect a child's response to pain. Each child is an individual with their own set of responses.
A child who is sleeping or playing is not in pain.	Sleep or play may be a coping strategy for the child in pain. Sleep may reflect exhaustion of the child who is coping with pain.
Children are truthful when they are asked if they are experiencing pain.	Often, children deny pain to avoid a painful situation or procedure, embarrassment, or loss of control. Children may assume that others know how they are feeling and will thus not verbalize their complaints.
Children learn to adapt to pain and painful procedures.	Repeated exposure to pain or painful procedures can result in an increase in behavioral manifestations.
Children experience more adverse effects of narcotic analgesics than adults do.	The risk of adverse effects of narcotic analgesics is the same for children as for adults.
Children are more prone to addiction to narcotic analgesics.	There is no increased risk of addiction to narcotics when used appropriately to treat children's pain.[b]

[a]Roué, J.-M. (2023). Assessment of neonatal pain. *UpToDate*. Retrieved March 13, 2023, from https://www.uptodate.com/contents/assessment-of-neonatal-pain

[b]Zeltzer, L. K., Krane, E. J., & Levy, R. L. (2020). Pediatric pain management. In R. M. Kleigman, J. W. St. Geme III, N. J. Blum, S. S. Shah, R. C. Tasker, K. M. Wilson, & R. E. Behrman (Eds.), *Nelson textbook of pediatrics* (21st ed., pp. 2915–3011). Elsevier.

Clinical Judgment and the Nursing Process

Nursing care of the child with pain includes nursing assessment, analysis, planning, interventions, and evaluation. Each step of this process must be individualized for each child. A general understanding of the physiology of pain, factors that influence pain, and effective pain management techniques can help to individualize the child's plan of care.

Assessment

Assessment of pain in children consists of both subjective and objective data collection. The acronym "QUESTT" is an excellent way to remember the key principles of pain assessment (Baker & Wong, 1987):

- *Q*uestion the child.
- *U*se a reliable and valid pain scale.
- *E*valuate the child's behavior and physiologic changes to establish a baseline and determine the effectiveness of the intervention. The child's behavior and motor activity may include irritability and protection as well as withdrawal of the affected painful area.
- *S*ecure the parent's involvement.
- *T*ake the cause of pain into account when intervening.
- *T*ake action.

TAKE NOTE!

Children do experience pain. Pain management techniques work just as well with children as they do with adults.

Health History

When assessing pain in children, tailor the assessment to the child's developmental level, and ask questions geared toward the child's cognitive ability. During the health history, determine the child's previous exposure to pain, if any, and how the child responded. This information will provide clues about how the child copes and their current response. Attempt to determine what word the child uses to denote pain. Some children may not understand the term "pain" but do understand terms such as "ouchie" or "boo-boo."

The health history also includes questioning the parents about their cultural beliefs related to pain and their child's usual responses. This information aids in planning developmentally and culturally appropriate family-centered care.

Questioning the Child

When questioning the child, phrase the questions in a manner that the child will be able to understand based on their developmental level. Some input from the child's family may be helpful in determining where best to focus the questions.

Ask the child what pain means to them. Use words that the child may comprehend more easily, such as "hurt," "boo-boo," or "ouch," as appropriate. Inquire about similar experiences in the past and how they responded. Determine whether the child let others know that they were hurting and how this message was conveyed (e.g., crying, acting out, or pointing to the hurting area).

Review the history of the pain and various influences such as cultural aspects, caregiver attitudes or expectations, previous experiences, and any education or teaching related to pain management. Continue to formulate questions to ascertain the following:

- Location, quality, severity, and onset of the pain, as well as the circumstances in which the child experiences the pain. Have the child point to the area where it hurts, or identify the location on a diagram or doll.
- Conditions, if any, that preceded the onset of pain and the conditions that followed the onset of pain
- Any associated symptoms, such as weight loss, fever, vomiting, or diarrhea, that may indicate a current illness.
- Any recent trauma, including any interventions that were used in an attempt to relieve the pain.

Continue the health history by inquiring about what the child wants others, including the nurse, to do when the child hurts. Conversely, ask the child what they don't want others to do. Finally, question the child about measures that seem to be most effective in relieving the pain. Ask if there is anything special the child wants to tell the nurse, such as a special pain relief technique or a specific comfort object.

If the child is experiencing chronic or recurrent pain, suggest the child and family record information in a symptom diary. Explain that this will be helpful in identifying the best ways to manage the pain.

Questioning the Parents

Parents play a key role in assessing pain in children. Often, it is the parents who provide information about the child's current and past experiences with pain. In addition, parents can provide information about how the child exhibits and responds to pain. Parents may be aware of subtle changes in the child's behavior that may precede the pain, occur with the pain, or indicate relief of pain. Including the parents in this process helps create a positive experience for all involved and promotes feelings of control over the situation.

The questions posed to the parents are similar in focus to those posed to the child. However, more detailed information may be obtained from the parents because they are usually able to describe events more fully or in greater detail owing to their higher cognitive level. Parents typically know their child best.

TAKE NOTE!

Parents may assume that nurses have greater expertise when it comes to assessing their child's pain and taking appropriate action. Thus, they may not always report when they notice changes suggesting that their child is uncomfortable. Emphasize the important role parents play in reporting any changes in their child so that pain relief measures can be instituted as soon as possible.

When questioning the parents, use the following examples as a guide for assessing the child's pain:

- Has your child ever been in pain before? If so, what was the cause of the pain? How long did they have the pain? Where was the pain located?
- How did your child react to the pain? What did you do to lessen the pain?
- Did your child let you know that they were in pain? Did they tell you or did you notice something?
- Are there any special signs that let you know that your child is hurting? If so, what are they?
- Is there anything that your child does or that you do when they are hurting that helps relieve the pain?
- Does one thing work better than another when your child is hurting?
- Is there any special information that you want to tell me about your child?

Using Pain Rating Scales

Various pain assessment, or pain rating, scales are available. These scales allow the child to report their pain, and the pain level is quantified. These standardized rating scales provide a greater alignment between the child's pain and the nurse's assessment of the severity of the pain. Self-report is the preferred source for the measurement of pain in verbal children (Gai et al., 2020). Self-report measures should be used in conjunction with observation and discussion with the child and family, especially in young children or in children with cognitive impairments (Hauer & Jones, 2021). Some children as young as 3 years of age can accurately use self-report tools to quantify their pain levels (Hauer & Jones, 2021). The reliability of these tools will increase as the child grows older and more cognitively mature. It is important to assess young children's ability to perform self-report tasks rather than rely solely on their chronologic age.

Many health care facilities have specific policies and procedures related to pain assessment, including the frequency of assessment, the rating tool to use, and nursing interventions to be instituted on the basis of the rating. For example, many facilities require assessment of the child using a specific tool with documentation at least once a shift and 30 minutes to 1 hour after a nonpharmacologic or pharmacologic pain relief intervention. This process provides a more objective method to determine whether the pain is increasing or decreasing and whether pain relief methods are effective.

TAKE NOTE!

Typically, different pain rating scales are appropriate for different developmental levels. However, children may regress when in pain, so a simpler tool may be needed to make sure that the child understands what is being asked. Regardless of the tool used, nurses need to be consistent in using the same tool so that appropriate comparisons can be made and effective interventions can be planned and implemented. Using the most appropriate tool consistently allows the most accurate assessment of the child's pain.

FACES Pain Rating Scale. The FACES pain rating scale (Fig. 14.3) is a self-report tool that is typically used in children 3 to 8 years of age (Hauer & Jones, 2021). The scale consists of six illustrations of faces arranged horizontally, with expressions ranging from smiling (indicating no hurt) to crying with frowning (indicating hurts worst). Under each face is a short description such as "hurts little bit" and a number. The number scale can be 0, 1, 2, 3, 4, and 5 or 0, 2, 4, 6, 8, and 10. The nurse explains the words associated with each face to the child. Then, the nurse asks the child to select the facial expression that best describes the level of pain they are feeling. The nurse then documents the number corresponding to the word description and face.

Oucher Pain Rating Scale. The Oucher pain rating scale is similar to the FACES scale in that it uses facial expressions to indicate increasing degrees of hurt. However, instead of illustrations, six photographs are used: "no hurt" is placed at the bottom of the arrangement and "most hurt" at the top. Alongside the photos is a scale ranging from 0 to 10 that corresponds to the facial expressions in the photographs (Fig. 14.4). After explaining the photos and numeric scale, the child is asked to point to the number that best describes their level of pain (Beyer et al., 1992).

This scale is useful for self-reporting of pain in children between 3 and 12 years of age (Beyer et al., 1992). Different versions have been developed for use with children of different racial and ethnic backgrounds (Beyer et al., 1992).

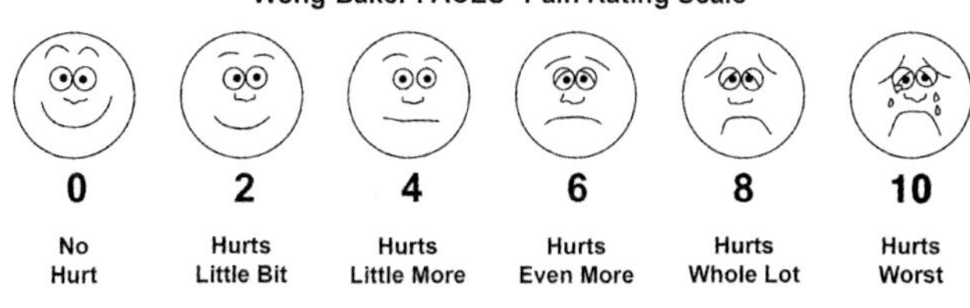

FIGURE 14.3 FACES pain rating scale. (© 1983 Wong-Baker FACES Foundation. www.WongBakerFACES.org. Used with permission. Originally published in Whaley & *Wong's Nursing Care of Infants and Children*. © Elsevier Inc.)

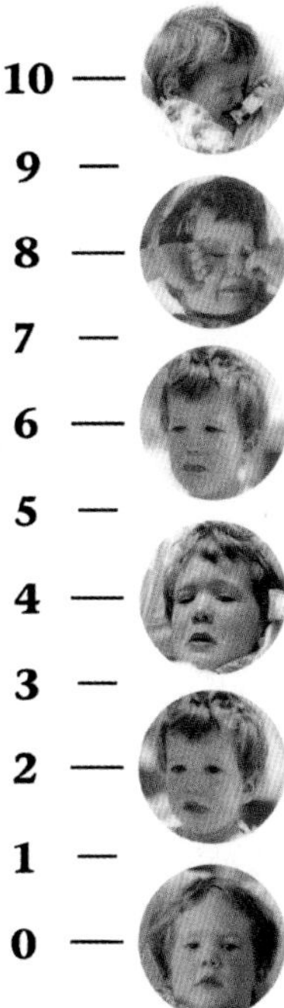

FIGURE 14.4 Oucher pain rating scale. (Reprinted with permission of Pain Associates in Nursing 2024.)

Poker Chip Tool. The poker chip tool, also known as the pieces of hurt tool, is a self-reporting pain assessment tool that uses four red poker chips to quantify the child's level of pain. The chips are arranged in a horizontal line on a surface in front of the child. Starting with the chip closest to the child's left side, the nurse points to the chip and explains that the first chip means a little hurt, the next chip means more hurt, the third chip means more hurt, and the fourth chip means the worst hurt ever. Then, the nurse asks the child how many "pieces of hurt" they are having (Fig. 14.5). If the child is not experiencing any pain, typically the child will state that they are not having any. When the child identifies the number of "pieces of hurt," the nurse follows up by asking the child to tell the nurse more about their hurt (Hester, 1979).

The poker chip tool is useful for assessing pain in preschool-age children and can be used in children 3 to 18 years of age (Thirion et al., 2015). Children may view this assessment tool as a game since it involves poker chips. However, the nurse needs to ensure that the child has the cognitive ability to distinguish the numbers.

TAKE NOTE!

Toddlers and preschoolers may not be used to being asked questions by strangers and may not understand quantitative ratings or estimation. Preschoolers will often construct an answer even if they do not understand the question. They will also often use extremes of scales, such as no pain or the worst pain (Thirion et al., 2015).

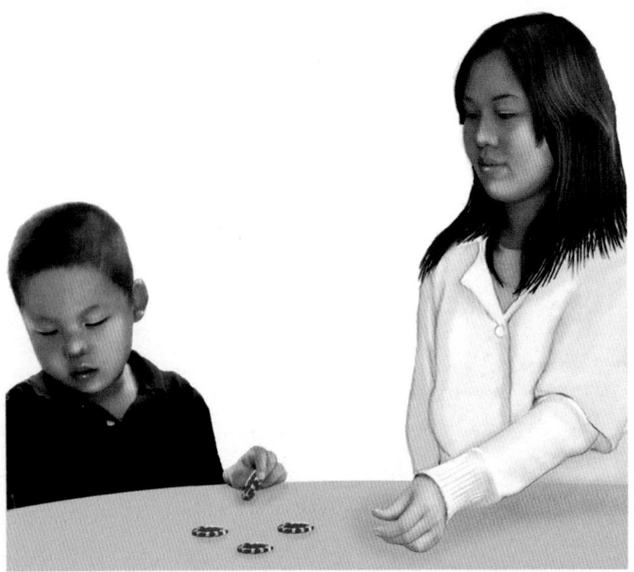

FIGURE 14.5 The poker chip tool. Here, the nurse asks the child to identify the number of chips that indicate their degree of "hurt."

Visual Analog and Numeric Scales. Visual analog and numeric scales involve a horizontal or vertical line with marked endpoints. With a visual analog scale, the endpoints are identified as no pain and worst pain. A numeric scale typically has endpoints of 0 and 10, reflecting no pain and worst pain, respectively (Fig. 14.6). The nurse explains the scale to the child. With the visual analog scale, the child makes a line that best describes the level of pain. The nurse then measures the distance from the "no pain" endpoint to the child's mark and records this as the pain score. With the numeric scale, the nurse asks the child to pick the number that best describes their level of pain.

The visual analog scale can be used in children 6 years or older (Zeltzer et al., 2020). The numeric scale can be used with children 7 years or older (Gai et al., 2020). Even though a younger child may be able to count and give numbers on the scale, they have not yet developed an understanding of the quantitative significance of the numbers.

Adolescent Pediatric Pain Tool. The Adolescent Pediatric Pain Tool is a multidimensional self-report type of tool useful for older children, usually between 8 and 17 years of age (Boitor et al., 2019). The tool involves three aspects of assessment. In the first assessment, the child identifies the location of the pain on two illustrations of the body—front and back views (Fig. 14.7).

The child is instructed to color the areas where they are hurting. The child is also instructed to color the area as big or as small as how much they are hurting. For example, if the hurt is mild or moderate, the child would color a moderate area of the location; if the pain is severe, they would color a much larger area. The second portion of the tool involves a scale that ranges from "no pain" to "worst possible pain." The nurse instructs the child to identify the severity of their pain. The third assessment is a list of words that may be used to describe pain, such as "throbbing,"

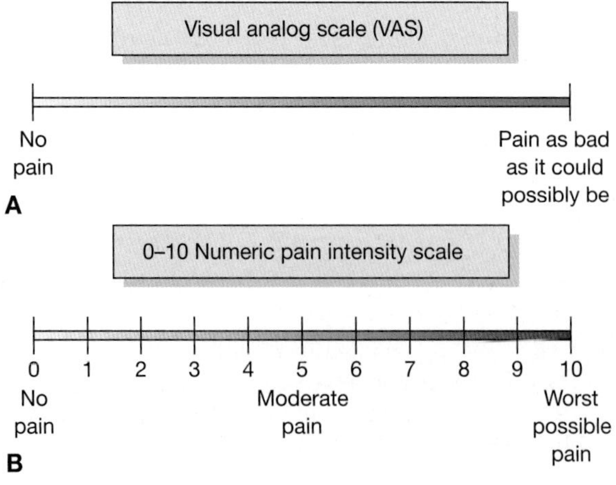

FIGURE 14.6 **A.** Visual analog scale. **B.** Numeric scale.

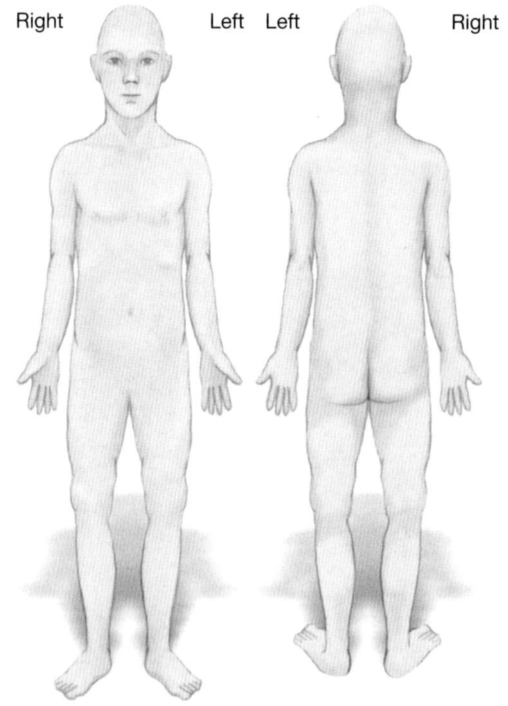

Sensory	Affective	Evaluative	Temporal
Aching ("pain all over")	Awful ("cannot do anything")	Annoying ("cannot sleep")	Always ("pain always there")
Hurting ("pain all over")	Crying ("hurts so bad")	Bad ("cannot stop the hurting")	Comes and goes ("always pain")
Sore ("like a cut")	Frightening ("scared it won't stop")	Miserable ("cannot sleep or do stuff")	Comes on all of a sudden ("no warning")
Beating (procedural pain "spots")	Screaming (afraid of "going to the hospital")	Terrible ("don't like it")	Constant ("never goes away")
Pounding ("gets on your nerves")	Terrifying ("cannot sleep," "really tired," "not going to live")	Uncomfortable ("can't stay in one spot")	Continuous ("pain not going away")
Cutting ("hurts more than a cut")		Uncontrollable ("cannot stop it")	Forever ("never will go away")
Like a sharp knife ("stabbing and sharp")	Dizzy ("don't know where I am")		Once in a while ("in a month sometimes pain; sometimes not")
Sharp (no meaning)			Sneaks up ("don't know when the pain will happen")
Stabbing (no meaning)			Sometimes ("goes away sometimes; sometimes not")
Cramping ("everywhere like a plane crash")			
Crushing (no meaning)			
Pressure ("pushing all over")			
Itching ("all over")			
Scratching ("helps sometimes")			
Shocking (pain "surprises" them)			
Splitting (body "splitting in half")			
Numb ("knows pain is there"/procedural pain)			
Stiff ("cannot move")			
Swollen ("meds do not help")			
Tight ("cannot move")			

FIGURE 14.7 Adolescent Pediatric Assessment Tool. (Top) Adolescent Pediatric Pain Tool (APPT): body outline. (Bottom) Pain Quality: Words chosen and meaning of words. (Used with permission from Crandall, M., & Savedra, M. [2005]. Multidimensional assessment using the adolescent pediatric pain tool: A case report. *Journal for Specialists in Pediatric Nursing, 10*[3], 115–123. https://doi.org/10.1111/j.1744-6155.2005.00023.x)

"pounding," "stabbing," or "sharp." The nurse asks the child to point to or circle the words that describe the current pain. Children with limited reading skills or vocabulary may have difficulty with some of the words listed to describe pain. Work with the child and encourage the parents to help the child understand the various descriptive words.

THINKING ABOUT **DEVELOPMENT**

Kaylee Cooper is a 4-year-old with a fractured femur. She has been in traction since arriving in the emergency room last night. When you enter her room at the beginning of your shift, you note she is quiet and withdrawn. How will Kaylee's developmental stage affect the use of self-report? What special considerations must the nurse think about when using self-report of pain with Kaylee? What is the most appropriate pain rating scale for Kaylee?

Physical Examination

Physical examination of the child for pain primarily involves the skills of observation and inspection. These skills are used to assess for physiologic and behavioral changes that indicate pain. Auscultation may also be used to assess for changes in vital signs, specifically heart rate and blood pressure.

OBSERVE FOR MANIFESTATIONS OF PAIN

Observe for physical signs and symptoms of pain, keeping in mind the child's developmental level. Look for facial expressions of discomfort, grimacing, or crying. Be alert for movements that may suggest pain. For example, an infant or toddler may pull on the ear when experiencing ear pain. The child may move the head from side to side, suggesting head pain. Typically, children with abdominal pain will lie on one side and draw their knees up to the abdomen. Inspect the child's gait; a limp or avoidance of weight bearing may suggest leg pain. Immobility, guarding of a particular body area, or refusal to move an area may be observed. Inspect the skin for flushing or diaphoresis, possible indicators of pain. Also monitor vital signs for changes. Pulse or heart rate, respiratory rate, and blood pressure may increase. Other physiologic parameters that suggest pain may include elevated intracranial pressure and pulmonary vascular resistance and decreased oxygen saturation levels.

The child may also exhibit behavioral changes indicating pain. Be alert for irritability and restlessness. Watch for clenching of teeth or fists, body stiffening, or increased muscle tension. Note any changes in the child's behavior. For example, a child who was previously talkative and playful may become quiet and withdrawn in response to pain. Remember, a child in pain may sleep or play in order to cope with the pain. In addition, pay close attention to the child's cultural background and how these beliefs may be affecting the behavioral response to pain.

Each child is an individual with unique responses to pain, so the nurse must ensure that observations of behavior do indeed reflect the child's pain level. To help ensure the accuracy of observations, several physiologic and behavioral assessment tools have been developed to help quantify the observations.

USING PHYSIOLOGIC AND BEHAVIORAL PAIN ASSESSMENT TOOLS

Use of physiologic and behavioral pain assessment tools allows measurement of specific parameters and changes that would indicate that the child is experiencing pain. These measurements aid in determining the intensity of the pain experience. Along with the self-report pain rating scales, measurement of these changes allows the nurse to objectively assess pain and the effectiveness of pain management measures.

Premature Infant Pain Profile. The Premature Infant Pain Profile (PIPP) is an assessment tool that is useful for measuring pain in term or preterm neonates. It looks at behavioral indicators, such as facial expressions, and physiologic changes, such as changes in heart rate and oxygen saturation. It also takes into account gestational age. See Table 14.2. Each parameter is scored as 0, 1, 2, or 3. The score is then totaled, and the maximum score that can be achieved is 21. The higher the total score, the more intense the pain.

Neonatal Infant Pain Scale. The Neonatal Infant Pain Scale (NIPS) is a behavioral assessment tool that is useful for measuring pain in term and preterm neonates (Lawrence et al., 1993). Six parameters are measured: facial expression, cry, breathing patterns, arms, legs, and state of arousal (Table 14.3). Each parameter, except for cry, is scored as 0 or 1; cry is scored as 0, 1, or 2. The scores are then totaled, and the maximum score that can be achieved is 7. A higher score indicates increased pain.

Riley Infant Pain Scale. The Riley Infant Pain Scale (RIPS) is a behavioral assessment tool useful for infants who lack verbal ability (Schade et al., 1996). Like NIPS, RIPS measures six parameters: facial expression, body movement, sleep, verbal or vocal ability, consolability, and response to movements and touch (Table 14.4). Each parameter is scored as 0, 1, 2, or 3. The score is then totaled, and the maximum score that can be achieved is 18. The higher the total score, the more intense the pain.

Pain Observation Scale for Young Children. The Pain Observation Scale for Young Children (POCIS) is a behavioral assessment tool designed for use in children between 1 and 4 years of age (Boelen-van der Loo et al., 1999). This tool measures seven parameters: facial expression, cry, breathing, torso, arms and fingers, legs and toes, and state of arousal (Table 14.5).

TABLE 14.2 • Premature Infant Pain Profile (PIPP)

Parameter	Finding		Score
Gestational age	36 weeks or more		0
	32–35 weeks + 6 days		1
	28–31 weeks + 6 days		2
	<28 weeks		3
Observe infant for 15 seconds	Behavioral state	Active, awake, eyes open, facial movements	0
		Quiet, awake, eyes open, no facial movements	1
		Active, awake, eyes closed, facial movements	2
		Quiet, asleep, eyes closed, no facial movements	3
Observe baseline heart rate and O_2 saturation for 30 seconds	Maximum heart rate	0–4 bpm increase	0
		5–15 bpm increase	1
		15–24 bpm increase	2
		24 bpm increase	3
	Oxygen saturation	92%–100%	0
		89%–91%	1
		85%–88%	2
		84% or less	3
Observe infant's facial action for 30 seconds	Brow bulge	None	0
		Minimum	1
		Moderate	2
		Maximum	3
	Eye squeeze	None	0
		Minimum	1
		Moderate	2
		Maximum	3
	Nasolabial furrow	None	0
		Minimum	1
		Moderate	2
		Maximum	3

Adapted with permission from Stevens, B., Johnston, C., Petryshen, P., & Taddio, A. (1996). Premature infant pain profile: Development and initial validation. *Clinical Journal of Pain, 12*(1), 13–22. https://doi.org/10.1097/00002508-199603000-00004

TABLE 14.3 • The Neonatal Infant Pain Scale (NIPS)

Parameter	Finding	Score
Facial expression	Relaxed (restful face; neutral expression)	0
	Grimace (tight facial muscles; furrowed brow, chin, or jaw; negative facial expression)	1
Cry	No cry (quiet; not crying)	0
	Whimper (mild intermittent moaning)	1
	Vigorous crying (loud screaming, shrill, continuous)	2
Breathing patterns	Relaxed	0
	Change in breathing (irregular; faster than usual; gagging; breath holding)	1
Arms	Relaxed (no muscular rigidity; occasional random movements of arm)	0
	Flexed/extended (tense, straight, rigid, or rapid flexion or extension)	1
Legs	Relaxed (no muscular rigidity; occasional random movements of leg)	0
	Flexed/extended (tense, straight, rigid, or rapid flexion or extension)	1
State of arousal	Sleeping/awake (quiet, peaceful; settled)	0
	Fussy (alert, restless, thrashing)	1

Copyright 1989, Children's Hospital of Eastern Ontario. Adapted with permission.

TABLE 14.4 • The Riley Infant Pain Scale

Parameter	Score
Facial expression	
• Neutral/smiling	0
• Frowning/grimacing	1
• Clenched teeth	2
• Full cry expression	3
Body movement	
• Calm, relaxed	0
• Restless, fidgeting	1
• Moderate agitation or mobility; thrashing, flailing, incessant agitation or strong voluntary mobility	2
• Voluntary immobility	3
Sleep	
• Sleeping quietly with easy respirations	0
• Restless while asleep	1
• Sleeping intermittently (sleep/awake)	2
• Sleeping for prolonged periods of time interrupted by jerky movements or inability to sleep	3
Verbal/vocal	
• No cry	0
• Whimpering, complaining	1
• Pain crying	2
• Screaming, high-pitched cry	3
Consolability	
• Neutral	0
• Easy to console	1
• Not easy to console	2
• Inconsolable	3
Response to movement/touch	
• Moves easily	0
• Winces when touched or moved	1
• Cries out when moved or touched	2
• High-pitched cry or scream when touched or moved	3

Adapted with permission from Schade, J. G., Joyce, B. A., Gerkensmeyer, J., & Keck, J. F. (1996). Comparison of three preverbal scales for postoperative pain assessment in a diverse pediatric sample. *Journal of Pain and Symptom Management, 12*(6), 348–359. https://doi.org/10.1016/S0885-3924(96)00182-0

Each parameter is scored as 0 or 1; the maximum score achievable is 7. The higher the score, the greater the pain being experienced by the child.

CRIES Scale for Neonatal Postoperative Pain Assessment. The CRIES scale is a behavioral assessment tool that also includes measures of physiologic parameters (Krechel & Bildner, 1995). It was developed to quantify postoperative pain in the newborn. The tool may also be used to monitor the infant's progress over time during recovery or after interventions. The tool assesses five parameters that create the "CRIES" acronym: *c*ry; oxygen *r*equired for saturation levels less than 95%; *i*ncreased vital signs; facial *e*xpression; and *s*leeplessness (Table 14.6). Each parameter is scored as 0, 1, or 2 and then totaled. As with other assessment tools, the higher the score, the greater the infant's pain.

TABLE 14.5 • The Pain Observation Scale for Young Children (POCIS)

Parameter	Finding	Score
Facial expression	Neutral Grimace (negative)	0 1
Cry	No cry Moan, scream	0 1
Breathing	Relaxed and regular Irregular and indrawn	0 1
Torso	At rest, inactive Tense, shivering	0 1
Arms and fingers	At rest, inactive Tense, restless	0 1
Legs and toes	At rest, inactive Tense, restless	0 1
State of arousal	Calm, sleepy Fussy	0 1

Reprinted with permission from Boelen-van der Loo, W. J. C., Scheffer, E., de Haan, R. J., & de Groot, C. J. (1999). Clinimetric evaluation of the pain observation scale for young children in children aged between 1 and 4 years after ear, nose, and throat surgery. *Developmental and Behavioral Pediatrics, 20*(4), 222–227. https://doi.org/10.1097/00004703-199908000-00004

r-FLACC Behavioral Scale for Pain in Nonverbal Young Children and Children With Cognitive Impairment. The original FLACC behavioral scale is a behavioral assessment tool that is useful in assessing a child's pain when the child cannot accurately report their level of pain (Merkel et al., 1997). It has been demonstrated to be a reliable tool for children from age 2 months to 7 years (Merkel et al., 1997). This tool measures five parameters that create the "FLACC" acronym: *f*acial expression, *l*egs, *a*ctivity, *c*ry, and *c*onsolability (Table 14.7). Observe the child with the legs and body uncovered. If the child is awake, observe them for 1 to 2 minutes; if sleeping, observe the child for 2 minutes or longer. Each parameter is scored as 0, 1, or 2. The scores are totaled, with a maximum achievable score of 10. As with other assessment tools, the higher the score, the greater the pain.

The revised FLACC (r-FLACC) is used in the same manner as the original FLACC, but it includes additional descriptors of behaviors most commonly associated with pain that have been validated in children with cognitive impairment (Hauer & Jones, 2021). Refer to Table 14.7. Pain assessment tools are a supplement to pain assessment and are not meant to replace caregiver or parent input. Review the descriptor terms with parents and caregivers, and individualize the scale by adding pain-related behaviors that are specific indicators of pain observed in the child in the appropriate categories (Hauer & Jones, 2021).

TABLE 14.6 • The Cries Scale for Neonatal Postoperative Pain Assessment

Assessment	0	1	2
Crying	No	High-pitched, but consolable	High-pitched, inconsolable
Oxygen required for saturation above 95%	No	<30%	>30%
Increased vital signs	Heart rate and blood pressure within 10% of preoperative values	Heart rate or blood pressure 11%–20% higher than preoperative values	Heart rate or blood pressure 21% or more above preoperative values
Expression	No grimace	Grimace	Grimace with grunt
Sleepless	No	Waking at frequent intervals	Constantly awake
Total infant score			

Reprinted with permission from Krechel, S. W., & Bildner, J. (1995). CRIES: A new neonatal postoperative pain measurement score. Initial testing of validity and reliability. *Paediatric Anaesthesia, 5*, 53–61. https://doi.org/10.1111/j.1460-9592.1995.tb00242.x

Nursing Analysis

After recognizing and analyzing cues from a thorough assessment, the nurse may identify several hypotheses. The most commonly identified nursing hypotheses would be acute pain and, in some cases, chronic pain, such as in a child with prolonged illness or injury, from effects of cancer on surrounding tissues or from treatment-related effects. However, the related factors and defining characteristics can vary widely. Nursing hypotheses will focus on the effects of pain on the child; for example, the stress incurred as a result of the pain or the fear or anxiety associated with the pain or events causing the pain. Moreover, pain can affect physiologic functions, such as sleep, nutrition, mobility, and elimination. Examples of common nursing hypotheses may include:

- Acute pain
- Anxiety

TABLE 14.7 • rFLACC Behavioral Scale

		SCORE (circle most appropriate)
FACE	0=No particular expression or smile	**0**
	1=Occasional grimace/frown; withdrawn or disinterested; **appears sad or worried**	**1**
	2=Consistent grimace or frown; Frequent/constant quivering chin, clenched jaw; **Distressed-looking face; Expression of fright or panic**	**2**
	Individual behavior: ____________	
LEGS	0=Normal position or relaxed; Usual tone & motion to limbs	**0**
	1=Uneasy, restless, tense; **occasional tremors**	**1**
	2=Kicking, or legs drawn up; **marked increase in spasticity, constant tremors or jerking**	**2**
	Individual behavior: ____________	
ACTIVITY	0=Lying quietly, normal position, moves easily; Regular, rhythmic respirations	**0**
	1=Squirming, shifting back and forth, tense or guarded movements; **mildly agitated (eg. head back & forth, aggression); Shallow, splinting respirations, intermittent sighs.**	**1**
	2=Arched, rigid or jerking; **severe agitation; head banging; shivering (not rigors); Breath holding, gasping or sharp intake of breaths, severe splinting**	**2**
	Individual behavior: ____________	
CRY	0=No cry	**0**
	1=Moans or whimpers; **occasional complaint; occasional verbal outburst or grunt**	**1**
	2=Crying steadily, screams or sobs, frequent complaints; **repeated outbursts, constant grunting**	**2**
	Individual behavior: ____________	
CONSOLABILITY	0=Content and relaxed	**0**
	1=Reassured by occasional touching, hugging or being talked to. Distractable	**1**
	2=Difficult to console or comfort; **pushing away caregiver, resisting care or comfort measures**	**2**
	Individual behavior: ____________	
		Total:

- Risk of constipation
- Deficient knowledge
- Sleep deprivation
- Risk of injury

The foregoing hypotheses provide suggestions for nursing care planning or concept mapping. The nurse will then generate solutions by planning interventions (suggested further on with rationales). The plan of care should be individualized, based on the child's and family's needs.

Goal/Outcome

When caring for a child experiencing pain, the ultimate goal is that the child will be free of pain, as evidenced by participation in age-appropriate activities of daily living and vital signs within age-appropriate parameters. However, at times, this may be unrealistic, especially if the child is experiencing chronic pain. Therefore, a more appropriate and realistic goal would be that the child reports that their pain has decreased to a tolerable level. Pain assessment tools can be used to quantify the amount by which the child's pain has decreased. For example, if the child has rated the pain as 7 out of 10, a realistic goal might be that the child reports a pain rating of no more than 4 out of 10. Additional goals would reflect improvement or resolution of the identified problem. For example, a short-term goal for a child experiencing disturbed sleep due to pain might be that the child sleeps for a minimum of 4 consecutive hours through the night. A long-term goal might be that the child sleeps for 7 to 8 hours undisturbed through the night.

Interventions

Various interventions can be used for pain management. These interventions include nonpharmacologic and pharmacologic measures. A guiding principle when caring for the child experiencing pain is the provision of atraumatic care (see Chapter 8 for more information). For example, cognitive and behavioral approaches are appropriate for pain management, including pain management related to procedures. In addition to nonpharmacologic measures, pharmacologic measures may be appropriate for pain management. For example, applying a topical anesthetic cream to a site early enough before a venipuncture can be effective. Another example is to use an intermittent infusion device to obtain multiple blood specimen samples rather than perform repeated venipunctures. In addition, it is a good idea to consider the use of sedation for more painful procedures.

Throughout the child's care, be sure to discuss specific goals and interventions with the child and family as appropriate. Include the family in developing appropriate interventions so they can continue to support the child. Education of the child and family about interventions, including various therapies, is key. Ongoing assessment is needed to determine the effectiveness of the pain relief measures in achieving the desired goals.

The previously listed hypotheses provide suggestions for nursing care planning or concept mapping. The nurse will then generate solutions by planning interventions (suggested next with rationales). The plan of care should be individualized, based on the child's and family's needs. Specific information related to pain management and the nurse's role will be discussed later in the chapter.

Nursing Analysis

Acute pain related to physical or biologic injury agents (such as invasive procedures, surgery, recent trauma, or infection) as evidenced by pain rating scale, facial grimacing, crying, irritability, withdrawal activity, or changes in vital signs.

Goal/Outcome

Child will achieve adequate comfort level, as evidenced by a decrease in rating number on a pain rating scale, quietness, calm resting behaviors, decrease in crying and irritability, and vital signs within acceptable parameters.

Promoting Pain Relief (interventions with *rationale*)

- Assess pain level using a developmentally appropriate pain rating tool *to establish a baseline.*
- Assess for verbal and nonverbal indicators of pain *to help determine child's pain level;* question parents about child's typical behaviors and previous experiences with pain *to determine factors that may be influencing child's response to pain.*
- Institute nonpharmacologic methods for pain control based on the child's age and cognitive level *to help decrease pain;* encourage parental participation in use of methods *to provide additional support and pain relief for the child.*
- Administer pharmacologic agents as ordered using the least traumatic route possible *to alter pain impulse transmission and minimize distress while promoting effective pain relief.*
- Explain the action of the drug and what the child should expect from the medication at a level that the child can understand *to promote trust and reduce fear while providing effective pain relief.*
- Give analgesics around the clock if pain is continuous and can be predicted *to maintain steady blood levels of the drug, thereby maximizing the drug's effect.*
- Perform atraumatic care at all times *to minimize the child's exposure to physical and psychological distress and pain.*
- Anticipate timing of procedures or situations that may lead to pain, and provide appropriate analgesic therapy as ordered *to ensure therapy is most effective at the time of the procedure.*
- Ensure the child's environment is quiet and conducive to rest, dim the lights, and close the door or

curtain *to reduce sensory overload that would increase the child's pain sensation.*

- Encourage the parents to stroke, touch, caress, and hold the child *to reduce discomfort and promote feelings of security.*
- Reassess the child's pain level after use of nonpharmacologic and pharmacologic methods *to determine effectiveness;* anticipate the need to modify or adapt nonpharmacologic methods or adjust analgesic dosage, route, or frequency *to promote maximum pain relief.*
- Perform nursing care activities after administering analgesics *to prevent exacerbating the child's pain.*
- Use diversional activities, distraction, and play appropriate to the child's age and cognitive level *to promote additional pain relief.*

Nursing Analysis

Anxiety related to stress and unmet needs (such as uncertainty of the situation; unknown cause of pain; lack of familiarity with procedures, testing, and health care facility; and painful procedures), as evidenced by crying, irritability, withdrawal, and/or stoic or aggressive behaviors

Goal/Outcome

Child and family will demonstrate a decrease in anxiety level, as evidenced by age-appropriate positive coping behaviors, verbalization of feelings, playing out of feelings, child and family cooperation with plan of care, and absence of signs and symptoms associated with escalating anxiety.

Minimizing Anxiety (interventions with *rationale*)

- Assess child's and parents' understanding of the situation, including their understanding of what may be causing the pain and the reasons for the procedures and testing *to provide baseline information about the child's and parents' knowledge and possible causes of anxiety.*
- Spend time with the child and parents discussing what they think might be happening, encouraging the child and parents to talk openly about their feelings to facilitate continued expressions and communication. Allow time for questions, and answer questions honestly *to establish rapport and build trust.*
- Approach the child and family in a calm, relaxed manner *to foster trust and communication and decrease anxiety.*
- Allow the child options related to interventions as much as possible, such as fluids to drink or snacks to eat, extremity to use for venipuncture (right or left), color of bandage, or holding tape or dressing, *to foster feelings of control.*
- Provide atraumatic care *to reduce exposure to distress, which would exacerbate the child's anxiety level.*
- Explain any procedures, tests, or activities at a level the child can understand *to reduce fear of the unknown.*
- Incorporate aspects of the child's routine at home as much as possible *to reduce feelings of separation and promote feelings of normalcy.*
- Ensure consistency in care *to facilitate trust and acceptance.*
- Encourage parents to use comfort measures such as stroking, cuddling, holding, and rocking *to promote feelings of security and minimize stress.*
- Provide positive reinforcement for choices, participation in activities, and use of appropriate coping methods *to foster self-esteem.*
- Encourage the child's participation in play (unstructured and therapeutic play as needed) *to promote expression of feelings and fears.*

Nursing Analysis

Risk of constipation; risk factors include decrease in GI motility (a side effect of some pain medications is decreased motility and hard, dry stools), and average daily physical activity is less than recommended for age (limited mobility due to pain).

Goal/Outcome

Child will pass soft bowel movements on a regular basis without pain or straining.

Preventing Constipation (interventions with *rationale*)

- Palpate for abdominal distention, percuss for dullness, and auscultate for bowel sounds *to assess for signs of constipation.*
- Encourage adequate fluid intake *to soften the stool.*
- Encourage adequate fiber intake: *fiber helps increase stool bulk and increase movement through the GI tract.*
- Administer medications as ordered *to keep stool moving on a regular basis.*
- Encourage activity as tolerated; *immobility contributes to constipation.*

Nursing Analysis

Deficient knowledge related to insufficient information or knowledge of resources (about current condition and appropriate methods for managing pain), as evidenced by crying, irritability, pushing away, and questions and verbalizations about pain and relief methods

Goal/Outcome

The child and parents will demonstrate adequate knowledge about the child's current condition and use of pain relief methods, as evidenced by statements about the cause of the child's pain, demonstration of chosen nonpharmacologic relief methods, use of pharmacologic agents, and statements related to signs and symptoms of increased and decreased pain.

Educating the Child and Family (interventions with *rationale*)

- Assess the child's and parents' knowledge and understanding of the child's current condition and current pain level *to establish a baseline for teaching.*
- Provide time for the child and parents to ask questions; answer questions honestly and in terms they can understand *to promote learning.*
- Explain in simplified terms how the child's condition is associated with pain or the rationale for procedures needed that may contribute to pain *to promote understanding and foster trust.*
- Teach in short sessions *to prevent overloading the child and parents with information.*
- Provide reinforcement and rewards *to help facilitate the teaching and learning process.*
- Use multiple modes of learning, such as written information, verbal instruction, demonstrations, and media when possible, *to facilitate learning and retention of information.*
- Instruct the parents and child as appropriate in nonpharmacologic methods for pain relief; encourage practice and participation by parents in methods chosen *to foster independence and use of method when necessary.*
- Teach the child as appropriate and parents about pharmacologic methods for pain relief; review specific information about the drug to be used, including action, duration, administration, possible adverse effects, and care necessary when the drug is used, *to promote learning;* have the child and parents report back information or demonstrate administration *to evaluate effectiveness of teaching.*
- Provide parents with written information about pain relief methods for use at home if indicated *to allow for reference at a later date.*

Nursing Analysis

Sleep deprivation related to prolonged discomfort (inability to manage pain effectively), as evidenced by frequent waking during the night; signs and symptoms of pain, including irritability and restlessness; statements about being tired; and pain rating scale remaining the same

Goal/Outcome

The child will exhibit increased ability to sleep during the night, as evidenced by increasing periods of calm and restfulness (initially starting at 2 hours and gradually increasing to 7 to 8 hours), decreased pain level on pain rating scale, and statements of decreased fatigue.

Promoting Sleep and Rest (interventions with *rationale*)

- Assist the child in using nonpharmacologic methods of pain relief, such as imagery, distraction, and muscle relaxation, *to promote relaxation.*
- Administer pharmacologic pain relief as ordered *to minimize pain interfering with sleep;* anticipate a change in drug therapy if pain relief is inadequate.
- Cluster nursing care activities *to minimize energy expenditure and disruptions in the child's ability to rest.*
- Help the child with a nighttime routine similar to one they use at home *to promote feelings of security.*
- Offer the child a back rub, warm bath, or warm liquids; reading a story; or listening to music *to facilitate relaxation;* provide stroking, hugging, cuddling, rocking, and light touch *to promote a sense of security and calm.*
- Dim the lights and close the curtain or door to the room *to provide a quiet, restful environment.*
- Ensure around-the-clock pain relief for the child through the night *to minimize the risk of pain.*

Nursing Analysis

Risk of injury; risk factors include unsafe mode of transport and alteration in cognitive and psychomotor functioning (possible adverse effects of analgesics).

Goal/Outcome

Child will remain free of any injury related to signs and symptoms of adverse effects of analgesic therapy, as evidenced by respiratory rate appropriate for age and no complaints of GI upset; dizziness; or sedation; or episodes of constipation, nausea, vomiting, or pruritus.

Promoting Safety (interventions with *rationale*)

- Ensure the child's call light is within reach *to allow for notification of health care personnel should the child need assistance.*
- Administer analgesic exactly as prescribed *to reduce the risk of error and development of adverse effects.*
- Assess the child's respiratory status closely for changes *to allow for early detection of respiratory depression.*
- If an opioid analgesic is being given, have naloxone readily available *to reverse the action of the narcotic if respiratory depression occurs.*
- Monitor appetite and assess bowel sounds for changes; note any abdominal distention or decreased bowel sounds, which would suggest decreased peristalsis, *to allow for early detection of constipation.*
- Ensure adequate fluid and fiber intake *to reduce risk of constipation.*
- Offer small frequent meals and give medication with food *to minimize the risk of GI upset.*
- Assess for nausea and vomiting; if necessary, withhold food and fluids *to rest the GI tract,* and administer antiemetics until nausea and vomiting resolve *to decrease nausea and vomiting.*
- Instruct the child to remain in bed after receiving analgesic, raise crib or side rails as appropriate, and instruct the child and parents to have someone

accompany the child to the bathroom, if allowed, *to reduce the risk of falls from sedation.*

- Assess for complaints of itching, and observe for rash or reddened areas; if pruritus occurs, urge the child not to scratch, and expect to administer an antihistamine as ordered *to reduce pruritus.*
- Provide the child with distraction *to assist in helping reduce the effects of pruritus.*

TAKE NOTE!

The National Database of Nursing Quality Indicators (NDNQI) was established by the American Nurses Association to evaluate nursing-sensitive care. One indicator that can help improve pain management is the pediatric pain assessment, intervention, and reassessment (AIR) cycle (NDNQI, n.d.).

Remember Aiden, the 6-year-old introduced at the beginning of the chapter? The nurse reporting off duty states, "Aiden's parents keep requesting pain medication for him. They say he's complaining of pain most of the time. I'm not sure if I believe them; when I see Aiden, he's playing video games or watching television and seems to be fine. I've tried to hold off on his pain medication as long as I can." When you enter Aiden's room, he is crying and says his leg hurts. What will be your initial action? What will be your plan of care to manage Aiden's pain (refer to the QUESTT assessment)? How would you address the statements made by the nurse in report? What approaches can you use to change staff behavior about pain management?

MANAGEMENT OF PAIN

Management of pain begins with assessment of the child's comfort level. If pain or the potential for pain, such as that caused by an invasive procedure, is identified, steps must be taken to minimize or treat the pain. Three general principles guide pain management in children:

1. Individualize interventions based on the amount of pain experienced and the child's characteristics, such as developmental level, temperament, previous pain experience, and coping strategies.
2. Use nonpharmacologic and pharmacologic approaches to ease or eliminate the pain.
3. Teach the child and family about pain relief interventions and techniques, and discuss with the child and family expectations of pain management.

Specific strategies for pain management include nonpharmacologic interventions, such as relaxation, distraction, and guided imagery, and pharmacologic interventions, such as analgesics, patient-controlled analgesia, local analgesia, epidural analgesia, and moderate sedation.

Nonpharmacologic Management

Various techniques may be available to assist in managing mild pain in children or to augment the effectiveness of medications for moderate or severe pain. Many of these nonpharmacologic techniques assist children in coping with pain and give them an opportunity to feel a sense of mastery or control over the situation. Two types of techniques are cognitive behavioral strategies and biophysical strategies. It is important to involve the parents in the process when using these techniques.

Behavioral Cognitive Strategies

Behavioral cognitive strategies for pain management involve measures that require the child to focus on a specific area rather than the pain. These strategies help change the interpretation of the painful stimuli, reducing pain perception or making pain more tolerable. In addition, these strategies help decrease negative attitudes, thoughts, and anxieties, thereby improving the child's coping mechanisms. Use of these strategies before procedures has resulted in decreased anxiety and has improved the transition to sedation and may result in a decreased amount of medication needed for sedation (Cravero & Roback, 2022). Typically, these interventions work well with older children, but younger children also benefit from these techniques if they are adapted to the child's age and developmental level. Common behavioral cognitive strategies include relaxation, distraction, imagery, biofeedback, thought stopping, and positive self-talk.

RELAXATION

Relaxation aids in reducing muscle tension and anxiety. A wide variety of techniques can be used. Relaxation can be as simple as holding an infant or young child closely while stroking the child or speaking in a soft soothing manner or having the child inhale and exhale slowly using rhythmically controlled deep breathing. It can also involve more sophisticated techniques such as progressive relaxation. With this technique, the child is asked to focus on one area of the body and let that body part go limp. Then, in an organized fashion, usually working from the toes to the head or vice versa, the child is asked to focus on another body part, making it go limp. Eventually, the exercises work through all body areas, leading to relaxation of the entire body.

DISTRACTION

Distraction involves having the child focus on another stimulus, thereby attempting to shield them from pain. Research has shown distraction to be associated with lower parental perception of pain and distress in younger children and decreased situational anxiety in older children (Cravero & Roback, 2022).

This technique does not eliminate the pain but can help to make it more tolerable. Various methods can be used for distraction, including:

- Counting
- Repeating specific phrases or words, such as "ouch"
- Listening to music or singing
- Playing games, including video games
- Blowing bubbles or blowing pinwheels or party favors
- Listening to or reading favorite stories (Fig. 14.8)
- Watching cartoons, television shows, or movies
- Playing on mobile devices
- Visiting with friends
- Humor

Humor has been demonstrated to be an effective distracting technique for pain management (Osincup, 2020; Strean, 2009). However, be sure to use an age-appropriate technique and to determine what or who will make the child laugh. If possible, allow the child and their family to choose the materials that they consider humorous.

The type of distraction used depends on the age of the child. For example, a younger child may enjoy blowing pinwheels and blowing bubbles. They also may enjoy listening to favorite stories or books. Older children may enjoy computer or video games, listening to favorite music, or visiting with friends.

ATRAUMATIC CARE

Play therapy may be helpful in allowing the child to express their feelings and adapt to the stressors of the current situation.

IMAGERY

Imagery involves the use of the imagination to create a mental image. This mental image is usually a positive, pleasurable image, but it doesn't need to be real. The child is encouraged to include details and sensations that are associated with the image, such as specific descriptions of the image, colors, sounds, feelings, and smells. In some instances, the child may write down or record the image on a tape or compact disc. When pain occurs, the child is encouraged to create the mental image or read or listen to the description.

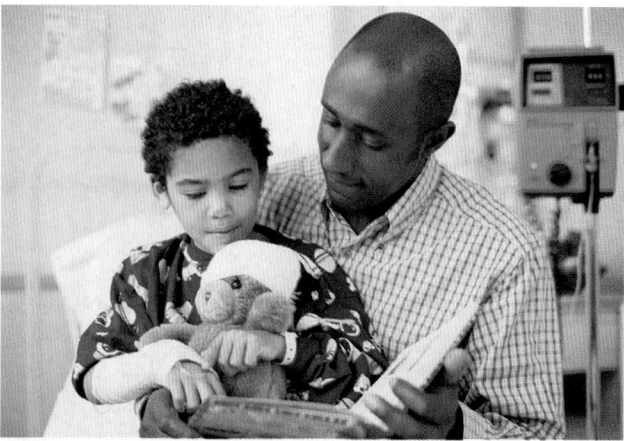

FIGURE 14.8 A child using distraction for pain management.

BIOFEEDBACK

Biofeedback involves having the child gain an awareness of their body functions and learn ways to modify them voluntarily. The child is usually taught specific skills about how to modify body functions using an apparatus that measures pain-related changes in muscle tone or physiologic data, such as blood pressure or pulse rate. This teaching is usually performed by a specialized health care provider and occurs over several sessions in advance of the pain experience. With practice, the child learns to control the changes without the apparatus. This technique can be used by older children, such as adolescents, who can concentrate for longer periods of time.

THOUGHT STOPPING

Thought stopping involves substituting a pleasurable or positive thought for the painful experience. Examples of positive thoughts might be, "It's only for a short time" or "It's important so I get better." The negative component of the pain is not ignored or suppressed; rather, it is transformed into something positive. Thought stopping can also involve the use of short, positive phrases. For example, the child may repeat "quick stick, feel better, go home soon" when they anticipate or experience pain.

Thought stopping is a useful method for reducing anxiety before and during events associated with pain. Children can be taught to use this technique anytime they experience anxiety related to a painful experience. Doing so helps promote the child's sense of control over the situation.

POSITIVE SELF-TALK

Positive self-talk is similar to thought stopping in that it involves the use of positive statements. With positive self-talk, the child is taught to say positive statements when they are experiencing pain. For example, the child may be taught to say, "I will feel better and be able to go home and play with my friends."

Biophysical Interventions

Biophysical interventions focus on interfering with the transmission of pain impulses reaching the brain. The interventions involve some type of cutaneous stimulation near the site of the pain. This stimulation decreases the ability of the A-delta and C fibers to transmit pain impulses. Examples of biophysical interventions include application of heat and cold, massage and pressure, and transcutaneous electrical nerve stimulation (TENS).

SUCKING AND SUCROSE

Sucking is a behavior from which infants derive satisfaction. Therefore, nonnutritive sucking (NNS) (e.g., sucking a pacifier) can be used to reduce pain behaviors in neonates undergoing painful procedures. In addition, infants show reduced pain behaviors after ingestion of sucrose or other sweet-tasting solutions, such as glucose, during single-event procedures, such as heel lancing (Roué, 2022). Optimal dosing for sucrose needs further research, and caution must be used in extremely low–birth-weight infants and infants with unstable blood glucose levels. Combining nonpharmacologic measures such as NNS, oral sucrose, skin-to-skin contact, and swaddling has been shown to increase the analgesic effectiveness of measures used alone (Roué, 2022). See Evidence-Based Practice 14.1.

• • • ATRAUMATIC CARE • • •

Breastfeeding is also a noninvasive, natural, and feasible way to use sucking to reduce pain in infants.

HEAT AND COLD APPLICATIONS

Heat and cold applications alter physiologic mechanisms associated with pain. Cold results in vasoconstriction and alters capillary permeability, leading to a decrease in edema at the site of the injury. Owing to vasoconstriction, blood flow is reduced, and the release of pain-producing substances such as histamine and serotonin is also decreased. Moreover, transmission of painful stimuli via peripheral nerve fibers is decreased.

Heat results in vasodilation and increases blood flow to the area. It also leads to a decrease in nociceptive stimulation and removal of chemical substances that can stimulate nociceptive fibers. The increase in blood flow alters capillary permeability, leading to a reduction in swelling and pressure on nociceptive nerve fibers. Heat may also trigger the release of endogenous opioids, which mediate the pain response.

MASSAGE AND PRESSURE

Massage and pressure, like other biophysical interventions, are believed to inhibit stimulation of the A-delta and C fibers. These methods are helpful in relaxing muscles and reducing tension. In addition, these techniques can aid in distracting the child. Massage can be as simple as rubbing a body part or pressing on an area such as an injection site for about 10 seconds. It can also be more involved, requiring the use of another person to perform the massage. Lotion or ointment can be used during the massage and may provide a comforting effect. Contralateral pressure or massage of the opposite area may be used, especially if the area of pain cannot be accessed or if the affected area is too painful to touch.

A more formal method of pressure application is acupressure. In acupressure, the fingertip, the thumb, or a blunt instrument is used to apply gentle, firm pressure to specifically designated sites to control pain. The pressure may be applied in one motion followed by releasing, in a circular motion for several minutes and then releasing, or with a vibrating motion using the fingertips. The motion of applying and then releasing pressure is thought to facilitate the release of endogenous endorphins and enkephalins.

EVIDENCE-BASED PRACTICE 14.1

What Is the Effect of the Use of Swaddling and Sucrose on the Intensity of Pain in Neonates During Venous Blood Sampling?

Neonates who are hospitalized undergo numerous painful experiences. It is well established that neonates feel pain. Pain in neonates has been found to have short- and long-term effects on the neonates' behavioral and neurologic development. Nonpharmacologic interventions used to decrease neonatal procedural pain include swaddling, NNS, sucrose, breastfeeding, and skin-to-skin contact. Some evidence has shown that combining sucrose with other nonpharmacologic interventions can be more effective than sucrose ingestion alone. This study aimed to evaluate the effectiveness of swaddling and sucrose ingestion on pain intensity during venous blood sampling.

STUDY

This study was a clinical trial. Sixty term infants were randomly divided into four groups. The first group was swaddled before blood sampling; the second group had sucrose administered; the third group was swaddled and given sucrose; and the fourth group was the control group.

Findings

The results showed that neonatal pain intensity mean scores during and after blood sampling were significantly different between the groups, with the control group having the highest scores. The results showed that pain intensity was lower in the intervention groups versus the control group and that the combined sucrose and swaddle group scores were lower than either intervention alone.

Nursing Implications

The use of swaddle and sucrose together is a safe and effective way to decrease procedural pain in neonates. Nurses should consider combining nonpharmacologic interventions with sucrose administration when performing painful procedures in neonates. More randomized controlled trials or well-designed studies are needed. Further research is warranted to determine safe and effective concentration, dosing, and dosing intervals of sucrose in the neonatal population.

Data from Talebi, M., Amiri, S. R. J., Roshan, P. A., Zabihi, A., Zahedpasha, Y., & Chehrazi, M. (2022). The effect of concurrent use of swaddle and sucrose on the intensity of pain during venous blood sampling in neonate: a clinical trial study. *BMC Pediatrics, 22*(1), 263. https://doi.org/10.1186/s12887-022-03323-0

The techniques of pressure and massage are easy to learn and use and can be taught to children and parents.

The Nurse's Role in Nonpharmacologic Pain Intervention

The nurse plays a major role in teaching the child and family about nonpharmacologic pain interventions. Help the child and family choose the most appropriate and most effective methods, and ensure that the child and parents use the methods before pain occurs as well as before the pain increases. Teaching Guidelines 14.1 lists some helpful instructions for the parents and child about nonpharmacologic pain management.

It is also important to assist the child and parents when using the technique in order to make sure that they are using the technique correctly. Offer suggestions for modifications or adaptations as necessary.

Parents are important to the pain management program. Give them the option to stay with the child, or let them know that someone else will support the child if they opt not to stay. Offer simple, concrete ways to assist and help the child manage pain. Many of the nonpharmacologic techniques can be done by parents, and children may respond better if their parents demonstrate the technique and encourage them to use it. Invite parents to participate in decisions as well as act as a coach to their child during procedures. Prepare the parents, and explain the most appropriate pain management approaches and strategies. Discuss the type and amount of pain expected as well as the potential complications associated with pain management approaches. Ask how the parent predicts the child will react to a painful situation. Finally, offer techniques and strategies to the parents as they act as the coach during these situations.

Although parents want to help their children and some are able to act as coaches, the responses of the child and parent to pain and stress and to different interventions are highly variable. Some children appear to be soothed by their parents' actions; others appear to become distressed. The nurse must be alert to these reactions and provide necessary support and education to ensure effectiveness of pain-relieving interventions.

TEACHING GUIDELINES **14.1** Teaching Nonpharmacologic Pain Management

- Review the methods available, and choose the method(s) that you and your child find best for your situation.
- Learn to identify the ways in which your child shows pain or demonstrates they are anxious about the possibility of pain. For example, do they get restless, make a face, or get flushed in the face?
- Begin using the technique chosen before your child experiences pain or when your child first indicates they are anxious about or beginning to experience pain.
- Practice the technique with your child, and encourage the child to use the technique when they feel anxious about pain or anticipate that a procedure or experience will be painful.
- Perform the technique with your child. For example, take the deep breath in and out or blow bubbles with them; listen to music or play a game with your child.
- Avoid using terms such as "hurt" or "pain" that suggest or cause your child to expect pain.
- Use descriptive terms like "pushing," "pulling," "pinching," or "heat."
- Avoid overly descriptive or biased statements such as "This will really hurt a lot" or "This will be terrible."
- Stay with your child as much as possible; speak softly and gently stroke or cuddle your child.
- Offer praise, positive reinforcement, hugs, and support for using the technique even if it was not effective.

Pharmacologic Management

Pharmacologic interventions involve the administration of drugs for pain relief. Administration may occur using a wide variety of methods. The selection of the method is determined by the drug being administered; the child's status; the type, intensity, and location of the pain; and any factors that may be influencing the child's pain. Research overwhelmingly supports the appropriate use of analgesics to reduce pain perception in children.

Medications Used for Pain Management

Analgesics (medications for pain relief) typically fall into one of two categories—nonopioid analgesics and opioid analgesics. The choice of analgesic medication is based on the child's pain intensity and the child's response to previously administered pain medications (Hauer & Jones, 2021). In general, mild pain can be treated with nonopioid medications, while moderate to severe pain may require opioid medications. Anesthetics may also be used. Drugs such as sedatives and hypnotics may be used as adjuvant medications to help minimize anxiety or provide or assist with pain relief when typical analgesics are ineffective.

NONOPIOID ANALGESICS

Nonopioid analgesics include acetaminophen and nonsteroidal antiinflammatory drugs (NSAIDs) such as ibuprofen, ketorolac, naproxen, and indomethacin (Drug Guide 14.1). These agents may be used to treat mild to moderate pain, often for conditions such as arthritis; joint, bone, and muscle pain; headache; dental pain; and menstrual pain. Acetaminophen and ibuprofen are also commonly used to treat fever in children.

DRUG GUIDE 14.1

COMMON DRUGS FOR PAIN MANAGEMENT

Drug	Actions/Indications	Nursing Implications
Acetaminophen (Tylenol)	Possible inhibition of cyclo-oxygenase in the central nervous system Direct action on hypothalamic heat-regulating center Mild to moderate pain, fever, arthritis, musculoskeletal pain, headache	• Administer orally, rectally, or intravenously. • Maximum daily dose ≤ 75 mg/kg/day in ≤ 5 divided doses (not to exceed 4,000 mg/day). • Do not exceed five intravenous doses or 60 mg/kg/day of drug in 24 hours. • Caution parents to read labels of other over-the-counter (OTC) drugs carefully; some may contain acetaminophen and, if given in conjunction, may lead to overdose and toxicity.
Ibuprofen (Motrin, Advil)	Inhibition of prostaglandin synthesis Mild to moderate pain, fever, treatment of inflammatory diseases	• Administer orally. • Give with food or after meals if GI upset occurs. • Assess for easy bruising, bleeding gums, or frank or occult blood in urine or stool. • Monitor for nausea, vomiting, GI upset, diarrhea or constipation, dizziness, or drowsiness. • Caution parents to read labels of OTC medications closely; some may contain ibuprofen or other NSAIDs and, if given in conjunction, may lead to overdose.
Other NSAIDs: ketorolac (Toradol), diclofenac (Voltaren), indomethacin (Indocin), naproxen (Naprosyn, Aleve)	Inhibition of prostaglandin synthesis Moderate to severe pain	• Administer oral form with food or after meals if GI upset occurs. • Monitor for headache, dizziness, nausea, vomiting, constipation, or diarrhea. • Assess for signs and symptoms of bleeding, such as bruising, epistaxis, gingival bleeding, or frank or occult blood in urine or stool. • Naproxen is also available in combination products (caution parents to read OTC labels carefully). • When administering indomethacin intravenously, report oliguria or anuria. • Diclofenac may also be given rectally.
Opioid agents: morphine, fentanyl (Sublimaze, Duragesic), hydromorphone (Dilaudid), oxycodone (OxyContin), methadone	Opioid agonist acting primarily at mu-receptor sites (morphine, fentanyl, hydromorphone, oxycodone, methadone) Moderate to severe acute and chronic pain Morphine: Intractable pain, preoperative sedation Fentanyl: Pain associated with short procedures such as bone marrow aspiration, fracture reductions, suturing	• Assess respiratory status frequently, noting any decrease in ventilatory rate or changes in breathing patterns; have naloxone readily available in case of respiratory depression (particularly with morphine, fentanyl, hydromorphone). • Monitor for sedation dizziness, lethargy, or confusion. • Educate parents and child that the drug may make the child sleepy, drowsy, or lightheaded. • Institute safety measures to prevent injury to the child. • Assess bowel sounds for decreased peristalsis; observe for abdominal distention. • Ensure adequate fiber intake and administer stool softeners as prescribed to minimize risk for constipation. • Monitor urine output for changes and report. • Morphine may cause itching, particularly of the face. • With fentanyl, observe for chest wall rigidity, which can occur with rapid intravenous infusion. • Oxycodone is the opioid component of brand-name products such as Tylox, Roxicet, and Percocet.

Data from Lexicomp. (2023b). Pediatric drug information. *UpToDate*. Retrieved April 5, 2023, from https://www.uptodate.com/contents/table-of-contents/drug-information/pediatric-drug-information

CLINICAL REASONING ALERT

Aspirin or products containing aspirin should not be used in infants or children for analgesic or antipyretic purposes because of the high risk of Reye syndrome.

Nonopioid agents are typically administered orally or rectally. In some cases, such as with postoperative pain, they may be administered intravenously as a continuous infusion or as bolus doses. Administration via intramuscular injection is not recommended because the injection can cause significant pain and the onset of pain relief is not increased.

Acetaminophen is a relatively safe medication, and it does not have the same GI or antiplatelet effects of NSAIDs; therefore, it is useful in children with cancer, with bleeding or clotting disorders, or children on anticoagulants. Acetaminophen toxicity and resulting hepatotoxicity can occur with misuse and overdosing. NSAIDs, owing to their antiinflammatory abilities, may be more effective in reducing pain caused by inflammatory conditions, such as musculoskeletal injuries and rheumatic diseases. Adverse effects associated with NSAIDs are uncommon but include GI irritation, blood clotting problems, and renal dysfunction. Nonopioids are relatively safe, have few incompatibilities with other medications, and do not depress the central nervous system. However, after a certain level, they do not provide increasing pain relief even when administered at increased doses. As a result, they may be combined with opioids for more effective pain relief.

OPIOID ANALGESICS

Opioid analgesics are typically used for moderate to severe pain. They are classified as either agonists (when they act as the neurotransmitter at the receptor site) or antagonists (when they block the action at the receptor site). Opioid agents that act as agonists include morphine, fentanyl, hydromorphone, oxycodone, and hydrocodone. Opioids that act as mixed agonists–antagonists include pentazocine, butorphanol, and nalbuphine. See Drug Guide 14.1. Opioids can be administered orally, rectally, intramuscularly, or intravenously. In addition, some agents such as fentanyl can be administered transdermally or transmucosally. Morphine is considered the "gold standard" and is the most commonly used of all opioid agonists; it is the drug to which all other opioids are compared and is the drug of choice for severe pain (Hauer & Jones, 2021).

> ***TAKE NOTE!***
>
> In 2017, the U.S. Food and Drug Administration (FDA) made the use of codeine or tramadol contraindicated in children younger than 12 years due to serious safety concerns related to the genetic variability in the metabolism of children (some children have slow metabolisms, while others have rapid metabolisms) (Hauer & Jones, 2021).

Opioid agonists, such as morphine, are associated with numerous adverse effects, resulting primarily from their depressant action on the central nervous system.

> **CLINICAL REASONING ALERT**
>
> When administering parenteral or epidural opioids, always have naloxone (Narcan) readily available to reverse the opioid's effects should respiratory depression occur.

Opioids stimulate the chemoreceptor trigger zone (CTZ), leading to nausea and vomiting. Moreover, **drug tolerance** (increased dosage required for the same pain relief previously achieved with a lower dose) and **physical dependence** (need for continued administration of the drug to prevent withdrawal symptoms) are commonly noted when opioids are given repeatedly (Yin, 2022). Drug Guide 14.1 gives additional information related to the opioid analgesics.

> **CLINICAL REASONING ALERT**
>
> Meperidine (Demerol), an opioid agonist, is not recommended as a first-choice agent for pain relief in children due to its toxicity on the central nervous system (Lexicomp, 2023a).

ADJUVANT DRUGS

Adjuvant drugs are drugs used to promote more effective pain relief, either alone or in combination with nonopioids or opioids. Their primary indications are for diagnoses other than pain. These agents are not classified as analgesics but may provide a coanalgesic effect or may treat side effects. Benzodiazepines, such as diazepam and midazolam, help relieve anxiety. Midazolam also produces amnesia. Anticonvulsants, such as gabapentin, and tricyclic antidepressants, such as amitriptyline and nortriptyline, may be used to treat neuropathic pain.

LOCAL ANESTHETICS

Local anesthetics are commonly used to provide analgesia for procedures. They are effective in providing successful pain relief, with only minimal risk of systemic adverse effects. However, local anesthetics such as lidocaine were not historically used in children because these drugs need to be injected. The belief was that children feared needles, and use of a local anesthetic subjected the child to two needlesticks instead of one. Advances in technology have led to the development of improved methods of delivery such as topical ointments and iontophoresis for administration of local anesthetics, thereby promoting atraumatic care. (For a more detailed discussion, see the next section on drug administration methods and later in the chapter on the nurse's role in managing procedure-related pain.)

Drug Administration Methods

With any medication administered for pain management, the timing of administration is vital. It is essential and more effective to stay ahead of pain and anticipate it, as opposed to treating it once it is present. Timing depends on the type of pain. For continuous or severe pain, administration of analgesia around the clock at scheduled intervals may be needed to achieve the necessary effect (Schechter, 2022). As-needed (PRN) dosing for continuous pain can lead to inadequate pain relief because of the delay before the drug reaches its peak effectiveness, and as a result, the child continues to experience pain, possibly necessitating a higher dose of analgesic to achieve relief. This then places the child at risk for overmedication and toxic effects.

For pain that can be predicted or considered temporary, such as with a procedure, analgesia is administered so that the peak action of the drug matches the time of the painful event.

There are various methods for administering pain medications to children. The preferred methods are the oral, rectal, intravenous, topical, or local nerve block routes. Epidural administration and moderate sedation may also be used.

ORAL METHOD

The oral method is often preferred because it is simple, easy, and convenient. The medication may be in the form of a pill, capsule, tablet, syrup, or elixir. Oral administration provides relatively steady blood levels of the drug when administered as a scheduled dose. Effectiveness typically occurs 1 to 2 hours after administration. As soon as possible, switch the child to oral dosing from parenteral dosing. However, keep in mind that higher doses of the oral medication may be needed to achieve the same effect.

RECTAL METHOD

The rectal method may be used when the child cannot take the medication orally, such as when the child has difficulty swallowing or is experiencing nausea and vomiting. It is a viable alternative for drug administration. Some analgesics are available in suppository form. For others that are not, the drug can be compounded into a suppository form. The absorption rate varies with rectal administration. Children may find insertion of a suppository uncomfortable and embarrassing.

INTRAVENOUS METHOD

Intravenous analgesia administration is the method of choice in emergency situations and when pain is severe and quick relief is needed. With intravenous administration, the drug usually takes effect within 5 minutes. Intravenous administration can be accomplished with bolus injections or continuous infusions. Continuous infusions may be preferred over bolus doses because steady blood levels are more easily maintained, thereby enhancing the drug's effect in relieving pain. Typically, opioids such as morphine, hydromorphone, and fentanyl are used due to their short half-life and decreased risk of toxicity.

PATIENT-CONTROLLED ANALGESIA

In **patient-controlled analgesia (PCA)**, a computerized pump is programmed to deliver an infusion of analgesics via a catheter inserted intravenously, epidurally, or subcutaneously. The analgesic may be given as a continuous infusion, as a continuous infusion supplemented by patient-delivered bolus doses, or as patient-delivered bolus doses only. Typically, the child presses a button to administer a bolus dose. The pump has a lockout function that is preset with the dose and time interval. If the child presses the button before the preset time, they will not receive an overdose of medication. By delivering small, frequent doses of opioids, the child can experience pain relief without the effects of oversedation. The child also experiences a sense of control over the pain experience.

The Institute for Safe Medication Practices (ISMP) has identified infants and young children as not being good candidates for PCA usage (2021). It may be appropriate for children starting around the age of 7 to 8 years (Schechter, 2022). It is essential to assess each child individually and consider the child's developmental level and psychosocial factors in determining appropriate PCA use. The child must have the necessary intellect, manual dexterity, and strength to operate the device.

PCA has been used to control postoperative pain and the pain associated with trauma, cancer, and sickle cell crisis. It can be used in acute care settings or in the home. Most commonly, morphine, hydromorphone, and fentanyl are the drugs used with PCA. The dosage is based on the child's response. Dosages for infusions depend on the child's age, the opioid used, and the type of pain.

The dangers and effectiveness of authorized agent–controlled analgesia, when family members or caregivers who are not authorized administer PCA doses "by proxy," warrant further research. In most circumstances, authorized agent–controlled analgesia by a family member should be avoided (Schechter, 2022). Health care providers who can assess pain and vital signs before and after each dose may be an alternative to activate the device. It is recommended that facilities develop specific criteria in any situation where authorized agent–activated PCA is being used (Schechter, 2022). Proper education and instruction are crucial in any situation in which someone other than the child may be administering PCA doses. Thorough assessment is necessary to ensure the child's pain is neither undertreated nor overtreated. To ensure safety with PCA use, each institution must have policies and procedures in place, appropriate education of health care staff, quality control measures, and quality machines.

LOCAL ANESTHETIC APPLICATION

A local anesthetic may sometimes be used to alleviate the pain associated with procedures such as venipuncture, injections, wound repair, lumbar puncture, or accessing of implanted ports. Local anesthesia is a type of regional analgesia that blocks or numbs specific nerves in a region of the body. Medications called local anesthetics include topical forms, such as creams, agents delivered by iontophoresis, vapocoolants, and skin refrigerants, as well as injectable forms.

Topical Forms

A common choice for effective, painless local anesthesia is a eutectic mixture of local anesthetics (EMLA). The mix is of lidocaine and prilocaine. It achieves anesthesia to a depth of 2 to 4 mm, so it reduces pain related to phlebotomy, venous cannulation, and intramuscular injections for up to 24 hours after the injection. However, it requires a 60- to 90-minute application time to intact skin using an occlusive dressing for superficial procedures and up to 2 to 3 hours for deeper, more invasive procedures (Box 14.1). EMLA is approved for use in infants born at 37 weeks' gestation or more (Lexicomp, 2023b). Maximum dosage and maximum area of application are based on the child's weight. Parents can be taught how to apply EMLA at home in preparation for a procedure (Fig. 14.9).

Sometimes, EMLA is not used due to the expense and the time needed to allow the drug to act. New approaches to EMLA delivery have been developed. Examples include other drug formulations and a patch delivery with a heat-activated system (Synera) that enhances the delivery of lidocaine and prilocaine. Synera is labeled for children older than 3 years and needs to be applied only 20 to 30 minutes before the procedure (Lexicomp, 2023b).

BOX 14.1 Applying Eutectic Mixture of Local Anesthetics (EMLA)

Follow these guidelines when applying EMLA:

- Explain the purpose of the medication to the child and parents, reinforcing that it will help the pain go away.
- Check the scheduled time for the procedure; plan to apply the cream 60 minutes before a superficial procedure such as an intramuscular injection or a venipuncture or 2 to 3 hours before a deeper procedure such as a lumbar puncture or bone marrow aspiration.
- Place a thick layer of the cream on the skin at the intended site of the procedure, making sure that the area where the cream is being applied is free of any breaks. Do not rub the cream in once it is applied to the skin.
- Cover the site with a transparent dressing, and secure it so that the dressing is occlusive. Alternatively, use plastic film wrap and tape the edges to secure the dressing.
- Instruct the child not to touch the dressing once it is secured. If necessary, cover the occlusive dressing with a protection device or a loosely applied gauze or elastic bandage.
- After the allotted time, remove the occlusive dressing, and wipe the cream from the skin. Inspect the skin for a change in color (blanching or redness), which indicates the medication has penetrated the skin adequately.
- Verify that sensation is absent by lightly tapping or scratching the area. Use this technique also to demonstrate to the child that the anesthetic is effective. If sensation is present, reapply the cream.
- Prepare the child for the procedure. Assess the child's pain after the procedure to evaluate for pain and to differentiate pain from fear and anxiety.

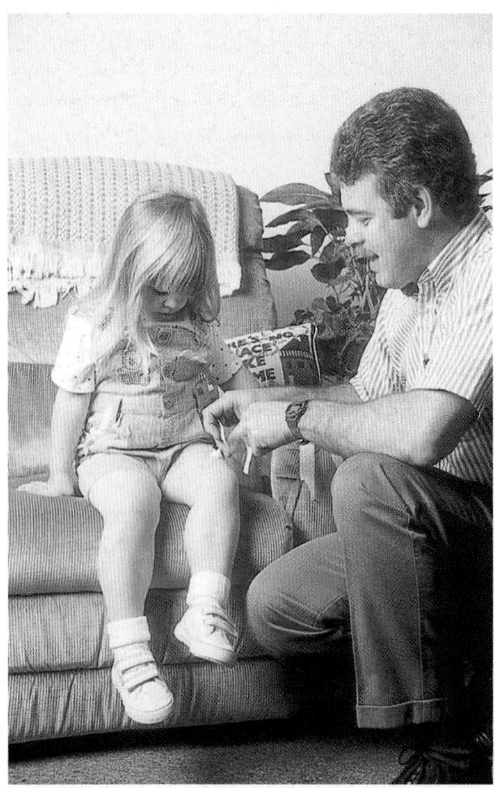

FIGURE 14.9 A parent applies EMLA cream to the child at home in preparation for a procedure. EMLA, eutectic mixture of local anesthetics.

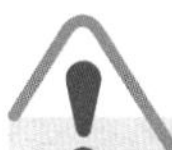

CLINICAL REASONING ALERT

EMLA is used with caution in children younger than 3 to 6 months and other susceptible patients because it may be associated with methemoglobinemia caused by prilocaine toxicity (Lexicomp, 2023b). It is contraindicated in children who have congenital or idiopathic methemoglobinemia (Lexicomp, 2023b). It must be used cautiously in children younger than 12 months who are receiving methemoglobin-inducing agents, such as sulfonamides, phenytoin, phenobarbital, and acetaminophen (Lexicomp, 2023b). Use of these agents in combination with EMLA increases the child's risk for methemoglobinemia, a condition that could lead to cyanosis and hypoxemia.

Other examples of topical anesthetics are tetracaine, epinephrine, cocaine (TAC) and lidocaine, epinephrine, tetracaine (LET). These are commonly used for lacerations that require suturing. The agent is applied directly to the wound with a cotton ball or swab for 20 to 30 minutes until the area is numb. These methods are not used in children with known sensitivity to any of these medications.

Lidocaine can also be dispersed in liposomes to allow for transcutaneous delivery (liposomal lidocaine). OTC lidocaine 4% (LMX4) or lidocaine 5% (LMX5), formerly called ELA-Max, is massaged into the skin without the use of an occlusive dressing. Anesthesia to the area is reached in 15 to 30 minutes and lasts about 60 minutes.

Needle-free powder lidocaine (Zingo or J-Tip) is another topical analgesic. It is labeled for use in children 3 to 18 years of age. It is a single-use, prefilled disposable system that provides analgesia in 1 to 3 minutes.

Another choice for local anesthesia is iontophoresis. Iontophoretic lidocaine (Numby Stuff) provides a deeper analgesia in a shorter duration (~10 to 25 minutes) and is used over intact skin. A mild electrical current from a small battery-powered generator and two iontophoretic drug-delivery electrodes push drug molecules (lidocaine hydrochloric acid 2% with epinephrine 1:100,000) into the skin. A mild tingling sensation may be felt during drug delivery, with an increase in tingling noted with higher currents. This type of local anesthesia is not recommended for use in children who have a history of allergy or sensitivity to these drugs, electrically sensitive equipment such as a pacemaker, or damaged skin or scar tissue. There is limited use of this anesthetic due to the discomfort associated with the procedure and local skin reactions, including blisters and burn-like reactions (Hsu, 2022).

Vapocoolant spray can be applied to the skin, but efficacy is highly dependent on spraying time, and it can cause discomfort (Hsu, 2022). The duration of analgesia is short, approximately 1 to 2 minutes, which may not allow enough time for a procedure to be completed.

TAKE NOTE!

Studies comparing lidocaine–prilocaine products to other topical anesthetics (such as liposomal lidocaine and heated lidocaine) have shown equal or better pain relief with a shorter onset of action (Hsu, 2022).

Injectable Forms

Injectable forms of lidocaine or procaine can be administered subcutaneously or intradermally around the procedural area approximately 5 to 10 minutes before the procedure. Common problems with this form of anesthetic include the pain associated with the subcutaneous injection and some burning associated with lidocaine administration, as well as blanching of the skin.

TAKE NOTE!

The burning that lidocaine causes on injection may be diminished by buffering lidocaine with sodium bicarbonate, using 10 parts lidocaine and one part sodium bicarbonate (1 mL of 1% to 2% lidocaine and 0.1 mL of 8.4% sodium bicarbonate). Then, inject 0.1 mL or less of the solution intradermally at the site of venipuncture. Anesthetic action is almost immediate. The solution is stable for only approximately 1 week if not refrigerated.

EPIDURAL ANALGESIA

For **epidural analgesia**, a catheter is inserted into the epidural space, usually between the lumbar (L3) and the thoracic (T3) areas. The drug, usually fentanyl or morphine, diffuses into the cerebrospinal fluid and crosses the dura mater to the spinal cord. Then, it binds with the opioid receptors located at the dorsal horn. The drugs can be administered as bolus injections (a one-time bolus or on an intermittent schedule), a continuous infusion, or PCA. Usually, an opioid such as morphine, fentanyl, or hydromorphone is given in conjunction with a long-acting local anesthetic such as bupivacaine.

Epidural analgesia is typically used postoperatively, providing analgesia to the lower body for approximately 12 to 14 hours. The small amount of medication used with this type of analgesia causes less sedation, thereby allowing the child to participate more actively in postoperative care activities. This type of analgesia is also effective for children undergoing upper or lower abdominal surgeries because it controls localized intense pain, somatic pain, and visceral pain.

When epidural analgesia is being administered, additional narcotic analgesics are not given in order to prevent complications such as respiratory depression, pruritus, nausea, vomiting, and urinary retention.

CLINICAL REASONING ALERT!

Respiratory depression, although rare when epidural analgesia is used, is always a possibility. When it does occur, it usually occurs gradually over a period of several hours after the medication is initiated. This allows adequate time for early detection and prompt intervention.

Constant assessment is essential because insertion of an epidural catheter and epidural analgesia can lead to infection at the site of the insertion, epidural hematoma, arachnoiditis, neuritis, spinal headache (rare) due to a cerebrospinal fluid leak, and respiratory depression. Frequent assessment, typically every 1 to 2 hours, of heart rate, respiratory rate, and depth of sedation, and every 2 to 4 hours of blood pressure, pain level, and motor function, is imperative. Assessing for adverse reactions such as nausea and vomiting and pruritus, checking the tubing and catheter site, and ensuring the occlusive dressing is intact are all important nursing interventions. The dermatome, which is the area of the body associated with supply by a particular nerve, that innervates the diaphragm can become suppressed during continuous epidural analgesia, resulting in respiratory depression. It is important to assess the child's sensory level frequently. Using cool water or an alcohol pad, bilaterally touch the child's body every 2 to 3 cm. The level at which the child states they feel the temperature change is the level of anesthesia. (Refer to Fig. 14.10 for dermatome levels.)

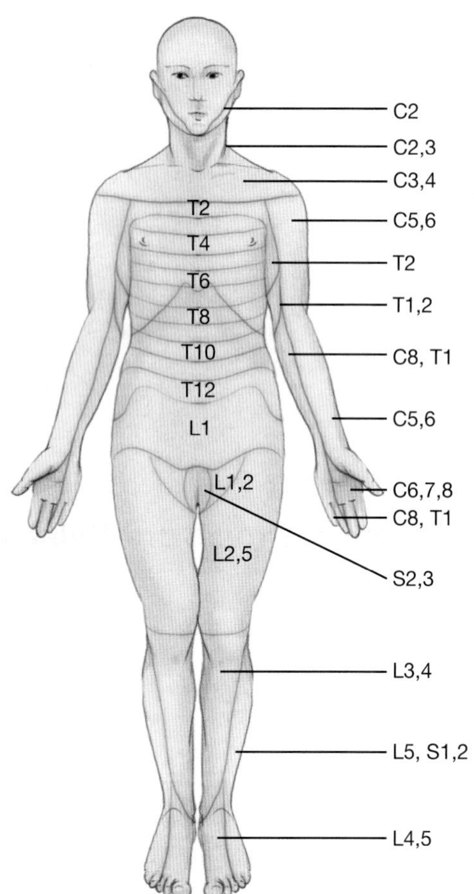

FIGURE 14.10 The level of anesthesia should not go higher than T4, the nipple line, in children.

MODERATE SEDATION

Moderate sedation used to be called conscious sedation, but the term "conscious" has been replaced since it can be misleading (Cravero & Roback, 2022). It is a medically controlled state of depressed consciousness that allows protective reflexes to be maintained so the child has the ability to maintain a patent airway and respond to physical or verbal stimulation.

Sedation in children is different than in adults as it is often administered to help control behavior in order to complete procedures or diagnostic studies. Moderate sedation requires adherence to specific protocols, and many regulatory bodies, such as The Joint Commission, and societies, including the AAP, American Academy of Pediatric Dentistry (AAPD), American Society of Anesthesiologists, and American College of Emergency Physicians, have published standards and guidelines to improve patient safety and outcomes. The depressed state is obtained by using various agents such as morphine, fentanyl, midazolam, ketamine, chloral hydrate, diazepam, pentobarbital, nitrous oxide, or propofol. The medication used will depend on the expected degree of pain and discomfort, amount of motion restriction needed, and individual factors such as age, ability to cooperate, and medical history.

Moderate sedation is used for procedures that are painful and stressful. For example, moderate sedation is suggested instead of restraints, especially for toddlers and preschool children undergoing frightening or invasive procedures who are manifesting extreme anxiety and behavioral upset. Other indications include situations involving:

- Evidence the child is experiencing a heightened stress reaction (e.g., attempting to flee, crying inconsolably, or flailing)
- Verbalization by the child that they are frightened and do not want to be touched
- Inability to remain immobilized, such as during laceration repair or computed tomography
- Any procedure that is painful and fear-provoking

The route of administering the medications for sedation should follow the guidelines of atraumatic care. Oral, topical, or an existing intravenous route should be used. The child may pass from the intended level of sedation to a deeper unintended level of sedation; therefore, personnel administering moderate sedation must be specially trained, with strong resuscitation and advanced pediatric life support skills, and emergency equipment and medications must be readily available (Cravero & Roback, 2022).

The Nurse's Role in Pharmacologic Pain Management

The nurse plays a major role in providing pharmacologic pain relief. As with any medication, the nurse is responsible for adhering to the rights of medication administration—right drug, right dose, right route, right time, right patient, and right approach. The nurse also adheres to additional rights, such as the right of the child and parents to be educated, the right of the child to refuse the medication, the right documentation, and the right form. The nurse must also have a solid knowledge base about the medications used for pain relief. This knowledge includes information about the drug's pharmacokinetics (absorption, distribution, metabolism, and excretion) and pharmacodynamics (mechanism of action, including adverse effects). Refer to Chapter 13 for further information.

Assessment is crucial when pharmacologic pain interventions are used. An initial assessment of pain provides a baseline from which options for relief can be chosen. Factors that can affect the choice of analgesic, such as the child's age, pain intensity, physiologic status, or previous experiences with pain, also need to be considered. The nurse acts as an advocate for the child and the family to ensure that the most appropriate pharmacologic agent is chosen for the situation.

Assessment is ongoing once the agent is administered. Monitor physiologic parameters such as level of consciousness, vital signs, oxygen saturation levels, and urinary output for changes that might indicate an adverse reaction to the agent. More intensive monitoring is needed when agents are administered intravenously or epidurally or by moderate sedation. For example, if the child is receiving moderate sedation, interventions include:

- Ensuring emergency equipment is readily available
- Maintaining a patent airway
- Monitoring the child's level of consciousness and responsiveness
- Assessing the child's vital signs (especially heart rate, blood pressure, and respiratory rate)
- Monitoring oxygen saturation levels

Typically, a specially trained health care provider is specifically designated to perform these activities during the administration of the sedation. Afterward, the nurse is responsible for ongoing monitoring of the child's status.

Monitor the child closely for evidence of adverse effects. Table 14.8 describes the interventions useful for responding to these adverse effects. Be alert for signs and symptoms of respiratory depression secondary to opioid administration. Have an opioid antagonist such as naloxone and the benzodiazepine antagonist flumazenil readily available should the child experience respiratory depression.

In addition to assessing physiologic parameters, assess the child's and parents' emotional status before and after the agent is administered. For example, increased anxiety and fear may necessitate a change in method of administration, such as topical application instead of an intradermal injection of a local anesthetic. Use nonpharmacologic methods to help lessen anxiety, thereby promoting more effective relief from the drug.

Nurses are also responsible for ensuring that the child and parents are adequately prepared for the use of the pharmacologic agent. Teach the child and parents about the drug, why it is being used, its intended effects, and possible adverse effects, tailoring the teaching to the child's cognitive level. Provide opportunities for the child and parents to ask questions, offering support and guidance throughout the experience. Provide a demonstration or use visual aids so that the child and parents know exactly what to expect. Encourage the use of play to help the child express fears and anxieties related to the administration.

TABLE 14.8 • Interventions for Common Opioid-Induced Adverse Effects

Adverse Effect	Nursing Interventions
Constipation	Encourage fluid intake unless contraindicated. Ensure intake of high-fiber foods, including fruits, if allowed. Encourage activity, including ambulation if possible. Obtain order for stool softener, and administer laxative as ordered.
Pruritus	Apply cool compresses and lotions. Administer antihistamine as ordered.
Nausea and vomiting	Inform child and parents that these symptoms usually subside in 1–2 days. Encourage small frequent meals with bland foods. Administer antiemetic if ordered. Notify health care provider for possible change in pain medication.

Management of Procedure-Related Pain

One of the most common causes of pain in children is procedure-related pain. The procedure may be minor, such as an intramuscular injection, heel stick, or venipuncture, or it may be more involved, such as lumbar puncture, bone marrow aspiration, or wound care. Regardless, pain is real for children, and painful procedures are often extremely distressing. Variables that affect pain include the intensity or length of the procedure and the skill of the health care provider performing it.

The Nurse's Role in Managing Procedure-Related Pain

Through the use of behavioral and pharmacologic approaches, nurses can significantly reduce the pain and distress of procedures. Use the guiding principles of atraumatic care, which include:

- Use topical EMLA or other topical analgesics such as liposomal lidocaine or tetracaine gel, iontophoretic lidocaine, vapocoolant spray, or buffered lidocaine at the intended site of a skin or vessel puncture.
- Incorporate the use of nonpharmacologic strategies for pain relief in conjunction with pharmacologic methods.
- Prepare the child and parents about the procedure, and then keep all equipment out of sight until it is ready to be used.
- Use therapeutic hugging (see Chapter 8) to secure the child.
- Use the smallest-gauge needle possible or an automated lancet device to puncture the skin.
- Use an intermittent infusion device or peripherally inserted central catheter (PICC) if multiple or repeated blood samples are necessary. Coordinate care so that several tests can be performed from one sample if possible.

- Opt for venipuncture in newborns instead of heel sticks if the amount of blood needed would require much squeezing.
- Use kangaroo care (skin-to-skin contact) for newborns before and after a heel stick.
- Provide NNS with sucrose solution, if appropriate; pacifier; or breastfeeding for newborns several minutes before the procedure.

TAKE NOTE!

Individualize interventions based on the painfulness of the procedure and the child's developmental age and personality. Use behavioral cognitive approaches and pharmacologic interventions. For example, encouraging the school-age child to assist during painful procedures in age-appropriate ways may help ease some of the pain related to a heightened state of anxiety or at least assist the child in coping with the situation. Always use appropriate pharmacologic treatment, especially for the first procedure, to provide as painless an experience as possible for the child.

Nursing care for the child with procedure-related pain includes the child as well as the parents. Be sure to prepare them for the procedure using an appropriate developmental approach. Promote environmental comfort, too. Ensure the child's privacy is maintained and the lighting is adequate for the procedure but not so bright as to cause the child discomfort.

Painful procedures performed in the child's room can lead to an association of pain or fear with the room or bed. Many hospitals have a special treatment room where procedures can be performed. These rooms are usually equipped with many activities, toys, and decorations to help distract the child. The use of a treatment room may not be feasible or desirable in all situations or for all procedures. The ultimate goal is to do what is best for the child; therefore, the nurse should consider the needs of the child, the demands of the procedures, and the conditions that would facilitate the best outcome.

Unless contraindicated, encourage the parents to be present before, during, and after the procedure to provide comforting support to the child. Also encourage the child and parents to use nonpharmacologic methods to help maximize pain relief and reduce anxiety. For example, nonpharmacologic methods that are helpful for the toddler and preschooler may include positioning the child on the lap and hugging the child, distracting the child with toys or interactive books, and blowing bubbles.

Play therapy can be useful when preparing children for painful procedures. Encourage children to make decisions about their care related to pain management if their condition or procedure allows. It is also helpful to anticipate and recognize painful situations and provide pain medication before the actual procedure to ensure comfort. Many nonpharmacologic strategies can be enhanced and better implemented with the help of the child life specialist or play therapist, who have specialized training in these techniques.

Recall Aiden from the beginning of the chapter. What are some interventions that may be helpful prior to, during, and after his dressing change?

Management of Chronic Pain

Typically, pain in children is acute, but chronic pain is a significant problem in the pediatric population as well. Chronic pain is ongoing and recurrent pain that persists beyond the expected healing time (World Health Organization [WHO], 2020). Chronic pain is the result of a complex interplay of biologic, psychological, and sociocultural factors. Children with chronic pain and their families may experience significant physical, emotional, and social consequences, including notable economic burdens from the pain and disability (WHO, 2020). Children with chronic pain have an increased risk of depression and anxiety, sleep problems, and problems with school functioning, and the experience of chronic pain in childhood may predispose the individual to chronic pain in adulthood (WHO, 2020).

The Nurse's Role in Managing Chronic Pain

The nurse's role in managing chronic pain in children is similar to that for the child experiencing acute pain or procedure-related pain. Assessment of the child's pain is key and should include a history of the present problem. Questions should focus on the onset of the pain; its intensity, duration, and location; and any factors that alleviate or exacerbate it. In addition, it is important to question the child and parents about the impact of the pain on the child's daily life, such as sleep; play; eating; school; and interactions with peers, other family members, and friends. Also address the impact of the child's chronic pain on the family's life.

Another key area of assessment is determining how the pain affects the child's and family's level of stress. Areas to address include the child's and parents' feelings of hopelessness, anxiety, and depression. Also question the child and parents about what they think has caused the pain and how they have coped with it. In addition, ascertain what methods the child and parents have used to alleviate the pain and the success of these methods. Inquire about any home remedies or alternative therapies that may have been used.

Review past physical examination findings for clues to the underlying problem. Observe the child's overall appearance, gait, and posture. Assess the child's cognitive level and emotional response, especially related to the experience of pain. Expect to complete a neurologic examination, and observe for muscle spasms, trigger points, and increased sensitivity to light touch. Abnormal body postures assumed by the child due to chronic pain may result in the development of secondary pain in the muscles and fascia. When children tense their muscles due to fear of examination, somatic pain may occur.

Various nonpharmacologic and pharmacologic strategies are used to manage chronic pain. Often, multiple strategies are combined to address pain relief as well as the pain's impact on other areas, such as sleep or school functioning. When pharmacologic agents are used, the oral form is the method of choice. As with any pain management strategy, education of the child and family is paramount. A referral to a pediatric pain specialist may be needed if the child's pain is not controlled effectively.

KEY CONCEPTS

- Pain is a highly individualized subjective experience affecting people of all ages. It is a universal experience and may be considered the fifth vital sign.
- Pain management is a critical element in a child's plan of care because children may lack the verbal capacity to describe their pain experience; caregivers and health care providers often have misconceptions about pain; assessment of the complex nature of the pain experience is difficult; if left unmanaged, pain in children can lead to serious physical and emotional consequences; and available resources and research related to pain relief strategies in children are limited.
- The sensation of pain involves a sequence of physiologic events: transduction, transmission, perception, and modulation.
- Pain can be classified by duration as acute or chronic, by etiology as nociceptive or neuropathic, or by source or location as somatic or visceral.
- Factors influencing a child's perception of pain include age and gender or sex, cognitive level, temperament, previous pain experiences, and family and cultural background, all of which cannot be changed. Situational factors involve behavioral, cognitive, and emotional aspects and can be changed.
- Infants, including preterm infants, experience pain. Behavioral and physiologic indicators are used to assess pain. Toddlers commonly react with intense emotional upset and physical resistance or aggression. Preschoolers may believe pain is a punishment for misbehaving or having bad thoughts. School-age children can communicate the type, location, and severity of pain but may deny having pain so as to appear brave or avoid further pain. Adolescents, with their focus on body image and fear of loss of control, often ask numerous questions and may attempt to remain stoic to avoid being viewed as childish.
- Assessment of pain in children includes both subjective and objective data. Nurses need to tailor the assessment to the child's developmental level and ask appropriate questions geared to the child's cognitive level. Parental questioning during the health history is also important.
- Self-report pain rating scales are valuable assessment tools that allow the child's level of pain to be quantified. Examples include the FACES pain rating scale, the Oucher pain rating scale, the poker chip tool, the visual analog and numeric scales, and the Adolescent Pediatric Pain Tool.
- Different pain rating scales are appropriate for different developmental levels. However, children may regress when in pain, so a simpler tool may be needed to make sure that the child understands what is being asked. Consistency in using the same tool is essential so that appropriate comparisons can be made and effective interventions can be planned and implemented.
- Physical examination of the child for pain primarily involves the skills of observation and inspection. These skills are used to assess for physiologic and behavioral changes that indicate pain. Auscultation may also be used to assess for changes in vital signs, specifically heart rate and blood pressure. Physiologic and behavioral pain assessment tools, such as the PIPP, NIPS, RIPS, Pain Observation Scale for Young Children, CRIES Scale for Neonatal Postoperative Pain Assessment, and r-FLACC Behavioral Scale, measure specific parameters and changes that would indicate the child is in pain.
- Nonpharmacologic pain management strategies aim to assist children in coping with pain and to give them a sense of mastery or control over the situation. These strategies may be categorized as behavioral cognitive, in which the child focuses on a specific area or aspect rather than the pain (e.g., relaxation, distraction, imagery, biofeedback, thought stopping, and positive self-talk), or biophysical, in which the focus is on interfering with the transmission of pain impulses reaching the brain (e.g., heat and cold applications, massage, and pressure).
- The nurse plays a major role in teaching the child and family about available nonpharmacologic pain interventions, helping them choose the most appropriate and most effective methods and ensuring the child and parents use the methods before the pain occurs as well as before it increases.
- Pharmacologic interventions involve the administration of drugs for pain relief, most commonly, nonopioids and opioid analgesics. The selection of the

method is determined by the drug being administered; the child's status; the type, intensity, and location of the pain; and any factors that may be influencing the child's pain. The preferred methods for administering analgesics include the oral, rectal, intravenous, or local nerve block routes; epidural administration; and moderate sedation.

- Nonopioid analgesics used to treat mild to moderate pain include acetaminophen and NSAIDs such as ibuprofen, ketorolac, naproxen, and, less commonly, indomethacin, diclofenac, and piroxicam.
- Morphine is considered the "gold standard" for all opioid agonists; it is the drug to which all other opioids are compared and is usually the drug of choice for severe pain (Hauer & Jones, 2021).
- Local anesthetics are commonly used to provide analgesia for procedures. They are effective in providing successful pain relief, with only minimal risk of systemic adverse effects. The first choice for the most effective, painless local anesthesia is EMLA. It achieves anesthesia to a depth of 2 to 4 mm, so it reduces pain associated with phlebotomy, venous cannulation, and intramuscular injections up to 24 hours after injection.
- Epidural analgesia involves the insertion of a catheter into the epidural space through which drugs can be administered as bolus injections (a one-time bolus or on an intermittent schedule), as a continuous infusion, or as PCA. Usually an opioid, such as morphine, fentanyl, or hydromorphone, is given in conjunction with a long-acting local anesthetic, such as bupivacaine.
- Moderate sedation is a medically controlled state of depressed consciousness that allows protective reflexes to be maintained so the child has the ability to maintain a patent airway and respond to physical or verbal stimulation.
- When providing pharmacologic pain relief, the nurse must adhere to the rights of medication administration and have a solid knowledge base about the medications used for pain relief and the drug's pharmacokinetics (absorption, distribution, metabolism, and excretion) and pharmacodynamics (mechanism of action, including adverse effects). Initial and ongoing assessment is crucial.
- The principles of atraumatic care guide nursing interventions for providing pain relief, especially for procedure-related pain.
- Chronic pain in children can significantly affect the child's daily life and activities as well as the family's life.

REFERENCES AND RECOMMENDED READINGS

American Academy of Pediatrics (AAP), Committee on Fetus and Newborn, & Section on Anesthesiology and Pain Medicine. (2016, reaffirmed 2020). Prevention and management of procedural pain in the neonate: An update. *Pediatrics, 137*(2). https://doi.org/ 10.1542/peds.2015-4271

American Pain Society. (1995). *Pain: The fifth vital sign*. Author.

Baker, C. M., & Wong, D. L. (1987). Q.U.E.S.T.: A process of pain assessment in children. *Orthopaedic Nursing, 6*(1), 11–21. https://doi.org/10.1097/00006416-198701000-00003

Beyer, J. E., Denyes, M. J., & Villarruel, A. M. (1992). The creation, validation, and continuing development of the Oucher: A measure of pain intensity in children. *Journal of Pediatric Nursing, 7*(5), 335–346.

Boelen-van der Loo, W. J., Scheffer, E., de Haan, R. J., & de Groot, C. J. (1999). Clinimetric evaluation of the pain observation scale for young children in children aged between 1 and 4 years after ear, nose, and throat surgery. *Journal of Developmental and Behavioral Pediatrics, 20*(4), 222–227. https://doi.org/10.1097/00004703-199908000-00004

Boitor, M., Gélinas, C., Rauch, F., Jacob, E., LeMay, S., Carrier, J. I., Bilodeau, C., & Tsimicalis, A. (2019). Validation of the adolescent pediatric pain tool for the multidimensional measurement of pain in children and adolescents diagnosed with osteogenesis imperfecta. *Canadian Journal of Pain, 3*(1), 148–156. https://doi.org/10.1080/24740527.2019.1626705

Crandall, M., & Savedra, M. (2005). Multidimensional assessment using the adolescent pediatric pain tool: A case report. *Journal for Specialists in Pediatric Nursing, 10*(3), 115–123. https://doi.org/10.1111/j.1744-6155.2005.00023.x

Cravero, J. P., & Roback, M. G. (2022). Procedural sedation in children: Approach. *UpToDate*. Retrieved March 22, 2023, from https://www.uptodate.com/contents/procedural-sedation-in-children-approach

Favaretto, E., Gögele, M., Bedani, F., Hicks, A. A., Erfurth, A., Perugi, G., Pramstaller, P. P., & Melotti, R. (2022). Pain sensitivity is modulated by affective temperament: Results from the population-based CHRIS Affective Disorder (CHRIS-AD) study. *Journal of Affective Disorders, 316*, 209–216. https://doi.org/10.1016/j.jad.2022.08.015

Gai, N., Naser, B., Hanley, J., Peliowski, A., Hayes, J., & Aoyama, K. (2020). A practical guide to acute pain management in children. *Journal of Anesthesia, 34*(3), 421–433. https://doi.org/10.1007/s00540-020-02767-x

Hauer, J., & Jones, B. L. (2021). Pain in children: Approach to pain assessment and overview of management principles. *UpToDate*. Retrieved March 13, 2023, from https://www.uptodate.com/contents/pain-in-children-approach-to-pain-assessment-and-overview-of-management-principles

Hester, N. K. (1979). The preoperational child's reaction to immunization. *Nursing Research, 28*(4), 250–255. https://doi.org/10.1097/00006199-197907000-00017

Hockenberry, M. J., & Wilson, D. (2009). *Wong's essentials of pediatric nursing* (8th ed., p. 162). Elsevier Mosby.

Horton, R. E., Pillai Riddell, R., Flora, D., Moran, G., & Pederson, D. (2015). Distress regulation in infancy: Attachment and temperament in the context of acute pain. *Journal of Developmental and Behavioral Pediatrics, 36*, 35–44. https://doi.org/10.1097/DBP.0000000000000119

Hsu, D. C. (2022). Clinical use of topical anesthetics in children. *UpToDate*. Retrieved April 8, 2023, from https://www.uptodate.com/contents/clinical-use-of-topical-anesthetics-in-children

Institute for Safe Medication Practices. (2021). *ISMP medication safety self-assessment for perioperative settings*. https://www.ismp.org/sites/default/files/attachments/2021-05/FAQs.pdf

International Association for the Study of Pain. (2011). *IASP pain terminology*. https://www.iasp-pain.org/Education/Content.aspx?ItemNumber=1698#Pain

Krechel, S. W., & Bildner, J. (1995). CRIES: A new neonatal postoperative pain measurement score. Initial testing of validity and reliability. *Paediatric Anaesthesia, 5*, 53–61. https://doi.org/10.1111/j.1460-9592.1995.tb00242.x

Lawrence, J., Alcock, D., McGrath, P., Kay, J., MacMurray, S. B., & Dulberg, C. (1993). The development of a tool to assess neonatal pain. *Neonatal Network, 12*(6), 59–66.

Lexicomp. (2023a). *Meperidine (pethidine): Pediatric drug information. UpToDate.* Retrieved April 5, 2023, from https://www.uptodate.com/contents/meperidine-pethidine-pediatric-druginformation

Lexicomp. (2023b). *Pediatric drug information. UpToDate.* Retrieved April 5, 2023, from https://www.uptodate.com/contents/table-of-contents/drug-information/pediatric-drug-information

Luo, F., Zhu, H., Mei, L., Shu, Q., Cheng, X., Chen, X., Zhao, Y., Chen, S., & Pan, Y. (2023). Evaluation of procedural pain for neonates in a neonatal intensive care unit: A single-centre study. *BMJ Paediatrics Open, 7*(1):e002107. https://doi.org/10.1136/bmjpo-2023-002107

McCaffery, M. (1968). *Nursing practice theories related to cognition, bodily pain and main environment interactions.* University of California, Los Angeles.

McGrath, P. A. (2005). Children—Not simply "little adults." In H. Merskey, J. D. Loeser, & R. Dubner (Eds.), *The paths of pain 1975–2005* (pp. 433–446). IASP Press.

Merkel, S. I., Voepel-Lewis, T., Shayevitz, J. R., & Malviya, S. (1997). The FLACC: A behavioral scale for scoring postoperative pain in young children. *Pediatric Nursing, 23*(3), 293–297.

Nath, J. (2023). *Applied pathophysiology* (4th ed.). Wolters Kluwer.

National Database of Nursing Quality Indicators. (n.d.). *NDNQI nursing-sensitive indicators.* Retrieved March 20, 2023, from https://nursingandndnqi.weebly.com/ndnqi-indicators.html

Osborne, N. R., & Davis, K. D. (2022). Chapter Eight—Sex and gender differences in pain. *International Review of Neurobiology, 164*: 277–307. https://doi.org/10.1016/bs.irn.2022.06.013

Osincup, P. (2020). How to use humor in clinical settings. *AMA Journal of Ethics, 22*(7):E588–E595. https://doi.org/10.1001/amajethics.2020.588

Roué, J.-M. (2022). Prevention and treatment of neonatal pain. *UpToDate.* Retrieved March 13, 2023, from https://www.uptodate.com/contents/prevention-and-treatment-of-neonatal-pain

Roué, J.-M. (2023). Assessment of neonatal pain. *UpToDate.* Retrieved March 13, 2023, from https://www.uptodate.com/contents/assessment-of-neonatal-pain

Schade, J. G., Joyce, B. A., Gerkensmeyer, J., & Keck, J. F. (1996). Comparison of three preverbal scales for postoperative pain assessment in a diverse pediatric sample. *Journal of Pain and Symptom Management, 12*(6), 348–359. https://doi.org/10.1016/S0885-3924(96)00182-0

Schechter, W. (2023). Pharmacologic management of acute perioperative pain in infants and children. *UpToDate.* Retrieved April 7, 2023, from https://www.uptodate.com/contents/pharmacologic-management-of-acute-perioperative-pain-in-infants-and-children

Strean, W. B. (2009). Laughter prescription. *Canadian Family Physician/Medecin de Famille Canadien, 55*(10), 965–967. https://www.cfp.ca/content/cfp/55/10/965.full.pdf

Talebi, M., Amiri, S. R. J., Roshan, P. A., Zabihi, A., Zahedpasha, Y., & Chehrazi, M. (2022). The effect of concurrent use of swaddle and sucrose on the intensity of pain during venous blood sampling in neonate: A clinical trial study. *BMC Pediatrics, 22*(1), 263. https://doi.org/10.1186/s12887-022-03323-0

Thirion, J., O'Riordan, M. A., & Stormorken, A. (2015). Commentary revisiting the pieces of hurt pain assessment tool—Do the pieces matter? *Pediatric Pain Letter, 17*(1), 1–4. http://childpain.org/ppl/issues/v17n1_2015/v17n1_thirion.pdf

World Health Organization. (2020). *Guidelines on the management of chronic pain in children.* https://www.who.int/publications/i/item/9789240017870

Yin, S. (2022). Opioid withdrawal in adolescents. *UpToDate.* Retrieved November 10, 2023, from https://www.uptodate.com/contents/opioid-withdrawal-in-adolescents

Zeltzer, L. K., Krane, E. J., & Levy, R. L. (2020). Pediatric pain management. In R. M. Kleigman, J. W. St. Geme III, N. J. Blum, S. S. Shah, R. C. Tasker, K. M. Wilson, & R. E. Behrman (Eds.), *Nelson textbook of pediatrics* (21st ed., pp. 2915–3011). Elsevier.

DEVELOPING CLINICAL JUDGMENT

PRACTICING FOR NCLEX

1. The nurse is preparing to assess the pain of a 3-year-old child who had surgery the day before. Which pain assessment methods would be most appropriate for the nurse to use? Select all that apply.
   a. FACES pain rating scale
   b. Numeric pain scale
   c. Asking the parents to report their child's pain scale
   d. Visual analog scale
   e. Observation of the child

2. When developing the plan of care for a child in pain, the nurse identifies appropriate strategies aimed at modifying which factors that influence pain? Select all that apply.
   a. Lack of control
   b. Cognitive level
   c. Previous pain experiences
   d. Anticipatory anxiety
   e. Gender
   f. Fear

3. An adolescent who is a competitive swimmer comes to the emergency department complaining of localized aching pain in their shoulder, stating, "I've been practicing really hard and long to get myself ready for my meet this weekend." The area is tender to the touch. The nurse determines that the adolescent is most likely experiencing which type of pain?
   a. Cutaneous pain
   b. Deep somatic pain
   c. Visceral pain
   d. Neuropathic pain

4. After teaching a child's parents about the different methods of distraction that can be used for pain management, which statement by the parents indicates a need for additional teaching?
   a. "We'll have her focus on her hand and count each finger slowly."
   b. "We'll read some of her favorite stories to her."
   c. "We'll have her imagine that she's at the beach this summer."
   d. "She likes to play video games, so we'll bring in some from home."

5. A child is scheduled for a bone marrow aspiration at 4 p.m. The nurse would plan to apply EMLA cream to the intended site at which time?
   a. 1:30 p.m.
   b. 3:00 p.m.
   c. 3:30 p.m.
   d. 4:00 p.m.

6. The patient is postoperative day 1 after cardiac surgery. The nurse understands that in a(n)____________ the most consistent indicator of pain is______________.
   Blank 1:
   a. infant
   b. preschooler
   c. adolescent
   d. school-age child
   Blank 2:
   e. increased heart rate
   f. high-pitched cry
   g. increased heart rate
   h. facial expression

CRITICAL THINKING EXERCISES

1. The nurse asks a 12-year-old if she is having pain. She denies pain, even though she is lying on her left side, holding her abdomen, with her knees flexed up to it. What might be some underlying factors leading the child to deny her pain? How would the nurse go about assessing this child's pain?

2. The nurse comes into the room of a 6-year-old who is sleeping. His parent states, "He's asleep, so he's not in pain." How should the nurse respond?

3. A child who is receiving ibuprofen is experiencing increased pain. The dosage of ibuprofen is increased but is no longer effective in providing adequate pain relief. What is occurring? What would be most likely to happen next?

STUDY ACTIVITIES

1. Interview nurses who work on a pediatric unit about their experiences with managing pain in children. Ask them how they assess pain in children and the major methods they use to assist the children in managing their pain.

2. Interview families of children with chronic illnesses who experience pain. Ask the parents how they assess their children's pain level and what methods they have used in assisting their children in managing pain.

3. Compare the drugs fentanyl and midazolam when used for moderate sedation in terms of onset of action, duration, primary effects, and antidotes.

4. A child is receiving epidural analgesia with morphine. The nurse would be alert for which adverse effects? Select all that apply.
   a. Respiratory depression
   b. Pruritus
   c. Constipation
   d. Vomiting
   e. Amnesia
   f. Hematoma

DOSAGE CALCULATION QUESTIONS

After you have performed your nonpharmacologic interventions, your patient, who is an infant, is exhibiting kicking, is not reaching for toys, and is occasionally crying. There is an order for morphine sulfate 1 mg IV every 3 to 4 hours. The safe dose range for morphine sulfate is 0.1 to 0.2 mg/kg/dose every 3 to 4 hours. Morphine sulfate is supplied as 1 mg/mL.

1. Is this a safe dose?

2. Describe how you will administer this medication and what you would assess for after giving it.

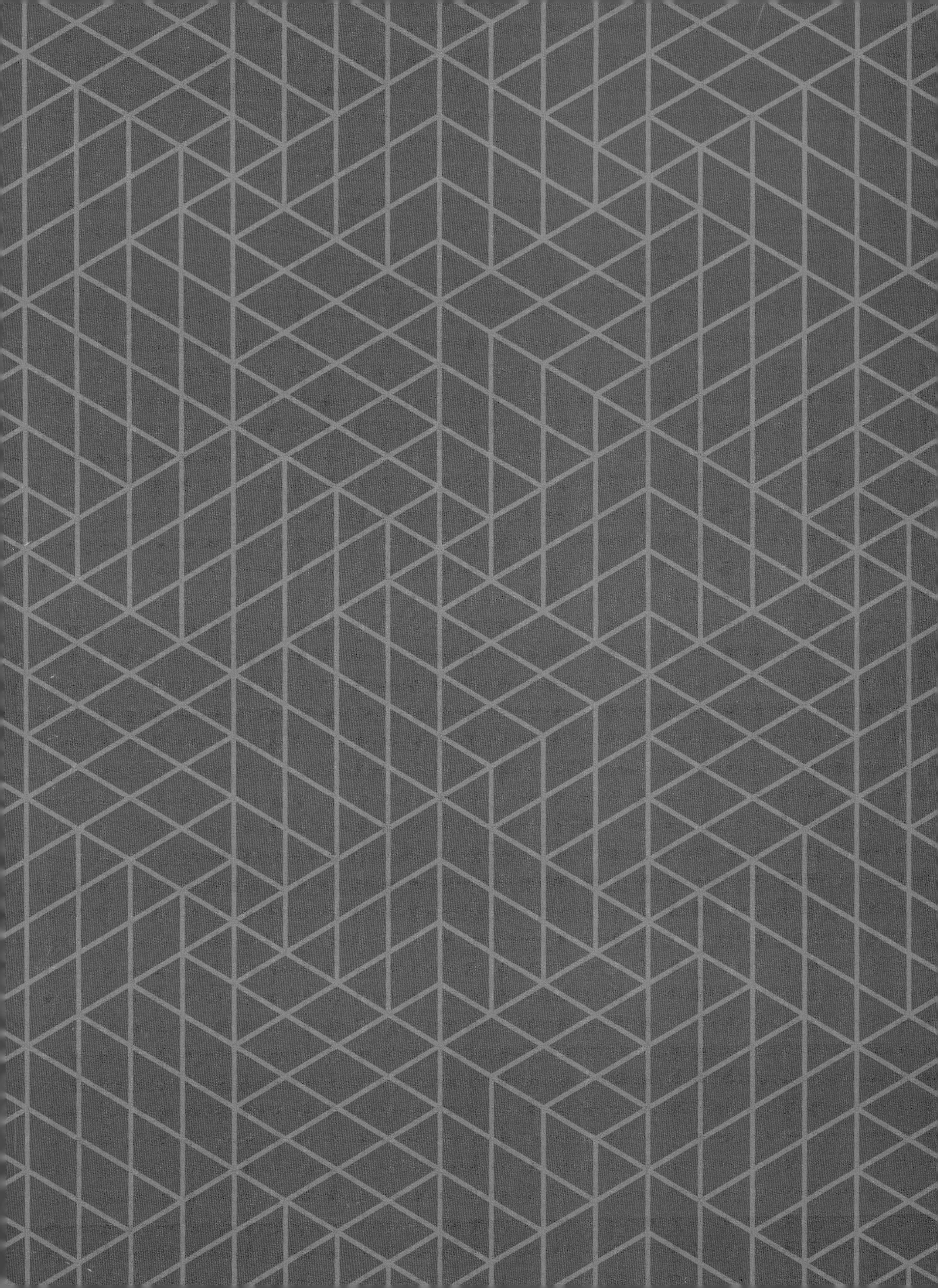

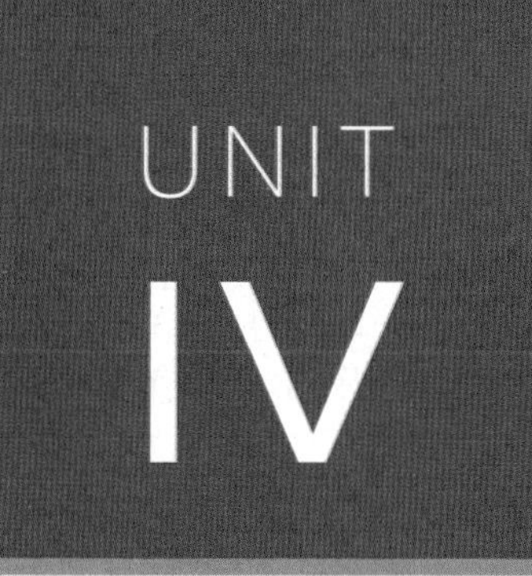

Nursing Care of the Child With a Health Disorder

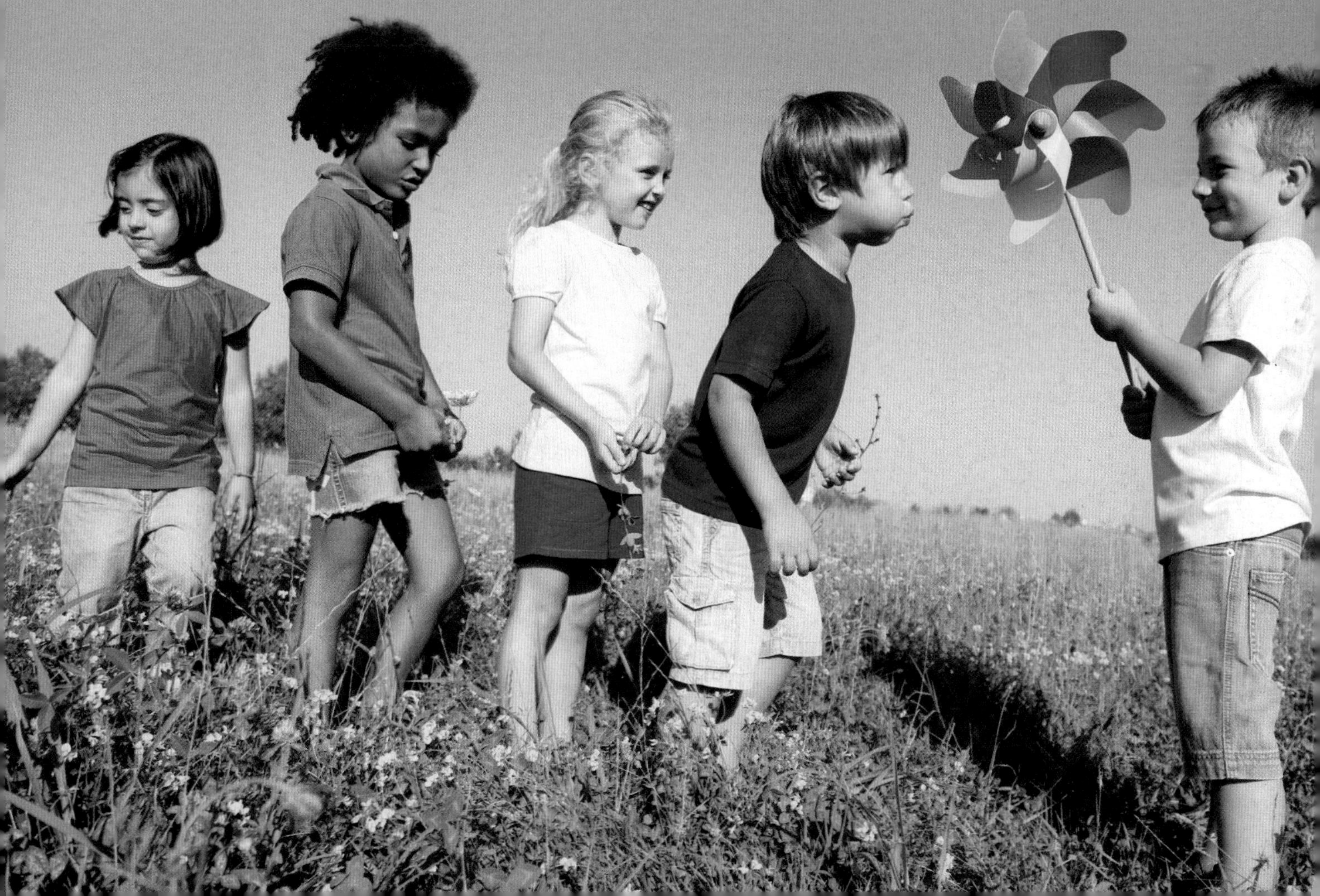

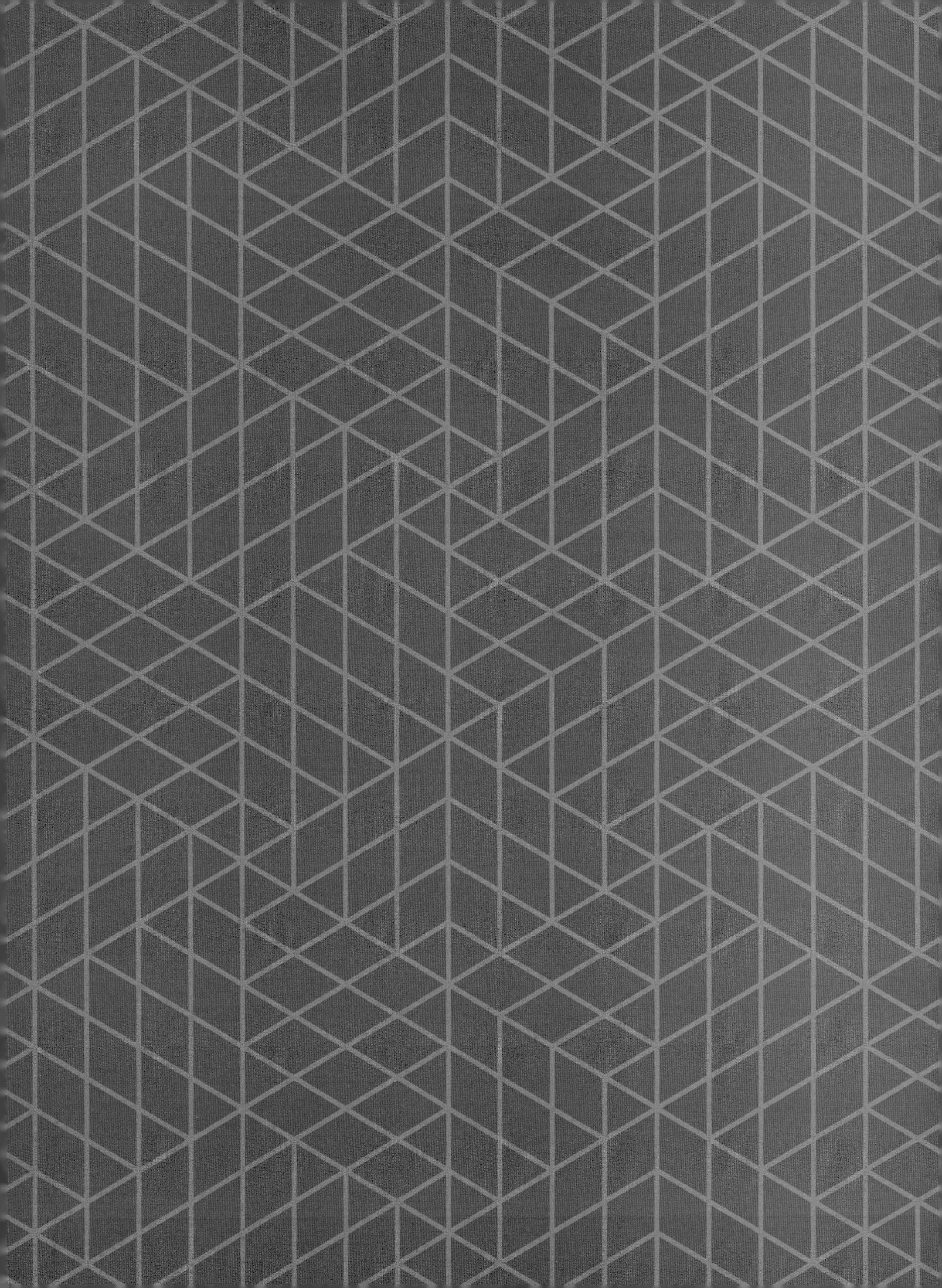

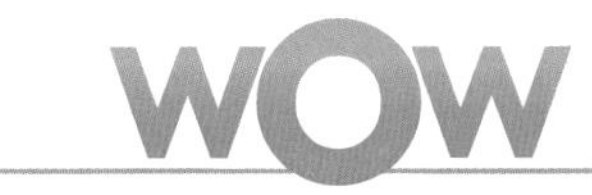

WORDS OF WISDOM

Complete and lasting freedom from infectious disease remains a dream, but one worth fighting a hard battle for.

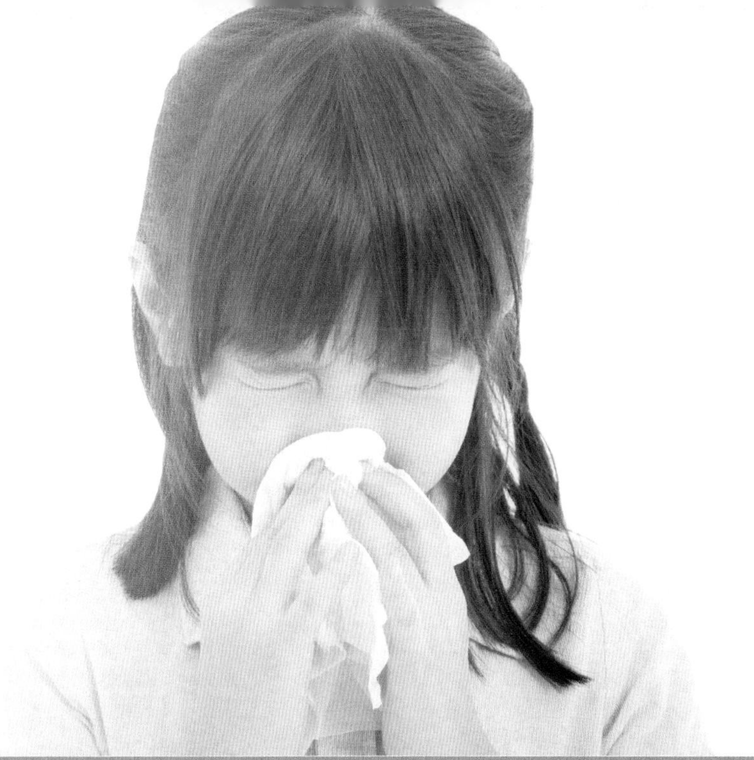

15

Nursing Care of the Child With an Infection

KEY TERMS

antibodies

antigen

chain of infection

communicability

endogenous pyrogens (en-doj´ĕ-nŭs pī´rō-jenz)

exanthem (eg-zan´thĕm)

phagocytosis (făg´ō-sī-tō´sis)

vector-borne

zoonotic (zō´ō-not´ik)

LEARNING OBJECTIVES

Upon completion of the chapter, you will be able to:

1. Discuss anatomic and physiologic differences in children versus adults in relation to the infectious process.
2. Identify nursing interventions related to common laboratory and diagnostic tests used in the diagnosis and management of infectious conditions.
3. Identify appropriate nursing assessments and interventions related to medications and treatments for childhood infectious and communicable disorders.
4. Distinguish various infectious illnesses occurring in childhood.
5. Devise an individualized plan of care for the child with an infectious or communicable disorder.
6. Develop child and family teaching plans for the child with an infectious or communicable disorder.

Samuel, 2 years old, is brought by his parent into the clinic. He presents with a history of fever and nasal congestion. His parent tells you, "He's been very irritable, crying more than usual and refusing to drink."

INTRODUCTION

Infection refers to the invasion of body cells and tissues by microorganisms with the potential to cause illness or disease (Nath, 2023). Nurses encounter potential or actual infections in all types of patients and must detect problems and intervene early to prevent life-threatening complications. Infections (infectious and communicable diseases) are one of the leading causes of death worldwide. As the world has become increasingly connected, infectious diseases have presented new challenges. Children are particularly vulnerable to these types of illnesses. Their immune systems are still developing and their natural curiosity, especially in infants and toddlers, leads to wide-range handling of objects and surfaces coupled with a tendency to place their hands and objects in their mouths without washing first. Infectious diseases in children can range in severity from mild with few or no symptoms to serious illness, such as damage to organs, and even death. Infectious and communicable diseases include bacterial infections (e.g., sepsis), viral infections (e.g., viral exanthems and rabies), zoonotic infections, vector-borne infections, parasitic and helminthic infections (e.g., roundworm and pediculosis capitis [head lice]), and sexually transmitted infections (STIs, e.g., chlamydia and gonorrhea).

There has been a dramatic decrease in the incidence and severity of infectious and communicable diseases since the advent of vaccines, antibiotics, antiviral drugs, and antitoxins. Some diseases have been effectively controlled, but the vast majority will not be eliminated. New diseases emerge and old diseases are reappearing, sometimes in a drug-resistant form. The Centers for Disease Control and Prevention (CDC) tracks certain infectious diseases. This list of nationally reportable diseases is revised periodically to add new pathogens or remove diseases as their incidence declines. Reporting by each state to the CDC is voluntary. Therefore, slight variations exist from state to state. Box 15.1 lists nationally reportable diseases.

Nurses, particularly those working in schools, child care centers, and outpatient settings, are often the first to see the signs of infectious or communicable diseases in children. These signs are often vague at first (e.g., a sore throat or rash). Therefore, nurses must have accurate assessment skills and be familiar with the signs and symptoms of common childhood infectious diseases so that they can provide prompt recognition, treatment, guidance, and support to families. Identifying the infectious agent is of primary importance to prevent further spread.

Many infectious diseases can be prevented through simple and inexpensive methods such as handwashing, adequate immunization, proper handling and preparation of food, and judicious antibiotic use. Nurses play a key role in educating parents and the community on ways to prevent infectious and communicable diseases.

BOX 15.1 Nationally Notifiable Diseases

- Botulism
- *Chlamydia trachomatis*
- COVID-19
- Diphtheria
- Ehrlichiosis
- Gonorrhea
- Hepatitis A, B, and C
- Influenza (pediatric mortality)
- Lyme disease
- Malaria
- Measles
- Meningococcal disease
- Mumps
- Pertussis
- Poliomyelitis, paralytic
- Poliovirus infection, nonparalytic
- Q fever
- Rabies
- Rocky Mountain spotted fever (spotted fever rickettsiosis)
- Rubella
- Syphilis
- Tetanus
- Tuberculosis
- Varicella (morbidity)
- Varicella (deaths only)

For a complete list of nationally notifiable diseases in the United States, go to https://ndc.services.cdc.gov/search-results-year.

HEALTHY PEOPLE 2030

Objective	Nursing Significance
Reduce the proportion of children who get no doses of recommended vaccines by age 2 years. Reduce cases of pertussis among infants. Maintain elimination of measles, rubella, congenital rubella syndrome (CRS), and acute paralytic poliomyelitis.	• Educate children and their families on the importance of proper immunizations. • Assess immunization status at every health encounter. • Provide families with a written record of immunizations given. • Promptly recognize infectious diseases, and provide child and family education regarding ways to prevent spread.

Healthy People Objectives retrieved from http://www.healthypeople.gov

INFECTIOUS PROCESS

Infection occurs when an organism enters the body and multiplies, causing damage to the tissues and cells. The body's response to this damage due to infection or injury is inflammation. The body delivers fluid, blood, and nutrients to the area of infection or injury and attempts to eliminate the pathogens and repair the tissues. The body does this through vascular and cellular reactions. The vascular response is an initial period of vasoconstriction followed by vasodilation. This vasodilation allows for the increase of fluids, blood, and nutrients to the area.

The cellular response involves the arrival of white blood cells (WBCs) to the area. WBCs are the body's defense against infection or injury. The types of WBCs are neutrophils, basophils, eosinophils, lymphocytes, and monocytes. Elevations in certain portions of the WBC count reflect different processes occurring in the body, such as infection, allergic reaction, or leukemia. Table 15.1 explains the function of each type of WBC. Each type is generally present in a balanced state; the types are reported as a percentage of the total WBC count or as the number per certain volume of blood.

TABLE 15.1 • Function of White Blood Cells by Leukocyte Type

Type of White Blood Cell	Function
Granulocytes • Neutrophils (polymorphonuclear leukocytes or PMNs, segs) • Eosinophils • Basophils	Phagocytic cells • First line of defense upon invasion of bacteria, fungus, cell debris, and other foreign substances • Respond to allergic disorders, parasitic infections, and chronic immune responses • Respond to allergic disorders and hypersensitivity reactions; used to study chronic inflammation
Lymphocytes (B lymphocytes, T lymphocytes, and natural killer cells)	Main source of producing an immune response; respond to viral infections (measles, rubella, chickenpox, infectious mononucleosis); tumors
Monocytes	Second line of defense; respond to larger and more severe infections than neutrophils by phagocytosis; leukemias and lymphomas; chronic inflammation

Data from Fischbach, F. T., Fischbach, M. A., & Stout, K. (2022). *A manual of laboratory and diagnostic tests* (11th ed.). Wolters Kluwer.

WBCs use **phagocytosis** to ingest and destroy the pathogen. If bacteria escape the action of phagocytosis, they enter the bloodstream and lymph system, and the immune system is activated. With activation of the immune system, B lymphocytes (humoral immunity) and T lymphocytes (cell-mediated immunity) are matured and activated. B and T cells recognize and attack infectious pathogens. B cells, which mature in the bone marrow, produce specific **antibodies** (specialized immune proteins) that bind to and neutralize a specific offending **antigen** (a substance that the body recognizes as foreign). T cells, which mature in the thymus, attack the antigen directly. Once B and T cells have been exposed to an antigen, some cells will remember the antigen. Therefore, if the particular antigen invades again, the body will act more quickly. A third type of lymphocyte, natural killer cells are a part of the innate immune system and function to destroy foreign material present.

Fever

Infection or inflammation caused by bacteria, viruses, or other pathogens stimulates the release of **endogenous pyrogens** (interleukins, tumor necrosis factor, and interferon). The pyrogens act on the hypothalamus, where they trigger prostaglandin production and increase the body's temperature set point. This triggers the cold response, resulting in shivering, vasoconstriction, and a decrease in peripheral perfusion to help decrease heat loss and allow the body's temperature to rise to the new set point, therefore resulting in fever. The definition of fever varies based on the age of the child, the method of temperature measurement, and the presence of any underlying conditions. There is no single value defined for fever due to individual variations, but Box 15.2 shows generally accepted guidelines based on measurement route in an otherwise healthy child. Refer to Chapter 10 for further information on measurement of temperature.

It is important to distinguish between fever and hyperthermia. Hyperthermia occurs when normal thermoregulation fails, resulting in an unregulated rise in core temperature. Hyperthermia may occur if the central nervous system of the child becomes impaired by disease, drugs, and abnormalities of heat production or thermal

BOX 15.2 General Guideline of Fever Based on Measurement Route

- Oral: >37.8°C (100°F)
- Rectal: >38°C (100.4°F)
- Axillary: >37.2°C (99°F)
- Tympanic: >38°C (100.4°F)
- Temporal: >38°C (100.4°F)

stressors, such as being left in a hot automobile or exertional heat stroke. In the absence of hyperthermia or neurologic impairment, the body does not allow fever to rise to lethal levels. The body actually produces a natural antipyretic, called cryogen. If there is no hyperthermic insult, it is rare to see a child's temperature rise above 41°C (105.8°F) (Ward, 2022).

Fever in their children is one of the most common reasons parents seek medical attention (Sullivan et al., 2011, reaffirmed 2023). Most infections or communicable diseases are accompanied by fever. Many parents have great concerns about fever. For example, they fear febrile seizures, neurologic complications, and a potential serious underlying disease. Many health care providers share these fears. This leads to the common recommendation to intervene and reduce fever. These fears and misconceptions about fever can lead to mismanagement of fever, such as inappropriate dosing of antipyretics, awakening the child during sleep to give antipyretics, or inappropriate use of nonpharmacologic treatments such as sponging the child with alcohol or cold water (Sullivan et al., 2011, reaffirmed 2023).

Fever is a protective mechanism the body uses to fight infection. Evidence exists that an elevated body temperature actually enhances various components of the immune response (Sullivan et al., 2011, reaffirmed 2023). Fever can slow the growth of bacteria and viruses and increase neutrophil production and T-cell proliferation (Sullivan et al., 2011, reaffirmed 2023). Another concern is that reducing fever may hide signs of serious bacterial illness (Sullivan et al., 2011, reaffirmed 2023).

TAKE NOTE!

Infants younger than 3 months with a rectal temperature greater than 38°C (100.4°F) should be seen by a health care provider or nurse practitioner.

Antipyretics are often used to lower fever and increase comfort. They decrease the temperature set point by inhibiting the production of prostaglandins. As a result, sweating and vasodilation occur, and there is heat loss and a drop in temperature. Antipyretics provide symptomatic relief but do not change the course of the infection. The major benefits of decreasing fever are increasing comfort in the child and decreasing fluid requirements, which helps to prevent dehydration. Children with certain underlying conditions, such as cardiovascular disease or pulmonary disease, also benefit from treating fever because such treatment decreases demands on the body. The use of acetaminophen or ibuprofen to reduce fever in children has been shown to be safe and effective when the appropriate dose is administered at the appropriate interval (Ward, 2022). However, some studies have shown that ibuprofen is superior in reducing fever and lasts longer than acetaminophen (Ward, 2022). Box 15.3 gives dosing recommendations for both medications.

BOX 15.3 Dose Recommendations for Oral Acetaminophen and Ibuprofen

Acetaminophen, 10–15 mg/kg/dose
- No more than every 4 hours
- No more than five doses in a 24-hour period
- Not to exceed 4,000 mg/day

Ibuprofen, 4–10 mg/kg/dose
- Only children older than 6 months of age
- Given every 6–8 hours; no more than four doses in a 24-hour period
- Maximum daily dose: 2,400 mg/day

Source: Lexicomp. (2023). Pediatric drug information. *UpToDate*. Retrieved April 5, 2023, from https://www.uptodate.com/contents/table-of-contents/drug-information/pediatric-drug-information

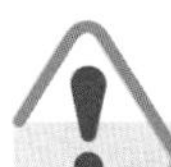

CLINICAL REASONING ALERT!

Never give aspirin or aspirin-containing products to children to reduce fever, due to the risk of Reye syndrome.

Acetaminophen is widely used and accepted, with a long track record of safety and efficacy when used according to the label directions, but overdose can lead to toxic reactions (Ward, 2022). Causes of acetaminophen toxicity include overdosing or incorrect dosing due to failure to read and understand the label instructions, use of an incorrect measuring device or concentration, and coadministration with an over-the-counter, fixed-dose combination medication (the parent may not recognize that it has acetaminophen in it).

Another factor that may cause acetaminophen toxicity is the controversial, but common, practice of alternating acetaminophen and ibuprofen to help reduce fever. Although insufficient evidence exists to support or refute alternating or combining acetaminophen with ibuprofen to treat fever, safety concerns remain (Sullivan et al., 2011, reaffirmed 2023). This practice can result in overdose or improper administration. It can be hard for parents to keep track of the time each medication is due. Parents may confuse which medication is given every 4 hours and which is given every 6 hours. They may exceed the recommended daily doses or may confuse the strength or dosage of the medicines. In some cases, alternating or combining acetaminophen and ibuprofen may be needed if the child's distress or discomfort persists or recurs before the next dose is due. In these cases, careful and thorough dosing instructions and intervals are imperative. See Evidence-Based Practice 15.1.

EVIDENCE-BASED PRACTICE 15.1

Which Is More Effective in Treating Fever in Children—Ibuprofen or Acetaminophen? Combined, Alternating, or Alone?

Fever is one of the most common health concerns seen in pediatrics, and it is an important component of the body's response to infection. Although ibuprofen (IBU) and acetaminophen (APAP) are the most widely used antipyretics and are recommended by the American Academy of Pediatrics (AAP), the question of safety and efficacy of one over the other and combining or alternating for fever reduction continues.

STUDY

This study was a narrative review of randomized, blinded, controlled studies assessing the effectiveness of IBU versus APAP, combined, alternating, or alone in reducing fever in children. This review compared health care provider dosing (IBU 10/mg; APAP 15 mg/kg) to over-the-counter (OTC) dosing (IBU 5 to 10 mg/kg; APAP 10 to 15 mg/kg) for both IBU and APAP.

Findings

This study suggests a modest improvement in fever reduction with IBU over APAP at OTC dosing but similar effectiveness in health care provider dosing. Combining or alternating IBU and APAP seems to provide a better reduction in fever and to be well tolerated.

Nursing Implications

According to the AAP, improvement of the child's overall comfort, not just reducing fever, should be the goal of antipyretic therapy. Therefore, future research is warranted focusing on this outcome. Future research also needs to focus on evaluating the effectiveness of combined versus alternating antipyretic therapy and safety concerns with these approaches. Nurses need to continue to educate parents regarding why fever occurs, fever facts and myths, when treatment of fever is necessary, and best treatment options.

Data from Paul, I. M., & Walson, P. D. (2021). Acetaminophen and ibuprofen in the treatment of pediatric fever: a narrative review. *Current Medical Research and Opinion, 37*(8), 1363–1375. https://doi.org/10.1080/03007995.2021.1928617

DOSAGE CALCULATION BOX 15.1

The nurse is caring for a toddler who is 2 years old and 28 lb. The order reads ibuprofen 100 mg po every 6 hours as needed for temperature greater than 38°C (100.4°F). Is this a safe and effective dose?

Stages of Infectious Disease

Infectious diseases follow a similar pattern. They progress through certain stages (Table 15.2) in which **communicability** (ability to spread to others) can be predicted. It is important for nurses to understand these stages to help control and manage infectious diseases.

TABLE 15.2 • Stages of Infectious Disease

Stage	Explanation
Incubation	Time from entrance of pathogen into the body to appearance of first symptoms; during this time, pathogens grow and multiply.
Prodrome	Time from onset of nonspecific symptoms such as fever, malaise, and fatigue to more specific symptoms
Illness	Time during which child demonstrates signs and symptoms specific to an infection type
Convalescence	Time when acute symptoms of illness disappear

Chain of Infection

The **chain of infection** is the process by which an organism is spread. Behaviors of infants and young children, mainly pertaining to hygiene, increase their risk for infection by promoting the chain of infection. Poor hygiene habits, including lack of handwashing, placing toys and hands in the mouth, drooling, and leaking diapers, all can contribute to the spread of infection and communicable diseases. Table 15.3 reviews the chain of infection and nursing implications related to it.

Preventing the Spread of Infection

Nurses play a key role in breaking the chain of infection and preventing the spread of diseases. It is important to follow infection control and prevention practices. It is also very important to educate parents and children on the measures they can take to prevent the spread of infection.

TAKE NOTE!

Frequent handwashing is the most important way to prevent the spread of infection.

Isolation precautions help nurses break the chain of infection and provide strategies to prevent the spread of pathogens among hospitalized children. Guidelines can be found on the CDC website (http://www.cdc.gov/hicpac/2007IP/2007isolationPrecautions.html). Additional guidelines are available from various infection control societies and regulatory agencies such as the

TABLE 15.3 • Chain of Infection

Chain Link	Explanation	Nursing Implications
Infectious agent	Any agent capable of causing infection; examples: bacteria, viruses, rickettsiae, protozoa, and fungi	Control or eliminate infectious agents through: • Handwashing • Wearing gloves • Cleaning, disinfecting, or sterilizing equipment
Reservoir	A place where the pathogen can thrive and reproduce; examples: human body, animals, insects, food, water, inanimate objects (e.g., stethoscopes)	• Control or eliminate reservoirs. • Control sources of body fluids, drainage, or solutions that may harbor pathogens. • Follow institutional guidelines for disposing of infectious wastes. • Provide proper wound care; change dressings or bandages when soiled. • Assist children to carry out appropriate skin and oral care. • Keep linens clean and dry.
Portal of exit	A way for the pathogen to exit the reservoir; examples: skin and mucous membranes, respiratory tract, urinary tract, gastrointestinal tract, reproductive tract	• Control portals of exit and educate children and families. • Cover mouth and nose when sneezing or coughing. • Avoid talking, coughing, or sneezing over open wounds or sterile fields. • Use personal protective equipment.
Modes of transmission	Direct transmission: body-to-body contact Indirect transmission: transferred by fomite or vector; spread by droplet or airborne transmission	• Wash hands before and after child contact, invasive procedures, or touching open wounds. • Use personal protective equipment when necessary. • Urge children and family to wash hands frequently, especially before eating or handling food, after eliminating, and after touching infectious material.
Portal of entry	A way for the pathogen to enter the host; examples: skin and mucous membranes, respiratory tract, urinary tract, gastrointestinal tract, reproductive tract	• Use proper sterile technique during invasive procedures. • Provide appropriate wound care. • Dispose of needles and sharps in puncture-resistant containers. • Provide all children with their own personal care items.
Susceptible host	Any person who cannot resist the pathogen	• Protect susceptible host by promoting normal body defenses against infection. • Maintain integrity of the child's skin and mucous membranes. • Protect normal defenses by regular bathing and oral care, adequate fluid intake and nutrition, and proper immunization.

Occupational Safety and Health Administration (OSHA) agency. The Joint Commission has also developed infection control standards. This leads to an array of complex guidelines that all health professionals need to be familiar with.

The Hospital Infection Control Practices Advisory Committee (HICPAC) has presented guidelines for hospitalized children that include two tiers (Siegel et al., 2007, updated 2022). Tier 1 is standard precautions, which are designed for the care of all children in the hospital regardless of their diagnosis. Tier 2 is transmission-based precautions, designed for children who are known, or suspected, to be infected with epidemiologically important pathogens. These pathogens can be spread by airborne, droplet, or contact transmission. Box 15.4 gives an overview of standard and transmission-based precautions.

TAKE NOTE!

Hand hygiene includes both handwashing with soap and water and the use of alcohol-based products (gels, rinses, foams) that do not require water. If there is no visible soiling of the hands, approved alcohol-based products are preferred because of their superior microbicidal activity, reduced drying of the skin, and convenience (Anderson, 2023; CDC, 2020a).

BOX 15.4 Standard Precautions and Isolation Precautions

Standard Precautions (Tier 1)

- Apply to all children.
- Apply to all body fluids, secretions, and excretions except sweat, nonintact skin, and mucous membranes.
- Designed to reduce the risk of transmission of microorganisms from recognized and unrecognized sources
- Techniques include:
  - Proper hand hygiene
  - Use of gloves (clean or sterile) when touching blood, body fluids, secretions or excretions, and contaminated items
  - Masks, eye protection, and face shields when patient care may include splashing or sprays of blood, body fluid secretions, or excretions, and during bronchoscopy, endotracheal intubation, and open suctioning of the respiratory tract
  - Fluid-resistant nonsterile gowns, to protect skin and clothing, when patient care may include splashing or sprays of blood, body fluid secretions, or excretions
  - Patient care equipment handled in a manner that prevents skin or mucous membrane exposure and contamination of clothing
  - All used linen is considered contaminated and needs to be handled and disposed of appropriately.
  - Mouthpieces, resuscitation bags with one-way valves, and other ventilation devices should be readily available.
  - Cleaning and disinfecting noncritical surfaces in patient care areas
  - Respiratory hygiene/cough etiquette: applies to any person with signs of illness including cough, congestion, rhinorrhea, or increased respiratory secretions that is entering a health care facility. It includes education regarding covering the mouth/nose with a tissue; prompt disposal of used tissues, along with surgical masks used by a person who is coughing when appropriate; hand hygiene after contact with respiratory secretions; and separation, ideally greater than 3 ft, of people with respiratory infections in common waiting areas when possible.
  - Safe injection practices: use of sterile single-use disposable needle. When possible, use of single-dose vials; precautions used to prevent injury when using, cleaning, or disposing of needles and sharps
  - Use of masks for insertion of catheters or injection into the spinal or epidural space via lumbar puncture procedures

Transmission-Based Precautions (Tier 2)

Designed for children with known or suspected infection with pathogens for which additional precautions are warranted to interrupt transmission

Airborne

- Designed to reduce the risk of infectious agents transmitted by airborne droplet nuclei or dust particles that may contain the infectious agent
- Examples of such illnesses include measles, varicella, and tuberculosis.
- Techniques include standard precautions as well as:
  - Room with negative air pressure ventilation, with air externally exhausted or high-efficiency particulate air filtered if recirculated; if unavailable, mask the child and place in private room with the door closed.
  - Wear a mask or respirator depending on specific recommendations based on disease, such as if infectious pulmonary tuberculosis is suspected or proven, wear a respiratory protective device, such as an N95 respirator, while in the child's room.
  - Susceptible health care personnel should not enter the room of children with measles or varicella zoster infections. Those with proven immunity to these viruses need not wear a mask.

Droplet

- Intended to prevent transmission of pathogens spread through close respiratory or mucous membrane contact with respiratory secretions. Designed to reduce the risk of infectious agents transmitted by contact of the conjunctivae or the mucous membranes of the nose or mouth of a susceptible person with large-particle droplets containing pathogens generated from a person (generally through coughing, sneezing, talking, or procedures such as suctioning) who has a clinical disease or who is a carrier of the disease
- Examples of such illnesses include diphtheria, pertussis, group A streptococcal disease, influenza, mumps, rubella, and scarlet fever.
- Techniques include standard precautions as well as:
  - Private room (if unavailable, consider cohorting children with the same disease. If this is not possible, separation of at least 3 ft between other children and visitors should be maintained.)
  - Wear a mask if within 3 ft of the child.

Contact

- Most important and most common route of transmission of health care–associated infections
- Designed to reduce the risk of infectious agents transmitted by direct or indirect contact. Direct-contact transmission involves skin-to-skin contact and physical transfer of pathogens between a susceptible host and an infected or colonized person. Examples include patient care activities that involve physical contact such as turning and bathing. Direct-contact transmission also can occur between two children, where one serves as the source of infectious pathogen and the other as a susceptible host. Indirect-contact transmission involves contact of a susceptible host with a contaminated intermediate object, usually inanimate, in the child's environment.
- Examples of such illnesses include diphtheria,[a] pediculosis, scabies, and multidrug-resistant bacteria.
- Techniques include standard precautions as well as:
  - Private room (if unavailable, consultation with infection control personnel is recommended. Consider cohorting children with the same disease. If this is not possible, separation of at least 3 ft between other children and visitors should be maintained.)
  - Gloves (clean or sterile) should be used at all times.
  - Proper hand hygiene after glove removal
  - Use gloves and gowns for all interactions that involve contact with the child or potentially contaminated areas. Don before entering and remove before leaving the child's room.

Prevention standards are applied in all health care settings and are modified to meet each setting's unique needs. Health care workers must practice within the specific institution's guidelines.

[a]Certain infections require more than one precaution.

Data from Siegel, J. D., Rhinehart, E., Jackson, M., Chiarello, L., & The Healthcare Infection Control Practices Advisory Committee. (2007, updated 2022). Guideline for isolation precautions: Preventing transmission of infectious agents in healthcare settings. https://www.cdc.gov/infectioncontrol/pdf/guidelines/isolation-guidelines-H.pdf

CLINICAL REASONING ALERT!

When caring for a child with suspected or confirmed norovirus or *Clostridioides* (formerly *Clostridium*) *difficile* ensure handwashing is performed using soap and water as alcohol does not kill these microorganisms (Anderson, 2023).

When caring for children, these guidelines may need to be modified. For instance, diaper changing is routine in the pediatric setting. Since it does not usually soil hands, it is not mandatory to wear gloves (except if gloves are required due to transmission-based precautions). According to the standard precaution guidelines, single rooms are required for those who are incontinent and cannot control bodily excretions. Since the majority of young children are incontinent, obviously this guideline is inappropriate in the pediatric setting. Pediatric units often have common rooms, such as playrooms and schoolrooms. Children placed on transmission-based isolation are not allowed to leave their rooms and therefore are not allowed to use these common rooms.

VARIATIONS IN PEDIATRIC ANATOMY AND PHYSIOLOGY

Normal immune function is an amazing protective response by the body. It involves complex responses including phagocytosis, humoral immunity, cellular immunity, and activation of the complement system. Blood and lymph are responsible for transporting the agents of the immune system. Due to the immature responses of the immune system, infants and young children are more susceptible to infection. The newborn displays a decreased inflammatory response to invading organisms, contributing to an increased risk for infection. Cellular immunity is generally functional at birth, and humoral immunity occurs when the body encounters and then develops immunity to new diseases. Since the infant has had limited exposure to disease and is losing the passive immunity acquired from maternal antibodies, the risk of infection is higher. Young children continue to have an increased risk for infection and communicable disorders because disease protection from immunizations is not complete. (Refer to Chapter 9 for further details.)

COMMON MEDICAL TREATMENTS

A variety of medications and other medical treatments are used to treat infectious disorders in children. Most of these treatments will require a health care provider's or nurse practitioner's order when the child is in the hospital. The most common treatments and medications are listed in Common Medical Treatments 15.1 and Drug Guide 15.1. The nurse caring for the child with an infectious disorder should be familiar with what the procedures are, how they work, and common nursing implications related to use of these modalities.

COMMON MEDICAL TREATMENTS 15.1

Treatment	Explanation	Indications	Nursing Implications
Hydration	Promoting proper fluid balance either orally or intravenously	Child who can't replace insensible loss due to fever, child who is vomiting or has diarrhea	• Encourage oral fluids, if possible. • Offer child preferred fluid; try popsicles or games to promote fluid intake. • If administering IV fluids, ensure proper fluid and rate per order and assess IV site and fluid intake every hour. • Maintain strict record of intake and output.
Fever reduction	Reducing temperature by use of antipyretics or nonpharmacologic interventions	Febrile child who is uncomfortable or who can't keep up with the increased metabolic demands associated with fever	• Administer antipyretics, such as ibuprofen and acetaminophen. • Avoid aspirin use in children and adolescents. • Use nonpharmacologic interventions such as dressing lightly, removing blankets, use of a fan, tepid bath, and cooling blanket. Make sure that nonpharmacologic measures do not induce shivering or discomfort. If they do, they should be stopped immediately.

IV, intravenous.

DRUG GUIDE 15.1

COMMON DRUGS FOR COMMUNICABLE DISORDERS

Medication	Actions/Indications	Nursing Implications
Antibiotics	Kill and prevent the growth of bacteria. Used for the treatment of bacterial infections such as sepsis	• Check for antibiotic allergies. • Give as prescribed for the length of time prescribed.
Antivirals (e.g., acyclovir)	Kill and prevent the growth of viruses. Used for the treatment of viral infections such as herpes simplex type 2	• Observe infusion site for signs of tissue damage. • If administering topically, clean and dry area before application and wear gloves. • Give as prescribed for the length of time prescribed.
Antipyretics (acetaminophen, ibuprofen)	Decrease the temperature set point (only in a child with a raised temperature) by inhibiting the production of prostaglandins, leading to heat loss (through vasodilation and sweating) and resulting in a reduction in fever. Used to decrease temperature in the febrile child who is uncomfortable or who can't keep up with the increased metabolic demands associated with fever	• Ensure proper dosing, concentration, and dosing interval. • Avoid aspirin use in children and adolescents. • Avoid ibuprofen use in children with a bleeding disorder. • Assess fever and any related symptoms such as tachycardia, shivering, or diaphoresis. • Properly educate caregivers on appropriate dosing, concentration, dosing interval, and use of accurate measuring device.
Antipruritics (usually antihistamines)	Given orally or topically to block the histamine reaction Used to relieve discomfort associated with itching	• When applying topically, wear gloves. • Do not apply to open wounds. • Oral antihistamines may cause drowsiness.

Adapted from Lexicomp. (2023). Pediatric drug information. *UpToDate*. Retrieved April 5, 2023, from https://www.uptodate.com/contents/table-of-contents/drug-information/pediatric-drug-information

Clinical Judgment and the Nursing Process for the Child With an Infection

Care of the child with an infectious or communicable disorder includes assessment, nursing analysis, planning, interventions, and evaluation. There are a number of general concepts related to the nursing process that may be applied to the care of children with infectious disorders. From a general understanding of the care involved for a child with an infectious disorder, the nurse can then individualize the care based on the child's specifics.

Assessment

Assessment of the child with a communicable or infectious disorder includes health history, physical examination, and laboratory and diagnostic testing.

Health History

The health history consists of the past medical history, including the birthing parent's pregnancy history; family history; and history of present illness (when the symptoms started and how they have progressed), as well as treatments used at home. The past medical history might be significant for lack of recommended immunizations, prematurity, infection during birthing parent's pregnancy or labor, prolonged difficult delivery, or immunocompromise. Family history might be significant for lack of immunization or recent infectious or communicable disease. When eliciting the history of the present illness, inquire about the following:

- Any known exposure to infectious or communicable disease
- Immunization history
- History of having any common childhood communicable diseases
- Fever
- Sore throat
- Lethargy
- Malaise
- Poor feeding or decreased appetite
- Vomiting
- Diarrhea
- Cough
- Rash (in the older child ask for a description [i.e., Is it painful? Does it itch?])

TAKE NOTE!

Many childhood infections and communicable diseases involve a rash. Rashes can be difficult to identify. Therefore, it is important to obtain a thorough description and history from the caregiver.

Physical Examination

Physical examination of the child with an infectious disorder includes inspection, observation, and palpation.

INSPECTION AND OBSERVATION

Begin the physical examination with inspection and observation. Assess the child's skin, mouth, throat, and hair for lesions or wounds. Note the color, shape, and distribution of any lesions or wounds. Assess whether there is any exudate from the lesions or wounds. A thorough and accurate description is important to assist in identifying the rash and causative organism. Observe for scratching, restlessness, avoidance of the use of a body part, or guarding of a body part. Observe the child's affect, energy level, and interaction with caregivers. Lethargy can indicate serious infection or sepsis. Observe if there is any discharge from the nose, cough, or respiratory difficulty.

Assess hydration status. Inspect the oral mucosa; dry and pale mucous membranes can indicate dehydration. Observe for other signs of dehydration, such as sunken eyes and no tears with crying.

Assessment of vital signs can provide more information about the child's condition. Elevated temperature can indicate infection. Often tachypnea and tachycardia accompany fever. Hypotension may also occur, but it is usually a late sign with sepsis.

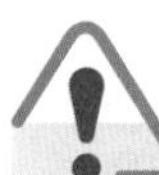

CLINICAL REASONING ALERT!

Neonates and young infants may not present with fever; some may present with normal or low temperatures and have serious infections (Cantey, 2023; Scarfone & Cho, 2022).

PALPATION

Palpate the skin to assess temperature, moisture, texture, and turgor. In a child with an infectious or communicable disease, the skin may be warm and moist due to fever. Turgor may be decreased secondary to dehydration. In infants, palpate the fontanels; if they are sunken, the infant may be dehydrated. Palpate the rash to determine if it is raised or flat. A thorough picture of the presenting rash can help identify the child's illness. Palpate the lymph nodes and note any that are swollen and tender.

Laboratory and Diagnostic Testing

Common Laboratory and Diagnostic Tests 15.1 discusses the tests used most commonly when communicable disorders are suspected. The tests can assist the health care provider or nurse practitioner in diagnosing the disorder and/or be used as guidelines in determining ongoing treatment. Laboratory or non-nursing personnel obtain some of the tests, while the nurse might obtain others. In either instance, the nurse should be familiar with how the tests are obtained, what they

COMMON LABORATORY AND DIAGNOSTIC TESTS 15.1

Test	Explanation	Indications	Nursing Implications
Complete blood count (CBC)	Evaluate white blood cell count (particularly the percentage of individual white cells).	Detect the presence of inflammation, infection.	• Normal values vary according to age and sex. • White blood cell count differential is helpful in differentiating source of infection. • May be affected by myelosuppressive drugs
Erythrocyte sedimentation rate (ESR)	Nonspecific test used in conjunction with other tests to determine presence of infection or inflammation	Detect the presence of inflammation, infection.	Send to laboratory quickly; specimens allowed to stand for longer than 24 hours may produce a falsely low result.
Standard C-reactive protein (CRP)	Nonspecific test that measures a type of protein produced in the liver that is present during episodes of acute inflammation or infection Usually used to diagnose acute infections	To detect the presence of infection, CRP is a more sensitive and rapidly responding indicator than ESR.	Do not confuse it with high-sensitivity CRP, which measures a different range and is used to evaluate cardiovascular risk.
Blood culture and sensitivity	Deliberate growing of microorganism in a solid or liquid medium. Once it has grown, it is tested against various antibiotics to determine which antibiotics will kill it.	Detect the presence of bacteria or yeast, which may have spread from a certain site in the body into the bloodstream. Determine which antibiotics the bacteria or yeast is sensitive to.	• Follow aseptic technique and hospital protocol to prevent contamination. • Two cultures obtained from two different sites are preferred. • Ideally obtain before administering antibiotics; if child is taking antibiotics, notify laboratory and draw specimen shortly before next dose. • Draw below intravenous line, if possible, to prevent dilution of sample.

COMMON LABORATORY AND DIAGNOSTIC TESTS 15.1

Test	Explanation	Indications	Nursing Implications
Stool culture (including stool for ova and parasites [O&P])	To determine if bacteria or parasite have infected the intestines	Detect pathogens, including parasites or overgrowth of normal flora in the bowel. Indicated for children with diarrhea, fever, or abdominal pain	• Stool must be free of urine, water, and toilet paper. • Do not retrieve out of toilet water. • Obtain freshly passed stool. • Deliver to laboratory immediately. • Mineral oil, barium, and bismuth interfere with the detection of parasites; specimen collection should be delayed for 7–10 days. • Often a minimum of three specimens on 3 separate days are required for adequate examination, since many parasites and worm eggs are shed intermittently.
Urine culture	Collection of urine to detect the presence of bacteria in the urine	Detect the presence of bacteria in the urinary tract. Indicated for children with fever of unknown origin, dysuria, frequency, or urgency, or if urinalysis suggests infection	• Should be obtained by midstream clean-catch, catheterization, or suprapubic aspiration. Avoid contamination with stool, vaginal secretions, hands, or clothing. • Placing bags on the perineum is not preferred due to high chance of contamination; if used, analyze specimen as soon as possible. • Obtain before antibiotics are administered. • Deliver to laboratory immediately (preferable) or refrigerate.
Wound culture	Allows for microbial growth and identification of specific organism	Identification of specific organism	• Do not take from exudate or eschar. • If moderate to heavy drainage is present, irrigate the wound with sterile saline. Disinfect the surface of the wound. • Specimens taken from wounds can harbor a variety of organisms. Pathogenicity depends on the quantity of organisms present. • Avoid touching intact skin at the wound edges. • Culture highly vascular granulation tissue.
Throat culture	Vigorous swabbing of the tonsillar area and posterior pharynx to detect the presence of invasive organisms	Most reliable method of detecting group A streptococcal pharyngitis Will also detect *Bordetella pertussis*, *Corynebacterium diphtheriae*; viral infections May be performed in those with fever of unknown origin	• Ensure specimen is of secretions in the pharyngeal or tonsillar area. Avoid touching tongue or lips with swab. • When performing on young children, have adult hold child in lap. • Health care worker needs to stabilize head by placing hand on the child's forehead.
Nasal swabs (nasopharyngeal)	Insertion of swabs into the nose until reaching the nasopharynx to detect the presence of invasive organisms	Optimal method for detecting *B. pertussis.* Also used to detect *Corynebacterium diphtheriae* and viral illnesses such as *respiratory syncytial virus* (RSV), *parainfluenza*	• The distance from the child's nose to ear gives an estimate of how far to insert the swab into the nostril to reach the nasopharynx. • Insert swab straight back, not up, and leave in nasopharynx for several seconds. • When performing on young children, have adult hold child in lap. • Health care worker needs to stabilize head as child will likely try to pull away.

Data from Fischbach, F. T., Fischbach, M. A., & Stout, K. (2022). *A manual of laboratory and diagnostic tests* (11th ed.). Wolters Kluwer.

are used for, and normal versus abnormal results. This knowledge will also be necessary when providing child and family education related to the testing.

OBTAINING BLOOD SPECIMENS

Giving a blood specimen may be frightening to children because of the fear of needles, pain, and blood loss. Provide atraumatic care when performing venipunctures and other needlesticks in children (refer to Chapter 8 for further information). Whether the laboratory technician or the nurse is drawing the blood, the procedure should be performed in an area other than the child's bed, such as the treatment room; the child's bed should be kept as a "safe" area. Provide teaching about the procedure based on the child's developmental level and readiness to learn. In infants and younger children, additional assistance with positioning and restraint will be needed to perform the procedure safely and to ensure proper collection. Use a topical anesthetic cream or gel (preferred), refrigerant spray, or iontophoresis before venipuncture. Refer to Chapter 14 for additional information about decreasing venipuncture-related pain in infants and children.

The usual sites for obtaining blood specimens via venipuncture are the superficial veins of the dorsal surface of the hand or the antecubital fossa, although other locations may also be used. In specific situations, the jugular or femoral vein may be used; in this case either the health care provider or the nurse practitioner will perform the venipuncture.

Capillary puncture of the child's fingertip, the great toe, or the infant's heel may also be used to obtain blood specimens. Fingertip puncture is similar to that in the adult, directed to the sides of the fingertip. Great toe puncture is performed in the same way. Capillary heel puncture must be performed in the proper location to avoid striking the medial plantar artery or periosteum (see Nursing Procedure 15.1). Automatic lancet devices can be used to deliver a more precise puncture depth.

ATRAUMATIC CARE

The young infant will benefit from the use of oral sucrose combined with nonnutritive sucking, skin-to-skin contact, and/or swaddling before and during the capillary puncture (Roué, 2022).

Occasionally, blood samples may be obtained from an artery rather than a vein or capillary. Blood gases in particular are usually obtained by arterial puncture. Arterial puncture requires additional training and in many institutions is performed only by the respiratory therapist, health care provider, or nurse practitioner.

Children with indwelling venous access devices may be spared the trauma of puncture for blood specimens. Follow your institution's guidelines for withdrawing blood from peripherally inserted venous

NURSING PROCEDURE 15.1 Capillary Heel Puncture

1. Choose the collection site and apply a commercial heel warmer or warm pack for several minutes prior to specimen collection.
2. Assemble equipment:
   - Gloves
   - Automatic lancet
   - Antiseptic wipe
   - Cotton ball or dry gauze
   - Capillary blood collection tube
   - Band-aid
3. Perform hand hygiene and don gloves. Remove the warm pack.
4. Cleanse the site with antiseptic prep pad and allow to dry.
5. Hold the dorsum of the foot with the nondominant hand; with the dominant hand, pierce the heel with the lancet. Place the extremity in the dependent position.
6. Wipe away the first drop of blood with the cotton ball or dry gauze.
7. Collect the blood specimen with a capillary specimen collection tube. Avoid squeezing the foot during specimen collection if possible, as it may contribute to hemolysis of the specimen.
8. Hold dry gauze over the site until bleeding stops, elevate extremity above the level of the heart, and then apply a Band-Aid.

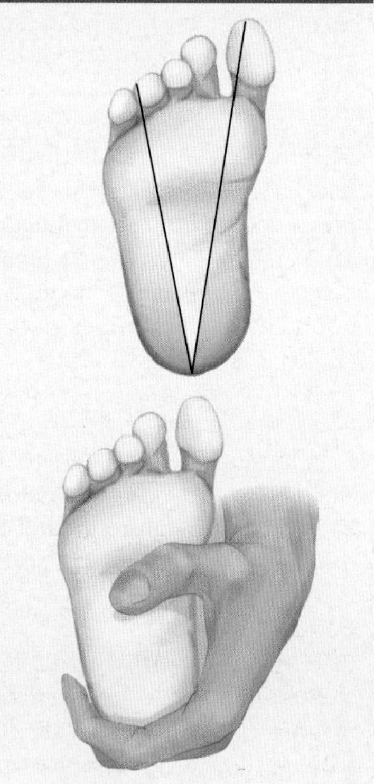

catheters or central venous catheters. The initial blood will be discarded to prevent contamination with intravenous fluids or medications such as heparin. The amount discarded depends on the size of the catheter, the weight of the child, and the institution's guidelines. After aspirating the specimen, flush the venous access device with normal saline to prevent clogging. The device may then be reconnected to the intravenous fluid or flushed according to the institution's protocol.

Remember Samuel, the child with fever, congestion, and irritability? What additional health history and physical examination assessment information should you obtain?

Nursing Analysis

After recognizing and analyzing cues from a thorough assessment, the nurse may identify several patient problems, including:

- Impaired comfort
- Infection risk
- Dehydration risk
- Social isolation
- Knowledge deficiency (specify)

After completing an assessment of Samuel, you note the following: rectal temperature of 39°C (102.2°F), poor sucking, and lethargy. Based on these assessment findings, what would your top three patient problems be for Samuel?

The patient problems provide suggestions for developing a nursing plan of care or concept mapping. The nurse will then generate solutions by planning interventions (suggested with rationales). The plan of care should be individualized, based on the child's and family's needs. Refer to Chapter 14 for the nursing process for pain management and to Chapter 11 for nursing interventions related to interrupted family processes and risk for caregiver role strain. Additional information will be included later in the chapter as it relates to specific disorders.

Nursing Analysis

Impaired comfort related to illness-related symptoms (infectious and/or inflammatory process) as evidenced by rectal temperature greater than 38°C (100.4°F), pruritus, rash or skin lesions, sore throat, or joint pain

Goal/Outcome

Pain or discomfort will be reduced to levels acceptable to the child. Child will verbalize absence or decrease of pain using a pain scale (FLACC, FACES, or linear pain scale), will verbalize or exhibit signs of comfort during febrile episode, will verbalize decrease in uncomfortable sensations such as itching and aches; infants will exhibit decreased crying and ability to rest quietly.

Improving Comfort (interventions with *rationale*)

- Assess pain and response to interventions frequently with use of pain scales or other pain measurement tools: *provides baseline of pain and allows for evaluation of effectiveness of interventions.*
- Administer analgesics and antipruritics as ordered *to relieve pain via interruption of central nervous system pathways and to decrease discomfort related to itching.*
- Administer antipyretics per health care provider order when the child is experiencing discomfort or cannot keep up with the metabolic demands of the fever. *Fever is a protective response of the body to fight infection. Antipyretics provide symptomatic relief but do not change the course of the infection. The major benefits to decreasing fever are increasing comfort in the child and decreasing fluid requirements, helping to prevent dehydration.*
- Keep linens and clothing clean and dry: *diaphoresis can leave clothing and linen soaked, increasing discomfort for the child.*
- Use of nonpharmacologic measures such as tepid bath and removal of clothing and blankets *to decrease temperature and increase comfort.* If used, discontinue if shivering begins *as this will increase temperature and increase discomfort.*
- Apply cool compresses to areas of pruritus or provide a cool bath *to decrease inflammation and soothe pruritus.*
- Keep child's fingernails short (use mitts, gloves, or socks over hands if necessary) to prevent injury *to the skin, which leads to increased pain.*
- Encourage child to press on rather than scratch the area of pruritus: *pressing on the area that itches can soothe the itching and prevent scratching, which can lead to skin injury.*
- Provide fluids frequently and offer warm fluids such as soup or cold foods such as popsicles *to ease the discomfort of a sore throat.*
- Provide cool mist humidification *to ease the discomfort of a sore throat.*
- Dress the child in light clothing: *restrictive clothing and diaphoresis can lead to increased pruritus.*
- Use diversional activities and distraction appropriate to developmental level: *distraction from pain can reduce the need for pharmacologic agents, and distraction from pruritus can minimize scratching.*

Nursing Analysis

Infection risk; risk factors include insufficient knowledge to avoid exposure to pathogens, inadequate vaccination, and exposure to disease outbreak.

Goal/Outcome

Child will exhibit no signs or symptoms of local or systemic infection. Child will not spread infection to others. Symptoms of infection will decrease over time; others will remain free of infection. Child and family will demonstrate appropriate hygiene measures using proper technique, such as handwashing, to prevent the spread of infection.

Preventing and Controlling Infection (interventions with *rationale*)

- Monitor vital signs: *elevation in temperature may indicate infection.*
- Monitor skin lesions for signs of local infection: redness, warmth, drainage, swelling, and pain at lesions: *can indicate infection.*
- Maintain aseptic technique and practice good handwashing: *to prevent introduction of further infectious agents and prevent transmission to others.*
- Administer antibiotics as prescribed: *to prevent or treat bacterial infection.*
- Encourage nutritious diet and proper hydration according to child's preferences and ability to feed orally: *to assist body's natural defenses against infection.*
- Isolate child as required based on transmission-based precautions: *to prevent nosocomial spread of infection.*
- Teach child and family preventive measures such as good handwashing, covering mouth and nose with cough or sneeze, and proper disposal of used tissues: *to prevent nosocomial or community spread of infection.*

Nursing Analysis

Dehydration risk due to insufficient fluid intake to meet fluid loss due to conditions such as increased metabolic demands and insensible loss due to fever, diaphoresis, vomiting, or poor feeding/fluid intake

Goal/Outcome

Fluid volume will be maintained and balanced. Oral mucosa is moist and pink, skin turgor is elastic, urine output is at least 1 to 2 mL/kg/hour.

Promoting Adequate Fluid Balance (interventions with *rationale*)

- Administer intravenous fluids if ordered *to maintain adequate hydration in children who are (nothing by mouth) NPO, unable to tolerate oral intake, or unable to keep up with fluid losses.*
- When oral intake is allowed and tolerated, encourage oral fluids *to promote intake and maintain hydration.*
- Assess for signs of adequate hydration such as pink and moist oral mucosa, elastic skin turgor, and adequate urine output *to detect fluid imbalance.*
- Monitor intake and output *to identify fluid imbalance.*
- Assess urine specific gravity, urine and serum electrolytes, blood urea nitrogen, creatinine, and osmolality and daily weights *to monitor fluid status.*

Nursing Analysis

Social isolation related to inability to engage in satisfying personal relationships (required isolation from peers secondary to transmission-based precautions) as evidenced by disruption in usual play secondary to inability to leave hospital room, activity intolerance, and fatigue

Goal/Outcome

Child will participate in stimulating activities. Child is able to verbalize reason for isolation and length of isolation (if developmentally appropriate); child verbalizes interest in activities.

Preventing Social Isolation (interventions with *rationale*)

- Explain reasons for transmission-based precautions and length of time: *this helps increase understanding and decrease anxiety about isolation. Children sometimes mistake isolation as punishment. Explaining length of time gives child an endpoint they can work toward.*
- Visit child frequently, at least every hour, and try to spend some uninterrupted time to play and allow child time to verbalize feelings about separation from others: *helps establish a therapeutic relationship and demonstrates caring.*
- Let child see caregiver's face before applying mask if appropriate: *to help child identify and relate to those caring for them and minimize anxiety about strangers and the unknown.*
- Consult child life specialist to arrange for stimulating activities child enjoys: *can help child to understand reasons for isolation and minimize feelings of social isolation.*
- Contact volunteers to spend time with child, if appropriate: *gives child attention and support, which will help child to cope and decrease stress.*

Nursing Analysis

Knowledge deficiency related to insufficient information (regarding medical condition, prognosis, and medical needs) as evidenced by verbalization, questions, or actions demonstrating lack of understanding regarding child's condition or care

Goal/Outcome

Child and family will verbalize accurate information and understanding about condition, prognosis, and medical needs. Child and family demonstrate knowledge of condition and prognosis and medical needs, including possible causes, contributing factors, and treatment measures.

Providing Child and Family Teaching (interventions with *rationale*)

- Assess the child's and family's willingness to learn: *child and family must be willing to learn in order for teaching to be effective.*
- Provide the family with time to adjust to diagnosis: *to facilitate adjustment and ability to learn and participate in child's care.*
- Repeat information: *to give family and child time to learn and understand.*
- Teach in short sessions: *many short sessions are more helpful and facilitate learning compared to one long session.*
- Gear teaching to level of understanding of the child and family (depends on age of child, physical condition, memory): *to ensure understanding.*
- Provide reinforcement and rewards: *to facilitate the teaching/learning process.*
- Use multiple modes of learning involving many senses (provide written, verbal, demonstration, and videos) when possible: *the child and family are more likely to retain information when it is presented in different ways using many senses.*

Managing Fever

Fever is typically managed at home, so it is important to give guidance and instruction at well-child visits and review this information at subsequent visits. Written and video materials about fever management may be effective in increasing caregivers' knowledge. Parents can refer to the written instructions when needed (see Teaching Guidelines 15.1).

Managing Skin Rashes

Skin rashes accompany many infectious or communicable diseases. These rashes can be uncomfortable and irritating for the child. Management often occurs at home, so it is important to educate parents on ways to relieve the discomfort and protect and maintain skin integrity. The health care provider may prescribe antipruritics, including oral medications or topical creams or ointments (see Drug Guide 15.1). Instruct parents on the importance of maintaining skin integrity to prevent infection or scarring. Teach parents to keep their child's fingernails short and hands clean. Explain the importance of discouraging scratching, and discuss distraction techniques they can use with the child. Cool compresses or cool baths can relieve itching. Encourage the child to press on rather than scratch the itchy area; this can relieve discomfort while maintaining skin integrity. Refer to Chapter 23 for more information on managing skin rashes.

TEACHING GUIDELINES 15.1 Fever Management

- Fever is a sign of illness, not a disease; it is the body's weapon to fight infection.
- Diurnal variation may allow temperature changes as much as 1°C (33.8°F) over a 24-hour period, peaking in the evening.
- Initially fever should be managed by trying to decrease the child's temperature by increasing fluid intake and decreasing activity.
- Antipyretics are used if the child demonstrates discomfort. Always check correct doses before administration. Never give aspirin or aspirin-containing products to a child younger than 19 years with a fever due to the risk of Reye syndrome.
- In some children fever can be associated with a seizure or dehydration, but this will not lead to brain damage or death. Discuss the facts about febrile seizures (see Chapter 16 for further information on febrile seizures).
- Watch for the signs and symptoms of dehydration; it is important to provide oral rehydration by increasing fluid intake.
- Dress the child lightly and avoid warm, binding clothing or blankets.
- The use of sponging with tepid water is controversial; if used, encourage the parent to give an antipyretic prior to sponging. Ensure the sponging does not produce shivering (which causes the body to produce heat and maintain the elevated set point), and reinforce the importance of using tepid water, not cold water or alcohol. Instruct the parent to stop if the child experiences discomfort.
- Call the provider for:
  - Any child younger than 3 months who has a rectal temperature above 38°C (100.4°F).
  - Any child who is lethargic or listless, regardless of temperature.
  - Fever lasting more than 3–5 days.
  - Fever greater than 40.6°C (105°F).
  - Any child who is immunocompromised by illness, such as cancer or human immunodeficiency virus (will need further evaluation and treatment).

THINKING ABOUT **DEVELOPMENT**

Lisa Hernandez is a 4-year-old with a history of fever and cold-like symptoms who presents currently with an itchy rash. Based on her developmental stage, how will you instruct her and her caregiver on managing her rash at home? How would your instructions change if the child was 12 years old?

Based on your top three nursing concerns for Samuel, describe appropriate nursing interventions.

SEPSIS

Sepsis is a systemic overresponse to infection resulting from bacteria and viruses (most commonly), fungi, viruses, rickettsiae, or parasites. It can lead to septic shock, which results in hypotension, low blood flow, and multisystem organ failure. Septic shock is a medical emergency, and children are usually admitted to an intensive care unit (see Chapter 29). The cause of sepsis may not be known, but common causative organisms in infants and children include *Escherichia coli*, group B streptococcus, *Staphylococcus aureus*, and *Streptococcus pneumoniae* (Pomerantz & Weiss, 2022). Sepsis can affect any age group, but infants less than 1 month of age, immunocompromised children, children with a debilitating chronic condition, children with a serious injury or large incision site, children with urinary tract abnormalities and frequent infections, and children with an indwelling vascular catheter are at higher risk (Pomerantz & Weiss, 2022).

Neonates and young infants have a higher susceptibility due to their immature immune system, inability to localize infections, and lack of immunoglobulin M (IgM), which is necessary to protect against bacterial infections.

The prognosis for sepsis is variable and depends on the child's age and the cause of the sepsis. Neonates are at highest risk for a poor outcome. Due to this high mortality rate, when an ill-appearing febrile neonate presents, a full workup is indicated (Kronman et al., 2023a). Usually, admission to the hospital to rule out sepsis is the standard of practice.

Pathophysiology

Sepsis results in the systemic inflammatory response syndrome (SIRS) due to infection. The pathophysiology of sepsis is complex. It results from the effects of circulating bacterial products or toxins, mediated by cytokine release, occurring as a result of sustained bacteremia. The pathogens cause an overproduction of proinflammatory cytokines, previously termed endotoxins. These cytokines are responsible for the clinically observable effects of the sepsis. Impaired pulmonary, hepatic, or renal function may result from excessive cytokine release during the septic process.

Therapeutic Management

Therapeutic management of sepsis in infants, especially neonates, is more aggressive than for older children. Neonates and infants with sepsis or even suspected sepsis are treated in the hospital. The infant or child with sepsis is admitted for close monitoring along with antibiotic therapy. Intravenous antibiotics are started immediately after the blood, urine, and cerebrospinal fluid cultures have been obtained. The length of therapy and the specific antibiotic used will be determined based on the source of the positive culture and the results of the culture and sensitivity. If final culture reports are negative and symptoms have subsided, antibiotics may be discontinued (usually after 72 hours of treatment). If the child is not responding to therapy and symptoms worsen, sepsis may be progressing to shock. Management of the child with septic shock is usually done in the intensive care unit.

Nursing Assessment

For a full description of the assessment phase of the nursing process, refer to the "Clinical Judgment and the Nursing Process" box earlier in this chapter. Assessment findings pertinent to sepsis are discussed further.

Health History

Elicit a description of the present illness and chief complaint. Signs of sepsis can vary with each child. Some common signs and symptoms reported during the health history might include:

- Child just does not look or act right.
- Crying more than usual, inconsolable
- Fever
- Hypothermia (in neonates and those with severe disease)
- Lethargic and less interactive or playful
- Increased irritability
- Poor feeding or poor suck
- Rash (e.g., petechiae, ecchymosis, diffuse erythema)
- Difficulty breathing
- Nasal congestion
- Diarrhea
- Vomiting
- Decreased urine output
- Hypotonia
- Changes in mental status (confused, anxious, excited)
- Seizures
- Older child may complain of heart racing.

Explore the child's current and past medical history for risk factors such as:

- Prematurity
- Lack of immunizations
- Immunocompromise
- Exposure to communicable pathogens

In neonates and young infants, seek pregnancy and labor risk factors such as:

- Premature rupture of membranes or prolonged rupture
- Difficult delivery
- Maternal infection or fever, including STIs
- Resuscitation and other invasive procedures
- Positive maternal group beta-streptococcal vaginosis

Sepsis may occur in the hospitalized child. Assess for risk factors such as:

- Intensive care unit stay
- Presence of central line or other invasive lines or tubes
- Immunosuppression

TAKE NOTE!

Listen to the parents' descriptions of their child's behavior and appearance, as well as changes they have observed. Many times, they are the first to notice when their child is not acting right, even before clinical signs of infection are seen.

Physical Examination

Perform a thorough physical examination of the infant or child with proven or suspected sepsis. Specific findings related to inspection and observation are noted further.

Inspection and Observation

Observe the child's general appearance, color, level of arousal, and hydration status. The child with sepsis may appear lethargic and pale and show signs of dehydration. In neonates and infants, observe the quality of their cry and reaction to parental stimulation, noting weak cry, lack of smile or facial expression, or lack of responsiveness. Inspect the skin for petechiae or other skin lesions. Petechiae may indicate a serious bacterial infection (often *Neisseria meningitidis*), and other skin lesion patterns may help identify the cause of the fever. Observe respiratory effort and rate. The infant or child with sepsis may demonstrate tachypnea and increased work of breathing, such as nasal flaring, grunting, and retractions.

Assess vital signs, noting abnormalities. Note elevation in temperature or hypothermia in the young infant. Note tachypnea or tachycardia in the child or apnea or bradycardia in the infant. Document blood pressure. Hypotension, especially when accompanied by signs of poor perfusion, can be a sign of worsening sepsis with progression to shock (refer to Chapter 29).

Laboratory and Diagnostic Tests

Symptoms of sepsis can be vague in infants. Therefore, laboratory tests play a crucial role in confirming or ruling out sepsis. Common laboratory and diagnostic studies ordered for the assessment of sepsis include:

- Complete blood count: WBC levels will be elevated; in severe cases they may be decreased (this is an ominous sign).
- C-reactive protein: elevated
- Blood culture: positive in septicemia, indicating bacteria is present in the blood
- Urine culture: may be positive, indicating presence of bacteria in the urine
- Cerebrospinal fluid analysis: may reveal increased WBCs and protein and low glucose
- Stool culture: may be positive for bacteria or other infectious organisms
- Culture of tubes, catheters, or shunts suspected to be infected: the fluid inside these tubes may be tested for bacteria.
- Chest radiograph: may reveal signs of pneumonia such as hyperinflation and patchy areas of atelectasis or infiltration

Nursing Management

Monitor the infant or child closely for changes in condition, especially the development of shock. Administer antibiotics as ordered. Refer to the "Clinical Judgment and the Nursing Process" section for patient problems and related interventions. In addition to these interventions, it is important to prevent infection and provide education to the child and family.

Preventing Infection

Sepsis is a potentially life-threatening illness, and prevention is important. Handwashing is the most effective intervention against nosocomial infection. Nurses play a key role in minimizing environmental sources by cleaning equipment, disposing of soiled linens and dressings properly, and adhering to proper aseptic technique with all invasive procedures. Follow your institution's policies, and use evidence-based practice guidelines for interventions such as invasive line dressing changes and intravenous tubing changes to reduce the risk of infection. Encourage immunization as recommended. To reduce group B streptococcus infection in neonates, screen pregnant patients. If the results are positive, administer intrapartum antibiotics.

TAKE NOTE!

There has been a dramatic reduction in invasive *Haemophilus influenzae* type B diseases since the widespread use of the Hib vaccine (CDC, 2022k).

Educating the Child and Family

Early recognition of the signs of sepsis is essential in preventing morbidity and mortality. Educate parents about the significance of fever, especially in neonates and infants younger than 3 months. Instruct parents to contact their health care provider or nurse practitioner if their infant or neonate has a fever. A health care provider or nurse practitioner should see any child with a fever accompanied by lethargy, poor responsiveness, or lack of facial expressions. Signs and symptoms of sepsis can be vague and vary from child to child. Encourage parents to contact their health care provider or nurse practitioner if they feel their febrile child is "just not acting right."

BACTERIAL INFECTIONS

Bacteria are one-celled organisms that can live, grow, and reproduce. They exist everywhere. Most are completely harmless and some are useful. Others can lead to disease either because they are in the wrong place in the body or they invade and cause disease in humans and animals. Children are at a high risk of developing bacterial infections, which can result in life-threatening illness. Fortunately, many bacterial diseases, such as diphtheria, pertussis, and tetanus, can be prevented by immunization (see Chapter 9 for more information on immunizations).

Community-Acquired Methicillin-Resistant *Staphylococcus aureus*

Community-acquired methicillin-resistant *Staphylococcus aureus* (CAMRSA) is a staphylococcal infection that is resistant to certain antibiotics. Methicillin-resistant *S. aureus* (MRSA) was originally a nosocomial acquired infection (hospital-acquired [HA]-MRSA) with few cases acquired in the community. However, community-acquired infection, in seemingly healthy individuals, is increasing in occurrence throughout the United States (Kaplan, 2023). These infections range from minor skin rashes to abscesses to serious, complicated, life-threatening infections. Serious and invasive infections, such as sepsis, necrotizing pneumonia, and osteomyelitis, often are secondary to a skin or soft tissue infection.

Transmission occurs through direct person-to-person contact, respiratory droplets, blood, or sharing personal items, such as hair brushes, towels, and sports equipment, and touching surfaces or items contaminated with MRSA. Clusters of MRSA have been found in day care centers and among athletic teams. Staphylococci are resistant to heat and drying and can be found on environmental surfaces months after contamination. Intact skin and mucous membranes, along with proper hand hygiene, are the best barriers to MRSA.

Nursing Assessment

In the child, skin and tissue infections are common infections caused by CAMRSA. Symptoms include a bump or skin area that is red, swollen, painful, and warm to touch. It may also include fever, fluctuance, and purulent drainage. The lesion may have appeared suddenly and be red and raised, resembling an insect bite. Necrotic areas may develop. Abscesses, especially abscessed hair follicles, and pimples are common presentations. Assessment needs to include a thorough past medical history to determine history of recurrent skin infections with or without complete resolution along with assessment for risk factors. Risk factors include frequent skin-to-skin contact; openings in the skin/skin trauma, such as abrasions and cuts; contact with potentially contaminated personal items, equipment, and surfaces; poor hygiene; limited access to health care; frequent exposure to antimicrobial agents; and crowded living conditions (Kaplan, 2023).

Diagnosis is determined through culture. Diagnostic tests include incision and drainage (I&D), aspiration of the abscess, and culturing the fluid or tissue. Antimicrobial susceptibility along with culture is critical.

Nursing Management

Care of the child with CAMRSA will typically occur at home. Antibiotics with microbial susceptibility will often be prescribed. Comprehensive wound care, which may include I&D, may occur. Follow-up for reassessment is key. Child and family education is crucial. Include the following in the teaching plan:

- Educate the family on the importance of taking the antibiotics as directed and finishing all the medicine. Emphasize that this will help slow the creation of antimicrobial-resistant organisms.
- Teach the child and parents proper hand hygiene and handwashing.
- Discourage family members from sharing personal items.
- Explain the risk factors involved in transmission.
- Explain the importance of keeping cuts and scrapes cleaned and covered.
- Review the signs of MRSA and emphasize the importance of early recognition and treatment.

Scarlet Fever

Scarlet fever is an infection resulting from group A streptococci. It usually occurs with a group A streptococci throat infection (i.e., strep throat) or rarely streptococcal skin infection. However, in the case of scarlet fever, the bacteria produce a toxin that causes a rash. Not all children with a group A streptococci infection will develop the rash of scarlet fever. Only children who are infected with streptococci that produce pyrogenic exotoxins and do not have antitoxin antibodies, making them sensitive to the bacterial toxin, will develop scarlet fever (Shulman & Reuter, 2020). Scarlet fever is usually seen in children 5 to 15 years of age and is rare in children younger than 3 years (CDC, 2022a). Transmission is through droplets and follows contact with respiratory tract secretions. Transmission is facilitated by the type of close contact that occurs in schools and child care centers. Food-borne outbreaks have occurred due to human contamination of food. After exposure, the incubation period is 2 to 5 days (Shulman & Reuter, 2020). Communicability is highest during acute infection, and the child is no longer contagious 24 hours after the initiation of appropriate antimicrobial therapy (Shulman & Reuter, 2020).

There has been a dramatic decrease in the mortality rate from scarlet fever due to antibiotic use, and scarlet fever today is seen less frequently and typically follows a benign course (Sotoodian, 2020). Rare but serious complications such as rheumatic fever, glomerulonephritis, skin infections, abscesses of the throat, pneumonia, and arthritis can still occur; therefore, prompt recognition and proper treatment are important (CDC, 2022a).

Nursing Assessment

Symptoms of scarlet fever begin abruptly. The health history may reveal a fever greater than 38.3°C (101°F), chills, body aches, loss of appetite, nausea, and vomiting. Inspect the pharynx, which is usually very red and swollen. The tonsils may have yellow or white specks of pus, and cervical lymph nodes may be swollen. Inspect the skin for the most striking symptom of scarlet fever, which is an erythematous rash appearing on the face, trunk, and extremities. The rash is typically absent from the palms and soles of the feet. It looks like a sunburn but feels like sandpaper (Fig. 15.1A). The rash lasts approximately 5 days and is followed by desquamation, typically on the fingers and toes. Early in the illness the tongue develops a thick coat with a strawberry appearance. The tongue will later lose the coating and become bright red (Fig. 15.1B).

Diagnosis is made by identification of group A streptococcus on throat culture. Several rapid tests for group A streptococcal pharyngitis are available. The accuracy of these tests depends on the quality of the specimen. It is important that the secretions obtained are pharyngeal or tonsillar (see Common Medical Treatments 15.1 for more information on throat cultures).

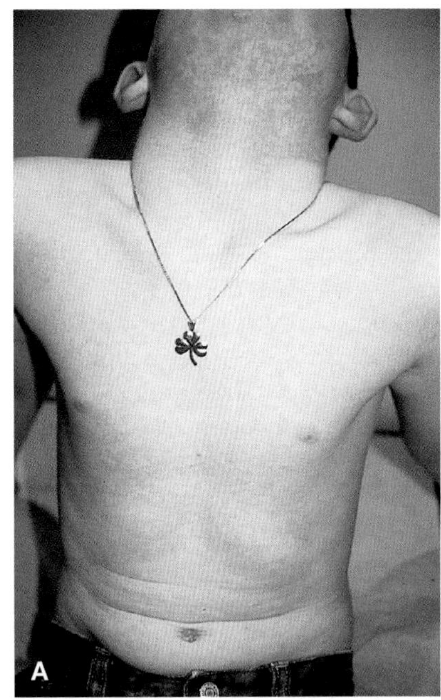

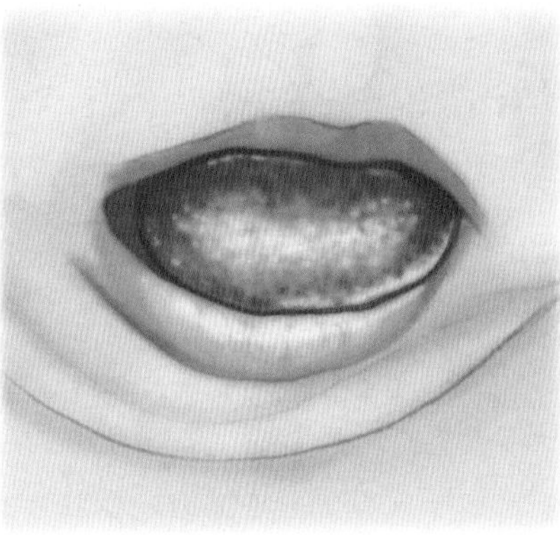

FIGURE 15.1 A. Rash of scarlet fever. **B.** Strawberry tongue.

Nursing Management

Children with scarlet fever are usually cared for at home. Penicillin and amoxicillin are the antibiotics of choice (Shulman & Reuter, 2020). In those sensitive to penicillin, erythromycin may be used. Educate the family on the importance of taking the antibiotic as directed and finishing all the medicine.

Encourage fluid intake to maintain adequate hydration due to fever. Teach parents ways to provide comfort for the child. A cool mist humidifier can soothe the child's sore throat. Soft foods, warm liquids like soup, or cold foods like popsicles may also be helpful. If the child is hospitalized, droplet precautions, along with standard precautions, are necessary.

Diphtheria

Diphtheria is caused by infection with *Corynebacterium diphtheriae* and may affect the nose, larynx, tonsils, or pharynx. Tonsillar and pharyngeal infections are the most common and will be the focus of this discussion. A pseudomembrane forms over the pharynx, uvula, tonsils, and soft palate (Fig. 15.2). The neck becomes edematous, and lymphadenopathy develops. The pseudomembrane causes airway obstruction and suffocation. Diphtheria is rare in developed countries but is reappearing in some regions and continues to be a serious disease worldwide due to lack of routine immunization (Barroso & Pegram, 2023). Risk factors include children and adults who are unimmunized or underimmunized, living in crowded or unsanitary living conditions, having a compromised immune system, and traveling to developing countries where diphtheria remains endemic (Barroso & Pegram, 2023). Routine infant immunization can prevent the disease. Therapeutic management involves administration of antibiotics and antitoxin, as well as airway management.

Nursing Assessment

Assess immunization history as children at risk for diphtheria are those who are unimmunized. Note history of sore throat and fever, usually less than 38.9°C (102°F). As the pseudomembrane forms, swallowing becomes difficult and signs of airway obstruction become apparent. A specimen of the membrane may be cultured for *C. diphtheriae*.

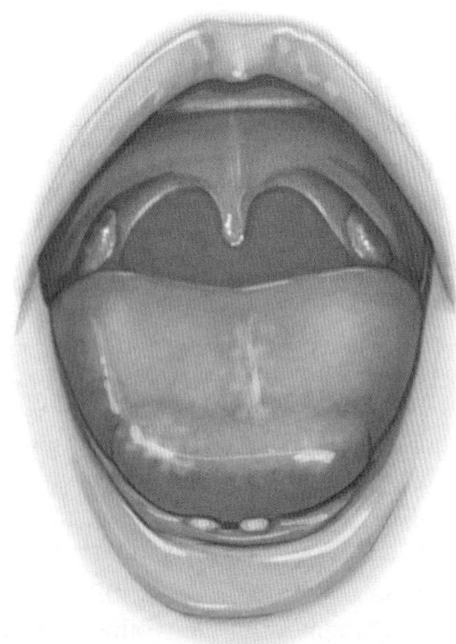

FIGURE 15.2 In diphtheria, a pseudomembrane forms over the pharynx, uvula, tonsils, and soft palate.

Nursing Management

Close observation of respiratory status is of utmost importance. Administration of antibiotics and the antitoxin is critical to encourage sloughing of the membrane. The child should remain on strict droplet precautions in addition to standard precautions and should maintain bed rest.

Pertussis

Pertussis is an acute respiratory disorder characterized by paroxysmal cough (whooping cough) and copious secretions. The highest incidence and the greatest risk for severe disease and death are seen in children younger than 1 year (Yeh & Mink, 2022). The disease is caused by *Bordetella pertussis*. The incubation period is 6 to 20 days, usually 7 to 10 days. Pertussis usually starts with 7 to 10 days of cold symptoms. The paroxysmal coughing spells then begin and can last 1 to 4 weeks. Convalescence occurs over the course of several weeks to months. Initially, immunization decreased the incidence of pertussis, but an increase has occurred since the 1990s (Yeh & Mink, 2022). Recent trends show pertussis as an increasing endemic with cycling epidemics and a shifting burden of disease to young infants, adolescents, and adults. Many factors contribute to this increase in pertussis such as changes in diagnostic testing, increase in recognition and reporting of pertussis, changes in the molecular makeup of the organism, and waning vaccine-induced immunity (CDC, 2021a). Infants and young children continue to be advised to get four doses of DTaP (diphtheria, tetanus, and pertussis) at 2, 4, 6, and 15 to 18 months; a fifth booster dose at 4 to 6 years before entering school; and an additional Tdap (tetanus, diphtheria, and acellular pertussis) booster at age 11. Complications of pertussis include hypoxia, apnea, secondary infections such as pneumonia and otitis media, seizures, encephalopathy, and death.

TAKE NOTE!

Rates of pertussis hospitalization in infants less than 2 months have decreased since the Advisory Committee on Immunization Practices (ACIP) advised pertussis immunization for pregnant people, preferably during their third trimester (Yeh & Mink, 2022).

Therapeutic Management

Therapeutic management of pertussis focuses on eradicating the bacterial infection and providing respiratory support. CDC guidelines recommend antimicrobial treatment early in the course of disease. Ideally, antibiotics are initiated during the first 1 to 2 weeks of illness prior to the occurrence of paroxysmal cough for the best treatment results (CDC, 2022b). For infants older than 1 month, macrolide drugs, including erythromycin, clarithromycin, and azithromycin, are the drugs of choice (CDC, 2022b). For younger infants, azithromycin should be used and erythromycin and clarithromycin avoided (CDC, 2022b). An alternative to macrolides in children older than 2 months is trimethoprim–sulfamethoxazole (TMP-SMZ) (CDC, 2022b). A course of macrolide antibiotics is also recommended to treat all close contacts regardless of age or immunization status (CDC, 2021a). Also, all close contacts who are younger than 7 years and who are unimmunized or underimmunized should have pertussis immunization initiated or the series completed according to the recommended dosing schedule (CDC, 2021a).

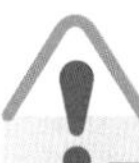

CLINICAL REASONING ALERT!

Monitor infants less than 1 month of age who receive macrolide antibiotics (particularly erythromycin) for signs of the development of infantile hypertrophic pyloric stenosis, such as projectile vomiting (Souder & Long, 2020).

Nursing Assessment

Assess for lack of immunization as this is the most important risk factor for the development of pertussis. Obtain history that may reveal cold and cough symptoms, progressing to paroxysmal coughing spells. During the paroxysms, the child might cough 10 to 30 times in a row, followed by a whooping sound. This might be accompanied by redness in the face, progressive cyanosis, and protrusion of the tongue. Saliva, mucus, and tears flow from the mouth, nose, and eyes. Between the paroxysmal episodes, the child might rest well and appear relatively unaffected. Assess oxygen levels, and auscultate the lungs to assess air exchange. The diagnosis may be confirmed by a variety of laboratory tests, such as culture, polymerase chain reaction, and serology, accompanied by clinical history.

Nursing Management

Nursing care will focus on providing a high-humidity environment and frequent suctioning to mobilize secretions. Observe for signs of airway obstruction and respiratory distress. Encourage fluids to keep secretions thin and maintain adequate hydration. Offer reassurance to the child and family; the coughing episodes can be very frightening. Droplet precautions along with standard precautions are necessary for the hospitalized child.

Tetanus

Tetanus is an acute, often fatal neurologic disease caused by the toxins produced by *Clostridium tetani*. Tetanus is rare in the United States but continues to be significant worldwide due to lack of routine immunization (Thwaites, 2022). It is characterized by increased muscle tone and spasm. *C. tetani* spores can live anywhere but are found most commonly in soil, dust, and feces from humans or animals, such as sheep, cattle, chickens, dogs, cats, and rats. The spores can enter the body through a wound that is contaminated, through a burn, or by injecting contaminated street drugs. Once it enters the body, an anaerobic environment allows it to multiply and a poisonous toxin is released.

There are four forms of tetanus. Neonatal tetanus affects newborns in the first week of life secondary to an infected umbilical stump in infants whose birthing parents were poorly immunized (CDC, 2021a). Most adults in the United States have been immunized and will pass the immunity to their fetus. Along with proper hygiene during delivery and adequate cord care, this makes this type rare in the United States, but in underdeveloped countries it remains a significant problem (CDC, 2021a). The second form is local tetanus. This rare form is characterized by local muscle spasms within the same area/extremity of the wound. The third type is cephalic tetanus, which is associated with recurrent otitis media or head trauma. It is also rare and affects the cranial nerves, especially facial nerves. Generalized tetanus is the most common and severe form, and patients will often present first with trismus (masseter muscle spasm or lockjaw) (CDC, 2021a). Symptoms then progress in a descending fashion with tonic contraction of the skeletal muscles and intermittent intense, painful muscular spasms. The most profoundly affected muscles are those of the neck and back.

The general incubation period is 1 to 21 days, with an average of 8 days (CDC, 2021a). Recovery can be long and difficult, and children with tetanus may have to spend several weeks in the hospital in an intensive care setting. It has been suggested that the shorter the incubation period, the higher the risk of more severe illness and poorer prognosis (CDC, 2021a). Complications associated with tetanus include breathing problems, fractures, elevated blood pressure, dysrhythmias, clotting in the blood vessels of the lung, pneumonia, and coma.

Therapeutic Management

Therapeutic management is directed toward supporting respiratory and cardiovascular function, stopping toxin production, neutralizing unbound toxins, and controlling muscle spasms. Tetanus immunoglobulin may be given as well as the tetanus vaccine. Removal of the offending organism, by debridement of the wound, may occur, and intravenous antibiotics such as metronidazole may be initiated. In severe cases, the child may require intensive nursing care with mechanical ventilation.

Nursing Assessment

Note history of initial signs such as headache, spasms, crankiness, and cramping of the jaw (lockjaw), which are followed by difficulty swallowing and a stiff neck. Tetanus progresses in a descending fashion to other muscle groups, causing spasms of the neck, arms, legs, and stomach; seizures may result. Document the presence of fever along with an elevated blood pressure and tachycardia. Opisthotonos (refer to Fig. 16.13 in Chapter 16) may be noted due to severe spasms of the neck and back. The spasms or muscle contractions in children may be strong enough to result in fractures. The diagnosis of tetanus is based on the clinical findings of the history and physical examination. There is no laboratory test to confirm tetanus.

Nursing Management

Nursing management focuses on observing for signs of respiratory distress. Provide a quiet environment with reduced external stimuli to decrease the incidence of spasms. Appropriately manage pain. Encourage adequate nutrition and hydration. Administer sedatives and muscle relaxants as ordered to reduce the pain associated with the muscle spasms and to prevent seizures. Encourage the parents to stay with their child. The child's mental status is unaffected by the disease, so the child is aware of what is happening. Efforts need to be made to reduce the child's anxiety and to provide reassuring, sympathetic care to the child and family. Tetanus is not contagious from person to person; therefore, standard precautions are sufficient.

Tetanus is a preventable but potentially fatal disease. Education is essential regarding the importance of receiving this routine immunization (refer to Chapter 9 for immunization schedule) as well as a booster every 10 years. Instructing parents on proper wound care can also help prevent tetanus. All wounds should be cleaned thoroughly and a proper antiseptic used. If a wound is deep and contamination is suspected, the child should be seen by a health care provider or nurse practitioner. If it has been more than 5 years since the last tetanus dose, a booster may be needed. This can help to neutralize the poison and prevent it from entering the nervous system.

Botulism

Botulism is a disease that is caused by a toxin produced in the immature intestines of young children resulting from infection with the bacterium *Clostridium botulinum*. It is rare but can cause serious paralytic illness. There are several types of botulism. Food-borne botulism results from ingestion of food contaminated with botulinum toxin. Wound botulism results from wounds infected with *C. botulinum*. Infant botulism is the most common in the United States and results from the ingestion of spores of *C. botulinum*, most often from environmental dust and soil. *C. botulinum* is common in soil and can also be found in a variety of foods, such as improperly preserved home-canned foods. Although recently thought to be a minor reservoir, *C. botulinum* spores can be found in raw honey. Botulism has been associated with feeding raw honey to infants; thus, this should be avoided in children younger than 1 year (CDC, 2022c; Pegram & Stone, 2023). The disease is not infectious; to become infected, the child must ingest the bacterial spores. These spores then multiply in the intestinal tract and produce the toxin, which is absorbed in the immature intestines of the infant. It is generally not a problem for older children because the bacteria do not grow well in mature intestines due to the presence of the normal intestinal flora. Prognosis is good, but if treatment is not initiated, paralysis of the arms, legs, trunk, and respiratory system can develop. Therapeutic management is usually supportive but may involve administration of botulinum immune globulin or botulism antitoxin.

Nursing Assessment

For a full description of the assessment phase of the nursing process, refer to the "Clinical Judgment and the Nursing Process" section earlier in this chapter. Assessment findings pertinent to botulism are discussed further.

HEALTH HISTORY

Elicit a description of the present illness and chief complaint. Signs and symptoms usually occur soon after ingestion of the bacteria. Common signs and symptoms in infants reported during the health history might include:

- Constipation
- Poor feeding
- Listlessness
- Generalized weakness
- Weak cry

Common signs and symptoms in older children reported during the health history might include:

- Double vision
- Blurred vision
- Drooping eyelids
- Difficulty swallowing
- Slurred speech
- Muscle weakness

PHYSICAL EXAMINATION AND LABORATORY AND DIAGNOSTIC TESTS

Assess for a diminished gag reflex, which is indicative of botulism. Diagnostic tests include cultures of stool and serum. Botulism is a rare disease and is difficult to diagnose since its symptoms are similar to those of other neuromuscular diseases. Therefore, assessment may include diagnostic tests to help rule out other diseases, such as Guillain–Barré syndrome, stroke, and myasthenia gravis.

Nursing Management

Treatment is mainly supportive and focuses on maintaining respiratory status and nutritional status. Administration of an antitoxin is the main therapeutic treatment and should occur as early as possible (Pegram & Stone, 2023). If ordered, administer botulinum immune globulin early in the disease to reduce its severity and progression.

Osteomyelitis

Osteomyelitis is a bacterial infection of the bone and soft tissue surrounding the bone. *S. aureus* is the most common infecting organism, with MRSA accounting for a third of these infections (Krogstad, 2022a). Additional causes in infants and children include group A and B streptococci, *E. coli, S. pneumoniae, Kingella kingae,* and *Haemophilus influenzae* (which is now rare due to improvements in immunizations) (Krogstad, 2022a). Children usually present for evaluation within a few days to a week of onset of symptoms, though some may present later.

Osteomyelitis acquired hematogenously (spread through the blood) is the most common mechanism in children (Kronman et al., 2023b). Bacteria from the bloodstream mainly invade the most rapidly growing portion of the bone. The invading bacteria trigger an inflammatory response, formation of pus and edema, and vascular congestion. Small blood vessels thrombose, and the infection extends into the metaphyseal marrow cavity. As the infection progresses, the inflammation extends throughout the bone and blood supply is disrupted, resulting in death of the bone tissues (Fig. 15.3).

Therapeutic Management

Aspiration is necessary to confirm diagnosis and identify specific microorganisms. Treatment includes a 4- to 6-week course of antibiotics. Some children may receive 1 to 2 weeks of intravenous antibiotics and then be switched to oral antibiotics for the remainder of the course. Surgical debridement is rarely necessary. Early treatment may prevent the complications of bone destruction, fracture, and growth arrest. Additional complications include recurrent infection, septic arthritis, and systemic infection.

Nursing Assessment

For a full description of the assessment phase of the nursing process, refer to the "Clinical Judgment and the Nursing Process" section earlier in this chapter. Assessment findings pertinent to osteomyelitis are discussed here.

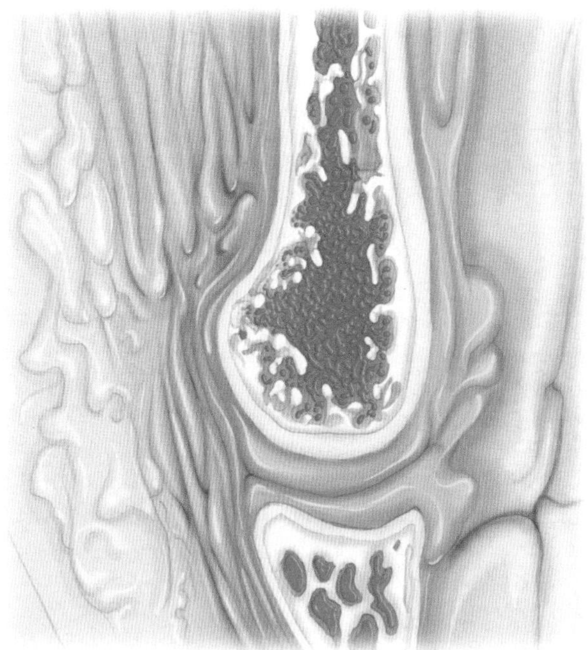

FIGURE 15.3 In osteomyelitis, bacterial invasion leads to infection within the bone.

Explore the health history for risk factors and symptoms. Risk factors include impetigo, infected varicella lesions, furunculosis, recent trauma, infected burns, prolonged intravenous line use, primary or acquired immune deficiency, and sepsis. Obtain history of current or recent antibiotic therapy and response. Note history of irritability, lethargy, possible fever, and onset of pain or change in activity level. The child usually refuses to walk and demonstrates decreased range of motion in the affected extremity. Inspect the affected extremity for swelling. Palpate for local warmth and tenderness. Note point tenderness over affected bone.

Laboratory and diagnostic testing may reveal:

- Elevated WBC count, erythrocyte sedimentation rate, and C-reactive protein level
- Positive blood cultures
- Deep soft tissue swelling on radiography
- Changes in ultrasound, computed tomography (CT) scan, or magnetic resonance imaging (MRI)

Nursing Management

Nursing management of the child with osteomyelitis focuses on assessment, pain management, and maintenance of intravenous access for administration of antibiotics. Individualize care based on the child's and family's response to the illness. Maintain bed rest initially to prevent injury and promote comfort. Administer antipyretics as ordered if the child is febrile in the initial stage of the illness. Encourage the use of unaffected extremities by providing developmentally appropriate toys and games.

Instruct the child and family on safe and proper use of crutches or walker if prescribed. Some children will be discharged home on intravenous antibiotics, while others will finish an oral antibiotic course. Teach parents proper administration of medications and maintenance of a peripherally inserted central catheter or central line at home if the child is finishing the antibiotic course intravenously.

Septic Arthritis

Acute septic arthritis is a condition in which bacteria invade the joint space, most often the hip or knee. It can occur at any age but usually occurs in children younger than 5 years (Krogstad, 2022b). Usually, bacteria gain access to the joint through the bloodstream but can also get access through direct puncture from injections, venipuncture, wound infection, surgery, or injury.

S. aureus is the most common causative organism with CAMRSA on the rise (Krogstad, 2022b). Various streptococci species, *K. kingae*, *N. meningitidis* (with or without an associated meningitis), *H. influenzae* (in unvaccinated children), and *Neisseria gonorrhoeae* are also responsible organisms (Krogstad, 2022b). Sepsis of the hip joint may cause avascular necrosis of the femoral head due to pressure on blood vessels and cartilage within the joint space. Septic arthritis is considered a medical emergency, as destruction of the joint cartilage may occur within just a few days. Additional complications of septic arthritis include permanent deformity, leg-length discrepancy, and long-term decreased range of motion and disability.

The goals of treatment of septic arthritis are to prevent destruction of the joint cartilage and maintain function, motion, and strength. Septic arthritis is treated rapidly with joint aspiration or arthrotomy, followed by intravenous antibiotic therapy while in the hospital and oral antibiotics at home.

Nursing Assessment

Note a history of predisposing factors such as respiratory infection or otitis media, skin or soft tissue infections, or, in the neonate, traumatic puncture wounds and femoral venipunctures. The history is usually significant for sudden onset of fever and moderate to severe pain.

Upon physical examination, the infant or child appears ill. Note extent of fever, reports of pain, refusal to bear weight or straighten the joint, and limited range of motion (the child usually maintains the joint in flexion and will not allow the leg to be straightened). The child will generally hold the joint in a position of comfort and the child or infant will appear without pain as long as the joint is immobile. Any attempt at passive range of motion will reveal pain. Palpate the affected joint for warmth and swelling.

Laboratory findings may include:

- WBC count normal or elevated with elevated neutrophil counts.
- Elevated erythrocyte sedimentation rate and C-reactive protein levels.
- Fluid from joint aspiration demonstrates elevated WBC count; culture determines responsible organism.
- Joint radiograph may show subtle soft tissue changes or increase in the joint space.
- Positive blood culture for the causative organism (40% of cases) (Krogstad, 2023).

Nursing Management

Assess aspiration wound for signs of infection. Monitor vital signs for resolution of fever. Pain management with ibuprofen or acetaminophen will be sufficient for some children; others may initially require an opioid, such as morphine. Assess the affected joint for a decrease in swelling, increasing range of motion, and decreasing or absent pain. The child may be discharged after 72 hours of intravenous antibiotics following joint aspiration if they are improving and can tolerate oral antibiotics. Some children may be discharged home on intravenous antibiotics. At discharge, if the child cannot ambulate, physical therapy may be consulted for short-term use of crutches or a wheelchair. Teach families how to assess for signs and symptoms of wound infection, how to administer oral antibiotics and pain medication, and how to assist their child with crutch walking.

VIRAL INFECTIONS

Viruses are very small particles that infect cells. They cannot multiply on their own and require a living host, such as humans, animals, or plants. They can reproduce only by invading and taking over the host cells. Young children are highly sensitive to viruses; their resistance is low and exposure is high. Viruses are hard to destroy without damaging or killing the living cells they infect. Therefore, drugs are not used to control them. However, many viral diseases can be prevented by immunization, such as measles, rubella, varicella, mumps, and poliomyelitis (see Chapter 9 for more information on immunizations).

Viral Exanthems

Many viral infections of the skin in childhood are called viral exanthems. **Exanthem** means rash or skin eruption. Viral exanthems of childhood often present with a distinct rash pattern that assists in the diagnosis of the virus. Table 15.4 discusses common childhood exanthems. Immunizations have led to a decrease in the incidence of certain viral exanthems, such as measles, rubella, and varicella.

TABLE 15.4 • Common Viral Exanthems of Childhood

Disease	Clinical Manifestations	Management/Complications	Nursing Implications
Rubella (German Measles)			
• Caused by rubella virus • Transmission: by direct or indirect contact with droplets, primarily by nasopharyngeal secretions, but also in blood, stool, and urine. Also transmitted from birthing parent to fetus • Peak incidence: late winter and early spring • Incubation period: 12–23 days (usually 14 days) • Communicable: 7 days before to 7 days after onset of rash 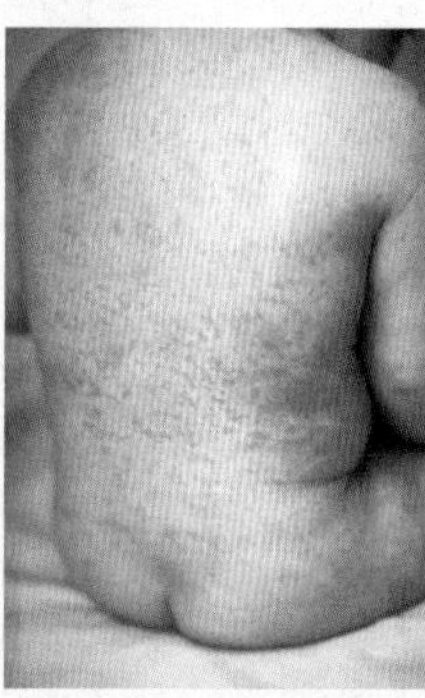 Rubella rash. (Courtesy of Centers for Disease Control and Prevention. [1978]. *Public health image library [PHIL]: Details.* https://phil.cdc.gov/Details.aspx?pid=712)	• Rash usually first sign. Maculopapular rash that begins on face and spreads head to foot; disappears in same order it spread, usually by the third day. On the second day, the rash may appear pinpoint. Desquamation is minimal. • In older children: lymphadenopathy (retroauricular, posterior cervical, postoccipital) 24 hours before the onset of the rash; lasting up to 1 week; low-grade fever, malaise, upper respiratory symptoms • Mild pruritus • Polyarthralgia and polyarthritis (rare in children but common in adolescents) • Half of cases may be subclinical or inapparent	• Usually mild and self-limiting • Treatment is mainly supportive. • Complications: encephalitis and thrombocytopenia (rare) • Maternal rubella during pregnancy can result in miscarriage, fetal death, or congenital malformations.	• Comfort measures such as antipyretics, antipruritics, and analgesics for joint pain • Droplet precautions until 7 days after onset of rash
Rubeola (Measles)			
• Caused by measles virus • Transmission: direct or indirect contact with droplets, primarily by nasopharyngeal secretions and airborne (virus can stay in air for up to 2 hours after infected person leaves the area); highly contagious • Peak incidence: late winter and spring • Incubation period: 6–21 days, usually 13 days • Communicable 1–2 days before the onset of symptoms (4 days before onset of rash) until 4 days after rash has appeared 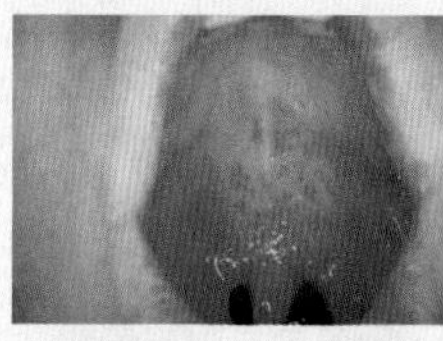 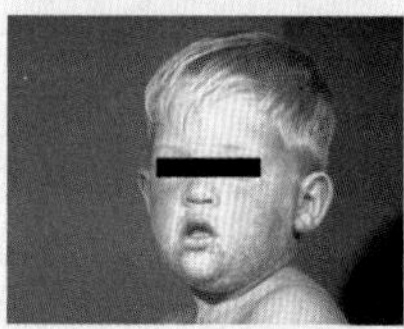 Koplik spots. (Courtesy of Centers for Disease Control and Prevention, & Eichenwald, H. F. [1958]. https://phil.cdc.gov/Details.aspx?pid=3187); (Courtesy of Centers for Disease Control and Prevention. [1963]. *Public health image library [PHIL]: Details.* https://phil.cdc.gov/Details.aspx?pid=1150)	• Prodromal phase: 2–4 days, consisting of fever, cough, coryza, conjunctivitis • Followed by Koplik spots (bright red spots with blue white centers on mucous membranes, mainly buccal mucosa; look like tiny grains of white sand surrounded by red rings) • Erythematous maculopapular, blanching rash appears 3–4 days after the onset of fever. Rash gradually proceeds from head downward and outward.	• Treatment is mainly supportive, including antipyretics, bed rest, adequate fluid intake, and antibiotics to treat secondary bacterial infections such as pneumonia and otitis media. • Postexposure vaccination of unimmunized child within 72 hours of exposure may prevent or reduce illness severity and duration. • Immune serum globulin (IG) given within 6 days of exposure may prevent or make symptoms less severe. • Possible vitamin A supplementation in children hospitalized for severe measles or its complications or those with immunodeficiency • Complications: diarrhea, otitis media, and pneumonia common in young children; acute encephalitis	• Comfort measures, such as antipyretics and antipruritics • Clean eyes with warm, moist cloth to remove secretions. • Cool mist humidification to alleviate coryza and cough • Airborne precautions until 4 days after the onset of rash

(continued)

TABLE 15.4 • Common Viral Exanthems of Childhood (*continued*)

Disease	Clinical Manifestations	Management/Complications	Nursing Implications
Varicella Zoster (Chickenpox)			
• Caused by varicella zoster virus, human herpes virus 3 • Transmission: direct contact with infected people's nasopharyngeal secretions or via airborne spread, to a lesser degree by contact with unscabbed lesions. Highly contagious. Also transmitted from birthing parent to fetus • Peak incidence: winter and early spring • Incubation period: 10–21 days, usually 14–16 days • Communicable 1–2 days before the onset of rash until all vesicles have crusted over (about 3–7 days after the onset of rash) 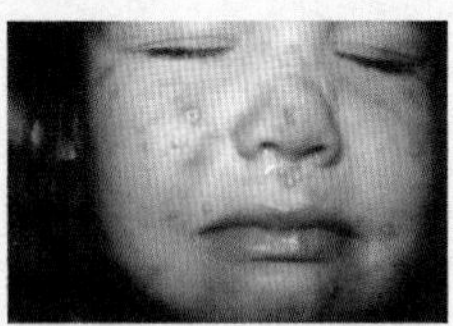 Varicella. (Courtesy of Centers for Disease Control and Prevention, & Noble, J. [1968]. *Public health image library [PHIL]: Details.* https://phil.cdc.gov/Details.aspx?pid=10486)	• Prodromal symptoms (fever, malaise, anorexia, headache, mild abdominal pain) may be present 24–48 hours before the onset of the rash. In children, rash is often the first sign of disease. • Lesions often appear first on scalp, face, trunk, then extremities; initially intensely pruritic erythematous macules that evolve to papules and then form clear, fluid-filled vesicles • Vesicles eventually erupt, and then lesions scab and crust. A variety of lesions are present at one time. • More severe in adolescents and adults than in young children	• Usually self-limiting; treatment is mainly supportive: fever reduction, antipruritics, and skin care to prevent infection of lesions • Antiviral therapy and varicella zoster IG may be used in those considered to be at high risk (immunocompromised, pregnant people, and newborns exposed to maternal varicella). Routine antiviral therapy is not recommended for the treatment of uncomplicated varicella infection in otherwise healthy children. • Complications: bacterial superinfection of skin lesions, thrombocytopenia, arthritis, hepatitis, cerebellar ataxia, encephalitis, meningitis, pneumonia, glomerulonephritis, congenital infection, and life-threatening perinatal infection • Lifelong latent infection occurs; reactivation results in herpes zoster (shingles), uncommon in childhood.	• Comfort measures, such as antipyretics and antipruritics • For those with exposure to susceptible people, airborne and contact precautions, from 8 to 21 days after exposure • Children may return to school or child care once lesions have crusted. • Airborne and contact precautions in the hospitalized child for a minimum of 5 days after the onset of rash and as long as vesicular lesions are present
Exanthem Subitum (Roseola Infantum or Sixth Disease)			
• Caused by B variant of human herpes virus 6 (HHV-6); (less frequently human herpes virus 7 [HHV-7], adenoviruses, enteroviruses, parainfluenza virus) • Transmission: little is known and depends on causative virus but HHV-6 suspected to be from saliva of infected person and enters the host through the oral, nasal, or conjunctival mucosa • Peak incidence: ages 7–13 months, spring and fall • Incubation period: 5–15 days, average of 10 days • Communicability is unknown, but most likely contagious before symptoms appear 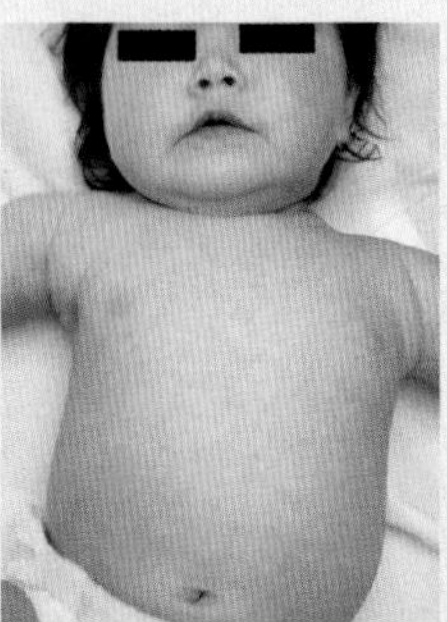 Exanthem subitum (roseola infantum).	• Prodromal phase: usually asymptomatic but may include upper respiratory signs • Clinical illness: high fever ranging from 37.9 to 40°C (101–106°F) for 3–5 days; resolves abruptly; rash appears 12–24 hours later, lasting about 1–3 days. Rash is pinkish red, flat or raised spots that blanch when touched.	• Course is generally benign. • In children who are uncomfortable or irritable or have a history of febrile seizures, antipyretics may be warranted. • Complications: HSV-6 may be responsible for some febrile seizures, encephalitis, aseptic meningitis, and thrombocytopenia purpura.	• Comfort measures, such as antipyretics, antipruritics • Standard precautions are sufficient in the hospitalized child.

TABLE 15.4 • Common Viral Exanthems of Childhood

Disease	Clinical Manifestations	Management/Complications	Nursing Implications
Erythema Infectiosum (Fifth Disease)			
• Caused by human parvovirus B19 • Transmitted by large droplet spread from nasopharyngeal viral shedding or percutaneous exposure to blood and blood products. Also transmitted from birthing parent to fetus • Peak incidence late winter and spring • Incubation period: 4–28 days, average 16–17 days • Communicability is uncertain, but most children are no longer infectious by the time the rash appears and diagnosis is made, so isolation or exclusion from school, once the child is diagnosed, is unnecessary (those with aplastic crisis may be communicable up to 1 week after the onset of symptoms and those who are immunosuppressed with chronic infection and severe anemia may be communicable for months to years). 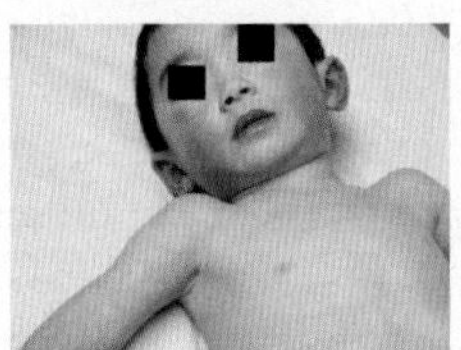 Erythema infectiosum (fifth disease).	• Prodromal phase: mild symptoms, low-grade fever, headache, mild upper respiratory infection • Characteristic rash occurs in three stages: • Begins with erythematous flushing often described as "slapped-cheek" appearance, often with circumoral pallor • Spreads to trunk • Moves peripherally, appearing as a maculopapular, lace-like appearance; often pruritic • Palms and soles are usually spared. Rash fluctuates in intensity and will disappear and reappear with environmental changes such as exposure to sunlight. • Resolves spontaneously over 1–3 weeks • Pain or swelling in joints may be present (more common in older adolescents). • Children with preexisting anemias may develop aplastic crisis (will have fever, malaise, myalgia, but usually no rash).	• Usually benign and self-limited; supportive treatment is all that is needed. • Blood transfusion may be necessary in children with aplastic crisis. • Intravenous immunoglobulin (IVIG) many be given if child is immunocompromised. • Complications: arthritis and arthralgia • May result in fetal loss, hydrops fetalis in pregnant person	• Comfort measures, such as antipyretics, antipruritics. • Inform pregnant people (including health care workers) of the potential risks to the fetus and preventive measures to decrease these risks (strict infection control practices, not caring for those likely to be contagious). The CDC does not recommend routine exclusion from a workplace where an outbreak is occurring. • Droplet precautions are required in the hospitalized child.
Hand, Foot, and Mouth Disease, or Herpangina (if Only Mouth Involvement)			
• Caused by viruses belonging to *Enterovirus* genus. Coxsackie A viruses (especially A16) is the most common. Transmitted by direct contact with infected fecal, oral secretions; spread mostly through saliva • Peak incidence during fall and summer, particularly in children who wear diapers and children <5 years old • Incubation period: 3–6 days • Communicable from time of infection until fever resolves; virus is shed for several weeks after the infection begins.	• High fever usually occurs first. • Vesicles on tongue and oral mucosa erode to shallow ulcers; vesicles on hands and feet are football shaped, with erythematous rims. • Extensive mouth lesions may lead to anorexia, dehydration, and drooling.	• Usually mild and self-limiting, resolving within 1 week • Treatment is mainly supportive. • Complications: dehydration, meningitis, encephalitis, and possible fingernail/toenail loss	• Encourage oral fluids of preference, such as popsicles. • Provide analgesics as needed. • Mouthwash or sprays to numb the mouth may be needed. • Standard precautions and good hand hygiene are necessary. Contact precautions for diapered or incontinent children

Data from Siegel, J. D., Rhinehart, E., Jackson, M., Chiarello, L., & The Healthcare Infection Control Practices Advisory Committee. (2007, updated 2022). Guideline for isolation precautions: Preventing transmission of infectious agents in healthcare settings. https://www.cdc.gov/infectioncontrol/pdf/guidelines/isolation-guidelines-H.pdf; Centers for Disease Control and Prevention. (2021a). In E. Hall, A. P. Wodi, J. Hamborsky, V. Morelli, & S. Schillie (Eds.), *Epidemiology and prevention of vaccine-preventable diseases* (14th ed.). Public Health Foundation. https://www.cdc.gov/vaccines/pubs/pinkbook/index.html; Centers for Disease Control and Prevention. (2020b). Measles (rubeola): For healthcare professionals. Retrieved April 27, 2023, from https://www.cdc.gov/measles/hcp/index.html; Centers for Disease Control and Prevention. (2022d). Chickenpox (varicella): For healthcare professionals. Retrieved April 27, 2023, from https://www.cdc.gov/chickenpox/hcp/; Tremblay, C., & Brady, M. T. (2023). Roseola infantum (exanthem subitum). *UpToDate*. Retrieved April 27, 2023, from https://www.uptodate.com/contents/roseola-infantum-exanthem-subitum; Koch, W. C. (2020). Parvoviruses. In R. M. Kleigman, J. W. St. Geme III, N. J. Blum, S. S. Shah, R. C. Tasker, K. M. Wilson, & R. E. Behrman (Eds.), *Nelson textbook of pediatrics* (21st ed., pp. 9133–9154). Elsevier; Centers for Disease Control and Prevention (CDC). (2021b). *Hand, foot and mouth disease (HFMD)*. Retrieved April 27, 2023, from https://www.cdc.gov/hand-foot-mouth/index.html#:~:text=Hand%2C%20Foot%2C%20and%20Mouth%20Disease%20(HFMD),-Espa%C3%B1ol%20(Spanish)&text=The%20illness%20is%20usually%20not,schools%20and%20day%20care%20centers.&text=Hand%2C%20foot%2C%20and%20mouth%20disease%20spreads%20easily.&text=Symptoms%20can%20include%20mouth%20sores%2C%20skin%20rash%2C%20and%20more

Typically, children with viral exanthems are cared for at home, but there are times when a child may be hospitalized or may develop the disease while being hospitalized. Appropriate transmission-based precautions must be taken. Therapeutic management of the viral exanthems focuses on fever management and relief of discomfort.

Nursing Assessment

Obtain the history of the present illness, noting the onset of rash in relation to the onset of fever. Note accompanying symptoms such as respiratory complaints. Document known exposure to childhood diseases. Note immunization status. Inspect the skin for rash, noting the distribution, type, and extent of lesions. Table 15.4 describes the rash as well as accompanying symptoms for each of the viral exanthems.

Nursing Management

Nursing management of viral exanthems focuses on fever reduction, relief of discomfort, and protection of skin integrity. Encourage hydration. Administer antipyretics and antipruritics as needed (refer to Drug Guide 15.1). Nonpharmacologic interventions to reduce fever, such as tepid sponging and cool compresses, may be used. Refer to the "Clinical Judgment and the Nursing Process" section earlier in the chapter. Care should be individualized based on the child's and family's response to the illness.

TAKE NOTE!

Trim the child's fingernails or cover hands with mitts, gloves, or socks (which work well with younger infants and children) if the rash itches to help prevent breaks in the skin, which can lead to discomfort and infection.

Mumps

Mumps, a contagious disease caused by Paramyxovirus, is characterized by fever and parotitis (inflammation and swelling of the parotid gland). Mumps is spread via airborne droplets or contact with infected droplets. The incubation period is 12 to 25 days, usually 16 to 18 days (Albrecht, 2021). Infected individuals are contagious several days prior to the onset of parotitis and for 6 to 9 days after parotid swelling begins (Albrecht, 2021). The most common complication in postpubertal boys is orchitis (inflammation of the testicle) (Albrecht, 2021). This may lead to some degree of testicular atrophy, but rarely sterility. In about 5% of females oophoritis (ovarian inflammation) occurs, with the relationship to fertility unknown (Albrecht, 2021). Complications of mumps include meningitis with or without encephalitis with seizures, pancreatitis, and auditory neuritis, which can result in hearing loss. Therapeutic management is supportive.

Since the recommendation of the two-dose MMR (measles, mumps, rubella) vaccine, the incidence of mumps has declined and made mumps a rare disease in the United States (CDC, 2021a). The AAP and the ACIP recommend immunization against mumps for all children (CDC, 2021a). Current recommendations include first mumps immunization between 12 and 15 months of age, followed by a second vaccine between 4 and 6 years of age (CDC, 2021a). According to the CDC (2021a), research shows that one dose of MMR prevents 78% of cases and two doses prevent approximately 88% of cases (see Chapter 9 for information on mumps vaccination).

Nursing Assessment

Note history of exposure to infected individuals as well as immunization status. Determine history of low-grade fever and onset and progression of parotid swelling. History may also include malaise, anorexia, headache, and abdominal pain. The parotid swelling is easily observed as swelling of the neck either bilaterally or unilaterally (Fig. 15.4). In boys, note orchitis. The diagnosis is usually based on the history and clinical presentation, but serum may be tested for the presence of mumps IgG or IgM antibody.

Nursing Management

Nursing management of mumps is primarily supportive. Acetaminophen or ibuprofen is used for fever management, and occasionally narcotic analgesics are required

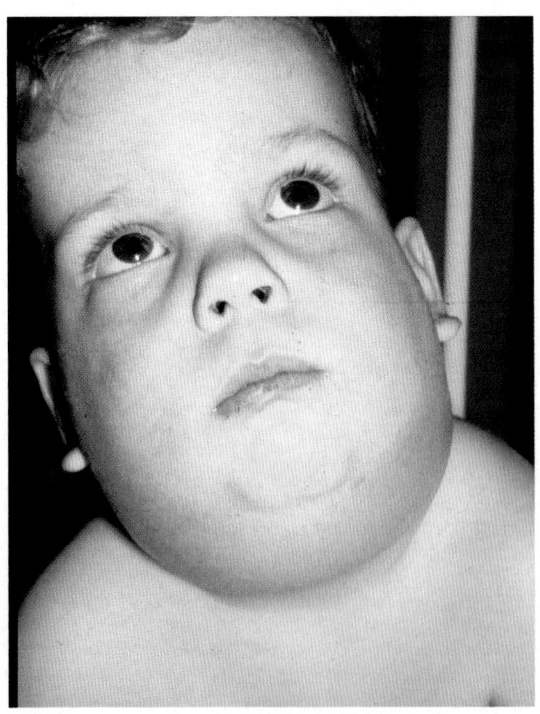

FIGURE 15.4 Parotitis associated with mumps.

for pain management. Oral fluids are encouraged to prevent dehydration. If orchitis is present, ice packs to the testicles and gentle testicular support may be helpful. Hospitalized children should be confined to respiratory isolation to prevent spread of the disease until 6 to 9 days following the onset of parotid swelling (Albrecht, 2021).

TAKE NOTE!

In recent years mumps outbreaks have occurred, mainly in settings where prolonged close contact with other people occurs, such as college campuses, camps, athletic teams, and worship groups (CDC, 2021a). The mumps vaccine is not 100% effective, and mumps infection can occur in vaccinated individuals. During an outbreak it is essential to define the population at risk and transmission setting, identify and isolate suspected cases, and identify and vaccinate susceptible individuals.

ZOONOTIC INFECTIONS

Zoonotic and **vector-borne** infections are diseases caused by infectious agents that are transmitted directly or indirectly from animals or vectors, such as ticks, mosquitoes, or other insect vectors, to humans. Zoonotic infections are responsible for about 75% of emerging infectious diseases, with approximately 60% of all human pathogens originating from animals (CDC, 2021c).

Children are at a particular risk for contracting zoonotic or vector-borne diseases. Young children are unaware of the health risks around them and cannot take protective measures. Their immature immune system leads to a decreased capacity to resist zoonotic or vector-borne diseases. These diseases can be severe and even fatal, although most are treatable if identified early. Many times, the child presents initially with nonspecific symptoms. Coupled with the fact that there are few definitive diagnostic tests available, this can lead to difficulty in promptly recognizing and treating these diseases. Tick-borne diseases are common vector-borne illnesses in the United States. Determining the incidence of zoonotic and vector-borne diseases is difficult due to the complexity of the transmission cycle and geographic climate variability. Table 15.5 discusses other zoonotic and vector-borne diseases. Nurses need to be aware of zoonotic and vector-borne diseases common in the area they are practicing as well as the impact of patient travel and the risk of these diseases. Nurses need to tap into state and local resources as well as national and international resources, such as the CDC and the World Health Organization (WHO).

TABLE 15.5 • Other Zoonotic and Vector-Borne Illnesses

Disease	Causative Organism	Geographic Distribution	Vector of Transmission	Manifestations
West Nile virus	*Flavivirus*	Throughout United States with higher rates found in Great Plains and mountain regions; seasonal epidemic from summer to fall	Mosquito bites Rare cases spread through blood transfusions, transplants, and birthing parent to baby during pregnancy and breastfeeding.	No symptoms in majority of cases Symptoms include febrile illness, headache, joint pain, body aches, vomiting, diarrhea, and rash; in rare cases serious symptoms such as meningitis, encephalitis, or acute flaccid paralysis are seen.
Dengue	*Dengue viruses (flaviviruses)*	Tropics and subtropics Asia, India, Southeast Asia, Latin America, the Pacific Islands, United States (mostly Florida and Texas), US territories (mostly Puerto Rico), and Africa	Mosquito	Sudden-onset high fever, headache, severe pain behind eyes, joint, muscle and bone pain, rash, mild bleeding such as nose or gums bleeding and bruising easily, leukopenia, thrombocytopenia, and hemorrhagic manifestations Symptoms can be mild to severe and life threatening.
Zika	*Flavivirus*	Americas, Caribbean, the Pacific, Africa, and Southeast Asia	Mosquito	Acute onset of low-grade fever, maculopapular rash, arthralgia, conjunctivitis Can be passed to fetus in utero Infection during pregnancy can lead to birth defects and neurologic complications of fetus.

(*continued*)

TABLE 15.5 • Other Zoonotic and Vector-Borne Illnesses (*continued*)

Disease	Causative Organism	Geographic Distribution	Vector of Transmission	Manifestations
Anaplasmosis	*Anaplasma phagocytophilum*	Mostly upper Midwest and northeast United States	Black-legged tick	Headache, fever, malaise, chills, muscle aches, nausea, abdominal pain, cough, and confusion Rash is rarely seen. Symptoms appear 1–2 weeks after infected tick bite.
Ehrlichiosis	Three pathogens: *Ehrlichia chaffeensis, Ehrlichia ewingii, Ehrlichia muris*	Mostly in southeastern and south-central United States	Black-legged and lone star tick	Fever, headaches, fatigue, muscle aches, chills, nausea, vomiting, diarrhea, confusion, red eyes. Clinical signs similar to Rocky Mountain spotted fever. Rash is less commonly associated but is more common in children. May also present with leukopenia, anemia, and hepatitis
Malaria	*Plasmodium* (five species exist that infect humans: *P. falciparum, P. vivax, P. ovale, P. malariae, P. knowlesi*)	Endemic in tropical areas of the world Highest incidence in Africa, Asia, and South America. Cases in the United States are usually in travelers and immigrants returning from countries where malaria transmission occurs.	Bite of *Anopheles* species of mosquito	High fever with chills, rigors, sweats, and headache, which may be paroxysmal Nausea, vomiting, diarrhea, cough, arthralgia, and abdominal and back pain may also occur. Anemia and thrombocytopenia with pallor and jaundice may be seen. May occur in a cyclic pattern, and depending on the species fever may occur every other day or every third day.

Adapted from Centers for Disease Control and Prevention. (2023a). West Nile virus. https://www.cdc.gov/westnile/index.html; Centers for Disease Control and Prevention. (2023d). Dengue. http://www.cdc.gov/Dengue/; Centers for Disease Control and Prevention. (2022h). Zika virus. https://www.cdc.gov/zika/index.html; Centers for Disease Control and Prevention. (2022i); Anaplasmosis. http://www.cdc.gov/anaplasmosis/; Centers for Disease Control and Prevention. (2022j). Ehrlichiosis. http://www.cdc.gov/ehrlichiosis/; Centers for Disease Control and Prevention. (2023e). Malaria. https://www.cdc.gov/parasites/malaria/index.html

TAKE NOTE!

The CDC lists the current infectious disease outbreaks that are being reported at http://www.cdc.gov/outbreaks.

TAKE NOTE!

In 2016 large outbreaks of Zika occurred with increasing cases in the United States. In 2017 cases in the United States began declining, and from 2018 to 2022 there were no reports of Zika virus in the United States (CDC, 2022h).

Cat-Scratch Disease

Cat-scratch disease is a relatively common and occasionally serious disease caused by the bacteria *Bartonella henselae*. It occurs in both children and adults but is more common in children (Orscheln, 2020). Cats can carry the bacteria in their saliva. In 87% to 99% of cases, the child has had a recent interaction with cats and often kittens (Orscheln, 2020). *B. henselae* is transmitted between cats via the cat flea. The incubation period is 7 to 12 days, with lymphadenopathy appearing in 1 to 4 weeks (Orscheln, 2020). Therapeutic management is supportive and is aimed at management of symptoms. The disease itself is usually self-limited, resolving on its own in 2 to 4 months. If lymphadenopathy persists or if the child is immunocompromised, antibiotics may be needed. Painful, swollen nodes may be treated with needle aspiration to provide symptom relief.

Nursing Assessment

Note history of headaches, fever, anorexia, and fatigue. The history may also include interaction or rough play with cats or kittens, resulting in a scratch. Document temperature, noting fever. Palpate for enlarged lymph nodes, noting their location. A skin papule or pustule may be present or reported at the site of the bite or scratch. Diagnostic tests are available to detect serum antibodies to antigens of *Bartonella* species.

Nursing Management

Administer antibiotics if ordered. No transmission-based isolation is required; standard precautions are sufficient. Educate the child and family about prevention and control measures. Teach children to avoid rough play with cats and kittens. Teach parents and children to immediately wash any bites or scratches with soap and running water. Explain that cats should never lick open wounds on the child. Control of fleas in cats is important to prevent the spread of *B. henselae*.

Rabies

Rabies is a preventable viral infection of the central nervous system. It is transmitted to other animals and humans through close contact with the saliva of a rabid animal, usually by a bite. It is rare in the United States and Western Europe due to routine vaccination of domestic animals, such as dogs, and the availability of effective postexposure prophylaxis (PEP). Now most cases of rabies in these areas are due to wild animals such as raccoons, skunks, bats, and foxes (Brown & DeMaria, 2022). Rabies continues to be a major health problem in other parts of the world, especially in areas where dogs are not controlled.

Most cases of rabies occur in children younger than 15 years, and most human deaths occur in Asia and Africa (Brown & DeMaria, 2022; WHO, 2023). Children have an increased susceptibility to rabies due to their fearlessness around animals, eagerness to play with animals, shorter stature, and inability to protect themselves. The incubation period for rabies is extremely variable. Typically, it is 1 to 3 months but can range from days to years (Brown & DeMaria, 2022). The incubation period tends to be shorter in children. Once symptoms of rabies have developed, the prognosis is poor. Death usually occurs within days of the onset of symptoms. Prevention is of paramount importance, and eliminating infection in animal vectors is essential. Successful animal vaccination and animal control campaigns in the United States have led to a very low rate of human rabies cases. Recently, rabies transmitted from other animals, especially bats, has become a cause for concern (WHO, 2023).

It is important to contact the local health department whenever there is an exposure, or suspected exposure, to rabies. Several factors need to be considered when deciding to provide PEP, such as local epidemiology, type of animal involved, availability of the responsible animal for testing or quarantine, and the circumstances of the exposure, such as a provoked versus an unprovoked attack. Algorithms are available to help health care providers decide if PEP is warranted (Brown & DeMaria, 2023). In a previously unvaccinated child, PEP should begin with a thorough cleansing of all wounds with soap and water followed by a virucidal agent, such as povidone–iodine solution, if available. Animal studies have shown a 90% reduction in the likelihood of developing rabies with proper wound cleaning (Brown & DeMaria, 2023). In the United States, concurrent use of passive (rabies immune globulin) and active (rabies vaccine) immunoprophylaxis is then recommended. It consists of a regimen of one dose of immune globulin and four doses of human rabies vaccine. Rabies immune globulin and the first dose of rabies vaccine should be given as soon as possible after exposure, ideally within 24 hours. Additional doses of rabies vaccine should be given on days 3, 7, and 14 after the first vaccination. Rabies immune globulin is infiltrated into and around the wound, with any remaining volume administered intramuscularly at a site distant from the vaccine inoculation. Human rabies vaccine is administered intramuscularly into the anterolateral thigh or deltoid, depending on the age and size of the child. Administration into the gluteus muscle should be avoided, since this site has been associated with vaccine failure (Brown & DeMaria, 2023). Preexposure vaccination can be given to prevent rabies in people at high risk, such as veterinarians, laboratory technicians working with the virus, and people exposed to wild animals (Brown & DeMaria, 2023).

Nursing Assessment

Note the history of an animal bite, especially if it was unprovoked, and exposure to bats. Document history of early symptoms of rabies infection, which are nonspecific and flu-like, such as fever, headache, and general malaise. The child may complain of pain, pruritus, and paresthesia at the bite site. As the virus spreads to the central nervous system, encephalitis develops. The disease will have progressive neurologic manifestations, which may include insomnia, confusion, anxiety, changes in behavior, agitation or excitation, hallucinations, hypersalivation, dysphagia, and hydrophobia, which results from aspiration when swallowing liquid or saliva. In some cases, progressive paralysis may be present. The child may have periods of lucidity alternating with these neurologic changes.

Laboratory testing may include hair and saliva specimens from which the virus may be isolated. Serum and cerebrospinal fluid can be tested for antibodies to the rabies virus. Direct fluorescent antibody testing can be done to diagnose rabies in a suspected animal. The test can only be done postmortem and requires brain tissue from the potentially rabid animal.

Nursing Management

Few people survive once symptomatic rabies infection develops. Intensive supportive care is required, but recovery is extremely rare. Therefore, it is vital to educate children and families about the importance of seeking medical care after any animal bite to prevent death from rabies infection. Also, teach children to avoid wild animals, stray animals, and any animal with unusual behavior. Teach children not to provoke or attempt to capture wild or stray animals.

TAKE NOTE!

There have been 17 survivors of rabies once symptoms developed using a treatment protocol developed by Dr. Rodney Willoughby, Jr. called the Milwaukee Protocol at the Children's Hospital of Wisconsin. In half of the survivors, neurologic outcomes were poor (Willoughby, 2020).

Regardless of whether immunoprophylaxis is initiated, appropriate wound management is necessary in all victims of a bite from a potentially rabid animal. This includes a thorough cleansing of all wounds with soap and water. Irrigation of wounds with large volumes of a virucidal agent, such as povidone–iodine solution, along with avoiding closure of the wound is recommended (Willoughby, 2020).

When caring for a child requiring PEP, provide support and education to the child and family. Due to the seriousness and urgency surrounding this disease and treatment, the child and family are often very frightened. Consider comfort measures, such as EMLA (eutectic mixture of local anesthetic) cream and positioning, when giving immunizations.

Lyme Disease

Lyme disease, the most commonly reported vector-borne disease in the United States, is caused primarily by the spirochete *Borrelia burgdorferi* (Mead, 2021). It is transmitted to humans via the bite of an infected black-legged (deer) tick. Ninety-three percent of reported Lyme disease cases occurred in 14 states, mainly in the northeast (Pennsylvania, New Jersey, New York, Massachusetts, Connecticut, Maryland, New Hampshire, Delaware, Maine, Rhode Island, Vermont, and Virginia) and the upper Midwest (Minnesota and Wisconsin) (Mead, 2021).

Lyme disease can affect any age group, but the incidence is highest among children between 5 and 14 years of age and adults 45 to 55 years old (Mead, 2021). The prognosis for recovery in children who are treated is excellent.

Therapeutic Management

In most cases Lyme disease can be cured by antibiotics, especially if they are started early in the illness. Doxycycline is the drug of choice for children followed by amoxicillin and cefuroxime (Hu & Shapiro, 2023). In the past doxycycline was not recommended in children less than 8 years of age due to the risk that it could cause permanent discoloration of the teeth. The AAP and CDC now support the use of doxycycline in young children if treatment duration is less than 21 days as studies have shown that short courses of doxycycline do not lead to tooth staining or weakening of tooth enamel (CDC, 2019). Duration of treatment is usually 10 to 28 days, depending on the stage of disease.

Nursing Assessment

The clinical signs of Lyme disease are divided into three stages—early localized, early disseminated, and late disease. Untreated children may progress through the three stages or may present with early disseminated or late disease without having any symptoms of the earlier stages. If children are treated in the early stage, it is uncommon to see them with late disease. Nursing assessment for Lyme disease includes an accurate health history as well as physical examination.

HEALTH HISTORY

Explore the health history for a tick bite. Document onset of rash. In early localized disease, the rash usually occurs 7 to 14 days after the tick bite (though it can appear 3 to 32 days after the bite). In early disseminated disease, the rash usually begins 3 to 5 weeks after the tick bite. Note complaints of fever, malaise, mild neck stiffness, headache, fatigue, myalgia, and arthralgia or pain in the joints. In late disease, note recurrent arthritis of the large joints, such as the knees, beginning weeks to months after the tick bite. The child with late disease may or may not have a history of earlier stages of the disease, including erythema migrans.

PHYSICAL EXAMINATION

Observe for a rash. A ring-like rash at the site of the tick bite (erythema migrans) characterizes early local disease (Fig. 15.5). If untreated, the rash gradually expands and will remain for 1 to 2 weeks. Suspect early disseminated disease if multiple areas of erythema migrans are found. The multiple lesions are usually smaller than the primary lesions. Note cranial nerve palsies (especially cranial nerve VII), conjunctivitis, or signs of meningeal irritation, which occur in early disseminated disease.

LABORATORY AND DIAGNOSTIC TESTING

When diagnosing Lyme disease health care providers need to consider presence of signs and symptoms of Lyme disease, likelihood of exposure, and other illnesses that may cause similar symptoms along with results of laboratory tests. Immunoglobulin-specific antibody tests may not be positive in the early stage of the disease but may be useful in the later stages. The CDC recommends a two-step test, where both steps are required and use the same blood sample (CDC, 2021d). If these are negative, no further testing is indicated.

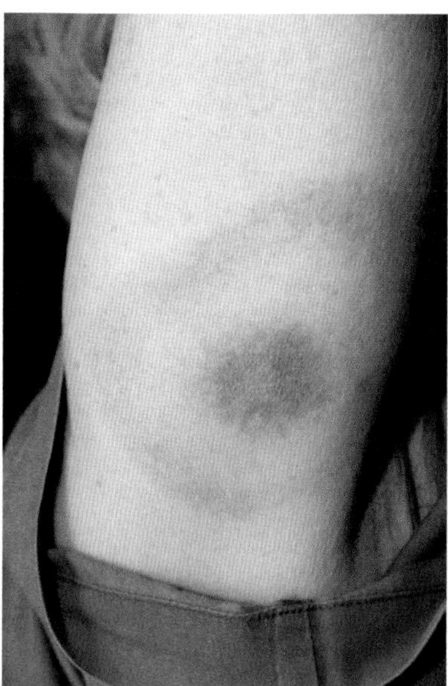

FIGURE 15.5 Erythema migrans, a ring-like rash at the site of the tick bite, occurs in Lyme disease. (Courtesy of CDC/James Gathany. [2007]. http://phil.cdc.gov/phil/details.asp?pid=9875)

Nursing Management

Administer antibiotics as ordered. In the hospitalized child, no transmission-based precautions are necessary. Educate the child and family on the importance of taking the antibiotic as directed and finishing all the medicine. Another important nursing function is educating the child, family, and community on prevention measures (Box 15.5). For infection to occur, typically the tick must be attached for 36 to 48 hours (CDC, 2023b). Therefore, prompt removal (within 24 hours) of ticks is essential to the prevention of Lyme disease. Teaching Guidelines 15.2 gives information on tick removal.

TEACHING GUIDELINES 15.2 Tick Removal

- Use clean, fine-tipped tweezers.
- Protect fingers with a tissue, paper towel, or latex gloves.
- Grasp tick as close to the skin as possible and pull upward with steady, even pressure.
- Do not twist or jerk the tick.
- Once the tick is removed, clean site with soap and water, rubbing alcohol, or iodine scrub and wash your hands.
- Save the tick for identification in case the child becomes sick. Place in a sealable plastic bag and put it in your freezer. Write date of bite on the bag.

Rocky Mountain Spotted Fever

Rocky Mountain spotted fever (RMSF) is the most severe and frequently reported rickettsial illness in the United States and is the second most common vector-borne disease after Lyme disease (Reller & Dumler, 2020). RMSF is caused by the bacteria *Rickettsia rickettsii*. The American dog tick and Rocky Mountain wood tick are the primary vectors, although others have been implicated. RMSF can be fatal without prompt and appropriate treatment (Reller & Dumler, 2020). Most cases occur between April and September (Reller & Dumler, 2020).

RMSF occurs throughout the United States. Its name is derived from the fact that it was discovered in the Rocky Mountain region, though few cases are found there today. It occurs in all age groups but most frequently in children, with the peak incidence in children older than 10 years (Reller & Dumler, 2020).

Complications of RMSF include noncardiogenic pulmonary edema, cerebral edema, and multiorgan damage. Long-term neurologic involvement, such as partial paralysis of the lower extremities, hearing loss, loss of bladder and bowel control, movement disorders, and language disorders, may be seen, especially in children with severe illness who require long hospital stays.

BOX 15.5 Prevention of Tick-Borne Illnesses

- Wear appropriate protective clothing when entering tick-infested areas. Clothing should fit tightly around wrists, waists, and ankles. Tuck pants into socks if possible.
- After leaving the area, do a full body check for ticks and remove them promptly.
- Examine gear, clothes, and pets for ticks. Tumble dry clothes and appropriate gear on high heat for an hour.
- Insect repellent may provide temporary relief but may produce toxicity, especially in children, if used frequently or in large doses.

Therapeutic Management

The fatality rate from RMSF has decreased with the widespread use of antimicrobial therapy (Reller & Dumler, 2020). However, delays in diagnosis and therapy are significant factors associated with severity of disease and death. In most cases RMSF resolves rapidly with appropriate antibiotic therapy, especially if it is started early. Treatment of choice for children of all ages is doxycycline (Sexton & McClain, 2021). Length of treatment is typically 5 to 7 days (Sexton & McClain, 2021).

Nursing Assessment

Note history of early signs of RMSF, such as sudden onset of fever, headache, malaise, nausea and vomiting, muscle pain, and anorexia. The incubation period varies from 2 to 14 days, with the average being around 7 days after the tick bite (Reller & Dumler, 2020). Other signs include a rash, usually seen 1 to 3 days after the onset of the fever, abdominal pain, joint pain, and diarrhea. Inspect

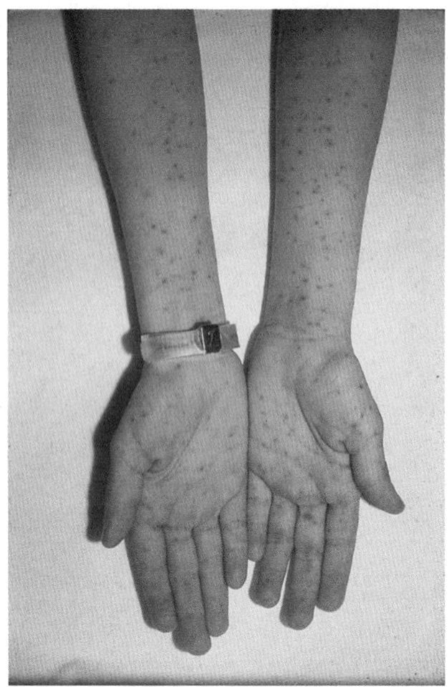

FIGURE 15.6 Rash associated with Rocky Mountain spotted fever.

the skin for a rash, which starts as small, pink, macular, nonitchy, blanchable spots on the wrists, forearms, and ankles. The rash then spreads rapidly over the entire body, including the soles and palms. After several days the rash will appear red, spotted, and petechial or hemorrhagic (Fig. 15.6). Approximately 3% to 5% of children with RMSF do not have a rash (Reller & Dumler, 20120). Laboratory findings may include a low leukocyte count, low or decreasing platelet count, and hyponatremia. Biopsy of the rash with immunofluorescent assay and serologic tests may also be used.

Nursing Management

Nursing management is similar to that for Lyme disease. Educate the family about completing the antibiotic course, preventing tick bites, and appropriate tick removal (refer to Box 15.5 and Teaching Guidelines 15.2).

> *TAKE NOTE!*
>
> Many folklore remedies exist for tick removal such as use of petroleum jelly, nail polish, or hot matches. These often do little to get the tick to detach and may actually irritate the tick and stimulate it to release more saliva or gut contents, therefore increasing the chance of disease. The goal of tick removal is to detach it as quickly as possible (CDC, 2022e).

PARASITIC AND HELMINTHIC INFECTION

Parasites are organisms larger than yeast or bacteria that can cause infection. They live in or on a host. Parasites receive nourishment from the host without benefiting or killing the host. Parasites frequently seen in children are scabies and head lice. A helminth is a parasitic intestinal worm. Helminthic infections seen in children include pinworms, roundworms, and hookworms. Children are at an increased risk for parasitic or helminthic infections due to poor hygiene practices. For example, children typically are more careless about handwashing and they tend to put things in their mouths and share toys and objects with other children.

Nursing Assessment and Management

Parents are often embarrassed when they find out that their child has a parasitic or helminthic infection. Reassure them that these infections can occur in any child. Tables 15.6 and 15.7 give nursing assessment and management information related to specific common parasitic and helminthic infections in children.

> *TAKE NOTE!*
>
> The head louse becoming resistant to pediculicides is a growing concern (Goldstein & Goldstein, 2022a).

> **CONSIDER THIS!**
>
> After cheerleading practice, I noticed my head was itchy. When I got home, I told my mom. She looked at my head and said she found lice. What am I going to do? Am I going to have to cut off all my hair? I love my hair! What are my friends on my team going to say if they find out? How could this happen to me?
>
> Thoughts: Why is this adolescent so upset?
>
> How does her developmental age affect her reaction to this discovery?
>
> How would you respond to her concerns?

> *TAKE NOTE!*
>
> Prescription-only treatments have been approved by the Food and Drug Administration (FDA) for the treatment of head lice, including spinosad, malathion, and ivermectin tablets. Over-the-counter permethrin or pyrethrins remain the first line of treatment, but the new medications may be helpful with difficult-to-get-rid-of cases or cases of resistant lice (Nolt et al., 2022).

SEXUALLY TRANSMITTED INFECTIONS

STIs, commonly called sexually transmitted diseases, are infectious diseases transmitted through sexual contact, including oral, vaginal, or anal intercourse. Certain infections can be transmitted in utero to the fetus or during childbirth to the newborn leading to miscarriage, stillbirth, ectopic pregnancy, preterm delivery, low birth weight, birth defects,

TABLE 15.6 • Common Parasitic Infections in Children

Infection/Causative Organism	Transmission	Clinical Manifestations	Diagnosis/Treatment	Isolation/Control Measures/Concerns
Pediculosis capitis (head lice) Caused by *Pediculus humanus capitis* (head louse)	Direct contact with hair of infested people, less commonly with personal belongings, such as combs and hats, of those infested Incubation period from laying of eggs to hatching of nymph is 6–10 days; adult lice will appear 2–3 weeks later.	Extreme pruritus is the most common symptom. Adult eggs (nits) or lice may be seen, especially behind the ears and at the nape of the neck.	Diagnosis by identification of eggs, nymph, and lice with the naked eye is possible; adult lice are rarely seen. Treatment: washing hair with a pediculicide such as pyrethroids (permethrin and pyrethrins) is preferred, or malathion, spinosad, and ivermectin. Wet combing (manual removal of lice) primarily used for young infants and patients who prefer to avoid pediculicides Careful instructions on proper use of any product should be given and strict adherence to application instructions encouraged. Retreatment is usually recommended 9 days after first treatment, depending on treatment used. Detection of living lice 24 hours after treatment suggests incorrect use, a very heavy infestation, reinfestation, or resistance to treatment.	Contact precautions After treatment check hair and comb nits and lice from hair shafts every 2–3 days to prevent reinfestation. Control measures: Household and other close contacts should be examined and if infested treated. Bedmates should be treated prophylactically. Head lice do not survive long once they have fallen off. Most children can be treated effectively without treating their clothing and bedding. But to help avoid reinfestation, disinfection of clothing, headgear, pillowcases, towels, and other items used by the individual within the past 2 days by washing in hot water and drying on the hot cycle may be helpful. Dry-cleaning nonwashable items or simply sealing them in a plastic bag for 10 days is effective. Soak combs and hairbrushes in pediculicide, shampoo, or hot water. Lice infestation is not a sign of poor hygiene; all socioeconomic groups are affected.
Pediculosis pubis (pubic lice) Caused by *Pthirus pubis*	Transmission usually occurs through sexual contact; also can be through contaminated items such as towels Adolescents and young adults most commonly affected	Pruritus of anogenital area; other hairy areas of the body, including eyelashes, eyebrows, axilla, legs, and beard, can be affected.	Diagnosis by identification of eggs, nymph, and lice with the naked eye is possible; adult lice are rarely seen. Same as treatment with pediculicides to treat head lice Retreat 9–10 days later. To treat eyelashes and eyebrows: if only a few nits are present, remove these with fingernails or a nit comb; if additional treatment is needed, apply ophthalmic-grade petrolatum ointment (prescription).	Standard precautions Control measures similar to head lice All sexual contacts should be treated simultaneously. Avoid sexual contact with partners until both they and their partners have been successfully treated and reevaluated. Evaluation for the presence of other sexually transmitted infections Bedding and clothing should be machine washed and dried at a high temperature or bagged for 2 weeks. If found on children, may be a sign of sexual exposure or abuse

(*continued*)

TABLE 15.6 • Common Parasitic Infections in Children (*continued*)

Infection/Causative Organism	Transmission	Clinical Manifestations	Diagnosis/Treatment	Isolation/Control Measures/Concerns
Scabies Caused by *Sarcoptes scabiei*	Incubation period from laying of eggs to hatching of nymph is 3–4 days; adult lice will appear 2–4 weeks later. Incubation period in those without previous exposure is 4–6 weeks. Usually no symptoms are present during this time but transmission to others can occur. People who were previously infested can develop symptoms in 1–4 days. Transmission usually occurs through prolonged, close personal contact.	Intense pruritus (especially at night) with the presence of erythematous, papular rash with excoriations. The lesions are generally distributed but often are concentrated on the hands and feet and in body folds. May be found on head and neck In infants and young children the rash is often heavy on palms, soles, and fingers, and it may include vesicles, pustules, or bullous lesions.	Diagnosis can be made by a history of itching (especially at night), classic rash, and reports of itching in household or sexual contacts. Mites can be seen on microscopic examination of skin scrapings to confirm diagnosis. Treatment: A scabicide, such as permethrin or lindane, should be applied to the entire body below the head. Treatment of infants and young children should include the head, neck, and body. In infants younger than 2 months, permethrin is not approved; therefore, a topical sulfur treatment cream is used and left on for a specified time (usually 8–14 hours) depending on the type of scabicide. Retreatment 1–2 weeks later may be needed. Oral ivermectin (cannot be used in children <15 kg) Careful instructions on proper use of any product should be given and strict adherence to application instructions should be urged. Itching may not subside for several weeks, even after successful treatment.	Contact precautions Prophylactic therapy for household members and sexual contacts Bedding and clothing used by infested person or household, sexual, or close contacts within 3–4 days before treatment should be laundered in hot water and dried on the hot cycle (mites do not survive more than 3–4 days without skin contact). Avoid direct skin-to-skin contact with person or items used by those infested. Room used by an infected person, especially if they have crusted scabies, should be thoroughly cleaned and vacuumed.

Data from Goldstein, A. O., & Goldstein, B. O. (2022a). Pediculosis capitis. *UpToDate*. Retrieved May 1, 2023, from https://www.uptodate.com/contents/pediculosis-capitis; Nolt, D., Moore, S., Yan, A. C., Melnick, L., & Committee on Infectious Diseases, Committee on Practice and Ambulatory Medicine, Section on Dermatology (2022). Head lice. *Pediatrics, 150*(4), e2022059282. https://doi.org/10.1542/peds.2022-059282; Goldstein, A. O., & Goldstein, B. G. (2023). Pediculosis pubis and pediculosis ciliaris. *UpToDate*. Retrieved May 1, 20123, from https://www.uptodate.com/contents/pediculosis-pubis-and-pediculosis-ciliaris; Goldstein, B. G., & Goldstein, A. O. (2022b). Scabies: Epidemiology, clinical features, and diagnosis. *UpToDate*. Retrieved May 1, 2023, from https://www.uptodate.com/contents/scabies-epidemiology-clinical-features-and-diagnosis; Goldstein, B. G., & Goldstein, A. O. (2022c). Scabies: Management. *UpToDate*. Retrieved May 1, 2023, from https://www.uptodate.com/contents/scabies-management; Siegel, J. D., Rhinehart, E., Jackson, M., Chiarello, L., & The Healthcare Infection Control Practices Advisory Committee. (2007, updated 2022). Guideline for isolation precautions: Preventing transmission of infectious agents in healthcare settings. Retrieved March 19, 2019, from https://www.cdc.gov/infectioncontrol/pdf/guidelines/isolation-guidelines-H.pdf

and congenital infection (Rietmeijer, 2023). Table 15.8 gives information on specific STIs and their effects on the fetus or newborn. Chapter 25 provides information related to human immunodeficiency virus (HIV).

STIs are a major health concern for adolescents. The rates of many STIs are highest in adolescents (Fortenberry, 2022). Adolescents are at a greater risk for developing STIs for a variety of reasons, including frequency of unprotected intercourse, being biologically more susceptible to infection, and engaging in partnerships of limited duration (Fortenberry, 2022).

Detection of STIs in infants and children is an important warning sign of potential sexual abuse. Due to the serious implications that a diagnosis of an STI can have in children, only tests that have high specificities and that can isolate an organism should be used. Also, treatment for the child with a suspected STI may be delayed until a definitive diagnosis can be made.

Nursing Assessment

Many health care providers fail to assess sexual behavior and STI risks, to screen for asymptomatic infection during clinic visits, or to counsel adolescents on STI risk reduction. Nurses need to remember that they play a key role in the detection, prevention, and treatment of STIs in adolescents and children. All states allow adolescents to give consent to confidential STI testing and treatment. Table 15.9 discusses common clinical manifestations of specific STIs in adolescents.

Nursing Management

Encourage the child or adolescent to complete the antibiotic prescription. Prevention of STIs among children and adolescents is critical. Health care providers have a unique opportunity to provide counseling and education in this setting. Adapt the style, content, and message to the child or adolescent's developmental level. Identify risk factors and risk behaviors and help the adolescent develop specific individualized actions for prevention. This conversation needs to be direct and nonjudgmental.

TABLE 15.7 • Common Helminthic Infections in Children

Infection/Causative Organism	Clinical Manifestations	Transmission	Diagnosis/Treatment	Isolation/Control Measures
Ascariasis Most commonly caused by *Ascaris lumbricoides*, common in temperate and tropical areas, especially in areas with unsanitary conditions	Most people are asymptomatic, may demonstrate slower growth and weight gain In more severe infections, loss of appetite, nausea, vomiting, and abdominal pain may be seen. Cough and difficulty breathing may be present as immature worms migrate through the lungs. In significant infestation, partial or complete intestinal obstruction may occur. The more worms, the worse the symptoms.	Human feces are the major source of infected eggs. Hand to mouth is the usual route of transmission. The eggs are swallowed due to unclean hands or contaminated food or water. They pass into the intestine; larvae then hatch, penetrate the intestinal wall, enter the circulatory system, and migrate to other body tissues, primarily the lungs first.	Diagnosis: once female worms are in the intestine, eggs can be visualized by microscopic evaluation of the stool. Occasionally a worm may be coughed up and visualized or seen in vomit, stool, or urine. Imaging can also be used. Mainstay of treatment is with mebendazole, albendazole, or pyrantel pamoate.	Standard precautions are sufficient. Sanitary disposal of feces Proper hand hygiene
Hookworm Caused by *Ancylostoma duodenale* (roundworm) and *Necator americanus* (roundworm); *Ancylostoma ceylanicum* (a hookworm found in cats and dogs that can cause human infections) common in tropics and subtropics especially in areas with unsanitary conditions; rare in areas with <40 in of annual rainfall	Most often people are asymptomatic until significant worms are established. May see pruritic erythematous papular rash at entry site (referred to as ground itch) or pulmonary symptoms as the larvae migrate One of the greatest concerns in chronic infection is anemia (microcytic hypochromic anemia) secondary to blood loss as the worms suck blood and juices from the intestines. This can lead to hypoproteinemia, edema, pica, and wasting. The infection may result in physical or intellectual disability in children.	Hookworms are found in soil and enter the host through pores, hair follicles, and even intact skin (hands and feet are major sites of entry). The maturing larvae travel through the circulatory system into the lungs and then up the bronchial tree and are swallowed with secretions. They then migrate into the intestinal tract and attach to the wall of the small intestines, where they feed and reproduce.	Diagnosis: through microscopic examination of feces that reveals hookworm eggs Treatment: albendazole (preferred), mebendazole, and pyrantel pamoate Iron supplementation and possible blood transfusion in severe cases	Standard precautions are sufficient. Proper sanitation and disposal of feces Treatment of all known infested people Screening of high-risk individuals Encourage the wearing of shoes and avoiding going barefoot

(continued)

TABLE 15.7 • Common Helminthic Infections in Children (*continued*)

Infection/Causative Organism	Clinical Manifestations	Transmission	Diagnosis/Treatment	Isolation/Control Measures
Pinworm Caused by *Enterobius vermicularis* (roundworm); found in tropical and temperate climates; most common helminthic infection found in the United States	Most people are asymptomatic. May cause anal itching (pruritus ani), especially at night Other clinical findings may include restlessness and teeth grinding at night, weight loss, enuresis, abdominal pain, nausea and vomiting. Most frequently seen in children 5–10 years of age	Fecal–oral route directly, indirectly, or inadvertently by contaminated hands or shared toys, bedding, clothing, toilet seats Incubation period is 1–2 months or longer.	Diagnosis: when adult worms are visualized in the perianal region; they are best viewed when the child is sleeping. Very few ova are present in stool, so examination of stool is not recommended. Transparent tape pressed to perianal area and then viewed under a microscope may reveal eggs. Three consecutive specimens should be obtained when the child first awakens in the morning. Treatment of choice is mebendazole, pyrantel pamoate, and albendazole, usually single doses and repeated in 2 weeks.	Standard precautions are sufficient. Reinfection occurs easily. Infected people should bathe, preferably in a shower, in the morning, which will remove a large portion of the eggs. Frequent changing of underclothes and bedding Personal hygiene measures such as keeping fingernails short, avoiding scratching of perianal area, and nail biting Good hand hygiene is the most effective preventive measure, especially after using the bathroom and before eating. All family members should be treated since transmission from person to person is very easy.

Data from Leder, K., & Weller, P. F. (2022a). Ascariasis. *UpToDate*. Retrieved May 1, 2023, from https://www.uptodate.com/contents/ascariasis; Weller, P. F., & Leder, K. (2021). Hookworm. *UpToDate*. Retrieved May 1, 2023, from https://www.uptodate.com/contents/hookworm-infection

Leder, K., & Weller, P. F. (2022b). Enterobiasis (pinworm) and trichuriasis (whipworm). In E. L. Baron (Ed.), *UpToDate*. Retrieved May 1, 2023, from https://www.uptodate.com/contents/enterobiasis-pinworm-and-trichuriasis-whipworm; Siegel, J. D., Rhinehart, E., Jackson, M., Chiarello, L. & The Healthcare Infection Control Practices Advisory Committee. (2007, updated 2022). Guideline for isolation precautions: Preventing transmission of infectious agents in healthcare settings. https://www.cdc.gov/infectioncontrol/pdf/guidelines/isolation-guidelines-H.pdf

TABLE 15.8 • Effects of Sexually Transmitted Infections (STIs) on the Fetus or Newborn

STI	Effects on Fetus or Newborn
Chlamydia	Newborn can be infected during delivery. Eye infections (neonatal conjunctivitis), pneumonia, low birth weight, increased risk of premature rupture of the membranes (PROM), and preterm birth
Gonorrhea	Newborn can be infected during delivery. Increased risk of miscarriage, PROM, low birth weight, preterm birth, and chorioamnionitis Gonococcal ophthalmia neonatorum can lead to blindness and sepsis (including arthritis and meningitis).
Herpes simplex virus (genital herpes)	Contamination can occur during birth. Newborn may develop skin or mouth sores. Intellectual disability, premature birth, low birth weight, blindness, death
Syphilis	Can be passed in utero Can result in fetal or infant death Congenital syphilis leads to problems in multiple organs including teeth and bones, and can lead to blindness, hearing loss, and brain damage.
Trichomoniasis	Low birth weight, increased risk of PROM and preterm birth
Venereal warts	Large warts on birthing parent can complicate vaginal delivery. Newborn may develop warts in throat (laryngeal papillomatosis); uncommon but life threatening

Data from Centers for Disease Control and Prevention. (2023c). Sexually transmitted diseases (STDs): STDs during pregnancy—CDC detailed fact sheet. https://www.cdc.gov/std/pregnancy/stdfact-pregnancy-detailed.htm

TABLE 15.9 • Sexually Transmitted Infections (STIs) Common in Adolescents

Disease	Causative Organism	Transmission Mode	Diagnostic Testing and Recommended Screening for Sexually Active Adolescents	Female Symptoms	Male Symptoms	Recommended Treatment
Chlamydia Curable STI Seen frequently among sexually active adolescents and young adults	*Chlamydia trachomatis* (bacteria)	Vaginal, anal, and oral sex and by childbirth	Preferred method: Noninvasive, non–culture-based testing is available using nucleic acid amplification and testing (NAAT) from urine—single test can test for chlamydia and gonorrhea. Culture fluid from urethral swabs in males or endocervical swabs for females. Conjunctival secretions in neonates Females (sexually active, <25 years old): screen annually. Males: screen high-risk adolescents.	May be asymptomatic Dysuria, urinary frequency, dyspareunia Cervical discharge (mucus or pus) Endocervicitis May lead to pelvic inflammatory disease, ectopic pregnancy, infertility Can cause inflammation of the rectum and conjunctiva Can infect the throat from oral sexual contact with an infected partner	May be asymptomatic Dysuria, urethral itching Penile discharge (mucus or pus) Urethral tingling May lead to epididymitis and sterility Can cause inflammation of the rectum and conjunctiva Can infect the throat from oral sexual contact with an infected partner	Preferred: Doxycycline (Vibramycin) Main Alternative: Azithromycin (Zithromax) Alternatives: Erythromycin (EES) Levofloxacin, Ofloxacin (Floxin) Sexual partners also need evaluation, testing, and treatment. Abstinence from sexual activity until therapy complete and symptoms no longer present Retesting in 3 months to rule out recurrence
Gonorrhea Curable STI Adolescent often coinfected with *Chlamydia trachomatis*	*Neisseria gonorrhoeae* (bacteria)	Vaginal, anal, and oral sex and by childbirth	Same noninvasive, non–culture-based test using NAAT from urine as chlamydia or Gram stain or culture directly for the bacterium Females (sexually active, <25 years old): screen annually. Males: screen high-risk adolescents.	May be asymptomatic or no recognizable symptoms until serious complications such as pelvic inflammatory disease Dysuria Urinary frequency Vaginal discharge (yellow and foul) Dyspareunia Endocervicitis Arthritis May lead to pelvic inflammatory disease, ectopic pregnancy, infertility Symptoms of rectal infection include discharge, anal itching, and occasional painful bowel movements with fresh blood.	Most produce symptoms, but can be asymptomatic Dysuria Penile discharge (pus) Arthritis May lead to epididymitis and sterility Symptoms of rectal infection include discharge, anal itching, and occasional painful bowel movements with fresh blood.	Intramuscular ceftriaxone Alternatives: Other cephalosporins and azithromycinother Sexual partners also need evaluation, testing, and treatment. Abstinence from sexual activity until therapy complete and symptoms no longer present Retesting in 3 months to rule out recurrence

(continued)

TABLE **15.9** • Sexually Transmitted Infections (STIs) Common in Adolescents (*continued*)

Disease	Causative Organism	Transmission Mode	Diagnostic Testing and Recommended Screening for Sexually Active Adolescents	Female Symptoms	Male Symptoms	Recommended Treatment
Herpes type 2 (genital herpes) Lifelong recurrent viral disease Most people have not been diagnosed. There is no cure.	Herpes simplex virus 1 and 2 (HSV-1 and HSV-2)	HSV-1 is spread through oral secretions; can be spread to genitals through poor hand-washing of infected person or oral–genital contact HSV-2 is spread by having sexual contact (vaginal, oral, or anal) with someone who is shedding the herpes virus either during an outbreak or during a period with no symptoms; can be spread to an infant through childbirth.	Visual inspection and symptoms or culture from swabs taken from lesions (success depends on stage of lesion—optimum is during vesicular stage) Polymerase chain reaction is more sensitive than culture. Serologic tests, such as antibody-based testing (herpes Western blot assay is the most sensitive) Type-specific laboratory testing important Routine screening not recommended	Initial symptoms include itching, tingling, and pain in genital area followed by small pustules and blister-like genital lesions that then crust over and gradually heal. Recurrence episodes are usually milder than the initial episode. Dysuria, dyspareunia, and urinary retention Fever, headache, malaise, muscle aches	Same as for females	Antivirals used to treat first episode, recurrence, and suppression Acyclovir, valacyclovir, and famciclovir mainstay in treatment Does not cure; just controls symptoms Counseling important to help adolescents cope and to prevent transmission Sexual partners benefit from evaluation and counseling. If symptomatic, need treatment If asymptomatic, offer testing and education.
Syphilis	*Treponema pallidum* (spirochete bacteria)	Sexual contact with an infected person	Serologic testing mainstay for diagnosis Venereal Disease Research Laboratory (VDRL), rapid plasma reagin (RPR), and treponemal tests (e.g., fluorescent treponemal antibody absorbed [FTA-ABS]) can lead to a presumptive diagnosis and are useful for screening. Use of two tests required Darkfield examination and direct fluorescent antibody tests of lesion exudate or tissue provide definitive diagnosis of early syphilis. New tests such as enzyme immunoassay are in development. Screen based on epidemiology and personal risk factors.	Course of disease divided into stages: **Primary infection:** • Chancre on place of entrance of bacteria (usually vulva or vagina but can develop in other parts of the body) **Secondary infection:** • Maculopapular rash (hands and feet) • Sore throat • Lymphadenopathy • Flu-like symptoms **Latent infection:** • No symptoms • Can be infective during first 1–2 years of latency • Many people if not treated will suffer no further signs and symptoms. • Some people will go on to develop tertiary or late syphilis. **Tertiary infections:** • Tumors of skin, bones, and liver • Central nervous system symptoms • Cardiovascular symptoms • Usually not reversible at this stage	Course of disease divided into stages: **Primary infection:** • Chancre on place of entrance of bacteria (usually on penis but can develop in other parts of the body) **Secondary, latent, and tertiary infections:** All similar to those of female symptoms	Benzathine penicillin G injection (if penicillin allergy, doxycycline, tetracycline, or azithromycin) Sexual partners need evaluation and testing.

Trichomoniasis	*Trichomonas vaginalis* (protozoa)	Vaginal intercourse with an infected partner May be picked up from direct genital contact with damp or moist objects, such as towels or wet clothing	Highly sensitive and specific testing, such as NAAT, available and recommended, Microscopic evaluation of vaginal secretions or culture still common but less sensitive	Many females have symptoms but some may be asymptomatic. Dysuria Frequency Vaginal discharge (yellow, green, or gray and foul odor) Dyspareunia Irritation or itching of genital area	Most males infected are asymptomatic. Dysuria Penile discharge (watery white)	Metronidazole (Flagyl) or tinidazole Sexual partners also need evaluation, testing, and treatment. Abstinence recommended until therapy complete
Venereal warts (condylomata acuminata) One of the most common STIs in the United States Could lead to cancers of the cervix, vulva, vagina, anus, or penis No cure; warts can be removed but virus remains	Human papillomavirus	Vaginal, anal, or oral sex with an infected partner	Visual inspection Abnormal Pap smear may indicate cervical infection of human papillomavirus (HPV)	Wart-like lesions that are soft, moist, or flesh colored and appear on the vulva and cervix, and inside and surrounding the vagina and anus Sometimes appear in clusters that resemble cauliflower-like bumps, and are either raised or flat, small or large	Wart-like lesions that are soft, moist, or flesh colored and appear on the scrotum or penis. They sometimes appear in clusters that resemble cauliflower-like bumps, and are either raised or flat, small or large.	May disappear without treatment Treatment is aimed at removing the lesions rather than HPV itself. No optimal treatment has been identified, but there are several ways to treat depending on size and location. Most methods rely on chemical or physical destruction of the lesion: Imiquimod cream 20% Podophyllin antimitotic solution 0.5% Podofilox solution 5% 5-fluorouracil cream Trichloroacetic acid (TCA) Small warts can be removed by: • Freezing (cryosurgery) • Burning (electrocautery) • Laser treatment • Surgical excision Large warts that have not responded to treatment may be removed surgically. Vaccination recommended starting around age 12 and may lead to decrease in cancer associated with HPV Abstinence from sexual activity during treatment to promote healing

Data from Burnstein, G. R. (2020). Sexually transmitted infections. In R. M. Kleigman, J. W. St. Geme III, N. J. Blum, S. S. Shah, R. C. Tasker, K. M. Wilson, & R. E. Behrman (Eds.), *Nelson textbook of pediatrics* (21st ed., pp. 6011-6057); Elsevier; Shafii, T., & Levine, D. (2020). Office-based screening for sexually transmitted infections in adolescents. *Pediatrics, 145* (Suppl_2), S219–S224. https://doi.org/10.1542/peds.2019-2056K

Encourage adolescents to postpone sexual intercourse for as long as possible, but explain the need to use barrier methods, such as male and female condoms, if they choose to have sexual intercourse. For adolescents who have already had sexual intercourse, encourage abstinence at this point. Also encourage them to minimize their lifetime number of sexual partners, to use barrier methods consistently and correctly, and to be aware of the connection between drug and alcohol use and sexual activity (see Teaching Guidelines 15.3, Table 15.10, and the Healthy People 2030 box).

TEACHING GUIDELINES 15.3 Proper Condom Use

- Use latex or polyurethane condoms.
- Use a new condom with each act of vaginal, anal, or oral sex. Never reuse a condom.
- Handle condoms with care to prevent damage from sharp objects such as fingernails and teeth.
- Ensure condom has been stored in a cool, dry place away from direct sunlight. Do not store condoms in wallet or automobile or anywhere they would be exposed to extreme temperatures.
- Do not use a condom if it appears brittle, sticky, or discolored. These are signs of aging.
- Put condom on before any genital contact.
- Ensure adequate lubrication during intercourse. If external lubricants are used, use water or silicone-based lubricants such as KY Jelly. Oil-based or petroleum-based lubricants, such as body lotion, massage oil, or cooking oil, can weaken latex condoms.

Male Condom Use

- Put condom on when penis is erect with rolled side out. Ensure it is placed so it will readily unroll.
- Hold the tip of the condom while unrolling. Ensure there is a space at the tip for semen to collect (about ½ in), but make sure no air is trapped in the tip (air bubbles can cause breakage).
- If you feel the condom break, stop immediately, withdraw, remove broken condom, and replace.
- Withdraw while penis is still erect, and hold condom firmly against base of penis. Remove carefully to ensure no semen spills out. Dispose of properly.

Female Condom Use

- Do not use a male condom with a female condom.
- The thick inner ring with the closed end goes into the vagina (similar to inserting a tampon); the thin outer ring remains outside the body.
- Ensure condom is not twisted, that penis does not slip between the condom and vaginal wall, and the outer ring does not get pushed into the vagina.

Adapted from Centers for Disease Control and Prevention. (2022f). Condom effectiveness: Male (external) condom use. https://www.cdc.gov/condomeffectiveness/external-condom-use.html?CDC_AA_refVal=https%3A%2F%2Fwww.cdc.gov%2Fcondomeffectiveness%2Fmale-condom-use.html; Centers for Disease Control and Prevention. (2022g). Condom effectiveness: Female (internal) condom use. https://www.cdc.gov/condomeffectiveness/internal-condom-use.html?CDC_AA_refVal=https%3A%2F%2Fwww.cdc.gov%2Fcondomeffectiveness%2FFemale-condom-use.html

TABLE 15.10 • Barriers to Condom Use and Means to Overcome Them

Perceived Barrier	Intervention Strategy
Decreases sexual pleasure (sensation) Note: often perceived by those who have never used a condom	• Encourage adolescent to try. • Put a drop of water-based lubricant or saliva inside the tip of the condom or on the glans of the penis before putting on the condom. • Try a thinner latex condom or a different brand or more lubrication.
Decreases spontaneity of sexual activity	• Incorporate condom use into foreplay. • Remind adolescent that peace of mind may enhance pleasure for self and partner.
Embarrassing, juvenile, "unmanly"	• Remind adolescent that it is "manly" to protect themselves and others.
Poor fit (too small or too big, slips off, uncomfortable)	• Smaller and larger condoms are available.

TABLE 15.10 • Barriers to Condom Use and Means to Overcome Them

Perceived Barrier	Intervention Strategy
Requires prompt withdrawal after ejaculation	• Reinforce the protective nature of prompt withdrawal and suggest substituting other postcoital sexual activities.
Fear of breakage may lead to less vigorous sexual activity.	• With prolonged intercourse, lubricant wears off and the condom begins to rub. Have a water-soluble lubricant available to reapply.
Nonpenetrative sexual activity	• Condoms have been advocated for use during fellatio; unlubricated condoms may prove best for this purpose due to the taste of the lubricant. • Other barriers, such as dental dams or an unlubricated condom, can be cut down the middle to form a barrier; these have been advocated for use during certain forms of nonpenetrative sexual activity (e.g., cunnilingus and anilingual sex).
Allergy to latex	• Polyurethane male and female condoms are available.A natural skin condom can be used together with a latex condom to protect partners from contact with latex.

HEALTHY PEOPLE 2030

Objective	Nursing Significance
Increase the proportion of sexually active adolescent and young females enrolled in Medicaid and commercial health plans who are screened for chlamydial infections. Reduce gonorrhea rates among adolescent and young males. Reduce the incidence of primary and secondary syphilis in females. Reduce the proportion of adolescents and young adults with herpes simplex virus 2. Reduce infections due to human papillomavirus (HPV) types prevented by the 9-valent vaccine in young adults.	• Provide confidential care to all adolescents. • Assess for sexual behaviors and sexually transmitted infection (STI) risks during clinic visits; take every opportunity to educate on risks of STIs and risk reduction. • Be direct and nonjudgmental and tailor your approach to the adolescent. • Encourage adolescents to postpone initiation of sexual intercourse for as long as possible. For adolescents who have already had sexual intercourse, encourage abstinence at this point. • Encourage adolescents to minimize their lifetime number of sexual partners. • Educate about the importance of correct and consistent condom use.

Healthy People Objectives retrieved from http://www.healthypeople.gov

KEY CONCEPTS

- Infants and young children are more susceptible to infection due to their immature immune system. Young children continue to have an increased risk for infections and communicable disorders because disease protection from immunizations is not complete.
- Health care providers need to remember to educate parents that fever is a protective mechanism the body uses to fight infection.
- When obtaining blood cultures, follow aseptic technique and hospital protocol to prevent contamination. Obtain the specimen before administering antibiotics.
- When administering antipyretics, proper education must be given to caregivers on appropriate dosing, concentration, dosing interval, and use of proper measuring device.
- Promoting proper fluid balance and reducing temperature in a febrile child are important nursing interventions when caring for a child with an infection or communicable illness.
- Many childhood infectious and communicable diseases involve a rash. Rashes can be difficult to identify, so a thorough description and history from the caregiver is important.
- Sepsis, a systemic overresponse to infection resulting from bacteria, fungi, viruses, or parasites, can lead to

septic shock. Any infant younger than 3 months with a fever or any child with a fever accompanied by extreme lethargy, unresponsiveness, or lack of facial expressions should be seen by a health care provider or nurse practitioner.

- Many bacterial and viral infections, such as diphtheria, tetanus, pertussis, mumps, measles, rubella, varicella, and poliomyelitis, can be prevented by vaccination.
- Viral exanthems of childhood often present with a distinct rash pattern that assists in the diagnosis of the virus. Common childhood exanthems include exanthem subitum (roseola infantum), rubella (German measles), rubeola (measles), varicella (chickenpox), and erythema infectiosum (fifth disease).
- Nurses play a key role in educating the public on the importance of immunizations.
- Zoonotic infections are diseases caused by infectious agents that are transmitted directly or indirectly from animals to humans. Cat-scratch disease and rabies are types of zoonotic infections.
- Children are at a particular risk for contracting vector-borne diseases, which are diseases transmitted by ticks, mosquitoes, or other insect vectors. Two of the most commonly seen are Lyme disease and RMSF.
- Parasites frequently seen in children are scabies and head lice. Helminthic infections seen in children include pinworms, roundworms, and hookworms.
- STIs are infectious diseases transmitted through sexual contact, including oral, vaginal, or anal intercourse. Certain infections can be transmitted in utero to the fetus or during childbirth to the newborn.
- STIs are a major health concern for adolescents. Adolescents are at a greater risk for developing STIs for a variety of reasons, including frequency of unprotected intercourse, being biologically more susceptible to infection, and engaging in partnerships of limited duration (Fortenberry, 2022).

REFERENCES AND RECOMMENDED READINGS

Albrecht, M. A. (2021). Mumps. *UpToDate*. Retrieved April 25, 2023, from https://www.uptodate.com/contents/mumps?search=mumps&source=search_result&selectedTitle=1~150&usage_type=default&display_rank=1

Anderson, D. J. (2023). Infection prevention: Precautions for preventing transmission of infection. *UpToDate*. Retrieved April 13, 2023, from https://www.uptodate.com/contents/infection-prevention-precautions-for-preventing-transmission-of-infection?search=Infection%20prevention:%20Precautions%20for%20preventing%20transmission%20of%20infection&source=search_result&selectedTitle=1~150&usage_type=default&display_rank=1

Barroso, L. F., & Pegram, P. S. (2023). Epidemiology and pathophysiology of diphtheria. *UpToDate*. Retrieved April 17, 2023, from https://www.uptodate.com/contents/epidemiology-and-pathophysiology-of-diphtheria?search=Epidemiology%20and%20pathophysiology%20of%20diphtheria&source=search_result&selectedTitle=1~150&usage_type=default&display_rank=1

Brown, C. M., & DeMaria, A., Jr. (2022). Clinical manifestations and diagnosis of rabies. *UpToDate*. Retrieved April 28, 2023, from https://www.uptodate.com/contents/clinical-manifestations-and-diagnosis-of-rabies?search=rabies&source=search_result&selectedTitle=3~86&usage_type=default&display_rank=2

Brown, C. M., & DeMaria, A., Jr. (2023). Rabies immune globulin and vaccine. *UpToDate*. Retrieved April 28, 2023, from https://www.uptodate.com/contents/rabies-immune-globulin-and-vaccine?search=rabies&source=search_result&selectedTitle=2~86&usage_type=default&display_rank=1

Burnstein, G. R. (2020). Sexually transmitted infections. In R. M. Kleigman, J. W. St. Geme III, N. J. Blum, S. S. Shah, R. C. Tasker, K. M. Wilson, & R. E. Behrman (Eds.), *Nelson textbook of pediatrics* (21st ed., pp. 6011–6057). Elsevier.

Cantey, J. B. (2023). Clinical features, evaluation, and diagnosis of sepsis in term and late preterm neonates. *UpToDate*. Retrieved April 13, 2023, from https://www.uptodate.com/contents/clinical-features-evaluation-and-diagnosis-of-sepsis-in-term-and-late-preterm-neonates?search=Approach%20to%20the%20ill-appearing%20infant%20(younger%20than%2090%20days%20of%20age)&topicRef=6467&source=see_link

Centers for Disease Control and Prevention. (2019). *Research on doxycycline and tooth staining*. https://www.cdc.gov/rmsf/doxycycline/index.html

Centers for Disease Control and Prevention. (2020a). *Hand hygiene in healthcare settings: Hand hygiene guidance*. https://www.cdc.gov/handhygiene/providers/guideline.html

Centers for Disease Control and Prevention. (2020b). *Measles (rubeola): For healthcare providers*. https://www.cdc.gov/measles/hcp/index.html

Centers for Disease Control and Prevention. (2021a). In E. Hall, A. P. Wodi, J. Hamborsky, V. Morelli, & S. Schillie (Eds.), *Epidemiology and prevention of vaccine-preventable diseases* (14th ed.). Public Health Foundation. https://www.cdc.gov/vaccines/pubs/pinkbook/index.html

Centers for Disease Control and Prevention. (2021b). *Hand, foot and mouth disease (HFMD)*. https://www.cdc.gov/hand-foot-mouth/index.html#:~:text=Hand%2C%20Foot%2C%20and%20Mouth%20Disease%20(HFMD),-Espa%C3%B1ol%20(Spanish)&text=The%20illness%20is%20usually%20not,schools%20and%20day%20care%20centers.&text=Hand%2C%20foot%2C%20and%20mouth%20disease%20spreads%20easily.&text=Symptoms%20can%20include%20mouth%20sores%2C%20skin%20rash%2C%20and%20more

Centers for Disease Control and Prevention. (2021c). *Zoonotic diseases*. https://www.cdc.gov/onehealth/basics/zoonotic-diseases.html

Centers for Disease Control and Prevention. (2021d). *Lyme disease: Diagnosis and Testing*. http://www.cdc.gov/lyme/diagnosistesting/LabTest/TwoStep/index.html

Centers for Disease Control and Prevention. (2022a). *Group A streptococcal (GAS) disease: Scarlet fever: All you need to know*. https://www.cdc.gov/groupastrep/diseases-public/scarlet-fever.html?CDC_AA_refVal=https%3A%2F%2Fwww.cdc.gov%2Ffeatures%2Fscarletfever%2Findex.html

Centers for Disease Control and Prevention. (2022b). *Pertussis (whooping cough)*. https://www.cdc.gov/pertussis/clinical/treatment.html

Centers for Disease Control and Prevention. (2022c). *Botulism*. Retrieved April 19, 2023, from https://www.cdc.gov/botulism/index.html

Centers for Disease Control and Prevention. (2022d). *Chickenpox (varicella): For healthcare professionals*. https://www.cdc.gov/chickenpox/hcp/

Centers for Disease Control and Prevention. (2022e). *Ticks: Tick removal*. http://www.cdc.gov/ticks/removing_a_tick.html

Centers for Disease Control and Prevention. (2022f). *Condom effectiveness: Male (external) condom use*. https://www.cdc.gov/condomeffectiveness/external-condom-use.html?CDC_AA_refVal=https%3A%2F%2Fwww.cdc.gov%2Fcondomeffectiveness%2Fmale-condom-use.html

Centers for Disease Control and Prevention. (2022g). *Condom effectiveness: Female (internal) condom use*. https://www.cdc.gov/condomeffectiveness/internal-condom-use.html?CDC_AA_refVal=https%3A%2F%2Fwww.cdc.gov%2Fcondomeffectiveness%2FFemale-condom-use.html

Centers for Disease Control and Prevention. (2022h). *Zika virus*. https://www.cdc.gov/zika/index.html

Centers for Disease Control and Prevention. (2022i); *Anaplasmosis*. http://www.cdc.gov/anaplasmosis/

Centers for Disease Control and Prevention. (2022j). *Ehrlichiosis*. http://www.cdc.gov/ehrlichiosis/

Centers for Disease Control and Prevention. (2022k). *Haemophilus influenzae disease (including Hib): For clinicians*. https://www.cdc.gov/hi-disease/clinicians.html

Centers for Disease Control and Prevention. (2023a). *West Nile virus* https://www.cdc.gov/westnile/index.html

Centers for Disease Control and Prevention. (2023b). *Lyme disease: Transmission*. Retrieved April 29, 2023, from http://www.cdc.gov/lyme/transmission/index.html

Centers for Disease Control and Prevention. (2023c). *Sexually transmitted diseases (STDs): STDs during pregnancy—CDC detailed fact sheet*. https://www.cdc.gov/std/pregnancy/stdfact-pregnancy-detailed.htm

Centers for Disease Control and Prevention. (2023d). *Dengue*. http://www.cdc.gov/Dengue/

Centers for Disease Control and Prevention. (2023e). *Malaria*. https://www.cdc.gov/parasites/malaria/index.html

Expert Working Group on the Canadian Guidelines for Sexually Transmitted Infections. (2008). *Canadian guidelines on sexually transmitted infections*. Public Health Agency of Canada.

Fischbach, F. T., Fischbach, M. A., & Stout, K. (2022). *A manual of laboratory and diagnostic tests* (11th ed.). Wolters Kluwer.

Fortenberry, J. D. (2022). Sexually transmitted infections: Issues specific to adolescents. *UpToDate*. Retrieved May 1, 2023, from https://www.uptodate.com/contents/sexually-transmitted-infections-issues-specific-to-adolescents?search=std%20and%20pregnancy&source=search_result&selectedTitle=5~150&usage_type=default&display_rank=5

Goldstein, A. O., & Goldstein, B. G. (2022a). Pediculosis capitis. *UpToDate*. Retrieved May 1, 2023, from https://www.uptodate.com/contents/pediculosis-capitis?search=Pediculosis%20capitis&source=search_result&selectedTitle=1~42&usage_type=default&display_rank=1

Goldstein, B. G., & Goldstein, A. O. (2022b). Scabies: Epidemiology, clinical features, and diagnosis. *UpToDate*. Retrieved May 1, 2023, from https://www.uptodate.com/contents/scabies-epidemiology-clinical-features-and-diagnosis?search=scabies&source=search_result&selectedTitle=1~100&usage_type=default&display_rank=1

Goldstein, B. G., & Goldstein, A. O. (2022c). Scabies: Management. *UpToDate*. Retrieved May 1, 2023 from https://www.uptodate.com/contents/scabies-management?search=scabies&source=search_result&selectedTitle=2~100&usage_type=default&display_rank=2

Goldstein, A. O., & Goldstein, B. G. (2023). Pediculosis pubis and pediculosis ciliaris. *UpToDate*. Retrieved May 1, 20123, from https://www.uptodate.com/contents/pediculosis-pubis-and-pediculosis-ciliaris?search=Pediculosis%20pubis%20and%20pediculosis%20ciliaris&source=search_result&selectedTitle=1~30&usage_type=default&display_rank=1#H15

Hu, L., & Shapiro, E. D. (2023). Treatment of Lyme disease. *UpToDate*. Retrieved April 29, 2023, from https://www.uptodate.com/contents/treatment-of-lyme-disease?-search=Epidemiology%20of%20Lyme%20disease&source=search_result&selectedTitle=4~150&usage_type=default&display_rank=4#H319783157

Kaplan, S. L. (2023). Methicillin-resistant *Staphylococcus aureus* infections in children: Epidemiology and clinical spectrum. *UpToDate*. Retrieved April 16, 2023, from https://www.uptodate.com/contents/methicillin-resistant-staphylococcus-aureus-infections-in-children-epidemiology-and-clinical-spectrum?search=Methicillin-resistant%20Staphylococcus%20aureus%20infections%20in%20children:&source=search_result&selectedTitle=1~150&usage_type=default&display_rank=1

Koch, W. C. (2020). Parvoviruses. In R. M. Kleigman, J. W. St. Geme III, N. J. Blum, S. S. Shah, R. C. Tasker, K. M. Wilson, & R. E. Behrman (Eds.), *Nelson textbook of pediatrics* (21st ed., pp. 9133–9154). Elsevier.

Krogstad, P. (2022a). Hematogenous osteomyelitis in children: Epidemiology, pathogenesis, and microbiology. *UpToDate*. Retrieved April 18, 2023, from https://www.uptodate.com/contents/hematogenous-osteomyelitis-in-children-epidemiology-pathogenesis-and-microbiology?search=Hematogenous%20osteomyelitis%20in%20children:%20Epidemiology,%20pathogenesis,%20and%20microbiology.&source=search_result&selectedTitle=1~54&usage_type=default&display_rank=1

Krogstad, P. (2022b). Bacterial arthritis: Epidemiology, pathogenesis, and microbiology in infants and children. *UpToDate*. Retrieved April 18, 2023, from https://www.uptodate.com/contents/bacterial-arthritis-epidemiology-pathogenesis-and-microbiology-in-infants-and-children?search=Bacterial%20arthritis:%20Epidemiology,%20pathogenesis,%20and%20microbiology%20in%20infants%20and%20children&source=search_result&selectedTitle=1~146&usage_type=default&display_rank=1

Krogstad, P. (2023). Bacterial arthritis: Clinical features and diagnosis in infants and children. *UpToDate*. Retrieved April 18, 2023, from https://www.uptodate.com/contents/bacterial-arthritis-clinical-features-and-diagnosis-in-infants-and-children?search=Bacterial%20arthritis:%20Epidemiology,%20 pathogenesis,%20and%20microbiology%20in%20infants%20and%20children&topicRef=6033&source=see_link

Kronman, M. P., Crowell, C. S., & Vora, S. B. (2023a). Section 16: Infectious diseases. Chapter 96: Fever without a focus. In K. J. Marcdante, R. M. Kleigman, & A. M. Schuh (Eds.), *Nelson essentials of pediatrics* (9th ed., pp. 386–390). Elsevier.

Kronman, M. P., Crowell, C. S., & Vora, S. B. (2023b). Section 16: Infectious diseases. Chapter 117: Osteomyelitis. In K. J. Marcdante, R. M. Kleigman, & A. M. Schuh (Eds.), *Nelson essentials of pediatrics* (9th ed., pp. 443–445). Elsevier.

Leder, K., & Weller, P. F. (2022a). Ascariasis. *UpToDate*. Retrieved May 1, 2023, from https://www.uptodate.com/contents/ascariasis?search=Ascariasis&source=search_result&selectedTitle=1~45&usage_type=default&display_rank=1#H498704788

Leder, K., & Weller, P. F. (2022b). Enterobiasis (pinworm) and trichuriasis (whipworm). In E. L. Baron (Ed.), *UpToDate*. Retrieved May 1, 2023, from https://www.uptodate.com/contents/enterobiasis-pinworm-and-trichuriasis-whipworm?search=pinworm&source=search_result&selectedTitle=1~31&usage_type=default&display_rank=1

Lexicomp. (2023). Pediatric drug information. *UpToDate*. Retrieved April 5, 2023, from https://www.uptodate.com/contents/table-of-contents/drug-information/pediatric-drug-information

Mead, P. (2021). Epidemiology of Lyme disease. *UpToDate*. Retrieved April 29, 2023, from https://www.uptodate.com/contents/epidemiology-of-lyme-disease?search=Epidemiology%20of%20Lyme%20disease&source=search_result&selectedTitle=1~150&usage_type=default&display_rank=1

Nath, J. (2023). *Applied pathophysiology* (4th ed.). Wolters Kluwer.

Nolt, D., Moore, S., Yan, A. C., Melnick, L., & Committee on Infectious Diseases, Committee on Practice and Ambulatory Medicine, Section on Dermatology. (2022). Head lice. *Pediatrics, 150*(4), e2022059282. https://doi.org/10.1542/peds.2022–059282

Orscheln, R. C. (2020). Cat-scratch disease (Bartonella henselae). In R. M. Kleigman, J. W. St. Geme III, N. J. Blum, S. S. Shah, R. C. Tasker, K. M. Wilson, & R. E. Behrman (Eds.), *Nelson textbook of pediatrics* (21st ed., pp. 8275–8288). Elsevier.

Paul, I. M., & Walson, P. D. (2021). Acetaminophen and ibuprofen in the treatment of pediatric fever: A narrative review. *Current Medical Research and Opinion*, *37*(8), 1363–1375. https://doi.org/10.1080/03007995.2021.1928617

Pegram, P. S., & Stone, S. M. (2023). Botulism. *UpToDate*. Retrieved April 18, 2023, from https://www.uptodate.com/contents/botulism?search=botulism&source=search_result&selectedTitle=1~88&usage_type=default&display_rank=1

Pomerantz, W. J., & Weiss, S. L. (2022). Systemic inflammatory response syndrome (SIRS) and sepsis in children: Definitions, epidemiology, clinical manifestations, and diagnosis. *UpToDate*. Retrieved April 16, 2023, from https://www.uptodate.com/contents/systemic-inflammatory-response-syndrome-sirs-and-sepsis-in-children-definitions-epidemiology-clinical-manifestations-and-diagnosis?search=Systemic%20inflammatory%20response%20syndrome%20(SIRS)%20and%20sepsis%20in%20children:%20Definitions,%20epidemiology,%20clinical%20manifestations,%20and%20diagnosis&source=search_result&selectedTitle=1~150&usage_type=default&display_rank=1

Reller, M. E., & Dumler, J. S. (2020). Rocky Mountain spotted fever (Rickettsia rickettsii). In R. M. Kleigman, J. W. St. Geme III, N. J. Blum, S. S. Shah, R. C. Tasker, K. M. Wilson, & R. E. Behrman (Eds.), *Nelson textbook of pediatrics* (21st ed., pp. 8693–8714). Elsevier.

Rietmeijer, K. (2023). Prevention of sexually transmitted infections. *UpToDate*. Retrieved March 13, 2023, from https://www.uptodate.com/contents/prevention-of-sexually-transmitted-infections?search=std%20and%20pregnancy&source=search_result&selectedTitle=3~150&usage_type=default&display_rank=3

Roué, J.-M. (2022). Prevention and treatment of neonatal pain. *UpToDate*. Retrieved March 13, 2023, from https://www.uptodate.com/contents/prevention-and-treatment-of-neonatal-pain?search=prevention%20and%20treatment%20of%20neonatal%20pain&source=search_result&selectedTitle=1~18&usage_type=default&display_rank=1

Scarfone, R. J., & Cho, C. (2022). Approach to the ill-appearing infant (younger than 90 days of age). *UpToDate*. Retrieved April 13, 2023, from https://www.uptodate.com/contents/approach-to-the-ill-appearing-infant-younger-than-90-days-of-age?search=approach-to-the-ill-appearing-infantyounger-than-90-days-of-age&source=search_result&selectedTitle=3~150&usage_type=default&display_rank=3

Sexton, D. J., & McClain, M. T. (2021). Treatment of Rocky Mountain spotted fever. *UpToDate*. Retrieved April 29, 2023, from https://www.uptodate.com/contents/treatment-of-rocky-mountain-spotted-fever?search=rocky%20mountain%20spotted%20fever&topicRef=7904&source=see_link

Shafii, T., & Levine, D. (2020). Office-based screening for sexually transmitted infections in adolescents. *Pediatrics*, *145*(Suppl_2), S219–S224. https://doi.org/10.1542/peds.2019-2056K

Shulman, S. T., & Reuter, C. H. (2020). Group A streptococcus. In R. M. Kleigman, J. W. St. Geme III, N. J. Blum, S. S. Shah, R. C. Tasker, K. M. Wilson, & R. E. Behrman (Eds.), *Nelson textbook of pediatrics* (21st ed., pp. 7617–7670). Elsevier.

Siegel, J. D., Rhinehart, E., Jackson, M., Chiarello, L., & The Healthcare Infection Control Practices Advisory Committee. (2007, updated 2022). *Guideline for isolation precautions: Preventing transmission of infectious agents in healthcare settings*. https://www.cdc.gov/infectioncontrol/pdf/guidelines/isolation-guidelines-H.pdf

Souder, E., & Long, S. S. (2020). Pertussis (*Bordetella pertussis* and *Bordetella parapertussis*). In R. M. Kleigman, J. W. St. Geme III, N. J. Blum, S. S. Shah, R. C. Tasker, K. M. Wilson, & R. E. Behrman (Eds.), *Nelson textbook of pediatrics* (21st ed., pp. 8020–8041). Elsevier.

Sotoodian, B. (2020). *Scarlet fever*. https://emedicine.medscape.com/article/1053253-overview#a6

Sullivan, J. E., Farrar, H. C., & The AAP's Section on Clinical Pharmacology and Therapeutics, and Committee on Drugs. (2011, reaffirmed 2023). Clinical report: Fever and antipyretic use in children. *Pediatrics*, *127*(3), 580–587. https://doi.org/10.1542/peds.2010-3852

Thwaites, L. (2022). Tetanus. *UpToDate*. Retrieved April 18, 2023, from https://www.uptodate.com/contents/tetanus?search=tetanus&source=search_result&selectedTitle=1~150&usage_type=default&display_rank=1

Tremblay, C., & Brady, M. T. (2023). Roseola infantum (exanthem subitum). *UpToDate*. Retrieved April 27, 2023, from https://www.uptodate.com/contents/roseola-infantum-exanthem-subitum?search=roseola%20infantum%20&source=search_result&selectedTitle=1~150&usage_type=default&display_rank=1https://www.uptodate.com/contents/roseola-infantum-exanthem-

U.S. Department of Health and Human Services. (n.d.). *Healthy People 2030*. https://health.gov/healthypeople

Ward, M. A. (2022). Fever in infants and children: Pathophysiology and management. *UpToDate*. Retrieved April 11, 2023, from https://www.uptodate.com/contents/fever-in-infants-and-children-pathophysiology-and-management?search=fever%20in%20infants%20and%20children&source=search_result&selectedTitle=2~150&usage_type=default&display_rank=2F

Weller, P. F., & Leder, K. (2021). Hookworm infection. *UpToDate*. Retrieved May 1, 2023, from https://www.uptodate.com/contents/hookworm-infection?search=Hookworm&source=search_result&selectedTitle=1~54&usage_type=default&display_rank=1

Willoughby, R. E., Jr. (2020). Rabies. In R. M. Kleigman, J. W. St. Geme III, N. J. Blum, S. S. Shah, R. C. Tasker, K. M. Wilson, & R. E. Behrman (Eds.), *Nelson textbook of pediatrics* (21st ed., pp. 9562–9576). Elsevier.

World Health Organization. (2023). *Rabies: Fact sheet*. http://www.who.int/mediacentre/factsheets/fs099/en/

Yeh, S., & Mink, C. M. (2022). Pertussis infection in infants and children: Clinical features and diagnosis. *UpToDate*. Retrieved April 17, 2023, from https://www.uptodate.com/contents/pertussis-infection-in-infants-and-children-clinical-features-and-diagnosis?search=Pertussis%20Infection%20in%20Infants%20and%20Children:%20Clinical%20features%20and%20diagnosis&source=search_result&selectedTitle=1~150&usage_type=default&display_rank=1

DEVELOPING CLINICAL JUDGMENT

PRACTICING FOR NCLEX

1. Compared with adults, why are infants and children at an increased risk for infectious and communicable diseases?
   a. The infant has had limited exposure to disease and is losing the passive immunity acquired from maternal antibodies.
   b. The infant demonstrates an increased inflammatory response.
   c. Cellular immunity is not functional at birth.
   d. Infants have an increased risk for infection until they receive their first set of immunizations.
2. A parent calls the clinic because their 2-year-old child has a rectal temperature of 37.8°C (100°F). The parent wonders how high a fever should be before they should give medications to reduce it. What is the best response by the nurse?
   a. "All fevers should be treated to prevent seizures."
   b. "Antipyretics should be used with any rise in temperature. They can help change the course of the infection."
   c. "Give your child aspirin when their fever is above 38°C (100.4°F)."
   d. "In a normal healthy child, if your child is not uncomfortable, fevers less than 39°C (102.2°F) do not require medication."
3. A neonate should be evaluated by a health care provider if which sign or symptom is present?
   a. Acting fussier than normal
   b. Refusing the pacifier
   c. Rectal temperature above 38°C (100.4°F)
   d. Mottling that is present during bathing
4. The public health nurse has been asked to provide information to local child care centers on controlling the spread of infectious diseases. What is the best information the nurse can provide?
   a. The etiology of common infectious diseases
   b. Proper handwashing techniques
   c. The physiology of the immune system
   d. Why children are at a higher risk of infection than adults
5. When teaching a group of adolescents about STIs, which of the following points are important to include? Select all that apply.
   a. Many people infected with chlamydia are unaware and have no symptoms.
   b. Gonorrhea is the least common of all STIs.
   c. Adolescent females who are sexually active should be screened annually for chlamydia.
   d. Genital herpes is a lifelong viral illness.
   e. Practicing good handwashing is the best way to prevent STIs.
   f. STIs are a major health concern for adolescents.
6. Parents of a 4-month-old infant tell the health care provider their child has had a mild fever, cough, and runny nose for the past 2 weeks and now the cough is worse. Upon assessment the nurse finds the infant's heart rate to be 152 bpm, respiratory rate 64, coughing spells with a whooping sound, and axillary temperature 38.3°C (101°F). Which two nursing actions are the priority?
   a. Promote mobility.
   b. Assess oxygen level.
   c. Assess pain level.
   d. Monitor elimination.
   e. Encourage rest.

DOSAGE CALCULATION QUESTIONS

1. The nurse is caring for a child who has a rash and is complaining of feeling itchy and is continually scratching. The child weighs 32 lb. The medication order reads: Diphenhydramine 6.25 mg po every 4 to 6 hours as needed for itching. Diphenhydramine is supplied as 12.5 mg/5 mL. How many milliliters will the nurse administer? Round to the nearest tenth.

CRITICAL THINKING EXERCISES

1. A 12-year-old child presents with a very sore throat and fever. On assessment you find an erythematous rash on the child's face that feels like sandpaper. You obtain a throat culture, which is positive for group A streptococcus. What instructions would you give the parents regarding the child's care at home?
2. A 1-month-old infant is admitted to the hospital to rule out sepsis. What would be your priority nursing interventions?

3. A 4-year-old child presents with a fever and rash. What three of the following items should the nurse obtain during the health history?
   a. Immunization history
   b. Any exposure to communicable or infectious diseases
   c. Whether the child takes a daily vitamin
   d. Thorough description and history of the rash
   e. Birthing parent's immunization history

STUDY ACTIVITIES

1. The 4-year-old presented in Question 3 of the Critical Thinking Exercises was diagnosed with varicella zoster virus. Write a nursing plan of care or concept map for a child with varicella.
2. You are asked to give a presentation to a group of adolescents on STIs, including transmission, symptoms, treatment, and prevention. What information would you include?
3. A child is brought to the school nurse with intense itching. Upon assessment the nurse finds an erythematous, papular rash with excoriations on the child's hands and feet. As suspected, the diagnosis of scabies is confirmed. What teaching is necessary for the parents, family, and classmates of the child?

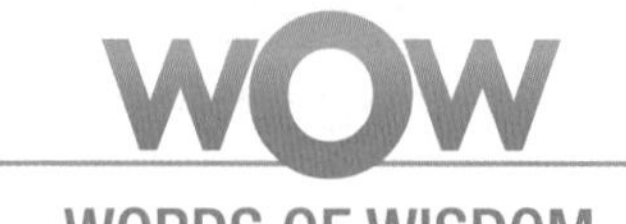

WORDS OF WISDOM

Listen to the parents of the children you care for; their insight and knowledge about their child is invaluable.

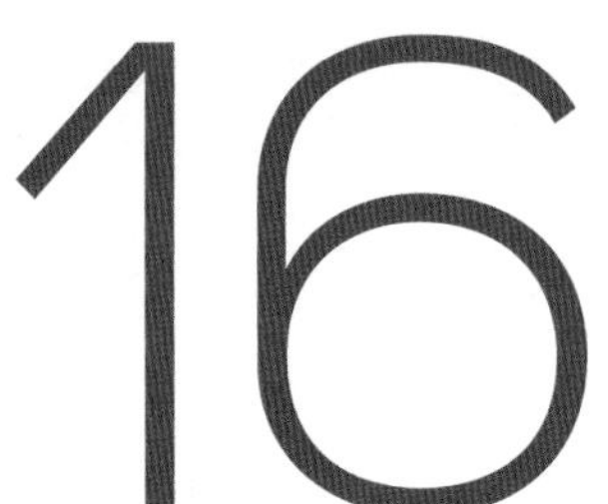

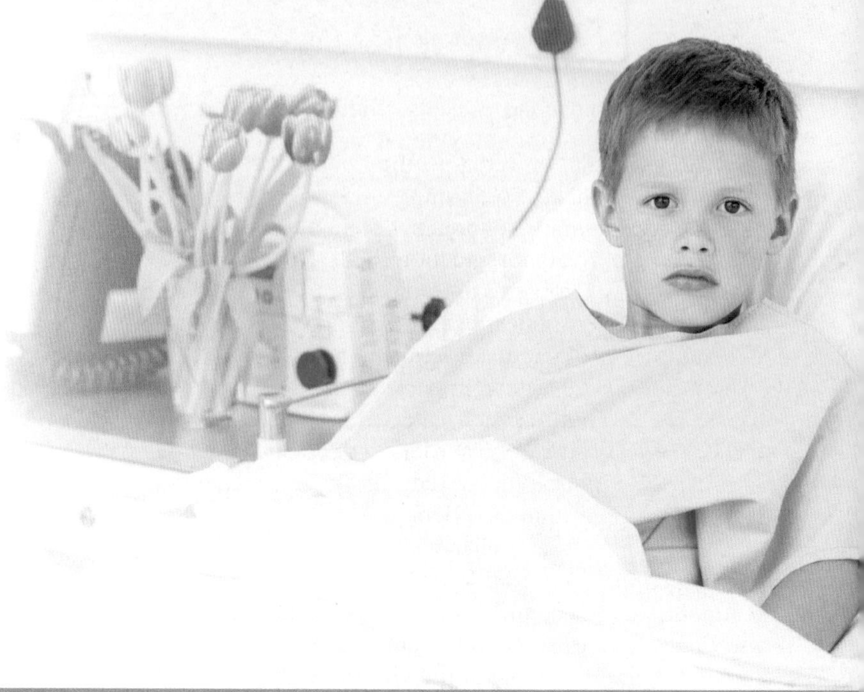

16 Nursing Care of the Child With an Alteration in Intracranial Regulation or Neurologic Disorder

KEY TERMS

central nervous system (CNS)

decerebrate posturing (dē-ser′ĕ-brăt pos′chŭr-ing)

decorticate posturing (dē-kōr′ti-kāt pos′chŭr-ing)

head circumference

intracranial pressure (ICP)

lumbar puncture (LP)

myelinization (mī′ĕ-li-nī-zā′shun)

neural tube

opisthotonic (ō′pis-thot′ŏ-nik)

postictal (post-ik′tăl)

teratogen (ter′ă-tō-jen)

LEARNING OBJECTIVES

Upon completion of the chapter, you will be able to:

1. Compare how the anatomy and physiology of the neurologic system in children differ from those of adults.
2. Identify various factors associated with neurologic disease in infants and children.
3. Discuss common laboratory and other diagnostic tests useful in the diagnosis of neurologic conditions.
4. Discuss common medications and other treatments used for treatment and palliation of neurologic conditions.
5. Recognize risk factors associated with various neurologic disorders.
6. Distinguish among different neurologic illnesses based on the signs and symptoms associated with them.
7. Discuss nursing interventions commonly used for neurologic illnesses.
8. Devise an individualized plan of care or concept map for the child with a neurologic disorder.
9. Develop child and family teaching plans for the child with a neurologic disorder.
10. Describe the psychosocial impact of chronic neurologic disorders on children.

Antonio Chapman, 3 months old, has had increased irritability, poor sucking and feeding, and a fever for the past 24 hours. Today, he is lethargic with a weak cry and is vomiting his feeds.

INTRODUCTION

Intracranial regulation refers to the ability of the cranial contents to maintain equilibrium and therefore neurologic function. Nurses encounter potential and actual alterations in intracranial regulation in all types of patients and must detect problems and intervene early to prevent life-threatening complications. Alterations in intracranial regulation (neurologic disorders) in children often have a devastating and lasting impact. Neurologic disorders can be divided into several categories, including structural disorders, seizure disorders, infectious disorders, trauma to the neurologic system, blood flow disruption disorders, and chronic disorders.

Nurses must be familiar with neurologic conditions affecting children in order to provide prevention, prompt treatment, guidance, and support to families. Neurologic disorders require acute interventions, but often have long-lasting implications for the child's health and development. Due to the potentially devastating effects that neurologic disorders can have on children and their families, nurses need to be skilled in assessment and interventions in this area and must be able to provide support throughout the course of the illness and beyond.

VARIATIONS IN PEDIATRIC ANATOMY AND PHYSIOLOGY

Neurologic disorders can result from congenital problems as well as from infections or traumas. Certain neurologic conditions occur in children more often than in adults, and these conditions will affect their growth and development. In addition, children are at an increased risk for different neurologic problems compared to adults due to anatomic and physiologic differences.

Brain and Spinal Cord Development

The brain and spinal cord make up the **central nervous system (CNS)**. Development of these structures occurs in the first 3 to 4 weeks of gestation from the **neural tube**. Infection, trauma, **teratogens** (any environmental substance that can cause physical defects in the developing embryo and fetus), and malnutrition during this period can result in malformations in brain and spinal cord development and may affect normal CNS development.

At birth, the cranial bones are not well developed and are not fused. Therefore, there is an increased risk for fracture. The brain is highly vascular, leading to an increased risk of hemorrhage. Premature infants are at greater risk for brain damage; the more premature the infant, the greater the risk. The premature infant has more capillaries in the periventricular area, which is the brain tissue that lines the outside of the lateral ventricles. These capillaries are fragile and at greater risk for rupture, leading to intracranial bleeding. Also, because the cranium is very soft in the preterm infant, external pressure can change its shape and cause increased pressure in areas of the brain and possible hemorrhage.

The sutures and fontanels present in the newborn help make the skull more flexible and help to accommodate for brain growth that continues after birth. Closure of the fontanels too early or too late can be indicative of problems with brain growth. The child's spine is very mobile, especially the cervical spine region, resulting in a high risk of cervical spine injury.

Nervous System

The development of the nervous system is complete but immature at birth. The infant is born with all the nerve cells that they will have throughout life. However, **myelinization**, the formation of myelin, which covers and protects the nerves, is incomplete. The speed and accuracy of nerve impulses increases as myelinization increases. This process accounts for the acquisition of fine and gross motor movements and coordination in early childhood. Myelinization proceeds in the cephalocaudal direction. For example, infants are able to control the head and neck before the trunk and extremities.

The immaturity of the CNS in preterm infants can result in delayed development of motor skills. Premature newborns may have difficulty coordinating sucking and swallowing, leading to feeding and growth issues. Also, episodes of apnea can be problematic in the preterm newborn due to the underdevelopment of the nervous system.

Head Size

The head of the infant and young child is large in proportion to the body. The head of an infant accounts for a quarter of the body height; in adults, it accounts for one eighth of the body height (Fig. 16.1). In addition, the infant's and child's neck muscles are not well developed. Both of these differences lead to an increased incidence of head injury from falls. The head is the fastest growing body part during infancy and continues to grow until the child is 5 years old.

COMMON MEDICAL TREATMENTS

A variety of interventions, including medical treatments and medications, are used to treat neurologic illness in children. Most of these treatments will require a health care provider's or nurse practitioner's order when the child is hospitalized. The most common treatments and medications used for neurologic disorders are listed in Common Medical Treatments 16.1 and Drug Guide 16.1.

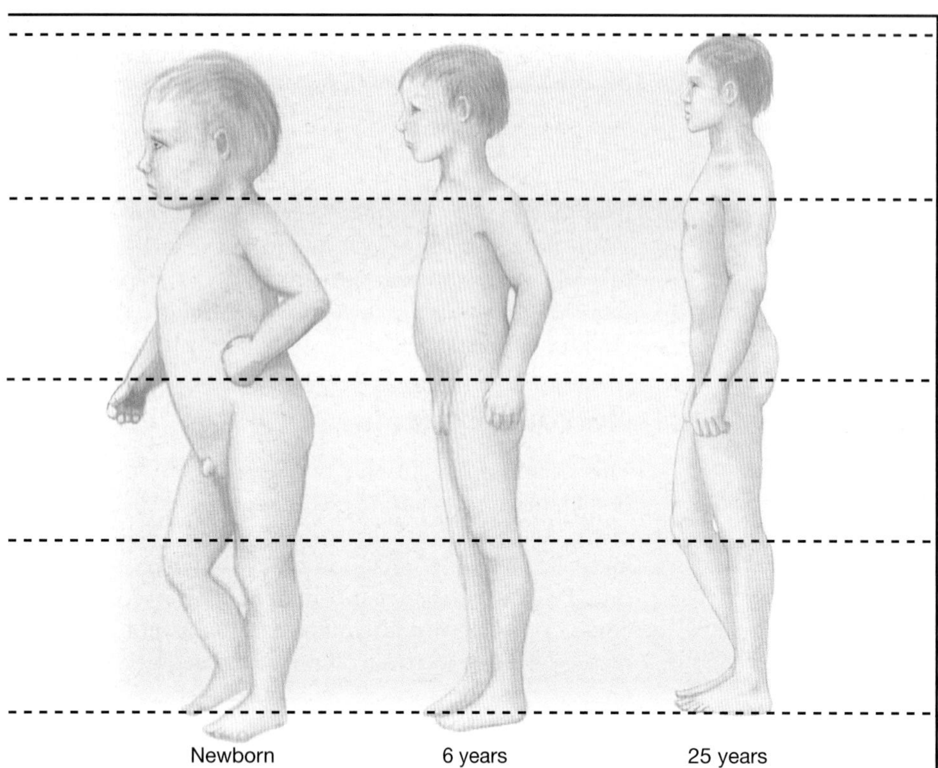

FIGURE 16.1 Proportion of head to body height in the newborn, child, and adult.

COMMON MEDICAL TREATMENTS 16.1

Treatment	Explanation	Indications	Nursing Implications
Shunt placement	A catheter is placed in the ventricle to pass the CSF to the peritoneal cavity, atrium of the heart, or pleural spaces. (Ventriculoperitoneal shunts are commonly used.)	Hydrocephalus, increased ICP	Monitor: • For signs and symptoms of increased ICP • Neurologic status closely • Level of consciousness and vital signs • For signs and symptoms of infection
Ventilation	Hyperventilation to decrease $PaCO_2$, which will result in vasoconstriction and therefore decrease in ICP Adequate oxygenation to prevent hypoxia and further damage to the brain	Increased ICP	Monitor: • Arterial blood gases • For signs and symptoms of increased ICP • Pulse oximetry
PT/OT/ST	Therapies are used to improve motor function and ability of children with neurologic disorders.	Head injury, intellectual disability	Ensure adequate communication exists within the interdisciplinary team.
External ventricular drainage (EVD)	A catheter is temporarily placed in the ventricle, and CSF is drained in a closed system to an external reservoir.	Most commonly used with shunt infections until CSF is sterile and shunt can be replaced; treats acute-onset hydrocephalus, meningitis, encephalitis, tumors that cause blockage of CSF, closed head injury, subarachnoid hemorrhage, increased ICP; also can be used to monitor ICP	Monitor: • For signs and symptoms of increased ICP • Neurologic status closely • Level of consciousness and vital signs • For signs and symptoms of infection • Level of collection container when drain is unclamped
Ventricular tap	To reduce accumulation of CSF and decrease ICP	Increased ICP	Monitor: • Level of consciousness • Neurologic status

COMMON MEDICAL TREATMENTS 16.1

Treatment	Explanation	Indications	Nursing Implications
Vagal nerve stimulator	A nerve stimulator is implanted, and a lead wire running under the skin is wrapped around the vagus nerve. The stimulator is programmed to provide the appropriate dose of stimulation at preset intervals; additional stimulation can be administered.	Short- and long-term seizure management in children over 12 years of age	Monitor: • For signs and symptoms of infection • For seizure activity
Ketogenic diet	Diet involving high intake of fats, adequate protein, and a very low intake of carbohydrates, resulting in a ketosis state. Child is kept in a mild state of dehydration.	Prevention, control, and reduction of seizures, in particular for children with difficult-to-control seizures	Monitor: • Input and output closely • For seizure activity • Growth and nutritional status • The diet is time-consuming, and many children find it unpalatable; therefore, all families and children do not accept it. • Recommended for a minimum of 3 months, reevaluate every 1–2 years • Alternative diets include: the medium chain triglyceride diet, modified Atkins diet, and a low glycemic index diet

CSF, cerebrospinal fluid; ICP, intracranial pressure; OT, occupational therapy; PT, physical therapy; ST, speech therapy.

Data from Kossoff, E. H. W. (2022). The ketogenic diet and other diet therapies for the treatment of epilepsy. *UpToDate*. Retrieved May 9, 2023, from https://www.uptodate.com/contents/ketogenic-dietary-therapies-for-the-treatment-of-epilepsy

DRUG GUIDE 16.1

Medication	Actions/Indications	Nursing Implications
Antibiotics (oral, parenteral, intrathecal)	Treatment of bacterial meningitis and shunt infections; kill and prevent the growth of bacteria.	Check for antibiotic allergies. Monitor serum levels to ensure therapeutic dosing, if indicated. Give as prescribed for the length of time prescribed.
Anticonvulsants (oral, parenteral)	Decrease hyperexcitability of nerves. Treatment and prevention of seizures	Maintain seizure precautions. Monitor for drug interactions and long-term adverse effects. Monitor and document all seizure activity. Many are used in combination, but patient and family need to be aware of interactions and long-term adverse effects. Stopping drug abruptly may precipitate seizures or even status epilepticus.
Benzodiazepines Diazepam (oral, rectal, IV, or IO) Lorazepam (oral, IV, or IO) Midazolam (IM, intranasal or buccal)	Minor sedative that prevents or stops seizures by slowing down the CNS, making abnormal electrical activity unlikely Treatment for status epilepticus	Diazepam is available in rectal form to stop prolonged seizures in children. Useful for home management; nurses must educate family members on administration and when to call health care provider or nurse practitioner. Monitor sedation level and for cessation of seizure activity.
Analgesics (acetaminophen, ibuprofen, ketorolac, morphine)	Block pain impulse in response to inhibition of prostaglandin synthesis Narcotic analgesics (i.e., morphine) act on receptors in the brain to alter perception of pain. Used to treat pain. Used to help avoid increase in ICP	Monitor for improvements in pain. Monitor sedation and respiratory status with narcotics. Monitor neurologic status closely. Used cautiously because loss of accurate neurologic evaluation can occur
Osmotic diuretics (i.e., mannitol)	Increase plasma osmolality, therefore inducing diffusion back into plasma and extravascular space/reduces ICP.	Monitor electrolytes. Monitor I/O closely. Monitor vital signs. Monitor for signs and symptoms of increased ICP.
Corticosteroids (i.e., dexamethasone)	Suppress inflammation and normal immune response/reduce cerebral edema.	Give oral doses with food. Dosage must be tapered before discontinuing.

I/O, intake/output; IO, intraosseous; IM, intramuscular; IV, intravenous

Data from Lexicomp. (2023). Pediatric drug information. *UpToDate*. Retrieved April 5, 2023, from https://www.uptodate.com/contents/table-of-contents/drug-information/pediatric-drug-information

Clinical Judgment and the Nursing Process for the Child With a Neurologic Disorder

Care of the child with a neurologic disorder includes assessment, nursing analysis, planning, intervention, and evaluation. There are a number of general concepts related to the nursing process that can be applied to the management of neurologic disorders. From an overall understanding of the care involved for a child with an alteration in intracranial regulation, the nurse can then individualize the care based on specifics for the particular child.

Assessment

Assessment of neurologic dysfunction in children includes health history, physical examination, and laboratory and diagnostic testing.

TAKE NOTE!

Neurologic assessment should proceed from least invasive to most invasive. The use of toys and familiar objects, as well as incorporating play, will help promote cooperation from the child.

Health History

The health history consists of past medical history, including the birthing parent's pregnancy history, family history, and history of present illness (when the symptoms started and how they have progressed), as well as treatments used at home. The past medical history might be significant for prematurity, difficult birth, infection during pregnancy, nausea, vomiting, headaches, changes in gait, falls, visual disturbances, or recent trauma. Family history might be significant for genetic disorders with neurologic manifestations, seizure disorders, or headaches. When eliciting the history of the present illness, inquire about the following:

- Nausea
- Vomiting
- Changes in gait
- Visual disturbances
- Complaints of headaches
- Recent trauma
- Changes in cognition
- Change in consciousness, including any loss of consciousness
- Poor feeding
- Lethargy
- Increased irritability
- Fever
- Pain
- Altered muscle tonicity
- Delays in growth and development
- Ingestion or inhalation of neurotoxic substances or chemicals

Physical Examination

Physical examination of the nervous system consists of inspection and observation, palpation, and auscultation.

Inspection and Observation

Specific areas to inspect and observe include:

- Level of consciousness (LOC)
- Vital signs
- Head, face, and neck
- Cranial nerve function
- Motor function
- Reflexes
- Sensory function
- Increased **intracranial pressure (ICP)** (a rise in the normal pressure within the skull)

Level of Consciousness. Begin the physical examination with inspection and observation. Observe the child's LOC, noting a decrease or significant changes. LOC is the earliest indicator of improvement or deterioration of neurologic status. Extreme irritability or lethargy is considered an abnormal finding. Consciousness consists of alertness, which is a wakeful state and includes the ability to respond to stimuli, and cognition, which includes the ability to process stimuli and demonstrate a verbal or motor response. Five different states constitute the levels of consciousness:

1. *Full consciousness* is defined as a state in which the child is awake and alert; is oriented to time, place, and person; and exhibits age-appropriate behaviors.
2. *Confusion* is defined as a state in which disorientation exists. The child may be alert but responds inappropriately to questions.
3. *Obtunded* is defined as a state in which the child has limited responses to the environment and falls asleep unless stimulation is provided.
4. *Stupor* exists when the child responds only to vigorous stimulation.
5. *Coma* defines a state in which the child cannot be aroused, even with painful stimuli.

CLINICAL REASONING ALERT!

Lack of response to painful stimuli is abnormal and can indicate a life-threatening condition. Report this finding immediately.

The Pediatric Glasgow Coma Scale is a popular scale used to standardize degree of consciousness. It consists of three parts: eye opening, verbal response, and motor response (Fig. 16.2). When assessing LOC in children, consider that the infant or child may not respond to unfamiliar voices in an unfamiliar environment. Therefore, it may be helpful to have a parent present to elicit the response.

TAKE NOTE!

Parents will often be the first to notice changes in their child's LOC. Listen to parents and respond to their concerns.

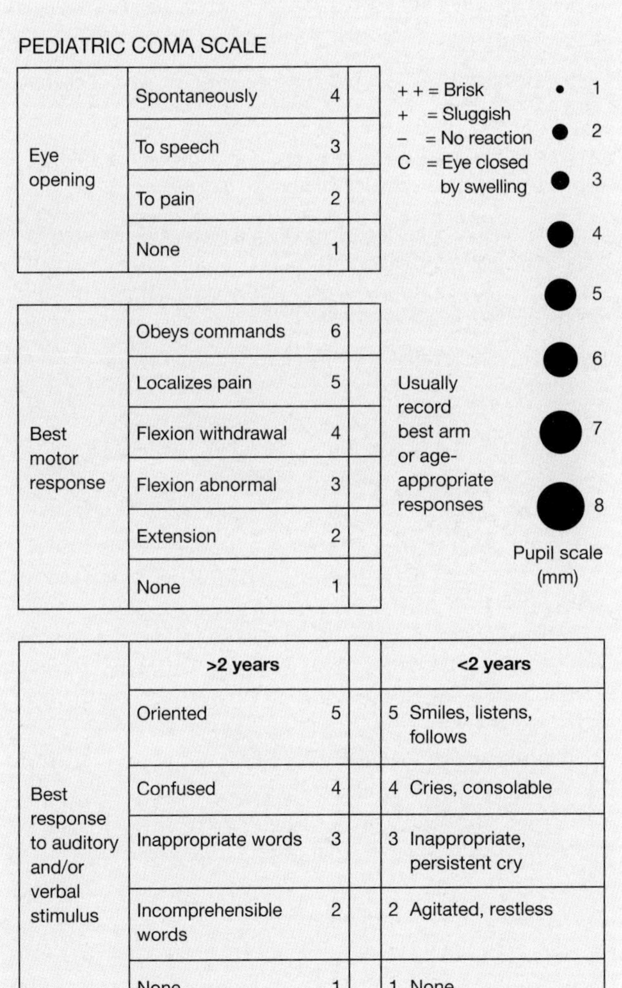

PEDIATRIC COMA SCALE

Eye opening	Spontaneously	4	
	To speech	3	
	To pain	2	
	None	1	

++ = Brisk
+ = Sluggish
– = No reaction
C = Eye closed by swelling

Best motor response	Obeys commands	6	
	Localizes pain	5	
	Flexion withdrawal	4	
	Flexion abnormal	3	
	Extension	2	
	None	1	

Usually record best arm or age-appropriate responses

Pupil scale (mm): 1, 2, 3, 4, 5, 6, 7, 8

	>2 years			<2 years
Best response to auditory and/or verbal stimulus	Oriented	5		5 Smiles, listens, follows
	Confused	4		4 Cries, consolable
	Inappropriate words	3		3 Inappropriate, persistent cry
	Incomprehensible words	2		2 Agitated, restless
	None	1		1 None
	Tracheal tube	T		T Tracheal tube

Pediatric coma scale total	

FIGURE 16.2 Pediatric Glasgow Coma Scale (GCS). The Pediatric GCS provides for developmentally appropriate cues to assess level of consciousness (LOC) in infants and children. Numeric values are assigned to the levels of response, and the sum provides an overall picture, as well as an objective measure, of the child's LOC. The lower the score, the less responsive the child.

Vital Signs. Assessment of vital signs can provide probable underlying causes for altered LOC as well as reveal the adequacy of oxygenation and circulation. Certain neurologic conditions like cerebral infections, increased ICP, coma, brain stem injury, or head injuries can cause alterations in the child's vital signs.

Head, Face, and Neck. Inspect and observe the head for size and shape. Abnormal skull shape can result from premature closure or widening of sutures. Inspect and observe the face for symmetry. Asymmetry may occur due to paralysis of certain cranial nerves, position in utero, or swelling caused by trauma. Assess range of motion (ROM) of the neck. Alterations in ROM can indicate CNS infections such as meningitis.

The most dramatic increase in brain volume occurs during the last 3 months of fetal development and the first 2 years of life. The relationship between head and brain growth explains why **head circumference** (measurement of the child's head around the largest area) is a standard assessment made in children younger than 3 years of age. All children younger than 3 years old, and any child whose head size is questionable, should have their head circumference measured and plotted on a growth chart (see Appendix A for growth charts).

Assessment of the growth trend of the head is important in detecting potential neurologic conditions. Report and investigate any variation in head circumference percentiles over time because variations may indicate abnormal brain or skull growth. A smaller than normal head circumference, which measures around the child's head at the largest area, may indicate microcephaly, and a larger than normal head circumference may indicate hydrocephalus.

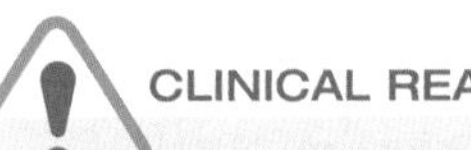

CLINICAL REASONING ALERT!

Do not attempt any assessment that involves movement of the head and neck in cases of trauma or suspected trauma until cervical injury is ruled out. Maintain complete immobilization of the cervical spine until that time.

Cranial Nerve Function. Techniques of assessment of cranial nerve function are similar to techniques for adult assessment. The method of obtaining responses may vary based on age and developmental level of the child. Certain elements of the adult assessment may be omitted. Alterations in cranial nerve function can be the result of compression of a specific nerve, infection, or trauma leading to brain injury. Refer to Table 16.1 for an explanation of cranial nerve assessment in children.

Use the doll's eyes maneuver to evaluate cranial nerves III, IV, and VI. This maneuver can be helpful when assessing an infant, uncooperative child, or comatose child. It examines horizontal and vertical eye movements by turning the head in one direction and

TABLE 16.1 • Assessment of Cranial Nerves in Infants and Children

Cranial Nerve	Function	Assessment Procedure
I (olfactory)	Sense of smell	Not evaluated in infants and young children. In children, assess child's ability to recognize common smells (i.e., an orange) while eyes are closed.
II (optic), III (oculomotor), IV (trochlear), VI (abducens)	Vision, motor control and sensation of eye muscles, movement of major eye muscles	Assess oculomotor ability by having child follow object (toy or brightly colored object). Assess vision fields and visual acuity in older child. Assess pupil reaction same as adult. May need to talk to child or have parent in visual field while applying light stimulus.
V (trigeminal)	Mastication muscles and facial sensation	Note strength of infant's suck on pacifier, examiner's thumb, or bottle. In children, assess strength of bite and ability to discern light touch on face.
VII (facial)	Facial muscles, salivation, and taste	Note symmetry of facial expressions; in infant, monitor during spontaneous cries or smiles. In older child, test as in adults. Assess taste by asking to discern certain common tastes (salt, sugar).
VIII (acoustic)	Hearing	In infant, note response to voice. In children, use whisper test or Weber or Rinne test.
IX (glossopharyngeal), X (vagus)	Motor impulses to heart and other organs, swallowing, and gag reflex	Gag reflex and swallowing tested as in adults. Check time of last feeding, especially in the infant, to avoid vomiting when gag reflex is tested.
XI (accessory)	Impulses to muscles of shoulders and pharynx	In infants, note symmetry of head position when placed in the sitting position. In children, same as adults.
XII (hypoglossal)	Motor impulses to tongue and skeletal muscles	In infants, note spontaneous tongue movements. In children, same as adults.

assessing if the eyes move symmetrically in the other direction. For example, if you suddenly turn the child's head to the right, the child's eyes should look to the left symmetrically. Assess vertical eye movements in a similar manner by flexing or extending the neck. Absence of expected eye movements may indicate increased ICP.

When assessing oculomotor function, be sure to note nystagmus or sunset appearance of the eyes. Observe for nystagmus by looking for involuntary, rapid, rhythmic eye movements that may be present at rest or with eye movement. Horizontal nystagmus may occur with lesions in the brain stem and can be the result of certain medications (phenytoin in particular). Vertical nystagmus indicates brain stem dysfunction. *Sunsetting* is when the sclera of the eyes is showing over the top of the iris (Fig. 16.3). Sunset eyes may indicate increased ICP as seen in hydrocephalus. Pupillary response is often abnormal when a neurologic disorder is present. Refer to Figure 16.4 for illustrations of varied pupillary responses.

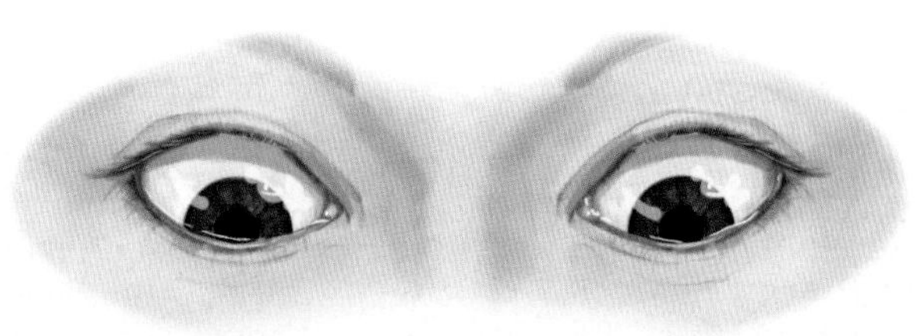

FIGURE 16.3 Sunsetting of the eyes is a sign of increased intracranial pressure.

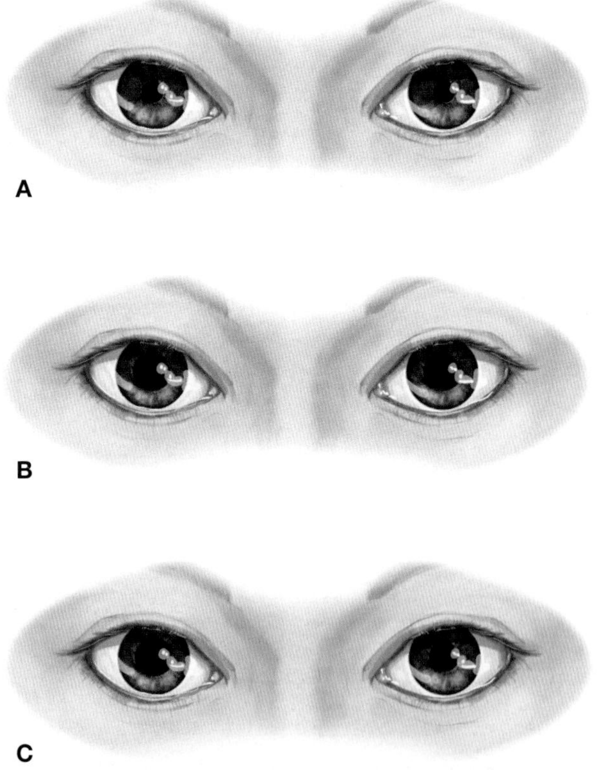

FIGURE 16.4 Assessing pupil size and reaction. **A.** *Pinpoint* is commonly observed in poisonings, brain stem dysfunction, and opiate use. **B.** *Dilated but reactive* is seen after seizures. *Fixed and dilated* is associated with brain stem herniation secondary to increased intracranial pressure. **C.** *One dilated (left eye) but reactive* is associated with intracranial mass.

CLINICAL REASONING ALERT!

Immediately report the sudden presence of fixed and dilated pupils.

Motor Function. Observe muscle strength, size, and tone in the infant or child. Assess bilaterally and compare. Observe spontaneous activity, posture, and balance, and assess for asymmetric movements. In the infant, observe resting posture, which will normally be a slightly flexed posture. The infant should be able to extend extremities to a normal stretch. Alterations in motor function, like changes in gait, muscle tone, or strength, may indicate certain neurologic problems such as increased ICP, head injury, and cerebral infections. Because cortical control of motor function is lost in certain neurologic disorders, postural reflexes reemerge and are directly related to the area of the brain that is damaged. Therefore, it is important to assess for two distinct types of posturing that may occur. **Decorticate posturing** occurs with damage of the cerebral cortex (Fig. 16.5A). **Decerebrate posturing** occurs with damage at the level of the brain stem (Fig. 16.5B). Both types of posturing are characterized by extremely rigid muscle tone.

Reflexes. Testing of deep tendon reflexes is part of the neurologic assessment, just as it is in adults. Testing of primitive and protective reflexes in the infant is important because infants cannot perform tasks on command. The Moro, tonic neck, and withdrawal reflexes are important in assessing neurologic health in infants. Refer to Chapter 3 for a further explanation of primitive and protective reflexes in infants (see Chapter 3, Table 3.1). Absence of certain reflexes, persistence of primitive reflexes after age of normal disappearance, or increases in reflexes may be present in specific neurologic conditions.

Sensory Function. When assessing the child, use techniques similar to those used in the adult assessment. Be sure to explain what you are doing to the child, especially before the pinprick test, to gain continued cooperation. When assessing sensory function, the child should be able to distinguish between light touch, pain, vibration, heat, and cold. When assessing an infant, limit the examination to responses to touch or pain. The normal response in a 4-month-old infant will be movement away from the stimulus. Alterations in sensory function can result from brain or spinal cord lesions.

Increased Intracranial Pressure. Observe for signs and symptoms associated with increased ICP while caring for a child with a potential or suspected neurologic disorder. Refer to Comparison Chart 16.1 for early versus late signs and symptoms of increased ICP. Increased ICP is a sign that may occur with many neurologic disorders. It may result from head trauma, birth trauma, hydrocephalus, infection, and brain tumors. As ICP increases, LOC decreases, and the signs and symptoms will become more pronounced. It is essential to recognize early signs and symptoms of increased ICP and intervene immediately to prevent long-term damage and possible death.

CLINICAL REASONING ALERT!

Presence of hypertension with a widening pulse pressure, bradycardia, and irregular respirations (referred to as Cushing triad) is a sign of impending herniation and a medical emergency.

Decorticate — Extremities flexed

A

Decerebrate — Extremities extended and pronated

B

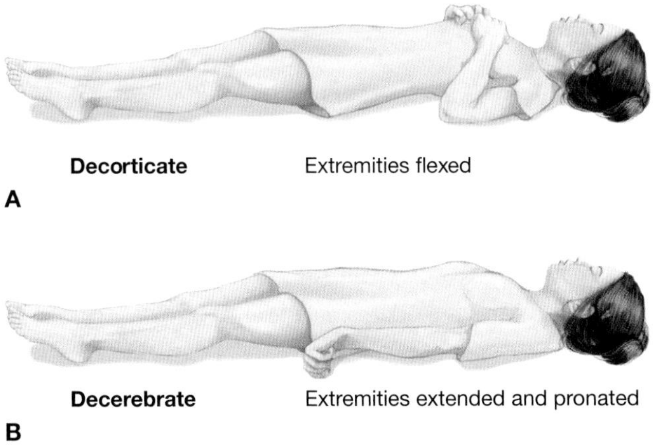

FIGURE 16.5 A. Decorticate posturing occurs with damage of the cerebral cortex and includes adduction of the arms, flexion at the elbows with arms held over chest, and flexion of the wrists with hands fisted. Lower extremities are adducted and extended. **B.** Decerebrate posturing occurs with damage to the midbrain and includes extension and pronation of the arms and legs.

Palpation

Palpation of the newborn and infant skull and fontanels is an important function of the neurologic examination. Changes in size or fullness of the fontanels may exist in certain neurologic conditions and must be noted. A bulging fontanel can be a sign of increased ICP and is seen in such neurologic disorders as hydrocephalus and head traumas. It is normal for the fontanels to be full or bulging during crying; take this into consideration during assessment.

Note any premature closure of fontanels, which can indicate skull deformities such as craniosynostosis. The posterior fontanel normally closes by 2 months of age, and the anterior fontanel normally closes by 12 to 18 months of age. In children with hydrocephalus, widening of the fontanels may be noted, along with a tense appearance and a resulting increase in head circumference.

Auscultation

Health care providers or nurse practitioners may perform auscultation of the skull. Soft, symmetric bruits may be found in children under 4 years of age or in children with acute febrile illness. A finding of a loud or localized bruit is usually significant and requires immediate further investigation. Increased ICP, resulting from conditions such as hydrocephalus, tumor, or meningitis, frequently produces intracranial bruits. Arterial venous malformations may also produce large bruits.

Laboratory and Diagnostic Testing

Common Laboratory and Diagnostic Tests 16.1 offers an explanation of the most commonly used laboratory and diagnostic tests utilized when considering neurologic disorders. The tests can assist the health care provider or nurse practitioner in diagnosing the disorder and/or serve as guidelines in determining ongoing treatment. Laboratory or nonnursing personnel obtain some of the tests, while the nurse might obtain others. In either instance, it is important to be familiar with how the tests are obtained, what they are used for, and normal versus abnormal results. This knowledge will also be necessary when providing child and family education related to the testing. Many of these tests, such as **lumbar puncture (LP)** (Fig. 16.6), can be frightening to parents and the child. Prepare the family and the child and provide support and reassurance during and after the test or procedure.

• • • ATRAUMATIC CARE • • •

During an LP, use distraction technique such as storytelling or music that will allow the child to remain in the proper position. Encourage parental involvement and enlist the help of a child life specialist, if possible.

COMMON LABORATORY AND DIAGNOSTIC TESTS 16.1

Test	Explanation	Indications	Nursing Implications
Lumbar puncture (LP)	Withdrawal of cerebrospinal fluid (CSF) from the subarachnoid space for analysis	To diagnose hemorrhage, infection, obstruction, tumor or malignancy, autoimmune disease, or multiple sclerosis Can obtain measurement of spinal fluid pressure	Assist with proper positioning (see Fig. 16.6). Help child maintain position and remain still. Maintain strict asepsis. Assist with collection and transport of specimen. Monitor respiratory status, changes in consciousness, heart rate, pain level. Encourage fluids after procedure, if not contraindicated. Keep child flat for 1 hour if ordered. Apply EMLA cream to puncture site 30–60 minutes before procedure to reduce pain, if ordered.
Head and neck x-ray	Radiographic image of the head and neck will show skull and spine structures	Detects skull and spinal fractures; shows location and course of ventricular catheters; reveals information about increased ICP and skull defects	Children may be afraid. Allow a parent or family member to accompany the child. If the child is unable or unwilling to stay still for the radiograph, restraint may be necessary. The time of restraint should be limited to the amount of time needed for the radiograph.
Fluoroscopy	Radiographic examination that uses continuous x-rays to show live up-to-date images	Can assess cervical spine for instability during movement	Same as head and neck radiographs. Child will need to cooperate with flexion and extension of neck.
Cerebral angiography	X-ray study of cerebral blood vessels. Involves injection of a contrast medium and use of fluoroscopy	Can assess for vessel defects or space-occupying lesions	Same as head and neck radiographs. Assess for allergy to contrast medium and possible NPO status. Push fluids following procedure, if not contraindicated, to help flush out contrast medium.

COMMON LABORATORY AND DIAGNOSTIC TESTS 16.1

Test	Explanation	Indications	Nursing Implications
Ultrasound	Use of sound waves to locate the depth and structure within soft tissues and fluid	Used to assess intracranial hemorrhage in newborns and ventricular size	Better tolerated by children who are not sedated than CT or MRI Can be performed portably at bedside
Computed tomography (CT)	Noninvasive x-ray study that looks at tissue density and structures. Images a "slice" of child's tissue	To diagnose congenital abnormalities, such as neural tube defects, hemorrhage, tumors, fractures	Machine is large and can be frightening to children. Procedure can be lengthy, and child must remain still. If unable to do so, sedation may be necessary. Can be performed with or without use of contrast medium; if used, assess for allergy and possible NPO status. Encourage fluids postprocedure, if not contraindicated.
Electroencephalogram (EEG)	Measures electrical activity of the brain	To diagnose seizures and brain death; to evaluate brain tumors, subdural hematomas, intracranial hemorrhages	Must remain still. If unable to do so, sedation may be necessary, but should be avoided, if possible, because sedatives can alter the EEG reading. Inform technician of what anticonvulsants the child is taking. Morning anticonvulsants may need to be held.
Magnetic resonance imaging (MRI)	Use of magnetic field to show different tissue compositions	Used to assess tumors and inflammation; used to diagnose congenital abnormalities, such as neural tube defects; shows normal versus abnormal brain tissue	Child may not have any metal devices, internal or external, while undergoing MRI (ensure hospital gown does not have metal snaps). Most new surgical implants are now MRI compatible; consult imaging center. Procedure can be lengthy, and child must remain still. Child is placed in long narrow tube, and the machine makes a booming noise when it is turned on and off during the procedure; therefore, can be difficult to gain cooperation. If the child is unable to remain still, sedation may be necessary. Can be performed with or without use of a contrast medium. If contrast medium is used, assess for allergy and possible NPO status. Encourage fluids postprocedure, if not contraindicated.
Positron emission tomography (PET)	Similar to CT or MRI, but radioisotope is added. Measures physiologic function	Provides information on brain functional development. Can assist in identifying seizure foci. Can assess tumors and brain metabolism	Procedure can be lengthy, and child must remain still. If unable to do so, sedation may be necessary. Intravenous access will be needed for the procedure. Encourage fluids postprocedure, if not contraindicated, to help body eliminate radioisotopes.
Single-photon emission computed tomography (SPECT)	Use of radiopharmaceuticals to provide three-dimensional splices; less expensive and more available than PET	Used to detect brain death, presence of encephalitis, hydrocephalus, to localize epileptic foci, assess metabolic activity, evaluate brain tumors, assessment of childhood development disorders	Similar to PET In children who are not cooperating, do not use sedation until after injection because it may affect brain activity Secure child's head. Sudden distractions or loud noises can alter the distribution of radionuclide.

(*continued*)

COMMON LABORATORY AND DIAGNOSTIC TESTS 16.1 *(continued)*

Test	Explanation	Indications	Nursing Implications
Cisternography	Radiopharmaceuticals injected intrathecally during a lumbar puncture to assess flow and reabsorption of CSF	Can assist in selection of type of shunt and pathway to use in treating hydrocephalus	Sterile LP performed and radionuclide injected into cerebrospinal circulation Imaging performed at specified times Child must lie flat after puncture.
Intracranial pressure (ICP) monitoring (intraventricular catheter, subarachnoid screw or bolt, epidural sensor, anterior fontanel pressure monitor)	A sensing device is placed in the head that monitors the pressure intracranially.	Used to monitor ICP resulting from hydrocephalus, acute head trauma, and brain tumors. Ventricular catheter also allows for draining of CSF to help reduce ICP.	Usually monitored in critical care setting Monitor for signs and symptoms of increased ICP. Monitor for infection. Keep head of bed elevated 15–30 degrees. Alarms for monitoring device should remain on at all times. Reduce stimulation and avoid interventions that may cause pain or stress and result in an increased ICP.
Video EEG	Measures electrical activity of the brain continuously along with recorded video of actions and behaviors	Can help determine precise localization of seizure area before surgery. Assists in diagnosis and management of seizures by correlating behaviors with abnormal EEG activity	Ensure that seizure precautions are in place. Parent or caregiver must be with child at all times. The child's movements are limited and usually confined to the room. When the child changes position, ensure they are still seen by video camera. Boredom can be a problem. Must notify nurse if seizure activity occurs; push the alert button to highlight attack on EEG recoding. Nurse must immediately go to the room, expose as much of the child as possible (remove covers; if at night, turn on light), and avoid blocking the camera. Ask questions (i.e., what is your name, can you raise your left arm, remember the word banana) to help assess responsiveness more accurately. Stay with the child until a full recovery has occurred. Ask the child what word you asked them to remember, and document all findings and time of the event.

Adapted from Fischbach, F. T., Fischbach, M. A., & Stout, K. (2022). *A manual of laboratory and diagnostic tests* (11th ed.). Wolters Kluwer.

Remember Antonio, the 3-month-old with lethargy, a weak cry, and vomiting? What additional health history and physical examination assessment information should the nurse obtain?

Nursing Analysis

After recognizing and analyzing cues from a thorough assessment, the nurse may identify several patient problems, including:

- Decreased intracranial adaptive capacity
- Altered tissue perfusion: cerebral
- Injury risk
- Infection risk
- Pain
- Activities of daily living (ADL) deficit (specify)
- Impaired physical mobility
- Delayed development risk
- Malnutrition
- Dehydration risk
- Knowledge deficiency
- Interrupted family processes

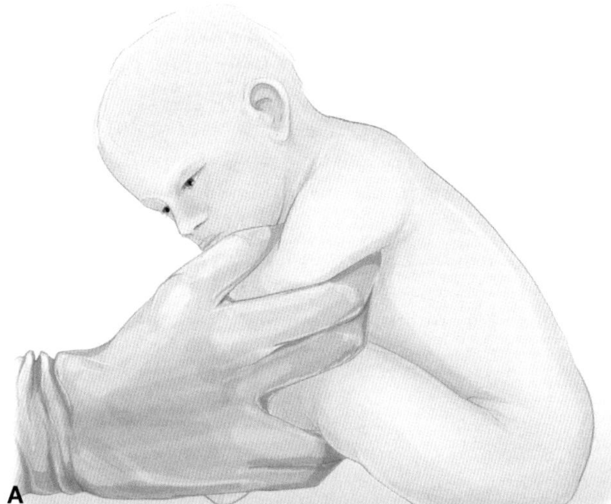

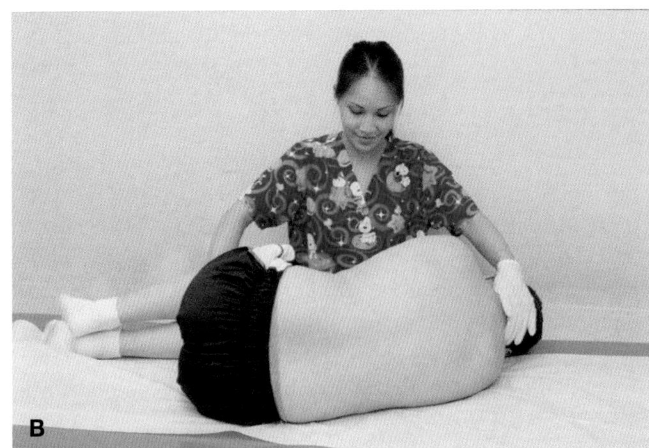

FIGURE 16.6 Proper positioning for a lumbar puncture. **A.** The newborn is positioned upright with head flexed forward. **B.** Child or older infant is positioned on the side with head flexed forward and knees flexed to abdomen.

After completing an assessment of Antonio, the nurse noted the following: a full anterior fontanel; when being held, Antonio was inconsolable; when lying still, he was calmer and in the opisthotonic position. Based on the assessment findings, what would be your top three prioritized patient problems for Antonio?

The previous patient problems or concerns provide suggestions for developing a nursing plan of care or concept mapping. The nurse will then generate solutions by planning interventions (suggested further on with rationales). The plan of care should be individualized, based on the child's and family's needs. Refer to Chapter 14 for the nursing process for pain management and to Chapter 11 for nursing interventions related to interrupted family processes and risk of caregiver role strain. Additional information will be included later in the chapter as it relates to specific disorders.

Nursing Analysis

Decreased intracranial adaptive capacity related to brain injury, sustained increase in ICP of 10 to 15 mm Hg (compression of brain tissue due to increased CSF or cerebral edema secondary to increased ICP resulting from brain injury, congenital structural defects, brain tumor, decreased reabsorption of CSF, or shunt malfunction) as evidenced by vomiting, headache, complaints of visual disturbances, elevated blood pressure, changes in LOC, increased head circumference, or bulging fontanel.

Goal/Outcome

Child will remain free of signs and symptoms of increased ICP, as evidenced by remaining free of headache, vomiting, vision disturbances, vital signs within parameters for age, no signs of altered levels of consciousness, able to maintain effective breathing pattern, free of excessive irritability or lethargy, head circumference within parameters for age.

Promoting Adequate Intracranial Adaptive Capacity (interventions with *rationale*)

- Assess neurologic status closely, and monitor for signs and symptoms of increased ICP; *changes in LOC, signs of irritability or lethargy, and changes in pupillary reaction can indicate changes in ICP.*
- Monitor vital signs; *decreased pulse and irregular respiratory rate and increased blood pressure or widening pulse pressure (Cushing triad) can indicate increased ICP and medical emergency.*
- Measure head circumference in children younger than 3 years of age; *increases in head circumference outside parameters for age can indicate increased ICP.*
- Elevate head of bed 15 to 30 degrees *to facilitate venous return and help to reduce ICP.*
- Minimize environmental stimuli and noise, and avoid pain-producing procedures, if possible; *these factors can increase ICP.*
- Have emergency equipment ready and available; *increased ICP can result in respiratory or cardiac failure.*
- Notify health care provider or nurse practitioner immediately if changes in assessment are noted; *early intervention is critical to prevent neurologic damage and death.*

Nursing Analysis

Altered (cerebral) tissue perfusion risk due to brain injury caused by increased ICP, alteration in blood flow secondary to hemorrhage, vessel malformation, or cerebral edema

Goal/Outcome

Child will exhibit adequate cerebral tissue perfusion through course of illness and childhood: child will remain alert and oriented with no signs of altered LOC; vital signs will be within parameters for age; motor, sensory, and cognitive function will be within parameters for age; head circumference will remain within parameters for age.

Promoting Adequate Tissue Perfusion (interventions with *rationale*)

- Assess neurologic status closely, and monitor for signs and symptoms of increased ICP. *Changes in LOC, signs of irritability or lethargy, and changes in pupillary reaction can indicate decreased cerebral tissue perfusion.*
- Monitor vital signs; *decreased pulse and irregular respiratory rate and increased blood pressure or widening pulse pressure (Cushing triad) can indicate increased ICP and a medical emergency, which can lead to decreased cerebral perfusion.*
- Have emergency equipment ready and available; *decreased cerebral perfusion can result in respiratory or cardiac failure.*
- Notify health care provider or nurse practitioner immediately if changes in assessment are noted; *early intervention is critical to prevent neurologic damage and death.*

Nursing Analysis

Injury risk; risk factors include alteration in cognitive functioning, alteration in psychomotor functioning (altered LOC, weakness, dizziness, ataxia, loss of muscle coordination secondary to seizure activity).

Goal/Outcome

Child will remain free of injury, as evidenced by no signs of aspiration or traumatic injury.

Preventing Injury (interventions with *rationale*)

- Ensure child has patent airway and adequate oxygenation (have suction, oxygen available at bedside) and place child in sidelying position, if possible. *A child with altered LOC may not be able to manage their secretions and is at risk for aspiration and ineffective airway clearance; providing suction and oxygenation can help ensure an open airway, and the sidelying position can help secretions drain and prevent obstruction of airway or aspiration.*
- Protect child from hurting self during seizures or changes in LOC by removing environmental obstacles, easing child to lying position, and padding side rails *to help keep the environment safe.*
- Institute seizure precautions for any child at risk for seizure activity (Box 16.1) *to help prevent injury that can result from acute seizure activity.*
- With seizure activity, do not insert a tongue blade or restrain child; *this can lead to injury to caregiver and child.*
- Administer anticonvulsant medications as ordered *to promote cessation and prevention of seizure activity.*
- Assist the child with ambulation *to help prevent injury in child with weakness, dizziness, or ataxia.*
- Allow for periods of rest *to prevent fatigue and decrease risk of injury.*

Nursing Analysis

Infection risk; risk factors include alteration in skin integrity, invasive procedure, malnutrition, stasis of body fluid (caused by surgical interventions, presence of foreign body like a shunt, trauma to the skull, nutritional deficiencies, stasis of pulmonary secretions and urine, and/or presence of infectious organisms).

Goal/Outcome

Child will exhibit no signs or symptoms of local or systemic infection and will not spread infection to others. Symptoms of infection will decrease over time; others will remain free of infection.

Preventing Infection (interventions with *rationale*)

- Monitor vital signs; *elevation in temperature can indicate presence of infection.*
- Monitor incision sites for signs of local infection; *redness, warmth, drainage, swelling, and pain at incision site can indicate presence of infection.*
- Maintain aseptic technique—practice good handwashing and use proper technique when managing postoperative incisions and external shunts *to prevent introduction of further infectious agents.*
- Administer antibiotics as prescribed *to prevent or treat bacterial infection.*

BOX **16.1** Seizure Precautions

- Padding of side rails and other hard objects
- Side rails raised on bed at all times when child is in bed
- Oxygen and suction at bedside
- Supervision, especially during bathing, ambulation, or other potentially hazardous activities
- Use of a protective helmet during activity may be appropriate
- Child should wear a medical alert bracelet.

- Encourage nutritious diet and proper hydration according to child's preferences and ability to feed orally *to assist body's natural defenses against infection.*
- Isolate the child as required *to prevent nosocomial spread of infection.*
- Teach the child and family preventive measures such as good handwashing, covering the mouth and nose upon cough or sneeze, and adequate disposal of used tissues *to prevent nosocomial or community spread of infection.*

Nursing Analysis

Bathing, dressing, feeding ADL deficit related to pain, alteration in cognitive functioning, neuromuscular impairments, as evidenced by an inability to perform hygiene care and transfer self independently.

Goal/Outcome

Child will demonstrate ability to care for themselves within age parameters and limits of disease: Child is able to feed, dress, and manage elimination within limits of disease and age.

Maximizing Self-Care (interventions with *rationale*)

- Introduce child and family to self-help methods as soon as possible *to promote independence from the beginning.*
- Encourage family and staff to allow child to do as much as possible *to allow child to gain confidence and independence.*
- Teach specific measures for bowel and urinary elimination as needed *to promote independence and increase self-care abilities and self-esteem.*
- Collaborate with physical therapy, occupational therapy, and speech therapy departments to provide child and family with appropriate tools to modify environment and methods to promote transferring and self-care *to allow for maximum functioning.*
- Praise accomplishments and emphasize child's abilities *to help improve self-esteem and encourage feeling of confidence and competence.*
- Balance activity with periods to rest so as *to reduce fatigue and increase energy for self-care.*

Nursing Analysis

Impaired physical mobility related to decrease in muscle control, mass and strength; contractures (hypertonicity), neuromuscular, musculoskeletal impairment (impaired coordination), as evidenced by an inability to move extremities, to ambulate without assistance, to move without limitations.

Goal/Outcome

Child will be able to engage in activities within age parameters and limits of disease: Child is able to move extremities, move about environment, and participate in exercise programs within limits of age and disease.

Maximizing Physical Mobility (interventions with *rationale*)

- Encourage gross and fine motor skill activities *to facilitate motor development.*
- Collaborate with physical therapy, occupational therapy, and speech therapy departments to strengthen muscles and promote optimal mobility *to facilitate motor development.*
- Utilize passive and active ROM, and teach child and family how to perform them so as *to prevent contractures and facilitate joint mobility and muscle development (active ROM) to help increase mobility.*
- Praise accomplishments and emphasize child's abilities *to help improve self-esteem and encourage feeling of confidence and competence.*

Nursing Analysis

Delayed development risk; risk factors include brain injury, chronic illness, and seizure disorder (physical disability, cognitive deficits, activity restrictions).

Goal/Outcome

Child will demonstrate developmental milestones within age parameters and limits of disease: child expresses interest in the environment and people around them and interacts with environment age appropriately.

Maximizing Development (interventions with *rationale*)

- Use therapeutic play and adaptive toys *to help facilitate developmental functioning.*
- Provide stimulating environment when possible *to maximize potential for growth and development.*
- Praise accomplishments and emphasize child's abilities *to help improve self-esteem and encourage feeling of confidence and competence.*

Nursing Analysis

Malnutrition risk related to insufficient dietary intake (vomiting and difficulty feeding secondary to increased ICP; difficulty sucking, swallowing, or chewing; surgical incision pain or difficulty assuming normal feeding position; inability to feed themselves), as evidenced by decreased oral intake, impaired swallowing, weight loss

Goal/Outcome

Child will exhibit signs of adequate nutrition: Weight will remain within parameters for age, skin turgor will be good, intake/output (I/O) will be within normal limits, adequate calories will be ingested, and vomiting will cease or decrease.

Promoting Adequate Nutrition (interventions with *rationale*)

- Monitor height and weight; *insufficient intake will lead to impaired growth and weight gain.*
- Monitor hydration status (moist mucous membranes, elastic skin turgor, adequate urine output); *insufficient intake can lead to dehydration.*
- Use techniques to promote caloric and nutritional intake and teach family (i.e., positioning, modified utensils, soft or blended foods, allow extra time) *to facilitate intake.*
- Assess respiratory system frequently *to assess for aspiration.*
- Monitor for nausea and vomiting, and medicate if ordered *to help reduce vomiting and increase intake.*
- Monitor for pain, and medicate if ordered *to help reduce pain related to surgical incisions and trauma, and increase intake.*
- Assist family to assume as normal a feeding position as possible *to help increase oral intake.*

Nursing Analysis

Dehydration risk; risk factors include insufficient fluid intake, active fluid volume loss, deviations affecting fluid intake from vomiting, altered LOC, poor feeding or intake, insensible loss due to fever, and/or failure of regulatory mechanisms (as in diabetes insipidus [DI]).

Goal/Outcome

Fluid volume will be maintained and balanced: oral mucosa moist and pink, skin turgor elastic, urine output at least 1 to 2 mL/kg/h.

Promoting Adequate Fluid Balance (interventions with *rationale*)

- Administer intravenous (IV) fluids, if ordered *to maintain adequate hydration in children who are nothing by mouth (NPO) or unable to tolerate oral intake.*
- When oral intake is allowed and tolerated, encourage oral (PO) fluids *to promote intake and maintain hydration.*
- Strict intake and output monitoring *can help identify fluid imbalance and also detect signs of abnormal pituitary secretions, resulting in conditions like syndrome of inappropriate antidiuretic hormone secretion (SIADH) and diabetes insipidus (DI)* (see Chapter 26 for further information).
- Maintain minimum hydration and avoid overhydration in children for whom cerebral edema is a concern; *fluid overload can contribute to cerebral edema.*
- Monitor urine specific gravity, urine and serum electrolytes (especially serum sodium), blood urea nitrogen, creatinine and osmolality, and daily weights as ordered; *these are reliable indicators of fluid status and can also detect signs of abnormal pituitary secretions, resulting in conditions such as SIADH and DI.*

Nursing Analysis

Knowledge deficiency related to insufficient information (regarding complex medical condition, prognosis, and medical needs), as evidenced by verbalization, questions, or actions demonstrating lack of understanding regarding child's condition or care

Goal/Outcome

Child and family will verbalize accurate information and understanding about condition, prognosis, and medical needs: child and family demonstrate knowledge of condition and prognosis and medical needs, including possible causes, contributing factors, and treatment measures.

Providing Child and Family Teaching (interventions with *rationale*)

- Assess child's and family's willingness to learn; *child and family must be willing to learn for teaching to be effective.*
- Provide family with time to adjust to diagnosis *to help facilitate adjustment and ability to learn and participate in child's care.*
- Repeat information *to allow family and child time to learn and understand.*
- Teach in short sessions; *many short sessions are found to be more helpful than one long session.*
- Gear teaching to a level of understanding of the child and also the family (depends on age of child, physical condition, memory) *to ensure understanding.*
- Provide reinforcement and rewards *to help facilitate the teaching–learning process.*
- Use multiple modes of learning involving many senses (provide written, verbal, demonstration, and videos) when possible; *the child and family are more likely to retain information when presented in different ways using many senses.*

Based on your top three patient problems for Antonio, describe appropriate nursing interventions.

SEIZURE DISORDERS

Approximately 4% to 10% of children experience one seizure, with a lifetime incidence of epilepsy being 3%, with half of these starting in childhood (Mikati & Tchapyjnikov, 2020). Most seizures are caused by disorders that originate outside of the brain such as a high fever, infection, head trauma, hypoxia, toxins, or cardiac dysrhythmias. Seizure disorders discussed further on include epilepsy, febrile seizures, and neonatal seizures.

Epilepsy

Epilepsy is a condition in which seizures are triggered recurrently from within the brain. Epilepsy is a common neurologic disorder discovered in childhood, although brain injury or infection can cause epilepsy at any age. The International League Against Epilepsy (ILAE) defines epilepsy by the presence of any of the following conditions:

- Two or more unprovoked (or reflex) seizures, which occur more than 24 hours apart
- One unprovoked (or reflex) seizure and a chance of further seizures the same as the general recurrence risk (at least 60%) after two unprovoked seizures, happening over the next 10 years
- Diagnosis of an epilepsy syndrome (Wilfong, 2022)

The prognosis for most children with seizures associated with epilepsy is good. Many children will outgrow epilepsy, but some children will have persistent seizures that are difficult to manage and may be unresponsive to pharmacologic interventions. Living with a seizure disorder may have a devastating impact on the quality of life of the child and family.

Pathophysiology

Epilepsy is a complex disorder of the CNS in which brain function is affected. Recurrent or unprovoked seizures are the clinical manifestation of epilepsy and result from a disruption of electrical communication among the neurons of the brain. This disruption results from an imbalance between the excitatory and inhibitory mechanisms in the brain, causing the neurons to either fire when they are not supposed to or not fire when they should. Epilepsy has numerous causes. It may be acquired and related to brain injury, or it may be a familial tendency, but in some cases the cause is unknown (Mikati & Tchapyjnikov, 2020).

The ILAE revised their system of classification in 2017 in the hopes of providing greater flexibility and transparency when classifying seizure types (Fisher et al., 2017; Wilfong, 2022). The ILAE classification is used by most neurologists to classify seizure types. There are three categories of seizures—focal (previously known as partial), generalized, and unknown seizures (i.e., epileptic spasms). In focal seizures, only one hemisphere of the brain is involved, while general seizures involve the entire brain. "Unknown" is used for epileptic spasms, tonic–clonic, and behavior arrest, where it is unclear whether the mode of onset is generalized or focal (Fisher et al., 2017; Wilfong, 2022). "Focal to bilateral tonic–clonic seizures" replaces the term "secondarily generalized seizures" to describe seizures that start on one side of the brain and spread to both sides (Fisher et al., 2017; Wilfong, 2022). There are many different types of seizures, and the classification of the type of seizure is crucial in assisting with the management and control of seizures. Not all cases are easily classified.

The new classification system is based on three key elements: where the seizure began within the brain (one side [focal], both sides [generalized], or unknown); LOC/awareness during the seizure (only for focal seizure classification as generalized seizures are assumed to affect consciousness in some way); and describing features of the seizure, including movement such as stiffening, jerking or automatisms (motor) or no movement (nonmotor) characteristics. The most common seizure types are discussed in Table 16.2.

TABLE 16.2 • Common Types of Seizures

Onset	Type	Description	Characteristics
Unknown	Motor: Tonic–clonic; Epileptic spasm Nonmotor: Behavior arrest	Mode of seizure onset unknown, whether focal or generalized Mode of seizure onset unknown, whether focal or generalized Type of epileptic spasm seen in infancy Usually seen between 3 and 12 months of age, peak incidence 3–7 months and rarely seen after the age of 18 months	Occurs in series or clusters Presents as symmetrical flexing or extending, in variant clinical patterns, of the neck, arms, legs, and trunk May see: • Extension of neck, trunk, arms, and legs • Flexion of neck, trunk, and extremities with contracting of abdominal muscles (may cause body to bend forward, often referred to as "jackknife seizures") • Cry may precede or follow. Majority of infants have some brain disorder before seizures begin. The infant seems to stop developing and may lose skills that they have already attained after the onset of infantile spasms. Hormonal therapy (mainly corticotropin) and anticonvulsants (most commonly, vigabatrin) are common forms of treatment. A decrease or ceasing of an ongoing motor activity during a seizure

(continued)

TABLE **16.2** • Common Types of Seizures (*continued*)

Onset	Type	Description	Characteristics
Generalized onset Nonmotor	Absence (formerly *petit mal*) • Typical • Atypical • Myoclonic • Eyelid myoclonic	Type of generalized seizure where motor activity is not prominent; presents with autonomic, behavior arrest, cognitive, emotional or sensory dysfunction	Abrupt onset and offset Sudden cessation of motor activity or speech with a blank facial expression or rhythmic twitching of the mouth, eyebrows, chin, eyelids, or other parts of the face Child may experience countless seizures in a day. Not associated with a postictal (after seizure) state May go unrecognized or mistaken for inattentiveness because of subtle change in child's behavior Myoclonic absence seizure consists of jerks of the shoulder and arms may result in lifting of the arms. Eyelid myoclonia brief (6 seconds) jerking of the eyelids with eyeballs rolling back; multiple seizures occur daily
Generalized onset Motor	Clonic	Type of generalized seizure that presents with repeated jerking movements	Muscles will spasm, jerk, then relax. Spasm/jerking cannot be stopped by restraining or repositioning. Clonic seizures alone are rare; may precede a tonic–clonic seizure
Generalized onset Motor	Tonic	Type of generalized seizures that present with stiffening of the muscles, typically the back, legs, arms	Consciousness usually preserved Tightening of chest muscles may lead to cyanosis; seen in children with Lennox–Gastaut syndrome
Generalized onset Motor	Tonic–clonic (formerly *grand mal*)	Extremely common generalized seizures; most dramatic seizure type	Associated with an aura Loss of consciousness occurs and may be preceded by a piercing cry. Presents with entire body experiencing tonic contractions followed by rhythmic clonic contractions alternating with relaxation of all muscle groups Cyanosis may be noted due to apnea. Saliva may collect in the mouth due to inability to swallow. Child may bite tongue. Loss of sphincter control, especially the bladder, is common. Postictal phase: child will be semicomatose or in a deep sleep for approximately 30 minutes–2 hours; usually responds only to painful stimuli Child will have no memory of the seizure; may complain of headache and feeling of fatigue Safety of the child is a primary concern. See Teaching Guidelines 16.1.
Generalized onset Motor	Myoclonic Myoclonic–tonic–clonic Myoclonic–atonic Epileptic spasm	Type of generalized seizure that involves the motor cortex of the brain. May occur along with other seizure forms	Sudden, brief, massive muscle jerks that may involve the whole body or one body part Child may or may not lose consciousness.
Generalized onset Motor	Atonic	Type of generalized seizure often referred to as "drop attacks." Seen in children with Lennox–Gastaut syndrome	Sudden loss of muscle tone. In children, may only be a sudden drop of the head. Child will regain consciousness within a few seconds to a minute. Can result in injury related to violent fall

TABLE 16.2 • Common Types of Seizures

Onset	Type	Description	Characteristics
Focal onset with retained consciousness/awareness (previously referred to as simple partial seizure)	Motor: Automatisms, atonic, clonic, hyperkinetic, myoclonic, tonic, epileptic spasm Nonmotor: autonomic, behavior arrest, cognitive, emotional, sensory	Seizure that occurs in one part of the brain. The symptoms seen will depend on which area of the brain is affected.	Motor activity characterized by clonic or tonic movements involving the face, neck, and extremities Can include sensory signs such as numbness, tingling, paresthesia, changes in vision and hearing, possible hallucinations, or pain Can include autonomic symptoms such as changes in blood pressure, heart rhythm, bowel function Can include psychic symptoms such as triggering emotions of fear, anxiety, joy, sadness Child remains conscious and may verbalize during the seizure. No postictal state
Focal seizure with impaired consciousness/awareness (previously known as complex partial seizure) Focal seizure may also be classified with unknown awareness (often seen with epileptic spasm)	Motor: Automatisms, atonic, clonic, hyperkinetic, myoclonic, tonic, epileptic spasm Nonmotor: autonomic, behavior arrest, cognitive, emotional, sensory	May begin with a focal seizure without impaired consciousness, then progress	May or may not have a preceding aura Consciousness will be impaired. Automatisms and complex purposeful movements are common features in infants and children. Infants will present with behaviors such as lip smacking, chewing, swallowing, and excessive salivation; can be difficult to distinguish from normal infant behavior In older children, will see picking or pulling at bed sheets or clothing, rubbing objects, or running or walking in a nondirective and repetitive fashion These seizures can be difficult to control.
Onset may be generalized, focal or absence	Status epilepticus	Common neurologic emergency in children. Can occur with any seizure activity. Febrile seizures are the most common type in young children. In children with epilepsy, it commonly occurs early in the course of epilepsy. Can be life threatening	Prolonged or clustered seizures where consciousness does not return between seizures The age of the child, cause of the seizures, and duration of status epilepticus influence prognosis. Prompt medical intervention is essential to reduce morbidity and mortality. Treatment: • Basic life support—ABCs (airway, breathing, circulation) • Administration of anticonvulsants to cease seizures is crucial. Common medications include benzodiazepines such as lorazepam and diazepam, and fosphenytoin (see Drug Guide 16.1 and Table 16.3). • Blood glucose levels and electrolytes along with evaluation of the underlying cause should be initiated.

Adapted from Fisher, R. S., Cross, J. H., French, J. A., Higurashi, N., Hirsch, E., Jansen, F. E., Lagae, L., Moshé, S. L., Peltola, J., Roulet Perez, E., Scheffer, I. E., & Zuberi, S. M. (2017). Operational classification of seizure types by the International League Against Epilepsy: Position paper of the ILAE Commission for Classification and Terminology. *Epilepsia, 58*, 522–530. https://doi.org/10.1111/epi.13670; Wilfong, A. (2022). Seizures and epilepsy in children: Classification, etiology, and clinical features. *UpToDate.* Retrieved May 4, 2023, from https://www.uptodate.com/contents/seizures-and-epilepsy-in-children-classification-etiology-and-clinical-features

Therapeutic Management

Management of epilepsy focuses on controlling seizures or reducing their frequency. Another focus of epilepsy management involves helping the child who has recurrent seizures and their family to learn to live with the seizures. The primary mode of treatment is the use of anticonvulsants. The goal for every child should be the use of the fewest drugs with the fewest possible side effects for the control of seizures. There have been significant advances in the treatment of epilepsy due to the many new anticonvulsant medications that have become available in recent years (see Table 16.3). Most anticonvulsants are taken orally and are often used in combination,

TABLE 16.3 • Common Anticonvulsant Medications

Medication	Nursing Implications
Phenytoin (IV and PO; IM administration is contraindicated)	Monitor serum levels to ensure therapeutic dosing. Be aware that gingival hyperplasia appears most commonly in children and adolescents. If on prolonged therapy, ensure adequate intake of vitamin D–containing foods. Monitor serum calcium, magnesium, folate, and vitamin B levels. IV form given in normal saline to prevent precipitation.
Fosphenytoin (IM or IV only)	Adverse effects are said to be less common than with phenytoin. It does not cause local irritation, but it is typically a more expensive drug than phenytoin. It is water-soluble, therefore allowing faster and easier administration than phenytoin. All dosing is in phenytoin sodium equivalents. It does not precipitate in commonly used IV diluents.
Phenobarbital	Assess for excessive sedation. Monitor serum levels to ensure therapeutic dosing. Monitor for drug interactions. Monitor folate, vitamin B, vitamin D, and calcium levels. Increase vitamin D–fortified foods or administer supplement, if prescribed. Withdrawal symptoms will occur if drug is stopped abruptly. Valproic acid interferes with this drug, causing increased phenobarbital levels.
Felbamate	Monitor for drug interactions, especially if child is taking barbiturates, phenytoin, or carbamazepine.
Valproic acid (divalproex sodium, sodium valproate, Depakote)	Monitor serum levels to ensure therapeutic dosing. Depakote sprinkles are available and useful for children who are unable to tolerate valproate suspension, tablets, or capsules. The contents can be sprinkled on food that does not require chewing.
Carbamazepine	Monitor serum levels to ensure therapeutic dosing; toxicity can occur even with levels slightly above therapeutic range. Monitor folate and vitamin B levels. Serum levels may be increased if taken with food and grapefruit juice. Plasma concentration decreased by phenytoin and may be increased by valproic acid.
Gabapentin	Do not administer within 2 hours of antacids. Rapidly absorbed in the gastrointestinal tract
Topiramate	Phenytoin, carbamazepine, and valproate products may decrease concentration of topiramate. Decreased bone mineral density may occur.
Oxcarbazepine	Monitor phenytoin levels, if administering concurrently. Monitor serum sodium.
Zonisamide	Phenobarbital may increase the metabolism of this drug and decrease serum concentration.
Lamotrigine	Severe and serious skin reactions have been noted. Valproate inhibits metabolism and enhances adverse effects; therefore, monitor serum blood values and decrease the dose, if necessary.
Levetiracetam	Increased incidence of psychiatric symptoms seen in children. Monitor for difficulty with gait or coordination. Plasma concentration decreased by phenytoin, phenobarbital, and carbamazepine.
Ethosuximide	Give with food if GI upset occurs. Monitor closely during periods of dosage adjustment or addition of new medications. Plasma concentration decreased by phenytoin and may be increased by valproate products.
Rufinamide	Give with food, helps increase absorption. Valproic acid may increase serum levels of rufinamide; phenytoin, carbamazepine, and phenobarbital may decrease serum levels of rufinamide.

GI, gastrointestinal; IM, intramuscular; IV, intravenous; PO, by mouth.

Data from Mikati, M. A., & Tchapyjnikov, D. (2020). Chapter 611. Seizures in childhood. In R. M. Kliegman, J. W. St. Geme III, N. J. Blum, S.S. Shah, R.C. Tasker, K.M. Wilson, & R. E. Behrman (Eds.), *Nelson textbook of pediatrics* (21st ed., pp. 16312–16492). Elsevier.

Lexicomp. (2023). Pediatric drug information. *UpToDate*. Retrieved April 5, 2023, from https://www.uptodate.com/contents/table-of-contents/drug-information/pediatric-drug-information

but the goal is single-drug therapy if possible. Different medications control different types of seizures, which may be due to individual variation. It can take time to find the right medication to best control an individual's seizures.

If seizures remain uncontrolled, another option for managing them is surgery. Depending on the area of the brain that is affected, it may be possible to remove the area that is responsible for the seizure activity or to interrupt the impulses from spreading and therefore stop or reduce the seizures. The adverse effects of surgery range from mild to severe, depending on the area of the brain that is affected. Other nonpharmacologic treatments that may be considered in children with intractable seizures include a ketogenic diet or placement of a vagal nerve stimulator. Refer to Common Medical Treatments 16.1.

Nursing Assessment

For a full description of the assessment phase of the nursing process, refer to the "Clinical Judgment and the Nursing Process" section earlier in the chapter. Assessment findings pertinent to epilepsy are discussed further on.

HEALTH HISTORY

Elicit a description of the present illness and chief complaint, which will usually involve a seizure episode. Gain information to help characterize the episode as a seizure or as a nonepileptic event (see Box 16.2 for a list of nonepileptic events). It is rare to actually observe the child having a seizure; therefore, a complete, accurate, and detailed history from a reliable source is essential. Questions should include:

- Where did the event occur—while sleeping, eating, playing, or just after waking?
- Description of child's behavior during the event—what types of movements, progression, length, respiratory status, apnea?
- How did the child act after the event?
- Have the episodes been recurrent? If so, how frequent?
- Any precipitating factors such as a fever, fall, activity, anxiety, infection, or exposure to strong stimuli such as flashing lights or loud noises?

BOX 16.2 Nonepileptic Events

- Syncope
- Breath holding
- Jitteriness
- Apnea
- Gastroesophageal reflux
- Cardiac conduction abnormalities
- Migraines
- Tics
- Night terrors
- Benign sleep movements

Explore the child's current and past medical history for risk factors such as:

- Family history of seizures or epilepsy
- Any complications during the prenatal, perinatal, or postnatal periods
- Changes in developmental status or delays in developmental milestones
- Any recent illness, fever, trauma, or toxin exposure

Children known to have epilepsy are often admitted to the hospital for other health-related issues or complications and treatment of their seizure disorder. The health history should include questions related to:

- Age of onset of seizures
- Seizure control—what medications is the child taking, and have they been able to take them; when was their last seizure?
- Description and classification of seizures—does the child lose consciousness; does the child become apneic?
- Precipitating factors that may contribute to onset of seizures
- Adverse effects related to anticonvulsant medications
- Compliance with medication regimen

PHYSICAL EXAMINATION

Perform a complete neurologic examination. Careful assessment of the child's mental status, language, learning, behavior, and motor abilities can help provide information about any neurologic deficits. If you observe seizure activity directly, provide a thorough and accurate description of the event. This description needs to include:

- Time of onset and length of seizure activity
- Alterations in behavior such as a cry or changes in facial expression, motor abilities, or sensory alterations before the seizure that may indicate an aura
- Precipitating factors such as fever, anxiety, just waking, or eating
- Description of movements and any progression
- Description of respiratory effort and any apnea noted
- Changes in color (pallor or cyanosis) noted
- Position of mouth, any injury to mouth or tongue, inability to swallow, or excessive salivation
- Loss of bladder or bowel control
- State of consciousness during seizure and **postictal** (after seizure) state—during the seizure, the nurse may ask the child to remember a word; after the seizure, assess if child is able to recall it, to help accurately establish current mental state
- Assess orientation to person, place, and time; motor abilities; speech; behavior; alterations in sensation postictally
- Duration of postictal state

LABORATORY AND DIAGNOSTIC TESTS

Laboratory and diagnostic tests are used to evaluate the cause of, and aid in identifying the type of, seizure activity (refer to Common Laboratory and Diagnostic Tests 16.1). Common laboratory and diagnostic studies ordered for the diagnosis and assessment of epilepsy include:

- Serum glucose, electrolytes, and calcium—to rule out metabolic causes such as hypoglycemia and hypocalcemia
- LP—to analyze cerebrospinal fluid (CSF) to rule out meningitis or encephalitis
- Skull x-ray examinations—to evaluate for the presence of fracture or trauma
- Computed tomography (CT) and magnetic resonance imaging (MRI) studies—to identify abnormalities and intracranial bleeds and rule out tumors
- Electroencephalographs (EEGs)—EEG findings may be noted with certain seizure types, but a normal EEG does not rule out epilepsy because seizure activity rarely occurs during the actual testing time. EEGs are useful in evaluating seizure type and assisting in medication selection. They can be useful in differentiating seizures from nonepileptic activity.
- Video EEGs—provide the opportunity to see the child's actual behavior on video, accompanied with EEG changes; can improve the chance of catching a seizure because the monitoring is done over a period of time.

Nursing Management

Nursing management focuses on preventing injury during seizures, administering appropriate medication and treatments to prevent or reduce seizures, and providing education and support to the child and family to help them cope with the challenges of living with a chronic seizure disorder. See Box 16.1 for a list of basic seizure precautions. In most cases, antiseizure medication should not be discontinued abruptly due to the possibility of increased seizure activity and the risk of status epilepticus. In addition to the patient problems and related interventions discussed in the "Clinical Judgment and the Nursing Process" section, earlier in the chapter, interventions common to epilepsy follow.

DOSAGE CALCULATION 16.1

Child's weight: 9.98 kg (22 lb)

Medication order: Phenobarbital 50 mg PO twice a day

As per the Pediatric Dosage Handbook, the recommended dose is 6 to 8 mg/kg/day in one to two divided doses. Is the ordered dose safe?

RELIEVING ANXIETY

Seizures produce fear and anxiety due to their unpredictable nature along with their uncontrolled, forceful, and, at times, violent appearance. Instruct parents and family members, along with those in the community who may care for the child, on how to respond in case of a seizure (see Teaching Guidelines 16.1). This will help to empower the parents, family, and other caregivers, and, in turn, alleviate some of the anxiety that they may feel.

TEACHING GUIDELINES 16.1 How to Respond When Your Child Has a Seizure

Instruct parents and caregivers:

- Remain calm.
- If child is standing or sitting, ease child to the ground, if possible.
- Time seizure episode.
- Tight clothing and jewelry around the neck should be loosened, if possible.
- Place child on one side and open airway, if possible.
- Do not restrain the child.
- Remove hazards in the area.
- Do not forcibly open jaw with a tongue blade or fingers.
- Document length of seizure, awareness level, and movements, also cyanosis or loss of bladder or bowel control and any other characteristics.
- Remain with child until fully conscious.
- Call emergency medical services (EMS) if:
  - The child stops breathing.
  - Any injury has occurred.
  - Seizure lasts for more than 5 minutes.
  - This is the child's first seizure.
  - Child is unresponsive to painful stimuli after seizure.

MANAGING TREATMENT

Provide child and family teaching and instruction regarding the administration of anticonvulsant therapy and its importance. Included in this discussion should be common adverse effects, the need to continue the medication unless instructed otherwise by the health care provider or nurse practitioner, and the need to call the health care provider or nurse practitioner if the child is ill and vomiting and unable to take their medication. Encourage parents to discuss unwanted adverse effects with the health care provider or nurse practitioner so that they can be addressed and noncompliance with the medication regimen can be reduced. A common cause of breakthrough seizures is medication noncompliance.

PROVIDING FAMILY SUPPORT AND EDUCATION

Having a child with a chronic seizure disorder can place stress and anxiety on the family. This stress and anxiety are often due to fears and misconceptions they may have. An important nursing function is to educate not only the child and family but also the community, including the child's teachers and caregivers, on the reality and facts of the disorder. Encourage parents to be involved in the management of their child's seizures, but encourage allowing the child to learn about the disorder and its management as soon as they are old enough. Encourage parents to treat the child with epilepsy just as they would treat a child without this disorder. Children who are brought up no differently than children without epilepsy will be more likely to develop a positive self-image and have increased self-esteem. Any activity restrictions, such as limiting swimming or participation in sports, will be based on the type, frequency, and severity of the seizures the child has. Educate parents and children on any restrictions, and encourage parents to place only the necessary restrictions on the child.

The needs of the child and family will change as the child grows and develops. The nurse needs to recognize these changes and provide appropriate education and support. Referral to support groups is appropriate.

CONSIDER THIS!

I am so worried about having a seizure at school. I think the other kids will tease me and not play with me if they see me having a seizure. I just don't want to go to school.

Thoughts: How would you respond to this child's concerns?

How can you work with the school, family, and child to help ease these concerns?

Febrile Seizures

Febrile seizures are the most common type of seizure seen in children under 5 years of age (Millichap, 2022a). They usually affect children who are under 5 years of age, with the peak incidence occurring in children between 12 and 18 months old (Millichap, 2022a). Febrile seizures are slightly more commonly seen in male children, and children who have a family history of febrile seizures are at an increased risk (Millichap, 2022a). Febrile seizures are associated with a fever that is not the result of an intracranial infection or metabolic imbalance and is usually related to a viral illness. These seizures are usually benign but can be frightening for both the child and the family. In most cases, the prognosis is excellent. However, febrile seizures may be a sign of a dangerous underlying infection, such as meningitis or sepsis. Although rare, complications associated with febrile seizures include status epilepticus, motor coordination deficits, intellectual disability, and behavioral problems.

Therapeutic Management

Therapeutic management includes determination and treatment of the cause of the fever and interventions to control the fever. The American Academy of Pediatrics (AAP) does not recommend long-term or intermittent anticonvulsant therapy for the child who has suffered one or more simple febrile seizures (American Academy of Pediatrics [AAP] et al., 2008; Millichap, 2022b). Due to the benign nature of febrile seizures, the risks of side effects from the antiepileptic agents outweigh the benefits (Millichap, 2022b). Rectal diazepam has been shown to be safe and effective in terminating febrile seizures and may be used in children at high risk for febrile seizures or in children whose parents are extremely anxious. Buccal and intranasal midazolam, if available, have also been found to be effective, and intranasal lorazepam is an additional option (Millichap, 2022b).

Nursing Assessment

A febrile seizure is usually associated with a rapid rise in core temperature to 39°C (102.2°F) or higher. The degree of fever seems to be the causing stimulus, as opposed to the rapid rate of the fever rising (Millichap, 2022a). A simple febrile seizure is the most common type and will be discussed here. It is defined as a generalized seizure lasting less than 15 minutes (usually a few seconds to 10 minutes) that occurs once in a 24-hour period and is accompanied by a fever without any CNS infection present (Millichap, 2022a). A brief postictal period is often seen when the child appears drowsy. The seizure is likely to have stopped by the time a child receives medical attention. Diagnosis is made based on a thorough history and physical examination, accompanied by a determination of the source of the fever. In some cases, an LP and/or neuroimaging may be performed to rule out meningitis or encephalitis. This will be based on the age and the clinical presentation of the child.

Risk factors for recurrence of a febrile seizure include young age at first febrile seizure and family history of febrile seizures and high fever. Children who experience one or more simple febrile seizures have a slightly greater risk of developing epilepsy than the general population (AAP et al., 2008; Millichap, 2022a). No evidence exists that febrile seizures cause structural damage or cognitive declines (AAP et al., 2008; Millichap, 2022b).

Nursing Management

Provide parental support and education regarding febrile seizures. Reassure parents of the benign nature of febrile seizures. Counsel parents on controlling fever, discuss how to keep a child safe during a seizure, and provide instruction and demonstration in the administration of rectal diazepam at the onset of a seizure (if applicable).

Instruct parents when to call their health care provider or nurse practitioner and when to take their child to the emergency room. Reinforce that any recurrent seizure activity will require prompt medical attention.

Neonatal Seizures

There is a high incidence of seizures during the neonatal period. The immature brain is more prone to seizure activity, and metabolic, infectious, structural, and toxic diseases are more likely to be seen in this age group (Mikati & Tchapyjnikov, 2020). Neonatal seizures are seizures that occur within the first 4 weeks of life and are most commonly seen within the first 10 days. Most seizures in newborns are associated with a specific underlying cause such as hypoxic ischemic encephalopathy (most common), metabolic disorders (hypoglycemia and hypocalcemia), neonatal infection (meningitis and encephalitis), cerebral infarction, and intracranial hemorrhage. The prognosis depends mainly on the underlying cause of the seizures and the severity of the insult. There is evidence that neonatal seizures have an adverse effect on neurodevelopment and may predispose the infant to cognitive, behavioral, or epileptic complications later in life (Shellhaas, 2022b). About 13% to 27% of neonates with seizures will go on to develop postnatal epilepsy (Shellhaas, 2022b). Neonatal epileptic syndromes are rare but are a well-recognized cause of neonatal seizures (Shellhaas, 2022b). Our discussion will focus on the more common symptomatic neonatal seizure related to a specific underlying cause.

Therapeutic Management

Acute neonatal seizures should be treated aggressively because repeated seizure activity may result in injury to the brain. Treatment focuses on addressing the underlying cause, such as correcting metabolic disturbances, treating CNS infections, ensuring adequate ventilation and cardiovascular support, and possibly administering anticonvulsant therapy. Phenobarbital is often used in the initial management of neonatal seizures, but efficacy remains uncertain. Antiepileptic medications may not be effective if the underlying cause is not treated (Shellhaas, 2022a). The dosage of anticonvulsants may be higher in the neonate because neonates metabolize drugs more rapidly than older infants.

Nursing Assessment

Neonatal seizures may be hard to recognize clinically and may be accompanied by a normal EEG, while in some cases, there may be no clinical signs but only EEG changes (Mikati & Tchapyjnikov, 2020). Neonatal seizures have to be distinguished from nonseizure behaviors seen in newborns, such as stretching, sudden random movements, and random sucking movements, coughing, or gagging (Shellhaas, 2023). Therefore, clinical recognition of newborn seizures is critical, and the use of EEG confirmation is now widely recognized. Assessment of neonatal seizures will include a detailed clinical characterization of the seizure activity, including appearance of the neonate; location and involvement of arms, legs, trunk, and face; sequence of clinical changes; and duration and frequency of seizure activity. If seizure activity is not witnessed by a health care provider a detailed history is essential. Assessment of the cause of the seizure is a priority.

Laboratory and diagnostic tests, including serum testing (e.g., serum glucose, electrolytes, calcium), LP (to analyze CSF), cranial ultrasound, CT, and MRI, may be performed to help determine the cause of the seizures. EEGs and video EEGs may assist in the characterization of neonatal seizures and their medical management.

Nursing Management

Nursing management will focus on carrying out interventions to cease seizure activity, monitoring neurologic status closely, recognizing the seizures, preventing injury during seizure activity, and providing support and education to the parents and family.

STRUCTURAL DEFECTS

Due to the sensitivity of the development of the neurologic system in the first few weeks of embryonic life, there exists a potential for defects to occur. These structural defects include neural tube defects (NTDs), microcephaly, Chiari malformation, hydrocephalus, intracranial arteriovenous malformation (AVM), and craniosynostosis.

Neural Tube Defects

NTDs account for the majority of congenital anomalies of the CNS (Kinsman & Johnston, 2020). NTDs are serious birth defects of the spine and the brain and include disorders such as spina bifida occulta, myelomeningocele, meningocele, anencephaly, and encephalocele. The neural tube closes between the third and fourth weeks in utero. The cause of NTDs is not known, but many factors such as drugs, malnutrition, chemicals, and genetics can adversely affect normal CNS development. It is well established that maternal preconception supplementation of folic acid can decrease the incidence of NTDs in pregnancies at risk by 50% (AAP & Committee on Genetics, 1999, reaffirmed 2017; Kinsman & Johnston, 2020). In 1992, the U.S. Public Health Service recommended that all people of childbearing age who are capable of becoming pregnant take 0.4 mg (400 mcg) of folic acid daily (Centers for Disease Control and Prevention [CDC], 2022a). Pregnant people with a history of pregnancies affected by NTDs are recommended to take a higher dosage. Prenatal screening of maternal serum for alpha-fetoprotein (AFP) and ultrasound examination can help identify fetuses at risk. Anencephaly and encephalocele are discussed further on. Refer to Chapter 22 for information on spina bifida occulta, meningocele, and myelomeningocele.

Anencephaly

Anencephaly is a defect in brain development resulting in small or missing brain hemispheres, skull, and scalp. It occurs when the cephalic or upper end of the neural tube fails to close during the third to fourth week of gestation. These infants are born without both a forebrain and a cerebrum, and the remaining brain tissue may be exposed. The condition is incompatible with life.

NURSING ASSESSMENT

Infants with anencephaly have a distinctive appearance, with a large defect noted in the vault of the skull (Fig. 16.7). The birthing parent may have had a difficult labor due to the malformation of the head not allowing it to engage in the cervix. The majority of infants will be stillborn. If not, most anencephalic infants die within hours to several days to weeks of birth (Tomita & Ogiwara, 2022). There have been a few cases in which the infant has lived for several months. The infant is usually blind, deaf, unconscious, and unable to feel pain. Some infants born with anencephaly may be born with a brain stem, but, due to the lack of a cerebrum, there is no possibility of gaining consciousness. Reflex actions such as respirations, reactions to sound and touch, and ability to suck may be present.

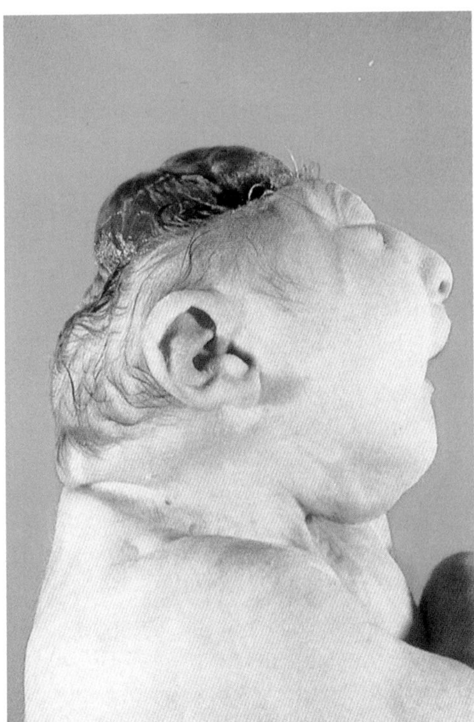

FIGURE 16.7 Anencephalic infant.

NURSING MANAGEMENT

The prognosis is extremely poor. Nursing management is supportive in nature and focuses on comfort measures for the dying infant. Some parents may have been aware of the diagnosis prenatally due to screening tests such as AFP and ultrasounds. Parents and family will need support and understanding from all health care professionals during this difficult time. Fear of what the child will look like may be overwhelming. Use of an infant cap can be helpful and allow parents to feel more comfortable holding and comforting their infant. Assisting with anticipatory grieving and decision making related to end-of-life care will also be key nursing interventions.

Encephalocele

Encephalocele is a protrusion of the brain and meninges through a skull defect. It results from failure of the anterior portion of the neural tube to close. The prognosis, including the extent of complications and cognitive deficits, will depend on the size and location of the encephalocele and involvement of other brain structures. Encephaloceles are often accompanied by craniofacial and other abnormalities such as hydrocephalus, microcephaly, spastic quadriplegia, ataxia, visual problems, developmental delay, mental and growth retardation, and seizures. Some children who are affected may display normal intelligence.

Therapeutic management consists of surgical repair, including placement of tissues back into the skull and removal of the sac; possible shunt placement to correct associated hydrocephalus; and corrective repair of any craniofacial abnormalities.

NURSING ASSESSMENT

Initial assessment after delivery will reveal a visible external sac protruding from the skull area. It occurs most commonly in the occipital region, but can occur elsewhere, such as frontally or nasofrontally. Generally, the lesion is covered by skin, but it may also be open. Therefore, assessment to ensure that the sac covering is intact remains important. Assess neurologic status carefully. Before surgical correction, the infant will be examined thoroughly to determine brain tissue involvement or associated anomalies. Diagnostic procedures such as CT, MRI, and ultrasound may be performed.

NURSING MANAGEMENT

Nursing management will consist of preoperative and postoperative care, along with symptomatic and supportive care. Preoperative and postoperative care will be similar to that for the child with myelomeningocele (refer to Chapter 22), with a focus on preventing rupture of the sac, preventing infection, and providing adequate nutrition and hydration. Infants with an encephalocele are at an increased risk for developing hydrocephalus. Therefore, monitor for signs and symptoms of increased ICP and head circumference.

Microcephaly

Microcephaly is defined as a head circumference that is more than three standard deviations below the mean for the age and sex of the infant (Kinsman & Johnston, 2020). It may be congenital, or it may be acquired and develop in the first few years of life. It generally results in intellectual disability due to the lack of functioning brain tissue. There are many causes. Microcephaly can be caused by abnormal development during gestation or follow intrauterine infections such as rubella, toxoplasmosis, and cytomegalovirus. It can also be caused by chromosomal abnormalities or be associated with other syndromes. Acquired microcephaly may occur due to severe malnutrition, perinatal infections, or anoxia in early infancy.

Nursing Assessment

Microcephalic infants will present at birth with a normal or reduced head size. As the child ages, head growth will fail, while the face will continue to grow at a normal rate. This results in a small head, a large face, and a loose, often wrinkled, scalp. As the child grows older, this smallness of the skull becomes more pronounced. Development of motor functions and speech may be delayed. The degree of intellectual disability varies, but it is a common occurrence. Convulsions may be present, and motor deficit ranges from clumsiness to spastic quadriplegia.

Nursing Management

There is no treatment. Nursing care will be supportive and focus on determining the extent of neurologic and cognitive deficits, as well as teaching parents how to care for a child with such impairments.

Chiari Malformation

Chiari malformations are classified into different groups and subgroups based on anatomic anomalies of the cerebellum, brain stem, and craniocervical junction along with downward displacement of the cerebellar structures (Khoury, 2023). The most common, type I and type II, are discussed here. Type I is usually not associated with hydrocephalus and is the more benign form. The deformity is a result of the cerebellar tonsils displacing into the upper cervical canal (Kinsman & Johnston, 2020). Type II (also referred to as Arnold–Chiari) is the most common and is usually associated with hydrocephalus and myelomeningocele. The deformity results from the cerebellum, the medulla oblongata, and the fourth ventricle displacing into the cervical canal, resulting in an obstruction of the CSF and causing hydrocephalus. The prognosis depends on the extent of the defect. Therapeutic management of the type II Chiari malformation includes surgical decompression.

Nursing Assessment

In type I, symptoms are typically seen in adolescence and adulthood. The patient will usually complain of neck pain; recurrent headaches that increase with physical activity or with Valsalva maneuvers such as coughing, laughing, or sneezing; and lower extremity spasticity (Khoury, 2023). Type II is almost always associated with myelomeningocele; therefore, it is typically detected prenatally or at birth. Symptoms seen in infancy include a weak cry, stridor, and apnea (Kinsman & Johnston, 2020). These symptoms require prompt medical treatment to reduce mortality. Gastrointestinal disturbances along with a history of chronic aspiration, choking, gagging, prolonged feeding times, and weight loss may also be present. In later infancy and childhood, progressive hydrocephalus is a common problem (Khoury, 2023). Assessment of shunt function is extremely important in the infant and older child presenting with type II Chiari malformation and associated hydrocephalus (refer to Hydrocephalus section). An MRI may be performed to help evaluate and diagnose Chiari malformations.

Nursing Management

Nursing management will focus on preoperative and postoperative care, prevention of infection, monitoring of blood loss, improvement of preoperative symptoms in the postoperative period, identification of any signs and symptoms of increased ICP, and identification of any resultant CNS injury.

Hydrocephalus

Hydrocephalus is not a specific illness but instead results from underlying brain disorders. It is a frequently seen disorder of the nervous system occurring in 0.5 to 0.8 per 1,000 live births (Haridas & Tomita, 2022a). It results from an imbalance in the production and absorption of CSF. In hydrocephalus, CSF accumulates within the ventricular system and causes the ventricles to enlarge and increases in ICP to occur.

Hydrocephalus may be congenital or acquired. Congenital hydrocephalus is present at birth and is often due to a genetic predisposition or environmental influences during fetal development. Causes of congenital hydrocephalus include abnormal intrauterine development, as is the case with myelomeningocele or other NTDs, or intrauterine infections. Acquired hydrocephalus develops at the time of birth or at some point after. It can occur at any age and can result from injury or disease. Acquired hydrocephalus can result from intentional or nonintentional trauma, intraventricular hemorrhage (IVH) in premature infants, neoplasms (e.g., posterior fossa brain tumor), infections (e.g., meningitis), or malformations (e.g., Chiari malformations).

Prognosis for the child with hydrocephalus depends mainly on the cause and whether or not brain damage has occurred prior to recognition and treatment. Children with hydrocephalus are at increased risk for developmental disabilities, visual problems, abnormalities in memory, and reduced intelligence. Long-term follow-up and multidisciplinary care are necessary.

Pathophysiology

CSF is formed primarily in the ventricular system by the choroid plexus. It flows because of the pressure gradient that exists between the ventricular system and the venous channels. CSF is absorbed primarily by the arachnoid villi. Hydrocephalus results when there is an obstruction in the ventricular system or obliteration or malfunction of the arachnoid villi. This results in impaired absorption or circulation of the CSF.

Hydrocephalus is classified as obstructive or noncommunicating versus nonobstructive or communicating. Obstructive or noncommunicating hydrocephalus occurs when the flow of CSF is blocked within the ventricular system. This is the most common type in children and is often associated with an increased ICP (Haridas & Tomita, 2022a). NTDs, neonatal meningitis, trauma, tumors, or Chiari malformations usually result in this type of hydrocephalus. One of the most common causes of obstructive or noncommunicating hydrocephalus in children is aqueductal stenosis, which results from the narrowing of the aqueduct of Sylvius (a passageway between the third and fourth ventricles in the middle brain) (Haridas & Tomita, 2022a). Nonobstructive or communicating hydrocephalus occurs when the flow of CSF is blocked after it exits from the ventricles. This form of hydrocephalus, in which the CSF can still flow between the ventricles, is most often caused by defective absorption of CSF. Examples include hydrocephalus that results from subarachnoid hemorrhage (most common), certain types of meningitis, and leukemia infiltrates (Kinsman & Johnston, 2020).

Therapeutic Management

Hydrocephalus must be identified early. Treatment needs to be initiated to prevent brain tissue damage that can result from the increased ICP that hydrocephalus creates. Specific treatment will depend on the underlying etiology. The goals of treatment include relieving hydrocephalus and managing complications associated with the disorder, such as growth and developmental delay. Most cases of hydrocephalus are treated with the surgical placement of an extracranial shunt. Most often, a ventriculoperitoneal (VP) shunt is placed. See Figure 16.8 for an illustration of a shunt. The shunt will need to be replaced as the child grows. Therefore, the child will undergo shunt revision surgery at various times during their life. It is important for health care professionals and parents to be able to recognize when a shunt needs replacing or when complications are occurring to decrease the possibility of death or disability that may occur due to increased ICP.

Although shunts have been the mainstay of treatment for hydrocephalus, they are not without complications such as infection, obstruction, and need for revision as the child grows. Endoscopic third ventriculostomy (EVT) is an alternative to shunt placement to treat hydrocephalus in select children. It has several advantages over VP shunts, such as fewer complications (infection and malfunction) and lower cost (Haridas & Tomita, 2022b). A small perforation is made in the thinned floor of the third ventricle, which allows for egress of CSF from the ventricle to the subarachnoid space. No permanently implanted hardware is needed. Success of the EVT depends on the child's age, cause of hydrocephalus, and history of previous complications.

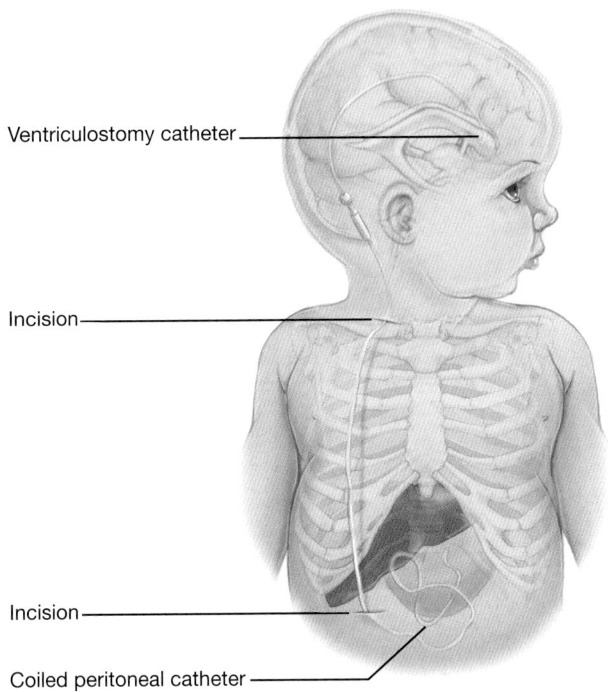

FIGURE 16.8 To treat hydrocephalus, a ventriculoperitoneal (VP) shunt catheter is placed in an enlarged ventricle. The shunt diverts the flow of cerebrospinal fluid (CSF) within the central nervous system to the peritoneum, where CSF is now absorbed across the peritoneal membrane into the body's circulation.

Nursing Assessment

For a full description of the assessment phase of the nursing process, refer to the "Clinical Judgment and the Nursing Process" section. Assessment findings pertinent to hydrocephalus are discussed further on.

Health History

Explore the pregnancy history and past medical history for:

- Intrauterine infections
- Prematurity with intracranial hemorrhage
- Meningitis
- Mumps encephalitis

Elicit a description of the present illness and chief complaint. Common signs and symptoms reported during the health history of the undiagnosed child might include:

- Irritability
- Lethargy
- Poor feeding
- Vomiting
- Complaints of headache in older children
- Altered, diminished, or changes in LOC

Children known to have hydrocephalus are often admitted to the hospital for shunt malfunctions or other complications of the disease. The health history should include questions related to:

- Neurologic status—have there been changes or decreases in LOC, changes in personality, or deterioration in school performance?
- Complaints of headache
- Vomiting
- Visual disturbances
- Any other changes in physical or cognitive state

Physical Examination

Physical examination of the infant or child with hydrocephalus will include inspection and observation, palpation, and percussion.

INSPECTION AND OBSERVATION

Observe general appearance and affect. Pay particular attention to the size of the skull, and note any asymmetry. Note LOC and motor function. Changes or decreases in LOC may be noted along with brisk reflexes and spasticity of the lower extremities. Symptoms seen vary by age, primarily because the infant's skull is able to accommodate the buildup of CSF because the sutures have not closed. In the infant, the most obvious indication is often a rapid increase in head circumference (Fig. 16.9). In the older child, loss of development and changes in personality may be seen. Signs and symptoms associated with increased ICP may be seen (refer to Comparison Chart 16.1).

PALPATION

In the infant, palpation of the fontanels may reveal wide-open, bulging fontanels. They will be nonpulsatile and feel tense and very full.

PERCUSSION

Upon percussion of the skull, by health care providers or nurse practitioners, a positive Macewen sign may be noted. This is when a "cracked pot" sound is heard during percussion and can indicate separation of the sutures.

Laboratory and Diagnostic Tests

Common laboratory and diagnostic tests ordered for the diagnosis and assessment of hydrocephalus include:

- Skull x-ray studies (may reveal separation of sutures)
- CT
- MRI

CT and MRI are used to evaluate for the presence of hydrocephalus and can also aid in identifying the cause of hydrocephalus. Refer to Common Laboratory and Diagnostic Tests 16.1.

Nursing Management

Nursing management of the child with hydrocephalus will focus on maintaining cerebral perfusion, minimizing

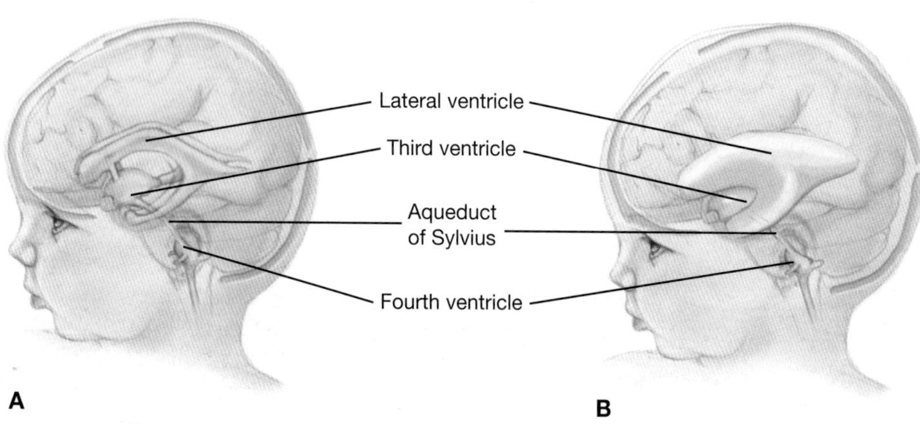

FIGURE 16.9 A. Infant without hydrocephalus. **B.** Infant with hydrocephalus. Note broadening of the forehead, bulging fontanel, and large head size.

COMPARISON CHART 16.1 Early Versus Late Signs of Increased Intracranial Pressure

Early Signs	Late Signs

• Headache
• Vomiting, possibly projectile
• Blurred vision, double vision (diplopia)
• Dizziness
• Increased blood pressure
• Pupil reaction time decreased and unequal
• Sunset eyes
• Changes in level of consciousness, irritability
• Seizure activity
• In infant, will also see:
  • Bulging, tense fontanel
  • Wide sutures and increased head circumference
  • Dilated scalp veins
  • High-pitched cry
	• Lowered level of consciousness
	• Decreased motor and sensory responses
	• Bradycardia
	• Irregular respirations
	• Hypertension and widening pulse pressure
	• Cheyne–Stokes respirations
	• Decerebrate or decorticate posturing
	• Fixed and dilated pupils

neurologic complications, maintaining adequate nutrition, promoting growth and development, and supporting and educating the child and family. In addition to the patient problems and related interventions discussed in the "Clinical Judgment and the Nursing Process" section earlier in the chapter, interventions common to hydrocephalus are discussed later.

PREVENTING AND RECOGNIZING SHUNT INFECTION AND MALFUNCTION

The major complications associated with shunts are infection and malfunction. Due to the serious nature and potentially devastating effects of shunt infection or malfunction, parents and health professionals need to be aware of the signs and symptoms to provide early recognition and prompt treatment. Signs and symptoms of a shunt infection include elevated vital signs, poor feeding, vomiting, decreased responsiveness, seizure activity, and signs of local inflammation along the shunt tract. Signs and symptoms of shunt malfunction include vomiting, drowsiness, and headache. Signs and symptoms of increased ICP, as listed in Comparison Chart 16.1, can also be indicative of shunt complications.

Infection can occur at any time but is more common 1 to 2 months after placement. Infection is treated with IV antibiotics, and, if the infection is persistent, the shunt will be removed and an external ventricular drainage (EVD) system put into place until the CSF is sterile (refer to Common Medical Treatments 16.1 and Box 16.3).

TAKE NOTE!

Rapid drainage of CSF, which may occur if the child sits up without the EVD system being clamped, will decrease ICP and can lead to extreme headache, collapse of the ventricles, formation of subdural hematomas, and neurologic deterioration.

A new shunt will be placed after the infection has cleared. Intrathecal administration of antibiotics may be performed by the health care provider or nurse practitioner. Keeping the peritoneal surgical incision free of feces and urine can help prevent infection. In addition, inspect surgical incisions after shunt placement for signs and symptoms of infection and any signs of leaking CSF.

Malfunction of the shunt can occur due to kinking, clogging, or separation of the tubing. Blockage is the most common reported complication. A shunt that has been placed within the past year is at higher risk of malfunction. Early recognition and operative intervention are essential to prevent neurologic deficits or possible death from occurring.

BOX 16.3 Nursing Management of External Ventricular Drainage (EVD) Device

- Ensure all connections are secure and label line as EVD.
- Regularly check that drip chamber of manometer is set at the height prescribed in relation to the child (i.e., zero at clavicle).
- Clamp the drain in the event of child movement or movement anticipated with care. Rezero and open clamps when done.
- Accurately document volume and color of cerebrospinal fluid (CSF) every hour (CSF is normally clear and colorless; cloudiness indicates infection). Notify health care provider, nurse practitioner, or charge nurse of any significant increase in amount of drainage (if exceeds 10 mL more than previous volumes).
- If minimal or no drainage, check tubing for kinks, blockage, or closed clamps. Check to see if CSF is oscillating in tubing. If blockage is suspected, notify neurosurgery department immediately.
- Dress the entry site into the skull with a sterile occlusive dressing; change the dressing if it is soiled or nonocclusive.
- Routine CSF samples may be sent for culture and analysis.
- Child may be taking prophylactic antibiotics due to increased risk of infection from the drain.

SUPPORTING AND EDUCATING THE CHILD AND FAMILY

Hydrocephalus is a serious and chronic illness. It will require lifelong follow-up and regular evaluations. It requires early recognition of complications to prevent neurologic damage. Children will require future surgeries and hospitalizations, which can place a strain on the family and its finances. Potential growth and developmental disabilities are an additional strain. The support of the family in establishing realistic goals and helping the child to achieve their developmental and educational potential is important.

The family should be involved in the child's care from the time of diagnosis. Initially, parents may be frightened because shunt placement involves entering the brain. Provide parents with accurate information regarding the procedure and be available to listen to parents' concerns and to answer questions that arise. Ongoing education about the illness and its treatment is important, including signs and symptoms of shunt complications. As the family becomes more comfortable with the diagnosis, treatment, and signs and symptoms of complications, they will become experts on the child's care and will often recognize subtle changes that may be indicative of shunt complications. Referral to support groups can be helpful for both the family and the child.

Intracranial AVM

Intracranial AVM is a rare congenital disorder. It is caused by an abnormal development of blood vessels and can occur in the brain, brain stem, or spinal cord. AVMs that hemorrhage can lead to serious neurologic deficits and even death. However, some cases of AVMs never cause problems.

Therapeutic Management

More aggressive treatment strategies are used in children. Treatment options include surgical excision; endovascular embolization, which involves closing off the vessels of the AVM by injecting glue into them; and radiosurgery, which involves focusing radiation on the AVM. The therapeutic management approach will be based on the age of the child and size and location of the malformation in the brain. The child will usually require at least 24 hours of intensive care monitoring following surgery.

Nursing Assessment

The most common symptoms include intracranial hemorrhage (children are more likely to present with hemorrhage than adults), seizures, headaches, and progressive neurologic deficits such as vision problems, loss of speech, problems with memory, and paralysis (Singer et al., 2022). In children under 2 years of age, presentation may include cardiac failure due to arteriovenous shunting in neonates and infants; a large head secondary to hydrocephalus; and seizure activity. Diagnosis is made using diagnostic imaging procedures such as MRI, CT, and arteriography.

Nursing Management

Nursing management for these children is aimed at supportive care. Monitor for changes in neurologic status, noting any seizure activity, signs or symptoms of increased ICP, or signs and symptoms of intracranial hemorrhage. Hydrocephalus may occur as a result of intracranial hemorrhage secondary to the AVM. An EVD and eventual shunt placement may be necessary (refer to the "Hydrocephalus" section).

Craniosynostosis

Craniosynostosis is premature closure of the cranial sutures (Fig. 16.10). Complete closure of all sutures does not normally occur until late in childhood. Premature closure can inhibit brain growth, and a distorted skull appearance will be evident. In cases where only one suture is fused, neurologic impairments are rarely seen. When two or more sutures are fused, neurologic complications such as hydrocephalus with increased ICP are more likely to occur. The incidence of craniosynostosis is approximately one in 2,000 births (Kinsman & Johnston, 2020). The cause is unknown, but in 10% to 20% of cases a genetic disorder such as Carpenter syndrome or Apert, Crouzon, or Pfeiffer disease is present (Kinsman & Johnston, 2020). There are numerous types of craniosynostosis; they are listed and illustrated in Table 16.4.

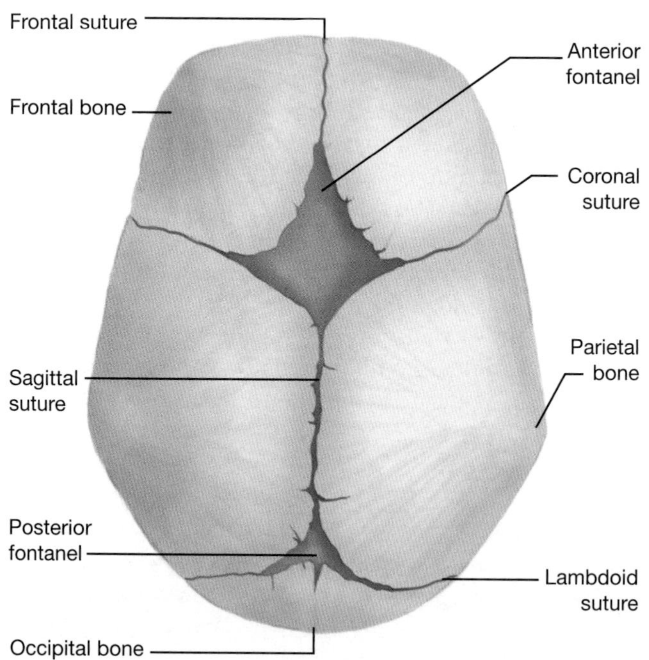

FIGURE 16.10 Skull sutures in the infant.

TABLE 16.4 • Types of Craniosynostosis

Types	Description	Illustration
Sagittal synostosis (scaphocephaly)	Sagittal suture is closed. Head grows long and narrow in anterior–posterior direction. Broad forehead and a prominent occiput are present. Most common form	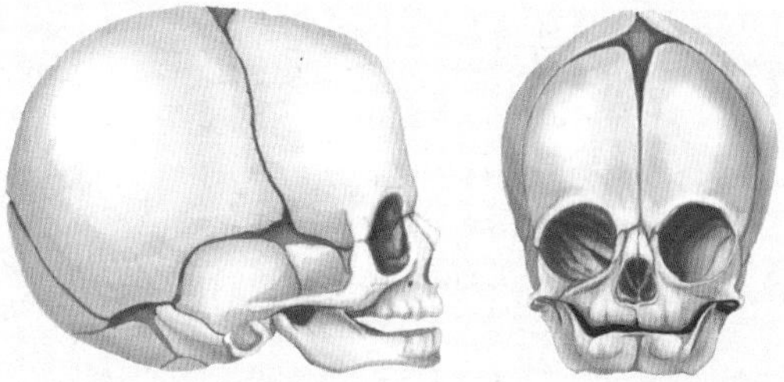
Metopic synostosis (trigonocephaly)	Metopic suture is closed. Usually a ridge down the forehead can be seen or felt. Triangular-shaped forehead Eyebrows may appear "pinched" on either side. Eyes may also appear close together.	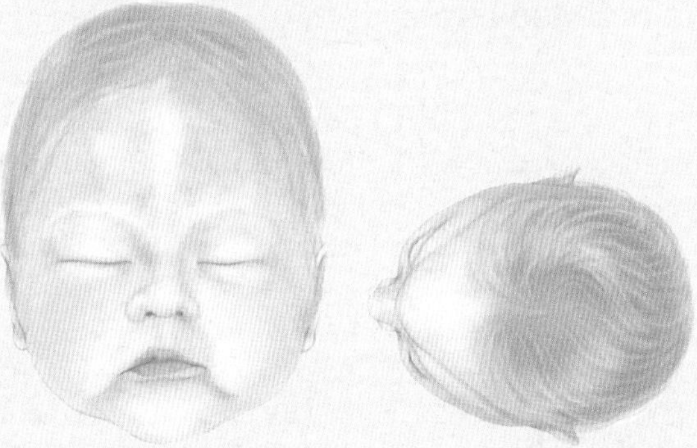
Unilateral coronal synostosis (anterior plagiocephaly)	Early closure of one side of the coronal suture Forehead and orbital rim (eyebrow) have a flattened appearance on that side. Eye on affected side has a different shape.	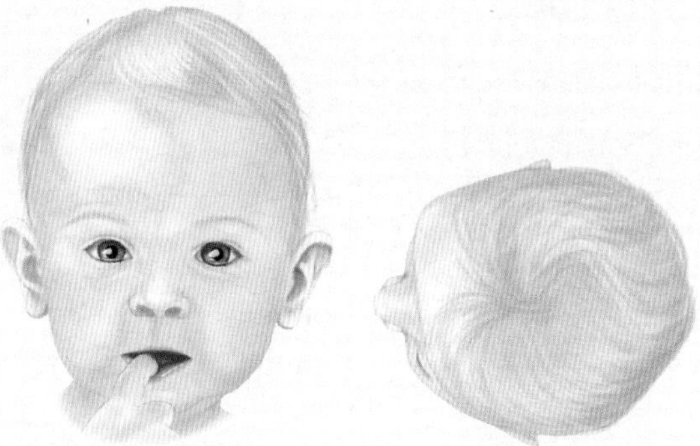
Bicoronal synostosis (brachycephaly)	Very flat, tall, recessed forehead Skull is shortened in the anterior–posterior direction. Wide-shaped head Commonly seen in Apert and Crouzon disease	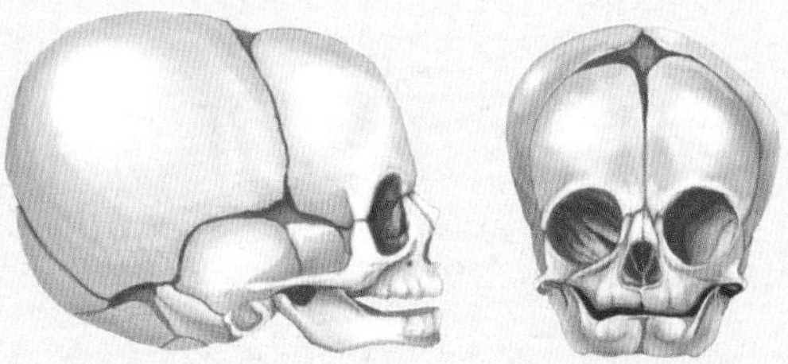
Lambdoid (posterior plagiocephaly)	Early closure of one lambdoid suture Flattening of back of head. Similar to shape found in positional molding or positional plagiocephaly	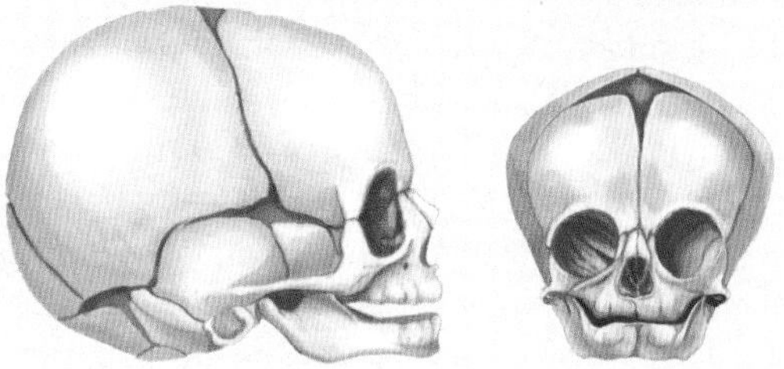

The prognosis is good for the majority of infants presenting with craniosynostosis, and normal brain development will occur. Exceptions to this are the infant or child who has associated genetic disorders that involve brain function and development.

Surgical correction may be done and allows for normal expansion of the brain and acceptable appearance of the head and skull. If one suture is fused, the surgical intervention is done mainly for cosmetic reasons. If more than one suture is fused, operative intervention is essential to prevent neurologic complications.

Nursing Assessment

Most cases of craniosynostosis are present at birth. Skull deformity is evident, and a prominent bony ridge can be palpated. X-ray studies can confirm fusion of the sutures. It is important that craniosynostosis be detected early if it is not evident at birth because premature closure of the suture lines will inhibit brain development. Therefore, measure head circumference in all children under 3 years old, and compare findings with normal head circumference parameters as well as past measurements of the infant or child.

Nursing Management

Nursing management focuses on postoperative care. This includes observing hemoglobin and hematocrit levels due to large volumes of blood loss that can occur and observing for pain, hemorrhage, fever, infection, and swelling. Due to the location of the surgery and incision line, large amounts of facial swelling may be present. This can result in an inability of the child to open their eyes for a few days postoperatively. Make sure that parents are aware of this. Encourage the parents to talk to, hold, and comfort their child during this time. Provide support and education to the parents before, during, and after the procedure.

Positional Plagiocephaly

Since the inception of the "back to sleep" program, which recommends placing all infants supine to sleep to decrease the risk of sudden unexplained infant death (SUID), there has been an increase in the incidence of positional plagiocephaly (Buchanan, 2021). Positional plagiocephaly refers to asymmetry in head shape without fused sutures. It results from gravitational force exertion on the developing cranium. Torticollis, which is when the neck muscles are too tight, have inadequate tone, or are shorter on one side, can contribute to plagiocephaly. Each condition, plagiocephaly and torticollis, exacerbates the other. Refer to Chapter 22 for further information on torticollis.

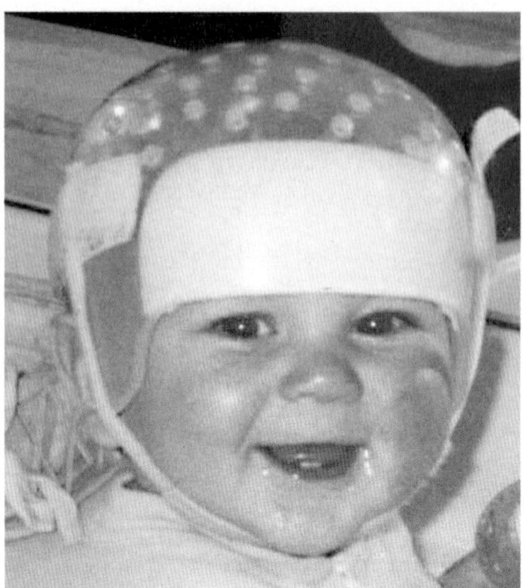

FIGURE 16.11 Molding helmet for positional plagiocephaly.

Therapeutic management for positional plagiocephaly is generally conservative, such as changing the infant's position, encouraging "tummy time," and avoiding excessive use of the car seat for infant seating outside of the automobile. Some infants may benefit from the use of a molding helmet (Fig. 16.11).

Nursing Assessment

View the infant's head from the top, noting asymmetry ranging from flattening on one side posteriorly to posterior flattening associated with anterior bulging (Fig. 16.12). Assess neck ROM to determine if torticollis

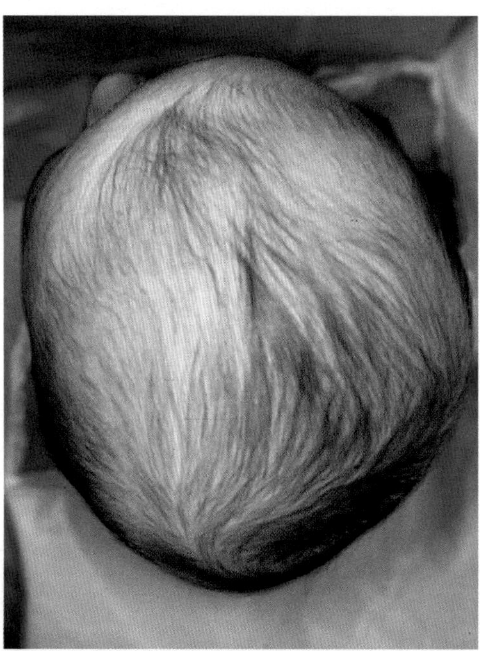

FIGURE 16.12 Note flattening of the right posterior parietal and occipital regions of the skull in this infant with positional plagiocephaly.

is also present. Palpate the cranial sutures, which will not feel overlapped as they do when they are fused. Skull x-ray examination or head CT scan will rule out craniosynostosis by demonstrating evidence of open sutures.

Nursing Management

Nursing management is directed toward repositioning the infant to decrease time spent with the flattened area in the dependent position. Position the infant so that turning away from the affected side is necessary for them to view objects of interest. Place the infant on the abdomen when awake and supervised. Discourage use of the car seat outside of the automobile. Place a rolled washcloth along the affected side of the head to discourage turning the head in that direction. Hold the child upright over the shoulder at times throughout the day, rotate feeding positions, and change the direction in which the infant lies in the crib. Following these recommendations may prevent positional plagiocephaly in the infant without congenital torticollis.

INFECTIOUS DISORDERS

Infectious disorders of the neurologic system include bacterial meningitis, aseptic meningitis, encephalitis, and Reye syndrome.

Bacterial Meningitis

Bacterial meningitis is an infection of the meninges, the lining that surrounds the brain and spinal cord. It is a serious illness in children and can lead to brain damage, nerve damage, deafness, stroke, and even death. It requires rapid assessment and treatment. See Table 16.5 for the most common types of meningitis seen in different age groups. In developed countries, disease resulting from *Haemophilus influenzae* type B, once the most common cause of meningitis in children, has decreased dramatically since the introduction of the Hib vaccine. In less developed countries, infection with *H. influenzae* type B remains a concern.

TABLE 16.5 • Common Causes of Meningitis in Different Age Groups

Age Affected	Causative Organism
Newborns and infants (birth–3 months)	*Escherichia coli; Streptococcus* group B*; Listeria monocytogenes; Streptococcus pneumonia*
Infants and children (3 months–6 years)	*S. pneumonia; Neisseria meningitides (meningococcal meningitis); Haemophilus influenzae* type B*; Streptococcus* group B*; Mycobacterium tuberculosis*
Older children and adolescents (6–16 years)	*S. pneumonia; N. meningitides (meningococcal meningitis)*

Data from Centers for Disease Control and Prevention. (2021a). *Meningitis: Bacterial meningitis.* http://www.cdc.gov/meningitis/bacterial.html

Pathophysiology

Bacterial meningitis causes inflammation, swelling, purulent exudates, and tissue damage to the brain. It can occur as a secondary infection to upper respiratory infections, sinus infections, or ear infections and can also be the result of direct introduction through LP; skull fracture or severe head injury; neurosurgical intervention; congenital structural abnormalities, such as spina bifida; or the presence of foreign bodies, such as a ventricular shunt or cochlear implants.

Therapeutic Management

Bacterial meningitis is a medical emergency and requires prompt hospitalization and treatment. Deterioration may be rapid and occur in less than 24 hours, leading to long-term neurologic damage and even death. IV antibiotics will be started immediately after the LP and blood cultures have been obtained if bacterial meningitis is suspected. The length of therapy and specific antibiotic will be determined based on the analysis and the culture and sensitivity of the CSF. Corticosteroids may be ordered to help reduce the inflammatory process. Specific medical treatment varies based on the suspected causative organism and will be determined by the health care provider or nurse practitioner.

Nursing Assessment

For a full description of the assessment phase of the nursing process, refer to the "Clinical Judgment and the Nursing Process" section. Assessment findings pertinent to bacterial meningitis are discussed further on.

Health History

Elicit a description of the present illness and chief complaint. Common signs and symptoms reported during the health history might include:

- Sudden onset of symptoms
- Preceding respiratory illness or sore throat
- Presence of fever, chills
- Headache
- Vomiting
- Photophobia
- Stiff neck
- Rash
- Irritability
- Drowsiness

- Lethargy
- Muscle rigidity
- Seizures

Symptoms in infants can be more subtle and atypical, but the history may reveal:

- Poor sucking and feeding
- Weak cry
- Lethargy
- Vomiting

Explore the child's current and past medical history for risk factors such as:

- Young age: 1 month to 5 years, with most cases in children younger than 1 year of age and young adults 15 to 24 years of age
- Any fever or illness during pregnancy or around delivery (for infants younger than 3 months of age)
- Exposure to ill people
- Exposure to tuberculosis
- Travel history
- History of maternal illness
- Recent neurosurgical procedure or head trauma
- Presence of a foreign body, such as a shunt or a cochlear implant
- Immunocompromised status
- Close-contact living spaces such as dormitories or military bases
- Day care attendance

Physical Examination

Observe the general appearance of the child. The infant with bacterial meningitis may rest in the **opisthotonic** position (Fig. 16.13), and the older child may complain of neck pain. In the infant, a bulging fontanel may be present, which is often a late sign, and the infant may be consolable when lying still as opposed to being held. Presence of positive Kernig and Brudzinski signs can indicate irritation of the meninges (Fig. 16.14). Inspect the child for presence of a rash; a petechial, vesicular, or macular rash may be seen.

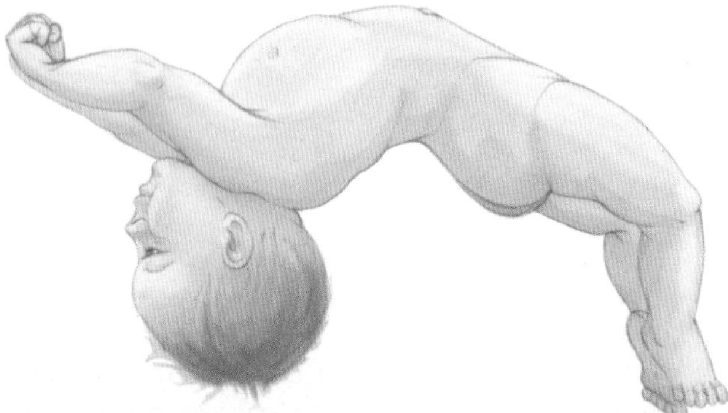

FIGURE 16.13 Infant in opisthotonic position: head and neck are hyperextended to relieve discomfort.

CLINICAL REASONING ALERT!

Abrupt eruption of a petechial or purplish rash can be indicative of meningococcemia (infection with *N. meningitidis*). Immediate medical attention is warranted.

Laboratory and Diagnostic Tests

Common laboratory and diagnostic studies ordered for the assessment of bacterial meningitis include:

- LP—Fluid pressure will be measured, and a sample is obtained for analysis and culture. CSF pressure will usually be elevated, and CSF will reveal increased white blood cells (WBCs) and protein and low glucose (the bacteria present feed on the glucose).
- Complete blood count (CBC)—WBCs will be elevated.
- Blood, urine, and nasopharyngeal culture—Performed to look for source of infection and to rule out sepsis. Blood culture will be positive in cases of septicemia.

Nursing Management

Administer prescribed antibiotics as soon as possible after obtaining cultures. Quickly initiate supportive measures to ensure proper ventilation, reduce the inflammatory response, and help prevent injury to the brain. Interventions are aimed at reducing ICP and maintaining cerebral perfusion along with treating fluid volume deficit, controlling seizures, and preventing injury that may result from altered LOC or seizure activity. Initiate appropriate isolation precautions. In addition to standard precautions, infants and children diagnosed with bacterial meningitis will be placed on droplet isolation until 24 hours of antibiotics have been received to help prevent transmission to others. Refer to the "Clinical Judgment and the Nursing Process" section earlier in the chapter for patient problems and related interventions. In addition to those problems and interventions, note any measures taken to reduce fever and prevent bacterial meningitis.

Reducing Fever

Increased body temperature; warm, flushed skin; and tachycardia may be present. Reducing fever is important to help maintain optimal cerebral perfusion by reducing the metabolic needs of the brain. Administer antipyretics such as acetaminophen and nonsteroidal antiinflammatory drugs (NSAIDs) such as ibuprofen, per order. Institute nonpharmacologic measures, if needed. Reduce environmental temperature and use cooling blankets, fans, cold compresses, and tepid baths to help reduce fever. Avoid measures that cause shivering because it increases heat production and is therefore counterproductive and uncomfortable for the child.

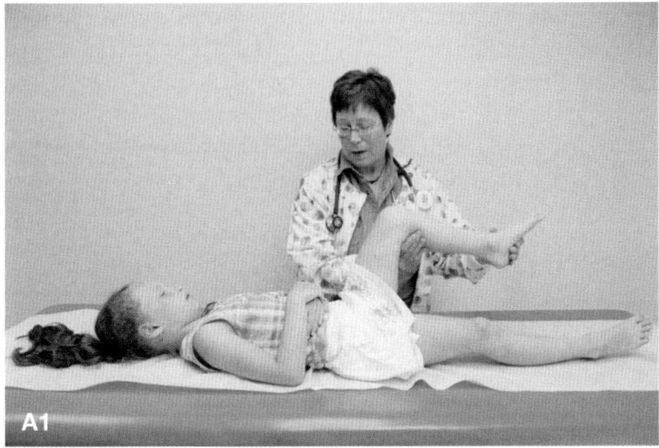

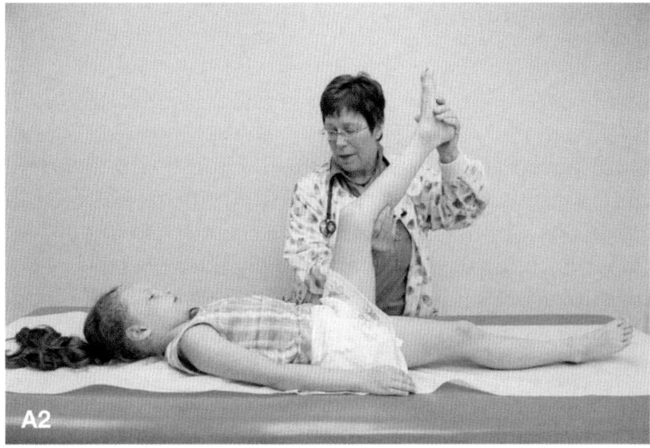

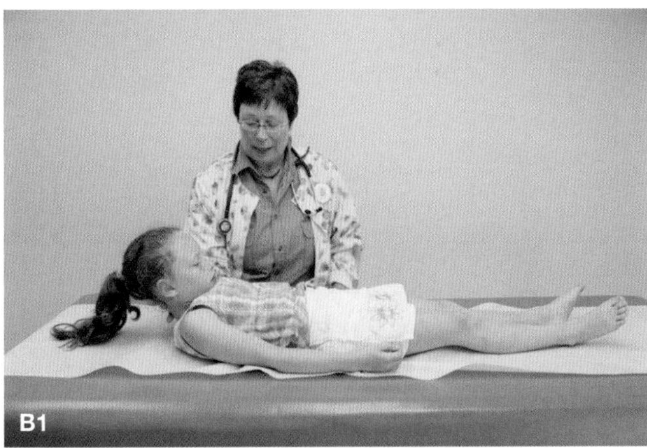

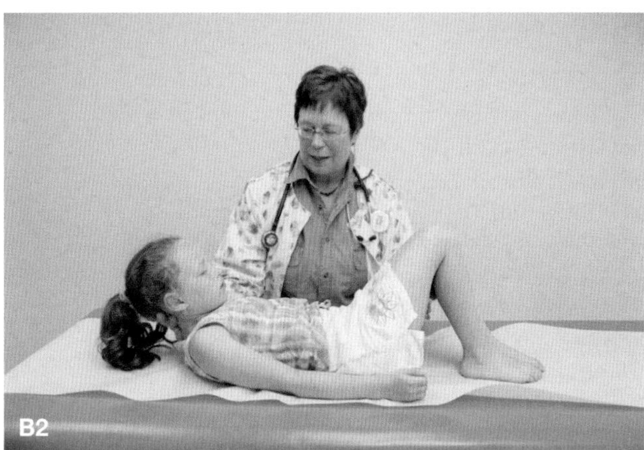

FIGURE 16.14 **A.** Kernig sign is tested by flexing legs at the hip and knee (**A1**), then extending the knee (**A2**). A positive report of pain along the vertebral column and/or inability to extend knee is a positive sign and indicates irritation of meninges. **B.** Brudzinski sign is tested by the child lying supine with the neck flexed (**B1**). A positive sign occurs if resistance or pain is met. The child may also passively flex hip and knees in reaction, indicating meningeal irritation (**B2**).

Preventing Bacterial Meningitis

Bacterial meningitis is a serious illness, and prevention is important. It is transmitted by direct close contact with respiratory droplets from the nose or throat. Most at risk are those living with the child or anyone with whom the child played or was in close contact. Postexposure prophylaxis and postexposure immunization may be effective. Control measures should be initiated in environments where risk exists. Disinfect toys and other shared objects to decrease transmission of the microorganisms to others.

To reduce group B streptococcus infection in neonates, screen pregnant people. If the screening results are positive, administer intrapartal antibiotics.

Vaccines are an important way to prevent bacterial meningitis and are available for some specific causative organisms, but complete vaccination prevention is not possible at this time. The Hib vaccine is routine, starting at 2 months of age, and all children should be immunized to continue the reduction of bacterial meningitis caused by *H. influenzae* type B. The pneumococcal vaccine is also routine for all children, starting at 2 months of age.

Meningococcal vaccination is routine for all children 11 to 12 years of age, with a booster at age 16. Adolescents aged 16 to 18 may be vaccinated with serogroup B meningococcal vaccines if they are part of certain at-risk groups. Refer back to Chapter 9 for further information regarding immunizations.

Aseptic Meningitis

Aseptic meningitis is the most common type of meningitis, and the majority of children affected are under 5 years of age (CDC, 2021b). If the causative organism can be identified, it is usually a virus. Enteroviruses, such as echovirus and coxsackievirus, account for the majority of cases of aseptic meningitis (CDC, 2021b). Less common causes include mumps; herpesviruses; measles; influenza; vector-borne viruses, such as West Nile virus; and lymphocytic choriomeningitis virus (CDC, 2021b).

Therapeutic Management

Prompt diagnosis and treatment are essential to improve outcomes. The child is treated aggressively as if they have bacterial meningitis until the diagnosis is confirmed. Antibiotics are administered and continued until the causative organism is recognized. If the cause is viral, antibiotics may be discontinued, and antiviral agents may be started at this time. After diagnosis is confirmed, treatment is mainly supportive in nature, and the illness is usually self-limiting, lasting 3 to 10 days.

Nursing Assessment

Elicit a description of the present illness and chief complaint. Common signs and symptoms reported during the health history might include:

- Fever
- General malaise
- Headache
- Photophobia
- Poor feeding
- Nausea
- Vomiting
- Irritability
- Lethargy
- Neck pain
- Positive Kernig and Brudzinski signs

The onset of symptoms may be abrupt or gradual. Assessment is similar to that of the child with bacterial meningitis. Signs and symptoms are similar to those seen in bacterial meningitis, but the child is usually less ill.

Nursing Management

Nursing management is similar to the nursing care of the child with bacterial meningitis and will focus on comfort measures to reduce pain and fever. Aseptic meningitis can be managed successfully at home if the child's neurologic status is stable and they are tolerating oral intake.

Encephalitis

Encephalitis is an inflammation of the brain that may also include an inflammation of the meninges. It is a rare complication and can be caused by protozoan, bacterial, fungal, or viral invasion. Viral illness and autoimmune disorders are the most commonly diagnosed cause in children, although in the majority of cases the cause remains unknown (Hardarson & Messacar, 2022). In the United States, common causative organisms include enteroviruses, such as poliovirus and coxsackievirus; herpes simplex virus 1 and 2; and vector-borne viruses. Recovery from encephalitis can occur in a few days or may be complicated and involve severe neurologic damage with residual effects. Prognosis depends on the age of the child and the causative organism. Prompt diagnosis and treatment are essential. The child suspected of having encephalitis should be hospitalized. Therapeutic management is mainly supportive in nature and focuses on maintaining optimal cerebral perfusion; hydration and nutrition; and injury prevention.

Nursing Assessment

Elicit a description of the present illness and chief complaint. Common signs and symptoms reported during the health history might include:

- Fever
- Flu-like symptoms
- Altered LOC
- Headache
- Lethargy
- Drowsiness
- Generalized weakness
- Seizure activity

Explore the child's current history for risk factors such as:

- Recent travel
- Recreational activities, such as hiking and camping
- Animal contacts

Physical Examination

Perform a neurologic examination to distinguish between encephalitis and viral meningitis. In encephalitis, a neurologic examination will reveal changes in sensorium and focal neurologic changes. Neurologic findings vary and reflect the areas of the brain that are involved.

Laboratory and Diagnostic Tests

An LP may be done, and the CSF may show an elevated leukocyte count and elevated protein and glucose levels. However, in some cases, levels may be normal. MRI, CT, and EEG procedures may be performed to help identify early changes and provide useful clues in developing a diagnosis.

Nursing Management

Nursing management is similar to nursing care for the child with meningitis. Specific antiviral therapy may be used for diseases caused by the herpes simplex virus. Teach children and their families how to prevent encephalitis. Encephalitis can result from complications of childhood illnesses such as measles, mumps, or chickenpox. Explain the importance of keeping children up-to-date in their immunizations. Effective vaccines are available for a few viral pathogens that cause encephalitis (such as rabies virus and Japanese encephalitis virus), but these vaccines are not routine; they are recommended for those at high risk. For example, postexposure rabies vaccines can be administered to a child who was bitten by a suspected rabid animal. Also, those traveling to areas where Japanese encephalitis is endemic, such as India and China, and planning a prolonged stay or extreme outdoor activity should receive the appropriate vaccine.

Vector control and avoiding mosquito and tick bites are the best prevention of vector-borne infection. Preventive measures include:

- Using insect repellent (repellents containing DEET [*N,N*-diethyl-meta-toluamide] should be used cautiously in children under 12 years of age and not at all in children under 1 year of age)
- Wearing clothing that covers the arms and legs
- Controlling mosquito populations by eliminating areas of standing water where mosquitoes can breed
- Using insect traps and public measures such as sprayed insecticides to reduce the mosquito population

Reye Syndrome

Reye syndrome is an extremely rare disease that primarily affects children under 15 years of age who are recovering from a viral illness. The exact cause of Reye syndrome is unknown. It has been found that Reye syndrome is a reaction that is triggered by the use of salicylates or salicylate-containing products to treat a viral infection. This reaction causes brain swelling, liver failure, and death in hours, if treatment in not initiated. In the 1980s, the adverse effects of salicylates used to treat viral illnesses began to be publicized, and the U.S. Food and Drug Administration (FDA) required warning labels to be placed on all salicylate-containing products, such as aspirin. Since then, there has been a dramatic decrease in the occurrence of Reye syndrome.

Nursing Assessment

Elicit a description of the present illness and chief complaint. Common signs and symptoms reported during the health history might include:

- Severe and continual vomiting
- Changes in mental status
- Lethargy
- Irritability
- Confusion
- Hyperreflexia

Explore the child's current and past medical history for risk factors such as:

- A prodromal viral illness, like chickenpox, croup, flu, or an upper respiratory infection
- Ingestion of salicylate-containing products within 3 weeks of the start of the viral illness

Elevated liver function tests and elevated serum ammonia levels can confirm diagnosis.

Nursing Management

Early recognition and treatment are the most important aspects of managing this illness. Nursing management is aimed at maintaining cerebral perfusion, managing and preventing increased ICP, providing safety measures due to changes in LOC and risk for seizures, and monitoring fluid status to prevent dehydration and overhydration.

Education is an important aspect of preventing this disease. Salicylates are found in many products, including many over-the-counter products, such as Alka-Seltzer and Pepto-Bismol. Recovery from Reye syndrome is dependent on the severity of swelling of the brain. Some children will make a full recovery, while others may suffer long-term neurologic damage.

TRAUMA

Trauma or injury is a leading cause of childhood morbidity and mortality in the United States (Gill & Kelly, 2022). The child faces significant risk of trauma to their developing neurologic system, often leading to neurologic disorders with life-threatening and lasting effects. Neurologic trauma may include head trauma, nonaccidental head trauma, birth injuries, and near-drowning.

Head Trauma

In the United States, injury causes more death in children than disease (CDC, 2021c). Of these injuries, head injury is a frequent cause of death and disability in childhood. Common causes of head trauma in children include falls, motor vehicle accidents, pedestrian and bicycle accidents, and child abuse (see next section, Nonaccidental Head Trauma). Many factors make children more susceptible to head trauma than adults. Larger head size in relation to the body, coupled with a higher center of gravity, causes the child to hit their head more readily when involved in motor vehicle accidents, bicycle accidents, and falls. Children are also at risk for injury related to psychosocial factors such as their high activity level, curiosity, incomplete motor development, and lack of knowledge and judgment skills.

Head trauma is a broad term that can include specific patterns of injury. Traumatic brain injury (TBI) occurs when a head trauma results in a disruption of the normal function of the brain. Not all head traumas result in a TBI. See Table 16.6 for descriptions of common head injuries seen in children. Head trauma in children is serious because it can cause an immediate threat to the child's life and many complications that can lead to lifelong impairment of an individual's physical, cognitive, and psychosocial functioning. Prognosis for the child who has suffered a head trauma depends on the extent and severity of the injury and any complications (see the Healthy People 2030 box).

TABLE 16.6 • Common Head Injuries Seen in Children

Types	Description	Characteristics
Skull fractures	A break in the bone surrounding the brain	In infants and children under 2 years old, a great deal of force is needed to produce a skull fracture. Due to the flexibility of the immature skull, it is able to withstand a great degree of deformation before a fracture will occur. Can result in little or no brain damage but may have serious consequences if the underlying brain tissue is injured
Linear skull fracture	A simple break in the skull that follows a relatively straight line	Most common skull fracture. Can result from minor head injuries such as being struck by a rock, stick, or other object; falls; or motor vehicle accidents. Not usually serious unless there is additional injury to the brain
Depressed skull fractures	The bone is locally broken and pushed inward, causing pressure on the brain.	Can result from forceful impact from a blunt object, such as a hammer or another heavy but fairly small object Surgery is often required to elevate the bony pieces and inspect the brain for evidence of injury.
Diastatic skull fracture	A fracture through the skull sutures	Most commonly occurs in the lambdoid sutures (refer to Fig. 16.10 for location of sutures) Usually, treatment is not required but observation will be necessary.
Compound skull fracture	A laceration of the skin and splintering of the bone	The fracture can be linear or depressed. Generally is the result of blunt force. Usually requires medical intervention, and surgery may be necessary
Basilar skull fracture	A fracture of the bones that form the base of the skull	Can result from severe blunt head trauma with significant force. Due to the proximity to the brain stem, this is a serious head injury. Findings include CSF rhinorrhea and otorrhea, bleeding from the ear, and orbital or postauricular ecchymosis (bruising behind ear is referred to as Battle sign), and these children are at increased risk for infection because the fracture may allow a portal of entry into the central nervous system.
Concussion	A type of traumatic brain injury that is caused by a bump, blow, jolt, jarring, or shaking and results in disruption or malfunction of the electrical activities of the brain	Most common head injury. Results from a blow or jolt to the head caused by sports injuries, motor vehicle accidents, and falls. Confusion and amnesia after the head injury are seen. Loss of consciousness may or may not occur. Noted symptoms may include increased distractibility and difficulty with concentration. Treatment includes rest and monitoring for neurologic changes that could indicate a more severe injury, such as increased sleepiness, worsening headache, increased vomiting, worsening confusion, difficulty walking or talking, changes in LOC, and seizures.
Contusion	Bruising of cerebral tissue	Results from a blow to the head from incidents such as a motor vehicle accident, falls, or abuse such as shaken baby syndrome. May cause focal disturbances in vision, strength, and sensation. The signs and symptoms will vary based on the extent of vascular injury and can range from mild weakness to prolonged unconsciousness and paralysis. Treatment includes close monitoring for neurologic changes. Surgery is usually not necessary.
Subdural hematoma	Collection of blood between the dura and cerebrum	Low incidence of fracture. Most common in children younger than 2 years old, especially infants. Results from birth trauma, falls, bicycle injuries, and abuse such as shaken baby syndrome. Usually consists of venous bleeding. Symptoms may occur within 3 days of trauma or as late as 20 days. Symptoms include vomiting, undernutrition, changes in LOC, seizures, and retinal hemorrhage. Treatment depends on clinical symptoms, size of clot, and area of the brain involved. In some cases, the bleed may be closely monitored for resolution. In other cases, treatment may include subdural taps in infants and surgical evacuation in older children. Close monitoring of neurologic status and for signs of increased ICP is indicated.
Epidural hematoma	Collection of blood located outside the dura but within the skull	Relatively uncommon. Often results from skull fracture. Seen when head trauma is severe. Usually arterial bleeding; therefore, brain compression occurs rapidly and can result in impairment of the brain stem and respiratory or cardiovascular function. Symptoms include vomiting, headache, and lethargy. Treatment depends on clinical symptoms, the size of the clot, and the area of the brain involved. Treatment includes prompt surgical evacuation and cauterization of the artery. The earlier the bleed is recognized and treated, the more favorable the outcome. Close monitoring of neurologic status is indicated.

HEALTHY PEOPLE 2030

Objective	Nursing Significance
Reduce fatal traumatic brain injuries.	• Educate children and families about safety such as helmet use when inline skating, skateboarding, bicycling, and playing football or other sports that may result in head injury. • Encourage appropriate child car seat and seat belt use. • Use every encounter with a child and family as an opportunity to provide education related to injury prevention.

Healthy People Objectives retrieved from http://www.healthypeople.gov

Nursing Assessment

For a full description of the assessment phase of the nursing process, refer to the "Clinical Judgment and the Nursing Process" section earlier in the chapter. Assessment findings pertinent to head trauma are discussed here.

HEALTH HISTORY

Take a detailed history, including past medical history along with details of the events surrounding the injury such as mental status at the time of the injury, any loss of consciousness, irritability, lethargy, abnormal behavior, vomiting (if so, how many times), any seizure activity, and any complaints of headache, visual changes, or neck pain.

PHYSICAL EXAMINATION

Perform a thorough physical examination. Initial physical assessment will focus on the ABCs (airway, breathing, and circulation) (refer to Chapter 29 for further information on emergency management). All children who experience head trauma need an assessment of their neurologic function as soon as they are seen. This includes LOC, pupillary response, and any seizure activity. Fixed and dilated pupils, fixed and constricted pupils, or sluggish pupillary reaction to light will warrant prompt intervention.

CLINICAL REASONING ALERT!

A child's spine must remain stabilized after a head injury until spinal cord injury is ruled out.

LABORATORY AND DIAGNOSTIC TESTS

Diagnostic tests that may be utilized include x-ray examinations of the head and neck and CT and MRI scans. These procedures can assist in providing a more definitive diagnosis of the severity and type of trauma.

CLINICAL REASONING ALERT!

If clear liquid fluid is noted draining from the ears or nose, notify the health care provider or nurse practitioner. If the fluid tests positive for glucose, this is indicative of leaking CSF.

Nursing Management

Nursing management of the child with head trauma depends on the seriousness of the injury. For all head trauma, however, the nurse provides support and education to the family and provides teaching on ways to prevent future head injuries.

CARING FOR THE CHILD WITH MILD TO MODERATE HEAD INJURY

Mild to moderate closed head injury is defined as brain injury without any penetrating injury to the brain, no loss of consciousness, no other injury to the head or body, normal behavior after the injury, and healthy status before the injury. Most children with this type of injury can be cared for and observed at home. Provide parents and caregivers with clear instructions regarding the care of their child at home. Explain that they must seek medical attention if the child's condition worsens at any time during the first several days after injury. See Teaching Guidelines 16.2.

TEACHING GUIDELINES 16.2 Monitoring the Child With Closed Head Injury at Home

Instruct parents and caregivers:

- Stay with the child for the first 24 hours, and be ready to take the child to the hospital, if necessary.
- Instructions for waking the child, if necessary, and at what frequency will be given based on child's symptoms and exam. If instructed, wake the child every 2–4 hours to ensure that they move normally, wake enough to recognize the caregiver, and respond to the caregiver appropriately.
- Closely observe the child for a few days.
- Call the medical provider or bring the child to the emergency room if the child exhibits any of the following:
  - Constant headache that gets worse
  - Slurred speech
  - Dizziness that does not go away or happens repeatedly

(continued)

TEACHING GUIDELINES 16.2 Monitoring the Child With Closed Head Injury at Home (*continued*)

- Extreme irritability or other abnormal behavior
- Vomiting more than two times
- Clumsiness or difficulty walking
- Oozing blood or watery fluid from ears or nose
- Difficulty waking up
- Unequal-sized pupils
- Unusual paleness that lasts longer than 1 hour
- Seizures
- Review signs and symptoms of increased intracranial pressure and provide parents with a number they can call if they have questions or concerns.

Adapted from Schutzman, S. (2021). Minor head trauma in infants and children: Management. *UpToDate*. Retrieved May 5, 2023, from https://www.uptodate.com/contents/minor-head-trauma-in-infants-and-children-management

Children with mild closed head injury may exhibit some cognitive and behavioral symptoms, such as difficulty paying attention, problems making sense of what has been seen or heard, and forgetting things, in the early days after the injury. The majority make a full recovery. However, some may experience ongoing cognitive and behavioral difficulties, including slow information processing and attention difficulties.

THINKING ABOUT DEVELOPMENT

Antonio Blackman is an 11-year-old who suffered a concussion during his soccer game. Based on his developmental stage, how will you instruct him and his caregivers on managing his head injury at home? How would your instructions change if the child were 5 years old?

CARING FOR THE CHILD WITH SEVERE HEAD INJURY

Severe head injuries can range from a temporary unconsciousness that resolves quickly to children who may remain in a comatose state for a prolonged time. Nursing management of the comatose child is similar to nursing care of the comatose adult.

Children with more severe head injury may require intensive care initially until stabilized. Focus will be on maintaining the child's airway; monitoring breathing, circulation, and neurologic status closely; preventing and ceasing any seizure activity; and treating any other injuries that may have occurred because of the trauma. Nursing management will continue to focus on evaluation of neurologic status and assessing for changes in LOC and signs and symptoms of increased ICP. Initiate seizure precautions as ordered.

Individualize care to the specific needs of the child. Maintain a quiet environment to help reduce restlessness and irritability. Manage pain and administer sedation as ordered. Observe the level of sedation closely to ensure that LOC will not become altered, which would hinder the ability to assess adequately for neurologic changes. Monitor for the development of complications, which include hemorrhage, infection, cerebral edema, and herniation.

TAKE NOTE!

Parents are extremely helpful resources in evaluating a child's behavior for changes or abnormalities. They can provide insight into whether a behavior seen is normal or abnormal for this child. Examples include the ease at which a child is normally aroused, how much the child normally sleeps during the day, and what is the child's normal visual and hearing acuity.

PROVIDING SUPPORT AND EDUCATION

Provide support and education for the family of a child who has suffered a head trauma. Encourage involvement in the child's care. The extent of residual neurologic damage and recovery may be unclear for the child with a head injury. This can be frustrating and stressful for parents and family. Encourage verbalization of their feelings and concerns. Rehabilitation of the child with permanent brain damage is an essential component of their care. It should begin as soon as possible in the hospital setting and may continue for months to years. This can place a strain on the family and its finances. Families need to be involved in the rehabilitation process. The nurse will be a key member in ensuring the parents and family are involved with the interdisciplinary team.

PREVENTING HEAD INJURIES

Prevention of head injuries provides the greatest benefit to children and the community. Nurses play a key role in educating the public on topics such as helmet use with certain sports; bicycle and motorcycle safety; car seat and seat belt use; and providing adequate supervision of children to help prevent injuries and accidents—and resultant head trauma—from occurring.

TAKE NOTE!

Sports-related traumatic brain injuries, including concussions, in children and adolescents are a growing concern, particularly related to the long-term effects of these injuries. Increasing education, awareness, and research about concussions will help to improve prevention, recognition, and treatment of this injury among school professionals, parents, coaches, and children and adolescents. See Evidence-Based Practice 16.1.

EVIDENCE-BASED PRACTICE **16.1**

How Does Screen Time Affect Recovery From Concussion?

The high incidence of concussion and the potential for short- and long-term complications make concussions in student athletes an important topic. General treatment protocol post sport-related concussion includes a period of cognitive and physical rest for the first 24 to 48 hours until symptom free and then a gradual, graded return to activity. Children and adolescents often spend several hours a day using screens, such as computers, tablets, and televisions. Parents and children frequently ask if screen time is permitted during the acute rest period post-concussion, and recommendations are often inconsistent. This study looks at what the evidence tells us about the effects of screen time on the duration of time until symptom recovery.

STUDY

This study was a randomized clinical trial involving 125 patients 12 to 25 years of age seen in an emergency department in a tertiary medical center.

Findings

This study found that avoiding screen time during the acute recovery phase may shorten the duration of concussion symptoms and lead to a faster recovery.

Nursing Implications

Nurses can educate children and their families on the benefits of cognitive and physical rest, which should include abstinence from screen time in the acute period, 48 hours post-concussion. Nurses can educate the child and families about signs and symptoms that would warrant further evaluation, treatment, and rehabilitation. Future clinical trials are needed on a larger scale. Further research is also needed on rest and active treatment and rehabilitation post sport-related concussion, preferably randomized controlled studies. The exact amount and duration of rest and the optimal timing, mode, duration, intensity, and frequency of active treatment warrant further studies.

Data from Macnow, T., Curran, T., Tolliday, C., Martin, K., McCarthy, M., Ayturk, D., Babu, K.M., & Mannix, R. (2021). Effect of screen time on recovery from concussion: A randomized clinical trial. *JAMA Pediatrics, 175*(11), 1124–1131. https://doi.org/10.1001/jamapediatrics.2021.2782

Nonaccidental Head Trauma

In the United States, inflicted or nonaccidental head trauma is the leading cause of traumatic death and morbidity resulting from physical abuse in childhood (Christian, 2023). Children's dependence on others to care for them places them at a high risk for injuries caused by child abuse.

The infant's large head size and weak neck muscles place them at an increased risk for head trauma due to violent shaking or cranial impacts compared with adults. In addition, children under 3 years of age have a very mobile spine, especially in the cervical region, along with immature neck muscles. This places them at a higher risk for injury from acceleration/deceleration injuries, which occur when the head receives a blow or is shaken. The sudden acceleration causes deformation of the skull and movement of the brain, allowing brain contents to strike parts of the skull. Bruising of the brain can occur at the point of impact or at that point distant from the impact where the brain collides with the skull. Another result of brain movement is hemorrhages in the brain, which are caused by the shearing forces that may tear small arteries. The child's thin skull places them at increased risk for skull fractures and penetrating injuries resulting from head trauma.

Causes of nonaccidental head trauma include violent shaking, referred to as shaken baby syndrome (SBS); blows to the head; and intentional cranial impacts against the wall, furniture, or the floor. SBS is a form of child abuse, and a significant number of head traumas result from it. However, it differs from many other forms of child abuse in that frequently, there was no intent to harm the child. Shaking happens when the parent or caregiver becomes frustrated or angry because they cannot get the baby to stop crying.

The full appearance of neurologic deficits resulting from nonaccidental head trauma may take several years to identify, and recovery can be slow. Long-term outcomes are not known, but many of these infants and children have poor outcomes and may suffer neurologic defects such as profound intellectual disability, spastic quadriplegia, severe motor dysfunction, and blindness. The majority of children with inflicted head injuries have some impairment of motor and cognitive abilities, language, vision, and behavior. These injuries may also contribute to later problems with education and social attainment.

Nursing Assessment

The infant who has been a victim of nonaccidental trauma can present in many ways. Symptoms and physical findings may be similar to those seen in children with accidental head trauma or increased ICP related to infection. Therefore, many nonaccidental traumas remain unidentified. Nurses are mandatory reporters of abuse (for further information on this, see Chapter 28). Early recognition of suspected child abuse is essential to prevent death and disability from repetitive inflicted head trauma.

HEALTH HISTORY

It is important to review the child's history closely and pay particular attention to the caregivers' explanation of the child's injury. Be alert to any discrepancies between the physical injuries and the history of injury given by the parent, especially if the stories are conflicting, or if the caregivers are unable to give an explanation for the injury. Also, note any previous intracranial or skeletal injuries that cannot be explained.

In less severe cases, common signs and symptoms may include:

- Poor feeding or sucking
- Vomiting
- Lethargy or irritability
- Undernutrition/malnutrition
- Increased sleeping
- Difficulty arousing

In more severe cases, the symptoms will be more acute and may consist of:

- Seizure activity
- Apnea
- Bradycardia
- Decreased LOC
- Bulging fontanel

PHYSICAL EXAMINATION

External bruising of the head and face may be evident in some inflicted head traumas. However, no evidence of external trauma, but the presence of intracranial or intraocular hemorrhages, is the classic presentation of SBS. Retinal hemorrhages are seen in most cases, which is a rare finding in accidental or nontraumatic events.

LABORATORY AND DIAGNOSTIC TESTS

Diagnostic tests, including CT, MRI, ophthalmologic examination to rule out retinal hemorrhages, and skeletal survey x-rays to rule out or confirm other injuries may be performed to help determine the extent and type of injury.

Nursing Management

Treatment and nursing management will be similar to that for the child with accidental head trauma (see earlier section, Head Trauma). Prevention of nonaccidental head trauma, including SBS, is a major concern for all health care professionals. Be aware of risk factors related to the potential for SBS to occur. Recognizing these risk factors will allow appropriate intervention and protection of the child to take place. See Box 16.4 for risk factors related to SBS.

Educating parents and caregivers on appropriate ways to handle stress and ways to cope with a crying infant can help to prevent nonaccidental head trauma (Teaching Guidelines 16.3). Many parents and caregivers may perceive shaking a child as a less violent way to react than other means of enforcing discipline. They need to be aware that shaking a baby, even for only a few seconds, can cause serious brain damage and death. Decreasing mortality and morbidity associated with SBS and nonaccidental injury through early preventive education is an essential nursing concern. Information about the dangers of shaking a baby should be a part of prenatal care and standard discharge teaching on postpartum units. In addition, this information should be provided to the community and in health education classes to reach young potential child care providers.

BOX 16.4 Risk Factors Associated With Abusive Head Trauma (Shaken Baby Syndrome)

- Single parent
- Young parent
- Substance misuse by a parent
- Any external factors present such as financial, social, or physical burdens that place stress on the parent
- Premature or sick infant
- Infant with colic

TEACHING GUIDELINES 16.3 Tips to Calm a Crying Baby

Instruct parents and caregivers:

- Try to figure out what is upsetting the baby.
  - Is the baby hungry?
  - Is the baby's diaper dry?
  - Is the baby cold or hot?
  - Is the baby overtired or overstimulated?
  - Is the baby in pain?
  - Is the baby sick or running a fever?
- Try to help the baby relax.
  - Turn down the lights.
  - Swaddle the baby.
  - Walk the baby.
  - Rock the baby.
  - Give the baby a breast, bottle, or pacifier.
  - Hush, talk to, or sing to the baby.
  - Take the baby for a stroller or car ride.
- Sometimes, the baby may continue to cry after all your efforts. If you feel overwhelmed, frustrated, or angry, focus on keeping the baby safe.
  - Stop what you are doing, take a deep breath, and count to 10.
  - Place the baby in a safe place, such as the crib or playpen.
  - Leave the room and shut the door, and find a quiet place for yourself.
  - Check on the baby every 5–15 minutes.
  - Do not be afraid to call for help; call a friend, relative, or neighbor.

COMPARISON CHART 16.2 Caput Succedaneum Versus Cephalohematoma

	Caput Succedaneum (Fig. 16.15A)	Cephalohematoma (Fig. 16.15B)
Description	An edematous area of the scalp of the newborn	Collection of blood between the skull bone and periosteum
Cause	Pressure from the uterus or vaginal wall during a head-first delivery, also as a result of vacuum extraction	Pressure against the birthing parent's pelvis results in bleeding. Common with forceps births
Characteristics	The swelling may be on any portion of the scalp and may cross the midline and suture lines. Mild discoloration may be present.	Does not cross the midline or suture lines. Typically, no discoloration; swelling not evident at birth
Treatment	None necessary (only observation)	In most cases, only observation is necessary, and resolution occurs within 2–9 weeks.
Complications	Usually heals spontaneously within a few days and without complication, but if extensive bruising is present, hyperbilirubinemia may occur.	Anemia; hypotension; underlying skull fracture; rarely leads to an infection such as meningitis. Due to the resolving hematoma, hemolysis of red blood cells occurs, and the infant may develop hyperbilirubinemia.

Data from Merhar, S. L., & Thomas, C. W. (2020). Chapter 120: Nervous system disorders. In R. M. Kliegman, J. W. St. Geme III, N. J. Blum, S. S. Shah, R. C. Tasker, K. M. Wilson, & R. E. Behrman (Eds.), *Nelson textbook of pediatrics* (21st ed., pp. 5148–5206). Elsevier.

Birth Trauma

Birth traumas are injuries sustained by the newborn during the birthing process. They may result from the pressure of birth, especially from a prolonged or abrupt labor, an abnormal or difficult presentation, cephalopelvic disproportion, or the use of mechanical forces such as forceps or vacuum during delivery. Newborns at risk include multiple deliveries, large-for-date infants, and those with extreme prematurity, a large fetal head, or congenital anomalies. Most injuries are minor and resolve without treatment.

Nursing Assessment

Inspect the head for lumps, bumps, or bruises. Note if swelling or bruising crosses the suture line. See Comparison Chart 16.2 and Figure 16.15 for a comparison of caput succedaneum and cephalohematoma (common types of head trauma resulting from the birth process).

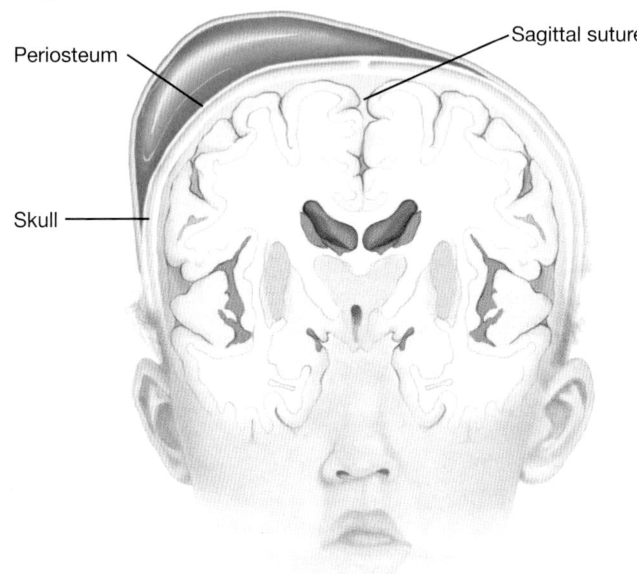

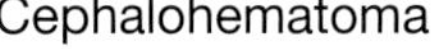

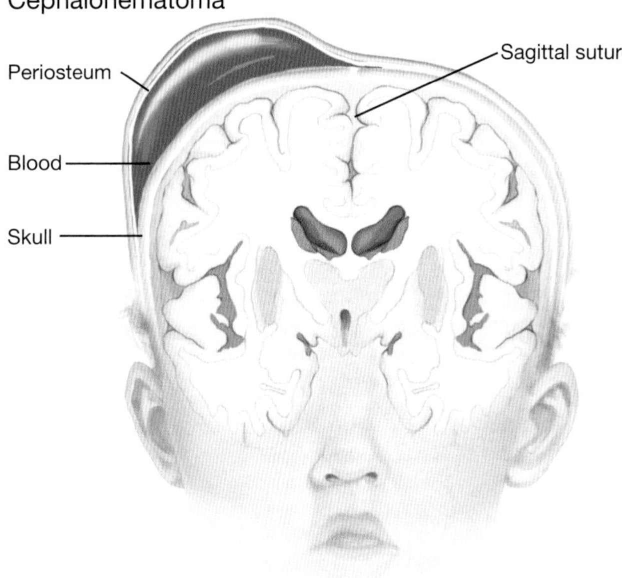

FIGURE 16.15 **A.** Infant with caput succedaneum. Edema is noted at birth and crosses the suture line. **B.** Infant with cephalohematoma. Bleeding appears within the first 2 to 3 days of birth and does not cross the suture line.

Nursing Management

Nursing management will be mainly supportive and will focus on assessing for resolution of the trauma or any associated complications, along with providing support and education to the parents. Provide parents with explanation and reassurance that these injuries are harmless. It can be very alarming and concerning to parents to see swelling or bruising on their child's head. Provide parents with education regarding the length of time until resolution and whether and when they need to seek further medical attention for the condition.

Nonfatal Drowning (Near-Drowning)

Drowning is a preventable problem that is far too common, especially in children. Drowning is the second leading cause of unintentional injury-related death in children between the ages of 1 and 14 years (CDC, 2022b). Those at greatest risk of drowning are children 1 to 4 years of age and adolescent males (CDC, 2022b).

Nonfatal or near-drowning is described as an incident in which a child has suffered a submersion injury and has survived for at least 24 hours. Nonfatal drowning events result in a significant number of injured children and can result in long-term neurologic deficits. Children under 1 year old most often drown in bathtubs, buckets, or toilets. Children between the ages of 1 and 4 years are more likely to drown or have a nonfatal drowning incident in residential swimming pools (CDC, 2022b). In children older than 15 years, most drownings occur in natural water settings, such as oceans or lakes (CDC, 2022b). Most incidents are accidental and result from inadequately supervising children who are in or near water, lack of use of personal flotation devices while on recreational water apparatus such as boats, and diving accidents.

Nursing Assessment

Hypoxia is the primary problem resulting from nonfatal drowning. Nursing assessment needs to begin with resuscitative measures. The child may be comatose, be hypothermic, lack spontaneous respirations, and present with hypoxia and hypercapnia. Gain information about the site of submersion (was it fresh or salt water?), the water temperature, the time of submersion, and how long it was until the child received interventions such as cardiopulmonary resuscitation (CPR) and EMS.

Nursing Management

Resuscitative measures should be started as soon as the child is pulled from the water, and the child should be transported to a hospital immediately. Management will be based on the degree of cerebral insult that has occurred. The child who has been successfully resuscitated will usually require intensive nursing care and monitoring. Promotion of oxygenation and monitoring for infection related to aspiration of water are primary nursing concerns. Chronic neurologic damage occurs in many nonfatal drownings secondary to hypoxia. The child may need rehabilitation and long-term follow-up. Provide parents with support and education relating to their child's condition. Educating children, families, and the community is an important nursing intervention to help prevent drowning (see Teaching Guidelines 16.4).

TEACHING GUIDELINES **16.4** Teaching to Prevent Drowning

Instruct parents and caregivers:

- Install proper pool fencing.
- Start water safety training at a young age.
- Have your child learn swimming skills.
- Never leave an infant or child without close adult supervision in or near water (this includes bathtubs).
- Empty water from all containers, such as 5-gallon buckets, immediately after use.
- Use proper-fitting, Coast Guard–approved personal flotation devices at all times when near water.
- Never allow children to walk, skate, or ride on thinning or thawing ice.
- Learn CPR and keep emergency numbers handy (make sure babysitters are CPR qualified).
- Know the depth of water before permitting a child to jump or dive.

BLOOD FLOW DISRUPTION

Pediatric cerebral vascular disorders occur less often than in adults, but they are still an important cause of mortality and chronic morbidity in children (Fox & Smith, 2023). Many children will develop lifelong cognitive and motor impairments. Childhood cerebral vascular disorders (stroke) are usually seen after the first month of life. Periventricular/intraventricular hemorrhage is seen in preterm infants and in infants up to 1 month of age.

Cerebral Vascular Disorders (Stroke)

A cerebral vascular disorder is a sudden disruption of the blood supply to the brain. It affects neurologic functioning, such as movement and speech. Two major types of adult cerebral vascular disorders are seen in children—ischemic stroke and hemorrhagic stroke. Ischemic stroke is more common than hemorrhagic stroke in children. In children, there are a wide array of risk factors and causes as compared with adults

COMPARISON CHART 16.3 Risk Factors and Causes of Stroke in Children and Adults

	Risk Factors and Causes in Children	Risk Factors and Causes in Adults
Ischemic stroke	Cardiac disorders and intracardiac defects (congenital such as ventricular septal defect, atrial septal defect, and aortic stenosis, or acquired such as rheumatic heart disease) Coagulation abnormalities that lead to thrombosis Sickle cell disease Infection, such as meningitis Arterial dissection Genetic disorders	Cardiac disease, including atherosclerosis Diabetes mellitus Hyperlipidemia Hypercoagulability states Polycythemia Sickle cell disease Smoking Increased age Male sex Obesity Excessive alcohol consumption
Hemorrhagic stroke	Vascular malformations such as intracranial arteriovenous malformation (AVM) Aneurysms Warfarin therapy Cavernous malformations Malignancy Trauma Coagulation disorders such as hemophilia Thrombocytopenia Liver failure Leukemia Intracranial tumors such as medulloblastomas	Hypertension Aneurysms Use of anticoagulant medications Smoking Increased age Male sex Obesity Excessive alcohol consumption

(see Comparison Chart 16.3), but in many cases the cause remains unidentified. The outcomes reported for cerebral vascular disorders in children vary, but many children will develop some neurologic or cognitive deficit.

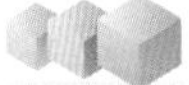
Concept Mastery Alert

Children are more likely to experience an ischemic stroke than a hemorrhagic stroke. If a child experiences a stroke, the symptoms are similar to those that an adult would experience.

Historically, children have been excluded from adult stroke studies. Therefore, many treatments used in children have had to be adapted from adult studies. Acute treatment is supportive and requires intensive care. The exact treatment will depend on the underlying cause.

Nursing Assessment

The clinical presentation will vary according to age, the underlying cause, and the location of the stroke. Signs and symptoms of acute stroke are similar to those seen in the adult and depend on the area of the brain that has been affected. Common signs include:

- Weakness on one side or hemiplegia
- Facial droop
- Slurred speech
- Speech deficits
- Seizures
- Headaches
- Lethargy

Strokes in children are diagnosed in the same manner as strokes in adults. However, further tests may need to be run in the child, such as metabolic studies, coagulation tests, echocardiogram, and LP to help identify the cause of the stroke.

Nursing Management

Nursing management will be similar to that for the adult patient who has suffered a stroke. Care will focus on assessing neurologic status, increasing mobility, providing adequate nutrition and hydration, and encouraging self-care. Rehabilitative care may be initiated, depending on the long-term deficits, to help the child attain optimal function. Parental support and education will be essential in helping them care for a child who has new disabilities.

Periventricular/Intraventricular Hemorrhage

Periventricular/intraventricular hemorrhage, which is bleeding into the ventricles, is most commonly seen in preterm infants (Merhar & Thomas, 2020). Due to the preterm infant's fragile capillaries in the periventricular area, immature cerebral vascular development, and poorly supported vascular bed, these infants are at an increased risk for intracranial bleeds. Causes of rupture of the capillaries leading to IVH vary and include fluctuations in systemic and cerebral blood flow, increases in cerebral blood flow from hypertension, IV infusion, seizure activity, increases in cerebral venous pressure due to vaginal delivery, hypoxia, and respiratory distress. The smaller the newborn is, and the more premature, the higher the risk of developing IVH.

Complications of IVH include development of hydrocephalus, periventricular leukomalacia (an ischemic injury resulting from inadequate perfusion of the white matter adjacent to the ventricles), cerebral palsy, and intellectual disability. The size and severity of the IVH is measured using a grading system. The system goes from grade I (mild) to grade IV (severe). In some settings, subcategories may be used to further distinguish the severity and extent of bleeding. Infants who experience mild IVH usually suffer no ill effects. Those with more severe grades of IVH are more likely to demonstrate neurologic and cognitive deficits.

Infants with a documented IVH will receive follow-up with scans to monitor the lesion for evidence of progression or resolution. Supportive care includes the correction of underlying medical disturbances that might be related to the development of IVH as well as cardiovascular, respiratory, and neurologic support. Correction of anemia, hypotension, and acidosis along with ventilatory support may be necessary in some cases. If hydrocephalus results, placement of a shunt may be necessary (see the "Hydrocephalus" section).

Nursing Assessment

The signs and symptoms seen with IVH vary significantly, and there may be no clinical signs evident. Closely monitor newborns who are at an increased risk, such as premature and low–birth-weight newborns. Some symptoms that may be seen include:

- Apnea
- Bradycardia
- Cyanosis
- Weak suck
- Seizure activity
- High-pitched cry
- Bulging fontanel
- Anemia

Premature and low–birth-weight newborns may have a head ultrasound in the first 10 days of life to assess for the presence of an IVH. Diagnostic tests such as CT and MRI scans may also be performed to document the presence of an IVH and provide more accurate assessment of the severity and size of the bleed.

Nursing Management

Nursing management will include monitoring for signs and symptoms of increased ICP, rapid increases in head circumference, neurologic changes, and delays in attainment of developmental milestones. In addition, provide education and support to the parents.

CHRONIC DISORDERS

Chronic disorders in children necessitate multidisciplinary care. Parents and children are in need of a large amount of education and support from the health care team. Chronic neurologic disorders commonly seen in children include headaches and breath holding.

Headaches

Acute and chronic headaches, including migraines, are common reasons why children miss school, visit their health care provider or nurse practitioner, and receive subsequent referrals to neurologists. Children with reports or symptoms of headaches need to be examined thoroughly. Headaches may result from sinusitis or eyestrain or can be indicative of more serious conditions such as brain tumors, acute meningitis, or increased ICP. Migraines are a specific type of headache. They are benign, recurrent, throbbing headaches often accompanied by nausea, vomiting, and photophobia. Acute migraines can occur in children as young as 3 to 4 years. The cause of migraine headaches is not well understood.

After other acute or chronic conditions are ruled out, management will focus on treating the child's pain. Pharmacologic measures may be utilized in the treatment of chronic headaches and migraines. Medications used in children to treat and prevent headaches are similar to the medications used to treat adults. Recent attention has been paid to headaches caused by medication overuse. The child may have a primary headache disorder that is exacerbated by the frequent use of medications. Although medication overuse headaches are common in children, they are frequently underrecognized and underdiagnosed.

Nursing Assessment

Elicit a description of the present illness and chief complaint. Important health history information to obtain is onset of the pain, aggravating and alleviating factors, frequency and duration of the pain, time of day the pain usually occurs, location of the pain, and quality and intensity of the pain.

In young children, symptoms of headache may be hard to recognize. However, common signs and symptoms may include:

- Irritability
- Lethargy
- Head holding

- Head banging
- Sensitivity to sound or light

Assessment also includes a thorough physical examination to rule out any life-threatening illness, such as a brain tumor or increased ICP. A detailed neurologic examination is warranted. Neuroimaging may be performed based on the child's history and physical examination, if needed, to rule out a brain tumor or mass as the cause of the headaches.

Nursing Management

Nursing measures will focus on support and education. After serious illness has been ruled out, reassure the child and family that no serious medical or neurologic disease is present. Because headaches are recurring and the cause may be unknown, pain management can be difficult. Provide education to help the child and parents gain control over the headaches. Teach the child and family to keep accurate records of headaches and activities surrounding the headaches to help establish a pattern of occurrence and identify triggering factors. Encourage parents and the child to recognize the triggering factors and to avoid them (Box 16.5). Teach the child and family about pain medications and how to use them. Teach other management techniques, which may include exercise, sleep regulation, proper diet with regularly spaced meals, avoiding caffeine, avoiding inadequate hydration, regular attendance at school, use of biofeedback, stress reduction techniques, and possible psychiatric assessment.

Breath Holding

Breath holding is a benign behavior of childhood, although it is extremely frightening for parents. It is normally seen in children 6 months to 6 years of age and is typically outgrown by 4 to 8 years of age (Nguyen et al., 2021). Breath holding is usually triggered by the child becoming angry or stressed after not getting their way and can also occur as a reflexive response to fear, pain, or being startled. The child stops inhaling and exhaling or hyperventilates, the brain becomes anoxic, and the child becomes cyanotic and may pass out. In some cases, a change in muscle tone, seizure-like activity, or hypoxic convulsions may be observed. This does not mean the child has a seizure disorder, but it must be ruled out. The spell usually resolves spontaneously. With the loss of consciousness, the child will begin breathing on their own and will often begin crying, screaming, and trying to catch their breath. The spells usually last only 30 to 60 seconds and, as long as the child does not sustain an injury while falling, have no consequences.

If no underlying condition is found, the child needs no therapy. The condition is self-limiting, and the child will outgrow it. Iron deficiency may play a role; therefore, iron supplementation may be prescribed (Nguyen et al., 2021).

Nursing Assessment

The first time a spell occurs, a primary care provider should evaluate the child because the event could indicate a seizure. Breath holding has also been shown to be aggravated by iron-deficiency anemia, and, in rare cases, it could indicate a more serious neurologic condition and therefore warrants a full evaluation. Elicit a full description of the episode and events leading up to it. Also, collect a thorough past medical history and perform a complete physical examination.

Nursing Management

Nursing management should focus on educating and supporting the parents. Breath holding is a scary event, and parents will want information on the effects of the behavior and how to prevent the behavior from recurring. Reinforce that the spells are involuntary and that they should not intervene to stop them. Encourage parents to maintain a safe environment when an episode is occurring, such as holding the child or placing them in the sidelying position. Reassure parents that the child will suffer no ill effects from breath holding and that they should not reinforce the breath-holding behavior or give in to the child. Children with breath-holding spells may benefit from structure and consistency to avoid unnecessary frustration and overtiredness.

BOX 16.5 Potential Headache Triggers

- Foods, such as chocolate, caffeine, or monosodium glutamate (MSG)–containing foods
- Changes in hormone levels, around menses and ovulation
- Changes in:
  - Weather
  - Season
  - Sleep patterns
  - Meal schedule
- Stress
- Intense activity
- Bright or flickering lights
- Odors, such as strong perfumes

Unfolding Patient Stories: Jackson Weber • Part 2

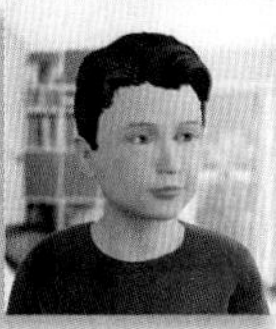

Think back to Chapter 4 where you met Jackson Weber. Jackson was diagnosed with generalized seizures 2 years ago at age 3. He had another seizure, and his parent brought him to the hospital. How would the nurse differentiate tonic–clonic seizures from other types of seizures? Compare and contrast the characteristics of each type of seizure.

Care for Jackson and other patients in a realistic virtual environment: ***vSim** for Nursing* (thepoint.lww.com/vSimPediatric). Practice documenting these patients' care in DocuCare (thePoint.lww.com/DocuCareEHR).

KEY CONCEPTS

- Development of the brain and spinal cord occurs early in gestation, in the first 3 to 4 weeks. Infection, trauma, teratogens, and malnutrition during this period can result in malformations and may affect normal CNS development.
- The brain of the newborn is highly vascular, leading to an increased risk of hemorrhage.
- The head of the infant and young child is large in proportion to the body, and the neck muscles are not well developed, placing the infant at an increased risk of head injury from falls and accidents.
- Neurologic disorders in children can result from congenital problems as well as infections or trauma.
- LP and CSF analysis can be useful in the diagnosis of hemorrhage, infection, or obstruction.
- CT and MRI studies can be useful in diagnosing congenital abnormalities such as NTDs, hemorrhage, tumors, fractures, demyelination, or inflammation.
- EEGs measure the electrical activity of the brain and can be used in diagnosing seizures or brain death.
- Antibiotics are utilized in the treatment of bacterial meningitis and shunt infections.
- Anticonvulsants are used in the treatment and prevention of seizures and are often used in combination.
- Corticosteroids are used to reduce cerebral edema and must be tapered before discontinuing.
- Risk factors associated with neurologic disorders include prematurity, difficult birth, infection during pregnancy, family history of genetic disorders with a neurologic manifestation, seizure disorders, and headaches.
- Alterations in motor function, such as changes in gait or muscle tone or strength, may indicate certain neurologic problems such as increased ICP, head injury, and cerebral infections.
- Increased ICP is a sign that may occur with many neurologic disorders. It may result from head trauma, birth trauma, hydrocephalus, infection, and brain tumors. It is essential that the nurse observes for signs and symptoms associated with increased ICP while caring for a child with a potential or suspected neurologic disorder.
- Sunset eyes may indicate increased ICP, as seen in hydrocephalus.
- A bulging fontanel can be a sign of increased ICP and is seen in such neurologic disorders as hydrocephalus and head traumas.
- Cortical control of motor function is lost in certain neurologic disorders; postural reflexes reemerge and are directly related to the area of the brain that is damaged. Decorticate posturing occurs with damage of the cerebral cortex. Decerebrate posturing occurs with damage at the level of the brain stem.
- Nursing management of seizures focuses on preventing injury during seizures, instituting seizure precautions, maintaining a patent airway, administering appropriate medication and treatments to prevent or reduce seizures, and providing education and support to the child and family to help them cope with the challenges of living with a chronic seizure disorder.
- Hydrocephalus results from an imbalance in the production and absorption of CSF. Key assessment findings include a rapid increase in head circumference seen in the infant or loss of development and changes in personality in the older child. Signs and symptoms associated with increased ICP may be seen.
- Nursing management of the child with hydrocephalus will focus on maintaining cerebral perfusion, minimizing neurologic complications, recognizing and preventing shunt infection and malfunction, maintaining adequate nutrition, promoting growth and development, and supporting and educating the child and family.
- Bacterial meningitis requires rapid assessment and treatment. On assessment, the nurse may find the infant with bacterial meningitis resting in the opisthotonic position, and the older child may complain of neck pain.
- Nursing management of the child with bacterial meningitis will include administration of IV antibiotics, reducing ICP, and maintaining cerebral perfusion along with treating fluid volume deficit, controlling seizures, and preventing injury that may result from altered LOC or seizure activity.
- Nurses play a key role in educating the public on topics such as helmet use with certain sports, bicycle and motorcycle safety, car seat and seat belt use, and provision of adequate supervision of children to help prevent injuries and accidents and resultant head trauma from occurring.
- Many neurologic disorders affect multiple body systems with lifelong deficits that require long-term rehabilitation. Adjusting to the demands this condition places on the child and family is difficult. Parents may need time to accept their child's condition, but as soon as possible they should be involved in the child's care.
- Children with neurologic disorders and their families often need large amounts of education and support throughout the child's lifetime. As the child grows, the needs of the family and child will change. The nurse needs to provide ongoing education and support.
- Some neurologic disorders require complete intensive daily care. Adjusting to these demands can be difficult for the family. Encourage respite care and provide meaningful education programs that emphasize independence for the child in the least restrictive educational environment. Refer caregivers to local resources, including education services and support groups.

REFERENCES AND RECOMMENDED READINGS

American Academy of Pediatrics & Committee on Genetics. (1999, reaffirmed 2017). Policy statement. Folic acid for the prevention of neural tube defects. *Pediatrics*. http://pediatrics.aappublications.org/content/104/2/325.full

American Academy of Pediatrics, Steering Committee on Quality Improvement and Management, & Subcommittee on Febrile Seizures. (2008). Febrile seizures: Clinical practice guideline for the long-term management of the child with simple febrile seizures. *Pediatrics, 121*(6), 1281–1286. https://doi.org/10.1542/peds.2008-0939

Buchanan, E. P. (2021). Overview of craniosynostosis. *UpToDate*. Retrieved May 6, 2023, from https://www.uptodate.com/contents/overview-of-craniosynostosis

Centers for Disease Control and Prevention. (2021a). *Meningitis: Bacterial meningitis*. http://www.cdc.gov/meningitis/bacterial.html

Centers for Disease Control and Prevention. (2021b). *Meningitis: Viral meningitis*. Retrieved May 8, 2023, from http://www.cdc.gov/meningitis/viral.html

Centers for Disease Control and Prevention. (2021c). *Injury prevention and control: Injuries among children and teens*. https://www.cdc.gov/injury/features/child-injury/index.html

Centers for Disease Control and Prevention. (2022a). *Folic acid recommendations*. http://www.cdc.gov/ncbddd/folicacid/recommendations.html

Centers for Disease Control and Prevention. (2022b). *Drowning facts*. https://www.cdc.gov/drowning/facts/index.html

Christian, C. (2023). Child abuse: Evaluation and diagnosis of abusive head trauma in infants and children. *UpToDate*. Retrieved May 8, 2023, from https://www.uptodate.com/contents/child-abuse-evaluation-and-diagnosis-of-abusive-head-trauma-in-infants-and-children

Fischbach, F. T., Fischbach, M. A., & Stout, K. (2022). *A manual of laboratory and diagnostic tests* (11th ed.). Wolters Kluwer.

Fisher, R. S., Cross, J. H., French, J. A., Higurashi, N., Hirsch, E., Jansen, F. E., Lagae, L., Moshé, S. L., Peltola, J., Roulet Perez, E., Scheffer, I. E., & Zuberi, S. M. (2017). Operational classification of seizure types by the International League Against Epilepsy: Position paper of the ILAE Commission for Classification and Terminology. *Epilepsia, 58*, 522–530. https://doi.org/10.1111/epi.13670

Fox, C., & Smith, S. E. (2023). Ischemic stroke in children and young adults: Epidemiology, etiology, and risk factors. *UpToDate*. Retrieved May 8, 2023, from https://www.uptodate.com/contents/ischemic-stroke-in-children-and-young-adults-epidemiology-etiology-and-risk-factors

Gill, A. C., & Kelly, N. R. (2022). Pediatric injury prevention: Epidemiology, history, and application. *UpToDate*. Retrieved May 8, 2023, from https://www.uptodate.com/contents/pediatric-injury-prevention-epidemiology-history-and-application

Hardarson, H. S., & Messacar, K. (2022). Acute viral encephalitis in children: Pathogenesis, incidence, and etiology. *UpToDate*. Retrieved May 8, 2023, from https://www.uptodate.com/contents/acute-viral-encephalitis-in-children-pathogenesis-epidemiology-and-etiology

Haridas, A., & Tomita, T. (2022a). Hydrocephalus in children: Physiology, pathogenesis, and etiology. *UpToDate*. Retrieved May 6, 2023, from https://www.uptodate.com/contents/hydrocephalus-in-children-physiology-pathogenesis-and-etiology

Haridas, A., & Tomita, T. (2022b). Hydrocephalus in children: Management & prognosis. *UpToDate*. Retrieved May 6, 2023, from https://www.uptodate.com/contents/hydrocephalus-in-children-management-and-prognosis

Khoury, C. (2023). *Chiari malformations. UpToDate*. Retrieved May 6, 2023, from https://www.uptodate.com/contents/chiari-malformations

Kinsman, S. L., & Johnston, M. V. (2020). Chapter 609: Congenital anomalies of the central nervous system. In R. M. Kliegman, J. W. St. Geme III, N. J. Blum, S. S. Shah, R. C. Tasker, K. M. Wilson, & R. E. Behrman (Eds.), *Nelson textbook of pediatrics* (21st ed., pp. 16200–16290). Elsevier.

Kossoff, E. H. W. (2022). The ketogenic diet and other diet therapies for the treatment of epilepsy. *UpToDate*. Retrieved May 9, 2023, from https://www.uptodate.com/contents/ketogenic-dietary-therapies-for-the-treatment-of-epilepsy

Lexicomp. (2023). Pediatric drug information. *UpToDate*. Retrieved April 5, 2023, from https://www.uptodate.com/contents/table-of-contents/drug-information/pediatric-drug-information

Macnow, T., Curran, T., Tolliday, C., Martin, K., McCarthy, M., Ayturk, D., Babu, K. M., & Mannix, R. (2021). Effect of screen time on recovery from concussion: A randomized clinical trial. *JAMA Pediatrics, 175*(11), 1124–1131. https://doi.org/10.1001/jamapediatrics.2021.2782

Merhar, S. L., & Thomas, C. W. (2020). Chapter 120: Nervous system disorders. In R. M. Kliegman, J. W. St. Geme III, N. J. Blum, S. S. Shah, R. C. Tasker, K. M. Wilson, & R. E. Behrman (Eds.), *Nelson textbook of pediatrics* (21st ed., pp. 5148–5206). Elsevier.

Mikati, M. A., & Tchapyjnikov, D. (2020). Chapter 611. Seizures in childhood. In R. M. Kliegman, J. W. St. Geme III, N. J. Blum, S. S. Shah, R. C. Tasker, K. M. Wilson, & R. E. Behrman (Eds.), *Nelson textbook of pediatrics* (21st ed., pp. 16312–16492). Elsevier.

Millichap, J. J. (2022a). Clinical features and evaluation of febrile seizures. *UpToDate*. Retrieved May 5, 2023, from https://www.uptodate.com/contents/clinical-features-and-evaluation-of-febrile-seizures

Millichap, J. J. (2022b). Treatment and prognosis of febrile seizures. *UpToDate*. Retrieved May 5, 2023, from https://www.uptodate.com/contents/treatment-and-prognosis-of-febrile-seizures

Nguyen, T. T., Kaplan, P. W., & Wilfong, A. (2021). Nonepileptic paroxysmal disorders in infancy. *UpToDate*. Retrieved on May 8, 2023, from https://www.uptodate.com/contents/nonepileptic-paroxysmal-disorders-in-infancy?sectionName=Breath-holding%20spells&search=Nonepileptic%20paroxysmal%20disorders%20in%20infancy&topicRef=6155&anchor=H8&source=see_link#H8

Schutzman, S. (2021). Minor head trauma in infants and children: Management. *UpToDate*. Retrieved May 5, 2023, from https://www.uptodate.com/contents/minor-head-trauma-in-infants-and-children-management

Shellhaas, R. (2022a). Treatment of neonatal seizures. *UpToDate*. Retrieved May 5, 2023, from https://www.uptodate.com/contents/treatment-of-neonatal-seizures

Shellhaas, R. (2022b). Etiology and prognosis of neonatal seizures. *UpToDate*. Retrieved May 5, 2023, from https://www.uptodate.com/contents/etiology-and-prognosis-of-neonatal-seizures

Shellhaas, R. (2023). Clinical features, evaluation and diagnosis of neonatal seizures. *UpToDate*. Retrieved on May 5, 2023, from https://www.uptodate.com/contents/clinical-features-evaluation-and-diagnosis-of-neonatal-seizures

Singer, R. J., Ogilvy, C. S., & Rordorf, G. (2022). Brain arteriovenous malformations. *UpToDate*. Retrieved May 5, 2023, from https://www.uptodate.com/contents/brain-arteriovenous-malformations

Tomita, T., & Ogiwara, H. (2022). Anencephaly. *UpToDate*. Retrieved May 6, 2023, from https://www.uptodate.com/contents/anencephaly

U.S. Department of Health and Human Services. (n.d.). *Healthy People 2030*. https://health.gov/healthypeople

Wilfong, A. (2022). Seizures and epilepsy in children: Classification, etiology, and clinical features. *UpToDate*. Retrieved May 4, 2023, from https://www.uptodate.com/contents/seizures-and-epilepsy-in-children-classification-etiology-and-clinical-features

DEVELOPING CLINICAL JUDGMENT

PRACTICING FOR NCLEX

1. When compared with adults, why are infants and children at an increased risk of head trauma? Select all that apply.
   a. The head of the infant and young child is large in proportion to the body.
   b. The development of the nervous system is complete at birth but remains immature.
   c. The spine is very immobile in infants and young children.
   d. The skull is more flexible due to the presence of sutures and fontanels.
   e. The neck muscles are not well developed.
   f. Infants and children have a high activity level.
2. At a well-child visit, hydrocephalus may be suspected in an infant if upon assessment the nurse finds:
   a. Narrow sutures
   b. Sunken fontanels
   c. A rapid increase in head circumference
   d. Increase in weight since last visit
3. A 10-year-old child is admitted to the hospital due to history of seizure activity. As the child's nurse, you are called into the room by their parent, who states the child is having a seizure. What would be the priority nursing intervention?
   a. Prevention of injury by removing the child from their bed
   b. Prevention of injury by placing a tongue blade in the child's mouth
   c. Prevention of injury by restraining the child
   d. Prevention of injury by placing the child on their side and opening their airway
4. A 6-month-old infant is admitted to the hospital with suspected bacterial meningitis. The child is crying, irritable, and lying in the opisthotonic position. The priority nursing intervention would be:
   a. Educate the family on ways to prevent bacterial meningitis.
   b. Initiate appropriate isolation precautions and begin intravenous antibiotics.
   c. Assess the infant's fontanels.
   d. Encourage the parent to hold the infant and feed the child.
5. The nurse is caring for an 8-year-old child involved in a bicycle accident. The child was not wearing a helmet, and a head injury has been diagnosed.

   Nurse's Notes

Time	Notes
1200	Spontaneously opens eyes, vomited x1, c/o headache and dizziness
1300	Sleeping, respiratory rate irregular

   Vital signs

Time	Temperature	Pulse	Respiratory Rate	Blood Pressure
1200	37.1°C (98.8°F)	76 beats per minute	16 breaths per minute	129/85
1300	36.9°C (98.4°F)	52 beats per minute	12 breaths per minute	148/92

   Which assessment findings indicate the child's condition is worsening? Select all that apply.
   a. Pulse of 52 bpm
   b. Dizziness
   c. Headache
   d. Irregular respiratory rate
   e. Vomited × 1
   f. BP 148/92 mm Hg
   g. Sleeping
   h. Spontaneously opens eyes
   i. 12 breaths per minute
6. The nurse is caring for a child in the emergency department. The parent reports the child had a seizure at home about an hour ago. Which assessment findings support a diagnosis of a simple febrile seizure? Select all that apply.
   a. A history of a respiratory illness for the past 24 hours
   b. No family history of seizures
   c. A fever of 39.5°C (103.1°F)
   d. Child is currently lethargic.
   e. The seizure lasted less than 2 minutes
   f. Child is 18 months old.

DOSAGE CALCULATION QUESTION

The nurse is caring for a child who is in status epilepticus. The child weighs 14.97 kg (33 lb). The medication order reads: Diazepam 3 mg IV push now. Per the Pediatric Dosage Handbook, the recommended dose is 0.1 to 0.3 mg/kg/dose. Diazepam is supplied as 5 mg/mL.

How many milliliters will the nurse administer? Round to the nearest tenth.

CRITICAL THINKING EXERCISES

1. A child is seen in the doctor's office after hitting their head while skateboarding. The child suffered no loss of consciousness and has no external injuries and no significant past medical history. The child is acting appropriately at this time. Their only complaint is a dull headache. What instructions would you give the parents regarding the child's care at home? Include when they should seek further medical care.

2. A 10-year-old child is admitted to the pediatric unit after experiencing a seizure. A complete, accurate, and detailed history from a reliable source is essential. What information would you ask for while obtaining the history?

3. A 6-year-old child is admitted to the hospital because of a possible seizure. The child's parent calls the nurse to the room because the child is "jerking all over" and won't respond when they call the child's name. List appropriate nursing interventions for this child. Prioritize the list of interventions.

4. Describe the impact of a cerebral vascular accident in the child as compared with the adult. How does it affect the child's future? How will the nurse provide care differently for the child stroke victim as compared with the adult?

STUDY ACTIVITIES

1. A 4-month-old child with a history of hydrocephalus has undergone surgery for placement of a VP shunt. What information would you include in the teaching plan?

2. Develop an example of a "headache log" that could be used by the family for chronicling the child's headaches, including triggers, relieving factors, and precipitating events. Ensure that the log is developed at a 6th-grade reading level to make it practical for parents with low literacy levels.

3. In the clinical setting, interview the parent of a child who has suffered significant brain trauma or injury (such as head trauma, IVH, or stroke). Talk with the family about the types of care the child requires. Reflect on this interview in your clinical journal, and compare how the ongoing care for this child compares with that for a typical child.

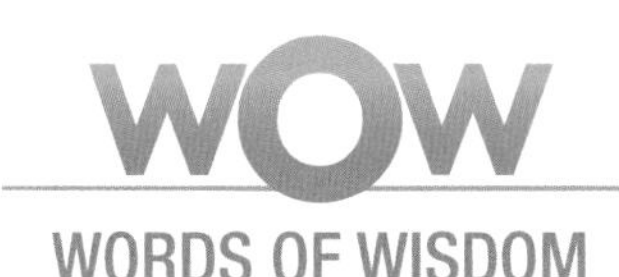

WORDS OF WISDOM
The child's senses provide an opportunity to explore the world.

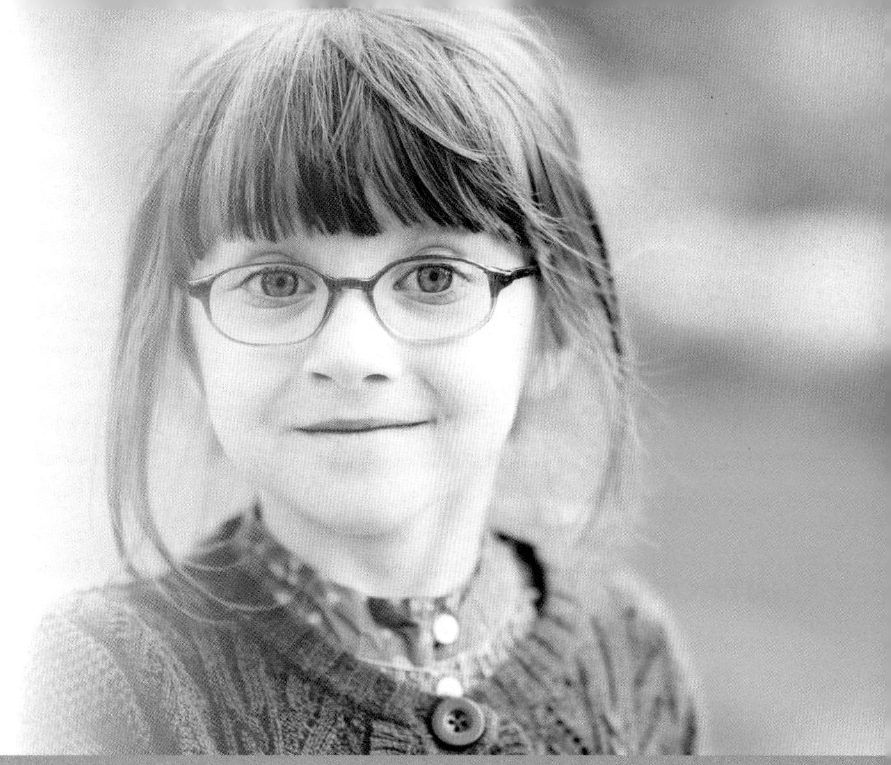

17

Nursing Care of the Child With an Alteration in Sensory Perception/ Disorder of the Eyes or Ears

LEARNING OBJECTIVES

Upon completion of the chapter, you will be able to:

1. Differentiate between the anatomic and physiologic differences of the eyes and ears in children as compared to adults.
2. Identify various factors associated with disorders of the eyes and ears in infants and children.
3. Discuss common laboratory and other diagnostic tests useful in the diagnosis of disorders of the eyes and ears.
4. Discuss common medications and other treatments used for treatment and palliation of conditions affecting the eyes and ears.
5. Recognize risk factors associated with various disorders of the eyes and ears.
6. Distinguish between different disorders of the eyes and ears based on the signs and symptoms associated with them.
7. Discuss nursing interventions commonly used in regard to disorders of the eyes and ears.

KEY TERMS

acuity
amblyopia (am′blē-ō′pē-ă)
blindness
conductive hearing loss
deafness
decibel (des′i-bĕl)
hearing impairment
nystagmus (nis-tag′mŭs)

pressure-equalizing (PE) tubes
ptosis (tō´sis)
sensorineural hearing loss (sen´sŏr-ē-nŭr´ăl hēr´ing laws)
sensory perception
strabismus (stră-biz´mŭs)
tympanometry (tim´pă-nom´ĕ-trē)
tympanostomy (tim´pă-nos´tŏ-mē)
vision impairment

8. Devise an individualized nursing care plan or concept map for the child with a sensory impairment or other disorders of the eyes or ears.
9. Develop child and family teaching plans for the child with a disorder of the eyes or ears.
10. Describe the psychosocial impact of sensory impairments on children.

Enrique Baxter, a 9-month-old, is brought to the clinic by his parent. His parent tells you, "Enrique has been fussy and not eating or sleeping well for the past 2 days."

INTRODUCTION

Sensory perception refers to receiving and interpreting stimuli. Disorders of the eyes or ears may lead to alterations in sensory perception. It is important for nurses to understand how to appropriately intervene for sensory perception alterations as well as other eye and ear disorders.

Children commonly suffer from disorders related to the eyes and ears. Conjunctivitis and otitis media are two common infectious and inflammatory disorders that affect the child's eyes or ears. Various alterations such as refractive error, strabismus, and amblyopia affect the development of visual acuity in children. Any alteration in the ear that contributes to the sensory perception alteration of hearing loss may have a significant impact on the child's language acquisition. It is important for the nurse to understand the impact of eye and ear disorders on the child's development.

Some children may be born with anomalies of the eyes or ears that will have a significant impact on vision and hearing, as well as psychomotor development. Disorders affecting the eyes or ears, particularly if chronic or recurrent, can have a significant impact on the development of visual acuity or may cause **hearing impairment** (varying degrees of hearing loss). In addition, the nurse may be caring for a child with another problem who is also either visually or hearing impaired. The nurse must take these developmental differences into account when planning care for these children.

VARIATIONS IN PEDIATRIC ANATOMY AND PHYSIOLOGY

The anatomy of children's eyes and ears differs somewhat from that of adults. In addition, visual **acuity** (sharpness of vision) develops from birth throughout early childhood. Hearing is intact at birth, but recurrent ear disorders may adversely affect the child's hearing.

Eyes

Light-skinned children are often born with blue eyes. The iris becomes pigmented over time, and eye color is determined by 6 to 12 months of age. The newborn's sclera may be slightly bluish tinged but becomes white within weeks. The eyeball of the infant and young child occupies a relatively larger space within the orbit than the adult's does, making it more susceptible to injury (Fig. 17.1).

Newborns have immature vision. The optic nerve is not fully myelinated until age 3 months, and the spherical shape of the newborn's lens negatively affects distance

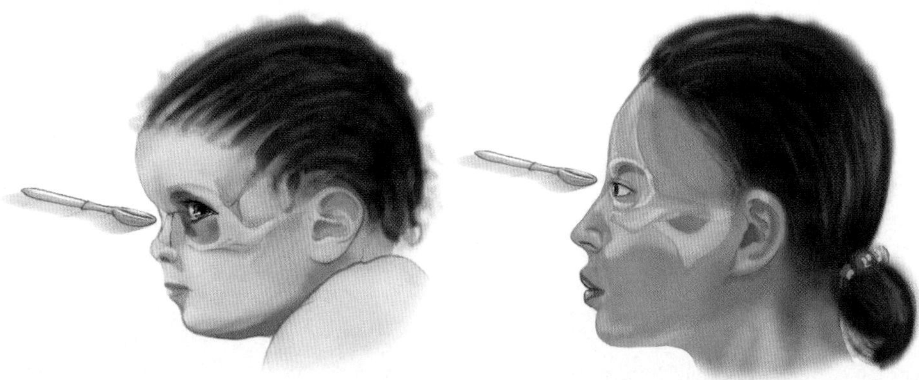

FIGURE 17.1 The relatively larger space that the infant's and young child's eyeball occupies within the orbit makes it more susceptible to injury as compared with the adult's eye.

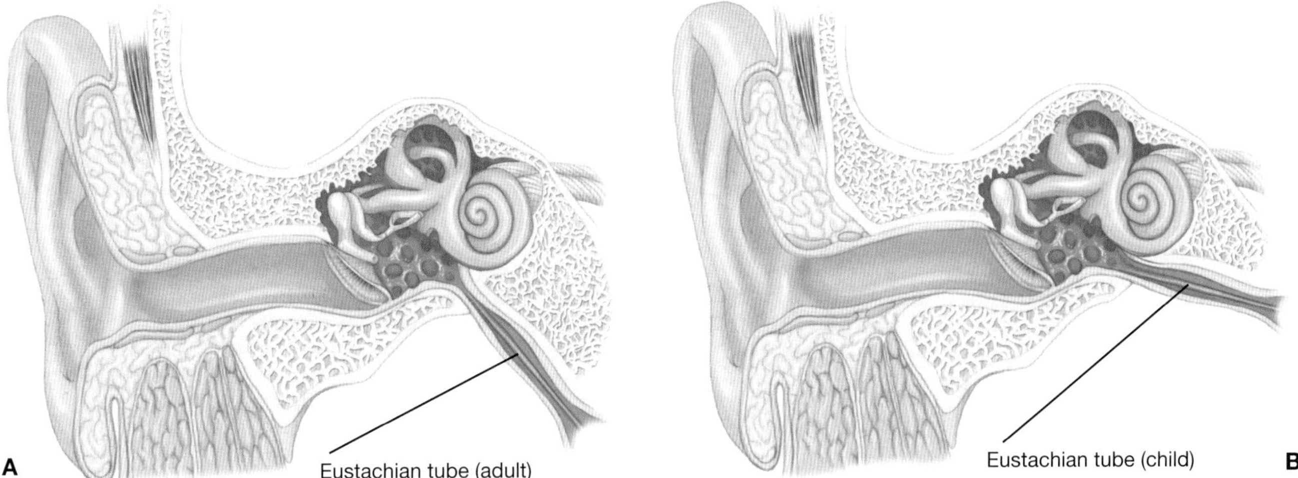

FIGURE 17.2 Note the child's relatively shorter, wider eustachian tubes and their horizontal positioning (**B**) as compared with the adult's (**A**).

accommodation (Olitsky & Marsh, 2020). At birth, visual acuity range is around 20/400. Visual acuity improves over the first few years of the child's life, with 20/20 usually achieved by age 5 years (Coats, 2023). The rectus muscles are uncoordinated at birth and mature over time so that binocular vision (the ability to focus with both eyes simultaneously) may be achieved between 3 and 7 months of age (Coats, 2023). In the preterm infant, retinal vascularization is incomplete, so visual acuity may be affected (Bhatt, 2023).

Ears

Congenital deformities of the ear are often associated with other body system anomalies and genetic syndromes. The presence of ear anomalies may lead to the search for, and subsequent diagnosis of, the other anomalies or syndromes. The infant's relatively short, wide, and horizontally placed eustachian tubes allow bacteria and viruses to gain access to the middle ear easily, resulting in increased numbers of ear infections as compared to the adult (Yoon et al., 2022). As the child matures, the tubes assume a more slanted position. Therefore, older children and adults generally have fewer cases of middle ear effusion and infection (Fig. 17.2). Sometimes enlargement of the adenoids contributes to obstruction of the eustachian tubes, leading to infection.

COMMON MEDICAL TREATMENTS

A variety of interventions are used to treat disorders of the eyes and ears in children. The treatments listed in Common Medical Treatments 17.1 and Drug Guide 17.1 usually require a health care provider's order when a child is hospitalized.

COMMON MEDICAL TREATMENTS 17.1

Treatment	Explanation	Indications	Nursing Implications
Warm compress	Warm, moist washcloth	Conjunctivitis	• Use very warm water from the tap (to avoid risk of burning, do not microwave).
Corrective lenses	In eyeglass form or as contact lenses	Correction of astigmatism, refractive error, strabismus	• Use a safety strap to help young children wear their eyeglasses.
Patching	An adhesive patch is applied to the healthier eye for several hours each day.	Strabismus, amblyopia, any other eye condition that results in one eye being weaker than the other	• Inform parents that though difficult to obtain, compliance with patching is critical. • A "pirate patch" may coax preschoolers into compliance.
Eye muscle surgery	Surgical alignment of the eyes	Strabismus	• Protect the operative site with patching. • Use elbow restraints if necessary.

(*continued*)

COMMON MEDICAL TREATMENTS 17.1 (*continued*)

Treatment	Explanation	Indications	Nursing Implications
Pressure-equalizing tubes (tympanostomy tubes)	Tiny plastic tubes inserted in the tympanic membrane	Chronic otitis media with effusion	• Teach parents dry ears precautions if prescribed or preferred by the surgeon. • Dry ears can be achieved by placing a cotton ball coated in petroleum jelly over the ear canal, in order to create a watertight seal.
Hearing aids	Amplification device worn in the ear	Hearing impairment	• Ensure appropriate fit and adequate amplification. • Direct families to outfitters that provide loaner aids of various brands and styles to determine best fit and amplification for the child.
Cochlear implants	Surgically inserted electronic prosthetic device	Sensorineural hearing loss	• Inform families that the usual minimum age for this procedure is 12 months.

Data from National Institute on Deafness and Other Communication Disorders. (2021). *Cochlear implants.* https://www.nidcd.nih.gov/health/cochlear-implants; Yoon, P. J., Scholes, M. A., & Herrmann, B. W. (2022). Ear, nose, & throat. In M. Bunik, W. W. Hay, M. J. Levin, & M. J. Abzug (Eds.), *Current diagnosis & treatment: Pediatrics* (26th ed.). McGraw-Hill Education.

DRUG GUIDE 17.1

COMMON DRUGS FOR EAR AND EYE DISORDERS

Medication	Actions	Indications	Nursing Implications
Antibiotics (oral, otic, ophthalmic)	Treatment of bacterial infections of the eyes and ears	Acute otitis media, otitis externa, conjunctivitis	Teach families to complete the entire course as prescribed. Check for drug allergies prior to administration.
Antihistamines	Block histamine reaction	Allergic conjunctivitis	Topical drops used. Oral agents usually prescribed if allergic rhinitis accompanies the conjunctivitis.
Analgesics	Pain relief	Otitis media, otitis externa, after eye or ear surgery	Narcotic analgesics may be necessary in some instances.

Data from UpToDate, Inc. (2024). *Lexicomp®* (Version 7.7.0) [Mobile app]. Wolters Kluwer. https://apps.apple.com/us/app/lexicomp/id313401238

COMMON LABORATORY AND DIAGNOSTIC TESTS 17.1

Test	Explanation	Indications	Nursing Implications
Culture of eye or ear discharge	Fluid draining from the eye or ear is cultured.	To determine specific bacteria present and appropriate antibiotic coverage	Easy to collect, relatively pain free. If drainage must be removed from within the ear canal, more likely to be painful
Tympanic fluid culture	Culture of fluid aspirated from the middle ear	To determine specific bacteria present and appropriate antibiotic coverage	Painful; usually performed only by specially trained health care providers
Tympanometry	Probe in ear canal measures movement of the eardrum.	Determines extent of effusion of the middle ear	Quick and easy to perform (seconds). Requires accurate-sized probe for adequate seal of the ear canal

Data from Yoon, P. J., Scholes, M. A., & Herrmann, B. W. (2022). Ear, nose, & throat. In M. Bunik, W. W. Hay, M. J. Levin, & M. J. Abzug (Eds.), *Current diagnosis & treatment: Pediatrics* (26th ed.). McGraw-Hill Education.

Clinical Judgment and the Nursing Process

Nursing care of the child with a disorder of the eyes or ears includes assessment, nursing analysis, planning, interventions, and evaluation. There are a number of general concepts related to the nursing process that can be applied to disorders of the eyes and ears. From an overall understanding of the care involved for a child with alterations in the eyes or ears, the nurse can then individualize care based on child and family specifics.

Assessment

Assessment of disorders of the eyes and ears in children includes health history, physical assessment, and laboratory or diagnostic testing.

Health History

The health history consists of past medical history, family history, history of present illness, and treatments used at home. The past medical history may be significant for prematurity, genetic defect, eye or ear deformities, visual acuity deficit or blindness, hearing impairment or **deafness** (the complete inability to hear sound), recurrent ear infections, or ear surgeries. Family history might be significant for eye or ear deformities or vision or hearing impairment or may reveal contacts for infectious exposure.

When eliciting the history of the present illness, inquire about its onset and progression and the presence of fever, nasal congestion, eye or ear pain, eye rubbing, ear pulling, headache, lethargy, or behavioral changes. Document if the child has corrective lenses or hearing aids prescribed and to what extent these devices are actually used.

Physical Examination

When assessing the eyes and ears, begin with inspection and observation. In addition, testing of visual activity and hearing may be performed.

INSPECTION AND OBSERVATION

Begin the physical examination with inspection and observation. Note whether the child uses eyeglasses, corrective lenses, or a hearing aid. Observe the eyes: note their positioning and symmetry and the presence of strabismus, nystagmus, and squinting. The eyelids should open equally (failure to open fully is termed **ptosis**). Note variations in eye slant and the presence of epicanthal folds. Assess the eyes for the presence of eyelid edema, sclera color, discharge, tearing, and pupillary equality, as well as the size and shape of the pupils.

Evert the eyelid to inspect the palpebral conjunctivae for redness. Test for extraocular movements and pupillary light response and accommodation. Note the symmetry of the corneal light reflex. Note the presence of the red reflex with an ophthalmoscope. Perform an age-appropriate visual acuity test. Refer to Chapter 9 for more detailed information related to visual acuity testing.

TAKE NOTE!

Attempts to inspect the palpebral conjunctivae may be frightening to children. Ask the older, cooperative child to evert the eyelid themselves while the nurse inspects the conjunctivae.

Inspect the ears: note their size and shape, position, and the presence of skin tags, dimples, or other anomalies (Fig. 17.3). Note that otoscopic examination is usually only performed by the advanced practice nurse. Upon otoscopic examination, note the presence of cerumen, discharge, inflammation, or a foreign body in the ear canal. Visualize the tympanic membrane and observe its color, landmarks, and light reflex, as well as the presence of perforation, scars, bulging, or retraction. Tympanic membrane mobility may be tested with

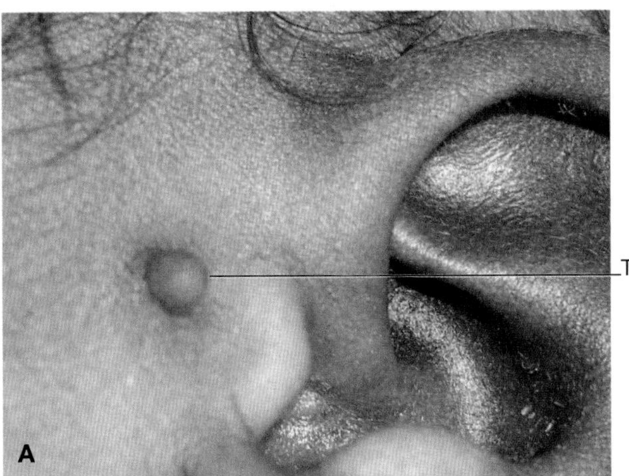

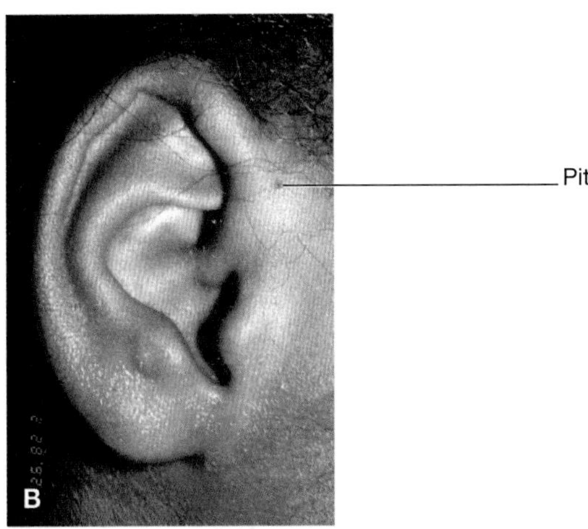

FIGURE 17.3 Note the skin tag (**A**) and preauricular pit (**B**) (in front of the ear).

pneumatic otoscopy. Auditory acuity is tested via the whisper test, audiometry, or other age-appropriate tests (refer to Chapter 9 for a more detailed explanation of hearing testing).

PALPATION

Usually, the eyes are not palpated. In the case of injury, the upper eyelid may be everted for examination purposes. Palpate the ear for tenderness over the tragus or pinna. Note the presence of tenderness over the mastoid area (tenderness may be present when otitis media progresses to mastoiditis). Palpate for enlarged cervical lymph nodes (this occurs when the eyes or ears are infected).

Laboratory and Diagnostic Testing

Common Laboratory and Diagnostic Tests 17.1 offers an explanation of the laboratory and diagnostic tests most commonly used for disorders of the eyes and ears. These tests can assist the health care provider or nurse practitioner in diagnosing the disorder and can be used as guidelines in determining ongoing treatment. Laboratory or nonnursing personnel obtain some of the tests, while the nurse may obtain others. In either instance, be familiar with how the tests are obtained, what they are used for, and normal versus abnormal results. This knowledge will also be necessary when providing child and family education related to the testing.

Remember Enrique, the 9-month-old with fussiness and poor feeding who was not sleeping well? What additional health history and physical examination assessment information should you obtain?

Nursing Analysis

After recognizing and analyzing cues from a thorough assessment, the nurse might identify several patient problems, including the following:

- Physical trauma risk
- Fear
- Delayed development risk
- Impaired verbal communication
- Deficient knowledge
- Pain
- Interrupted family processes

After completing an assessment of Enrique, the nurse noted the following: fever, tugging at his ears, and increased crying when lying down. Based on the assessment findings, what would your top three problems be for Enrique?

The preceding nursing analyses provide suggestions for nursing care planning or concept mapping. Suggested interventions with rationales are provided further. Care planning or concept mapping should be individualized, based on the child's and family's needs. Refer to Chapter 14 for the nursing care plan for pain management and to Chapter 11 for nursing interventions related to interrupted family processes. Additional information will be included later in the chapter as it relates to nursing management of children with specific disorders, as well as specific nursing interventions for deficient knowledge depending upon the disorder.

Nursing Analysis

Physical trauma risk related to insufficient vision

Goal/Outcome

The infant or child will remain free from physical trauma.

Preventing Physical Trauma (interventions with *rationale*)

- Orient the child to hospital surroundings *because awareness is the first step to preventing injury.*
- Encourage parent to be at bedside *so that the child feels more comfortable.*
- Encourage use of assistive devise *to promote safety.*

Nursing Analysis

Fear related to sensory deficit (severe visual impairment or blindness) and unfamiliar setting as evidenced by apprehensiveness or verbalization of feeling of alarm

Goal/Outcome

Child will experience decreased fear: child will verbalize comfort with environment or react calmly to interventions.

Decreasing Fear (interventions with *rationale*)

- Allow the verbal child to share their feelings *to promote coping in the child.*
- For the child who is severely impaired or the child who is blind, identify yourself via voice, and name items in the environment for the child *so that the child is aware of their surroundings.*
- Engage the parents in bedside caregiving *because the parents' voice and presence are reassuring to the child.*
- Encourage nutritious diet according to child's preferences *to assist body's natural infection-fighting mechanisms.*
- Isolate the child as required *to prevent nosocomial spread of infection.*
- Teach child and family preventive measures such as good handwashing, covering mouth and nose when coughing or sneezing, and adequate disposal of used tissues *to prevent nosocomial or community spread of infection.*

Nursing Analysis

Delayed development risk related to impaired vision or hearing impairment

Goal/Outcome

Child will achieve optimum independence for age: child participates in age-appropriate developmental activities.

Encouraging Development (interventions with *rationale*)

- Encourage attainment of developmental milestones with use of assistive devices as needed *for timely developmental achievements.*
- Foster independence in activities of daily living (ADLs) *to promote sense of accomplishment.*
- Encourage participation in play with another child or within a group *to promote socialization.*
- Assist family to set limits and apply discipline *because structure and routine provide a secure environment in which the developing child can grow.*
- Encourage friendships with other children with a sensory impairment *to promote socialization and let the child know that they are not the only one with these challenges.*

Nursing Analysis

Impaired verbal communication related to physiologic condition (hearing loss) as evidenced by difficulty verbalizing or inappropriate verbalization

Goal/Outcome

The child will communicate effectively with the method chosen by the family (this may be sign language, oral/deaf speech, cued speech, or augmentative alternative communication device).

Improving Communication (interventions with *rationale*)

- Encourage choice of and attendance at communication habilitation program *to promote continued learning.*
- Provide consistency between home and hospital in regard to communication style/devices *to optimize communication.*
- Support the child's efforts at correct speech *to promote speech development through reinforcement and praise.*
- Encourage family to use spoken language and read books at home *to continue to promote appropriate language development.*

Nursing Analysis

Deficient knowledge related to insufficient information or knowledge of resources (about sensory impairment)

Goal/Outcome

Parents express understanding of medical diagnosis and care of child: parents verbalize understanding, demonstrate use of assistive devices, or independently perform medical treatments.

Educating the Family (interventions with *rationale*)

- Review medical diagnosis and plan of care with the parents *to promote understanding of the disease process.*
- Refer family to resources available for children with sensory impairment *to provide further education and support to the parents.*
- Demonstrate medical treatments prescribed or use of assistive devices, requiring a return demonstration, *which shows the parents' ability to provide the prescribed care for the child.*
- Encourage exploration of different communication and learning modes available for the child with sensory impairment *to allow the child and family to find the right educational and communication style fit.*

Based on your top three problems for Enrique, describe appropriate nursing interventions.

INFECTIOUS AND INFLAMMATORY DISORDERS OF THE EYES

Infectious and inflammatory disorders of the eyes include conjunctivitis, nasolacrimal duct obstruction, eyelid lesions, and periorbital cellulitis.

Conjunctivitis

Inflammation of the bulbar or palpebral conjunctiva is referred to as conjunctivitis. It can be infectious, allergic, or chemical in nature. Viruses or bacteria may cause infectious conjunctivitis. Adenoviruses and influenza account for the bulk of cases of viral conjunctivitis. The most common bacterial causes are *Staphylococcus aureus*, *Streptococcus pneumoniae*, and *Haemophilus influenzae* (Howard & de St. Maurice, 2021). In the newborn, *Chlamydia trachomatis* and *Neisseria gonorrhoeae* are more common causes. Infectious conjunctivitis is very contagious, so epidemics are common, particularly in young children. Risk factors for acute infectious conjunctivitis include age younger than 2 weeks; day care, preschool, or school attendance; concomitant viral upper respiratory infection; pharyngitis; or otitis media. Concurrent acute otitis media (AOM) may occur depending on the bacterial cause. Complications from simple infectious conjunctivitis are uncommon. Neonates with chlamydial conjunctivitis may be at risk for the development of chlamydial pneumonia.

Allergic conjunctivitis results from exposure to particular allergens. Allergic conjunctivitis may be a seasonal or year-round complaint. A genetic predisposition to allergic conjunctivitis exists, just as it does for asthma, allergic rhinitis, and atopic dermatitis. Allergic conjunctivitis occurs more frequently in school-age children and adolescents than it does in infants and young children because of repeat exposure to allergens over time. In the case of seasonal allergic conjunctivitis, the severity of symptoms and the number of children affected are directly related to the pollen count in the area.

Pathophysiology

When bacteria or viruses come in contact with the bulbar or palpebral conjunctiva, they are recognized as foreign antigens and an antigen–antibody immune reaction occurs, resulting in inflammation. Allergic conjunctivitis occurs through a different mechanism. Contact with the allergen results in an allergic response (overreaction of the immune response). The mast cell and histamine mediators are then activated, resulting in inflammation.

Therapeutic Management

Therapeutic management of conjunctivitis is prescribed depending on the cause. Bacterial conjunctivitis is generally treated with an ophthalmic antibiotic preparation (drops or ointment). Viral conjunctivitis is a self-limiting disease and does not require topical medication. Eye drops with an antihistamine or mast cell stabilization effect may be helpful in alleviating symptoms of allergic conjunctivitis. If other allergy signs and symptoms are also present, an oral antihistamine may also be prescribed. Table 17.1 compares bacterial, viral, and allergic conjunctivitis.

Nursing Assessment

Nursing assessment of the child with conjunctivitis, regardless of the cause, is similar. It includes health history, physical examination, and, in rare instances, laboratory testing.

Health History

Elicit a description of the present illness and chief complaint. Common signs and symptoms reported during the health history might include the following:

- Redness
- Edema
- Tearing
- Discharge
- Eye pain
- Itching of the eyes (usually with allergic conjunctivitis)

Determine the onset of symptoms and their progression as well as response to treatments used at home. Assess for risk factors for infectious conjunctivitis, such as day care or school attendance. Note any history of an upper respiratory infection, sore throat, or earache. Question parents about possible infectious exposure. Review the health history for risk factors for allergic conjunctivitis, such as a family history and a history of asthma, allergic rhinitis, or atopic dermatitis. Determine seasonality related to the symptoms and whether the symptoms occur after exposure to particular allergens, such as pollen, hay, or animals.

Physical Examination

Observe for eyelid swelling or redness. Inspect the conjunctivae for redness (Fig. 17.4). Note quantity, color, and consistency of discharge. Bacterial infections generally result in a thick, colored discharge, whereas a clear or white discharge is generally seen with viral conjunctivitis. Allergic conjunctivitis often results in a watery discharge, sometimes profuse, which is usually present bilaterally. Contact with an allergen rubbed into one of the eyes may result in unilateral symptoms. Observe the child for other signs of allergic or atopic disease and document the presence of a runny nose or cough as well.

Laboratory and Diagnostic Tests

Cases of bacterial, viral, and allergic conjunctivitis are generally diagnosed based on history and clinical presentation. Cases of viral and allergic conjunctivitis do not warrant laboratory testing. If bacterial conjunctivitis is suspected, then a bacterial culture of the eye drainage may be performed to determine the exact causative organism, thus allowing the most appropriate antibiotic to be prescribed.

Nursing Management

Nursing management of the various types of conjunctivitis focuses on alleviating symptoms and, for infectious causes, preventing spread.

TABLE 17.1 • Types of Conjunctivitis

Type of Conjunctivitis	Conjunctivae	Discharge	Additional Findings	Eyelid Edema	Treatment
Bacterial	Inflamed	Purulent, mucoid	Mild pain	Occasional	Antibiotic drops or ointment
Viral	Inflamed	Watery, mucoid	Lymphadenopathy, photophobia, tearing	Usually present	Symptom relief; antiherpetic agent if cause is herpes
Allergic	Inflamed	Watery or stringy	Itching	Usually present	Antihistamine and/or mast cell stabilizer drops

Data from Mehner, L., & Jung, J. L. (2022). Eye. In M. Bunik, W. W. Hay, M. J. Levin, & M. J. Abzug (Eds.), *Current diagnosis & treatment: Pediatrics* (26th ed.). McGraw-Hill Education.

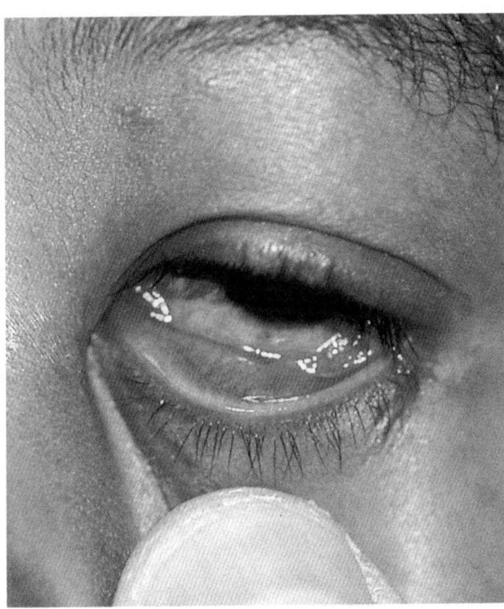

FIGURE 17.4 Note redness of conjunctiva.

Alleviating Symptoms

Teach parents how to apply eye drops or ointment (antibiotic for bacterial causes and antihistamine or mast cell stabilizer for allergic causes). Warm compresses may be used to help loosen the crust that accumulates on the eyelids overnight when drainage is copious, particularly with bacterial conjunctivitis.

ATRAUMATIC CARE

When instilling ear drops in the young child, use distraction (a song, a favorite toy) to decrease perceived trauma to the child.

The child with allergic conjunctivitis may experience perennial or seasonal allergies (or both). Encourage the child to avoid perennial allergens once the offending allergen is determined (refer to Chapter 18 for additional information related to education about perennial allergen avoidance). Seasonal allergies may include tree pollen in the winter or spring, grass pollen in the summer, and ragweed or flower pollen in the fall.

It is impossible to completely eliminate seasonal allergic responses, partly because it is important for children to participate in physical activity outdoors. Teach families to minimize seasonal allergens on the child's skin and hair. Educate families to:

- Encourage the child not to rub or touch the eyes.
- Rinse the child's eyelids periodically with a clean washcloth and cool water.
- Wash the child's face and hands when the child comes in from outdoors.
- Ensure that the child showers and shampoos before bedtime.

TAKE NOTE!

The itching of allergic conjunctivitis may be relieved with cool compresses. An easy way to accomplish this is to have the child hold a tube of yogurt over the affected eye.

Preventing Infectious Spread

Because infectious conjunctivitis is extremely contagious, the parent must wash hands diligently after caring for the child. Teach parents and children about appropriate handwashing and discourage them from sharing towels and washcloths. Children with viral conjunctivitis may return to school or day care when symptoms lessen. When mucopurulent drainage is no longer present (usually after 24 to 48 hours of treatment with a topical antibiotic), the child with bacterial conjunctivitis may safely return to day care or school (Jacobs, 2023a).

TAKE NOTE!

Avoid the use of vasoconstricting eye drops such as Visine to rid the eyes of redness. Rebound vasodilation may occur, and with it the redness returns. This leads to repeated frequent use of the drops to keep the eyes from being red but does not treat the actual cause of the redness (Lexicomp, 2024).

THINKING ABOUT DEVELOPMENT

Raisa Jordan is a 3-year-old who has been diagnosed with bacterial conjunctivitis and prescribed antibiotic eye drops. Based on her developmental stage, how will you assist her caregivers to administer the eye drops? How would this assistance change if the child was 12 years old?

Nasolacrimal Duct Obstruction

Stenosis or simple obstruction of the nasolacrimal duct is a common disorder of infancy, occurring in about 6% of newborns and infants (Paysse & Coats, 2023). Chronic tearing occurs, and buildup in the lacrimal sac causes a mucoid or mucopurulent drainage. About 66% of all cases resolve spontaneously by 6 months of age (Paysse & Coats, 2023). No apparent risk factors exist for the development of nasolacrimal duct obstruction or stenosis. Therapeutic management involves a watchful waiting approach. Massage may be prescribed, and if secondary bacterial infection is suspected or confirmed, antibiotic ointment or drops may be ordered. If the obstruction does not resolve spontaneously, then the pediatric ophthalmologist may probe the duct to relieve the obstruction (a brief outpatient procedure) (Paysse & Coats, 2023).

Nursing Assessment

Tearing or discharge from one or both eyes is often first noted at the 2-week check-up. Obtain a thorough history about the eye drainage to distinguish it from neonatal conjunctivitis. Determine the onset and progression of symptoms, as well as the newborn's response to any interventions attempted so far. Upon physical examination, note redness of the lower lid of the affected eye. If drainage is present, note its consistency, color, and quantity. Nasolacrimal duct obstruction is usually a diagnosis based on clinical presentation, but culture of the eye drainage may be used to rule out conjunctivitis or secondary bacterial infection (Fig. 17.5).

Nursing Management

Teach parents to clean the eye area frequently with a moist cloth. In addition, teach parents to massage the nasolacrimal duct, which may change the pressure and cause it to open, allowing drainage to occur. Refer to Teaching Guidelines 17.1 for appropriate nasolacrimal duct massage technique. Ensure that parents are educated about when and how to administer antibiotic eye drops if ordered.

Eyelid Disorders

Disorders of the eyelid include hordeolum (stye), chalazion, and blepharitis. Hordeolum is a localized infection of the sebaceous gland of the eyelid follicle, usually caused by bacterial invasion. Chalazion is a chronic painless infection of the meibomian gland. Blepharitis refers to chronic scaling and discharges along the eyelid

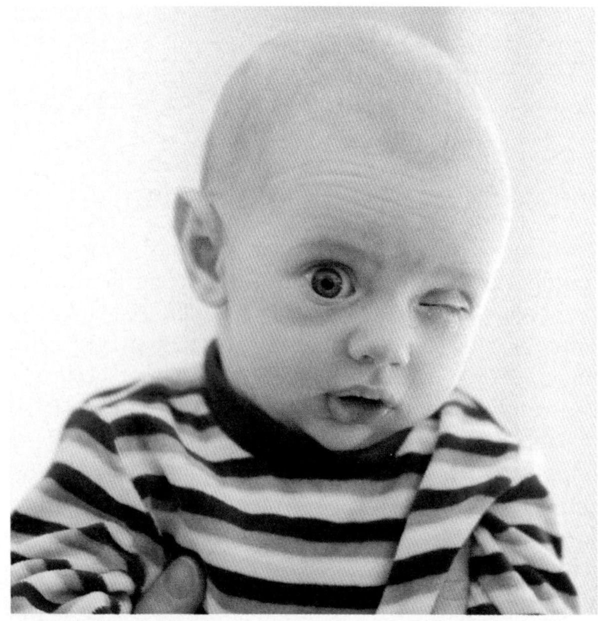

FIGURE 17.5 Mild eyelid redness and crusting are present in the infant with nasolacrimal duct stenosis.

TEACHING GUIDELINES **17.1** Nasolacrimal Duct Massage

- Using the forefinger or little finger, push on top of the bone (the puncta must be blocked).

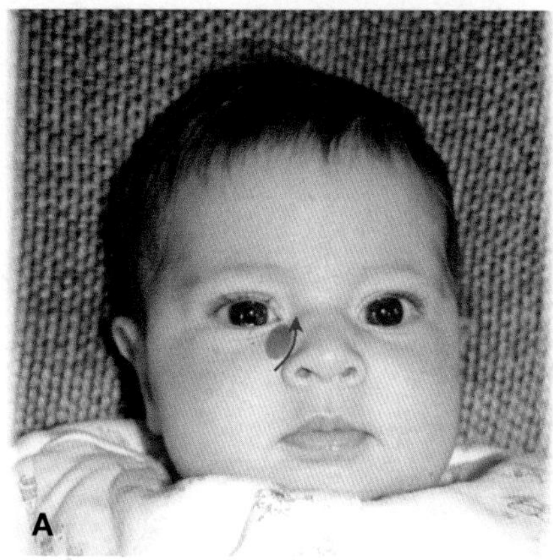

- Gently push in and up.

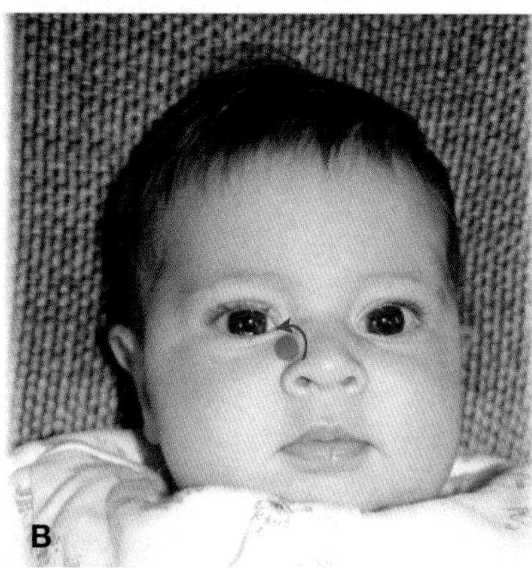

- Then gently push downward along the side of the nose.

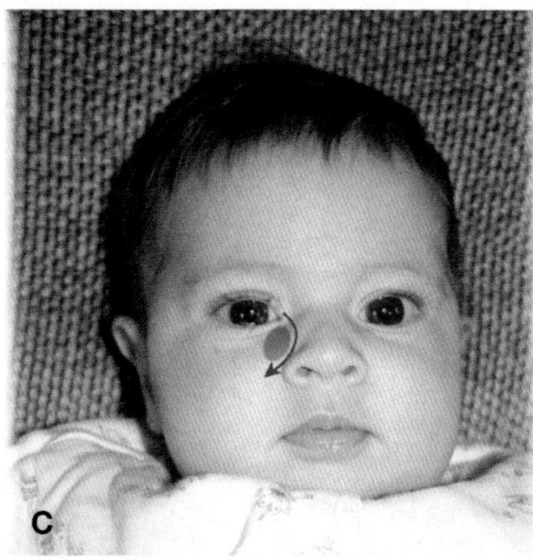

Adapted from Paysse, E. A., & Coats, D. K. (2023). Nasolacrimal duct obstruction (dacryostenosis) and dacryocystocele. *UpToDate*. Retrieved January 23, 2024, from https://www.uptodate.com/contents/congenital-nasolacrimal-duct-obstruction-dacryostenosis-and-dacryocystocele

margin. Chalazion may resolve spontaneously. Therapeutic management of hordeolum and blepharitis usually involves the use of antibiotic ointment.

Nursing Assessment

Determine the child's health history, noting onset of symptoms, extent and character of eye discharge, and presence of pain (hordeolum is usually painful). Inspect the eyelids, noting redness along the eyelid margin and presence of eyelid edema (hordeolum, blepharitis). Hordeolum may also be quite visible as an enlarged lesion along the lid margin, with purulent drainage present (Fig. 17.6). Chalazion may be visible as a small nodule on the lid margin. The conjunctivae remain clear with all three of these disorders.

Nursing Management

For hordeolum and blepharitis, instruct parents on how to administer antibiotic ointment. Encourage the use of hot, moist compresses. Inform parents that the stye may require several weeks to resolve completely. Also inform parents that chalazion will usually resolve spontaneously; if it does not, it may require minor surgical drainage.

EYE INJURIES

As mentioned earlier, infants and young children are more susceptible to eye injuries than adults since the eyeball is relatively larger in relation to the space within the orbit. Developmental maturity may also play a part in eye injuries. For example, as infants and toddlers learn to walk and run, they do not have the awareness and maturity to avert disaster. Older children involved in sports and school science experiments are also at risk for eye injuries. A few of the more common eye injuries are eyelid injuries, contusion, scleral hemorrhage, corneal abrasion, a foreign body in the eye, and chemical injury (Mehner & Jung, 2022).

Therapeutic management depends on the type of injury. Eyelid lacerations may require suturing. Deep lacerations may result in ptosis at a later date, so these children should be referred to an ophthalmologist. Simple contusions (black eye) usually need only observation, ice, and analgesics. Scleral hemorrhages resolve gradually without intervention over a few weeks. Corneal abrasions may be allowed to self-heal, or antibiotic ointment may be prescribed. Foreign bodies in the eye require removal to prevent further irritation or abrasion. Chemical injuries require irrigation and vision evaluation.

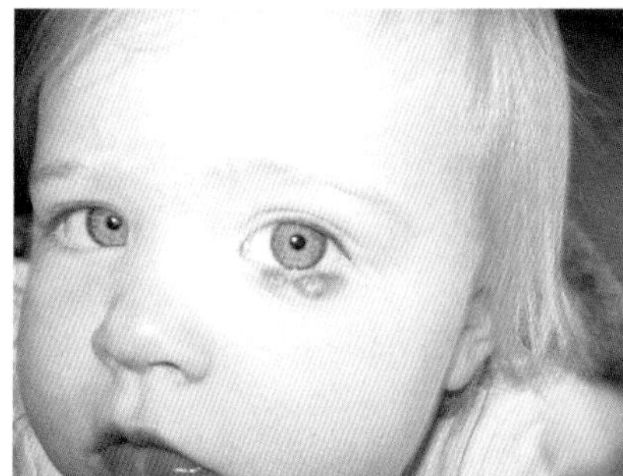

FIGURE 17.6 Hordeolum.

Nursing Assessment

When a child presents with an eye injury, it is important to obtain an accurate history related to the injury. Follow the history by performing a focused physical examination, which consists mostly of inspection and observation. It is important to determine whether an eye injury is nonemergent or emergent in order to provide rapid and appropriate treatment in the case of an emergency so that vision may be preserved.

Health History

Obtain an accurate history. Determine the mechanism of injury, and obtain as much detail about the injury as possible. Questions to ask during the health history include the following:

- When did the injury occur?
- What exactly happened?
- Was an object involved? If so, what type of object, and how fast was it going?
- Was it a splash injury?
- Was the child wearing eye protective gear or eyeglasses when the injury occurred?

Determine the extent of pain if present. Document photosensitivity, sensation of a foreign body in the eye, and blurry or lost vision. Inquire about past medical history, including previous eye injury or surgery or vision problems. Determine the child's immunization status.

Physical Examination

Regardless of the type of eye injury, the examination of the child's eye can be difficult. The nurse plays an important role in assisting the child and family to cope with the examination. Children with an eye injury often are in acute pain. The area surrounding the eye swells quickly after blunt trauma. Edema and tearing make the eye examination more difficult. Children are very frightened because of the pain and difficulty seeing. Approach the child in a calm and gentle manner. Soothe and coax the child as the eye is examined. Younger children may need to be restrained briefly in order for the examination to proceed safely.

Note the eyelid placement and look for signs of trauma such as bleeding, edema, and eyelid malformation. Evaluate the child's ability to open the eyes. Use a penlight to evaluate the pupils' response to light and

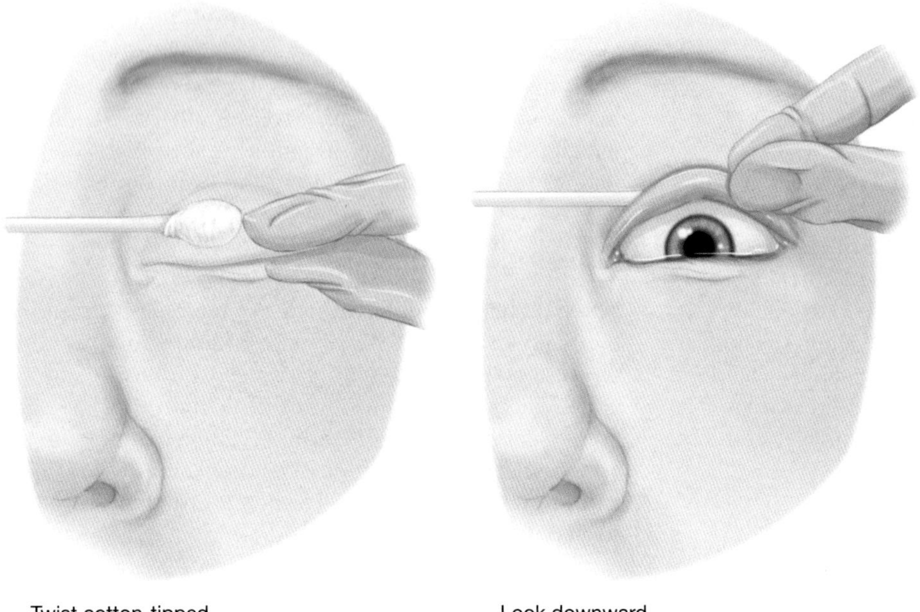

FIGURE 17.7 Eversion of the eyelid for examination. Place a cotton-tipped applicator over the eyelid. Pull the eyelid outward and up over the applicator.

accommodation (in the case of nonemergent eye trauma, the pupils should remain equally round and reactive to light and accommodation [PERRLA]). Note redness or irritation of the sclerae and/or conjunctivae. Observe for excessive tearing. Figure 17.7 shows the appropriate technique for eversion and examination of the interior of the eyelid.

In a nonemergent situation, evaluate visual acuity via the use of an age-appropriate vision screening tool (refer to Chapter 9 for additional information related to visual acuity screening). Table 17.2 provides assessment information specific to eyelid laceration, simple contusion, scleral hemorrhage, corneal abrasion, and foreign body in the eye.

TABLE **17.2** • Assessment of Eye Injuries

Description of Injury	Nursing Assessment
Eyelid injuries: May occur as laceration to the eyelid	• Laceration is noted at any point along the lid. • Vision is unaffected.
Simple contusion (black eye): Occurs as a result of blunt trauma to the eye area	• Bruising and edema of lids or area surrounding eye • PERRLA • Extraocular movements intact • Visual acuity intact • No diplopia or blurred vision • Pain surrounding eye but not within the eye
Scleral hemorrhage: Caused by blunt trauma or increased pressure such as with coughing	• Painless • Appears as erythema in the sclera; can be quite large initially • Vision unaffected
Corneal abrasion: Results from foreign body such as sand, grit, or other small object scratching the cornea	• May have tearing • Eye pain • PERRLA • Vision may be blurry. • Photophobia may be present.
Foreign body: May be dirt, glass, or other small particle	• Tearing • Complaint of "something in the eye" • PERRLA • Vision may be blurry.

PERRLA, pupils equally round and reactive to light and accommodation.

Data from Howard, L. M., & Annabelle de St. Maurice, A. (2021). Unraveling the impact of pneumococcal conjugate vaccines on bacterial conjunctivitis in children. *Clinical Infectious Diseases, 72*(7), 1208–1210. https://doi.org/10.1093/cid/ciaa202; Mehner, L., & Jung, J. L. (2022). Eye. In M. Bunik, W. W. Hay, M. J. Levin, & M. J. Abzug (Eds.), *Current diagnosis & treatment: Pediatrics* (26th ed.). McGraw-Hill Education.

TAKE NOTE!

If pupillary reaction is abnormal, vision is affected (decreased acuity from the child's norm, diplopia, or blurriness), or extraocular movements are affected, the child should be immediately referred to an ophthalmologist for further evaluation (Mehner & Jung, 2022).

Nursing Management

Refer children with urgent or emergent conditions to an ophthalmologist immediately to preserve vision. Non-emergent eye injuries usually need only simple management. Assist the health care provider or nurse practitioner with positioning and distraction of the child for eyelid laceration suturing. The child may require sedation or pain medication for this procedure.

To decrease edema in the child with a black eye (simple contusion), instruct the parent to apply an ice pack to the area for 20 minutes, then remove it for 20 minutes, and continue to repeat the cycle as often as possible during the first 24 hours. Tell the parents and child that bruising of the surrounding eye area may take up to 3 weeks to resolve.

Instruct the parents and child about the benign nature of the scleral hemorrhage (the appearance may be frightening). Educate parents about the natural history of resolution of the scleral hemorrhage without intervention over a period of a few weeks.

If the child with a corneal abrasion has pain, administer analgesics as needed. Tell parents that most corneal abrasions heal on their own. If an antibiotic ointment is prescribed, instruct the parents on how to administer the ointment appropriately.

TAKE NOTE!

Patching of the eye with a small, uncomplicated corneal abrasion or abrasion from a contact lens is not recommended. Patching does not result in decreased pain nor promote faster healing. In addition, it may place the child at risk for injury due to visual field loss while patched (Jacobs, 2023b).

Foreign bodies may be removed from the eye by gently everting the eyelid and wiping the foreign body away with a sterile cotton-tipped applicator. Irrigation with normal saline may also wash the foreign body away.

For chemical injury, irrigate the eye with copious amounts of water. Consult ophthalmology for further evaluation and management.

CLINICAL REASONING ALERT!

Refer the child with a large foreign body in the eye or one that is embedded in the globe of the eye to the ophthalmologist for appropriate, safe removal.

Eye injuries can be prevented, and nurses play a vital role in educating the public about prevention of eye injuries and use of appropriate safety equipment. See Evidence-Based Practice 17.1.

VISUAL DISORDERS

Adequate visual development requires appropriate sensory stimulation to both eyes over the first few years of life (Coats, 2023). When one or both eyes are deprived of this stimulation, visual development does not progress appropriately, and visual impairment or blindness may result. This may occur when the eyes are not aligned properly, visual acuity between the eyes is disparate, or other problems with the eyes exist (Coats, 2023). If vision disorders are diagnosed at an early age and treatment is begun, then vision may progress normally. However, when these disorders go untreated, the young child's developing vision may be reduced significantly. Therefore, it is important to appropriately screen children for these disorders. Common visual disorders in childhood include refractive errors, strabismus, amblyopia, nystagmus, glaucoma, and cataracts.

Refractive Errors

The most common cause of visual difficulties in children is refractive errors. When the light that enters the lens does not bend appropriately to allow it to fall directly

EVIDENCE-BASED PRACTICE **17.1**

Antibiotic Ointment for Corneal Abrasions

STUDY

Simple corneal abrasions are a common eye complaint. Antibiotic ointment is often used for treatment. The authors reviewed randomized controlled trials comparing antibiotic use to other antibiotics and to placebo. Two trials with a total of 527 participants were included in the review.

Findings

The authors found the evidence lacking. The review did not demonstrate prevention of ocular infection nor acceleration of corneal abrasion healing with ophthalmic antibiotic use. It also did not find ill effects from antibiotic use.

Nursing Implications

Parents worry significantly when their child experiences even a very mild eye injury. Teach parents about the ability of the cornea to heal quickly from a minor abrasion.

Data from Algarni, A., Guyatt, G. H., Turner, A., & Alamri, S. (2022). Antibiotic patching for corneal abrasion. *Cochrane Database of Systematic Reviews, 5,* CD014617. https://doi.org/10.1002/14651858.CD014617.pub2

on the retina, a refractive error occurs. Infants and young children naturally have mild hyperopia (farsightedness) because the depth of the eye globe is not fully developed until about 5 years of age (Coats & Paysse, 2023c). These children may have blurriness at close range, but by school age this blurriness usually resolves. When the light entering the eye focuses in front of the retina, it results in myopia (nearsightedness). Children who are nearsighted may see well at close range but have difficulty focusing on the blackboard or other objects at a distance.

Therapeutic management for both hyperopia and myopia is prescription eyeglasses or contact lenses. Generally, a child 12 years of age can demonstrate the responsibility necessary to wear and care for contact lenses. Contact lenses may be used in younger children but are lost or damaged more readily. Because of the continuing refractive development in the child's vision through adolescence, laser surgery for vision correction is not recommended for most children (Mehner & Jung, 2022).

Nursing Assessment

Elicit the health history, noting blurred vision, complaints of eye fatigue with reading, or complaints of eye strain (headache, pulling sensation, or eye burning). Note complaints of difficulty concentrating on or maintaining a clear focus on objects up close, avoidance of up close work, or poor work performance (hyperopia). Note the risk factor of family history of myopia. Observe for squinting when the child looks at objects at a distance. Observe the hyperopic child for the presence of esotropia. Readily observable physical findings are not noted in the myopic child. Test visual acuity using an age-appropriate screening tool (for more information related to visual acuity screening, refer to Chapter 9). Hyperopia is usually not identified with visual acuity screening alone; it usually requires a retinal examination by an ophthalmologist.

Nursing Management

Nursing management of the child with a refractive error focuses on providing education about corrective lens use and monitoring for the need for new eyeglasses or contact lenses.

EDUCATING ABOUT EYEGLASS USE

Encourage the child with newly prescribed eyeglasses to wear them by having the parent spend "special time" with the child doing an activity that requires the glasses (such as reading or drawing). Provide positive reinforcement for wearing the glasses. Teach the parent and child to remove eyeglasses with both hands and to lay them on their side (not directly on the lens on any surface). Instruct the child and family about cleaning the glasses daily with mild soap and water or a commercial cleansing agent provided by the optometrist. Use a soft cloth to clean the glasses, not paper towels, tissues, or toilet paper.

CONSIDER THIS!

I can't believe I have to start wearing glasses! I have heard the other kids mock my classmates and call them "four-eyes." I'm old enough now to start wearing makeup and how will that look with glasses? I'll look like a nerd....

Thoughts: How will you respond to her worries? With this early adolescent, what will your approach be to ensure she wears her glasses as prescribed?

EDUCATING ABOUT CONTACT LENS USE

Teach the older child or adolescent how to care for the contact lenses properly, including lens hygiene and lens insertion and removal. Inform the child and parents that protective eyewear should be worn when the child is participating in contact sports. If the eye becomes inflamed, remove the contact lens and wear eyeglasses until the eye is improved. Consult with the child's eye care provider to determine if medications prescribed for an eye problem can be used while the contact lens is in.

MONITORING FOR FIT AND VISUAL CORRECTION

Encourage the family to complete visual assessments as scheduled. Since the child's vision is continuing to develop and refraction is not stable, the corrective lens prescription may change more frequently than it does in an adult. As the young child in particular is continuing to grow at a rapid rate, the head size is also changing (American Association for Pediatric Ophthalmology and Strabismus [AAPOS], 2023). Eyeglass frames may hurt or pinch the child as the child's head becomes larger. Teach families to check the fit of the glasses monthly. Monitor for signs of ill fit, such as constant removal of the glasses in an older child or rubbing at the glasses or eyes in the very young child. Monitor for squinting, eye fatigue or strain, and complaints of headache or dizziness, which may indicate the need for a change in the lens prescription. See the Healthy People 2030 box.

HEALTHY PEOPLE 2030

Objective	Nursing Significance
Increase the proportion of children aged 3–5 years who receive vision screening. Reduce visual loss from refractive errors. Reduce vision loss in children and adolescents.	• Ensure that visual acuity testing begins with an age-appropriate screening tool by 3 years of age and continues yearly throughout childhood and adolescence. • Refer for an eye evaluation any children with complaints of difficulty seeing the front of the classroom or complaints of eye strain or difficulty with close work. • Screen infants and children for asymmetric corneal light reflex for early detection of amblyopia.

Healthy People Objectives retrieved from http://www.healthypeople.gov

Strabismus

Strabismus refers to misalignment of the eyes. It is common and occurs in up to 4% of the population (Coats & Paysse, 2023b). The most common types of strabismus are exotropia and esotropia. In exotropia, the eyes turn outward; in esotropia, they turn inward. Because of this unequal alignment, visual development in each eye may proceed at different rates. Diplopia (double vision) may result, so vision in one eye may be "turned off" by the brain to avoid diplopia. Many infants have strabismus intermittently, but this usually resolves by 3 to 6 months of age. Persistent esotropia that persists past 4 months of age or constant strabismus at any age warrants referral to an ophthalmologist for further evaluation (Coats & Paysse, 2023b).

It is extremely important to treat strabismus appropriately in the developing years so that equal visual acuity may be achieved in both eyes. Therapeutic management of strabismus may include patching of the stronger eye or eye muscle surgery. Corrective lenses are also used for strabismus. Complications of strabismus include amblyopia and visual deficits.

Nursing Assessment

Parents may be the first people to notice that the child's eyes do not face in the same direction. Question parents about the onset of the problem and whether it is continuous or intermittent. If intermittent, does it occur more often when the child is tired? Elicit the health history, noting complaints of blurred vision, tired eyes, squinting or closing one eye in bright sunlight, tilting the head to focus on an object, or a history of bumping into objects (depth perception may be limited).

Observe the child's eyes for obvious exotropia or esotropia. In the absence of an obvious finding, assessment of the symmetry of the corneal light reflex is extremely helpful (Fig. 17.8). The "cover test" is also a useful tool for the identification of strabismus.

True strabismus should not be confused with pseudostrabismus. In pseudostrabismus, the eyes may appear slightly crossed (as in the child with a wide nasal bridge and epicanthal folds), but the corneal light reflex remains symmetric (Coats & Paysse, 2023b).

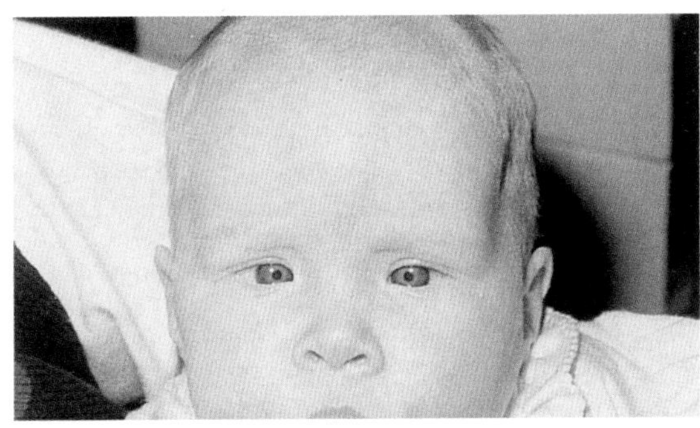

FIGURE 17.8 Esotropia. Test for strabismus by observing symmetry of the corneal light reflex. The reflex falls to the left of one pupil and to the right of the other.

Nursing Management

When patching is prescribed, encourage the family to comply with this modality. Encourage eyeglass wearing if prescribed. Provide appropriate postoperative care by protecting the operative site with eye patching.

Amblyopia

Amblyopia refers to poor visual development in the otherwise structurally normal eye. It develops within the first decade of life and, if left untreated, is the most common cause of vision loss in children and young adults, occurring in about 1% to 4% of children (Coats & Paysse, 2022). The vision in one eye is reduced because the eye and the brain are not working together properly. While the eyes are fighting to focus differently because of their differences in visual acuity, one eye is stronger than the other. This is why amblyopia is often referred to as "lazy eye."

Amblyopia may be caused by any disorder that affects normal visual development, including strabismus, differences in visual acuity between the two eyes, or astigmatism (cornea or lens is not perfectly spherical). It may also result from eye trauma, ptosis, or cataract. If untreated, children with amblyopia will have worsening acuity of the poorer eye and strain in the better eye, which may also lead to worsening of acuity in that eye. Eventually, blindness will result in one or both eyes.

It is important for children with amblyopia to receive appropriate treatment during the early years of visual development. Therapeutic management of amblyopia focuses on strengthening the weaker eye. This may be achieved through patching for several hours per day, using atropine drops in the better eye (once daily), vision therapy, or eye muscle surgery if the cause is strabismus. Patching the better eye for several hours each day encourages the eye with poorer vision to be used appropriately and promotes visual development in that eye. The once-daily use of atropine drops in the better eye results in blurring in that eye, similarly encouraging use and development of the weaker eye (Coats & Paysse, 2023a).

Nursing Assessment

One of the most important functions of the nurse is to identify the preschool child with amblyopia on screening. Begin visual acuity testing using an age-appropriate tool by 3 years of age. Observe for asymmetry of the corneal light reflex in the child of any age. This may be the only sign in the preverbal child.

Nursing Management

Support and encourage children and parents to comply with the patching protocol or atropine drop use. Promoting eye safety is extremely important for the child with amblyopia; if the better eye suffers a serious injury, both eyes may become blind.

Nystagmus

Nystagmus refers to a rapid, irregular eye movement. It is described by some as "bouncing" of the eyes. It may occur in children with congenital cataracts, but the most common cause is a neurologic problem. It is difficult for the brain and eyes to communicate when the eyes are in continuous motion; thus, visual development may be affected. Children with nystagmus must receive further evaluation by an ophthalmologist and possibly a neurologist.

Infantile Glaucoma

Infantile glaucoma is an autosomal recessive disorder that is more common in interrelated parents. It is often associated with other genetic disorders. It occurs in about one of 10,000 live births (Reynolds & Reynolds, 2023). Infantile glaucoma is characterized by obstruction of aqueous humor flow and increased intraocular pressure that results in large, prominent eyes. Vision loss may occur as a result of corneal scarring, optic nerve damage, or, most commonly, amblyopia.

Unlike adult glaucoma, in which medical management is the first step, therapeutic management of infantile glaucoma is focused on surgical intervention. Infantile glaucoma is treated surgically via goniotomy (removal of obstruction of the aqueous humor). Laser surgery is being used as well. Sometimes several surgeries may be necessary to correct the problem. Ongoing medication therapy may also be required.

Nursing Assessment

Note any family history of infantile glaucoma or other genetic disorders. Elicit the health history, noting history of the infant keeping the eyes closed most of the time or rubbing the eyes. Observe the eye for corneal enlargement and clouding; the eye may appear enlarged. Photophobia may occur, so bright light may bother the infant. Tearing or conjunctivitis and eyelid squeezing or spasm may also occur. The pediatric ophthalmologist may use a tonometer to measure the intraocular pressure during the diagnostic phase.

Nursing Management

The main goals of nursing care for the infant with glaucoma are providing postoperative care and educating the family. Postoperatively, focus on protection of the surgical site. Maintain eye patching and ensure the child remains on bedrest. If necessary, for infants and toddlers, use elbow restraints to prevent them from rubbing the affected eye. Use a calm and soothing approach, as well as distraction and developmentally appropriate play activities to calm the anxiety associated with being unable to see while patched.

Before the first surgery occurs, prepare parents for the possibility that three or four operations may be necessary. Postoperatively, teach families how to administer medications. Instruct parents and children to make sure the child avoids roughhousing and contact sports for at least 2 weeks after surgery. Encourage parents to comply with ongoing recommended visual assessments.

Congenital Cataract

A congenital cataract is an opacity of the lens of the eye that is present at birth. Sensory amblyopia will result if the infant goes untreated. Complications include visual developmental delay related to amblyopia. The disruption in visual development makes cataracts one of the leading causes of visual impairment in children (McCreery, 2023). Bilateral cataracts may be associated with metabolic or genetic syndromes. Surgery to remove the opaque lens can be done as early as 2 weeks of age. An intraocular lens implant is used, or the infant is fitted with a contact lens (McCreery, 2023). The best visual outcomes occur when cataracts are removed prior to 3 months of age. Glaucoma may occur as a complication after cataract surgery.

Nursing Assessment

Note history of lack of visual awareness. Observe the eyes for apparent cloudiness of the cornea (not always visible). Upon ophthalmoscopic examination, the red reflex will not be observed in the affected eye.

Nursing Management

Postoperative care focuses on protecting the operative site and providing developmentally appropriate activities. Ensure that the protective eye patch is secure. Elbow restraints may be necessary in the older infant to prevent accidental injury to the operative site. Teach families how to administer antibiotic or corticosteroid ophthalmic drops if prescribed for postoperative use. Once the surgical site is healed, the healthy eye may be patched for several hours a day to promote visual development in the eye with the intraocular lens or contact. Remind parents that regular visual assessments are critical for determining the adequacy of visual development after cataract removal. Instruct parents about the importance of using sunglasses that block ultraviolet rays in the child who has had a lens removed. See the Healthy People 2030 box.

HEALTHY PEOPLE 2030

Objective	Nursing Significance
Reduce visual impairment due to glaucoma.	• Appropriately screen infants and children for glaucoma or cataract.
Reduce visual impairment due to cataract.	• Refer suspected cases to a pediatric ophthalmologist for further evaluation.

Healthy People Objectives retrieved from http://www.healthypeople.gov

Retinopathy of Prematurity

Retinopathy of prematurity (ROP) is a disorder characterized by rapid growth of retinal blood vessels in the premature infant. In the fetus, retinal vascularization begins at 4 months and progresses until completion at 9 months or shortly after birth. The premature infant is born with incomplete retinal vascularization, yet new vessels continue to grow between the vascularized and nonvascularized retina. Risk factors include low birthweight, early gestational age, sepsis, high light intensity, and hypothermia. Changes in oxygen tension resulting from hypoxia, oxyhemoglobin dissociation curve changes that occur when adult blood is transfused to the premature infant, and the duration/concentration of supplemental oxygen are thought to play an important role in the development of ROP.

Premature infants should have serial examinations by an ophthalmologist until the ROP has regressed and normal vascularization is seen. If ROP continues to progress, laser surgery may be necessary to prevent blindness. Complications of ROP include myopia, glaucoma, and blindness. Strabismus may occur even in cases of regressed (resolved) ROP. Refractive errors and amblyopia may occur as early as 3 months corrected age. In the first year of life, ophthalmologic examinations should occur frequently so that if corrective lenses are needed, they may be prescribed at the earliest possible time. After 1 year corrected age, former premature infants should continue to have yearly ophthalmologic examinations to detect and treat visual deficits early.

Nursing Assessment

Ensure that all former premature infants are routinely screened for visual deficits. Discuss developmental progress with the parents. Observe for the development of strabismus, manifested by an asymmetric corneal light reflex.

Nursing Management

Nursing management of infants with ROP mainly focuses on ensuring that the family is compliant with the ophthalmologist's follow-up recommendations. Recurrent illness or rehospitalization of premature infants may interfere with scheduled eye follow-up appointments. Ensure that these appointments are rescheduled and that the family understands the importance of them. Many children who have regressed ROP or who require cryotherapy have refractive errors, so even when the ROP is considered resolved, these children should still maintain appropriate ophthalmology follow-up.

Visual Impairment

Vision impairment in children refers to acuity between 20/60 and 20/200 in the better eye on examination. "Legal **blindness**" is a term used to refer to vision of less than 20/200 or peripheral vision less than 20 degrees. In most cases, vision may be augmented with corrective lenses. Some children with blindness can differentiate light versus dark, while others live in total darkness.

Visual impairment in children may result from a number of different causes. In the United States, visual impairment and blindness may be caused by a number of disorders including but not limited to refractive error, astigmatism, strabismus, amblyopia, nystagmus, infantile glaucoma, congenital cataract, and ROP (Bregman et al., 2023). Factors that increase the risk for developing visual impairment include prematurity, developmental delay, genetic syndrome, family history of eye disease, African American heritage, previous serious eye injury, diabetes, human immunodeficiency virus (HIV), and chronic corticosteroid use. Trauma is also an important cause of blindness in children. Visual impairments are associated with many other syndromes. For example, many children with genetic syndromes have visual impairments, and albinism is associated with blindness (Bregman et al., 2023).

Children with visual impairments often exhibit motor and cognitive delays as well (World Health Organization [WHO], 2023b). With one less sense with which to experience their environment, these children may lag behind in developmental milestones. Children with blindness, since they lack the visual stimulation that children usually receive, may develop self-stimulatory actions in compensation, often called blindisms. Examples of blindisms are eye pressing, rocking, spinning, bouncing, and head banging. These repetitive behaviors may indicate an effort to communicate, and they may interfere with the child's ability to socialize (Hammer, n.d.).

TAKE NOTE!

Laser pointers pose a risk of retinal damage in infants and young children. Damage occurs if the child stares at the red light for longer than 10 seconds. They should not be used as toys (U.S. Food and Drug Administration, 2023).

Nursing Assessment

Nursing assessment for visual impairment includes a careful health history, physical examination, and visual acuity testing.

HEALTH HISTORY

Parents and nurses alike should be alert to signs of potential visual impairment. One of the most important functions of the nurse is to recognize signs of visual impairment as early as possible. These signs may include:

- At any age, a dull, vacant stare
- Infants:
  - Do not "fix and follow"
  - Do not make eye contact
  - Are unaffected by bright light
  - Do not imitate facial expression
- Toddlers and older children:
  - Rub, shut, and cover eyes
  - Squinting
  - Frequent blinking
  - Hold objects close or sit close to television
  - Bumping into objects
  - Head tilt or forward thrust

PHYSICAL EXAMINATION

Assess for symmetry or asymmetry of the corneal light reflex. Perform the "cover test." Use an age-appropriate visual acuity screening tool (refer to Chapter 9 for additional information on visual acuity screening).

Nursing Management

For the child with visual impairment, encourage the use of corrective lenses for enhancement of vision (if applicable). Encourage parents to comply with vision screening appointments in order to determine visual acuity progression or problems. Support the family's efforts at vision therapy and other habilitation programs to promote vision enhancement. Important nursing functions in relation to visual impairment and blindness are supporting the child and family and promoting socialization, development, and education. In addition, when the child with a visual impairment is hospitalized for any reason, the nurse must plan appropriate care for that child, taking into consideration the child's level of disability. Box 17.1 provides tips on working with the visually impaired child. It is important to teach these tips to families.

Supporting the Child and Family

Provide emotional support to the family with a visually impaired child. Ensure that the child's environment provides familiarity and security. Encourage activities that stimulate development; these activities will vary from child to child depending on whether the child also demonstrates impairment in other areas, such as hearing or motor skills. The infant with blindness will not provide the eye contact that parents are looking for, so educate the parents about other indicators that the infant is acknowledging the parents' presence, such as:

- Increased motor activity
- Eyelid movement
- Changes in breathing pattern
- Making sounds

Encourage the family of a child with visual impairment to display affection through touch and tone of voice. Refer families to support networks and other resources for people with blindness and visual impairment.

BOX 17.1 Tips for Interacting With the Child With Visual Impairment

- Use the child's name to gain attention.
- Identify yourself and let the child know you are there before you touch the child.
- Encourage the child to be independent while maintaining safety.
- Name and describe people/objects to make the child more aware of what is happening.
- Discuss upcoming activities with the child.
- Explain what other children or individuals are doing.
- Make directions simple and specific.
- Allow the child additional time to think about the response to a question or statement.
- Use touch and tone of voice appropriate to the situation.
- Use parts of the child's body as reference points for the location of items.
- Encourage exploration of objects through touch.
- Describe unfamiliar environments and provide reference points.
- Use the sighted-guide technique when walking with a visually impaired child.

Data from VisionServe Alliance. (2023). *Interacting with children who are visually impaired.* https://visionservealliance.org/interacting-with-children-who-are-visually-impaired/

Promoting Socialization, Development, and Education

Work with the parents to determine whether a strategy for the development of alternative behaviors specific to the individual child would be helpful. Refer the child with blindness or visual impairment who is younger than 3 years to the local district of Early Intervention to establish case management services for the child's developmental needs. After age 3, state laws provide for public education and related services for children with disabilities. An individualized education plan (IEP) should be developed to maximize the child's learning ability. Nurses may be one of the professionals involved in the development of the IEP. Refer the child with severe visual impairment or blindness for Braille training and for education on navigation of the environment with the use of a cane or other method.

INFECTIOUS AND INFLAMMATORY DISORDERS OF THE EARS

Infectious and inflammatory disorders of the ears include otitis externa and types of otitis media. Otitis media is defined as inflammation of the middle ear with the presence of fluid. It can be subdivided into two categories: AOM and otitis media with effusion (OME). AOM refers to an acute infectious process of the middle ear that may produce a rapid onset of ear pain and possibly fever. OME refers to a collection of fluid in the middle ear space without signs and symptoms of infection. Chronic OME is defined as OME lasting longer than 3 months. Otitis externa refers to inflammation of the external ear canal.

Acute Otitis Media

AOM is a common illness in children, resulting from infection (bacterial or viral) of fluid in the middle ear. Increased susceptibility in infants and young children may be partly explained by the short length and horizontal positioning of the eustachian tube, limited response to antigens, and lack of previous exposure to common pathogens (Yoon et al., 2022). AOM occurs mostly in the fall through spring, with the highest incidence in the winter. AOM often recurs in infants and young children when the fluid in the middle ear becomes reinfected. The most significant risk factors for otitis media are eustachian tube dysfunction and susceptibility to recurrent upper respiratory infections.

Pathophysiology

An upper respiratory infection frequently precedes AOM. Fluid and pathogens travel upward from the nasopharyngeal area, invading the middle ear space. Fluid behind the eardrum has difficulty draining back out toward the nasopharyngeal area because of the horizontal positioning of the eustachian tube. A viral upper respiratory infection may cause AOM or may place the child at risk for bacterial invasion. Pathogens gain access to the eustachian tube, where they proliferate and invade the mucosa. Fever and pain occur acutely. Increased pressure behind the tympanic membrane may result in perforation. This may result in decreased pain and drainage in the ear canal. Most perforations heal spontaneously and are completely benign.

AOM is most commonly caused by viral pathogens, *Streptococcus pneumoniae*, *Haemophilus influenzae*, and *Moraxella catarrhalis*. Viral causes of AOM resolve spontaneously.

After clearance of the infection, fluid remains in the middle ear space behind the tympanic membrane, sometimes for several months (OME). This may occur because of the positioning of the eustachian tubes, resulting in difficulty in draining fluid back to the nasopharyngeal area. OME may also occur because of the high frequency of upper respiratory infections in infants and young children, which again result in backup of fluid from the nasopharyngeal area.

The most common complications of AOM include:

- Hearing loss
- Expressive speech delay
- Tympanosclerosis (scarring of the tympanic membrane; usually has no effect on hearing)
- Tympanic membrane perforation (acute with resolution or chronic)
- Chronic suppurative otitis media (chronic drainage via perforation or tympanostomy tubes)
- Acute mastoiditis (infection of the mastoid process)
- Intracranial infections, including bacterial meningitis and abscesses

Therapeutic Management

Viral causes of AOM usually resolve spontaneously, but bacterial causes may require treatment with an antibiotic. It is unreasonable to obtain a culture of middle ear fluid with every episode of AOM to determine the specific cause. Scientific studies of fluid obtained via **tympanostomy** (creation of a hole in the tympanic membrane) in children with AOM have been performed, and clinical decision making is based on this research. Antibiotic resistance develops due to the overuse of antibiotics (WHO, 2023a). For this reason, clinical practice guidelines have been developed for a number of disorders based on large quantities of research.

Certain diagnosis of AOM is based on:

- Signs of fluid in the middle ear: moderate to severe bulging of the tympanic membrane, or mild bulging of the tympanic membrane with recent (within 48 hours) complaint of ear pain, and presence of middle ear infusion noted on pneumatic otoscopy or tympanometry

and

- Signs or symptoms of inflammation in the middle ear: complaint of ear pain or intense erythema of the tympanic membrane

or

- New-onset otorrhea in the absence of otitis externa (Yoon et al., 2022)

The choice of antibiotic will depend on the timing, the child's age, and whether the episode is a first or subsequent infection. The current recommendations by the American Academy of Pediatrics (AAP) allow for a period of observation or watchful waiting in certain children. This allows for natural resolution of AOM related to viral causes and decreases the overuse of antibiotics in the pediatric population (Yoon et al., 2022) (see Dosage Calculation Box 17.1).

DOSAGE CALCULATION 17.1

Child's weight: 12 lb, 4 oz

Medication order: cefuroxime 100 mg PO twice a day

Per the Pediatric Dosage Handbook, the recommended dose is 20–30 mg/kg/day in two divided doses.

Is the ordered dose safe?

Recommendations for AOM treatment in previously healthy children are found in Table 17.3. Pain management is also an important component of AOM treatment, as is appropriate follow-up to ensure disease resolution.

Nursing Assessment

Nursing assessment of the child with AOM consists of health history and physical examination.

HEALTH HISTORY

Elicit a description of the present illness and chief complaint. Note acute, abrupt onset of signs and symptoms. Common signs and symptoms reported during the health history might include:

- Fever (may be low grade or higher)
- Complaints of otalgia (ear pain)
- Fussiness or irritability
- Crying inconsolably, particularly when lying down
- Batting or tugging at the ears (may also occur with teething or OME, or may be a habit)
- Rolling the head from side to side
- Poor feeding or loss of appetite
- Lethargy
- Difficulty sleeping or awakening crying in the night
- Fluid draining from the ear

Determine the child's response to any treatments used thus far. Explore the child's current and past medical history for risk factors such as:

- Young age
- Day care attendance
- Previous history of AOM or OME
- Antecedent or concurrent upper respiratory infection
- Other risk factors (Box 17.2)

BOX 17.2 Risk Factors for AOM

- Eustachian tube dysfunction
- Recurrent upper respiratory infection
- First episode of AOM before 3 months of age
- Day care attendance (increases exposure to viruses causing upper respiratory infections)
- Previous episodes of AOM
- Family history
- Passive smoking
- Crowding in the home or large family size
- Native American, Inuit, or Aboriginal Australian ethnicity
- Absence of infant breastfeeding
- Immunocompromise
- Poor nutrition
- Craniofacial anomalies
- Presence of allergies (possibly)

AOM, acute otitis media.

Data from Yoon, P. J., Scholes, M. A., & Herrmann, B. W. (2022). Ear, nose, & throat. In M. Bunik, W. W. Hay, M. J. Levin, & M. J. Abzug (Eds.), *Current diagnosis & treatment: Pediatrics* (26th ed.). McGraw-Hill Education.

PHYSICAL EXAMINATION

The child may complain of pain when the ear is examined. On otoscopic examination, the tympanic membrane will have a dull or opaque appearance and is bulging and/or red (Fig. 17.9). Sometimes pus (greenish or yellowish) may be visible behind the eardrum. Upon

TABLE 17.3 • Treatment Recommendations for AOM

Age	Unilateral or Bilateral AOM?	Severe Signs and Symptoms?[a]	Otorrhea Present?	Treatment
6 months–2 years	Either		Yes	Antibiotics
6 months–2 years	Either	Yes		Antibiotics
6 months–2 years	Bilateral	No	No	Antibiotics
6 months–2 years	Unilateral	No	No	Antibiotics or observation[b]
>2 years	Either		Yes	Antibiotics
>2 years	Either	Yes		Antibiotics
>2 years	Bilateral	No	No	Antibiotics or observation[b]
>2 years	Unilateral	No	No	Antibiotics or observation[b]

AOM, acute otitis media.

[a]Severe illness is defined as temperature 39°C (102.2°F) or higher or moderate to severe otalgia or otalgia for at least 48 hours. Nonsevere illness is defined as mild otalgia for less than 48 hours and fever less than 39°C (102.2°F).

[b]Observation is appropriate when follow-up can be ensured in order that antibiotic therapy may begin if the child fails to improve or worsens within 48 to 72 hours.

Data from Yoon, P. J., Scholes, M. A., & Herrmann, B. W. (2022). Ear, nose, & throat. In M. Bunik, W. W. Hay, M. J. Levin, & M. J. Abzug (Eds.), *Current diagnosis & treatment: Pediatrics* (26th ed.). McGraw-Hill Education.

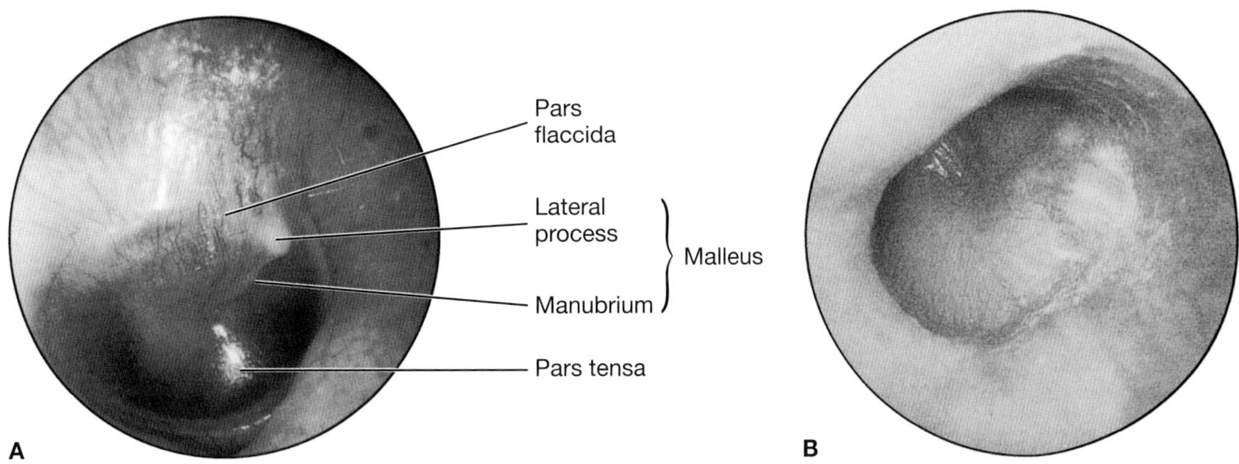

FIGURE 17.9 **A.** Normal tympanic membrane. **B.** Acute otitis media: note opacity of the tympanic membrane.

pneumatic otoscopy, the eardrum will be immobile. (A health care provider or nurse practitioner usually performs the otoscopic examination.) If the tympanic membrane has become perforated, drainage may be present in the ear canal, but the canal will otherwise appear normal. Palpate for possible cervical lymphadenopathy. Tympanometry is used to determine the presence of middle ear effusion (Yoon et al., 2022).

Nursing Management

Nursing management of the child with AOM is mainly supportive in nature. It focuses on pain management, family education, and prevention of AOM.

MANAGING PAIN ASSOCIATED WITH AOM

Administer analgesics such as acetaminophen and ibuprofen as they have been shown to be effective at managing mild to moderate pain associated with AOM and have the added benefit of reducing fever. Occasionally, narcotic analgesics may be prescribed for severe pain. Apply a warm or cool compress if helpful to the child. Instruct the family to have the child lie on the affected side with the heating pad or a covered ice pack in place against that ear.

EDUCATING THE FAMILY

If the treatment selected for AOM is observation or watchful waiting, explain the rationale for this to the family. Ensure that the family understands the importance of returning for reevaluation if the child is not improving within 48 to 72 hours or if the AOM progresses to severe illness. When antibiotics are prescribed, ensure the family understands the importance of completing the entire course of antibiotics. Families are tempted to stop giving the antibiotic because the child is usually vastly improved after taking the medication for 24 to 48 hours. Follow-up for resolution of AOM is necessary for all children and the health care provider or nurse practitioner will determine the timing of that follow-up. Emphasize the importance of follow-up to the parents, educating them about OME and its potential impact on hearing and speech. See the Healthy People 2030 box.

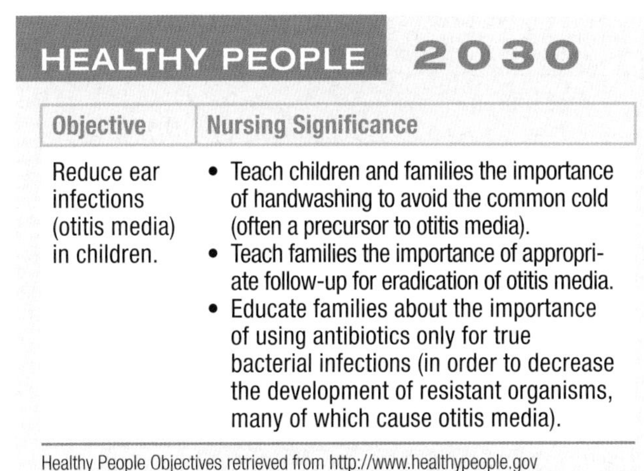

HEALTHY PEOPLE 2030

Objective	Nursing Significance
Reduce ear infections (otitis media) in children.	• Teach children and families the importance of handwashing to avoid the common cold (often a precursor to otitis media). • Teach families the importance of appropriate follow-up for eradication of otitis media. • Educate families about the importance of using antibiotics only for true bacterial infections (in order to decrease the development of resistant organisms, many of which cause otitis media).

Healthy People Objectives retrieved from http://www.healthypeople.gov

PREVENTING AOM

Encourage breastfeeding for at least 6 to 12 months, as breastfed infants have a lower incidence of AOM than formula-fed infants, and breast milk's immunologic benefits are well known (Yoon et al., 2022). Instruct families to avoid excess exposure to individuals with upper respiratory infections to decrease the incidence of these infections in their child. Educate families that infants and children should not be exposed to second-hand smoke. Encourage parents to stop smoking. If quitting smoking is not possible, then instruct parents not to smoke inside the house or automobile. Encourage the parents to have the child immunized with Prevnar and the influenza vaccine. When families question the protective benefits of xylitol, educate them that studies thus far have been inconclusive, and with excessive dosing, xylitol can cause diarrhea (Pelton & Marchisio, 2023).

Otitis Media With Effusion

OME refers to the presence of fluid within the middle ear space, without signs or symptoms of infection. It may occur independent of AOM or may persist after the infectious process of AOM has resolved. Risk factors for OME include passive smoking, absence of breastfeeding, frequent viral upper respiratory infections, allergy, young age, male sex, adenoid hypertrophy, eustachian tube dysfunction, and certain congenital disorders (Yoon et al., 2022). Complications of OME include AOM, hearing loss, and deafness.

Nursing Assessment

Nursing assessment of the child with OME includes health history, physical examination, and diagnostic testing.

HEALTH HISTORY

Determine the extent of symptoms. Children may be asymptomatic or may experience a popping sensation or fullness behind the eardrum. Explore the health history for risk factors such as passive smoking, absence of breastfeeding, frequent viral upper respiratory infections, allergy, or recent history of AOM.

PHYSICAL EXAMINATION AND DIAGNOSTIC TESTING

Otoscopic examination may reveal a dull, opaque tympanic membrane that may be white, gray, or bluish (Fig. 17.10). If the tympanic membrane is not opaque, a fluid level or air bubble may be visualized. Mobility may be absent or diminished upon pneumatic otoscopy. Tympanometry may be used to confirm the diagnosis of OME.

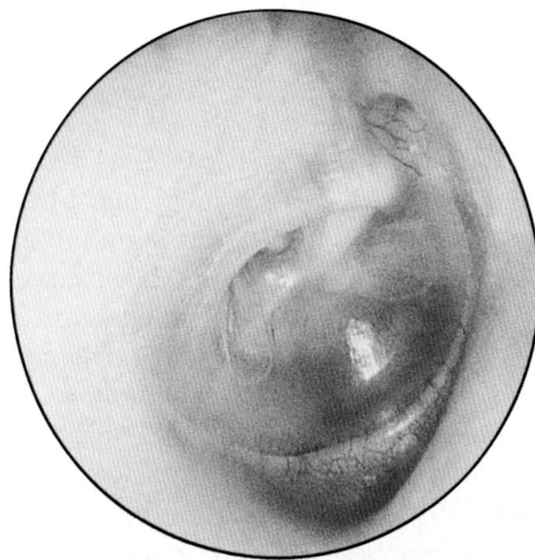

FIGURE 17.10 Otitis media with effusion; note dull white tympanic membrane.

Nursing Management

OME may take several months to resolve. Nursing management during the resolution phase focuses on education and monitoring for hearing loss.

EDUCATING THE FAMILY

Educate the family about the natural history of OME and the anatomic differences in young children that contribute to OME. Inform parents that antihistamines, decongestants, antibiotics, and corticosteroids have not been proven to hasten the resolution of OME and thus are not recommended. OME usually resolves spontaneously, but children should be rechecked every 4 weeks while this resolution is occurring. Teach parents not to feed infants in a supine position and to avoid bottle propping.

MONITORING FOR HEARING LOSS

When OME persists, the primary concern is its effect on hearing. In the infant or toddler who should be experiencing rapid language development, impaired hearing can depress language acquisition significantly (Yoon et al., 2022). Children with OME who are at risk for speech, language, or learning problems may be referred for evaluation of hearing earlier than a child with OME who is not at risk (Box 17.3). Children with chronic OME (persistent OME of 3 months' duration or longer) should be referred to a specialist for hearing evaluation (Pelton & Marom, 2022). Children who are not already at risk for speech concerns and are not experiencing difficulty with language acquisition may be reassessed every 3 to 6 months as long as hearing loss is not identified. At-risk children may require treatment earlier.

To communicate more effectively with children with OME who have hearing loss:

- Turn off music or television.
- Position yourself within 3 ft of the child before speaking.
- Face the child while speaking.
- Use visual cues.

BOX 17.3 Children at Risk for Speech, Language, or Learning Difficulties

- Permanent hearing loss (without otitis media with effusion)
- Speech/language delay (suspected or diagnosed)
- Craniofacial disorder that may interfere with speech
- Any pervasive developmental disorder
- Genetic disorders or syndromes associated with speech or learning problems
- Cleft palate
- Blindness or significant visual impairment

Data from Pelton, S., & Marom, T. (2022). Otitis media with effusion (serous otitis media) in children: Management. *UpToDate*. Retrieved January 23, 2024, from https://www.uptodate.com/contents/otitis-media-with-effusion-serous-otitis-media-in-children-management

- Increase the volume of your speech only slightly.
- Speak clearly.
- Request preferential classroom seating.

TAKE NOTE!

Evaluation of hearing is recommended when OME lasts 3 months or more if language delay, hearing loss, or a learning problem is suspected (Pelton & Marom, 2022).

PROVIDING POSTOPERATIVE CARE FOR THE CHILD WITH PRESSURE-EQUALIZING TUBES

Educate parents about the surgical insertion of **pressure-equalizing (PE) tubes** into the tympanic membrane (via myringotomy). Cover the following:

- PE tubes equalize the pressure behind the eardrum, allowing for tympanic membrane movement. This allows for adequate hearing, which in turn encourages speech development.
- The procedure is usually done as an outpatient surgery and the child returns home in the evening.
- The tubes stay in place for at least several months and generally fall out on their own (Fig. 17.11).
- Teach the parents to administer ear drops postoperatively if prescribed.
- Advise parents to have the child wear earplugs when swimming in potentially contaminated water such as lakes or rivers.
- Teach parents if the middle ear becomes infected with PE tubes in place, the tubes allow infected fluid to drain from the ear (if this occurs, they should contact their health care provider or nurse practitioner).

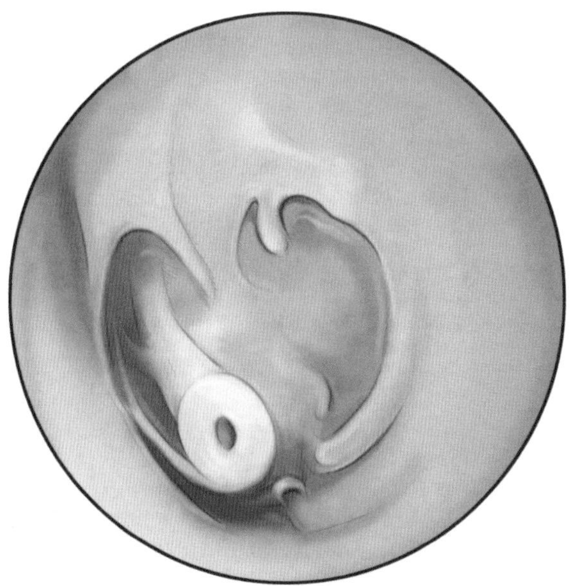

FIGURE 17.11 Pressure-equalizing tube in place in the tympanic membrane.

Otitis Externa

Otitis externa is defined as an infection and inflammation of the skin of the external ear canal. *Pseudomonas aeruginosa* and *Staphylococcus aureus* are typical causative agents, though fungi such as *Aspergillus* and other bacteria also may be implicated. Moisture in the canal contributes to pathogen growth (Yoon et al., 2022). Otitis externa is commonly known as "swimmer's ear" since it occurs more frequently in those who swim often (and thus have wet ear canals). Changing the pH in the ear canal contributes to the inflammatory process.

Nursing Assessment

Nursing assessment of the child with otitis externa focuses on the health history and physical examination.

HEALTH HISTORY

Elicit a description of the present illness and chief complaint. Note history of ear itching or pain, ear drainage, or a feeling of fullness in the ear canal, with possible difficulty hearing. Note onset and progression of symptoms, as well as the child's response to treatments. Explore the child's current and past medical history for risk factors such as previous episodes of otitis externa or history of recent swimming in a pool, lake, or ocean.

TAKE NOTE!

The child with otitis externa usually has significant ear pain. Pressure on the tragus should be avoided, as it can worsen the pain.

PHYSICAL EXAMINATION

Typically, a white or colored discharge can be seen in the ear canal or running from the ear. On otoscopy, the canal is red and edematous, often too swollen for insertion of the speculum and viewing of the tympanic membrane (Fig. 17.12). Diagnosis is based on clinical findings. Occasionally the ear drainage is cultured for bacteria or fungus, particularly if otitis externa is not improving with treatment.

Nursing Management

The primary goals of nursing management for otitis externa are pain relief, treatment of the infection, and prevention of recurrence.

MANAGING PAIN

Administer analgesics (possibly narcotics) to manage the pain. Apply a warm compress or heating pad to the affected ear as it is helpful in some children.

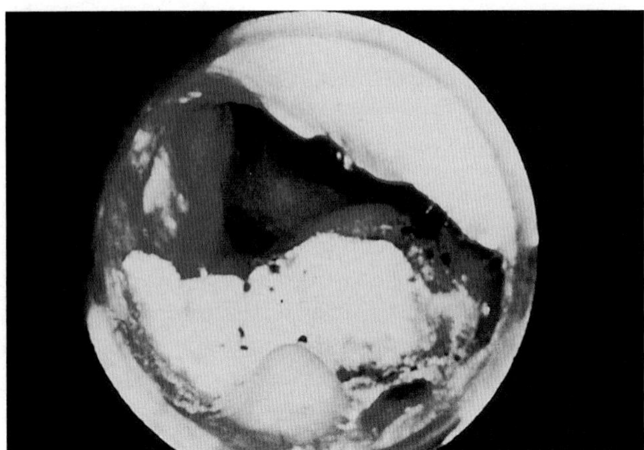

FIGURE 17.12 Note edema and erythema of the ear canal as well as purulent discharge in the child with otitis externa.

TREATING THE INFECTION

Administer antibiotic or antifungal eardrops as prescribed. If a wick is placed in the ear canal, teach the parents that it keeps the antibiotic drops in contact with the skin of the ear canal and promotes healing. Assist with wick insertion as it can be extremely painful, and younger children will need to be restrained during insertion for their safety.

PREVENTING REINFECTION

Teach children and their parents about prevention of further episodes once the infection has resolved. Since moisture contributes to otitis externa, explain the importance of keeping the ear canals dry. Encourage the child and parents to use one of the methods described in Teaching Guidelines 17.2 after swimming or showering.

TEACHING GUIDELINES 17.2 Preventing Otitis Externa

- Avoid the use of cotton swabs, headphones, and earphones.
- Wear earplugs when swimming.
- Promote ear canal dryness and alternate pH. Use one or more of the following methods:
  - Dry the ear canals using a hair dryer set on a lower setting.
  - Administer solutions that have a drying effect on the auditory canal skin and change the pH of the canal to discourage organism growth in susceptible children. The following solutions can be used:
    - A few drops of Domeboro solution can be placed in the canal and then allowed to run out.
    - A mixture of half rubbing alcohol and half vinegar (squirted into the canal and then allowed to run out). The alcohol solution should be used only when the ear canals are healthy. Using it while the canals are inflamed will cause stinging and increased pain.

Adapted from Johns Hopkins Medicine. (2023). *Swimmer's ear.* https://www.hopkinsmedicine.org/health/conditions-and-diseases/swimmers-ear

HEARING LOSS AND DEAFNESS

Infants are ordinarily born with the sense of hearing fully developed. Language development in infancy and early childhood is dependent upon adequate hearing, and even the fluctuating hearing loss associated with intermittent bouts of AOM can hinder language development (Pelton & Marom, 2022). Hearing loss may be unilateral (involving one ear) or bilateral (involving both ears). The extent of hearing loss is defined based on the softest intensity of sound that is perceived, described in **decibels** (dB). Levels of hearing loss are:

- 0 to 20 dB: normal
- 20 to 40 dB: mild loss
- 40 to 60 dB: moderate loss
- 60 to 80 dB: severe loss
- Greater than 80 dB: profound loss (American Speech-Language-Hearing Association [ASHA], 2024b)

Hearing loss may be congenital or acquired. Most congenital hearing loss is inherited through a single gene, or associated with a syndrome, though it also occurs as a result of prenatal infection (ASHA, 2024c). Premature infants and those with persistent pulmonary hypertension of the newborn are at increased risk for hearing loss compared with other infants. A variety of newborn universal hearing screening mandates have been passed by legislation in 43 states, thus allowing for earlier identification of infants with congenital hearing loss (National Center for Hearing Assessment and Management, 2024). See the Healthy People 2030 box.

HEALTHY PEOPLE 2030

Objective	Nursing Significance
Increase the proportion of newborns who are screened for hearing loss no later than age 1 month. Increase the proportion of infants who did not pass the hearing screening test who get evaluated for hearing loss no later than age 3 months. Increase the proportion of infants with confirmed hearing loss who are enrolled for intervention services no later than age 6 months.	• Encourage appropriate hearing assessments. • Refer children who are diagnosed with a hearing deficit to appropriate local services.

Healthy People Objectives retrieved from http://www.healthypeople.gov

Delayed-onset (acquired) hearing loss may be conductive, sensorineural, or mixed. **Conductive hearing loss** results when transmission of sound through the middle ear is disrupted, as in the case of OME. When fluid fills the middle ear, the tympanic membrane is unable to move properly, and partial or complete hearing loss occurs. **Sensorineural hearing loss** is caused by damage to the hair cells in the cochlea or along the auditory pathway. This may result from kernicterus, use of ototoxic medication, intrauterine infection with cytomegalovirus or rubella, neonatal or postnatal infection such as meningitis, severe neonatal respiratory depression, or exposure to excess noise. Mixed hearing loss occurs when the cause may be attributed to both conductive and sensorineural problems. Regardless of the cause of hearing loss, early intervention can make a difference in the child's ability to communicate. Once the hearing loss has been determined, intervention can begin. Hearing aids, cochlear implants, communication devices, and speech education may enable these children to communicate verbally. Improved communication beginning in infancy and early childhood may also improve the child's school achievement.

Nursing Assessment

Nursing assessment of the child with hearing loss or impairment focuses on the health history, physical examination, and diagnostic hearing testing.

Health History

Common symptoms reported during the health history might include:

- Infant:
  - Wakes only to touch, not environmental noises
  - Does not startle to loud noises
  - Does not turn to sound by 4 months of age
  - Does not babble at 6 months of age
  - Does not progress with speech development
- Young child:
  - Does not speak by 2 years of age
  - Communicates needs through gestures
  - Does not speak distinctly, as appropriate for their age
  - Displays developmental (cognitive) delays
  - Prefers solitary play
  - Displays immature emotional behavior
  - Does not respond to ringing of the telephone or doorbell
  - Focuses on facial expressions when communicating
- Older child:
  - Often asks for statements to be repeated
  - Is inattentive or daydreams
  - Performs poorly at school
  - Displays monotone or other abnormal speech
  - Gives inappropriate answers to questions except when able to view face of speaker
- At any age:
  - Speaks loudly
  - Sits close to the TV or radio or turns volume up too loud
  - Responds only to moderate or loud voices

Investigate signs of hearing loss as early as possible in order for appropriate intervention to begin. Explore the child's current and past medical history for risk factors such as congenital anomalies, genetic syndrome, infection, family history, kernicterus, neonatal ventilator use, ototoxic medication, or exposure to excess noise. Note whether newborn hearing screening was done and, if so, what the results were.

Physical Examination and Diagnostic Testing

Determine the child's level of interaction with the environment. For preschoolers and older children, administer the whisper test, keeping in mind that this is a gross screening test only. Perform the Weber and Rinne tests (refer to Chapter 9 for further explanation). If further evaluation is needed, the nurse may be responsible for administering an otoacoustic emissions test or auditory brain stem evoked response test, either in the hospital or in the outpatient office.

Nursing Management

The primary goal of nursing care for the child with a hearing impairment is to provide education and support to the family and child. Individualize care for the child with a hearing impairment and the family based on their specific responses to the hearing impairment.

Augmenting Hearing

Educate the family that compliance with hearing aids and communication curricula is critical so that the child can develop hearing and speech. Teach the child and family that hearing aids should be cleaned daily with a damp cloth and to change batteries weekly. For safety purposes, ensure parents understand that hearing aid batteries are a serious aspiration risk and should always be kept out of reach of young children. Teach parents when inserting the aid, the volume should be turned down, then adjusted to the appropriate level after insertion. Also teach families that as the infant or child grows, the hearing aid will need to be reassessed for proper fit. Many deaf schools and other organizations provide loaner hearing aids so that the best fit and amplification may be determined prior to purchase. Assist the family to explore this type of option in the local community. When cochlear implants are used, the nurse focuses on postoperative care of the incision site and pain management.

Promoting Communication and Education

Talk with families about how they need to learn how to communicate effectively with their child. If the child learns American Sign Language, for instance, the parents and siblings should as well. Table 17.4 provides information on communication options for hearing-impaired children and their families. Teach families that communication may also be enhanced by the use of text telephone service in the home, closed-caption television, and lights rather than bells or alarms to alert the child. Provide a sign language interpreter for the child at health care visits if the parent is not present for interpretation.

TABLE 17.4 • Comparing Communication Options for the Hearing Impaired

Spoken Language	
Oral deaf education (auditory-verbal therapy)	Uses technology to boost auditory potential; teaches children to notice sound and give it meaning. Develops oral speech
Cued speech	A system using hand signs to clarify lip-reading; gives the person clues about the sounds the speaker is making
Signed Language	
American Sign Language (ASL)	Entirely communicated through hand signs, gestures, and facial expressions. Has its own grammar and syntax
Combination: total communication	Combines auditory training and teaching of spoken language with "signing exact English" (corresponds to the words and syntax of English)
Augmentative and Alternative Communication (AAC)	
May use gestural communication	Can also include physical devices such as notebooks, communication boards, charts, or computers. Ranges from very low-tech to technologically complex

Data from American Speech-Language-Hearing Association. (2024a). *Augmentative and alternative communication.* http://www.asha.org/public/speech/disorders/AAC.htm

Encouraging Education

Refer the child younger than 3 years to the local district of Early Intervention for case management of developmental needs. Educate families that at 3 years of age and beyond, state laws provide for public education and related services for children with disabilities. Communicate to families that an IEP should be developed to maximize the child's learning ability. Contribute to the development of the IEP as appropriate.

Refer families to schools specifically geared toward deaf students depending upon the family's preferences and resources.

Providing Support

Encourage families to express their feelings as the diagnosis of a significant disability can be extremely stressful. Provide emotional support. Ensure that the needs of any siblings are also attended to. When the family is ready, encourage them to network with other families who have children with similar needs. Educate the family about the child's prescribed plan of care. Refer families to resources and support groups.

KEY CONCEPTS

- Though hearing is fully developed at birth, visual development continues to progress until about age 7 years.
- Binocular vision develops by age 4 months; visual acuity progresses to 20/50 by age 3 years and usually reaches 20/20 by about age 5 years.
- The relatively short and horizontally positioned eustachian tubes of infants and young children make them more susceptible to otitis media than adults.
- To maximize speech and language development, hearing loss should be identified early, and intervention begun immediately.
- Children with genetic syndromes or family history are at increased risk of visual and hearing impairments.
- The corneal light reflex test and cover test are useful tools for identifying strabismus and amblyopia.
- Tympanometry is used to determine the presence of fluid behind the eardrum (such as with OME).
- Topical ophthalmic medications are used to treat certain infectious eye disorders.
- Appropriate handwashing is the single most important factor to reduce the spread of acute viral or bacterial conjunctivitis.
- Systemic antibiotics are used for the treatment of periorbital cellulitis.
- Strabismus, glaucoma, and cataracts may all lead to visual impairment if left untreated.
- Asymmetry of the corneal light reflex occurs with true strabismus.
- Amblyopia must be identified early and treated with patching, corrective lenses, or surgery to prevent visual deterioration and promote appropriate vision development.
- A cloudy cornea indicates the presence of cataract.
- Very premature infants are at high risk of developing visual deficits related to ROP and are also at increased risk of hearing impairment compared to other infants.
- Eye strain, eye rubbing, and headaches may indicate a visual deficit.
- Children with visual disorders should be encouraged to use prescribed corrective lenses.
- Recurrent episodes of AOM may negatively affect the child's hearing.
- Recurrent or constant nasal congestion contributes to OME.
- Otitis externa can be prevented by keeping the ear canal dry and altering canal pH.
- The fluctuating hearing loss associated with recurrent otitis media and the hearing loss associated with

chronic OME can both significantly hinder language development in the infant and toddler.

- The child with hearing loss should receive early intervention with hearing aids or other augmentative devices.

REFERENCES AND RECOMMENDED READINGS

Algarni, A., Guyatt, G. H., Turner, A., & Alamri, S. (2022). Antibiotic patching for corneal abrasion. *Cochrane Database of Systematic Reviews, 5*, CD014617. https://doi.org/10.1002/14651858.CD014617.pub2

American Association for Pediatric Ophthalmology and Strabismus. (2023). *Glasses fitting for children*. https://aapos.org/viewdocument/glasses-fitting-for-children

American Speech-Language-Hearing Association. (2024a). *Augmentative and alternative communication*. https://www.asha.org/practice-portal/professional-issues/augmentative-and-alternative-communication/

American Speech-Language-Hearing Association. (2024b). *Degree of hearing loss*. https://www.asha.org/public/hearing/degree-of-hearing-loss/

American Speech-Language-Hearing Association. (2024c). *Hearing loss at birth (congenital hearing loss)*. https://www.asha.org/public/hearing/congenital-hearing-loss/

Bhatt, A. (2023). Retinopathy of prematurity: Risk factors, classification, and screening. *UpToDate*. Retrieved January 23, 2024, from https://www.uptodate.com/contents/retinopathy-of-prematurity-rop-risk-factors-classification-and-screening

Bregman, J., Sohal, P., Mishra, S., deBeaufort, H., Prakalapakorn, G., Bregman, J., Kumar, P., & Rodriguez, S. (2023). *Pediatric low vision*. https://eyewiki.aao.org/Pediatric_Low_Vision#Causes_of_Pediatric_Low_Vision

Coats, D. K. (2023). Vision screening and assessment in infants and children. *UpToDate*. Retrieved January 23, 2024, from https://www.uptodate.com/contents/vision-screening-and-assessment-in-infants-and-children

Coats, D. K., & Paysse, E. A. (2022). Amblyopia in children: Classification, screening, and evaluation. *UpToDate*. Retrieved January 23, 2024, from https://www.uptodate.com/contents/amblyopia-in-children-classification-screening-and-evaluation

Coats, D. K., & Paysse, E. A. (2023a). Amblyopia in children: Management and outcome. *UpToDate*. Retrieved January 23, 2024, from https://www.uptodate.com/contents/amblyopia-in-children-management-and-outcome

Coats, D. K., & Paysse, E. A. (2023b). Evaluation and management of strabismus in children. *UpToDate*. Retrieved January 23, 2024, from https://www.uptodate.com/contents/evaluation-and-management-of-strabismus-in-children

Coats, D. K., & Paysse, E. A. (2023c). Refractive errors in children. *UpToDate*. Retrieved January 23, 2024, from https://www.uptodate.com/contents/refractive-errors-in-children

Hammer, E. (n.d.). *Self-stimulation: Dr. Hammer responds*. http://www.nfb.org/images/nfb/Publications/fr/fr17/Issue3/F170308.htm

Howard, L. M., & Annabelle de St. Maurice, A. (2021). Unraveling the impact of pneumococcal conjugate vaccines on bacterial conjunctivitis in children. *Clinical Infectious Diseases, 72*(7), 1208–1210. https://doi.org/10.1093/cid/ciaa202

Jacobs, D. S. (2023a). Conjunctivitis. *UpToDate*. Retrieved January 23, 2024, from https://www.uptodate.com/contents/conjunctivitis

Jacobs, D. S. (2023b). Corneal abrasions and corneal foreign bodies: Management. *UpToDate*. Retrieved January 23, 2024, from http://www.uptodate.com/contents/corneal-abrasions-and-corneal-foreign-bodies-management

Johns Hopkins Medicine. (2023). *Swimmer's ear*. https://www.hopkinsmedicine.org/health/conditions-and-diseases/swimmers-ear

Lexicomp®. (2024). *Lexi-Drugs/tetrahydrozoline (ophthalmic)*. (Version 7.7.0) [Mobile app]. Wolters Kluwer. https://apps.apple.com/us/app/lexicomp/id313401238

McCreery, K. M. (2023). Cataract in children. *UpToDate*. Retrieved January 23, 2024, from https://www.uptodate.com/contents/cataract-in-children

Mehner, L., & Jung, J. L. (2022). Eye. In M. Bunik, W. W. Hay, M. J. Levin, & M. J. Abzug (Eds.), *Current diagnosis & treatment: Pediatrics* (26th ed.). McGraw-Hill Education.

National Center for Hearing Assessment and Management. (2024). *EDHI legislation: Overview*. http://www.infanthearing.org/legislation/

National Institute on Deafness and Other Communication Disorders. (2021). *Cochlear implants*. https://www.nidcd.nih.gov/health/cochlear-implants

Olitsky, S. E., & Marsh, J. D. (2020). Growth and development of the eye. In R. M. Kliegman, J. W. St. Geme, N. J. Blum, S. S. Shah, R. C. Tasker, & K. M. Wilson (Eds.), *Nelson textbook of pediatrics* (21st ed.). Elsevier Health Sciences.

Paysse, E. A., & Coats, D. K. (2023). Nasolacrimal duct obstruction (dacryostenosis) and dacryocystocele. *UpToDate*. Retrieved January 23, 2024, from https://www.uptodate.com/contents/congenital-nasolacrimal-duct-obstruction-dacryostenosis-and-dacryocystocele

Pelton, S., & Marchisio, P. (2023). Acute otitis media: Prevention of recurrence. *UpToDate*. Retrieved January 23, 2024, from https://www.uptodate.com/contents/acute-otitis-media-in-children-prevention-of-recurrence

Pelton, S., & Marom, T. (2022). Otitis media with effusion (serous otitis media) in children: Management. *UpToDate*. Retrieved January 23, 2024, from https://www.uptodate.com/contents/otitis-media-with-effusion-serous-otitis-media-in-children-management

Reynolds, J. D., & Reynolds, A. L. (2023). Primary infantile glaucoma. *UpToDate*. Retrieved November 17, 2023, from https://www.uptodate.com/contents/primary-infantile-glaucoma

UpToDate, Inc. (2024). *Lexicomp®* (Version 7.7.0) [Mobile app]. Wolters Kluwer. https://apps.apple.com/us/app/lexicomp/id313401238

U.S. Department of Health and Human Services. (n.d.). *Healthy People 2030*. https://health.gov/healthypeople

U.S. Food and Drug Administration. (2023). *Laser toys: How to keep kids safe*. https://www.fda.gov/consumers/consumer-updates/laser-toys-how-keep-kids-safe

VisionServe Alliance. (2023). *Interacting with children who are visually impaired*. https://visionservealliance.org/interacting-with-children-who-are-visually-impaired/

World Health Organization. (2023a). *Antibiotic resistance*. https://www.who.int/news-room/fact-sheets/detail/antimicrobial-resistance

World Health Organization. (2023b). *Blindness and vision impairment*. https://www.who.int/news-room/fact-sheets/detail/blindness-and-visual-impairment

Yoon, P. J., Scholes, M. A., & Herrmann, B. W. (2022). Ear, nose, & throat. In M. Bunik, W. W. Hay, M. J. Levin, & M. J. Abzug (Eds.), *Current diagnosis & treatment: Pediatrics* (26th ed.). McGraw-Hill Education.

DEVELOPING CLINICAL JUDGMENT

PRACTICING FOR NCLEX

1. Which situation would cause the nurse to become concerned about possible hearing loss?
   a. A 12-month-old who babbles incessantly, making no sense
   b. An 8-month-old who says only "da"
   c. A 3-month-old who startles easily to sound
   d. A 3-year-old who drops the letter "s"

2. A 4-year-old complains of extreme pain when the tragus is touched. Though not diagnostic, this sign is most indicative of which disorder?
   a. AOM
   b. Acute tympanic effusion
   c. Otitis interna
   d. Otitis externa

3. The nurse is caring for an infant who has undergone surgery for infantile glaucoma. What is the priority nursing intervention?
   a. Place the child prone postoperatively for comfort.
   b. Teach the family use of the contact lens.
   c. Place elbow restraints on the infant.
   d. Provide a mobile for optical stimulation.

4. A 2-year-old has been prescribed eye patching for strabismus 6 hours per day. What teaching does the nurse provide for the parent?
   a. Try to patch 6 hours per day, but if you miss some it is okay.
   b. Patching is necessary to strengthen vision in the weaker eye.
   c. Patching will keep the eye from turning in.
   d. Since the child is so young, patching can be delayed until school age.

5. The nurse is caring for a toddler with recurrent AOM. Which are risk factors for AOM? Select all that apply.
   a. Recurrent upper respiratory infection
   b. African American ethnicity
   c. Passive smoking
   d. Day care avoidance
   e. Absence of infant breastfeeding
   f. First episode of AOM after 12 months of age

6. A 16-month-old toddler was treated with amoxicillin for otitis media at 14 months of age. After non-resolution of the infection, the toddler was then prescribed amoxicillin-clavulanate. Two weeks later the toddler had OME. One month following that, OME persisted. Today, the toddler has a cold, is irritable and febrile, and is diagnosed with AOM. The toddler is at risk for ___ and ___ as a result of ___.

   Blanks 1 and 2:
   a. tympanic membrane perforation
   b. hearing impairment
   c. antibiotic resistance
   d. speech delay

   Blank 3:
   a. otitis externa
   b. upper respiratory infection
   c. persistent middle ear effusion
   d. lack of antibiotic adherence

DOSAGE CALCULATION QUESTION

The nurse is caring for a child with AOM. The child weighs 22 lb. The medication order reads: amoxicillin 160 mg PO every 8 hours. Amoxicillin is supplied as 200 mg/5 mL. How many milliliters will the nurse administer? Round to the nearest whole number.

CRITICAL THINKING EXERCISES

1. A 16-month-old toddler is being seen for his sixth ear infection. What particular information about his growth and development must the nurse ask about? Be specific about the questions you would ask.

2. How would you distinguish allergic conjunctivitis from acute bacterial conjunctivitis?

3. A 13-month-old has been diagnosed with severe visual impairment. Develop a list of sample nursing problems or concerns for this situation.

STUDY ACTIVITIES

1. Develop a sample plan for teaching a low-literacy parent about the etiology, treatment, and complications of recurrent AOM.

2. While in the pediatric clinical setting, compare the play styles of a sighted child with those of a visually impaired child.

3. Research hearing and vision resources in your local community.

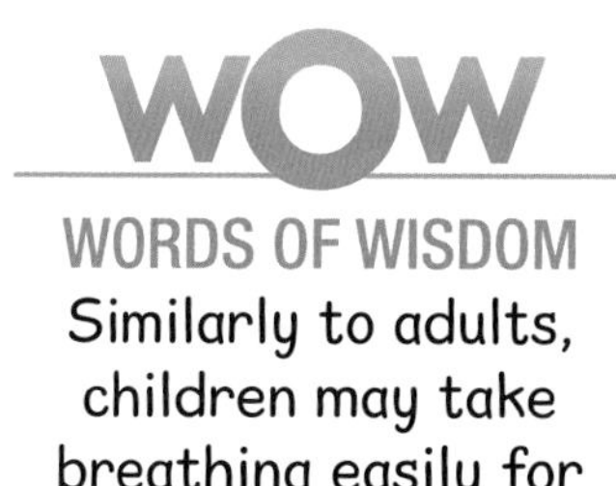

Similarly to adults, children may take breathing easily for granted.

18

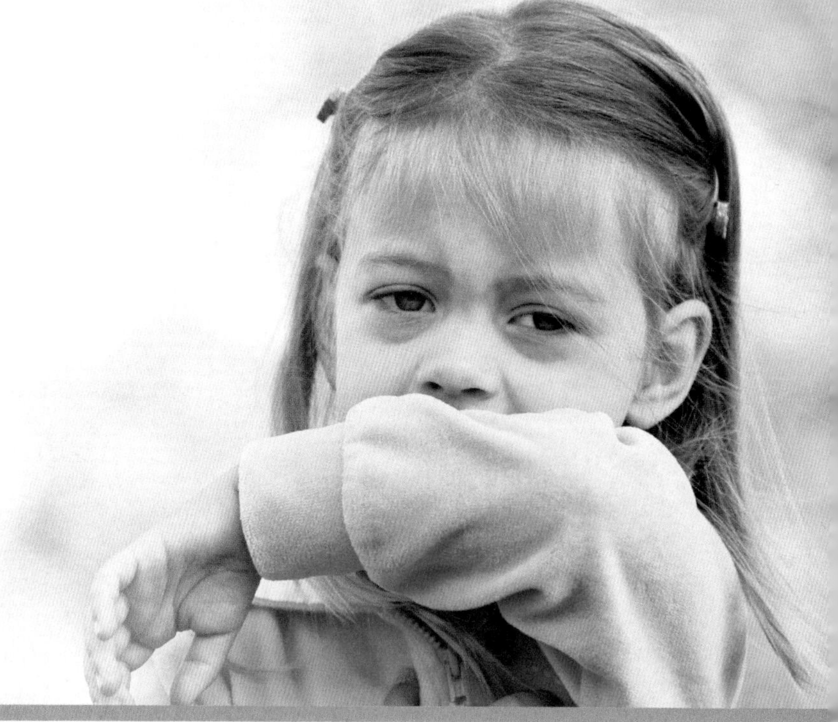

Nursing Care of the Child With an Alteration in Gas Exchange/ Respiratory Disorder

KEY TERMS

atelectasis (at′ĕ-lek′tă-sis)
atopy (at′ŏ-pē)
clubbing
coryza (kō-rī′ză)
cyanosis
hypoxemia
hypoxia
infiltrates
oxygenation
pulse oximetry
rales (rahlz)
retractions
rhinorrhea
stridor

LEARNING OBJECTIVES

Upon completion of the chapter, you will be able to:

1. Distinguish differences between the anatomy and the physiology of the respiratory system in children versus adults.
2. Identify various factors associated with respiratory illness in infants and children.
3. Discuss common laboratory and other diagnostic tests useful in the diagnosis of respiratory conditions.
4. Describe nursing care related to common medications and other treatments used for management and palliation of respiratory conditions.
5. Recognize risk factors associated with various respiratory disorders.
6. Distinguish different respiratory disorders based on their signs and symptoms.
7. Discuss nursing interventions commonly used for respiratory illnesses.
8. Devise an individualized nursing care plan or concept map for the child with a respiratory disorder.

suctioning
tachypnea (tak′ip-nē′ă)
tracheostomy
ventilation
wheezing
work of breathing

9. Develop child and family teaching plans for the child with a respiratory disorder.
10. Describe the psychosocial impact of chronic respiratory disorders on children.

Alexander Roberts, a 4-month-old, is brought into the clinic. He has a cold and has been coughing a great deal for 2 days. Today, he has had difficulty taking his bottle and is breathing very quickly. His parent says he seems tired.

INTRODUCTION

Gas exchange refers to the process by which oxygen is transported to cells and carbon dioxide is transported from cells (Giddens, 2021). Nurses encounter potential and actual alterations in gas exchange in all types of patients and must detect problems and intervene early to prevent life-threatening complications.

Alterations in gas exchange (respiratory disorders) are the most common causes of illness and hospitalization in children. These illnesses range from mild, nonacute disorders (such as the common cold or sore throat) to serious life-threatening conditions (such as epiglottitis). Chronic disorders, such as allergic rhinitis or asthma, can affect quality of life, but frequent acute or recurrent infections can also interfere significantly with the well-being of some children.

Children experience numerous respiratory infections. The child's age, socioeconomic status, and general health status can influence both the development of respiratory disorders and the course of the illness. Infants and younger children are more likely to deteriorate quickly from a respiratory illness, and children with chronic disorders such as diabetes, congenital heart disease, sickle cell anemia, cystic fibrosis (CF), and cerebral palsy tend to be more severely affected with respiratory disorders.

In addition, the season of the year can influence the development of respiratory disorders and the course of the illness. For example, certain viruses are more prevalent in the winter, whereas allergen-related respiratory diseases are more prevalent in the spring and fall.

Parents may have difficulty determining the severity of their child's condition and might either seek care early in the course of the illness (when it is still mild) or wait, presenting to the health care setting when the child is ill. Nurses must be familiar with respiratory conditions affecting children so that they can provide guidance and support to families. Difficulty with breathing can be frightening for both the child and the parents. Nurses must be able to ask questions that can help establish the severity of the child's illness and determine whether the family should seek care at a health care facility.

Since respiratory illnesses account for the majority of pediatric admissions to general hospitals, nurses caring for children need to have expert assessment and intervention skills in this area. Detection of worsening respiratory status early in the course of deterioration allows for timely treatment and the chance to prevent a minor problem from becoming a critical illness. Nurses are also in a unique position to provide education about respiratory illnesses and to promote efforts to prevent these illnesses.

VARIATIONS IN PEDIATRIC ANATOMY AND PHYSIOLOGY

Alterations in gas exchange/respiratory conditions often affect both the upper and the lower respiratory tract, although some affect primarily one or the other. Respiratory dysfunction in children tends to be more severe than in adults, and several differences in the infant's or child's respiratory system account for this increased severity.

Nose

Newborns are preferential nose breathers until at least 4 weeks of age. The young infant cannot automatically open their mouth to breathe if the nose is obstructed. The nares must be patent for breathing to be successful while feeding. Newborns breathe through their mouths only while crying.

The upper respiratory mucus serves as a cleansing agent, yet newborns produce very little mucus, making them more susceptible to infection. However, the newborn and young infant have very small nasal passages, so when excess mucus is present, airway obstruction is more likely (D. Smith, 2022).

Infants are born with maxillary and ethmoid sinuses present. The frontal sinuses (most often associated with sinus infection) and the sphenoid sinuses develop by age 6 to 8 years. Therefore, younger children are less apt to acquire sinus infections compared to adults.

Throat

The tongue of the infant relative to the oropharynx is larger than in adults. Posterior displacement of the tongue can quickly lead to severe airway obstruction.

Through early school age, children tend to have enlarged tonsillar and adenoidal tissue even in the absence of illness. This can contribute to an increased incidence of airway obstruction.

Trachea

The airway lumen is smaller in infants and children than in adults. The infant's trachea is approximately 4 mm wide, compared with that of adults, which is 20 mm. When edema, mucus, or bronchospasm is present, the capacity for air passage is greatly diminished. A small reduction in the diameter of a child's airway (resulting from the presence of edema or mucus) will result in an exponential increase in resistance to airflow (Fig. 18.1). Increased **work of breathing** (effort or labor associated with respiration) then occurs.

In adolescents and adults, the larynx is cylindrical and fairly uniform in width. In infants and children younger than 10 years old, the cricoid cartilage is underdeveloped, resulting in laryngeal narrowing (Nagler, 2022). Thus, in infants and children, the larynx is funnel-shaped. In addition, the larynx and glottis are located higher in the neck, increasing the chance of aspiration of foreign material into the lower airways. Congenital laryngomalacia occurs in some infants and results in the laryngeal structure being weaker than normal, yielding greater collapse on inspiration. Box 18.1 discusses congenital laryngomalacia.

The child's airway is highly compliant, making it quite susceptible to dynamic collapse in the presence of airway obstruction (Nagler, 2022). The muscles supporting the airway are less functional than those in the adult. Children have a large amount of soft tissue surrounding the trachea, and the mucous membranes lining the airway are less securely attached as compared with adults. This increases the risk for airway edema and obstruction. Upper airway obstruction resulting from a foreign body, croup, or epiglottitis can result in tracheal collapse during inspiration.

BOX 18.1 Congenital Laryngomalacia

- Inspiratory stridor is present and is intensified with certain positions.
- Suprasternal retractions may be present, but the infant exhibits no other signs of respiratory distress.
- Congenital laryngomalacia is generally a benign condition that improves as the cartilage in the larynx matures. It usually disappears by age 1 year.
- The crowing noise heard with breathing can make parents very anxious. Reassure parents that the condition will improve with time.
- Parents become very familiar with the "normal" sound their infant makes and are often able to identify intensification or change in the stridor. Airway obstruction may occur earlier in infants with this condition, so intensification of stridor or symptoms of respiratory illness should be evaluated early by the primary health care provider or nurse practitioner.

A

B

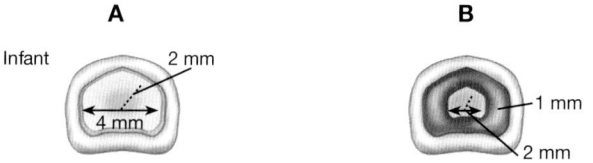

1 mm circumferential edema causes 50% reduction of diameter and radius, increasing pulmonary resistance by a factor of 16.

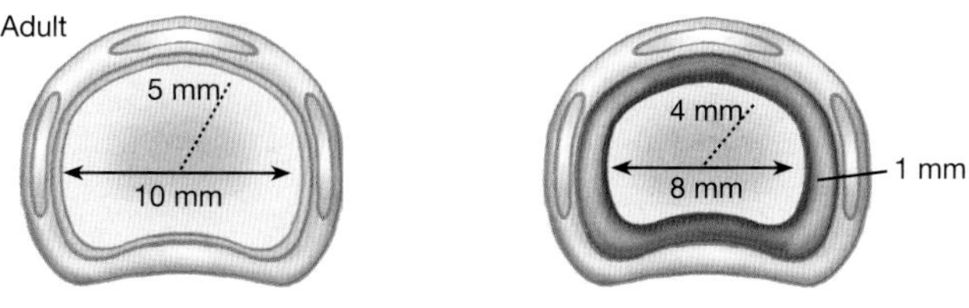

1 mm circumferential edema causes 20% reduction of diameter and radius, increasing pulmonary resistance by a factor of 2.4.

FIGURE 18.1 A. Note the smaller diameter of the child's airway under normal circumstances. **B.** With 1 mm of edema present, note the exponential decrease in airway lumen diameter as compared with the adult.

Lower Respiratory Structures

The bifurcation of the trachea occurs at the level of the third thoracic vertebra in children, compared with the level of the sixth thoracic vertebra in adults (Nagler, 2022). This anatomic difference is important when suctioning children and when endotracheal intubation is required (see Chapter 29 for further discussion). This difference in placement also contributes to the risk of foreign material aspiration. The bronchi and bronchioles of infants and children are narrower in diameter than the adult's, placing them at increased risk for lower airway obstruction (see Fig. 18.1). Lower airway obstruction during exhalation often results from bronchiolitis or asthma or is caused by foreign body aspiration into the lower airway.

Alveoli are developed at approximately 24 weeks' gestation. Term infants are born with about 150 million alveoli. At some point between 3 and 8 years of age, the child has developed the adult number of alveoli of around 300 million (Moore et al., 2020). Alveoli make up most of the lung tissue and are the major sites for gas exchange. Oxygen moves from the alveolar air to the blood, while carbon dioxide moves from the blood into the alveolar air. Smaller numbers of alveoli, particularly in the premature and/or young infant, place the child at a higher risk of hypoxemia (deficiency in the concentration of oxygen in arterial blood) and carbon dioxide retention.

Chest Wall

In older children and adults, the ribs and sternum support the lungs and help keep them well expanded. The movement of the diaphragm and intercostal muscles alters volume and pressure within the chest cavity, resulting in air movement into the lungs. Infants' chest walls are highly compliant (pliable) and fail to support the lungs adequately. Functional residual capacity can be greatly reduced if respiratory effort is diminished. This lack of lung support also makes the tidal volume of infants and toddlers almost completely dependent on movement of the diaphragm. If diaphragm movement is impaired (as in states of hyperinflation, such as asthma), the intercostal muscles cannot lift the chest wall, and respiration is further compromised.

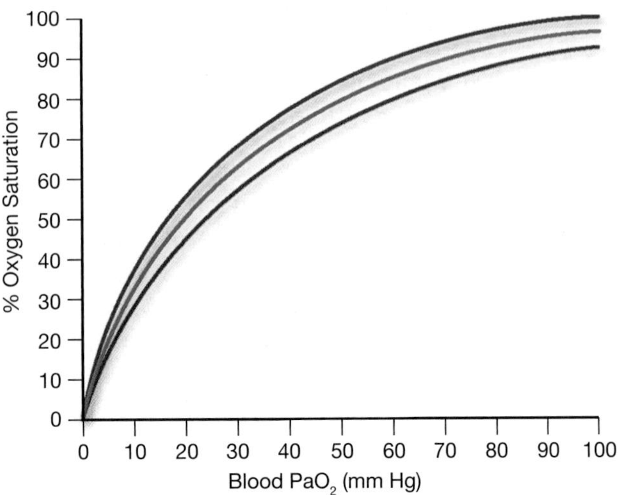

FIGURE 18.2 Normal hemoglobin dissociation curve (green), shift to the right (red), and shift to the left (blue).

Metabolic Rate and Oxygen Need

Children have a significantly higher metabolic rate than adults. Their resting respiratory rates are faster, and their demand for oxygen is higher. Adult oxygen consumption is 3 to 4 L per minute, while infants consume 6 to 8 L per minute. In any situation of respiratory distress, infants and children will develop hypoxemia more rapidly than adults (Weiner, 2022). This may be attributed not only to the child's increased oxygen requirement but also to the effect that certain conditions have on the oxyhemoglobin dissociation curve.

Normal oxygen transport relies on binding of oxygen to hemoglobin in areas of high partial pressure of oxygen (paO_2) (pulmonary arterial beds) and release of oxygen from hemoglobin when the paO_2 is low (peripheral tissues). Normally, a paO_2 of 95 mm Hg results in an oxygen saturation of 97%. A decrease in oxygen saturation results in a disproportionate (much larger) decrease in pO_2 (Fig. 18.2). Thus, a small decrease in oxygen saturation reflects a larger decrease in paO_2. Conditions such as alkalosis, hypothermia, hypocarbia, anemia, and fetal hemoglobin cause oxygen to become more tightly bound to hemoglobin, resulting in the curve shifting to the left. Common pediatric conditions such as acidosis, hyperthermia, and hypercarbia cause hemoglobin to decrease its affinity for oxygen, shifting the curve further to the right.

COMMON MEDICAL TREATMENTS

A variety of interventions are used to treat respiratory illness in children. The treatments listed in Common Medical Treatments 18.1 and Drug Guide 18.1 usually require a primary health care provider or nurse practitioner's order when a child is hospitalized.

COMMON MEDICAL TREATMENTS 18.1 Respiratory Disorders

Treatment	Explanation	Indications	Nursing Implications
Oxygen	Supplemented via mask, nasal cannula, hood, or tent or via endotracheal or nasotracheal tube	Hypoxemia, respiratory distress	Monitor response via work of breathing and pulse oximetry.
High humidity	Addition of moisture to inspired air	Common cold, croup, tonsillectomy	Infant may require extra blankets with cool mist and frequent changes of bedclothes under oxygen hood or tent as they become damp.
Suctioning	Removal of secretions via bulb syringe or suction catheter	Excessive airway secretions (common cold, flu, bronchiolitis, pertussis)	Should be done carefully and only as far as recommended for age or tracheostomy tube size or until cough or gag occurs
Chest physiotherapy (CPT) and postural drainage	Promotes mucus clearance by mobilizing secretions with the assistance of percussion or vibration accompanied by postural drainage	Bronchiolitis, pneumonia, cystic fibrosis, or other conditions resulting in increased mucus production; not effective in inflammatory conditions without increased mucus	May be performed by respiratory therapist in some institutions, by nurses in others; in either case, nurses must be familiar with the technique and able to educate families on its use.

COMMON MEDICAL TREATMENTS 18.1 Respiratory Disorders

Treatment	Explanation	Indications	Nursing Implications
Saline gargles	Relieves throat pain via saltwater gargle	Pharyngitis, tonsillitis	Recommended for children old enough to understand the concept of gargling (to avoid choking)
Saline lavage	Normal saline introduced into the airway, followed by suctioning	Common cold, flu, bronchiolitis, any condition resulting in increased mucus production in the upper airway	Helpful for loosening thick mucus; child may need to be in semi-upright position to avoid aspiration.
Chest tube	Insertion of a drainage tube into the pleural cavity to facilitate removal of air or fluid and allow full lung expansion	Pneumothorax, empyema	Should tube become dislodged from container, the chest tube must be clamped immediately or the open end placed into a container of sterile water to avoid further air entry into the chest cavity.
Bronchoscopy	Introduction of a bronchoscope into the bronchial tree for diagnostic purposes; also allows for bronchiolar lavage	Removal of foreign body, cleansing of bronchial tree	Watch for postprocedure airway swelling, complaints of sore throat.

DRUG GUIDE 18.1

COMMON DRUGS FOR RESPIRATORY DISORDERS

Medication	Actions/Indications	Nursing Implications
Expectorant (guaifenesin)	Reduces viscosity of thickened secretions by increasing respiratory tract fluid Used for the common cold, pneumonia, and other conditions requiring mobilization and subsequent expectoration of mucus	Encourage deep breathing before coughing to mobilize secretions. Maintain adequate fluid intake. Assess breath sounds frequently.
Cough suppressants (dextromethorphan, codeine, hydrocodone)	Relieve irritating, nonproductive cough by direct effect on the cough center in the medulla, which suppresses the cough reflex Used for the common cold, sinusitis, pneumonia, bronchitis	Should be used only with nonproductive coughs in the absence of wheezing
Antihistamines	Treatment of allergic conditions such as allergic rhinitis, asthma	May cause drowsiness or dry mouth
Antibiotics (oral, parenteral)	Treatment of bacterial infections of the respiratory tract such as pharyngitis, tonsillitis, sinusitis, bacterial pneumonia, cystic fibrosis, empyema, abscess, tuberculosis	Check for antibiotic allergies. Should be given as prescribed for the length of time prescribed
Antibiotics (inhaled)	Treatment of bacterial infections of the respiratory tract in children with cystic fibrosis	Can be given via nebulizer
Beta$_2$-adrenergic agonists (short acting) (i.e., albuterol, levalbuterol, pirbuterol)	Relax airway smooth muscle, resulting in bronchodilation Used for acute and chronic treatment of wheezing and bronchospasm in asthma, bronchiolitis, cystic fibrosis, chronic lung disease; also used to prevent wheezing in exercise-induced asthma	Administered via inhalation Can be used for acute relief of bronchospasm May cause nervousness, tachycardia, and jitteriness Inhaled agents result in fewer systemic side effects.
Beta$_2$-adrenergic agonists (long acting) (i.e., formoterol, salmeterol)	Long-acting bronchodilator used in chronic asthma management and for prevention of exercise-induced asthma Long-term control in chronic asthma Prevention of exercise-induced asthma	Administered via inhalation Used only for long-term control or for exercise-induced asthma. Not for relief of bronchospasm in an acute wheezing episode
Racemic epinephrine	Produces bronchodilation Indicated for croup	Assess lung sounds and work of breathing. Observe for rebound bronchospasm.

(continued)

DRUG GUIDE 18.1 (*continued*)

COMMON DRUGS FOR RESPIRATORY DISORDERS

Medication	Actions/Indications	Nursing Implications
Anticholinergic (ipratropium)	Produces bronchodilation in asthma or chronic lung disease	In children, generally used as an adjunct to beta$_2$-adrenergic agonists for treatment of bronchospasm
Antiviral agents (oral: amantadine, rimantadine, oseltamivir: inhaled zanamivir)	Treatment and prevention of influenza A	Amantadine, rimantadine: monitor for confusion, nervousness, and jitteriness. Oseltamivir, zanamivir: well tolerated but expensive
Corticosteroids (inhaled) (beclomethasone, budesonide, fluticasone, mometasone)	Exert a potent, locally acting antiinflammatory effect to decrease the frequency and severity of asthma attacks; may also delay pulmonary damage that occurs with chronic asthma; also used for chronic lung disease and croup syndromes	Not for treatment of acute wheezing Rinse mouth after inhalation to decrease incidence of fungal infections, dry mouth, and hoarseness. Minimal systemic absorption makes inhaled steroids the treatment of choice for asthma maintenance program.
Corticosteroids (oral, parenteral) (prednisolone, prednisone)	Suppress inflammation and normal immune response Used for acute asthma exacerbations, wheezing with chronic lung disease, and severe croup	May cause hyperglycemia May suppress reaction to allergy tests Consult health care provider if vaccinations are ordered during course of systemic corticosteroid therapy. Short courses of therapy are generally safe. Although effective, long-term or chronic use can result in peptic ulceration, altered growth, and numerous other side effects. Children on long-term dosing should have growth assessed.
Decongestants (e.g., pseudoephedrine)	Treatment of runny or stuffy nose associated with the common cold, sinusitis, or allergic rhinitis in children older than age 6	Assess child periodically for nasal congestion. Some children react to decongestants with excessive sleepiness or increased activity.
Leukotriene receptor antagonists (montelukast, zafirlukast)	Decrease inflammatory response by antagonizing the effects of leukotrienes to control asthma in children age 1 year and older Montelukast: for allergic rhinitis in children 6 months and older	Given once daily, in the evening Not for relief of bronchospasm during an acute wheezing episode, but may be continued during the episode
Mast cell stabilizers (cromolyn, nedocromil)	Prevent release of histamine from sensitized mast cells, resulting in decreased frequency and intensity of allergic reactions in children with asthma or chronic lung disease; also used as preexposure treatment for allergens	Administered via inhalation For prophylactic use, not to relieve bronchospasm during an acute wheezing episode; can be used 10–15 minutes prior to exposure to allergen, to decrease reaction to allergen
Respiratory stimulants (methylxanthines: theophylline, aminophylline, caffeine)	To provide for continuous airway relaxation in moderate or severe asthma to achieve long-term control (methylxanthines)	Administered orally or intravenously; sustained-release oral preparation can be used to prevent nocturnal symptoms. Monitor drug levels routinely. Report signs of toxicity immediately: tachycardia, nausea, vomiting, diarrhea, stomach cramps, anorexia, confusion, headache, restlessness, flushing, increased urination, seizures, arrhythmias, insomnia.
Inhaled pulmonary enzyme (dornase alfa)	Enzyme that hydrolyzes the DNA in sputum, reducing sputum viscosity in children with cystic fibrosis	Administered via nebulizer Monitor for dysphonia and pharyngitis.

Data from UpToDate, Inc. (2023). *Lexi-comp®* (Version 7.7.0) [Mobile app]. Wolters Kluwer. https://apps.apple.com/us/app/lexicomp/id313401238

COMMON LABORATORY AND DIAGNOSTIC TESTS 18.1

Alterations in Oxygenation/Respiratory Disorders

Test	Explanation	Indications	Nursing Implications
Allergy skin testing	Suggested allergen is applied to skin via scratch, pin, or prick. A wheal response indicates allergy to the substance.	Allergic rhinitis, asthma	Antihistamines must be discontinued before testing, as they inhibit the test. Close observation for anaphylaxis is necessary. Epinephrine and emergency equipment should be readily available. Some children react to the skin test almost immediately; others take several minutes.
Arterial blood gases	Invasive method (requires blood sampling) of measuring arterial pH, partial pressure of oxygen and carbon dioxide, and base excess in blood	Usually reserved for severe illness, the intubated child, or suspected carbon dioxide retention	Hold pressure for several minutes after a peripheral arterial stick to avoid bleeding. Radial arterial sticks are common and can be very painful. Note if the child is crying excessively during the blood draw, as this affects the carbon dioxide level.
Chest radiograph	Radiographic image of the expanded lungs: can show hyperinflation, atelectasis, pneumonia, foreign body, pleural effusion, abnormal heart or lung size	Bronchiolitis, pneumonia, tuberculosis, asthma, cystic fibrosis, bronchopulmonary dysplasia	Children may be afraid of the x-ray equipment. If a parent or familiar adult can accompany the child, often the child is less afraid. If the child is unable or unwilling to hold still for the x-ray, restraint may be necessary. Restraint should be limited to the amount of time needed for the x-ray.
Fluorescent antibody testing	Determines presence of respiratory syncytial virus (RSV), adenovirus, influenza, parainfluenza, or *Chlamydia* in nasopharyngeal secretions	Bronchiolitis, pneumonia	To obtain a nasopharyngeal specimen, instill 1–3 mL of sterile normal saline into one nostril, aspirate the contents using a small sterile bulb syringe, place the contents in sterile container, and immediately send them to the lab.
Fluoroscopy	Radiographic examination that uses a fluorescent screen for real-time imaging	Identification of masses, abscesses	Requires the child to lie still. Equipment can be frightening. Children may respond to presence of parent or familiar adult.
Gastric washings for AFB	Determines presence of AFB (acid-fast bacilli) in stomach (children often swallow sputum)	Tuberculosis	Nasogastric tube is inserted, and saline is instilled and suctioned out of the stomach to obtain the specimen.
Peak expiratory flow	Measures the maximum flow of air (in L/s) that can be forcefully exhaled in 1 second	Daily use can indicate adequacy of asthma control.	It is important to establish the child's "personal best" by taking twice-daily readings over a 2-week period while well. The average of these is termed "personal best." Charts based on height and age are also available to determine expected peak expiratory flow.
Pulmonary function tests	Measure respiratory flow and lung volumes	Asthma, cystic fibrosis, chronic lung disease	Usually performed by a respiratory therapist trained to do the full spectrum of tests. Spirometry can be obtained by the trained nurse in the outpatient setting.
Pulse oximetry	Noninvasive method of continuously (or intermittently) measuring oxygen saturation	Can be useful in any situation in which a child is experiencing respiratory distress	Probe must be applied correctly to finger, toe, foot, hand, forehead, or ear for the machine to appropriately pick up the pulse and oxygen saturation.
Rapid flu test	Rapid test for detection of influenza A or B	Influenza	Should be done in first 24 hours of illness so that medication administration can begin Have the child gargle with sterile normal saline and then spit into a sterile container. Send immediately to the lab.
Rapid strep test	Instant test for presence of streptococcus A antibody in pharyngeal secretions	Pharyngitis, tonsillitis	Results in 5–10 minutes; negative tests should be backed up with throat culture.

(*continued*)

COMMON LABORATORY AND DIAGNOSTIC TESTS 18.1 (*continued*)

Alterations in Oxygenation/Respiratory Disorders

Test	Explanation	Indications	Nursing Implications
RAST (radioallergosorbent test)	Measures minute quantities of immunoglobulin E in the blood Carries no risk of anaphylaxis but is not as sensitive as skin testing	Asthma (food allergies)	Blood test that is usually sent out to a reference laboratory
Sinus radiographs, computed tomography (CT), or magnetic resonance imaging (MRI)	Radiologic tests that may show sinus involvement	Sinusitis, recurrent colds	X-ray results are usually received more quickly than CT or MRI results.
Sputum culture	Bacterial culture of invasive organisms in the sputum	Pneumonia, cystic fibrosis, tuberculosis	Must be true sputum, not mucus from the mouth or nose; child can deep breathe, cough, and spit, or specimen may be obtained via suctioning of the artificial airway.
Sweat chloride test	Collection of sweat on filter paper after stimulation of skin with pilocarpine Measures concentration of chloride in the sweat	Cystic fibrosis	May be difficult to obtain sweat in a young infant
Throat culture	Bacterial culture (minimum of 24–48 hours required) to determine presence of streptococcus A or other bacteria	Pharyngitis, tonsillitis	Can be obtained on separate swab at same time as rapid strep test to decrease trauma to the child (swab both applicators at once); do not perform immediately after the child has had medication or something to eat or drink.
Tuberculin skin test	Mantoux test (intradermal injection of purified protein derivative)	Tuberculosis, chronic cough	Must be given intradermally; not a valid test if injected incorrectly

Data from Corbett, J. A., & Banks, A. D. (2019). *Laboratory tests and diagnostic procedures with nursing diagnoses* (9th ed.). Pearson Education Inc.; Medtronic. (2023). *Pulse oximetry.* https://www.medtronic.com/covidien/en-us/products/pulse-oximetry.html

Clinical Judgment and the Nursing Process for the Child With a Respiratory Disorder

Care of the child with a respiratory disorder includes assessment, nursing analysis, planning, interventions, and evaluation. There are several general concepts related to the nursing process that can be applied to respiratory disorders. From an overall understanding of the care involved for a child with an alteration in gas exchange, the nurse can then individualize the care based on specifics for the particular child.

Assessment

Assessment of respiratory dysfunction in children includes health history, physical examination, and laboratory or diagnostic testing.

Health History

The health history consists of the past medical history, family history, and history of present illness (when the symptoms started and how they have progressed), as well as treatments used at home. Ascertain immunization history. The past medical history might be significant for recurrent colds or sore throats, **atopy** (genetic tendency toward asthma, allergic rhinitis, or atopic dermatitis), prematurity, respiratory dysfunction at birth, poor weight gain, or history of recurrent respiratory illnesses or chronic lung disease. Family history might be significant for chronic respiratory disorders such as asthma or might reveal contacts for infectious exposure. When eliciting the history of the present illness, inquire about onset and progression; fever; nasal congestion; noisy breathing; presence and description of cough; rapid respirations; increased work of breathing; ear, nose, sinus, or throat pain; ear pulling; headache; vomiting with coughing; poor feeding; and lethargy. Also inquire about exposure to second-hand smoke. Children exposed to environmental smoke have an increased incidence of respiratory infections, acute otitis media, and asthma exacerbations (Centers

HEALTHY PEOPLE 2030

Objective	Nursing Significance
Reduce the proportion of people exposed to second-hand smoke.	• Educate the family about the effects that passive smoking has on children. • Encourage families to join smoking cessation programs.

Healthy People Objectives retrieved from http://www.healthypeople.gov

for Disease Control and Prevention [CDC], 2022). See the Healthy People 2030 box.

Physical Examination

Physical examination of the respiratory system includes inspection and observation, auscultation, percussion, and palpation.

Inspection and Observation

Inspection and observation of the respiratory system includes assessing color, overall appearance, respiratory rate, and hydration status; inspecting the nose and oral cavity as well as the nail beds for clubbing; observing work of breathing; and audibly listening for cough and other airway noises.

COLOR

Observe the child's skin color, noting pallor or cyanosis (circumoral or central). Pallor (pale appearance) occurs as a result of peripheral vasoconstriction in an effort to conserve oxygen for vital functions. **Cyanosis** (a bluish tinge to the skin and mucous membranes) occurs as a result of hypoxia (oxygen deficiency). It might first present circumorally (just around the mouth) and progress to central cyanosis. In darker-skinned individuals, areas with the least amount of pigment may demonstrate cyanosis. Check the conjunctiva, oral mucosa, nail beds, palms, or soles for a bluish tint or the lips and tongue for a gray or white color (Pusey-Reid et al., 2023).

Newborns might have blue hands and feet (acrocyanosis), a normal finding. The infant might have pale hands and feet when cold or when ill, as peripheral circulation is not well developed in early infancy. It is important, then, to note if the cyanosis is central (involving the midline), as this is a true sign of hypoxia. Children with low red blood cell counts might not demonstrate cyanosis as early in the course of hypoxemia as children with normal hemoglobin levels. Therefore, absence of cyanosis or the degree of cyanosis present is not always an accurate indication of the severity of respiratory involvement.

Note the rate and depth of respiration as well as work of breathing. Often, the first sign of respiratory illness in infants and children is **tachypnea** (increased respiratory rate for age).

> **TAKE NOTE!**
>
> A slow or irregular respiratory rate in an acutely ill infant or child is an ominous sign (Weiner, 2022). See Chapter 29.

NOSE AND ORAL CAVITY

Inspect the nose and oral cavity. Note nasal drainage and redness or swelling in the nose. Note the color of the pharynx, presence of exudate, tonsil size, and status and presence of lesions anywhere in the oral cavity.

COUGH AND OTHER AIRWAY NOISES

Note the sound of the cough (Is it wet or productive, dry and hacking, tight? When does the cough occur? Is it only or mainly at night?). Also note if noises associated with breathing are present (e.g., grunting, stridor, or audible wheeze). Grunting occurs on expiration and is produced by premature glottic closure. It is an attempt to preserve or increase functional residual capacity. Grunting might occur with alveolar collapse or loss of lung volume, such as in **atelectasis** (a collapsed or airless portion of the lung), pneumonia, and pulmonary edema. **Stridor**, a high-pitched, readily audible inspiratory noise, is a sign of upper airway obstruction. Sometimes, wheezes can be heard with the naked ear; these are referred to as audible wheezes.

RESPIRATORY EFFORT

Assess respiratory effort for depth and quality. Is breathing labored? Infants and children with significant nasal congestion may have tachypnea, which usually resolves when the nose is cleared of mucus. Mouth breathing may occur when a large amount of nasal congestion is present. Increased work of breathing, particularly if associated with restlessness and anxiety, usually indicates lower respiratory involvement. Assess for the presence of nasal flaring, retractions, or bobbing of the head with each breath. Nasal flaring can occur early in the course of respiratory illness and is an effort to inhale greater amounts of oxygen.

RETRACTIONS

Retractions (the inward pulling of soft tissues with respiration) can occur in the intercostal, subcostal, substernal, supraclavicular, or suprasternal regions

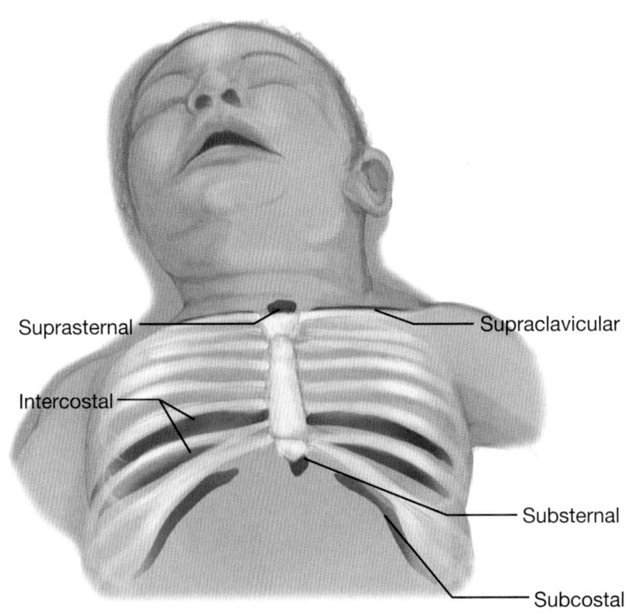

FIGURE 18.3 Location of retractions.

(Fig. 18.3). Document the severity of the retractions: mild, moderate, or severe. Also note the use of accessory neck muscles. Note the presence of paradoxical breathing (lack of simultaneous chest and abdominal rise with the inspiratory phase).

TAKE NOTE!

Seesaw (or paradoxical) respirations are very ineffective for **ventilation** (gas exchange) and **oxygenation** (binding of oxygen). The chest falls on inspiration and rises on expiration.

ANXIETY AND RESTLESSNESS

Is the child anxious or restless? Restlessness, irritability, and anxiety result from difficulty in securing adequate oxygen. These might be early signs of respiratory distress, especially if accompanied by tachypnea. Restlessness might progress to listlessness and lethargy if the respiratory dysfunction is not corrected.

CLUBBING

Inspect the fingertips for the presence of **clubbing**, an enlargement of the terminal phalanx of the finger, resulting in a change in the angle of the nail to the fingertip (Fig. 18.4). Clubbing might occur in children with a chronic respiratory illness. It is the result of increased capillary growth as the body attempts to supply more oxygen to distal body cells.

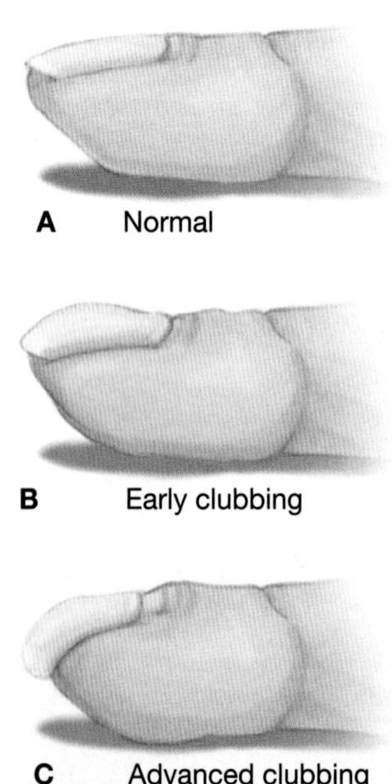

FIGURE 18.4 Normal fingertip (**A**). Early clubbing (**B**) may progress eventually to advanced clubbing (**C**) as a result of chronic hypoxemia.

HYDRATION STATUS

Note the child's hydration status. Palpate the infant's fontanels to determine if sunken. Assess the oral mucosa for color and moisture. Note skin turgor, presence of tears, and adequacy of urine output. The child with a respiratory illness is at risk for dehydration. Pain related to sore throat or mouth lesions may prevent the child from drinking properly. Nasal congestion interferes with the infant's ability to suck effectively at the breast or bottle. Tachypnea and increased work of breathing interfere with the ability to safely ingest fluids.

Palpation

Palpate the sinuses for tenderness in the older child. Assess for enlargement or tenderness of the lymph nodes of the head and neck. Document alterations in tactile fremitus detected on palpation. Increased tactile fremitus might occur in the case of pneumonia or pleural effusion. Fremitus might be decreased in the case of barrel chest, as with CF. Absent fremitus might be noted with pneumothorax or atelectasis.

Compare central and peripheral pulses. Note the quality of the pulse as well as the rate. With significant respiratory distress, perfusion often becomes compromised. Poor perfusion might be reflected in weaker peripheral pulses (radial, pedal) when compared with central pulses.

Percussion

When percussing, note sounds that are not resonant in nature. Flat or dull sounds might be percussed over partially consolidated lung tissue, as in pneumonia. Tympany might be percussed with a pneumothorax. Note the presence of hyperresonance (as might be apparent with asthma).

Auscultation

Assess lung sounds via auscultation. Evaluate breath sounds over the anterior and posterior chest, as well as in the axillary areas. Note the adequacy of aeration. Breath sounds should be equal bilaterally. The intensity and pitch should be equal throughout the lungs; document diminished breath sounds. In the absence of concurrent lower respiratory illness, the breath sounds should be clear throughout all lung fields. During normal respiration, the inspiratory phase is usually softer and longer than the expiratory phase. Prolonged expiration is a sign of bronchial or bronchiolar obstruction. Bronchiolitis, asthma, pulmonary edema, and an intrathoracic foreign body can cause prolonged expiratory phases.

Infants and young children have thin chest walls. When the upper airway is congested (as in a severe cold), the noise produced in the upper airway might be transmitted throughout the lung fields. When upper airway congestion is transmitted to the lung fields, the congested sounding noise heard over the trachea is the same type of noise heard over the lungs but is much louder and more intense. To ascertain if these sounds are truly adventitious lung sounds or if they are transmitted from the upper airway, auscultate again after the child coughs or their nose has been suctioned. Another way to discern the difference is to compare auscultatory findings over the trachea to the lung fields to determine if the abnormal sound is truly from within the lung or is actually a sound transmitted from the upper airway.

Note adventitious sounds heard on auscultation. **Wheezing**, a high-pitched sound that usually occurs on expiration, results from obstruction in the lower trachea or bronchioles. Wheezing that clears with coughing is most likely a result of secretions in the lower trachea. Wheezing resulting from obstruction of the bronchioles, as in bronchiolitis, asthma, chronic lung disease, or CF, does not clear with coughing. **Rales** (crackling sounds) result when the alveoli become fluid filled, such as in pneumonia. Note the location of the adventitious sounds as well as the timing (on inspiration, expiration, or both). Tachycardia might also be present. An increase in heart rate often initially accompanies hypoxemia.

Laboratory and Diagnostic Testing

Common Laboratory and Diagnostic Tests 18.1 explains the laboratory and diagnostic tests most commonly used for a child with a respiratory disorder. The tests can assist the primary health care provider or nurse practitioner in diagnosing the disorder and/or be used as guidelines in determining ongoing treatment. Laboratory or nonnursing personnel obtain some of the tests, while the nurse might obtain others. In either instance, it is important for the nurse to be familiar with how the tests are obtained, what they are used for, and normal versus abnormal results. This knowledge will also be necessary when providing child and family education related to the testing.

> Remember Alexander, the 4-month-old with the cold, cough, fatigue, feeding difficulty, and fast breathing? What additional health history and physical examination assessment information should the nurse obtain?

Nursing Analysis

After recognizing and analyzing cues from a thorough assessment, the nurse might identify several patient problems, including:

- Ineffective airway clearance
- Ineffective breathing pattern
- Impaired gas exchange
- Deficient fluid volume risk
- Imbalanced nutrition (less than body requirements)
- Activity intolerance
- Fear
- Pain
- Interrupted family processes
- Caregiver role strain risk
- Deficient knowledge

> After completing an assessment of Alexander, what would your top three patient problems be?

The preceding patient problems or concerns provide suggestions for nursing care planning or concept mapping. Suggested interventions with rationales are provided further on. Care planning should be individualized, based on the child's and family's needs. Refer to Chapter 14 for the nursing process for pain management and to Chapter 11 for nursing interventions related to interrupted family processes and for caregiver role strain risk. Additional information will be included later in the chapter as it relates to nursing management of children with specific disorders, as well as nursing interventions for deficient knowledge.

Nursing Analysis

Ineffective airway clearance related to excessive mucus, exudate in the alveoli, foreign body in airway, or presence of artificial airway as evidenced by adventitious breath sounds, alteration in respiratory pattern or rate, dyspnea, or excessive sputum.

Goal/Outcome

Child will maintain patent airway, free from secretions or obstruction, with easy work of breathing, and respiratory rate within parameters for age.

Maintaining a Patent Airway (interventions with *rationale*)

- Position with airway open (sniffing position if supine) and/or elevate head of bed *to allow for adequate ventilation.*
- Humidify oxygen or room air and ensure adequate fluid intake (intravenous or oral) *to liquefy secretions for ease in clearance.*
- Suction with bulb syringe or via nasopharyngeal catheter as needed, particularly prior to bottle-feeding, *to promote clearance of secretions.*
- If tachypneic, maintain nothing by mouth (NPO) status *to avoid aspiration.*
- In the older child, encourage expectoration of sputum with coughing *to promote airway clearance.*
- Perform chest physiotherapy (CPT) if ordered *to mobilize secretions.*
- Ensure emergency equipment is readily available *to avoid delay should airway become unmaintainable.*

Nursing Analysis

Ineffective breathing pattern related to respiratory muscle fatigue as evidenced by abnormal breathing pattern, bradypnea, nasal flaring, tachypnea, use of accessory muscles to breathe, dyspnea, or prolonged expiratory phase.

Goal/Outcome

Child will demonstrate effective breathing pattern: respiratory rate within parameters for age, easy work of breathing (absence of retractions, accessory muscle use, grunting, and nasal flaring), or appropriate expiratory phase.

Promoting Effective Breathing Patterns (interventions with *rationale*)

- Assess respiratory rate, breath sounds, and work of breathing frequently *to ensure progress with treatment and so that deterioration can be noted early.*
- Position for comfort with open airway and room for lung expansion (usually with head of bed elevated). Use pillows or padding, if necessary, to maintain position *to ensure optimal ventilation via maximum lung expansion.*
- Allow for adequate sleep and rest periods *to conserve energy.*
- Administer antibiotics as ordered: *may be indicated in the case of bacterial respiratory infection*
- Encourage incentive spirometry and coughing with deep breathing (can be accomplished through play) *to maximize ventilation (play enhances the child's participation).*

Nursing Analysis

Impaired gas exchange related to airway plugging, hyperinflation, or atelectasis, as evidenced by abnormal skin color (duskiness or cyanosis), hypoxia, irritability, restlessness, or alterations in arterial blood gases

Goal/Outcome

Gas exchange will be adequate: Pulse oximetry reading on room air is within normal parameters for age, blood gases within normal limits, absence of cyanosis, irritability, restlessness.

Promoting Adequate Gas Exchange (interventions with *rationale*)

- Monitor oxygen saturation via pulse oximetry *to detect alterations in oxygenation.*
- Administer oxygen as ordered *to improve oxygenation.*
- Encourage clearance of secretions via coughing, expectoration, CPT, and suctioning *to improve gas exchange.*
- Administer bronchodilators if ordered (albuterol, levalbuterol, or racemic epinephrine) *to treat bronchospasm and improve gas exchange.*
- Provide frequent contact and support to the child and family *to decrease anxiety, which increases the child's oxygen demands.*
- Assess and monitor mental status (confusion, lethargy, restlessness, combativeness): *hypoxemia can lead to changes in mental status.*

Nursing Analysis

Deficient fluid volume risk related to insufficient fluid intake and factors influencing fluid needs (insensible losses via fever, tachypnea, or diaphoresis)

Goal/Outcome

Fluid volume will be maintained: oral mucosa moist and pink, skin turgor elastic, urine output at least 1 to 2 mL/kg/hour.

Maintaining Adequate Fluid Volume (interventions with *rationale*)

- Administer intravenous fluids if ordered *to maintain adequate hydration in NPO state.*
- When allowed oral intake, encourage oral fluids. Popsicles, favorite fluids, and games can be used *to promote intake.*
- Assess for signs of *adequate hydration* (flat fontanels, elastic skin turgor, moist mucosa, adequate urine output).
- Monitor intake and output *to identify fluid imbalance.*
- Monitor urine specific gravity, urine and serum electrolytes, blood urea nitrogen, creatinine, and osmolality *to determine fluid status.*

Nursing Analysis

Imbalanced nutrition (less than body requirements) related to insufficient dietary intake as evidenced by food intake less than daily recommended allowance

Goal/Outcome

Child will maintain adequate nutritional intake: Weight is gained or maintained. Child consumes adequate diet for age.

Promoting Adequate Nutritional Intake (interventions with *rationale*)

- Weigh on same scale at same time daily *so that measurements are consistent.*
- Perform calorie counts over a 3-day period *to determine whether caloric intake is sufficient.*
- Encourage child to choose higher-calorie, protein-rich foods *to optimize growth potential.*
- Coax young children to eat better by playing games and offering favorite foods *to improve intake.*

Nursing Analysis

Activity intolerance related to imbalance between oxygen supply and demand as evidenced by exertional dyspnea (need for frequent rest while playing), fatigue, or generalized weakness

Goal/Outcome

Child will resume normal activity level: Activity is tolerated without difficulty breathing. Pulse oximetry readings and vital signs are within parameters for age and activity level.

Increasing Activity Tolerance (interventions with *rationale*)

- Provide rest periods balanced with periods of activity, and group nursing activities and visits *to allow for sufficient rest.*
- Provide small, frequent meals *to prevent overtiring (energy is expended while eating).*
- Encourage quiet activities that do not require exertion *to prevent boredom.*
- Allow gradual increase in activity as tolerated, keeping pulse oximetry reading within normal parameters, *to minimize risk of further respiratory compromise.*

Nursing Analysis

Fear related to unfamiliar setting or learned response to threat (difficulty breathing) as evidenced by apprehensiveness (clinging, crying, fussing, lack of cooperation) or feeling of alarm (verbalization)

Goal/Outcome

Fear will be reduced: decreased episodes of crying or fussing, happy and playful at times.

Relieving Fear (interventions with *rationale*)

- Establish trusting relationship with child and family *to decrease anxiety and fear.*
- Utilize play *to gain child's cooperation and trust.*
- Explain procedures to child at developmentally appropriate level *to decrease fear of unknown.*
- Provide favorite blanket or bear as well as comfort measures preferred by child such as rocking or music *for added security.*
- Involve parents in care *to give child reassurance and decrease fear.*

Based on the top three patient problems for Alexander, describe appropriate nursing interventions.

Providing Oxygen Supplementation

Oxygen may be delivered to the child by a variety of methods (Fig. 18.5). Since oxygen administration is considered a drug, it requires a primary health care provider or nurse practitioner's order, except when following emergency protocols outlined in a health care facility's policies and procedures. Many health care settings develop specific guidelines for oxygen administration that are often coordinated by respiratory therapists, yet the nurse remains responsible for ensuring that oxygen is administered properly.

Oxygen sources include wall-mounted systems as well as cylinders. The supply of oxygen available from a wall-mounted source is limitless, but use of a wall-mounted source restricts the child to the hospital room. Cylinders are portable oxygen tanks; the D-cylinder holds a little less than 400 L of oxygen, and the E-cylinder holds about 650 L of oxygen. Cylinders turn on with a gauge attached to the top of the tank. The

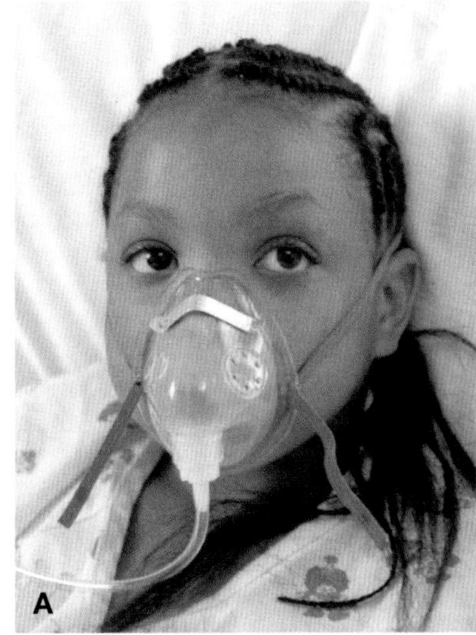

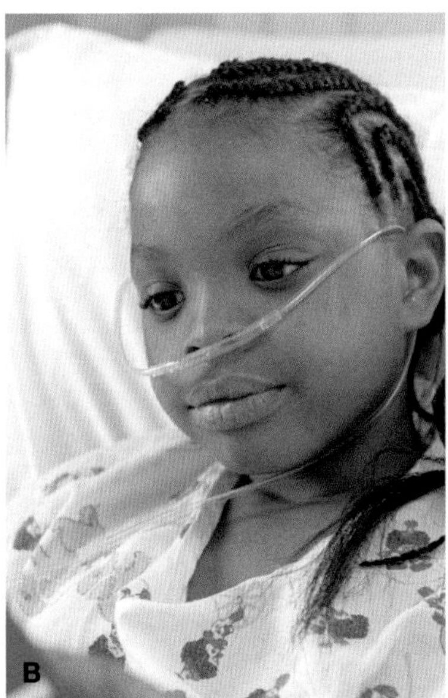

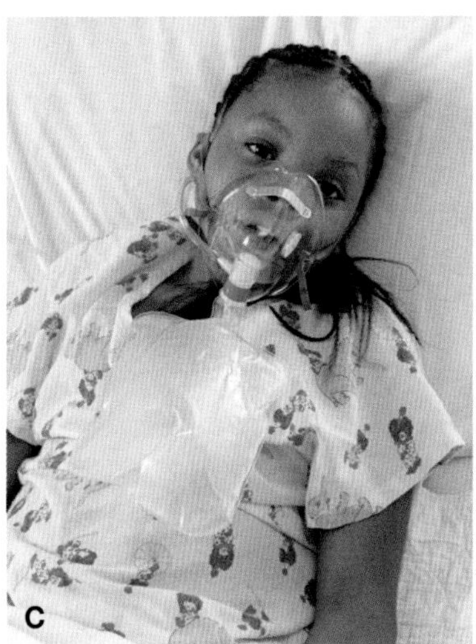

FIGURE 18.5 A. Simple oxygen mask provides about 40% oxygen. **B.** The nasal cannula provides an additional 4% oxygen per 1 L of oxygen flow (i.e., 1 L will deliver 25% oxygen). **C.** The nonrebreather mask provides 80% to 100% oxygen.

cylinder is useful for the child on low-flow oxygen because it allows for mobility.

The tank empties relatively quickly if the child requires a high flow of oxygen, so this is not the best oxygen source in an emergency. Respiratory therapists usually maintain the respiratory equipment that is found in the emergency room or hospital. However, in an outpatient setting, the nurse may be responsible for maintaining respiratory equipment and checking the level of oxygen in the office's oxygen tanks each day.

TAKE NOTE!

Oxygen is highly flammable, so use safety precautions. Post signs ("Oxygen in Use"); inform the family to avoid matches, lighters, and flammable or volatile materials; and use only facility-approved equipment.

The efficiency of oxygen delivery systems is affected by several variables, including the child's respiratory effort, the liter flow of oxygen delivered, and whether the equipment is being used appropriately. In general, oxygen facemasks come in infant, child, and adult sizes. Select the mask that best fits the child. In addition, ensure that the mask is sealed properly to decrease the amount of oxygen that escapes from the mask. Ensure that the liter flow is set according to the manufacturer's recommendations for use with that particular delivery method. The oxygen flow rate or concentration is usually determined by the primary health care provider or nurse practitioner's order. Whichever method of delivery is used, provide humidification during oxygen delivery to prevent drying of nasal passages and to assist with liquefying secretions. Table 18.1 provides details on oxygen delivery methods.

TABLE 18.1 • Oxygen Delivery Methods

Delivery Method	Description	Nursing Implications
Simple mask	Provides 35%–60% oxygen with a flow rate of 6–10 L/min. Oxygen delivery percentage is affected by respiratory rate, inspiratory flow, and adequacy of mask fit.	• Must maintain oxygen flow rate of at least 6 L/min to maintain inspired oxygen concentration and prevent rebreathing of carbon dioxide. • Mask must fit snugly to be effective but should not be so tight as to irritate the face.
Venturi mask	Provides 24%–50% oxygen by using a special gauge at the base of the mask that allows mixing of room air with oxygen flow	• Set oxygen flow rate according to percentage of oxygen desired as indicated on the gauge/dial. • As with simple mask, must fit snugly
Nasal cannula	Provides low oxygen concentration (22%–44%)	• Must be used with humidification to prevent drying and irritation of airways • Can provide very small amounts of oxygen (as low as 25 mL/min) • Maximum recommended liter flow in children is 4 L/min. • Children can eat or talk while on oxygen. • Inspired oxygen concentration affected by mouth breathing • Requires patent nasal passages
Oxygen tent	Provides high-humidity environment with up to 50% oxygen concentration	• Oxygen level drops when tent is opened. • Must change linen frequently as it becomes damp from the humidity • Secure edges of tent with blankets or by tucking edges under mattress. • Young children may be fearful and resistant. • Mist may interfere with visualization of child inside tent.
Oxygen hood	Provides high concentration (up to 80%–90%) for infants only. Allows easy access to chest and lower body	• Liter flow must be set at 10–15 L/min. • Good method for infant but need to remove for feeding • Can and should be humidified
Partial rebreathing mask	Simple facemask with an oxygen reservoir bag; provides 50%–60% oxygen concentration	• Must set liter flow rate at 10–12 L/min to prevent rebreathing of carbon dioxide • The reservoir bag does not completely empty when child inspires if flow rate is set properly.
Nonrebreathing mask	Simple facemask with valves at the exhalation ports and an oxygen reservoir bag with a valve to prevent exhaled air from entering the reservoir; provides 95% oxygen concentration	• Must set liter flow rate at 10–12 L/min to prevent rebreathing of carbon dioxide • The reservoir bag does not completely empty when child inspires if flow rate is set properly.

Data from American Heart Association. (2020). *Pediatric advanced life support: Provider manual.* https://www.amazon.com/Pediatric-Avanced-Support-Provider-Advanced/dp/1616695595?asin=B08KPFWYJ9&revisionId=&format=4&depth=1; Wolters Kluwer. (2023). *Lippincott nursing procedures* (9th ed.). Author.

CLINICAL REASONING ALERT!

Monitor vital signs, color, respiratory effort, pulse oximetry, and level of consciousness before, during, and after oxygen therapy to evaluate its effectiveness.

ACUTE INFECTIOUS DISORDERS

Acute infectious disorders include the common cold, sinusitis, influenza, pharyngitis, tonsillitis, laryngitis, croup syndromes, respiratory syncytial virus (RSV), pneumonia, and bronchitis.

Common Cold

The common cold is also referred to as a viral upper respiratory infection (URI) or nasopharyngitis. Colds can be caused by rhinoviruses, parainfluenza, RSV, enteroviruses, adenoviruses, and human metapneumovirus. Viral particles spread through the air or from person-to-person contact. Colds occur more frequently in the winter. They affect children of all ages and have a higher incidence among children who attend day care and school-age children (Yoon et al., 2022). It is not unusual for a child to have six to nine colds per year. Spontaneous resolution of the common cold occurs after about 7 to 10 days. Potential complications include secondary bacterial infections of the ears, throat, sinuses, or lungs.

Therapeutic management of the common cold is directed toward symptom relief. Nasal congestion may be relieved via humidity and use of normal saline nasal wash or spray followed by suctioning. Antihistamines are not indicated, as they dry secretions further. Over-the-counter cold preparations are available singly and in combinations. These preparations have not been proven to reduce the length or severity of the cold but may offer symptomatic relief in some children older than 6 years (they are not recommended in children younger than 4 years due to side effects) (Yoon et al., 2022). See the Healthy People 2030 box.

HEALTHY PEOPLE 2030

Objective	Nursing Significance
Reduce inappropriate antibiotic use in outpatient settings.	• Appropriately educate families that the cause of the common cold is a number of viruses and that antibiotics are inappropriate for the treatment of viral infections. • Encourage families to use measures such as normal saline nasal washes to decrease symptoms associated with the common cold more quickly.

Healthy People Objectives retrieved from http://www.healthypeople.gov

TAKE NOTE!

Over-the-counter cold preparations containing decongestants intended for use in infants and toddlers are no longer on the market. The products are labeled "not for use in children under 4 years of age" (U.S. Food and Drug Administration, 2023).

Nursing Assessment

The child may have either a stuffy or a runny nose. Nasal discharge is usually thin and watery at first but may become thicker and discolored. The color of nasal discharge is not an accurate indicator of viral versus bacterial infection. The child may be hoarse and complain of a sore throat. Cough usually produces very little sputum. Fever, fatigue, watery eyes, and appetite loss may also occur. Symptoms are generally at their worst over the first few days and then decrease over the course of the illness.

Assess for risk factors such as day care or school attendance. Inspect for edema and vasodilation of the mucosa. Diagnosis is based on clinical presentation rather than laboratory or x-ray studies. Comparison Chart 18.1 differentiates causes of nasal congestion.

COMPARISON CHART 18.1 Causes of Nasal Congestion

Sign or Symptom	Allergic Rhinitis	Common Cold	Sinusitis
Length of illness	Varies; may have year-round symptoms	10 days or less	Longer than 10–14 days
Nasal discharge	Thin, watery, clear	Thick, white, yellow, or green; can be thin	Thick, yellow, or green
Nasal congestion	Varies	Present	Present
Sneezing	Varies	Present	Absent
Cough	Varies	Present	Varies
Headache	Varies	Varies	Varies
Fever	Absent	Varies	Varies
Bad breath	Absent	Absent	Varies

Nursing Management

Nursing management of the child with a common cold consists of promoting comfort, providing family education, and preventing spread of the cold.

PROMOTING COMFORT

Provide supportive measures such as normal saline nose drops and bulb syringe suctioning for the relief of nasal congestion in infants and toddlers. Teach older children to use a normal saline nose spray to mobilize secretions. A cool mist humidifier also helps with nasal congestion. If over-the-counter nose sprays are used in children, remind parents they are only for short-term use. Promote adequate oral fluid intake to liquefy secretions.

Educate parents about the use of cold and cough medications. Although they may offer some symptomatic relief, they have not been proven to shorten the length of cold symptoms. Counsel parents to use the appropriate product depending on the symptom relief desired, rather than a combination product. Products containing acetaminophen combined with other "cold symptom" medications may mask a fever in the child who is developing a secondary bacterial infection. As with all viral infections in children, teach parents that aspirin use should be avoided because of its association with Reye syndrome (Stanford Children's Health, 2023).

PROVIDING FAMILY EDUCATION

Currently, there are no medications available to treat the viruses that cause the common cold, so symptomatic treatment is all that is necessary. Antibiotics are not indicated unless the child also has a bacterial infection. Explain to parents the importance of reserving antibiotic use for appropriate illnesses. Provide education about the use of normal saline nose drops and bulb suctioning to clear the infant's nose of secretions. Normal saline nasal wash using a bulb syringe to instill the solution is also helpful for children of all ages with nasal congestion. Although normal saline for nasal administration is available commercially, parents can also make it at home (Box 18.2). Teaching Guidelines 18.1 gives instructions on use of the bulb syringe.

Counsel parents about how to recognize complications of the common cold, which include:

- Prolonged fever
- Increased throat pain or enlarged, painful lymph nodes
- Increased or worsening cough, cough lasting longer than 10 days, chest pain, difficulty breathing
- Earache, headache, tooth, or sinus pain
- Unusual irritability or lethargy
- Skin rash

If complications do occur, tell parents to notify the primary health care provider or nurse practitioner for further instructions or reassessment.

BOX 18.2 Homemade Saltwater Nose Drops

Mix 8-oz distilled water, a half-teaspoon sea salt, and a quarter-teaspoon baking soda. Keep for 24 hours in the refrigerator but allow it to come to room temperature prior to use.

PREVENTING THE COMMON COLD

Teaching about ways to prevent the common cold is a vital nursing intervention. Explain that frequent handwashing helps to decrease the spread of viruses that cause the common cold. Teach parents and family to avoid second-hand smoke as well as crowded places, especially during the winter. Avoid close contact with individuals known to have a cold. Encourage parents and families to consume a healthy diet and get enough rest.

CONSIDER THIS!

Corey Davis, a 3-year-old, is brought to the clinic by her parent. She presents with a runny nose, congestion, and a nonproductive cough. Her parent says, "She's miserable. I just don't know what to do. Ever since I put her in day care she gets sick every few weeks. This is all my fault."

How should the nurse respond? How would you feel if your child was healthy until entering day care? What type of support can the nurse provide to Corey's parent?

Sinusitis

Sinusitis (also called rhinosinusitis) generally refers to a bacterial infection of the paranasal sinuses. The disease may be either acute or chronic in nature. In young children, the maxillary and ethmoid sinuses are the main sites of infection. After age 10 years, the frontal sinuses may be more commonly involved (Yoon et al., 2022). Mucosal swelling, decreased ciliary movement, and thickened nasal discharge all contribute to bacterial invasion of the nose. Nasal polyps also place the child at risk for bacterial sinusitis. Complications include orbital cellulitis and intracranial infections, such as subdural empyemas.

Symptoms lasting less than 30 days generally indicate acute sinusitis, whereas symptoms persisting longer than 4 to 6 weeks usually indicate chronic sinusitis. Sinusitis is managed with antibiotic treatment. The therapeutic management approach varies with chronicity. The course of treatment is usually 14 days. Naturally, chronic sinusitis requires a longer course of treatment than acute sinusitis. Surgical therapy may be indicated for children with chronic sinusitis, particularly if it is recurrent or if nasal polyps are present.

Nursing Assessment

The most common presentation of sinusitis is persistent signs and symptoms of a cold. Rather than improving

TEACHING GUIDELINES 18.1 Using the Bulb Syringe to Suction Nasal Secretions

1. Hold the infant on your lap or on the bed with the head tilted slightly back.

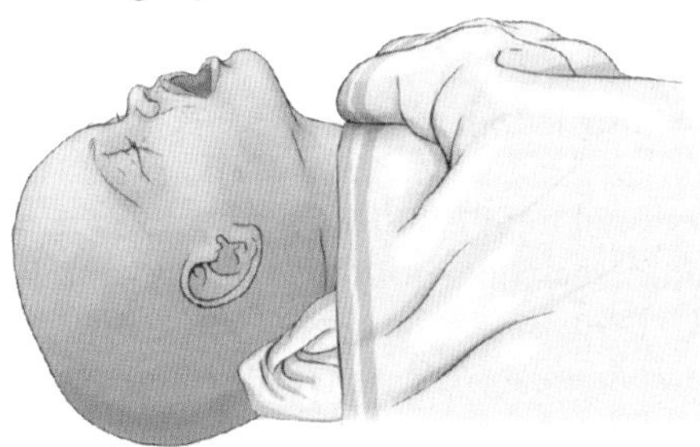

2. If using saline, instill several drops of saline solution in one of the infant's nostrils.

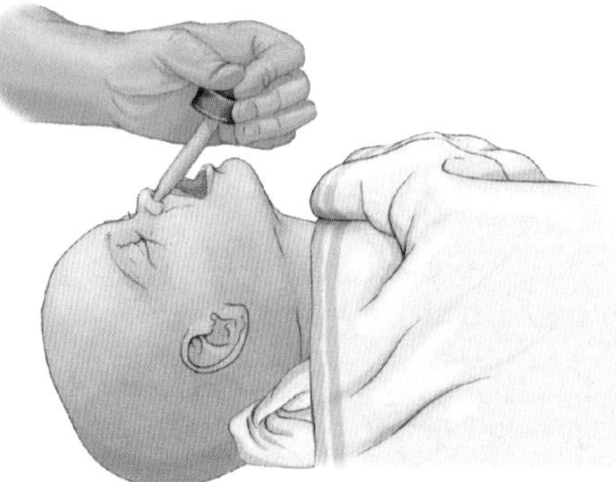

3. Compress the sides of the bulb syringe completely. Use only a rubber-tipped bulb syringe. Place the rubber tip in the infant's nose.

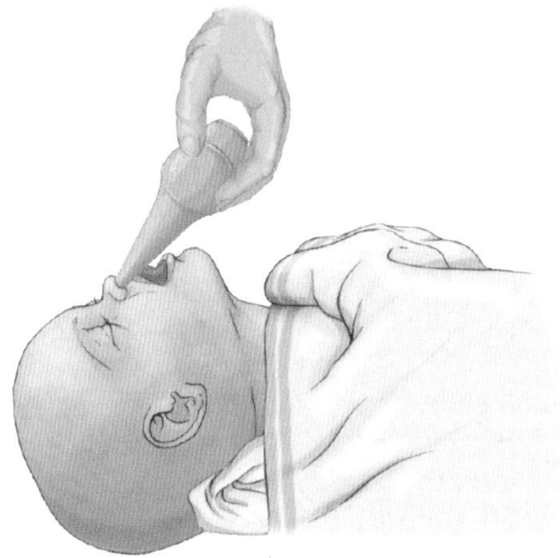

4. Release pressure on the bulb.

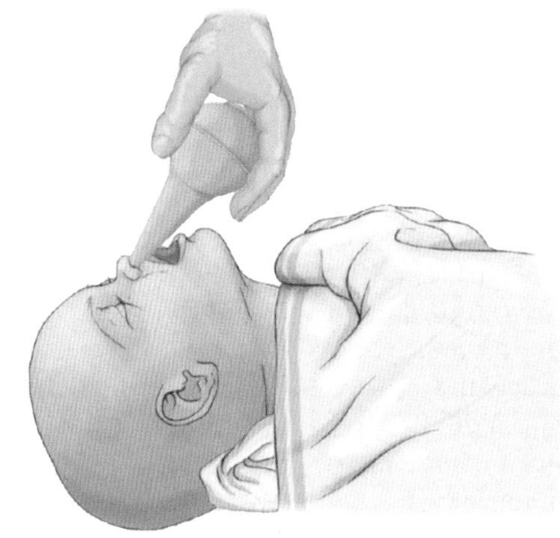

5. Remove the syringe and squeeze bulb over tissue or the sink to empty it of secretions.

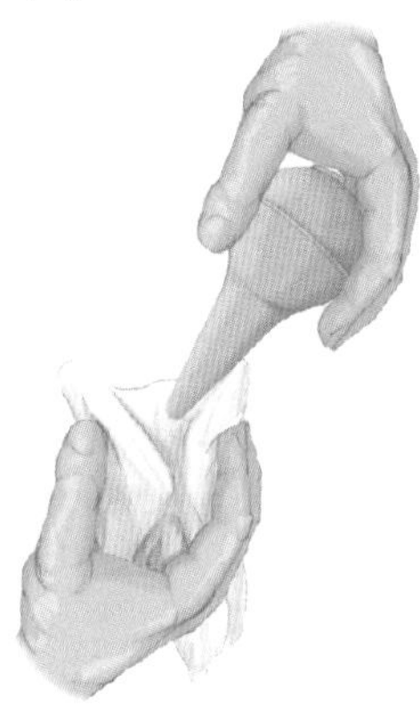

6. Repeat on other nostril if necessary. Using a bulb syringe prior to bottle-feeding or breastfeeding may relieve congestion enough to allow the infant to suck more efficiently.
7. Clean the bulb syringe thoroughly with warm water after each use, and allow to air dry.

after 7 to 10 days, nasal discharge persists. Explore the history for:

- Cough
- Fever
- Halitosis (bad breath) in preschoolers or older children
- Facial pain may or may not be present, so it is not a reliable indicator of disease.
- Eyelid edema (in the case of ethmoid sinus involvement)
- Irritability
- Poor appetite

Assess for risk factors such as a history of recurrent cold symptoms or a history of nasal polyps.

On physical examination, note eyelid swelling, extent of nasal drainage, and halitosis. Inspect the throat for postnasal drainage. Inspect the nasal mucosa for erythema. Palpate the sinuses, noting pain with mild pressure. The diagnosis may be made based on the history and clinical presentation. The use of x-ray, computed tomography scan, or magnetic resonance imaging is not necessary as they are not specific and do not distinguish viral from bacterial infection (Yoon et al., 2022). (Refer to Comparison Chart 18.1, which differentiates the causes of nasal congestion.)

Nursing Management

Normal saline nose drops or spray, cool mist humidifiers, and adequate oral fluid intake are recommended for children with sinusitis. Teach families the importance of continuing the full course of antibiotics to eradicate the cause of infection. Also educate the family that the use of decongestants and antihistamines as adjuncts in the treatment of sinusitis has not been shown to be beneficial, although intranasal steroids may benefit those with allergic rhinitis (Yoon et al., 2022). Advise parents that normal saline nose spray or nasal washes may promote drainage.

Influenza

Influenza viral infection (known commonly as the "flu") occurs primarily during the winter. It is spread through inhalation of droplets or contact with fine-particle aerosols. Infected children shed the virus for 1 to 2 days before symptoms begin and may continue shedding the virus in increased amounts (as compared with adults) for as long as 2 weeks. Average annual infection rates in children range from 10% to 40% (Munoz & Edwards, 2023). Influenza viruses primarily affect the upper respiratory epithelium but can cause systemic effects as well. Children with chronic heart or lung conditions, diabetes, chronic kidney disease, or immune deficiency are at higher risk for more severe influenza infection compared with other children.

Bacterial infections of the respiratory system commonly occur as complications of influenza infection, severe pneumococcal pneumonia, in particular. Otitis media occurs in 10% to 50% of children with influenza (Munoz & Edwards, 2023). Rarely, Reye syndrome occurs in children with influenza who have taken aspirin. Acute myositis is a rare and severe complication, which is particular to children. A sudden onset of severe pain and tenderness in both calves causes the child to refuse to walk. Due to the potential for complications, a prolonged fever or a fever that returns during convalescence should be investigated.

> *TAKE NOTE!*
>
> Current recommendations are for all children older than 6 months of age to be immunized yearly against influenza (CDC, 2023b).

Nursing Assessment

Children who attend day care or school are at higher risk for influenza infection than those who are routinely at home. Note the presence of risk factors for severe disease, such as chronic heart or lung disease (such as asthma), diabetes, chronic kidney disease, or immune deficiency, or children with cancer receiving chemotherapy. School-age children and adolescents experience the illness similarly to adults. Abrupt onset of fever, facial flushing, chills, headache, myalgia, and malaise are accompanied by cough and **coryza** (nasal discharge). About half of infected individuals have a dry or sore throat. Ocular symptoms such as photophobia, tearing, burning, and eye pain are common.

Infants and young children exhibit symptoms similar to other respiratory illnesses. Fever greater than 39.5°C is common. Infants may be mildly toxic in appearance and irritable and have a cough, coryza, and pharyngitis. Wheezing may occur, as influenza can also cause bronchiolitis. An erythematous rash may be present, and diarrhea may also occur. The diagnosis may be confirmed by a rapid assay test.

Nursing Management

Nursing management of influenza is mainly supportive. Provide symptomatic treatment of cough and fever. Instruct parents on the maintenance of hydration. Administer antiviral drugs as prescribed as they can reduce the symptoms associated with influenza if they are started within the first 48 hours of the illness (UpToDate, Inc., 2023).

Pharyngitis

Inflammation of the throat mucosa (pharynx) is referred to as pharyngitis. A sore throat may accompany nasal congestion and is often viral in nature. A bacterial sore throat most often occurs without nasal symptoms. Group A streptococci account for 20% to 30% of cases, with the remainder being caused by other viruses or bacteria (Yoon et al., 2022).

Suppurative complications of group A streptococcal infection include peritonsillar or retropharyngeal abscess. Peritonsillar abscess may be noted by asymmetric swelling of the tonsils, shifting of the uvula to one side, and palatal edema. Retropharyngeal abscess may progress to the point of airway obstruction, hence requiring careful evaluation and appropriate treatment. Additional complications include acute rheumatic fever (see Chapter 19) and acute glomerulonephritis (see Chapter 21).

Viral pharyngitis is usually self-limited and does not require therapy beyond symptomatic relief. Group A streptococcal pharyngitis requires antibiotic therapy. If either the rapid diagnostic test or throat culture (described further on) is positive for group A streptococci, penicillin is generally prescribed. Appropriate alternative antibiotics include amoxicillin and, for those allergic to penicillin, macrolides, and cephalosporins.

TAKE NOTE!

A "strep carrier" is a child who has a positive throat culture for streptococci when asymptomatic. Strep carriers are not at risk for complications from streptococci, as are those who are acutely infected with streptococci and are symptomatic (Yoon et al., 2022).

Nursing Assessment

Inquire about sudden onset of pharyngitis. The history may include a fever, sore throat and difficulty swallowing, headache, and abdominal pain. Ask about recent incidence of viral or strep throat in the family, day care center, or school.

Inspect the pharynx and tonsils, which may demonstrate varying degrees of inflammation (Fig. 18.6). Exudate may be present but is not diagnostic of bacterial infection. Note the presence of petechiae on the palate. Inspect the tongue for a strawberry appearance. Palpate for enlargement and tenderness of the anterior cervical nodes. Inspect the skin for a fine, red, sandpaper-like rash (called scarlatiniform), particularly on the trunk or abdomen, a common finding with streptococcus A infection.

The nurse may obtain a throat swab for rapid diagnostic testing and throat culture. The rapid strep test is a sensitive and reliable measure, rarely resulting in false-positive readings (Yoon et al., 2022). If the rapid strep test is negative, the second swab may be sent for a throat culture.

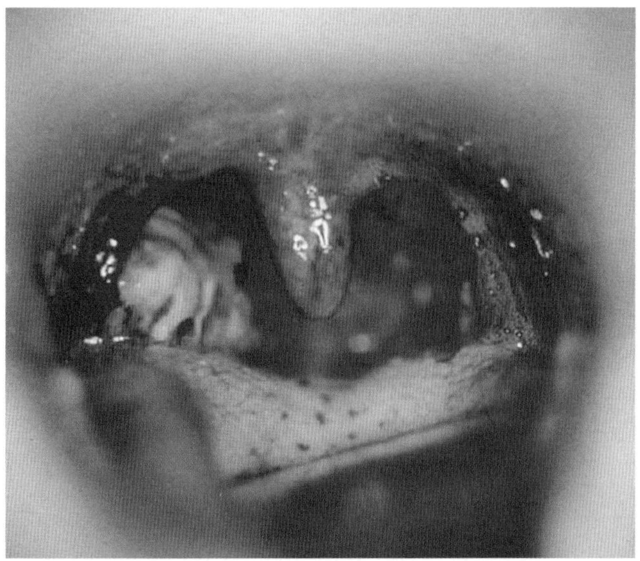

FIGURE 18.6 Note the redness of the pharynx, tonsillar exudate, and white strawberry tongue coating.

ATRAUMATIC CARE

When obtaining two swabs for rapid strep testing and throat culture, swab the applicators simultaneously to decrease perceived trauma to the child.

Nursing Management

Nursing management of the child with pharyngitis focuses on promoting comfort and providing family education.

PROMOTING COMFORT

Teach families that saline gargles (made with 8 oz of warm water and a half-teaspoon of table salt) are soothing for children old enough to cooperate. Administer analgesics such as acetaminophen and ibuprofen to ease fever and pain. Educate families that sucking on throat lozenges or hard candy may also ease pain. Provide cool mist humidity to keep the mucosa moist in the event of mouth breathing. Encourage the child to ingest Popsicles, cool liquids, and ice chips to maintain hydration.

PROVIDING FAMILY EDUCATION

Parents may often need additional education about treatments as they may be accustomed to "sore throats" being treated with antibiotics. However, teach parents that in the case of a viral cause, antibiotics will not be necessary and that the pharyngitis will resolve in a few days. For the child with streptococcal pharyngitis, urge parents to have the child complete the entire prescribed course of antibiotics. After 24 hours of antibiotic therapy, instruct the parents to discard the child's toothbrush to avoid reinfection. Educate parents that children may return to day care or school after they have been receiving antibiotics for 24 hours; they are considered noncontagious at that point.

Tonsillitis

Inflammation of the tonsils often occurs with pharyngitis and, thus, may also be viral or bacterial in nature. Viral infections require only symptomatic treatment. Treatment for bacterial tonsillitis is the same as for bacterial pharyngitis. Occasionally, surgical intervention is warranted. Tonsillectomy (surgical removal of the palatine tonsils) may be indicated for the child with recurrent streptococcal tonsillitis or massive tonsillar hypertrophy or for other reasons. When hypertrophied adenoids obstruct breathing, adenoidectomy (surgical removal of the adenoids) may be indicated.

Nursing Assessment

Note whether fever is present currently or by history. Inquire about the history of recurrent pharyngitis or tonsillitis. Note whether the child's voice sounds muffled or hoarse. Inspect the pharynx for redness and enlargement of the tonsils. As the tonsils enlarge, the child may experience difficulty breathing and swallowing. When tonsils touch at the midline ("kissing tonsils" or 4+ in size), the airway may become obstructed. Also, if the adenoids are enlarged, the posterior nares become obstructed. The child may breathe through the mouth and may snore. Palpate the anterior cervical nodes for enlargement and tenderness. Rapid test or culture may be positive for streptococcus A.

Nursing Management

Tonsillitis that is medically treated requires the same nursing management as pharyngitis. Nursing care for the child after tonsillectomy is described here.

PROMOTING AIRWAY CLEARANCE

Until fully awake, place the child in a sidelying or prone position to facilitate safe drainage of secretions. Once alert, the child may prefer to sit up or have the head of the bed elevated. Suctioning, if necessary, should be done carefully to avoid trauma to the surgical site. Note that dried blood may be present on the teeth and the nares, with old blood present in emesis. Since the presence of blood can be very frightening to parents, alert them to this possibility.

MAINTAINING FLUID VOLUME

Although unusual postoperatively, monitor for hemorrhage as it may occur any time from the immediate postoperative period to as late as 10 days after surgery. Inspect the throat for bleeding. Mucus tinged with blood may be expected, but fresh blood in the secretions indicates bleeding. Watch for continuous swallowing of small amounts of blood while awake or sleeping as this may indicate early bleeding. Monitor for other signs of hemorrhage, including tachycardia, pallor, restlessness, frequent throat clearing, and emesis of bright red blood.

To avoid trauma to the surgical site, discourage the child from coughing, clearing the throat, blowing the nose, and using straws. Upon discharge, instruct the parents to immediately report any sign of bleeding to the primary health care provider or nurse practitioner. To maintain fluid volume postoperatively, encourage children to take any fluids they desire; Popsicles and ice chips are particularly soothing. Citrus juice and brown or red fluids should be avoided; the acid in citrus juice may irritate the throat, and red or brown fluids may be confused with blood if vomiting occurs.

RELIEVING PAIN

Educate families that for the first 24 hours after surgery, the throat is very sore. Provide adequate pain relief (may be with or without narcotics) to establish adequate oral fluid intake. Apply an ice collar if prescribed. Counsel parents to maintain pain control on discharge from the facility, not only for the child's comfort but also to enable the child to continue to drink fluids.

Infectious Mononucleosis

Infectious mononucleosis is a self-limited illness caused by the Epstein–Barr virus. It is characterized by fever, malaise, sore throat, and lymphadenopathy. Mononucleosis is commonly called the "kissing disease" since it is transmitted by oropharyngeal secretions. It can occur at any age but is most often diagnosed in adolescents and young adults (Aronson & Auwaerter, 2023). Some infected individuals may have concomitant streptococcal pharyngitis. Complications include splenic rupture, Guillain–Barré syndrome, and aseptic meningitis.

Nursing Assessment

Note any history of exposure to infected individuals. Determine history of fever and onset and progression of sore throat, malaise, and other complaints. Observe for periorbital edema. Inspect the pharynx and tonsils for inflammation and patches of gray exudate. Petechiae may be present on the palate. Palpate for bilateral nontender enlargement of the posterior cervical lymph nodes. After 3 to 5 days of illness, the pharynx may become edematous and the tonsillar exudate more extensive. Lymphadenopathy may progress to include the anterior cervical nodes, which may become tender. Palpate the abdomen for splenomegaly or hepatomegaly. An erythematous maculopapular rash may appear as the illness progresses. Definitive diagnosis may be made by Monospot or Epstein–Barr virus titers.

TAKE NOTE!

The heterophile antibodies test may demonstrate a false negative if obtained within the first 7 days of illness with infectious mononucleosis. Epstein-Barr virus titer is reliable at any point in the illness (Aronson & Auwaerter, 2023).

Nursing Management

Nursing management of mononucleosis is primarily symptomatic. The throat may be very sore, so encourage families to administer analgesics and provide the child with saltwater gargles. Encourage bed rest while the child is febrile. Instruct the child and family that frequent rest periods may be necessary for several weeks after the onset of illness, as fatigue may persist as long as 6 weeks. During the acute phase, if tonsillar or pharyngeal edema threatens to obstruct the airway, administer corticosteroids as prescribed to decrease the inflammation. When children or teens have splenomegaly or hepatomegaly, educate the child and family that strenuous activity and contact sports should be avoided. Ensure parents understand that the appearance of a rash or jaundice should be reported to the primary health care provider or nurse practitioner.

Laryngitis

Inflammation of the larynx is termed laryngitis. It may occur alone or in conjunction with other respiratory symptoms. It is characterized by a hoarse voice or loss of the voice (so soft as to make it difficult to hear). Oral fluids might offer relief, but resting the voice for 24 hours will allow the inflammation to subside. Laryngitis alone requires no further intervention.

Croup

Croup most frequently affects children between 3 months and 3 years of age and rarely affects children over 6 years of age (Woods, 2023). Croup is also referred to as laryngotracheobronchitis because inflammation and edema of the larynx, trachea, and bronchi occur as a result of viral infection. Parainfluenza is responsible for the majority of cases of croup, although other viruses may also be implicated (Woods, 2023). The inflammation and edema obstruct the airway, resulting in symptoms. Mucus production also occurs, further contributing to obstruction of the airway. Narrowing of the subglottic area of the trachea results in audible inspiratory stridor. Edema of the larynx causes hoarseness. Inflammation in the larynx and trachea causes the characteristic barking cough of croup.

Symptoms occur most often at night, presenting suddenly, with resolution of symptoms in the morning. Croup is usually self-limited, lasting only about 3 to 5 days. Complications of croup are rare but may include worsening respiratory distress, hypoxia, or bacterial superinfection (as in the case of bacterial tracheitis).

Croup is usually managed on an outpatient basis, with affected children rarely requiring hospitalization. Corticosteroids (usually a single dose) are used to decrease inflammation, and racemic epinephrine aerosols demonstrate the alpha-adrenergic effect of mucosal vasoconstriction, helping to decrease edema. Children with croup may be hospitalized if they have significant stridor at rest or severe retractions after a several-hour period of observation. Comparison Chart 18.2 compares croup with epiglottitis.

Nursing Assessment

Note the age of the child; children between 3 months and 3 years of age are most likely to present with viral croup (laryngotracheobronchitis). History may reveal a cough that developed during the night (most common presentation) and that sounds like barking (of a seal). Inspect for the presence of mild URI symptoms. Temperature may be normal or mildly elevated. Listen for inspiratory stridor and observe for suprasternal retractions. Auscultate the lungs for adequacy of breath sounds. Croup is usually diagnosed based on history and clinical presentation, but a lateral neck radiograph may be obtained to rule out epiglottitis.

CLINICAL REASONING ALERT!

The child with fever, a toxic appearance, and increasing respiratory distress despite appropriate croup treatment may have bacterial tracheitis (Woods, 2023). Notify the primary health care provider or nurse practitioner of these findings in a child with croup.

COMPARISON CHART 18.2 Croup Versus Epiglottitis

	Spasmodic Croup	Epiglottitis
Preceding illness	None or minimal coryza	None or mild upper respiratory infection
Age group usually affected	3 months to 3 years	1–8 years
Onset	Usually sudden, often at night	Rapid (within hours)
Fever	Variable	High
Barking cough, hoarseness	Yes	No
Dysphagia	No	Yes
Toxic appearance	No	Yes
Cause	Viral	*Haemophilus influenzae* type b

Nursing Management

If the child's care is being managed at home, advise parents about the symptoms of respiratory distress, and instruct them to seek treatment if the child's respiratory condition worsens. Teach parents to expose their child to humidified air (via a cool mist humidifier or steamy bathroom). Although never clinically proven, use of humidified air has long been recommended for alleviating coughing jags and has anecdotally been reported as helpful (particularly exposure to cooler air). Administer dexamethasone if ordered or teach parents about home administration. Explain to parents that the effects of racemic epinephrine last about 2 hours and that the child must be observed closely as occasionally a child will worsen again, requiring another aerosol. Teaching Guidelines 18.2 provides information about home care of croup.

TEACHING GUIDELINES 18.2 Home Care of Croup

- Keep the child quiet and discourage crying.
- Allow the child to sit up (in your arms).
- Encourage rest and fluid intake.
- If stridor occurs, take the child into a steamy bathroom for 10 minutes.
- Administer medication (corticosteroid) as directed.
- Watch the child closely. Call the primary health care provider or nurse practitioner if:
  - The child breathes faster, has retractions, or has any other difficulty breathing.
  - The nostrils flare or the lips or nails have a bluish tint.
  - The cough or stridor does not improve with exposure to moist air.
  - Restlessness increases or the child is confused.
  - The child begins to drool or cannot swallow.

Adapted from Schare, R. S. (2021). *Croup.* http://kidshealth.org/parent/infections/lung/croup.html

Epiglottitis

Epiglottitis (inflammation and swelling of the epiglottis) is most often caused by *Haemophilus influenzae* type b and has become a rare occurrence with the extensive use of the Hib vaccine since the 1980s (Houin et al., 2022). Respiratory arrest and death may occur if the airway becomes completely occluded. Additional complications include pneumothorax and pulmonary edema. Therapeutic management focuses on airway maintenance and support. Intravenous antibiotic therapy is necessary. The child will be managed in the intensive care unit. See Comparison Chart 18.2 for information comparing croup with epiglottitis.

Nursing Assessment

Carefully assess the child with suspected epiglottitis. Note sudden onset of symptoms and high fever. The child has an overall toxic appearance. They may refuse to speak or may speak only with a very soft voice. The child may refuse to lie down and may assume the characteristic position: sitting forward with the neck extended. Drooling may be present. Note anxiety or a frightened appearance. Note the child's color. Cough is usually absent. A lateral neck radiograph may be performed to determine whether epiglottitis is present. This is done cautiously so as not to induce airway obstruction with changes in position of the child's neck.

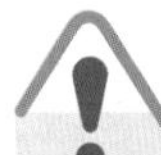

CLINICAL REASONING ALERT!

Do not, under any circumstances, attempt to visualize the throat: reflex laryngospasm may occur, precipitating immediate airway occlusion.

Nursing Management

Do not leave the child unattended. Keep the child and parents as calm as possible. Allow the child to assume a position of comfort. Do not place the child in a supine position, as airway occlusion may occur. Provide 100% oxygen in the least invasive manner that is acceptable to the child. If the child with epiglottitis experiences complete airway occlusion, an emergency **tracheostomy** (incision in trachea to permit breathing) may be necessary. Ensure that emergency equipment is available and that personnel trained in intubation of the pediatric occluded airway and percutaneous tracheostomy are notified of the child's presence in the facility.

CLINICAL REASONING ALERT!

Epiglottitis is characterized by dysphagia, drooling, anxiety, irritability, and significant respiratory distress. Prepare for the event of sudden airway occlusion.

Bronchiolitis

Bronchiolitis is an acute inflammatory process of the bronchioles and small bronchi. Nearly always caused by a viral pathogen, RSV accounts for the majority of cases of bronchiolitis, with adenovirus, parainfluenza, and human meta-pneumovirus also being important causative agents. This discussion will focus on RSV bronchiolitis.

The peak incidence of bronchiolitis is in the fall and winter, coinciding with RSV season, which in the United States and Canada generally begins in September or October and continues through the spring. Virtually all children will contract RSV infection within the first few years of life. RSV bronchiolitis occurs most often in infants and toddlers (Piedra, 2023). The severity of disease is related inversely to the age of the child. The frequency and severity of RSV infection decrease with age. Repeated RSV infections occur throughout life but are usually localized to the upper respiratory tract after toddlerhood.

Pathophysiology

RSV is a highly contagious virus and may be contracted through direct contact with respiratory secretions or from particles on objects contaminated with the virus. RSV invades the nasopharynx, where it replicates and then spreads down to the lower airway via aspiration of upper airway secretions. RSV infection causes necrosis of the respiratory epithelium of the small airways, peribronchiolar mononuclear infiltration, and plugging of the lumens with mucus and exudate. The small airways become variably obstructed; this allows adequate inspiratory volume but prevents full expiration. This leads to hyperinflation and atelectasis. Serious alterations in gas exchange occur, with arterial hypoxemia and carbon dioxide retention resulting from mismatching of pulmonary ventilation and perfusion. Hypoventilation occurs secondary to markedly increased work of breathing.

Therapeutic Management

Management of RSV focuses on supportive treatment: supplemental oxygen, nasal and/or nasopharyngeal suctioning, and oral or intravenous hydration. Many infants are managed at home with close observation and adequate hydration. Hospitalization is required for children with more severe disease. The infant with tachypnea, significant retractions, poor oral intake, or lethargy can deteriorate quickly, to the point of requiring ventilatory support, and thus warrants hospital admission.

Nursing Assessment

For a full description of the assessment phase of the nursing process, refer to the "Clinical Judgment and the Nursing Process" section. Assessment findings pertinent to RSV bronchiolitis are discussed further on.

HEALTH HISTORY

Elicit a description of the present illness and chief complaint. Common signs and symptoms reported during the health history might include:

- Onset of illness with a clear runny nose (sometimes profuse)
- Pharyngitis
- Low-grade fever
- Development of cough 1 to 3 days into the illness, followed by a wheeze shortly thereafter
- Poor feeding

Explore the child's current and past medical history for risk factors such as:

- Young age (younger than 2 years old), more severe disease in a child younger than 6 months old
- Prematurity
- Multiple births
- Birth during April to September
- History of chronic lung disease (bronchopulmonary disease)
- Cyanotic or complicated congenital heart disease
- Immunocompromise
- Male sex
- Exposure to passive tobacco smoke
- Crowded living conditions
- Day care attendance
- School-age siblings
- Low socioeconomic status
- Lack of breastfeeding

PHYSICAL EXAMINATION

Examination of the child with RSV involves inspection, observation, and auscultation.

Inspection and Observation

Observe the child's general appearance and color (centrally and peripherally). The infant with RSV bronchiolitis might appear air-hungry, exhibiting various degrees of cyanosis and respiratory distress, including tachypnea, retractions, accessory muscle use, grunting, and periods of apnea. Cough and audible wheeze might be heard. The infant might appear listless and uninterested in feeding, surroundings, or parents.

Auscultation

Auscultate the lungs, noting adventitious sounds and determining the quality of aeration of the lung fields. Earlier in the illness, wheezes might be heard scattered throughout the lung fields. In more serious cases, the chest might sound quiet and without wheeze. This is due to significant hyperexpansion with poor air exchange.

LABORATORY AND DIAGNOSTIC TESTS

Common laboratory and diagnostic studies ordered for the assessment of RSV bronchiolitis include:

- Pulse oximetry: oxygen saturation might be decreased significantly.
- Chest radiograph: might reveal hyperinflation and patchy areas of atelectasis or infiltration
- Blood gases: might show carbon dioxide retention and **hypoxemia** (low oxygen concentration in blood)
- Nasal–pharyngeal washings: positive identification of RSV can be made via enzyme-linked immunosorbent assay (ELISA) or immunofluorescent antibody (IFA) testing.

Nursing Management

RSV infection is usually self-limited, and goals and interventions for the child with bronchiolitis are aimed at supportive care. Children with less severe disease might require only antipyretics, adequate hydration, and close observation. They can often be successfully managed at home, provided the primary caregiver is reliable and comfortable with close observation. Teach parents or caregivers to watch for signs of worsening and to seek care quickly should the child's condition deteriorate.

Hospitalization is required for children with more severe disease, and children admitted with RSV bronchiolitis warrant close observation. In addition to the patient problems and related interventions discussed in the "Clinical Judgment and the Nursing Process" section earlier in this chapter, interventions common to bronchiolitis follow.

MAINTAINING PATENT AIRWAY

Position the child with the head of the bed elevated to facilitate an open airway. Frequently assess airway patency and suction as needed. Use a Yankauer or tonsil-tip suction catheter to suction the mouth or pharynx of older infants or children, rinsing the catheter after each suctioning. Nasal bulb suctioning may be sufficient to clear the airway in some infants, while others will require nasopharyngeal suctioning with a suction catheter. Nursing Procedure 18.1 gives further information. Adjust the pressure ranges for suctioning infants and children between 60 and 100 mm Hg (40 and 60 mm Hg for premature infants).

NURSING PROCEDURE 18.1 Nasopharyngeal or Artificial Airway Suction Technique

1. Make sure the suction equipment works properly before starting.
2. After washing your hands, assemble the equipment needed:
   - Appropriate-size sterile suction catheter
   - Sterile gloves
   - Supplemental oxygen
   - Sterile water-based lubricant
   - Sterile normal saline if indicated
3. Don sterile gloves, keeping dominant hand sterile and nondominant hand clean.
4. Preoxygenate the infant or child if indicated.
5. Apply lubricant to the end of the suction catheter.
6. If indicated for loosening of secretions, instill sterile saline.
7. Maintaining sterile technique, insert the suction catheter into the child's nostril or airway:
   - Insert only to the point of gagging if inserting via the nostril.
   - Insert only 0.5 cm further than the length of the artificial airway.
8. Intermittently apply suction for no longer than 10 seconds while twisting and removing the catheter.
9. Supplement with oxygen after suctioning.

PROMOTING ADEQUATE GAS EXCHANGE

Assess work of breathing, respiratory rate, and oxygen saturation as infants and children with RSV bronchiolitis might deteriorate quickly as the disease progresses. Adjust the percentage of inspired oxygen (FiO_2) as needed to maintain oxygen saturation within the prescribed range. Position the infant with the head of the bed elevated to improve gas exchange. Frequent assessment is necessary for the hospitalized child with bronchiolitis.

CLINICAL REASONING ALERT!

In the tachypneic infant, slowing of the respiratory rate does not necessarily indicate improvement: often, a slower respiratory rate is an indication of tiring, and carbon dioxide retention may soon be followed by apnea (Weiner, 2022).

REDUCING RISK FOR INFECTION

Since RSV is easily spread through contact with droplets, isolate inpatients according to hospital policy to decrease the risk of nosocomial spread to other children. Safely cohort children with RSV. Maintain attention to handwashing, as droplets might enter the eyes, nose, or mouth via the hands.

PROVIDING FAMILY EDUCATION

Educate parents so they can recognize signs of worsening distress. Tell parents to call the primary health care provider or nurse practitioner if the child's breathing becomes rapid or more difficult or if the child cannot eat secondary to tachypnea. Inform families that children who are younger than 1 year or who are at higher risk (those who were born prematurely or who have chronic heart or lung conditions) might have a longer course of illness. Instruct parents that cough can persist for several days to weeks after resolution of the disease but that infants usually act well otherwise.

PREVENTING RESPIRATORY SYNCYTIAL VIRUS DISEASE

Teach strict adherence to handwashing policies in day care centers and when exposed to individuals with cold symptoms for all age groups. It is recommended that all pregnant people receive the RSV vaccine between 32 and 36 weeks of gestation for protection of newborns and infants through 6 months of age (CDC, 2023c). The vaccine provides 5 months of protection against serious RSV disease. If the birthing parent did not receive the RSV vaccine during pregnancy, the infant 8 months or younger should receive one dose of nirsevimab (Barr & Graham, 2023). During their second RSV season, infants at increased risk for severe RSV infection who are 8 to 19 months of age should receive a second dose of nirsevimab. Those at high risk include infants and toddlers with chronic lung disease of prematurity, immunocompromise, or CF as well as Alaska Natives and Native Americans (Barr & Graham, 2023). Children who are not high risk and who are older than 8 months do not require a second dose.

Pneumonia

Pneumonia is an inflammation of the lung parenchyma. It can be caused by a virus, bacteria, *Mycoplasma,* or fungus. Respiratory viruses are the most common cause of pneumonia in younger children and the least common cause in older children. Viral pneumonia is usually better tolerated in children of all ages. Children with bacterial pneumonia are more apt to present with a toxic appearance, but they generally recover rapidly if appropriate antibiotic treatment is instituted early. *Streptococcus pneumoniae* is a common cause of bacterial pneumonia in all ages of children, and *Mycoplasma pneumoniae* is a common causative agent in the school-age child and adolescent. Fungal infection may also result in pneumonia. Aspiration pneumonia may result from aspiration of foreign material into the lower respiratory tract. Pneumonia occurs more often in winter and early spring. It is common in children but is seen most frequently in infants and young toddlers.

TAKE NOTE!

Community-acquired pneumonia (CAP) refers to pneumonia in a previously healthy person that is contracted outside of the hospital setting (Barson, 2022).

Pneumonia is usually a self-limited disease. A child who presents with recurrent pneumonia should be evaluated for chronic lung disease such as asthma or CF. Potential complications of pneumonia include bacteremia, pleural effusion, empyema, lung abscess, and pneumothorax. Excluding bacteremia, these complications are often treated with thoracentesis and/or chest tubes as well as antibiotics if appropriate. Pneumatoceles (thin-walled cavities developing in the lung) might occur with certain bacterial pneumonias and usually resolve spontaneously over time.

Therapeutic management of children with less severe disease includes antipyretics, adequate hydration, and close observation. Even bacterial pneumonia can be successfully managed at home if the work of breathing is not severe and oxygen saturation is within normal limits. However, hospitalization is required for children with more severe disease. The child with tachypnea, significant retractions, poor oral intake, or lethargy might require hospital admission for the administration of supplemental oxygen, intravenous hydration, and antibiotics.

Nursing Assessment

For a full description of the assessment phase of the nursing process, refer to the "Clinical Judgment and the Nursing Process" section. Assessment findings pertinent to pneumonia are discussed further on.

HEALTH HISTORY

Elicit a description of the present illness and chief complaint. Note onset and progression of symptoms. Common signs and symptoms reported during the health history include:

- Antecedent viral URI
- Fever
- Cough (note type and whether productive or not)
- Increased respiratory rate
- History of lethargy, poor feeding, vomiting, or diarrhea in infants
- Chills, headache, dyspnea, chest pain, abdominal pain, and nausea or vomiting in older children

Explore the child's past and current medical history for risk factors known to be associated with an increase in the severity of pneumonia, such as:

- Prematurity
- Malnutrition
- Passive smoke exposure
- Low socioeconomic status
- Day care attendance
- Underlying cardiopulmonary, immune, or nervous system disease (Houin et al., 2022)

PHYSICAL EXAMINATION

Observe the child's general appearance and color (centrally and peripherally), as the child with bacterial pneumonia may appear ill and cyanosis might accompany coughing spells. Assess work of breathing, noting substernal, subcostal, or intercostal retractions. Tachypnea and nasal flaring may be present. Describe cough and quality of sputum if produced.

Auscultate the lungs for wheezes or rales in the younger child, or local or diffuse rales in the older child. Document diminished breath sounds. Percuss for local dullness over a consolidated area in the older child (percussion is much less valuable in the infant or younger child). Palpate for tactile fremitus, which may be increased with pneumonia.

LABORATORY AND DIAGNOSTIC TESTS

Common laboratory and diagnostic studies ordered for the assessment of pneumonia include:

- Pulse oximetry: oxygen saturation might be decreased significantly or within normal range.
- Chest radiograph: varies according to child age and causative agent; in infants and young children, bilateral air trapping and perihilar **infiltrates** (collection of inflammatory cells, cellular debris, and foreign organisms) are the most common findings. Patchy areas of consolidation might also be present. In older children, lobar consolidation is seen more frequently.

- Sputum culture: may be useful in determining causative bacteria in older children and adolescents
- White blood cell count: might be elevated in the case of bacterial pneumonia

Nursing Management

Patient problems, goals, and interventions for the child with pneumonia are primarily aimed at providing supportive care and education about the illness and its treatment. Prevention of pneumococcal infection is also important. Children with more severe disease will require hospitalization. Refer to the "Clinical Judgment and the Nursing Process" section for patient problems and related interventions. In addition to the interventions listed there, the following should be noted.

PROVIDING SUPPORTIVE CARE

Ensure adequate hydration and assist in thinning of secretions by encouraging oral fluid intake in the child whose respiratory status is stable. Provide intravenous fluids as ordered to children with increased work of breathing to maintain hydration. Allow and encourage the child to assume a position of comfort, usually with the head of the bed elevated to promote aeration of the lungs. If pain due to coughing or pneumonia itself is severe, administer analgesics as prescribed. Provide supplemental oxygen to the child with respiratory distress or **hypoxia** (low oxygen concentration in the tissues) as needed.

PROVIDING FAMILY EDUCATION

Educate the family about the importance of adhering to the prescribed antibiotic regimen. Antibiotics may be given intravenously if the child is hospitalized. Oral antibiotics are used on discharge or if the child is managed on an outpatient basis.

Teach the parents of a child with bacterial pneumonia to expect that for 1 to 2 weeks following resolution of the acute illness, the child might continue to tire easily and that the infant might continue to need small, frequent feedings. Cough may also persist after the acute recovery period but should lessen over time.

If the child is diagnosed with viral pneumonia, provide parents with an explanation that antibiotics are not utilized to treat viral infections (pneumonia is often perceived by the public as a bacterial infection). As with bacterial pneumonia, the child may experience a week or two of weakness or fatigue following resolution of the acute illness.

Teach parents of young children about the risk of the development of aspiration pneumonia. Parents need to understand that the child might be at risk for injury related to their age and developmental stage. To prevent recurrent or further aspiration, teach the parents the safety measures in Teaching Guidelines 18.3.

TEACHING GUIDELINES 18.3 Preventing Aspiration

- Keep toxic substances such as lighter fluid, solvents, and hydrocarbons out of reach of young children. Toddlers and preschoolers cannot distinguish safe from unsafe fluids due to their developmental stage.
- Avoid oily nose drops and oil-based vitamins or home remedies to avoid lipid aspiration into the lungs.
- Avoid oral feedings if the infant's respiratory rate is 60 or greater to minimize the risk of aspiration of the feeding.
- Discourage parents from "force feeding" in the event of poor oral intake or severe illness to minimize the risk of aspiration of the feeding.
- Position infants and ill children on their right side after feeding to minimize the risk of aspirating emesis or regurgitated feeding.

PREVENTING PNEUMOCOCCAL INFECTION

Provide immunization to children at high risk for severe pneumococcal infection. This includes all children between 0 and 23 months of age, as well as children between 24 and 59 months of age who either never received the vaccine before age 2 or did not receive a booster dose between 12 and 23 months of age. In addition, children between 24 and 59 months of age with certain conditions such as immune deficiency, sickle cell disease, asplenia, chronic cardiac conditions, chronic lung problems, cerebrospinal fluid leaks, chronic renal insufficiency, diabetes mellitus, and organ transplants should receive the vaccine (CDC, 2023a). For additional information on immunization, refer to Chapter 9.

Bronchitis

Bronchitis is an inflammation of the trachea and major bronchi. It is often associated with a URI. Bronchitis is usually viral in nature, although *M. pneumoniae* and other bacterial organisms are causative in about 10% of cases (Carolan, 2023). Recovery usually occurs within 5 to 10 days. Therapeutic management involves mainly supportive care. Expectorant administration and adequate hydration are important. If bacterial infection is the cause, antibiotics are indicated.

Nursing Assessment

Ascertain the history, which usually begins with a mild URI. Note the development of fever, followed by a dry, hacking cough that might become productive in older children. Determine if the cough wakes the child at night. Auscultate the lungs to determine if coarse rales are present. Note that respirations remain unlabored. The chest radiograph might show diffuse alveolar hyperinflation and perihilar markings.

Nursing Management

Nursing management is aimed at providing supportive care. Teach parents that expectorants will help loosen secretions and that antipyretics will help reduce the fever, making the child more comfortable. Encourage adequate hydration. Inform parents that antibiotics are prescribed only in cases believed to be bacterial in nature (infrequent). Discourage the use of cough suppressants: it is important for accumulated sputum to be raised.

Tuberculosis

Tuberculosis (TB) is a highly contagious disease caused by inhalation of droplets of *Mycobacterium tuberculosis* or *Mycobacterium bovis*. Children usually contract the disease from an immediate household member. Children experiencing homelessness and poverty are at higher risk, as are those exposed to an adult with TB infection (Batra & Ang, 2022). After exposure to an infected individual, the incubation period is 2 to 10 weeks. The inhaled tubercle bacilli multiply in the alveoli and alveolar ducts, forming an inflammatory exudate. The bacilli are spread by the bloodstream and lymphatic system to various parts of the body. Although pulmonary TB is the most common, children may also have infection in other parts of the body, such as the gastrointestinal tract or central nervous system. Children who test positive for TB but who do not have symptoms or radiographic/laboratory evidence of disease are considered to have latent infection.

In the case of drug-sensitive TB, the American Academy of Pediatrics (AAP) recommends a 4-month course of oral therapy. The first 2 months consist of isoniazid, rifampin, pyrazinamide, and ethambutol given daily. This is followed by twice-weekly isoniazid and rifampin; administration must be observed directly (usually by a public health nurse). In the case of multidrug-resistant TB, a TB specialist is consulted, and intramuscular injection may be given (Kimberlin et al., 2021). Children with latent TB are treated with isoniazid or other drugs to prevent progression to active disease. See the Healthy People 2030 box.

HEALTHY PEOPLE 2030

Objective	Nursing Significance
Reduce tuberculosis (TB).	• Assess the health history of all infants, children, and adolescents for risk factors for TB infection. • Provide TB screening as recommended. • Refer all TB infections to the local public health department. • Educate families about the importance of completing medication therapy as prescribed for active and latent TB and the need for appropriate follow-up and retesting for TB infection.

Healthy People Objectives retrieved from http://www.healthypeople.gov

Nursing Assessment

Children considered to be at high risk for contracting TB should be screened using the Mantoux test. High-risk children are those who:

- Are infected with HIV
- Are incarcerated or institutionalized
- Have a positive recent history of latent TB infection
- Are immigrants from or have a history of travel to endemic countries
- Are exposed at home to people who have an HIV infection, are experiencing homelessness, use illicit drugs, were recently incarcerated, are migrant farm workers, or are nursing home residents

Evaluate the health history for symptoms such as fever, malaise, weight loss, anorexia, pain, and tightness in the chest, and rarely hemoptysis. Note whether cough is present or not and, if present, whether it has progressed slowly over several weeks to months. As TB progresses, note an increase in respiratory rate, diminished breath sounds, and crackles with poor aeration in the affected lung. Percussion may reveal dullness. Keep in mind that some children are asymptomatic. Diagnosis is confirmed with a positive Mantoux test, positive gastric washings for acid-fast bacillus, interferon-gamma release assay (IGRA), and/or a chest radiograph consistent with TB.

Nursing Management

Hospitalization of children with TB is necessary only for the most serious cases. Nursing management is aimed at providing supportive care and encouraging adherence to the treatment regimen. Most nursing care for childhood TB is provided in outpatient clinics, schools, or a public health setting. Supportive care includes ensuring adequate nutrition and adequate rest, providing comfort measures such as fever reduction, preventing exposure to other infectious diseases, and preventing reinfection. Isolate hospitalized children with TB according to hospital policy to prevent nosocomial spread of TB infection.

TAKE NOTE!

Administration of Bacille Calmette–Guérin (BCG) vaccine can provide incomplete protection against tuberculosis, and it is not widely used in the United States (Kimberlin et al., 2021).

COVID-19

URIs have long been known to be caused by the Coronaviridae family of viruses, among many others. In 2020, the SARS CoV-2 (COVID-19) virus quickly spread worldwide, causing a significant amount of morbidity and mortality, particularly in certain populations (S. Smith, 2022).

Infection may be mild, lead to respiratory failure, or result in multisystem inflammatory syndrome (MIS-C) 4 to 6 weeks after an initial mild or unidentified infection (Zachariah, 2022). A vaccine was made available, first to older adults or those vulnerable to severe infection, later to all adults, then, finally, to children as young as 6 months. The CDC recommends every person 6 months of age and older complete the initial COVID-19 immunization series and receive boosters at the appropriate time (Regan et al., 2023).

Quarantines implemented nationwide (and across most parts of the world) in early 2020 resulted in income and job losses, as well as academic and social consequences for children who were unable to attend day care or school. As the COVID-19 pandemic has eased, morbidity and mortality rates have decreased significantly. Thus, quarantines and social distancing requirements have been lifted, and people have returned to work and school as they did prior to the pandemic. In 2023, some states still required certain populations (i.e., those who work in health care and/or certain state agencies) either to be vaccinated against COVID-19 or to submit to regular testing for the infection (Rough & Markowitz, 2023).

Nursing Assessment

About 50% of children with COVID-19 are asymptomatic (Zachariah, 2022). Evaluate the health history for symptoms such as fever (may or may not be present), cough, runny nose, sore throat, nausea, vomiting, or diarrhea. The infected infant may be apneic, and the older child or adolescent may experience loss of the senses of smell and taste. Headache may be present in the older child. Determine the child's immunization status.

Nursing Management

Provide supportive care to the child with mild COVID-19. Antipyretics and symptomatic relief of other clinical manifestations will make the child more comfortable. Educate families about handwashing, social distancing (6 ft apart), and the proper use of masks if the child is 2 years of age or older (Rabinowicz et al., 2020). Refer families to the World Health Organization's (WHO) website for continually updated information regarding COVID-19 (WHO, 2023).

ACUTE NONINFECTIOUS DISORDERS

Acute noninfectious disorders include epistaxis, foreign body aspiration, respiratory distress syndrome (RDS), acute RDS, and pneumothorax.

Epistaxis

Epistaxis (a nosebleed) occurs most frequently in children before adolescence. Bleeding of the nasal mucosa occurs most often from the anterior portion of the septum. Epistaxis may be recurrent and idiopathic (meaning there is no known cause). The majority of cases are benign, but in children with bleeding disorders or other hematologic concerns, epistaxis should be further investigated and treated.

Nursing Assessment

Explore the child's history for initiating factors such as local inflammation, mucosal drying, or local trauma (usually nose picking). Inspect the nasal cavity for blood.

Nursing Management

Remain calm, and encourage the parents to do so as well since the presence of blood often frightens children and their parents. Have the child sit up and lean forward (lying down may allow aspiration of the blood). Apply continuous pressure to the anterior portion of the nose by pinching it closed. Encourage the child to breathe through the mouth during this portion of the treatment. Ice or a cold cloth applied to the bridge of the nose may also be helpful. The bleeding usually stops within 10 to 15 minutes. Apply water-soluble gel to the nasal mucosa with a cotton-tipped applicator to moisten the mucosa and prevent recurrence.

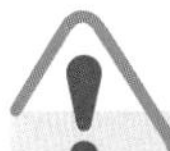

CLINICAL REASONING ALERT!

The child with recurrent epistaxis or epistaxis that is difficult to control should be further evaluated for underlying bleeding or platelet concerns.

Foreign Body Aspiration

Foreign body aspiration occurs when any solid or liquid substance is inhaled into the respiratory tract. It is common in infants and young children and can present in a life-threatening manner. The object may lodge in the upper or lower airway, causing varying degrees of respiratory difficulty. Small, smooth objects such as peanuts are the most frequently aspirated, but any small toy, article, or piece of food smaller than the diameter of the young child's airway can be aspirated (Safe Kids, 2024).

TAKE NOTE!

Items smaller than 1.25 in (3.2 cm) can be aspirated easily. A simple way for parents to estimate the safe size of a small item or toy piece is to gauge its size against a standard toilet paper roll (not double roll), which is generally about 1.5 in in diameter.

Foreign body aspiration occurs most frequently in children between 6 months and 3 years of age (Houin et al., 2022). Children at this age are growing and developing rapidly. They tend to explore things with their mouths and can easily aspirate small items.

The child often coughs out foreign bodies from the upper airway. If the foreign body reaches the bronchus, then it may need to be surgically removed via bronchoscopy. Postoperative antibiotics are used if an infection is also present. Complications of foreign body aspiration include pneumonia or abscess formation, hypoxia, respiratory failure, and death.

Nursing Assessment

Evaluate the history of the infant or young child for usually sudden onset of cough, wheeze, or stridor, although the onset of respiratory symptoms can be more gradual. Stridor suggests that the foreign body is lodged in the upper airway. Auscultate the lungs for wheezing, rhonchi, and decreased aeration, which can be heard on the affected side. A chest radiograph will demonstrate the foreign body only if it is radiopaque (Fig. 18.7).

Nursing Management

The most important nursing intervention related to foreign body aspiration is prevention. Anticipatory guidance for families with 6-month-olds should include a discussion of aspiration avoidance. Repeat this information at each subsequent well-child visit through age 5. Tell parents to avoid letting their child play with toys with small parts and to keep coins and other small objects out of the reach of children. Teach parents not to feed peanuts and popcorn to their child until they are at least 4 years old (Durani, 2023). When children progress to table food, teach parents to chop all foods so that they are small enough to pass down the trachea should the child neglect to chew them up thoroughly. Carrots, grapes, and hot dogs should be cut into small pieces. Harmful liquids should be kept out of the reach of children.

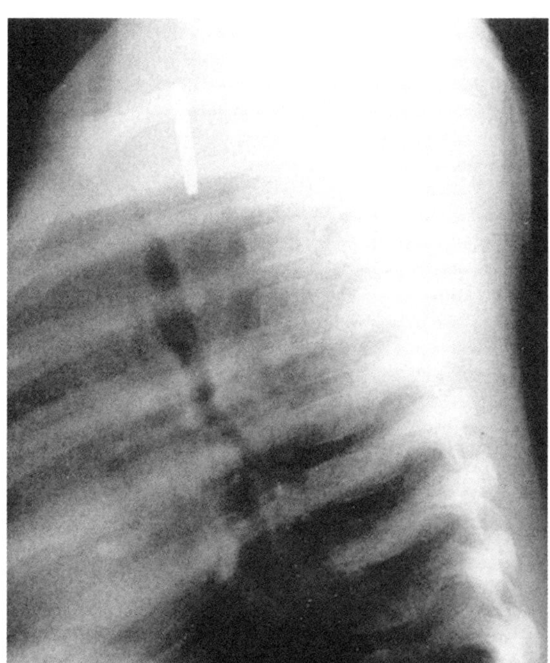

FIGURE 18.7 Foreign body is noted in the bronchus on a chest radiograph.

TAKE NOTE!

Prevent young children from playing with latex balloons. When popped, small pieces pose an aspiration danger.

Respiratory Distress Syndrome

RDS is a respiratory disorder that is specific to neonates. It results from lung immaturity and a deficiency in surfactant, so it is seen most often in premature infants. Other infants who might experience RDS include infants of birthing parents with diabetes, those delivered via cesarean birth without preceding labor, and those experiencing perinatal asphyxia (Pramanik, 2020). It is believed that each of these conditions has an impact on surfactant production, thus resulting in RDS in the term infant.

Pathophysiology

The lack of surfactant in the affected newborn's lungs results in stiff, poorly compliant lungs with poor gas exchange. Right-to-left shunting and hypoxemia result. As the disease progresses, fluid and fibrin leak from the pulmonary capillaries, causing a hyaline membrane to form in the bronchioles, alveolar ducts, and alveoli. Presence of the membrane further decreases gas exchange. If untreated, RDS progresses to seesaw respirations, respiratory failure, and shock.

Complications of RDS include air leak syndrome, chronic lung disease of prematurity (formerly termed "bronchopulmonary dysplasia"), patent ductus arteriosus and congestive heart failure, intraventricular hemorrhage, retinopathy of prematurity, necrotizing enterocolitis, complications resulting from intravenous catheter use (infection, thrombus formation), and developmental delay or disability.

Therapeutic Management

The administration of surfactant via an endotracheal tube shortly after delivery helps to decrease the incidence and severity of RDS. Therapeutic management of RDS focuses on intensive respiratory care, usually with mechanical ventilation. Newer techniques for ventilatory support are also available (Table 18.2).

TABLE 18.2 • Alternatives to Traditional Mechanical Ventilation

Mode	Description	Additional Information
High-frequency ventilators (high-frequency, oscillating, or jet)	Provide very high respiratory rates (up to 1,200 breaths per min) and very low tidal volumes	May decrease risk of barotrauma associated with ventilator pressures
Nitric oxide	Causes pulmonary vasodilation, helping to increase blood flow to alveoli	Safe; no long-term developmental risks
Liquid ventilation	Perfluorocarbon liquid acts as a surfactant. Provides an effective medium for gas exchange and increases pulmonary function	Virtually no reported physiologic sequelae
Extracorporeal membrane oxygenation (ECMO)	Blood is removed from body via catheter, warmed and oxygenated in the ECMO machine, and then returned to infant.	Labor-intensive; risk of bleeding is great.

Nursing Assessment

Assess the infant for the onset of RDS, which usually occurs within several hours of birth. Note signs of respiratory distress, including tachypnea, retractions, nasal flaring, grunting, and varying degrees of cyanosis. Auscultation reveals fine rales and diminished breath sounds.

Nursing Management

Closely observe the neonate placed on the ventilator after surfactant administration; although rare, mucus plugging can occur. Watch for adequate lung expansion. In addition to expert respiratory intervention, other crucial nursing goals include maintenance of normothermia, prevention of infection, maintenance of fluid and electrolyte balance, and promotion of adequate nutrition (parenterally or via gavage feeding). Nursing care of the infant with RDS generally occurs in the intensive care unit.

Acute Respiratory Distress Syndrome

Acute respiratory distress syndrome (ARDS) occurs following a primary insult such as sepsis, infectious or aspiration pneumonia, and COVID-19 in infants and children with previously healthy lungs (Purohit, 2023; Zachariah, 2022). The alveolar–capillary membrane becomes more permeable, and pulmonary edema develops. Hyaline membrane formation over the alveolar surfaces and decreased surfactant production cause lung stiffness. Mucosal swelling and cellular debris lead to atelectasis. Gas diffusion is impaired significantly. Some children have residual lung disease, and some recover completely. However, ARDS can progress to respiratory failure and death.

Therapeutic management is aimed at improving oxygenation and ventilation. Mechanical ventilation is used, with special attention to lung volumes and positive end-expiratory pressure (PEEP). Newer treatment modalities show promise for improving outcomes of ARDS.

Nursing Assessment

Note tachycardia and tachypnea occurring over the first few hours of the illness. Observe for significantly increased work of breathing, nasal flaring, and retractions. Auscultate the breath sounds, which might range from normal to high-pitched crackles throughout the lung fields. Note decreased oxygen saturation. Bilateral infiltrates can be seen on a chest radiograph.

Nursing Management

Nursing care of the child with ARDS is mainly supportive and occurs in the intensive care unit. Closely monitor respiratory and cardiovascular status. Comfort measures such as hygiene and positioning as well as pain and anxiety management, maintenance of nutrition, and prevention of infection are also key nursing interventions. Soothe the child's fears as the acute phase of worsening respiratory distress can be frightening for a child of any age. As the disease worsens and progresses, especially when ventilatory support is required, it is especially important to provide psychological support of the family as well as education about the intensive care unit procedures.

Pneumothorax

A collection of air in the pleural space is called a pneumothorax. It can occur spontaneously in an otherwise healthy child or because of chronic lung disease, cardiopulmonary resuscitation (CPR), surgery, or trauma. Trapped air consumes space within the pleural cavity, and the affected lung suffers at least partial collapse. Needle aspiration and/or placement of a chest

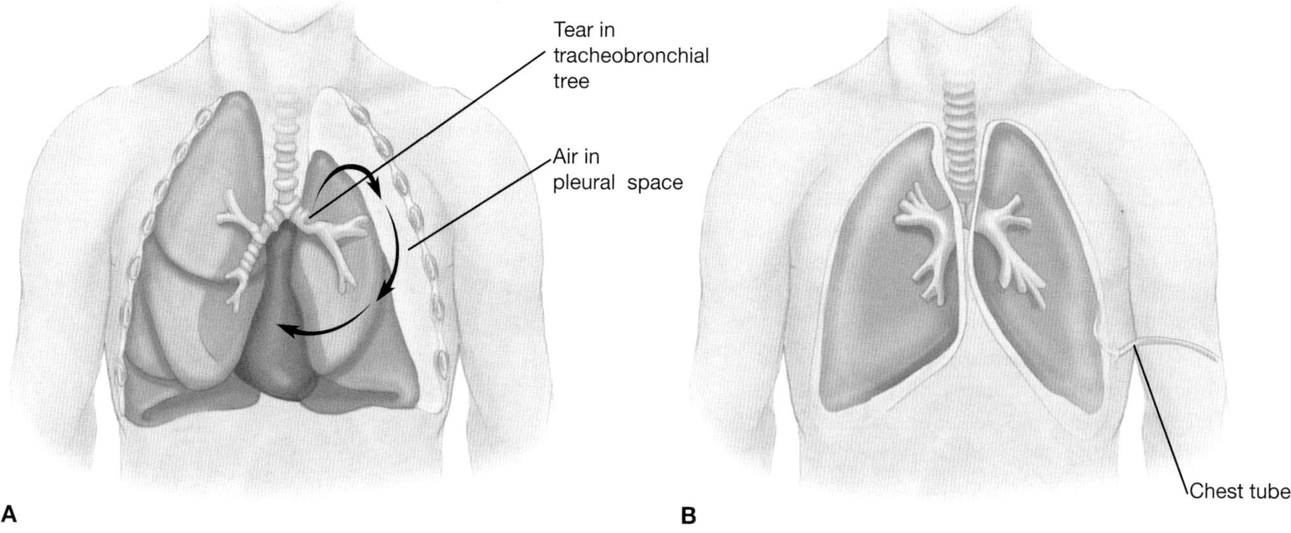

FIGURE 18.8 **A.** Pneumothorax. **B.** Note reinflation of the lung when the chest tube is present.

tube are used to evacuate the air from the chest. Some small pneumothoraces resolve independently, without intervention.

Nursing Assessment

The infant or child with a pneumothorax might have a sudden or gradual onset of symptoms. Determine risk factors for acquiring a pneumothorax, including chest trauma or surgery, intubation and mechanical ventilation, or a history of chronic lung disease such as CF. Note the presence of chest pain, tachypnea, retractions, nasal flaring, grunting, pallor, or cyanosis. Auscultate for tachycardia and absent or diminished breath sounds on the affected side. The radiograph reveals air within the thoracic cavity (Fig. 18.8).

Nursing Management

Frequently assess the child's respiratory status. Administer 100% oxygen as ordered as it hastens the reabsorption of air (generally used only for a few hours) (Janahi, 2022). Assist with needle aspiration and/or chest tube insertion. If a chest tube is connected to a dry suction or water seal apparatus, provide care of the drainage apparatus as appropriate (Fig. 18.9). Keep a pair of hemostats at the bedside to clamp the tube should it become dislodged from the drainage container, or the open end may be placed in a container of sterile water. The dressing around the chest tube is occlusive and is not routinely changed. If the tube becomes dislodged from the child's chest, apply Vaseline gauze and an occlusive dressing, immediately perform appropriate respiratory assessment, and notify the primary health care provider or nurse practitioner.

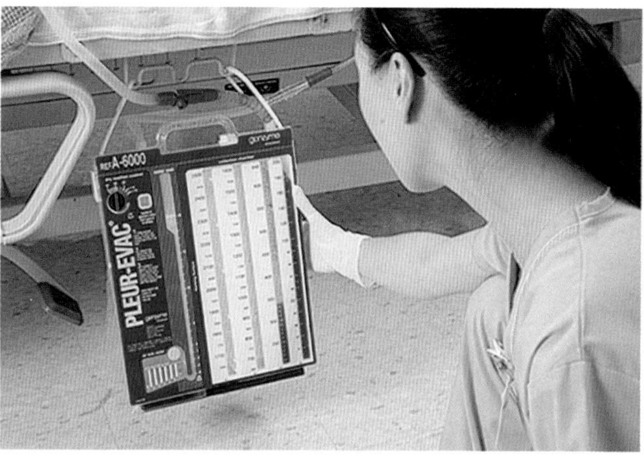

FIGURE 18.9 The chest tube is connected to a suction or water seal via a drainage container.

CHRONIC RESPIRATORY DISORDERS

Chronic respiratory disorders include allergic rhinitis, asthma, chronic lung disease (bronchopulmonary dysplasia), CF, and apnea.

Allergic Rhinitis

Allergic rhinitis is a common chronic condition in childhood, affecting a significant number of children. Allergic rhinitis is associated with atopic dermatitis and asthma. Perennial allergic rhinitis occurs year-round and is associated with indoor environments. Allergens commonly implicated in perennial allergic rhinitis include dust mites, pet dander, cockroach antigens, and molds. Seasonal allergic rhinitis is caused by elevations in outdoor levels of allergens. It is typically caused by certain pollens, trees, weeds, fungi, and molds. Complications from allergic rhinitis include exacerbation of asthma symptoms, recurrent sinusitis and otitis media, and dental malocclusion.

Pathophysiology

Allergic rhinitis is an intermittent or persistent inflammatory state that is mediated by immunoglobulin E (IgE). In response to contact with an airborne allergen protein, the nasal mucosa mounts an immune response. The antigen (from the allergen) binds to a specific IgE on the surface of mast cells, releasing the chemical mediators of histamine and leukotrienes. Shortly thereafter, various white blood cells release chemical mediators, and inflammation results. IgE binds to receptors on the surfaces of mast cells and basophils, creating the sensitization memory that causes the reaction with subsequent allergen exposures. Allergen exposure then results in the inflammatory response. Histamine and other factors cause nasal vasodilation, watery **rhinorrhea** (runny nose), nasal congestion, pruritus, and sneezing. Treatment of allergic rhinitis is aimed at decreasing response to these allergic mediators as well as treating inflammation.

Nursing Assessment

For a full description of the assessment phase of the nursing process, refer to the "Clinical Judgment and the Nursing Process" section. Assessment findings pertinent to allergic rhinitis are discussed here.

HEALTH HISTORY

Elicit a description of the present illness and chief complaint. Common signs and symptoms reported during the health history might include:

- Mild, intermittent, to chronic nasal stuffiness
- Thin, runny nasal discharge
- Sneezing
- Itching of nose, eyes, palate
- Mouth breathing and snoring

Determine the seasonality of symptoms. Are they perennial (year-round) or do they occur during certain seasons only? What types of medications or other treatments have been used, and what was the child's response?

Explore the history for the presence of risk factors such as:

- Family history of atopic disease (asthma, allergic rhinitis, or atopic dermatitis)
- Known allergy to dust mites, pet dander, cockroach antigens, pollens, or molds
- Early childhood exposure to indoor allergens
- Early introduction to foods or formula in infancy
- Exposure to tobacco smoke

PHYSICAL EXAMINATION

Physical examination of the child with allergic rhinitis includes inspection, observation, and auscultation.

Inspection and Observation

Observe the child's facies for red-rimmed eyes or tearing, mild eyelid edema, "allergic shiners" (bluish or grayish cast beneath the eyes), and "allergic salute" (a transverse nasal crease between the lower and middle thirds of the nose that results from repeated nose rubbing) (Fig. 18.10). Inspect the nasal cavity. The turbinates may be swollen and gray/blue. Clear mucoid nasal drainage may be observed. Inspect the skin for rash. Listen for nasal phonation with speech.

Auscultation

Auscultate the lungs for adequate aeration and clarity of breath sounds. In the child who also has asthma, exacerbation with wheezing often occurs with allergic rhinitis.

LABORATORY AND DIAGNOSTIC TESTS

The initial diagnosis is often made based on the history and clinical findings. Common laboratory and diagnostic studies ordered for the assessment of allergic rhinitis may include:

- Nasal smear (positive for eosinophilia)
- Positive allergy skin test
- Positive radioallergosorbent test (RAST)

To distinguish between the causes of nasal congestion, refer to Comparison Chart 18.1.

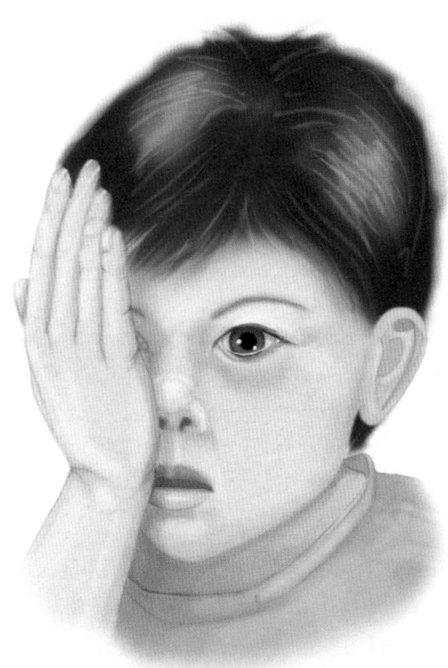

FIGURE 18.10 Allergic shiners beneath the eyes and allergic salute across the nose.

Nursing Management

In addition to the nursing patient problems and related interventions discussed in the "Clinical Judgment and the Nursing Process" section, interventions common to allergic rhinitis follow.

MAINTAINING PATENT AIRWAY

Perform nasal washes with normal saline to keep the nasal mucus from becoming thickened and lessen nasal obstruction. Thickened, immobile secretions often lead to a secondary bacterial infection. The nasal wash also decongests the nose, allowing for improved nasal airflow. Administer antiinflammatory (corticosteroid) nasal sprays as prescribed to decrease the inflammatory response to allergens and/or mast cell stabilizing nasal spray such as cromolyn sodium to decrease the intensity and frequency of allergic responses. Teach families about nasal medications as well as other recommended drugs such as once-daily oral antihistamines, combined antihistamine/nasal decongestants, or leukotriene modifiers such as montelukast. See Dosage Calculation Box 18.1.

DOSAGE CALCULATION BOX 18.1

Child's weight: 30 lb

Medication order: cetirizine 2.5 mg PO every morning

Cetirizine is supplied as 5 mg/5 mL.

How many milliliters will the nurse administer? Round to the nearest tenth.

PROVIDING FAMILY EDUCATION

One of the most important tools in the treatment of allergic rhinitis is learning to avoid known allergens. Teaching Guidelines 18.4 gives information on educating families about avoidance of allergens. Children may be referred to a specialist for allergen desensitization (allergy shots). Products helpful with control of allergies are available from several vendors.

Asthma

Asthma is a chronic inflammatory airway disorder characterized by airway hyperresponsiveness, airway edema, and mucus production. Airway obstruction resulting from asthma might be partially or completely reversed. Severity ranges from long periods of control with infrequent acute exacerbations in some children to the presence of persistent daily symptoms in others. It is the most common chronic illness of childhood with 5 million American children diagnosed before age 18 years (Volkman & Chiu, 2023). The incidence and severity of asthma are increasing; this might be attributed to increased urbanization, increased air pollution, and more accurate diagnosis. See the Healthy People 2030 box.

TEACHING GUIDELINES 18.4 Controlling Exposure to Allergens

Tobacco
- Avoid all exposure to tobacco smoke.
- No parental smoking inside the home or car.

Dust Mites
- Use pillow and mattress covers.
- Wash bed linen once a week in 130°F water.
- Use blinds rather than curtains in bedroom.
- Remove stuffed animals from bedroom or minimize number and wash weekly.
- Reduce indoor humidity to <50%.
- Remove carpet from bedroom.
- Clean solid-surface floors with wet mop each week.

Pet Dander
- Remove pets from home permanently.
- If unable to remove them, keep them out of bedroom and off carpet and upholstered furniture.

Cockroaches
- Keep kitchen clean.
- Avoid leaving food or drinks out.
- Use pesticides if necessary, but ensure that the asthmatic child is not inside the home when the pesticide is sprayed.

Indoor Molds
- Repair water leaks.
- Use dehumidifier to keep basement dry.
- Reduce indoor humidity to <50%.

Outdoor Molds, Pollen, and Air Pollution
- Avoid going outdoors when mold and pollen counts are high.
- Avoid outdoor activity when pollution levels are high.

Adapted from Houin, P., Stillwell, P., Deboer, E. M., & Hoppe, J. (2022). Respiratory tract & mediastinum. In M. Bunik, W. W. Hay, M. J. Levin, & M. J. Abzug (Eds.), *Current diagnosis and treatment: Pediatrics* (26th ed.). McGraw-Hill Education; Volkman, K. K., & Chiu, A. M. (2023). Allergy. In K. J. Marcdante & R. M. Kliegman (Eds.), *Nelson's essentials of pediatrics* (9th ed.). Elsevier.

HEALTHY PEOPLE 2030

Objective	Nursing Significance
Reduce asthma deaths, hospitalizations for asthma, hospital emergency department visits for asthma.	• Appropriately educate children with asthma and their families about the ongoing management of asthma. • Provide appropriate education and triage to families of children with asthma, particularly when the child is experiencing symptoms or a decreased peak flow rate.

Healthy People Objectives retrieved from http://www.healthypeople.gov

Severity ranges from symptoms associated only with vigorous activity (exercise-induced bronchospasm) to daily symptoms that interfere with quality of life (such as severe persistent asthma resulting in nighttime symptoms occurring every day). Although uncommon, childhood death related to asthma is also on the rise worldwide. Many children with asthma also have gastroesophageal disease, although the relationship between the two diseases is not clearly understood. Children with asthma are more susceptible to serious bacterial and viral respiratory infections. Acute complications include status asthmaticus and respiratory failure.

Pathophysiology

In asthma, the inflammatory process contributes to increased airway activity. Thus, control or prevention of inflammation is the core of asthma management. Asthma results from a complex variety of responses in relation to a trigger. When the process begins, mast cells, T lymphocytes, macrophages, and epithelial cells are involved in the release of inflammatory mediators. Eosinophils and neutrophils migrate to the airway, causing injury. Chemical mediators such as leukotrienes, bradykinin, histamine, and platelet-activating factor also contribute to the inflammatory response. The presence of leukotrienes contributes to prolonged airway constriction. Autonomic neural control of airway tone is affected, airway mucus secretion is increased, mucociliary function changes, and airway smooth muscle responsiveness increases. As a result, acute bronchoconstriction, airway edema, and mucus plugging occur (Fig. 18.11).

In most children, this process is considered reversible and until recently was not considered to have long-standing effects on lung function. Current research and scientific thought, however, recognize the concept of airway remodeling as a significant long-term complication. Over time, with repeat asthma exacerbations, irreversible structural airway changes occur, and pulmonary function decreases with this remodeling (Volkman & Chiu, 2023). In some individuals with poorly controlled asthma, these changes may be permanent, resulting in decreased responsiveness to therapy.

Therapeutic Management

Current goals of medical therapy are avoidance of asthma triggers and reduction or control of inflammatory episodes. The most recent recommendations by the National Asthma Education and Prevention Program (NAEPP) and the Global Initiative for Asthma (GINA) suggest a stepwise approach to medication management as well as control of environmental factors (allergens) and comorbid conditions that affect asthma. The NAEPP and GINA guidelines stress periodic assessment of asthma control. Treatment decisions may then be made based on the individual's level of asthma control, rather than on the severity at diagnosis. The stepwise approach to asthma treatment involves increasing medications as the child's condition worsens, then backing off treatment as they improve (Box 18.3).

Short-acting bronchodilators may be used in the acute treatment of bronchoconstriction, and long-acting forms may be used to prevent bronchospasm. Exercise-induced bronchospasm may occur in any child with asthma or as the only symptom in the child with mild intermittent asthma. Most children may avoid exercise-induced bronchospasm by using a longer warm-up period prior to vigorous exercise and, if necessary, inhaling a short-acting bronchodilator just prior to exercise. Long-term prevention usually involves inhaled steroids. Leukotriene modifiers may be used as an alternative but are not preferred for mild persistent asthma (Covar et al., 2022).

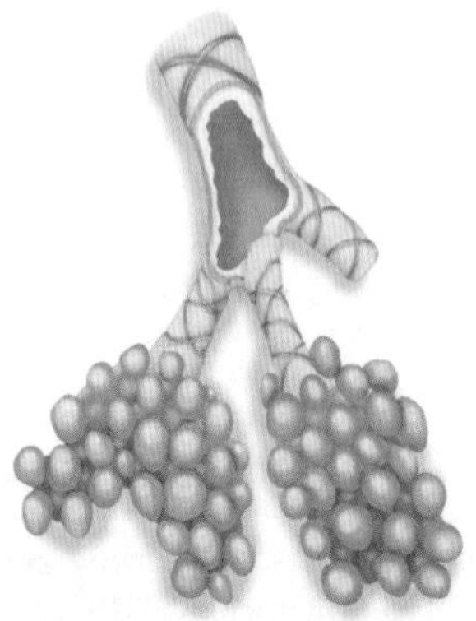

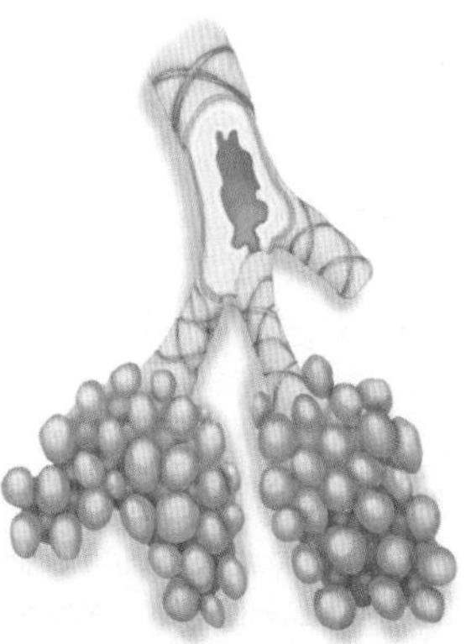

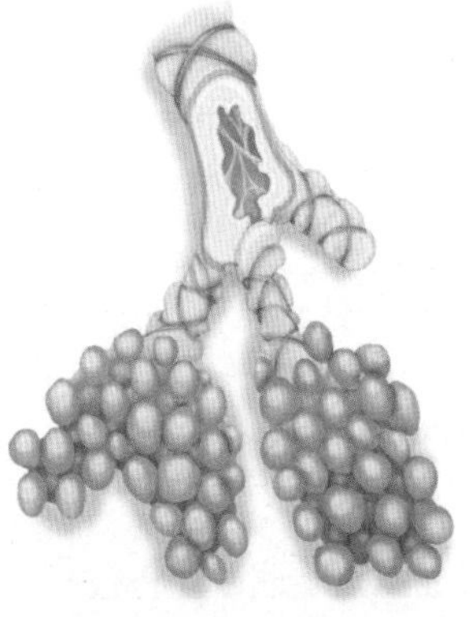

FIGURE 18.11 Note airway edema, mucus production, and bronchospasm occurring with asthma.

BOX 18.3 Stepwise Approach to Asthma Management

All children: child education, environmental control, and management of comorbidities at each step; consider referral to asthma specialist at step 3. (Step 2 and beyond are persistent asthma.)

Step 1 (Intermittent Asthma)

Preferred: short-acting beta$_2$-agonist PRN

Step 2

Preferred: low-dose inhaled corticosteroid
Alternative: cromolyn or leukotriene modifier

Step 3

Preferred: medium-dose inhaled corticosteroid (all ages) OR low-dose inhaled corticosteroid and leukotriene modifier or long-acting beta$_2$-agonist (children older than 4 years)

Step 4

Preferred: medium-dose inhaled corticosteroids and long-acting beta$_2$-agonist (can use leukotriene modifier in children younger than 4 years)

Step 5

Preferred: high-dose inhaled corticosteroids and long-acting beta$_2$-agonist (or leukotriene modifier or theophylline)

Step 6

Preferred: high-dose inhaled corticosteroids, long-acting β_2-agonist, and oral systemic corticosteroids

Adapted from Houin, P., Stillwell, P., Deboer, E. M., & Hoppe, J. (2022). Respiratory tract & mediastinum. In M. Bunik, W. W. Hay, M. J. Levin, & M. J. Abzug (Eds.), *Current diagnosis and treatment: Pediatrics* (26th ed.). McGraw-Hill Education; Volkman, K. K., & Chiu, A. M. (2023). Allergy. In K. J. Marcdante & R. M. Kliegman (Eds.), *Nelson's essentials of pediatrics* (9th ed.). Elsevier.

Nursing Assessment

For a full description of the assessment phase of the nursing process, refer to the "Clinical Judgment and the Nursing Process" section. Assessment findings pertinent to asthma are discussed here.

HEALTH HISTORY

Elicit a description of the present illness and chief complaint. Common signs and symptoms reported during the health history might include:

- Cough, particularly at night: hacking cough that is initially nonproductive, becoming productive of frothy sputum
- Difficulty breathing: shortness of breath, chest tightness or pain, dyspnea with exercise
- Wheezing

Explore the child's current and past medical history for risk factors such as:

- History of allergic rhinitis or atopic dermatitis
- Family history of atopy (asthma, allergic rhinitis, atopic dermatitis)
- Recurrent episodes diagnosed as wheezing, bronchiolitis, or bronchitis
- Known allergies
- Seasonal response to environmental pollen
- Tobacco smoke exposure
- Poverty

PHYSICAL EXAMINATION

Physical examination of the child with asthma includes inspection, auscultation, and percussion.

Inspection

Observe the child's general appearance and color. During mild exacerbations, the child's skin color or the conjunctivae, palms, nail beds, or soles might remain pink. As the child worsens, cyanosis might result. Assess work of breathing, which is variable, ranging from mild retractions to significant accessory muscle use and eventually head bobbing if not treated effectively. Note lethargy, irritability, or the appearance of anxiety or fearfulness. An audible wheeze might be present. Children with persistent severe asthma may have a barrel chest and routinely demonstrate mildly increased work of breathing.

Auscultation and Percussion

A thorough assessment of lung fields is necessary. Wheezing is the hallmark of airway obstruction and might vary throughout the lung fields. Coarseness might also be present. Assess the adequacy of aeration. Breath sounds might be diminished in the bases or throughout. A quiet chest in an asthmatic child can be an ominous sign. With severe airway obstruction, air movement can be so poor that wheezes might not be heard on auscultation. Percussion may yield hyperresonance.

LABORATORY AND DIAGNOSTIC TESTS

Laboratory and diagnostic studies commonly ordered for the assessment of asthma include:

- Pulse oximetry: oxygen saturation may be decreased significantly or normal during a mild exacerbation.
- Chest radiograph: usually reveals hyperinflation
- Blood gases: might show carbon dioxide retention and hypoxemia
- Pulmonary function tests (PFTs): can be useful in determining the degree of disease but are not useful during an acute attack; children as young as 5 or 6 years might be able to comply with spirometry.
- Peak expiratory flow rate (PEFR): is decreased during an exacerbation
- Allergy testing: skin test or RAST can determine allergic triggers for the asthmatic child.

Nursing Management

Initial nursing management of the child with an acute exacerbation of asthma is aimed at restoring a clear airway and effective breathing pattern as well as promoting adequate oxygenation and ventilation (gas exchange). Ongoing management focuses on adherence with the maintenance treatment plan and supporting the child and family. Refer to the "Clinical Judgment and the Nursing Process" section for suggested patient problems and interventions. Additional specific considerations are reviewed further on.

• • • ATRAUMATIC CARE • • •

When caring for a young child who must receive a nebulizer treatment by mask, play make-believe about the mask, and utilize other distraction techniques, such as reading a book. Making activities into games and utilizing distraction both help to minimize trauma when providing necessary care to young children.

EDUCATING THE CHILD AND FAMILY

Teach families of children with asthma, and the children themselves, how to care for the disease; they need to understand the chronicity of asthma. Help families to understand that symptom-free periods (often long) are interspersed with episodes of exacerbation. Educate parents and children about the importance of maintenance medications for long-term control. Teach them that the episodes of exacerbation (sometimes requiring hospitalization or emergency room visits) should not be viewed as an acute illness. While parents may be relieved when an episode resolves, they should not view the child as disease-free during the periods between acute episodes. Educate families that the long-term maintenance schedules must be maintained during those periods as well. Inform families that the prolonged inflammatory process occurring in the absence of symptoms, primarily in children with moderate to severe asthma, can lead to airway remodeling and eventual irreversible disease.

Educate the child and family about the management plan in place to determine when to step up or step down treatment. Figure 18.12 provides an example of an action plan that may be helpful to families in the management of asthma. Instruct parents to ensure the action plan is kept on file at the child's school and that relief medication is always available to the child. Children who experience exercise-induced bronchospasm may still participate in physical education or athletics but

AAAAI
AMERICAN ACADEMY OF ALLERGY ASTHMA & IMMUNOLOGY
www.aaaai.org

ASTHMA ACTION PLAN

Name: ______ Date: ______
Emergency Contact: ______ Relationship: ______
Cell phone: ______ Work phone: ______
Health Care Provider: ______ Phone number: ______
Personal Best Peak Flow: ______

GREEN ZONE:
Doing Well
✓ No coughing, wheezing, chest tightness, or difficulty breathing
✓ Can work, play, exercise, perform usual activities without symptoms
OR
✓ Peak flow ____ to ____
(80% to 100% of personal best)

Take these medicines every day for control and maintenance:

Medicine	How much to take	When and how often

YELLOW ZONE:
Caution/Getting Worse
✓ Coughing, wheezing, chest tightness, or difficulty breathing
✓ Symptoms with daily activities, work, play, and exercise
✓ Nighttime awakenings with symptoms
OR
✓ Peak flow ____ to ____
(50% to 80% of personal best)

CONTINUE your Green Zone medicines PLUS take these quick-relief medicines:

Medicine	How much to take	When and how often

Call your doctor if you have been in the Yellow Zone for more than 24 hours.

Also call your doctor if: ______

RED ZONE:
Alert!
✓ Difficulty breathing, coughing, wheezing not helped with medications
✓ Trouble walking or talking due to asthma symptoms
✓ Not responding to quick relief medication
OR
✓ Peak flow is less than ____
(50% of personal best)

FOR EXTREME TROUBLE BREATHING/SHORTNESS OF BREATH GET IMMEDIATE HELP!

Take these quick-relief medicines:

Medicine	How much to take	When and how often

CALL your doctor NOW.
GO to the hospital/emergency department or CALL for an ambulance NOW!

This information is for general purposes and is not intended to replace the advice of a qualified health professional. For more information on asthma, visit www.aaaai.org.

FIGURE 18.12 Asthma action plan. (Used with permission from the American Academy of Allergy, Asthma & Immunology. Visit AAAAI.org for additional information and updates.)

may need to be allowed to use their medicine before the activity. Provide appropriate education to the child and family based on the child's individualized stepwise treatment plan. Stress the concept of maintenance medications for the prevention of future serious disease in addition to controlling or preventing current symptoms.

Educate families and children on the appropriate use of nebulizers, metered-dose inhalers, spacers, dry-powder inhalers, and Diskus, as well as the purposes, functions, and side effects of the medications they deliver. Require return demonstrations of equipment use to ensure that children and families can use the equipment properly (Teaching Guidelines 18.5).

TAKE NOTE!

It is recommended to use an age-appropriate spacer or holding chamber with metered-dose inhalers to increase the bioavailability of medication in the lungs (Volkman & Chiu, 2023).

In children who have more severe asthma, the use of the PEFR helps to determine daily control. PEFR measurements obtained via a home peak flow meter can be helpful if the meter is used appropriately (Volkman & Chiu, 2023). Teaching Guidelines 18.6 gives instructions

TEACHING GUIDELINES 18.5 Using Asthma Medication Delivery Devices

Nebulizer

1. Plug in the nebulizer and connect the air compressor tubing. 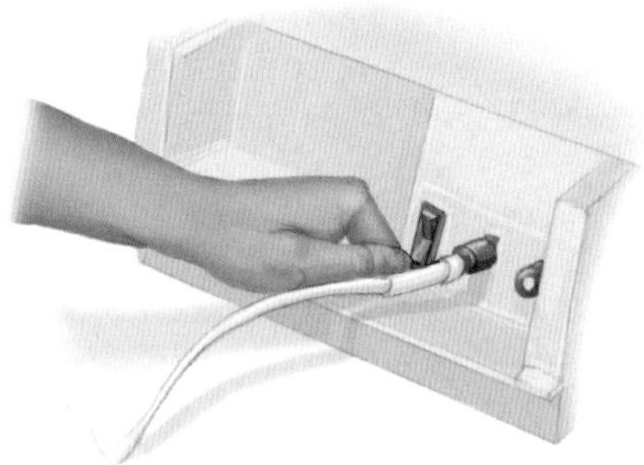
2. Add the medication to the medicine cup. 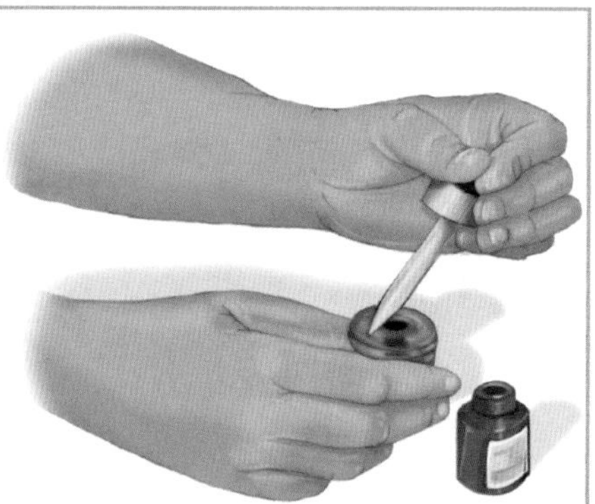
3. Attach the mask or the mouthpiece and hose to the medicine cup. 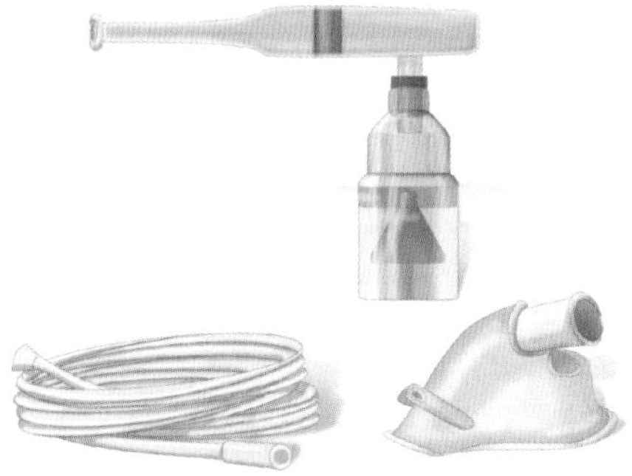
4. Place the mask on the child *or* (see step 5). 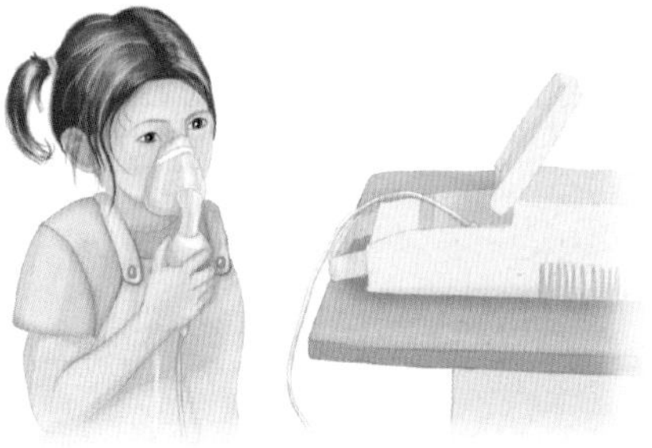
5. Instruct the child to close the lips around the mouthpiece and breathe through the mouth. 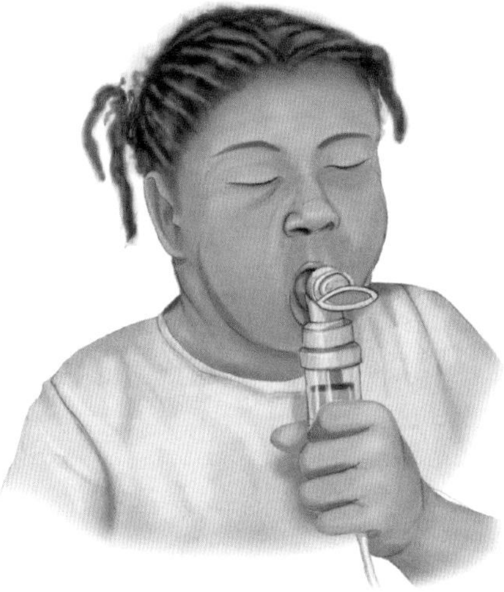
6. After use, wash the mouthpiece and medicine cup with water and allow to air dry.

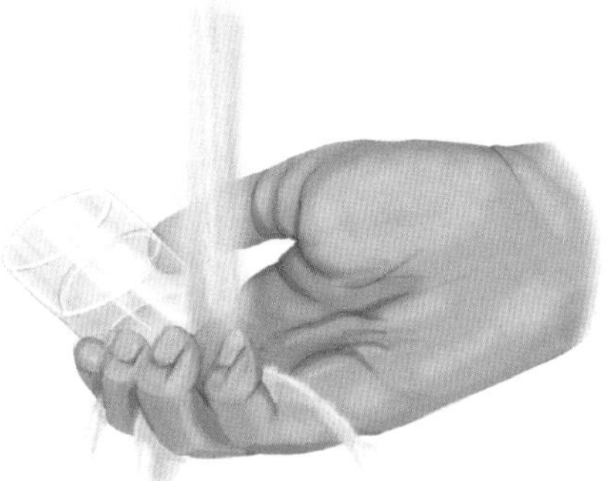

(*continued*)

TEACHING GUIDELINES 18.5 Using Asthma Medication Delivery Devices (*continued*)

Metered-Dose Inhaler

1. Shake the inhaler and take off the cap.

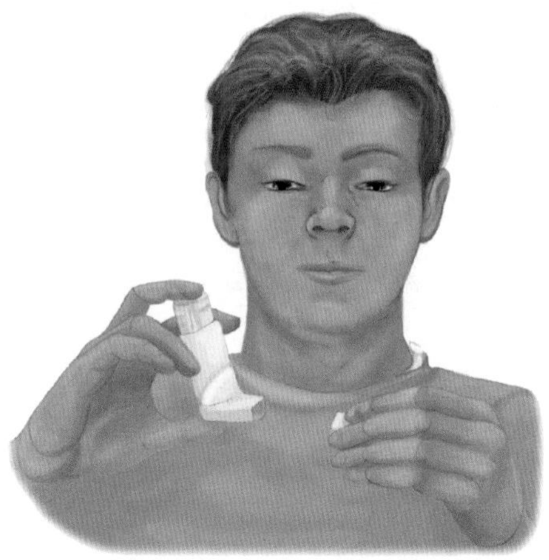

2. Attach the inhaler to the spacer or holding chamber.
3. Breathe out completely.

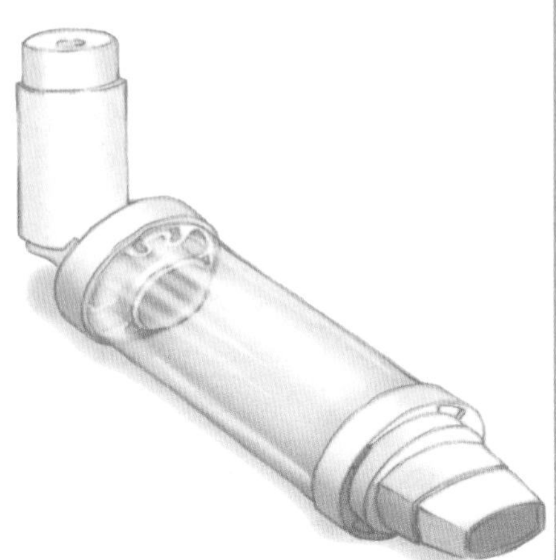

4. Put the spacer mouthpiece in the mouth (or place the mask over the child's nose and mouth, ensuring a good seal).

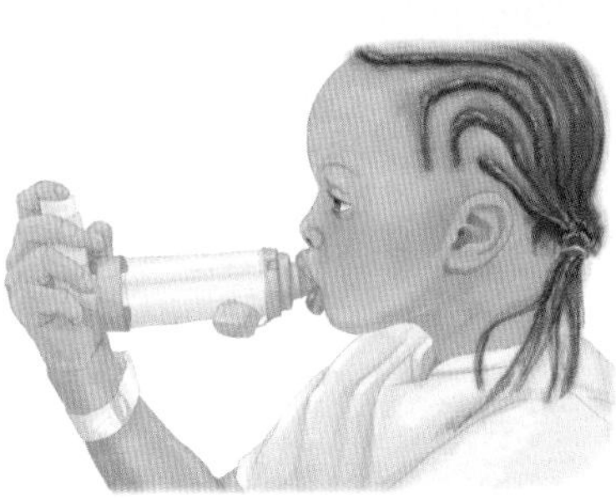

5. Compress the inhaler and inhale slowly and deeply. Hold the breath for a count of 10.
6. Wait 1 full minute before second inhalation, if prescribed.

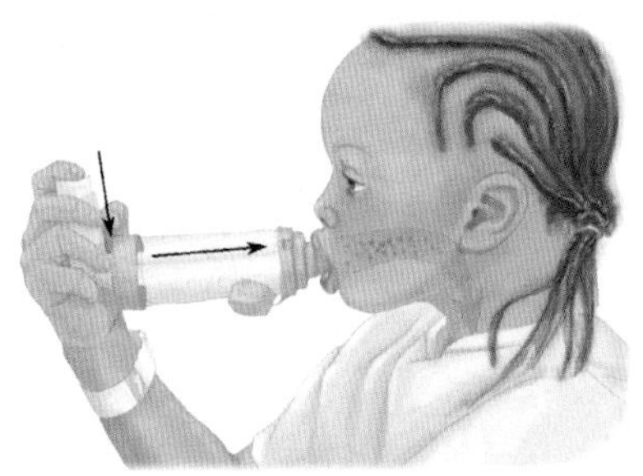

Diskus

1. Hold the Diskus in a horizontal position in one hand, and push the thumb grip with the thumb of your other hand away from you until mouthpiece is exposed.

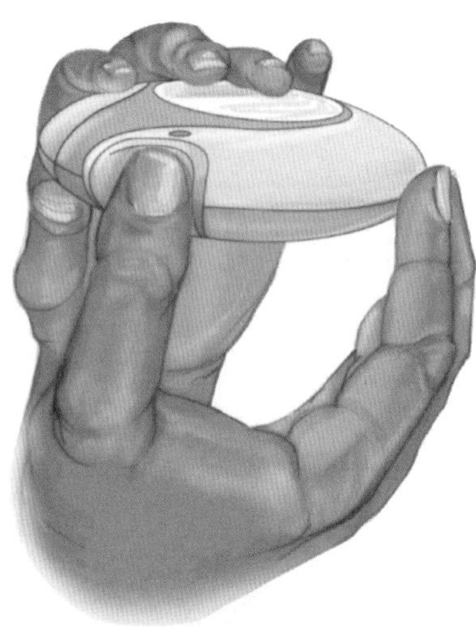

2. Push the lever until it clicks (the dose is now loaded).
3. Breathe out fully.

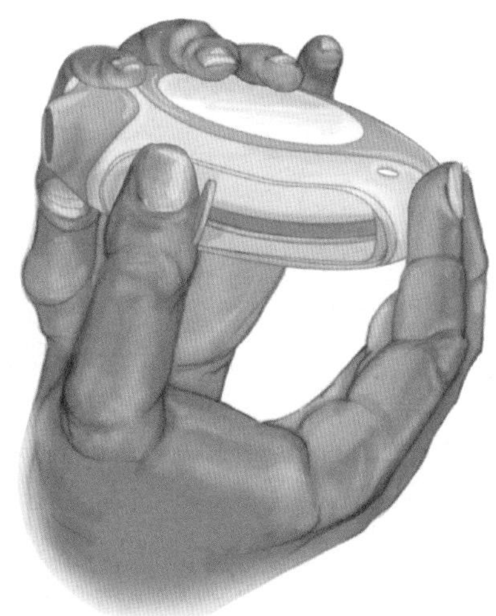

4. Place your mouth securely around the mouthpiece, then inhale.

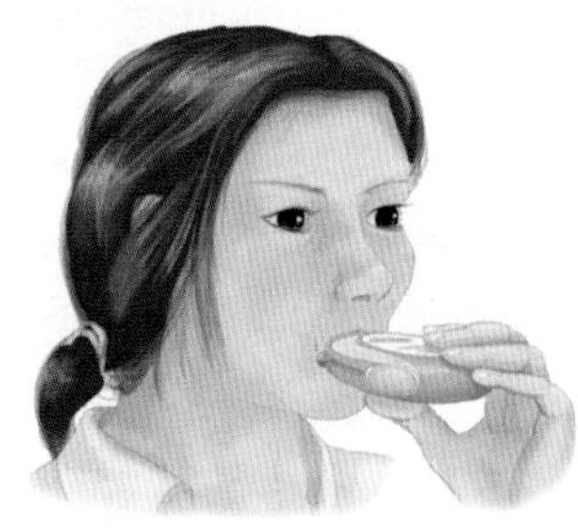

5. Remove the Diskus, hold the breath for 10 seconds, and then breathe out.

TEACHING GUIDELINES 18.5 Using Asthma Medication Delivery Devices

Turbuhaler

1. Hold the Turbuhaler upright. Load the dose by twisting the brown grip fully to the right.

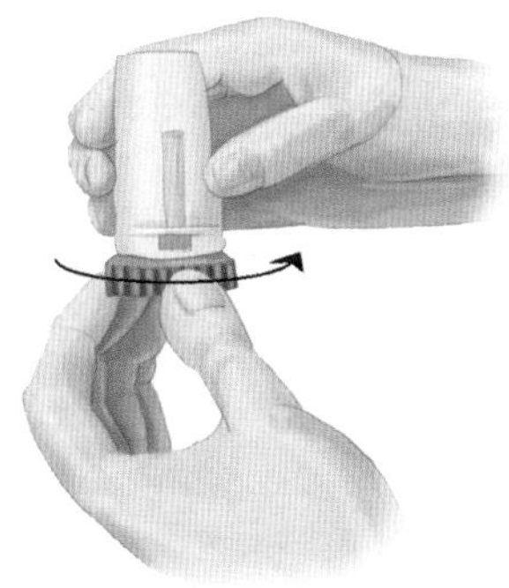

2. Then twist it to the left until you hear it click.
3. Breathe out fully.

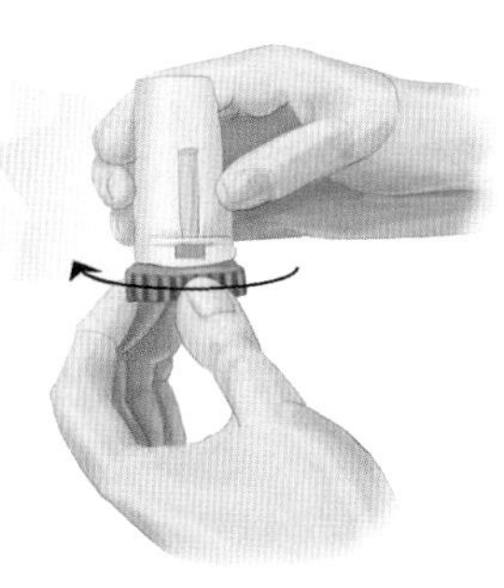

4. Holding the Turbuhaler horizontally, place the mouth firmly around the mouthpiece, and inhale deeply and forcefully.

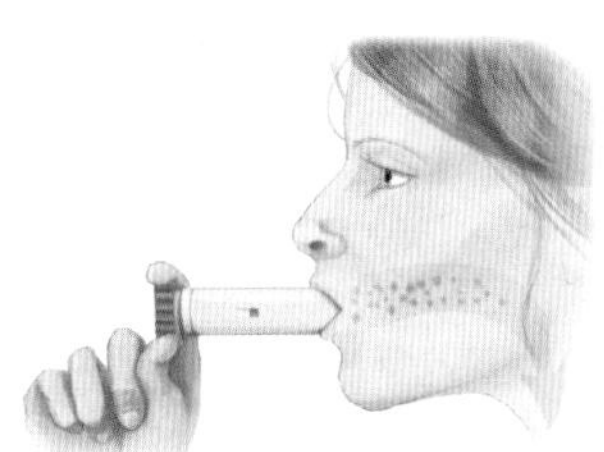

5. Remove the Turbuhaler from the mouth and then breathe out.

TEACHING GUIDELINES 18.6 Using a Peak Flow Meter

- Slide the arrow down to "zero."
- Stand up straight.
- Take a deep breath, and close the lips tightly around the mouthpiece.
- Blow out hard and fast.
- Note the number the arrow moves to.
- Repeat three times and record the highest reading.
- Keep a record of daily readings, being sure to measure peak flow at the same time each day.

Data from Gerald, L. B., & Carr, T. (2022). Patient education: How to use a peak flow meter (beyond the basics). *UpToDate*. Retrieved March 24, 2023, from https://www.uptodate.com/contents/how-to-use-a-peak-flow-meter-beyond-the-basics

on peak flow meter use. The child's "personal best" is determined collaboratively with the primary health care provider or nurse practitioner during a symptom-free period. PEFR is measured daily at home using the peak flow meter. The asthma management plan then gives specific instructions based on the PEFR measurement (Table 18.3).

TAKE NOTE!

Young children with asthma receiving inhaled medications via a nebulizer should use a snugly fitting mask to ensure accurate deposition of medication to the lungs and reduce loss of medication to the ambient air (Volkman & Chiu, 2023).

TABLE 18.3 • Assessment of Peak Expiratory Flow Rate (PEFR)

Zone[a]	PEFR	Symptoms	Action
Green: Good control	>80% personal best	None	Take usual medications.
Yellow: Caution	50%–80% personal best	Possibly present	Take short-acting inhaled beta$_2$-agonist right away. Talk to your primary health care provider or nurse practitioner.
Red: Medical alert	<50% personal best	Usually present	Take short-acting inhaled beta$_2$-agonist right away. Go to office or emergency department.

[a]The National Asthma Education and Prevention Program recommended the "traffic light" approach for educating individuals on PEFRs and management plans.

Data from Houin, P., Stillwell, P., Deboer, E. M., & Hoppe, J. (2022). Respiratory tract & mediastinum. In M. Bunik, W. W. Hay, M. J. Levin, & M. J. Abzug (Eds.), *Current diagnosis and treatment: Pediatrics* (26th ed.). McGraw-Hill Education; Volkman, K. K., & Chiu, A. M. (2023). Allergy. In K. J. Marcdante & R. M. Kliegman (Eds.), *Nelson's essentials of pediatrics* (9th ed.). Elsevier.

Avoidance of allergens is another key component of asthma management. Avoiding known triggers helps to prevent exacerbations as well as long-term inflammatory changes. This can be a difficult task for most families, particularly if the affected child suffers from several allergies. Refer to Teaching Guidelines 18.4 for strategies of allergen avoidance.

TAKE NOTE!

Teach the child and family that exposure to cigarette smoke increases the need for medications in children with asthma as well as the frequency of asthma exacerbations. Both indoor air quality and environmental pollution contribute to asthma in children.

Asthma education is a critical component for ensuring optimal health in children with asthma. This education is not limited to the hospital or clinic setting. Nurses can become involved in community asthma education: community-centered education in schools, churches, and day care centers or through peer educators has been shown to be effective. Education should include pathophysiology, asthma triggers, and prevention and treatment strategies. With such a large number of children affected with this chronic disease, community education has the potential to make a broad impact.

School nurses must also become experts in asthma management as well as being committed to ongoing education of the child and family. See Evidence-Based Practice 18.1. Resources for schools include:

- Open Airways for Schools: This educational program, presented by the American Lung Association, focuses on increasing asthma awareness and adherence with asthma action plans and decreasing asthma emergencies. Contact the local lung association or call 1-800-LUNG-USA.
- Indoor AIRepair at Home, School & Play: This free download, available from Allergy and Asthma Network, provides tips for improving indoor air quality.
- The Environmental Protection Agency (2023) offers many resources for creating and maintaining healthy school environments.

PROMOTING THE CHILD'S SELF-ESTEEM

The importance of education in the use of controller medications is well known, as increased use leads to decreased emergency room visits (Carey et al., 2019). In addition to the provision of quality asthma education, offer emotional support to children with asthma and their families. As children transition to assuming more control over their asthma, provide additional support to the child in their efforts and to the parent in trusting their child's abilities. Shared management of asthma care changes over time in a developmental fashion, as the child becomes more capable of taking responsibility for their own health. The school-age years, in particular, are known to be a transition time (Sonney et al., 2019). An agreement related to asthma management being shared between the child and the parent my result in higher quality asthma control (Sonney et al., 2019).

In addition to coping with a chronic illness, the child with asthma must often also cope with school-related issues. As compared with other children, children with asthma often experience impaired sleep and participate less often in physical activity. They also experience increased stress and anxiety (Lack et al., 2020). Performing yoga increases physical activity in children with asthma and has been shown to improve lung function over time. Mindfulness training may also be beneficial, as increased mindfulness in people with asthma leads to improved quality of life because of increased asthma control (Lack et al., 2020).

Through education and support, the child can gain a sense of control. Children need to learn to master their

EVIDENCE-BASED PRACTICE **18.1**

School-Based Interventions for Asthma

STUDY

Asthma is a common respiratory condition in children and adolescents. Theoretically, acquisition of skills for self-management of asthma could occur within the school (a place where children already participate in learning). The review included 55 studies, with over 20,000 child and adolescent participants. The objectives of the review were to identify intervention features aligned with successful intervention and to determine effectiveness in school-based interventions in relation to child/adolescent asthma self-management.

Findings

Compared with no school intervention, school-based interventions mildly decreased the numbers of hospitalizations and emergency department visits for participants. In addition, the intervention may be responsible for slightly increasing the participants' quality of life.

Nursing Implications

Nurses should consider the results of this review. School nurses could implement interventions for self-management. Nurses outside of the school system have the opportunity to reinforce the self-management interventions as structured by the school.

Data from Harris, K., Kneale, D., Lasserson, T., McDonald, V. M., Grigg, J., & Thomas, J. (2019). School-based self-management interventions for asthma in children and adolescents: A mixed methods systematic review. *Cochrane Database of Systematic Reviews, 1*(1), CD011651. https://doi.org/10.1002/14651858.CD011651.pub2

disease. Accurate evaluation of asthma symptoms and improvement of self-esteem may help the child to experience less panic with an acute episode. Improved self-esteem might also help the child cope with the disease, in general, and with being different from their peers. The school-age child has the cognitive ability to begin taking responsibility for asthma management, with continued involvement on the part of the parents. Transferring control of asthma care to the child is an important developmental process that will increase the child's feeling of control over the illness.

PROMOTING FAMILY COPING

Parent denial is an issue in many families. The family, through education and encouragement, can become the experts on the child's illness as well as advocates for the child's well-being. The resilient child is better able to cope with the challenges facing them, including asthma. Cohesiveness and warmth in the family environment can improve a child's resiliency as well as contribute to family hardiness. Parents need to be allowed to ask questions and voice their concerns. A nurse who understands the family's issues and concerns is better able to plan for support and education. Provide culturally sensitive education and interventions that focus on increasing the family's commitment to, and control of, asthma management. As the child and parents become confident in their ability to recognize asthma symptoms and cope with asthma and its periodic episodes, the family's ability to cope will improve.

> **THINKING ABOUT DEVELOPMENT**
>
> Ryan Jennings is a 13-year-old with a history of moderate asthma. He has been prescribed a long-term control medication to be taken routinely and a rescue medicine to be used as needed and before exercise. He is a talented pitcher and would like to participate with his school's baseball team.
>
> How will Ryan's developmental stage affect self-care related to his asthma? What is the most appropriate approach for the nurse to take to educate Ryan about his medications and disease process?
>
> How will the nurse foster compliance in Ryan?

Chronic Lung Disease

Chronic lung disease (formerly termed bronchopulmonary dysplasia) is often diagnosed in infants who have experienced RDS and who continue to require oxygen at 28 days of age. It is a chronic respiratory condition seen most commonly in premature infants. It results from a variety of factors, including pulmonary immaturity, acute lung injury, barotrauma, inflammatory mediators, and volutrauma. Epithelial stretching, macrophage and polymorphonuclear cell invasion, and airway edema affect the growth and development of lung structures. Cilia loss and airway lining denudation reduce the normal cleansing abilities of the lung. The number of normal alveoli is reduced by one third to one half. Lower birth weights, White race, and male sex pose increased risk of development of chronic lung disease. Complications include pulmonary artery hypertension, cor pulmonale, congestive heart failure, and severe bacterial or viral pneumonia.

Antiinflammatory inhaled medications are used for maintenance, and short-acting bronchodilators are used as needed for wheezing episodes. Supplemental long-term oxygen therapy may be required in some infants.

Nursing Assessment

In the infant or toddler, observe for tachypnea and increased work of breathing as they are characteristic of chronic lung disease. Determine level of dyspnea associated with activity or oral feeding. Note growth parameters, often identifying failure to thrive. Auscultate the breath sounds, noting if they are diminished in the bases, with wheezing present during times of reactive airway episodes. Rales may be heard if fluid overload develops.

Nursing Management

If the infant is oxygen-dependent, provide education to the parents about oxygen tanks, nasal cannula use, pulse oximetry use, and nebulizer treatments. Instruct families on the use of increased calorie formulas if recommended. Teach families about fluid restrictions and/or diuretics if prescribed. Encourage follow-up echocardiograms to determine resolution of pulmonary artery hypertension prior to weaning from oxygen. Encourage developmentally appropriate activities. It might be difficult for the infant or toddler who is dependent on oxygen to reach gross motor milestones or explore the environment because the length of the oxygen tubing limits them.

Parental support is also a key nursing intervention. After a long and trying period of ups and downs with their newborn in the intensive care unit, parents find themselves exhausted caring for their medically fragile infant at home.

Cystic Fibrosis

CF is an autosomal recessive disorder that affects 40,000 children and adults in the United States (Cystic Fibrosis Foundation, n.d.). A deletion occurring on the long arm of chromosome 7 at the cystic fibrosis transmembrane conductance regulator (CFTR) is the responsible gene mutation. DNA testing can be used prenatally and in newborns to identify the presence of the mutation. The American College of Obstetricians and Gynecologists (2023) currently recommends screening for cystic fibrosis to any person seeking preconception or prenatal care. At present, all states include testing for CF as part of newborn screening.

CF is the most common debilitating disease of childhood among those of European descent. Medical advances in recent years have greatly increased the length and quality of life for affected children, with median age for survival being 39.3 years (Katkin, 2023). Complications include hemoptysis, pneumothorax, bacterial colonization, cor pulmonale, volvulus, intussusception, intestinal obstruction, rectal prolapse, gastroesophageal reflux disease, diabetes, portal hypertension, liver failure, gallstones, and decreased fertility.

Pathophysiology

In CF, the CFTR mutation causes alterations in epithelial ion transport on mucosal surfaces, resulting in generalized dysfunction of the exocrine glands. The epithelial cells fail to conduct chloride, and water transport abnormalities occur. This results in thickened, tenacious secretions in the sweat glands, gastrointestinal tract, pancreas, respiratory tract, and other exocrine tissues. The increased viscosity of these secretions makes them difficult to clear. The sweat glands produce a larger amount of chloride, leading to a salty taste of the skin and alterations in electrolyte balance and dehydration. The pancreas, intrahepatic bile ducts, intestinal glands, gallbladder, and submaxillary glands become obstructed by viscous mucus and eosinophilic material. Pancreatic enzyme activity is lost, and malabsorption of fats, proteins, and carbohydrates occurs, resulting in poor growth and large, malodorous stools. Excess mucus is produced by the tracheobronchial glands. Abnormally thick mucus plugs the small airways, and then bronchiolitis and further plugging of the airways occur. Secondary bacterial infection with *Staphylococcus aureus*, *Pseudomonas aeruginosa*, and *Burkholderia cepacia* often occurs. This contributes to obstruction and inflammation, leading to chronic infection, tissue damage, and respiratory failure. Nasal polyps and recurrent sinusitis are common. Males have tenacious seminal fluid and experience blocking of the vas deferens, often making them infertile. In females, thick cervical secretions might limit penetration of sperm (Katkin, 2023). Table 18.4 gives further details of the pathophysiology and resulting respiratory and gastrointestinal clinical manifestations of CF.

TABLE **18.4** • Pathophysiology of Cystic Fibrosis and Resultant Respiratory and Gastrointestinal Clinical Manifestations

Defect in the CFTR Gene Effects	Pathophysiology	Clinical Manifestations
Respiratory tract	• Infection leads to neutrophilic inflammation. • Cleavage of complement receptors and immunoglobulin G leads to opsonophagocytosis failure. • Chemoattractant interleukin-8 and elastin degradase contribute to inflammatory response. • Thick, tenacious sputum that is chronically colonized with bacteria results. • Air trapping related to airway obstruction occurs. • Pulmonary parenchyma is eventually destroyed.	• Airway obstruction • Difficulty clearing secretions • Respiratory distress and impaired gas exchange • Chronic cough • Barrel-shaped chest • Decreased pulmonary function • Clubbing • Recurrent pneumonia • Hemoptysis • Pneumothorax • Chronic sinusitis • Nasal polyps • Cor pulmonale (right-sided heart failure)
Gastrointestinal tract	• Decreased chloride and water secretion into the intestine (causing dehydration of the intestinal material) and into the bile ducts (causing increased bile viscosity) • Reduced pancreatic bicarbonate secretion • Hypersecretion of gastric acid • Insufficiency of pancreatic enzymes (amylase, lipase, pancreas) necessary for digestion and absorption • Pancreas secretes thick mucus.	• Meconium ileus • Retention of fecal matter in distal intestine, resulting in vomiting; abdominal distention; and cramping, anorexia, right lower quadrant pain • Sludging of intestinal contents may lead to fecal impaction, rectal prolapse, bowel obstruction, and intussusception. • Obstructive cirrhosis with esophageal varices and splenomegaly • Gallstones • Gastroesophageal reflux disease (compounded by postural drainage with chest physiotherapy) • Inadequate protein absorption • Altered absorption of iron and vitamins A, D, E, and K • Failure to thrive • Hyperglycemia and development of diabetes later in life

CFTR, cystic fibrosis transmembrane conductance regulator

Data from Houin, P., Stillwell, P., Deboer, E. M., & Hoppe, J. (2022). Respiratory tract & mediastinum. In M. Bunik, W. W. Hay, M. J. Levin, & M. J. Abzug (Eds.), *Current diagnosis and treatment: Pediatrics* (26th ed.). McGraw-Hill Education; Katkin, J. P. (2023). Cystic fibrosis: Clinical manifestations and diagnosis. *UpToDate*. Retrieved December 1, 2023, from https://www.uptodate.com/contents/cystic-fibrosis-clinical-manifestations-and-diagnosis

Therapeutic Management

Therapeutic management of CF is aimed toward minimizing pulmonary complications, maximizing lung function, preventing infection, and facilitating growth. All children with CF who have pulmonary involvement require CPT with postural drainage (or an alternate method) several times daily to mobilize secretions from the lungs. Physical exercise is encouraged. Dornase alfa is given daily using a nebulizer to decrease sputum viscosity and help clear secretions. Inhaled bronchodilators and anti-inflammatory agents are prescribed for some children. Aerosolized antibiotics are often prescribed and may be given at home as well as in the hospital. Choice of antibiotic is determined by sputum culture and sensitivity results. Pancreatic enzymes and supplemental fat-soluble vitamins are prescribed to promote adequate digestion and absorption of nutrients and optimize nutritional status. Increased-calorie, high-protein diets are recommended, and supplemental high-calorie formula, either orally or via feeding tube, is sometimes needed. Some children require total parenteral nutrition to maintain or gain weight. Lung transplantation has been successful in some children with CF.

TAKE NOTE!

Children 6 years and older who have particular mutations of the CF gene may be prescribed a CFTR modulator such as ivacaftor or lumacaftor. Use of the CFTR modulator results in thinning of lung mucus, resulting in easier airway clearance via coughing (Simon, 2023).

Nursing Assessment

For a full description of the assessment phase of the nursing process, refer to the "Clinical Judgment and the Nursing Process" section. Assessment findings pertinent to CF are discussed further on.

HEALTH HISTORY

Elicit a description of the present illness and chief complaint. Common signs and symptoms reported during the health history in the undiagnosed child might include:

- A salty taste to the child's skin (resulting from excess chloride loss via perspiration)
- Meconium ileus or late, difficult passage of meconium stool in the newborn period
- Abdominal pain or difficulty passing stool (infants or toddlers might present with intestinal obstruction or intussusception at the time of diagnosis)
- Bulky, greasy stools
- Poor weight gain and growth despite good appetite
- Chronic or recurrent cough and/or upper or lower respiratory infections

Children known to have CF are often admitted to the hospital for pulmonary exacerbations or other complications of the disease. The health history should include questions related to:

- Respiratory status: has cough, sputum production, or work of breathing increased?
- Appetite and weight gain
- Activity tolerance
- Increased need for pulmonary or pancreatic medications
- Presence of fever
- Presence of bone pain
- Any other changes in physical state or medication regimen

PHYSICAL EXAMINATION

The physical examination includes inspection, percussion, palpation, and auscultation.

Inspection

Observe the child's general appearance and color. Check the nasal passages for polyps. Note respiratory rate, work of breathing, use of accessory muscles, position of comfort, frequency and severity of cough, and quality and quantity of sputum produced. The child with CF often has a barrel chest (anterior–posterior diameter approximates transverse diameter) (Fig. 18.13). Clubbing of the nail beds might also be present. Note whether

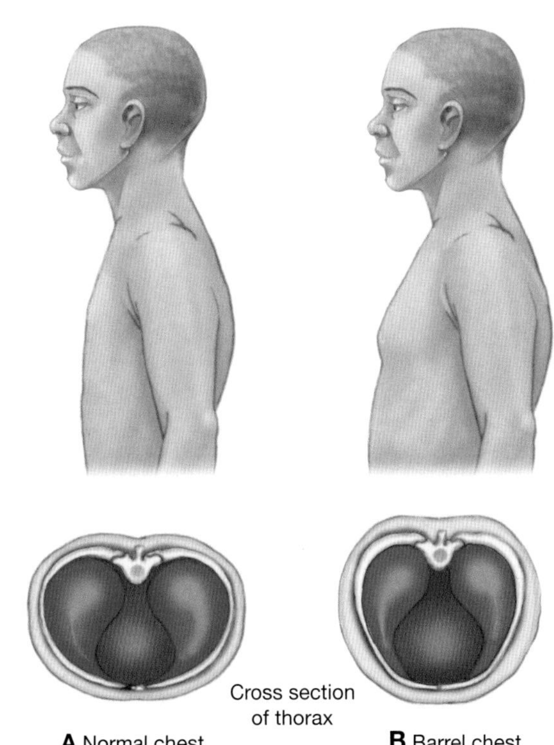

FIGURE 18.13 A. Normal chest shape—transverse diameter is greater than anterior–posterior diameter. **B.** Barrel chest—transverse diameter equals anterior–posterior diameter.

rectal prolapse is present. Does the child appear small or thin for their age? The child might have a protuberant abdomen and thin extremities, with decreased amounts of subcutaneous fat. Observe for the presence of edema (sign of cardiac or liver failure). Note distended neck veins or the presence of a heave (signs of cor pulmonale).

Percussion and Palpation

Percussion over the lung fields usually yields hyperresonance due to air trapping. Diaphragmatic excursion might be decreased. Percussion of the abdomen might reveal dullness over an enlarged liver or mass related to intestinal obstruction. Palpation might yield a finding of asymmetric chest excursion if atelectasis is present. Tactile fremitus may be decreased over areas of atelectasis. Note whether tenderness is present over the liver (might be an early sign of cor pulmonale).

Auscultation

Auscultation may reveal a variety of adventitious breath sounds. Fine or coarse crackles and scattered or localized wheezing might be present. With progressive obstructive pulmonary involvement, breath sounds might be diminished. Tachycardia might be present. Note the presence of a gallop (might occur with cor pulmonale). Note the adequacy of bowel sounds.

LABORATORY AND DIAGNOSTIC TESTS

Common laboratory and diagnostic studies ordered for the diagnosis and assessment of CF include:

- Sweat chloride test: considered suspicious if the level of chloride in collected sweat is above 50 mEq/L and diagnostic if the level is above 60 mEq/L
- Pulse oximetry: oxygen saturation might be decreased, particularly during a pulmonary exacerbation.
- Chest radiograph: may reveal hyperinflation, bronchial wall thickening, atelectasis, or infiltration
- PFTs: might reveal a decrease in forced vital capacity and forced expiratory volume, with increases in residual volume

Nursing Management

Management of CF focuses on minimizing pulmonary complications, promoting growth and development, and facilitating coping and adjustment by the child and the family. In addition to the patient problems and related interventions discussed in the "Clinical Judgment and the Nursing Process" section, interventions common to CF follow.

MAINTAINING PATENT AIRWAY

Provide CPT, use of the vest airway clearance system, use of the flutter-valve device, and/or positive expiratory pressure therapy to clear secretions and maintain airway patency. For children with CF, CPT is a critical intervention. CPT involves percussion, vibration, and postural drainage, and either it or another bronchial hygiene therapy must be performed several times a day to assist with mobilization of secretions. Nursing Procedure 18.2 gives instructions on the CPT technique. The vest airway clearance system provides high-frequency chest wall oscillation to increase airflow velocity to create repetitive cough-like shear forces and to decrease the viscosity of secretions (Hill-Rom, 2021).

For older children and adolescents, the flutter-valve device provides high-frequency oscillation to the airway as the child exhales into a mouthpiece that contains a steel ball. Positive expiratory pressure therapy involves exhaling through a flow resistor, which creates positive expiratory pressure. The cycles of exhalation are repeated until coughing yields expectoration of secretions. Breathing exercises are also helpful in promoting mucus clearance. Encourage physical exercise, as it helps to promote mucus secretion as well as providing cardiopulmonary conditioning. Ensure that dornase alfa is administered, as well as inhaled bronchodilators and antiinflammatory agents, if prescribed.

PREVENTING INFECTION

Ensure that parents and older children understand that vigorous pulmonary hygiene to mobilize secretions is critical to prevent infection. Administer aerosolized antibiotics as prescribed in the hospital, or teach parents to provide them at home. Children with frequent or severe respiratory exacerbations might require lengthy courses of intravenous antibiotics.

MAINTAINING GROWTH

Administer pancreatic enzyme supplements (pancrelipase) with all meals and snacks to promote adequate digestion and absorption of nutrients. The number of capsules required depends on the extent of pancreatic insufficiency and the amount of food being ingested. The dosage can be adjusted until an adequate growth pattern is established and the number of stools is consistent at one or two per day. Children will need additional enzyme capsules when high-fat foods are being eaten. In the infant or young child, the enzyme capsule can be opened and sprinkled on cereal or applesauce. Provide a well-balanced, high-calorie, high-protein diet to ensure adequate growth. Some children require up to one and a half times the recommended daily allowance of calories for children their age. A number of commercially available nutritional formulas and shakes are available for diet supplementation.

In infants, breastfeeding should be continued with enzyme administration. Some infants will require fortification of breast milk or supplementation with high-calorie formulas. Commercially available infant formulas can continue to be used for the formula-fed infant and can be mixed to provide a larger number of

NURSING PROCEDURE 18.2 Performing Chest Physiotherapy

May be preceded by an inhalation treatment; should not be performed after eating

1. Provide percussion via a cupped hand or an infant percussion device. Appropriate percussion yields a hollow sound, not a slapping sound.

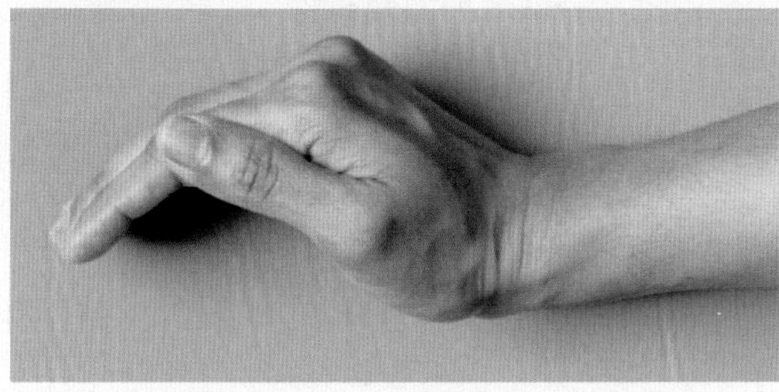

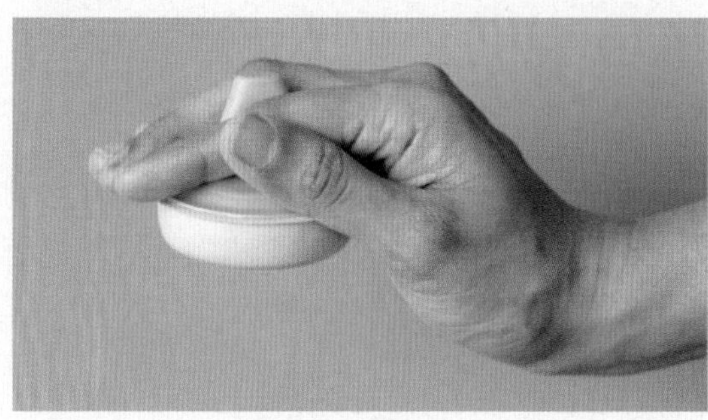

2. Percuss each segment of the lung for 1 to 2 minutes.

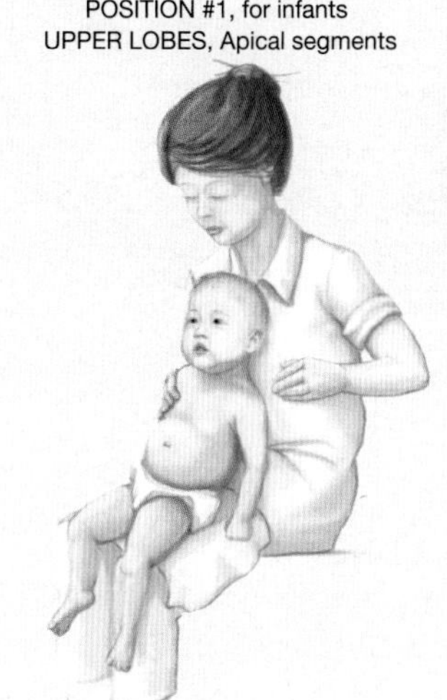

POSITION #1
UPPER LOBES, Apical segments

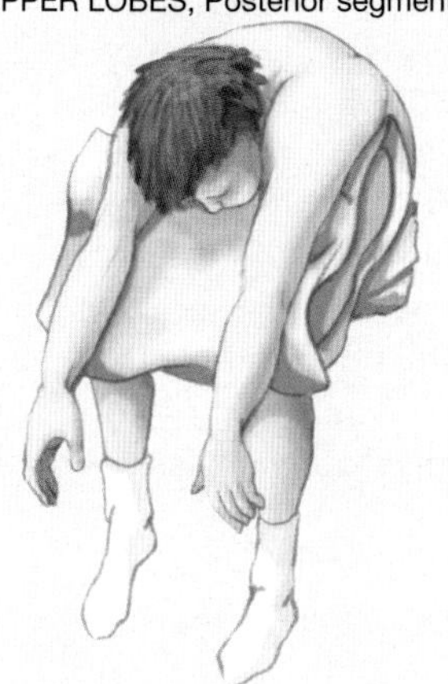

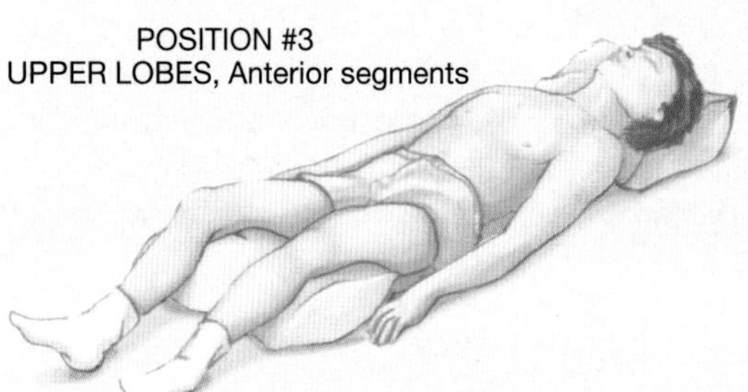

(continued)

NURSING PROCEDURE 18.2 Performing Chest Physiotherapy (*continued*)

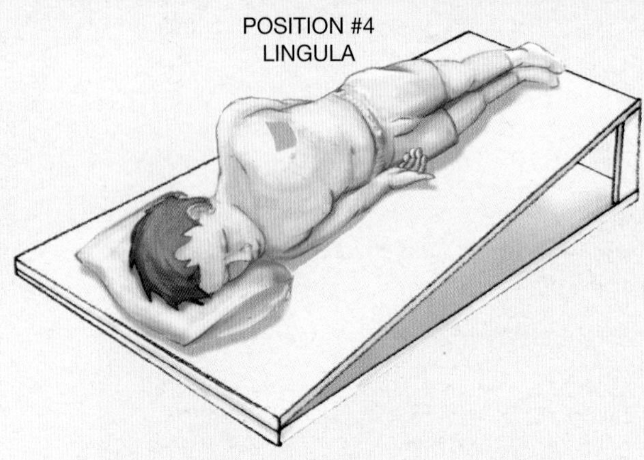

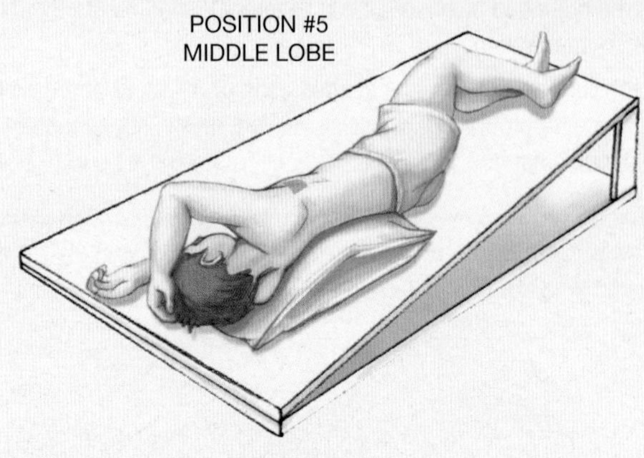

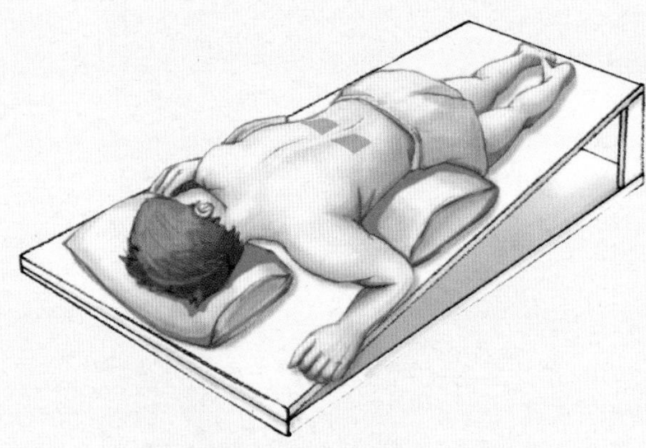

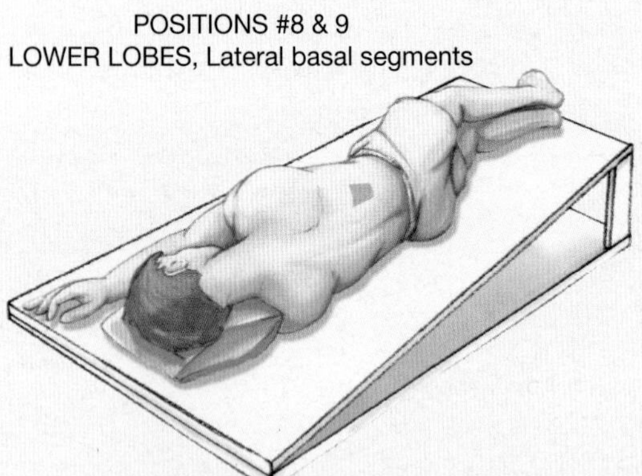

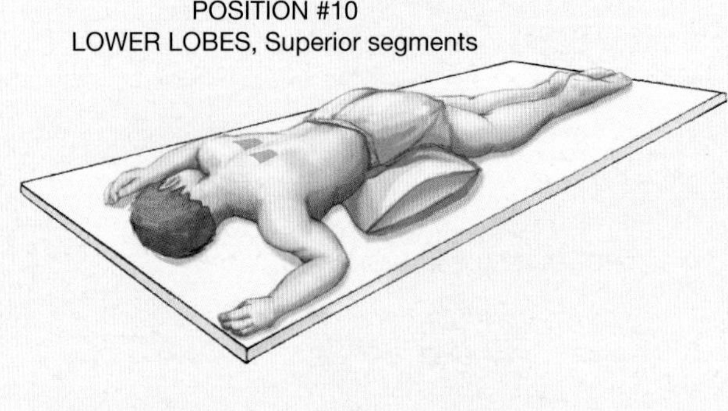

3. Place the ball of the hand on the lung segment, keeping the arm and shoulder straight. Vibrate by tensing and relaxing your arms during the child's exhalation. Vibrate each lung segment for at least five exhalations.
4. Encourage the child to deep breathe and cough.
5. Change drainage positions, and repeat percussion and vibration.

calories if necessary. Administer vitamin A, D, E, and K supplementation. Administer gavage feedings or total parenteral nutrition as prescribed to provide for adequate growth.

PROMOTING FAMILY COPING

Assist families in learning to cope with the daily interventions required for the serious chronic illness of CF. Help families to develop a schedule for provision of pulmonary hygiene several times daily as well as to pay close attention to appropriate diet and enzyme supplementation. Adjusting to the demands that the illness places on the child and the family is difficult. Continual adjustments within the family must occur. Children are frequently hospitalized, and this may place an additional strain on the family and its finances. Children with CF may express fear or feelings of isolation, and siblings may be worried or jealous. Encourage the family to lead a normal life through involvement in activities and school attendance during periods of wellness.

Starting at the time of diagnosis, families often demonstrate significant stress as the severity of the diagnosis and the significance of disease chronicity become real for them. Involve the family in the child's care from the time of diagnosis, whether in the outpatient setting or in the hospital. Ongoing education about the illness and its treatments is necessary. Once the initial shock of diagnosis has passed and the family has adjusted to initial care, the family usually learns how to manage the requirements of care. Powerlessness gives way to adaptation. As family members become more comfortable with their understanding of the illness and the required treatments, they will eventually become the experts on the child's care. It is important for the nurse to recognize and respect the family's changing needs over time.

Providing daily intense care can be tiring, and noncompliance on the part of the family or child might occur as a result of this fatigue. Hypervigilance may also occur as parents attempt to control the difficult situation and protect the child. Families welcome support and encouragement. Most families eventually progress past the stages of fear, guilt, and powerlessness to a way of living that is different than what they anticipated yet something that they can manage.

Refer parents to a local support group for families of children with CF. The Cystic Fibrosis Foundation has chapters throughout the United States. With appropriate treatment and minimal complications, children with CF are currently living into adulthood. Yet some children may experience significant complications, and parents might face the death of their child at an earlier age than expected. In this case, assisting with anticipatory grieving and making decisions related to end-of-life care are other important nursing interventions.

Preparing the Child and Family for Adulthood With Cystic Fibrosis

With current technologic and medication advances, and the use of lung transplantation, children with CF are living well into adulthood. Children with CF should have the goal of independent living as an adult, as other children do. Making the transition from a pediatric medical home to an adult medical home should be viewed as a normal part of growing up, similarly to completing school or finding a first job. Pediatric clinics are focused on family-centered care that heavily involves the child's parents, but adults with CF need a different focus, one that views them as independent adults.

Those with CF can make the transition from pediatric to adult care with thoughtful preparation and coordination. They desire and deserve a smooth transition in care that will result in appropriate ongoing medical management of CF in an environment that is geared toward adults rather than children.

Adults with CF are able to find rewarding work and pursue relationships. People with CF might have difficulty conceiving, and when they do, birthing parents with CF should be cautioned about the additional respiratory strain that pregnancy causes. All children of parents with CF will be carriers of the gene.

Apnea

Apnea is defined as absence of breathing for longer than 20 seconds; it might be accompanied by bradycardia. Sometimes, apnea presents in the form of brief, resolved, unexplained event (BRUE), an event in which the infant or child exhibits some combination of apnea, color change, muscle tone alteration, coughing, or gagging. Apnea may also occur acutely at any age because of respiratory distress. This discussion will focus on apnea that is chronic or recurrent in nature or that occurs as part of a BRUE.

Apnea in infants may be central (unrelated to any other cause) or may occur with other illnesses such as sepsis and respiratory infection. Apnea in newborns might be associated with hypothermia, hypoglycemia, infection, or hyperbilirubinemia. Apnea of prematurity occurs secondary to an immature respiratory system. Apnea should not be considered a predecessor to sudden unexplained infant death (SUID). Current research has not proven this theory, and SUID generally occurs in otherwise healthy young infants (Moon et al., 2022). Box 18.4 gives more information about SUID and its prevention.

Therapeutic management of apnea varies depending on the cause. When apnea occurs as a result of another disorder or infection, treatment is directed toward that cause. In the event of apnea, stimulation may trigger the infant to take a breath. If breathing does not

BOX 18.4 Sudden Unexplained Infant Death (SUID)

Definition

Sudden death of a previously healthy infant younger than 1 year

Prevention

- Place all infants in the supine position to sleep.
- Provide a firm sleep surface, avoiding soft bedding, bumper pads, excess covers, pillows, and stuffed animals in the crib.
- Avoid maternal prenatal smoking and exposure of the infant to second-hand smoke.
- Avoid maternal prenatal alcohol and illicit drug exposure.
- Ensure the infant sleeps in a separate bed from the parents for the first 6 months.
- Avoid overbundling or overdressing the infant.
- Encourage pacifier use during naps and at bedtime if the infant is receptive to it (Moon et al., 2022).

Support and Information

- American Sudden Infant Death Syndrome Institute: www.sids.org
- National SUID/SIDS Resource Center: www.sidscenter.org
- SIDS Alliance: www.sidsalliance.org
- Sudden Infant Death Syndrome Network, Inc.: http://sids-network.org/

resume, rescue breathing or bag-valve-mask ventilation is necessary. Infants and children who have experienced a BRUE or who have chronic apnea may require ongoing cardiac/apnea monitoring. Caffeine citrate is sometimes administered, primarily in premature infants, to stimulate respirations (S. Smith, 2022).

Nursing Assessment

Question the parents about the infant's position and activities preceding the apneic episode. Did the infant experience a color change? Did the infant self-stimulate (breathe again on their own), or did they require stimulation from the caregiver? Assess risk factors for apnea, which may include prematurity, anemia, and history of metabolic disorders. Apnea may occur in association with cardiac or neurologic disturbances, respiratory infection, sepsis, child abuse, or poisoning.

In the hospitalized infant, note absence of respiration, position, color, and other associated findings, such as emesis on the bedclothes. If an infant who is apneic fails to be stimulated and does not breathe again, pulselessness will result.

Nursing Management

When an infant is noted to be apneic, gently stimulate them to take a breath again. If gentle stimulation is unsuccessful, then rescue breathing or bag-valve-mask ventilation must be started. To avoid apnea in the newborn, maintain a neutral thermal environment. Administer caffeine or theophylline if prescribed and teach families about the use of these medications.

Infants with recurrent apnea or BRUE may be discharged on a home apnea monitor (Fig. 18.14). Provide education on use of the monitor, guidance about when to notify the primary health care provider or nurse practitioner or monitor service about alarms, and training in infant CPR. The monitor is usually discontinued after 3 months without a significant event of apnea or bradycardia. In some ways the monitor gives parents peace of mind, but in others it can make them more nervous about the well-being of their child. When apnea monitors are used in the home, parental sleep may be disrupted by machine alarms. Parents often express increased fear, anxiety, and depressive symptoms associated with home monitoring (Corwin, 2023). Providing appropriate education to the parents about the nature of the child's disorder as well as action to take in the event of apnea may give the family a sense of mastery over the situation, thus decreasing their anxiety. Refer families to local support groups such as those offered by Parent to Parent and Parents Helping Parents.

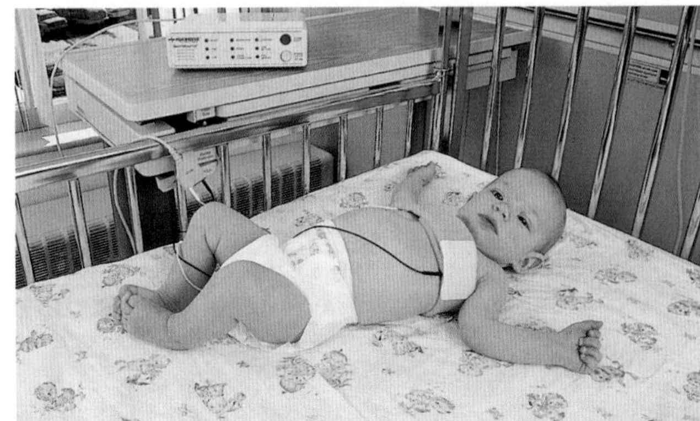

FIGURE 18.14 The home apnea monitor uses a soft belt with a Velcro attachment to hold two leads in the appropriate position on the chest.

TRACHEOSTOMY

A tracheostomy is an artificial opening in the airway; usually, a plastic tracheostomy tube is in place to form a patent airway. Tracheostomies are performed to relieve airway obstruction, such as with subglottic stenosis (narrowing of the airway sometimes resulting from long-term intubation). They are also used for pulmonary hygiene and in the child who requires chronic mechanical ventilation. The tracheostomy facilitates secretion removal, reduces work of breathing, and increases the child's comfort. In some cases, the tracheostomy facilitates mechanical ventilation weaning. It may be permanent or temporary, depending on the indication. The tracheostomy tube varies in size and type depending on the child's airway size and health and the length of time the child will require the tracheostomy. Silastic tracheostomy tubes are soft and flexible; they are available with a single lumen or may have an outer and inner lumen. Both types have an obturator (the guide used during tube changes). Uncuffed tubes are used more often in the pediatric population. Figure 18.15 shows various types of tracheostomy tubes.

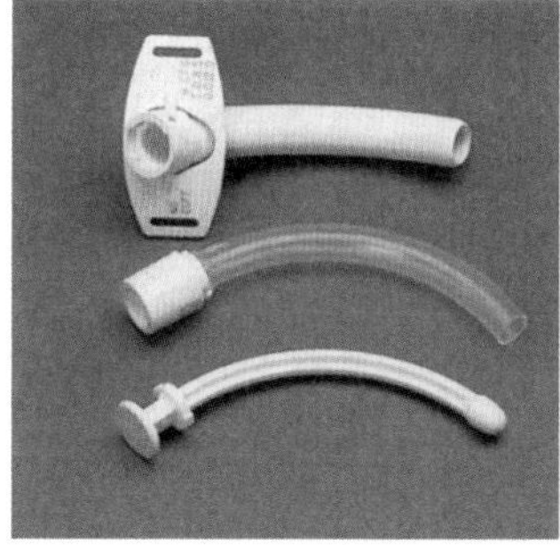

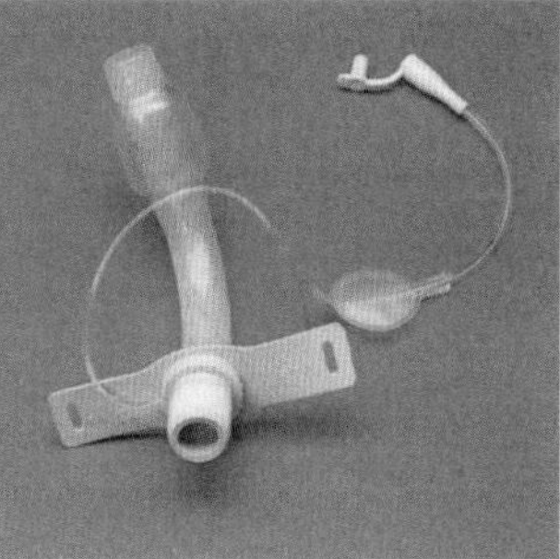

FIGURE 18.15 Note smaller size and absence of inner cannula on particular brands of pediatric tracheostomy tubes.

Complications immediately after surgery include hemorrhage, air entry, pulmonary edema, anatomic damage, and respiratory arrest. At any point in time the tracheostomy tube may become occluded, which compromises ventilation. Complications of chronic tracheostomy include infection, cellulitis, and formation of granulation tissue around the insertion site.

Nursing Assessment

When obtaining the history for a child with a tracheostomy, note the reason for the tracheostomy, as well as the size and type of tracheostomy tube. Inspect the site. The stoma should appear pink and without bleeding or drainage. The tube itself should be clean and free from secretions. The tracheostomy ties should fit securely, allowing one finger to slide beneath the ties. Inspect the skin under the ties for rash or redness. Observe work of breathing.

When caring for the infant or child with a tracheostomy, whether in the hospital, home, or community setting, a thorough respiratory assessment is necessary. Note the presence of secretions and their color, thickness, and amount. Auscultate for breath sounds, which should be clear and equal throughout all lung fields. Measure pulse oximetry. When infection is suspected or secretions are discolored or have a foul odor, a sputum culture may be obtained.

TAKE NOTE!

Keep small toys (risk of aspiration), plastic bibs or bedding (risk of airway occlusion), and talcum powder (risk of inhalation injury) out of reach of the child with a tracheostomy.

Nursing Management

In the immediate postoperative period, the infant or child may require restraints to avoid inadvertent dislodgment of the tracheostomy tube. Infants and children who have had a tracheostomy for a certain period become accustomed to it and usually do not attempt to remove the tube. Since air inspired via the tracheostomy tube bypasses the upper airway, it lacks humidification, and this lack of humidity can lead to a mucus plug in the tracheostomy and resultant hypoxia. Provide humidity to either room air or oxygen via a tracheostomy collar or ventilator, depending on the child's need (Fig. 18.16). Box 18.5 lists the equipment that should be available at the bedside of any child who has a tracheostomy.

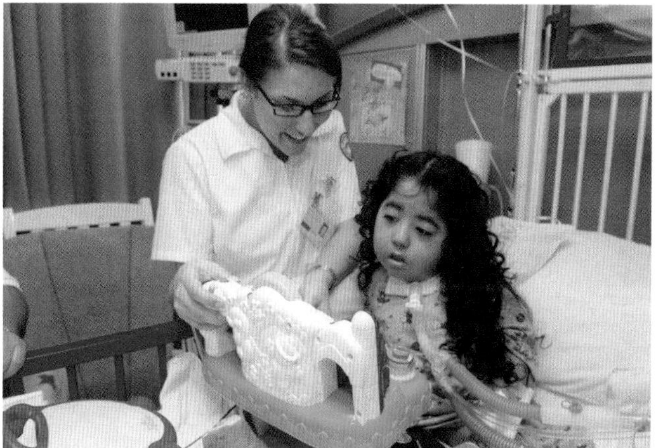

FIGURE 18.16 The trach collar allows for humidification of inspired air or supplemental oxygen.

Tracheostomies require frequent suctioning to maintain patency. The appropriate length for insertion of the suction catheter depends on the size of the tracheostomy and the child's needs. Place a sign at the head of the child's bed indicating the suction catheter size and the length (in centimeters) that it should be inserted for suctioning. Keep an extra tracheostomy tube of the same size and one size smaller at the bedside in the event of an emergency.

Many pediatric tracheostomy tubes do not have an inner cannula that requires periodic removal and cleaning, so periodic removal and replacement of the chronic tracheostomy tube is required. Clean the removed tracheostomy tube with half-strength hydrogen peroxide and pipe cleaners. Rinse with distilled water and allow it to dry. The tracheostomy tube can be reused many times if adequately cleaned between uses.

BOX 18.5 Emergency Equipment (Available at Bedside)

- Two spare tracheostomy tubes (one the same size and one a size smaller)
- Suction equipment
- Stitch cutter (new tracheostomy)
- Spare tracheostomy ties
- Lubricating jelly
- Bag-valve-mask device
- Call bell within child's/parent's reach

NURSING PROCEDURE 18.3 Tracheostomy Care

1. Gather the necessary equipment:
    - Cleaning solution
    - Gloves
    - Precut gauze pad
    - Cotton-tipped applicators
    - Clean tracheostomy ties
    - Extra tracheostomy tube in case of inadvertent dislodgment
2. Position the infant or child supine with a blanket or towel roll to extend the neck.
3. Open all packaging and cut tracheostomy ties to appropriate length if necessary.
4. Cleanse around the tracheostomy site with prescribed solution (half-strength hydrogen peroxide or acetic acid, normal saline or soap and water if at home) and cotton-tipped applicators, working from just around the tracheostomy tube outward.
5. Rinse with sterile water and cotton-tipped applicator in similar fashion.
6. Place the precut sterile gauze under the tracheostomy tube.
7. With the assistant holding the tube in place, cut the ties and remove from the tube.
8. Attach the clean ties to the tube, and tie or secure in place with Velcro (Fig. 18.17).

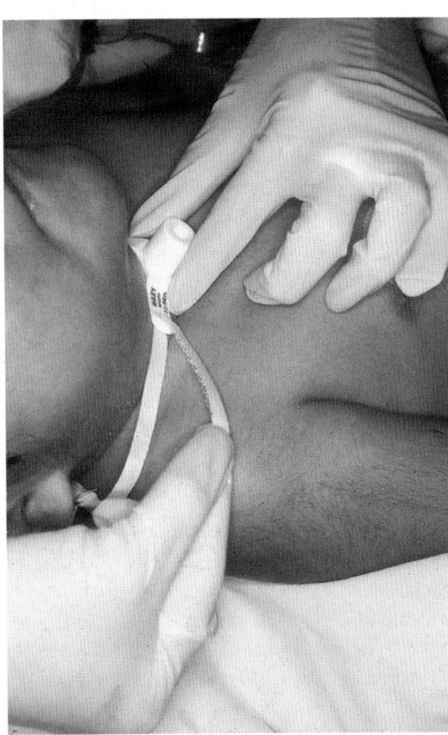

FIGURE 18.17 Trach ties are attached to the tube and secured in place with Velcro.

Perform tracheostomy care every 8 hours or per institution protocol. Change the tracheostomy tube only as needed or per institution protocol. Nursing Procedure 18.3 gives information about tracheostomy care. Always change tracheostomy ties with an assistant to avoid inadvertent dislodgment of the tube.

If the older child or adolescent has a tracheostomy tube with an inner cannula, care of the inner cannula is similar to that of an adult. Involve parents in the care of the tracheostomy, and begin education about caring for the tracheostomy tube at home as soon as the child is stable. The child with a tracheostomy often qualifies for a Medicaid waiver that will provide a certain amount of home nursing care. Refer the family to local support groups.

Unfolding Patient Stories: Sabina Vasquez • Part 2

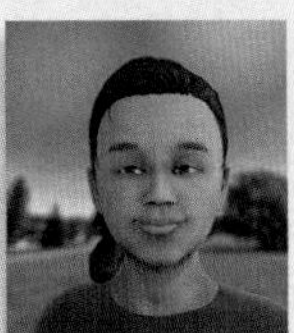

Recall Sabina Vasquez from Chapter 5, a 5-year-old diagnosed with asthma who uses an albuterol inhaler. What questions and assessments help the nurse evaluate her current respiratory status during a routine clinic visit? What methods can the nurse use to guide asthma management, and determine how well Sabina's asthma is managed at home?

Care for Sabina and other patients in a realistic virtual environment: ***vSim** for Nursing* (thepoint.lww.com/vSimPediatric). Practice documenting these patients' care in DocuCare (thePoint.lww.com/DocuCareEHR).

KEY CONCEPTS

- Respiratory infections account for the majority of acute illnesses in children.
- The upper and lower airways are smaller in children than adults, making them more susceptible to obstruction in the presence of mucus, debris, or edema.
- Newborns are preferential nose breathers.
- The child's highly compliant airway is quite susceptible to dynamic collapse in the presence of airway obstruction.
- Because they have fewer alveoli, children have a higher risk of hypoxemia than adults.
- Generally, disorders of the nose and throat do not result in increased work of breathing or affect the lungs. Thus, if the lungs are involved, lower respiratory disease must be considered.
- Wheezing may be associated with a variety of lower respiratory disorders, such as asthma, bronchiolitis, and CF.
- Pulse oximetry is a useful tool for determining the extent of hypoxia. Findings should be correlated with the child's clinical presentation.

- Rapid streptococcus and rapid influenza tests are very useful for the quick diagnosis of strep throat or influenza so that appropriate treatment may be instituted early in the illness.
- Supplemental oxygen is often necessary in the child who is hospitalized (particularly with lower respiratory disease). Oxygen should be humidified to prevent drying of secretions.
- Suctioning, whether with a bulb syringe or suction catheter, is effective at maintaining airway patency, especially in the younger child or infant.
- Normal saline nasal wash is an inexpensive, simple, and safe method for decongesting the nose in the case of the common cold, allergic rhinitis, and sinusitis.
- Infants who were born prematurely; children with a chronic illness such as diabetes, congenital heart disease, sickle cell anemia, or CF; and children with developmental disorders such as cerebral palsy tend to be more severely affected with respiratory disorders.
- Passive cigarette smoke exposure increases the infant's and child's risk of respiratory disease.
- Continual swallowing while awake or asleep is an indication of bleeding in the postoperative tonsillectomy child.
- Positioning to ease work of breathing and maintaining a patent airway are priorities for the child with a respiratory disorder.
- To avoid Reye syndrome, aspirin should not be given to treat fever or pain in the infant or child with a viral infection.
- Infants and children at high risk for serious RSV disease should be immunized with palivizumab each RSV season. Children older than 6 months of age should be immunized against influenza yearly.
- Children at high risk for exposure to TB should be screened for infection.
- Many children with COVID-19 remain asymptomatic.
- Promoting airway clearance and maintenance, effective breathing patterns, and adequate gas exchange is the priority focus of nursing intervention in pediatric respiratory disease.
- Children with any degree of respiratory distress require frequent assessment and early intervention to prevent progression to respiratory failure.
- Avoidance of allergens is critical in the treatment plan for the child with allergic rhinitis.
- Avoidance of allergic triggers, control of the inflammatory process, and education of the child and the family are the focus of asthma management.
- CPT is extremely useful for mobilizing secretions in any condition resulting in an increase in mucus production and is required in children with CF.
- Children with chronic respiratory disorders and their families often need large amounts of education and psychosocial support: children often experience fear and isolation, while families must learn to balance care of the child with chronic illness with other family life.

REFERENCES AND RECOMMENDED READINGS

American Academy of Allergy, Asthma and Immunology. (2011). *Asthma action plan.* http://www.aaaai.org/Aaaai/media/MediaLibrary/PDF%20Documents/Libraries/NEW-WEBSITE-LOGO-asthma-action-plan_HI.pdf

American College of Obstetricians and Gynecologists. (2023). *Cystic fibrosis: Prenatal screening and diagnosis.* https://www.acog.org/womens-health/faqs/cystic-fibrosis-prenatal-screening-and-diagnosis

American Heart Association. (2020). *Pediatric advanced life support: Provider manual.* https://www.amazon.com/Pediatric-Avanced-Support-Provider-Advanced/dp/1616695595?asin=B08KPFWYJ9&revisionId=&format=4&depth=1

Aronson, M. D., & Auwaerter, P. G. (2023). *Infectious mononucleosis. UpToDate.* Retrieved December 1, 2023, from https://www.uptodate.com/contents/infectious-mononucleosis

Barr, F. E., & Graham, B. S. (2023). *Respiratory syncytial virus infection: Prevention in infants and children. UpToDate.* Retrieved December 1, 2023, from https://www.uptodate.com/contents/respiratory-syncytial-virus-infection-prevention-in-infants-and-children

Barson, W. J. (2022). *Community-acquired pneumonia in children: Outpatient treatment. UpToDate.* Retrieved December 1, 2023, from https://www.uptodate.com/contents/community-acquired-pneumonia-in-children-outpatient-treatment

Batra, V., & Ang, J. Y. (2022). *Pediatric tuberculosis. Medscape.* Retrieved December 1, 2023, from https://emedicine.medscape.com/article/969401-overview

Carey, S. K., Edds-McAfee, C., Martinez, V., Gutierrez de Blume, A. P., & Thornton, K. M. (2019). An examination of factors affecting quality of life for children with asthma and their caregivers in southeastern Georgia. *Journal of Pediatric Health Care, 33*(5), 529–536. https://doi.org/10.1016/j.pedhc.2019.01.008

Carolan, P. L. (2023). *Pediatric bronchitis. Medscape.* Retrieved December 1, 2023, from https://emedicine.medscape.com/article/1001332-overview

Centers for Disease Control and Prevention. (2022). *Health problems caused by secondhand smoke.* https://www.cdc.gov/tobacco/secondhand-smoke/health.html

Centers for Disease Control and Prevention. (2023a). *Pneumococcal vaccination.* https://www.cdc.gov/vaccines/vpd/pneumo/index.html

Centers for Disease Control and Prevention. (2023b). *Seasonal influenza vaccination resources for health professionals.* https://www.cdc.gov/flu/professionals/vaccination/index.htm

Centers for Disease Control and Prevention. (2023c). *Respiratory syncytial virus (RSV) vaccine VIS.* https://www.cdc.gov/vaccines/hcp/vis/vis-statements/rsv.html

Corbett, J. A., & Banks, A. D. (2019). *Laboratory tests and diagnostic procedures with nursing diagnoses* (9th ed.). Pearson Education Inc.

Corwin, M. J. (2023). *Use of home cardiorespiratory monitors in infants. UpToDate.* Retrieved December 1, 2023, from https://www.uptodate.com/contents/use-of-home-cardiorespiratory-monitors-in-infants

Covar, R. A., Fleisher, M., Cho, C., & Boguniewicz, M. (2022). Allergic disorders. In M. Bunik, W. W. Hay, M. J. Levin, & M. J. Abzug (Eds.), *Current diagnosis and treatment: Pediatrics* (26th ed.). McGraw-Hill Education.

Cystic Fibrosis Foundation. (n.d.). *About cystic fibrosis.* https://www.cff.org/What-is-CF/

Durani, Y. (2023). *Preventing choking*. https://kidshealth.org/en/parents/safety-choking.html

Environmental Protection Agency. (2023). *Healthy school environments*. https://www.epa.gov/schools

Gerald, L. B., & Carr, T. (2022). *Patient education: How to use a peak flow meter (beyond the basics)*. *UpToDate*. Retrieved December 1, 2023, from https://www.uptodate.com/contents/how-to-use-a-peak-flow-meter-beyond-the-basics

Giddens, J. F. (2021). *Concepts for nursing practice* (3rd ed.). Elsevier.

Harris, K., Kneale, D., Lasserson, T., McDonald, V. M., Grigg, J., & Thomas, J. (2019). School-based self-management interventions for asthma in children and adolescents: A mixed methods systematic review. *Cochrane Database of Systematic Reviews, 1*(1), CD011651. https://doi.org/10.1002/14651858.CD011651.pub2

Hill-Rom, Inc. (2021). *Comparison guide*. https://respiratorycare.hill-rom.com/en/patients/comparison/

Houin, P., Stillwell, P., Deboer, E. M., & Hoppe, J. (2022). Respiratory tract & mediastinum. In M. Bunik, W. W. Hay, M. J. Levin, & M. J. Abzug (Eds.), *Current diagnosis and treatment: Pediatrics* (26th ed.). McGraw-Hill Education.

Janahi, I. A. (2022). *Spontaneous pneumothorax in children*. *UpToDate*. Retrieved December 1, 2023, from https://www.uptodate.com/contents/spontaneous-pneumothorax-in-children

Katkin, J. P. (2023). *Cystic fibrosis: Clinical manifestations and diagnosis*. *UpToDate*. Retrieved December 1, 2023, from https://www.uptodate.com/contents/cystic-fibrosis-clinical-manifestations-and-diagnosis

Kimberlin, D. W., Barnett, E. D., Lynfield, R., & Sawyer, M. H. (Eds.). (2021). Tuberculosis. In D. W. Kimberlin, E. D. Barnett, R. Lynfield, & M. H. Sawyer (Eds.), *Red book 2021–2024: Report of the committee on infectious diseases* (32nd ed.). American Academy of Pediatrics.

Lack, S., Brown, R., & Kinser, P. A. (2020). An integrative review of yoga and mindfulness-based approaches for children and adolescents with asthma. *Journal of Pediatric Nursing, 52*, 76–81. https://doi.org/10.1016/j.pedn.2020.03.006

Medtronic. (2023). *Pulse oximetry*. https://www.medtronic.com/covidien/en-us/products/pulse-oximetry.html

Moon, R. Y., Carlin, R. F., Hand, I., & the Task Force on Sudden Infant Death Syndrome and The Committee on Fetus and Newborn. (2022). Sleep-related infant deaths: Updated 2022 Recommendations for reducing infant deaths in the sleep environment. *Pediatrics, 150*(1), e2022057990. https://doi.org/10.1542/peds.2022-057990

Moore, K. L., Persaud, T. V. N., & Torchia, M. G. (2020). *The developing human: Clinically oriented embryology* (11th ed.). Elsevier.

Munoz, F. M., & Edwards, M. S. (2023). *Seasonal influenza in children: Clinical features and diagnosis*. *UpToDate*. Retrieved December 1, 2023, from https://www.uptodate.com/contents/seasonal-influenza-in-children-clinical-features-and-diagnosis

Nagler, J. (2022). *Emergency airway management in children: Unique pediatric considerations*. *UpToDate*. Retrieved December 1, 2023, from https://www.uptodate.com/contents/emergency-airway-management-in-children-unique-pediatric-considerations

Piedra, P. A. (2023). *Bronchiolitis in infants and children: Clinical features and diagnosis*. *UpToDate*. Retrieved December 1, 2023, from https://www.uptodate.com/contents/bronchiolitis-in-infants-and-children-clinical-features-and-diagnosis

Pramanik, A. K. (2020). *Respiratory distress syndrome*. *Medscape*. Retrieved December 1, 2023, from https://emedicine.medscape.com/article/976034-overview#a5

Purohit, P. (2023). *Pediatric acute respiratory distress syndrome*. *Medscape*. Retrieved December 1, 2023, from https://emedicine.medscape.com/article/803573-overview#a7

Pusey-Reid, E., Quinn, L., Samost, M. E., & Reidy, P. (2023). Skin assessment in patients with dark skin tone. *American Journal of Nursing, 123*(3), 36–43. https://doi.org/10.1097/01.NAJ.0000921800.61980.7e

Rabinowicz, S., Leshem, E., & Pessach, I. M. (2020). COVID-19 in the pediatric population—Review and current evidence. *Current Infectious Disease Reports, 22*, Article 29. https://doi.org/10.1007/s11908-020-00739-6

Regan, J. J., Moulia, D. L., Link-Gelles, R., Godfrey, M., Mak, J., Najdowski, M., Rosenblum, H. G., Shah, M. M., Twentyman, E., Meyer, S., Peacock, G., Thornburg, N., Havers, F. P., Saydah, S., Brooks, O., Talbot, H. K., Lee, G. M., Bell, B. P., Mahon, B. E., … Wallace, M. (2023). Use of updated COVID-19 vaccines 2023–2024 formula for persons aged ≥6 months: Recommendations of the Advisory Committee on Immunization Practices—United States, September 2023. *Morbidity and Mortality Weekly Report, 72*(42), 1140–1146. https://www.cdc.gov/mmwr/volumes/72/wr/mm7242e1.htm

Rough, J., & Markowitz, A. (2023). *List of coronavirus-related restrictions in every state*. https://www.aarp.org/politics-society/government-elections/info-2020/coronavirus-state-restrictions.html#Florida

Safe Kids. (2024). *Choking and strangulation*. http://www.safekids.org/safety-basics/safety-resources-by-risk-area/choking-suffocation-and-strangulation/

Schare, R. S. (2021). *Croup*. https://kidshealth.org/en/parents/croup.html

Simon, R. H. (2023). *Cystic fibrosis: Treatment with CFTR modulators*. *UpToDate*. Retrieved December 1, 2023, from https://www.uptodate.com/contents/cystic-fibrosis-treatment-with-cftr-modulators

Smith, D. (2022). The newborn infant. In M. Bunik, W. W. Hay, M. J. Levin, & M. J. Abzug (Eds.), *Current diagnosis and treatment: Pediatrics* (26th ed.). McGraw-Hill Education.

Smith, S. (2022). Management of lower respiratory disorders. In T. Kyle (Ed.), *Primary care pediatrics for the nurse practitioner: A practical approach*. Springer.

Sonney, J., Segrin, C., & Kolstad, T. (2019). Parent- and child-reported asthma responsibility in school-age children: Examining agreement, disagreement, and family functioning. *Journal of Pediatric Health Care, 33*, 386–393. https://doi.org/10.1016/j.pedhc.2018.11.005

Stanford Children's Health. (2023). *Reye syndrome in children*. https://www.stanfordchildrens.org/en/topic/default?id=reye-syndrome-90-P02620

UpToDate, Inc. (2023). *Lexi-comp®* (Version 7.7.0) [Mobile app]. Wolters Kluwer. https://apps.apple.com/us/app/lexicomp/id313401238

U.S. Department of Health and Human Services. (n.d.). *Healthy People 2030.* https://health.gov/healthypeople

U.S. Food and Drug Administration. (2023). *Should you give kids medicine for coughs and colds?* https://www.fda.gov/consumers/consumer-updates/should-you-give-kids-medicine-coughs-and-colds

Volkman, K. K., & Chiu, A. M. (2023). Allergy. In K. J. Marcdante & R. M. Kliegman (Eds.), *Nelson's essentials of pediatrics* (9th ed.). Elsevier.

Weiner, D. L. (2022). *Acute respiratory distress in children: Emergency evaluation and initial stabilization. UpToDate.* Retrieved December 1, 2023, from https://www.uptodate.com/contents/acute-respiratory-distress-in-children-emergency-evaluation-and-initial-stabilization

Woods, C. R. (2023). *Croup: Clinical features, evaluation, and diagnosis. UpToDate.* Retrieved December 1, 2023, from https://www.uptodate.com/contents/croup-clinical-features-evaluation-and-diagnosis

World Health Organization. (2023). *Coronavirus disease (COVID-19) advice for the public: Mythbusters.* https://www.who.int/emergencies/diseases/novel-coronavirus-2019/advice-for-public/myth-busters

Yoon, P. J., Scholes, M. A., & Herrmann, B. W. (2022). Ear, nose, & throat. In M. Bunik, W. W. Hay, M. J. Levin, & Abzug, M. J. (Eds.), *Current diagnosis & treatment: Pediatrics* (26th ed.). McGraw-Hill Education.

Zachariah, P. (2022). COVID-19 in children. *Infectious Disease Clinics of North America, 36*(1), 1–14. https://doi.org/10.1016/j.idc.2021.11.002

DEVELOPING CLINICAL JUDGMENT

PRACTICING FOR NCLEX

1. A 5-month-old infant with RSV bronchiolitis is in respiratory distress. The baby has copious secretions, increased work of breathing, cyanosis, and a respiratory rate of 78. What is the most appropriate initial nursing intervention?
   a. Attempt to calm the infant by placing the infant in the parent's lap and offering them a bottle.
   b. Alert the primary health care provider or nurse practitioner to the situation and ask for an order for a stat chest radiograph.
   c. Suction secretions, provide 100% oxygen via mask, and anticipate respiratory failure.
   d. Bring the emergency equipment to the room and begin bag-valve-mask ventilation.

2. A toddler has moderate respiratory distress, is mildly cyanotic, and has increased work of breathing, with a respiratory rate of 40. What is the priority nursing intervention?
   a. Airway maintenance and 100% oxygen by mask
   b. 100% oxygen and pulse oximetry monitoring
   c. Airway maintenance and continued reassessment
   d. 100% oxygen and provision of comfort

3. The nurse is caring for a child with cystic fibrosis who receives pancreatic enzymes. Which statement by the child's parent indicates an understanding of how to administer the supplemental enzymes?
   a. "I will stop the enzymes if my child is receiving antibiotics."
   b. "I will decrease the dose by half if my child is having frequent, bulky stools."
   c. "Between meals is the best time for me to give the enzymes."
   d. "The enzymes should be given at the beginning of each meal and snack."

4. Which of these factors contributes to infants' and children's increased risk of upper airway obstruction as compared with adults?
   a. Underdeveloped cricoid cartilage and narrow nasal passages
   b. Small tonsils and narrow nasal passages
   c. Cylinder-shaped larynx and underdeveloped sinuses
   d. Underdeveloped cricoid cartilage and smaller tongue

5. The school nurse is presented with a child whose nose began bleeding a few moments ago. Which is the appropriate nursing intervention?
   a. Have the child lie down and breathe through their mouth; then apply pressure to the bridge of the nose.
   b. Have the child lie down and breathe through their mouth; then pinch the lower third of the nose closed.
   c. Instruct the child to sit up and lean forward; then apply pressure to the bridge of the nose.
   d. Instruct the child to sit up and lean forward; then pinch the lower third of the nose closed.

6. The nurse is caring for a toddler who was admitted for observation because of respiratory changes. The parent states the child doesn't want to eat and seems tired.

Nurses' Notes

Time	Notes
1200	Alert, fearful of RN, resists examination. Color pink. Skin warm, dry, intact. Heart rate regular without murmur. Minimal intercostal retractions. Harsh cough.
1400	Parent called RN to room as toddler is restless. Does not resist examination. Color pink. Skin warm, diaphoretic. Heart rate regular with murmur. Moderate intercostal retractions, with mild nasal flaring. Harsh cough.

Vital Signs

Time	Temperature	Pulse	Respiratory Rate	Blood Pressure
1200	37.4°C (99.4°F)	100 bpm	28 bpm	118/70 mm Hg
1400	37.2°C (99.0°F)	110 bpm	34 bpm	Not taken

Which assessment findings indicate the toddler is progressing to respiratory distress? Select all that apply.
   a. Cough
   b. Diaphoresis
   c. Heart rate
   d. Malaise
   e. Nasal flaring
   f. Respiratory rate
   g. Restlessness
   h. Retraction

7. A young infant has been diagnosed with bronchiolitis in the clinic. The infant will be cared for at home. What should the nurse include when teaching the parent about home care? Select all that apply.
   a. Offer small amounts of fluids frequently.
   b. Use the nebulizer machine as instructed.
   c. Allow the infant to sleep prone for comfort.
   d. Call the clinic if the infant vomits.
   e. Perform chest physiotherapy every 4 hours.
   f. Watch for difficulty breathing.

DOSAGE CALCULATION QUESTION

The nurse is caring for a child with acute asthma. The child weighs 37.5 lb. The medication order reads: methylprednisolone 20 mg IV twice a day. The *Pediatric Dosage Handbook* provides a recommended dose for acute asthma of 1 to 2 mg/kg/day in two divided doses. Is the ordered dose safe?

CRITICAL THINKING EXERCISES

1. A 10-month-old infant is admitted to the pediatric unit with a history of recurrent pneumonia and failure to thrive. The sweat chloride test confirms the diagnosis of cystic fibrosis. The infant is frail in appearance with thin extremities and a slightly protuberant abdomen. The infant is tachypneic, has retractions, and coughs frequently. Based on the limited information given here and your knowledge of cystic fibrosis, choose three of the following categories as priorities to focus on when planning the infant's care:
   a. Prevention of bronchospasm
   b. Promotion of adequate nutrition
   c. Education of the child and family
   d. Prevention of pulmonary infection
   e. Balancing fluid and electrolytes
   f. Management of excess weight gain
   g. Prevention of spread of infection
   h. Promoting adequate sleep and rest
2. A child with asthma is admitted to the pediatric unit for the fourth time this year. The parent expresses frustration that the child is getting sick so often. Besides information about onset of symptoms and events leading up to this present episode, what other types of information would you ask for while obtaining the history?
3. The parent of the child in the previous question tells you that they smoke (but never around the child), the family has a cat that comes inside sometimes, and they always give the child the medication prescribed. The parent gives salmeterol and budesonide as soon as the child starts to cough. When the child is not having an episode, the parent gives them albuterol before baseball games. Diphenhydramine helps the runny nose in the springtime. Based on this new information, what advice/instructions would you give the parent?
4. A 7-year-old presents with a history of recurrent nasal discharge. The child sneezes every time they visit their cousins, who have pets. The child lives in an older home that is carpeted. Tobacco smokers live in the home. The parent reports that the child snores and is a mouth breather. They say the child has symptoms nearly year-round but that they are worse in the fall and the spring. The parent reports that diphenhydramine is somewhat helpful with the symptoms but does not like to give it to the child on school days because it makes them drowsy. Based on the foregoing history, develop a teaching plan for this child.
5. The nurse is caring for a 4-year-old who returned from the recovery room after a tonsillectomy 3 hours ago. The child has cried off and on over the past 2 hours and is now sleeping. What areas should the nurse assess and focus on for this child?

STUDY ACTIVITIES

1. While caring for children in the pediatric setting, compare the signs and symptoms of a child with asthma with those of an infant with bronchiolitis. What are the most notable differences? How does the history of the two children differ?
2. A child with asthma has been prescribed fluticasone and salmeterol, albuterol, and prednisone. Develop a sample teaching plan for the child and the family. Include appropriate use of the devices used to deliver the medications, as well as important information about the medications (uses and adverse effects).
3. While caring for children in the pediatric setting, compare the signs and symptoms and presentation of a child with the common cold with those of a child with either sinusitis or allergic rhinitis.
4. While caring for children in the pediatric setting, review the census of children, and identify those at risk for severe influenza and thus those who would benefit from annual influenza vaccination.
5. Compare the differences in oxygen administration between a young infant and an older child.

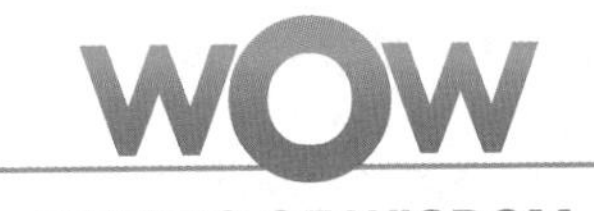

WORDS OF WISDOM

The heart of the matter is healing the child's heart so they can embrace life to its fullest.

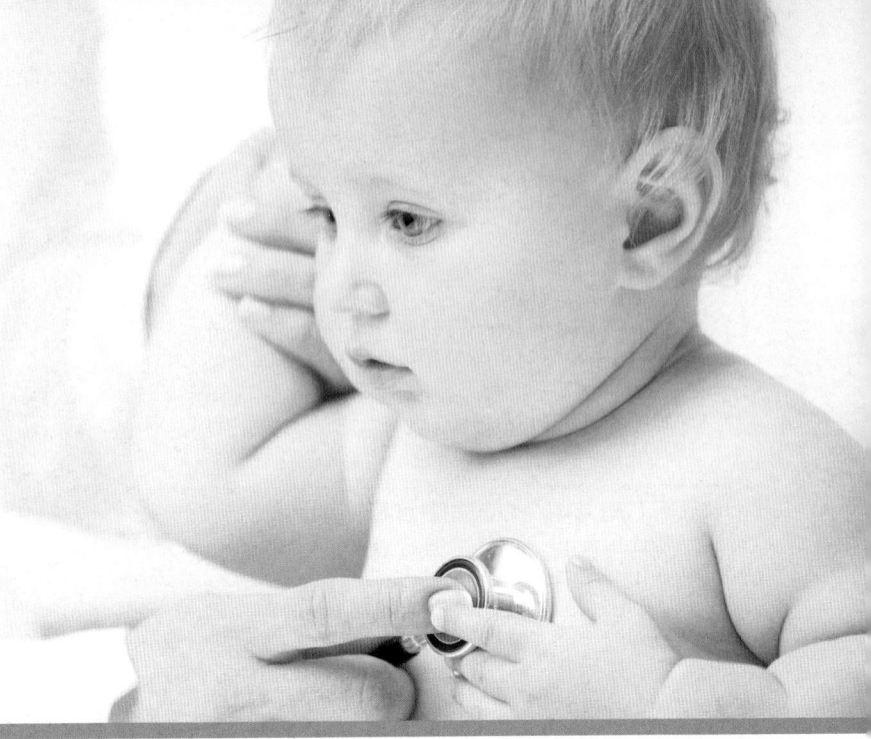

19 Nursing Care of the Child With an Alteration in Perfusion/Cardiovascular Disorder

LEARNING OBJECTIVES

Upon completion of the chapter, you will be able to:

1. Compare anatomy and physiology of the cardiovascular system in infants and children with that of adults.
2. Describe nursing care related to common laboratory and diagnostic tests used in the medical diagnosis of pediatric cardiovascular conditions.
3. Distinguish cardiovascular disorders common in infants, children, and adolescents.
4. Identify appropriate nursing assessments and interventions related to medications and treatments for pediatric cardiovascular disorders.
5. Develop an individualized nursing care plan or concept map for the child with a cardiovascular disorder.
6. Describe the psychosocial impact of chronic cardiovascular disorders on children.
7. Devise a nutrition plan for the child with cardiovascular disease.
8. Develop child and family teaching plans for the child with a cardiovascular disorder.

KEY TERMS

arrhythmia

cardiomegaly (kahr´dē-ō-meg´ă-lē)

clubbing

echocardiography

electrocardiogram

heart failure

orthotopic (ōr´thō-tō´pik)

polycythemia (pol´ē-sī-thē´mē-ă)

Logan Bernstein, 6 weeks old, is brought to the clinic by his parent. He presents with poor feeding. His parent states, "Logan falls asleep while feeding, and he's always sweaty during feedings."

INTRODUCTION

Perfusion refers to the mechanisms that facilitate blood through tissue. Nurses may encounter alterations in perfusion in children and should be familiar with various cardiovascular disorders that children experience. Alterations in perfusion, or cardiovascular disease, are a significant cause of chronic illness and death in children. Typically, cardiovascular disorders in children are divided into two major categories—congenital heart defects (CHDs) and acquired heart disease.

CHD is defined as structural anomalies that are present at birth, although they are often not diagnosed until later in life. About 40,000 babies are born annually with CHD, accounting for the largest percentage of all birth defects (American Heart Association [AHA], 2022). CHD may result from a genetic abnormality or be associated with a genetic syndrome. About 40% to 50% of children with Down syndrome have a CHD (Nees & Chung, 2020). Many CHDs result in **heart failure** (inability of the heart to pump blood sufficiently) and chronic cyanosis, leading to failure to thrive.

Acquired heart disease includes disorders that occur after birth. These disorders develop from a wide range of causes, or they can occur as a complication or long-term effect of CHD.

The diagnosis of a cardiovascular disorder in any person can be extremely frightening and overwhelming. Early on, children learn that the heart is necessary for life, so knowing that there is a heart problem can promote feelings of dread. These feelings are compounded by the child's age, the view of the child as being vulnerable and defenseless, and the stressors associated with the disorder itself. The child and parents need much support and reassurance (Gaskin & Kennedy, 2019).

Nurses need to have a sound knowledge base about cardiovascular conditions affecting children so that they can provide appropriate assessment, intervention, guidance, and support to the child and family. Cardiovascular disorders require acute interventions that often have long-term implications for the child's health and growth and development. Due to the potentially overwhelming and devastating effects that cardiovascular disorders can have on children and their families, nurses need to be skilled in assessment and interventions in this area and able to provide support throughout the course of the illness and beyond.

VARIATIONS IN PEDIATRIC ANATOMY AND PHYSIOLOGY

The cardiovascular system undergoes numerous changes at birth. Structures that were vital to the fetus are no longer needed. Circulation via the umbilical arteries and vein is replaced with the child's own closed independent circulation. Changes in the size of the heart, pulse rate, and blood pressure (BP) also occur.

Circulatory Changes From Gestation to Birth

The fetal heart rate is present on about postconceptual day 17. The four chambers of the heart and arteries are formed during gestational weeks 2 through 8, with maturation of the structures occurring throughout the remainder of gestation. During fetal development, oxygenation of the fetus occurs via the placenta; the lungs, although perfused, do not perform oxygenation and ventilation. The foramen ovale, an opening between the atria, allows blood flow from the right to the left atrium. The ductus arteriosus allows blood flow between the pulmonary artery and the aorta, shunting blood away from the pulmonary circulation (Cunningham et al., 2022). Figure 19.1 illustrates fetal circulation.

With the newborn's first breath, several changes occur in the cardiopulmonary system that enable the newborn to make the transition from fetal circulation to normal circulation. As the newborn breathes for the first time, the lungs inflate, reducing pulmonary vascular resistance to blood flow. As a result, pulmonary artery pressure drops. Subsequently, pressure in the right atrium decreases. Blood flow to the left side of the heart increases the pressure in the left atrium. This change in pressure leads to closure of the foramen ovale. The drop in pressure of the pulmonary artery promotes closure of the ductus arteriosus, which is located between the aorta and the pulmonary artery. The ductus venosus, located between the left umbilical vein and the inferior vena cava, closes because of a lack of blood flow and vasoconstriction. The closed ductus arteriosus and ductus venosus eventually become ligaments. With the lack of blood flow to the umbilical arteries and vein, these structures atrophy (Cunningham et al., 2022).

Structural and Functional Differences

The structure and function of the infant's and child's cardiovascular system differ from those of adults, depending on age. In infants and children younger than 7 years, the heart lies more horizontally, resulting in the apex lying higher in the chest, below the fourth intercostal space. As the lungs grow over time, the heart is displaced downward. Between ages 1 and 6 years, the heart is four times the birth size. Between 6 and 12 years of age, the child's heart is 10 times the size it was at birth. However, the heart is smaller proportionally at this time than at any other stage in life. During the school-age years, the heart

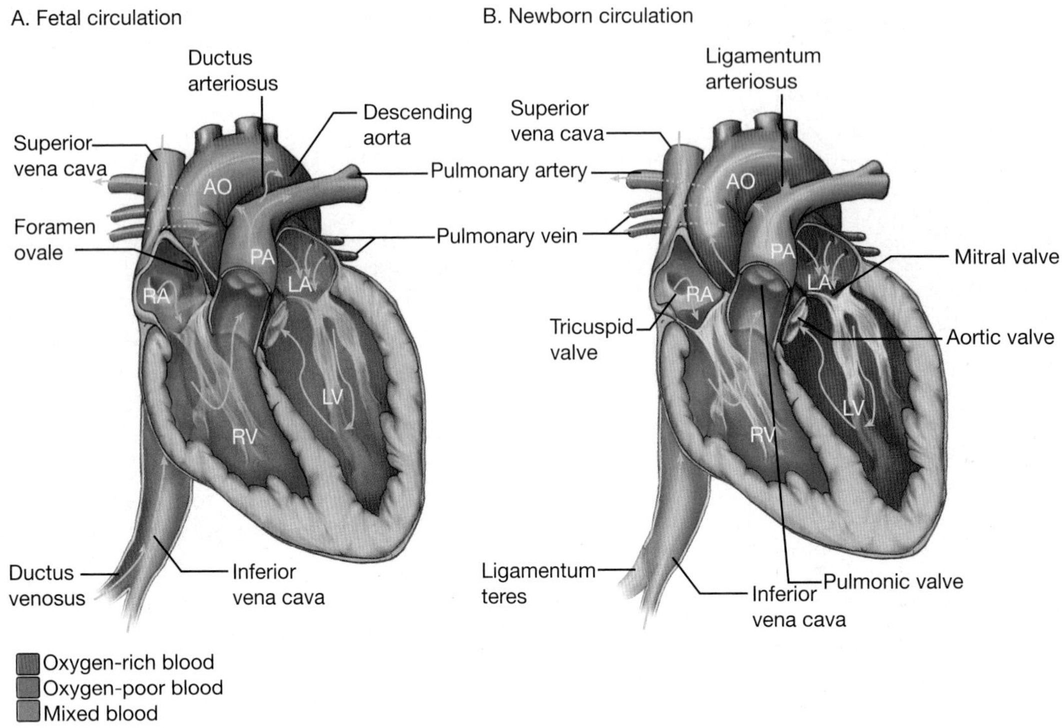

FIGURE 19.1 Fetal and newborn circulation.

grows more vertically within the thoracic cavity. During adolescence, the heart continues to grow in relation to the adolescent's rapid growth.

At birth, the ventricle walls are similar in thickness, but with time the left ventricular wall thickens. The immature myocytes of the infant's heart are thinner and less compliant than those of the adult. Right ventricular function dominates at birth, and over the first few months of life, left ventricular function becomes dominant. The infant's heart at rest exhibits a greater resting tension than the adult's, so volume loading or increased stretch may actually lead to decreased cardiac output. The infant's sarcoplasmic reticulum is less well organized than the adult's, making the infant dependent on serum calcium for contraction. Inotropic response to calcium in the actin and myosin (contractile proteins) increases with age.

The normal heart rate is higher in infancy than in adulthood, limiting the infant's ability to increase cardiac output by increasing the heart rate. The heart's efficiency increases as the child ages and the heart rate drops over time. The normal infant heart rate ranges from 90 to 160 beats per minute (bpm), the toddler's or preschooler's is 80 to 115 bpm, and the school-age child's and the adolescent's ranges from 60 to 100 bpm. Innocent murmurs and physiologic splitting of heart sounds may be noted in infancy or childhood. These findings are related to the change in the size of the heart in relation to the thoracic cavity. The infant's and child's blood vessels widen and increase in length over time. The average infant's BP is about 80/55 mm Hg; BP is usually lower in the younger infant and can be slightly higher in the older infant. The BP increases over time to the adult level. The toddler or preschooler's BP averages 90 to 110/55 to 75 mm Hg, the school-age child's 100 to 120/60 to 75 mm Hg, and the adolescent's 100 to 120/70 to 80 mm Hg (Kleinman et al., 2021).

COMMON MEDICAL TREATMENTS

A variety of medications as well as other medical treatments and surgical procedures are used to treat cardiovascular problems in children. Most of these treatments will require a health care provider's order when the child is in the hospital. The most common treatments and medications are listed in Common Medical Treatments 19.1 and Drug Guide 19.1. The nurse caring for the child with a cardiovascular disorder should be familiar with what the procedures and medications are and how they work as well as common nursing implications related to use of these modalities.

TAKE NOTE!

Give digoxin at regular intervals, every 12 hours, such as at 8 a.m. and 8 p.m., 1 hour before or 2 hours after a feeding. If a digoxin dose is missed, give the dose as soon as it is realized the dose was missed. If it is close to the next dose's time, hold the missed dose. Monitor potassium levels, as a decrease enhances the effects of digitalis, causing toxicity (UpToDate, Inc., 2024).

COMMON MEDICAL TREATMENTS 19.1

Treatment	Explanation	Indications	Nursing Implications
Oxygen	Supplemented via mask, nasal cannula, hood, tent, or endotracheal/nasotracheal tube	Hypoxemia, respiratory distress, heart failure	Monitor response via work of breathing and pulse oximetry.
Chest physiotherapy (CPT) and postural drainage	Promotes mucus clearance by mobilizing secretions with the assistance of percussion or vibration accompanied by postural drainage (refer to Chapter 18 for additional information related to CPT and postural drainage)	Mobilization of secretions, particularly in postoperative period or with heart failure	May be performed by respiratory therapist in some institutions, by nurses in others; in either case, nurses must be familiar with the technique and able to educate families on its use.
Chest tube	Drainage tube is inserted into the pleural cavity to facilitate removal of air or fluid and allow full lung expansion.	After open heart surgery, pneumothorax	If tube becomes dislodged from container, the chest tube must be clamped immediately to avoid further air entry into the chest cavity. Alternatively, the end may be immediately placed into a container of sterile water or saline to create a water seal.
Pacing	External wiring connected to a small generator used to electrophysiologically correct cardiac arrhythmias or heart block (temporary).Permanent pacing achieved with an implantable internal pacemaker.	Bradyarrhythmias, heart block, cardiomyopathy, sinoatrial or atrioventricular node malfunction	Provide close observation of the child, pacing unit, and ECG. Maintain asepsis at pacing lead insertion site. Explain to the child and family that the permanent pacemaker may be felt under the skin. Advise against participation in contact sports.[a]

ECG, electrocardiogram

[a]Children's Hospital of Wisconsin. (2024). *Living with a pediatric pacemaker.* https://childrenswi.org/medical-care/herma-heart/conditions/living-with-a-pacemaker

DRUG GUIDE 19.1

Medication	Actions/Indications	Nursing Implications
Alprostadil (prostaglandin)	Direct vasodilation of the ductus arteriosus smooth muscle Indicated for temporary maintenance of ductus arteriosus patency in infants with ductal-dependent congenital heart defects	• Apnea occurs in 10%–20% of neonates within first hour of infusion. • Monitor arterial BP, respiratory rate, heart rate, ECG, temperature, and pO2; watch for abdominal distention. • Fresh IV solution required every 24 hours. • Reposition catheter if facial or arm flushing occurs. • Use with caution in neonate with bleeding tendency. • Contraindicated in respiratory distress syndrome or persistent fetal circulation
Digoxin (cardiac glycoside, antiarrhythmic agent)	Increases contractility of the heart muscle by decreasing conduction and increasing force Used for heart failure, atrial fibrillation, atrial flutter, supraventricular tachycardia	• Prior to administering each dose, count apical pulse for one full minute, noting rate, rhythm, and quality. Withhold if apical pulse is <60 in an adolescent, <90 in an infant. • Avoid giving oral form with meals, as altered absorption may occur. • Monitor serum digoxin levels (therapeutic range: 0.8–2 ng/mL). • Note signs of toxicity: nausea, vomiting, diarrhea, lethargy, and bradycardia. • Ginseng, hawthorn, and licorice intake increase risk of drug toxicity. • Note contraindications (ventricular fibrillation and hypersensitivity to digitalis). • Avoid rapid IV administration, as this may lead to systemic and coronary artery vasoconstriction.

(*continued*)

DRUG GUIDE 19.1 (*continued*)

Medication	Actions/Indications	Nursing Implications
Furosemide (loop diuretic)	Inhibits resorption of sodium and chloride Used to manage edema associated with heart failure, and hypertension in combination with antihypertensives	• Administer with food or milk to decrease GI upset. • Monitor BP, kidney function, electrolytes (particularly potassium), and hearing. • May cause photosensitivity
Heparin (anticoagulant)	Interferes with conversion of prothrombin to thrombin, preventing clot formation Indicated for the prophylaxis and treatment of thromboembolic disorders, especially after cardiac surgery	• Administer SQ, not IM. • Dose is adjusted according to coagulation test results. • Monitor for signs of bleeding, platelet counts. • Ensure that the antidote, protamine sulfate, is available. • Do not administer with uncontrolled bleeding or if subacute bacterial endocarditis is suspected.
Indomethacin (nonsteroidal antiinflammatory agent)	Inhibits prostaglandin synthesis in order to close patent ductus arteriosus	• Monitor heart rate, BP, ECG, and urine output; monitor for murmur. • Monitor serum sodium, glucose, platelet count, BUN, creatinine, potassium, and liver enzymes. • May mask signs of infection • Note development of edema.
Spironolactone (potassium-sparing diuretic)	Competes with aldosterone to result in increased water and sodium excretion (spares potassium) Used to manage edema due to heart failure and for treatment of hypertension	• Administer with food. • Monitor serum potassium, sodium, and kidney function. • May cause drowsiness, headache, and arrhythmia • May cause false elevations in digitalis level • Teach children to avoid high-potassium diets, salt substitutes, and natural licorice. • Contraindicated in hyperkalemia, kidney failure, and anuria
Antibiotics		
Penicillin G benzathine Penicillin V potassium	Inhibits bacterial wall synthesis in susceptible organisms. Indicated in mild to moderate infections, for prophylaxis of endocarditis and rheumatic fever	• Contraindications include hypersensitivity to penicillins. • Report hypersensitivity reactions (chills, fever, wheezing, pruritus, anaphylaxis) immediately. • PCN-G: administer IM. • Pen-VK: administer orally on empty stomach 1 hour before or 2 hours after a meal.
Erythromycin (macrolide)	Inhibits ribonucleic acid transcription in susceptible organisms. Used in children with penicillin allergy, mild to moderate infections, or endocarditis, and for rheumatic fever prophylaxis	• Contraindicated in preexisting liver disease • IV administration may result in CV abnormalities. • Abdominal distress common with oral use. • Fever, dizziness, and rash may occur.
Antihypertensive Drugs		
Angiotensin-converting enzyme (ACE) inhibitors (captopril, enalapril)	Competitive inhibition of ACE for management of hypertension Heart failure management in conjunction with digitalis and diuretics	• Monitor BP, kidney function, WBC count, and serum potassium. • Discontinue if angioedema occurs. • Captopril: administer orally on empty stomach 1 hour before or 2 hours after meals. • Enalapril: may administer orally without regard to food
Beta-adrenergic blockers (propranolol, atenolol, sotalol)	Competitively block response to beta-adrenergic stimulation, decreasing heart rate, and force of contraction. Used for management of hypertension, arrhythmias, and prevention of myocardial infarction	• Monitor ECG and BP. • Propranolol: administer with food. • Atenolol, sotalol: administer without regard to food. Do not stop drug abruptly. • May result in bradycardia, dizziness, nausea and vomiting, dyspnea, and hypoglycemia (propranolol) • Contraindications: heart block, uncompensated heart failure, cardiogenic shock, asthma, or hypersensitivity
Hydralazine (vasodilator)	Direct vasodilation of arterioles to manage moderate to severe hypertension, heart failure	• Monitor heart rate and BP. • Closely monitor BP with IV use. • Administer oral dose with food. • May cause palpitations, flushing, tachycardia, dizziness, nausea, and vomiting • Notify health care provider or nurse practitioner if flu-like symptoms occur. • Contraindicated in rheumatic valvular disease

BP, blood pressure; BUN, blood urea nitrogen; CV, cardiovascular; ECG, electrocardiogram; GI, gastrointestinal; IM, intramuscularly; IV, intravenous; pO2, partial pressure of oxygen; SQ, subcutaneously; WBC, white blood cell.

Source: UpToDate, Inc. (2024). *UpToDate® Lexidrug™* (Version 8.2.0) [Mobile app]. Wolters Kluwer. https://apps.apple.com/us/app/lexicomp/id313401238

COMMON LABORATORY AND DIAGNOSTIC TESTS 19.1

Test	Explanation	Indications	Nursing Implications
Arteriogram (angiogram: visualization of arteries or veins)	Radiopaque contrast solution is injected through a catheter and into the circulation. Radiographs are then taken to visualize the structure of the heart and blood vessels.	To observe blood flow to parts of body and detect lesions; to confirm a diagnosis Catheters can be used to remove plaques.	• Make sure the parent signs a consent form. • Administer premedication as ordered. • Obtain child's weight to determine amount of dye needed. • Keep the child NPO before the procedure according to institutional protocol. • After the procedure, maintain the child on bed rest. • Observe the puncture site for bleeding. • Monitor vital signs frequently and check the pulse distal to the site.
Ambulatory electrocardiographic monitoring (Holter)	Monitoring of the heart's electrical patterns for 24 hours using a portable compact unit	To identify and quantify arrhythmias in a 24-hour period during normal daily activities	• Instruct the child and parent to push the "event button" whenever chest pain, syncope, or palpitations occur. • Normal daily activities should be carried out during the testing period. • Having the child wear a snug undershirt over the leads helps to keep them in place.
Chest radiograph	A radiographic film of the chest area; will determine size of the heart and its chambers and pulmonary blood flow	Serves as a baseline for comparison with films taken after surgery; used to identify abnormalities of the lungs, heart, and other structures in the chest	• Instruct child not to wear jewelry or any metal around neck or on the hospital gown. • Explain to the child and family that no pain or discomfort should result. • If a portable radiograph at bedside is done, remove electrodes temporarily.
Echocardiogram	Noninvasive ultrasound procedure used to assess heart wall thickness, size of heart chambers, motion of valves and septa, and relationship of great vessels to other cardiac structures	Specific diagnosis of structural defects; determines hemodynamics and detects valvular defects	• Assure the child that the echo does not hurt. • Instruct the child about ECG lead placement and use of gel on the scope's wand during the procedure. • Encourage the child to lie still throughout the test.
Electrocardiogram (ECG)	A graphic record produced by an electrocardiograph (device used to record the electrical activity of the myocardium to detect transmission of the cardiac impulse through the conductive tissues of the muscle) Facilitates evaluation of the heart rate, rhythm, conduction, and musculature.	To detect heart rhythm and chamber overload; also serves as a baseline for measuring postoperative complications.	• Assure the child that monitoring is a painless procedure. • Place electrodes in the appropriate location. • The child must lie still during the ECG recording period (usually about 5 minutes). • Wipe electrode paste or jelly off after procedure.
Exercise stress test	Monitoring of heart rate, blood pressure, ECG, and oxygen consumption at rest and during exercise	Quantifies exercise tolerance; can be used to provoke symptoms or arrhythmias	• Child should be NPO for 4 hours prior to test. • Obtain baseline ECG and vital signs. • Instruct child to verbalize symptoms during testing. • Usually takes about 45 minutes.
Hemoglobin (Hgb) and hematocrit (Hct)	Measures the total amount of hemoglobin in the blood and indirectly measures the red blood cell number and volume.	To detect anemia or polycythemia (may occur with CHD resulting in cyanosis)	• False elevations occur with dehydration. • May be obtained quickly via capillary puncture • Normal values vary with age.
Partial pressure of oxygen (pO2)	Measures the amount of oxygen in the blood.	To determine the presence and degree of hypoxia	• Most accurate result is with arterial specimen (venous and capillary specimens demonstrate lower levels). • Observe child for cyanosis. • Supplement with oxygen per protocol.
Pulse oximetry screening	Noninvasive method of measuring oxygen saturation in the blood	To detect critical congenital heart disease in the newborn	• Take measurements in the right hand and in either foot. Apply the probe correctly and securely, being sure to minimize movement and ambient light interference.

CHD, congenital heart defect; NPO, nothing by mouth

Data from Children's Heart Institute. (2023). *Heart tests? When do* you *need them?* https://www.childrensheartinstitute.org/health-library/health-wise/?DOCHWID=aba5713; Corbett, J. A., & Banks, A. D. (2019). *Laboratory tests and diagnostic procedures with nursing diagnoses* (9th ed.). Pearson Education Inc; Oster, M. (2023). Newborn screening for critical congenital heart disease using pulse oximetry. *UpToDate*. Retrieved March 31, 2023, from https://www.uptodate.com/contents/newborn-screening-for-critical-congenital-heart-disease-using-pulse-oximetry

CARDIAC CATHETERIZATION

Cardiac catheterization is the definitive study for infants and children with cardiac disease. It has become almost a routine diagnostic procedure and may be performed on an outpatient basis. However, it is highly invasive and not without risks, especially in sick infants and children. Indications for cardiac catheterization include:

- Cardiovascular disease, causing cyanosis in infants; these infants need to be catheterized as soon as they are in a reasonably stable condition.
- Severe heart failure or progressive problems such as pulmonary edema
- Questionable anatomic or physiologic abnormalities
- Planned cardiac surgery
- Progressive monitoring related to pulmonary hypertension
- Periodic assessment after repair of a cardiac defect
- Therapeutic interventions such as septostomy or balloon valvotomy

Cardiac catheterization may be categorized as diagnostic or interventional. The type of catheterization performed varies based on the individual needs of the child. The procedure lasts from 2 to 5 hours (UPMC, 2024).

In cardiac catheterization, a radiopaque catheter is inserted into a blood vessel and is then guided through the vessel to the heart with the aid of fluoroscopy. For a right-sided catheterization, the catheter is threaded to the right atrium via a major vein such as the femoral vein. With a left-sided catheterization, the catheter is threaded to the aorta and heart via an artery. Once the tip of the catheter is in the heart, contrast material is injected via the catheter, and radiographic images are taken.

While the catheter is in the heart, several procedures can be performed. The BP, changes in cardiac output or stroke volume, and oxygen saturation in each heart chamber and major blood vessels are recorded. With the injection of contrast material, information is revealed about the heart anatomy, ventricular wall motion and ejection fraction, intracardiac pressures and hemodynamic parameters, cardiac valve function, and structural abnormalities. The movement of the contrast material is filmed so that the details of the cardiac procedure are recorded. Samples of heart tissue to evaluate for infection, muscular dysfunction, or rejection after a transplant may also be obtained (UPMC, 2024).

Clinical Judgment and the Nursing Process

Care of the child with a cardiovascular disorder includes all steps of the nursing process: assessment, nursing analysis, planning, interventions, and evaluation. There are a number of general concepts related to the nursing process that may be applied to any child with a cardiovascular disorder. The nurse should be knowledgeable about the procedures, treatments, and medications as well as familiar with the nursing implications related to these interventions. With an understanding of these concepts, the nurse can individualize the care based on the child's and family's needs.

Assessment

When assessing a child with a cardiovascular disorder, expect to obtain a health history, perform a physical examination, and prepare the child for laboratory and diagnostic testing.

Health History

The health history consists of a history of the present illness, past medical history, and family history. Depending on their age, the child should be included in the health history interview; the child's age will determine the degree of involvement and the terminology used. Table 19.1 gives examples of typical questions that can be used when obtaining the child's health history.

HISTORY OF PRESENT ILLNESS

Elicit the history of the present illness, which addresses when the symptoms started and how they have progressed. Inquire about any treatments and medications used at home. Ask parents about history of orthopnea, dyspnea, easy fatigability, growth delays, squatting, edema, dizziness, and/or frequent occurrences of pneumonia, which can be significant signs of pediatric heart disease. The history of present illness may reveal a history of poor feeding, including fatigue, lethargy, and/or vomiting, or failure to thrive, even with adequate caloric intake. The parents may report diaphoresis, which is often seen in early heart failure. The parent or caregiver may also report delays in gross motor development, cyanosis (possibly reported by the parents as more of a gray color than blue), and tachypnea (indicative of heart failure).

PAST MEDICAL HISTORY

The past medical history includes information about the child and the birthing parent's pregnancy history. Assess the child's past medical history for:

- Problems occurring after birth (history of the child's condition after birth may reveal evidence of an associated congenital malformation or other disorder.)
- Frequent infections
- Chromosomal abnormalities
- Prematurity
- Autoimmune disorders
- Use of medications, such as corticosteroids

Assess the birthing parent's pregnancy, labor, and delivery history. Be sure to include information about the status of the neonate at birth. Also inquire about the birthing parent's use of medications, including illicit

TABLE 19.1 • Examples of Questions for Obtaining a Child's Health History

Questions	Provides Information About
• What types and amounts (dosages) of medications has the child received? What were they used for?	• Possible underlying conditions that may be related to the child's current status
• Who prescribed them?	• Other healthcare personnel involved in the child's care as well as the parents' health care beliefs and patterns
• Were they effective? Did the child experience any adverse effects?	• How the medications may be affecting the child's health
• To whom does the child go for medical evaluation? How often? Were the visits for regular health check-ups or for situational problems? Were there previous hospitalizations? What for?	• The child's health status and the parents' healthcare knowledge, practices, and beliefs
• Has the child experienced any growth delay? Does the child have any problems with activity and coordination?	• Problems that may result from impaired cardiac output, adequacy of tissue oxygenation, and concomitant disorders associated with heart disease
• Does the child's skin color change when crying? If so, what color do you see?	• Effectiveness of tissue oxygenation. A blue or gray skin color may be due to cyanosis.
• Does the child stop frequently during play to sit or squat?	• The child's exercise tolerance and tissue oxygenation
• Does the child have feeding difficulty? Does the child tire easily or sleep excessively?	• The child's energy expenditure, ability to tolerate activity, and tissue oxygenation
• Does the child frequently develop strep throat?	• The child's risk for developing rheumatic fever and heart disease

Data from Hueckel, R. M. (2019). Pediatric patient with congenital heart disease. *Journal for Nurse Practitioners, 15*(1), 118–124. https://doi.org/10.1016/j.nurpra.2018.10.017

or over-the-counter drugs and alcohol; exposure to radiation; presence of hypertension; and viral illnesses such as coxsackievirus, cytomegalovirus, influenza, mumps, or rubella. A history of significant problems related to labor and delivery is also important: stress or asphyxia at birth may be related to cardiac dysfunction and pulmonary hypertension in the newborn.

Assess for additional risk factors such as:

- Family history of heart disease or CHD (investigate the history further if heart disease occurred in a first-degree relative)
- Hyperlipidemia
- Diabetes mellitus
- Obesity
- Inactivity
- Stress
- High-cholesterol diet

PHYSICAL EXAMINATION

Physical examination of the child with a cardiovascular condition consists of inspection, palpation, and auscultation. In addition, obtain the child's vital signs and measure the child's height and weight. Plot this information on a standard growth chart to evaluate nutritional status and growth. If the child is younger than 3 years, measure and plot the head circumference also.

INSPECTION

Assess the child's overall appearance. Inspect the color of the skin, noting cyanosis. Inspect the skin for edema. In infants, peripheral edema occurs first in the face, then the presacral region, and then the extremities. Edema of the lower extremities is characteristic of right ventricular heart failure in older children.

CLINICAL REASONING ALERT!

Suspect CHD in the cyanotic newborn who does not improve with oxygen administration (Weiner et al., 2021).

Inspect the fingers and toes for clubbing. Clubbing (which usually does not appear until after 1 year of age) implies chronic hypoxia due to severe CHD. The first sign of **clubbing** is softening of the nail beds, followed by rounding of the fingernails, followed by shininess and thickening of the nail ends (see Fig. 18.5 in Chapter 18). Obtain the child's temperature; fever would suggest infection. Assess respirations, including rate, rhythm, and effort. Note location and severity of retractions if present. Inspect the chest configuration, noting any prominence of the precordial chest wall, which is often seen in infants and children with **cardiomegaly** (abnormal heart enlargement). Note visible pulsations, which may indicate increased heart activity. Also inspect the neck veins for engorgement or abnormal pulsations. Note abdominal distention.

CLINICAL REASONING ALERT!

Children with cardiac conditions resulting in cyanosis will often have baseline oxygen saturations that are relatively low because of the mixing of oxygenated with deoxygenated blood.

PALPATION

Palpate the right and left radial or brachial pulse to assess cardiac rate and rhythm. Throughout infancy and childhood, the rate may vary. Palpate the femoral pulse; it should be readily palpable and equal in amplitude and strength to the brachial or radial pulse. A femoral pulse that is weak or absent in comparison to the brachial pulse is associated with coarctation of the aorta. Significant variations in pulse occur with activity, so the most accurate heart rate may be determined during sleep. In older children, exercise and emotional factors may influence the heart rate. A bounding pulse is characteristic of patent ductus arteriosus (PDA) or aortic regurgitation. Narrow or thready pulses may occur in children with heart failure or severe aortic stenosis (Driscoll, 2022). Note tachycardia, bradycardia, rhythm irregularities, diminished peripheral pulses, or thready pulse. Palpate the child's abdomen for hepatomegaly, a sign of right-sided heart failure in the infant and child.

AUSCULTATION

Auscultate the apical pulse for a full minute to determine heart rate and rhythm. Note irregularities in rhythm, tachycardia, or bradycardia. Auscultate the heart for murmurs. Many children have functional or innocent murmurs, but all murmurs must be evaluated on the basis of the following characteristics:

- Location
- Relation to the heart cycle and duration
- Intensity: grade I, soft and hard to hear; grade II, soft and easily heard; grade III, loud without thrill; grade IV, loud with a precordial thrill; grade V, loud with a precordial thrill, audible with a stethoscope partially off chest; grade VI, very loud, audible with a stethoscope or with the naked ear
- Quality: harsh, musical, or rough; high, medium, or low pitch
- Variation with position (sitting, lying, standing) (Driscoll, 2022)

Auscultate for the character of heart sounds. Note distinct, muffled, or distant heart sounds. Abnormal splitting or intensifying of S_2 sounds occurs in children with major heart problems. Ejection clicks, which are high pitched, are related to problems with dilated vessels and/or valve abnormalities. Heard throughout systole, they can be early, moderate, or late. Clicks on the upper left sternal border are related to the pulmonary area. Aortic clicks are best heard at the apex and can be mitral or aortic in origin. A mild to late ejection click at the apex is typical of a mitral valve prolapse. The S_3 heart sound may be heard in children, diminishing when moving from supine to upright, and a pathologic S_3 may occur with poor cardiac function. The S_4 heart sound is not normally audible and is associated with cardiomyopathy or diastolic dysfunction (Jone et al., 2022).

Auscultate the BP in the upper extremities and lower extremities, and compare the findings; there should be no major differences between the upper and lower extremities. Determine the pulse pressure by subtracting the diastolic pressure from the systolic pressure. The pulse pressure is less than 50 mm Hg, or less than half the systolic pressure. A widened pulse pressure, which is usually accompanied by a bounding pulse, is associated with PDA, aortic insufficiency, fever, anemia, or complete heart block. A narrowed pulse pressure is associated with aortic stenosis. Note hypotension or hypertension.

TAKE NOTE!

Alert children and parents if a heart murmur is detected, even if it is benign.

Laboratory and Diagnostic Testing

Common Laboratory and Diagnostic Tests 19.1 explains the laboratory and diagnostic tests most commonly used when considering cardiovascular disorders in children. The tests can assist the health care provider in diagnosing the disorder or can be used as guidelines in determining ongoing treatment. Laboratory or nonnursing personnel obtain some of the tests, while the nurse might obtain others. In either instance, the nurse should be familiar with how the tests are obtained, what they are used for, and normal versus abnormal results. This knowledge will also be necessary when providing child and family education related to the testing.

Remember Logan, the 6-week-old with poor feeding? What additional health history and physical examination assessment information should the nurse obtain?

Nursing Analysis

After recognizing and analyzing cues from a thorough assessment, the nurse might identify several patient problems, including:

- Decreased cardiac output
- Excess fluid volume
- Activity intolerance
- Imbalanced nutrition, less than body requirements
- Risk of delayed development
- Pain
- Interrupted family processes
- Deficient knowledge

After completing Logan's assessment, the nurse noted the following: poor weight gain, tachypnea with occasional nasal flaring, crackles heard on auscultation, and edema noted in the face, presacral area, and extremities. Based on these assessment findings, what would your top three concerns be for Logan?

The foregoing patient issues provide suggestions for nursing care planning or concept mapping. Suggested interventions with rationales are provided later. Care planning should be individualized, based on the child's and family's needs. Refer to Chapter 14 for the nursing process for pain management and to Chapter 11 for nursing interventions related to interrupted family processes. Additional information will be included later in the chapter as it relates to nursing management of children with specific disorders, as well as particular nursing interventions for deficient knowledge.

ATRAUMATIC CARE

When a child is diagnosed with congenital heart disease, involve the child life specialist early in the course of treatment. The child will likely have been undergoing diagnostic procedures such as electrocardiograms and echocardiograms, as well as open heart surgery. The child life specialist can be very helpful with providing atraumatic care.

Nursing Analysis

Decreased cardiac output related to structural defect, congenital anomaly, or ineffective heart pumping as evidenced by arrhythmias, edema, murmur, abnormal heart rate, or abnormal heart sounds

Goal/Outcome

Child or infant will demonstrate adequate cardiac output as evidenced by elastic skin turgor, brisk capillary refill, demonstrate pink color, pulse, and BP within normal limits for age, regular heart rhythm, adequate urinary output.

Increasing Cardiac Output (interventions with *rationale*)

- Monitor vital signs closely, especially BP and heart rate, *to detect increases or decreases.*
- Monitor cardiac rhythm via cardiac monitor *to detect arrhythmias quickly.*
- Observe for signs of hypoxia such as tachypnea, cyanosis, tachycardia, bradycardia, dizziness, and/or restlessness *to identify this change early.*
- Administer oxygen as needed *to correct hypoxia.*
- Place child in knee-to-chest or squatting position as needed *to increase systemic vascular resistance.*
- Administer antiarrhythmics, vasopressors, angiotensin-converting enzyme (ACE) inhibitors, beta-blockers, corticosteroids, or diuretics as prescribed *to improve cardiac output.*
- Monitor for signs of thrombosis such as restlessness, seizure, coma, oliguria, anuria, edema, hematuria, or paralysis *to identify this condition early.*
- Administer adequate hydration *to decrease possibility of thrombosis formation.*
- Cluster nursing care and other activities *to allow adequate periods of rest.*
- Anticipate child's needs *to decrease the child's stress, thereby decreasing oxygen consumption requirement.*

Nursing Analysis

Excess fluid volume related to compromised regulatory mechanism (ineffective cardiac muscle function) as evidenced by weight gain, edema, jugular vein distention, dyspnea, or adventitious breath sounds

Goal/Outcome

Child will attain appropriate fluid balance, will lose weight (fluid), edema or bloating will decrease, lung sounds will be clear, and heart sounds will be normal.

Encouraging Fluid Loss (interventions with *rationale*)

- Weigh daily on the same scale in a similar amount of clothing; *in children, weight is the best indicator of changes in fluid status.*
- Monitor location and extent of edema (measure abdominal girth daily if ascites is present); *a decrease in edema indicates positive increase in oncotic pressure.*
- Protect edematous areas from skin breakdown; *edema leads to increased risk for alterations in skin integrity.*
- Auscultate lungs carefully *to identify crackles, indicating pulmonary edema.*
- Assess work of breathing and respiratory rate; increased *work of breathing is associated with pulmonary edema.*
- Assess heart sounds for gallop; *the presence of* S_3 *may indicate fluid overload.*
- Maintain fluid restriction as ordered *to decrease intravascular volume and workload on the heart.*
- Strictly monitor intake and output *to quickly note discrepancies and provide intervention.*
- Provide sodium-restricted diet as ordered; *restricting sodium intake allows better kidney excretion of extra fluid.*
- Administer diuretics as ordered, and monitor for adverse effects *to encourage excretion of fluid and elimination of edema, reduce cardiac filling pressures, and increase kidney blood flow. Adverse effects include electrolyte imbalance as well as orthostatic hypotension.*

Nursing Analysis

Activity intolerance related to imbalanced oxygen supply and demand (ineffective cardiac muscle function, increased energy expenditure) as evidenced by exertional discomfort (squatting position), exertional dyspnea, weakness, or fatigue

Goal/Outcome

Child will increase activity level as tolerated: Child participates in play and activities (specify particular activities and level as individualized for each child).

Promoting Activity (interventions with *rationale*)

- Assess level of fatigue and activity tolerance *to determine baseline for comparison.*

- Note extent of dyspnea, oxygen requirement, or color change with exertion *to provide baseline for comparison.*
- Cluster care activities, allowing rest periods in between, *to conserve child's energy.*
- Work with the parent and child to determine a mutually satisfactory daily schedule *to allow adequate rest and energy conservation.*
- Instruct family and child in prescribed activity restrictions *to prevent fatigue while allowing some activity.*
- In the infant, avoid long periods of crying or prolonged nipple feeding; *these expend excessive calories.*
- Provide neutral thermal environment *to avoid increased oxygen and energy needs associated with excessive heat or cold.*

Nursing Analysis

Imbalanced nutrition (less than body requirements) related to the inability to increase adequate calories (due to increased energy expenditure and fatigue) as evidenced by food intake less than recommended daily allowance, weight loss or length/height and weight below accepted standards

Goal/Outcome

Child will improve nutritional intake, resulting in steady increase in weight and length/height and will feed without tiring easily.

Promoting Adequate Nutrition (interventions with *rationale*)

- Determine body weight and length/height norm for age *to determine a goal to work toward.*
- Assess child for food preferences that fall within dietary restrictions; *the child will be more likely to consume adequate amounts of foods that they like.*
- Weigh the child daily or weekly (according to health care provider order or institutional standard), and measure length/height weekly *to monitor for increased growth.*
- Offer highest-calorie meals at the time of day when the child's appetite is the greatest *to increase likelihood of increased caloric intake.*
- Provide increased-calorie shakes or puddings within diet restriction; *high-calorie foods increase weight gain.*
- Consult with the pediatric dietician *to provide optimal caloric intake within dietary restrictions.*
- Provide small, frequent feedings *to discourage tiring with feeding.*
- Feed infants with special nipple as needed *to decrease amount of energy expended for sucking.*
- Administer vitamin and mineral supplements as prescribed *to attain/maintain vitamin and mineral balance in the body.*

Nursing Analysis

Delayed development risk related to congenital disorder or chronic illness (effects of cardiac disease and necessary treatments, inadequate nutrition, or frequent separation from caregivers secondary to illness)

Goal/Outcome

Child will display development appropriate for age with evidence of cognitive and motor function within normal limits (individualized for each child)

Promoting Appropriate Development (interventions with *rationale*)

- Promote adequate caloric intake *to stimulate growth and provide adequate energy.*
- Provide age-appropriate developmental activities *to stimulate development.*
- Consult with the physical or occupational therapist or child life specialist *to determine activities most appropriate for the child within the constraints of the child's illness.*
- Schedule daily activities to allow for essential rest periods *for energy conservation.*
- Encourage parents, teachers, and playmates to be sensitive to child's self-image, using positive comments *to improve the child's self-concept.*
- As energy allows, encourage participation in all activities as feasible *to allow the child to feel normal.*

Based on your top three issues for Logan, describe appropriate nursing interventions.

Cardiac Catheterization

Nursing management of the child undergoing cardiac catheterization includes preprocedure nursing assessment and preparation of the child and family, postprocedural nursing care, and discharge teaching.

Assessment Before the Procedure

Obtain a thorough history and physical examination to establish a baseline. Measure vital signs. Note fever or other signs and symptoms of infection, which may necessitate rescheduling the procedure. Obtain the child's height and weight to aid in determining medication dosages. Assess the child for any allergies, especially to iodine and shellfish, because some contrast materials contain iodine as a base. Review the child's medications; medications such as anticoagulants are typically withheld for several days or longer prior to the procedure to reduce the child's risk for bleeding. Check the results of any laboratory tests, such as hemoglobin and hematocrit levels.

Perform a complete physical examination. Pay particular attention to assessing the child's peripheral pulses, including pedal pulses. Use an indelible pen to mark the location of the child's pedal pulses so they can be easily assessed after the procedure. Document the location and quality in the child's medical record.

Educating the Child and Family Before the Procedure

Teach the parents and, if age-appropriate, the child, about all aspects of the procedure in order to decrease their anxiety. Let them know the procedure is commonly performed on an outpatient basis but that some health care providers or nurse practitioners require the child to be admitted for an overnight stay for observation. Include information about what the procedure involves, how long it will take, and any special instructions from the health care provider or nurse practitioner. Use a variety of teaching methods as appropriate, such as videos, books, and pamphlets.

Adapt these teaching methods to the child's developmental stage. For example, introduce the younger child to equipment through play therapy. For school-age and older children and their parents, offer a tour of the cardiac catheterization laboratory. Mention sounds and sights they may experience during the procedure. Explain the use of intravenous (IV) fluid therapy, sedation, and, if ordered, anesthesia to the child and parents. Tell the child that they may feel a sensation of the heart racing when the catheter is inserted. Also warn the older child that they may experience a feeling of warmth or stinging when the contrast material is injected. Encourage the child to use familiar ways to relax. If necessary, teach the child simple relaxation measures.

Tell families to withhold food and fluid for 4 to 6 hours before the procedure (as ordered). The parent should administer prescribed medications with a sip of water. On the day of the procedure, check to ensure that a signed informed consent form is on the child's medical record and that all necessary assessment data have been included. Just before the procedure, ask the child to void, and administer a sedative, as ordered. If appropriate and permitted, allow the parents to accompany the child to the catheterization area.

Teach the child and family what to expect after the procedure is completed. Inform the parents of the possible complications that might occur, such as bleeding, low-grade fever, loss of pulse in the extremity used for the catheterization, and development of **arrhythmia** (abnormal heart rhythm). Explain to the child that they will have a dressing over the catheter site and that they will need to keep the leg straight for several hours after the procedure. Teach the child and parent that frequent monitoring will be required after the procedure.

Assessment After the Procedure

Throughout the postprocedure period, closely monitor the child for complications of bleeding, arrhythmia, hematoma, and thrombus formation and infection. Evaluate the child's vital signs, the neurovascular status of the lower extremities, and the pressure dressing over the catheterization site every 15 minutes for the first hour and then every 30 minutes for 1 hour. Vital signs should remain within acceptable parameters. Hypotension may signify hemorrhage due to perforation of the heart muscle or bleeding from the insertion site. Expect to monitor cardiac rhythm and oxygen saturation levels via pulse oximetry for the first few hours after the procedure to help identify possible complications.

Assess the child's distal pulses bilaterally for presence and quality. The pulse of the affected extremity may be slightly less than that of the other extremity in the initial postprocedure period, but it should gradually return to baseline. Also assess the color and temperature of the extremity; pallor or blanching would indicate an obstruction in blood flow. Check capillary refill and sensation to evaluate blood flow to the area.

Nursing Interventions Following Cardiac Catheterization

Maintain bed rest in the immediate postprocedure period. Ensure that the child maintains the extremity in a straight position for approximately 4 to 8 hours, depending on the approach used and the facility's policy. Inspect the pressure dressing frequently. Check to make sure that it is dry and intact, without evidence of bleeding. Reinforce the dressing as necessary and report any evidence of drainage on the dressing. If there is a risk of the dressing becoming soiled or wet, cover it with plastic.

> ***TAKE NOTE!***
>
> If bleeding occurs after a cardiac catheterization, apply pressure 1 in above the site to create pressure over the vessel, thereby reducing the blood flow to the area.

Monitor the child's intake and output closely to ensure adequate hydration. The contrast material has a diuretic effect, so assess the child for signs and symptoms of dehydration and hypovolemia. Typically, the child resumes oral intake as tolerated, beginning with sips of clear liquids and progressing to their preprocedure diet. Continue IV fluids as ordered, and encourage oral fluid intake as allowed and ordered to promote elimination of the contrast material. Allow the child to talk about the experience and how and what they felt. Provide positive reinforcement for the child's actions.

Educating About Home Care Following Cardiac Catheterization

Provide child and family education before the child is discharged home (see Teaching Guidelines 19.1). Areas

TEACHING GUIDELINES 19.1 Providing Care After a Cardiac Catheterization

- Change the pressure dressing on the day after the procedure. Apply a dry sterile dressing or adhesive bandage for the next several days. Keep the dressing dry; cover it with plastic if there is a chance that the dressing could become wet or soiled.
- When changing the dressing, inspect the insertion site for redness, irritation, swelling, drainage, and bleeding. Report any of these to the health care provider or nurse practitioner.
- Check the temperature, color, sensation, and pulses on the child's extremities and compare. Report any changes to the health care provider or nurse practitioner.
- Resume the child's usual diet after the procedure; report any nausea or vomiting.
- Check the child's temperature at least once a day for approximately 3 days after the procedure. Report any temperature elevation of 100.4°F or greater.
- Avoid giving the child a tub bath for approximately 3 days after the procedure; use sponge baths or showers instead.
- Discourage strenuous exercise or activity for approximately 3 days after the procedure.
- Watch for changes in the child's appearance, such as changes in skin color, reports of the heart "fluttering" or "skipping a beat," fever, or difficulty breathing.
- Give acetaminophen (Tylenol) or ibuprofen (Motrin) for complaints of pain.
- Schedule a follow-up appointment with the health care provider or nurse practitioner in the time specified.

Based on KidsHealth Medical Experts. (2023). *Cardiac catheterization*. https://kidshealth.org/en/parents/cardiac-catheter.html; UCSF Benioff Children's Hospital. (2024). *Cardiac catheterization*. https://www.ucsfbenioff-childrens.org/education/cardiac_catheterization/

to address include site care, signs and symptoms of complications (especially within 24 hours after the catheterization, such as fever; bleeding or bruising at the catheterization site; or changes in color, temperature, or sensation in the extremity used), diet, and activity level.

THINKING ABOUT **DEVELOPMENT**

Jeremy Titus is a 2-year-old with congenital heart disease. He is having a cardiac catheterization today. How will the nurse encourage Jeremy to stay in bed and keep his leg straight for several hours following the catheterization? What types of activities would be appropriate for occupying Jeremy while he is confined to bed? How would the nurse's approach differ if Jeremy were an older child?

CONGENITAL HEART DEFECTS

In North America, more than 1% of newborn infants have CHD resulting from numerous causes. The prevalence of CHD ranges from six to 13 per 1,000 live births; premature infants have a higher rate (Altman, 2022). About one third of infants with CHD will have disease serious enough to result in death or will require cardiac catheterization or cardiac surgery within the first year of life. Complications of CHD include heart failure, hypoxemia, growth delay, developmental delay, and pulmonary vascular disease. Children with severe anomalies frequently experience failure to thrive.

With advances in palliative and corrective surgery over the past 60 years, many more children are now able to survive into adulthood. About 90% of children with CHD grow to be adults (Jone et al., 2022). As compared to healthy children, children with CHD tend to have poorer health overall and more frequently have additional morbidities either physical or neurodevelopmental in nature (Centers for Disease Control and Prevention [CDC], 2022). Due to the potential long-term effects that CHD may have on these children, nurses must be expertly equipped to care for them.

Pathophysiology

The exact cause of CHD is unknown. However, the belief is that it results from the interplay of several factors, including genetics (e.g., chromosomal alterations) and exposure during pregnancy to environmental factors (e.g., toxins, infections, chronic illnesses, and alcohol).

CHDs result from some interference in the development of the heart structure during fetal life. Subsequently, the septal walls or valves may fail to develop completely, or vessels or valves may be stenotic, narrowed, or transposed. Structures that formed to allow fetal circulation may fail to close after birth, altering the pressures necessary to maintain adequate blood flow.

After birth, with the change from fetal to newborn circulation, pressures within the chambers of the right side of the heart are less than those of the left side, and pulmonary vascular resistance is less than that for the systemic circulation. These normal pressure gradients are necessary for adequate circulation to the lungs and the rest of the body. However, these pressure gradients become disrupted if a structure has failed to develop, a fetal structure has failed to close, or a narrowing, stenosis, or transposition of a vessel has occurred. For example, blood typically flows from an area of higher pressure to one of lower pressure. If the ductus arteriosus fails to close, blood will move from the aorta to the pulmonary artery, ultimately increasing right atrial pressure. With this shunting of blood, highly oxygenated blood can mix with less oxygenated blood, interfering with the amount available to the tissues via the systemic circulation. Some of the defects may result in significant hypoxemia, the sequelae of which include clubbing, **polycythemia** (excess amount of red blood cells [RBCs]), exercise intolerance, hypercyanotic spells, brain abscess, and cerebrovascular accident (CVA) (Jone et al., 2022; Schneider, 2023).

CHDs are categorized based on hemodynamic characteristics (blood flow patterns in the heart):

- Disorders with decreased pulmonary blood flow: tetralogy of Fallot and tricuspid atresia
- Disorders with increased pulmonary blood flow: PDA, atrial septal defect (ASD), and ventricular septal defect (VSD)
- Obstructive disorders: coarctation of the aorta, aortic stenosis, and pulmonic stenosis
- Mixed disorders: transposition of the great arteries (TGA), total anomalous pulmonary venous return (TAPVR), truncus arteriosus, and hypoplastic left heart syndrome (HLHS)

Therapeutic Management

Prenatal education about avoiding certain substances or preventing infection is essential to promote optimal outcomes for the fetus. Encourage parents of children with CHD to receive genetic counseling because of the probability of having subsequent children with a CHD. Children with small septal defects are urged to lead normal lives and often require no medical intervention. Therapeutic management of other forms of CHDs focuses on palliative care or a surgical corrective approach necessary for most of the defects. In newborns and very young infants with severe cyanosis (tricuspid atresia, TGA), a prostaglandin infusion will maintain patency of the ductus arteriosus, improving pulmonary blood flow. Definitive correction of structural disorders requires surgical intervention. Table 19.2 describes the surgical procedures used for the various CHDs and the relevant nursing measures. Nursing management for the child with CHD will be provided following the disorders section.

Disorders With Decreased Pulmonary Blood Flow

Defects involving decreased pulmonary blood flow occur when there is some obstruction of blood flow to the lungs. As a result of the obstruction, pressure in the right side of the heart increases and becomes greater than that in the left side of the heart. Blood from the higher-pressure right side of the heart then shunts to the lower-pressure left side through a structural defect. Subsequently, deoxygenated blood mixes with oxygenated blood on the left side of the heart. This mixed blood, which is low in oxygen, is pumped via the systemic circulation to the body tissues.

Defects with decreased pulmonary blood flow are characterized by mild to severe oxygen desaturation. Typically, the child exhibits oxygen saturation levels ranging from 50% to 90%, which can produce severe cyanosis. To compensate for low blood oxygen levels, the kidneys produce the hormone erythropoietin to stimulate the bone marrow to produce more RBCs. This increase in RBCs is called polycythemia. Polycythemia can lead to an increase

TABLE 19.2 • Common Surgical Procedures and Nursing Measures for Congenital Heart Defects

Disorder	Surgical Procedure	Nursing Measures
Tetralogy of Fallot	Palliation with systemic-to-pulmonary anastomoses: • Blalock–Taussig shunt: an end-to-side anastomosis (or connection with a small Gore-Tex tube) of the subclavian artery and the pulmonary artery • Waterston shunt: anastomosis of the ascending aorta and the pulmonary artery • Definitive correction involves patch closure of the VSD and repair of the pulmonary valve and right ventricular outflow tract	• Avoid BP measurements and venipunctures in the affected arm after a Blalock–Taussig shunt. Pulse will not be palpable in that arm because of use of the subclavian artery for the shunt. • Monitor for ventricular arrhythmias after corrective repair.
Tricuspid atresia	• Palliation with Blalock–Taussig shunt or pulmonary artery banding may be performed. • At 3–6 months of age, the superior vena cava is detached from the heart and connected to the pulmonary artery (Glenn procedure). • By age 2–5 years, a modified Fontan procedure may be performed. Systemic venous return is redirected to the pulmonary artery directly.	• Monitor for atrial arrhythmias, left ventricular dysfunction, and protein-losing enteropathy. • Some children may eventually require a pacemaker.
Atrial septal defect (ASD)	• If small, the defect may be sutured closed. Larger defects may require a patch of pericardium or synthetic material. • Ostium secundum ASD may be repaired percutaneously via cardiac catheterization with a septal occluder.	• Monitor for atrial arrhythmias (lifelong) after surgical closure. • With the septal occluders, strenuous activity should be avoided for 2 weeks after the procedure.[a]

(continued)

TABLE 19.2 • Common Surgical Procedures and Nursing Measures for Congenital Heart Defects (*continued*)

Disorder	Surgical Procedure	Nursing Measures
Ventricular septal defect (VSD)	• If surgical closure is required, it should be performed before permanent pulmonary vascular changes develop. • Surgical closure may be in the form of suture closure of the VSD, transcatheter placement of a device in the defect, or Dacron patch closure.	• Monitor for ventricular dysrhythmias or atrioventricular block. • With the clamshell occluding or Amplatzer device, strenuous activity should be avoided for 1 month after the procedure.[b]
Atrioventricular canal defect	• Pulmonary artery banding as palliation in very young infants • Surgical correction by 3–18 months of age • Patch closure of the septal defects and suturing of the valve leaflets or valve reconstruction are performed.	• Monitor for complete heart block postoperatively. • Teach parents that mitral regurgitation is a long-term complication and may require valve replacement.
Patent ductus arteriosus (PDA)	• PDA is closed by coil embolization or device via cardiac catheterization. • May also be surgically ligated	• Monitor for bleeding and laryngeal nerve damage.
Coarctation of the aorta	• Balloon angioplasty via cardiac catheterization is possible in some children. • Most common surgical repair is resection of the narrowed portion of the aorta, followed by end-to-end reanastomosis.	• Preoperatively, administer prostaglandin medications as ordered to relax the ductal tissue. • Postoperatively, measure and compare BP in all four extremities and quality of upper vs. lower pulses.
Aortic stenosis	• Balloon dilation is accomplished via the umbilical artery in the newborn or the femoral artery via cardiac catheterization in the older child.	• Provide routine postcatheterization care. • Teach parents that long-term aortic regurgitation requiring valve replacement may occur.
Pulmonic stenosis	• Balloon dilation valvuloplasty is performed via cardiac catheterization to dilate the valve. This is effective in all but the most severe of cases, which will require surgical valvotomy.	• Provide routine postcatheterization care for balloon dilation. • Explain to parents that prognosis is excellent.
Transposition of the great vessels (arteries)	• Balloon atrial septotomy is usually done as soon as the diagnosis is made. A balloon-tipped catheter is passed through the atrial septum to enlarge the atrial septum. • Surgical correction involves switching the arteries into their normal anatomic positions.	• Administer prostaglandin to maintain the open state of the ductus arteriosus, which will allow the mixing of poorly oxygenated blood with well-oxygenated blood. • Monitor for rapid respirations and cyanosis. • Administer oxygen as needed preoperatively.
Total anomalous pulmonary venous return	• The pulmonary vein is repositioned to the back of the left atrium, and the ASD is closed.	• Monitor for dysrhythmias, heart block, and persistent heart failure.
Truncus arteriosus	• VSD repair, separation of the pulmonary arteries from the aorta, with subsequent connection to the right ventricle with a valve conduit	• Preoperatively, administer prostaglandin infusion to prevent closing of the ductus arteriosus.
Hypoplastic left heart syndrome	• Heart transplantation is the treatment of choice. • Palliative staged treatment. First, Norwood procedure, reconstruction of the aorta and pulmonary arteries, includes a cardiac transplant. Second, bidirectional Glenn procedure, connection of the superior vena cava to the right pulmonary artery to increase the blood flow to the lungs. Third, modified Fontan procedure	• Preoperatively, administer prostaglandin infusion to prevent closing of the ductus arteriosus. • After palliative repairs, monitor for dysrhythmias or worsening ventricular function.
Valve disorders	• The incompetent valve is replaced with valve prosthesis.	• Lifelong anticoagulation therapy is necessary with prosthetic valves. • Monitor prothrombin times. • Monitor heart sounds for alterations.

[a]Cleveland Clinic. (2023). *Cardiac closure devices.* https://my.clevelandclinic.org/health/treatments/16838-cardiac-implant-closure-devices-in-adults
[b]Abbott. (2023). *Amplatzer septal occluder.* https://www.myamplatzer.com/hcp/congenital-heart-defect-solutions/ventricular-septal-defects-vsd/
Based on Jone, P.-N., Kim, J. S., Burkett, D., Jacobsen, R., & VonAlvensleben, J., (2022). Cardiovascular disease. In M. Bunik, W. W. Hay, M. J. Levin, & M. J. Abzug (Eds.), *Current diagnosis and treatment: Pediatrics* (26th ed.). McGraw-Hill Education; Schneider, D. S. (2023). The cardiovascular system. In K. J. Marcdante & R. M. Kliegman (Eds.), *Nelson's essentials of pediatrics* (8th ed.). Elsevier.

in blood volume and possibly blood viscosity, further taxing the workload of the heart. Although the number of RBCs increases, there is no change in the amount of blood that reaches the lungs for oxygenation. Disorders within this classification include tetralogy of Fallot and tricuspid atresia.

Tetralogy of Fallot

Tetralogy of Fallot is a CHD composed of four heart defects: pulmonic stenosis (a narrowing of the pulmonary valve and outflow tract, creating an obstruction of blood flow from the right ventricle to the pulmonary artery); VSD; overriding aorta (enlargement of the aortic valve to the extent that it appears to arise from the right and left ventricles rather than the anatomically correct left ventricle); and right ventricular hypertrophy (the muscle walls of the right ventricle increase in size due to continued overuse as the right ventricle attempts to overcome a high-pressure gradient). Surgical intervention is usually required during the first year of life (Jone et al., 2022; Schneider, 2023).

Pathophysiology

With pulmonic stenosis, the blood flow from the right ventricle is obstructed and slowed, resulting in a decrease in blood flow to the lungs for oxygenation and a decrease in the amount of oxygenated blood returning to the left atrium from the lungs. The obstructed flow also increases the pressure in the right ventricle. This blood, which is poorly oxygenated, is then shunted across the VSD into the left atrium. Poorly oxygenated blood also travels through the overriding aorta (if it extends to both ventricles). In some cases when the VSD is large, the pressure in the right ventricle may be equal to that of the left ventricle. In this case, the path of blood shunting depends on which circulation is exerting the higher pressure, pulmonary or systemic.

Regardless of which way shunting occurs, a mixing of oxygenated and poorly oxygenated blood occurs, with this blood ultimately being pumped into the systemic circulation. The oxygen saturation of the blood in the systemic circulation is reduced, leading to cyanosis. The degree of cyanosis depends on the extent of the pulmonic stenosis, the size of the VSD, and the vascular resistance of the pulmonary and systemic circulations.

Tetralogy of Fallot is usually diagnosed during the first few weeks of life due to the presence of a murmur and/or cyanosis. Some newborns may be acutely cyanotic, while others may exhibit only mild cyanosis that gradually becomes more severe, particularly during times of stress as the child grows older. Most often, infants with tetralogy of Fallot have a PDA at birth, providing additional pulmonary blood flow and thereby decreasing the severity of the initial cyanosis. Later, as the ductus arteriosus closes, such as within the first few days of life, more severe cyanosis can occur (Fig. 19.2) (Jone et al., 2022; Schneider, 2023).

Nursing Assessment

Nursing assessment consists of the health history, physical examination, and laboratory and diagnostic tests.

HEALTH HISTORY AND PHYSICAL EXAMINATION

Obtain the health history, noting a history of color changes associated with feeding, activity, or crying. Determine if the infant or child is demonstrating hypercyanotic spells. Hypercyanosis develops suddenly and is manifested as increased cyanosis, hypoxemia, dyspnea, and agitation. If the infant's oxygen demand is greater than the supply, such as with crying or during feeding, then the spell progresses to anoxia. When the degree of cyanosis is severe and persistent, the infant may become unresponsive. As the infant gets older, they may use specific postures, such as bending at the knees or assuming the fetal position, to relieve a hypercyanotic spell. The walking infant or toddler may squat periodically. These positions improve pulmonary blood flow by increasing systemic vascular resistance. Ask the parents if they have noticed any of these unusual positions. Note history of irritability, sleepiness, or difficulty breathing.

During the physical examination, observe the skin color and note any evidence of cyanosis. Also observe for changes in skin color with positional changes, and inspect the fingers for clubbing. Note if the child has a hypercyanotic spell during the assessment. Count the child's respiratory rate and observe work of breathing, noting retractions, shortness of breath, or noisy breathing. Document oxygen saturation via pulse oximetry; it will likely be decreased. Auscultate the chest for adventitious breath sounds, which may suggest the development of heart failure. Auscultate the heart, noting a loud, harsh murmur characteristic of this disorder.

LABORATORY AND DIAGNOSTIC TESTS

Note increased hematocrit, hemoglobin, and RBC count associated with polycythemia. Additional testing may include:

- **Echocardiography** (ultrasound study of structure and motion of heart), possibly revealing right ventricular hypertrophy, decreased pulmonary blood flow, and reduced size of the pulmonary artery
- Electrocardiogram (ECG), indicating right ventricular hypertrophy
- Cardiac catheterization and angiography, which reveal the extent of the structural defects

Tricuspid Atresia

Tricuspid atresia is a CHD in which the valve between the right atrium and right ventricle fails to develop. As a result, there is no opening to allow blood to flow from the right atrium to the right ventricle and subsequently through the pulmonary artery into the lungs (Jone et al., 2022; Schneider, 2023).

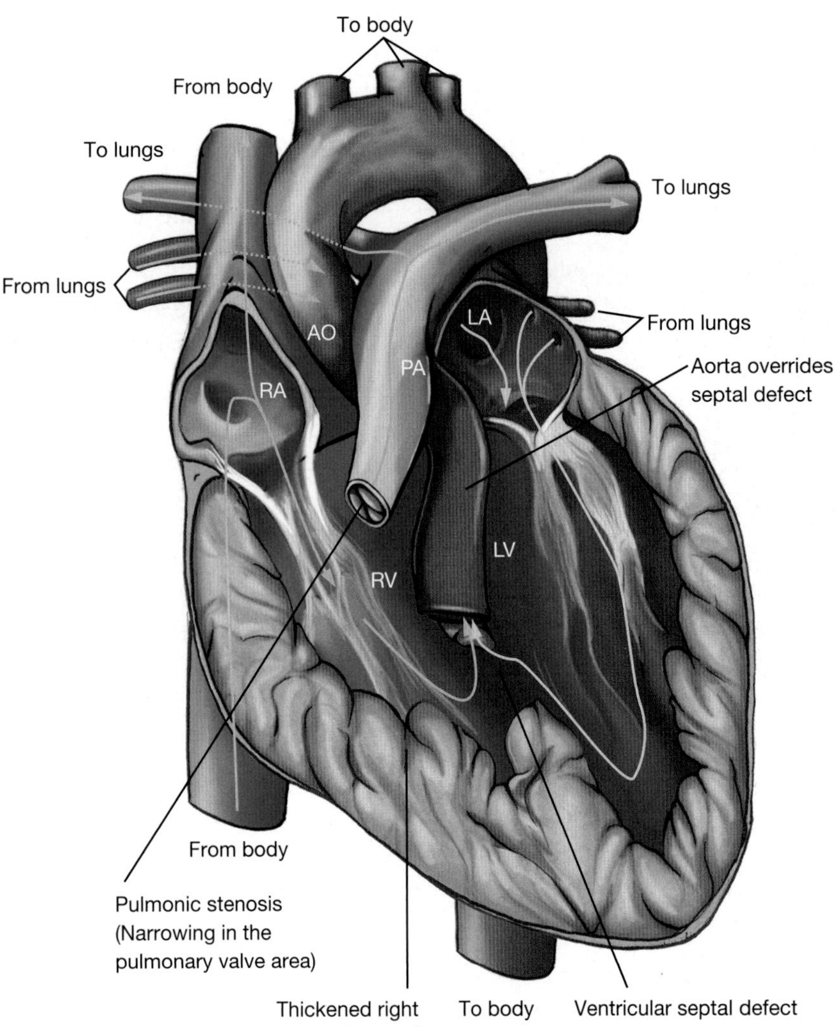

FIGURE 19.2 Tetralogy of Fallot.

> **CONSIDER THIS!**
>
> Ava Gardener, 2 weeks old, is brought to the clinic by her parent. She presents with trouble feeding. Her parent states, "When Ava eats, she seems to have trouble breathing, and a couple of times she has looked a little bluish." As the nurse takes Ava into her arms, Ava has a hypercyanotic spell.
>
> Ava is to be admitted to the hospital secondary to suspected tetralogy of Fallot. Ava's parent is very upset about the diagnosis. They say, "My poor baby, she'll never ever be able to run and play like a normal child."
>
> How should the nurse respond? How would you feel if your young baby was diagnosed with a serious disorder? What type of support can the nurse provide to Ava's parent?

Pathophysiology

In tricuspid atresia, blood returning from the systemic circulation to the right atrium cannot directly enter the right ventricle due to agenesis of the tricuspid valve. Subsequently, deoxygenated blood may pass through an opening in the atrial septum (patent foramen ovale) into the left atrium, never entering the pulmonary vasculature. Thus, deoxygenated blood mixes with oxygenated blood in the left atrium. The blood then travels to the lungs through a PDA. Most cases of tricuspid atresia are associated with a VSD, and the newborn receives inadequately oxygenated blood (Fig. 19.3) (Jone et al., 2022; Schneider, 2023).

Nursing Assessment

Nursing assessment consists of the health history, physical examination, and laboratory and diagnostic tests.

HEALTH HISTORY AND PHYSICAL EXAMINATION

Note the infant's history since birth. Document history of cyanosis either at birth or a few days later when the ductus arteriosus closed. Note history of rapid respirations and difficulty with feeding. Inspect the skin for cyanosis or a pale gray color. Observe the apical impulse, noting overactivity. Evaluate the baby's sucking strength (will usually have a weak or poor suck). Count the respiratory rate, noting tachypnea. Note increased work

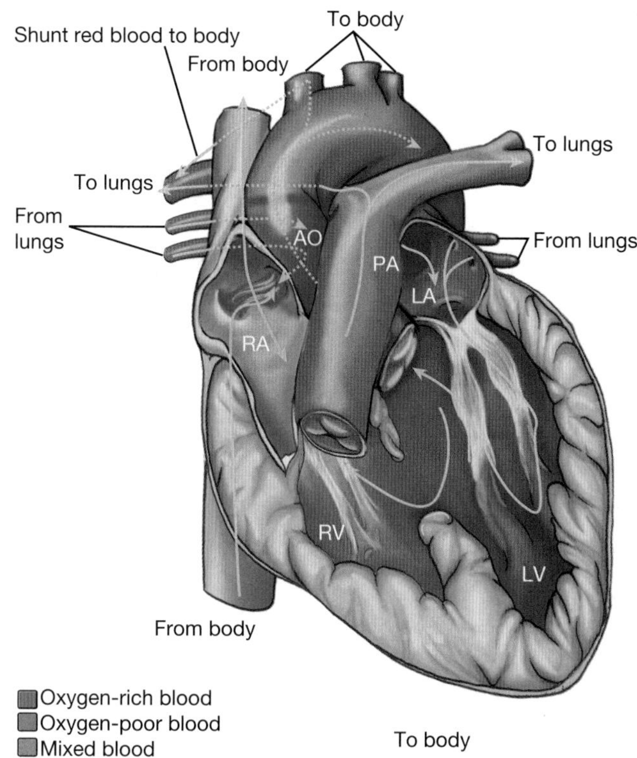

FIGURE 19.3 Tricuspid atresia.

of breathing. Auscultate the lungs, noting crackles or wheezes if heart failure is beginning to develop. Auscultate the heart, noting a murmur. Palpate the skin, noting coolness and clamminess of the extremities. Document the presence of clubbing in the older infant or child.

LABORATORY AND DIAGNOSTIC TESTING

Laboratory and diagnostic testing is similar to that for tetralogy of Fallot. A complete blood cell (CBC) count is needed to assess compensatory increases in hematocrit, hemoglobin, and erythrocyte (RBC) count, indicating the development of polycythemia. Pulse oximetry or arterial blood gas tests may be used to determine oxygen saturation levels (typically reduced). Additional testing may include:

- Echocardiography, revealing absence of tricuspid valve or underdeveloped right ventricle
- ECG, indicating possible heart failure
- Cardiac catheterization and angiography, which reveal the extent of the structural defects

Disorders With Increased Pulmonary Flow

Most CHDs involve increased pulmonary blood flow. Normally, the left side of the heart has a higher pressure than the right side. Defects with connections involving the left and right sides will shunt blood from the higher-pressure left side to the lower-pressure right side. Even a small pressure gradient such as a 1- to 3-mm difference between the left and the right sides will produce a movement of blood from the left to the right. In turn, the increase in blood on the right side of the heart will cause a greater amount of blood to move through the heart. If the amount of blood flowing to the lungs is large, the child may develop heart failure early in life. In addition, right ventricular hypertrophy may result. Sometimes, with ventricular hypertrophy, the right side of the heart pumps so forcefully that left-to-right shunting is reversed to right-to-left shunting. If this occurs, deoxygenated blood mixes with oxygenated blood, thereby lowering the overall blood oxygen saturation level.

Excessive blood flow to the lungs can produce a compensatory response such as tachypnea or tachycardia. Tachypnea increases caloric expenditure; poor cellular nutrition from decreased peripheral blood flow leads to feeding problems. Subsequently, the infant experiences poor weight gain, which delays overall growth and development. Increased pulmonary blood flow results in decreased systemic blood flow, so sodium and fluid retention may occur. Increased pulmonary blood flow also places the child at higher risk for pulmonary infections. As the child grows, the continuous increased pulmonary blood flow will cause vasoconstriction of the pulmonary vessels, actually decreasing the pulmonary blood flow. This may lead to pulmonary hypertension. For children with congenital defects with increased pulmonary blood flow, oxygen supplementation is not helpful. Oxygen acts as a pulmonary vasodilator. If pulmonary dilation occurs, pulmonary blood flow is even greater, causing tachypnea, increasing lung fluid retention, and eventually causing a much greater problem with oxygenation. Over time, continuous increased pulmonary blood flow may cause pulmonary vasoconstriction and pulmonary hypertension. Therefore, preventing the development of pulmonary disease via early surgical correction is essential.

Examples of defects with increased pulmonary blood flow are ASD, VSD, atrioventricular canal defect, and PDA.

Atrial Septal Defect

An ASD is a passageway or hole in the wall (septum) that divides the right atrium from the left atrium (Fig. 19.4). Three types of ASDs are identified based on the location of the opening:

- Ostium primum (ASD1): The opening is at the lower portion of the septum.
- Ostium secundum (ASD2): The opening is near the center of the septum.
- Sinus venosus defect: The opening is near the junction of the superior vena cava and the right atrium.

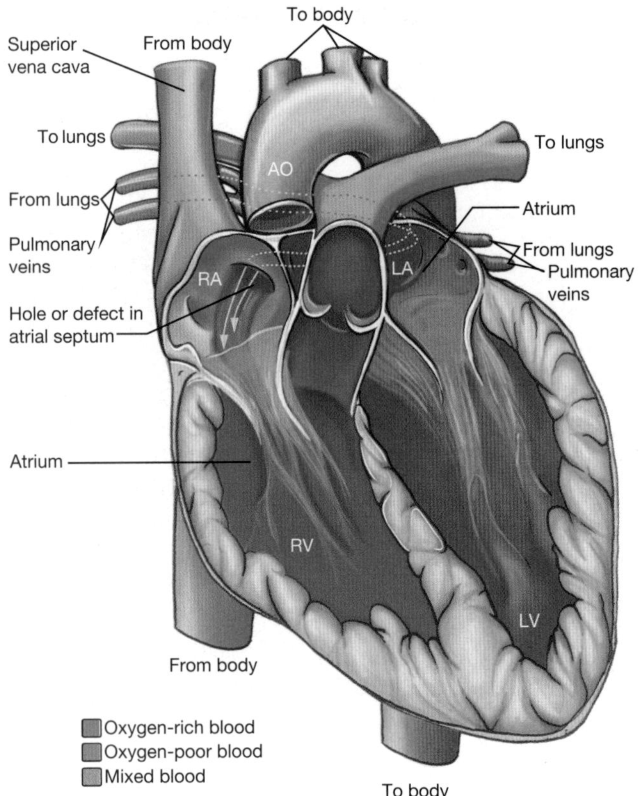

FIGURE 19.4 Atrial septal defect; note the opening between the two atria.

When the ASD is small, most infants may have a spontaneous closure within the first 18 months of life. If it does not spontaneously close by age 3, the child will most likely need corrective surgery (Jone et al., 2022; Schneider, 2023).

Pathophysiology

With ASD, blood flows through the opening from the left atrium to the right atrium due to pressure differences. The shunting increases the blood volume entering the right atrium. This, in turn, leads to increased blood flow into the lungs. If untreated, the defect can cause problems such as pulmonary hypertension, heart failure, atrial arrhythmias, or stroke (Jone et al., 2022; Schneider, 2023).

Nursing Assessment

Most children with ASDs are asymptomatic. However, a very large defect can cause increased blood flow, leading to heart failure, which results in shortness of breath, easy fatigability, or poor growth.

HEALTH HISTORY AND PHYSICAL EXAMINATION

Obtain the health history, noting poor feeding as an infant, decreased ability to keep up with peers, or history of difficulty growing. Observe the child's chest, noting a hyperdynamic precordium. Auscultate the heart, noting a fixed split-second heart sound and a systolic ejection murmur, best heard in the pulmonic valve area. Palpate along the left sternal border for a right ventricular heave.

LABORATORY AND DIAGNOSTIC TESTS

Echocardiography is done to confirm the diagnosis. An **electrocardiogram** (graphic recording of the heart's electrical activity) may show normal sinus rhythm or prolonged PR intervals. The chest radiograph may show enlargement of the heart and increased vascularity of the lungs.

Ventricular Septal Defect

A VSD is an opening between the right and left ventricular chambers of the heart (Fig. 19.5). It is one of the most common CHDs and accounts for about 30% of all CHDs. Spontaneous closure of small VSDs occurs in about half of children by age 2 years. Long-term outcomes for surgically repaired VSDs are good. Repair of larger defects by 2 years of age is recommended to prevent the development of pulmonary vascular disease (Jone et al., 2022; Schneider, 2023).

Pathophysiology

In VSD, there is an abnormal opening between the right and the left ventricles. The opening varies in size, from

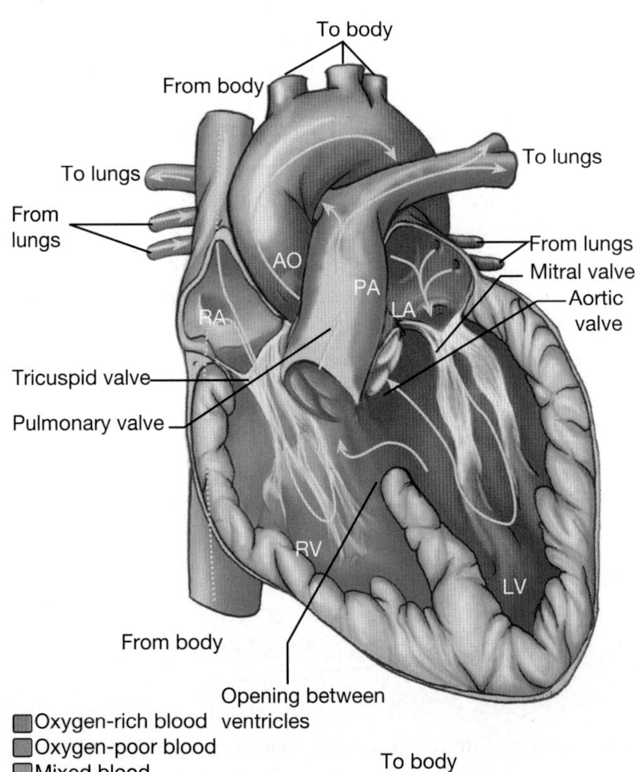

FIGURE 19.5 Ventricular septal defect; note the opening between the ventricles.

as small as a pinhole to a complete opening between the ventricles so that the right and the left sides are as one. Children with small VSDs may remain asymptomatic. In other children, blood shunts across the opening in the septum. Pulmonary vascular resistance and systemic vascular resistance determine the direction of blood flow. A left-to-right shunt results when pulmonary vascular resistance is low. Increased amounts of blood flowing into the right ventricle are then pumped to the pulmonary circulation, eventually causing an increase in pulmonary vascular resistance. Increased pulmonary vascular resistance leads to increased pulmonary artery pressure (pulmonary hypertension) and right ventricular hypertrophy. When the pulmonary vascular resistance exceeds the systemic vascular resistance, right-to-left shunting of blood across the VSD occurs, resulting in Eisenmenger syndrome (pulmonary hypertension and cyanosis). Heart failure commonly occurs in children with moderate to severe unrepaired VSDs. Children with VSDs are also at risk for the development of aortic valve regurgitation as well as infective endocarditis (Jone et al., 2022; Schneider, 2023).

Nursing Assessment

Initially, the newborn may not exhibit any signs and symptoms at birth because left-to-right shunting is most likely minimal due to the high pulmonary resistance common after birth.

HEALTH HISTORY AND PHYSICAL EXAMINATION

Determine the health history, which commonly reveals signs of heart failure around 4 to 8 weeks of age. Note history of tiring easily, particularly with exertion or feeding. Document the child's growth history, noting difficulty thriving. Ask the parent about color change or diaphoresis with nipple feeding in the infant. Note history of frequent pulmonary infections, shortness of breath, and possibly edema. Inspect the extremities for edema, noting whether pitting is present. Note mild tachypnea.

Auscultate the heart, noting a characteristic holosystolic harsh murmur along the left sternal border. In some instances, a murmur may be noted only with excessive blood flow across the opening. Adventitious lung sounds may be auscultated if the child is experiencing heart failure. Palpate the chest for a thrill.

LABORATORY AND DIAGNOSTIC TESTS

Magnetic resonance imaging (MRI) or echocardiogram with color flow Doppler may reveal the opening as well as the extent of left-to-right shunting. These studies may also identify right ventricular hypertrophy and dilation of the pulmonary artery resulting from the increased blood flow. Cardiac catheterization may be used to evaluate the extent of blood flow being pumped to the pulmonary circulation and to evaluate hemodynamic pressures.

Atrioventricular Septal Defect

Atrioventricular septal defect (AVSD) accounts for 4% of CHD. Thirty-five to forty percent of children with Down syndrome and CHD have this defect (Jone et al., 2022).

Pathophysiology

AVSD occurs because of failure of the endocardial cushions to fuse (Fig. 19.6). These cushions are needed to separate the central parts of the heart near the tricuspid and mitral (AV) valves. The complete AVSD involves ASDs and VSDs as well as a common AV orifice and a common AV valve. Partial and transitional forms of AVSD also occur, involving variations of the complete form.

The complete AVSD permits oxygenated blood from the lungs to enter the left atrium and ventricle, crossing over the atrial or ventricular septum and returning to the lungs via the pulmonary artery. This recirculation problem, which typically involves a left-to-right shunt, is inefficient because the left ventricle must pump blood back to the lungs and also meet the body's peripheral demand for oxygenated blood. Subsequently, the left ventricle must pump two to three times more blood than in a normal heart. Therefore, this specific type of cardiac defect causes a large left-to-right shunt; an increased workload of the left ventricle; and high pulmonary arterial pressure, resulting in an increased amount of blood in the lungs and causing pulmonary edema (Jone et al., 2022; Schneider, 2023).

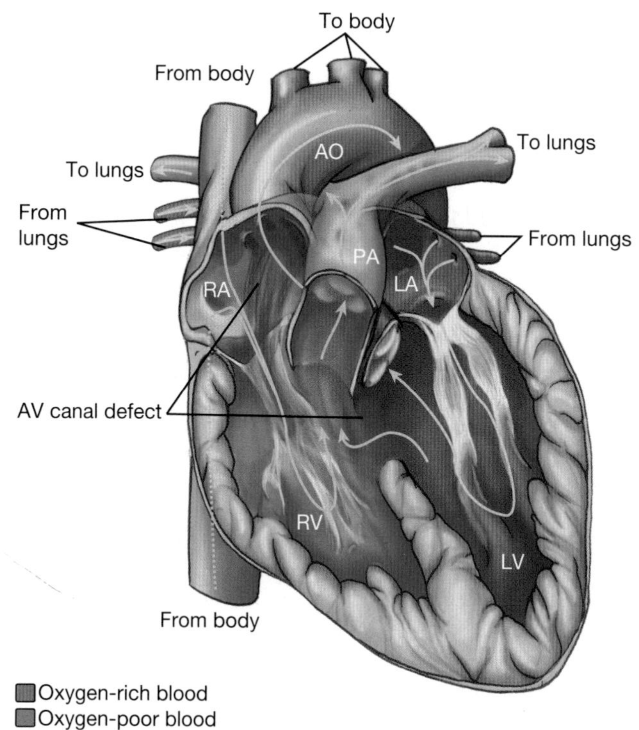

FIGURE 19.6 Atrioventricular canal defect.

Nursing Assessment

The infant with a complete AVSD commonly exhibits moderate to severe signs and symptoms of heart failure. However, for infants with a partial or transitional AVSD, the signs and symptoms will be subtler.

HEALTH HISTORY AND PHYSICAL EXAMINATION

Obtain the health history, noting frequent respiratory infections and difficulty gaining weight. Ask the parent if the infant has been experiencing difficulty feeding or increased work of breathing.

Inspect the skin, fingernails, and lips for cyanosis. Observe for retractions, tachypnea, and nasal flaring. Auscultate the lungs and heart, noting rales and a loud murmur. The murmur is commonly noted within the first 2 weeks of life. Infants with a partial or transitional AVSD defect may display more subtle signs.

LABORATORY AND DIAGNOSTIC TESTS

Echocardiography will reveal the extent of the defect and shunting as well as right ventricular hypertrophy. ECG may indicate right ventricular hypertrophy and possible first-degree heart block due to impulse blocking before reaching the AV node.

Patent Ductus Arteriosus

PDA is failure of the ductus arteriosus, a fetal circulatory structure, to close within the first few weeks of life (Fig. 19.7).

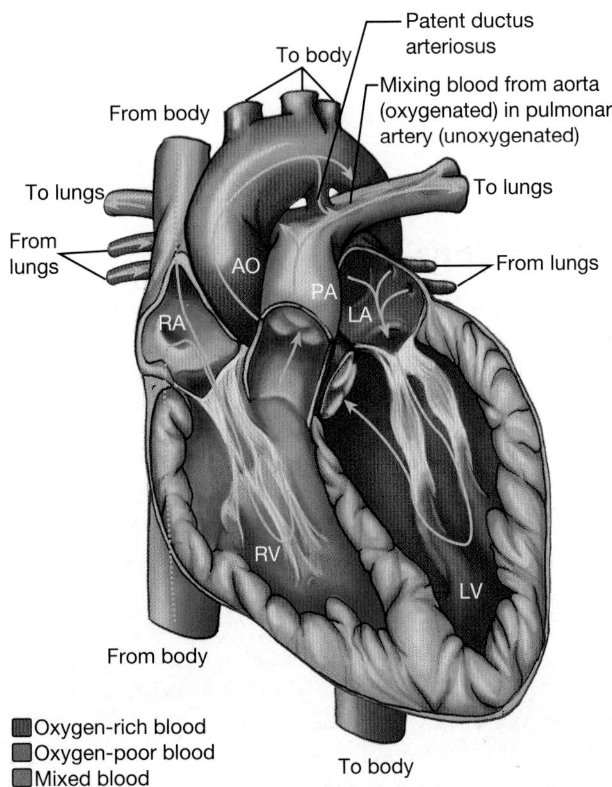

FIGURE 19.7 Patent ductus arteriosus.

As a result, there is a connection between the aorta and pulmonary artery. PDA is the second most common CHD and accounts for 10% of CHD cases (Jone et al., 2022). PDA occurs much more frequently in premature than in term infants and in infants born at high altitudes compared with those born at sea level. Infants with other CHDs that result in right-to-left shunting of blood and cyanosis may additionally display a PDA. In these infants, the PDA allows for some level of oxygenated blood to reach the systemic circulation (Jone et al., 2022; Schneider, 2023).

Pathophysiology

Failure of the ductus arteriosus to close leads to continued blood flow from the aorta to the pulmonary artery. Blood returning to the left atrium passes to the left ventricle, enters the aorta, and then travels to the pulmonary artery via the PDA instead of entering the systemic circulation. This altered blood flow pattern increases the workload of the left side of the heart. Pulmonary vascular congestion occurs, causing an increase in pressure. Right ventricular pressure increases in an attempt to overcome this increase in pulmonary pressure. Eventually, right ventricular hypertrophy occurs (Jone et al., 2022; Schneider, 2023).

Nursing Assessment

The symptoms of PDA depend on the size of the ductus arteriosus and the amount of blood flow it carries. If it is small, the infant may be asymptomatic. Some infants demonstrate signs and symptoms of heart failure.

HEALTH HISTORY AND PHYSICAL EXAMINATION

Determine the health history, which may reveal frequent respiratory infections, fatigue, and poor growth and development. On physical examination, note tachycardia, tachypnea, bounding peripheral pulses, and a widened pulse pressure. The diastolic BP typically is low due to the shunting. Auscultate the lungs and heart, noting rales if heart failure is present. Note a harsh, continuous, machine-like murmur, usually loudest under the left clavicle at the first and second intercostal spaces.

LABORATORY AND DIAGNOSTIC TESTS

Echocardiogram reveals the extent of the defective opening and confirms the diagnosis. ECG may be normal, or it may indicate ventricular hypertrophy, especially if the defect is large. Chest radiography demonstrates cardiomegaly.

Obstructive Disorders

Another group of CHDs is classified as obstructive disorders. These disorders involve some type of narrowing of a major vessel, interfering with the ability of the blood to flow freely through the vessel. As a result, peripheral circulation or blood flow to the lungs is affected. Increased pressure backing up toward the heart causes an increased workload on the heart. Examples of defects in this group include coarctation of the aorta, aortic stenosis, and pulmonic stenosis (PS).

Coarctation of the Aorta

Coarctation of the aorta is narrowing of the aorta, the major blood vessel carrying highly oxygenated blood from the left ventricle of the heart to the rest of the body (Fig. 19.8). It accounts for about 10% of CHDs (Schneider, 2023).

Pathophysiology

Coarctation of the aorta occurs most often in the area near the ductus arteriosus. The narrowing can be preductal (between the subclavian artery and the ductus arteriosus) or postductal (after the ductus arteriosus). As a result of the narrowing, blood flow is impeded, causing pressure to increase in the area proximal to the defect and to decrease in the area distal to it. Thus, BP is increased in the heart and the upper portions of the body and decreased in the lower portions of the body. Left ventricular afterload is increased, and in some children, this may lead to heart failure. Collateral circulation may also develop as the body attempts to ensure adequate blood flow to the descending aorta. Due to the elevation in BP, the child is also at risk for aortic rupture, aortic aneurysm, and CVA (Jone et al., 2022; Schneider, 2023).

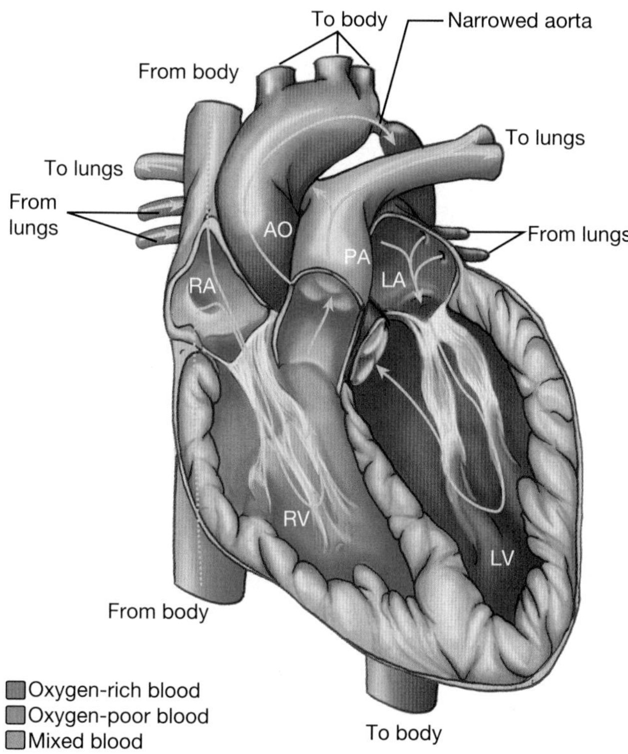

FIGURE 19.8 Coarctation of the aorta.

Nursing Assessment

The extent of the symptoms depends on the severity of the coarctation. Some children with coarctation of the aorta grow well into the school-age years before the defect is discovered.

HEALTH HISTORY AND PHYSICAL EXAMINATION

Determine the health history, noting problems with irritability and frequent epistaxis. In older children, there may also be reports of leg pain with activity, dizziness, fainting, and headaches. Assess pulses throughout, noting full, bounding pulses in the upper extremities with weak or absent pulses in the lower extremities. Determine BP in all four extremities. BP in the upper extremities may be 20 mm Hg or higher than that in the lower extremities. Inspect the school-age child's chest, noting notching of the ribs. Auscultate the heart for a soft or moderately loud systolic murmur, most often heard at the base of the heart (on the back or in the left axilla) (Jone et al., 2022).

LABORATORY AND DIAGNOSTIC TESTS

Diagnosis of coarctation of the aorta is based primarily on the history and physical examination. In addition, an echocardiogram may disclose the extent of narrowing and evidence of collateral circulation. Chest radiography may reveal left-sided cardiac enlargement and rib notching, indicative of collateral arterial enlargement. Other tests, such as ECG, computed tomography, or MRI, may be done to provide additional evidence about the extent of the coarctation and subsequent effects.

Aortic Stenosis

Aortic stenosis is a condition causing obstruction of the blood flow between the left ventricle and the aorta. The incidence of aortic stenosis is about 5% of all CHDs (Schneider, 2023).

Pathophysiology

Aortic stenosis can be caused by a muscle obstruction below the aortic valve, an obstruction at the valve itself, or an aortic narrowing just above the valve (Fig. 19.9). The most common type is an obstruction of the valve itself, called aortic valve stenosis. The aortic valve consists of three very pliable leaflets. Normally, the leaflets of the aortic valve spread open easily when the left ventricle ejects blood into the aorta. Aortic stenosis occurs when the aortic valve narrows, causing an obstruction between the left ventricle and the aorta. As a result, cardiac output

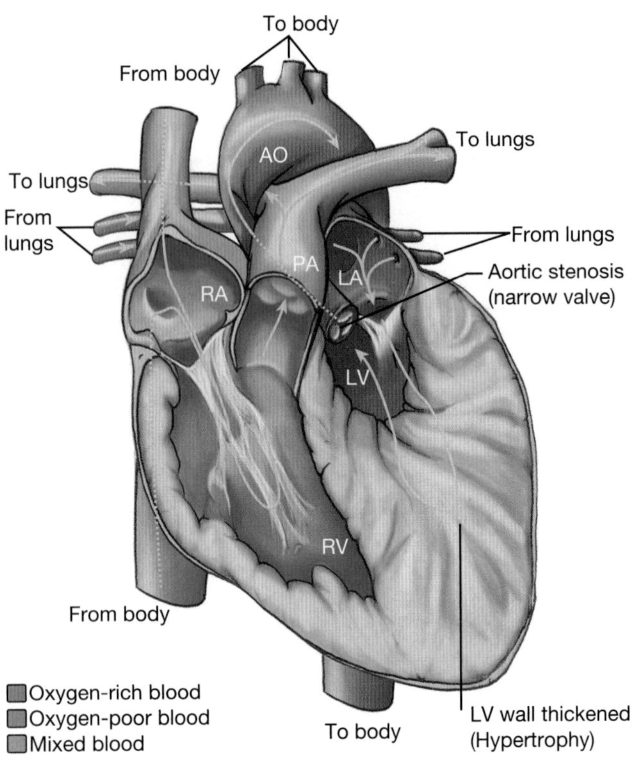

FIGURE 19.9 Aortic stenosis.

decreases. When the aortic valve does not function properly, the left ventricle must work harder to pump blood into the aorta. Because of the increased workload, the left ventricular muscle hypertrophies. If this continues, left ventricular failure can occur, leading to a backup of pressure in the pulmonary circulation and pulmonary edema. Heart failure may occur, but this is more commonly seen in the infant (Jone et al., 2022; Schneider, 2023).

Nursing Assessment

Typically, the child with aortic stenosis is asymptomatic. However, it is important to obtain an accurate health history and perform a physical examination.

HEALTH HISTORY AND PHYSICAL EXAMINATION

Obtain the child's health history, noting easy fatigability or complaints of chest pain similar to anginal pain when active. Dizziness with prolonged standing may also be reported. In the infant, note difficulty with feeding. Palpate the child's pulse; if aortic stenosis is severe, the pulses may be faint. Palpate the child's chest, noting a thrill at the base of the heart. Auscultate the heart, noting a systolic murmur best heard along the left sternal border with radiation to the right upper sternal border.

LABORATORY AND DIAGNOSTIC TESTS

The echocardiogram is the most important noninvasive test to identify aortic stenosis. An ECG may be normal in children with mild to moderate forms of aortic stenosis. For children with severe aortic stenosis, left ventricular hypertrophy may be determined from the ECG. For children experiencing easy fatigability and chest pain, an exercise stress test may be done to evaluate the degree of cardiac compromise.

Pulmonic Stenosis

PS is a condition that causes an obstruction in blood flow between the right ventricle and the pulmonary arteries. Pulmonic stenosis occurs in 0.6 to 0.8 per 1,000 live births (Peng, 2022). It is often associated with other heart anomalies and with genetic syndromes. Children may be asymptomatic, although some children with severe pulmonic stenosis may demonstrate cyanosis (Peng, 2022).

Pathophysiology

Pulmonic stenosis may occur as a muscular obstruction below the pulmonary valve, an obstruction at the valve, or a narrowing of the pulmonary artery above the valve (Fig. 19.10). Valve obstruction is the most common form of PS. Normally, the pulmonary valve is constructed with three thin and pliable valve leaflets; they spread apart easily, allowing the right ventricle to eject blood freely into the pulmonary artery. The most common problem

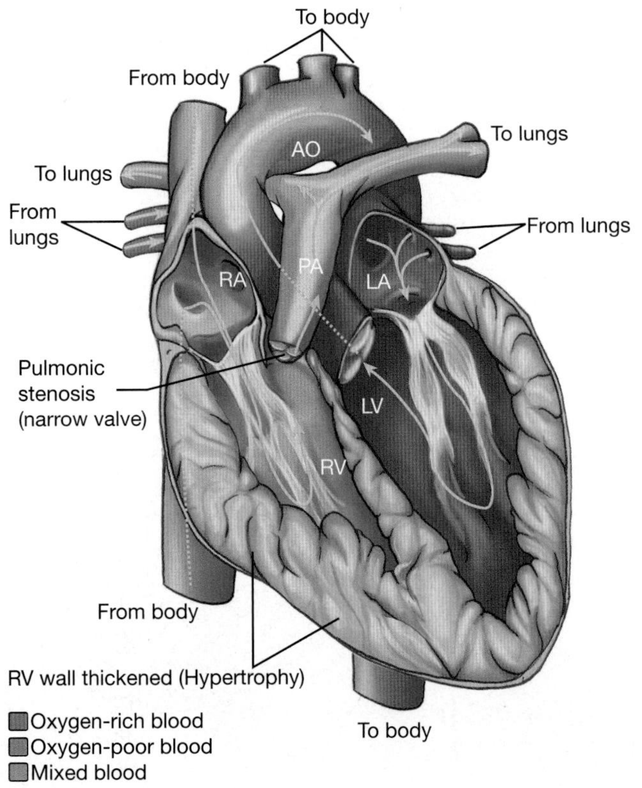

FIGURE 19.10 Pulmonic stenosis.

causing pulmonic stenosis is that the pulmonary valve leaflets are thickened and fused together along their separation lines, causing the obstruction to blood flow. The right ventricle has an additional workload, causing the muscle to thicken, resulting in right ventricular hypertrophy and decreased pulmonary blood flow. When the pulmonary valve is severely obstructed, the right ventricle cannot eject sufficient blood into the pulmonary artery. As a result, pressure in the right atrium increases, which could lead to a reopening of the foramen ovale. If this occurs, deoxygenated blood would pass through the foramen ovale into the left side of the heart and would then be pumped to the systemic circulation. In some cases, a PDA may be present, thus allowing for some compensation by shunting blood from the aorta to the pulmonary circulation for oxygenation (Peng, 2022).

Nursing Assessment

The child with pulmonic stenosis may be asymptomatic or may exhibit signs and symptoms of mild heart failure. If the stenosis is severe, the child may demonstrate cyanosis. Therefore, it is important for the nurse to obtain an accurate health history and physical examination.

HEALTH HISTORY AND PHYSICAL EXAMINATION

Elicit the health history, noting mild dyspnea or cyanosis with exertion. Document the child's growth history, which is typically normal. Carefully palpate the sternal border for a thrill (not always present). Auscultate the heart, noting a high-pitched click following the second heart sound and a systolic ejection murmur loudest at the upper left sternal border.

LABORATORY AND DIAGNOSTIC TESTS

An echocardiogram reveals the extent of obstruction present at the valve, as well as right ventricular hypertrophy. An ECG also helps to detect right ventricular hypertrophy.

Mixed Defects

Mixed defects are CHDs that involve a mixing of well-oxygenated blood with poorly oxygenated blood. As a result, systemic blood flow contains a lower oxygen content. Cardiac output is decreased, and heart failure occurs. Examples of mixed defects include TGA, total anomalous pulmonary venous connection (TAPVC), truncus arteriosus, and HLHS.

Transposition of the Great Arteries

TGA is a CHD in which the pulmonary artery and the aorta are transposed from their normal positions. The aorta arises from the right ventricle instead of the left ventricle, and the pulmonary artery arises from the left ventricle instead of the right ventricle. TGA accounts about 5% of all CHD cases (Schneider, 2023). It is most often diagnosed in the first few days of life when the infant manifests cyanosis, which indicates decreased oxygenation. As the ductus arteriosus closes, the symptoms will worsen. Corrective surgery is usually performed by age 4 to 7 days.

PATHOPHYSIOLOGY

TGV creates a situation in which poorly oxygenated blood returning to the right atrium and ventricle is then pumped out to the aorta and back to the body (Fig. 19.11). Oxygenated blood returning from the lungs to the left atrium and ventricle is then sent back to the lungs through the pulmonary artery. Unless there is a connection somewhere in the circulation where the oxygen-rich and oxygen-poor blood can mix, all the organs of the body will be poorly oxygenated. Often, the ductus arteriosus remains patent, allowing for some mixing of blood. Similarly, if a VSD is also present, mixing of blood may occur, and cyanosis will be delayed. However, these associated defects can lead to increased pulmonary blood flow that increases pressure in the pulmonary circulation. This predisposes the child to heart failure (Jone et al., 2022; Schneider, 2023).

NURSING ASSESSMENT

Significant cyanosis without a murmur in the newborn period is highly indicative of TGA. In some infants, cyanosis will not develop until several days of age as the PDA closes. In infants with septal defects, cyanosis may be further delayed.

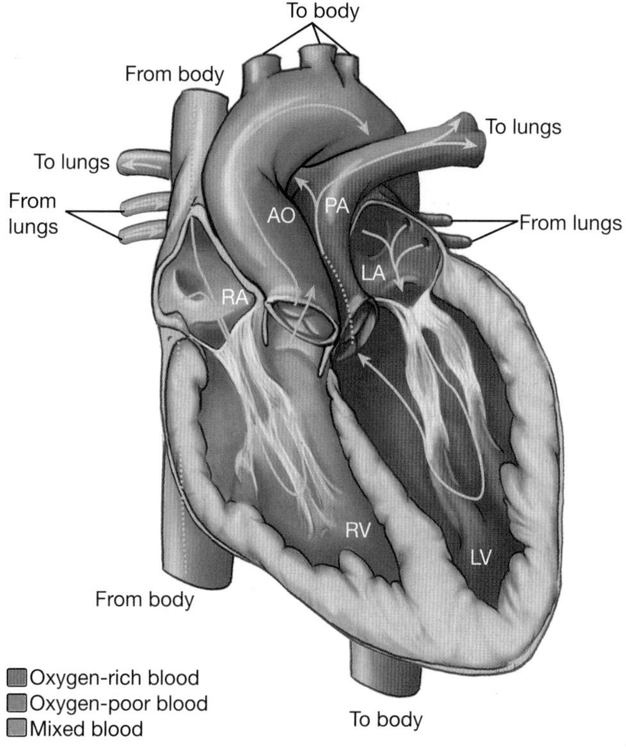

FIGURE 19.11 Transposition of the great vessels.

Health History and Physical Examination

Elicit the health history, noting onset of cyanosis with feeding or crying. Observe the infant for cyanosis while active and at rest. Observe the chest, noting a prominent ventricular impulse. Auscultate the heart, noting a loud second heart sound. A murmur may be heard if the ductus remains open or a septal defect is present. If heart failure is present, note edema, tachypnea, and adventitious lung sounds.

Laboratory and Diagnostic Tests

Echocardiography clearly reveals evidence of the transposition. Cardiac catheterization may be performed to determine whether oxygen saturation levels are low due to the mixing of the blood.

Total Anomalous Pulmonary Venous Connection

TAPVC is a CHD in which the pulmonary veins do not connect normally to the left atrium. Instead, they connect to the right atrium, often by way of the superior vena cava. Relatively rare, it accounts for up to 1.5% of all CHD (Soriano & Fulton, 2022). TAPVC may also be referred to as TAPVR.

PATHOPHYSIOLOGY

Oxygenated blood that would normally enter the left atrium now enters the right atrium and passes to the right ventricle. As a result, the pressure on the right side of the heart increases, leading to hypertrophy. TAPVC is incompatible with life unless there is an associated defect present that allows for shunting of blood from the highly pressured right side of the heart. A patent foramen ovale or an ASD is usually present. Since none of the pulmonary veins connect normally to the left atrium, the only source of blood to the left atrium is blood that is shunted from the right atrium across the defect to the left side of the heart (Fig. 19.12). The highly oxygenated blood from the lungs completely mixes with the poorly oxygenated blood returning from the systemic circulation. This causes an overload of the right atrium and right ventricle. The increased blood volume going into the lungs can lead to pulmonary hypertension and pulmonary edema (Soriano & Fulton, 2022).

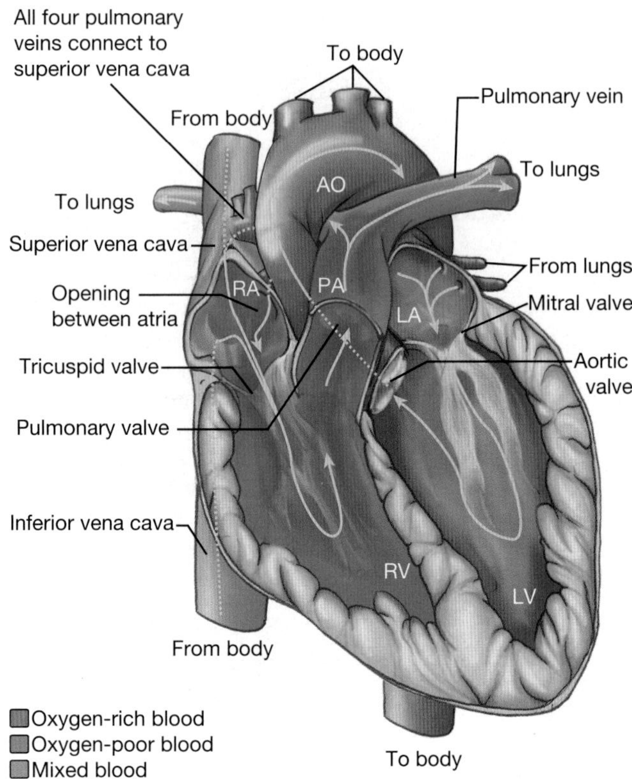

FIGURE 19.12 Total anomalous pulmonary venous connection.

NURSING ASSESSMENT

The degree of cyanosis present with TAPVC depends on the extent of the associated defects. For example, if the foramen ovale closes or the ASD is small, significant cyanosis will be present. The physical examination findings will vary depending on the type of TAPVC the infant has, whether obstruction is present, and whether other associated cardiac anomalies are present.

Health History and Physical Examination

Note history of cyanosis, tiring easily, and difficulty feeding. Observe the chest for prominence of the right ventricular impulse and retractions with tachypnea. Auscultate the heart, noting fixed splitting of the second heart sound and a murmur. Palpate the abdomen for hepatomegaly.

Laboratory and Diagnostic Tests

An echocardiogram will reveal the abnormal connection of the pulmonary veins, enlargement of the right atrium and right ventricle, and an ASD if present. The chest radiograph will demonstrate an enlarged heart and pulmonary edema. Cardiac catheterization can also be useful to visualize the abnormal connection of the pulmonary veins, particularly if an obstruction is present.

Truncus Arteriosus

Truncus arteriosus is a CHD in which only one major artery leaves the heart and supplies blood to the pulmonary and systemic circulations. It accounts for less than 1% of all CHD cases (Jone et al., 2022; Schneider, 2023). A VSD is almost always present as well.

PATHOPHYSIOLOGY

The one great vessel contains one valve. This valve consists of two to five leaflets and is positioned over both the left and the right ventricles (Fig. 19.13). Due to the location of the valve, blood from the left ventricle mixes with blood from the right ventricle. Pressure

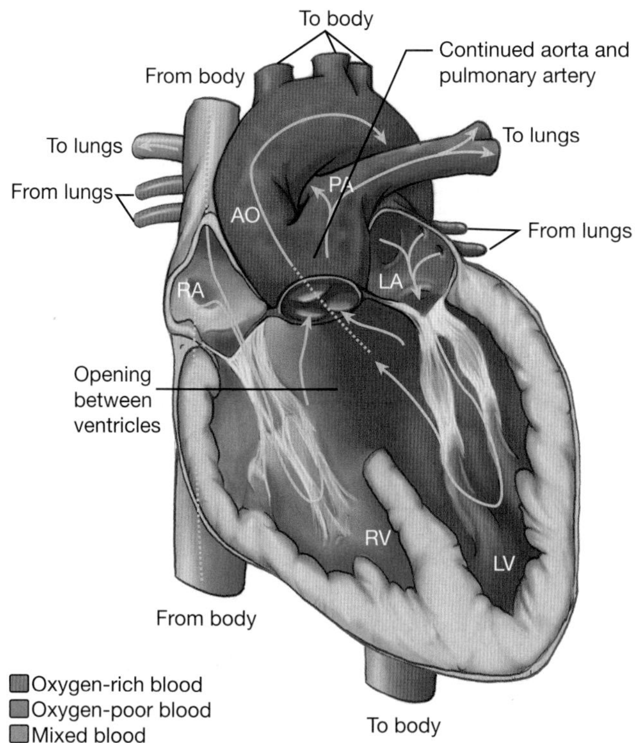

FIGURE 19.13 Truncus arteriosus.

in the pulmonary circulation is typically less than that of the systemic circulation, leading to increased blood flow to the lungs. As a result, systemic blood flow is decreased. Over time, the increased pulmonary blood flow can lead to pulmonary vascular disease (Jone et al., 2022; Schneider, 2023).

NURSING ASSESSMENT

Typically, the infant demonstrates cyanosis in varying degrees, depending on the extent of compromise in the systemic circulation. Obtain an accurate health history and perform a physical examination.

Health History and Physical Examination

Elicit the health history, noting history of cyanosis that increases with periods of activity such as feeding. Also note history of tiring easily, difficulty in feeding, and poor growth. Count the respiratory rate, which may be elevated. Observe for nasal flaring, grunting or noisy breathing, retractions, and restlessness. Auscultate the lungs, noting adventitious breath sounds, and the heart, noting a murmur associated with a VSD.

Laboratory and Diagnostic Tests

An echocardiogram will confirm the presence of truncus arteriosus as the anatomy of the great vessels, the single truncal valve, and the VSD will be seen. On rare occasions, a cardiac catheterization may be done to determine pressures in the pulmonary arteries.

Hypoplastic Left Heart Syndrome

HLHS is a CHD in which all structures on the left side of the heart are severely underdeveloped (Fig. 19.14). The mitral and aortic valves are completely closed or very small. The left ventricle is nonfunctional. Thus, the left side of the heart is completely unable to supply blood to the systemic circulation. HLHS is the fourth most common CHD. It appears to have a multifactorial and autosomal recessive inheritance pattern and occurs in 1.4% to 3.8% of cases of CHD (Jone et al., 2022). The options for treatment include palliative care, cardiac transplantation within the first few weeks of life, or palliative reconstructive surgery consisting of three stages, beginning within days to weeks of birth.

PATHOPHYSIOLOGY

With HLHS, the right side of the heart is the main working part of the heart. Blood returning from the lungs into the left atrium must pass through an ASD to the right side of the heart. The right ventricle must then pump blood to the lungs and to the systemic circulation through the PDA. A few days after birth, when the ductus arteriosus closes, the heart cannot pump blood into the systemic circulation, causing poor perfusion of the vital organs and shock. Death will occur rapidly without intervention (Jone et al., 2022; Schneider, 2023).

NURSING ASSESSMENT

Initially after birth, the newborn may be asymptomatic because the ductus arteriosus is still patent. However, as

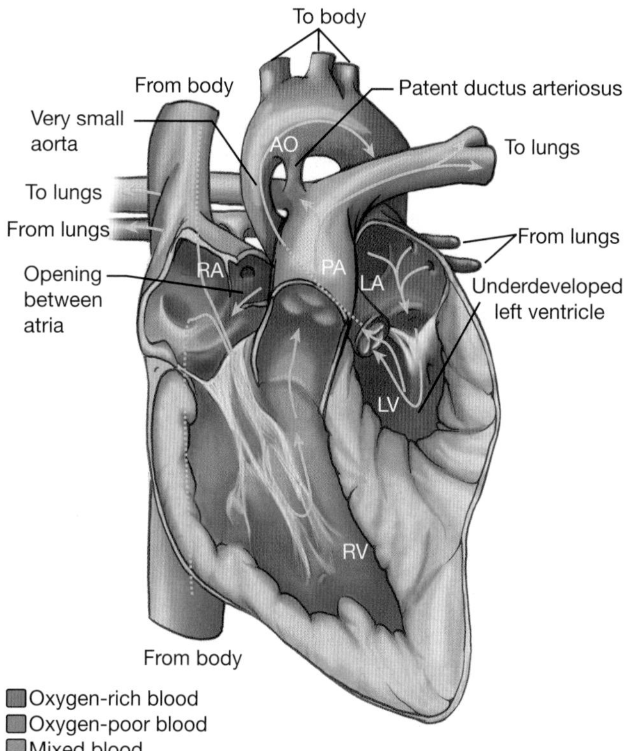

FIGURE 19.14 Hypoplastic left heart syndrome.

the ductus begins to close at a few days of age, the newborn will begin to exhibit cyanosis. Some infants may present with circulatory collapse (shock) and must be resuscitated emergently.

Health History and Physical Examination

Obtain the health history, noting onset of cyanosis. Note poor feeding and history of tiring easily. Evaluate the vital signs, noting tachycardia, tachypnea, and hypothermia. Observe for increased work of breathing and gradually increasing cyanosis. Note pallor of the extremities and decreased oxygen saturation via pulse oximetry. Auscultate the heart and lungs. Note adventitious breath sounds, a gallop rhythm, a single second heart sound, and a soft systolic ejection or holosystolic murmur.

Laboratory and Diagnostic Tests

Prenatally, a fetal echocardiogram can diagnose this syndrome, as can an ultrasound of the pregnant person. After birth, the echocardiogram illustrates the defect.

Nursing Management of the Child With a Congenital Heart Defect

The child with a CHD has multiple needs and requires comprehensive, multidisciplinary care. Nurses play a key role in helping the child and family during this intensely stressful time. Nursing care focuses on improving oxygenation, promoting adequate nutrition, assisting the child and family with coping, providing postoperative nursing care, preventing infection, and providing child and family education. An important component of education involves preparing the child and parents for discharge. In addition to the nursing management presented further on, refer to the "Clinical Judgment and the Nursing Process" section for additional interventions appropriate for the child with CHD. Individualize nursing care specific to the child's needs.

Improving Oxygenation

Provide frequent ongoing assessment of the child's cardiopulmonary status as oxygenation status varies due to the hemodynamic changes accompanying the underlying structural defect. Assess airway patency and suction as needed. Position the child in the Fowler or semi-Fowler position to facilitate lung expansion. Monitor vital signs, especially heart and respiratory rates. Monitor the child's color and oxygen saturation levels closely, using these to guide oxygen administration. Observe for tachypnea and other signs of respiratory distress, such as nasal flaring, grunting, and retractions. Auscultate the lungs for adventitious sounds. Provide humidified supplemental oxygen as ordered, warming it to prevent wide temperature fluctuations. Anticipate the need for assisted ventilation if the child has difficulty maintaining the airway or experiences deterioration in oxygenation capacity. Box 19.1 lists interventions related to relief of hypercyanotic spells.

BOX 19.1 Relieving Hypercyanotic Spells

- Use a calm, comforting approach.
- Place the infant or child in a knee-to-chest position.
- Provide supplemental oxygen.
- Administer morphine sulfate (0.1 mg/kg IV, IM, or SQ).
- Supply IV fluids.
- Administer propranolol (0.1 mg/kg IV).

IM, intramuscularly; IV, intravenously; SQ, subcutaneously.

Data from Doyle, T., & Kavanaugh-McHugh, A. (2023). Management and outcome of tetralogy of Fallot. *UptoDate*. Retrieved January 12, 2024, from http://www.uptodate.com/contents/management-and-outcome-of-tetralogy-of-fallot

DOSAGE CALCULATION BOX 19.1

Child's weight: 12 lb 12 oz

Medication order: digoxin 60 mcg by mouth every 12 hours.

Per the Pediatric Dosage Handbook, the recommended dose is 10–15 mcg/kg/day in two divided doses.

Is the ordered dose safe?

Promoting Adequate Nutrition

Provide nutrition orally, enterally, or parenterally in order to foster growth and development as well as to reduce the risk of infection. The nutritional method will vary depending on the individual child's energy expenditure associated with increased cardiac and respiratory workloads. In addition, for example, for the newborn or infant, nutrition via breast milk or formula may be provided orally or via gavage feedings. Breastfeeding is usually associated with decreased energy expenditure during the act of feeding, yet some infants in intensive care are not stable enough to breastfeed. Gavage with breast milk is possible, and the use of human milk fortifier (either with breastfeeding or added to the gavage feed) adds additional calories that the infant requires. Formula-fed infants may also require increased-calorie formula, which may be achieved by more concentrated mixing of the formula or through the use of additives such as Polycose or vegetable oil. Consult the nutritionist to determine the individual infant's caloric needs and prescription of appropriate feeding.

Cutting a larger hole in the nipple or cross-cutting the nipple decreases the work of feeding for some infants. Generally, nipple feedings should be limited to a 20-minute duration, as feeding for longer periods results in excess caloric expenditure. Many infants may feed orally for 20 minutes, receiving the remainder of that feeding via orogastric or nasogastric tube. Offer older children small, frequent feedings to reduce the amount of energy required to feed or eat and to prevent overtiring the child. When needed, administer and monitor total parenteral nutrition as prescribed.

TAKE NOTE!

Breastfeeding a child before and after cardiac surgery may boost the infant's immune system, which can help fight postoperative infection. If breastfeeding is not possible, pumped breast milk may be given via bottle, dropper, or gavage feeding.

Assisting the Child and Family With Coping

Support the family's efforts to cope with the diagnosis of CHD as it can be overwhelming for the child and the parents. The numerous examinations, diagnostic tests, and procedures are sources of stress for the infant or child regardless of age and for the parents. The parents may fear long-term disability or death or may worry that allowing the child to engage in any activity will worsen their status. Thus, the parents may tend to overprotect the child. It is important for the parents to continue parenting the child, even when the child requires extended hospitalizations or intensive care. Explain all that is happening with the child, using language the parents and child can understand. Allow the parents and child to voice their feelings, concerns, or questions. Provide ample time to address these questions and concerns. Encourage the parents and the child, as developmentally appropriate, to participate in the child's care.

If the child is a newborn or infant, encourage attachment and bonding. Emphasize the child's positive attributes, including the normal aspects of the infant. Help the parents to experience the joy of a new infant and see the beauty of the child, no matter how ill the infant is. Urge the parents to touch, stroke, pat, and talk to the infant. Encourage them to hold the infant close, using kangaroo care as appropriate. If the child is older, offer suggestions as to how the parents can meet the child's emotional needs. For example, encourage them to bring a favorite toy or object from home while the child is hospitalized.

Provide developmentally appropriate explanations to the child. Encourage play therapy to help the child understand what is happening.

Preventing Infection

Teach parents proper hand hygiene. Provide appropriate dental care. Make sure the child receives prophylaxis for infective endocarditis as needed. Ensure that children 24 months or younger who are undergoing heart transplantation during respiratory syncytial virus (RSV) season receive appropriate prophylaxis via vaccination with palivizumab (Kimberlin et al., 2021).

Providing Care for the Child Undergoing Cardiac Surgery

Cardiac surgery may be necessary to correct a congenital defect or to provide symptomatic relief. The surgery may be planned as an elective procedure or done as an emergency. Open heart surgery involves an incision of the heart muscle to repair the internal structures. This may require cardiopulmonary bypass. Closed heart surgery involves structures related to the heart but not the heart muscle itself and may be performed with or without cardiopulmonary bypass.

PROVIDING PREOPERATIVE CARE

Complete the preoperative assessment to provide important baseline information for comparison during the postoperative period. Establish a relationship with the child and parents. Identify problems that may require particular nursing interventions during the postoperative period. Before cardiac surgery, interview the parents and, if age appropriate, the child. Focus the interview on the history of the present illness, cardiac risk factors, the child's present physical and functional status, additional medical problems, current medications and drug allergies, the child's and family's understanding of the illness and planned procedure, and the family support system.

The preoperative physical assessment includes:

- Temperature and weight measurements
- Examination of extremities for peripheral edema, clubbing, and evaluation of peripheral pulses
- Auscultation of the heart (rate, rhythm, heart sounds, murmurs, clicks, and rubs)
- Respiratory assessment, including respiratory rate, work of breathing, and auscultation of the lungs for breath sounds

Obtain any necessary laboratory and diagnostic tests to establish a baseline. In addition, review the results of any tests done previously. Testing may include CBC count, electrolyte levels, clotting studies, urinalysis, cultures of blood and other body secretions, kidney and hepatic function tests, chest radiography, ECG, echocardiogram, and cardiac catheterization.

In most nonemergent cases, preoperative assessment is performed in an outpatient setting, and the child is admitted to the hospital on the day of surgery. Nursing care during this phase focuses on thorough child and parent education. If the surgery is an emergency, teaching must be done quickly, emphasizing the most important elements of the child's care (Beke et al., 2021).

Child and parent education typically includes the following topics:

- Heart anatomy and its function, including what area is involved with the defect that is to be corrected
- Events before surgery, including any testing or preparation such as a skin scrub
- Location of the child after surgery, such as a pediatric intensive care unit, which may include a visit to the unit, if appropriate, and explanation of the sights and sounds that may be present
- Appearance of the child after surgery (equipment or devices used for monitoring, such as oxygen

administration, ECG leads, pulse oximeter, chest tubes, mechanical ventilation, or IV lines)
- Approximate location of the incision and coverage with dressings
- Postoperative activity level, including measures to reduce the risk of complications, such as coughing and deep-breathing exercises, incentive spirometry, early ambulation, and leg exercises
- Nutritional restrictions, such as nothing by mouth for a specified time before surgery and use of IV fluids
- Medications, such as anesthesia, sedation, and analgesics as well as medications the child is taking now that need to be continued or withheld (Beke et al., 2021)

Prepare and educate the child at an age- and developmentally appropriate level. Advise parents to read books with their child about CHD and hospitalization such as:

- *Clifford Visits the Hospital* by N. Bridwell, 2000 (Scholastic Inc.)
- *Franklin Goes to the Hospital* by P. Bourgeois, 2000 (Scholastic Paperbacks)
- *Pump the Bear* by G. O. Whittington, 2000 (Brown Books)
- *Blue Lewis and Sasha the Great* by C. D. Newell, 2005 (Cally Press)
- *Cardiac Kids: A Book for Families Who Have a Child with Heart Disease* by V. Elder, 1994 (Dayton Area Heart and Cancer Association)
- *When Molly Was in the Hospital: A Book for Brothers and Sisters of Hospitalized Children* by D. Duncan, 1994 (Rayve Productions) (siblings)
- *A Night Without Stars* by J. Howe, 1993 (Camelot) (older children)

In addition, parents may order *It's My Heart,* a parent resource book, free of charge from the Children's Heart Foundation via this link: https://www.childrensheartfoundation.org/about-chds/resources.html.

Parents may also help their child by buying a small thrift store suitcase, spray painting it, and allowing the child to decorate it with their name, pictures of family, stickers, or favorite story characters. This will be the child's "hospital suitcase" that the child may pack with toys and videos to bring to the hospital. Hospital tours are appropriate for school-age children, and older children and adolescents may benefit from an intensive care unit tour before surgery.

Instruct parents to stop food and liquids at the designated time, depending on the child's age, and to give all medications as directed. Some medications may be withheld before surgery. If the child's nutritional status is poor or questionable, nutritional supplementation may be ordered for a period preoperatively to ensure that the child has the best possible nutritional status before surgery. When it is time for the child to be transported to the surgical area, allow the parents to accompany the child as far as possible, depending on the institution's policy. Also reinforce with the child that their parents will be present at the bedside when they awaken from surgery (Beke et al., 2021).

PROVIDING POSTOPERATIVE CARE

Postoperative nursing care for the child after cardiac surgery includes the following measures:

- Assess vital signs frequently, as often as every 1 hour, until stable.
- Assess the color of the skin and mucous membranes, check capillary refill, and palpate peripheral pulses.
- Observe cardiac rate and rhythm via electronic monitoring, and auscultate heart rate and rhythm and heart sounds frequently.
- Monitor hemodynamic status via arterial and/or central venous lines (left and right atrial and pulmonary artery pressures, pulmonary artery oxygen saturation).
- Provide site care and tubing changes according to the institution's policy.
- Auscultate lungs for adventitious, diminished, or absent breath sounds.
- Assess oxygen saturation levels via pulse oximetry and arterial blood gases as well as work of breathing and level of consciousness frequently.
- Administer supplemental oxygen as needed.
- Monitor mechanical ventilation and suction as ordered.
- Inspect chest tube functioning, noting amount, color, and character of drainage.
- Inspect the dressing (incision and chest tube) for drainage and intactness. Reinforce or change the dressing as ordered.
- Assess the incision for redness, irritation, drainage, or separation.
- Monitor intake and output hourly.
- Maintain accurate IV infusion rate; restrict fluids as ordered to prevent hypervolemia.
- Assess for changes in level of consciousness. Report restlessness, irritability, or seizures.
- Obtain ordered laboratory tests, such as CBC, coagulation studies, cardiac enzyme levels, and electrolyte levels. Report abnormal results.
- Administer medications, such as digoxin or inotropic or vasopressor agents, as ordered, watching the child closely for possible adverse effects.
- Encourage the child to turn, cough, deep breathe, use the incentive spirometer, and splint the incisional area with pillows.
- Assess the child's pain level and administer analgesics as ordered. Allow time for the child to rest and sleep.
- Assist the child to get out of bed as soon as possible and as ordered.
- Assess daily weights.
- Administer small, frequent feedings or meals when oral intake is allowed.

BOX **19.2** **Possible Complications After Cardiac Surgery**

- Atelectasis
- Bacterial endocarditis
- Cardiac arrhythmias
- Cardiac tamponade
- Cerebrovascular accident
- Heart failure
- Hemorrhage
- Pleural effusion
- Pneumonia
- Pneumothorax
- Postperfusion syndrome
- Postcardiac surgery syndrome
- Pulmonary edema
- Seizures
- Wound infection

Data from Fleitman, J. (2023). Postoperative complications among patients undergoing cardiac surgery. *UpToDate*. Retrieved January 12, 2024, from https://www.uptodate.com/contents/postoperative-complications-among-patients-undergoing-cardiac-surgery

- Position the child in a comfortable position, one that maximizes chest expansion. Change position frequently.
- Assess the child for complications (Box 19.2).
- Provide emotional and physical support to the child and family, making appropriate referrals, such as to social services for assistance.
- Prepare the child and family for discharge (Beke et al., 2021).

TAKE NOTE!

Abrupt cessation of chest tube output accompanied by an increase in heart rate and increased filling pressure (right atrial) may indicate cardiac tamponade (Beke et al., 2021).

Providing Child and Family Education

Provide child and family education throughout the child's stay. Initially, teaching focuses on the underlying defect and measures to treat or control the problem. If the child requires surgery, teaching shifts to preoperative and postoperative events. Emphasize discharge teaching for each admission. Teaching Guidelines 19.2 highlights the major areas to be addressed in child and family education.

TEACHING GUIDELINES **19.2** Caring for the Child With a Congenital Heart Disease

- Give medications, if ordered, exactly as prescribed.
- Weigh the child at least once a week or as ordered at approximately the same time of the day with the same scale and wearing the same amount of clothing.
- Allow the child to engage in activity as directed. Provide time for the child to rest frequently throughout the day to prevent overexertion.
- Provide a nutritious diet, taking into account any restrictions for fluids or foods.
- Use measures to prevent infection, such as frequent handwashing, prophylactic antibiotics, and skin care.
- Adhere to schedule for follow-up diagnostic tests and procedures.
- Support the child's growth and development needs.
- Use available community support services.
- Notify the health care provider or nurse practitioner if the child has increasing episodes of respiratory distress, cyanosis, or difficulty breathing; fever; increased edema of the hands, feet, or face; decreased urinary output; weight loss or difficulty eating or drinking; increased fatigue or irritability; decreased level of alertness; or vomiting or diarrhea (Gaskin & Kennedy, 2019; Hueckel, 2019).

ACQUIRED CARDIOVASCULAR DISORDERS

Acquired cardiovascular disorders occur in children because of an underlying cardiovascular problem or may refer to other cardiac disorders that are not congenital. The most common type of acquired cardiovascular disorder in children is heart failure. Other acquired disorders include rheumatic fever, cardiomyopathy, infective endocarditis, hyperlipidemia, hypertension, and Kawasaki disease.

Heart Failure

Heart failure refers to a set of clinical signs and symptoms that reflect the heart's inability to pump effectively to provide adequate blood, oxygen, and nutrients to the body organs and tissues (Kusumoto, 2019). Heart failure occurs most often in children with CHD and is the most common reason for admission to the hospital for children with CHD. The estimated number of children experiencing heart failure annually is 12,000 to 25,000 (Singh & Singh, 2022). Heart failure also occurs secondary to other conditions such as myocardial dysfunction following surgical intervention for CHD, cardiomyopathy, myocarditis, fluid volume overload, hypertension, anemia, or sepsis or as a toxic effect of certain chemotherapeutic agents used in the treatment of cancer.

The child experiencing heart failure requires a multidisciplinary approach to care. Collaboration is necessary to achieve improved cardiac function, restored fluid balance, decreased cardiac workload, and improved oxygen delivery to the tissues.

Pathophysiology

Cardiac output is controlled by preload (diastolic volume), afterload (ventricular wall tension), myocardial contractility (inotropic state), and heart rate. Protracted alterations in any of these factors may lead to heart failure. In the event of reduced cardiac output, multiple compensatory mechanisms are activated. When the ventricular contraction is impaired (systolic dysfunction), reduced ejection of blood occurs, and therefore cardiac output is reduced. Diminished ability to receive venous return (diastolic dysfunction) occurs when high venous pressures are required to support ventricular function. As a result of decreased cardiac output, the renin–angiotensin–aldosterone system is activated as a compensatory mechanism. Fluid and sodium retention as well as improved contractility and vasoconstriction then occur. Initially, BP is supported, and organ perfusion is maintained, but increased afterload worsens systolic dysfunction. As the heart chambers dilate, myocardial oxygen consumption increases, and cardiac output is limited by excessive wall stretch. Over time, the capacity of the heart to respond to these compensatory mechanisms fails, and cardiac output is further decreased (Kusumoto, 2019). Figure 19.15 shows the clinical manifestations that occur related to the mechanisms of heart failure.

Therapeutic Management

Management of heart failure is supportive. Promotion of oxygenation and ventilation is of utmost importance. Digitalis, diuretics, inotropic agents, vasodilators, antiarrhythmics, and antithrombotics have been widely used in children for palliation of symptoms. Many children with heart failure require management in the intensive care unit until they are stabilized. Augmenting nutrition and ensuring adequate rest are also key components of management.

Nursing Assessment

For a full description of the assessment phase of the nursing process, refer to the "Clinical Judgment and the

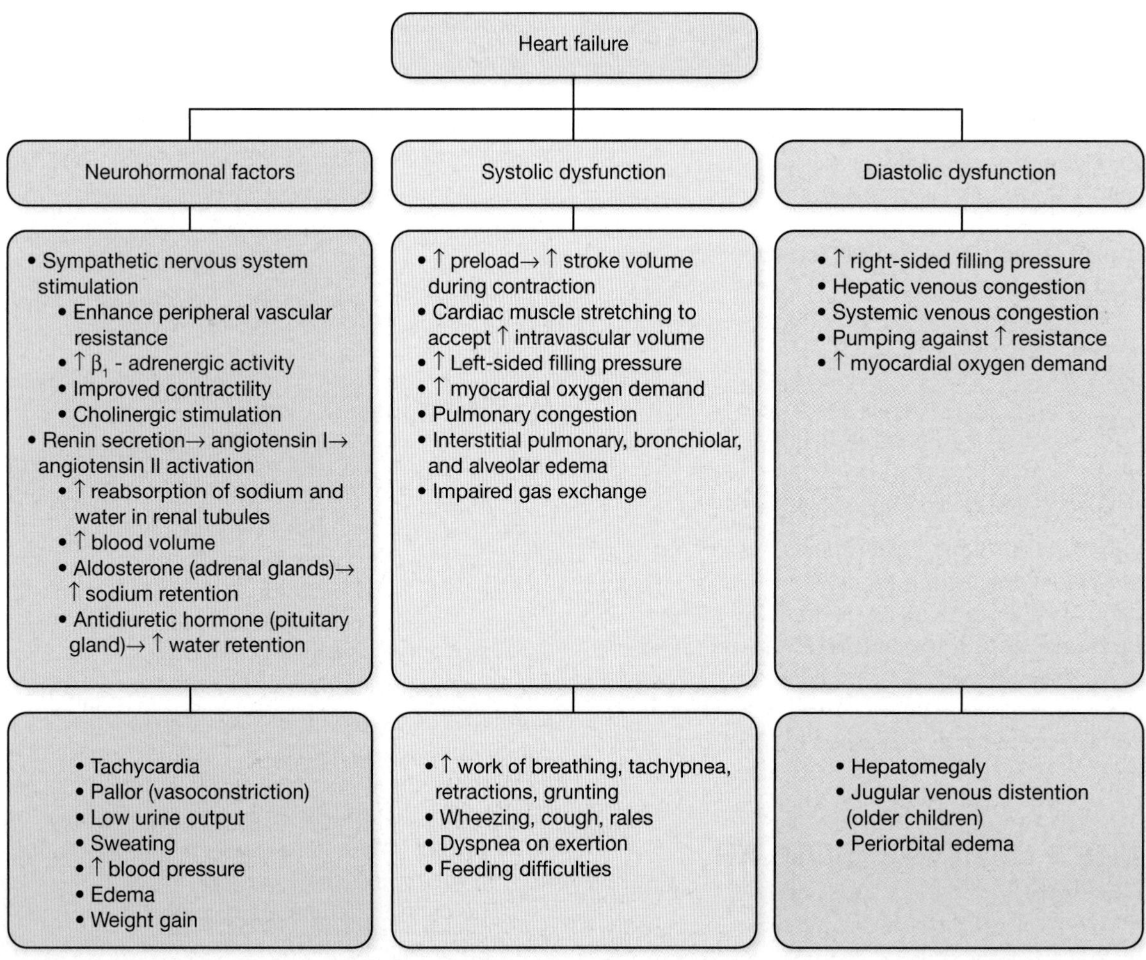

FIGURE 19.15 Pathophysiology of heart failure. (Data from Kusumoto, F. M. [2019]. Cardiovascular disorders: Heart disease. In G. D. Hammer & S. J. McPhee [Eds.], *Pathophysiology of disease: An introduction to clinical medicine* [8th ed.]. McGraw-Hill Education.)

Nursing Process" section earlier in the chapter. Specific assessment findings related to heart failure are discussed further on.

HEALTH HISTORY

When obtaining the health history, elicit a description of the present illness and chief complaint. Common complaints reported during the health history might include:

- Failure to gain weight or rapid weight gain
- Failure to thrive
- Difficulty feeding
- Fatigue
- Dizziness, irritability
- Exercise intolerance
- Shortness of breath
- Sucking and then tiring quickly
- Syncope
- Decreased number of wet diapers

Infants with heart failure often display subtle signs such as difficulty feeding and tiring easily. Pay close attention to reports of these problems from the parents. Also be alert for statements such as "The baby drinks a small amount of breast milk (or formula) and stops but then wants to eat again very soon afterwards;" "The baby seems to perspire a lot during feedings;" or "The baby seems to be more comfortable when he's sitting up or on my shoulder than when he's lying flat." In addition, the parents may report episodes of rapid breathing and grunting.

The child's current and past medical history also provide additional clues. Question the parents about any history of CHDs and treatments such as surgery to repair the defect. Determine the current medication regimen. Also ask about any recent or past infections, such as streptococcal infections or fever.

PHYSICAL EXAMINATION

Weigh the child and note recent rapid weight gain or lack of weight gain. Obtain the child's vital signs, noting tachycardia or tachypnea. These findings are often the first indicators of heart failure in an infant or older child. Measure the BP in the upper and lower extremities, comparing the findings for differences. Note decreased BP, which may be due to impaired cardiac muscle function. Inspect the skin color, noting pallor or cyanosis. Also observe for diaphoresis (profuse sweating). Inspect the face, hands, and lower extremities for edema. Observe for increased work of breathing, such as nasal flaring or retractions. Note the presence of a cough, which may be productive with bloody sputum.

Auscultate the apical pulse, noting its location and character. Listen for a murmur, which may suggest a CHD, a gallop rhythm, or an accentuated third heart sound, suggesting sudden ventricular distention. Auscultate the lungs, noting crackles or wheezes suggestive of pulmonary congestion. Palpate the peripheral pulses, noting weak or thready pulses. Note the temperature and color of the extremities; they may be cool, clammy, and pale. Assess the child's abdomen, looking for distention indicative of ascites. Gently palpate the abdomen to identify hepatomegaly or splenomegaly.

LABORATORY AND DIAGNOSTIC TESTS

The diagnosis of heart failure is based on the child's signs and symptoms and is confirmed with several laboratory and diagnostic tests. These include:

- Chest radiograph, revealing an enlarged heart and/or pulmonary edema
- ECG, indicating ventricular hypertrophy
- Echocardiogram, revealing the underlying cause of heart failure, such as a CHD

Other tests may be done to support the diagnosis. For example, the CBC count may show evidence of anemia or infection. Electrolyte levels may reveal hyponatremia secondary to fluid retention and hyperkalemia secondary to tissue destruction or impaired kidney function. Arterial blood gas results may demonstrate respiratory alkalosis in mild heart failure or metabolic acidosis. Tissue hypoxia may be evidenced by increased lactic acid and decreased bicarbonate levels.

Nursing Management

Nursing management of the child with heart failure focuses on promoting oxygenation, supporting cardiac function, providing adequate nutrition, and promoting rest.

PROMOTING OXYGENATION

Position the infant or child in a semi-upright position to decrease work of breathing and lessen pulmonary congestion. Suction as needed. Chest physiotherapy and postural drainage may also be beneficial. Administer supplemental oxygen as ordered and monitor oxygen saturation via pulse oximetry. Oxygen also serves the function of vasodilator and decreases pulmonary vascular resistance. Occasionally, the infant or child with heart failure may require intubation and positive-pressure ventilation to normalize blood gas tension.

CLINICAL REASONING ALERT!

In a child with a large left-to-right shunt, oxygen will decrease pulmonary vascular resistance while increasing the systemic vascular resistance, which leads to increased left-to-right shunting. Monitor the child carefully and use oxygen only as prescribed.

SUPPORTING CARDIAC FUNCTION

Administer digitalis, ACE inhibitors, and diuretics as prescribed. Digoxin therapy begins with a digitalizing dose divided into several doses (oral or IV) over a

24-hour period to reach maximum cardiac effect. During digitalization, monitor the ECG for a prolonged PR interval and decreased ventricular rate. Doses are then administered every 12 hours. Monitor the child for signs of digoxin toxicity. Measure BP before and after administration of ACE inhibitors, holding the dose and notifying the health care provider if the BP falls more than 15 mm Hg. Observe for signs of hypotension such as lightheadedness, dizziness, or fainting. Weigh the child daily to determine fluid loss. Maintain accurate records of intake and output, restricting fluid intake if ordered. Carefully monitor potassium levels, administering potassium supplements if prescribed. Sodium intake is not usually restricted in the child with heart failure.

PROVIDING ADEQUATE NUTRITION

Due to the increased metabolic rate associated with heart failure, the infant may require as much as 150 calories/kg/day. Older children will also require higher caloric intake than typical children. Offer small, frequent feedings if the child can tolerate them. During the acute phase of heart failure, many infants in particular will require continuous or intermittent gavage feeding to maintain or gain weight. Concentrate infant formula to 24 to 28 calories/oz as instructed by the nutritionist.

PROMOTING REST

Minimize metabolic needs to decrease cardiac demand. The infant or older child with heart failure will usually limit activities based on energy level. Ensure adequate time for sleep, and attempt to limit disturbing interventions. Provide age-appropriate activities that can be performed quietly or in bed, such as books, coloring or drawing, and video or board games. The older child or adolescent with significant heart failure may require home schooling. As the child improves, a rehabilitation program may be helpful for maximizing activity within the child's cardiovascular status limits.

Infective Endocarditis

Infective endocarditis is a microbial infection of the endothelial surfaces of the heart's chambers, septum, or valves (most common). Children with CHDs (septum or valve defects) or prosthetic valves are at increased risk for acquiring bacterial endocarditis, which is potentially fatal in these children. Other risk factors for endocarditis include central venous catheters and IV drug use. Infective endocarditis occurs when bacteria or fungi gain access to a damaged epithelium. Turbulence in blood flow associated with narrowed or incompetent valves or with a communication between the systemic and pulmonary circulation leads to damage of the endothelium. Thrombi and platelets then adhere to the endothelium, forming vegetations. When a microbe gains access to the bloodstream, it colonizes the vegetation, using the thrombi as a breeding ground. Clumps may separate from the vegetative patch and travel to other organs of the body, causing significant damage (septic emboli). Bacteria (particularly alpha-hemolytic streptococcus or *Staphylococcus aureus*) are the most common pathogens responsible for infective endocarditis, and, although rare, *Candida* species may also be found (O'Brien, 2023).

Complete antibiotic or antifungal treatment of the causative organism is necessary, and treatment generally lasts 4 to 6 weeks. Prevention of infective endocarditis in the susceptible child with CHD or a valvular disorder undergoing an invasive procedure is of the utmost importance (O'Brien, 2023).

Nursing Assessment

For a full description of the assessment phase of the nursing process, refer to "Clinical Judgment and the Nursing Process" section. Assessment findings related to endocarditis are discussed further on.

HEALTH HISTORY

Obtain the health history, noting intermittent, unexplained low-grade fever. Document history of fatigue, anorexia, weight loss, or flu-like symptoms (e.g., arthralgia, myalgia, chills, night sweats). Note history of CHD, valve disorder, or heart failure.

PHYSICAL EXAMINATION

Measure the child's temperature, noting low-grade fever. Observe for edema if heart failure is also present. Note petechiae on the palpebral conjunctiva, the oral mucosa, or the extremities. Inspect for signs of extracardiac emboli:

- Roth spots: splinter hemorrhages with pale centers on sclerae, palate, buccal mucosa, chest, fingers, or toes
- Janeway lesions: painless, flat, red or blue hemorrhagic lesions on the palms or the soles
- Osler nodes: small, tender nodules on the pads of the toes or fingers
- Black lines (splinter hemorrhages) under the nails (O'Brien, 2023)

Evaluate the ECG for a prolonged PR interval or dysrhythmias. Auscultate the heart for a new or changing murmur. Auscultate the lungs for adventitious breath sounds. Palpate the abdomen for splenomegaly.

LABORATORY AND DIAGNOSTIC TESTS

Diagnosis is usually based on the clinical presentation. Laboratory tests may reveal the following:

- Blood culture: bacteria or fungus
- CBC: anemia, leukocytosis
- Urinalysis: microscopic hematuria
- Echocardiogram: cardiomegaly, abnormal valve function, area of vegetation

Nursing Management

Nursing management focuses on maintaining IV access for at least 4 weeks to appropriately administer the antibiotic or antifungal course of therapy. Monitor the child's temperature and subsequent blood culture results.

Ideally, infective endocarditis in children should be prevented. Children at increased risk for the development of infective endocarditis include those with:

- Prosthetic cardiac valve or prosthetic material used for cardiac valve repair
- Previous endocarditis
- Unrepaired cyanotic CHD
- Completely repaired CHD with prosthetic material or device within the first 6 months after the procedure
- Repaired CHD with residual defects at the site or adjacent to the site of a prosthetic patch or prosthetic device
- Cardiac transplantation recipients who develop cardiac valve abnormalities (AHA, 2021)

Children at high risk should practice good oral hygiene, including regular toothbrushing and flossing. Instruct parents or the older child to carry emergency medical identification at all times (wallet card is available from the AHA). The card may be presented to any health care provider or nurse practitioner and includes the recommended antibiotic prophylactic regimen (AHA, 2024a). Instruct the parents to notify the primary care provider or cardiologist if the child develops flu-like symptoms or a fever.

High-risk children (as noted previously) who are undergoing dental procedures should receive prophylaxis as recommended by the AHA. Antibiotics typically used for prophylaxis may include ampicillin, amoxicillin, gentamicin, or vancomycin.

Acute Rheumatic Fever

Acute rheumatic fever (ARF) is a delayed sequela of group A streptococcal pharyngeal infection. In the United States, this disease occurs more often in school-age children between 5 and 15 years of age in areas where streptococcal pharyngitis is more prevalent, especially during the colder months. It usually develops 2 to 4 weeks after the initial streptococcal infection. Current understanding of the disease process of ARF is that the child develops an antibody response to surface proteins of the bacteria. The antibodies then cross-react with antigens in cardiac muscle and neuronal and synovial tissues, causing carditis, arthritis, and chorea (involuntary random, jerking movements). ARF affects the joints, central nervous system, skin, and subcutaneous tissue and causes chronic, progressive damage to the heart and valves. Most episodes of ARF resolve, but rheumatic fever may recur with subsequent streptococcal infections (Jone et al., 2022).

Diagnosis of ARF is based on the modified Jones criteria (Box 19.3). Therapeutic management is directed toward managing inflammation and fever, eradicating the bacteria, preventing permanent heart damage, and preventing recurrences. A full 10-day course of penicillin therapy (or equivalent) is used along with corticosteroids and nonsteroidal antiinflammatory drugs. Children without valvular disease will receive continued prophylaxis with monthly intramuscular injections of penicillin G benzathine or daily oral doses of penicillin or erythromycin following the initial illness to prevent a new streptococcal infection and recurrent ARF. Prophylaxis is usually continued until age 21 years (Jone et al., 2022).

Nursing Assessment

Elicit a description of the present illness and chief complaint, noting fever and joint pain. Explore the child's recent medical history for risk factors, such as documented streptococcal infection or sore throat within the past 2 to 3 weeks, or for history of ARF. Observe the child for Sydenham chorea, a movement disorder of the face and upper extremities. Inspect the skin for evidence of the classic rash, erythema marginatum, a maculopapular red rash with central clearing and elevated edges. Auscultate the heart, noting a murmur. Palpate the surfaces of the wrist, elbows, and knees for firm, painless, subcutaneous nodules. Note prolonged PR interval on the ECG. Throat culture will provide definitive diagnosis of current streptococcal infection, while streptococcal antibody tests may yield evidence of recent infection. Echocardiogram is required to determine if carditis is present.

Nursing Management

Nursing management of the child with ARF focuses on ensuring compliance with the acute course of antibiotics

BOX 19.3 Modified Jones Criteria

Diagnosis of ARF requires the presence of either two major criteria or one major plus two minor criteria.

Major Criteria

- Carditis
- Migratory polyarthritis
- Subcutaneous nodules
- Erythema marginatum
- Sydenham chorea

Minor Criteria

- Polyarthralgia
- Elevated ESR or CRP
- Prolonged PR interval (unless carditis is a major criterion)

ARF, acute rheumatic fever; CRP, C-reactive protein; ESR, erythrocyte sedimentation

Data from Jone, P.-N., Kim, J. S., Burkett, D., Jacobsen, R., & VonAlvensleben, J. (2022). Cardiovascular diseases. In M. Bunik, W. W. Hay, M. J. Levin, & M. J. Abzug (Eds.), *Current diagnosis and treatment: Pediatrics* (26th ed.). McGraw-Hill Education.

as well as prophylaxis following initial recovery from ARF. Allow the child to verbalize the frustration they may be feeling in relation to chorea symptoms. Offer support for dealing with the abnormal movements. Educate the child and others that the sudden jerky movements of chorea will eventually disappear, although they may last as long as several months. Some children may require a neuroleptic agent such as haloperidol (Haldol) for management of chorea. Administer corticosteroids or nonsteroidal antiinflammatory agents for control of joint pain and swelling.

Cardiomyopathy

Cardiomyopathy is a condition in which the myocardium cannot contract properly. The incidence of cardiomyopathy among children is increasing; it occurs at a rate of one per 100,000 (AHA, 2024b). Cardiomyopathy may occur in children with genetic disorders or CHDs, as a result of an inflammatory or infectious process or hypertension, or after cardiac transplantation or surgery, but most commonly, it is idiopathic. Cardiomyopathy occurs predominantly in clusters in infancy and adolescence. Three types of cardiomyopathy exist—restrictive, dilated, and hypertrophic. Restrictive cardiomyopathy is rare in children and results in atrial relaxation. Dilated cardiomyopathy is the most common type in childhood and may result in heart failure (it may be their presentation) because of ventricular dilation with decreased contractility (Jone et al., 2022). There is also some familial tendency toward dilated cardiomyopathy (Cooper, 2022). Hypertrophic cardiomyopathy is more common in adolescence and results in hypertrophy of the heart muscle, particularly the left ventricle, affecting the heart's ability to fill. About two-thirds of all cases of hypertrophic cardiomyopathy are familial, with some inherited in an autosomal dominant fashion (Cooper, 2022).

There is no cure for cardiomyopathy, meaning that currently, heart muscle function cannot be restored. Therapeutic management is directed toward improving heart function and BP. Mechanical ventilation and vasoactive medications are needed in many children. ACE inhibitors, beta-blockers, or calcium channel blockers may be used. Pacemakers or surgery may be helpful in some children. For children in whom medical management is unsuccessful, heart transplantation is the only viable long-term treatment option (Jone et al., 2022).

Nursing Assessment

Explore the health history for risk factors such as:

- CHD, cardiac transplantation, or surgery
- Duchenne or Becker muscular dystrophy
- History of myocarditis, HIV infection, or Kawasaki disease
- Hypertension
- Drugs, alcohol, or radiation exposure
- Connective tissue, autoimmune, or endocrine disease
- Maternal diabetes
- Familial history of sudden death

Inquire about a history of respiratory distress, fatigue, poor growth (dilated), chest pain, dizziness, or syncope (hypertrophic). Observe the child for extremity edema and abdominal distention. Note increased work of breathing. Auscultate the heart, noting tachycardia and irregular rhythm. Evaluate heart rhythm via ECG, noting dysrhythmias or indications of left ventricular hypertrophy.

Chest radiography may reveal cardiomegaly or congested lungs. Echocardiogram demonstrates increased heart size, poor contractility, decreased ejection fraction, or asymmetric septal hypertrophy. Cardiac catheterization is usually performed to aid in the diagnosis.

Nursing Management

Many children with cardiomyopathy require intensive care initially. Monitor for complications such as blood clots or arrhythmias, which could lead to cardiac arrest. Refer to the previous section on heart failure for nursing interventions related to heart failure, which may be present with dilated cardiomyopathy. Administer vasoactive and other medications as prescribed, monitoring the child closely for response to these therapies as well as for complications. Support the child in choosing activities that fit within the prescribed restrictions. Provide extensive emotional support to the child and family, who may experience significant stress as they realize the severity of this illness.

Hypertension

Hypertension has seen a rise in prevalence among children and adolescents. It has been found to be independently associated with body mass index and waist circumference. Childhood or adolescent hypertension often leads to long-term health consequences such as cardiovascular disease and left ventricular hypertrophy (Mattoo, 2023). In children, acceptable BP values are based on sex, age, and height. For children age 1 to 13 years, stage 1 hypertension is defined as BP persistently greater than or equal to the 95th percentile for sex, age, and height or less than the 95th percentile plus 12 mm Hg (whichever is lower). Stage 2 hypertension in children is identified as BP greater than or equal to the 95th percentile plus 12 mm Hg or 140/90, whichever is lower. For adolescents 13 years and older, stage 1 hypertension is defined as BP 130/80 to 139/89, while stage 2 hypertension is identified as BP greater than or equal to 140/90. The term "elevated blood pressure" refers to BP that is persistently between the 90th and 95th percentiles or 130/80 (whichever is lower) in children up to age 13 years. In adolescents 13 years of age or older, elevated BP refers to systolic blood pressure of 120 to 129, with diastolic BP less than 80. BP is considered normal when the systolic and diastolic values are less than the 90th percentile for sex, age, and height in the child 1 to 13 years of age or less than 120/80 in the adolescent 13 years and older (Flynn et al., 2017).

Childhood hypertension may be further defined as primary or secondary. Primary hypertension in children is found more commonly in non-Hispanic African Americans and children with overweight or obesity (Mattoo, 2023). Secondary hypertension in children most frequently occurs with an underlying medical problem such as kidney or cardiac disease (Mattoo, 2023). Mild to moderate hypertension in childhood is usually asymptomatic and is usually determined only upon BP screening during a well-child visit or during follow-up for known risk factors. Refer to Box 9.5 in Chapter 9 for a synopsis of childhood hypertension guidelines.

It is important to screen for and treat prehypertension and hypertension in children and adolescents, as they are more likely to experience hypertension as adults progressing to further cardiovascular disease (Mattoo, 2021). Therapeutic management depends on the extent of the hypertension and the length of time it has existed. Weight reduction, appropriate diet (including sodium restriction in some children), and increased physical activity are important components of management of prehypertensive and asymptomatic hypertensive children. Some children are candidates for and require antihypertensive medications or diuretics (Mattoo, 2021).

Pathophysiology

The balance between cardiac output and vascular resistance determines the BP. An increase in either of these variables, in the absence of a compensatory decrease in the other, increases the mean BP. Factors regulating cardiac output and vascular resistance include changes in electrolyte balance, particularly sodium, calcium, and potassium.

Nursing Assessment

Nursing assessment consists of the health history, physical examination, and laboratory and diagnostic tests.

HEALTH HISTORY

Elicit the health history, determining the presence of risk factors for hypertension such as:

- Family history
- Obesity
- Hyperlipidemia
- Kidney disease (including frequent urinary tract infections)
- Systemic lupus erythematosus
- CHD
- Neurofibromatosis, Turner syndrome, and other genetic disorders
- Prematurity
- Prolonged neonatal ventilation
- Umbilical artery catheterization
- Diabetes mellitus
- Increased intracranial pressure
- Malignancy
- Solid organ transplant
- Medications known to raise BP

Signs and symptoms reported during the health history might include:

- Growth delays (with certain chronic medical conditions)
- Obesity
- Signs and symptoms seen particularly in older children
- Headache
- Subtle behavioral or school performance changes
- Fatigue
- Blurred vision
- Nosebleed
- Bell palsy

PHYSICAL EXAMINATION

Determine the child's weight and height/length. Plot these growth parameters on the sex-appropriate chart for the child's age. Note the percentile for height/length, as it will be used to determine the BP percentile (see Appendix B, "Blood Pressure Charts for Children and Adolescents"). Measure the BP in all four extremities (to rule out coarctation of the aorta). Ensure that the child is relaxed and sitting or reclined. Refer to Chapter 10 for specific information related to accurate BP measurement in children.

Inspect the skin for:

- Acne, hirsutism, or striae (associated with anabolic steroid use)
- Café-au-lait spots (associated with neurofibromatosis)
- Malar rash (associated with lupus)
- Pallor, diaphoresis, or flushing (associated with pheochromocytoma)

Observe the extremities for edema (kidney disease) or joint swelling (lupus). Inspect the chest for apical heave (ventricular hypertrophy) or wide-spaced nipples (Turner syndrome). Auscultate heart sounds, noting tachycardia (associated with primary hypertension) or murmur (associated with coarctation of the aorta). Palpate the abdomen for a mass or enlarged kidney.

LABORATORY AND DIAGNOSTIC TESTING

Although diagnosis of hypertension is based on BP measurements, additional laboratory or diagnostic tests may be used to evaluate the underlying cause of secondary hypertension, including:

- Urinalysis, blood urea nitrogen, and serum creatinine: may determine the presence of kidney disease
- Renal ultrasound or angiography: may reveal kidney or genitourinary tract abnormalities
- Echocardiogram: may show left ventricular hypertrophy
- Lipid profile: determines the presence of hyperlipidemia

Nursing Management

Salt restriction and potassium or calcium supplements have not been scientifically shown to decrease BP in children. However, children with obesity may benefit from salt restriction, as those children seem to be sensitive to salt intake. Assist the child and family to develop a plan for weight reduction if the child has overweight or obesity. Encourage the child and family to control portion sizes, decrease the intake of sugary beverages and snacks, eat more fresh fruits and vegetables, and eat a healthy breakfast. Consult the nutritionist for additional assistance with meal planning. To increase physical activity, encourage the child to find a sport or type of exercise in which they are interested. Aerobic activities involving running, walking, or cycling are particularly helpful. When a child requires antihypertensive therapy, teach the child and family how to administer the medication. Caution the parents about side effects related to antihypertensives. Teach the parent to measure the child's BP as determined by the health care provider or nurse practitioner, as well as to keep appointments for BP follow-up.

Kawasaki Disease

Kawasaki disease is an acute systemic vasculitis occurring mostly in children 6 months to 5 years of age. It is the leading cause of acquired heart disease among children and in the United States, occurs more than 19 times per year per 100,000 children (Lo et al., 2025). Although Kawasaki disease affects all ethnic groups, it occurs more frequently in those of Asian or Pacific descent. It is a self-limited syndrome but can cause cardiovascular complications, such as coronary artery aneurysm and cardiomyopathy (Lo et al., 2025).

Therapeutic management of acute Kawasaki disease focuses on reducing inflammation in the walls of the coronary arteries and preventing coronary thrombosis. Chronic management of children developing aneurysms during the initial phase is directed toward preventing myocardial ischemia. In the acute phase, high-dose aspirin in four divided doses daily and a single infusion of intravenous immunoglobulin (IVIG) are used (Lo et al., 2025). See Evidence-Based Practice 19.1.

Pathophysiology

Although the etiology is still unknown, current thought is that some infectious organism (as yet unidentified) causes disease in genetically susceptible people. Kawasaki disease appears to be an autoimmune response mediated by cytokine-induced endothelial cell surface antigens that leads to vasculitis in the medium-size arteries, including the coronary arteries. Neutrophils, mononuclear cells, T lymphocytes, and immunoglobulin A–producing plasma cells infiltrate the vessels. Then, elastin and collagen fibers fragment, and the structural integrity of the vessel wall are impaired. Generalized systemic vasculitis occurs in the blood vessels throughout the body due to the inflammation and edema and can lead to coronary dilation or aneurysm. Some children never develop coronary artery changes, while others develop an aneurysm in either the acute phase or as a long-term sequela (Lo et al., 2025).

EVIDENCE-BASED PRACTICE **19.1**

Treating Kawasaki Disease With Intravenous Immunoglobulin (IVIG)

STUDY

Coronary artery abnormalities remain the most serious complication of the acute vasculitis occurring in Kawasaki disease. Historically, IVIG of varying doses and other medications such as aspirin and corticosteroids have been used to reduce the risk of coronary artery anomaly (CAA) development. The study explored the use of IVIG in the acute phase. In their review, the authors included 31 studies with 4,609 participants.

Findings

It was determined that high-dose IVIG provided during the acute phase probably reduced the risk of development of CAA as compared to the use of moderate- or low-dose IVIG, aspirin, or corticosteroids. The occurrence of adverse effects was low for all treatment regimens.

Nursing Implications

The study results are consistent with the current recommendations for treatment of Kawasaki disease. Teach families that administration of IVIG is safe and that it is used to reduce the risk of CAA development. Refer to Chapter 25 for additional information related to IVIG administration.

Based on Broderick, C., Kobayashi, S., Suto, M., Ito, S., & Kobayashi, T. (2023). Intravenous immunoglobulin for the treatment of Kawasaki disease. *Cochrane Database of Systematic Reviews*, *1*, CD014884. https://doi.org/10.1002/14651858.CD014884.pub2

Nursing Assessment

Nursing assessment consists of determining the health history, physical examination, and laboratory and diagnostic testing.

HEALTH HISTORY

Elicit the health history, noting any:

- Fever
- Chills
- Headache
- Malaise
- Extreme irritability
- Vomiting
- Diarrhea
- Abdominal pain
- Joint pain

Of note is a history of high fever (39.9°C [103.8°F]) of at least 5 days' duration that is unresponsive to antibiotics.

PHYSICAL EXAMINATION

Observe for significant bilateral conjunctivitis without exudate. Inspect the mouth and throat for dry, fissured lips; strawberry (cracked and reddened) tongue; and pharyngeal and oral mucosa erythema. Note hyperdynamic precordium. Evaluate the skin for:

- Diffuse, erythematous, polymorphous rash
- Edema of the hands and feet
- Erythema and painful induration of the palms and soles
- Desquamation (peeling) of the perineal region, fingers, and toes, extending to the palms and soles
- Possible jaundice

Palpate the neck for cervical lymphadenopathy (usually unilateral) and the joints for tenderness. Palpate the abdomen for liver enlargement. Auscultate the heart, noting tachycardia, gallop, or murmur.

LABORATORY AND DIAGNOSTIC TESTING

The CBC may reveal mild to moderate anemia, an elevated white blood cell count during the acute phase, and significant thrombocytosis (elevated platelet count [500,000 to 1 million]) in the later phase. The erythrocyte sedimentation rate (ESR) and the C-reactive protein (CRP) level are elevated. Echocardiogram is performed as soon as possible after the diagnosis is confirmed to provide a baseline of a healthy heart or to evaluate for coronary artery involvement. Echocardiograms may be repeated during the illness and as part of long-term follow-up. Occasionally, cardiac involvement warrants cardiac catheterization.

Nursing Management

In addition to the administration of aspirin and immunoglobulin, nursing management of the child with Kawasaki disease focuses on monitoring cardiac status, promoting comfort, and providing family education.

MONITORING CARDIAC STATUS

Administer IV and oral fluids as ordered, evaluating intake and output carefully. Prepare the child for the echocardiogram. Assess frequently for signs of developing heart failure such as tachycardia, gallop, decreased urine output, or respiratory distress. Evaluate quality and strength of pulses. Provide cardiac monitoring as ordered, reporting arrhythmias.

PROMOTING COMFORT

Provide acetaminophen for fever management, and apply cool cloths as tolerated. Keep the environment quiet, and cluster nursing care activities to decrease stimulation and hence irritability. Teach parents that irritability is a prominent feature of Kawasaki disease, and support their efforts to console the child. Apply petrolatum jelly or another lubricating ointment to the lips. Encourage the older child to suck on ice chips; the younger child may suck on a cool, moist washcloth. Popsicles are also soothing. Provide comfortable positioning, particularly if the child has joint pain or arthritis.

PROVIDING CHILD AND FAMILY EDUCATION

Teach parents to continue to monitor the child's temperature after discharge until the child has been afebrile for several days. Children with prolonged or recurrent fever may require a second dose of IVIG. Inform parents that irritability may last for up to 2 months after initial diagnosis with Kawasaki disease. Report any toxic effects of aspirin therapy, such as headache, confusion, dizziness, or tinnitus to the health care provider or nurse practitioner. It is important to avoid nonsteroidal antiinflammatory agents while aspirin therapy is ongoing. For children with continued arthritis (which resolves in several weeks), range-of-motion exercises with a morning bath may help to decrease stiffness. Instruct parents to avoid measles and varicella vaccination for 11 months after high-dose IVIG administration. It is critical that the family comply with regularly scheduled cardiology follow-up appointments to determine development or progression of coronary artery ectasia or aneurysm. If the child has severe cardiac involvement, teach the parents about infant and/or child cardiopulmonary resuscitation before discharge from the hospital.

Dyslipidemia

Dyslipidemia refers to high levels of lipids (fats/cholesterol) in the blood. High lipid levels are a risk factor for the development of atherosclerosis, which can result in coronary artery disease, a serious cardiovascular disorder occurring in adults. Children with high lipid levels, although remaining asymptomatic, are likely to have high levels as adults, which increases their risk for coronary artery disease. Therefore, detection, screening, and early intervention are important, especially if there is a family tendency toward heart disease (de Ferranti & Newburger, 2023b).

Pathophysiology

Cholesterol is a building block for hormones and cell membranes. It occurs naturally in foods derived from animals such as eggs, dairy products, meat, poultry, and seafood. Cholesterol is also manufactured in the body. Together, cholesterol and triglycerides are known as lipids. Very low–density lipoprotein (VLDL) is a lipoprotein composed mainly of triglycerides with only small amounts of cholesterol, phospholipid, and protein. VLDLs are easily converted to low-density lipoproteins (LDLs). Cholesterol is expressed in terms of LDL cholesterol or high-density lipoprotein (HDL) cholesterol. LDLs contain relatively more cholesterol and triglycerides than they do protein. HDLs contain about 50% protein, with the rest being cholesterol, triglyceride, and phospholipid. High levels of cholesterol and triglycerides place a person at risk for atherosclerosis. Elevated VLDL and LDL levels and decreased HDL levels produce a particular increase in the risk for atherosclerosis (de Ferranti & Newburger, 2023b).

Therapeutic Management

Screening children for hyperlipidemia is of prime importance for early detection, intervention, and subsequent prevention of adult atherosclerosis. The American Academy of Pediatrics recommends universal screening for dyslipidemia between 9 and 11 years of age and again between 18 and 21 years of age (Hagan et al., 2017). Performing a risk assessment screening at 24 months and at 4, 6, 8, and 12 through 17 years of age is also recommended. Selectively screening children at high risk for hyperlipidemia can reduce their lifelong risk of coronary artery disease. The risk assessment focuses on the child's family history. Screen if parents, grandparents, aunts and uncles, or siblings, have or have had documented:

- Coronary atherosclerosis
- Myocardial infarction
- Angina pectoris
- Peripheral vascular disease
- Cerebrovascular disease/stroke
- Coronary artery bypass graft/stent/angioplasty at less than 55 years of age in males and less than 65 years in females
- Sudden cardiac death
- Blood cholesterol level of 240 mg/dL or higher

The child should be screened at the health care provider's discretion if the parental history is unobtainable, the child has diabetes or hypertension, or the child has any lifestyle risk factors (cigarette smoking, obesity, sedentary lifestyle, or high-fat dietary intake) (de Ferranti & Newburger, 2023b).

All children should eat a diet with the appropriate amount of fats (see the section on nursing management further on) and should participate in physical activity. When diet and exercise are not enough to lower cholesterol to appropriate levels, medications such as statins may be used (Jone et al., 2022).

Nursing Assessment

Elicit the health history, noting risk factors such as family history of hyperlipidemia, early heart disease, hypertension, diabetes or other endocrine abnormality, cerebral vascular accident, or sudden death. Note prior lipid levels if available. Measure the child's height and weight, plotting them on standardized growth charts. Note if the child has overweight or obesity, as these are risk factors associated with hyperlipidemia. Typically, there are no other particular physical findings associated with hyperlipidemia. Table 19.3 gives details about the interpretation of cholesterol levels.

Nursing Management

Instruct families that the child must fast for 12 hours before lipid screening (initially and on follow-up samples). Dietary management is the first step in the prevention and management of hyperlipidemia in children older than 2 years. The diet should consist primarily of fruits, vegetables, low-fat dairy products, whole grains, beans, lean meat, poultry, and fish. As in adults, fat should account for no more than 30% of daily caloric intake. Fat intake may vary over a period of days, as many young children are picky eaters. Limit saturated fats by choosing lean meats; removing skin from poultry before cooking; and avoiding palm, palm kernel, and coconut oils as well as hydrogenated fats. Teach families to read nutrition labels to determine the content of the food. Limit intake of processed or refined foods as well as high-sugar drinks; these products provide minimal nutrition and significant

TABLE 19.3 • Interpretation of Cholesterol Levels for Children and Adolescents

Total Cholesterol (mg/dL)	Interpretation	LDL (mg/dL)	Interpretation	HDL (mg/dL)	Interpretation
<170	Desirable	<110	Optimal	35	Desirable
170–199	Borderline			110–129	Borderline
≥200	High			>130	High

HDL, high-density lipoprotein; LDL, low-density lipoprotein

Data from de Ferranti, S. D., & Newburger, J. W. (2023b). Dyslipidemia in children and adolescents: Definition, screening, and diagnosis. *UpToDate*. Retrieved January 12, 2024, from https://www.uptodate.com/contents/dyslipidemia-in-children-and-adolescents-definition-screening-and-diagnosis

calories. Children 5 to 10 years of age need vigorous play or physical activity for 1 hour per day, three times per week, while children older than 10 years of age should participate in vigorous activity 60 minutes daily (de Ferranti & Newburger, 2023a). Refer parents to "Healthy Habits for Healthy Kids—A Nutrition and Activity Guide for Parents" published by the American Dietetic Association and available at http://www.clocc.net/wp-content/uploads/Healthy_Habits_Healthy_Kids.pdf.

If medications are required, teach the child and family about the dose, administration, and possible adverse effects. Assist the family to develop a medication-dosing plan that is compatible with school and work schedules to increase compliance.

HEART TRANSPLANTATION

Heart transplantation is indicated in children with inoperable CHD or with end-stage heart disease related to cardiomyopathy or palliated CHD. Worldwide, 600 to 700 children receive a heart transplant each year (Bock & Chinnock, 2022). The 5-year survival rate is greater than 70%, and 20-year survival has been achieved in some instances (Bock & Chinnock, 2022).

A comprehensive evaluation is performed to determine whether the child is a candidate for heart transplant. The evaluation includes:

- Chest radiograph, ECG, echocardiogram, exercise stress test, cardiac catheterization, and pulmonary function tests
- CBC with differential, prothrombin and partial thromboplastin time, serum chemistries and electrolytes, blood urea nitrogen, and creatinine
- Urinalysis and urine creatinine clearance
- Blood, throat, urine, stool, and sputum cultures for bacteria, viruses, fungi, and parasites
- Epstein–Barr virus, cytomegalovirus, varicella, herpes, hepatitis, and HIV titers
- Human leukocyte antigen (HLA) typing and panel reactive antibody typing and titer
- Computed tomography or MRI scan and electroencephalogram
- Consults with neurology, psychology, genetics, social work, nutritionist, physical and occupational therapy, and financial coordinator or case manager (Bock & Chinnock, 2022)

Children with irreversible lung, liver, kidney, or central nervous system disease; recent malignancy (past 5 years); or chronic viral infection may be excluded as candidates.

Once candidacy is determined, the transplant center registers the child as a potential recipient with the United Network for Organ Sharing (UNOS). Blood type, body size, length of time on the waiting list, and medical urgency are used to evaluate compatibility. Children awaiting transplantation may need continuous or intermittent hospitalization. Coordination of organ procurement and the transplantation procedure is essential.

Surgical Procedure and Postoperative Therapeutic Management

Most transplantation procedures are **orthotopic**, which means that the recipient's heart is removed and the donor heart is implanted in its place in the normal anatomic position. Cardiopulmonary bypass and hypothermia are used to maintain circulation, protect the brain, and oxygenate the recipient during the procedure. Postoperatively, the child may have near-normal heart function and capacity for exercise and may be able to return to school.

Immunosuppressive therapy is necessary for the rest of the child's life to avoid rejection of the transplanted heart. Usually, a three-drug regimen is used that includes calcineurin inhibitors (cyclosporine, tacrolimus), cell toxins (mycophenolate mofetil, azathioprine), and corticosteroids. The cardiologist and transplant surgeon provide ongoing follow-up. Complications of heart transplantation include infection, pulmonary hypertension, arrhythmia, heart failure, hypertension, kidney dysfunction, and organ rejection. Neoplasm may occur as a result of chronic immunosuppression.

Nursing Management

Preoperative nursing care for the child undergoing a heart transplant is similar for children undergoing other types of heart surgery. In addition, the nurse should assist with the comprehensive pretransplant evaluation. Care for the child in the posttransplant period is intense and complex. Evaluate the family's ability to perform the tasks that will be necessary. Teach families about the evaluation and transplantation process, as well as the waiting period. In the immediate preoperative period, perform a thorough history and physical examination, and obtain last-minute blood work. Provide preoperative teaching similar to other cardiac surgeries. Older children, adolescents, and parents may enjoy the book *Future Conditional* by J. Hatton (1996, Yorkshire Art Circus), which was written by one of the first heart transplant survivors.

Postoperatively, provide frequent assessments and routine care for children who have had cardiac surgery. In addition, monitor the child closely for infection or signs of rejection. Acute rejection may be indicated by low-grade fever, fatigue, tachycardia, nausea, vomiting, abdominal pain, and decreased activity tolerance, although some children will be asymptomatic. Maintain strict handwashing techniques and isolate the child from other children with infections. Although live vaccines are contraindicated in children with immunosuppression, inactivated vaccines should be given as recommended (CDC, 2020). Teach children and families that the child may return to school and usual activities about 3 months after the transplant. Provide emotional support to the child related to body image changes such as hair growth, gum hyperplasia, weight gain, moon facies, acne, and rashes that occur due to long-term immunosuppressive therapy.

KEY CONCEPTS

- At birth, when the umbilical cord is cut and the neonate's first breath occurs, the ductus venosus closes with the foramen ovale, and the ductus arteriosus closes shortly thereafter. Pulmonary vascular resistance decreases, and systemic vascular resistance increases.
- The infant's heart rate averages 120 to 130 bpm and decreases throughout childhood, reaching the adult rate in adolescence. Conversely, the infant's and child's BP is significantly lower than the adult's, increasing as the child ages.
- Check the infant's apical pulse prior to digoxin administration, and hold the dose if the heart rate is less than 90.
- Poor weight gain, failure to thrive, and increased fatigability commonly occur with congestive heart failure.
- Clubbing of the fingernails occurs because of chronic hypoxia in the child with severe CHD.
- Children with cardiac conditions resulting in cyanosis often have baseline oxygen saturations that are relatively low, because of the mixing of oxygenated with deoxygenated blood.
- Document the presence of a murmur by grading its intensity (I through IV), describing where it occurs within the cardiac cycle, and noting the location where the murmur is best heard.
- CHD should be suspected in the cyanotic newborn who does not improve with oxygen administration.
- Cardiac catheterization postprocedure care focuses on evaluation of the child's vital signs and condition of the pressure dressing, as well as assessment of the distal pulses bilaterally for presence and quality.
- Congenital heart disorders resulting in decreased pulmonary blood flow (tetralogy of Fallot, tricuspid atresia) result in cyanosis.
- Disorders with increased pulmonary blood flow (PDA, ASD, and VSD) may result in pulmonary edema if the defect is severe.
- A decrease in the lower extremity pulses or BP as compared with the upper extremities may be indicative of coarctation of the aorta.
- It is important to remain calm when an infant or child demonstrates a hypercyanotic spell. Place the child in a knee-chest position, administer oxygen and/or morphine or propranolol, and supply IV fluids.
- Children with certain CHDs and/or heart failure require additional calories to display adequate growth.
- Children with hypertrophic cardiomyopathy, certain CHDs, valve dysfunction, or prosthetic valves require prophylaxis for infective endocarditis when undergoing procedures or invasive dental work.
- Hypertension in the child or adolescent often leads to long-term health consequences such as cardiovascular disease and left ventricular hypertrophy.
- Kawasaki disease may result in severe cardiac sequelae, so these children need ongoing cardiac follow-up to screen for development of problems.
- It is important to screen for hyperlipidemia in high-risk children.
- Abrupt cessation of chest tube output, accompanied by an increase in the heart rate and increased filling pressure, may indicate cardiac tamponade.

REFERENCES AND RECOMMENDED READINGS

Abbott. (2023). *Amplatzer septal occluder*. https://www.myamplatzer.com/hcp/congenital-heart-defect-solutions/ventricular-septal-defects-vsd/

Altman, C. A. (2022). Identifying newborns with critical congenital heart disease. *UpToDate*. Retrieved January 12, 2024, from http://www.uptodate.com/contents/identifying-newborns-with-critical-congenital-heart-disease

American Heart Association. (2021). *Infective endocarditis*. https://www.heart.org/en/health-topics/infective-endocarditis

American Heart Association. (2022). *Understand your risk for congenital heart defects*. https://www.heart.org/en/health-topics/congenital-heart-defects/understand-your-risk-for-congenital-heart-defects

American Heart Association. (2024a). *Infective endocarditis wallet card*. https://www.heart.org/en/health-topics/consumer-healthcare/order-american-heart-association-educational-brochures/infective-bacterial-endocarditis-wallet-card

American Heart Association. (2024b). *Pediatric cardiomyopathies*. https://www.heart.org/en/health-topics/cardiomyopathy/pediatric-cardiomyopathies

Beke, D., Jowa, M., & Rummell, M. (2021). *Nurse curriculum*. The Pediatric Cardiac Intensive Care Society.

Bock, M., & Chinnock, R. E. (2022). Pediatric heart transplantation. *Medscape*. Retrieved March 31, 2023, from http://emedicine.medscape.com/article/1011927-overview

Broderick, C., Kobayashi, S., Suto, M., Ito, S., & Kobayashi, T. (2023). Intravenous immunoglobulin for the treatment of Kawasaki disease. *Cochrane Database of Systematic Reviews*, *1*, CD014884. https://doi.org/10.1002/14651858.CD014884.pub2

Centers for Disease Control and Prevention. (2020). *Who should not get vaccinated with these vaccines?* https://www.cdc.gov/vaccines/vpd/should-not-vacc.html

Centers for Disease Control and Prevention. (2022). *Long term outcomes in children with congenital heart disease*. https://www.cdc.gov/ncbddd/heartdefects/features/keyfinding-chd-longterm-outcomes.html

Children's Hospital of Wisconsin. (2024). *Living with a pediatric pacemaker*. https://childrenswi.org/medical-care/herma-heart/conditions/living-with-a-pacemaker

Cleveland Clinic. (2023). *Cardiac closure devices*. https://my.clevelandclinic.org/health/treatments/16838-cardiac-implant-closure-devices-in-adults

Cooper, L. T. (2022). Definition and classification of the cardiomyopathies. *UpToDate*. Retrieved January 12, 2024, from https://www.uptodate.com/contents/definition-and-classification-of-the-cardiomyopathies

Corbett, J. A., & Banks, A. D. (2019). *Laboratory tests and diagnostic procedures with nursing diagnoses* (9th ed.). Pearson Education Inc.

Cunningham, F. G., Leveno, S. L., Dashe, J. S., Hoffman, B. L., Spong, C. Y., & Casey, B. M. (2022). *Williams obstetrics* (26th ed.). McGraw-Hill Education.

de Ferranti, S. D., & Newburger, J. W. (2023a). Dyslipidemia in children and adolescents: Management. *UpToDate*. Retrieved January 12, 2024, from https://www.uptodate.com/contents/dyslipidemia-in-children-and-adolescents-management

de Ferranti, S. D., & Newburger, J. W. (2023b). Dyslipidemia in children and adolescents: Definition, screening, and diagnosis. *UpToDate*. Retrieved January 12, 2024, from https://www.uptodate.com/contents/dyslipidemia-in-children-and-adolescents-definition-screening-and-diagnosis

Doyle, T., & Kavanaugh-McHugh, A. (2023). Management and outcome of tetralogy of Fallot. *UpToDate*. Retrieved January 12, 2024, from http://www.uptodate.com/contents/management-and-outcome-of-tetralogy-of-fallot

Driscoll, D. (2022). History and physical examination. In R. E. Shaddy, D. J. Penny, T. F. Feltes, F. Cetta, & S. Mital (Eds.), *Moss and Adams' heart disease in infants, children, and adolescents: Including the fetus and young adult* (10th ed., pp. 243-250). Wolters Kluwer Health.

Fleitman, J. (2023). Postoperative complications among patients undergoing cardiac surgery. *UpToDate*. Retrieved January 12, 2024, from https://www.uptodate.com/contents/postoperative-complications-among-patients-undergoing-cardiac-surgery

Flynn, J. T., Kaelber, D. C., Baker-Smith, C. M., Blowey, D., Carroll, A. E., Daniels, S. R., de Ferranti, S. D., Dionne, J. M., Falkner, B., Flinn, S. K., Gidding, S. S., Goodwin, C., Leu, M. G., Powers, M. E., Rea, C., Samuels, J., Simasek, M., Thaker, V. V., Urbina E. M., & the Subcommittee on Screening and Management of High Blood Pressure in Children. (2017). Clinical practice guideline for screening and management of high blood pressure in children and adolescents. *Pediatrics*, *140*(3), e20171904. https://doi.org/10.1542/peds.2017-1904

Gaskin, K., & Kennedy, F. (2019). Care of infants, children and adults with congenital heart disease. *Nursing Standard*, *34*(8), 37–42. https://doi.org/10.7748/ns.2019.e11405

Hagan, J. F., Shaw, J. S., & Duncan, P. M. (Eds.). (2017). *Bright futures: Guidelines for health supervision of infants, children, and adolescents* (4th ed.). American Academy of Pediatrics.

Hueckel, R. M. (2019). Pediatric patient with congenital heart disease. *Journal for Nurse Practitioners*, *15*(1), 118–124. https://doi.org/10.1016/j.nurpra.2018.10.017

Jone, P.-N., Kim, J. S., Burkett, D., Jacobsen, R., & VonAlvensleben, J. (2022). Cardiovascular diseases. In M. Bunik, W. W. Hay, M. J. Levin, & M. J. Abzug (Eds.), *Current diagnosis and treatment: Pediatrics* (26th ed., pp. 541-604). McGraw-Hill Education.

KidsHealth Medical Experts. (2023). *Cardiac catheterization*. https://kidshealth.org/en/parents/cardiac-catheter.html

Kimberlin, D. W., Barnett, E. D., Lynfield, R., & Sawyer, M. H. (Eds.). (2021). *Red book 2021-2024: Report of the committee on infectious diseases* (32nd ed.). American Academy of Pediatrics.

Kleinman, K., McDaniel, L., & Malloy, M. (2021). *The Harriet Lane handbook* (22nd ed.). Elsevier.

Kusumoto, F. M. (2019). Cardiovascular disorders: Heart disease. In G. D. Hammer & S. J. McPhee (Eds.), *Pathophysiology of disease: An introduction to clinical medicine* (8th ed.). McGraw-Hill Education.

Lo, M. S., Son, M. B. F., & Newburger, J. W. (2025). Chapter 208: Kawasaki disease. In R. M. Kliegman, J. W. St Geme, N. J. Blum, R. C. Tasker, K. M. Wilson, A. M. Schuh, & C. L. Mack, *Nelson textbook of pediatrics* (22nd ed., pp. 1540-1548). Elsevier.

Mattoo, T. K. (2021). Nonemergent treatment of hypertension in children and adolescents. *UpToDate*. Retrieved January 12, 2024, from https://www.uptodate.com/contents/nonemergent-treatment-of-hypertension-in-children-and-adolescents

Mattoo, T. K. (2023). Epidemiology, risk factors, and etiology of hypertension in children and adolescents. *UpToDate*. Retrieved January 12, 2024, from http://www.uptodate.com/contents/epidemiology-risk-factors-and-etiology-of-hypertension-in-children-and-adolescents

Nees, S. N., & Chung, W. K. (2020). Genetic basis of human congenital heart disease. *Cold Spring Harbor Perspectives in Biology*, *12*(9), a036749. https://doi.org/10.1101/cshperspect.a036749

O'Brien, S. E. (2023). Infective endocarditis in children. *UpToDate*. Retrieved January 12, 2024, from https://www.uptodate.com/contents/infective-endocarditis-in-children

Oster, M. (2023). Newborn screening for critical congenital heart disease using pulse oximetry. *UpToDate*. Retrieved January 12, 2024, from https://www.uptodate.com/contents/newborn-screening-for-critical-congenital-heart-disease-using-pulse-oximetry

Peng, L. F. (2022). Pulmonic stenosis in infants and children: Clinical manifestations and diagnosis. *UpToDate*. Retrieved January 12, 2024, from https://www.uptodate.com/contents/pulmonic-stenosis-in-infants-and-children-clinical-manifestations-and-diagnosis

Schneider, D. S. (2023). The cardiovascular system. In K. J. Marcdante & R. M. Kliegman (Eds.), *Nelson's essentials of pediatrics* (9th ed.). Elsevier.

Singh, R. K., & Singh, T. P. (2022). Heart failure in children: Etiology, clinical manifestations, and diagnosis. *UpToDate*. Retrieved January 12, 2024, from https://www.uptodate.com/contents/heart-failure-in-children-etiology-clinical-manifestations-and-diagnosis

Soriano, B. D., & Fulton, D. R. (2022). Total anomalous pulmonary venous connection. *UpToDate*. Retrieved January 12, 2024, from https://www.uptodate.com/contents/total-anomalous-pulmonary-venous-connection

UCSF Benioff Children's Hospital. (2024). *Cardiac catheterization*. https://www.ucsfbenioffchildrens.org/education/cardiac_catheterization/

University of Pittsburgh Medical Center. (2024). *Heart catheterization*. https://www.chp.edu/our-services/heart/patient-procedures/catheterization

UpToDate, Inc. (2024). *UpToDate® Lexidrug™* (Version 8.2.0) [Mobile app]. Wolters Kluwer. https://apps.apple.com/us/app/lexicomp/id313401238

Weiner, G. M., Zaichkin, J., Kattwinkel, J., Byrne, B., Escobedo, M., Finan, E., Foglia, E., Goldsmith, J., Gupta, A., Halamek, L. P., Illuzi, J., Kapadia, V., Lakshminrusimha, S., Lee, H. C., Leone, T., Perlman, J. M., Rhein, M. D., Sawyer, T., Strand, M. L., … Olech Smith, M. J. (2021). *Textbook of neonatal resuscitation* (8th ed.). American Academy of Pediatrics.

DEVELOPING CLINICAL JUDGMENT

PRACTICING FOR NCLEX

1. The nurse is caring for a 5-year-old child with a congenital heart anomaly causing chronic cyanosis. When performing the history and physical examination, what is the nurse least likely to assess?
   a. Obesity from overeating
   b. Clubbing of the nail beds
   c. Squatting during play activities
   d. Exercise intolerance
2. A 2-day-old infant was just diagnosed with aortic stenosis. What is the most likely nursing assessment finding?
   a. Gallop and rales
   b. Blood pressure discrepancies in the extremities
   c. Right ventricular hypertrophy on ECG
   d. Heart murmur
3. Sam, age 11, has a diagnosis of rheumatic fever and has missed school for a week. What is the most likely cause of this problem?
   a. Previous streptococcal throat infection
   b. History of open heart surgery at 5 years of age
   c. Playing too much soccer and not getting enough rest
   d. Exposure to a sibling with pneumonia
4. The nurse is caring for a child after a cardiac catheterization. What is the nursing priority?
   a. Allow early ambulation to encourage activity participation.
   b. Check pulses above the catheter insertion site for strength and quality.
   c. Assess extremity distal to the insertion site for temperature and color.
   d. Change the dressing to evaluate the site for infection.
5. While assessing a 4-month-old infant, the nurse notes that the baby experiences a hypercyanotic spell. What is the priority nursing action?
   a. Provide supplemental oxygen by face mask.
   b. Administer a dose of IV morphine sulfate.
   c. Begin cardiopulmonary resuscitation.
   d. Place the infant in a knee-to-chest position.
6. The nurse is providing discharge instructions to the parent of a 2-month-old infant who has been prescribed digoxin to be administered every 12 hours orally. Which instructions should the nurse include in the discharge instructions? Select three items.
   a. Notify the health care provider or nurse practitioner if more than two consecutive doses are missed.
   b. Mix the medication with a small amount of formula or breast milk.
   c. If the infant demonstrates poor feeding or vomiting, notify the health care provider or nurse practitioner.
   d. If the child vomits immediately after administration, repeat the dose.
   e. As soon as it is noted that a dose has been missed, give the medication.
   f. Always give the medication at regular intervals.
7. An adolescent patient was admitted with a sore throat, a red rash on the trunk, swollen and painful joints, and aimless movements of the extremities. The diagnosis of ARF is made.

Vital Signs

Time	Temperature	Apical Heart Rate	Respiratory Rate	Blood Pressure
0800	38.0°C	94	22	110/80
1200	37.1°C	142	24	120/84

   What should the nurse do first?
   a. Administer prescribed acetaminophen.
   b. Apply moisturizer to the adolescent's rash.
   c. Notify the health care provider or nurse practitioner of the vital signs change.
   d. Splint the affected joints to relieve pain.

DOSAGE CALCULATION QUESTION

The nurse is caring for an infant with a VSD who has heart failure. The infant weighs 11 lb. The medication order reads: spironolactone 5 mg PO every 12 hours. Spironolactone is provided by the pharmacy in a solution of 2.5 mg/1 mL. How many milliliters will the nurse administer? Round to the nearest whole number.

CRITICAL THINKING EXERCISES

1. A baby was born at 26 weeks' gestation to 15-year-old parents with substance use disorder. The infant weighed 1.5 kg at birth and was diagnosed with AV canal defect and Down syndrome. Discuss some of the major issues in planning for care. Include a care plan and a list of teaching needs for the family.
2. A 4-year-old has parents with less than a high school education, and the child has Medicaid coverage. Another child is 7 years old and has parents with advanced degrees and private insurance coverage. Both children need a heart transplant, and a heart is available that is a good match for both children. Discuss some of the issues involved in deciding which child should receive the heart.
3. A 13-year-old was diagnosed with hypertension more than 2 years ago. He is nonadherent to his antihypertensive medication regimen.

He is 5 ft tall and weighs 170 lb. His favorite activity is video games. Develop a teaching plan for this adolescent, providing creative approaches at the appropriate developmental level.

STUDY ACTIVITIES

1. Teach a class of sixth graders about healthy activities to prevent high cholesterol levels, hypertension, and heart disease. Use visual materials.
2. Spend the day with a nurse practitioner in the pediatric cardiology clinic. Report to the clinical group your observations about the children's quality of life, growth, and development.
3. Observe in the pediatric cardiothoracic intensive care unit or telemetry unit. Note the different cardiac rhythms displayed by children with a variety of cardiovascular disorders.

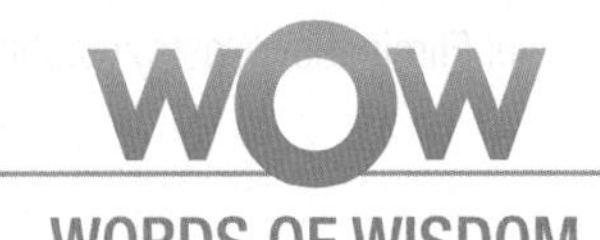

WORDS OF WISDOM

Children instinctively eat to live, and the nurse can help them devour the joys that life brings.

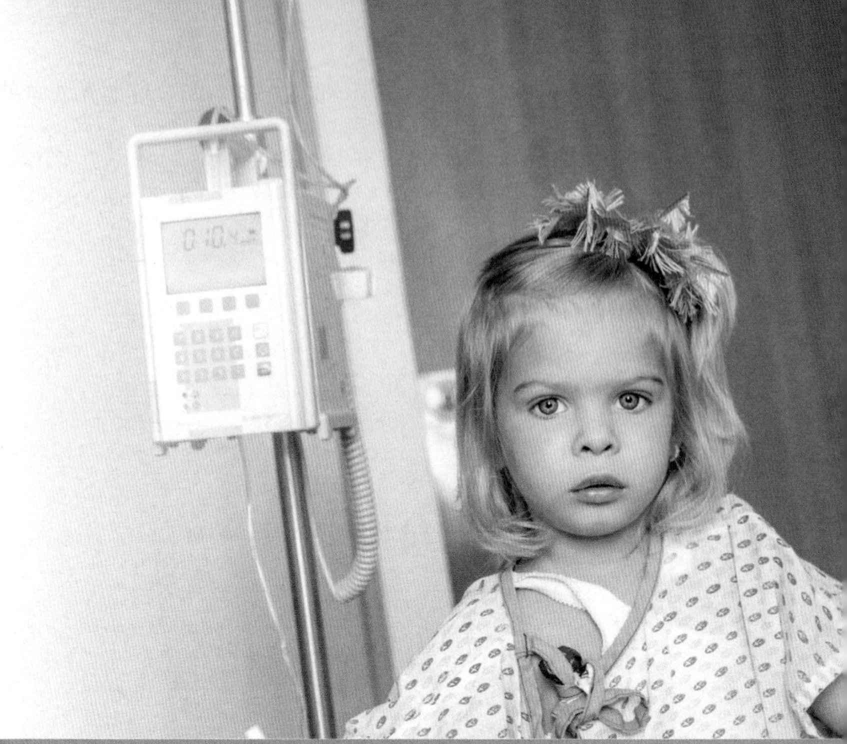

20

Nursing Care of the Child With an Alteration in Bowel Elimination/ Gastrointestinal Disorder

KEY TERMS

cholestasis (kōl′ĕ-stā′sis)
dysphagia (dis-fā′zē-ă)
fecal impaction
guarding
icteric (ik-ter′ik)
lethargy
protuberant
rebound tenderness
regurgitation
steatorrhea (stē′ă-tŏr-ē′ă)

LEARNING OBJECTIVES

Upon completion of the chapter, you will be able to:

1. Compare the differences in the anatomy and physiology of the gastrointestinal system between children and adults.
2. Discuss common medical treatments for infants and children with alterations in bowel elimination (gastrointestinal disorders).
3. Distinguish common laboratory and diagnostic tests used to identify disorders of the gastrointestinal tract.
4. Discuss medication therapy used in infants and children with alterations in bowel elimination (gastrointestinal disorders).
5. Recognize risk factors associated with various gastrointestinal illnesses.
6. Differentiate between acute and chronic gastrointestinal disorders.
7. Distinguish common gastrointestinal illnesses of childhood.
8. Discuss nursing interventions commonly used for gastrointestinal illnesses.
9. Devise an individualized nursing care plan or concept map for the infant or child with an alteration in bowel elimination or gastrointestinal disorder.
10. Develop teaching plans for family and child education for children with gastrointestinal illnesses.
11. Describe the psychosocial impact that chronic gastrointestinal illnesses have on children.

Ethan Richardson, 2 months old, is brought to the clinic by his parent. He has been vomiting for the past 3 days. His parent states that they switched formula to see if that would help, but the vomiting worsened. Since last night they have attempted to feed him only Pedialyte. Ethan's parent says, "He can't keep anything down and he's very irritable." His weight at birth was 8 lb 9 oz, length 21 in, and head circumference 37 cm. At his 2-month checkup last week he weighed 13 lb.

INTRODUCTION

Bowel elimination refers to the secretion and excretion of body waste through the intestinal system. Nurses who may encounter children with alterations in bowel elimination should be familiar with various gastrointestinal (GI) disorders that children experience. Alterations in bowel elimination or GI disorders affect children of all ages. GI illnesses range from acute to chronic and from non–life-threatening to life-threatening problems. Even acute, non–life-threatening illnesses (e.g., diarrhea or vomiting) can become life threatening without proper nursing assessment and interventions. The most common result of a GI illness is dehydration, requiring fluid therapy at home or, in more extreme cases, in a hospital setting. It is important to take all GI disorders seriously until symptoms are well controlled.

Child and family education related to the treatment of GI disorders is often the key to preventing the illness from progressing to an emergency. Therefore, the nurse's knowledge of the disorders that affect the GI system is crucial. Most often, the parents or child, if the child is older, will contact the health care provider or nurse practitioner in an outpatient setting to seek help. The nurse is usually the person to triage the phone call to determine the next step in the situation, which may be determining whether the child should be managed at home, brought to the office for assessment, or sent directly to an emergency room for evaluation. Most GI disorders can be handled in an outpatient setting to avoid unnecessary hospitalization. However, some life-threatening problems (e.g., bowel obstruction) require emergency care in the hospital. The knowledge base of the nurse is instrumental in obtaining the proper information by taking a thorough and accurate health history from the parents or child (if the child is older).

VARIATIONS IN PEDIATRIC ANATOMY AND PHYSIOLOGY

The GI tract includes all structures from the mouth to the anus. The primary functions of the GI system are the digestion and absorption of nutrients and water, elimination of waste products, and secretion of various substances required for digestion. Babies are born with immature GI tracts that are not fully mature until age 2. Due to this immaturity, there are many differences between the digestive tract of the young child and that of the older child or adult.

Mouth

The mouth is highly vascular, making it a common entry point for infectious invaders. In addition, infants and young children repeatedly bring objects to their mouths and explore them in that fashion. This behavior increases the infant's and young child's risk for contracting infections via the mouth.

Esophagus

The esophagus provides a passageway from the mouth to the stomach for food. The lower esophageal sphincter (LES) prevents **regurgitation** (backflow) of stomach contents up into the esophagus and/or oral cavity. The muscle tone of the LES is not fully developed until age 1 month, so infants younger than 1 month of age frequently regurgitate after feedings. Many children younger than 1 year of age continue to regurgitate for several months, but this usually disappears with age. If edema or narrowing of the esophagus occurs in a child with undeveloped esophageal muscle tone, **dysphagia** (difficult or painful swallowing) may occur.

Stomach

Newborns have a stomach capacity of only 10 to 20 mL. At 2 months of age, an infant has the capacity to hold up to 200 mL, though most young infants cannot tolerate 200-mL feedings. By age 16, the stomach capacity is 1,500 mL; by adulthood it is 2,000 to 3,000 mL. Hydrochloric acid, which is found in gastric contents to aid in digestion, reaches the adult level by the time the child is 6 months old.

Intestines

The small intestine is not functionally mature at birth. A full-term infant has approximately 250 cm of small intestine; an adult has up to 600 cm. Infants who have small bowel loss during early infancy have more problems with absorption and diarrhea than adults who have the same amount of small bowel loss.

Biliary System

The liver is relatively large at birth, allowing for the smooth edge of the liver to be easily palpated in infancy, as much as 2 cm below the costal margin. The pancreatic enzymes continue to develop postnatally, reaching adult levels around 2 years of age.

Fluid Balance and Losses

Compared with adults, children exhibit differences in how fluid volume is maintained. These differences are evident in body fluid balance and insensible fluid losses.

Body Fluid Balance

Infants and children have a proportionately greater amount of body water than do adults. Infants and young children require a larger relative fluid intake than adults and excrete a relatively greater amount of fluid. This places them at increased risk for fluid loss with illness compared to adults. Until age 2 years, the extracellular fluid, with its larger proportion of sodium and chloride, makes up about half of the child's total body water. Therefore, when potential fluid loss states occur, water loss occurs more rapidly and in larger amounts than in adults.

Insensible Fluid Losses

Fever increases fluid loss at a rate of about 7 mL/kg/24-hour period for every sustained 1°C rise in temperature. Since children become febrile with illness more readily and their fevers are higher than those of adults, infants and young children are more apt than adults to experience insensible fluid loss with fever when ill.

Fluid loss via the skin accounts for about two thirds of insensible fluid loss. Infants have a larger body surface area (BSA) relative to their body mass as compared to older children and adults. The newborn's BSA to body mass ratio is about two or three times greater than the adult's, and the preterm infant's is about five times greater than the adult's. This places infants, especially young infants, at increased risk of insensible fluid loss as compared to older children and adults.

The basal metabolic rate in infants and children is higher than that of adults to support growth. This higher metabolic rate, even in states of wellness, accounts for increased insensible fluid loss and increased need for water for excretory functions. The young infant's renal immaturity does not allow the kidneys to concentrate urine as well as in older children and adults. This puts infants at risk for dehydration or overhydration, depending on the circumstances.

COMMON MEDICAL TREATMENTS

There are many different forms of medical treatment for GI disorders. In the hospital setting, most medical treatments will require a health care provider's order. The most common treatments and medications used for GI disorders are listed in Common Medical Treatments 20.1 and Drug Guide 20.1. Both boxes provide essential information about medical treatments and medications used in pediatric GI disorders. Refer to these boxes as needed while completing the remainder of the chapter.

COMMON MEDICAL TREATMENTS 20.1 Gastrointestinal Disorders

Treatment	Explanation	Indications	Nursing Implications
Cleansing enema	Insertion of fluid into the rectum to soften the stool and stimulate bowel activity	Fecal impaction, severe constipation	Explain procedure to child prior to enema. With multiple enemas, observe for electrolyte imbalances.
Bowel preparation	Use of highly osmotic fluids to induce severe diarrhea to cleanse the entire bowel	Preparation for colonoscopy or bowel surgery	Some children may need to have a nasogastric tube placed so they can consume the needed amounts of fluids. Observe for signs and symptoms of dehydration/electrolyte imbalance.
Feeding tubes	Flexible tubes used for enteral feeding when the infant or child is incapable of swallowing safely or for augmenting nutrition. May be orogastric, nasogastric, gastrostomy, or jejunostomy	Feeding difficulties, failure to thrive, gastroesophageal reflux disease (GERD), chronic illness	Orogastric and nasogastric tubes must be checked for placement prior to each use. If required long term, use a softer, flexible tube intended for long-term use. Stomahesive or DuoDERM applied to the cheek may decrease risk of skin breakdown from tape. Gastrostomy tubes vary in type. Keep insertion site clean and dry.
Intravenous therapy	Administration of fluids via a catheter that delivers electrolytes and fluids into the venous system	Dehydration, bowel rest, NPO status	Monitor intravenous site for redness, swelling, and pain. Assess urine output to evaluate hydration status.

COMMON MEDICAL TREATMENTS 20.1 Gastrointestinal Disorders

Treatment	Explanation	Indications	Nursing Implications
Ostomy	A portion of the intestine is brought to the level of the skin to allow passage of stool.	Imperforate anus, gastroschisis, omphalocele, Hirschsprung disease, necrotizing enterocolitis, Crohn disease, ulcerative colitis	Ostomy contents may be acidic and irritate the skin. Use Stomahesive or DuoDERM under the pouch to avoid tape irritation to the skin. The pouch should fit the stoma correctly. Assess the stoma for pinkness and moist appearance.
Oral rehydration therapy	Administration by mouth of fluids that contain certain amounts of electrolytes and glucose to prevent dehydration and/or promote rehydration	Diarrhea, acute gastroenteritis, vomiting	Fluid administration should begin prior to the onset of dehydration. Urine output should be monitored to evaluate hydration status.
Probiotics (lactobacillus, acidophilus)	Food supplement containing dormant bacteria that when activated may alter the intestinal microflora	Treatment/prevention of diarrhea	Particularly helpful in the prevention of or decreasing incidence of antibiotic-induced diarrhea
Total parenteral nutrition (TPN)	Intravenous complete nutrition that provides glucose, protein, lipids, vitamins, and minerals	Long-term NPO status, swallowing difficulties, difficulties tolerating enteral feeding (short bowel syndrome, necrotizing enterocolitis)	Higher glucose and protein concentrations and solutions containing calcium require central venous access. Monitor blood glucose levels with initiation, rate changes, and discontinuation. Blood chemistries should be monitored on a regular basis.

DRUG GUIDE 20.1

COMMON DRUGS FOR GI DISORDERS

Classification	Actions/Indications	Nursing Implications
Histamine-2 blockers (ranitidine, famotidine, cimetidine, nizatidine)	Decrease histamine production, thereby reducing gastric acid secretion Used for heartburn, esophagitis, GERD, benign duodenal or gastric ulcers	May cause drowsiness or dizziness
Proton pump inhibitors (omeprazole, lansoprazole, esomeprazole, pantoprazole, rabeprazole)	Block the pump that produces gastric acids Indicated for erosive esophagitis, symptomatic GERD, *Helicobacter pylori* eradication	Adverse effects include headache, nausea, abdominal pain, and diarrhea.
Prokinetics (metoclopramide, cisapride)	Stimulate GI motility to help empty the stomach faster and promote intestinal motility	Metoclopramide may have central nervous system adverse effects. Cisapride is available only in limited-access protocol studies.
Antibacterials/antibiotics (metronidazole, vancomycin)	Treatment of bacterial infections of the GI tract Used for suspected or proven bacterial infections of the GI tract, such as *Clostridium difficile* or parasitic infections	May cause GI upset, diarrhea; important to finish entire course of treatment
Immunosuppressants (6-mercaptopurine, azathioprine)	Suppress the immune system to keep autoimmune disorders in remission such as Crohn disease, ulcerative colitis, autoimmune hepatitis	Drug levels should be checked to determine drug metabolite levels and potential for hepatotoxicity or bone marrow suppression.
Stimulants (senna, docusate sodium)	Stimulate peristalsis in the large intestine to produce a bowel movement Used to relieve constipation	May cause cramping or diarrhea; stool patterns should be constantly assessed
Laxatives (polyethylene glycol, milk of magnesia, lactulose)	Soften the stool to allow for easier passage through the colon Used to relieve constipation	Stool patterns should be monitored. Doses may need to be readjusted frequently to find the correct dose for the child.

(*continued*)

DRUG GUIDE 20.1 (*continued*)

COMMON DRUGS FOR GI DISORDERS

Classification	Actions/Indications	Nursing Implications
Antidiarrheals (loperamide, diphenoxylate/atropine)	Decrease peristalsis, thus prolonging transit time of stool through the intestines Indicated to treat diarrhea related to short bowel syndrome, chronic nonspecific diarrhea, irritable bowel syndrome	May cause drowsiness or constipation
Corticosteroids (prednisone)	Act systemically to reduce inflammation and suppress the normal immune response Used in inflammatory bowel disease, autoimmune disorders	Systemic adverse effects include hirsutism, osteoporosis, GI upset, cushingoid appearance, increased intraocular pressure, irritability, and personality changes. Should be taken as directed. Stopping the medication suddenly may cause adrenal insufficiency.
Antiemetics (promethazine, metoclopramide)	Act on the central nervous system transmitters to prevent nausea and vomiting	May have central nervous system adverse effects, such as drowsiness or irritability
Anticholinergic/antispasmodics (hyoscyamine, dicyclomine, glycopyrrolate)	Used to control abdominal spasms and cramping associated with irritable bowel syndrome, functional bowel disorders	May cause excessive thirst or dizziness. Encourage plenty of fluids while taking these medications.
Antiinflammatories (mesalamine, balsalazide, hydrocortisone enemas/suppositories, olsalazine, sulfasalazine)	Reduce inflammation in the colon associated with ulcerative colitis, proctitis	Stool output should be monitored to assess for presence of oral medications (indicating poor absorption).

GERD, gastroesophageal reflux disease; GI, gastrointestinal.

Source: UpToDate, Inc. (2024). *UpToDate® Lexidrug™* (Version 8.2.0) [Mobile app]. Wolters Kluwer. https://apps.apple.com/us/app/lexicomp/id313401238

COMMON LABORATORY AND DIAGNOSTIC TESTS 20.1

Test	Explanation	Indications	Nursing Implications
Abdominal ultrasonography	Visualizes abdominal organs and related vessels	Abdominal pain, vomiting, pregnancy, abnormal liver tests, abdominal mass, enlarged organs on palpation	Barium decreases visualization of organs on ultrasound.
Abdominal radiograph (KUB)	Plain radiograph of the abdomen without contrast media	Constipation, abdominal pain, abdominal distention, ascites, foreign body, palpable mass	Usually ordered as flat and upright to allow for free air and fluid levels in the bowel to be detected
Amylase (serum)	An enzyme that changes starch to sugar, which enters the blood with inflammation of the pancreas	Acute pancreatitis, pancreatic trauma, acute cholecystitis	Increased levels are seen after 3–6 hours of the onset of abdominal pain.
Barium enema	After instillation of barium, it fluoroscopically allows visualization of the colon.	Constipation, rectal prolapse, bleeding	Bowel preparation prior to examination may be ordered. Stool will be light colored due to barium for a few days.
Electrolytes (serum)	Sodium, potassium, CO_2, chloride, BUN, creatinine	To determine extent of dehydration	BUN and creatinine may be elevated with dehydration. Sodium, potassium, chloride, and CO_2 levels can be greatly affected with dehydration.
Barium swallow/upper GI series	Visualizes the form, position, mucosal folds, peristaltic activity, and motility of the esophagus, stomach, and upper GI tract	Foreign body ingestion, abdominal pain, vomiting, dysphagia, malrotation	People who may become pregnant should be screened for pregnancy. Infants may need to be given barium via syringe.

COMMON LABORATORY AND DIAGNOSTIC TESTS 20.1

Test	Explanation	Indications	Nursing Implications
Small bowel series	Done in conjunction with upper GI series to visualize the small intestine contour, position, and motility	Suspected inflammatory bowel disease (bowel wall thickening), intussusception	Important to encourage large amounts of water/fluids after test to avoid barium-induced constipation
Endoscopic retrograde cholangiopancreatography (ERCP)	A fiberoptic endoscope is used to view the hepatobiliary system by instilling contrast to outline the pancreatic and common bile ducts.	Pancreatitis, jaundice, pancreatic tumors, common duct stones, biliary tract disease	Monitor for infection, urinary retention, cholangitis, or pancreatitis after the procedure. It is done only occasionally in children.
Esophageal manometry	Tests the esophagus for normal contractile activity and effectiveness of swallowing by measurement of intraluminal pressures and acid sensors	Abnormal esophageal muscle function, dysphagia, chest pain of unknown cause, esophagitis, vomiting	Often done in conjunction with pH probe. The manometric catheter is placed through the nose into the esophagus. May cause nasal irritation/sore throat.
Esophageal pH probe	A single- or double-channeled probe placed into the esophagus to monitor the pH of the contents that are regurgitated into the esophagus from the stomach	Vomiting, gastroesophageal reflux, correlation of symptoms to gastroesophageal reflux events and high risk for problems, as in asthma, apparent life-threatening event, sinusitis, or choking/gagging episodes	24-hour study is most accurate. A special diet during the study is often used. Accurate diary of symptoms and feedings during the study is essential. May cause nasal irritation/sore throat
Gastric emptying scan	Assesses the rate at which the stomach empties food into the small intestine by adding isotopes to food and visualizing with scans	Unexplained nausea, vomiting, diarrhea, abdominal cramping	Medications may alter gastric emptying times. Crying or stress during the examination may cause delay in emptying and should be documented.
Hemoccult	Checks for occult blood in the stool	Crohn disease, ulcerative colitis, malabsorption syndromes, diarrhea, abdominal pain	Indicates bleeding in the GI tract
Hepatobiliary scan (HIDA scan)	Visualizes the gallbladder and determines patency of the biliary system by use of a radionuclide. The amount of radionuclide ejected from the gallbladder (ejection fraction) is calculated.	Differentiate biliary atresia and neonatal hepatitis; assess liver trauma, right upper quadrant pain, and congenital malformations	An intravenous line will be established to give radionuclide. Pain during injection should be assessed and documented.
Lactose tolerance test	After ingesting lactose, this tests the hydrogen levels in the breath, which will increase with lactose buildup in the intestines.	Postprandial diarrhea, gassiness, bloating, abdominal pain	May produce similar symptoms during the test itself. A positive test will require diet modification and education regarding lactose intolerance.
Lipase (serum)	An enzyme that changes fat to fatty acids and glycerol appearing in the blood with pancreatic change	Pancreatitis, pancreatic carcinoma, cholecystitis, peritonitis	Lipase levels stay elevated longer with acute pancreatitis.
Liver biopsy	A test done to evaluate the microscopic hepatic structures	Hyperbilirubinemia, jaundice, chronic liver disease, hepatitis	Monitor after procedure for bleeding complications; must maintain strict bed rest for up to 8 hours
Liver function tests (LFTs) (AST/ALT/GGT)	Enzymes that have high concentrations in the liver	Elevations may indicate the severity of liver disease.	May be affected by drugs or viral illnesses

(continued)

COMMON LABORATORY AND DIAGNOSTIC TESTS 20.1 *(continued)*

Test	Explanation	Indications	Nursing Implications
Lower endoscopy (colonoscopy)	Allows visualization and biopsies of the lower GI tract from the anus to the terminal ileum with a fiberoptic instrument	Rectal bleeding, lower abdominal pain, suspected tumors or strictures, foreign body removal	The child must undergo a bowel cleansing prior to the examination. Encourage fluids to prevent dehydration. Conscious sedation or anesthesia care; monitor for possible complications of perforation, bleeding, and increased abdominal pain
Meckel scan	A gamma camera is used to identify gastric mucosa seen in the distal portion of the ileum after injection of radiopharmaceuticals.	Rectal bleeding, anemia, used only to identify a Meckel diverticulum	Gloves are worn by nurse during and after scan when radiopharmaceuticals are given.
Oropharyngeal motility study (OPMS)	A study done with different textures to evaluate the dynamics of swallowing and reveal transient abnormalities	Dysphagia, recurrent aspiration	Usually done in collaboration with therapists and nutritionist
Rectal suction biopsy	Biopsy of the rectum is taken at different levels to assess for the presence of ganglion cells.	Absence of ganglion cells indicates Hirschsprung disease.	Infants/children should be assessed for rectal bleeding after examination.
Stool culture	Stool is smeared on culture medium and assessed for growth of bacteria over a period of days.	To determine bacterial cause of diarrhea	Requires minimum of 48 hours for growth, several days to weeks in some cases. Can be done with a small amount of stool
Stool for ova and parasites (O&P)	Checks for the presence of parasites or their eggs in the stool	To determine cause of diarrhea or abdominal pain	Requires about 2 tbsp of stool
Upper endoscopy (EGD)	Allows visualization and biopsies of the upper GI tract (mouth to upper jejunum) with a fiberoptic instrument	Dysphagia, foreign body removal, epigastric/abdominal pain, suspected celiac disease	Conscious sedation or anesthesia care; monitor for complications of perforation/bleeding
Urea breath test	Used to detect the presence of *Helicobacter pylori* in the exhaled breath	*H. pylori* infection	Child must not take proton pump inhibitors for 5 days, all antibiotic therapy and Pepto-Bismol for 14 days

ALT, alanine transaminase; AST, aspartate aminotransferase; BUN, blood urea nitrogen; EGD, esophagogastroduodenoscopy; GGT, gamma-glutamyl transferase; GI, gastrointestinal; HIDA, hepatobiliary iminodiacetic acid; KUB, kidney, ureter, and bladder.

Data from Corbett, J. A., & Banks, A. D. (2019). *Laboratory tests and diagnostic procedures with nursing diagnoses* (9th ed.). Pearson Education Inc.; and CHOC. (2023). *Stool tests.* https://www.choc.org/programs-services/gastroenterology/digestive-disorder-diagnostics/stool-tests/

Clinical Judgment and the Nursing Process

Nursing care of the child with a GI disorder or alteration in bowel elimination includes nursing assessment, nursing analysis, planning, interventions, and evaluation. It is important to individualize each step of this process for each child.

Assessment

The assessment of the child with a GI disorder includes a health history, physical examination, and laboratory and diagnostic testing.

Health History

A thorough health history is important in the assessment of a child with a GI disorder. In the health history include past history (previous illnesses/surgeries), past family history, present illness (when the symptoms began and how this differs from the child's normal status), and how the child's symptoms have been managed up to this point (relevant medical records/home treatments). Determine the child's historical growth patterns. Assess the family history to identify common genetic or familial GI symptoms or disorders such as irritable bowel syndrome (IBS), inflammatory bowel disease (IBD), or food allergies. Detail within the history of the present illness can often distinguish chronic problems from acute disorders. Ask descriptive questions of the child and family.

Physical Examination

Perform the physical examination of the child from the least invasive part of the examination to the most invasive. It is important for the child to remain as relaxed as possible during this part of the assessment.

Inspection and Observation

Inspect and observe the child's color, hydration status, abdominal size and shape, and mental status.

COLOR

First observe the child's skin, eye, and lip color, as pallor may be a sign of anemia or dehydration. Note the presence of jaundiced skin or **icteric** (yellowed in color) sclerae, which indicate elevated bilirubin levels related to liver dysfunction. Inspect the abdomen for distended veins, indicating abdominal or vascular obstruction or distention. As in any part of a physical assessment, watch for areas of ecchymosis (bruising), which may be a sign of abuse.

HYDRATION STATUS

Carefully assess the child's hydration status as it may indicate how severe the current GI illness is. Decreased turgor and skin turgor tenting indicate dehydration. During crying, especially in infants, the absence of tears may indicate dehydration. Assess the amount of urine output the child has had in the past 24 hours.

ABDOMINAL SIZE AND SHAPE

Inspect the size and shape of the abdomen while the child is standing and while the child is lying supine. The abdomen should be flat when the child is supine. An especially **protuberant** (bulging outward) abdomen suggests the presence of ascites, fluid retention, gaseous distention, or even a tumor. A depressed or concave abdomen could indicate a high abdominal obstruction or dehydration. Inspect the umbilicus for color, odor, discharge, inflammation, and herniation.

MENTAL STATUS

Perform a brief mental status examination as mental status changes can occur with severe dehydration, anaphylactic reactions to foods or medicines, and elevated ammonia levels. Irritability and restlessness are usually the early signs of mental status changes. **Lethargy** (sluggishness or abnormal drowsiness) and listlessness can occur much more rapidly in children than in adults. It is important to identify this promptly and treat it emergently.

Auscultation

Auscultate bowel sounds in all four quadrants. Hyperactive bowel sounds may be noted in children with diarrhea or gastroenteritis. Hypoactive or absent bowel sounds may signify an obstructive process. The nurse can determine the absence of bowel sounds after a 5-minute period of auscultation. This can be extremely difficult to perform with children and infants, who may be uncooperative during the examination.

CLINICAL REASONING ALERT!

Immediately report hypoactive or absent bowel sound findings to the health care provider or nurse practitioner.

Percussion

Percuss the abdomen to reveal the expected finding of dullness or flatness along the right costal margin and 1 to 3 cm below the costal margin of the liver. The area above the symphysis pubis may be dull in young children with full bladders, which is an expected finding. Percussion of the remainder of the abdomen should reveal tympany. Note any unexpected findings.

Palpation

Reserve palpation for last in the sequence of an abdominal examination. First, lightly palpate the abdomen to assess for areas of tenderness, lesions, muscle tone, turgor, and cutaneous hyperesthesia (a finding in acute peritonitis). Then perform deep palpation from the lower quadrants upward to best feel the liver edge, which should be firm and smooth. In infants and children, palpate the liver during inspiration below the right costal margin. The tip of the spleen may also be palpated during inspiration; it should be 1 to 2 cm below the left costal margin. Palpable kidneys, except in neonates, may indicate tumor or hydronephrosis. The sigmoid colon can be palpated in the left lower quadrant. The cecum may be felt in the right lower quadrant as a soft mass. Areas of firmness or masses may indicate tumor or stool in the abdomen.

Tenderness in the abdomen is not an expected physical finding. Right upper quadrant tenderness could indicate liver enlargement. Right lower quadrant pain, including **rebound tenderness** (pain upon release of pressure during palpation), can be a warning sign of appendicitis; immediately report any positive findings to a health care provider. Palpate the external inguinal canals for the presence of inguinal hernias, often elicited by having the child turn the head and cough or blow up a balloon.

Laboratory and Diagnostic Testing

Common Laboratory and Diagnostic Tests 20.1 gives information about the tests most often ordered by health care providers for children with GI illnesses. Some of these tests are ordered in the hospital setting; others are done on an outpatient basis. Typically, the nurse may be directly involved in specimen collection while a specifically trained person performs the diagnostic tests. Regardless of who performs the test, nurses must be familiar with preparation guidelines for the child, how each test is performed, and expected and unexpected findings and their significance to provide appropriate child and family education. Box 20.1 gives tips on collecting stool specimens.

Remember Ethan, the 2-month-old with vomiting and irritability? What additional health history and physical examination assessment information should you obtain?

Nursing Analysis, Goals, Interventions, and Evaluation

After recognizing and analyzing cues from a thorough assessment, the nurse might identify several patient problems, including:

- Deficient fluid volume risk
- Diarrhea
- Constipation
- Imbalanced nutrition (less than body requirements)
- Impaired skin integrity risk
- Ineffective breathing pattern
- Disturbed body image
- Pain
- Interrupted family processes
- Caregiver role strain risk

After completing an assessment on Ethan, you note the following: weight 10 lb, length 23.5 in, head circumference 40.75 cm. Head is round with sunken anterior fontanel, eyes appear sunken, mucous membranes are dry, heart rate 158, breath sounds clear with respiratory rate of 42, positive bowel sounds in all four quadrants, difficulty palpating abdomen due to crying. Based on these assessment findings, what would your top three patient problems be for Ethan?

The abovementioned patient problems provide suggestions for nursing care planning or concept mapping. Suggested interventions with rationales are provided further. Care planning should be individualized, based on the child's and family's needs. Refer to Chapter 14 for the nursing process for pain management and to Chapter 11 for nursing interventions related to interrupted family processes and caregiver role strain risk. Additional information will be included later in the chapter as it relates to nursing care for children with specific disorders, as well as particular nursing interventions for deficient knowledge.

BOX **20.1** Stool Specimen Collection Variations

- If the child is in diapers, use a tongue blade to scrape a specimen into the collection container.
- If the child has runny stool, a piece of plastic wrap in the diaper may catch the stool specimen. Very liquid stool may require application of a urine bag to the anal area to collect the stool.
- The older ambulatory child may first urinate in the toilet, and then the stool specimen may be retrieved from the new or clean collection container that fits under the seat at the back of the toilet.
- For the bedridden child, collect the stool specimen from a clean bedpan (do not allow urine to contaminate the stool specimen).
- Send the specimen to the laboratory immediately for accurate results.

Nursing Analysis

Deficient fluid volume risk related to active fluid volume loss (vomiting or diarrhea) or insufficient fluid intake (possible nothing by mouth [NPO] status)

Goal/Outcome

Child will maintain adequate fluid volume as evidenced by elastic skin turgor; moist, pink oral mucosa; presence of tears; urine output 1 mL/kg/h or more.

Maintaining Fluid Balance (interventions with *rationale*)

- Weigh child daily; *accurate weight is one of the best indicators of fluid volume status in children.*
- Maintain IV line and administer IV fluid as ordered *to maintain fluid volume.*
- Offer small amounts of oral rehydration solution (ORS) frequently *to maintain fluid volume. Small amounts are usually well tolerated by children with diarrhea and vomiting.*
- When symptoms have lessened or resolved, reintroduce regular diet *to reduce number of stools, provide adequate nutrition, and shorten duration of effects of illness.*
- Avoid high-carbohydrate fluids such as Kool-Aid and fruit juice, *as they are low in electrolytes, and increased simple carbohydrate consumption can decrease stool transit time.*
- Assess hydration status (skin turgor, oral mucosa, presence of tears) every 4 to 8 hours *to evaluate maintenance of adequate fluid volume.*
- Assess adequacy of urine output *to assess end-organ perfusion.*
- Maintain strict intake and output record and weigh child daily *to evaluate effectiveness of rehydration.*
- Discourage milk products and fluids that contain high levels of sugar during the acute phase of illness, *as these products may worsen diarrhea.*

Nursing Analysis

Diarrhea related to GI inflammation, infection, or exposure to toxin, as evidenced by loose liquid stools, hyperactive bowel sounds, or abdominal cramping

Goal/Outcome

Child will experience decrease in diarrhea and Child will have bulkier stool as per normal routine.

Relieving Diarrhea (interventions with *rationale*)

- Maintain clear liquid diet no longer than 24 hours, *as prolonged clear liquids will result in continued liquid ("starvation") stools.*
- Avoid milk products until diarrhea improves; *temporary poor absorption from villus injury follows viral diarrhea.*
- Encourage complex carbohydrate foods *to bulk up the stools.*
- Add fat to carbohydrates to increase intestinal transit time *to encourage water absorption (bulks up stool).*

Nursing Analysis

Constipation related to irregular defecation, decrease in GI motility (obstructive lesion), or insufficient fluid or fiber intake as evidenced by abdominal pain, decrease in stool frequency or volume, distended abdomen, liquid stool, pain with defecation, hard, formed stool, or palpable abdominal mass

Goal/Outcome

Child will experience improvement in constipation by passing daily soft bowel movement without pain or straining.

Relieving Constipation (interventions with *rationale*)

- Palpate for abdominal distention, percuss for dullness, and auscultate for bowel sounds *to assess for signs of constipation.*
- Encourage adequate fluid intake *to soften the stool.*
- Administer medications as ordered *to keep stool moving on daily basis.*
- Encourage activity as tolerated; *immobility contributes to constipation.*
- The child with stool withholding should sit on the toilet twice daily, preferably after breakfast and dinner, *to maximize chances for successful stool passage by taking advantage of the gastrocolic reflex.*
- For behavioral stool holding, use rewards or stickers *to encourage appropriate toileting.*

Nursing Analysis

Imbalanced nutrition (less than body requirements) related to insufficient dietary intake; inability to ingest or digest food, inability to absorb nutrients; or psychological disorder as evidenced by lack of appropriate weight gain or growth, weight loss, food aversion, insufficient muscle tone, or food intake less than recommended daily allowance

Goal/Outcome

Nutritional status will be maximized: Child will maintain or gain weight appropriately.

Maintaining Appropriate Nutrition (interventions with *rationale*)

- Encourage favorite foods (within prescribed diet restrictions if present) *to maximize oral intake.*
- Administer enteral tube feedings as ordered *to maximize caloric intake.*
- Add butter, gravy, or cheese as appropriate to foods (if allowed within diet restrictions) *to increase caloric intake.*
- Encourage high-quality, high-calorie snacks between meals, *so as not to interfere with meal intake.*
- Document response to feeding *to determine feeding tolerance.*
- Limit intake of calorie-free beverages; *beverages should contain nutrients and calories.*
- Consult nutritionist *for appropriate diet supplementation recommendations.*

Nursing Analysis

Impaired skin integrity risk related to moisture (frequent loose stools, or presence of stoma or gastrostomy tube)

Goal/Outcome

Child's skin will remain intact; the skin of the buttocks will be free from rash and excoriation. In the child with an ostomy or gastrostomy, the skin surrounding the stoma or tube will remain intact and free from redness, rash, and excoriation.

Maintaining Skin Integrity (interventions with *rationale*)

- Change diapers frequently *to limit acidic stool content contact with skin.*
- Use barrier diaper cream *to protect skin.*
- Assess skin integrity at every diaper change to recognize skin changes early *so that corrective measures can begin.*
- Leave diaper area open to air several times a day if redness is present *so that air can circulate and skin healing can be facilitated.*
- Use plain water or only mild soap to cleanse the skin with diaper changes *to avoid pH changes that contribute to diaper area skin breakdown.*
- Avoid diaper wipes that contain fragrance or alcohol if the skin is red or has a rash, *as both alcohol and perfume cause stinging if used on nonintact skin and can worsen skin breakdown.*

For the child with an ostomy:

- Ensure proper fit of the ostomy appliance/pouch *to avoid acidic stool contact with skin.*
- Use a barrier wafer (e.g., Stomahesive or DuoDERM) to attach the appliance to avoid *repeated pulling of adhesive tape from skin.*
- If redness occurs, use barrier/healing cream or paste on the skin around the stoma *to promote healing and prevent further skin breakdown.*
- Consult enterostomal therapy nurse as needed *to provide additional support.*

Nursing Analysis

Ineffective breathing pattern related to pain, or body posture inhibiting lung expansion (postoperative immobility) as evidenced by bradypnea, dyspnea, tachypnea, nasal flaring, or use of accessory muscles to breathe

Goal/Outcome

Child will demonstrate effective breathing pattern: Child respiratory rate normal for age, absence of accessory muscle use, adequate aeration with clear breath sounds throughout all lung fields.

Promoting Effective Breathing Patterns (interventions with *rationale*)

- Have the child turn, cough, and deep breathe every 2 hours *to encourage adequate aeration and discourage fluid pooling in lungs.* In the infant or toddler, turn every 2 hours and use percussor or chest physiotherapy *to prevent pooling of secretions.*
- Play games to encourage deep breathing (blow out penlight, blow cotton ball across bedside table with straw, etc.): *Children are more likely to cooperate with interventions if play is involved.*
- In the developmentally able child, encourage incentive spirometer use every 2 hours *to improve lung aeration.*
- Demonstrate/encourage use of pillow splinting with coughing *to decrease abdominal pain and stress on incision.*

Nursing Analysis

Disturbed body image related to surgical procedure (presence of stoma, scars), alteration in body function (loss of control of bowel elimination), or treatment regimen as evidenced by negative feeling about body or avoiding looking at body (refusal to look at stoma).

Goal/Outcome

Child or adolescent will demonstrate acceptance of change in body image by verbalization of adjustment; looking at, touching, and caring for their body; and returning to previous social involvement.

Promoting Proper Body Image (interventions with *rationale*)

- Observe child's coping mechanisms *to reinforce their use in times of stress.*
- Acknowledge denial, anger, and other feelings as normal *to support child/teen through difficult transition.*
- Allow child gradual introduction to stoma *to ease transition.*
- Encourage child/adolescent to participate in care, *as this sense of control will contribute to positive self-esteem.*

Based on your top three patient problems for Ethan, describe appropriate nursing interventions.

Stool Diversions

Children may undergo stool diversions for a variety of GI disorders. Surgical procedures involve the creation of an ostomy, primarily an *ileostomy* or *colostomy*, by bringing a portion of the small or large intestine to the surface of the abdomen (Fig. 20.1). Ostomy pouches are worn over the ostomy site to collect stool. The pouch must be of an appropriate size and it should fit around the stoma properly (Fig. 20.2). The pouch may be tucked inside the diaper or underwear or angled to fit outside of the diaper/underwear. Contemporary pouches cannot be seen under most clothing because they are designed to lie flat against the body.

Providing Ostomy Care

Empty the ostomy pouch and measure for stool output several times per day. The stool may be semisolid to liquid in consistency depending on the location of the stoma. Liquid stool output can be acidic, causing irritation and severe burn-like areas on the surrounding skin, so special attention to skin care around the ostomy site is essential. Products such as powders and pastes are available to help protect the skin. The stoma should be moist and pink or red, demonstrating proper circulation to the intestine (Fig. 20.3). Notify the provider if the volume of stool output is greatly increased or if the stoma is prolapsed or retracted.

Perform ostomy care as needed; pouches usually need to be changed every 1 to 4 days. Refer to Nursing Procedure 20.1 for an explanation of the steps for changing an ostomy pouch.

CLINICAL REASONING ALERT!

Immediately notify the provider if the stoma is not moist and pink or red.

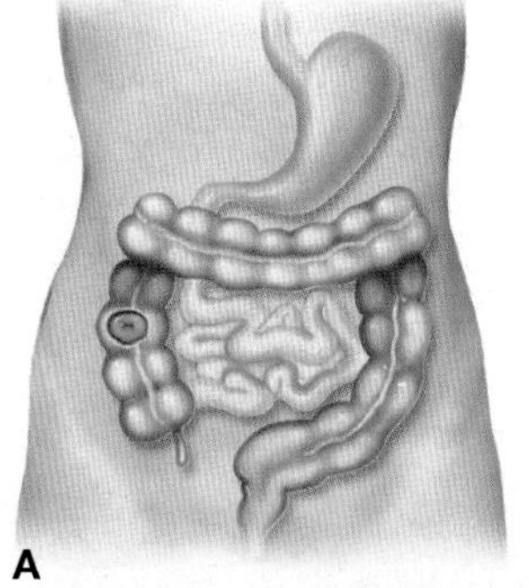

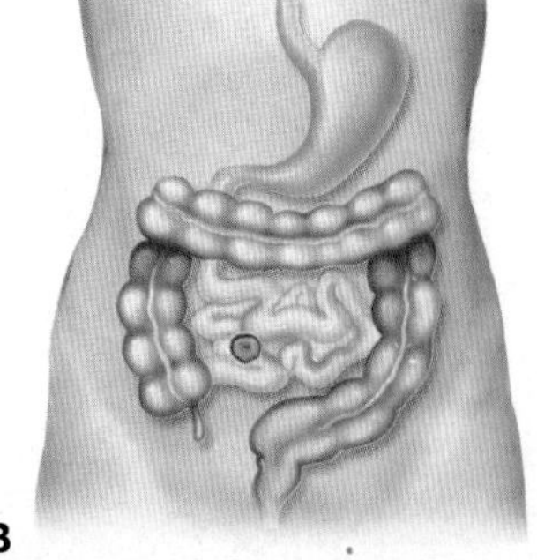

A B

FIGURE 20.1 A colostomy is a stoma from the colon (**A**); an ileostomy is a stoma from the ileum (**B**).

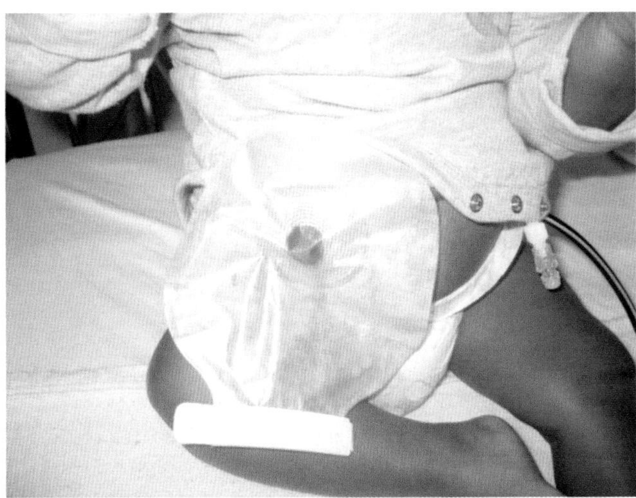

FIGURE 20.2 Ensure that the ostomy pouch fits closely around the stoma to prevent irritation of the surrounding skin.

Educating the Child and Family About Ostomy Care

Educate the child and parent to avoid tight or constricting clothing around the stoma site. Teach families to store ostomy supplies in a cool, dry place. Educate parents to inform school staff that the child should be allowed to use the water fountain and the bathroom without restriction, and the school nurse should have extra ostomy supplies available.

STRUCTURAL ANOMALIES OF THE GI TRACT

Structural anomalies of the GI tract include cleft lip and palate, omphalocele and gastroschisis, hernias (inguinal and umbilical), and anorectal malformations.

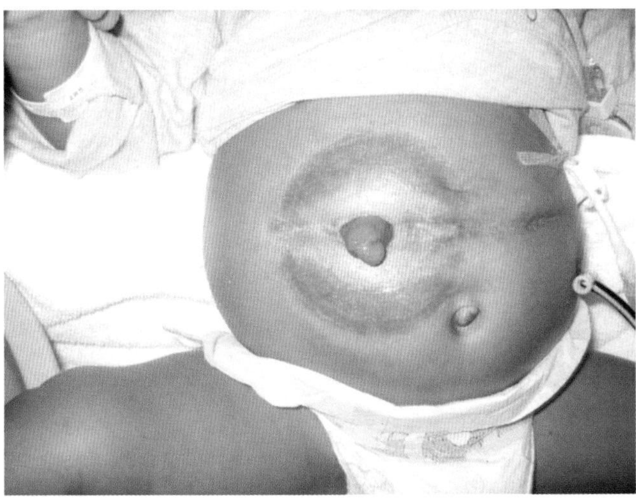

FIGURE 20.3 The healthy stoma is pink and moist.

NURSING PROCEDURE 20.1
Performing Ostomy Care

1. Set up the equipment:
    - Warm, wet washcloths or paper towels
    - Clean pouch and clamp
    - Skin barrier powder, paste, and/or sealant
    - Pencil or pen
    - Scissors
    - Pattern to measure stoma size
2. Take off the pouch (may need to use adhesive remover or wet washcloth to ease pouch removal).
3. Observe the stoma and surrounding skin. Clean the stoma and skin as needed, allowing it to dry thoroughly.
4. Measure the stoma, mark the new pouch backing, and cut the new backing to size.
5. Apply the new pouch.

Based on University of California San Francisco. (2024). *Colostomy (pediatric)*. https://surgery.ucsf.edu/procedure/colostomy-pediatric

Cleft Lip and Palate

Cleft lip and palate (Fig. 20.4) is the most common congenital craniofacial anomaly, occurring once in every 700 births worldwide (Bishop & Ebach, 2023). Cleft palate with and without cleft lip often occur in association with other anomalies and appear in about 200 syndromes (Phalke & Goldman, 2023).

Complications of cleft lip and palate include feeding difficulties, altered dentition, delayed or altered speech development, and otitis media. The infant with cleft lip may have difficulty forming an adequate seal around a nipple in order to create the necessary suction for feeding and may also experience excessive air intake. Gagging, choking, and nasal regurgitation of milk may occur in babies with cleft palate. Excessive feeding time, inadequate intake, and fatigue contribute to insufficient growth. Primary or permanent teeth may be missing, malformed, or unusually positioned. Children with cleft palate may have a nasal quality to the speech as well as delays in speech development. Optimally, speech articulation should be clear by 4 years of age, or additional surgical intervention may be necessary. The opening in the cleft palate contributes to buildup of fluid in the middle ear (otitis media with effusion), which can lead to an acute infection (acute otitis media). Otitis media with effusion leads to intermittent hearing and language delays (Meeks et al., 2022).

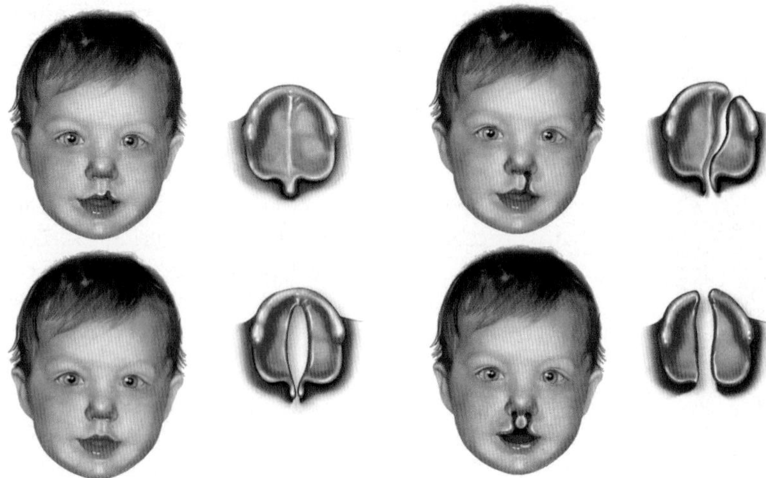

FIGURE 20.4 The cleft lip may extend all the way through the vermilion border and up into the nostril, or it may be significantly smaller. The cleft palate may be a small opening or may involve the entire palate.

Pathophysiology

Development of the cleft occurs early in pregnancy. Cleft lip results from failure of the mesenchymal tissue to properly fuse during the embryonic stage, usually by week 5, and cleft palate results when there is absence of midline fusion by week 7 (Meeks et al., 2023). Cleft lip or cleft palate may occur in isolation from one another or may co-occur. The cleft may be unilateral or bilateral.

Therapeutic Management

Babies with cleft lip and cleft palate are usually managed by a specialized team that may include a plastic surgeon or craniofacial specialist, oral surgeon, dentist or orthodontist, prosthodontist, psychologist, otolaryngologist, nurse, social worker, audiologist, and speech-language pathologist. Many children's hospitals offer these services in one location, such as a craniofacial specialty center. Cleft lip is usually surgically repaired by the age of 3 months and cleft palate around 12 months of age (Bishop & Ebach, 2023). Early repair of the cleft lip restores a normal appearance to the child's face and may improve parent–infant bonding. Regardless of the timing of the surgical repair, however, surgical revision of the palate may be required as the child grows.

Nursing Assessment

For a full description of the assessment phase of the nursing process, refer to the assessment section of the Nursing Process Overview earlier in the chapter. Assessment findings pertinent to cleft lip and palate are discussed further.

HEALTH HISTORY

For the newborn, explore pregnancy history for risk factors for development of cleft lip and cleft palate, which include:

- Birthing parent who smokes
- Prenatal infection
- Advanced age of birthing parent
- Use of anticonvulsants, steroids, and other medications during early pregnancy

When an infant or child with cleft lip or palate returns for a clinic visit or hospitalization, inquire about feeding difficulties, respiratory difficulties, speech development, and otitis media.

PHYSICAL EXAMINATION

Observe the infant for the presence of the characteristic physical appearance of cleft lip. The cleft may involve the lip only or extend up into the nostril (Fig. 20.5). Cleft palate may be visualized on examination of the mouth. Palpate with a gloved finger to discover mild clefts.

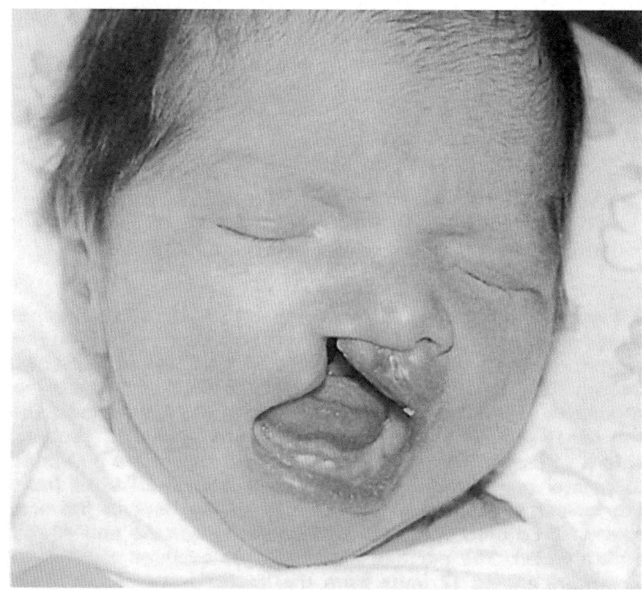

FIGURE 20.5 Cleft lip.

CONSIDER THIS!

The nurse is caring for a 2-week-old infant with a cleft lip who presents for a well-child check. The parent states, "I can't believe she looks like this; I always wanted a perfect baby girl. I feel like I can't go anywhere with her, other people will look at her like she's a monster. And after her surgery she's going to have an ugly scar over her lip." The parent then begins crying.

How will you respond as the nurse? Are you concerned about anything other than the parent's feelings in the situation? What would you feel like if you had a baby with a facial deformity? Think about the best ways to respond to this parent in a therapeutic manner.

Nursing Management

Refer to the "Clinical Judgment and the Nursing Process" section for patient problems and interventions related to fluid balance promotion and restoration of family processes, and to Chapter 14 for pain management. These should be individualized for the particular child. In addition to the patient problems and related interventions discussed in the "Clinical Judgment and the Nursing Process" section, interventions common to cleft lip and cleft palate follow.

PREVENTING INJURY TO THE SUTURE LINE

It is critical to prevent injury to the facial suture line or to the palatal operative sites. Do not allow the infant to rub the facial suture line. To prevent this, position the infant in a supine or side-lying position. It may be necessary to use arm restraints to stop the hands from touching the face or entering the mouth. Clean the suture line as ordered by the surgeon. Possible care options include using petroleum jelly on the facial suture line or a lip-protective device such as a Logan bow (curved thin metal apparatus) or a butterfly adhesive, both of which protect and maintain the suture line. Protect the palate operative site. Avoid putting items in the mouth that might disrupt the sutures (e.g., suction catheter, spoon, straw, pacifier, or plastic syringe).

Prevent vigorous or sustained crying in the infant because this may cause tension on either suture line. Ways to prevent crying include administering medications as needed for pain and providing other comfort or distraction measures, such as cuddling, rocking, and anticipation of needs.

PROMOTING ADEQUATE NUTRITION

Preoperatively, the baby with a cleft lip may demonstrate enhanced growth patterns if breastfed. The contour and softness of the breast against the lip may allow for a better seal to be maintained for adequate sucking in some infants (Cleft Lip & Palate Association [CLAPA], 2024). Some infants will be fed with a special cleft lip nipple (Fig. 20.6). Parent and surgeon preference will determine the method of feeding. Burp the infant well to expel excess air taken in due to difficulty with sucking.

The infant with unrepaired cleft palate is at risk for aspiration with oral feeding. In some instances, a prosthodontic device may be created to form a false palate covering. This device may prevent breast milk or formula from being aspirated. Breastfeeding may be effective in the infant with a small cleft palate due to the pliability of the breast and the fact that soft breast tissue may cover the opening in the palate (CLAPA, 2024). In the bottle-fed infant special nipples or feeders may have to be used. When the suture line is healed, ordinary feeding may resume.

ENCOURAGING INFANT–PARENT BONDING

For some parents, the appearance of a cleft lip is appalling. Encourage parents to hold the medically stable

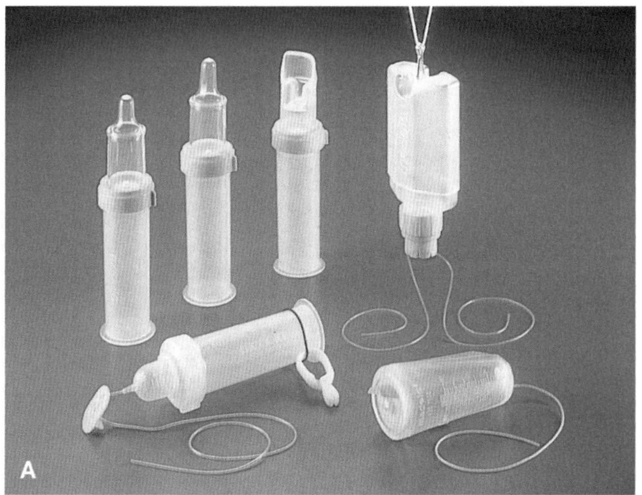

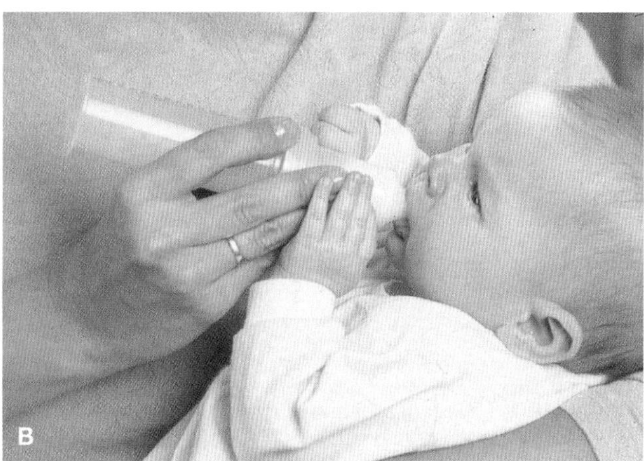

FIGURE 20.6 **A.** Specialty feeding devices used for infants with cleft lip and cleft palate. **B.** An infant uses a Haberman feeder.

infant immediately after delivery to encourage bonding. Acknowledge normal feelings of guilt, anger, and sadness. Support the parents in providing care for the infant, particularly feeding, which is viewed as a significant nurturing function. Provide education about the anticipated surgical procedure and eventual normal appearance of the infant's lip.

PROVIDING EMOTIONAL SUPPORT

Many families will benefit from support in addition to that received from the craniofacial team.

Esophageal Atresia and Tracheoesophageal Fistula

Esophageal atresia and tracheoesophageal fistula are GI anomalies in which the esophagus and trachea do not separate normally during embryonic development. Esophageal atresia refers to a congenitally interrupted esophagus where the proximal and distal ends do not communicate; the upper esophageal segment ends in a blind pouch and the lower segment ends a variable distance above the diaphragm (Fig. 20.7).

Tracheoesophageal fistula is an abnormal communication between the trachea and esophagus. When associated with esophageal atresia, the fistula most commonly occurs in the distal esophageal segment (Smith, 2022). Both defects are thought to be the result of incomplete separation of the lung bed from the foregut during early fetal development. A large percentage of newborns with either of these defects also have other congenital anomalies (Smith, 2022).

Nursing Assessment

Review the birthing parent's history for polyhydramnios, which commonly occurs as the fetus cannot swallow and absorb amniotic fluid in utero, leading to accumulation (Smith, 2022). Soon after birth, the newborn may exhibit copious, frothy bubbles of mucus in the mouth and nose, accompanied by drooling. Note abdominal distention as air builds up in the stomach. In esophageal atresia, a gastric tube cannot be inserted beyond a certain point because the esophagus ends in a blind pouch. The newborn may have rattling respirations, excessive salivation and drooling, and "the three C's" (coughing, choking, and cyanosis) if feeding is attempted. The presence of a fistula increases the risk of respiratory complications such as pneumonitis and atelectasis due to aspiration of food and secretions. Diagnosis is made by radiograph showing either an inserted gastric tube appearing coiled in the upper esophageal pouch (indicating esophageal atresia) or air in the GI tract (indicating the presence of a fistula between the trachea and esophagus).

Nursing Management

Nursing management focuses on preparing the newborn and parents for surgery and providing meticulous postoperative care.

PROVIDING PREOPERATIVE CARE

Preoperative nursing interventions include:

- Initiate nothing by mouth (NPO) status.
- Elevate the head of the bed 30 to 45 degrees to prevent reflux and aspiration.

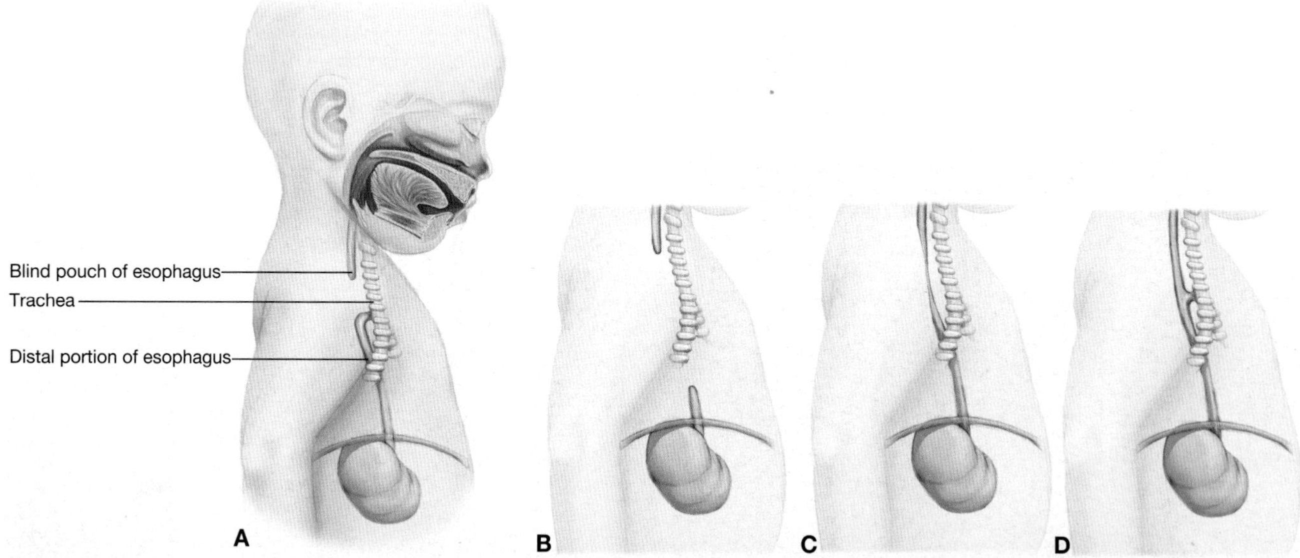

FIGURE 20.7 Esophageal atresia and tracheoesophageal fistula. **A.** The most common type of esophageal atresia, in which the esophagus ends in a blind pouch and a fistula connects the trachea with the distal portion of the esophagus. **B.** The upper and distal portions of the esophagus end in a blind pouch. **C.** The esophagus is one segment, but a portion of it is narrowed. **D.** The upper portion of the esophagus connects to the trachea via a fistula.

- Monitor hydration status and fluid and electrolyte balance; administer and monitor parenteral intravenous (IV) fluid infusions.
- Assess and maintain the patency of the orogastric tube; monitor the functioning of the tube, which is attached to low continuous suction; and avoid irrigation of the tube to prevent aspiration.
- Have oxygen and suctioning equipment readily available should the newborn experience respiratory distress.
- Assist with diagnostic studies to rule out other anomalies.
- Use comfort measures to minimize crying and prevent respiratory distress; provide nonnutritive sucking.
- Inform the parents about the rationales for the aspiration prevention measures.
- Document frequent observations of the newborn's condition.

PROVIDING POSTOPERATIVE CARE

Surgery consists of closing the fistula and joining the two esophageal segments. Postoperative care involves closely observing all of the newborn's body systems to identify any complications. Expect to administer total parenteral nutrition (TPN) and antibiotics until the esophageal anastomosis is proven intact and patent. Then begin oral feedings, usually within a week after surgery. Keep the parents informed of their newborn's condition and progress. Closely assess the newborn during feeding and report any difficulty with swallowing. Provide parent teaching. Demonstrate and reinforce all teaching prior to discharge.

Omphalocele and Gastroschisis

Omphalocele and gastroschisis are congenital anomalies of the anterior abdominal wall. An omphalocele is a defect of the umbilical ring that allows evisceration of the abdominal contents into an external peritoneal sac. Defects vary in size; they may be limited to bowel loops or may include the entire GI tract and liver (Fig. 20.8). Bowel malrotation is common, but the displaced organs are usually normal. Omphaloceles occur in 2 in 10,000 live births (Smith, 2022).

Gastroschisis is a herniation of the abdominal contents through an abdominal wall defect, usually to the left or right of the umbilicus. The incidence of gastroschisis has been increasing worldwide and occurs in up to 1% of live births (Smith, 2022). Gastroschisis differs from omphalocele in that there is no peritoneal sac protecting the herniated organs, and thus exposure to amniotic fluid makes them thickened, edematous, and inflamed. Both of these diagnoses require that a pediatric surgeon be available at delivery to determine the extent of the defect and complications.

Nursing Assessment

Review the birthing parent's history for factors associated with high-risk pregnancies, such as illness and infection, drug use, smoking, and genetic abnormalities. They contribute to placental insufficiency and the birth of a small-for-gestational-age or preterm newborn, the populations in which both of these abdominal defects most commonly occur.

Omphalocele and gastroschisis are observed readily. Note the appearance of the protrusion on the abdomen and evidence of a sac. Inspect the sac closely for the presence of organs, most commonly the intestines but sometimes the liver. Also inspect the contents for any twisting of the intestines. Note the color of the organs within the sac and measure the size of the omphalocele.

Also perform a complete physical examination of the newborn. These congenital conditions may be associated with other congenital anomalies, such as those involving the cardiovascular, genitourinary, and central nervous systems.

Nursing Management

Nursing care for newborns with omphalocele or gastroschisis focuses on preventing hypothermia,

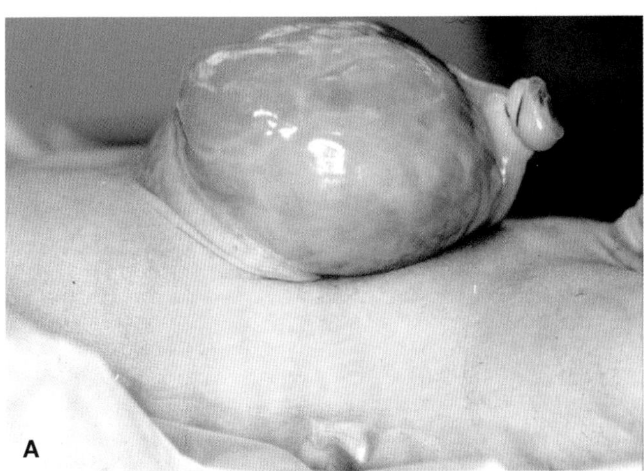

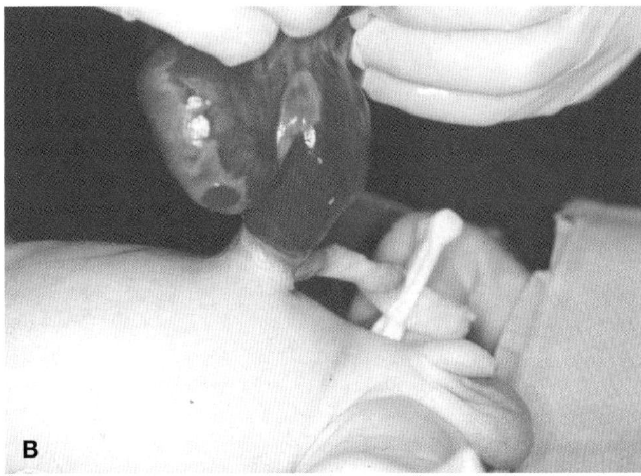

FIGURE 20.8 A. Omphalocele: a membranous sac covers the exposed organs. **B.** In gastroschisis, the organs are not covered by a membrane.

maintaining perfusion to the eviscerated abdominal contents by minimizing fluid loss, and protecting the exposed abdominal contents from trauma and infection. The abdominal contents are covered with a nonadherent sterile dressing in such a fashion so as to avoid causing trauma to the contents. Strict sterile technique is necessary to prevent contamination. A radiant warmer is necessary to maintain the newborn's temperature. Covering the dressing with plastic wrap may help to decrease heat and fluid loss (Stephenson et al., 2023).

Maintain low suction to an orogastric tube to prevent intestinal distention. Establish an IV line to maintain fluid and electrolyte balance and provide a route for antibiotic therapy. As much as two to three times maintenance may be required to maintain perfusion to the exposed organs and tissues (Stephenson et al., 2023). Monitor the newborn's fluid status frequently. Closely observe the exposed bowel for vascular compromise, such as changes in color or a decrease in temperature, and report these immediately.

PROVIDING POSTOPERATIVE CARE

Surgical repair of both defects occurs after initial stabilization and comprehensive evaluation for any other anomalies. It may have to occur in stages, depending on the defect.

Postoperative care involves providing pain management, monitoring respiratory and cardiac status, monitoring intake and output, assessing for vascular compromise, maintaining the orogastric tube to suction, documenting the amount and color of drainage, and administering ordered medications and treatments. Also be alert for complications, such as short bowel syndrome (see the "Short Bowel Syndrome" section later in the chapter).

PROMOTING PARENT–NEWBORN INTERACTION

Give the parents continued support and progress reports on their newborn. They may be distraught at the sight of the anomaly, and they may be frightened to touch their newborn. Encourage the parents to touch the newborn and participate in care as much as possible. Because of the nature of this defect, bonding opportunities will be limited initially. However, strongly encourage frequent visiting. In addition, provide information to the parents about the defect, treatment modalities, and prognosis. After surgery, instruct the parents in care measures and provide them with home care instructions. Anticipate the need for a referral to a home health care agency and community resources for support.

Anorectal Malformations

Imperforate anus is a congenital malformation of the anorectal opening. The defect is identified in the newborn period and occurs in 1 in 5,000 live births and may occur with other congenital anomalies (Singh & Mehra, 2023). The level (high or low) of the defect significantly influences the outcome in terms of fecal continence as well as management (Fig. 20.9). The nurse may encounter the infant with imperforate anus and an ostomy when the child is admitted to the hospital at several months of age for corrective surgery. Infants often require a staged repair in which the bowel is connected to the anal opening or an anal opening is created. When the final repair is achieved, the stoma will be closed, and the infant will pass stool through the anal opening.

Anomalies Associated With Anorectal Malformations

- VACTERL syndrome: vertebral, anorectal, cardiovascular, tracheoesophageal, renal, and limb
- Esophageal atresia
- Intestinal atresia
- Malrotation
- Renal agenesis
- Hypospadias
- Vesicoureteral reflux
- Bladder exstrophy
- Cardiac anomalies
- Skeletal anomalies

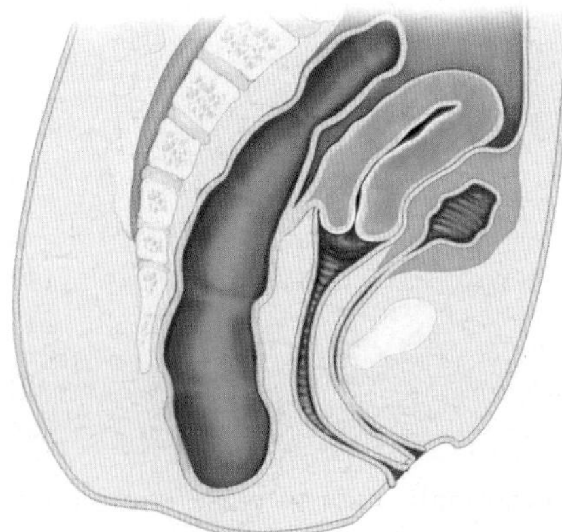

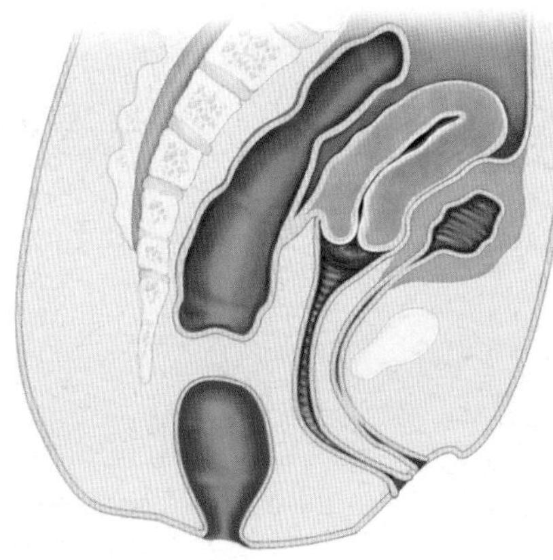

FIGURE 20.9 Imperforate anus, in which the rectum ends in a blind pouch.

Surgical intervention is needed for both high and low types of imperforate anus. Surgery for a high type of defect involves a colostomy in the newborn period, with corrective surgery performed in stages to allow for growth. Surgery for the low type of anomaly, which frequently includes a fistula, involves closure of the fistula, creation of an anal opening, and repositioning of the rectal pouch into the anal opening. A major challenge for either type of surgical repair is finding, using, or creating adequate nerve and muscle structures around the rectum to provide for normal evacuation.

Nursing Assessment

In the newborn, observe for an appropriate anal opening. If the anal opening exists, observe for passage of meconium stool within the first 24 hours of life (generally not passed in the infant with imperforate anus). Assess urine output to identify accompanying genitourinary problems. Assess for signs of intestinal obstruction, which may occur as a result of the malformation. These include abdominal distention and bilious vomiting.

Nursing Management

Nursing management focuses on preparing the newborn for surgery and providing postoperative care. Preoperatively, maintain the newborn's NPO status and provide gastric decompression. Administer IV therapy and antibiotic therapy as ordered and monitor the newborn's hydration status. It is important to provide the parents with a full explanation of the defect, surgical options, potential complications, typical postoperative course, and long-term care needed. Prepare the parents for the possibility that the newborn may require an ostomy. Provide support to the parents and family.

Postoperative care includes ensuring adequate pain relief, maintaining NPO status and gastric decompression until normal bowel function is restored, and providing colostomy care if applicable. After the intestinal pull-through procedure is completed, it will be the first time that stool has passed through the anal sphincter. The stool may be quite loose depending on the severity of the imperforate anus. The perianal skin is at significant risk for breakdown. Therefore, use a barrier cream on the area and clean it once daily with soap and water. Otherwise, wipe liquid stool off the barrier cream with mineral oil and cotton balls. Most of the barrier cream will remain intact, protecting the infant's perianal area.

TAKE NOTE!

To decrease the drying associated with frequent cleaning, avoid baby wipes and frequent use of soap and water.

Meckel Diverticulum

Meckel diverticulum is the result of an incomplete fusion of the omphalomesenteric duct during embryonic development. This causes a fibrous band to connect the small intestine to the umbilicus, known as a Meckel diverticulum. It is the most common congenital anomaly of the GI tract, occurring in 1.5% of the population (Brumbaugh et al., 2022). Complications associated with Meckel diverticulum include bleeding, anemia, and intestinal obstruction such as volvulus and intussusception, half of which occur within the first 2 years of life (Brumbaugh et al., 2022). Surgical correction of the Meckel diverticulum is necessary in children who have complications. The surgery is usually done to remove the diverticulum itself. At times, ileal resection is necessary.

Nursing Assessment

Elicit a description of the present illness and chief complaint. Common signs and symptoms reported during the health history might include bleeding, anemia, or severe colicky abdominal pain (in children with associated intestinal obstruction). Assess the child for an acute abdomen. Observe for abdominal distention, auscultate for hypoactive bowel sounds, and then palpate for an abdominal mass, **guarding** (tensing of the abdominal wall muscles), and rebound tenderness. Stool for occult blood is usually positive, and a complete blood count (CBC) may reveal anemia. A positive Meckel scan is conclusive.

Nursing Management

If anemia is significant, administer ordered blood products (packed red blood cells) to stabilize the child before surgery. Administer IV fluids and maintain NPO status for symptomatic children while further evaluation is being performed. Immediately report an acute abdomen to a health care provider or nurse practitioner. Postoperative care will vary depending on the surgery that was performed. Provide child and family education as necessary to relieve anxiety related to the diagnosis and surgical intervention. Refer to the "Clinical Judgment and the Nursing Process" section for additional information.

Inguinal and Umbilical Hernias

Inguinal and umbilical hernias are defects that occur during fetal development. Either may be visible at birth, and inguinal hernias may be noted later in life (Brumbaugh et al., 2022).

Inguinal Hernia

When the processus vaginalis fails to close completely during embryonal development, an inguinal hernia may occur. This allows the abdominal or pelvic viscera to travel through the internal inguinal ring into the inguinal canal. The hernia sacs that develop most often contain bowel in males and fallopian tubes or ovaries in females. Males are more likely than females to develop inguinal hernia, and premature infants demonstrate an increased incidence overall (Brumbaugh et al., 2022). Surgical correction of the inguinal hernia is usually performed when the infant is several weeks old and has been thriving.

NURSING ASSESSMENT

Assess infants and children with an inguinal hernia for the presence of a bulging mass in the lower abdomen or groin area (Fig. 20.10). It may be possible to visualize the mass, but often the mass is seen only during crying or straining, making it difficult to identify in the clinic setting.

NURSING MANAGEMENT

If a mass is felt upon palpation, the health care provider or nurse practitioner may attempt to reduce the hernia by pushing it back through the external inguinal ring. The health care provider or nurse practitioner may ask the nurse to assist in a reduction, most likely helping to hold the child in a position that will allow the health care provider or nurse practitioner to reduce the hernia. Reduction is only a temporary method of managing inguinal hernias; they must be corrected surgically. If reduction is not possible even with sedation, the hernia could be incarcerated (Brumbaugh et al., 2022). An incarcerated hernia could eventually lead to bowel strangulation.

The hernia should be manually reduced as needed until the time of the surgery, so teach the family how to reduce the hernia. Instruct the family to contact the surgeon immediately if the hernia becomes irreducible. Provide routine preoperative and postoperative care during inguinal hernia surgical repair, including child and family education to relieve anxiety.

CLINICAL REASONING ALERT!

Tell the parents that if the child's inguinal hernia becomes hard, discolored, or painful (evidenced by inconsolable crying), they should immediately call the health care provider or nurse practitioner to determine the next course of action (office visit or emergency room visit).

Umbilical Hernia

Umbilical hernia occurs commonly in full-term infants and much more frequently in Black infants compared to White infants (Brumbaugh et al., 2022). An umbilical hernia is caused by an incomplete closure of the umbilical ring, allowing intestinal contents to herniate through the opening. Most children will have spontaneous closure of the umbilical hernia by 4 to 5 years of age, and those without spontaneous closure may have surgical correction at that time (Brumbaugh et al., 2022).

NURSING ASSESSMENT

Assess whether the hernia can be reduced. Notify the surgeon if the hernia will not reduce. Incarceration is extremely rare, but when it does occur, the child will report abdominal pain, tenderness, or redness at the umbilicus (see Fig. 20.10).

NURSING MANAGEMENT

Since operative repair is not as likely with umbilical hernias as with inguinal hernias, the aim of nursing management is education. Teach the child and family how to reduce the hernia. The child may have some self-esteem issues related to the large protrusion of the unrepaired umbilical hernia. Teach the child coping skills to help relieve anxiety.

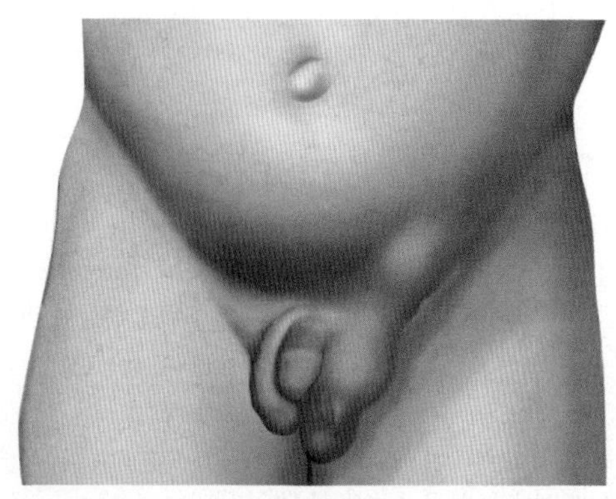

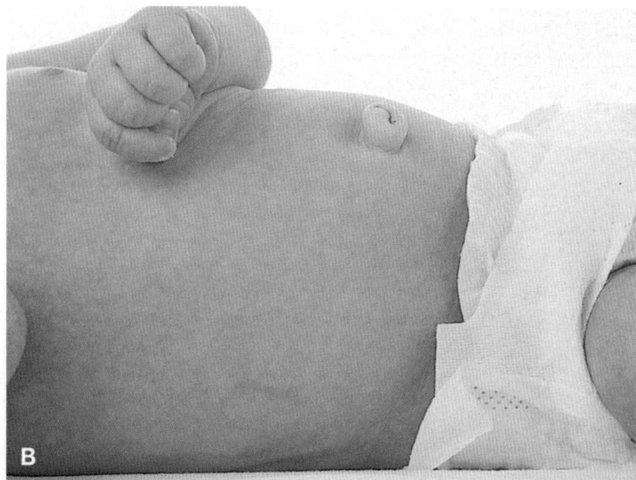

FIGURE 20.10 **A.** Inguinal hernia: note the bulge in the inguinal (groin) area. **B.** Umbilical hernia: note the protrusion in the umbilical area.

TAKE NOTE!

The use of home remedies to reduce an umbilical hernia should be discouraged because of the risk of skin maceration. This includes taping a quarter over a reduced umbilical hernia and the use of "belly bands" (Palazzi & Brandt, 2023).

ACUTE GI DISORDERS

Acute GI disorders include dehydration, vomiting, diarrhea, oral candidiasis, oral lesions, hypertrophic pyloric stenosis, necrotizing enterocolitis, intussusception, malrotation and volvulus, and appendicitis.

Dehydration

Dehydration occurs more readily in infants and young children than it does in adults. The risk is increased in infants and young children because they have an increased extracellular fluid percentage and a relative increase in body water compared to adults. Increased basal metabolic rate, increased ratio of BSA to body mass, immature renal function, and increased insensible fluid loss through temperature elevation also contribute to the increased risk for dehydration in infants and young children as compared to adults. Dehydration left unchecked leads to shock, so early recognition and treatment of dehydration is critical to prevent progression to hypovolemic shock. The goals of therapeutic management of dehydration are to restore appropriate fluid balance and to prevent complications.

Nursing Assessment

For a full description of the assessment phase of the nursing process, refer to "Clinical Judgment and the Nursing Process" section. Assessment findings pertinent to dehydration are discussed further.

HEALTH HISTORY

Elicit a description of the present illness and chief complaint. Common signs and symptoms reported during the health history are included in Comparison Chart 20.1, which compares the clinical manifestations of mild, moderate, and severe dehydration.

Explore the child's current and past medical history for risk factors for dehydration such as:

- Diarrhea
- Vomiting
- Decreased oral intake
- Sustained high fever
- Diabetic ketoacidosis
- Extensive burns

CLINICAL REASONING ALERT!

Nurses must be able to assess a child's hydration status accurately and intervene quickly. Children are at higher risk than adults for hypovolemic shock. Dehydrated children may deteriorate very quickly and experience shock.

COMPARISON CHART 20.1 Dehydration

	Mild	Moderate	Severe
Mental status	Alert	Alert to listless	Alert to comatose
Fontanels	Soft and flat	Sunken	Sunken
Eyes	Normal	Mildly sunken orbits	Deeply sunken orbits
Oral mucosa	Pink and moist	Pale and slightly dry	Dry
Skin turgor	Elastic	Decreased	Tenting
Heart rate	Normal	May be increased	Increased, progressing to bradycardia
Blood pressure	Normal	Normal	Normal, progressing to hypotension
Extremities	Warm, pink, brisk capillary refill	Delayed capillary refill	Cool, mottled, or dusky, significantly delayed capillary refill
Urine output	May be slightly decreased	<1 mL/kg/h	Significantly <1 mL/kg/h

Data from Kleinman, K., McDaniel, L., & Malloy, M. (2023). *The Harriet Lane handbook* (22nd ed.). Elsevier; Hanna, M. G., & Bock, M. (2022). Fluid, electrolyte, and acid-base disorders & therapy. In M. Bunik, W. W. Hay, M. J. Levin, & M. J. Abzug (Eds.), *Current pediatric diagnosis and treatment* (26th ed.). McGraw-Hill Education.

PHYSICAL EXAMINATION

Assess the child's hydration status, including heart rate, blood pressure, skin turgor, fontanels, oral mucosa, eyes, temperature and color of extremities, mental status, and urine output. Children usually compensate well initially; their heart rate increases in moderate dehydration, but blood pressure remains normal until it decreases in severe dehydration.

Nursing Management

Nursing goals for the infant or child with dehydration are aimed at restoring fluid volume and preventing progression to hypovolemia. Provide oral rehydration to children for mild-to-moderate states of dehydration (see Teaching Guidelines 20.1). Children with severe dehydration should receive IV fluids. Initially, administer 20 mL/kg of normal saline or lactated Ringer's, and then reassess the hydration status (refer to Chapter 29 for further specifics regarding hypovolemic shock).

Once initial fluid balance is restored, the health care provider or nurse practitioner may order IV fluids at the maintenance rate or as much as 1.5 times maintenance. Maintenance fluid requirements refer to the amount needed under conditions of normal hydration. Maintenance fluid requirements may be determined with the use of the formula found in Box 20.2. In the example provided in Box 20.2, a 23-kg child will need maintenance fluid equivalent to 65 mL/h.

The same anatomic and physiologic differences that make infants and young children susceptible to dehydration also make them susceptible to overhydration. Thus, continuously evaluate hydration status and be aware of the appropriateness of IV fluid orders.

Vomiting

Vomiting is the forceful expulsion of gastric contents through the mouth. It occurs as a reflex with three different phases:

TEACHING GUIDELINES 20.1 Oral Rehydration Therapy

- Oral rehydration solution (ORS) should contain 75 mmol/L sodium chloride and 13.5 g/L glucose (standard ORS solutions include Pedialyte, Infalyte, and Ricelyte).
- Tap water, milk, undiluted fruit juice, soup, and broth are NOT appropriate for oral rehydration.
- Children with mild-to-moderate dehydration require 50–100 mL/kg of ORS over 4 hours.
- After reevaluation, oral rehydration may need to be continued if the child is still dehydrated.
- When rehydrated, the child can resume a regular diet.

Data from Freedman, S. (2023). Oral rehydration therapy. *UpToDate*. Retrieved January 12, 2024, from http://www.uptodate.com/contents/oral-rehydration-therapy

BOX 20.2 Formula for Fluid Maintenance

- 100 mL/kg for first 10 kg
- 50 mL/kg for next 10 kg
- 20 mL/kg for remaining kg
- Add together for total mL needed per 24-hour period.
- Divide by 24 for mL/h fluid requirement.

Thus, for a 23-kg child:

- $100 \times 10 = 1{,}000$
- $50 \times 10 = 500$
- $20 \times 3 = 60$
- $1{,}000 + 500 + 60 = 1{,}560$

$1{,}560/24 = 65$ mL/h

Data from Kleinman, K., McDaniel, L., & Malloy, M. (2023). *The Harriet Lane handbook* (22nd ed.). Elsevier.

- Prodromal period: nausea and signs of autonomic nervous system stimulation
- Retching
- Vomiting

Vomiting in infants and children has many different causes and is considered to be a symptom of some other condition. Table 20.1 lists common causes of vomiting.

Therapeutic management of vomiting most often involves slow oral rehydration and at times may require administration of antiemetics.

Nursing Assessment

For a full description of the assessment phase of the nursing process, refer to the "Clinical Judgment and the Nursing Process" section. Assessment findings pertinent to vomiting are discussed further.

HEALTH HISTORY

Elicit a description of the present illness and chief complaint. Note onset and progression of symptoms. Determine timing of the vomiting episodes as vomiting several hours after a meal could signify delayed gastric emptying and vomiting in middle of the night or upon awakening may be associated with an intracranial lesion. Ask whether the vomiting seems effortless (as seen with gastroesophageal reflux [GER]) or if it is projectile (such as with pyloric stenosis). Inquire about the contents and character of the emesis. Bilious vomiting is never considered normal and suggests an obstruction, whereas bloody emesis can signify esophageal or GI bleeding (Brumbaugh et al., 2022). Note any events associated with the vomiting, such as diarrhea or pain.

Assess the child's past medical history to identify preexisting illnesses, drug misuse, trauma, prescribed medications, and previous abdominal surgery. Risk factors for vomiting include exposure to viruses, certain medication use, and overfeeding in an infant.

TABLE 20.1 • Causes of Vomiting by Temporal Pattern

Category	Acute	Chronic	Cyclic
Infectious	Gastroenteritis, otitis media, pharyngitis, sinusitis (acute), hepatitis, pyelonephritis, meningitis	*Helicobacter pylori, Giardia,* sinusitis (chronic)	Chronic sinusitis
Gastrointestinal	Intussusception, malrotation with volvulus, appendicitis, cholecystitis, pancreatitis	GERD, gastritis, peptic ulcer disease	GERD, malrotation with volvulus
Genitourinary	Ureteropelvic junction obstruction, pyelonephritis	Pregnancy, pyelonephritis	Hydronephrosis
Endocrine/metabolic	Diabetic ketoacidosis	Adrenal hyperplasia	Diabetic ketoacidosis, Addison disease, acute intermittent porphyria
Neurologic	Concussion, subdural hematoma, brain tumor	Brain tumor, Arnold–Chiari malformation	Migraines, Arnold–Chiari malformation, brain tumor
Other	Food poisoning, toxic ingestion	Bulimia, rumination	Cyclic vomiting syndrome

GERD, gastroesophageal reflux disease.

PHYSICAL EXAMINATION

Perform a physical examination, noting the child's general appearance. Note hydration status, as well as mental status changes. Note the quality of bowel sounds upon auscultation. Palpate the abdomen for the presence of abdominal masses, tenderness, or signs of trauma.

Nursing Management

Nursing management focuses on promoting fluid and electrolyte balance. Oral rehydration is accomplished successfully in most outpatient cases of simple vomiting. Teach the primary caregiver about oral rehydration (refer to Teaching Guidelines 20.1). In the child with mild-to-moderate dehydration resulting from vomiting, withhold oral feeding for 1 to 2 hours after emesis, after which time oral rehydration can begin. Give the infant or child 0.5 to 2 oz of ORS every 15 minutes, depending on the child's age and size. Most infants and children can retain this small amount of fluid if fed the restricted amount every 15 minutes. As the child improves, larger amounts will be tolerated.

TAKE NOTE!

Homemade ORS can be made by combining 1 quart of water (can be water poured from cooking rice if desired), 8 teaspoons sugar, and 1 teaspoon salt.

If oral rehydration is not possible due to continued nausea and vomiting, IV fluids will likely be ordered. In some cases, antiemetics may be used to help control the vomiting, and ondansetron is preferred over promethazine due to lesser side effects. Educate the family regarding the prevention of vomiting and use of antiemetic therapy.

TAKE NOTE!

Ginger capsules (10 mg), ginger tea, and candied ginger are generally useful in reducing nausea, are safe for use in children over age 2 years, and usually produce no side effects (Canani, 2018).

Diarrhea

Diarrhea is either an increase in the frequency or a decrease in the consistency of stool. Diarrhea in children can either be acute or chronic. In resource-abundant regions, viruses cause most cases of diarrhea (Bishop & Ebach, 2023).

Pathophysiology

Acute diarrhea in children is most commonly caused by viruses, but it may also be related to bacterial or parasitic enteropathogens. Viruses injure the absorptive surface of mature villous cells, resulting in decreased fluid absorption and disaccharidase deficiency. Bacteria produce intestinal injury by directly invading the mucosa, damaging the villous surface, or releasing toxins. Acute diarrhea may be bloody or nonbloody. The viral, bacterial, and parasitic causes of acute infectious diarrhea are discussed in Box 20.3. Diarrhea may also occur in relation to antibiotic use. Risk factors for acute diarrhea include

BOX 20.3 Acute Infectious Diarrhea

Causes	Manifestations	Distinguishing Features	Treatment
Viruses: Rotavirus, adenovirus, norovirus, parvovirus, pestivirus, calicivirus, astrovirus, cytomegalovirus	Loose, watery stools, fever, vomiting	Rotavirus most common, especially in young children Norovirus more common in older children	Supportive care includes oral rehydration, electrolyte replacement in some cases, and early refeeding of diet. Antidiarrheals are not effective.
Bacteria: *Salmonella, Shigella, Escherichia coli* 0157:H7, *Campylobacter, Clostridium difficile, Yersinia enterocolitica*	Stools may be bloody or contain mucus.	*Salmonella* may be shed for a year. *E. coli* 0157:H7 causes hemolytic anemia. *C. difficile* results from antibiotic use.	Care includes rehydration and early refeeding of diet. Some but not all cases require antibiotic therapy.
Parasites: *Giardia lamblia, Entamoeba histolytica, Cryptosporidium*	Fever, watery stools	Oral–fecal transmission, *Cryptosporidium* spread by farm animals	Some cases require antiparasitic therapy.

Data from Brumbaugh, D., Furuta, G. T., Hoffenberg, E., Kobak, G., Kramer, R., Walker, T., Septer, S., Shull, M., Soden, J., & Walker, T. (2022). Gastrointestinal tract. In M. Bunik, W. W. Hay, M. J. Levin, & M. J. Abzug (Eds.), *Current diagnosis and treatment: Pediatrics* (26th ed.). McGraw-Hill Education; Thiagarajah, J. R., & Martin, M. G. (2023). Pathogenesis of acute diarrhea in children. *UpToDate*. Retrieved January 12, 2024, from http://www.uptodate.com/contents/pathogenesis-of-acute-diarrhea-in-children

recent ingestion of undercooked meats, foreign travel, day care attendance, and well water use.

Since most cases of diarrhea are acute and viral in nature, therapeutic management of diarrhea is usually supportive (maintaining fluid balance and nutrition). Probiotic supplementation may be useful in the prevention of diarrhea but has not been shown to be effective in its treatment (Levy, 2022).

Though most cases of diarrhea in children are of acute origin, diarrhea may also occur chronically. Chronic diarrhea is diarrhea that lasts for more than 2 weeks. This type of diarrhea is not usually caused by serious illnesses. The causes of chronic diarrhea are listed according to age group in Box 20.4.

Nursing Assessment

For a full description of the assessment phase of the nursing process, refer to the assessment section of the Nursing Process Overview earlier in the chapter. Assessment findings pertinent to diarrhea are discussed further.

BOX 20.4 Causes of Chronic Diarrhea by Age

Infants	Toddlers	School-Age Children
Intractable diarrhea of infancy Milk and soy protein intolerance Infectious enteritis Hirschsprung disease Nutrient malabsorption	Chronic nonspecific diarrhea Viral enteritis *Giardia* Tumors (secretory diarrhea) Ulcerative colitis Celiac disease	Inflammatory bowel disease Appendiceal abscess Lactase deficiency Constipation with encopresis

HEALTH HISTORY

Elicit a description of the present illness and chief complaint. Important information related to the course of the diarrhea includes:

- Number and frequency of stools
- Duration of symptoms
- Stool volume
- Associated symptoms (abdominal pain, cramping, nausea, vomiting, fever)
- Presence of blood or mucus in the stool

Ask about the child's urine output (decreased with dehydration). Explore the child's current and past medical history for risk factors such as:

- Likelihood of exposure to infectious agents (well water, farm animals, day care attendance)
- Dietary history
- Family history of similar symptoms
- Recent travel
- Child's age (to identify common etiology for that age group)

PHYSICAL EXAMINATION

Note the child's general appearance and color. Note decreased tear production, sunken orbits, or dry mucous membranes with moderate to severe dehydration. Determine mental status; listlessness or lethargy may occur with moderate to severe dehydration. Evaluate skin turgor noting that nonelasticity or tenting may occur with moderate to severe dehydration. Note abdominal distention or concavity. Stool output may be available to assess for color and consistency. Inspect the anal area for presence of redness or rash related to increased stool volumes and increased frequency.

Auscultate bowel sounds to assess for the presence of hypoactive (obstruction or peritonitis) or hyperactive bowel sounds (diarrhea or gastroenteritis). Percuss the abdomen, noting any abnormality as it could indicate a pathologic process. Note tenderness to palpation in the lower quadrants, though rebound tenderness should not be present.

LABORATORY AND DIAGNOSTIC TESTS

Common laboratory and diagnostic studies ordered for the assessment of diarrhea include:

- Stool culture: may indicate presence of bacteria
- Stool for ova and parasites (O&P): may indicate the presence of parasites
- Stool viral panel or culture: to determine the presence of rotavirus or other viruses
- Stool for occult blood: may be positive if inflammation or ulceration is present in the GI tract
- Stool for leukocytes: may be positive in cases of inflammation or infection
- Stool pH/reducing substances: to see if the diarrhea is caused by carbohydrate intolerance
- Electrolyte panel: may indicate dehydration
- Abdominal radiographs (kidney, ureter, and bladder [KUB]): presence of stool in colon may indicate constipation or **fecal impaction** (hardened immobile bulk of stool); air–fluid levels may indicate intestinal obstruction

Nursing Management

Nursing management of diarrhea focuses on restoring fluid and electrolyte balance and providing family education.

RESTORING FLUID AND ELECTROLYTE BALANCE

Continue the child's regular diet if the child is not dehydrated. Initial nursing management of the dehydrated child with diarrhea is focused on fluid and electrolyte balance restoration. After rehydration is achieved, it is important to encourage the child to consume a regular diet to maintain energy and growth.

TAKE NOTE!

Avoid fluids high in sugar, such as fruit juice, gelatin, and soda, which may worsen diarrhea.

PROVIDING FAMILY EDUCATION

Teach the parents the importance of oral rehydration therapy (see Teaching Guidelines 20.1). The health care provider may order medication therapy. In such instances, teach the importance of finishing all prescribed antibiotic therapy. After the cause of the diarrhea is known, teach the child and family how to prevent further occurrences. As most cases of acute diarrhea are infectious, provide education about proper handwashing techniques and transmission route. Chronic diarrhea is often a result of excessive intake of formula, water, or fruit juice, so teach the parents about appropriate fluid intake.

Oral Candidiasis (Thrush)

Oral candidiasis (thrush) is a fungal infection of the oral mucosa. It is most common in newborns and infants. Children at risk for thrush include those with immune disorders, those using corticosteroid inhalers, and those receiving therapy that suppresses the immune system (e.g., chemotherapy for cancer). Antibiotic use may also contribute to thrush. In addition, fungal infection may be transmitted from the chest- or breastfeeding parent to the infant (Campbell & Palazzi, 2023).

Therapeutic management includes treatment with oral antifungal agents such as nystatin or fluconazole.

Nursing Assessment

Assess for risk factors for oral candidiasis such as young age, immune suppression, antibiotic use, use of corticosteroid inhalers, or presence of fungal infection in the birthing parent. Inspect the oral mucosa. Thrush appears as thick white patches on the tongue, mucosa, or palate, resembling curdled milk (Fig. 20.11). Unlike milk retained in the mouth, the patches do not easily wipe off with a swab or washcloth. Also assess for the presence of candidal diaper rash (beefy-red rash with satellite lesions). Determine the extent to which the presence of the lesions is interfering with the infant's ability to feed. The lesions may cause significant discomfort.

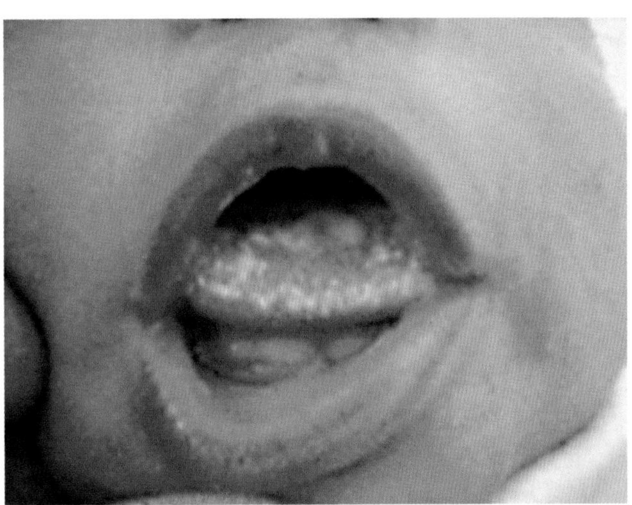

FIGURE 20.11 Thick white patches in the infant with oral candidiasis (thrush).

Diagnosis is usually based on clinical presentation. However, a careful scraping of the lesions can be sent out for fungal culture.

Nursing Management

Nursing management of the child with thrush includes administering medications and providing family education.

ADMINISTERING MEDICATIONS

Ensure appropriate administration of oral antifungal agents. Administer nystatin suspension four times per day following feeding to allow the medication to remain in contact with the lesions. In the younger infant, apply nystatin to the lesions with a cotton-tipped applicator. The older infant or child can easily swallow the pleasantly flavored suspension. An advantage of fluconazole is its once-daily dosing, but monitor infants and children receiving it for hepatotoxicity. Unlike nystatin, it is important to administer fluconazole with food to decrease the side effects of nausea and vomiting.

EDUCATING THE FAMILY

If the chest- or breastfeeding parent is also infected, they must receive antifungal treatment. Fungal infection of the breast can cause a great deal of pain with nursing, but if appropriately treated breastfeeding can continue without interruption. Stress appropriate handwashing. It is important to keep bottle nipples and pacifiers clean. Infants and young children often mouth their toys, so it is important to clean them appropriately. Explain to parents of infants with thrush the importance of reporting diaper rash because fungal infections in the diaper area often occur concomitantly with thrush and also need to be treated.

TAKE NOTE!

Geographic tongue is a benign, noncontagious condition. A reduction in the filiform papillae (bumps on the tongue) occurs in patches that migrate periodically, thus giving a map-like appearance to the tongue, with darker and lighter, higher and lower patches. Do not confuse the lighter patches of geographic tongue with the thick white plaques that form on the tongue with thrush.

Oral Lesions

A number of oral lesions may affect infants and children. A few of the most common are aphthous ulcers, gingivostomatitis (from herpes simplex virus [HSV]), and herpangina. Table 20.2 lists the causes of common oral lesions. Regardless of type, oral lesions are often painful and can interfere with the child's ability to eat. Therapeutic management of oral lesions varies depending on the cause.

Nursing Assessment

Explore the health history for the presence of risk factors such as immune deficiency, cancer chemotherapy treatment, exposure to infectious agents, trauma, stress, or celiac or Crohn disease. Note the onset of the lesion(s) and progression over time. Question the parent or child about the presence of sore throat or dysphagia (occurs with herpangina). Inspect the oral cavity, including the tongue, buccal mucosa, palate, and hypoglossal area. Note the presence of lesions and their distribution. Refer to Table 20.2 for descriptions and illustrations of various oral lesions. Inspect the pharynx, which may be red

TABLE **20.2** • Oral Lesions

	Aphthous Ulcers	Gingivostomatitis	Herpangina
Cause	Trauma, vitamin deficiency, celiac disease, Crohn disease	Herpes simplex virus	Enterovirus (Coxsackie)
Appearance	Erythematous border, often yellow appearance to the ulcer, anywhere on the oral mucosa or lips	Vesicular lesions on erythematous base, anywhere in the oral cavity, including lips	Bright red ulcers, generally in the posterior oral cavity
Fever	Generally absent	May have high fever with initial outbreak	Abrupt onset of high fever (up to 39.4–40.6°C), lasting 1–4 days
Length of illness	Generally heal within 7–14 days; may recur	10–12 days initially; may recur with stress, febrile illness, or intense sunlight exposure (as virus lies dormant in system)	Generally resolves within 5–7 days
Therapeutic management	Topical corticosteroid in dental paste may help	Acyclovir	Supportive treatment only

Data from Kyle, T. (2022). Management of mouth disorders. In T. Kyle (Ed.), *Primary care pediatrics for the nurse practitioner: A practical approach*. Springer.

with herpangina. Generally, the diagnosis is based on the history and clinical presentation, but occasionally oral lesions are cultured for HSV.

Nursing Management

The primary concerns with oral lesions are pain management and maintenance of hydration. A corticosteroid-containing dental paste used for aphthous ulcers is formulated to "stick" to mucous membranes, so the lesion area should be as dry as possible prior to application of the paste. Children do not care for having the paste applied and will often resist. Older children with herpangina or stomatitis can "swish and spit" various formulations of "magic mouthwash" (typically a combination of liquid diphenhydramine, liquid acetaminophen, and milk of magnesia) that may offer some pain relief. Common over-the-counter medications such as Anbesol, Orajel, and Kank-A may be helpful for topical pain relief, though oral analgesics are often necessary.

The child with herpangina is typically an infant or young child (Kyle, 2022). It may be very difficult to coach a young child to drink fluids when their mouth is hurting. Playing games and offering favorite fluids and popsicles may encourage adequate oral intake. It is important to avoid carbonated beverages and citrus juices when oral lesions are present as they can cause further stinging and burning.

TAKE NOTE!

Viscous lidocaine should be used with caution in younger children as a topical treatment for numbing the lesions or as a swish-and-spit treatment because the child may swallow the lidocaine (UpToDate, Inc., 2024).

Hypertrophic Pyloric Stenosis

In hypertrophic pyloric stenosis, the circular muscle of the pylorus becomes hypertrophied, causing thickness in the luminal side of the pyloric canal (Fig. 20.12). This thickness creates a gastric outlet obstruction, causing nonbilious vomiting that presents between weeks 3 and 6 of life. The vomiting becomes more frequent and forceful as time goes on and is often projectile. The incidence is 1 to 3.5 per 1,000 live births, and it occurs more in males than females (5:1), with first-born infants being affected up to 1.5 times more often (Endom et al., 2023). The cause of pyloric stenosis is probably multifactorial.

Pyloric stenosis requires surgical intervention. A pyloromyotomy is performed to cut the muscle of the pylorus and relieve the gastric outlet obstruction (see Fig. 20.12). Postoperative complications are rare.

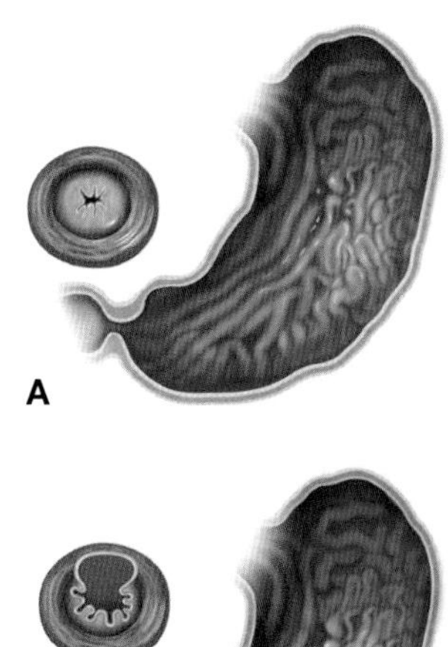

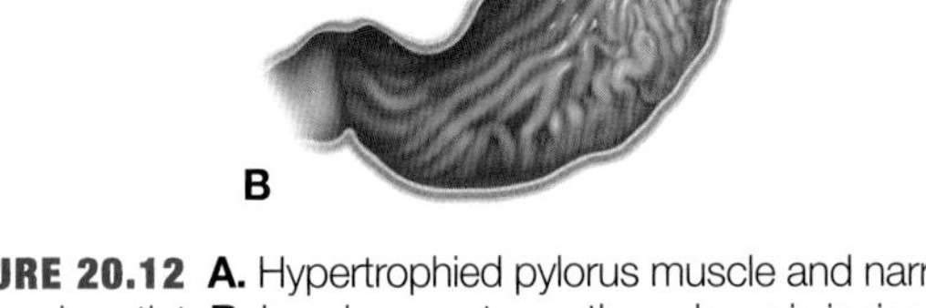

FIGURE 20.12 A. Hypertrophied pylorus muscle and narrowed stomach outlet. **B.** In pyloromyotomy, the pylorus is incised, thus increasing the diameter of the pyloric outlet.

Nursing Assessment

For a full description of the assessment phase of the nursing process, refer to "Clinical Judgment and the Nursing Process" section.

Elicit a description of the present illness and chief complaint. Common symptoms reported during the health history might include:

- Forceful, nonbilious vomiting, unrelated to feeding position
- Hunger soon after vomiting episode
- Weight loss due to vomiting
- Progressive dehydration with subsequent lethargy
- Possible positive family history

Palpate for a hard, movable "olive" in the right upper quadrant (hypertrophied pylorus). If an easily palpable mass is felt, no further testing is necessary, and a surgical consult is called. If no mass is identified, a pyloric ultrasound may be ordered to identify a thickened hypoechoic ring in the region of the pylorus. Assess laboratory values to determine if the infant has metabolic alkalosis resulting from dehydration.

TAKE NOTE!

It may be difficult to examine the infant's abdomen when pyloric stenosis is suspected because of the infant's extreme irritability. A pacifier or nipple dipped in glucose water may soothe the infant long enough to perform the abdominal examination.

Nursing Management

Preoperative management of pyloric stenosis is aimed at fluid management and correcting abnormal electrolyte values. Family anxiety is high during this time because of the impending surgery for an otherwise healthy infant. Provide emotional support to the family. Teach them about the surgical procedure and what to expect postoperatively. After surgery, infants usually resume oral feedings after 1 to 2 days.

Intussusception

Intussusception is a process that occurs when a proximal segment of bowel "telescopes" into a more distal segment, causing edema, vascular compromise, and, ultimately, partial or total bowel obstruction (Fig. 20.13). Most cases occur in toddlers 1 to 2 years of age (Bishop & Ebach, 2023). A lead point (i.e., pathologic point) may cause the telescoping. Examples of lead points are Meckel diverticulum, duplication cysts, polyps, hemangiomas, tumors, or the appendix. Typically, symptoms flare and then regress. Between episodes, children may have no symptoms of intussusception. This return to a normal state is due to the intussusception reducing on its own. The child may be asymptomatic and may appear well when presenting to the health care provider or nurse practitioner or emergency room. Again, this may be a sign that the bowel has reduced spontaneously. A pneumatic (air) enema is successful at reducing up to 90% of intussusception cases; other cases are reduced surgically (Bishop & Ebach, 2023). If surgical reduction is unsuccessful or bowel necrosis has occurred, a portion of the bowel must be resected.

Nursing Assessment

Elicit a description of the present illness and chief complaint. Common symptoms reported during the health history might include:

- Sudden onset of intermittent, crampy abdominal pain
- Severe pain (children usually draw up their knees and scream)

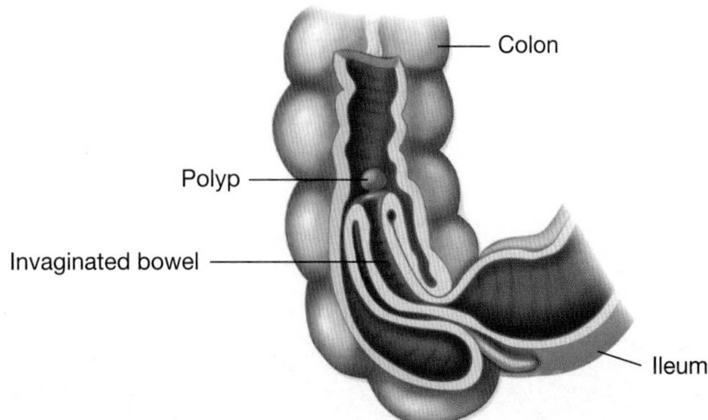

FIGURE 20.13 In intussusception, the intestine telescopes upon itself.

- Vomiting
- Diarrhea
- Currant jelly stools, gross blood, or hemoccult-positive stools
- Lethargy

Determine risk factors such as cystic fibrosis or celiac disease. Determine the severity of pain, length of time the symptoms have been present, presence of vomiting, and stool patterns and color.

Palpate the abdomen for the presence of a sausage-shaped mass in the upper midabdomen (a hallmark sign of intussusception). Note any mental status changes. Intussusception is usually diagnosed with a pneumatic (air) enema. White blood cell elevation may occur, and electrolytes may show signs of dehydration.

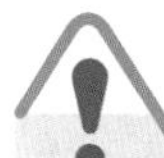

CLINICAL REASONING ALERT!

Immediately report the presence of bilious vomiting, which occurs only in an obstructive situation.

Nursing Management

Administer IV fluids and antibiotics before the diagnostic laboratory and radiograph studies are performed. Refer to the "Clinical Judgment and the Nursing Process" section for nursing care for the postoperative child. Offer emotional support to the parents as they may be very fatigued after dealing with a crying child and quite anxious about surgery in an otherwise healthy child. Provide appropriate preoperative and postoperative education to the family.

Malrotation and Volvulus

Intestinal malrotation results from a disruption in embryonic development. When malrotation occurs, the intestine is abnormally attached and the mesentery narrows, twisting on itself (volvulus). If the volvulus involves the entire small bowel, it is termed a midgut volvulus.

The main symptom of malrotation is bilious vomiting. Many children also have abdominal pain, shock symptoms, abdominal distention, tachycardia, and bloody stools. Most cases of malrotation will present in the first few weeks of life, but symptoms may occur in the older infant, child, or adult (Bishop & Ebach, 2023).

Therapeutic management of malrotation and volvulus is accomplished surgically. A Ladd procedure is performed, during which the intestine is straightened out and bands contributing to the misalignment are divided. If bowel necrosis has occurred (rare), then an ostomy may be necessary.

Nursing Assessment

Elicit a description of the present illness and chief complaint. Common symptoms reported during the health history might include vomiting and abdominal pain. Note severity of pain, auscultate for hypoactive bowel sounds, and palpate for abdominal guarding or rebound tenderness. A KUB may reveal obstruction. An upper GI series can identify the location of the duodenojejunal junction and corkscrew appearance of the twisted bowel.

Nursing Management

When diagnostic testing reveals malrotation/volvulus, administer ordered IV fluids and IV antibiotics. Place a nasogastric tube to decompress the stomach if ordered. Prepare the child and parents for surgery as it is performed as soon as possible. After surgery, provide postoperative care of the child. Provide continuous emotional support and family education.

Appendicitis

Appendicitis is an acute inflammation of the appendix. It is the most common cause of emergent abdominal surgery in children and peaks in prevalence at 15 to 30 years of age (Brumbaugh et al., 2022). If left untreated, the appendix may rupture.

Pathophysiology

Appendicitis is due to a closed-loop obstruction of the appendix (Fig. 20.14). It is thought that the obstruction is due to fecal material impacted into the relatively narrow appendix, though other causes such as ingested foreign bodies may exist. This causes a subsequent increase in the intraluminal pressure of the appendix, resulting in mucosal edema, bacterial overgrowth, and eventual perforation. Due to the fecal material in the appendix, perforation causes inflammatory fluid and bacterial contents to leak into the abdominal cavity, resulting in peritonitis. Diffuse peritonitis is more likely in younger children. Older children and adolescents have a more developed omentum, which walls off the inflamed or perforated appendix, often causing a focal abscess.

Therapeutic Management

Appendicitis is considered a surgical emergency due to the likelihood of perforation if left uncorrected. Surgical removal of the appendix is necessary and is often accomplished via a minimally invasive laparoscopic technique. In the case of perforation, an open surgical procedure is

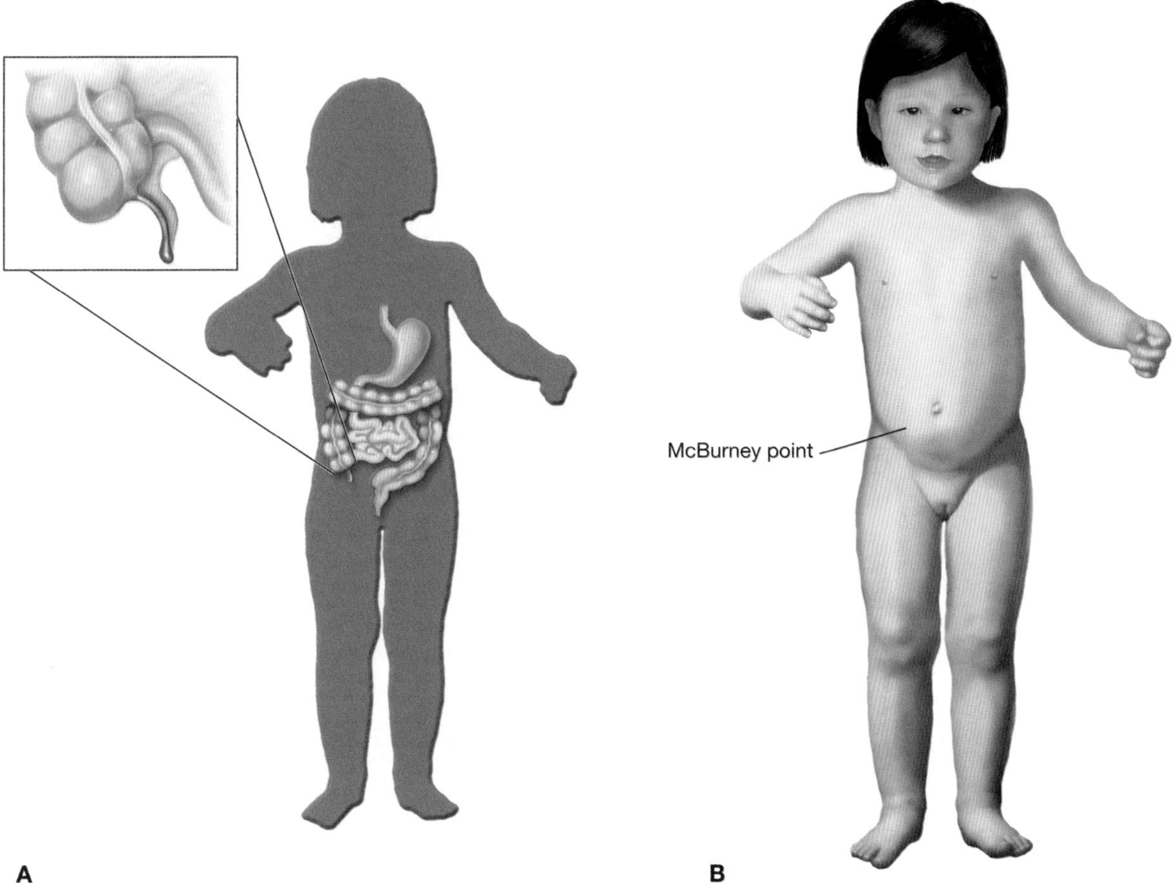

FIGURE 20.14 **A.** In appendicitis, the lumen of the appendix is obstructed, resulting in edema and compressed blood vessels. **B.** As appendicitis progresses, pain may become localized at McBurney point (a point midway between the anterior superior iliac crest and the umbilicus).

usually required, and lavage of the abdominal cavity may be performed to cleanse it of the infected fluid released from the appendix.

Nursing Assessment

Early diagnosis and intervention are the key elements to avoid perforation. For a full description of the assessment phase of the nursing process, refer to "Clinical Judgment and the Nursing Process" section. Assessment findings pertinent to appendicitis are discussed further.

HEALTH HISTORY

Elicit a description of the present illness and chief complaint. Appendicitis may be gradual, but symptoms usually do not come and go; they remain persistent and intensify. Common symptoms reported during the health history might include:

- Vague abdominal pain in the initial stages, localizing to the right lower quadrant over a few hours
- Nausea and vomiting (which usually develop after the onset of pain)
- Small-volume, frequent, soft stools, often confused with diarrhea
- Fever (usually low grade unless perforation occurs, which results in high fever)

THINKING ABOUT DEVELOPMENT

Children with appendicitis often experience referred pain. How will you accurately assess pain location in a school-age child, as compared with a toddler?

PHYSICAL EXAMINATION

Note an ill appearance to the child. The child often cannot walk or climb up onto the examination table without assistance. Upon palpation, maximal tenderness occurs over McBurney point in the right lower quadrant (see Fig. 20.14). Diffuse abdominal tenderness or distention may indicate peritonitis.

CLINICAL REASONING ALERT!

If the child's abdominal pain is suddenly relieved without intervention, suspect perforation and notify the health care provider immediately.

LABORATORY AND DIAGNOSTIC TESTS

Common laboratory and diagnostic studies ordered for the assessment of appendicitis include:

- Abdominal computed tomography (CT) scan: performed to visualize the appendix for further evaluation
- Laboratory testing: may reveal an elevated white blood cell count
- C-reactive protein: may be elevated

Nursing Management

Provide pre- and postoperative care and child and family education (see "Clinical Judgment and the Nursing Process" section). A nonruptured, nongangrenous appendix usually requires no antibiotic therapy, so provide routine postsurgical care. In addition to routine postoperative care, administer 48 to 72 hours of ordered antibiotics to the child with a suppurative or gangrenous (nonperforated) appendix to decrease the risk of postoperative infection. The child with a perforated appendix may require 7 to 14 days of IV antibiotic therapy in addition to normal postoperative care. Provide family teaching, because the child is often discharged home while still receiving IV antibiotic therapy.

• • • ATRAUMATIC CARE • • •

For the child requiring a postsurgical dressing change, make sure to premedicate the child with prescribed pain medication. Employ distraction techniques appropriate for age and/or personal preference. For a complex dressing change, it may be necessary to additionally consult the child life specialist to determine how best to proceed with the dressing change in the most atraumatic fashion possible.

CHRONIC GI DISORDERS

Chronic GI disorders include GER, peptic ulcer disease (PUD), constipation/encopresis, Hirschsprung disease, short bowel syndrome, IBD, celiac disease, functional abdominal pain, failure to thrive, and chronic feeding problems.

Gastroesophageal Reflux Disease

GER is passage of gastric contents into the esophagus. It is considered a normal physiologic process that occurs in healthy infants and children. However, when complications develop from the reflux of gastric contents back into the esophagus or oropharynx, it becomes more of a pathologic process known as gastroesophageal reflux disease (GERD). GER occurs frequently during the first year of life, is considered benign, and usually resolves by 12 to 18 months of age (Brumbaugh et al., 2022). GER is particularly common in premature infants.

Pathophysiology

The process of GER occurs during episodes of transient relaxation of the LES, which can occur during swallowing, crying, or other Valsalva maneuvers that increase intra-abdominal pressure. Delayed esophageal clearance and gastric emptying, highly acidic gastric contents, hiatal hernia (protrusion of the stomach upward into the mediastinal cavity through the esophageal hiatus of the diaphragm), or neurologic disease may also be contributing factors associated with reflux.

The signs and symptoms of GERD are often seen as a result of the damaging components of the refluxate (the pH of the gastric contents, bile acids, and pepsin). GERD may cause esophagitis, esophageal stricture, Barrett esophagus (a precancerous condition), or anemia from chronic esophageal erosion. In addition, complications such as laryngitis, recurrent pneumonia, or asthma may occur.

Therapeutic Management

Conservative medical management begins with appropriate positioning, such as elevating the head of the bed and keeping the infant or child upright for 30 minutes after feeding. Smaller, more frequent feedings may be helpful. If reflux does not improve with these measures, medications such as histamine blockers or proton pump inhibitors are prescribed to decrease acid production and stabilize the pH of the gastric contents (Brumbaugh et al., 2018) (Dosage Calculation Box 20.1).

DOSAGE CALCULATION BOX 20.1

Infant's weight: 11 lb, 8 oz

Medication order: omeprazole 4 mg PO once a day

Per the Pediatric Dosage Handbook, the recommended dose is 0.7 mg/kg/dose.

Is the ordered dose safe?

If the GERD cannot be medically managed effectively or requires long-term medication therapy, surgical intervention may be necessary. A Nissen fundoplication is the most common surgical procedure performed for antireflux therapy. The gastric fundus is wrapped around the lower 2 to 3 cm of the esophagus (Fig. 20.15). Laparoscopic fundoplications are being performed as a way to minimize the recovery period and reduce potential complications.

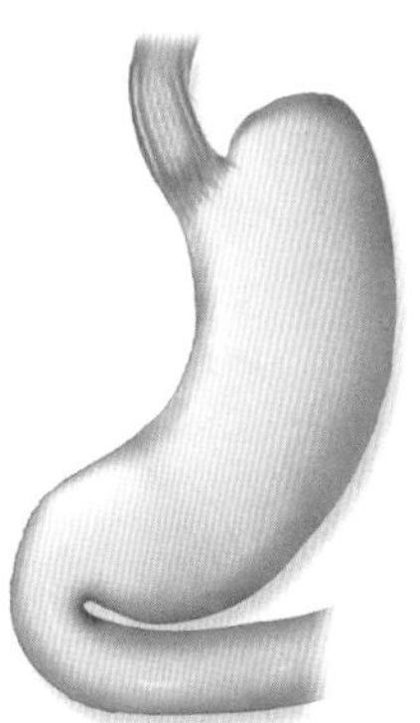

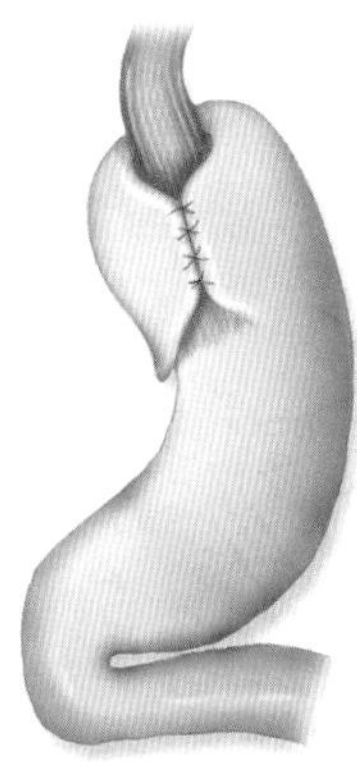

FIGURE 20.15 In Nissen fundoplication, the fundus (upper portion of the stomach) is wrapped around the lower segment of the esophagus.

Nursing Assessment

A full description of the assessment phase of the nursing process was presented in the "Clinical Judgment and the Nursing Process" section. Assessment findings pertinent to GER and GERD are discussed further.

HEALTH HISTORY

Elicit a description of the present illness and chief complaint. Note onset and progression of symptoms. Common symptoms reported during the health history include:

- Recurrent vomiting or regurgitation
- Weight loss or poor weight gain
- Irritability in infants
- Respiratory symptoms (chronic cough, wheezing, stridor, asthma, apnea)
- Hoarseness/sore throat
- Halitosis (mostly in older children)
- Heartburn or chest pain
- Abdominal pain
- Abnormal neck posturing (Sandifer syndrome)
- Hematemesis
- Dysphagia or feeding refusal
- Chronic sinusitis, otitis media
- Poor dentition (caused by acid erosion)

Explore the child's current and past medical history for risk factors such as:

- Prematurity, noting prolonged ventilator use or chronic lung disease
- Dietary habits (e.g., chocolate, coffee, spicy or fatty foods, caffeine, formula-fed or chest- or breastfed, overeating or overfeeding)
- Current medications
- Smoking or alcohol use in older children
- Food allergies
- Other GI disorders (gastric outlet dysfunction/hiatal hernia) or congenital abnormalities
- Feeding positions and patterns (especially important in infants)
- Sleeping positions or patterns
- Other medical history, such as asthma or recurrent infections/pneumonia

PHYSICAL EXAMINATION

Note an underweight or malnourished appearance in infants and children with uncontrolled GER for a period of time. Determine if the infant is irritable due to painful regurgitation/reflux events. Note breathing patterns, because reflux-induced asthma may have developed. Observe the child for cyanosis, altered mental status, and alterations in tone. Inspect emesis for blood or bile. Auscultate the lung fields for the presence of adventitious breath sounds related to GERD complications. Use caution when palpating the abdomen, especially in infants with GERD, because it may induce vomiting. No abnormalities should be identified on palpation.

CLINICAL REASONING ALERT!

Not all children with GERD actually vomit. Some may only demonstrate irritability associated with feeding or posturing (arching back during or after feeding [termed Sandifer syndrome]) and grimacing (Winter, 2023).

LABORATORY AND DIAGNOSTIC TESTS

Common laboratory and diagnostic studies ordered for the assessment of GER include:

- Upper GI series: though not sensitive or specific to GER, may show some reflux; studies are used to narrow down the differential diagnosis
- Esophageal pH probe study: quantifies GER episodes as they correlate to symptoms
- Esophagogastroduodenoscopy (EGD): shows esophageal and gastric tissue damage from GERD
- CBC: may demonstrate anemia if chronic esophagitis or hematemesis is present
- Hemoccult: may be positive if chronic esophagitis is present

Nursing Management

As with most GI disorders, initial nursing management is aimed at restoring proper fluid balance and nutrition. Refer to the "Clinical Judgment and the Nursing Process" section to individualize care. Additional considerations are reviewed further.

PROMOTING SAFE FEEDING TECHNIQUES AND POSITIONING

Feeding adjustments are an essential part of reflux management. Give infants smaller, more frequent feedings using a nipple that controls flow well. Frequently burp the infant during feeds to control reflux. Thickening of the formula with products such as rice or oatmeal cereal can significantly help keep the formula and gastric contents down. Positioning after feedings is important. Keep infants upright for 30 to 45 minutes after feeding by holding them and/or elevating the head of the crib 30 degrees. Placing in infant seats or swings is not recommended as this increases intra-abdominal pressure (Winter, 2023). For older children, elevate the head of the bed as much as possible and restrict meals for several hours before bedtime.

MAINTAINING A PATENT AIRWAY

GERD symptoms often involve the airway. Maximize reflux precautions to keep the risk of airway involvement to a minimum. If GERD causes apnea or there is a history of brief resolved unexplained event (BRUE), use an apnea or bradycardia monitor to monitor for such episodes. The monitor requires a health care provider's order and can be ordered through a home health company. Teach parents how to deal with these episodes, as their anxiety may be high. Provide cardiopulmonary resuscitation (CPR) instruction to all parents whose children have had a BRUE previously.

EDUCATING THE FAMILY AND CHILD

The goals for the infant or child with GERD are a decrease in symptoms, a decrease in the frequency and duration of reflux episodes, healing of the injured mucosa, and prevention of further complications of GERD. Teach the parents the signs and symptoms of complications. Explain that reflux is usually limited to the first year of life, though in some cases it persists. If medications are prescribed, thoroughly explain their use and their side effects (see Drug Guide 20.1).

PROVIDING POSTOPERATIVE CARE

If the child requires fundoplication, a gastrostomy tube is often placed for use in the immediate postoperative period or for long-term feeding. In the immediate postoperative period, assess for pain, abdominal distention, and return of bowel sounds. If a gastrostomy tube is placed, it is often open to straight drain for a period of time postoperatively to keep the stomach empty and allow for the internal incision to heal. When bowel sounds have returned and the infant or child is stable, introduce feedings slowly (typically via the gastrostomy tube). Assess for tolerance of feedings (absence of abdominal distention or pain, minimal residual, and passage of stool). If the abdomen does become distended or the child has discomfort, open the gastrostomy tube to air to decompress the stomach. Assess the insertion site of the gastrostomy tube for redness, edema, or drainage. Keep the site clean and dry per surgeon or hospital protocol. Teach the parents how to care for the gastrostomy tube and insertion site and how to use the tube for feeding.

PROMOTING FAMILY AND CHILD COPING

Parents may experience a great deal of anxiety. Teach the family about all aspects of GERD to help promote coping. School-age children often have reflux episodes exhibited by postprandial vomiting, which can be very embarrassing for the children. Notify the school about the medical issues related to GER to minimize the situations for the child.

Peptic Ulcer Disease

PUD is a term used to describe a variety of disorders of the upper GI tract that result from the action of gastric secretions (Fig. 20.16). Mucosal inflammation and subsequent ulceration occur as a result of either a primary or

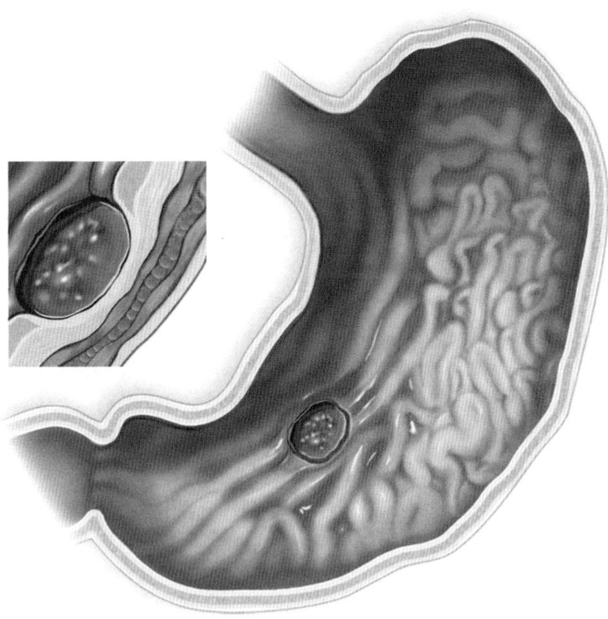

FIGURE 20.16 Peptic ulcer disease.

a secondary factor. Primary ulcers are usually associated with *Helicobacter pylori*, a Gram-negative organism that causes mucosal inflammation and in some cases more severe disease (Bishop & Ebach, 2023). *H. pylori* is found mostly in the duodenum. Secondary peptic ulcers may occur as a result of an identifiable factor, such as excess acid production, stress, medications, or the presence of other underlying conditions. Secondary ulcers tend to be gastric in location as opposed to duodenal.

Therapeutic Management

PUD may be treated with antibiotics (if *H. pylori* is verified), histamine agonists, and/or proton pump inhibitors. If the child presents with a severe esophageal or gastric hemorrhage, a nasogastric tube may be placed to decompress the stomach. The child may require IV infusion of a histamine-2 receptor antagonist or a proton pump inhibitor initially until the bleeding has stopped and the disease is stabilized.

Nursing Assessment

Elicit a description of the present illness and chief complaint. Common symptoms reported during the health history might include abdominal pain (most common), vomiting, or GI bleeding. The pain of PUD tends to be dull and vague, be mostly epigastric or periumbilical, worsen after meals, and/or wake the child at night. Explore the child's current and past medical history for risk factors such as a family history of PUD or other GI diseases, or chronic salicylate or prednisone use.

Palpate the abdomen for the location of the pain, which is usually epigastric or periumbilical. Note the presence of blood in emesis or stools, as GI bleeding may occur. Diagnostic studies used to identify *H. pylori* include antibody testing, urea breath test, or biopsy. An upper GI series or upper endoscopy may detect the presence of ulcerations.

Nursing Management

Hemodynamic stabilization should be the focus of nursing management if significant GI bleeding occurs. Once children are stabilized and tolerating oral feeds, they may be discharged to home. Provide discharge instructions on the following topics:

- Medications
- Dietary management (especially when allergic gastroenteropathy is found)
- Safety precautions (in cases of ingested substances)
- Stressors
- Prevention of disease recurrence

Constipation and Encopresis

Constipation is a common problem among children, affecting up to 30% of the pediatric population and accounting for 3% to 5% of all pediatric outpatient visits (Sood, 2023b). It may be defined as failure to achieve complete evacuation of the lower colon. Chest- or breastfed infants may produce a stool with each feeding, though some will skip a few days between stools. Most bottle-fed babies will produce a stool one or two times per day, but they may go 2 to 3 days without producing a stool. The bowel habits of both infants and children vary widely, so assess and treat each child on an individual basis.

Functional constipation may be defined by the presence of at least two of the following over the course of 1 month:

- Fewer than three bowel movements weekly
- At least one episode of fecal incontinence weekly (after toilet trained)
- Excessive stool retention history
- Hard or painful bowel movements
- Large fecal rectal mass
- Stool passage of a volume to clog the toilet
- Stool withholding behavior (retentive posturing) (children age 4 years or older)

Encopresis is a term used to describe soiling of fecal contents into the underwear beyond the age of expected toilet training (4 to 5 years of age). Encopresis is often seen as a result of chronic constipation and withholding of stool. As stool is withheld in the rectum, the rectal muscle can stretch over time, and this stretching of the rectum causes fecal impactions. Children who have a stretched rectal vault may experience liquid stool leakage around a fecal mass. This is often an embarrassing issue that occurs with school-age children, and the child may hide their underwear to avoid punishment.

Pathophysiology

As stool passes through the colon, water is reabsorbed into the colon, resulting in a formed stool by the time it reaches the rectum. At this point, the anal sphincter relaxes to allow the passage of stool from the anus. In constipation, however, this relaxation does not occur.

Most causes of constipation are functional in nature (inorganic) (Sood, 2023b). Children with functional constipation usually present with this problem during the toilet-training years or in the preschool period. Children have a painful experience during defecation, which in turn creates a fear of defecation, resulting in further withholding of stool. Organic causes of constipation rarely occur in children. When they do occur, they may be a sign of a disease such as spina bifida or sacral agenesis.

Therapeutic Management

Once any organic process is ruled out as a cause, constipation may initially be managed with dietary manipulation such as increasing fiber and fluids. However, behavior modification is necessary for most children. Children need to relearn to allow bowel evacuation when stool is present. Children with severe constipation and withholding behaviors may not benefit from dietary management and may require laxative therapy. Sometimes mechanical disimpaction is required initially, followed by the above measures.

Nursing Assessment

For a full description of the assessment phase of the nursing process, refer to the assessment section in the "Clinical Judgment and the Nursing Process" section. Assessment findings pertinent to constipation/encopresis are discussed further.

HEALTH HISTORY

Elicit a description of the present illness and chief complaint. Note the onset of symptoms as described by the parent/child. Common symptoms reported during the health history may include:

- Altered stooling patterns (size, frequency, amount, and color)
- Pain with defecation
- Withholding behaviors (postures to try to withhold the stool, such as crossing the legs, squatting or hiding in a corner, or "dancing")
- Complaints of abdominal pain and cramping and poor appetite
- Diarrhea leakage
- Soiling of undergarments

It is important to note the duration of the symptoms to determine an acute onset versus a chronic disorder. Explore the child's past and current medical history for risk factors such as:

- Family history of GI disorders
- History of rectal bleeding or anal fissures
- Report of first meconium stool after 24 hours of age
- History of sexual abuse

Determine the child's dietary habits, history of fluid intake, and current medication or laxative use.

PHYSICAL EXAMINATION

Note whether the abdomen appears distended or rounded. Observe the lower back for a deep pilonidal dimple with hair tuft, which is suggestive of spina bifida occulta, or for flat buttocks suggestive of sacral agenesis. Inspect the anus for signs of fissures or soiling. Inspect the child's underwear for stains or smears, which are indicative of soiling. Auscultate bowel sounds to determine the possibility of an obstruction (hypoactive or absent bowel sounds) in the child with an acute case of constipation. Percuss the abdomen to reveal dullness, indicating a fecal mass. Palpate the abdomen for any tenderness or masses. The nurse may assist the health care provider or nurse practitioner with the performance of a rectal examination to assess for rectal tone and rectal vault size.

LABORATORY AND DIAGNOSTIC TESTS

Laboratory and diagnostic tests are not routine with the diagnosis of functional constipation, but if an organic cause is suspected, the following laboratory and diagnostic tests may be ordered:

- Stool for occult blood: The presence of blood could indicate some other disease process.
- Abdominal radiograph: Large quantities of stool may be seen in the colon.
- Sitz marker study: to detect colonic dysmotility
- Barium enema: to rule out a stricture or Hirschsprung disease
- Rectal manometry: to evaluate rectal musculature dysfunction
- Rectal suction biopsy: to rule out Hirschsprung disease

Nursing Management

Nursing management for constipation during infancy or childhood is aimed at educating the child and family and promoting child and family coping. Individualize care based on the patient problems and interventions presented earlier in the chapter in the "Clinical Judgment and the Nursing Process" section. Additional considerations are reviewed here.

EDUCATING THE FAMILY AND CHILD

Teach parents how to assess for signs of constipation and withholding behaviors. Also provide guidelines on scheduling and supervising bowel habits in reconditioning the child to use the toilet regularly. Teach parents to use positive reinforcement techniques. For example, when the child produces an adequate-volume bowel movement, reward them with stickers, extra playtime or television time, and so on.

Educate parents that dietary changes may help some children as high-fiber diets help to regulate bowel activity. Encourage the parent to increase the child's fluid intake to aid in bringing extra water into the bowel, thereby softening the stool. If a formula or milk change is recommended for the infants or toddler, educate the family that the change may result in better bowel habits. Teach families about the importance of adherence to medication use, if medication is ordered. Parents often are very anxious about the use of these medications, but stress to them that adherence is essential.

Many children present to their health care provider or nurse practitioner with fecal impaction or partial impaction. Teach parents how to disimpact their children at home; this often requires an enema or stimulation therapy. Nursing Procedure 20.2 gives instructions on enema administration in children. Explain the procedure to the child in developmentally appropriate terms. Enema administration can be uncomfortable, but calming measures, such as distraction and praise, provide a comforting environment. After the impaction is removed, promote regular bowel habits to keep the impaction from recurring.

NURSING PROCEDURE 20.2
Administering an Enema

1. Gather supplies (enema bag, lubricant, enema solution).
2. Wash hands and apply gloves.
3. Position the child:
   - Infant or toddler on abdomen with knees bent
   - Child or adolescent on left side with right leg flexed toward chest
4. Clamp the enema tubing, remove the cap, and apply lubricant to the tip.
5. Insert the tube into the rectum:
   - 2.5–4 cm (1–1.5 in) in the infant
   - 5–7.5 cm (2–3 in) in the child
6. Unclamp the tubing and administer the prescribed volume of enema solution at a rate of about 100 mL/min. Recommended volumes:
   - 250 mL or less for the infant
   - 250–500 mL for the toddler or preschooler
   - 500–1,000 mL for the school-age child
7. Hold the child's buttocks together if needed to encourage retention of the enema for 5–10 minutes.

Data from Cincinnati Children's. (2022). *How is an enema administered?* http://www.cincinnatichildrens.org/health/e/enema/

PROMOTING CHILD AND FAMILY COPING

Childhood constipation can be a stressful process for both the child and family. Behavior modification is necessary for many children. To facilitate daily bowel evacuation, the child should sit on the toilet twice a day (after breakfast and dinner) for 5 to 15 minutes with their feet on a stool as necessary. Instruct the family to keep a "star" or reward chart to encourage adherence. Parents should award the star for adherence to time sitting on the toilet and should not reserve rewards for successful bowel movements only. Weeks to months may be required to change the stooling pattern (Sood, 2023a).

Many parents seek counselors to help the entire family deal with the issues. Counseling is geared toward allaying the fears of a child who is afraid to defecate due to pain. Also, children who are older may have behavioral issues that need to be addressed. Psychological evaluation and possible behavioral therapy may need to be implemented if constipation becomes a power struggle.

Hirschsprung Disease (Congenital Aganglionic Megacolon)

Hirschsprung disease is a disorder of motility of the intestinal track resulting in obstruction (Fig 20.17; Bishop & Ebach, 2023). The disease is most commonly characterized by failure to pass a stool (meconium) within the first 24 hours of life. This is due to a lack of ganglion cells in the intestine, which causes inadequate motility in part of the intestine. These ganglion cells can be absent from the rectosigmoid colon all the way into the small intestine. Hirschsprung disease occurs in 1 of every 5,000 live births, being about four times more common in males than in females (Brumbaugh et al., 2022).

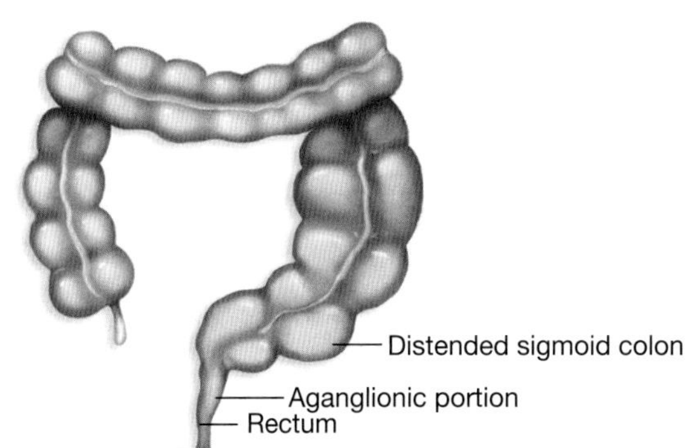

FIGURE 20.17 Enlarged megacolon of Hirschsprung disease.

Therapeutic Management

Surgical resection of the aganglionic bowel and reanastomosis of the remaining intestine are necessary to promote proper bowel function. There are several types of surgical procedures to correct this, usually performed in stages. The surgical resection requires the child to have an ostomy to divert the stool through a stoma on the abdomen. This allows the area of the resected bowel and anastomosis to heal before it is used. The ostomy is closed at a later date.

Nursing Assessment

When eliciting the history of the present illness, keep in mind that newborn stool patterns are a key element related to this diagnosis. Assess whether the newborn passed a meconium stool within the first 24 to 48 hours of life. Determine if the newborn required rectal stimulation to pass their first meconium stool or passed a meconium plug. Explore the child's current and past medical history for risk factors such as Down syndrome or other chromosomal abnormality, or a family history of Hirschsprung disease or Down syndrome (Brumbaugh et al., 2022).

Inspect the abdomen for distention. Palpate the abdomen for the presence of stool masses. Perform a rectal examination to assess for rectal tone and the presence of stool in the rectum. Often with Hirschsprung disease, no stool is present in the rectum. However, at the end of the rectal examination, when the finger is being withdrawn, a child with Hirschsprung disease may have a forceful expulsion of fecal material. Barium enema may reveal intestinal narrowing.

Rectal suction biopsy will demonstrate an absence of ganglion cells and provides the definitive diagnosis.

Nursing Management

Nursing management includes providing postoperative care, performing ostomy care, and providing child and family education.

PROVIDING POSTOPERATIVE AND OSTOMY CARE

Provide routine postoperative care and observe for the possible complication of enterocolitis. The child with Hirschsprung disease may have either a colostomy or ileostomy, depending on the extent of disease in the intestine. In either case, perform proper ostomy care to avoid skin breakdown. Accurately measure stool output to assess the child's fluid volume status.

Observe for the following signs and symptoms of enterocolitis: fever, abdominal distention, chronic diarrhea or explosive stools, rectal bleeding, or straining. If any of the above symptoms are noted, immediately notify the health care provider or nurse practitioner, maintain bowel rest, and administer IV fluids and antibiotics to prevent the development of shock and possibly death.

PROVIDING CHILD AND FAMILY EDUCATION

The family may be anxious and fearful about upcoming surgeries and possible complications. Help to relieve their anxiety by providing information about the diagnosis and the stages of surgical procedures the child will undergo. Provide postoperative teaching to educate parents on proper stoma care as well as medication management (to avoid dehydration, most children with Hirschsprung disease will be prescribed medications to slow stool output). Arrange for the family to consult with a wound care nurse to help them deal with the anxieties and care of newly placed stomas. Provide education about possible postsurgical problems, emphasizing the importance of prompt medical treatment for signs of enterocolitis.

Short Bowel Syndrome

Short bowel syndrome is a clinical syndrome of nutrient malabsorption and excessive intestinal fluid and electrolyte losses that occurs following massive small intestinal loss or surgical resection. The degree of malabsorption is usually related to the extent of resection of small bowel, absence of ileocecal valve or colon, and small bowel bacterial overgrowth (Brumbaugh et al., 2022). If the terminal ileum is lost, vitamin B_{12} deficiency and bile salt malabsorption may occur. The most common causes of short bowel syndrome are necrotizing enterocolitis, small intestinal atresia, gastroschisis, malrotation with volvulus, and trauma to the small intestine.

Therapeutic Management

The child with short bowel syndrome is at risk for chronic complications. The goals of therapeutic management are to minimize bacterial overgrowth and to maximize the child's nutritional status. Antibiotics may be used to control bacterial overgrowth. Vitamin and mineral supplementation is necessary because the small intestine is usually where fat-soluble vitamins, calcium, magnesium, and zinc are absorbed. Antidiarrheal agents such as loperamide and gastric acid–suppressive medications may be used to decrease stool output. Many children with short bowel syndrome require TPN for extended periods to achieve adequate growth. Progression to enteral feeding may occur extremely slowly, depending on the intestine's response. Despite a markedly improved prognosis for these children, some will not do as well and may ultimately require intestinal and liver transplantation due to irreversible liver damage from long-term use of TPN.

Nursing Assessment

Elicit the health history, noting diarrhea, which is the primary symptom of short bowel syndrome. Note past history of bowel loss or resection as noted earlier. Assess the child's hydration state. Inspect the stool for consistency, color, odor, and volume. Review laboratory results, particularly chemistries, to evaluate hydration status, and liver function tests, which may reveal evolving **cholestasis** (impairment of bile flow) secondary to long-term TPN use.

Nursing Management

Nursing management focuses on encouraging adequate nutrition and promoting effective family coping.

ENCOURAGING ADEQUATE NUTRITION

Treatment for short bowel syndrome can be a slow and tedious process. Most children will require TPN until they can tolerate enteral feeds without significant malabsorption. TPN is usually required for a lengthy time, so most children will require long-term IV access. Long-term IV access places the child at high risk for infection and resulting sepsis. Therefore, closely monitor for signs and symptoms of infection. Immediately report to the health care provider or nurse practitioner any fevers or redness or drainage at the IV site.

When started, enteral feeding must be administered very slowly to avoid further malabsorption. Usually the feeding is started continuously, 24 hours per day, via a feeding pump. Most children have long-term feeding tubes, usually gastrostomy tubes. Most of these children will require special formulas to promote absorption. Assess for feeding tube residuals and abdominal distention or discomfort. Strictly monitor intake and output to avoid dehydration. Assess the stool for signs of carbohydrate malabsorption. Administer vitamin and mineral supplementation, antidiarrheals, and antibiotics as ordered. Teach the family about use of enteral feeding tubes, feeding pumps, and medication administration.

PROMOTING EFFECTIVE FAMILY COPING

Children with short bowel syndrome are considered to be medically fragile for a lengthy period. There can be much anxiety related to the initial bowel resection that resulted in short bowel. Long-term hospitalization is almost always required, causing parents to miss work and cutting down on the time they have to spend with other children. This can lead to even more anxiety about finances and relationships. Encourage families to become the experts on their child's needs and condition via education and participation in care. Provide teaching so that the family is better able to care for the child in an outpatient setting. Education focuses on information about TPN and central line care, enteral feedings, assessing for hydration status, and managing medications.

TAKE NOTE!

Maintaining long-term central venous access for TPN in infants can present a challenge. One-piece clothing with the central venous line (CVL) tubing exiting and secured on the back of the outfit can help discourage the infant from pulling on (and subsequently dislodging) the line.

Inflammatory Bowel Disease

Crohn disease and ulcerative colitis are the two major idiopathic IBDs of children. The causes are unknown. However, they may be due to an abnormal or uncontrolled genetically determined immunologic or inflammatory response to an environmental antigenic trigger, possibly a virus or bacterium (Bishop & Ebach, 2023). The features of Crohn disease and ulcerative colitis are listed in Comparison Chart 20.2.

COMPARISON CHART 20.2 Features of Crohn Disease and Ulcerative Colitis

Feature	Crohn Disease	Ulcerative Colitis
Age at onset	10–20 years	10–20 years
Incidence	4–6 per 100,000	3–15 per 100,000
Area of bowel affected	Oropharynx, esophagus, and stomach, rare: small bowel only, 25%–30%; colon and anus only, 25%; ileocolitis, 40%; diffuse disease, 5%	Total colon, 90%; proctitis, 10%
Distribution	Segmental; disease-free skip areas common	Continuous; distal to proximal
Pathology	Full-thickness, acute, and chronic inflammation; noncaseating granulomas (50%), extraintestinal fistulas, abscesses, stricture, and fibrosis may be present	Superficial, acute inflammation of mucosa with microscopic crypt abscess
Radiography findings	Segmental lesions; thickened, circular folds; cobblestone appearance of bowel wall secondary to longitudinal ulcers and transverse fissures; fixation and separation of loops; narrowed lumen; "sting sign;" fistulas	Superficial colitis; loss of haustra; shortened colon and pseudopolyps (islands of normal tissue surrounded by denuded mucosa) are late findings

(continued)

COMPARISON CHART 20.2 Features of Crohn Disease and Ulcerative Colitis (*continued*)

Feature	Crohn Disease	Ulcerative Colitis
Intestinal symptoms	Abdominal pain, diarrhea (usually loose with blood if colon involved), perianal disease, enteroenteric or enterocutaneous fistula, abscess, anorexia	Abdominal pain, bloody diarrhea, urgency, tenesmus
Extraintestinal Symptoms		
Arthritis/arthralgia	15%	9%
Fever	40%–50%	40%–50%
Stomatitis	9%	2%
Weight loss	90% (mean 5.7 kg)	68% (mean 4.1 kg)
Delayed growth and sexual development	30%	5%–10%
Uveitis, conjunctivitis	15% (in Crohn colitis)	4%
Sclerosing cholangitis	—	4%
Renal stones	6% (oxalate)	6% (urate)
Pyoderma gangrenosum	1%–3%	5%
Erythema nodosum	8%–15%	4%
Laboratory findings	High erythrocyte sedimentation rate; microcytic anemia; low serum iron and total iron-binding capacity; increased fecal protein loss; low serum albumin; antineutrophil cytoplasmic antibodies present in 10%–20%; *Saccharomyces cerevisiae* antibodies positive in 60%	High erythrocyte sedimentation rate; microcytic anemia; high white blood cell count with left shift; antineutrophil cytoplasmic antibodies present in 80%

Data from Bishop, W. P., & Ebach, D. R. (2023). Digestive system. In K. J. Marcdante, R. M. Kliegman, & A. M. Schuh (Eds.). *Nelson's essentials of pediatrics* (9th ed.) [Kindle version]. Elsevier; Brumbaugh, D., Furuta, G. T., Hoffenberg, E., Kobak, G., Kramer, R., Walker, T., Septer, S., Shull, M., Soden, J., & Walker, T. (2022). Gastrointestinal tract. In M. Bunik, W. W. Hay, M. J. Levin, & M. J. Abzug (Eds.), *Current diagnosis and treatment: Pediatrics* (26th ed.). McGraw-Hill Education.

Therapeutic Management

Medication is used to control inflammation and symptoms. Medications commonly used include 5-aminosalicylates (ASA), antibiotics, immunomodulators, immunosuppressives, and anti–tumor necrosis antibody therapy. Dietary manipulation is also very important.

Failure to respond to medical therapy may result in surgical intervention. Many children with ulcerative colitis eventually undergo a total proctocolectomy, with resulting ostomy, as a curative measure. Children or adolescents with Crohn disease may require surgery to relieve obstruction, drain an abscess, or relieve intractable symptoms.

Nursing Assessment

For a full description of the assessment phase of the nursing process, refer to the "Clinical Judgment and the Nursing Process" section. Assessment findings pertinent to Crohn disease and ulcerative colitis are discussed further.

HEALTH HISTORY

Elicit a description of the present illness and chief complaint. Common symptoms reported during the health history include:

- Abdominal cramping
- Nighttime symptoms, including waking due to abdominal pain or urge to defecate
- Fever
- Weight loss
- Poor growth
- Delayed sexual development

Children may be reluctant or unwilling to talk about their bowel movements, so explain the importance of doing so. Assess stool pattern history, including frequency, presence of blood or mucus, and duration of symptoms. Explore the child's family history for risk factors such as IBD, colon cancer, or immunologic disorders.

PHYSICAL EXAMINATION

Assess the child's growth using growth charts to identify any poor growth patterns. Perform a full abdominal examination, noting tenderness, masses, or fullness. Inspect the perianal area to look for skin tags or fissures, which would be highly suspicious for Crohn disease. Assist the health care provider in performing a rectal examination to further assess the rectal area for blood or other lesions. Laboratory test results may be normal. Results for children with Crohn disease and ulcerative colitis are found in Comparison Chart 20.2. An upper GI series with small bowel series may identify evidence of intestinal inflammation, estimate distribution and extent of disease, and help distinguish between Crohn disease and ulcerative colitis. An upper endoscopy or colonoscopy may rule out affected mucosal tissue and/or diagnose IBD. A CT scan may be used to rule out suspected abscess.

Nursing Management

Nursing management focuses on teaching about disease management, teaching about nutritional management, teaching about medication therapy, and promoting family and child coping.

TEACHING ABOUT DISEASE MANAGEMENT

The diagnosis of Crohn disease or ulcerative colitis can be very difficult for the child and family to comprehend. Provide teaching about the disease process and medication therapy to help the child and family understand the seriousness of the disease. The health care provider may discuss surgical options during uncontrolled flare-ups, but the nurse may be the person to whom the family members or child addresses their questions regarding surgery. Provide the family with information to help answer some of their questions and allay fears.

TEACHING ABOUT NUTRITIONAL MANAGEMENT

Teach the child and family about nutritional management of the disease. For example, adequate nutrition with a high-protein and high-carbohydrate diet may be recommended. When the disease is active, lactose may be tolerated poorly, and vitamin and iron supplements will most likely be recommended. Explain that in severe cases enteral feeding tubes or TPN may be needed; this is rare but often induces remission.

TEACHING ABOUT MEDICATION THERAPY

Medications are extremely important in controlling IBD. Provide information about the following common medications used to control the disease:

- 5-ASA: used to prevent relapse (usually used in ulcerative colitis)
- Antibiotics (usually metronidazole and ciprofloxacin): typically used in children who have perianal Crohn disease
- Immunomodulators (usually 6-mercaptopurine [6-MP] or azathioprine): used to help maintain remission. Monitor children for neutropenia and hepatotoxicity.
- Cyclosporine or tacrolimus: used occasionally in conjunction with 6-MP or azathioprine to maintain remission in fulminant ulcerative colitis
- Methotrexate: sometimes used to manage severe Crohn disease
- Anti–tumor necrosis antibody therapy: widely used for children with Crohn disease; occasionally used for children with ulcerative colitis

PROMOTING FAMILY AND CHILD COPING

IBD is a chronic and often debilitating illness. Many children with this diagnosis can lead normal lives, but frequent illnesses can cause school absences, which in turn add stress to the situation. Because schools have become much less tolerant of absences and tardiness, it may be necessary to write letters to the school explaining the frequent absences or in-school needs. Bathroom privileges should be very flexible for children during flare-ups. Affected children and adolescents may experience stunted growth and delayed puberty so will need additional emotional support. Children with ostomies as a result of surgical resection may have self-esteem issues related to the presence and care of the ostomy. Arrange for counseling for both the child and family to discuss fears and anxiety related to a chronic disease.

Celiac Disease

Celiac disease, also known as celiac sprue, is an immunologic disorder in which gluten, a product most commonly found in grains, causes damage to the small intestine. The villi of the small intestine are damaged due to the body's immunologic response to the digestion of gluten. The function of the villi is to absorb nutrients into the bloodstream. When the villi are blunted or damaged, malnutrition occurs.

Celiac disease is a common disorder in the United States, with a prevalence of 0.3% to 0.9% with recent increasing incidence (Bamberger et al., 2022). Increased incidence occurs in those with a family history of celiac disease and in people with autoimmune or genetic disorders.

The only current treatment for celiac disease is a strict gluten-free diet. Eliminating gluten will cause the villi of the intestines to heal and function normally, with subsequent improvement of symptoms. Even very small amounts of gluten introduced back into the diet can cause damage to the villi, so the child must adhere to the diet throughout life.

Nursing Assessment

The child with symptoms of celiac disease often presents for evaluation by age 2, though diagnosis in older children is increasingly occurring.

Elicit a description of the present illness noting the classic symptoms of celiac disease:

- Diarrhea
- **Steatorrhea** (fatty stools)
- Constipation
- Failure to thrive or weight loss
- Abdominal distention or bloating
- Poor muscle tone
- Irritability and listlessness
- Dental disorders
- Anemia
- Delayed onset of puberty or amenorrhea
- Nutritional deficiencies

Explore the child's current and past medical history for risk factors such as genetic predisposition (presence of HLS-DQ2 or DQ8 gene) and first-degree relative with celiac disease. Assess for the typical appearance of children with celiac disease: distended abdomen, wasted buttocks, and very thin extremities (Fig. 20.18). Tissue transglutaminase immunoglobulin A (IgA) is a sensitive screening test, yet if the result is negative, the endomysial antibodies test is specific for celiac disease. Small bowel biopsy may reveal partial or subtotal villous atrophy or blunting of the villi of the small intestine. Genetic testing for celiac disease includes DQ2 and/or DQ8 human leukocyte antigen (HLA) haplotypes (Bamberger et al., 2022).

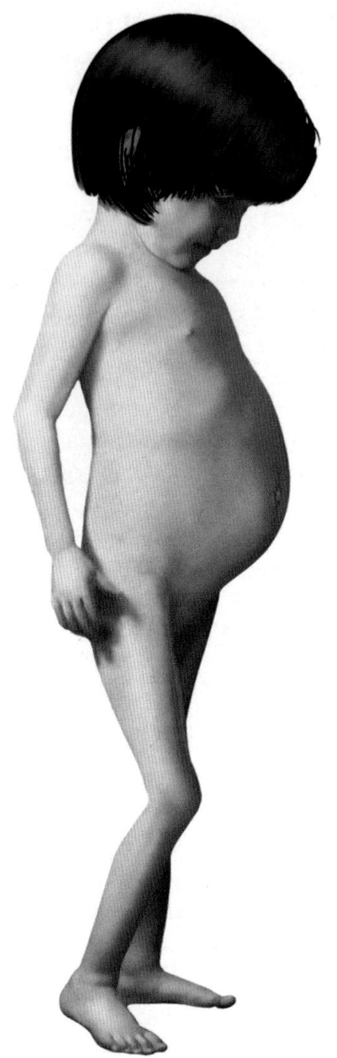

FIGURE 20.18 The child with celiac disease typically displays a distended abdomen and wasted extremities.

Nursing Management

Providing child and family education is the key nursing role in caring for children with celiac disease. The child must adhere to a strict gluten-free diet for their entire life. This is often very challenging, because gluten is found in most wheat products, rye, barley, and possibly oats. Encourage the parents and child to maintain this gluten-free diet. Often, families consult a dietitian to learn about the gluten-free diet (Teaching Guidelines 20.2).

Provide educational materials and resources to the parents. Many resources are available today about celiac disease because it is becoming more commonly diagnosed. These resources can offer information on all aspects of celiac disease, including dietary guidelines and resources for food shopping and eating in restaurants. A reading source appropriate for school-age children is *Gluten-Free Friends: An Activity Book for Kids* by Nancy Patin Falini.

Functional Abdominal Pain Disorders

Functional abdominal pain is a common GI complaint of children and adolescents. It affects children of all ages, and about 2% to 4% of all pediatric outpatient visits are related to recurrent abdominal pain (Brumbaugh et al., 2022). The etiology remains unclear. Functional abdominal pain in children should not be confused with IBS. Box 20.5 outlines the Rome Committee's criteria for IBS and information on treatment of IBS.

Pathophysiology

The etiology of functional abdominal pain is likely multifactorial, involving regulatory factors in both the enteric and central nervous systems. Functional abdominal pain may occur as referred pain following rectal distention,

TEACHING GUIDELINES **20.2** Dietary Considerations in a Gluten-Free Diet

Foods Allowed	Foods to Avoid
Potato, soy, rice, or bean flour; rice bran, cornmeal, arrowroot, corn or potato starch, sago, tapioca, buckwheat, millet, flax, teff, sorghum, amaranth, quinoa	All wheat products; rye, triticale, barley, oats, or oat bran; graham, gluten, spelt, or durum flour; bulgur, farina, or kamut; malt extract; hydrolyzed vegetable protein
Plain, fresh, frozen, or canned vegetables made with allowed ingredients	Any creamed or breaded vegetables, canned baked beans, some French fries
All fruits and fruit juices	Some commercial fruit pie fillings and dried fruit
All milk and milk products except those made with gluten additives, aged cheese	Malted milk, flavored or frozen yogurt
All meat, poultry, fish, and shellfish; dried peas and beans, nuts; peanut butter; soybean; cold cuts, frankfurters or sausage without fillers	Any meats or poultry prepared with wheat, rye, oats, barley, gluten stabilizers, or fillers for meats; canned meats; self-basting turkey; some egg substitutes
Butter, margarine, salad dressings, sauces, soups, and desserts with allowable ingredients; sugar, honey, jelly, jam, hard candy, plain chocolate, coconut, molasses, marshmallows, meringues, pure instant or ground coffee, tea, carbonated drinks, wine (from the United States)	Commercial salad dressings, prepared soups, condiments, sauces, and seasonings made with avoided products; nondairy cream substitutes, flavored instant coffee, alcohol distilled from cereals, licorice

Source: Celiac Disease Foundation. (2023). *Gluten-free foods*. http://celiac.org/live-gluten-free/glutenfreediet/

impaired gastric relaxation response to pain, or heightened sensitivity to visceral pain. Psychological symptoms may occur as a result of persistent or recurrent pain experiences. Therapeutic management focuses on avoidance of triggers and increasing the child's coping skills. Returning to normal activity is an important component of management (Chacko & Chiou, 2023). See Evidence-Based Practice 20.1.

BOX **20.5** **Rome Committee Criteria for Irritable Bowel Syndrome**

All of the following occur at least once per week minimum for at least 2 months before diagnosis:

- Abdominal pain relieved 25% of the time by defecation
- Onset of discomfort associated with a change in frequency of stool
- Onset of discomfort associated with a change in appearance of the stool
- No structural, neoplastic, inflammatory, or metabolic explanation for this abdominal pain

Treatment of IBS

For some children, dietary manipulation or medications may help to control diarrhea.

Data from Bishop, W. P., & Ebach, D. R. (2023). Digestive system. In K. J. Marcdante, & R. M. Kliegman (Eds.), *Nelson's essentials of pediatrics* (9th ed.) [Kindle version]. Elsevier. https://www.amazon.com/Nelson-Essentials-Pediatrics-Book-Marcdante-ebook/dp/B09TFSS9V9/ref=tmm_kin_swatch_0?_encoding=UTF8&qid=1679658509&sr=8-1; Brumbaugh, D., Furuta, G. T., Hoffenberg, E., Kobak, G., Kramer, R., Walker, T., Septer, S., Shull, M., Soden, J., & Walker, T. (2022). Gastrointestinal tract. In M. Bunik, W. W. Hay, M. J. Levin, & M. J. Abzug, & (Eds.), *Current diagnosis and treatment: Pediatrics* (26th ed.). McGraw-Hill Education.

Nursing Assessment

Determine the details of the pain, which is usually periumbilical and described as attacks of pain. The pain does not cause night awakening. Obtain a dietary history and a detailed medication history. Identifying social and school stressors is essential. Note the child's body positioning and facial expressions. Interactions with family members during the interview may provide more details regarding social stressors. Palpate the abdomen for tenderness. Laboratory and diagnostic testing may be performed to rule out organic causes of abdominal pain.

Nursing Management

Once the diagnosis of functional abdominal pain with no organic cause is made, the majority of the nursing management is focused on promoting coping skills. Often the health care provider or nurse practitioner performs a battery of tests to rule out organic causes, especially when the child's and family's anxiety is high. After these tests are complete, teach the family about the factors that exacerbate the pain and how to deal with these factors. If a specific dietary trigger is identified, teach the child and family to avoid the trigger, offering suggestions for an alternate food.

Arrange for behavioral therapies as ordered and support the child's and family's efforts to follow through with those. Help families determine a plan for school management if pain occurs, in order to normalize the child's life and ensure they are returned to school in a timely fashion (Chacko & Chiou, 2023).

EVIDENCE-BASED PRACTICE **20.1**

Probiotics for Diarrhea

STUDY

Acute diarrhea in children is a worldwide problem. The authors reviewed the published literature to determine how supplementation with probiotics affects the length of the diarrheal episode. They reviewed 82 studies involving over 12,000 participants who were mostly children.

Findings

The authors were unable to find a difference in length of diarrhea when comparing probiotics to placebo to no treatment. Additionally, for those hospitalized with diarrhea, the use of probiotics did not shorten the length of stay. No serious side effects from probiotics were noted.

Nursing Implications

While probiotics are likely not harmful to infants, children, and adolescents with diarrhea, the evidence does not warrant their use. Educate families to follow the health care provider's or nurse practitioner's recommendations for treatment of diarrhea, in particular focusing on maintaining hydration, rather than attempting to shorten the course of diarrhea with probiotics.

Data from Collinson, S., Deans, A., Padua-Zamora, A., Gregorio, G. V., Li, C., Dans L. F., & Allen, S.J. (2020). Probiotics for treating acute infectious diarrhoea (Review). *Cochrane Database of Systematic Reviews, 12,* CD003048. https://doi.org/10.1002/14651858.CD003048.pub4

HEPATOBILIARY DISORDERS

Hepatobiliary disorders include pancreatitis, gallbladder disease, jaundice, biliary atresia, hepatitis, cirrhosis and portal hypertension, and liver transplantation.

Pancreatitis

Pancreatitis is increasingly being recognized as a childhood problem (Sokol et al., 2022). It is classified into two categories—acute and chronic. Acute pancreatitis is an acute inflammatory process that occurs within the pancreas, with variable involvement of localized tissues and remote organ systems. Most common causes of acute pancreatitis include abdominal trauma, drugs and alcohol (though probably rare in children), multisystem disease (such as IBD or systemic lupus erythematosus), infections (usually viruses such as cytomegalovirus [CMV] or hepatitis), congenital anomalies (ductal or pancreatic malformations), obstruction (most likely gallstones or tumors in children), and metabolic disorders. Chronic pancreatitis is defined based on the structural and/or functional permanent changes that occur in the pancreas.

When pancreatitis is suspected, the child is placed on immediate bowel rest (NPO). Often, a nasogastric tube placed for suction will be needed to keep the stomach decompressed. Serial monitoring of serum amylase levels will determine when oral feeding may be restarted.

Nursing Assessment

Refer to the "Clinical Judgment and the Nursing Process" section for a full description of the assessment process. Assessment findings pertinent to pancreatitis are discussed further.

HEALTH HISTORY

Elicit a description of the present illness and chief complaint. Common symptoms reported during the health history include:

- Acute onset of persistent midepigastric and periumbilical abdominal pain, often with radiation to the back or chest
- Vomiting, especially after meals
- Fever

Explore the child's current and past medical history for risk factors such as cystic fibrosis, history of gallstones, traumatic injury, or family history of hereditary pancreatitis.

PHYSICAL EXAMINATION

Upon auscultation, the bowel sounds may be diminished, suggesting peritonitis. The abdomen may be tender, and distention may occur in younger children and infants. In severe cases, jaundice, ascites, or pleural effusions may occur. Bluish discoloration around the umbilicus or flanks is seen in the most severe cases of pancreatitis when hemorrhage is present.

LABORATORY AND DIAGNOSTIC TESTS

Common laboratory and diagnostic studies ordered for the assessment and monitoring of pancreatitis include:

- Serum amylase and/or lipase: Levels three times the normal values are extremely indicative of pancreatitis.
- Liver profile: often done to check for increased liver functions and/or bilirubin levels
- Blood work: Leukocytosis is common with acute pancreatitis. Hyperglycemia and hypocalcemia may also be noted.
- C-reactive protein: Levels may be elevated.

Diagnostic imaging studies performed to identify malformations or cysts on the pancreas include:

- Plain abdominal radiograph: may show a localized ileus
- Ultrasound: allows direct visualization of the pancreas and the surrounding structures
- Endoscopic retrograde cholangiopancreatography (ERCP): used in some children who may have ductal anomalies, usually with chronic pancreatitis

Nursing Management

Maintain NPO status and nasogastric tube suction and patency. Administer IV fluids to keep the child hydrated and correct any alterations in fluid and electrolyte balance. Pain management is crucial in children with pancreatitis. If hemorrhagic pancreatitis has occurred, blood products and/or IV antibiotics may be needed. Oral feedings are restarted only after the serum amylase level has returned to normal (usually in 2 to 4 days). Often, pancreatic enzymes are given with oral feedings if pain occurs after oral feeds are restarted.

Surgery is rarely needed in children with pancreatitis, except in those with severe abdominal trauma or major ductal abnormalities. Though chronic pancreatitis is rare in children, provide child and family education regarding the signs and symptoms of recurrence and complications.

Gallbladder Disease

Cholelithiasis is the presence of stones in the gallbladder. Cholesterol stones are usually associated with hyperlipidemia, obesity, pregnancy, birth control pill use, or cystic fibrosis (Schwarz & Hebra, 2023). They are seen more often in females than males, and increased risk occurs with age and onset of puberty (Schwarz & Hebra, 2023). These stones occur in the gallbladder and may be found in the common bile duct. Pigment stones are found in prepubertal children and occur about equally in males and females. They are usually found in the common bile duct (associated with bacterial or parasitic infections) or the gallbladder itself (associated with hemolytic anemia or liver cirrhosis).

Cholecystitis is an inflammation of the gallbladder that is caused by chemical irritation due to the obstruction of bile flow from the gallbladder into the cystic ducts. This inflammation is typically associated with gallstones in children. The most common complication in children with gallstone disease is pancreatitis. If cholelithiasis results in symptomatic cholecystitis, then surgical removal of the gallbladder (cholecystectomy) will be necessary. This is often accomplished laparoscopically.

Nursing Assessment

Common symptoms reported during the health history include right upper quadrant pain, often radiating substernally or to the right shoulder, nausea and vomiting, and jaundice and fever (with cholecystitis). Pain episodes usually occur postprandially, especially after the ingestion of fatty or greasy foods. Younger children may present with more nonspecific symptoms, most often due to their lack of ability to communicate their symptoms to others. Explore the child's current and past medical history for risk factors such as chronic TPN use or sickle cell disease.

Palpate the abdomen for tenderness localized in the area of the gallbladder. Assess skin and sclerae color for jaundice. Determine the presence of fever. Note elevated liver function tests, serum bilirubin, and C-reactive protein. Ultrasound, ERCP, or hepatobiliary iminodiacetic acid (HIDA) scan may be performed to evaluate the function of the gallbladder and determine presence of stones.

Nursing Management

The child with symptomatic cholecystitis will usually be hospitalized. Administer IV fluids, maintain NPO status and gastric decompression, and administer pain medications. If ordered, administer IV antibiotics to treat clinically worsening symptoms of cholecystitis, such as persistent fever. Provide routine postoperative care after cholecystectomy is performed. Provide pre- and postoperative teaching for families of children undergoing gallbladder removal.

Biliary Atresia

Biliary atresia is an absence of some or all of the major biliary ducts, resulting in obstruction of bile flow. The ensuing obstruction to bile flow causes cholestasis resulting in jaundice and eventual progressive fibrosis with end-stage cirrhosis of the liver. Biliary atresia affects 1 in 12,000 infants (Sokol et al., 2022). The etiology of biliary atresia is unknown, but there are several theories, including infectious, autoimmune, or ischemic causes.

Therapeutic Management

If there is a high suspicion of biliary atresia, the infant will undergo exploratory laparotomy. If biliary atresia is found, a Kasai procedure (hepatoportoenterostomy) is performed to connect the bowel lumen to the bile duct remnants found at the porta hepatis. This procedure is most successful for infants 30 to 45 days of age, as bile flow restoration after this age is minimal (Sokol et al., 2022). Infants who are not identified early enough or those who have failed to respond to the Kasai procedure will need to undergo liver transplantation (Sokol et al., 2022).

Nursing Assessment

Determine history of persistent or recurring jaundice in the young infant. Note jaundice of the skin and sclerae (yellow discoloration caused by bile pigment deposition). Palpate the abdomen for a hardened and enlarged liver and possibly splenomegaly. Note stools to be acholic (chalky and white due to the lack of bile pigment). Serum bilirubin, alkaline phosphatase, liver enzymes, and gamma-glutamyl transferase (GGT) will be elevated. Ultrasound, biliary scan, and liver biopsy may be performed.

Nursing Management

Nursing management of biliary atresia will focus on vitamin and caloric support. Administer fat-soluble vitamins A, D, E, and K. Special formulas containing medium-chain triglycerides are used because significant fat malabsorption occurs when cholestasis is present. Administer feedings via nasogastric tube as needed to ensure increased caloric intake. Identify infections as quickly as possible and administer IV antibiotics as ordered. Manage ascites with diuretics and dietary restrictions. Preoperative management before a Kasai procedure is focused on preparation for surgery; infants who have suspected biliary atresia require immediate surgery to optimize outcomes. Provide extensive emotional support if the family is likely to have extreme anxiety due to the implications of the diagnosis and outcomes.

Hepatitis

Hepatitis is an inflammation of the liver that is caused by a variety of agents, including viral infections, bacterial invasion, metabolic disorders, chemical toxicity, and trauma. The most common viral causes of hepatitis are listed in Table 20.3. Other viruses that may cause hepatitis are CMV, Epstein–Barr virus (EBV), and adenovirus. Fulminant hepatitis is thought to be caused by a non-A, non-B, or non-C virus. Children who present with fulminant hepatitis have acute massive hepatic necrosis. The disease progresses rapidly to severe jaundice, coagulopathy, elevated ammonia levels, significantly elevated liver enzyme levels (aspartate aminotransferase [AST] and alanine aminotransferase [ALT]), and progressive coma, resulting in death without liver transplantation. Autoimmune hepatitis is a chronic disorder, affecting mostly adolescent females. The clinical presentation of a child with autoimmune hepatitis includes hepatosplenomegaly, jaundice, fever, fatigue, and right upper quadrant pain.

Therapeutic Management

Acute hepatitis is treated with rest, hydration, and nutrition. Control of bleeding may also be necessary. Chronic hepatitis often eventually requires liver transplantation. Corticosteroids and immunosuppressants may be used for autoimmune hepatitis. The child with fulminant hepatitis usually requires intensive care with cardiorespiratory support. See the Healthy People 2030 box.

HEALTHY PEOPLE 2030

Objective	Nursing Significance
Reduce hepatitis A and hepatitis B infection.	• Educate families about hepatitis B and its transmission. • Encourage routine infant and childhood vaccination against hepatitis A and hepatitis B as recommended. • For hepatitis A prevention, educate families about appropriate hygiene and handwashing.

Healthy People Objectives retrieved from http://www.healthypeople.gov

TABLE 20.3 • Hepatitis Viruses A–E

	Hepatitis A (HAV)	Hepatitis B (HBV)	Hepatitis C (HCV)	Hepatitis D (HDV)	Hepatitis E (HEV)
Transmission route	Oral–fecal route, poor sanitation, waterborne	Sexual, intravenous drug use, blood transfusion, perinatally transmitted from birthing parent to infant	Blood product transfusion, intravenous drug use	Same as HBV; HBV markers in serum must be present	Oral–fecal
Incubation period	15–30 days	50–150 days	30–160 days	50–150 days	15–65 days
Signs and symptoms	Flu-like symptoms Pre-icteric phase: headache, fatigue, fever, anorexia Icteric phase: jaundice, dark urine, tender liver (right upper quadrant pain)	Some cases are asymptomatic; others present with anorexia, abdominal pain, fatigue, rash, slight fever, visible jaundice, enlarged liver	Chronic cases usually present asymptomatically; others with flu-like symptoms, jaundice, hepatosplenomegaly	Same as HBV	Same as HAV, more severe in pregnant people
Prognosis	Rarely develops into fulminant liver failure; 95% of children recover without sequelae	Chronic disease state likely; increased risk of hepatic cancer	Many will develop chronic hepatitis and cirrhosis	Same as HBV, but increased likelihood of chronic active hepatitis and cirrhosis	Same as HAV; high mortality in pregnant people

Data from Sokol, R. J., Mark, J. A., Mack, C. L., Felman, A.G., & Sundaram, S. S. (2022). Liver & pancreas. In M. Bunik, W. W. Hay, M. J. Levin, & M. J. Abzug (Eds.), *Current diagnosis and treatment: Pediatrics* (26th ed.). McGraw-Hill Education.

Nursing Assessment

Elicit the health history, noting likely symptoms of fever, fatigue, abdominal pain, and jaundice.

Explore the child's current and past medical history for risk factors such as:

- Recent foreign travel
- Sick contacts
- Medication use
- Abdominal trauma
- Sexual activity
- IV drug use
- Blood product transfusion

Observe the skin for jaundice and the sclerae for icterus. Palpate the abdomen to reveal abnormal liver and spleen size or tenderness. Laboratory studies may reveal elevated liver enzymes, GGT, and ammonia level (in the presence of encephalopathy). Prothrombin time (PT)/partial thromboplastin time (PTT) will be prolonged. Viral and autoimmune studies may be used to identify the cause of the hepatitis. An ultrasound or liver biopsy may also be performed.

Nursing Management

Acute hepatitis requires rest, hydration, and nutrition. If the child develops vomiting, dehydration, elevated bleeding times (PT/PTT), or mental status changes (encephalopathy), hospitalization may be required. When caring for children with infectious hepatitis, provide education about transmission and prevention, including proper hygiene, safe sexual activity, careful handwashing techniques, and blood/bodily fluid precautions.

Fulminant hepatitis treatment is aggressive and will require NPO status, nasogastric tube administration of lactulose to decrease ammonia levels that lead to encephalopathic conditions, TPN administration, vitamin K injections to help with coagulopathies, and, ultimately, liver transplantation. Fear and anxiety of the child and parents will likely be very high. Teach the child and family about the diagnosis and what to expect during treatment. Provide immunoglobulin therapy and vaccinations to close contacts of children with infectious hepatitis.

Cirrhosis and Portal Hypertension

Cirrhosis of the liver occurs as a result of the destructive processes that occur during liver damage, leading to the formation of nodules. These nodules can be small (micronodular [less than 3 mm]) or large (macronodular [greater than 3 mm]) and distort the vasculature of the liver, leading to further complications. Causes of cirrhosis in children include biliary malformations, α_1-antitrypsin deficiency, Wilson disease, galactosemia, tyrosinemia, and chronic active hepatitis (Sokol et al., 2022).

Major complications may exist due to cirrhosis of the liver, including portal hypertension. In portal hypertension, the blood flow to, through, or from the liver meets resistance, causing portal blood flow pressures to rise. As these pressures rise, collateral veins form between the portal and systemic venous circulations. The most significant complication of portal hypertension is GI bleeding, from shunting to submucosal veins (varices) in the stomach and esophagus. Esophageal varices may be treated with sclerotherapy during endoscopy to stop acute bleeding. Often blood product administration and vasopressive drugs are needed. In the long term, the only cure for cirrhosis is liver transplantation.

Nursing Assessment

During the health history, note the common symptoms of nausea and vomiting, weakness, jaundice, swelling, and weight loss. Explore the child's current and past medical history for risk factors such as hepatitis, cystic fibrosis, Wilson disease, hemochromatosis, and biliary atresia.

Inspect for jaundice, ascites, spider angiomas, and palmar erythema. Note gynecomastia in males. Palpate the liver; typically, it is enlarged and hard, but occasionally it is small and shrunken. Evaluate mental status to determine the presence of hepatic encephalopathy. Laboratory and diagnostic testing will be similar to that for a child with hepatitis.

Nursing Management

Care is very similar to that for the child with hepatitis. In cases of cirrhosis causing portal hypertension and bleeding varices, GI bleeding must be controlled. This is usually done by replacing blood loss and providing vasopressive therapy to constrict the shunted blood flow. As with all liver disorders and GI bleeding, address and manage family and child anxiety. Be honest about the child's treatment plan and prognosis. Involve the family in the care of the child and educate them as needed.

Liver Transplantation

Hepatobiliary disorders that result in failure of the liver to function result in the need for liver transplantation. Liver transplantation in children has become increasingly successful in the past several years due to advances in immunosuppression, better selection of transplant candidates, and improvements in surgical techniques and postoperative care (Sokol et al., 2018). Transplant centers now offer both cadaveric and living-related liver transplants for children. Rejection of the transplanted liver is the most significant complication. Most children will require immunosuppressive therapy for their lifetime, putting them at risk for infections.

Nursing Assessment

Many children will be admitted to a transplant center for a preoperative workup to determine the best possible tissue and blood match for the child. There is much anxiety among family members when a cadaveric transplant is the only possibility for survival. This puts a child on a waiting list that is prioritized based on several criteria. Because there are a limited number of pediatric liver transplant centers throughout the country, there may be many issues regarding transportation, finances, job loss, and lodging. Assess the need for social work intervention; a social worker is almost always involved with these children. A liver transplant coordinator will assist with coordinating the care for pretransplant and posttransplant children.

Nursing Management

Preoperatively, assist with the transplant workup and teach the child and family what to expect during and after the liver transplantation. Postoperatively, the child will be in the intensive care unit for several days until they are stabilized from the actual surgery. After the child is sent to a regular unit in the hospital, monitor the child for several days to weeks for signs and symptoms of rejection and infection, including fever, increasing liver function test results and GGT, and increasing pain, redness, and swelling at the incision site. Child and family education is an important element of nursing management in the posttransplant child. Assess and reassess medication knowledge throughout the entire hospitalization, as these children usually require medications for their lifetime.

Unfolding Patient Stories: Eva Madison • Part 2

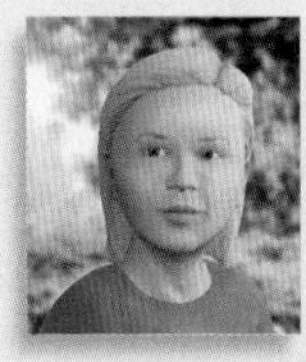

Recall Eva Madison, the 5-year-old child you met in Chapter 10. She is diagnosed with bacterial gastroenteritis. How would the nurse prepare Eva and her parents for hospitalization? What nursing actions can promote a more favorable hospital experience in this age group?

Care for Eva and other patients in a realistic virtual environment: ***vSim** for Nursing* (thepoint.lww.com/vSimPediatric). Practice documenting these patients' care in DocuCare (thePoint.lww.com/DocuCareEHR).

KEY CONCEPTS

- The esophagus of the young child exhibits underdeveloped muscle tone compared with the adult.
- A major difference between children and adults is the reduced stomach capacity in the child and the significantly shorter length of the small intestine (250 cm in the child versus 600 cm in the adult).
- Infants and children have a proportionately greater amount of body water than adults, resulting in a relatively greater fluid intake requirement than adults and placing infants and children at higher risk for fluid loss as compared with adults.
- The most common result of GI illnesses in infants and children is dehydration.
- The mildly or moderately dehydrated child must be identified and receive rehydration therapy to prevent progression to hypovolemic shock.
- Rehydration is a key medical treatment for dehydration as a result of many different GI disorders. Oral rehydration is most common, but in cases requiring hospitalization IV fluid therapy is key.
- Promotion of adequate nutrition is another significant treatment component. The child with a chronic GI disorder may require IV TPN or enteral tube feedings to exhibit appropriate growth.
- Surgical intervention is necessary for many acute or congenital GI disorders, such as pyloric stenosis, omphalocele, gastroschisis, cleft lip and palate, appendicitis, Hirschsprung disease, and intestinal malrotation.
- Monitoring the blood count, electrolyte levels, and liver function tests is necessary in many pediatric GI disorders.
- Histamine-2 blockers, proton pump inhibitors, and prokinetic agents are used to treat disorders in which gastric acid is a problem, such as esophagitis, GERD, and ulcers.
- Close monitoring for infection is important in children with IBD, autoimmune hepatitis, or liver transplant who are being treated with immunosuppressants and/or corticosteroids.
- GI stimulants and laxatives may be necessary for treating constipation and encopresis.
- Diarrhea, vomiting, decreased oral intake, sustained high fever, diabetic ketoacidosis, and extensive burns place the infant or child at risk for the development of dehydration.
- Risk factors for vomiting include exposure to viruses, use of certain medications, and overfeeding in the infant.
- Risk factors for acute diarrhea include recent ingestion of undercooked meats, foreign travel, day care attendance, and well water ingestion.
- Vomiting is a symptom and should be characterized in terms of volume, color, relation to meals, duration, and associated symptoms.
- Bleeding may occur as a result of a GI disorder, particularly from the intestine with Meckel diverticulum and from esophageal varices with portal hypertension.
- Acute GI disorders are those that usually have a rapid onset and a short course, which at times may be severe. Examples include dehydration, vomiting, diarrhea, hypertrophic pyloric stenosis, and appendicitis.

- Chronic GI disorders are those that are long lasting or recur over time. Examples include constipation, GERD, IBD, functional abdominal pain, and failure to thrive.
- Right lower quadrant pain and rebound tenderness of the abdomen found on physical examination are telltale signs of appendicitis, which is considered a surgical emergency.
- Bilious vomiting is the main symptom of conditions resulting in bowel obstruction, such as malrotation with volvulus.
- The focus of nursing management of diarrhea or vomiting is restoring proper fluid and electrolyte balance through oral rehydration therapy or IV fluids if necessary.
- Reduction of inguinal and umbilical hernias should be attempted; if reduction of the hernia is impossible, immediately notify the health care provider.
- Small, frequent, and thickened feedings and proper positioning after feedings are key elements in the treatment of GER.
- A crucial nursing intervention related to cleft lip and palate repair is protection of the surgical site while it is healing.
- Palpation of the abdomen should be the last part of the physical examination of an infant or child.
- A key element of nursing care for the child with a GI disorder is promotion of appropriate bowel elimination.
- Maximizing nutritional status is a critical nursing function for the child with a GI disorder.
- For the child who has undergone surgical repair for correction of a GI disorder, promoting effective breathing patterns and managing pain are important nursing goals.
- Counseling families about how to manage the child with vomiting or diarrhea at home, including oral rehydration therapy, is a key component of child/family education.
- Education of the child and family regarding the importance of medication adherence for management of IBD is critical.
- Behavioral therapy and counseling may be necessary for children who have functional constipation and stool withholding.
- The child or adolescent with ineffective bowel control, poor growth, or an ostomy may have poor self-esteem and body image.

REFERENCES AND RECOMMENDED READINGS

Bamberger, J. M., Nelson, S. S., & Westry, M. F. G. (2022). Management of nutritional disorders. In T. Kyle (Ed.), *Primary care pediatrics for the nurse practitioner: A practical approach*. Springer.

Bishop, W. P., & Ebach, D. R. (2023). Digestive system. In K. J. Marcdante, R. M. Kliegman, & A. M. Schuh (Eds.), *Nelson's essentials of pediatrics* (9th ed.) [Kindle version]. Elsevier.

Brumbaugh, D., Furuta, G. T., Hoffenberg, E., Kobak, G., Kramer, R., Walker, T., Septer, S., Shull, M., Soden, J., & Walker, T. (2022). Gastrointestinal tract. In M. Bunik, W. W. Hay, M. J. Levin, & M. J. Abzug (Eds.), *Current diagnosis and treatment: Pediatrics* (26th ed.). McGraw-Hill Education.

Campbell, J. R., & Palazzi, D. L. (2023). Candida infections in children. *UpToDate*. Retrieved January 12, 2024, from https://www.uptodate.com/contents/candida-infections-in-children

Canani, R. B. (2018). *Abstract G-O-053. Presented at ESPGHAN 51st Annual Meeting, Geneva, Switzerland*. https://www.healio.com/gastroenterology/therapeutics-diagnostics/news/online/%7B2723f19c-6f91-4656-a80b-d6d6125f7e37%7D/ginger-effective-for-treating-vomiting-in-children-with-acute-gastroenteritis

Celiac Disease Foundation. (2023). *Gluten-free foods*. https://celiac.org/gluten-free-living/gluten-free-foods/

Chacko, M. R., & Chiou, E. (2023). Functional abdominal pain in children and adolescents: Management in primary care. *UpToDate*. Retrieved January 12, 2024, from https://www.uptodate.com/contents/functional-abdominal-pain-in-children-and-adolescents-management-in-primary-care

CHOC. (2023). *Stool tests*. https://www.choc.org/programs-services/gastroenterology/digestive-disorder-diagnostics/stool-tests/

Cincinnati Children's. (2022). *How is an enema administered?* https://www.cincinnatichildrens.org/health/e/enema

Cleft Lip & Palate Association. (2024). *Breastfeeding*. https://www.clapa.com/treatment/feeding/breastfeeding/

Collinson, S., Deans, A., Padua-Zamora, A., Gregorio, G. V., Li, C., Dans L. F., & Allen, S.J. (2020). Probiotics for treating acute infectious diarrhoea (Review). *Cochrane Database of Systematic Reviews*, *12*, CD003048. https://doi.org/10.1002/14651858.CD003048.pub4

Corbett, J. A., & Banks, A. D. (2019). *Laboratory tests and diagnostic procedures with nursing diagnoses* (9th ed.). Pearson Education Inc.

Endom, E. E., Dorfman, S. R., & Olivé, A. P. (2023). Infantile hypertrophic pyloric stenosis. *UpToDate*. Retrieved January 12, 2024, from https://www.uptodate.com/contents/infantile-hypertrophic-pyloric-stenosis

Freedman, S. (2023). *Oral rehydration therapy. UpToDate*. Retrieved January 12, 2024, from https://www.uptodate.com/contents/oral-rehydration-therapy

Hanna, M. G., & Bock, M. (2022). Fluid, electrolyte, and acid-base disorders & therapy. In M. Bunik, W. W. Hay, M. J. Levin, & M. J. Abzug (Eds.), *Current diagnosis & treatment: Pediatrics* (26th ed.). McGraw-Hill Education.

Kleinman, K., McDaniel, L., & Malloy, M. (2023). *The Harriet Lane handbook* (22nd ed.). Elsevier.

Kyle, T. (2022). Management of mouth disorders. In T. Kyle (Ed.), *Primary care pediatrics for the nurse practitioner: A practical approach*. Springer.

Levy, J. (2022). Diagnostic approach to diarrhea in children in resource-rich countries. *UpToDate*. Retrieved January 12, 2024, from https://www.uptodate.com/contents/diagnostic-approach-to-diarrhea-in-children-in-resource-rich-countries

Meeks, N. J. L., Kochlar, A., Duis, J., & Saenz, M. (2022). Genetics & dysmorphology. In M. Bunik, W. W. Hay, M. J. Levin, & M. J. Abzug (Eds.), *Current diagnosis and treatment: Pediatrics* (26th ed.). McGraw-Hill Education.

Palazzi, D. L., & Brandt, M. L. (2023). Care of the umbilicus and management of umbilical disorders. *UpToDate*. Retrieved

January 12, 2024, from https://www.uptodate.com/contents/care-of-the-umbilicus-and-management-of-umbilical-disorders

Phalke, N., & Goldman, J. J. (2023). *Cleft palate*. StatPearls. https://www.ncbi.nlm.nih.gov/books/NBK563128/

Schwarz, S. M., & Hebra, A. (2023). Pediatric cholecystitis. *Medscape*. Retrieved January 12, 2024, from https://emedicine.medscape.com/article/927340-overview

Singh, M., & Mehra, K. (2023). *Imperforate anus*. StatPearls. https://www.ncbi.nlm.nih.gov/books/NBK549784/

Smith, D., & Grover, T. (2022). The newborn infant. In M. Bunik, W. W. Hay, M. J. Levin, & M. J. Abzug (Eds.), *Current diagnosis and treatment: Pediatrics* (26th ed.). McGraw-Hill Education.

Sokol, R. J., Mark, J. A., Mack, C. L., Felman, A.G., & Sundaram, S. S. (2022). Liver & pancreas. In M. Bunik, W. W. Hay, M. J. Levin, & M. J. Abzug (Eds.), *Current diagnosis and treatment: Pediatrics* (26th ed.). McGraw-Hill Education.

Sood, M. R. (2023a). Chronic functional constipation and fecal incontinence in infants, children, and adolescents: Treatment. *UpToDate*. Retrieved January 12, 2024, from https://www.uptodate.com/contents/chronic-functional-constipation-and-fecal-incontinence-in-infants-children-and-adolescents-treatment

Sood, M. R. (2023b). Functional constipation in infants, children, and adolescents: Clinical features and diagnosis. *UpToDate*. Retrieved January 12, 2024, from https://www.uptodate.com/contents/functional-constipation-in-infants-children-and-adolescents-clinical-features-and-diagnosis

Stephenson, C. D., Lockwood, C. J., & MacKenzie, A. P. (2023). Gastroschisis. *UpToDate*. Retrieved January 12, 2024, from https://www.uptodate.com/contents/gastroschisis

Thiagarajah, J. R., & Martin, M. G. (2023). Pathogenesis of acute diarrhea in children. *UpToDate*. Retrieved January 12, 2024, from http://www.uptodate.com/contents/pathogenesis-of-acute-diarrhea-in-children

University of California San Francisco. (2024). *Colostomy (pediatric)*. https://surgery.ucsf.edu/procedure/colostomy-pediatric

UpToDate, Inc. (2024). *UpToDate® Lexidrug™* (Version 8.2.0) [Mobile app]. Wolters Kluwer. https://apps.apple.com/us/app/lexicomp/id313401238

U.S. Department of Health and Human Services. (n.d.). *Healthy People 2030*. https://health.gov/healthypeople

Winter, H. S. (2023). Gastroesophageal reflux in infants. *UpToDate*. Retrieved January 12, 2024, from https://www.uptodate.com/contents/gastroesophageal-reflux-in-infants

DEVELOPING CLINICAL JUDGMENT

PRACTICING FOR NCLEX

1. A parent brings their 6-month-old infant to the clinic. The child has been vomiting since early morning and has had diarrhea since the day before. The child's temperature is 38°C (100.4°F), pulse 140, and respiratory rate 38. The infant has lost 6 oz since their well-child visit 4 days ago, cries before passing a bowel movement, and refuses to feed today. Which is the priority patient issue?
   a. Thermoregulation alteration
   b. Pain (abdominal) related to diarrhea
   c. Fluid volume deficit related to excessive losses and inadequate intake
   d. Alteration in nutrition (less than body requirements) related to decreased oral intake

2. A child presents with a 2-day history of fever, abdominal pain, occasional vomiting, and decreased oral intake. Which finding would the nurse prioritize for immediate reporting to the health care provider?
   a. The child has a temperature of 38.3°C (100.9°F).
   b. The child has rebound tenderness and abdominal guarding.
   c. The parents will be leaving the child alone in the hospital.
   d. The child can tolerate only sips of fluid without nausea.

3. A 3-day-old infant presenting with physiologic jaundice is hospitalized and placed under phototherapy. Which response indicates to the nurse that the parent needs more teaching?
   a. "These lights place my infant at risk for dehydration."
   b. "My infant needs to stay under the lights, except during feeding time."
   c. "I will be able to continue to breastfeed during this time."
   d. "I am so upset my infant has a serious liver disease."

4. A 3-month-old infant presents with a history of vomiting after feeding. The plan for the infant is to rule out GERD. What information from the history would lead the nurse to believe that this infant may need further intervention?
   a. Poor weight gain
   b. Small "spits" after feeding
   c. Sleeps through the night
   d. Difficult to burp

5. The nurse is caring for a child who has had diarrhea and vomiting for the past several days. What is the priority nursing assessment?
   a. Determine the child's weight.
   b. Ask if the family has traveled outside of the country.
   c. Assess circulation and perfusion.
   d. Send a stool specimen to the laboratory.

6. The nurse is caring for a 2-year-old with dehydration secondary to rotavirus infection who was admitted at 2:00 p.m. the day prior. The child is not toilet trained, and their weight is 15 kg. The child's IV line fell out during the night. After reviewing the intake and output chart, the nurse uses the situation, background, assessment, recommendation (SBAR) communication technique to call the health care provider with the recommendation for which prescription?

Intake and Output Record

Date	Time	Oral	Type	IV	Type	Urine	Stool	Emesis
Total 6/12		120	Pedialyte	500	D5 ¼ NS with 20 mEq KCl/L	440	X2	0
6/13	0100	15	Pedialyte	50				
6/13	0200			50		30		Mod.
6/13	0300			0				Mod.
6/13	0400			0			Large	
6/13	0500			0				Mod.
6/13	0600			0		Diaper dry		

   a. Indwelling urinary catheter
   b. IV antibiotic
   c. Normal saline IV fluid bolus
   d. One-time dose of loperamide

7. An infant has vomited six times in the past 24 hours. The parent attempted to feed the infant Pedialyte without success. The infant's stools are watery and coat the entire diaper, sometimes with leakage. The infant is at risk for ______ related to ______.
   Blank 1:
   a. impaired urinary elimination
   b. deficient fluid volume
   c. impaired parenting
   d. pain
   Blank 2:
   e. excessive losses from severe diarrhea
   f. infant refusing feeding
   g. vomiting and diarrhea

DOSAGE CALCULATION QUESTION

A child is NPO during the preoperative period and requires IV fluid maintenance. The child weighs 31 lb 4 oz. What is the child's recommended hourly IV fluid rate?

CRITICAL THINKING EXERCISES

1. A 6-month-old child is brought to the health care provider's office with a history of diarrhea. The infant has had six watery stools in the past 18 hours and is vomiting the formula. The parent states the infant has had no fever.

a. Upon completion of the history and physical examination, what signs and symptoms would you expect to find that would indicate that the baby is experiencing mild dehydration?
b. What is the priority patient problem for this infant?
c. Identify a plan for this patient problem; include a teaching plan for the parent.

2. A 14-kg child with moderate dehydration has received two boluses of normal saline in the emergency room prior to being admitted to the pediatric nursing unit. The health care provider orders D5 ½ NS at 1½ maintenance.
   a. What would the IV fluid rate be?
   b. What will the nurse assess for to determine whether the child is becoming overhydrated?
3. An infant requires a temporary colostomy. What discharge instructions would you provide to the parents about how to take care of the colostomy and when to call their child's health care provider or nurse practitioner?

STUDY ACTIVITIES

1. In the clinical setting, compare the growth records of a child with celiac disease to those of a similar-aged child without disease.
2. While caring for children in the clinical setting, compare and contrast the medical history, signs and symptoms of illness, and prescribed treatment for a child with Crohn disease and one with ulcerative colitis.
3. In the clinical setting, observe the behavioral responses of an infant or young child with inorganic failure to thrive.

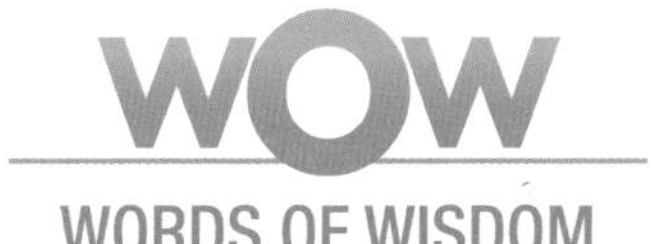

WORDS OF WISDOM

A child's essential bodily processes of elimination can be a major event of wonder and creative accomplishment.

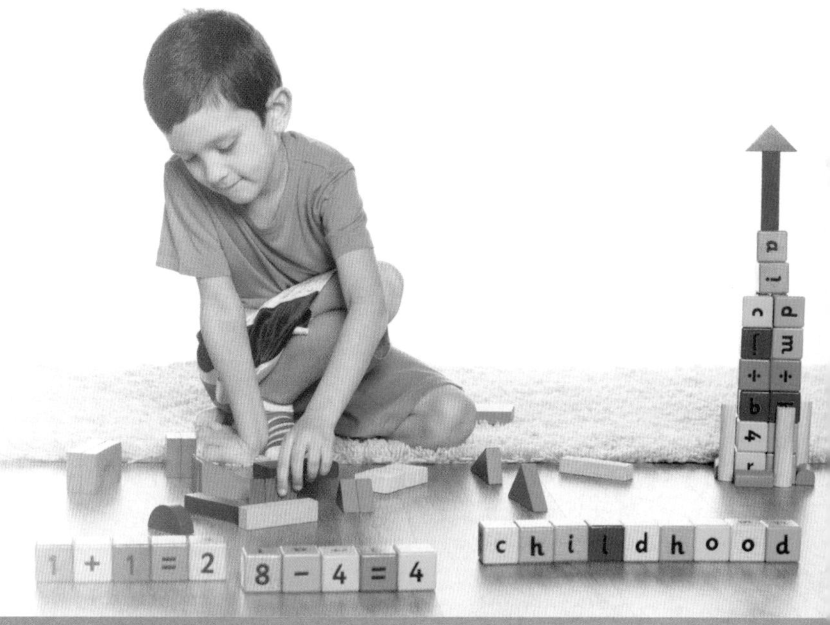

21 Nursing Care of the Child With an Alteration in Urinary Elimination/ Genitourinary Disorder

KEY TERMS

amenorrhea
anasarca
anuria
bacteriuria (bak-tēr′ē-yūr′ē-ă)
dysmenorrhea (dis-men′ōr-ē′ă)
dysuria
hematuria
oliguria (ol′i-gyūr′ē-ă)
proteinuria
urgency
urinary frequency

LEARNING OBJECTIVES

Upon completion of the chapter, you will be able to:

1. Compare the anatomy and physiology of the genitourinary system of infants and children with those of adults.
2. Describe nursing care related to common laboratory and diagnostic testing used in the medical diagnosis of pediatric genitourinary and reproductive system conditions.
3. Distinguish alterations in urinary elimination and genitourinary disorders common in infants, children, and adolescents.
4. Identify appropriate nursing assessments and interventions related to medications and treatments for alterations in urinary elimination, genitourinary, and reproductive system disorders in children.
5. Develop an individualized nursing care plan or concept map for the child with an alteration in urinary elimination or genitourinary disorder.
6. Describe the psychosocial impact of chronic genitourinary disorders on children.
7. Devise a nutrition plan for the child with renal insufficiency.
8. Develop child and family teaching plans for the child with an alteration in urinary elimination or genitourinary disorder.

Corey Bond, 5 years old, is brought to the clinic by her parent. She presents with fever and lethargy for the past 24 hours. Her parent states, "Corey has had a few accidents in her pants over the past few days, which is unusual for her. She also has been getting up at night more often to use the bathroom."

INTRODUCTION

Urinary elimination refers to the secretion and excretion of body waste through the urinary/renal system. Nurses may encounter children with alterations in urinary elimination and should be familiar with various genitourinary (GU) disorders that children experience. Alterations in urinary elimination or GU disorders in children and adolescents may occur because of abnormalities in fetal development, infectious processes, trauma, neurologic deficit, genetic influences, or other causes.

Congenital disorders account for a large proportion of GU disorders in infants. External GU malformations are easily identified at birth, but internal structural defects may not be identified until later in infancy or childhood when symptoms or complications arise. Enuresis and urinary tract infection (UTI) also occur in a significant number of children.

Some alterations in urinary elimination directly involve the kidney from the outset, while others involve other parts of the urinary tract and may have a long-term effect on the kidneys and renal function, particularly if left untreated or treated inadequately. Disorders affecting the reproductive organs often require early diagnosis and management to preserve future reproductive capabilities.

Nurses must be knowledgeable about pediatric GU conditions to provide prompt recognition, nursing care, education, and support to children and their families. Although some disorders are acute and resolve quickly, many have a long-term effect on quality of life and will require more intense, extended support. Management of acute or common pediatric GU disorders may be provided in the pediatric or family practice outpatient setting, while specialists such as pediatric nephrologists or urologists usually manage chronic or involved GU disorders.

VARIATIONS IN PEDIATRIC ANATOMY AND PHYSIOLOGY

Although the urinary tract and reproductive organs are present at birth, their initial functioning is immature. The infant or child is at increased risk for the development of certain urinary elimination alterations because of the anatomic and physiologic differences between children and adults.

Structural Differences

The kidney is large in relation to the size of the abdomen until the child reaches adolescence. Due to this increased size, the kidneys of the child are less well protected from injury by the ribs and fat padding than they are in the adult. The urethra is naturally shorter in all ages of females compared with males, placing them at increased risk for the entrance of bacteria into the bladder via the urethra. In the female infant or child, this risk is compounded by the physical proximity of the urethral opening to the rectum. The male urethra is much shorter in childhood than in adulthood, placing the young male at increased risk for UTI compared with the adult male.

Urinary Concentration

Blood flow through the kidneys (glomerular filtration rate [GFR]) is slower in the infant and young toddler compared with the adult. The kidney is less able to concentrate urine and reabsorb amino acids, placing the infant and young toddler at increased risk for dehydration during times when fluid loss or decreased fluid intake occurs. The normal range for serum blood urea nitrogen (BUN) and creatinine of the healthy infant or young toddler is usually less than the older child's or adult's. The renal system usually reaches functional maturity at around 2 years of age.

Urine Output

Bladder capacity is about 30 mL in the newborn; it increases to the expected adult capacity of about 270 mL by 1 year of age. The expected urine output in the infant and child is 0.5 to 2 mL/kg/h, with the average 1-year-old voiding about 400 to 500 mL per day. The average urine output for an adolescent is about 800 to 1,400 mL per day. The infant and toddler may void as often as 9 or 10 times per day. By age 3, the average number of voids per day is the same as that of an adult (3 to 8).

Reproductive Organ Maturity

The reproductive organs are also immature at birth. The gonads are not mature until adolescence in most children. The hormonal changes that occur with puberty account for some of the reproductive concerns, particularly for female adolescents.

COMMON MEDICAL TREATMENTS

A variety of medications as well as other medical treatments and surgical procedures are used to treat urinary elimination alterations and GU problems in children. Most of these treatments will require a health care provider's or nurse practitioner's order when the child is in the hospital. The most common treatments and medications are listed in Common Medical Treatments 21.1 and Drug Guide 21.1. The nurse caring for the child with a GU disorder should be familiar with what the procedures are, how the treatments and medications work, and common nursing implications related to use of these modalities.

COMMON MEDICAL TREATMENTS 21.1 Genitourinary Disorders

Treatment	Explanation	Indications	Nursing Implications
Urinary diversion	Surgical diversion of ureters to the abdominal wall; continent diversion uses a piece of intestine to create a bladder that can be catheterized. Noncontinent diversion involves a stoma on the abdominal wall that requires use of an ostomy pouch.	Any situation in which the bladder needs to be removed or does not function correctly (bladder exstrophy or prune belly)	Meticulous skin care is necessary to prevent breakdown around the stoma. Teach families how to care for the ostomy pouch or how to catheterize the continent stoma. Expect mucus in the urine if intestine is used for the urinary reservoir. Monitor for signs of urinary tract infection.
Foley catheter	An indwelling urinary catheter stays in place by means of an inflated balloon.	Usually used only during the postoperative period	Monitor for urethral drainage or irritation. Keep the area clean and dry. Monitor color, consistency, clarity, and amount of urine in drainage bag. Monitor for infection, checking results of urinalysis and urine cultures.
Ureteral stent	A thin catheter temporarily placed in the ureter to drain urine; removed via cystoscopy when it is time for discontinuation	Urinary tract anomalies	Monitor urine output carefully. Check for bleeding postoperatively.
Nephrostomy tube	Tube placed directly into the kidney to drain urine externally to a bag	Urinary tract anomalies	Monitor urine output carefully.
Suprapubic tube	Catheter placed in the bladder via the abdominal wall above the symphysis pubis	Postoperative urine drainage with reconstructive surgeries	Monitor for blood in the urine and adequate urine output. Minimize manipulation of the suprapubic tube to avoid triggering bladder spasms.
Vesicostomy	Stoma in the abdominal wall to the bladder	Urinary tract anomalies, neurogenic bladder	Constant urine drainage requires diaper use. Monitor urine output. Assess skin around the stoma for breakdown.
Appendicovesicostomy (Mitrofanoff procedure)	Uses appendix to create a stoma on the abdominal wall that allows for catheterization of the bladder	Urinary tract anomalies, neurogenic bladder	Allows for urinary continence, which improves the child's self-esteem. Teach the family and child how to catheterize the stoma.
Bladder augmentation	Uses a piece of stomach or intestine to enlarge bladder capacity	Decreased bladder capacity	Since a portion of the gastrointestinal tract is used,the urine is often mucuslike.

DRUG GUIDE 21.1

COMMON DRUGS FOR GU DISORDERS

Medication	Actions/Indications	Nursing Implications
Anticholinergic agents (oxybutynin, propantheline bromide, belladonna, and opium suppository)	Cause smooth muscle relaxation of the bladder, used for urinary tract spasms or contractions related to surgical procedure or use of catheters; control of nocturnal enuresis	Increase fluid intake (limit to during the day in the child with nocturnal enuresis). Avoid use in a febrile child.
Antibiotics (oral, parenteral)	Kill bacteria or arrest their growth; used for urinary tract infection	Check for antibiotic allergies. Should be given as prescribed for the length of time indicated
Desmopressin	Antidiuretic hormone; causes renal tubule to absorb more water, decreasing volume of urine in children with nocturnal enuresis	Nasal spray may cause nasal irritation, nausea, flushing, or headache. Administer at bedtime; alternate nares. Associated with a high relapse rate
Human chorionic gonadotropin (hCG)	Stimulates production of gonadal steroids to precipitate testicular descent	Monitor for signs of precocious puberty if used long term.

(*continued*)

DRUG GUIDE 21.1 (*continued*)

COMMON DRUGS FOR GU DISORDERS

Medication	Actions/Indications	Nursing Implications
Corticosteroids	Antiinflammatory and immunosuppressive action to induce remission and promote diuresis in nephrotic syndrome; high-dose intravenous therapy used when nephrotic syndrome is resistant to conventional doses	Administer with food to decrease GI upset. May mask signs of infection Do not stop treatment abruptly, or acute adrenal insufficiency may occur. Monitor for Cushing syndrome.
Cytotoxic drugs (cyclophosphamide and chlorambucil)	Interfere with normal function of DNA by alkylation; used to induce prolonged remission in nephrotic syndrome	Doses may be tapered over time. Monitor for hypertension during infusion. Causes bone marrow suppression. Monitor for signs of infection. Cyclophosphamide: Administer in the morning; provide adequate hydration; have the child void frequently during and after infusion to decrease risk of hemorrhagic cystitis. Chlorambucil: Administer with nonspicy, nonacidic foods; seizures occur rarely.
Immunosuppressant drugs (cyclosporine A [CyA], azathioprine, tacrolimus, mycophenolate)	Cause immune suppression to prevent rejection of kidney transplants; CyA and tacrolimus may be used for steroid-dependent nephrotic syndrome.	Monitor complete blood count, serum creatinine, potassium, and magnesium. Monitor blood pressure and observe for signs of infection. Blood levels should be drawn prior to morning dose. CyA: do not give with grapefruit juice. Azathioprine and mycophenolate: Give on an empty stomach; do not open capsule or crush tablet. Tacrolimus: Give on an empty stomach; assess for development of hyperglycemia. Relapse of nephrotic syndrome may occur after withdrawal of CyA or tacrolimus therapy.
Muromonab-CD3	Removal of all CD3 molecules from T-lymphocyte surface so it has inability to act; used for treatment of acute kidney transplant rejection	Monitor for development of pulmonary edema. First-dose effect may cause fever, chills, chest tightness, wheezing, nausea, and vomiting.
Angiotensin-converting enzyme (ACE) inhibitors (captopril, enalapril)	Potent vasoconstrictors, prevent conversion of angiotensin I to angiotensin II; used to treat renal causes of hypertension	Monitor blood pressure frequently; may cause cough, hyperkalemia Captopril: Administer on an empty stomach. Enalapril: Administer without regard to food.
Imipramine (tricyclic antidepressant)	Increases the synaptic concentration of serotonin and/or norepinephrine; treatment of enuresis	Monitor for urinary retention; may cause decreased appetite
Diuretics: furosemide, hydrochlorothiazide	Inhibit resorption of sodium and chloride leading to increased excretion of water and electrolytes; used in nephrotic syndrome, acute glomerulonephritis, hemolytic uremic syndrome, or other instances of fluid overload with renal sufficiency	Administer with food or milk to decrease GI upset. Monitor blood pressure, kidney function, and electrolytes (particularly potassium). May cause photosensitivity
Vasodilators: hydralazine, minoxidil	Direct vasodilation of arterioles, resulting in decreased systemic resistance; used to treat renal causes of hypertension	May cause fluid retention Hydralazine: Administer with food. Monitor heart rate and blood pressure (closely with intravenous use). Minoxidil: may be administered without regard to food; may cause dizziness
Calcium channel blocker: nifedipine	Prevents calcium from entering voltage-sensitive channels, resulting in coronary vasodilation; used to treat renal causes of hypertension	Administer with food; avoid grapefruit juice. Insoluble shell of extended-release tablet may pass in stool. Use caution when administering liquid-filled capsule sublingually or by bite-and-swallow method, as significant hypotension may occur.
Albumin (intravenous)	Increases intravascular oncotic pressure, resulting in movement of fluid from interstitial to intravascular space; indicated for fluid volume excess associated with nephrotic syndrome	May require a filter depending on brand used Rapid infusion can result in vascular overload. Monitor vital signs; observe for pulmonary edema and cardiac failure.

GI, gastrointestinal.

Source: UpToDate, Inc. (2023). *Lexi-comp*® (Version 7.7.0) [Mobile app]. Wolters Kluwer. https://apps.apple.com/us/app/lexicomp/id313401238

Clinical Judgment and the Nursing Process for the Child With an Alteration in Urinary Elimination or Genitourinary Disorder

Care of the child with an alteration in urinary elimination or GU disorder includes assessment, nursing analysis, planning, interventions, and evaluation. It is important to individualize each step of this process for each child.

Assessment

Assessment of urinary tract, renal, or reproductive dysfunction includes health history, physical examination, and laboratory and diagnostic testing.

Health History

The health history consists of the birthing parent's pregnancy history, family history, and history of present illness (when the symptoms started and how they have progressed), as well as medications and treatments used at home. The medical history may be significant for maternal polyhydramnios, oligohydramnios, diabetes, hypertension, or alcohol or cocaine ingestion. Neonatal history may include the presence of a single umbilical artery or an abdominal mass, chromosome abnormality, or congenital malformation. Document medical history of UTI or other problems with the GU tract.

Family history may be significant for kidney disease or uropathology, chronic UTIs, renal calculi, or a history of parental enuresis. Determine age of successful toilet training, pattern of incontinent episodes (having "accidents"), and toileting hygiene self-care routines. Note myelomeningocele or other spinal disturbance that may affect the child's ability to urinate. Note previous urologic surgeries or ongoing renal interventions (e.g., dialysis). For the adolescent female, obtain a thorough menstrual history, including sexual behavior and pregnancy history.

When determining the history of the present illness, inquire about the following:

- Burning on urination
- Changes in voiding patterns
- Foul-smelling urine
- Vaginal or urethral discharge
- Genital pain, irritation, or discomfort
- Blood in the urine
- Edema
- Masses in the groin, scrotum, or abdomen
- Flank or abdominal pain
- Cramps
- Nausea and/or vomiting
- Poor growth
- Weight gain
- Fever
- Infectious exposure (particularly *Streptococcus* A or *Escherichia coli*)
- Trauma

Record medications used for acute or chronic conditions or for contraception.

Physical Examination

Physical examination of the GU system includes inspection and observation, auscultation, percussion, and palpation.

INSPECTION AND OBSERVATION

Observe the child's general appearance, noting growth retardation or unusual weight gain. Inspect the skin for the presence of pruritus, edema (generalized or periorbital), or bruising. Note pallor of the skin or dysmorphic features (associated with genetic conditions). Document the presence of lethargy, fatigue, rapid respirations, confusion, or developmental delay. Observe the external genitalia area for infant diaper rash, constant urine dribble, displaced urethral opening, reddened urethral opening, or discharge. Note vaginal irritation or labial fusion; inspect the scrotal sac for enlargement or discoloration. Note the condition of a urinary stoma or diversion if present. With the child lying flat, observe the abdomen for distention, ascites, or slack abdominal musculature.

AUSCULTATION

Listen carefully to heart sounds, as a flow murmur may be present in the anemic child with a kidney disorder (Klabunde, 2023). Note elevated heart rate. Auscultate blood pressure with the appropriate-size cuff, noting elevation or depression. In the edematous child, carefully auscultate the lungs, noting the presence of adventitious sounds. Note the absence of bowel sounds, as this may indicate peritonitis. In the child who receives chronic hemodialysis, auscultate the fistula for the presence of a bruit (desired expected finding).

TAKE NOTE!

Use the bell of the stethoscope when auscultating the infant's or child's blood pressure so that you can hear the softer Korotkoff sounds more accurately.

PERCUSSION

Percuss the abdomen. Note unusual dullness or flatness (dullness is usually heard over the spleen at the right costal margin, over the kidneys, and 1 to 3 cm below the left costal margin). A full bladder may yield dullness above the symphysis pubis.

PALPATION

Palpate the abdomen. Note the presence of palpable kidneys (indicating enlargement or mass, as they are usually difficult to palpate in the older infant or child). Note the presence of abdominal masses or a distended bladder. Document tenderness to palpation or along the costovertebral angle. Palpate the scrotum for the presence of descended testicles, masses, or other abnormalities. Note whether the foreskin is present, but do not forcibly retract the foreskin. In the child who receives chronic hemodialysis, palpate the fistula or graft for the presence of a thrill (desired expected finding).

Laboratory and Diagnostic Testing

Common Laboratory and Diagnostic Tests 21.1 explains the most commonly used laboratory and diagnostic tests for a child suspected of having a GU disorder. The test results can help the health care provider or nurse practitioner to diagnose the disorder or to determine treatment. Laboratory or nonnursing personnel obtain some of the tests, while the nurse might obtain others. In either instance, the nurse should be familiar with how the tests are obtained, what they are used for, and expected versus unexpected results. This knowledge will also be necessary when providing child and family education related to the tests and results.

Remember Corey, the 5-year-old with fever and lethargy? What additional health history and physical examination assessment information should you obtain?

COMMON LABORATORY AND DIAGNOSTIC TESTS 21.1

Test	Explanation	Indications	Nursing Implications
Complete blood count	Evaluates hemoglobin and hematocrit, white blood cell count, and platelet count	Any condition in which anemia, infection, or thrombocytopenia is suspected	Expected values vary according to age and sex. White blood cell count differential is helpful in evaluating source of infection.
Blood urea nitrogen (BUN) (serum)	Indirect measurement of kidney function and glomerular filtration in the presence of adequate liver function	Nephrotic syndrome, hemolytic uremic syndrome, kidney failure, acute glomerulonephritis, or other kidney diseases	BUN may be elevated with high-protein diet or dehydration; may be decreased with overhydration or malnutrition
Creatinine (serum)	This is a more direct measurement of kidney function, only minimally affected by liver function. Generally, doubling of the creatinine level is suggestive of a 50% reduction in glomerular filtration rate.	Used to diagnose impaired kidney function	A diet high in meat may cause a transient, though not pronounced, increase in creatinine. There are also slight diurnal variations in levels. Draw at the same time each day if serial evaluations are ordered.
Creatinine clearance (urine and serum)	A 24-hour urine collection is evaluated for the presence of creatinine, then compared with the serum creatinine level to determine creatinine clearance.	Used to diagnose impaired kidney function	Discard the first void, and then begin the 24-hour urine collection. Keep the specimen on ice during the collection period. Collect *all* urine passed in the 24-hour period. Ensure that a venous blood sample is drawn during the 24-hour period. The urine specimen should be sent promptly to the laboratory at the end of the 24-hour period.
Potassium (serum)	Measures the concentration of potassium in the blood	Any suspected kidney disease; followed routinely in kidney failure	Avoid hemolysis and allow the child to open and close the hand with a tourniquet in place, as these can cause elevation in potassium levels. Evaluate the child with increased or decreased potassium levels for cardiac arrhythmias. Immediately notify the health care provider or nurse practitioner of critically high potassium levels.
Total protein, globulin, albumin (serum)	Protein electrophoresis separates the various components into zones according to their electrical charge.	Used to diagnose, evaluate, and monitor chronic kidney disease	Significantly low levels of albumin contribute to extent of edema, as albumin is necessary in the blood to maintain colloidal osmotic pressure.
Calcium (serum)	Measurement of calcium level in the blood; half of all calcium is protein bound, so the level will decrease with hypoalbuminemia.	Kidney diseases associated with hypoalbuminemia and edema	Avoid prolonged tourniquet use during blood draw, as this may falsely increase the calcium level.

COMMON LABORATORY AND DIAGNOSTIC TESTS 21.1

Test	Explanation	Indications	Nursing Implications
Phosphorus (serum)	Measurement of phosphate level in the blood; phosphorus levels are inversely related to calcium levels (they increase when calcium levels decrease).	Kidney disease, ongoing monitoring, particularly in the child with hypocalcemia	Child should be NPO past midnight prior to the morning of the blood draw. Avoid hemolysis, as it can falsely elevate the phosphate level.
Urinalysis (urine)	Evaluates color, pH, specific gravity, and odor of urine; also assess for presence of protein, glucose, ketones, blood, leukocyte esterase, red and white blood cells, bacteria, crystals, and casts.	Reveals preliminary information about the urinary tract; useful in children with fever, dysuria, flank pain, urgency, or hematuria; proteinuria may be noted in kidney disorders.	Be aware of the many drugs affecting urine color, and notify laboratory if the child is taking one. Notify laboratory if the patient is menstruating. Refrigerate the specimen if not processed promptly. While proteinuria may occur with various kidney disorders, it may also occur as either transient or orthostatic proteinuria, both of which are benign events.
Cystoscopy	Endoscopic visualization of the urethra and bladder	Evaluate hematuria and recurrent urinary tract infection; determine ureteral reflux; measure bladder capacity.	Encourage fluids. Monitor vital signs. The child may feel burning with voiding after the procedure. A pink tinge to the urine is common after the procedure.
Urine culture and sensitivity	Urine is plated in the laboratory and evaluated every day for the presence of bacteria. A final report is usually issued after 48–72 hours. Sensitivity testing is performed to determine the best choice of antibiotic.	Used to diagnose urinary tract infection	Obtain a culture specimen prior to starting antibiotics if possible. Avoid contamination of the specimen with stool. The sample may be obtained by catheterization, clean-catch specimen, or sterile U-bag; in some institutions, suprapubic tap is performed in neonates and young infants by the health care provider or nurse practitioner.
Urodynamic studies	Measure the urine flow during micturition via a urine flow meter.	Dysfunctional voiding	The child must have a full bladder. The child then urinates into the urine flow meter. There is no discomfort associated with the test.
Voiding cystourethrogram (VCUG)	The bladder is filled with contrast material via catheterization. Fluoroscopy is performed to demonstrate filling of the bladder and collapsing after emptying.	Hematuria, urinary tract infections, vesicoureteral reflux, suspected structural anomalies	Just prior to the test, insert the Foley catheter. Ensure that the adolescent is not pregnant. After the test, encourage the child to drink fluids to prevent bacterial accumulation and aid in dye elimination.
Intravenous pyelogram (IVP)	Radiopaque contrast material is injected intravenously and filtered by the kidneys. X-ray films are obtained at set intervals to show passage of the dye through the kidneys, ureters, and bladder.	Urinary outlet obstruction, hematuria, trauma to the renal system, suspected kidney tumor	Contraindicated in children allergic to shellfish or iodine. If the dye infiltrates at the intravenous site, hyaluronidase may be used to speed absorption of the iodine. Ensure adequate hydration before and after the test. Some institutions require enema or laxative evacuation of the bowel prior to the study to ensure adequate visualization of the urinary tract.
Kidney biopsy	Usually, a percutaneous specimen is obtained by inserting a needle through the skin and into the kidney. The sample of kidney tissue obtained is then microscopically examined.	Diagnosis of kidney disease or assessment of kidney transplant rejection	After the biopsy, carefully assess for signs or symptoms of bleeding: increased heart rate, pale color, flank pain or backache, shoulder pain, or lightheadedness. Inspect the urine for gross hematuria. The child will be on bed rest, preferably supine, for 24 hours.
Kidney ultrasound	Reflected sound waves allow visualization of the kidneys, ureters, and bladder.	Useful in determining kidney size (as with hydronephrosis and polycystic kidney), presence of cysts or tumors, or rejection of kidney transplant	No fasting is required prior to the procedure, which does not require contrast material. The child should feel no discomfort during the ultrasound.

NPO, nothing by mouth.

Data from Corbett, J. A., & Banks, A. D. (2019). *Laboratory tests and diagnostic procedures with nursing diagnoses* (9th ed.). Pearson Education Inc.

Nursing Analysis and Related Interventions

After recognizing and analyzing cues from a thorough assessment, the nurse might identify several patient problems, including:

- Fluid volume excess
- Imbalanced nutrition, less than body requirements
- Impaired urinary elimination
- Activity intolerance
- Disturbed body image
- Pain
- Interrupted family processes
- Deficient knowledge

After completing an assessment of Corey, you note the following: foul-smelling urine; abdominal tenderness; redness in her perineal area; and slightly blood-tinged, cloudy urine. Based on these assessment findings, what would your top three patient problems be for Corey?

The foregoing patient problems provide suggestions for nursing care planning or concept mapping. Suggested interventions with rationales are provided further on. Care planning should be individualized, based on the child's and family's needs. Refer to Chapter 14 for the nursing process for pain management and to Chapter 11 for nursing interventions related to interrupted family processes. Additional information will be included later in the chapter as it relates to nursing management of specific disorders, as well as particular nursing interventions for deficient knowledge.

Nursing Analysis

Excess fluid volume related to compromised regulatory mechanism (decreased protein in the bloodstream, decreased urine output, sodium retention) or possible inappropriate fluid intake, as evidenced by edema, anasarca, weight gain, oliguria, azotemia, pulmonary congestion, or presence of S_3 heart sound.

Goal/Outcome

Child will attain appropriate fluid balance, will lose weight (fluid), edema or anasarca will decrease, lung sounds will be clear, and heart sounds as expected.

Encouraging Fluid Loss (interventions with *rationale*)

- Weigh child daily on same scale in similar amount of clothing; *in children, weight is the best indicator of changes in fluid status.*
- Monitor location and extent of edema (measure abdominal girth daily if ascites present); *decrease in edema indicates positive increase in oncotic pressure.*
- Auscultate lungs carefully to determine presence of crackles (*indicating pulmonary edema*).
- Assess work of breathing and respiratory rate; *increased work of breathing is associated with pulmonary edema.*
- Assess heart sounds for presence or absence of gallop; *presence of S_3 may indicate fluid overload.*
- Maintain fluid restriction as ordered *to decrease intravascular volume and workload on the heart.*
- Strictly monitor intake and output *to quickly note discrepancies and provide intervention.*
- Provide sodium-restricted diet as ordered; *restricting sodium in the diet allows for better renal excretion of extra fluid.*
- Administer diuretics as ordered, and monitor for side effects of those medications. *Diuretics encourage excretion of fluid and elimination of edema, reduce cardiac filling pressures, and increase renal blood flow. Side effects include electrolyte imbalance and orthostatic hypotension.*

Nursing Analysis

Imbalanced nutrition (less than body requirements) related to biologic factors (protein loss) or insufficient dietary intake (anorexia) as evidenced by weight, length/height, and/or body mass index (BMI) below average for age.

Goal/Outcome

Child will improve nutritional intake, resulting in steady increase in weight and length/height.

Promoting Adequate Nutrition (interventions with *rationale*)

- Determine expected body weight and length/height for age *to determine goal to work toward.*
- Assess child for food preferences that fall within dietary restrictions, *as the child will be more likely to consume adequate amounts of foods that they like.*
- Weigh daily or weekly (according to health care provider or nurse practitioner's order or institutional standard) and measure length/height weekly *to monitor for increased growth.*
- Offer highest-calorie meals at the time of day when the child's appetite is the greatest *to increase likelihood of increased caloric intake.*
- Provide increased-calorie shakes or puddings within diet restriction: *High-calorie foods increase weight gain.*
- Administer vitamin and mineral supplements as prescribed *to attain/maintain vitamin and mineral balance in the body.*

Nursing Analysis

Impaired urinary elimination related to pathologic process, anatomic obstruction, sensory motor impairment, or dysfunctional voiding as evidenced by dysuria, or urinary retention or incontinence or urgency.

Goal/Outcome

Child's bladder will empty adequately, according to preestablished quantities and frequencies individualized for the child (usual urine output is 0.5 to 2 mL/kg/h).

Promoting Adequate Urinary Elimination and Successful Bladder Emptying (interventions with *rationale*)

- Assess the child's usual voiding pattern and success within that pattern *to determine baseline.*
- Assess the child's ability to adequately empty their bladder via history focused on character and duration of lower urinary symptoms *to determine baseline.*
- Develop a schedule for bladder emptying *to decrease bladder overdistention and to encourage voiding in the toilet.*
- Maintain adequate hydration *to avoid irritating effects of dehydration on the bladder.*
- Avoid constipation, encopresis, or fecal impaction *as alterations in bowel elimination may have a negative impact on urinary elimination.*
- Assess for bladder distention by palpation or urinary retention by postvoid residual obtained via catheterization or bladder ultrasound *to determine extent of retention.*
- Teach the parents to restrict the child's fluid intake after dinner *to avoid bedwetting.*
- Ensure the child voids prior to going to bed *to avoid bedwetting.*
- Teach bladder-stretching exercises as prescribed per the care provider *to increase bladder capacity.*
- In the child with significant urinary retention, teach the parents and child the technique of clean intermittent catheterization, *which allows for regular complete bladder emptying.*

Nursing Analysis

Activity intolerance related to physical deconditioning (generalized edema, weakness) or imbalance between oxygen supply/demand (anemia) as evidenced by abnormal heart rate response with activity, exertional discomfort or dyspnea (elevated respiratory rate, complaint of shortness of breath with play or activity), fatigue, or generalized weakness.

Goal/Outcome

Child will display increased activity tolerance and desire to play without developing symptoms of exertion.

Promoting Activity (interventions with *rationale*)

- Encourage activity or ambulation per the health care provider's or nurse practitioner's orders: *Early mobilization results in better outcomes.*
- Observe the child for symptoms of activity intolerance such as pallor, nausea, lightheadedness, or dizziness or changes in vital signs *to determine level of tolerance.*
- If the child is on bed rest, perform range-of-motion exercises and frequent position changes *as negative changes to the musculoskeletal system occur quickly with inactivity and immobility.*
- Cluster nursing care activities and plan for periods of rest before and after exertional activities *to decrease oxygen need and consumption.*
- Refer the child to physical therapy *for exercise prescription to increase skeletal muscle strength.*

Nursing Analysis

Disturbed body image related to alteration in self-perception, alteration in body function (short stature, or effects of long-term corticosteroid use) as evidenced by negative feeling about body.

Goal/Outcome

Child or adolescent will display appropriate body image, will look at self in mirror, and will participate in social activities.

Promoting Body Image (interventions with *rationale*)

- Acknowledge feelings of anger over body changes and illness: *Venting feelings is associated with less body image disturbance.*
- Support the child's or adolescent's choices of comfortable, fashionable clothing *that may disguise anatomic abnormalities and dialysis tubing.*
- Involve the child, and especially the adolescent, in the decision-making process *as a sense of control of their own body will improve body image.*
- Encourage children or adolescents to spend time with others of their own age who have short stature or other effects of kidney disorders: *A peer's opinions are often better accepted than those of people in authority, such as parents or health care professionals.*

Based on your top three patient problems for Corey, describe appropriate nursing interventions.

Collecting Urine Specimens in Children

Urine specimens may be collected using a variety of methods in infants and children. Suprapubic aspiration is a useful method for obtaining a sterile urine specimen from the neonate or young infant. A sterile needle is inserted into the bladder through the anterior wall of the abdomen, and the urine is then aspirated. The health care provider or nurse practitioner generally performs this method. Infants and toddlers who are not toilet trained may require a urine bag for urine collection. A sterile urine bag is required for a urine culture, a clean bag for routine urinalysis. A 24-hour urine collection bag is also available. Nursing Procedure 21.1 gives details on the use of the urine bag.

NURSING PROCEDURE 21.1 Applying the Urine Bag

1. Cleanse the perineal area well and pat dry (Fig. A). If a culture is to be obtained, cleanse the genital area with povidone-iodine (Betadine) or per institutional protocol.

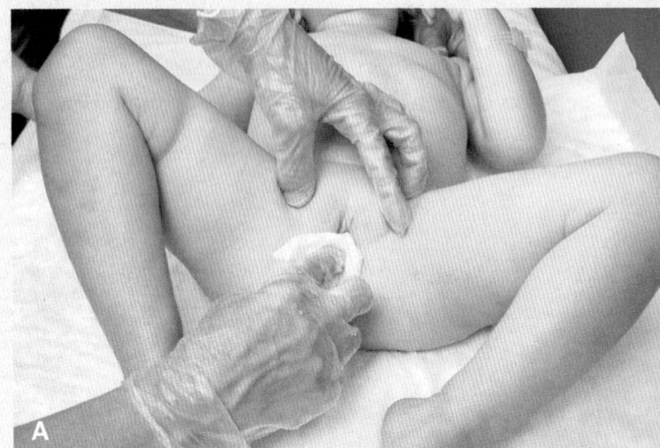

A

2. Apply benzoin around the scrotum or the vulvar area to aid with urine bag adhesion.
3. Allow the benzoin to dry.
4. Apply the urine bag.
   - Ensure that the penis is fully inside the bag; a portion of the scrotum may or may not be inside the bag, depending on scrotal size.
   - Apply the narrow portion of the bag on the perineal space between the anal and vulvar areas first for best adhesion, and then spread the remaining adhesive section (Fig. B).

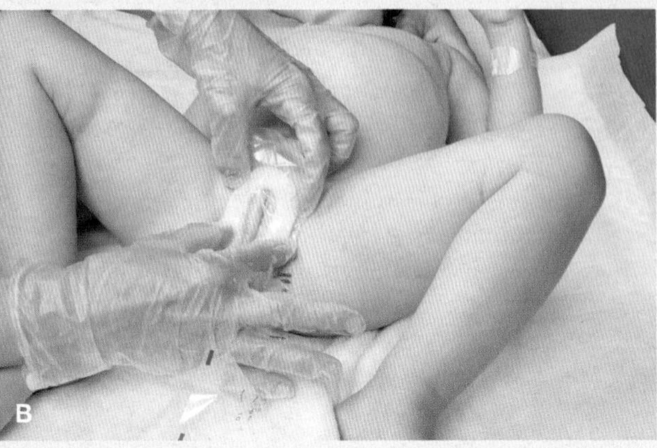

B

5. Tuck the bag downward inside the diaper to discourage leaking.
6. Check the bag frequently for urine (Fig. C).

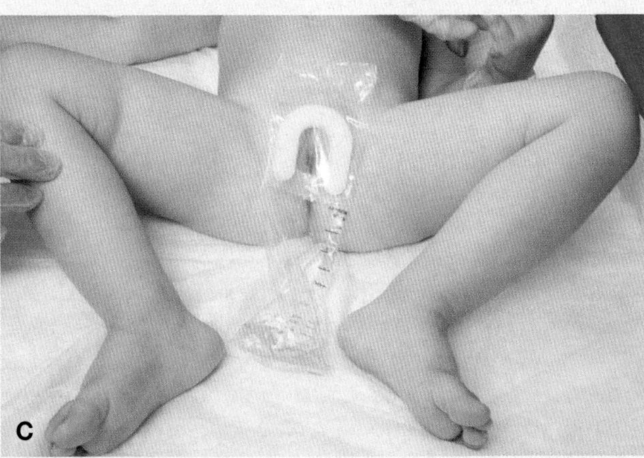

C

Nationwide Children's Hospital. (2024). *U-bag urine collection guidelines* for males and females. https://www.nationwidechildrens.org/family-resources-education/health-wellness-andsafety-resources/helping-hands/ubag-urine-collectionguidelines-for-males-and-females

Sterile urinary catheterization is performed like that in adults. The size of the catheter varies depending on the size of the child. General size recommendations are:

- 6 to 8 French: Birth to 1 year old
- 8 to 10 French: 1 to 8 years old
- 10 to 12 French: 8 to 12 years old
- 12 to 14 French: 12 years and older (Hucker & Lawson-Wood, 2023)

• • • ATRAUMATIC CARE • • •

When examining the genital area or performing urinary catheterization of the young female, allow them to sit with their parent on the examination table to decrease anxiety. Have the child lie back on their parent's chest, seated on the table between the parent's legs. Encourage the parent to console and hug the child while the invasive examination or procedure is being performed.

TAKE NOTE!

Use familiar terms such as "pee-pee," "tinkle," or "potty" to explain to the child what is needed and to gain their cooperation.

URINARY TRACT AND KIDNEY DISORDERS

The urinary tract and kidney disorders discussed in what follows include structural disorders, UTI, enuresis, and acquired disorders that result in altered kidney function.

Structural Disorders

Numerous urologic conditions are congenital (present at birth) and occur as a result of altered fetal development. Many of these defects are apparent at birth, yet some are not recognized until later in infancy or childhood when symptoms or complications arise.

Bladder Exstrophy

In classic bladder exstrophy, a midline closure defect occurs during the embryonic period of gestation, leaving the bladder open and exposed outside of the abdomen. The bony pelvis may also be malformed, resulting in an opening in the pelvic arch. Bladder exstrophy may be diagnosed by prenatal ultrasound. Complications include UTI from ascending organisms. Treatment of bladder exstrophy involves surgical repair.

Nursing Assessment

On physical examination of the infant or child, note the red appearance to the bladder seen on the abdominal wall (Fig. 21.1). Draining urine will be visible. Note excoriation of abdominal skin around the bladder resulting from contact with urine. A malformed urethra may be present in females, while males may have an unformed or malformed penis or an expected penis with an epispadias.

Nursing Management

Nursing management consists of preventing infection and skin breakdown, providing postoperative care, and catheterizing the stoma.

PREVENTING INFECTION AND SKIN BREAKDOWN

Bladder exstrophy requires surgical repair. In the preoperative period, care is focused on protecting the exstrophied bladder and preventing infection. Keep the infant in a supine position; keep the bladder moist and cover it with a sterile plastic bag. Change soiled diapers immediately to prevent contamination of the bladder with feces. Sponge-bathe the infant rather than immersing them in water to prevent pathogens in the bath water from entering the bladder. Prevent breakdown of the surrounding abdominal skin by applying protective barrier creams. In some instances, it may be necessary to consult the ostomy nurse for advice on dealing with abdominal skin excoriation. If an orthopedic surgeon is involved due to the malformed pubic arch, follow through with recommended positioning or bracing to prevent further separation of the pubic arch.

PROVIDING POSTOPERATIVE CARE

Nursing management in the postoperative period focuses on preventing infection. Keep the infant supine, and quickly change soiled diapers to prevent contamination of the incision with stool. Surgical reconstruction of the bladder within the pelvic cavity and reconstruction of the urethra are done if enough bladder tissue is present. An indwelling urethral catheter or suprapubic tube will allow urinary drainage, allowing the bladder to rest in the initial postoperative period. Ensure that catheters drain freely and do not become kinked. Sometimes, tubes or catheters used in the postoperative period require irrigation. Refer to the institution's policy and the surgeon's orders for specifics related to urinary catheter irrigation.

Manage bladder spasms with oxybutynin or belladonna and opioid suppositories as ordered. Note blood-tinged urine upon return from surgery, with clearing of urine within hours to days.

CATHETERIZING THE STOMA

If bladder tissue is insufficient for repair, then the bladder is removed, and a continent urinary reservoir is created. The ureters are connected to a portion of the small intestine that is separated from the gastrointestinal (GI) tract, thus creating a urinary reservoir. The intestines are reanastomosed to leave the GI tract intact and separate from the GU tract. A stoma is created on the abdominal wall; it provides access to the urinary reservoir (Fig. 21.2). The stoma is catheterized about four times per day to empty the reservoir of urine. Urine from an intestine-based urinary reservoir tends to be mucuslike

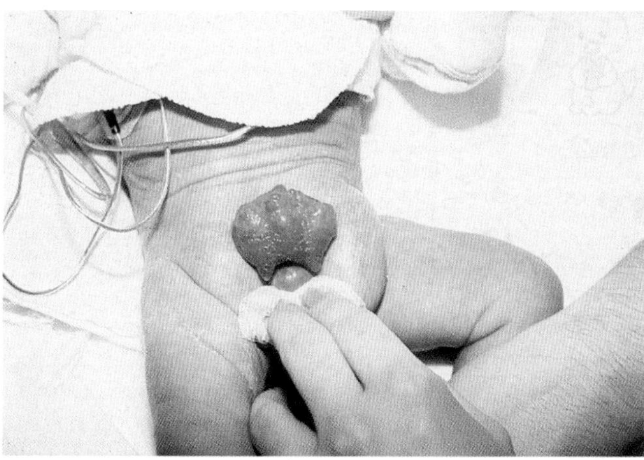

FIGURE 21.1 Note the bright-red color of the bladder exstrophy.

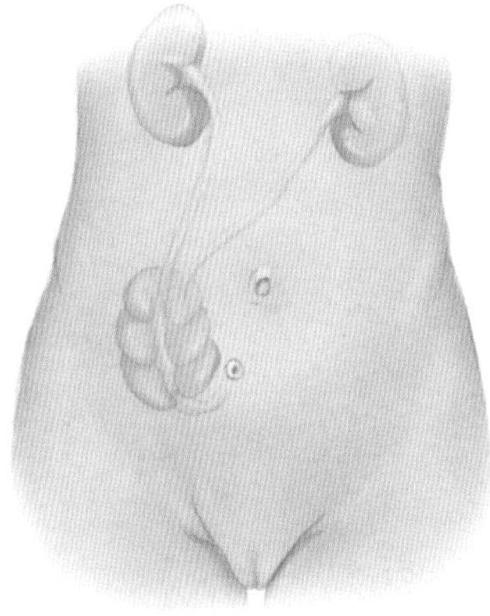

FIGURE 21.2 The abdominal stoma allows for urinary continence and requires catheterization.

and is often cloudier than urine from a urinary bladder. Teach parents the procedure for catheterizing the urinary reservoir, and instruct them to call the child's urologist or health care provider or nurse practitioner if signs or symptoms of UTI occur.

TAKE NOTE!

Children with congenital urologic malformations are at high risk for the development of latex allergy (Hamilton, 2023). Latex allergy can result in anaphylaxis. Primary prevention of latex allergy is warranted in all children with urologic malformations, so use latex-free gloves, tubes, and catheters when caring for these children.

Hypospadias/Epispadias

Hypospadias is a urethral defect in which the opening of the penis is on the ventral surface rather than at the end of it (Fig. 21.3). Epispadias is a urethral defect in which the opening is on the dorsal surface of the penis. In either case, the opening may be near the glans of the penis, midway along the penis, or near the base. If left uncorrected, the child may not be capable of appropriately aiming a urinary stream from a standing position. In addition, the abnormal placement of the urethral opening may result in erectile dysfunction or interfere with the deposition of sperm during intercourse, causing infertility. For these reasons, the defect is usually repaired between 6 months and 1 year of age (Baskin, 2023a). The goal of surgical correction for either condition is to provide for an appropriately placed meatus that allows for normal voiding and ejaculation. The meatus is moved to the glans penis, and the urethra is reconstructed as needed. Most repairs are accomplished in one surgery. More extensive reconstructions may require two stages.

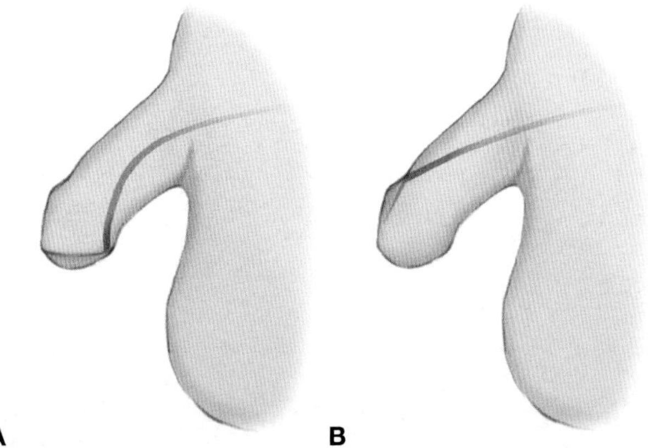

FIGURE 21.3 A. Hypospadias: The urethral opening is located on the ventral side of the penis. **B.** Epispadias: The urethral opening is located on the dorsal side of the penis.

Nursing Assessment

Note history of an unusual urine stream. Inspect the penis for placement of the urethral meatus: It may be slightly off center of the glans or may be present somewhere along the shaft of the penis. Inspect for chordee, a fibrous band causing the penis to curve downward. Palpate for the presence or absence of testicles in the scrotal sac because cryptorchidism (undescended testicles) often occurs with hypospadias, as do hydrocele and inguinal hernia.

Nursing Management

The newborn with hypospadias or epispadias should not undergo circumcision until after surgical repair of the urethral meatus. In more extreme cases, the surgeon may need to use some of the excess foreskin while reconstructing the meatus. Nursing care for the infant who has undergone a hypospadias or epispadias repair focuses on providing routine postoperative care and parent education.

PROVIDING POSTOPERATIVE CARE

Postoperatively, assess urinary drainage from the urethral stent or drainage tube, which allows for discharge of urine without stress along the surgical site. Ensure that the urinary drainage tube remains carefully taped, with the penis in an upright position to prevent stress on the urethral incision. The penile dressing is usually a compression type, used to decrease edema and bruising. Administer antibiotics if prescribed. Assess for pain, which is usually not extensive, and administer analgesics or antispasmodics (oral oxybutynin or belladonna and opium [B&O] suppository) as needed for bladder spasms. See Dosage Calculation Box 21.1. Bladder spasms may also be managed effectively through the use of epidural analgesia.

DOSAGE CALCULATION BOX 21.1

Child's weight: 17 lb, 12 oz

Medication order: oxybutynin 1.6 mg PO three times a day.

Per the Pediatric Dosage Handbook, the recommended dose is 0.2 mg/kg/dose two to three times daily.

Is the ordered dose safe?

Double diapering is a method used to protect the urethra and stent or catheter after surgery; it also helps keep the area clean and free from infection. The inner diaper contains stool, and the outer diaper contains urine, allowing separation between the bowel and bladder output. Nursing Procedure 21.2 details the double-diapering technique. Change the outside (larger) diaper when the child is wet; change both diapers when the child has a bowel movement.

NURSING PROCEDURE 21.2 Double Diapering

1. Cut a hole or a cross-shaped slit in the front of the smaller diaper.
2. Unfold both diapers, and place the smaller diaper (with the hole) inside the larger one.
3. Place both diapers under the child.
4. Carefully bring the penis (if applicable) and catheter/stent through the hole in the smaller diaper, and close the diaper.
5. Close the larger diaper, making sure the tip of the catheter/stent is inside the larger diaper.

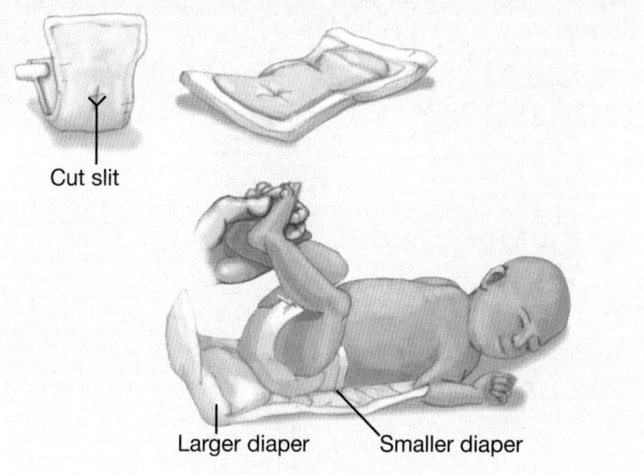

Text adapted from St. Lukes. (n.d.). *When your child needs surgery for hypospadias.* https://www.saintlukeskc.org/health-library/when-your-child-needs-surgery-hypospadias

EDUCATING THE FAMILY

If the child is to be discharged with the urinary catheter in place (which is common), teach the parents how to care for the catheter and drainage system. Have parents demonstrate their ability to irrigate the catheter should a mucus plug occur. Tub baths are generally prohibited until it is time to remove the penile dressing. Roughhousing, ride-on toys, and any activity involving straddling are not allowed for 4 weeks (Baskin, 2023a).

Obstructive Uropathy

Obstructive uropathy is an obstruction at any level along the upper or lower urinary tract. This discussion will focus on congenital structural defects, although obstruction can also occur as a result of other disease processes (acquired obstructive uropathy). The most common sites of obstruction are listed in Table 21.1. The defect may be unilateral or bilateral and can cause partial or complete

TABLE 21.1 • Common Sites of Obstructive Uropathy

Disorder	Site	Illustration
Ureteropelvic junction (UPJ) obstruction	Junction of the upper ureter with the pelvis of the kidney	Urinary tract with unilateral hydronephrosis and narrowing of the UPJ on that side Renal pelvis Site of obstruction Kidney Ureter Bladder
Ureterovesical junction (UVJ) obstruction	Junction of the lower ureter and the bladder	Urinary tract with unilateral hydronephrosis and dilated ureters with narrowing of the UVJ on that side Kidney Bladder Ureter Obstruction

(continued)

TABLE 21.1 • Common Sites of Obstructive Uropathy (*continued*)

Disorder	Site	Illustration
Ureterocele	Ureter swells into the bladder	Bladder with cystic pouch where ureters insert (unilateral) Hydroureter Ureterocele
Posterior urethral valves (males only)	Flaps of tissue in the proximal urethra	Distended proximal urethra, bladder, ureters, and hydronephrosis Kidney Renal pelvis Ureter Thickened bladder walls with dilated bladder Posterior valves

Data from Elder, J. R. (2020). Chapter 555: Obstruction of the urinary tract. In R. M. Kliegman, J. W. St Geme, N. J. Blum, S. S. Shah, R. C. Tasker, & K. M. Wilson (Eds.), *Nelson textbook of pediatrics* (21st ed.). Elsevier.

obstruction of urine flow, resulting in dilation of the affected kidney (hydronephrosis). Complications include recurrent UTI, kidney insufficiency, and progressive damage to the kidney, resulting in kidney failure.

Nursing Assessment

For a full description of the assessment phase of the nursing process, refer to the "Assessment" section of the "Clinical Judgment and the Nursing Process" section earlier in the chapter. Assessment findings pertinent to obstructive uropathy are discussed further on.

HEALTH HISTORY

Elicit a description of the present illness and chief complaint. Common symptoms reported during the health history might include:

- Recurrent UTI
- Incontinence
- Fever
- Foul-smelling urine
- Flank pain
- Abdominal pain
- **Urinary frequency** (needing to void often)
- Urinary **urgency** (urge to void immediately)
- **Dysuria** (difficulty or pain with voiding)
- **Hematuria** (blood in the urine)

Explore the child's current and past medical history for risk factors such as:

- "Prune belly" syndrome
- Chromosome abnormalities
- Anorectal malformations
- Ear defects

PHYSICAL EXAMINATION AND LABORATORY AND DIAGNOSTIC TESTS

Palpate the abdomen for the presence of an abdominal mass (hydronephrotic kidney). Assess the blood pressure; elevation may occur if kidney insufficiency is present. Many cases of obstructive uropathy may be diagnosed with prenatal ultrasound if the obstruction has been significant enough to cause hydronephrosis or dilation elsewhere along the urinary tract.

Nursing Management

Surgical correction is specific to the type of obstruction and generally consists of removal of the obstruction, reimplantation of the ureters as necessary, and, occasionally, creation of a urinary diversion. Postoperatively, assess urine output via vesicostomy, nephrostomy, suprapubic tube, or urethral catheter for color, clots, clarity, and amount. Encourage fluids once the child can tolerate them orally. Administer analgesics and/or antispasmodics as needed for bladder spasms. Teach parents care of vesicostomy or drainage tubes, with which the child may be discharged.

CLINICAL REASONING ALERT!

Upon return from surgery, most children have intravenous fluids without added potassium infusion. Potassium is withheld from the intravenous fluid until adequate urine output is established postoperatively to avoid the development of hyperkalemia should the kidneys fail to function properly (UTMB Health, 2024).

Hydronephrosis

Hydronephrosis is a condition in which the pelvis and calyces of the kidney are dilated (Fig. 21.4). Hydronephrosis may occur as a congenital defect, as a result of obstructive uropathy, or secondary to vesicoureteral reflux (VUR). Congenital hydronephrosis may be revealed on prenatal ultrasound. Complications of hydronephrosis include kidney insufficiency; hypertension; and, eventually, kidney failure.

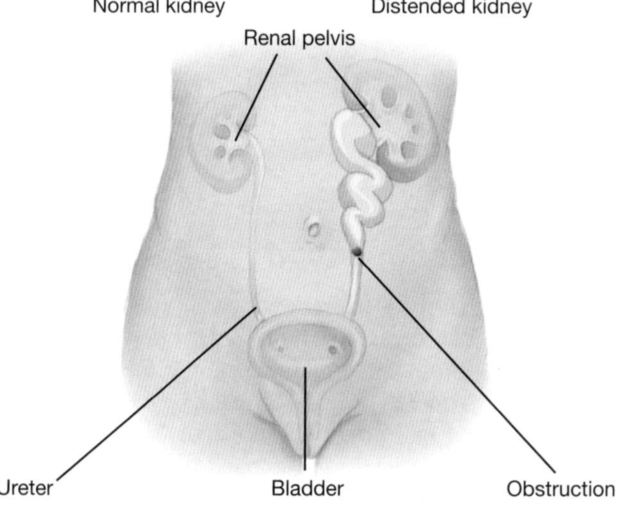

FIGURE 21.4 Hydronephrosis.

Nursing Assessment

The infant may be asymptomatic, but symptoms reported during the health history might include failure to thrive; intermittent hematuria; presence of an abdominal mass; or symptoms associated with a UTI such as fever, vomiting, poor feeding, and irritability.

Explore the child's current and past medical history for risk factors for congenital hydronephrosis such as a birthing parent with oligohydramnios or polyhydramnios or elevated levels of serum alpha-fetoprotein.

Monitor the blood pressure of infants and children suspected of having hydronephrosis. Palpation of the abdomen may reveal enlarged kidney(s) or a distended bladder. A voiding cystourethrogram (VCUG) will be performed to determine the presence of a structural defect that may be causing the hydronephrosis. Other diagnostic tests, such as a kidney ultrasound or an intravenous pyelogram, may also be performed to clarify the diagnosis.

Nursing Management

Teach the parents signs and symptoms of UTI and sepsis, as these complications may occur. Explain to the parents that they should observe the child for adequacy of urine output and hydration status. Teach the parents to perform appropriate perineal hygiene and to avoid using irritants in the genital area. The infant or child with hydronephrosis will need follow-up with a pediatric nephrologist or urologist.

Vesicoureteral Reflux

VUR is a condition in which urine from the bladder flows back up the ureters. This reflux of urine occurs during bladder contraction with voiding (Fig. 21.5). Reflux may occur in one or both ureters. If reflux occurs when the urine is infected, the kidney is exposed to bacteria, and pyelonephritis may result. The increased pressure placed

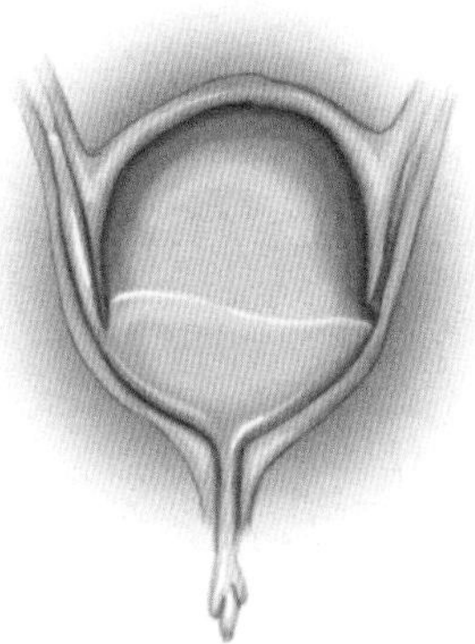

FIGURE 21.5 Note retrograde flow of urine up the ureter on bladder contraction.

upon the kidney with reflux can cause renal scarring and lead later in life to hypertension and, if severe, renal insufficiency or failure.

Primary VUR results from a congenital abnormality at the VUR junction that results in incompetence of the valve. Secondary VUR is related to other structural or functional problems such as neurogenic bladder, bladder dysfunction, or bladder outlet obstruction. About 30% to 40% of children diagnosed with a febrile UTI have VUR (Estrada & Cendron, 2021). VUR is graded according to its severity from grade I, which is characterized by minor dilation of the proximal ureter, to grade V, which is characterized by severe dilation of the ureter and pelvis of the kidney. Grades I through III usually resolve spontaneously by age 5, but grade IV or V VUR may be associated with recurrent UTI and kidney issues, necessitating surgical repair (Estrada & Cendron, 2021).

The goal of therapeutic management of VUR is prevention of pyelonephritis and subsequent renal scarring, which may contribute to the development of hypertension later in life. Management includes antibiotic prophylaxis to prevent breakthrough UTI (Estrada & Cendron, 2021). Additionally, hygiene and voiding practices are used to assist with prevention of UTI. Serial urine cultures are used to determine recurrence of UTI. Biannual, annual, or biennial radionuclide VCUGs are performed to determine the status of VUR. Grade III, IV, and V VUR usually warrants surgical intervention. The ureters are resected from the bladder and reimplanted elsewhere in the bladder wall to regain functionality.

TAKE NOTE!

The keys to prevention of long-term sequelae such as hypertension in children with urologic conditions are early diagnosis and intervention, prevention of infection, and close clinical follow-up. Nurses play a key role in monitoring and education.

Nursing Assessment

Common symptoms reported during the health history might include:

- fever
- dysuria
- frequency or urgency
- nocturia
- hematuria
- back, abdomen, or flank pain.

Explore the child's current and past medical history for risk factors such as history of UTI, congenital defect, or family history of VUR. For the child who is receiving ongoing follow-up for VUR, determine whether UTIs have occurred since the last visit, as well as the name and dose of prophylactic antibiotic.

Monitor the blood pressure for elevation. Palpate the abdomen for presence of a mass (if hydronephrosis is present). VCUG may be used to diagnose VUR.

Nursing Management

Nursing management of VUR includes preventing infection and providing postoperative care.

PREVENTING INFECTION

When VUR is present, the goal is to avoid urine infection so that infected urine cannot gain access to the kidneys. Initially, most cases of VUR are managed medically. Teach the child to empty the bladder completely. Teach the child and parents appropriate perineal hygiene as well as toileting hygiene to prevent recurrence of UTI. Teach parents about the antibiotic therapy prescribed; the child will be maintained on a low daily dose to prevent UTI. The drug is most effective when given at bedtime because of urinary stasis overnight. Inform parents of the schedule for serial urine cultures and follow-up VCUG.

PROVIDING POSTOPERATIVE CARE

If VUR is severe or if UTI is recurrent, surgical correction will be necessary. In the first 24 to 48 hours after surgery, maintain the intravenous fluid rate at 1.5 times maintenance to encourage a high urinary output. Monitor urine output via the Foley catheter; urine should be bloody initially, clearing within 2 to 3 days. If ureteral stents are present, monitor urine output from those as well. Administer analgesics for incisional pain relief and antispasmodics or B&O suppositories as needed for bladder spasms. Encourage ambulation and advancement of diet as ordered to promote return of appropriate bowel function. Teach parents that prophylactic antibiotics will be given until 1 to 2 months after surgery, when the VCUG demonstrates absence of reflux.

TAKE NOTE!

When caring for the child who has undergone urologic surgery, avoid manipulating the Foley or suprapubic catheter. Catheter manipulation contributes to bladder spasms.

Urinary Tract Infection

UTI is an infection of the urinary tract, most commonly affecting the bladder. UTI occurs most often because of bacteria ascending to the bladder via the urethra. About 8% of females and 2% of males will experience at least one UTI during childhood (Bock et al., 2022). One explanation for the more common occurrence in females is that the female's shorter urethra allows bacteria to have easier access to the bladder. The urethra is also located quite close to the vagina and anus in females, allowing spread of bacteria from those areas. The sexually active female adolescent is at risk for the development of UTI, as bacteria may be forced into the urethra by pressure from intercourse. The adolescent male may be somewhat protected from UTI by the antibacterial properties of prostate secretions.

UTI presents differently in infants than it does in children. Infants may exhibit fever, irritability, vomiting, failure to thrive, or jaundice. Children may also experience fever and vomiting but may also have dysuria, frequency, hesitancy, urgency, and/or pain.

Pathophysiology

Escherichia coli most commonly causes UTI, as it is usually found in the perineal and anal regions, close to the urethral opening. Other organisms include *Klebsiella, Staphylococcus aureus, Proteus, Pseudomonas,* and *Haemophilus*. Numerous factors may contribute to bacterial proliferation. Urinary stasis contributes to the development of a UTI once the bacteria have gained entry. Urine that remains in the bladder after voiding allows bacteria to grow rapidly. A decreased fluid intake also contributes to bacterial growth, as the bacteria become more concentrated. If the urine is alkaline, bacteria are better able to flourish. Untreated bladder infection may allow reflux of infected urine up the ureters to the kidneys and result in pyelonephritis, a more serious infection.

Therapeutic Management

UTIs are treated with either oral or intravenous antibiotics, depending on the severity of the infection. Urine culture and sensitivity determine the appropriate antibiotic. A 7- to 14-day course of antibiotics is often prescribed, although 2- to 5-day courses may be as effective. Adequate fluid intake is necessary to flush the bacteria from the bladder. Fever management may also be needed.

Nursing Assessment

For a full description of the assessment phase of the nursing process, refer to the "Assessment" section of the "Clinical Judgment and the Nursing Process" section earlier in the chapter. Assessment findings pertinent to UTI are discussed further on.

HEALTH HISTORY

Elicit a description of the present illness and chief complaint. Common symptoms reported during the health history might include:

- Fever
- Nausea or vomiting
- Chills
- Abdomen, back, or flank pain
- Lethargy
- Jaundice (in the neonate)
- Poor feeding or "just not acting right" (in the infant)
- Urinary urgency or frequency
- Burning or stinging with urination (signs: crying with urination [infant], grabbing the diaper [toddler])
- Foul-smelling urine
- Poor appetite (child)
- Enuresis or incontinence in a previously toilet-trained child
- Blood in the urine

Explore the child's current and past medical history for risk factors such as:

- Previous UTI
- Obstructive uropathy
- Inadequate toileting hygiene (often occurs with preschoolers)
- VUR
- Constipation
- Urine holding or dysfunctional voiding
- Neurogenic bladder
- Uncircumcised male
- Sexual intercourse
- Pregnancy
- Chronic illness

PHYSICAL EXAMINATION

In the neonate or young infant, observe for jaundice or increased respiratory rate. In infants and children, inspect the perineal area for redness or irritation. Observe the urine for visible blood, cloudiness, dark color, sediment, mucus, or foul odor. Note pallor, edema, or elevated blood pressure. Palpate the abdomen. Note distended bladder; abdominal mass; or tenderness, particularly in the flank area.

LABORATORY AND DIAGNOSTIC TESTS

Common laboratory and diagnostic studies ordered for the assessment of UTI include:

- Urinalysis (clean-catch, suprapubic, or catheterized): may be positive for blood, nitrites, leukocyte esterase, white blood cells, or bacteria (**bacteriuria**)
- Urine culture: will be positive for infecting organism
- Kidney ultrasound: may show hydronephrosis if the child also has a structural defect
- VCUG: This is not usually performed until the child has been treated with antibiotics for at least 48 hours, as infected urine tends to reflux up the ureters anyway. VCUG performed once the urine has regained sterility may be positive for VUR.

Kidney ultrasound or VCUG may be indicated in certain populations. The health care provider or nurse practitioner will determine the need for radiologic testing.

Nursing Management

Goals for nursing management include eradicating infection, promoting comfort, and preventing recurrence of infection.

ERADICATING INFECTION

The child who can tolerate oral intake will be prescribed an oral antibiotic. The child who has protracted vomiting related to the UTI or who has suspected pyelonephritis will require hospitalization and intravenous antibiotics. Children younger than 3 months and those with dehydration, a toxic appearance, or sepsis should also be hospitalized for administration of intravenous antibiotics (Bock et al., 2022). Administer oral or intravenous antibiotics as prescribed. Urge the parent to complete the entire course of oral antibiotic at home, even after the child is feeling better. Administer intravenous fluids as ordered or encourage generous oral fluid intake to help flush the bacteria from the bladder.

PROMOTING COMFORT

Administer antipyretics such as acetaminophen or ibuprofen to reduce fever. A heating pad or warm compress may help relieve abdomen or flank pain. If the child is afraid to urinate due to burning or stinging, encourage voiding in a warm sitz or tub bath.

PREVENTING RECURRENCE OF INFECTION

Encourage the parents to return as ordered for a repeat urine culture after completion of the antibiotic course to ensure eradication of bacteria. Refer to Teaching Guidelines 21.1 for further information on preventing UTI.

Enuresis

Enuresis is continued incontinence of urine past the age of toilet training. Nocturnal enuresis refers to bedwetting and occurs in about 15% of children at age 5 years, decreasing to 5% of children by 10 years of age (Paul & Wallace, 2023). Nocturnal enuresis may persist in some children into late childhood and adolescence, causing significant distress for the affected child and family. Occasional daytime wetting or dribbling of urine is usually not a cause for concern, but frequent daytime wetting concerns both the child and the parents.

In some children, enuresis may occur secondary to a physical disorder such as diabetes mellitus or insipidus, sickle cell anemia, ectopic ureter, or urethral obstruction. Other causes common to both diurnal and nocturnal enuresis include a urine-concentrating defect, UTI, constipation, and emotional distress (sometimes serious). The most frequent cause of daytime enuresis is dysfunctional voiding or holding of urine, although giggle incontinence and stress incontinence also occur. Nocturnal enuresis may be related to a high fluid intake in the evening, obstructive sleep apnea, sexual abuse, a family history of enuresis, or inappropriate family expectations. Physical causes of enuresis must be treated; further management of the disorder focuses on behavioral training, which may be augmented with the use of enuresis alarms or medications.

TEACHING GUIDELINES 21.1 Preventing Urinary Tract Infection in Females

- Drink enough fluid to keep urine flushed through bladder.
- Drink cranberry juice to acidify the urine.
- Avoid colas and caffeine, which irritate the bladder.
- Urinate frequently and do not "hold" urine (to discourage urinary stasis).
- Avoid bubble baths, which contribute to vulvar and perineal irritation.
- Wipe from front to back after voiding to avoid contaminating the urethra with rectal material.
- Wear cotton underwear to decrease the incidence of perineal irritation.
- Avoid wearing tight jeans or pants.
- Wash the perineal area daily with soap and water.
- While menstruating, change sanitary pads frequently to discourage bacterial growth.
- Void immediately after sexual intercourse.

Nursing Assessment

Elicit a description of the present illness and chief complaint. Determine the age of toilet training and when or if the child achieved successful daytime and nighttime dryness. Inquire about urine-holding behaviors such as squatting, dancing, or staring as well as rushing to the bathroom (diurnal enuresis). Inquire about the amount and types of fluid the child typically consumes before bedtime (nocturnal enuresis). Assess for risk factors such as:

- Family disruption or other stressors
- Chronic constipation (carefully assess bowel movement patterns)
- Excessive family demands related to toileting patterns
- History of being difficult to arouse from sleep
- Family history of enuresis

Assess the child's cognitive status: Developmentally delayed children may take significantly longer to achieve urine continence than their typical same-age peers. Assess for short stature or elevated blood pressure, as these may occur when kidney abnormalities are present.

Nursing Management

For the child with diurnal enuresis, encourage them to increase the amount of fluid consumed during the day in order to increase the frequency of the urge to void. Set a fixed schedule for the child to attempt to void throughout the day. These practices will usually be sufficient to retrain the child's voiding patterns. See Evidence-Based Practice 21.1.

EVIDENCE-BASED PRACTICE 21.1

Interventions for Enuresis

STUDY

Nocturnal enuresis (bedwetting) may affect the child's psychosocial well-being and relationship with the parents. Parents and children seek resolution of this problem, although most cases of nocturnal enuresis spontaneously resolve by age 15 years. In their critical review, the authors included 4 studies with a total of 269 child participants (aged 5 to 15 years). The studies compared monotherapy (bedwetting alarms) with combined therapy (bedwetting alarms and medication).

Findings

Use of a bedwetting alarm is as effective as the use of an alarm with a medication. The only difference noted was that with combined therapy there was slightly quicker resolution of enuresis with the combined therapy, although the result was not statistically significant.

Nursing Implications

Educate the child and parents about appropriate use of the bedwetting alarm as this treatment results in the best long-term resolution. Even when medications are prescribed, the alarm should still be used. Families may see a quicker response with combination therapy, so it may be the choice of some families.

Data from Aksakall, T., Cinislioğlu, A. E., & Aksoy, Y. (2022). The efficacy of combined alarm therapy versus alarm monotherapy in the treatment of monosymptomatic nocturnal enuresis: A review of current literature. *Eurasian Journal of Medicine, 54*(Suppl. 1), S164–S167. http://doi.org/10.5152/eurasianjmed.2022.22311

EDUCATING THE CHILD AND FAMILY ABOUT NOCTURNAL ENURESIS

Teach the family that the child is not lazy, nor do they wet the bed intentionally. Encourage the child and family to read books such as *Dry All Night: The Picture Book Technique That Stops Bedwetting* by Alison Mack or *Waking Up Dry: A Guide to Help Children Overcome Bedwetting* by Dr. Howard Bennett. Encourage the parents to limit intake of bladder irritants such as chocolate and caffeine. Teach parents to limit fluid intake after dinner and ensure that the child voids just before going to bed. Waking the child to void at 11 p.m. may also be helpful. Teach the parents to use bed pads and to make the bed with two sets of sheets and pads to decrease the workload in the middle of the night. When sleeping at home, the child should wear their usual underwear or pajamas. If away on a family vacation, pull-ups may decrease the stress on both the child and the parents.

PROVIDING SUPPORT AND ENCOURAGEMENT

Enuresis may be a source of shame for children and adolescents. It is important for the child to understand that they are not alone. Depending on the child's developmental level, explain that as many as 5 million people have enuresis. (This can be done in terms the child can relate to, such as a proportion within a school or 100 times the number of children in one school, etc.) It is not only "little kids" who wet the bed, and all kids who wet the bed need help overcoming this problem. Parents should include the child in plans for nighttime urinary control; this helps to increase the child's motivation to become dry. Parents should set up a reward system for dry nights. Parents should include the child in bed linen changes when they wet the bed but should do so in a matter-of-fact manner rather than in a punitive way; in fact, it is important to always avoid punishment for bedwetting. Although enuresis may cause family disruption, with patience, consistency, and time, dryness will be achieved. Provide ongoing emotional support and positive reinforcement to the child and family.

DECREASING NIGHTTIME VOIDING

Teach the family using an enuresis alarm system how to use the alarm as well as the previously mentioned techniques (Fig. 21.6). Most of these devices work by sounding an alarm when the first few drops of urine appear; the child then awakens and stops the urine flow. Over time, the child becomes conditioned to either awaken when the bladder is full or stop the urine flow when sleeping.

When behavioral and motivational therapies are unsuccessful, particularly in the older child, medications may be prescribed. Teach the child and parents about the use of medications such as oxybutynin, imipramine, and desmopressin if these are prescribed (refer to Drug Guide 21.1).

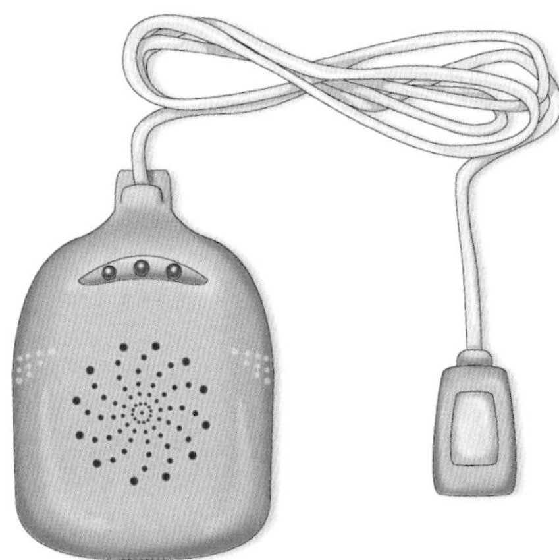

FIGURE 21.6 Some children and families find great success with the use of an enuresis alarm. The alarm wakes the child at the first sign of wetness. Over time, the child learns to awaken at night in response to the sensation of a full bladder.

Acquired Disorders Resulting in Altered Kidney Function

A number of acquired disorders are responsible for alterations in kidney function. They may occur as an autoimmune response or in relation to a bacterial infection. Kidney dysfunction may also occur as a result of obstructive disorders or repeated VUR, as discussed earlier. Left untreated, these disorders may lead to kidney failure. Even when treated appropriately, the appropriate response is sometimes not achieved, and acute or chronic kidney disease develops. Kidney disorders are the most frequent cause of hypertension in children.

CLINICAL REASONING ALERT!

Severe ambulatory hypertension (blood pressure higher than the 95th percentile for age and sex) places the child at risk for damage to the eyes or vital organs (kidney, brain, or heart) (Flynn, 2023). Nurses must be adept at accurately measuring blood pressure in children.

Nephrotic Syndrome

Nephrotic syndrome occurs as a result of increased glomerular basement membrane permeability, which allows abnormal loss of protein in the urine. Nephrotic syndrome generally occurs in three forms—congenital, idiopathic, and secondary.

Congenital nephrotic syndrome is an inherited disorder; it is rare and occurs primarily in families of Finnish descent. The prognosis is poor, although some success has occurred with early, aggressive treatment and with the advances in kidney transplantation in infants (Bock et al., 2022). Nephrotic syndrome may also occur secondary to another condition such as systemic lupus erythematosus, Henoch–Schönlein purpura, or diabetes.

Idiopathic nephrotic syndrome is the most commonly occurring type in children and is also called minimal change disease (MCD). Idiopathic nephrotic syndrome most often has its onset in children by age 10 years (Bock et al., 2022). This discussion will focus primarily on minimal change nephrotic syndrome (MCNS). Complications of nephrotic syndrome include anemia, infection, poor growth, peritonitis, thrombosis, and kidney failure.

Pathophysiology

Increased glomerular permeability results in the passage of larger plasma proteins through the glomerular basement membrane. This results in excess loss of protein (albumin) in the urine (**proteinuria**) and decreased protein and albumin (hypoalbuminemia) in the bloodstream. Protein loss in nephrotic syndrome tends to be almost exclusively albumin. Hypoalbuminemia results in a change in osmotic pressure, and fluid shifts from the bloodstream into the interstitial tissue (causing edema). This decrease in blood volume triggers the kidneys to respond by conserving sodium and water, leading to further edema. The liver senses the protein loss and increases production of lipoproteins. Hyperlipidemia then develops as the excess lipids cannot be excreted in the urine. Hyperlipidemia associated with nephrotic syndrome may be quite severe, yet cholesterol levels may decrease when the nephrotic syndrome is in remission, only to rise significantly again with a relapse.

Children with nephrotic syndrome are at increased risk for clotting (thromboembolism) because of the decreased intravascular volume. They are also at increased risk for the development of serious infection, most commonly pneumococcal pneumonia, sepsis, or spontaneous peritonitis. Steroid-resistant nephrotic syndrome may result in acute kidney injury.

Therapeutic Management

Medical management of MCD usually involves the use of corticosteroids. Intravenous albumin may be used in the severely edematous child. Diuretics are also required in the edematous phase. Long-term therapy is usually required to induce remission. The nephrologist will determine the length of therapy based on the child's response. Children who have steroid-responsive MCD generally have a favorable prognosis. Some children with MCD exhibit a minimal response to steroid therapy or experience remissions, and the MCD is steroid resistant (Bock et al., 2022). Immunosuppressive therapy such as cyclophosphamide, cyclosporine A, or mycophenolate mofetil may be necessary.

Nursing Assessment

For a full description of the assessment phase of the nursing process, refer to the "Clinical Judgment and the Nursing Process" section earlier in the chapter. Assessment findings pertinent to MCD are discussed further on.

HEALTH HISTORY

Elicit a description of the present illness and chief complaint. Common symptoms reported during the health history might include:

- Nausea or vomiting (may be related to ascites)
- Recent weight gain
- History of periorbital edema upon waking, progressing to generalized edema throughout the day
- Weakness or fatigue
- Irritability or fussiness

PHYSICAL EXAMINATION

Observe the child for edema (periorbital, generalized [**anasarca**], or abdominal ascites). As the disease progresses, the edema also progresses to become more generalized, eventually becoming severe. Inspect the skin for a stretched, tight appearance; pallor; or skin breakdown related to significant edema (Fig. 21.7). Document height (or length) and weight. Note increased respiratory rate or increased work of breathing related to ascites and edema.

Note the blood pressure; it may be elevated in the child with nephrotic syndrome, although it is most often either normal or decreased unless the child is progressing to kidney failure. Auscultate heart and lung sounds, noting abnormalities related to fluid overload. Palpate the skin, noting tautness. Palpate the abdomen, and document the presence of ascites.

LABORATORY AND DIAGNOSTIC TESTS

Urine dipstick will reveal marked proteinuria. Infrequently, mild hematuria is also present. Serum protein and albumin levels will be low (often markedly so). Serum cholesterol and triglyceride levels are elevated. With continued nephrotic syndrome, creatinine and BUN may become elevated.

Nursing Management

Goals for nursing management include promoting diuresis, preventing infection, promoting adequate nutrition, and educating the parents about ongoing care at home. As with other chronic disorders, provide ongoing emotional support to the child and family.

PROMOTING DIURESIS

Administer corticosteroids as ordered. Tapering or weaning doses are required when the time comes to stop corticosteroid therapy. Administer diuretics if ordered, usually furosemide. Children may develop hypokalemia because of potassium loss as an adverse effect of furosemide. Those children may require potassium supplementation or a diet higher in potassium-containing foods. Monitor urine output and the amount of protein in the urine (by dipstick). Weigh the child daily on the same scale either naked or wearing the same amount of clothing. Assess for resolution of edema. Measure pulse rate and blood pressure every 4 hours to detect hypovolemia resulting from excessive fluid shifts. Enforce oral fluid restrictions if ordered.

In cases of severe hypoalbuminemia, intravenous albumin may be administered. Increases in the serum albumin level cause fluid to shift from the subcutaneous spaces back into the bloodstream. A diuretic such as furosemide administered immediately after the albumin infusion allows for optimal diuresis and prevents fluid overload. Refer to Drug Guide 21.1 for the nursing implications related to use of these medications.

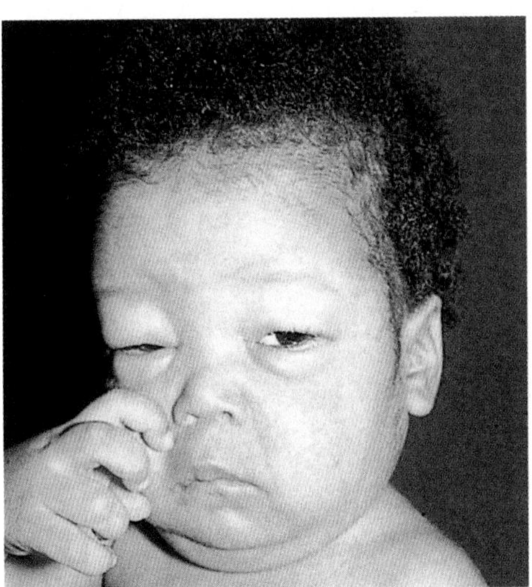

FIGURE 21.7 Note marked edema associated with nephrotic syndrome.

> **CONSIDER THIS!**
>
> Thirteen-year-old Jimmy Sanderson has a history of steroid-responsive nephrotic syndrome. In the clinic today he tells you, "I am not going to take those steroids anymore!" "I am shorter than everyone in my class; my 11-year-old brother is taller than me." "It's just not fair; I'll never get a girlfriend if I'm a shorty."
>
> Think back to when you were an adolescent. How did you feel or how would you have felt if you had a chronic illness and your necessary medications stunted your growth? As the nurse, how can you help Jimmy in this situation?

PREVENTING INFECTION

Monitor the child's temperature. Administer pneumococcal vaccine as prescribed (see Chapter 9 for information on immunizations). Administer prophylactic antibiotics, if prescribed. Delay administering live vaccines until at least 2 weeks after corticosteroid or other immunosuppressive medication therapy ceases. Teach parents that if the child is unimmunized and is exposed to chickenpox, the parents should notify the child's pediatrician, nurse practitioner, or nephrologist immediately so that the child may receive varicella zoster immunoglobulin.

ENCOURAGING ADEQUATE NUTRITION AND GROWTH

Encourage a nutrient-rich diet within prescribed restrictions. Fluid restriction is reserved for children with massive edema. Sodium intake may be restricted in the edematous child in an effort to prevent further fluid retention. Consultation with the dietitian is often helpful in meal planning because many of the foods that children like are high in sodium. Encourage protein-rich snacks. Consult with the child and family in planning meals and snacks that the child likes and will be likely to consume. Use of nutritional supplement shakes may be helpful for some children.

EDUCATING THE FAMILY

Teach parents how to give medications and monitor for adverse effects. Demonstrate the urine dipstick technique for detecting protein, and encourage the family to keep a chart of dipstick results. The child may return to school but should avoid contact with sick playmates. If the child is exposed to another child with an infectious illness, explain to the parents that they should monitor temperature and urine dipstick results more frequently to identify a relapse in nephrotic syndrome early so that treatment can begin.

PROVIDING EMOTIONAL SUPPORT

Nephrotic syndrome is often a chronic condition, and children who are responsive to steroid treatment may enter remission only to experience relapse. This cycle of relapse and remission takes an emotional toll on the child and family. Frequent hospitalizations require the child to miss school and the parents to miss work; this creates further stress for the family. The child may experience social isolation because they must avoid exposure to infections or because of self-esteem problems. The child may be dissatisfied with their appearance because of edema and weight gain, short stature, and the classic "moon face" associated with chronic steroid use.

Provide emotional support to the child and family. Encourage them in their efforts to maintain the treatment plan. Introduce the child to other youngsters with chronic kidney conditions.

Acute Poststreptococcal Glomerulonephritis

Acute poststreptococcal glomerulonephritis (APSGN) is a condition in which immune processes injure the glomeruli. Immune mechanisms cause inflammation, which results in altered glomerular structure and function in both kidneys. It often occurs following an infection, usually an upper respiratory or skin infection. APSGN is caused by an antibody–antigen reaction secondary to an infection with a nephritogenic strain of group A beta-hemolytic streptococcus (Flores, 2020). The most serious complication is progression to uremia and kidney failure (either acute or chronic).

There is no specific medical treatment for APSGN. Treatment is aimed at maintaining fluid volume and managing hypertension. If there is evidence of a current streptococcal infection, antibiotic therapy will be necessary.

Nursing Assessment

Refer to the "Clinical Judgment and the Nursing Process" section for a full description of the assessment phase of the nursing process. Assessment findings pertinent to acute glomerulonephritis are discussed further on.

HEALTH HISTORY

Elicit a description of the present illness and chief complaint. Common symptoms reported during the health history might include:

- Fever
- Lethargy
- Headache
- Decreased urine output
- Abdominal pain
- Vomiting
- Anorexia

Assess the child's current and past medical history for risk factors such as a recent episode of pharyngitis or other streptococcal infection, age older than 3 years, or male sex.

PHYSICAL EXAMINATION AND LABORATORY AND DIAGNOSTIC TESTS

Assess the child's blood pressure for elevation, which is common. Note the presence of mild edema. Observe for signs of cardiopulmonary congestion such as increased work of breathing or cough. Auscultate the lungs for crackles and the heart for gallop. The urine dipstick test will reveal proteinuria as well as hematuria. Inspect the urine for gross hematuria, which will cause the urine to appear tea-colored, cola-colored, or even a dirty green color. Serum creatinine and BUN may be normal or elevated, the serum complement level is depressed, and the erythrocyte sedimentation rate is elevated. Laboratory findings specific to streptococcus include an elevated antistreptolysin O (ASO) titer and an elevated DNAase B antigen titer.

Nursing Management

Administer antihypertensives such as labetalol or nifedipine and diuretics as ordered. Monitor blood pressure frequently. Maintain sodium and fluid restrictions as prescribed during the initial edematous phase. Weigh the child daily on the same scale wearing the same amount of clothing. Monitor increasing urine output, and note improvement in the urine color. Document resolution of edema. Provide a careful neurologic evaluation, as hypertension may cause encephalopathy and seizures. Children with APSGN are generally fatigued and choose bed rest during the acute phase. Provide the child with age-appropriate activities and cluster care to allow rest periods.

Some children may receive care at home if edema is mild and they are not hypertensive. Teach the family to monitor urine output and color, take blood pressure measurements, and restrict the diet as prescribed. The child cared for at home should not participate in strenuous activity until proteinuria and hematuria are resolved. If kidney involvement progresses, dialysis may become necessary.

TAKE NOTE!

Avoid use of nonsteroidal antiinflammatory drugs (NSAIDs) in children with questionable kidney function, as they worsen kidney disease (Solomon, 2022).

Hemolytic Uremic Syndrome

Hemolytic uremic syndrome (HUS) is defined by three features—hemolytic anemia, thrombocytopenia—and acute kidney injury. Typical HUS features an antecedent diarrheal illness. Other causes of HUS include idiopathic, inherited, drug-related, association with malignancies, transplantation, and malignant hypertension. This discussion will focus on typical HUS, the type preceded by a diarrheal illness. Watery diarrhea progresses to hemorrhagic colitis, then to the triad of HUS. The features of HUS, as well as effects on other organs, are caused primarily by microthrombi and ischemic changes within the organs. The thrombotic events in the small blood vessels of the glomerulus lead to occlusion of the glomerular capillary loops and glomerulosclerosis, resulting in kidney failure.

A verotoxin-producing strain of *E. coli,* O157:H7, causes the majority of cases, though *Streptococcus pneumoniae, Shigella dysenteriae,* and other bacteria may also be the cause (Tan & Silverberg, 2021). It is thought that antibiotic treatment for the bacteria may contribute to release of the verotoxin. Undercooked ground beef accounts for most cases of *E. coli* O157:H7 infection, but it is also transmitted via the feces of numerous animals as well as unpasteurized dairy and fruit products. Transmission also occurs via human feces, and cases have been linked to public swimming pools. HUS occurs most often in children up to age 5 years (Tan & Silverberg, 2021). Complications include chronic kidney disease, seizures and coma, pancreatitis, intussusception, rectal prolapse, cardiomyopathy, congestive heart failure, and acute respiratory distress syndrome.

Therapeutic management of HUS is directed toward maintaining fluid balance; correcting hypertension, acidosis, and electrolyte abnormalities; replenishing circulating red blood cells; and providing dialysis if needed. Recently, the monoclonal antibody eculizumab has been successful in terminating the microangiopathic process associated with HUS (Tan & Silverberg, 2021). Children receiving this medication are at high risk for meningococcal infection and so should receive the meningococcal vaccine.

Nursing Assessment

Elicit a description of the present illness and chief complaint. Common symptoms reported during the health history might include watery diarrhea accompanied by cramping and sometimes vomiting. After several days, the diarrhea becomes bloody and eventually improves.

Explore the child's current and past medical history for risk factors such as ingestion of ground beef, visits to a water park or to a petting zoo before the onset of the diarrheal illness, or use of antidiarrheal medications or antibiotics.

Observe the child for pallor, toxic appearance, edema, **oliguria** (decreased urine output), or **anuria** (absent urine output). Assess for elevated blood pressure and tenderness in the abdomen. Assess the child for neurologic involvement, which may include irritability, altered level of consciousness, seizures, posturing, or coma.

LABORATORY AND DIAGNOSTIC TESTS

Urinalysis may reveal the presence of blood, protein, pus, and/or casts. Serum laboratory abnormalities are numerous and may include:

- Elevated BUN and creatinine
- Moderate to severe anemia (with the presence of Burr cells, schistocytes, spherocytes, or helmet cells), mild to severe thrombocytopenia
- Increased reticulocyte count
- Increased bilirubin and lactic dehydrogenase (LDH) levels
- Negative Coombs test (except in cases of *S. pneumoniae* infection)
- Leukocytosis with left shift
- Hyponatremia
- Hyperkalemia
- Hyperphosphatemia
- Metabolic acidosis

Nursing Management

Nursing management of HUS focuses on close observation and monitoring of the child's status. Institute and maintain contact precautions to prevent spread of *E. coli* O157:H7 to other children (bacteria are shed for up to 17 days after resolution of the diarrhea). Close attention must be paid to fluid volume status. Prevention of HUS is also an important nursing function.

MAINTAINING APPROPRIATE FLUID VOLUME BALANCE

Maintain strict intake and output monitoring and recording to evaluate the progression toward kidney failure. Carefully monitor intravenous infusions and blood chemistries. Administer diuretics as ordered. Assess blood pressure frequently and report elevations to the health care provider or nurse practitioner. Administer antihypertensives as ordered and monitor their effectiveness. Encourage adequate nutritional intake within the constraints of prescribed dietary restrictions. Monitor for bleeding as well as for fatigue and pallor. Follow the institutional protocol for transfusion of packed red blood cells and/or platelets (platelets are usually transfused only if active bleeding or severe thrombocytopenia occurs). Report progressive deterioration in laboratory findings to the health care provider or nurse practitioner. Some children with HUS will require dialysis for at least several days.

PREVENTING HUS

Proper handwashing is necessary. Teach children to wash their hands after using the bathroom, before eating, and after petting farm animals. Encourage the use of "swim diapers," which catch feces, for children who are not toilet trained. Teach parents to thoroughly cook all meats to a core temperature of 68°C (155°F), or until the meat is gray or brown throughout and the juices from the meat are clear rather than pink. Wash all fruits and vegetables thoroughly. Ensure that drinking water and water used for recreation are treated appropriately. Avoid unpasteurized dairy products and fruit juices (including cider).

Kidney Failure

Kidney failure is a condition in which the kidneys cannot concentrate urine, conserve electrolytes, or excrete waste products. As in adults, kidney failure in children may occur as an acute or chronic condition. Some cases of acute kidney injury resolve without further complications, while dialysis is necessary in other children. When acute kidney injury continues to progress, it becomes chronic kidney disease and later, end-stage kidney disease (ESKD). Dialysis and kidney transplantation are treatment modalities used for ESKD.

Acute Kidney Injury

Acute kidney injury is defined as a sudden, often reversible, decline in kidney function that results in the accumulation of metabolic toxins (particularly nitrogenous wastes) as well as fluid and electrolyte imbalance. Fluid overload may lead to hypertension, pulmonary edema, and congestive heart failure. Additional complications include hyperkalemia, metabolic acidosis, hyperphosphatemia, and uremia. In children, acute kidney injury most commonly occurs as a result of decreased renal perfusion, as occurs in hypovolemic or septic shock. It may also occur in children with hemolytic anemia or as a result of nephrotoxicity from medications. Complications include anemia, hyperkalemia, hypertension, pulmonary edema, cardiac failure, and altered level of consciousness or seizures. In addition, acute kidney injury may also progress to a chronic state.

Therapeutic management is aimed at treating the underlying cause, managing the fluid and electrolyte disturbances, and decreasing blood pressure.

TAKE NOTE!

Medications commonly used in children can reduce kidney function. Cephalosporins may cause a transient increase in BUN and creatinine. Truly nephrotoxic drugs often used in children include aminoglycosides, sulfonamides, vancomycin, and NSAIDs. Make sure that potentially nephrotoxic drugs are administered according to published safe guidelines (dosage, frequency, rate of administration) (UpToDate, Inc., 2023).

Nursing Assessment

The health history may reveal the following common symptoms: nausea, vomiting, diarrhea, lethargy, fever, and decreased urine output. Assess the child's current and past medical history for risk factors such as history of shock, trauma, burns, urologic abnormalities, kidney disease, use of nephrotoxic medications, or severe blood transfusion reaction.

Note decreased skin elasticity, dry mucous membranes, or edema. Auscultate the lungs for crackles, which may occur with pulmonary edema. Document tachypnea. Note cardiac rhythm disturbances. Evaluate the child's level of consciousness. Laboratory tests will reveal increased serum creatinine levels and possible electrolyte disturbances, such as hyperkalemia or hypocalcemia. Urinalysis may reveal proteinuria or hematuria.

CLINICAL REASONING ALERT!

Monitor the infant or child with kidney failure carefully for signs of congestive heart failure, such as edema accompanied by bounding pulse, presence of an S_3 heart sound, adventitious lung sounds, and shortness of breath.

Nursing Management

Nursing care focuses on managing hypertension, restoring fluid and electrolyte balance, and educating the family.

MANAGING HYPERTENSION

Carefully monitor the child's blood pressure. Administer antihypertensives as prescribed. When a fast-acting drug such as nifedipine sublingually or labetalol intravenously is used, stay with the child and frequently monitor blood pressure. Immediately notify the health care provider or nurse practitioner if high blood pressure is resistant to medication and the blood pressure remains elevated.

RESTORING FLUID AND ELECTROLYTE BALANCE

Monitor vital signs frequently, and assess urine specific gravity. Maintain strict records of intake and output.

Administer diuretics as ordered. When urine output is restored, diuresis may be significant. Monitor for signs of hyperkalemia (weak, irregular pulse; muscle weakness; abdominal cramping) and hypocalcemia (muscle twitching or tetany). Administer polystyrene sulfonate as ordered orally, rectally, or through a nasogastric tube to decrease potassium levels. Polystyrene sulfonate removes potassium primarily by exchanging sodium for it, which is then eliminated in the feces. Administer packed red blood cell transfusions as ordered (may need to be followed by a dose of diuretic). Dialysis may become necessary if oliguria is sustained and leads to significant fluid overload, the electrolyte imbalance reaches dangerous levels, or uremia results in depression of the central nervous system.

PROVIDING FAMILY EDUCATION

Educate the family about the plan of care and the need for fluid restriction, if ordered. Instruct the family to save all voids for observation and measurement by the nurse. Provide education about the use of dialysis if relevant.

End-Stage Kidney Disease

ESKD is chronic kidney disease (CKD) requiring long-term dialysis or kidney transplantation. CKD in children most often results from congenital structural defects such as obstructive uropathy. It may also be caused by an inherited condition such as familial nephritis or may result from an acquired problem such as glomerulonephritis or HUS (Patel & Vogt, 2023). This is in contrast to CKD in adults, which results primarily from diabetes or hypertension.

Uremia, hypocalcemia, hyperkalemia, and metabolic acidosis occur. Complications of ESKD are many. Uremic toxins deplete erythrocytes, and the failing kidneys cannot produce erythropoietin, so severe anemia results. Hypertension is common and heart failure may occur. Hypocalcemia results in renal rickets (brittle bones). Growth is delayed, and sexual maturation may be delayed or absent. Children with ESKD may experience increased rates of depression as compared to children without ESKD (Stahl et al., 2022). See the Healthy People 2030 box.

HEALTHY PEOPLE 2030

Objective	Nursing Significance
Reduce the rate of new cases of end-stage kidney disease.	Encourage adherence to medical regimens related to urinary tract disorders in order to prevent progression to CKD.

Healthy People Objectives retrieved from http://www.healthypeople.gov

Nursing Assessment

Explore the health history for low birth weight (associated with kidney dysfunction and anatomic alterations), poor growth (weight, length/height, and head circumference), and regimen of dialysis. Note decreased appetite or energy level, dry or itchy skin, or bone or joint pain.

Perform a thorough physical assessment, noting any abnormalities (may vary from child to child). If present, assess the peritoneal catheter site for absence of drainage, bleeding, or redness. If the child undergoes hemodialysis, assess the fistula or graft site for the presence of a bruit and a thrill. Laboratory tests may reveal low hemoglobin and hematocrit; increased serum phosphorus and potassium levels; and decreased sodium, calcium, and bicarbonate levels. BUN, uric acid, and creatinine levels will be elevated. A 24-hour urine creatinine clearance test will show increased amounts of creatinine in the urine, reflecting decreasing kidney function.

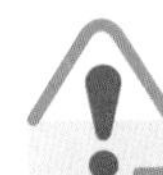

CLINICAL REASONING ALERT!

Carefully assess children with ESKD for worsening uremia or metabolic acidosis. Uremia may result in central nervous system symptoms such as headache or coma, or GI or neuromuscular disturbances. Metabolic acidosis causes lethargy, dull headache, and confusion.

Nursing Management

Nursing goals for the child with ESKD include promoting growth, removing waste products and maintaining fluid balance via dialysis, encouraging psychosocial well-being, and supporting and educating the family.

PROMOTING GROWTH

Encourage the child to choose foods they like that are within the imposed dietary restrictions. Daily protein requirements for adequate growth range from 0.9 to 1.5 g of protein per kilogram of weight. Sodium and/or potassium restrictions may also be necessary. Enforce fluid restrictions if prescribed. Administer medications such as erythropoietin, growth hormone, and vitamin and mineral supplements to augment nutritional status and promote growth. Table 21.2 lists medications and supplements used to support growth.

ENCOURAGING PSYCHOSOCIAL WELL-BEING

Refer children and their families to the hospital social worker or counselor as needed for depression or anxiety issues. The chronic need for dialysis (daily with peritoneal dialysis or three or four times per week with hemodialysis) confers long-term stress on the child and family. The child usually demonstrates poor growth and often suffers from body image disturbance. Frequent medical appointments and hospitalizations interfere with the

TABLE 21.2 • Medications and Supplements Commonly Used to Treat End-Stage Kidney Disease Complications

Medication or Supplement	Purpose
Vitamin D and calcium	Correct hypocalcemia and hyperphosphatemia
Ferrous sulfate	Treat anemia
Bicitra or sodium bicarbonate tablets	Correct acidosis
Multivitamin	Augment nutritional status
Erythropoietin injections	Stimulate red blood cell growth
Growth hormone injections	Stimulate growth in stature

Data from UpToDate, Inc. (2023). *Lexi-comp®* (Version 7.7.0) [Mobile app]. Wolters Kluwer. https://apps.apple.com/us/app/lexicomp/id313401238

child's scholastic achievements. Introduce the child to other children with ESKD. (This often happens anyway at the hemodialysis center.)

Ensure that the family is aware of financial and support resources within the community, and refer them to the National Kidney Foundation. Also suggest the American Kidney Fund, which provides financial aid and access to summer camps for children with kidney problems. Camp is an excellent way for children to demonstrate that they have mastered some of the loss-of-control issues related to their disease.

Several websites provide forums for children and adolescents with kidney failure or transplantation so they can learn about their disease, access resources, and/or communicate with other children.

Dialysis and Transplantation

Peritoneal dialysis or hemodialysis is required on a long-term basis for children with CKD or ESKD. Once the child has progressed to ESKD, kidney transplantation is needed in order for the child to progress with normal growth and development.

Peritoneal Dialysis

Peritoneal dialysis uses the child's abdominal cavity as a semipermeable membrane to help remove excess fluid and waste products (Figs. 21.8 and 21.9). The parent or caregiver performs peritoneal dialysis at home after completing a training course. The process is either completed overnight with the use of a machine (continuous cyclic peritoneal dialysis) or in increments throughout the day for a total of 4 to 8 hours (continuous ambulatory peritoneal dialysis). Comparison Chart 21.1 compares these two methods of peritoneal dialysis.

The advantages of peritoneal dialysis over hemodialysis include improved growth as a result of more dietary freedom, increased independence in daily activities, and a steadier state of electrolyte balance. However, the risk of infection (peritonitis and sepsis) is a continual concern with peritoneal dialysis (Chua & Warady, 2024). Dialysate exchange protocols, care of the catheter in the abdomen, and dressing changes must all be performed using sterile technique to avoid introducing microorganisms into the peritoneal cavity. Box 21.1 lists additional risks associated with peritoneal dialysis.

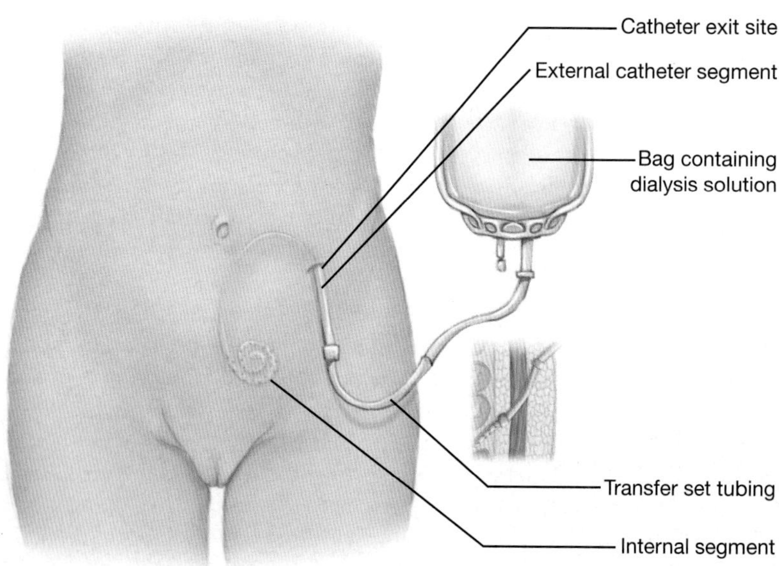

FIGURE 21.8 The peritoneal dialysis catheter is tunneled under the skin into the peritoneal cavity.

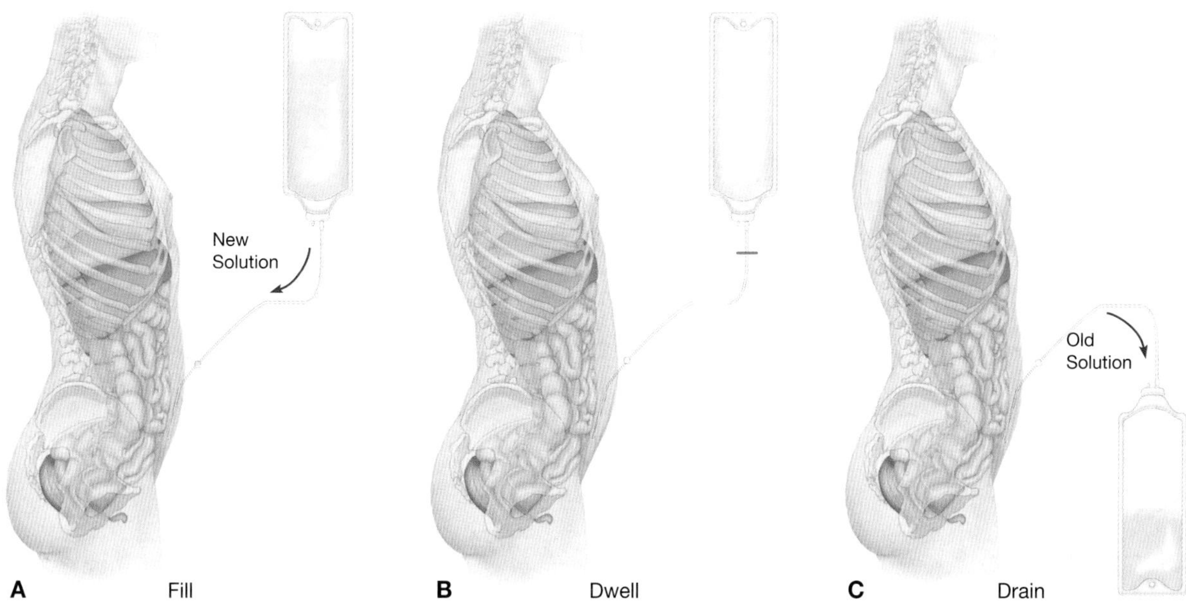

FIGURE 21.9 **A.** During the "fill" phase of peritoneal dialysis, dialysate fluid is instilled into the peritoneal cavity. **B.** During the "dwell" phase, the child may be up out of bed with the empty dialysate bag folded up with the tubing under their clothing. **C.** During the "drain" phase, the old dialysate is drained from the peritoneum by gravity, bringing with it waste products and excess fluid. The dialysate bags are weighed prior to filling and after draining to determine the amount of fluid removed from the child.

Hemodialysis

Hemodialysis removes toxins and excess fluid from the blood by pumping the child's blood through a hemodialysis machine and then reinfusing the blood into the child. Needles to remove and reinfuse the blood are inserted into an arteriovenous fistula or graft, usually located in the child's arm (Figs. 21.10 and 21.11).

Hemodialysis frees the parent from the need to perform daily dialysis, but the procedure, which takes 3 to 6 hours, must be done two to four times per week (usually three) at a pediatric hemodialysis center. This requires time away from school and other activities for the child and from work and other family responsibilities for the parent. Since hemodialysis is usually performed only every other day, larger amounts of waste products build up in the child's blood (uremia), placing the child at higher risk for seizures. The access site may become infected, and occlusion is also possible. The child must follow a stricter diet between hemodialysis treatments, although dietary restrictions are usually lifted while the child is actually undergoing the treatment.

Nursing Assessment

Refer to the "Clinical Judgment and the Nursing Process" section on nursing assessment of the child with CKD/ESKD, as it is similar to assessment of the child undergoing dialysis. Assess for alterations in blood pressure and laboratory values following dialysis. Monitor for signs and symptoms of infection.

Assess the child receiving peritoneal dialysis for toleration of the fluid volume instilled within the peritoneum.

COMPARISON CHART 21.1 Methods of Peritoneal Dialysis

	Continuous Ambulatory Peritoneal Dialysis (CAPD)	Continuous Cyclic Peritoneal Dialysis (CCPD)
When performed	Throughout the day, with exchanges every 3–6 hours; fluid is usually allowed to dwell overnight to allow the child to sleep.	Usually overnight while the child is sleeping
Method	Manual instillation and draining and changing of dialysate bags with each exchange	Automated via CCPD machine; bags and tubing are attached when started, then disconnected in the morning.
Dwell time	3–6 hours	Usually 30 minutes to 1 hour
Mobility	Allows for mobility and permits the child to participate in activities between exchanges	The child is confined to bed during the night while CCPD is ongoing but completely mobile while off CCPD during the day.

BOX 21.1 Risks Associated With Peritoneal Dialysis

- Hypertension and other cardiac complications
- Seizures
- Obstructed catheter
- Dialysate leakage
- Hyperglycemia
- Increased triglyceride levels
- Increased protein loss
- Parental stress and burnout related to repetitive nature of daily intervention

The abdomen will remain distended while the fluid is indwelling and will be significantly flatter when the fluid is drained. Assess the Tenckhoff catheter site for signs of infection. Monitor the child's temperature. Inspect the dialysate effluent for fibrin or cloudiness, which may indicate infection. Weigh the child daily (in the drain phase if on peritoneal dialysis).

For the child who receives hemodialysis, assess the arteriovenous fistula or graft site with each set of vital signs. Auscultate the site for the presence of a bruit, and palpate for the presence of a thrill. Notify the health care provider or nurse practitioner immediately if either is absent.

TAKE NOTE!

Avoid taking blood pressure, performing venipuncture, or using a tourniquet in the extremity with the arteriovenous fistula or graft; these procedures may cause occlusion and subsequent malfunction of the fistula or graft. Teach parents and children to inform all health care providers they come in contact with about the presence of the fistula or graft.

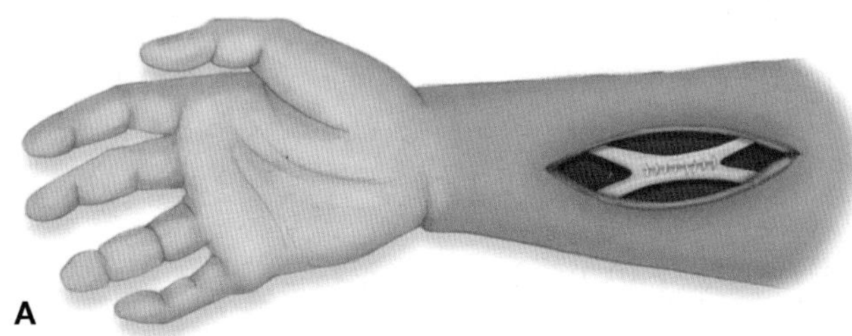

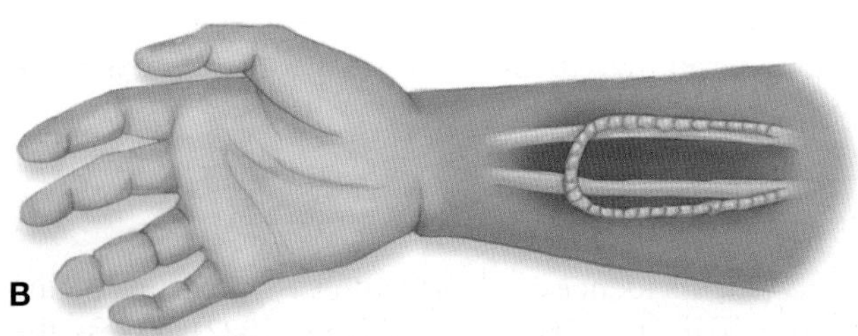

FIGURE 21.10 **A.** Arteriovenous fistula. **B.** Arteriovenous graft.

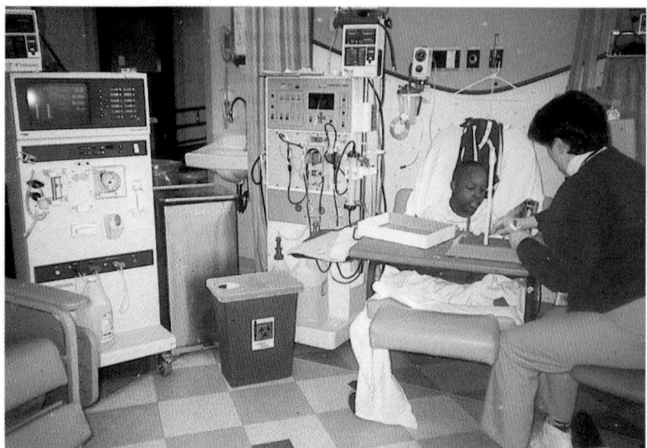

FIGURE 21.11 Pediatric hemodialysis.

Nursing Management

Specially trained and certified nurses perform both peritoneal dialysis and hemodialysis. The general pediatric nurse's role is related to the ongoing care of the child. The child undergoing peritoneal dialysis is usually allowed a more liberal diet and intake of fluid than the child undergoing hemodialysis. Peritoneal dialysis removes waste and excess fluids on a daily basis, whereas hemodialysis occurs about every other day. Most routine medications are withheld on the morning that hemodialysis is scheduled, since they would be filtered out through the dialysis process anyway. Administer these medications as soon as the child returns from the dialysis unit.

THINKING ABOUT DEVELOPMENT

Trevon Smith is a 17-year-old male football player who was on track for a college scholarship. Following an episode of acute glomerulonephritis, Trevon has progressed to CKD and is dependent on hemodialysis. He is listed for a kidney transplant.

How will Trevon's developmental stage affect his desire to adhere to the medical regimen? What types of psychosocial issues might Trevon be experiencing, and how can the nurse best support Trevon at this time?

How will the nurse educate Trevon about self-care?

Kidney Transplantation

Kidney transplantation is the optimal treatment for ESKD and offers the best opportunity for the child to live a normal life. Vigilant medication administration is necessary after the transplant to prevent organ rejection. The child achieves improved kidney function with the transplant and may demonstrate improved growth, enhanced cognitive development, and improved psychosocial development and quality of life.

Kidneys are obtained from a cadaver (a patient declared brain-dead who had previously given consent to organ donation) or from a blood relative (living-related). The transplanted kidney must match the child's blood type and the child's human leukocyte antigens (HLAs). The cadaver kidney or living-related kidney is implanted surgically in the abdomen, and the blood vessels are anastomosed to the aorta and superior vena cava.

Generally, living-related transplants have a lower rejection rate compared to cadaver transplants (McDonald, 2023). Living-related kidney donation and subsequent transplantation can be planned ahead and scheduled in advance. In contrast, cadaver kidneys become available suddenly, leaving less time for preoperative preparation. For either type, last-minute blood tissue typing is required before the final decision is made to move forward with transplantation. Often the child's native kidneys are removed before or at the time of the kidney transplant because of their association with hypertension in the child (McDonald, 2023).

TAKE NOTE!

Cadaver kidneys are allocated to potential recipients based on the recipient's age, the time that they have been awaiting a transplant, blood type, HLA antibody matching, panel reactive antibodies, and region of the country (so that the donated kidney can be received expeditiously; UNOS [2024]).

Nursing Assessment

A thorough physical assessment is warranted for any child undergoing kidney transplant, whether in the initial postoperative period, at a clinic visit, or when admitted to the hospital, to rule out transplant rejection. Note recent health history, medications and their doses, and any symptoms the child has been having. In the initial postoperative period, assess the incision for redness, edema, or drainage. If any of these signs of infection or rejection occur, notify the transplant surgeon and nephrologist immediately. Monitor blood pressure and other vital signs closely. Document resolution of edema. Record intake and output accurately. Assess for signs and symptoms of transplant rejection such as malaise, fever, unexplained weight gain, or pain over the transplant area.

Nursing Management

Postoperative care focuses on preventing rejection, monitoring kidney function, maintaining fluid and electrolyte balance, and educating the child and family.

TAKE NOTE!

Encourage the child with a kidney transplant to wear a medical alert necklace or bracelet, and urge the parents to inform community emergency services of the child's transplant status.

PREVENTING REJECTION AND PROMOTING KIDNEY FUNCTION

Administer immunosuppressants accurately and in a timely fashion. Obtain and monitor serum levels of these medications per protocol. Immediately report significant alterations in vital signs or edema at the surgical site, as they may indicate transplant rejection. Maintain strict documentation of intake and output. Once adequate urine output is established, intake is usually liberalized.

EDUCATING THE CHILD AND FAMILY

Develop a schedule to cluster care so that the child may receive the rest needed for recovery despite the many and frequent assessments and interventions. With the family, develop a medication schedule that will be compatible with the family's life at home as well as the restrictions related to some medications. Begin teaching with the family as soon as the child's condition is stable. Accurate medication administration and home monitoring are necessary to prevent rejection. The child may return to school when discharged from the hospital, but the family will need to communicate closely with the school nurse about the child's immunosuppressed status. The American Nephrology Nurses Association (2021) has developed a kidney transplant fact sheet that can be shared with the school nurse.

TAKE NOTE!

Tell the parents to inform their child's health care provider or nurse practitioner about the child's long-term corticosteroid use and/or immunosuppressed status, as the child should not receive any live vaccines.

REPRODUCTIVE ORGAN DISORDERS

A number of disorders may occur within the genitalia and internal reproductive organs in children. These problems may be structural, infectious, or menstrual.

Labial Adhesions

Labial adhesion or labial fusion is partial or complete adherence of the labia minora (Fig. 21.12). UTI may result from urinary stasis behind the labia. If the adhesions are left untreated, the vaginal orifice may become inaccessible, presenting difficulty with sexual intercourse in the future.

Nursing Assessment

The peak incidence of labial adhesions occurs in the second year of life (Laufer & Emans, 2022). Assess the history for dysuria or urinary frequency. Inspect the genitalia for fusion or adherence of the labia minora.

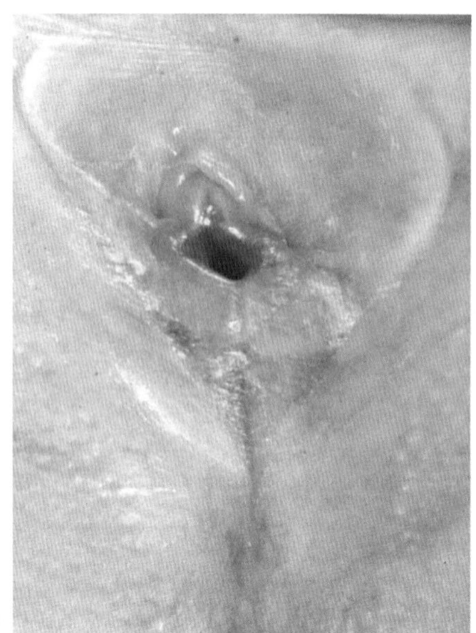

FIGURE 21.12 Labial adhesions: Note fusion of the labia minora. (Reprinted with permission from Emans, S. J., Laufer, M. R., & DiVasta, A. [2019]. *Emans, Laufer, Goldstein's pediatric and adolescent gynecology* [7th ed.]. Wolters Kluwer.)

Nursing Management

Administer topical estrogen cream as prescribed, usually once or twice daily. Teach the parents to continue cream application until the labia separate. Encourage use of petroleum jelly daily for 1 month following labial separation to prevent recurrence of adhesion.

Vulvovaginitis

Vulvovaginitis is inflammation of the vulva and vagina. Inflammation may occur as a result of bacterial or yeast overgrowth or from chemical factors such as bubble bath, soaps, or perfumes found in personal care products. Poor hygiene may also cause vulvovaginitis. Tight clothing may cause a heat rash in the perineal area. Persistent scratching of the irritated area may result in the complication of superficial skin infection.

Nursing Assessment

Eliciting the health history may reveal the common symptoms of itching or burning in the perineal area. Explore the child's current and past medical history for risk factors, which may include young age (toilet-trained preschooler), poor hygiene, sexual activity, immune disorders, or diabetes mellitus. Inspect the perineum for redness, edema, irritation, rash, or vaginal discharge (note color, consistency, and odor).

Nursing Management

Teach appropriate hygiene (daily and toileting). Children or their parents should wash the genital area thoroughly on a daily basis with mild soap and water. Rinse the area well. Encourage them to wipe in a front-to-back motion after urinating and after bowel movements. The child should wear cotton underwear and should change it at least once a day. Administer topical or oral medications as ordered. Table 21.3 lists treatments related to specific types of vulvovaginitis.

Pelvic Inflammatory Disease

Pelvic inflammatory disease (PID) is an inflammation of the upper female genital tract and nearby structures. The fallopian tubes, ovaries, or peritoneum may be involved, and endometriosis may also be present. PID results from bacterial invasion through the cervix and

TABLE 21.3 • Vulvovaginitis: Types and Treatments

Cause	Assessment Findings	Treatment
Unhygienic practices	Irritation of labia and vaginal opening May have foul brownish-green discharge if infected with bacteria from the rectum	Good hygiene Sometimes, a mild antiinflammatory cream is prescribed. Assess for signs and symptoms of UTI, which may occur as a complication.
Candida albicans	Red bumpy perineal rash in infants White cottage-cheese–like discharge Intense itching	Antifungal cream or vaginal suppository Prevent by ingesting probiotics (found in yogurt and kefir) daily and supplementing with a probiotic such as Lactinex when taking antibiotics.
Bordetella, Gardnerella	Thin gray vaginal discharge with fishy odor	Metronidazole orally
Trichomonas vaginalis	Foul yellow-gray or green vaginal discharge	Metronidazole orally; sexually transmitted, so can be prevented with the use of condoms

Data from Bauman, D. (2019). Chapter 38: Pediatric & adolescent gynecology and Bernstein, J. (2019). Chapter 40: Benign disorders of the vulva and vagina. In A. H. DeCherney, L. Nathan, N. Laufer, & A. S. Roman (Eds.), *Current diagnosis & treatment: Obstetrics & gynecology* (12th ed.). McGraw-Hill Education.

vagina, ascending into the uterus and fallopian tubes. The most common causes of PID are *Chlamydia trachomatis* and *Neisseria gonorrhoeae,* although other bacteria and normal vaginal flora may be implicated (Ross, 2023). PID may result in fever, abdominal pain, pain with intercourse, **dysmenorrhea** (painful menstrual cycles), and abnormal uterine bleeding. Long-term complications include chronic pelvic pain, ectopic pregnancy, and infertility related to scarring.

Nursing Assessment

For a full description of the assessment phase of the nursing process, refer to the "Clinical Judgment and the Nursing Process" section earlier in the chapter. When discussing any problem related to the reproductive organs or menstruation with the preadolescent or adolescent, it is necessary to discuss sexuality. The adolescent may be reluctant to share this information with the nurse. The following approaches to discussing sexuality with the adolescent may increase the likelihood of obtaining a truthful history:

- Discuss general health, menarche, and menstrual cycle first, and then work toward discussing sexual behavior.
- Start with questions about friends and social life, moving the conversation toward sexual behavior.
- Always discuss sexual behavior one on one with the adolescent (without the parent present), and then ask the adolescent's permission to discuss concerns with the parent. If the adolescent does not consent to parental involvement, then confidentiality must be maintained.

Assessment findings pertinent to PID are discussed in the following sections.

HEALTH HISTORY

Elicit a description of the present illness and chief complaint. Common symptoms reported during the health history might include:

- Abdominal pain (ranging from mild to severe)
- Prolonged or increased menstrual bleeding
- Dysmenorrhea
- Dysuria
- Painful sexual intercourse
- Nausea
- Vomiting

Explore current and past medical health history for risk factors such as:

- Multiple sexual partners
- Lack of consistent condom use
- Lack of contraceptive use
- History of prior sexually transmitted infection
- Douching
- Sex work or victimization
- Alcohol or drug use (particularly if associated with sexual activity)

PHYSICAL EXAMINATION

Inspect for fever (usually over 38°C [101°F]) or vaginal discharge. Palpate the abdomen, noting tenderness over the uterus or ovaries. An elevated C-reactive protein level and an elevated erythrocyte sedimentation rate indicate an inflammatory process. Cervical culture reveals the causative bacterial organism.

Nursing Management

Antibiotics are needed to eradicate the infection. PID is often treated in the outpatient setting with intramuscular or oral antibiotic regimens (Wiesenfeld, 2022). If the adolescent is severely ill or has a very high fever or protracted vomiting, then they may be hospitalized. Maintain hydration via intravenous fluids if necessary, and administer analgesics as needed for pain. Semi-Fowler positioning promotes pelvic drainage. A key element in treatment of PID is education to prevent recurrence (see the Healthy People 2030 box and Teaching Guidelines 21.2).

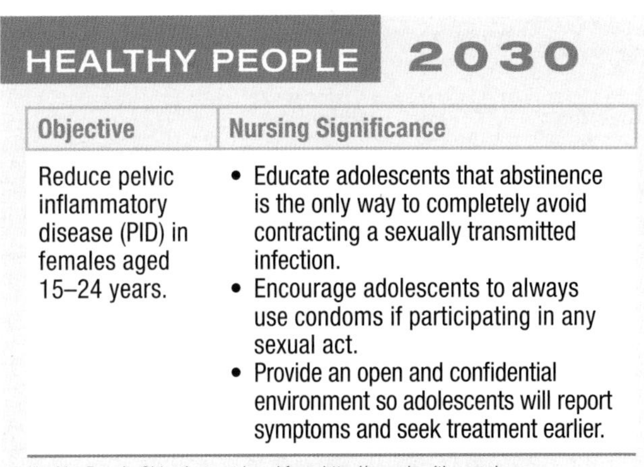

HEALTHY PEOPLE 2030

Objective	Nursing Significance
Reduce pelvic inflammatory disease (PID) in females aged 15–24 years.	• Educate adolescents that abstinence is the only way to completely avoid contracting a sexually transmitted infection. • Encourage adolescents to always use condoms if participating in any sexual act. • Provide an open and confidential environment so adolescents will report symptoms and seek treatment earlier.

Healthy People Objectives retrieved from http://www.healthypeople.gov

Menstrual Disorders

Menstruation typically begins about 2 years after breast development starts, around the time of Tanner stage 4 breast and pubic hair development and on average at around 12 to 13 years of age. Menstruation has many effects, including emotional and self-image issues. Adolescents may suffer from a variety of menstrual disorders, including

TEACHING GUIDELINES 21.2 Preventing PID

- Insist that sexual partners use condoms.
- Do not use a vaginal douche routinely, as this may lead to bacterial overgrowth.
- Get screened regularly for sexually transmitted infections.
- Make sure that each sexual partner also receives antibiotic treatment.

premenstrual syndrome and several different disorders related to menstrual bleeding and cramping (Table 21.4).

In healthy adolescents, the menstrual period varies in the heaviness of flow. Periods may occur irregularly for up to 2 years after menarche (the onset of menstruation), but after that the regular menstrual cycle should be established. A healthy cycle can vary from 21 to 45 days in length, with the period usually lasting 2 to 7 days. People who take oral contraceptives often have regular 28-day cycles with lighter bleeding than those who do not take contraceptives.

Pathophysiology

Premenstrual syndrome is a collection of physical and/or affective symptoms that occur predictably during the luteal phase of the menstrual cycle. Symptoms begin 5 to 10 days before each period and usually resolve by the time the period begins or shortly thereafter (the timing may vary by adolescent but is consistent with each cycle). Disorders of bleeding and cramping are summarized in Table 21.4.

Nursing Assessment

Refer to the "Clinical Judgment and the Nursing Process" section for a full description of the assessment phase of the nursing process. When patients present for evaluation of menstrual concerns, a focused yet thorough nursing assessment is necessary.

HEALTH HISTORY

Obtain a thorough and accurate menstrual history; determine age at menarche, usual length of menstrual period, usual menstrual flow, number of pads or tampons used per day, date of last normal menstrual period, premenstrual symptoms, and any pain related to the menstrual cycle. Obtain a description of the pain, what relief measures have been tried, and what the success of those measures has been. If pain occurs with menstrual periods, assess for associated symptoms such as nausea, vomiting, dizziness, or loose stools. Explore the history for symptoms of bloating, water retention, weight gain, headache, muscle aches,

TABLE 21.4 • Common Menstrual Disorders

Disorder	Definition	Cause
Primary amenorrhea	Lack of menarche within 2 years after reaching Tanner stage 4 breast development or by 16 years of age	• Imperforate hymen • Agenesis of vulva or vagina • Turner syndrome • Chronic illness associated with delayed pubertal development (e.g., cystic fibrosis, Crohn disease, sickle cell disease) • Suppressed levels of follicle-stimulating hormone (FSH) or luteinizing hormone (LH), as occurs with eating disorders, intense athletics, severe psychological stress, or extreme weight loss
Secondary amenorrhea	Absence of menses for 6 months in the patient who has been menstruating regularly	• Pregnancy (most common cause) • Anovulation (resulting from lack of hypothalamic–pituitary axis maturity) • Polycystic ovary syndrome (PCOS) • Suppressed levels of FSH or LH, as occurs with eating disorders, intense athletics, severe psychological stress, or extreme weight loss
Mittelschmerz	Abdominal pain, usually unilateral, that varies from a few sharp cramps to several hours of crampy pain	Usually occurs midway through the menstrual cycle, around the time of ovulation; is thought to be a result of egg release from the ovary
Dysmenorrhea	Pain associated with menstruation, usually abdominal cramps ranging from mild to severe	• Prostaglandin release is responsible for the smooth muscle contraction of the uterus during menstruation (primary). • Fibroids, adenomyosis, endometriosis, scar tissue (secondary)
Menorrhagia	Excessive menstrual bleeding	• Anovulatory cycles • Endometriosis • Blood dyscrasias, bleeding disorders, or use of anticoagulants • Reproductive system neoplasms
Metrorrhagia	Bleeding between menstrual periods	• Improper use of oral contraceptives • Intrauterine device • Endometriosis • Reproductive system neoplasms • Miscarriage or ectopic pregnancy

Data from Katzman, D. K., Gordon, C. M., Callahan, S. T., Chung, R. J., Joffe, A., Rosenthal, S. L., & Trent, M. E. (2023). *Neinstein's adolescent and young adult health care: A practical guide* (7th ed.). Wolters Kluwer Health.

abdominal pain, food cravings, or breast tenderness. Determine the extent of emotional symptoms related to the menstrual cycle, such as anxiety, insomnia, mood swings, tension, crying spells, or irritability. Note the timing of these symptoms within the menstrual cycle.

Note past medical history, including any chronic illnesses and family history of gynecologic concerns. Elicit a sexual behavior history, including the type of sexual activity (oral, anal, or vaginal), number and sex of sexual partners, frequency and most recent sexual contact, history of molestation or sexual abuse, and use of contraceptives (noting type) and/or condoms. Take a medication history, including prescription medications and contraceptives, and determine whether the patient uses anabolic steroids, tobacco, cannabis, cocaine, or other recreational drugs.

PHYSICAL EXAMINATION

Inspect the breasts and pubic hair distribution to determine Tanner stage. Observe the external genitalia for vaginal discharge, redness, or irritation. Note pallor or weight gain. Document presence and extent of clots in menstrual flow. Measure orthostatic blood pressure and orthostatic pulse; decreases with position change may occur with anemia. Palpate the abdomen, noting distention or tenderness. The bimanual pelvic examination and Papanicolaou (Pap) smear are usually indicated only for more severe menstrual disorders and are usually performed by the health care provider or nurse practitioner. A complete blood count (CBC) may determine the presence of anemia with menorrhagia or metrorrhagia. Human chorionic gonadotropin may be obtained to assess for pregnancy with **amenorrhea** (absence of menses).

Nursing Management

Nursing goals for the patient with a menstrual disorder focus on normalizing menstrual flow and restoring blood volume, providing comfort, and encouraging independence in self-care.

NORMALIZING MENSTRUAL FLOW AND RESTORING BLOOD VOLUME

For the patient with mild anemia related to menorrhagia, administer iron supplements as ordered. For moderate menorrhagia, oral contraceptives may also be prescribed, since altering hormone levels decrease menstrual flow. If the contraceptive contains a high dose of estrogen, the patient may experience nausea. Administer antiemetics as ordered, and encourage the patient to eat small, frequent meals to alleviate nausea. Adolescents with severe anemia may require hospitalization and blood transfusion.

PROVIDING COMFORT

Provide a heating pad or warm compress to help alleviate menstrual cramps. Administer NSAIDs such as ibuprofen or naproxen to inhibit prostaglandin synthesis, which contributes to menstrual cramps. Advise adolescents that beginning NSAID therapy at the first sign of menstrual discomfort is the best way to minimize discomfort. If NSAIDs are unsuccessful, oral contraceptives may be ordered; teach the appropriate use of oral contraceptives.

The adolescent experiencing premenstrual syndrome should keep a diary of their symptoms, their severity, and when they occur in the menstrual cycle. Like all adolescents, patients with premenstrual syndrome should eat a balanced diet that includes nutrient-rich foods so they can avoid hypoglycemia and associated mood swings. Encourage adolescents to participate in aerobic exercise three times a week to promote a sense of well-being, decrease fatigue, and reduce stress. Administer calcium (1,000 to 1,200 mg per day), magnesium (200 to 360 mg per day), and vitamin B_6 as prescribed. NSAIDs may be useful for painful physical symptoms, and spironolactone may help reduce bloating and water retention. Herbs such as chasteberry or ginkgo may be recommended.

TAKE NOTE!

Adolescents who experience more extensive emotional symptoms with premenstrual syndrome should be evaluated for premenstrual dysphoric disorder, as they may require antidepressant therapy (Shushan, 2019).

ENCOURAGING INDEPENDENCE IN SELF-CARE

Establishing a trusting relationship with the adolescent may make education about self-care more successful. Some adolescents have open relationships with their parents and can discuss issues related to menses and sexuality with them, but many others cannot discuss such "embarrassing" issues with their parents, and the nurse or other health care provider may be the only source of reliable information. Provide the adolescent with accurate information about menstruation and sexuality. Educate them about normal menstruation, the menstrual cycle, and the risk for pregnancy if sexual intercourse occurs. Refer the adolescent for contraception if sexually active. Refer them to reliable websites if they are not comfortable with receiving information from the nurse. Encourage the patient to call or visit the office if they have additional questions.

Phimosis and Paraphimosis

In phimosis, the foreskin of the penis cannot be retracted. Although this is normal in the newborn, it can be pathologic later. Over time, the prepuce (foreskin) naturally becomes retractable. Local irritation, balanitis, or UTI may occur if urine is retained within the foreskin after voiding. Paraphimosis (Fig. 21.13) is a more serious disorder

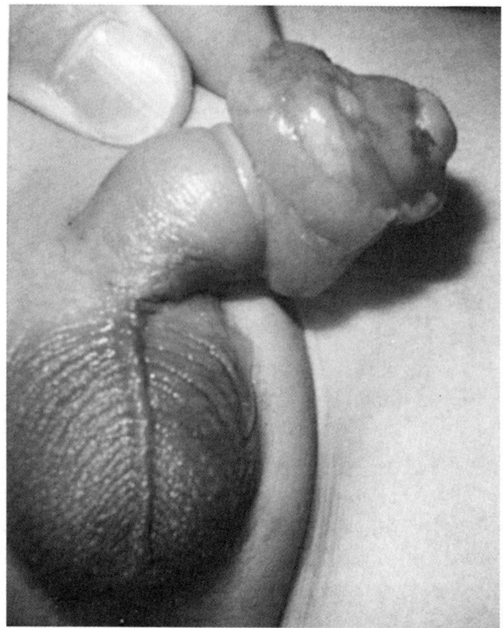

FIGURE 21.13 Paraphimosis: Note the swollen prepuce. (Reprinted with permission from Shaw, K. N., & Bachur, R. G. [2020]. *Fleisher & Ludwig's textbook of pediatric emergency medicine* [8th ed.]. Wolters Kluwer.)

characterized by retraction of the phimotic prepuce, which causes a constricting band behind the glans of the penis and results in incarceration if left untreated (Tews, 2024).

Topical steroid cream applied twice a day for 1 month may be prescribed for phimosis. Paraphimosis requires reduction of the prepuce or a small dorsal incision to release the foreskin. Circumcision may be used to treat either condition.

Nursing Assessment

Common symptoms reported during the health history might include irritation or bleeding from the opening of the prepuce or dysuria (with phimosis), or pain and swollen penis (with paraphimosis). Determine the onset of symptoms and inspect the penis for irritation, erythema, edema, or discharge (Tews, 2024).

CLINICAL REASONING ALERT!

A swollen, reddened penis (paraphimosis) is a medical emergency and can quickly result in necrosis of the tip of the penis if left untreated.

Nursing Management

Apply topical steroid medication as prescribed for phimosis, following gentle retraction to stretch the foreskin back. Topical vitamin E cream may also help to soften the phimotic ring. When surgical intervention is necessary, provide routine postprocedural care and pain management (refer to the "circumcision" section further on). Teach the parents and uncircumcised child proper hygiene, which will help to prevent phimosis and paraphimosis (Teaching Guidelines 21.3).

TEACHING GUIDELINES 21.3 Hygiene in the Uncircumcised Child

- The foreskin does not normally retract in the newborn, so do not force it to do so.
- Change the diaper frequently, and wash the penis daily with water and mild soap.
- When the child is older and the foreskin easily retracts, gently retract the foreskin and clean around the glans with water and mild soap once a week.
- Dry the area prior to replacing the foreskin.
- Always replace the foreskin after retraction.
- Teach the child to clean the penis during each bath or shower, including under the foreskin after it retracts.

Circumcision

Circumcision is the removal of the foreskin of the penis. Although it is procedure, and not a disorder, relevant nursing assessment and management will be discussed here. Some newborns are circumcised shortly after birth before going home from the hospital. Some parents elect not to have their newborn circumcised at that time but may desire it later. Neonatal circumcision may be performed in the newborn nursery, hospital unit treatment room, or outpatient office. Circumcision is indicated later for the conditions of phimosis and paraphimosis. Circumcision done after the newborn period usually requires general anesthesia.

The benefits of circumcision include a decreased incidence of UTI, sexually transmitted infections, AIDS, and penile cancer, and in female partners, a decreased occurrence of cervical cancer (Baskin, 2023b). Complications of circumcision are rare and include bleeding, penile adhesions, imperfect amount of foreskin removal, and meatal stenosis (Baskin, 2023b). Whether to circumcise or not is a personal decision that is often based on religious beliefs or social or cultural customs. Nurses should support and educate the parents in either case.

Nursing Assessment

Prior to the procedure, assess for normal placement of the urinary meatus on the glans penis (with hypospadias, circumcision should be delayed until evaluation by the pediatric urologist). After the circumcision, assess for redness, edema, or active bleeding. Note signs of infection, such as purulent drainage. Assess pain level.

Nursing Management

Nursing care of the patient undergoing circumcision focuses on managing pain, providing postprocedural care, and educating the parents.

MANAGING PAIN

Whether circumcision is performed in the obstetric area of the hospital before newborn discharge or in the outpatient setting at a few days of age, pain management during the procedure must not be neglected. Advocate for appropriate pain management for the infant undergoing circumcision. Pain management techniques during the procedure may include a subcutaneous ring block with lidocaine, local anesthetic with lidocaine/prilocaine, or a dorsal nerve block to the penis. Playing calming music during the procedure may also help to soothe the infant, providing distraction. A sucrose-dipped pacifier may also be used as adjuvant therapy for pain management.

• • • ATRAUMATIC CARE • • •

Restrain the infant in a padded circumcision chair, with blankets covering the legs and upper body to provide a sense of comfort. If a padded restraint chair is not available, provide atraumatic care by padding the circumcision board and covering the infant as previously described.

PROVIDING POSTPROCEDURAL CARE

Usual care after circumcision depends on the type of appliance used (Gomco or Mogen clamp or Plastibell apparatus). Cleanse the penis with clear water for the first few days, and avoid using alcohol-containing wipes. To avoid irritation to the penis, fasten diapers loosely. Notify the health care provider or nurse practitioner if excessive redness, active bleeding, or purulent discharge occurs. Assess for the first void following the procedure, or if performed in the outpatient setting, instruct parents to call the health care provider or nurse practitioner if the infant has not voided by 6 to 8 hours after the circumcision. Apply antibiotic ointment or petroleum jelly to the penile head with each diaper change as prescribed, based on the circumcision method used and the preference of the health care provider or nurse practitioner.

CLINICAL REASONING ALERT!

If excess bleeding occurs after the circumcision, apply direct pressure and notify the health care provider or nurse practitioner immediately.

EDUCATING THE PARENTS

Instruct the parents to give sponge baths until the circumcision is healed. Describe the normal granulation tissue that will be present during the healing process. Teach the parents to apply ointment or petroleum jelly if indicated. Instruct the parents to call the health care provider or nurse practitioner if any of the following occur:

- The infant does not urinate within 6 to 8 hours after the procedure.
- Heavy bleeding occurs (more than small spots on the diaper or bleeding that requires direct pressure to stop it).
- There is purulent or serous drainage from the circumcised area.
- There is redness or swelling of the penile shaft.

Cryptorchidism

Cryptorchidism (also known as undescended testicles) occurs when one or both testicles do not descend into the scrotal sac. Ordinarily, the testes, which in the fetus develop in the abdomen, make their descent into the scrotal sac during the seventh month of gestation. The cause of this failure to descend may be mechanical, hormonal, chromosomal, or enzymatic. The disorder may occur unilaterally or bilaterally. Up to 3.4% of term male infants exhibit cryptorchidism (Patel & Vogt, 2023).

Complications associated with cryptorchidism that is allowed to progress into the school-age years include sterility and an increased risk of testicular cancer in adolescence or the young adult years. Therapeutic management is surgical. An orchiopexy is performed to release the spermatic cord, and the testes are then pulled into the scrotum and tacked into place.

Nursing Assessment

Explore the health history for risk factors such as prematurity, first-born child, cesarean birth, low birth weight, or hypospadias. Palpate for the presence (or absence) of both testes in the scrotal sac.

TAKE NOTE!

A retractile testis is one that may be brought into the scrotum, remains for a time, and then retracts back up the inguinal canal. This should not be confused with true cryptorchidism.

Nursing Management

If the testes are not descended by 12 months of age, the infant should be referred for surgical repair. Postoperatively, observe the incision for signs of bleeding or infection.

Hydrocele and Varicocele

Hydrocele (fluid in the scrotal sac) is usually a benign and self-limiting disorder. It is usually noted early in infancy and often resolves spontaneously by 1 year of age. Varicocele (a venous varicosity along the spermatic cord) is often noted as a swelling of the scrotal sac. Complications of varicocele include low sperm count or reduced sperm motility, which can result in infertility.

Nursing Assessment

Elicit a description of the present illness and chief complaint. The patient with hydrocele will have an enlarged scrotum that may decrease in size when lying down. Inspect the scrotum for a fluid-filled appearance.

The patient with varicocele will have a mass on one or both sides of the scrotum and bluish discoloration. Inspect the scrotum for masses; the spermatic vein feels worm-like on palpation. The patient with varicocele may have pain.

Nursing Management

Both hydrocele and painless varicocele require watchful waiting, as these conditions will usually resolve spontaneously. If they do not resolve, or if the difference in testicular volume is marked in the child with varicocele, refer them to a urologist, as surgery may be indicated. Reassure parents that hydrocele is not associated with the development of infertility. Varicocele may lead to infertility if left untreated, so instruct parents to seek care if pain occurs or if there is a large difference in testicular size. Either condition may be surgically corrected on an outpatient basis. Provide routine postoperative care following either surgery.

Testicular Torsion

In testicular torsion, a testicle is abnormally attached to the scrotum and twisted. It requires immediate attention because ischemia can result if the torsion is left untreated, leading to infertility. Testicular torsion may occur at any age but most commonly occurs in children aged 12 to 18 years (Brenner & Ojo, 2023).

Nursing Assessment

Symptoms of testicular torsion include sudden, severe scrotal pain. Inspect the affected side for significant swelling, which may appear hemorrhagic or blue-black.

Nursing Management

Surgical correction is necessary immediately. Administer pain medication prior to surgery. Reassure the child and family that surgery will alleviate the problem and is performed to restore adequate blood flow to the testicle. After surgical repair, provide routine postoperative care.

TAKE NOTE!

Testicular torsion is considered a surgical emergency, as necrosis of the testis may occur, and gangrene may set in.

Epididymitis

Epididymitis (inflammation of the epididymis) is caused by infection with bacteria. It is the most common cause of pain in the scrotum. It rarely occurs before puberty, but if it does, it may occur as a result of a urethral or bladder infection related to a urogenital anomaly. Therapeutic management is directed toward eradicating the bacteria. If left untreated, a scrotal abscess, testicular infarction, or infertility may occur.

Nursing Assessment

Note history of painful swelling of the scrotum, which may be gradual or acute. If the patient is sexually active, explore history of sexual encounters prior to the onset of symptoms. Document history of dysuria or urethral discharge. Note fever, which may last from days to weeks. On inspection, note edema and erythema of the scrotum. Gently palpate the scrotum for a hardened and tender epididymis. Note urethral discharge if present. Palpate the inguinal lymph nodes for enlargement. Urinalysis may be positive for bacteria and white blood cells. The culture of urethral discharge may be positive for a sexually transmitted infection such as gonorrhea or *Chlamydia*. The CBC may reveal an elevated white blood cell count.

Nursing Management

Encourage the child to rest in bed with the scrotum elevated. Ice packs to the scrotum may help with pain relief. Administer pain medications such as NSAIDs or other analgesics as needed. Administer antibiotics as prescribed. Educate the child and family to complete the entire course of antibiotics as prescribed to eradicate the infection. Advise the child and family to notify the health care provider or nurse practitioner if the condition is not improving or if the pain and swelling worsen.

KEY CONCEPTS

- Although present at birth, the reproductive organs do not reach functional maturity until puberty.
- The short length of the urethra in females and its proximity to the vagina and anus place the young female at higher risk for the development of UTIs compared with the adult.
- The urinary tract is immature in infants and young children, with a slower GFR and a decreased ability to concentrate urine and reabsorb amino acids compared with the adult.
- The expected urine output in the infant and child is 0.5 to 2 mL/kg/h.
- Obtaining a clean or sterile urine specimen is necessary for accurate urine culture results.
- A urinary catheter must be inserted just prior to the VCUG.
- Close monitoring of serum blood counts and electrolytes is a critical component of nursing care related to kidney disorders.

- Certain congenital urologic anomalies may require multiple surgeries as well as urinary diversion; urine drains through a stoma on the abdominal wall that is either pouched or catheterized.
- The treatment for nocturnal enuresis may include the use of desmopressin nasal spray and/or an enuresis alarm to train the child to awaken to the sensation of a filling bladder.
- Nephrotic syndrome results in significant proteinuria and edema.
- Acute glomerulonephritis most often follows a group A streptococcal infection and commonly results in hematuria, proteinuria, and hypertension.
- The most common cause of HUS is infection with *E. coli* O157:H7. It can be prevented by adequately cooking ground meat, washing hands and produce well, and making sure that an appropriate chemical balance is maintained in public recreational water sources such as swimming pools and water parks.
- Corticosteroids can cause GI upset. If used on a long-term basis, they should be tapered rather than discontinued abruptly to avoid adrenal crisis.
- In children, CKD is most often the result of congenital structural defects, or infectious, inflammatory, or immune processes that damage the kidney, whereas in adults it usually results from hypertension or diabetes.
- Children taking immunosuppressants for nephrotic syndrome or for kidney transplant are at increased risk for the development of overwhelming infection.
- Peritoneal dialysis may be accomplished at home by the parent. Close attention to sterile technique is needed.
- Hemodialysis requires an arteriovenous fistula or graft that is accessed with needles three or four times per week at a hemodialysis center. This is disruptive to the child's academic, social, and family lives.
- Kidney transplantation is the best option for the treatment of ESKD in children, but vigilant medication administration is needed to prevent organ rejection.
- Children with kidney failure experience anemia, poor growth, depression, anxiety, and low self-esteem.
- The diet for a child with a kidney disorder must be individualized according to prescribed sodium, fluid, and protein restrictions.
- Postoperative care for the child undergoing urologic surgery includes pain management, avoidance or treatment of bladder spasms, and monitoring of urine output.

REFERENCES AND RECOMMENDED READINGS

Aksakall, T., Cinislioğlu, A. E., & Aksoy, Y. (2022). The efficacy of combined alarm therapy versus alarm monotherapy in the treatment of monosymptomatic nocturnal enuresis: A review of current literature. *Eurasian Journal of Medicine, 54*(Suppl. 1), S164–S167. http://doi.org/10.5152/eurasianjmed.2022.22311

American Nephrology Nurses' Association. (2021). *Pediatric ESRD renal transplant fact sheet.* https://www.annanurse.org/download/reference/practice/pedTransplantFactSheet.pdf

Baskin, L. S. (2023a). Hypospadias: Management and outcome. *UpToDate.* Retrieved April 12, 2024, from https://www.uptodate.com/contents/hypospadias-pathogenesis-diagnosis-and-evaluation

Baskin, L. S. (2023b). Patient education: Circumcision in baby boys (beyond the basics). *UpToDate.* Retrieved April 12, 2024, from https://www.uptodate.com/contents/circumcision-in-baby-boys-beyond-the-basics#H15

Bauman, D. (2019). Chapter 38: Pediatric & adolescent gynecology. In A. H. DeCherney, L. Nathan, N. Laufer, & A. S. Roman (Eds.), *Current diagnosis & treatment: Obstetrics & gynecology* (12th ed.). McGraw-Hill Education.

Bock, M. E., Blanchette, E., & Hanna, M. G. (2022). Chapter 24: Kidney & urinary tract. In M. Bunik, W. W. Hay, M. J. Levin, & M. J. Abzug (Eds.), *Current diagnosis & treatment: Pediatrics* (26th ed.). McGraw-Hill Education.

Brenner, J. S., & Ojo, A. (2023). Causes of scrotal pain in children and adolescents. *UpToDate.* Retrieved April 12, 2024, from https://www.uptodate.com/contents/causes-of-scrotal-pain-in-children-and-adolescents

Corbett, J. A., & Banks, A. D. (2019). *Laboratory tests and diagnostic procedures with nursing diagnoses* (9th ed.). Pearson Education Inc.

Chua, A., & Warady, B. A. (2024). Chronic peritoneal dialysis in children. *UpToDate.* Retrieved April 12, 2024, from https://www.uptodate.com/contents/chronic-peritoneal-dialysis-in-children

Elder, J. R. (2020). Chapter 555: Obstruction of the urinary tract. In R. M. Kliegman, J. W. St Geme, N. J. Blum, S. S. Shah, R. C. Tasker, & K. M. Wilson (Eds.), *Nelson textbook of pediatrics* (21st ed.). Elsevier.

Estrada, C. R., & Cendron, M. (2021). *Vesicoureteral reflux treatment & management.* Medscape. https://emedicine.medscape.com/article/439403-overview

Flores, F. X. (2020). Chapter 537: Isolated glomerular diseases associated with recurrent gross hematuria. In R. M. Kliegman, J. W. St Geme, N. J. Blum, S. S. Shah, R. C. Tasker, & K. M. Wilson (Eds.), *Nelson textbook of pediatrics* (21st ed.). Elsevier.

Flynn, J. T. (2024). Ambulatory blood pressure monitoring in children. *UpToDate.* Retrieved April 12, 2024, from https://www.uptodate.com/contents/ambulatory-blood-pressure-monitoring-in-children

Hamilton, R. G. (2023). Latex allergy: Epidemiology, clinical manifestations, and diagnosis. *UpToDate.* Retrieved April 12, 2024, from http://www.uptodate.com/contents/latex-allergy-epidemiology-clinical-manifestations-and-diagnosis

Hucker, J., & Lawson-Wood, H. (2023). Indwelling urinary catheter insertion 1: Children and young people. *Nursing Times* [online] *119,* 3. https://www.nursingtimes.net/roles/childrens-nurses/indwelling-urinary-catheter-insertion-1-children-and-young-people-20-02-2023/#

Katzman, D. K., Gordon, C. M., Callahan, S. T., Chung, R. J., Joffe, A., Rosenthal, S. L., & Trent, M. E. (2023). *Neinstein's adolescent and young adult health care: A practical guide* (7th ed.). Wolters Kluwer Health.

Klabunde, P. (2023). *Functional cardiac murmurs*. https://www.cvphysiology.com/Heart%20Disease/HD006

Laufer, M. R., & Emans, S. J. (2022). Overview of vulvovaginal complaints in the prepubertal child. *UpToDate*. Retrieved April 12, 2024, from https://www.uptodate.com/contents/overview-of-vulvovaginal-complaints-in-the-prepubertal-child

McDonald, R. A. (2023). Kidney transplantation in children: General principles. *UpToDate*. Retrieved April 12, 2024, from https://www.uptodate.com/contents/general-principles-of-renal-transplantation-in-children

Nationwide Children's Hospital. (2024). *U-bag urine collection guidelines for males and females*. https://www.nationwidechildrens.org/family-resources-education/health-wellness-and-safety-resources/helping-hands/ubag-urine-collection-guidelines-for-males-and-females

Patel, H. P., & Vogt, B. A. (2023). Section 22: Nephrology and urology. In K. J. Marcdante, R. M. Kliegman, & A. M. Schuh (Eds.), *Nelson's essentials of pediatrics* (9th ed.). Elsevier.

Paul, C. R., & Wallace, C. M. (2023). Chapter 14: Control of elimination. In K. J. Marcdante, R. M. Kliegman, & A. M. Schuh (Eds.), *Nelson's essentials of pediatrics* (9th ed.). Elsevier.

Ross, J. (2023). Pelvic inflammatory disease: Clinical manifestations and diagnosis. *UpToDate*. Retrieved April 12, 2024, from https://www.uptodate.com/contents/pelvic-inflammatory-disease-clinical-manifestations-and-diagnosis

Shushan, A. (2019). Chapter 39: Complications of menstruation & abnormal uterine bleeding. In A. H. DeCherney, L. Nathan, N. Laufer, & A. S. Roman (Eds.), *Current diagnosis & treatment: Obstetrics & gynecology* (12th ed.). McGraw-Hill Education.

Solomon, D. H. (2022). Patient information: Nonsteroidal anti-inflammatory drugs (NSAIDs) (beyond the basics). *UpToDate*. Retrieved April 11, 2024, from https://www.uptodate.com/contents/nonsteroidal-antiinflammatory-drugs-nsaids-beyond-the-basics

Stahl, J. L., Wightman, A. G., Flythe, J. E., Noel S., Weiss, N. S., Hingorani, S. R., & Vander Stoep, A. (2022). Psychiatric diagnoses in children with CKD compared to the general population. *Kidney Medicine*, *4*(6), 100451. https://doi.org/10.1016/j.xkme.2022.100451

St. Lukes. (n.d.). *When your child needs surgery for hypospadias*. https://www.saintlukeskc.org/health-library/when-your-child-needs-surgery-hypospadias

Tan, A. J., & Silverberg, M. A. (2021). Hemolytic uremic syndrome in emergency medicine. *Medscape*. https://emedicine.medscape.com/article/779218-overview

Tews, M. (2024). Paraphimosis: Clinical manifestations, diagnosis, and treatment. *UpToDate*. Retrieved April 11, 2024, from https://www.uptodate.com/contents/paraphimosis-clinical-manifestations-diagnosis-and-treatment

UNOS. (2024). *How we match organs*. https://unos.org/transplant/how-we-match-organs/

UpToDate, Inc. (2023). *Lexi-comp®* (Version 7.7.0) [Mobile app]. Wolters Kluwer. https://apps.apple.com/us/app/lexicomp/id313401238

U.S. Department of Health and Human Services. (n.d.). *Healthy people 2030*. https://health.gov/healthypeople

UTMB Health. (2024). *Replacement fluid therapy*. https://www.utmb.edu/Pedi_Ed/CoreV2/Fluids/Fluids10.html

Wiesenfeld, H. C. (2024). Pelvic inflammatory disease: Treatment in adults and adolescents. *UpToDate*. Retrieved April 11, 2024, from https://www.uptodate.com/contents/pelvic-inflammatory-disease-treatment-in-adults-and-adolescents

DEVELOPING CLINICAL JUDGMENT

PRACTICING FOR NCLEX

1. The nurse is performing education for the parents of an infant with bladder exstrophy. Which statement by the parents would indicate an understanding of the child's future care?
   a. "Care will be no different than that of any other infant."
   b. "My infant will only need this one surgery."
   c. "My child will wear diapers their whole life."
   d. "We will need to care for the urinary diversion."

2. A 4-year-old presents with recurrent UTI. A prior workup did not reveal any urinary tract abnormalities. What is the priority nursing action?
   a. Obtain a sterile urine sample after completion of antibiotics.
   b. Teach appropriate toileting hygiene.
   c. Prepare the child for surgery to reimplant the ureters.
   d. Administer antibiotics intramuscularly.

3. A 5-year-old who had a kidney transplant 9 months ago and has no history of chickenpox presents to the pediatric clinic for vaccinations. Which is the most appropriate set to give?
   a. DTaP, IPV
   b. DTaP, IPV, MMR, varicella
   c. DTaP, IPV, varicella
   d. IPV only

4. When the nurse is caring for a child with HUS or acute glomerulonephritis and the child is not yet toilet trained, which action by the nurse would best determine fluid retention?
   a. Test urine for specific gravity.
   b. Weigh the child daily.
   c. Weigh the wet diapers.
   d. Measure abdominal girth daily.

5. An 8-year-old had a cold and sore throat that resolved about a week and a half ago. The parent is concerned that the child does not seem to be urinating as frequently as usual, has been tired, and looks pale. The child ordinarily does well in school and is active. On physical examination, the nurse notes periorbital edema and blood pressure of 134/88 mm Hg. hypertension, decreased urine output, pallor, and fatigue. The child is admitted to the pediatric unit Choose the correct options for each of the blanks in the following statements. Patients presenting with acute ________________ glomerulonephritis may have a history of a(n) ________________ infection. Urine laboratory testing will reveal ________________.

   Blank 1
   a. postpneumococcal
   b. poststaphylococcal
   c. poststreptococcal
   d. lupus erythematosus

   Blank 2
   a. group A beta-hemolytic streptococcus
   b. group B beta-hemolytic streptococcus
   c. acute lung
   d. respiratory syncytial viral

   Blank 3
   a. increased glucose
   b. increased white blood cells
   c. high leukocyte esterase
   d. increased red blood cells

6. A 4-year-old says it hurts "when I tinkle." The child has been toilet-trained since age 28 months. The parent reports the child felt warm today and the urine is strong-smelling, with frequency and pain on urination. A urinalysis with culture is ordered. Which of the following does the nurse consider as true regarding obtaining the specimen? Select all that apply.
   a. Obtaining a clean voided urine sample is appropriate in children who are toilet trained.
   b. To maintain sterility, the urine specimen should be obtained through suprapubic aspiration.
   c. Since the child has a fever, an antibiotic should be started prior to obtaining the specimen.
   d. Painful urination can be resolved if the child drinks a large amount of fluid.
   e. Have the child begin urinating in the toilet, then collect the urine midway in a sterile container.

7. The nurse is caring for a 9-month-old who has had surgical correction for hypospadias. The infant will have a stent in place to drain urine for the next 5 to 10 days. Which of the following should the nurse include in the discharge teaching? Select all that apply.
   a. "The catheter will allow urine to drain into the diaper."
   b. "Administer pain medication around the clock for 10 days."
   c. "Use the double-diapering method while the stent is in place."
   d. "To prevent infection, be sure to give the antibiotic as prescribed."
   e. "Allowing tub baths may help with the child's pain control."
   f. "Avoid ride-on toys and roughhousing until cleared by the surgeon."

DOSAGE CALCULATION QUESTION

The nurse is caring for a child who has had a kidney transplant. The child weighs 47 lb. The medication order reads: cyclosporine 96 mg PO every 12 hours. Cyclosporine is supplied as 100 mg/mL. How many milliliters will the nurse administer? Round to the nearest whole number.

CRITICAL THINKING EXERCISES

1. Devise a meal plan for a 5-year-old child with a kidney disorder who requires a 2-g sodium restriction per day. Keep in mind the child's developmental level and feeding idiosyncrasies at this age.
2. Develop a discharge teaching plan for a 3-year-old with nephrotic syndrome who will be taking corticosteroids long term.
3. Devise a developmental stimulation plan for an 11-month-old who has had significant urinary tract reconstruction surgery and is facing a prolonged period of confinement to the crib.

STUDY ACTIVITIES

1. In the clinical setting, compare the growth and development of two children of the same age, one with CKD and one who has been healthy.
2. While caring for children in the clinical setting, compare and contrast the medical history, signs and symptoms of illness, and prescribed treatments for a child with nephrotic syndrome and one with acute glomerulonephritis.
3. Observe peritoneal dialysis in the hospital or hemodialysis in a hospital or outpatient center. Record observations about the children's psychosocial and developmental status.

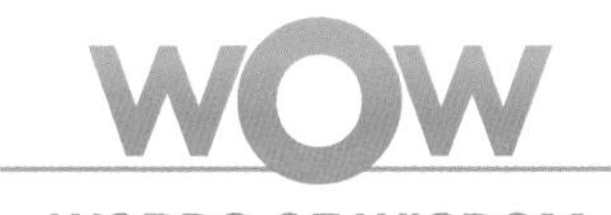

WORDS OF WISDOM
Enhancing a child's abilities may enhance their strength to overcome anything.

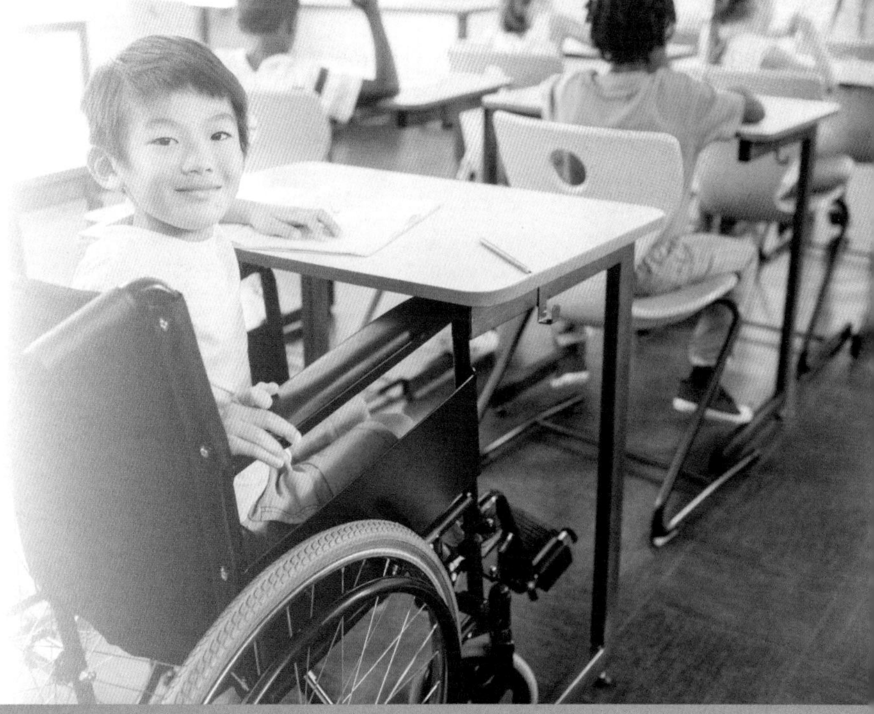

22

Nursing Care of the Child With an Alteration in Mobility/Neuromuscular or Musculoskeletal Disorder

KEY TERMS

ataxia (ă-tak´sē-ă)
clonus (klō´nŭs)
contracture (kŏn-trak´shŭr)
epiphysis (e-pif´i-sis)
external fixation
hypertonia
hypotonia
kyphosis (kī-fō´sis)
lordosis (lōr-dō´sis)
ossification (os´i-fi-kā´shŭn)
spasticity
traction
Trendelenburg gait

LEARNING OBJECTIVES

Upon completion of the chapter, you will be able to:

1. Compare the anatomy and physiology of the neuromuscular and musculoskeletal systems in children with those of adults.
2. Identify nursing interventions related to common laboratory and diagnostic tests used in the diagnosis and management of neuromuscular and musculoskeletal conditions.
3. Identify appropriate nursing assessments and interventions related to medications and treatments used for childhood neuromuscular and musculoskeletal conditions.
4. Distinguish various neuromuscular and musculoskeletal disorders occurring in childhood.
5. Devise an individualized plan of care or concept map for the child with a neuromuscular or musculoskeletal disorder.
6. Develop child and family teaching plans for the child with a neuromuscular or musculoskeletal disorder.
7. Describe the psychosocial impact of chronic neuromuscular and musculoskeletal disorders on the growth and development of children.

Frederick Stevens, 4 years old, seems to be falling often and has started to have difficulty climbing the stairs on his own. His parent states, "Recently he hasn't been able to keep up with his 6-year-old sister when we're playing at the park. He usually ends up sitting on the bench with me." The parent is concerned about the changes they have seen in their child.

INTRODUCTION

Mobility refers to mechanisms that facilitate or impair a person's ability to move. Nurses encounter potential or actual alterations in mobility in all types of patients and must detect problems and intervene early to prevent complications. A variety of alterations in mobility (neuromuscular or musculoskeletal disorders) may affect children, but the result of each is muscular and/or skeletal dysfunction. Some of the disorders result from a neurologic insult such as trauma or hypoxia to the brain or spinal cord. Others occur as a result of genetic dysfunction or structural abnormality that is present from birth but may not be identified until later in childhood or adolescence. Infants and young children have resilient soft tissue, so sprains and strains are less common in this age group. Older school-age children and adolescents often participate in sports, resulting in an increased risk of injuries such as sprains, fractures, and torn ligaments.

The immobility associated with most neuromuscular and musculoskeletal disorders may affect the child's development and acquisition of motor skills, leading to motor dysfunction. Many neuromuscular and musculoskeletal disorders are chronic, lasting the child's entire life and resulting in disability.

The nurse caring for a child with altered mobility plays an important role in the management of these disorders. Not only must the nurse provide direct intervention in response to health alterations that result, but also the nurse is often part of the larger multidisciplinary team and may serve as the coordinator of many specialists or interventions. Understanding the most common responses to these disorders gives the nurse the foundation required to plan care for any child with any neuromuscular or musculoskeletal disorder.

VARIATIONS IN PEDIATRIC ANATOMY AND PHYSIOLOGY

The neuromuscular system is the combination of the nervous system and the muscles working together to create movement. The musculoskeletal system provides the body with form, support, stability, protection, and the ability to move. It is made up of bones, muscles, cartilage, tendons, ligaments, joints, and connective tissue. Anatomic and physiologic differences in infants and children, such as the immaturity of the neurologic and musculoskeletal systems, place them at increased risk for the development of a neuromuscular or musculoskeletal disorder and may hinder the child's growth and movement.

Brain and Spinal Cord Development

Early in gestation, around 3 to 4 weeks, the neural tube of the embryo begins to differentiate into the brain and spinal cord. If the fetus suffers infection, trauma, malnutrition, or teratogen exposure during this critical period of growth and differentiation, brain or spinal cord development may be altered. The premature infant's central nervous system is less mature than the term newborn's. Such immaturity in the preterm infant places them at higher risk for central nervous insult within the neonatal period, which may result in delayed motor skill attainment or cerebral palsy. Compared with the adult, the child's spine is very mobile, especially the cervical spine region, resulting in a higher risk of cervical spine injury.

Myelinization

Although the development of the structures of the nervous system is complete at birth, myelinization is incomplete. Myelinization continues to progress and is complete by about 2 years of age. Myelinization proceeds in a cephalocaudal and proximodistal fashion, allowing the infant to gain head and neck control before becoming able to control the trunk and the extremities. As myelinization proceeds, the speed and accuracy of nerve impulses increase. Primitive reflexes are replaced with voluntary movement.

Muscular Development

The muscular system, including tendons, ligaments, and cartilage, arises from the mesoderm in early embryonic development. At birth (term or preterm), the muscles, tendons, ligaments, and cartilage are all present and functional. The newborn infant is capable of spontaneous movement but lacks purposeful control. Full range of motion (ROM) is present at birth. Healthy infants and children demonstrate normal muscle tone; **hypertonia** (increased muscle tone) or **hypotonia** (low muscle tone) is an abnormal finding. Deep tendon reflexes are present at birth and are initially brisk in the newborn and progress to average over the first few months. Sluggish deep tendon reflexes indicate an abnormality. As the infant matures and becomes mobile, the muscles develop further and become stronger. The infant's muscles account for approximately 25% of total body weight, while the adult's account for about 40% of total body weight (Neudauer, 2019). Muscles grow rapidly in adolescence; this contributes to clumsiness, which places the adolescent at increased risk for injury. In response to testosterone release, the adolescent male experiences a growth spurt, particularly in the trunk and legs, and develops bulkier muscles. Female infants tend to have laxer ligaments than male infants, possibly due to the presence of female hormones, placing them at increased risk for developmental dysplasia of the hip (DDH) (Sankar et al., 2020).

Skeletal Development

The infant's skeleton is not fully ossified at birth. The infant's and young child's bones are more flexible and more porous and have a lower mineral content than the adult's. These structural differences of a young child's bones allow for greater shock absorption, so the bones will often bend rather than break when an injury occurs. The thick, strong periosteum of the child's bones allows for a greater absorption of force than is seen in adults. As a result, the cortex of the bone does not always break, but sometimes only buckles or bends. The skeleton contains increased amounts of cartilage compared with adolescents and adults. **Ossification**, the conversion of cartilage to bone, continues throughout childhood and is complete at adolescence.

During fetal development the spine displays **kyphosis**, an outward curvature. Cervical **lordosis**, inward curvature, develops as the infant starts to hold the head up. When the infant or toddler assumes an upright position, the primary and secondary curves of the spine begin to develop. The balance of the curves allows the head to be centered over the pelvis. During the toddler years, the period of early walking, lumbar lordosis may be significant (also termed toddler lordosis), and the toddler appears quite swaybacked and potbellied. As the child develops, the spine takes on more adult-like curves. During adolescence, thoracic kyphosis may become evident. This is most often a postural effect, and as the adolescent matures, the posture appears similar to that of an adult.

Growth Plate

The ends of the bones in young children are composed of the **epiphysis**, the end of a long bone, and the physis, in combination termed the growth plate. In infants, the epiphyses are cartilaginous and ossify over time. In children, the epiphysis is the secondary ossification center at the end of the bone. The physis is a cartilaginous area between the epiphysis and the metaphysis. Growth of the bones occurs primarily in the epiphyseal region. This area is vulnerable and structurally weak. Traumatic force applied to the epiphysis during injury may result in fracture in that area of the bone. Epiphyseal injury may result in early, incomplete, or partial closure of the growth plate, leading to deformity or shortening of the bone. Epiphyseal growth continues until skeletal maturity is reached during adolescence. Production of androgens in adolescence gradually causes the growth plates to fuse, and thus long bone growth is complete (Fig. 22.1).

Bone Healing

The child's bones have a thick, strong periosteum with an abundant blood supply. Bone healing occurs in the same fashion as in the adult, but because of the rich nutrient supply to the periosteum, it occurs more quickly in children. Children's bones produce callus more rapidly and in larger quantities than do adults. As new bone cells quickly form, a bulge of new bone growth occurs at the site of the fracture. The younger the child, the more quickly the bone heals. Also, the closer the fracture is to the growth plate (epiphysis), the more quickly the fracture heals. The capacity for remodeling (the process of breaking down and forming new bone) is increased in children as compared with adults. This means that straightening of the bone over time occurs more easily in children.

Positional Alterations

The lower extremities of the infant tend to have a bowed appearance, attributable to in utero positioning. In utero, the fetus's hips are usually flexed, abducted, and externally rotated, with the knees also flexed and the lower limbs inwardly rotated. This normal developmental variation is termed internal tibial torsion. The legs straighten

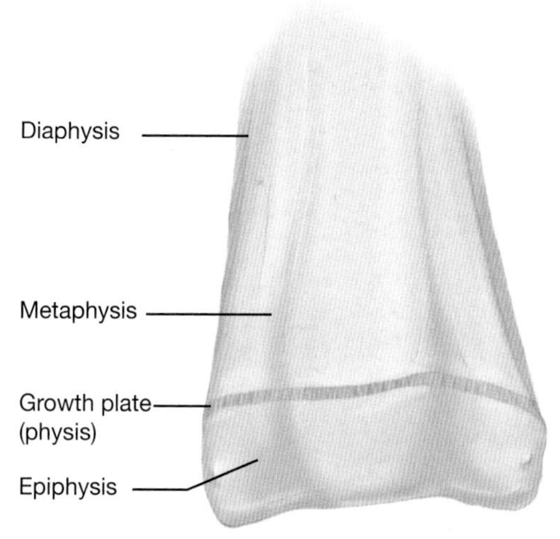

FIGURE 22.1 Anatomic areas of growing bone.

with passive motion, and internal tibial torsion should not be confused with "bowlegs" (Fig. 22.2). Internal tibial torsion usually resolves independently within the second or third year of life as the toddler bears weight and the lower extremity muscles and bones mature. The bowlegged appearance is sometimes also referred to as genu varum. As internal tibial torsion or genu varum resolves, physiologic genu valgum occurs. Children usually demonstrate symmetric genu valgum (knock-knees) by the age of 2 to 3 years. In genu valgum, when the knees are touching, the ankles are significantly separated, with the lower portion of the legs angled outward (Fig. 22.3). By age 7 or 8 years, genu valgum gradually resolves in most children.

The newborn's feet also display in-toeing (metatarsus adductus) as a result of in utero positioning (see Fig. 22.2). The feet remain flexible and may be passively moved to midline and in a straight position. This also resolves as the infant's musculoskeletal system matures. Pes planus (flat feet) is noted in infants when they begin to walk. The long arch of the foot is not yet developed and makes contact with the floor, resulting in a medial bulge. As the child grows and the muscles become less lax, the arch generally develops. Some children may continue with flexible flat feet, and this is considered an expected variation.

COMMON MEDICAL TREATMENTS

A variety of medications as well as other medical treatments are used to treat neuromuscular and musculoskeletal disorders in children. Most of these treatments will require a health care provider's or nurse practitioner's order when the child is in the hospital. The most common treatments and medications are listed in Common Medical Treatments 22.1 and Drug Guide 22.1. The nurse caring for the child with a neuromuscular or musculoskeletal disorder should become familiar with what these procedures are and how they work as well as common nursing implications related to use of these modalities. The treatment of musculoskeletal disorders often involves immobilization via casting, bracing, splinting, or traction to allow healing with the bones in appropriate alignment. The length of treatment with these immobilization methods varies from weeks to months depending on the type of disorder being treated and its severity. Complications related to casting and traction include neurovascular compromise, skin integrity impairment, soft tissue injury, compartment syndrome, and, with skeletal traction, pin site infection or osteomyelitis.

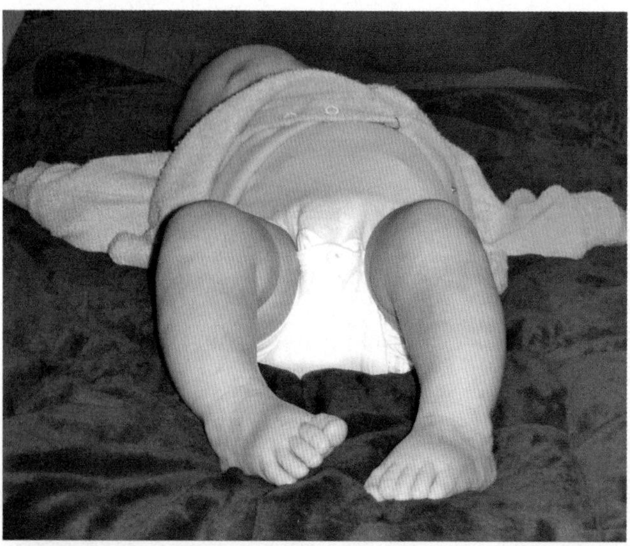

FIGURE 22.2 Internal tibial torsion with metatarsus adductus—expected findings in the infant.

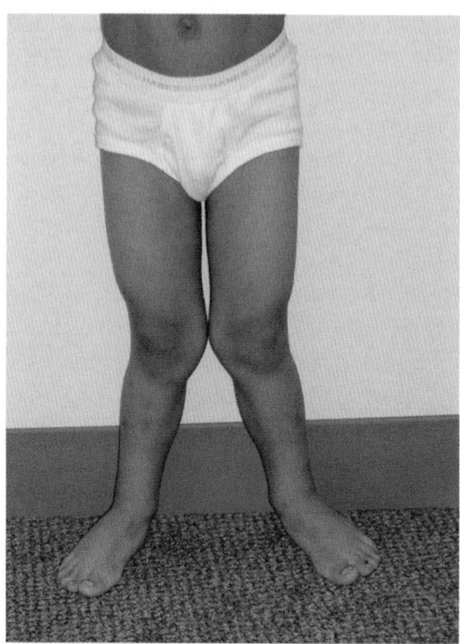

FIGURE 22.3 Genu valgum (knock-knees): note knees touching at midline and outward angle of the lower half of the legs.

Casts

Casts are used to immobilize a bone that has been injured or a diseased joint. When a fracture has occurred, a cast serves to hold the bone in reduction, thus preventing deformity as the fracture heals. Casts are constructed of a hard material, traditionally plaster but now more commonly fiberglass. The hard nature of the cast keeps the bone aligned so that healing may occur more quickly. In a fracture that would heal on its own without specific immobilization, a cast may be used to reduce pain and to allow the child increased mobility. The choice of cast material and type of cast will be determined by the health care provider or nurse practitioner or orthopedic surgeon. Figure 22.4 shows selected casts used in children.

COMMON MEDICAL TREATMENTS 22.1

Treatment	Explanation	Indications	Nursing Implications
Casting	Application of plaster or fiberglass material to form a rigid apparatus to immobilize a body part	Fracture reduction, dislocations, correction of deformities	Assess frequently for neurovascular compromise, skin impairment at cast edges. Protect the cast from moisture. Teach the family how to care for the cast at home.
Splinting	Temporary stiff support of injured area	Temporary fracture reduction, immobilization and support of sprains	Similar to cast care; some splints are removable and are replaced when the child is up out of bed. Teach the family appropriate use of splints.
Fixation	Surgical reduction of a fracture or skeletal deformity with an internal or external pin or fixation device	Fractures, skeletal deformities	No additional care for internal fixation External fixation: Perform pin care as prescribed by the surgeon. Assess for excess drainage or pin slippage; notify the health care provider or nurse practitioner if this occurs. Velcro or snaps on sleeves and pant legs help with dressing.
Cold therapy	Application of ice bags, commercial cold packs, or cold compresses	Most often used in acute injuries to cause vasoconstriction, thereby decreasing pain and swelling	Apply for 20–30 minutes, then remove for 1 hour, and reapply for 20–30 minutes. Discontinue when numbness occurs. Place a towel between the cold pack and the skin to prevent thermal injury.
Crutches	Ambulatory devices that transfer body weight from lower to upper extremities	Used whenever weight bearing is contraindicated	The top of the crutch should reach 2–3 fingerbreadths below the axillae to prevent nerve palsy. Teach the child appropriate ambulation with crutches or reinforce teaching if performed by a physical therapist.
Skeletal or cervical traction	Traction is an application of a pulling force on an extremity or body part.	To minimize or prevent trauma to the spinal cord; fracture reduction, dislocations, correction of deformities	To maintain even, constant traction: • Ensure weights hang free at all times and ropes remain in the pulley grooves. • Keep weights out of the child's reach. • Maintain prescribed weight. • Elevate the head or foot of bed only with health care provider order. Monitor for complications: • Perform neurovascular checks at least every 4 hours. • Monitor neurologic status closely. • Assess for signs and symptoms of infection or impaired skin integrity. • Provide appropriate pin site care.
Physical therapy, occupational therapy, or speech therapy	Physical therapy focuses on attainment or improvement of gross motor skills. Occupational therapy focuses on refinement of fine motor skills, feeding, and activities of daily living. Speech therapy is warranted for the child with a speech impairment or feeding difficulty related to oral muscular issues.	Cerebral palsy, spina bifida, spinal cord injury, muscular dystrophy, spinal muscular atrophy; restore function after injury or surgery; promote developmental activities when limb use is compromised, as in limb deficiency	Provide follow-through with prescribed exercises or supportive equipment. Success of the therapy is dependent on continued adherence to the prescribed regimen. Ensure that adequate communication exists within the interdisciplinary team.
Orthotics, braces	Adaptive positioning devices specially fitted for each child by the physical or occupational therapist or orthotist; used to maintain proper body or extremity alignment, improve mobility, and prevent contractures	Cerebral palsy, spinal cord injury, spina bifida, muscular dystrophy, spinal muscular atrophy; used to immobilize a body part or prevent deformity through positioning; used to treat developmental dysplasia of the hip and scoliosis; may also be used for a period of time after cast removal	Provide frequent assessments of skin covered by the device to avoid skin breakdown. A cotton undergarment worn under the brace helps to maintain skin integrity. Follow the therapist's schedule of recommended "on" and "off" times. Encourage the family to comply with use.

DRUG GUIDE 22.1

COMMON DRUGS FOR NEUROMUSCULAR DISORDERS

Medication	Actions/Indications	Nursing Implications
Benzodiazepines (diazepam, lorazepam)	Anticonvulsant; enhance the inhibition of GABA Used adjunctively for relief of skeletal muscle spasm associated with cerebral palsy, paralysis resulting from spinal cord injury, traction, and casting	Monitor sedation level. May cause dizziness Paradoxical excitement may occur. Assess for improvements in spasticity.
Baclofen (oral or intrathecal)	Central-acting skeletal muscle relaxant; precise mechanism unknown Used to treat painful spasms and decrease spasticity in children with motor neuron lesions, such as cerebral palsy and spinal cord injury	Assess motor function. Monitor for a decrease in spasticity. Observe for mental confusion, depression, or hallucinations. Dosage must be tapered before discontinuing because withdrawal symptoms may occur.
Corticosteroids	Antiinflammatory and immunosuppressive action Duchenne muscular dystrophy, myasthenia gravis, dermatomyositis	Administer with food to decrease GI upset. May mask signs of infection Do not stop treatment abruptly, or acute adrenal insufficiency may occur. Monitor for Cushing syndrome. Dosage may be tapered over time.
Botulin toxin	Neurotoxin produced by *Clostridium botulinum* that blocks neuromuscular conduction Relief of spasticity in cerebral palsy, occasionally for torticollis	Injected into the muscle by an advanced provider May cause dry mouth
Acetaminophen	Blocks pain impulses in response to inhibition of prostaglandin synthesis. Relief of mild pain if used alone; moderate or severe pain if used with a narcotic analgesic	Often combined with a narcotic such as codeine or oxycodone for increased analgesic effect Monitor pain levels and response to medication.
Narcotic analgesics	Act on receptors in the brain to alter perception of pain; relief of moderate to severe pain associated with injuries, orthopedic procedures	Assess pain location, quality, intensity, and duration. Assess respiratory rate prior to and periodically after administration. Monitor sedation level. May cause nausea, vomiting, constipation, pupil constriction
Nonsteroidal antiinflammatory drugs (NSAIDs: ibuprofen, ketorolac)	Inhibit prostaglandin synthesis, having a direct inhibitory effect on pain perception; relief of mild to moderate pain, treatment of Legg–Calvé–Perthes disease	Monitor for nausea, vomiting, diarrhea, and constipation. Administer with water or food to decrease GI upset.
Bisphosphonate: IV—pamidronate, zoledronic acid; oral—alendronate, risedronate	Increase bone mineral density, decrease incidence of fractures in moderate to severe osteogenesis imperfecta	IV: given at 4-month intervals, causes a decrease in serum calcium level, influenza-like reaction with first IV dose Oral: Side effects include heartburn, regurgitation, and upper abdominal discomfort.

GABA, γ-aminobutyric acid; GI, gastrointestinal; IV, intravenously.

Lexicomp (2023). Pediatric drug information. *UpToDate*. Retrieved May 10, 2023, from https://www.uptodate.com/contents/table-of-contents/drug-information/pediatric-drug-information

TAKE NOTE!

Gore-Tex is a special material that can be used to line casts and make them waterproof. These casts can get completely wet in the bath, in the shower, or during swimming. These casts cannot be used for all types of fractures, and they have an increased cost that may not be covered by insurance.

Traction

Traction, another common method of immobilization, may be used to reduce and/or immobilize a fracture, to align an injured extremity, and to allow the extremity to be restored to its normal length. Traction may also reduce pain by decreasing the incidence of muscle spasm. In running traction, the weight pulls directly on the extremity in only one plane. This may be achieved

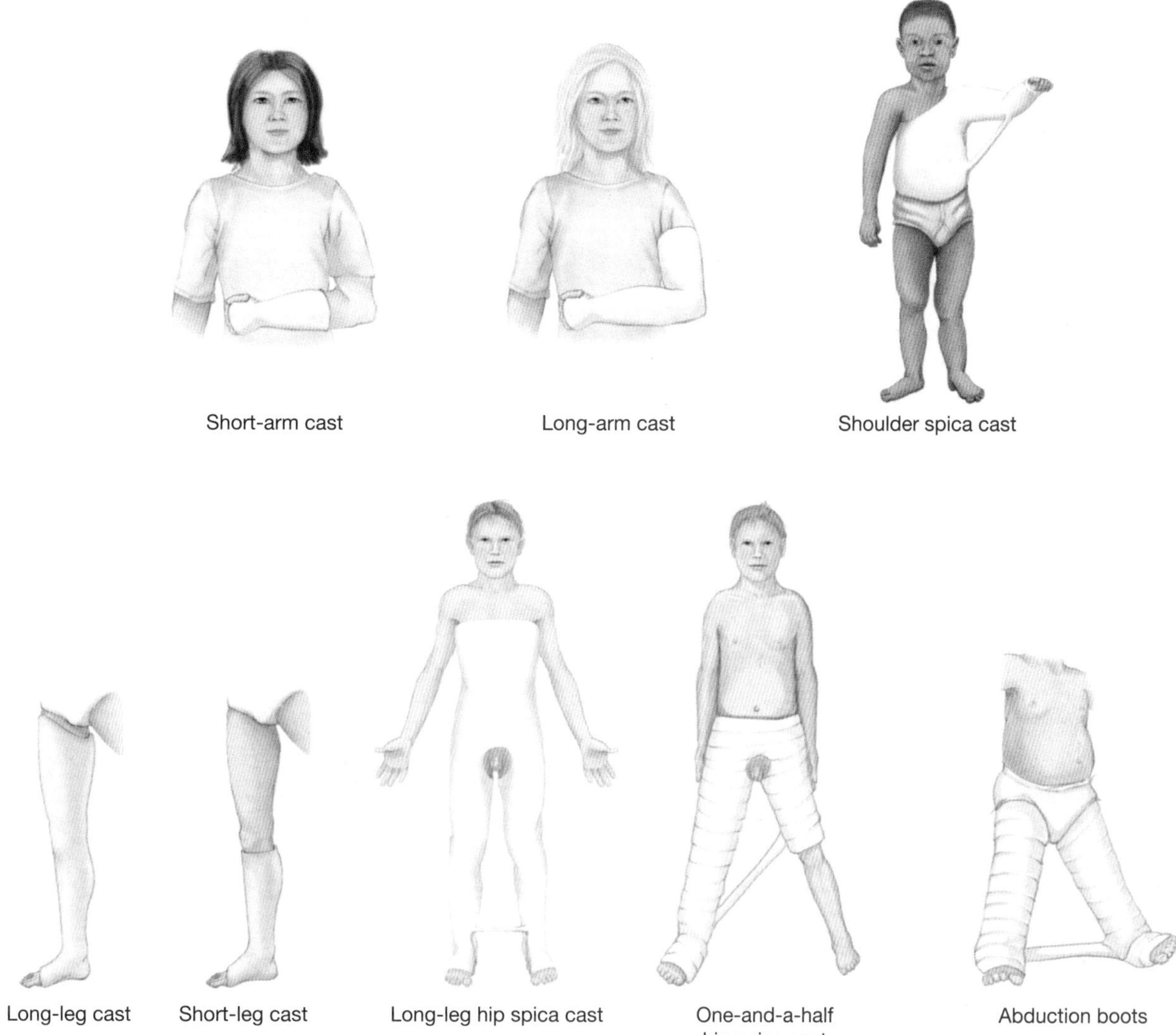

FIGURE 22.4 Selected casts used in children.

with either skin or skeletal traction. In balanced suspension traction, additional weights are used to provide a counterbalance to the force of traction. This allows for constant pull on the extremity even if the child changes position somewhat. Comparison Chart 22.1 discusses skin versus skeletal traction.

External Fixation

External fixation may be used for complicated fractures, especially open fractures with soft tissue damage. A series of pins or wires are inserted into bone and then attached to an external frame. The fixator apparatus may be adjusted as needed by the health care provider or

COMPARISON CHART 22.1 Skin Versus Skeletal Traction

	Skin Traction	Skeletal Traction
Application of force	To the skin via strips or tapes secured with Ace bandages or traction boots	To the body part directly by fixation into or through the bone
Length of treatment	Usually limited	Allows for longer periods of traction
Amount of force	Less	More

nurse practitioner. Once the desired level of correction is achieved, no further adjustment occurs, and the bone is allowed to heal. Advantages of external fixation include increased comfort for the injured child and improved function of muscles and joints when complicated fracture occurs.

Clinical Judgment and the Nursing Process for the Child With a Neuromuscular or Musculoskeletal Disorder

Care of the child with a neuromuscular or musculoskeletal disorder includes assessment, nursing analysis, planning, interventions, and evaluation. There are many general concepts related to the nursing process that may be applied to neuromuscular and musculoskeletal dysfunction in children. From an overall understanding of the care involved for a child with an alteration in mobility, the nurse can then individualize the care based on specifics particular to that child. The nursing care of immobilized children is similar to that of adults, yet developmental and age-appropriate effects must be taken into account. Prevention of complications is a key nursing function.

Assessment

Assessment of neuromuscular and musculoskeletal dysfunction in children includes health history, physical examination, and laboratory and diagnostic testing.

Health History

The health history consists of the past medical history, including the birthing parent's pregnancy history, family history, and history of present illness (when the symptoms started and how they have progressed), as well as treatments used at home. The past medical history might be significant for prematurity, difficult birth, infection during pregnancy, changes in gait, falls, delayed development, poor growth, musculoskeletal congenital anomaly, or orthopedic injury during the birthing process. Breech delivery may be associated with developmental DDH. Inquire about the child's usual level of physical activity, participation in sports, and use of protective equipment. Family history might be significant for neuromuscular disorders that are genetic or orthopedic problems. Determine the child's history of attainment of developmental milestones. Note the age at which milestones such as sitting, crawling, and walking were attained, and determine whether the pace of attainment of milestones has decreased. Some children may progress normally at first and then demonstrate decreased velocity of development of achievements or even loss of abilities. Obtain a clear description of weakness: Is it fatigue, or is the child truly not as strong as they were in the past?

When eliciting the history of the present illness, inquire about the following:

- Changes in gait or limp
- Recent trauma (determine the mechanism of injury)
- Recent strenuous exercise
- Poor feeding
- Lethargy
- Fever
- Weakness
- Alteration in muscle tone
- Areas of redness or swelling

Physical Examination

Physical examination of the nervous and musculoskeletal systems consists of inspection, observation, and palpation. It should also include auscultation of the heart and lungs, as the function of these organs may be affected by certain neuromuscular conditions.

INSPECTION AND OBSERVATION

Observe the infant or child playing with toys, crawling, or walking to obtain significant information about cranial nerve, cerebellar, and motor function. Observe the child's general appearance, noting any asymmetry in muscle development. Observe the child's posture and alignment of the trunk. Inspect the extremities for symmetry and positioning and for absence, duplication, or webbing of any digits. Note any obvious extremity deformity or limb-length discrepancy. When extremities are not used, muscular atrophy develops, so a shortened limb may indicate chronic hemiparesis. Observe gait in the child who has achieved the developmental skill of walking. Note refusal to walk, limping, in-toeing, out-toeing, or foot slap. Inspect injured joints for ecchymosis or swelling. In the injured extremity, note the color of the fingertips or toes. Observe spontaneous ROM. Perform scoliosis screening to determine spinal alignment. Note symmetry of thigh folds. Note symmetry of spontaneous movement of extremities as well as facial muscles. Determine cranial nerve function (refer back to Chapter 16 for a complete description of assessment of cranial nerves). Inspect the skin for redness, warmth, bruises, and puncture sites. Inspect the spine for cutaneous abnormalities such as dimples or hair tufts, which may be associated with spinal cord abnormalities. Observe the child's level of consciousness (LOC), noting a decrease or significant changes. Note the presence of lethargy. Refer to Chapter 16 for a complete description of evaluation of LOC.

Motor Function. Observe spontaneous activity, posture, and balance, and assess for asymmetric movements. In the infant, observe resting posture, which will normally be a slightly flexed posture. The infant should be able to extend extremities to an expected stretch. Note position of comfort of the infant's or child's neck.

Reflexes. Note sluggish or brisk deep tendon reflexes. Note persistence of primitive reflexes in the older infant or child, such as Moro or tonic neck. Assess for development of protective reflexes, which is often delayed in infants with motor disorders.

Sensory Function. Alterations in sensory function accompany many neuromuscular disorders. Assess sensory function in a similar fashion to that used in the adult. The sensory functions of light touch, pain, vibration, heat, and cold are distinguishable by a child. In the infant, assess for response to light touch or pain. The usual response to pain will be withdrawal from the stimulus. Always prepare the child for the sensory examination in order to gain cooperation. The pinprick test may be particularly frightening, but most children will cooperate if educated appropriately.

PALPATION

Assess muscle strength and tone in the infant or child. Compare strength and tone bilaterally. Evaluate neck tone by pulling the infant from a supine position to a sitting position (Fig. 22.5). By 4 to 5 months, the infant should be able to maintain the head in a neutral position. Perform passive ROM of the neck. Alterations in ROM may indicate a neuromuscular disorder or torticollis. Note trunk tone in the infant by holding the infant under the axillae and palpating for trunk tone. The hypotonic infant will feel as though they are slipping through the examiner's hands. Generalized hypotonia is a common sign of neuromuscular disease in the infant and young child (Sarant, 2020). The hypertonic infant will feel rigid, extending the trunk and legs. Assess leg tone in the infant by placing the infant in the vertical position with the feet on a flat surface; the 4-month-old infant should be able to momentarily support their weight (Fig. 22.6). Assess the strength of the infant or young child by noting ability to move the muscles against gravity. In older children, have the child push against the examiner's hand with the sole of the foot to determine muscle strength (Fig. 22.7). Note any hypertonia or **spasticity**, which is involuntary muscle contractions that are not coordinated with other muscles (e.g., when you stretch out your forearm, the triceps contract and the biceps stretch; in spasticity,

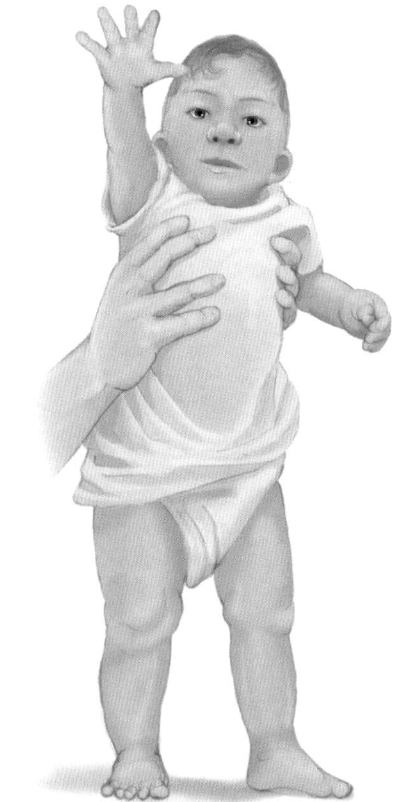

FIGURE 22.6 Assessing leg tone in an infant.

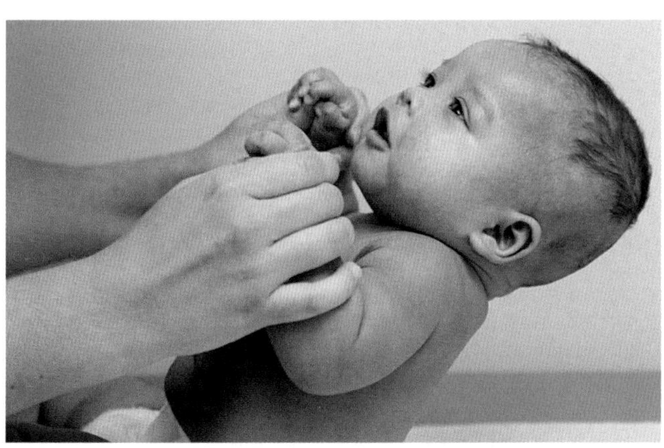

FIGURE 22.5 Assessing neck tone in an infant.

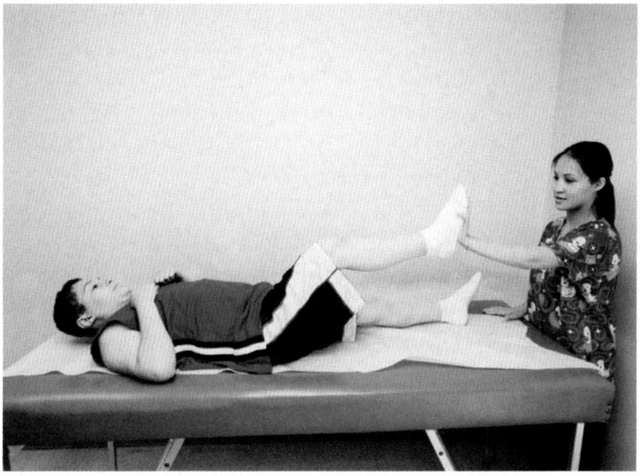

FIGURE 22.7 Assessing leg strength of the child.

they both contract at the same time). These may be an early indication of cerebral palsy or another neuromuscular disorder.

CLINICAL REASONING ALERT!

In cases of trauma or suspected trauma, do not perform any assessment that involves movement of the head and neck until cervical injury is ruled out. Maintain complete immobilization of the cervical spine until that time.

Palpate the clavicles in the newborn or young infant for tenderness or a bump that indicates callus formation with clavicle fracture. Perform active ROM to determine if a joint position is fixed (e.g., clubfoot). Palpate the affected joint or extremity to detect warmth or tenderness. In the injured child or the child with a cast or splint, thoroughly assess the neurovascular status of the affected extremities. Palpate the fingers or toes for warmth. Determine the capillary refill time. Note the presence of sensation or motion. Evaluate muscle strength. Palpate pulses distal to the injury, noting their strength and quality. Perform the Ortolani and Barlow maneuvers (see the "Developmental Dysplasia of the Hip" section later in this chapter) to assess for DDH.

TAKE NOTE!

Assess the injured site last and do so gently.

AUSCULTATION

Auscultate the child's lungs; adventitious sounds are often present when respiratory muscle function is impaired.

Laboratory and Diagnostic Testing

Common Laboratory and Diagnostic Tests 22.1 offers an explanation of the laboratory and diagnostic tests most commonly used in neuromuscular and musculoskeletal disorders. The tests can assist the health

COMMON LABORATORY AND DIAGNOSTIC TESTS 22.1

Test	Explanation	Indications	Nursing Implications
Radiographs (x-rays)	Radiographic image; usually, two views are obtained of the affected extremity (lateral and anteroposterior).	To detect fractures and other anomalies	The child must hold still. Enlist the family's help in calming the child. In the patient who has experienced trauma, the cervical spine should remain immobilized until cleared after cervical spine radiographs.
Fluoroscopy	Radiographic examination that uses continuous x-rays to show live, real-time images	Assessment of cervical spine instability during movement	The child may be afraid of the x-ray machine but will need to cooperate with flexion and extension of the neck. Allow a parent or family member to accompany the child.
Myelography	X-ray study of the spinal cord allowing visualization of the cord, nerve roots, and surrounding meninges	Detection of space-occupying lesions of the spinal cord; visualization of neural tube defects; evaluation of traumatic injury	This involves injection of contrast medium into the CSF via lumbar puncture. Postprocedure interventions vary based on type of contrast medium; therefore, determine which one was used. After the procedure, bed rest is necessary for 4–24 hours; keep the head of bed elevated for several hours. Encourage hydration. Observe for signs of meningeal irritation.
Ultrasound	Use of sound waves to locate the depth and structure within soft tissues and fluid	Assessment of spinal abnormalities; to diagnose Legg–Calvé–Perthes disease, slipped capital femoral epiphysis, fractures, ligament or soft tissue injuries Monitoring and follow-up of fractures and remodeling	Better tolerated by children who are not sedated than CT or MRI Can be performed with a portable unit at bedside.

COMMON LABORATORY AND DIAGNOSTIC TESTS 22.1

Test	Explanation	Indications	Nursing Implications
Computed tomography (CT)	Noninvasive x-ray study that looks at tissue density and structures; images a "slice" of tissue	Evaluation of congenital abnormalities such as neural tube defects, fractures, demyelinization, or inflammation; to evaluate the extent of Legg–Calvé–Perthes disease or slipped capital femoral epiphysis or to rule out other problems	The machine is large and can be frightening to children. The procedure can be lengthy, and the child must remain still. If they are unable to do so, sedation may be necessary. If performed with contrast medium, assess for allergy. Encourage fluids after the procedure if not contraindicated.
Magnetic resonance imaging (MRI)	Based on how hydrogen atoms behave in a magnetic field when disturbed by radiofrequency signals; does not require ionizing radiation; provides a 3D view of the body part being scanned	Assessment of inflammation, congenital abnormalities such as neural tube defects; to assess hard and soft tissue, as well as bone marrow; to evaluate the extent of Legg–Calvé–Perthes disease or slipped capital femoral epiphysis or to rule out other problems	Remove all metal objects from the child. The child must remain motionless for the entire scan; the parent can stay in the room with the child. Younger children will require sedation in order to be still. A loud thumping sound occurs inside the machine during the procedure; this can be frightening to children. Most new surgical implants are now MRI-compatible; consult the imaging center.
Creatine kinase	Reflects muscle damage; leaks from muscle into plasma as muscles deteriorate	Diagnosis of muscular dystrophy, spinal muscular atrophy	Draw the sample before electromyogram or muscle biopsy, as those tests may lead to release of creatine kinase.
Electromyography (EMG)	A recording electrode is placed in the skeletal muscle, and electrical activity is recorded.	Differentiates muscular disorders from those that are neurologic in origin	EMG requires insertion of short needles into the muscles. Sedation or analgesia may be ordered.
Nerve conduction velocity	Measures the speed of nerve conduction. Patch-like electrodes are attached to the skin at various nerve locations.	Differentiation of muscular disorders	Feels like mild electric shocks EMG often performed at the same time
Muscle biopsy	Removal of a piece of muscular tissue either by needle or by open biopsy	Determination of type of muscular dystrophy or spinal muscular atrophy	Postbiopsy care is similar to that for other types of biopsies. Involves a small incision with one or two sutures
Complete blood count	Evaluates hemoglobin and hematocrit, white blood cell count, platelet count	To evaluate hemoglobin and hematocrit with fracture with potential bleeding; to determine toxic synovitis	Expected values vary according to age and sex. A white blood cell count differential is helpful in evaluating for infection. May be affected by myelosuppressive drugs
Arthrography	Multiple radiographic images of a joint after direct injection with a radiopaque substance	To assess ligaments, muscles, tendons, and cartilage, particularly after injury	It should not be performed if joint infection is present. The joint should be rested for 12 hours. Apply cold therapy afterward, and assess for swelling and pain. Crepitus may be present in the joint for 1–2 days after procedure.
Genetic testing	Tests for presence of the gene for the disease or for carrier status	Determination of disease or carrier status of inherited muscular disorder	The entire family should be tested, even those unaffected, because carrier status should be determined, and genetic counseling related to reproduction should be provided.

Data from Fischbach, F. T., Fischbach, M. A., & Stout, K. (2022). *A manual of laboratory and diagnostic tests* (11th ed.). Wolters Kluwer.

care provider or nurse practitioner in diagnosing the disorder and/or can be used as guidelines in determining ongoing treatment. Laboratory or nonnursing personnel perform some of the tests, while the nurse might perform others. In either instance, the nurse should be familiar with how the tests are performed, what they are used for, and expected versus unexpected results. This knowledge will also be necessary when providing child and family education related to the testing.

Remember Frederick, the 4-year-old child who has been falling and having difficulty climbing stairs and who seems to tire easily when playing with his sibling? What additional health history and physical examination assessment information should the nurse obtain?

Nursing Analysis

After recognizing and analyzing cues from a thorough assessment, the nurse might identify several patient problems, including:

- Pain
- Impaired physical mobility
- Malnutrition risk
- Urinary retention
- Constipation risk
- Activities of daily living (ADLs) deficit (specify)
- Altered skin integrity risk
- Chronic sorrow
- Injury risk
- Knowledge deficiency (specify)
- Delayed development risk
- Family processes, interrupted

After completing an assessment of Fredrick, the nurse noted the following: He started walking at 2 years of age, he has difficulty jumping, his gait has a waddling appearance, and he does not rise from the floor in the usual fashion. Based on these assessment findings, what would your top three patient problems be for Fredrick?

These patient problems or concerns provide suggestions for developing a nursing plan of care or concept map. The nurse will then generate solutions by planning interventions (suggested following with rationales). The plan of care should be individualized, based on the child's and family's needs. Refer to Chapter 14 for the nursing process for pain management and to Chapter 11 for nursing interventions related to interrupted family processes and risk for caregiver role strain. Additional information will be included later in the chapter as it relates to specific disorders.

Nursing Analysis

Impaired physical mobility related to decrease in muscle control, mass, and/or strength; pain; joint stiffness; contractures; musculoskeletal or neuromuscular impairment as evidenced by an inability to move extremities, to ambulate without assistance, to move without limitations.

Goal/Outcome

The child will be able to engage in activities within age parameters and limits of injury or disease; the child is able to move their extremities, move about the environment, assist with transfers and positioning in bed, and/or participate in exercise programs within the limits of age and disease.

Maximizing Physical Mobility (interventions with *rationale*)

- Assess the child's ability to move based on the injury or disease and within limits of prescribed treatment *to determine baseline.*
- Prior to prescribed exercise or major position changes, ensure that pain medication is given; *relief of pain increases the child's ability to tolerate and participate in activity.*
- Encourage gross and fine motor activities *to facilitate motor development.*
- Collaborate with physical therapy, occupational therapy, and speech therapy to strengthen muscles and promote optimal mobility. Support therapy activities by using the same equipment and technique *to help rehabilitate musculoskeletal deficits, improve mobility, facilitate motor development, and allow for maximum functioning.*
- Use passive and active ROM exercises and teach the child and family how to perform them *to prevent contractures, facilitate joint mobility and muscle development (active ROM), and help increase mobility.*
- Praise accomplishments and emphasize the child's abilities *to improve self-esteem and encourage feelings of confidence and competence.*
- Teach the child and family necessary care related to mobility issues *so the family can continue with these measures at home.*

Nursing Analysis

Malnutrition risk related to insufficient dietary intake (difficulty feeding secondary to deficient sucking, swallowing, or chewing; difficulty assuming normal feeding position; inability to feed self) as evidenced by decreased oral intake, impaired swallowing, weight loss, or plateau.

Goal/Outcome

The child will exhibit signs of adequate nutrition as evidenced by appropriate weight gain, intake and output within normal limits, and adequate ingestion of calories.

Promoting Adequate Nutrition (interventions with *rationale*)

- Monitor height and weight: *Insufficient intake will lead to impaired growth and weight gain.*

- Monitor hydration status (moist mucous membranes, elastic skin turgor, adequate urine output): *Insufficient intake can lead to dehydration.*
- Use techniques to promote caloric and nutritional intake, and teach the family about these techniques (e.g., positioning, modified utensils, soft or blended foods, allowing extra time) *to facilitate intake.*
- Assess the respiratory system frequently *to assess for aspiration.*
- Assist the family to help the child assume as normal a feeding position as possible *to help increase oral intake.*

Nursing Analysis

Urinary retention related to sensory motor impairment as evidenced by dribbling, inadequate bladder emptying.

Goal/Outcome

The child's bladder will empty adequately, according to preestablished quantities and frequencies individualized for the child (usual urine output is 0.5 to 2 mL/kg/h).

Promoting Successful Bladder Emptying (interventions with *rationale*)

- Assess the child's ability to empty their bladder via history focused on character and duration of lower urinary symptoms *to establish baseline.*
- Assess for history of fecal impaction or constipation, *as alterations in bowel elimination may hinder urinary elimination.*
- Assess for bladder distention by palpation or urinary retention by postvoid residual obtained via catheterization or bladder ultrasound *to determine the extent of retention.*
- Maintain adequate hydration *to avoid irritating effects that dehydration has on the bladder.*
- Schedule voiding *to decrease bladder overdistention.*
- Teach the family and the child (if old enough) with significant urinary retention the technique of clean intermittent catheterization *to allow regular, complete bladder emptying.*

Nursing Analysis

Constipation risk (risk factors: average daily physical activity is less than recommended for sex and age, decreased gastrointestinal motility [immobility, loss of sensation, and/or use of narcotic analgesics]).

Goal/Outcome

Child will demonstrate adequate stool passage: will pass soft, formed stool every 1 to 3 days without straining or other adverse effects.

Promoting Appropriate Bowel Elimination (interventions with *rationale*)

- Assess usual pattern of stooling *to determine baseline and identify potential problems with elimination.*
- Palpate for abdominal fullness and auscultate for bowel sounds *to assess for bowel function and presence of constipation.*
- Encourage fiber intake *to increase frequency of stools.*
- Ensure adequate fluid intake *to prevent formation of hard, dry stools.*
- Encourage activity within the child's limits or restrictions: *even minimal activity increases peristalsis.*
- Administer medications or enemas as ordered *to promote bowel training/evacuation (especially in the child with myelomeningocele or spinal cord injury).*

Nursing Analysis

Difficulty with ADLs, bathing, dressing, feeding; deficit related to muscular, skeletal, and/or neuromuscular impairments; alteration in cognitive functioning; weakness, pain, or fatigue as evidenced by an inability to perform hygiene care and transfer self independently.

Goal/Outcome

The child will demonstrate ability to care for themselves within age parameters and limits of injury or disease; the child is able to feed, dress, and manage elimination within limits of injury, disease, and age.

Maximizing Self-Care (interventions with *rationale*)

- Introduce the child and family to self-help methods as soon as possible *to promote independence from the beginning.*
- Encourage the family and staff to allow the child to do as much as possible *to allow the child to gain confidence and independence.*
- Teach specific measures for bowel and urinary elimination as needed *to promote independence and increase self-care abilities and self-esteem.*
- Collaborate with physical therapy, occupational therapy, and speech therapy to provide the child and family with appropriate tools to modify the environment and methods to promote transferring and self-care *to allow for maximum functioning.*
- Praise accomplishments and emphasize the child's abilities *to improve self-esteem and encourage feelings of confidence and competence.*
- Balance activity with periods of rest *to reduce fatigue and increase energy for self-care.*

Nursing Analysis

Altered skin integrity risk; risk factors include pressure over bony prominences, alteration in sensation, impaired circulation (immobility, casting, traction, use of braces or adaptive devices).

Goal/Outcome

The child's skin will remain intact, without evidence of redness or breakdown.

Promoting Skin Integrity (interventions with *rationale*)

- Monitor the condition of the entire skin surface at least daily *to provide a baseline and to allow for early identification of areas at risk.*
- Avoid excessive friction or harsh cleaning products *that may increase risk of skin breakdown in the child with susceptible skin.*
- Keep the child's skin free from stool and urine *to decrease risk of breakdown.*
- Keep linen clean, dry, and free from food crumbs and wrinkles *to prevent pressure areas from forming.*
- Change the child's position frequently *to decrease pressure to susceptible areas.*
- Monitor skin condition affected by braces or adaptive equipment frequently *to prevent skin breakdown related to poor fit.*

For the child in traction:

- Pad bony prominences with cotton padding before applying traction *to protect skin from injury.*
- Gently massage the child's back and sacrum with lotion *to stimulate circulation.*

For the child in a spica cast:

- Apply plastic wrap to the perineal edges of the cast *to prevent soiling of cast edges, which can contribute to cast breakdown.*
- Use a fracture bedpan *to facilitate toileting without soiling the cast.*
- For the child still in diapers, tuck a smaller diaper under the perineal edges of the cast, and cover it with a larger diaper *to prevent cast soiling.*

Nursing Analysis

Chronic sorrow related to presence of chronic disability, missed milestones, missed opportunities as evidenced by child's or family's expression of sadness, anger, disappointment, or feeling overwhelmed.

Goal/Outcome

The child and family will accept the situation; the child and family will appropriately identify feelings, function at a normal developmental level, and plan for the future.

Easing Sorrow (interventions with *rationale*)

- Assess degree of sorrow *to provide baseline for intervention.*
- Identify problems with eating or sleeping; *these are often affected when grief or sorrow is present.*
- Spend time with the child and family: *An empathetic presence is valued by suffering families.*
- Encourage the use of positive coping techniques: *Taking action, expressing feelings, and intentional attempts at coping are helpful techniques.*
- Refer the family to appropriate support groups: *It can be helpful to talk to others in similar situations.*
- Refer the family spiritual counseling as desired: *Many families experience grief resolution in a timelier fashion if their spiritual needs are addressed.*

Nursing Analysis

Injury risk; risk factors include unsafe mode of transport (muscle weakness).

Goal/Outcome

The child will remain free from injury; the child will not fall or experience other injury.

Preventing Injury (interventions with *rationale*)

- Ensure that the side rails of bed are elevated when the caregiver is not directly at bedside *to prevent a fall from bed.*
- Use appropriate safety restraints with adaptive equipment and wheelchairs *to prevent a fall or slipping from equipment.*
- Do not leave the child unattended in the tub *as weakness may cause the child to slip under the water.*
- Avoid restraint use if at all possible. Close observation is more appropriate. *It is in the best interest of the child to use the least restrictive measure while maintaining the child's safety.*

Nursing Analysis

Knowledge deficiency related to insufficient information regarding cast care, activity restrictions, complex medical condition, prognosis, and/or medical needs as evidenced by verbalization, questions, or actions demonstrating lack of understanding regarding the child's condition or care.

Goal/Outcome

The child and family will verbalize accurate information and understanding about the condition, prognosis, and medical needs; the child and family will demonstrate knowledge of the condition, prognosis, and medical needs, including possible causes, contributing factors, and treatment measures, through verbalization and return demonstration.

Providing Child and Family Teaching (interventions with *rationale*)

- Assess the child's and family's willingness to learn: The *child and family must be willing to learn for teaching to be effective.*
- Provide the family with time to adjust to the diagnosis *to facilitate adjustment and ability to learn and participate in the child's care.*
- Repeat information *to allow the family and child time to learn and understand.*
- Teach in short sessions: *Multiple short sessions are more helpful than one long session.*
- Gear teaching to the level of understanding of the child and family as appropriate for the age of child, physical condition, and memory *to ensure understanding.*

- Provide reinforcement and rewards *to facilitate the teaching and learning process.*
- Use multiple modes of learning involving multiple senses (provide written, verbal, demonstration, and videos) when possible: The *child and family are more likely to retain information when it is presented in different ways using multiple senses.*

Nursing Analysis

Delayed development risk; risk factors include treatment regimen, chronic illness (immobility, alterations in extremities).

Goal/Outcome

Development will be enhanced; the child will make continued progress toward developmental milestones and will not show regression in abilities.

Promoting Development (interventions with *rationale*)

- Screen for developmental capabilities *to determine the child's current level of functioning.*
- Offer age-appropriate toys, play, and activities (including gross motor) *to encourage further development.*
- Perform exercises or interventions as prescribed by the physical or occupational therapist: *Repeat participation in those activities helps to promote function and acquisition of developmental skills.*
- Provide support to the child and family: Immobility *and extremity deficits may lead to slow progress in achieving developmental milestones, so ongoing motivation is needed.*

Assisting With Cast Application

Before cast or splint application, perform baseline neurovascular assessment for comparison after immobilization. Include:

- Color (note cyanosis or other discoloration)
- Movement (note inability to move fingers or toes)
- Sensation (note whether loss of sensation is present)
- Edema
- Quality of pulses

Enlist the cooperation of the child, and reduce their fear by showing the child the cast materials and using an age-appropriate approach to describe cast application. Premedicate as ordered to reduce pain when manual traction is applied to align the bone. Use distraction throughout cast application, and assist with application of the cast or splint (Fig. 22.8).

TAKE NOTE!

Modern fiberglass cast materials are available in a variety of colors, as well as a few patterns. Allowing the child to choose the color will increase the child's cooperation with the procedure.

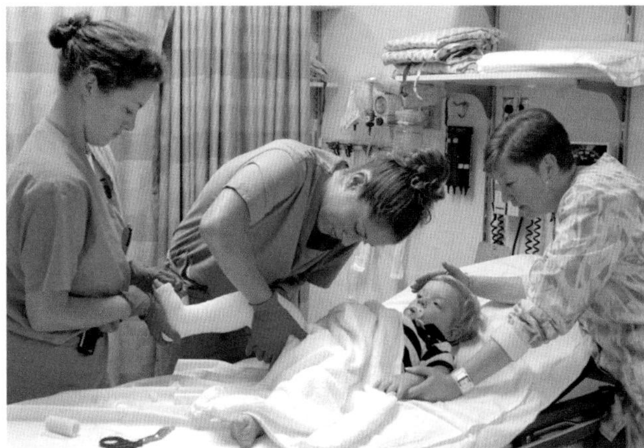

FIGURE 22.8 Assist with cast application by distracting or comforting the child.

After the cast or splint is applied, drying time will vary based on the type of material used. Splints and fiberglass casts usually take only a few minutes to dry and will cause a very warm feeling inside the cast, so warn the child that it will begin to feel warm. Plaster requires 24 to 48 hours to dry. Take care not to cause depressions in the plaster cast while drying, as those may cause skin pressure and breakdown. Instruct the child and family to keep the cast still, positioning it with pillows as needed.

Caring for the Child With a Cast

Perform frequent neurovascular checks of the casted extremity to identify signs of compromise early. These signs include:

- Increased pain
- Increased edema
- Pale or blue color
- Skin coolness
- Numbness or tingling
- Prolonged capillary refill
- Decreased pulse strength (or absence of pulse)

Notify the health care provider or nurse practitioner of changes in neurovascular status or odor or drainage from the cast.

Fiberglass casts usually have a soft fabric edge, so they usually do not cause skin rubbing at the edges of the cast. On the other hand, plaster casts require special treatment of the cast edge to prevent skin rubbing. This may be accomplished through a technique called petaling: cut rounded-edge strips of moleskin or another soft material with an adhesive backing and apply them to the edge of the cast, as shown in Figure 22.9.

TAKE NOTE!

If a cast is lined with Gore-Tex, do not petal it.

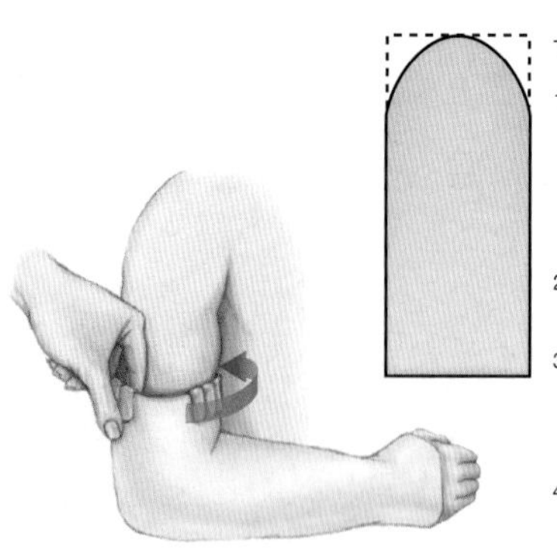

To petal a cast:

1. Cut several strips of adhesive tape or Moleskin 3 to 4 in in length. Use 1 in tape for smaller areas (e.g., infant's foot) and 2 in tape for larger areas (e.g., adolescent's waist).
2. Round one end of each strip to keep the corners from rolling.
3. Apply the first strip by tucking the straight end inside the cast and by bringing the rounded end over the cast edge to the outside.
4. Repeat the procedure, overlapping each additional strip, until all rough edges are completely covered.

FIGURE 22.9 Petaling the cast.

Position the child with the casted extremity elevated on pillows. Ice may be applied during the first 24 to 48 hours after casting if needed. Teaching the child to use crutches is an important nursing intervention for any child with lower extremity immobilization so that the child can maintain mobility (Fig. 22.10). Provide home care instructions to the family about cast care (see Teaching Guidelines 22.1).

CLINICAL REASONING ALERT!

Persistent complaints of pain may indicate compromised skin integrity under the cast.

Assisting With Cast Removal

Children may be frightened by cast removal. Prepare the child using age-appropriate terminology:

- The cast cutter will make a loud noise (Fig. 22.11).
- The skin or extremity will not be injured. (Demonstrate by touching the cast cutter lightly to your palm.)
- The child will feel warmth or vibration during cast removal.

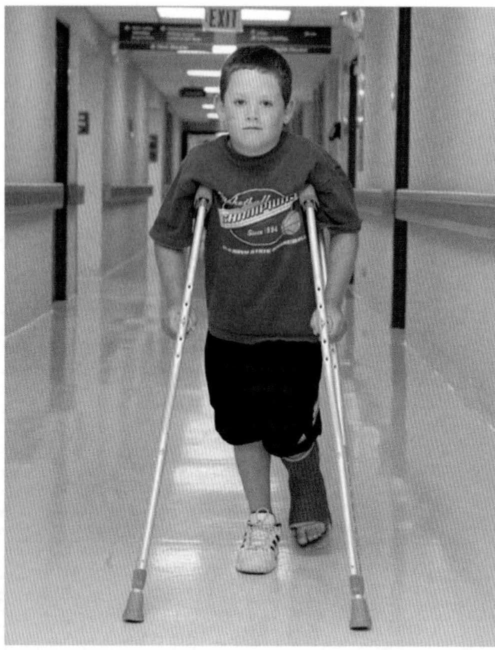

FIGURE 22.10 Reinforce appropriate crutch walking for children with lower extremity immobilization.

TEACHING GUIDELINES **22.1** Home Cast Care

- For the first 48 hours, elevate the extremity above the level of the heart and apply cold therapy for 20 minutes, then off for 2 hours, and repeat while awake.
- Take your prescribed pain medication for at least the first 48 hours.
- Assess for swelling, and have the child wiggle the fingers or toes frequently (hourly while awake).
- For itching inside the cast:
  - Never insert anything into the cast for the purposes of scratching.
  - Blow cool air in from a hair dryer set on the lowest setting or tap lightly on the cast.
  - Do not use lotions or powders.
- Do not pull padding out from the inside of the cast.
- Protect the cast from wetness.
  - Apply two plastic bags around the cast, and tape each bag separately and securely for bathing or showering. Continue to avoid placing the cast directly in water (unless it is Gore-Tex lined).
  - Waterproof cast covers are available through medical supply stores, but remain cautious about submerging the cast in water.
  - Cover the cast when your child eats or drinks.
  - If the cast becomes soiled, it can be wiped clean with a slightly damp clean cloth.
  - If the cast gets wet, dry it with a blow dryer on the cold setting. (If the warm setting is used, the child could get burned). Use of a vacuum cleaner with a hose attachment to pull air through may speed drying; be careful to avoid skin.
- If the child has a large cast, change position every 2 hours during the day; while sleeping, change position as often as possible.
- Check the skin for irritation.
  - Press the skin back around edges of the cast.
  - Use a flashlight to look for reddened or irritated areas.
  - Feel for blisters or sores.
- Call the health care provider or nurse practitioner if:
  - The casted extremity is cool to the touch, pale, blue, or very swollen.
  - The child cannot move the fingers or toes.
  - Severe pain occurs when the child attempts to move the fingers or toes.
  - Persistent numbness or tingling occurs.
  - Drainage or a foul smell comes from under the cast.
  - Severe itching occurs inside the cast.
  - The child runs a fever greater than 101.5°F for longer than 24 hours.
  - Skin edges are red and swollen or exhibit breakdown.
  - The child complains of rubbing or burning under the cast.
  - The cast gets wet and does not dry or is cracked, split, or softened.

Data from Schweich, P. (2021). Patient education: Cast and splint care (Beyond the Basics). *UpToDate*. Retrieved May 11, 2023, from https://www.uptodate.com/contents/cast-and-splint-care-beyond-the-basics

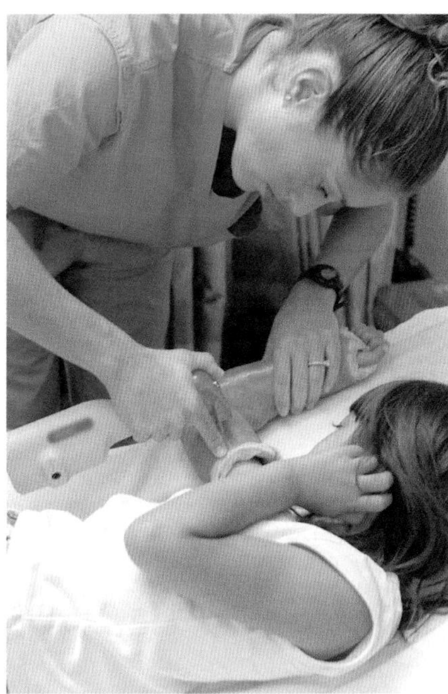

FIGURE 22.11 The loud noise of the cast saw may frighten the child.

Teaching Guidelines 22.2 gives instructions related to skin care after cast removal.

Caring for the Child in Traction

Nursing care of the child in any type of traction focuses not only on appropriate application and maintenance of traction but also on promoting normal growth and development and preventing complications (Table 22.1). Apply skin traction over intact skin only so that the pull of the traction is effective. Prepare the skin with an appropriate adhesive before applying the traction tapes to ensure that the tapes adhere well, preventing skin friction. After application of the traction tapes, apply the elastic bandage or use the foam boot. Attach the traction spreader block, and then apply the prescribed amount of weight via a rope attached to the spreader block. Ensure that the rope moves without obstruction and that the weights hang freely without touching the floor.

In skeletal traction, apply weight via ropes attached to the skeletal pins. Treat the pin sites as surgical wounds (see "The Providing Pin Care" section). Protect the exposed ends of the pins to avoid injury. Whether skin or skeletal traction is used, be sure that constant and even traction is maintained.

TEACHING GUIDELINES 22.2 Skin Care After Cast Removal

- Brown, flaky skin is normal and occurs as dead skin, and secretions accumulate under the cast.
- New skin may be tender.
- Soak with warm water daily.
- Wash with warm soapy water, avoiding excessive rubbing, which may traumatize the skin.
- Discourage the child from scratching the dry skin.
- Apply moisturizing lotion to relieve dry skin.
- Encourage activity to regain strength and motion of extremity.

TAKE NOTE!

Avoid sudden bumping or movement of the bed; this can disturb traction alignment, and cause additional pain to the child as the weights are jostled.

Preventing Complications

Refer to the "Clinical Judgment and the Nursing Process" section in Chapter 14 for interventions related to pain management, and refer to earlier discussions in this chapter for interventions related to prevention of complications of immobility such as skin integrity impairment. To prevent **contractures** (the shortening and hardening of muscles, tendons, or tissues leading to fixated and stiff joints) and atrophy that may result from disuse of muscles, ensure that unaffected extremities are exercised. Assist the child to exercise the unaffected joints and to use the unaffected extremity if this does not disrupt traction alignment. Promote use of a trapeze if not contraindicated to involve the child in repositioning and assist with movement. Encourage deep-breathing exercises to prevent the pulmonary complications of long-term immobilization.

Promote normal growth and development by:

- Placing age-appropriate toys within the child's reach
- Encouraging visits from friends
- Providing diversional activities such as drawing, coloring, or video games (Fig. 22.12)

CLINICAL REASONING ALERT!

Ongoing, careful neurovascular assessments are critical in the child with a cast or in skeletal traction. Notify the health care provider or nurse practitioner immediately if these signs of compartment syndrome occur: extreme pain (out of proportion to the situation), pain with passive ROM of digits, distal extremity pallor, inability to move digits, or loss of pulses.

Caring for the Child With an External Fixator

Care of the child with an external fixator involves maintaining skin integrity, preventing infection, and preventing injury. Routine neurovascular and skin assessment is essential. Skin care is similar to that for the child in skeletal traction and includes pin care daily. Elevation of the extremity can help prevent swelling. The fixator may be moved by grasping the frame, as the fixator can tolerate ordinary movement. Encourage weight bearing as prescribed. Provide appropriate education to the child and family. Encourage the child to look at the apparatus. Teach the child not to pick or manipulate the pins. Baggy or loose clothing can be worn over the device. Velcro sewn into the seams can be helpful and allows clothes to slip over the device.

TABLE 22.1 • Types of Traction and Nursing Implications

Type of Traction	Description	Nursing Implications
Bryant traction 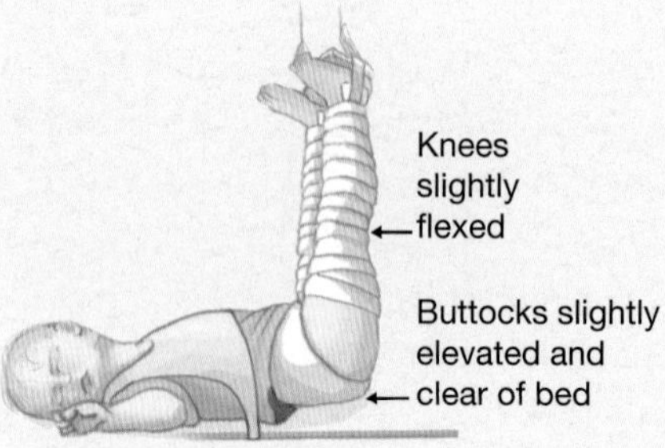 Knees slightly flexed Buttocks slightly elevated and clear of bed	Both legs are extended vertically, with the child's weight serving as countertraction. Skin traction is applied to both legs. Bryant traction is used to reduce femur fracture in children younger than 2 years or with developmental dysplasia of the hip.	Maintain appropriate position. Ensure the heels and ankles are free from pressure. Assess the condition and position of the elastic bandages every shift, and rewrap the elastic bandages as ordered.
Russell traction 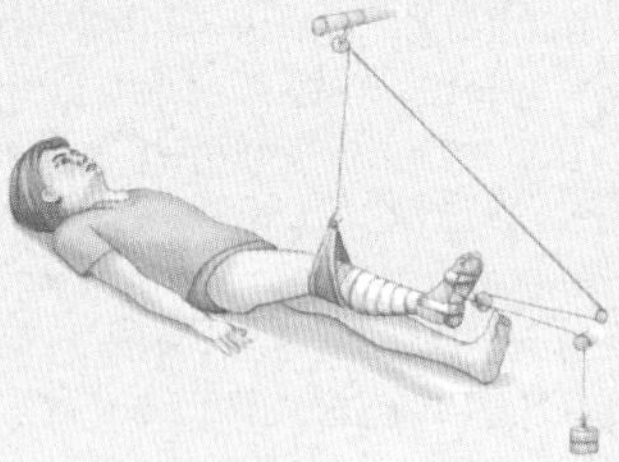	Skin traction for femur fracture, hip, and specific types of knee injuries or contractures. Uses a knee sling. In split Russell traction, a portion of the traction weight may be redistributed via a pulley from the sling to the head of the bed (used for femur fracture, Legg–Calvé–Perthes disease, and slipped capital femoral epiphysis).	Wrap bandages from the ankle to thigh on children younger than age 2 years and from the ankle to knee on children older than 2 years. Use a foot support to prevent foot drop. Ensure the heel is free from the bed. Assess the popliteal region for skin breakdown from the sling. Mark the leg to ensure proper replacement of sling.
Buck traction 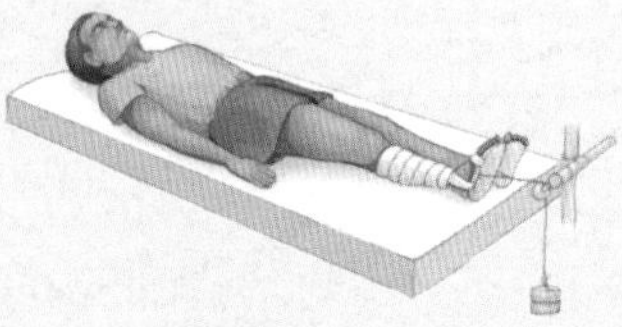	Skin traction for hip and knee contractures, Legg–Calvé–Perthes disease, and slipped capital femoral epiphysis. Used to rest an injured limb or to prevent spasms of injured muscles or joints Traction force delivered in straight line	Remove the traction boot every 8 hours to assess skin. The leg may be slightly abducted.
Cervical skin traction 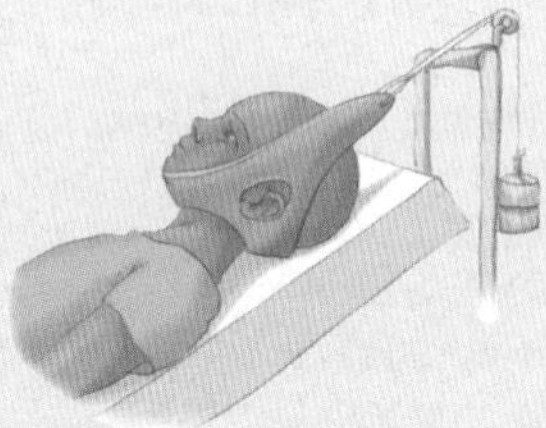	Skin traction applied with a skin strap (head halter). Used for neck sprains/strains, torticollis, or nerve trauma	Ensure that the head halter or skin strap does not place pressure on the ears or throat. Limit of 5 to 7 lb of weight
Side-arm 90–90 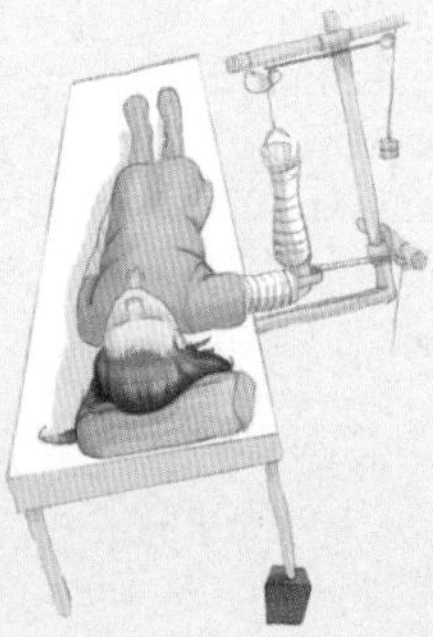	Skin traction used to treat fractures of the humerus and injuries in or around the shoulder girdle	Maintain elbow flexed at 90 degrees. The fingers and hand may feel cool because of elevation. The child may turn to the affected side only.

TABLE 22.1 • Types of Traction and Nursing Implications

Type of Traction	Description	Nursing Implications
Dunlop side-arm 00–90 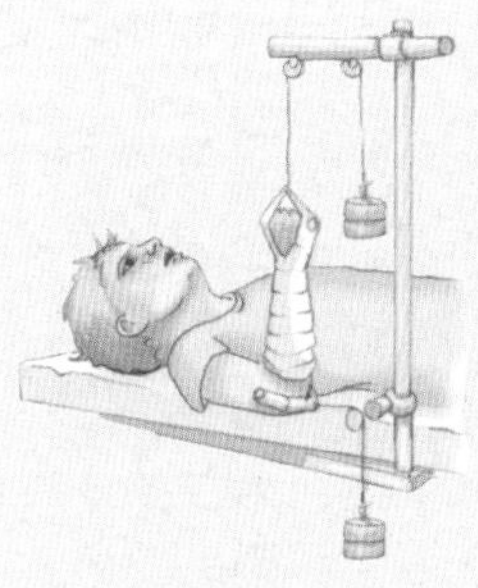	Skeletal traction through an olecranon screw or pin in distal humerus. The lower arm is held in balanced suspension.	See side-arm 90–90. In addition, provide appropriate pin site care.
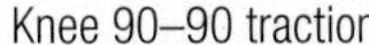 Knee 90–90 traction 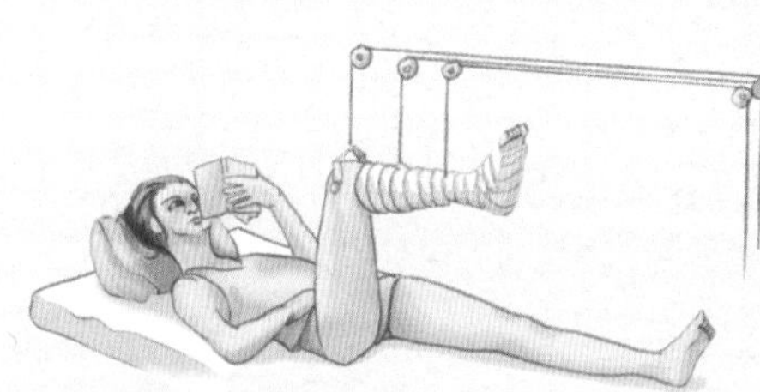	For femur fracture reduction when skin traction is inadequate. Skeletal traction with force is applied through a pin in distal femur.	A foam boot may be used for suspension of the lower leg. Force of traction is applied to the femur via the pin. The amount of weight used is just enough to hold the lower limb suspended.
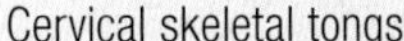 Cervical skeletal tongs 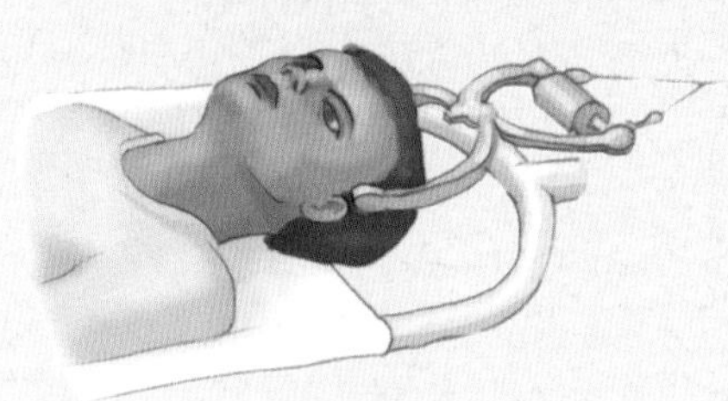	Tongs attached to skull via pins. Used with fractures or dislocations of the cervical or high thoracic vertebrae	Assess frequently for increased pain; respiratory distress; and spinal cord, cranial nerve, or brachial plexus injury. Place the child on a Stryker frame or specially equipped bed to ease positioning without disruption of alignment.
Halo traction 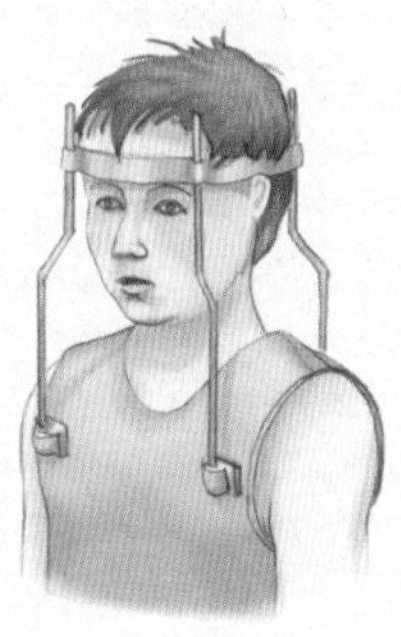	Metal halo attached to skull via pins. Used for cervical or high thoracic vertebrae fracture or dislocation and for postoperative immobilization following cervical fusion	Refer to nursing implications for cervical tongs. Tape a small wrench to the front of the brace so that the front panel can be quickly removed in an emergency. May become ambulatory in this type of traction; will be top-heavy so may need assistance with balance Assess pin sites and provide pin care as ordered.
Balanced suspension traction 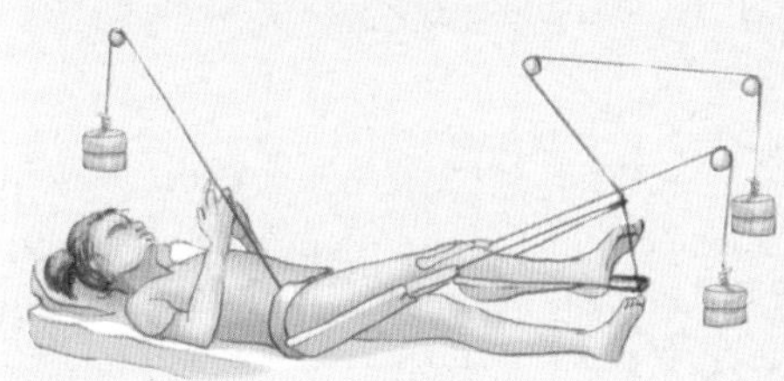	Used for femur, hip, or tibial fracture. The Thomas splint suspends the thigh, while the Pearson attachment allows knee flexion and supports the leg below the knee.	Avoid pressure to the popliteal area.

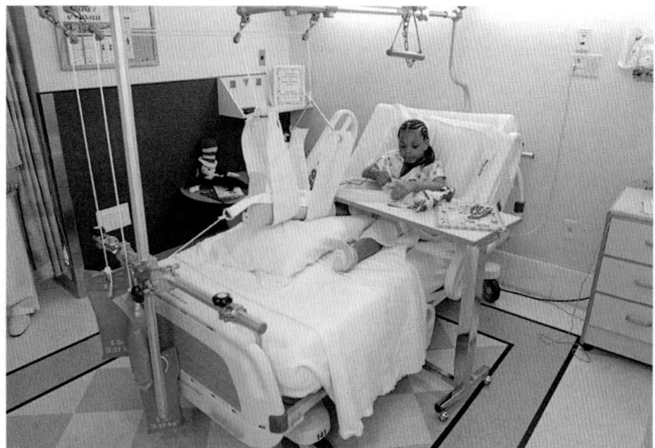

FIGURE 22.12 Provide age-appropriate diversional activities and school work for children confined to bed in traction.

Providing Pin Care

Whether pins are inserted for skeletal traction or as part of an external fixator (see the "Fractures" section), keeping the pin sites clean is important to prevent infection. Cleaning of the pin sites prevents infection by promoting comfort and preventing healing skin from adhering to the metal pin. Notify the orthopedic surgeon if signs of pin site infection are present or if pin slippage occurs.

Thus far, there is insufficient evidence to support a particular strategy of pin care, and more randomized trials are needed (Iobst, 2017; Shields et al., 2022). The National Association of Orthopaedic Nurses has published minimal guidelines, which include:

- Perform pin care weekly after the first 48 to 72 hours. Perform earlier if a large amount of drainage is present, dressing becomes wet, or infection is suspected.
- The most effective solution for pin site care may be chlorhexidine 2 mg/mL in alcohol. If the child has sensitivity to this, use normal saline.
- Use a nonshedding material for cleaning.
- Cover pin sites with a nonshedding dressing.
- Teach the child and their family pin site care along with instructions on the signs and symptoms of infection before discharge (Holmes et al., 2005; Walker, 2018).

Since the research available is minimal, these recommendations are made tentatively (Holmes et al., 2005). Therefore, interventions for pin care need to be individualized based on the child's condition and response to treatment and according to institutional policy or the health care provider's or nurse practitioner's orders. Certain health care providers or nurse practitioners prefer the site to be cleaned with normal saline; others choose a solution with antibacterial properties. Some institutions recommend removal of all crusts formed on the skin around the pin; others do not. The rationale for crust removal is to promote free drainage and prevent the surrounding skin from adhering to the pin. A keyhole dressing may be necessary around the pin if drainage is present. No matter which procedure is ordered or preferred, perform pin care as necessary to prevent infection at the pin site. The Ilizarov fixator uses wires that are thinner than ordinary pins, so simply cleansing by showering is usually sufficient to keep the pin site clean. If drainage is present, cleanse the skin around the wires with a dry gauze pad.

TAKE NOTE!

When caring for children in the hospital, particularly those with complex medical needs, follow their home care routines as much as possible.

Based on your top three patient problems for Fredrick, describe appropriate nursing interventions.

CONGENITAL AND DEVELOPMENTAL DISORDERS

Several disorders with neuromuscular and musculoskeletal effects are congenital in nature. These include neural tube defects and genetic neuromuscular disorders. The structural disorders are spina bifida occulta, meningocele, and myelomeningocele (neural tube defects). Congenital anomalies of the musculoskeletal system are usually readily identified at birth. Congenital structural anomalies involving the skeleton include pectus excavatum, pectus carinatum, limb deficiencies, polydactyly or syndactyly, metatarsus adductus, congenital clubfoot, and osteogenesis imperfecta (OI). A developmental anomaly that may be diagnosed at birth or later in life is DDH. A muscular condition, torticollis, most often presents as a congenital condition but may also develop after birth. Tibia vara is a developmental disorder affecting young children. Rarely, a developmental positional alteration such as genu varum, genu valgum, or pes planus will persist past the usual age of resolution or cause the child pain. If those situations occur, bracing, orthotics, or surgical correction may become necessary. The genetic neuromuscular disorders include the various types of muscular dystrophy and spinal muscular atrophy (SMA). These disorders are not always recognized at birth because signs and symptoms are not evident until months or even years after birth. However, they are still considered to be congenital as they have a genetic basis.

NEURAL TUBE DEFECTS

Neural tube defects account for the majority of congenital anomalies of the central nervous system. The neural tube closes between the third and fourth weeks of gestation. The cause of neural tube defects is not known, but many factors, such as drugs, malnutrition, chemicals, and genetics, can hinder normal central nervous system development. It is well established that preconception supplementation of folic acid by the birthing parent can decrease the incidence of neural tube defects in pregnancies by 50% or more (American Academy of Pediatrics [AAP], Committee on Genetics, 1999, reaffirmed 2017; Kinsman & Johnston, 2020). Since 1992, the U.S. Public Health Service, along with the Centers for Disease Control and Prevention (CDC), has recommended that anyone of childbearing age who is capable of becoming pregnant take 0.4 mg (400 mcg) of folic acid daily (CDC, 2022a). Pregnant people who had a previous child with a neural tube defect are recommended to take a higher dosage and should consult with their health care provider or nurse practitioner (AAP, Committee on Genetics, 1999, reaffirmed 2017). Prenatal screening of the pregnant parent's serum for alpha-fetoprotein (AFP) and ultrasound examination can help identify fetuses at risk. Neural tube defects primarily affecting spinal cord development include spina bifida occulta, meningocele, and myelomeningocele (Fig. 22.13). Neural tube defects primarily affecting brain development are discussed in Chapter 16.

Spina Bifida Occulta

Spina bifida is a term that is often used to refer to all neural tube disorders that affect the spinal cord. This can be confusing and a cause of concern for parents. There are well-defined degrees of spinal cord involvement, and it is important for health care professionals to use the correct terminology.

Spina bifida occulta is a defect of the vertebral bodies without protrusion of the spinal cord or meninges. This defect is not visible externally and, in most cases, has no adverse effects (see Fig. 22.13). Children with spina bifida occulta need no immediate medical intervention. Complications are rare but may include more significant abnormalities of the spinal cord such as tethered cord, syringomyelia, or diastematomyelia.

Nursing Assessment

In most cases, spina bifida occulta is benign and asymptomatic and produces no neurologic signs. The defect, which is usually present in the lumbosacral area, often goes undetected. However, there may be noticeable dimpling, abnormal patches of hair, or discoloration of skin at the defect site. If so, further investigation, including magnetic resonance imaging (MRI), may be warranted.

Nursing Management

Nursing care will focus on educating the family. Inform parents of its presence and what the diagnosis means. Parents will often confuse this diagnosis with spina bifida cystica, a much more serious defect. Occasionally, children with spina bifida occulta eventually need surgical intervention due to degenerative changes or involvement of the spine and nerve roots resulting in complications such as tethered cord, syringomyelia, or diastematomyelia. When these associated problems occur, the condition is often termed "occult spinal dysraphism" to avoid confusion.

Meningocele

Meningocele, the less serious form of spina bifida cystica, occurs when the meninges herniate through a defect in the vertebrae. The spinal cord is usually normal, and there are typically minor or no associated neurologic deficits. Treatment for meningocele involves surgical correction of the lesion (see Fig. 22.13).

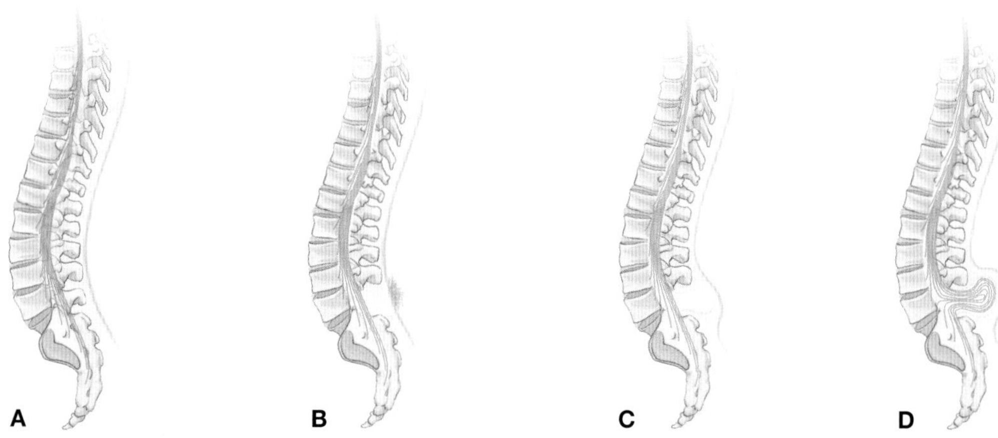

FIGURE 22.13 **A.** Normal spine. **B.** Spina bifida occulta. **C.** Meningocele. **D.** Myelomeningocele.

Nursing Assessment

Initial assessment after delivery will reveal a visible external sac protruding from the spinal area. It is most often seen in the lumbar region but can be anywhere along the spinal canal. Most are covered with skin and pose no threat to the child. However, assessment to ensure that the sac covering is intact remains important. Assess neurologic status carefully. Before surgical correction, the infant will be thoroughly examined to determine whether any neural involvement or associated anomalies exist. Diagnostic procedures such as computed tomography (CT), MRI, and ultrasound may be performed.

Nursing Management

Surgical correction may be delayed if the skin covering the sac is intact and the child has normal neurologic functioning (Kinsman & Johnston, 2020). However, as in a child with myelomeningocele, immediately report any evidence of leaking cerebrospinal fluid (CSF) to ensure prompt intervention to prevent infection. A child with leaking CSF or a thin skin covering will require immediate surgical correction (Kinsman & Johnston, 2020). Nursing management will be supportive. Provide pre- and postoperative care similar to that for the child with myelomeningocele to prevent rupture of the sac, to prevent infection, and to provide adequate nutrition and hydration. Monitor for symptoms of constipation or bladder dysfunction that may result due to increasing size of the lesion. Resulting hydrocephalus has been associated with some cases of meningocele (Kinsman & Johnston, 2020). Therefore, monitor head circumference and watch for signs and symptoms of increased intracranial pressure (ICP).

Myelomeningocele

Myelomeningocele, the most severe form of neural tube defect, occurs in approximately 1 in 4,000 live births (Kinsman & Johnston, 2020). Myelomeningocele is a type of spina bifida cystica, and, clinically, the term "spina bifida" is often used to refer to myelomeningocele. It may be diagnosed in utero via ultrasound. Otherwise, it is visually obvious at birth. The newborn with myelomeningocele is at increased risk for meningitis, hypoxia, and hemorrhage.

In myelomeningocele, the spinal cord often ends at the point of the defect, resulting in absent motor and sensory function beyond that point (Fig. 22.14). Therefore, the long-term complications of paralysis, orthopedic deformities, and bladder and bowel incontinence are often seen in children with myelomeningocele. The presence of neurogenic bladder and frequent catheterization put the child at an increased risk for urinary tract infections, pyelonephritis, and hydronephrosis, which may result in long-term renal damage if managed inappropriately.

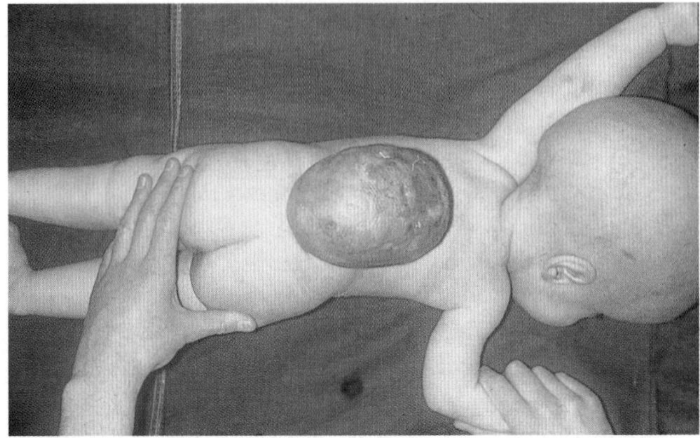

FIGURE 22.14 Usually, a sac covers the deformity of myelomeningocele and is visible at birth.

Accompanying hydrocephalus associated with type II Chiari defect is seen in 80% of children with myelomeningocele (Kinsman & Johnston, 2020). Due to the improper development and the downward displacement of the brain into the cervical spine, CSF flow is blocked, resulting in hydrocephalus. The lower the deformity is on the spine, the lower the risk of developing hydrocephalus is (Kinsman & Johnston, 2020).

Children with myelomeningocele usually require multiple surgical procedures. In addition, due to frequent catheterizations, these children are at an increased risk for developing a latex allergy (Kinsman & Johnston, 2020). Learning problems and seizures are common among these children, but the majority of those surviving with myelomeningocele have average intelligence (Kinsman & Johnston, 2020). Ambulation is possible for some children, depending on the level of the lesion.

Pathophysiology

The cause of myelomeningocele is unknown, but risk factors are consistent with other neural tube defects, such as drug use by the pregnant parent, malnutrition, and genetic predisposition (Kinsman & Johnston, 2020). In myelomeningocele, the neural tube fails to close at the end of the fourth week of gestation. As a result, an external sac-like protrusion that encases the meninges, spinal fluid, and, in some cases, nerves is present on the spine (see Fig. 22.13). A myelomeningocele can be located anywhere along the spinal cord, but the highest incidence occurs in the lumbosacral region (Kinsman & Johnston, 2020). The degree of neurologic deficit will depend on the location and size of the lesion (Kinsman & Johnston, 2020). An increase in neurologic deficit is seen with higher lesions as more nerves are affected.

Therapeutic Management

Surgical closure will be performed as soon as possible after birth, especially if a CSF leak is present or if there is a danger of the sac rupturing. The goal of early surgical intervention is to prevent infection and to minimize further loss of function, which can result from the stretching of nerve roots as the meningeal sac expands after birth. In utero fetal surgery to repair the myelomeningocele has been successful, showing improved outcomes for the fetus, such as improved psychomotor function and lower need for shunt placement, but is not without risks to the pregnant person and fetus (Bowman, 2022). Ongoing management of this disorder remains complex. A multidisciplinary approach is needed, involving specialists in neurology, neurosurgery, urology, orthopedics, therapy, and rehabilitation along with intense nursing care. The chronic nature of this disorder necessitates lifelong follow-up.

Nursing Assessment

For a full description of the assessment phase of the nursing process, refer to the "Clinical Judgment and the Nursing Process" section earlier in the chapter. Assessment findings pertinent to myelomeningocele are discussed further on.

HEALTH HISTORY

High-risk deliveries should be identified. Explore the pregnancy history and past medical history for risk factors such as:

- Lack of prenatal care
- Lack of preconception and/or prenatal folic acid supplementation
- Previous child born with neural tube defect or family history of neural tube defects
- Consumption by the pregnant parent of certain drugs that antagonize folic acid, such as anticonvulsants (carbamazepine and phenobarbital)

The older infant or child with a history of myelomeningocele requires numerous surgical procedures and lifelong follow-up. In an infant or child returning for a clinic visit or hospitalization, the health history should include questions related to:

- Current mobility status and any changes in motor abilities
- Genitourinary function and regimen
- Bowel function and regimen
- Signs or symptoms of urinary infections
- History of hydrocephalus with presence of shunt
- Signs or symptoms of shunt infection or malfunction (refer to "Hydrocephalus" section in Chapter 16)
- Latex sensitivity
- Nutritional status, including changes in weight
- Any other changes in physical or cognitive state
- Resources available and used by the family

PHYSICAL EXAMINATION

Initial assessment after delivery will reveal a visible external sac protruding from the spinal area (see Fig. 22.14). Observe the baby's general appearance, and assess whether the sac covering is intact. Assess neurologic status and look for associated anomalies. Assess for movement of extremities and anal reflex, which will help determine the level of neurologic involvement. Flaccid paralysis, absence of deep tendon reflexes, lack of response to touch and pain stimuli, skeletal abnormalities such as club feet, constant dribbling of urine, and a relaxed anal sphincter may be found.

In the older infant or child, perform a thorough physical examination, and focus on the functional assessment. Note the level of paralysis or paresthesia. Inspect the skin for breakdown. Determine the child's motor capabilities.

LABORATORY AND DIAGNOSTIC TESTS

A myelomeningocele may be detected prenatally around 16 to 18 weeks' gestation by ultrasound, by a blood test that detects AFP increases, or by analysis of amniotic fluid for AFP increases. Common laboratory and diagnostic studies ordered for the assessment of myelomeningocele include:

- MRI
- CT
- Ultrasound
- Myelography

These diagnostic tests are used to evaluate brain and spinal cord involvement (refer to Common Laboratory and Diagnostic Tests 22.1).

Nursing Management

Initial nursing management of the child with myelomeningocele involves preventing trauma to the meningeal sac and preventing infection before surgical repair of the defect. Refer to the "Clinical Judgment and the Nursing Process" section earlier in this chapter. Additional considerations are reviewed further on.

PREVENTING INFECTION

Risk of infection related to the presence of the meningeal sac and potential for rupture is a central nursing concern in the newborn with myelomeningocele. Until surgical intervention occurs, the goal is to prevent rupture or leakage of CSF from the sac. Keeping the sac from drying out is important, as is preventing trauma or pressure on the sac. Use sterile saline-soaked nonadhesive gauze or antibiotic-soaked gauze to keep the sac moist. Immediately report any seepage of clear fluid from the lesion, as this could indicate an opening in the sac and provide a portal of entry for microorganisms. Position the infant in the prone position or supported on the side to avoid pressure on the sac. To keep the infant warm, place the infant in a warmer or isolette to avoid the use of blankets, which could exert too much pressure on the sac. Pay special attention while the infant is in a warmer or isolette because the radiant heat can cause drying and cracking of the sac.

Keep the lesion free of feces and urine to help avoid infection. Position the infant so that urine and feces flow away from the sac (e.g., prone position, or place a folded towel under the abdomen) to help prevent infection. Placing a piece of plastic wrap below the meningocele is another way of preventing feces from coming into contact with the lesion. After surgery, position the infant in the prone or side-lying position to allow the incision to heal. Continue with precautions to prevent urine or feces from coming into contact with the incision.

PROMOTING URINARY ELIMINATION

Children with myelomeningocele often have bladder incontinence, although some children may achieve normal urinary continence. The level of the lesion will influence the amount of dysfunction. Myelomeningocele remains one of the more common causes of neurogenic bladder in children. Therefore, evaluation of renal function by a pediatric urologist should be performed on the child with myelomeningocele. Refer to Chapter 21 for further information regarding neurogenic bladder and appropriate nursing interventions, including clean intermittent catheterization.

PROMOTING BOWEL ELIMINATION

Children with myelomeningocele often have bowel incontinence as well; the level of the lesion affects the amount of dysfunction. Many children with myelomeningocele can achieve some degree of bowel continence. Bowel training with the use of timed enemas or suppositories along with diet modifications can allow for defecation at predetermined times once or twice a day. Although bowel incontinence can be difficult for children as they grow older, due to social concerns and self-esteem and body image disturbances, it does not pose the same health risks as urinary incontinence.

PROMOTING ADEQUATE NUTRITION

The risk of altered nutrition related to the restrictions on positioning of the infant before and after surgery is another nursing concern. Assist the family in assuming as normal a feeding position as possible. Preoperatively, the risk of rupture may be too high to warrant holding. Therefore, the infant's head can be turned to the side, or the infant can be placed in the side-lying position to facilitate feeding. If the infant is held, special care needs to be taken to avoid pressure on the sac or postoperative incision. Encourage the parents to interact as much as possible with the infant by talking to and touching the infant during feeding to help promote intake. If the parent was planning on chest or breastfeeding the infant, assist them in meeting this goal, if possible. If the infant can be held, encourage the parent to do this, or assist them in pumping and saving breast milk to be given to the infant via bottle until the infant is able to be held. Feeding an infant in an unusual position can be difficult, and it is the nurse's role to provide support, education, and modeling for the parents and family when needed.

PREVENTING LATEX ALLERGIC REACTION

Sensitivity to latex or natural rubber is common among children with myelomeningocele. They are at an increased risk for developing an allergy to latex related to the multiple exposures to latex products during surgical procedures and bladder catheterizations. A latex-free environment should be created for all procedures performed on children with myelomeningocele to prevent latex allergy. Also, children with a known latex allergy must be identified and managed in a latex-free environment. The nurse must ensure that these children do not come into direct contact with latex or equipment and supplies that contain latex. Be familiar with those products and equipment at your facility that contain latex and those that are latex free. The Food and Drug Administration (FDA) requires that all medical supplies be labeled if they contain latex (U.S. Food and Drug Administration, 2014), but this is not the case for consumer products. Many resources exist that list products that are latex free, and each hospital should have such a list readily available to health care professionals.

Children who are at a high risk for latex sensitivity should wear medical alert identification. Education programs regarding latex sensitivity and ways to prevent it need to be directed at those who care for high-risk children, including teachers, school nurses, relatives, babysitters, and all health care professionals.

MAINTAINING SKIN INTEGRITY

Address the risk for altered skin integrity related to the infant's prone position and impaired mobility. The prone position puts constant pressure on the knees and elbows, and it may be difficult to keep the infant clean of urine and feces. Diapering may be contraindicated preoperatively to avoid pressure on the sac. Therefore, ensure that the infant is kept as clean and dry as possible. This is made more difficult by the constant dribbling of stool and urine that may be present. Placing a pad beneath the diaper area and changing it frequently are important. Perform meticulous skin care. Place the infant on a special care mattress, and place synthetic sheepskin under the infant to help reduce friction. Special attention to the infant's legs needs to occur when positioning them, since paralysis may be present. Using a folded diaper between the legs can help reduce pressure and friction from the legs rubbing together.

EDUCATING AND SUPPORTING THE CHILD AND FAMILY

Myelomeningocele is a serious disorder that affects multiple body systems and produces varying degrees of deficits. It is a disorder that has lifelong effects. Thanks to medical advances and technology, most children born with myelomeningocele can expect to live a normal life, but challenges remain for the family and child as they learn to cope and live with this physical condition. Adjusting to the demands this condition places on the child and family is difficult. Parents may need time to accept their infant's condition, but as soon as possible, they should be involved in the infant's care.

Teaching should begin immediately in the hospital. Teaching should include positioning, preventing infection, feeding, promoting urinary elimination through clean intermittent catheterization, preventing latex allergy, and identifying the signs and symptoms of complications such as increased ICP. Due to the chronic nature of this condition, long-term planning needs to begin in the hospital. These children usually require multiple surgical procedures and hospitalizations, and this can place stress on the family and their finances. The nurse has an important role in providing ongoing education about the illness and its treatments and the plan of care. As the family becomes more comfortable with the condition, they will become the experts in the child's care. Respect and recognize the family's changing needs. Providing intense daily care can take its toll on a family, and continual support and encouragement are needed. Referral to the Spina Bifida Association and a local support group for families of children with myelomeningocele is appropriate. See the Healthy People 2030 box.

HEALTHY PEOPLE 2030

Objective	Nursing Significance
Increase the proportion of students with disabilities who spend at least 80% of their time in regular education programs.	Become familiar with local schools' offerings and capabilities so that you can refer families to an educational site appropriate for their child.

Healthy People Objectives retrieved from http://www.healthypeople.gov

CONSIDER THIS!

After learning that our new baby will be born with spina bifida, I felt so alone. I feel scared and sad; I am angry too. I wish I knew how this could happen.

Thoughts: How would you respond to their concerns? What local resources could you refer them to?

Pectus Excavatum

Pectus excavatum and pectus carinatum are anterior chest wall deformities. Pectus excavatum, a funnel-shaped chest, accounts for greater than 90% of all congenital chest wall deformities (Boas, 2020). A depression that sinks inward is apparent at the xiphoid process (Fig. 22.15). Pectus carinatum, a protuberance of the chest wall, accounts for only 5% to 15% of anterior chest wall deformities (Boas, 2020). The remainder are mixed deformities. Male predominance is evident in both types (Boas, 2020).

Pectus excavatum does not resolve as the child grows; rather, it progresses with growth. The chest depression may be minimal or marked. When the pectus is more pronounced, cardiac and pulmonary compression occurs. Symptoms of this compression most often present during puberty, when the pectus quickly worsens. The child may complain of shortness of breath, withdraw from physical activities, and have a poor body image.

Therapeutic Management

Therapeutic management of pectus excavatum is based on the severity and physiologic compromise. Options include observation; use of physical therapy to work on musculoskeletal compromise; and surgical correction, preferably before puberty, when the skeleton is more pliable. Various surgical techniques may be used and generally involve either the placement of a surgical steel bar or using a piece of bone in the rib cage to lift the depression. This discussion will focus on care of the child who undergoes surgical steel bar placement for pectus correction. This procedure, referred to as the Nuss procedure, is performed more often and is considered minimally invasive (Mayer, 2022).

Nursing Assessment

Elicit the health history, noting progression of the defect and effects on the child's cardiopulmonary function. Note shortness of breath, exercise intolerance, or chest

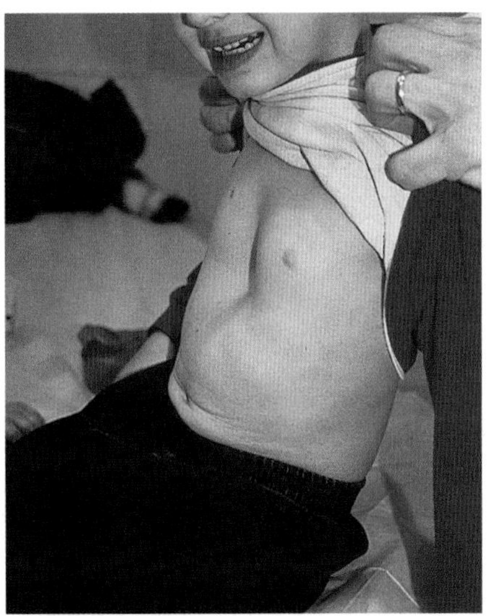

FIGURE 22.15 Pectus excavatum: note the depression in the chest wall at the xiphoid process.

pain. Observe the child's chest for anterior wall deformity, noting depth and severity. Auscultate the lungs to determine the adequacy of aeration. Radiographs, CT, or MRI may be used to determine the extent of the anomaly and compression of inner structures.

Nursing Management

Prepare the child preoperatively by allowing a tour of the surgical area and the pediatric intensive care unit. Introduce the child to the pain scale that will be used in the postoperative period.

Postoperatively, nursing management focuses on assessment, protection of the surgical site, and pain management. Auscultate lung sounds frequently to determine the adequacy of aeration and to monitor for development of the complication of pneumothorax. Assess for signs of wound infection that would necessitate removal of the curved bar. During the first few postoperative days, positioning is challenging; do not allow the child to roll in bed, lie on either side, or rotate or flex the spine (these positions may disrupt the bar's position). Administer analgesics as needed either intravenously or via the epidural catheter. Teach the family that the child will not be allowed to lie on their side at home for 4 weeks after the surgery to ensure that the band does not shift. Encourage aerobic activity at home after being cleared by the surgeon (this will increase the child's vital capacity, previously hindered by the pectus). The bar will be removed 2 to 4 years after the initial placement.

Limb Deficiencies

Limb deficiencies, either deformity or complete absence of a limb or a portion of it, occur as the fetus is developing. The limb either fails to form normally or does not form at all. The cause is unknown. Certain behaviors and exposures can increase the risk of limb deficiencies such as exposure to certain chemicals, viruses, medications, and possible exposure of the pregnant parent to tobacco smoke (CDC, 2022b). These defects can be attributed to an amniotic band constricting the limb, resulting in either incomplete development or amputation of the limb. Many children born with limb deformities also have congenital anomalies such as craniofacial abnormalities and cardiac and abdominal wall defects (CDC, 2022b).

Therapeutic management is aimed at improving the child's functional ability. Physical therapy and occupational therapy may be helpful. Adaptive equipment such as a prosthesis may also be prescribed.

Nursing Assessment

Note the extent of limb deformity, providing an accurate description of the presence or absence of a portion of the arm or leg, or missing fingers or toes. Assess the child's ability to use the extremity as a helper (arms) or in ambulation (legs). Determine status of acquisition of developmental skills.

Nursing Management

Reinforce prescribed activities that are meant to improve the child's function. Provide activities in which the child is capable of participating. If the limb deficiency is significant, refer the infant to the local early intervention office as soon as possible after birth. Early intervention, available in all 50 states, is designed to promote development from birth to age 3 years. Absence of a limb or a significant portion of a limb will have a considerable impact on the child's ability to meet developmental milestones as expected.

Polydactyly and Syndactyly

Polydactyly is the presence of extra digits on the hand or foot (Fig. 22.16). One third of the time, polydactyly occurs in both the hand and the foot, and 50% of the time it is seen bilaterally (Winell & Davidson, 2020). It usually involves digits at the border of the hand or foot but can also occur by a central digit (Winell & Davidson, 2020). Syndactyly is webbing of the fingers and toes. Both polydactyly and syndactyly can be normal variants in the newborn and can also be inherited and associated with other genetic syndromes (Winell & Davidson, 2020).

Therapeutic management includes surgical removal of the digit. No treatment is usually required for syndactyly, although surgical repair is sometimes performed for cosmetic reasons.

Nursing Assessment

Inspect the hands and feet for the presence of extra digits. Note whether the additional digits are soft (without

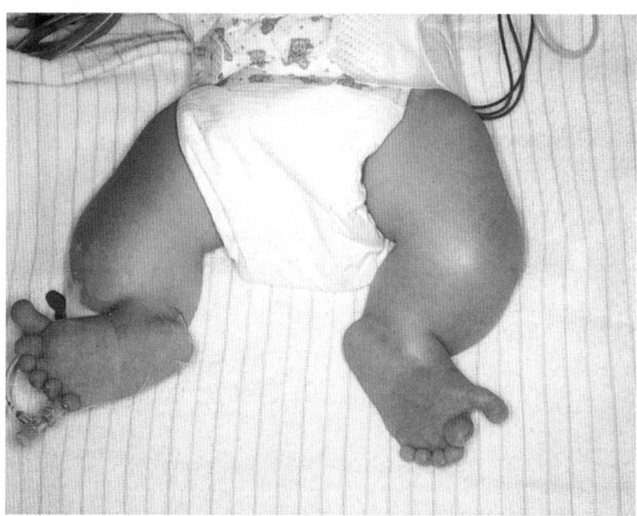

FIGURE 22.16 Note additional digits (toes) of polydactyly.

bone) or are full or whether partial digits with bone are present. Note the location of webbing.

Nursing Management

When surgical removal is necessary, provide routine preoperative and postoperative care as appropriate.

Metatarsus Adductus

Metatarsus adductus, a medial deviation of the forefoot, is one of the more common foot deformities of childhood (Fig. 22.17). It occurs most commonly as a result of in utero positioning (Winell & Davidson, 2020). Half of all cases occur bilaterally (Winell & Davidson, 2020). The degree of flexibility is important and determines treatment. If the forefoot is flexible past neutral manipulation passively, observation is often sufficient. If the forefoot is flexible only to neutral manipulation, stretching exercises may be beneficial. If the forefoot is rigid and is not flexible to neutral manipulation, serial casting, preferably before the age of 8 months, may be required (Winell & Davidson, 2020). Surgical intervention is rarely needed.

Nursing Assessment

The deformity is usually noted at birth. Note inward deviation of the forefoot with the hindfoot remaining in normal position. The great and second toes might be separated. Determine forefoot flexibility. ROM of the ankle, hindfoot, and midfoot is as expected.

Nursing Management

Most cases will resolve without treatment, and nursing care is aimed at education and reassurance of the parents. Nursing care for the child with severe metatarsus adductus is similar to that of the child with clubfoot (see the next section).

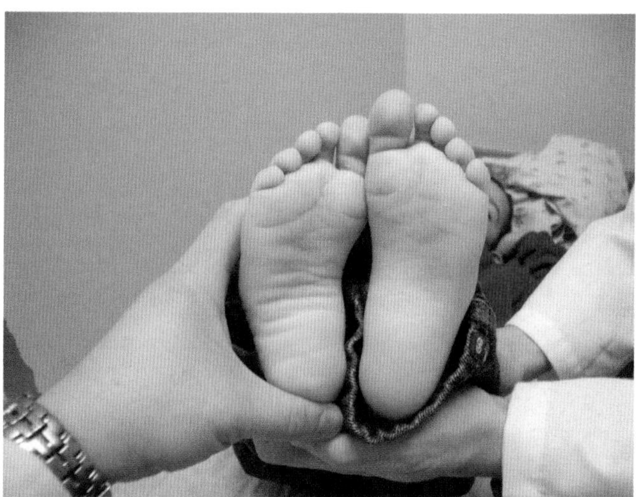

FIGURE 22.17 Metatarsus adductus: Note medial deviation of the forefoot.

Congenital Clubfoot

Congenital clubfoot (also termed congenital talipes equinovarus) is a congenital anomaly that occurs in about 1 of 1,000 live births (Winell & Davidson, 2020). Clubfoot consists of:

- Talipes varus (inversion of the heel)
- Talipes equinus (plantarflexion of the foot; the heel is raised and would not strike the ground in a standing position)
- Cavus (plantarflexion of the forefoot on the hindfoot)
- Forefoot adduction with supination (the forefoot is inverted and turned slightly upward)

The foot resembles the head of a golf club (Fig. 22.18). Half of all cases occur bilaterally, and males are affected more frequently than females (Winell & Davidson, 2020). The exact etiology of clubfoot is unknown.

Clubfoot may be classified into four categories: postural, neurogenic, syndromic, and idiopathic. Postural clubfoot often resolves with a short series of manipulative casting. Neurogenic clubfoot occurs in infants with myelomeningocele. Clubfoot in association with other syndromes (syndromic) is often resistant to treatment. Idiopathic clubfoot occurs in otherwise healthy infants. The approach to treatment is similar regardless of the classification.

Therapeutic Management

The goal of therapeutic management of clubfoot is achievement of a functional foot; treatment starts as soon after birth as possible. Weekly manipulation with serial cast changes is performed; later, cast changes occur

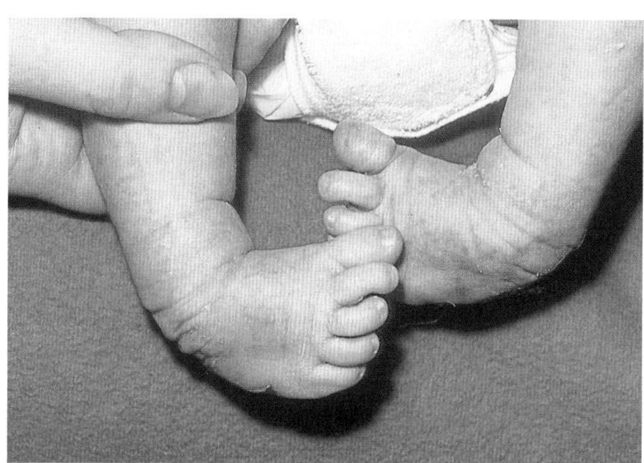

FIGURE 22.18 Note inverted heel, ankle equinus, and forefoot adduction in this infant with bilateral clubfoot.

every 2 weeks. Other infants require corrective shoes or bracing. In some infants, surgical release of soft tissue may be necessary. Following surgery, the foot is immobilized with a cast for up to 12 weeks, and then ankle–foot orthoses (AFOs) or corrective shoes are used for several years.

Complications of clubfoot and its treatment include residual deformity, rocker-bottom foot, awkward gait, weight bearing on the lateral portion of the foot if uncorrected, and disturbance to the epiphysis.

Nursing Assessment

Note family history of foot deformities and obstetric history of breech position. Inspect the foot for position at rest. Perform active ROM, noting inability to move foot into normal positioning at midline. X-rays are obtained to determine bony abnormality and note progress during treatment.

Nursing Management

Perform neurovascular assessment and cast care for infants requiring casting. Provide emotional support, as treatment often begins in the newborn period and the family may have a difficult time adjusting to the diagnosis and treatment required for their new baby. Teach the family cast care and about the use of orthotics or braces as prescribed.

Osteogenesis Imperfecta

OI is a genetic bone disorder that results in low bone mass, increased fragility of the bones, and other connective tissue problems such as joint hypermobility, resulting in instability of the joints. All of these contribute to fracture occurrence. Dentinogenesis imperfecta may also occur. This is characterized by the tooth enamel wearing easily and brittle and discolored teeth.

The disorder usually occurs as a result of a defect in the collagen type 1 gene, usually through an autosomal dominant inheritance pattern, but some types are inherited in a recessive manner (Balasubramanian, 2022). The types of OI range from mild to severe connective tissue and bone involvement. Originally, OI was classified into four types based on observable clinical characteristics. Since then, over 20 types have been defined (Balasubramanian, 2022). Table 22.2 discusses several types and their characteristic findings. Subtypes A and B exist depending on (A) the absence or (B) the presence of dentinogenesis imperfecta (Marini, 2020). In children with moderate to severe disease, fractures are more likely to occur, and short stature is common. In addition to multiple fractures, additional complications include early hearing loss, acute and chronic pain, scoliosis, and respiratory problems.

TABLE 22.2 • Classification of Osteogenesis Imperfecta

Classification	Characteristics
I	Mild Accounts for 70%–75% of OI cases Blue sclera Hearing loss Frequent shoulder and elbow dislocations Recurrent fractures in childhood After growth is complete, incidence of fractures diminishes dramatically. Average or slightly shorter stature compared to family members Gross motor development delays
II	Most severe form Lethal in perinatal period or within first year of life Low birth weight, very short limbs, small chest, and soft skull Intrauterine fractures evident Very dark blue/gray sclera
III	Most severe nonlethal form Sclera ranges from white to blue. Fractures in utero and at birth with progressive deformity Bone fragility and fracture rate vary Results in significant disability Marked short stature
IV	Moderately severe Sclera may be light blue in infancy and lighten to white during childhood. Fragile bones May present at birth with in utero fractures or bowing of lower long bones Height may be less than average for age.
V and VI	Clinically within type IV, but microscopic studies reveal distinct bone patterns that do not involve deficits of type I collagen. Moderate in severity Similar to type IV in degree of fractures and skeletal deformity Type VI is extremely rare.
VII, VIII, and IX	Recessive inheritance patterns Types VII and VIII resemble types II or III, except infants have white sclera. Stature is short. IX is very rare; the severity ranges from moderate to lethal.

OI, osteogenesis imperfecta.

Adapted from Marini, J. C. (2020). Osteogenesis imperfecta. In R. M. Kleigman, J. W. St. Geme III, N. J. Blum, S. S. Shah, R. C. Tasker, K. M. Wilson, & R. E. Behrman (Eds.), *Nelson textbook of pediatrics* (21st ed., pp. 19520–19539). Elsevier; Balasubramanian, M. (2022). Osteogenesis imperfecta: An overview. *UpToDate*. Retrieved May 14, 2023, from https://www.uptodate.com/contents/osteogenesis-imperfecta-an-overview

TAKE NOTE!

Blue/gray sclera is not diagnostic of OI, but it is a common finding (Balasubramanian, 2022). However, there are some individuals with blue sclerae who do not have OI. Keep in mind that the sclerae of newborns tend to be bluish, progressing to white over the first few weeks of life.

Therapeutic Management

The goal of medical and surgical management is to decrease the incidence of fractures and maintain mobility. Bisphosphonate administration is used for moderate to severe disease. Fracture care is often required. Physical therapy and occupational therapy prevent contractures and maximize mobility. Standing with bracing is encouraged. Lightweight splints or braces may allow the child to bear weight earlier. Severe cases may require surgical insertion of rods into the long bones.

Nursing Assessment

Elicit a health history, which may reveal a family history of OI, a pattern of frequent fractures, or screaming associated with routine care and handling of the newborn. Inspect the eyes for sclerae that have a blue, purple, or gray tint. Note abnormalities of the primary teeth. Inspect skin for bruising, and note joint hypermobility with active ROM. Laboratory tests may include a skin biopsy (which reveals abnormalities in type 1 collagen) or DNA testing (locating the genetic mutation).

Nursing Management

Handle the child carefully, and teach the family to avoid trauma (Teaching Guidelines 22.3).

Encourage safe mobility. Reinforce physical and occupational therapists' recommendations for promotion of fine motor skills and independence in ADLs, as well as use of adaptive equipment and appropriate promotion of mobility. Adapted physical education is important to promote mobility and maintain bone and muscle mass. If the child is ambulatory, even with adaptive equipment use, walking is a good form of exercise. Swimming and water therapy are appropriate, allowing independent movement with little fracture risk.

TEACHING GUIDELINES 22.3 Preventing Injury in Children With Osteogenesis Imperfecta

- Never push or pull on an arm or leg.
- Do not bend an arm or a leg into an awkward position.
- Lift a baby by placing one hand under the legs and buttocks and one hand under the shoulders, head, and neck.
- Do not lift a baby's legs by the ankles to change the diaper.
- Do not lift a baby or small child from under the armpits.
- Provide supported positioning.
- If fracture is suspected, handle the limb minimally.

TAKE NOTE!

Use caution when inserting an intravenous line or taking a blood pressure measurement, as pressure on the arm or leg can lead to bruising and fractures.

Developmental Dysplasia of the Hip

DDH refers to abnormalities of the developing hip that include dislocation, subluxation, and dysplasia of the hip joint. In DDH, the femoral head has an abnormal relationship to the acetabulum. Frank dislocation of the hip may occur, in which there is no contact between the femoral head and acetabulum. Subluxation is a partial dislocation, meaning that the acetabulum is not fully seated within the hip joint. Dysplasia refers to an acetabulum that is shallow or sloping instead of cup shaped. DDH may affect just one or both hips. The dysplastic hip may be provoked to subluxation or dislocated and then reduced again (Fig. 22.19).

Pathophysiology

While dislocation may occur during a growth period in utero, the laxity of the newborn's hip allows dislocation and relocation of the hip to occur. The hip can develop normally only if the femoral head is appropriately and deeply seated within the acetabulum. If subluxation and periodic or continued dislocation occur, then structural changes in the hip's anatomy occur. Continued dysplasia of the hip leads to limited abduction of the hip and contracture of muscles. DDH is more common in females, probably due to the greater susceptibility of the female newborn to hormones in the pregnant parent that contribute to laxity of the ligaments (Sankar et al., 2020). Mechanical factors such as breech positioning, the presence of oligohydramnios, or large birth weight also contribute to the development of DDH. Genetic factors also play a role. There is an increased incidence of DDH among people of Native American and Eastern Europe

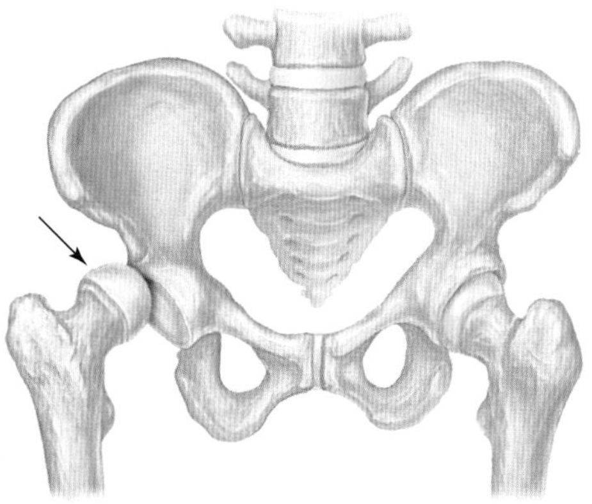

FIGURE 22.19 Developmental dysplasia of the hip.

an descent, with very low rates among people of African or Chinese heritage (Sankar et al., 2020). Complications of DDH include avascular necrosis of the femoral head, loss of ROM, recurrently unstable hip, femoral nerve palsy, leg-length discrepancy, and early osteoarthritis.

Therapeutic Management

The goal of therapeutic management is to maintain the hip joint in reduction so that the femoral head and acetabulum can develop properly.

Treatment varies based on the child's age and the severity of DDH. In newborns younger than 4 weeks, the hip will often stabilize on its own in a few weeks, requiring only observation (Sankar et al., 2020). Infants younger than 6 months may be treated with a Pavlik harness, which reduces and stabilizes the hip by preventing hip extension and adduction and maintaining the hip in flexion and abduction (Sankar et al., 2020). The Pavlik harness is successful in the treatment of DDH in the majority of infants younger than 6 months if it is used on a full-time basis and applied properly (Sankar et al., 2020). Children from 6 months to 2 years of age often require closed reduction (Sankar et al., 2020). Skin or skeletal traction may be used first to gradually stretch the associated soft tissue structures. Closed reduction occurs under general anesthesia, with the hip being gently maneuvered back into the acetabulum. A spica cast worn for 12 weeks maintains reduction of the hip. After the cast is removed, the child may wear an abduction brace full time (except for baths) (Sankar et al., 2020). Then, the brace is worn at night and during naps until development of the acetabulum is as expected. Children older than 2 years of age or those who have failed to respond to prior treatment require an open surgical reduction followed by a period of casting (Sankar et al., 2020). Follow-up continues until the age of skeletal maturity.

Nursing Assessment

Nursing assessment of children with DDH includes obtaining a health history and inspecting, observing, and palpating for findings common to DDH.

HEALTH HISTORY

Assess the health history for risk factors such as:

- Family history of DDH
- Female sex
- Oligohydramnios, high birth weight, or breech birth
- Native American or Eastern European descent
- Associated lower limb deformity, metatarsus adductus, hip asymmetry, torticollis, or other congenital musculoskeletal deformity

Previously undiagnosed older children may complain of hip pain.

PHYSICAL ASSESSMENT

The physical examination for DDH includes inspection, observation, and palpation. Since DDH is a developmental process, ongoing screening assessments are required throughout at least the first several months of the infant's life.

Inspection and Observation

Ensure that the infant is on a flat surface and is relaxed. Note asymmetry of thigh or gluteal folds with the infant in a prone position. Document shortening of the affected femur observed as limb-length discrepancy. Older children may exhibit **Trendelenburg gait**; due to the weakness of the hip abductors, the child's trunk is shifted over the affected hip during ambulation. Figure 22.20 illustrates these assessments.

Palpation

Note limited hip abduction while performing passive ROM. Abduction should ordinarily occur to 75 degrees and adduction to within 30 degrees with the infant's pelvis stabilized. Perform Barlow and Ortolani tests, feeling for, or noting, a "clunk" as the femoral head dislocates (positive Barlow) or reduces (positive Ortolani) back into the acetabulum. Force is not necessary when performing the Barlow and Ortolani maneuvers (see Fig. 22.20 and Nursing Procedure 22.1).

TAKE NOTE!

A higher-pitched "click" may occur with flexion or extension of the hip. When assessing for DDH, do not confuse this benign, adventitial sound with a true "clunk."

LABORATORY AND DIAGNOSTIC TESTING

Ultrasound of the hip allows for visualization of the femoral head and the outer edge of the acetabulum. Plain hip x-rays may be used in the infant or child older than 6 months of age.

Nursing Management

Earlier recognition of hip dysplasia with earlier harness use results in better correction of the anomaly. Excellent assessment skills and reporting of any abnormal findings are critical. Initially, the infant will need to wear the Pavlik harness continuously (Fig. 22.21). The health care provider or nurse practitioner makes all appropriate adjustments to the harness when applied so that the hips are held in the optimal position for appropriate development. Teach parents use of the harness and assessment of the baby's skin. If started early, harness use usually continues for about 3 months (Teaching Guidelines 22.4). Chest or breastfeeding can continue throughout the harness treatment period, but creative positioning of the infant may be needed.

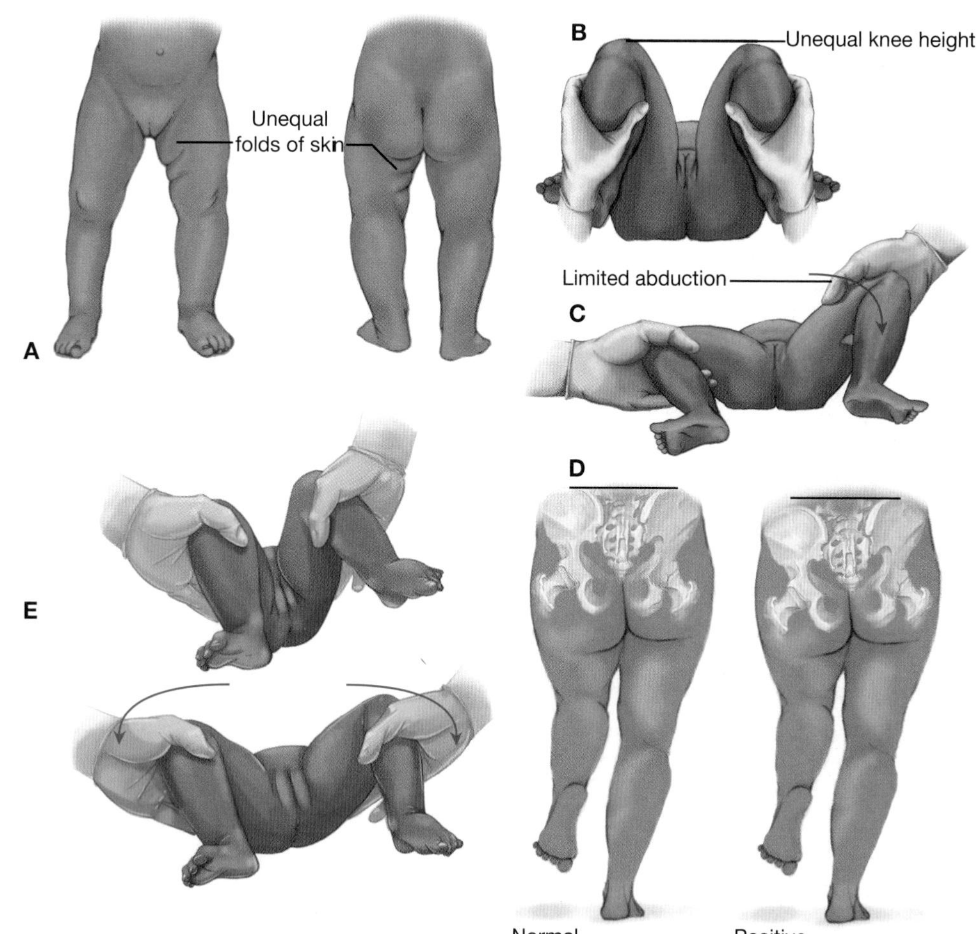

FIGURE 22.20 Assessment techniques for developmental dysplasia of the hip. **A.** Assess for asymmetry of thigh and gluteal folds. **B.** Assess for unequal knee height related to femur shortening. **C.** Note limitation in hip abduction. **D.** Positive Trendelenburg sign: Note pelvis/hip drops when the leg is raised. **E.** Feel for "clunk" when adduction and depression of femur dislocates hip (Barlow test). Assess for "clunk" when the dislocated hip is abducted and relocated (Ortolani sign).

NURSING PROCEDURE 22.1 Performing Ortolani and Barlow Maneuvers

Purpose: To Detect Congenital Developmental Dysplasia of the Hip

Ortolani Maneuver

1. Place the newborn in the supine position, and flex the hips and knees to 90 degrees at the hip.
2. Grasp the inner aspect of the thighs and abduct the hips (usually to approximately 180 degrees) while applying upward pressure.

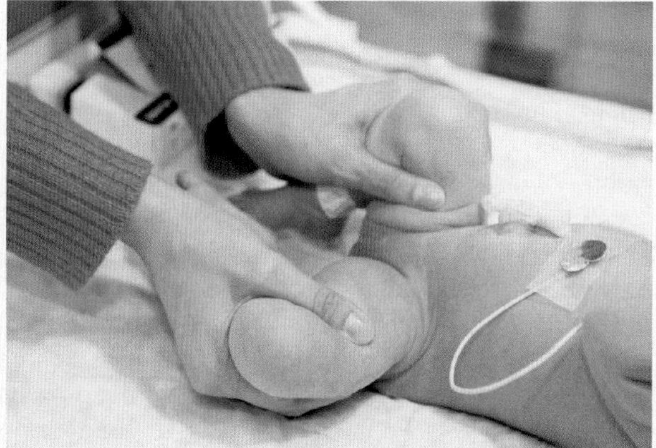

3. Listen for any sounds during the maneuver. There should be no "clunk" heard or felt when the legs are abducted. Such a sound indicates the femoral head hitting the acetabulum as the femoral head reenters the area. This suggests developmental hip dysplasia.

Barlow Maneuver

4. With the newborn still lying supine and grasping the inner aspect of the thighs (as just mentioned), adduct the thighs while applying outward and downward pressure to the thighs.

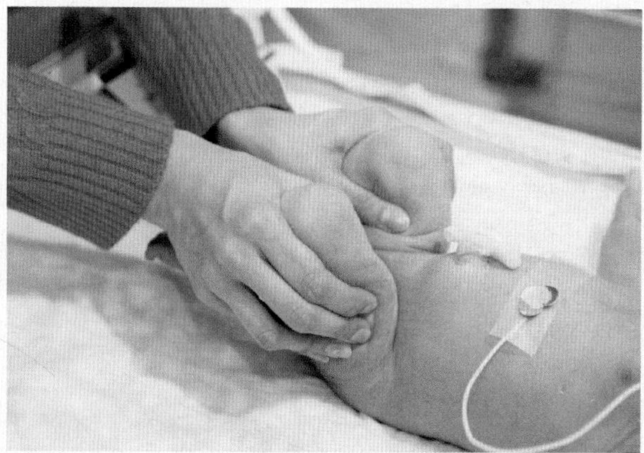

5. Feel for the femoral head slipping out of the acetabulum; also listen and feel for a "clunk."

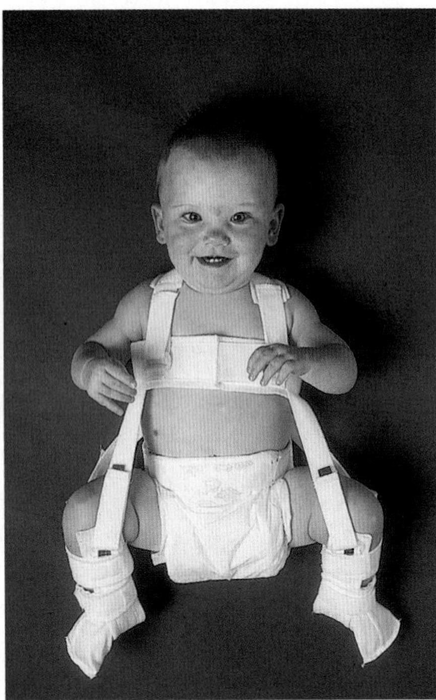

FIGURE 22.21 Pavlik harness used to keep the knees flexed and hips abducted to allow the hips to grow normally in a child with developmental dysplasia of the hip.

TEACHING GUIDELINES 22.4 Caring for a Child in a Pavlik Harness

- Do not adjust the straps without checking with the health care provider or nurse practitioner first.
- Until your health care provider or nurse practitioner instructs you to take the harness off for a period of time each day, it must be used continuously (for the first week or sometimes longer).
- Change your baby's diaper while they are in the harness.
- Place your baby to sleep on their back.
- Check skin folds, especially behind the knees and diaper area, for redness, irritation, or breakdown. Keep these areas clean and dry.
- Once the baby is permitted to be out of the harness for a short period, you may bathe your baby while the harness is off.
- Long knee socks and an undershirt are recommended to prevent rubbing of the skin against the brace.
- Note the location of the markings on the straps for appropriate placement of the harness.
- Wash the harness with mild detergent by hand and air dry. If using the dryer, use *only* the air fluffing setting (no heat).
- Call the doctor if:
  - Your baby's feet are swollen or bluish.
  - The harness appears too small.
  - Your baby's skin is raw or a rash develops.
  - Your baby is unable to actively kick their legs.

For infants or children diagnosed later than 6 months of age or those who do not improve with harness use, surgical reduction may be performed (Sankar et al., 2020). Postoperative casting followed by bracing or orthotic use is common. Caring for the child in the postoperative period is similar to care of any child in a cast. Pain management and monitoring for bleeding are priority activities. Teach families care of the cast at home.

Torticollis

Torticollis is a painless muscular condition presenting in infants or in children with certain syndromes. Congenital muscular torticollis may result from in utero positioning or difficult birth. Preferential turning of the head to one side while in the supine position after birth may also lead to torticollis. Torticollis results from tightness of the sternocleidomastoid muscle, resulting in the infant's head being tilted to one side.

Therapeutic management involves passive stretching exercises. These exercises should be effective in 90% of cases of congenital torticollis, especially if treatment is started within the first 3 months of life (Mistovich & Spiegel, 2020a). Physical therapy may be prescribed, and a tubular orthosis for torticollis (TOT) collar may also be used. Surgery is not common but may be done in the preschool years if other methods have been unsuccessful. Plagiocephaly may result from the continued pressure on the side of the skull to which the neck is turned.

Nursing Assessment

Note history of head tilt and the infant's lack of desire to turn the head in the opposite direction. Observe the infant for wryneck (tilting of the head to one side; Fig. 22.22). Note limited movement of the neck while performing passive ROM. Palpate the neck, noting a mass in the sternocleidomastoid muscle on the affected side. Examine the head for evidence of plagiocephaly. Accompanying hip dysplasia is seen in 8% to 20% of cases. Therefore, careful examination of the hips is warranted (Mistovich & Spiegel, 2020a).

Nursing Management

Teach parents gentle neck-stretching exercises to be performed several times a day. While immobilizing the shoulder on the affected side, gently sustain a side-to-side stretch toward the unaffected side, holding the stretch for 10 to 30 seconds. Repeat 10 to 15 times per session. Perform an ear-to-shoulder stretch in a similar fashion. To prevent the development of torticollis in the unaffected infant, prevent positional plagiocephaly. Prevent flatness of one side of the head by varying the infant's head position, and do not always turn the infant's head to one side while they are in the infant seat, in the swing, or lying supine.

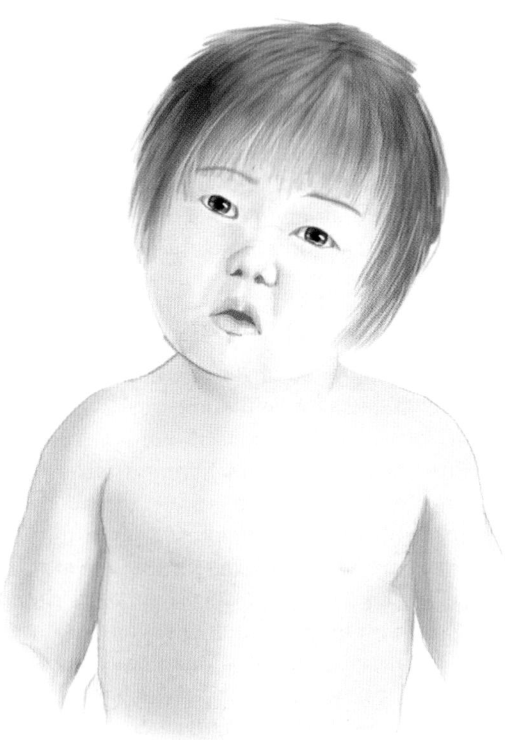

FIGURE 22.22 Note wryneck or head tilt in the infant with torticollis.

Tibia Vara (Blount Disease)

Tibia vara (Blount disease) is a developmental disorder affecting young children. There are three types: infantile (1 to 3 years), juvenile (4 to 10 years), and adolescent (11 years or older) (Winell et al., 2020). Infantile is the most common and is discussed here (Winell et al., 2020). The normal physiologic bowing or genu varum becomes more pronounced in the child with tibia vara. The cause of tibia vara is unknown, but it is considered to be a developmental disorder because it occurs most frequently in children who are early walkers. Most cases occur in Black females, and both extremities are affected (Winell et al., 2020). In addition to early walking, higher body weight is also a risk factor. If left untreated, the growth plate of the upper tibia ceases bone production. Asymmetric growth at the knee then occurs, and the bowing progresses. Severe degenerative arthritis of the knee is an additional long-term complication.

Therapeutic management is aimed at stopping the progression of the disease through bracing or surgical treatment. Medical or surgical treatment should begin early, before 4 years of age.

Nursing Assessment

Elicit a health history, and determine the age at which the child started walking. Assess growth parameters to determine whether the risk factor of higher body weight is present. Note significant bowing of the legs while the child is standing and ambulating (Fig. 22.23).

Nursing Management

Bracing may include a modified knee–ankle–foot orthosis that relieves the compression forces on the growth plate, allowing bone growth resumption and correction of bowlegs. To be successful, bracing must be continued for months to years, and the brace must be worn 23 hours per day. Adherence is the most significant barrier to successful treatment. Parents have a difficult time forcing their toddler to stay in a brace that inhibits mobility for the bulk of the day (particularly a bilateral brace). Support parents by encouraging and praising their adherence to bracing. Teach parents to assess for potential skin impairment from brace rubbing.

When surgical treatment is required, the leg(s) will be immobilized in a long-leg bent knee or spica cast after the osteotomy is performed. Perform routine cast care. Refer to the Clinical Judgment and the Nursing Process section earlier in the chapter for additional interventions related to care of the immobilized child.

Muscular Dystrophy

Muscular dystrophy refers to a group of inherited conditions that result in progressive muscle weakness and wasting. The muscles affected are primarily the skeletal (voluntary) muscles. Various types of muscular dystrophy

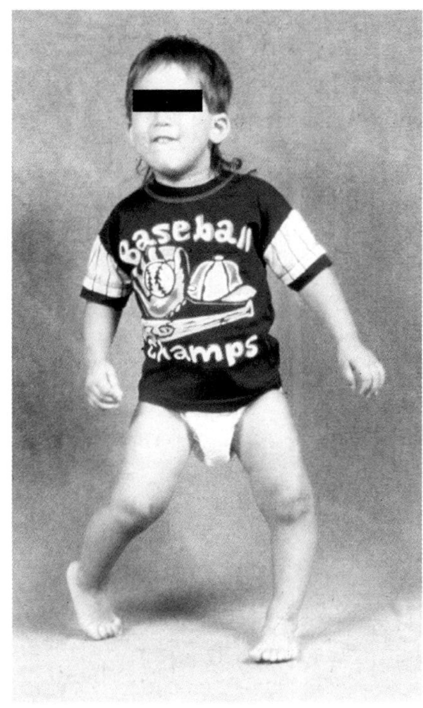

FIGURE 22.23 Note extreme bowing of the legs in tibia vara.

exist. All include muscle weakness over the lifetime; it is progressive in all cases but more severe in others. The various muscular dystrophies are most often diagnosed in childhood and affect a variety of muscle groups. The inheritance pattern for muscular dystrophy differs for each type but may be X-linked, autosomal dominant, or recessive. The genetic mutation in muscular dystrophy results in absence or decrease of a specific muscle protein that prevents normal function of the muscle. The skeletal muscle fibers are affected, yet there are no structural abnormalities in the spinal cord or the peripheral nerves. Table 22.3 gives specifics related to the common types of muscular dystrophy.

Duchenne muscular dystrophy, the most common neuromuscular disorder of childhood, results in a shortened life expectancy (Darras, 2022). Due to advances in medical care, such as improvements in noninvasive mechanical ventilation, better management of cardiac dysfunction using angiotensin-converting enzymes (ACE) inhibitors, and the use of steroids, survival into the person's 30s—and in some cases into their 40s or 50s—is becoming more common (Darras, 2021). The incidence is about 1 in 3,600 live male births (Bharucha-Goebel, 2020). For these reasons, this discussion will focus on Duchenne muscular dystrophy.

Pathophysiology

The gene mutation in Duchenne muscular dystrophy results in the absence of dystrophin, a protein that is critical for maintenance of muscle cells. The gene is X-linked recessive, meaning that mainly males are affected, and they receive the gene from their female parent (females are carriers but have mild to no symptoms). Absence of dystrophin leads to generalized weakness of voluntary muscles, and the weakness progresses over time. The hips, thighs, pelvis, and shoulders are affected initially; as the disease progresses, all voluntary muscles as well as cardiac and respiratory muscles are affected.

Children with Duchenne muscular dystrophy are often late in learning to walk. As toddlers, they may display pseudohypertrophy (enlarged appearance) of the calves. During the preschool years, they fall often and are quite clumsy. The affected child has difficulty climbing stairs and running and cannot get up from the floor in the usual fashion. The school-age child walks on the toes or balls of

TABLE **22.3** • Types of Muscular Dystrophy

Type	Onset	Inheritance	Muscle Involvement
Duchenne (pseudohypertrophic)	Early childhood (usually 3–6 years)	X-linked recessive (primarily only males; female carriers may show mild symptoms)	Generalized weakness, muscle wasting; limb and trunk first
Becker	2–16 years	X-linked recessive (primarily only males; female carriers may show mild symptoms)	Similar but less severe than Duchenne
Congenital (severe involvement at birth)	At birth to 2 years	Most forms are autosomal recessive (primarily affects males).	Generalized muscular weakness, possible joint deformities, contractures and hypotonia noted at birth
Emery–Dreifuss	Childhood to early adolescence (usually by 10 years)	Most often X-linked recessive (primarily affects males)	Weakness; wasting of shoulder, upper arm, and shin muscles
Limb-girdle	Late adolescence to middle age	Most often autosomal recessive but may be dominant (primarily affects males)	Weakness, wasting of shoulder and pelvic girdles first
Facioscapulohumeral	Usually, late childhood to early adulthood (usually by age 20)	Autosomal dominant	Facial muscles weaken first, then shoulders and upper arms.
Myotonic	Infancy to adult years	Autosomal dominant	Generalized weakness; wasting of face, feet, hands, and neck first Delayed relaxation of muscles after contraction

Data from Bharucha-Goebel, D. X. (2020). Muscular dystrophies. In R. M. Kleigman, J. W. St. Geme III, N. J. Blum, S. S. Shah, R. C. Tasker, K. M. Wilson, & R. E. Behrman (Eds.), *Nelson textbook of pediatrics* (21st ed., pp. 17216–17284). Elsevier; Darras, B. T. (2021). Patient education: Overview of muscular dystrophies (Beyond the Basics). *UpToDate*. Retrieved May 16, 2023, from https://www.uptodate.com/contents/overview-of-muscular-dystrophies-beyond-the-basics

the feet with a rolling or waddling gait. Balance is disturbed significantly, and the child's belly may stick out when the shoulders are pulled back to stay upright and keep from falling over. During the school-age years, it also becomes difficult for the child to raise their arms. Sometime between the ages of 7 and 12 years, nearly all children with Duchenne muscular dystrophy lose the ability to ambulate, and by adolescence any activity of the arms, legs, or trunk requires assistance or support (Darras, 2022). Most children with Duchenne muscular dystrophy have some degree of intellectual impairment. Although their intelligence level is often expected, many may exhibit a specific learning disability (Bharucha-Goebel, 2020).

Therapeutic Management

There is no cure for Duchenne muscular dystrophy. However, the use of glucocorticoids may slow the progression of the disease (Darras, 2023). The side effects of glucocorticoids are many, including weight gain, short stature, osteoporosis, hirsutism, cushingoid appearance, and mood changes (Darras, 2023). Calcium supplements and vitamin D are prescribed to prevent osteoporosis, and antidepressants may be helpful when depression occurs related to the chronicity of the disease and/or as an effect of corticosteroid use (Darras, 2022). Medications to decrease the workload of the heart, such as beta-blockers and ACE inhibitors, may be prescribed.

TAKE NOTE!

Researchers continue to search for a way to stop or reverse this disease. Gene therapy, exon skipping or codon read through, and gene repair are some new strategies being investigated. The FDA has approved some medications, such as eteplirsen, golodirsen, viltolarsen, and ataluren, that have shown the ability to increase dystrophin. Studies are underway to establish clinical benefit (Darras, 2023).

Braces or orthoses and mobility and positioning aids are necessary. As the muscles deteriorate, joints may become fixated, resulting in contractures. Contractures restrict flexibility and mobility and cause discomfort. Sometimes, contractures require surgical tendon release. Spinal curvatures result over time. The child with Duchenne muscular dystrophy who can still walk may develop lordosis. More frequently, scoliosis or kyphosis develops with this disorder. Surgical spinal fixation with rod implantation is often required by adolescence (Darras, 2022). Additional complications include pulmonary, urinary, or systemic infections; depression; learning or behavioral disorders; aspiration pneumonia (as oropharyngeal muscles become affected); cardiac dysrhythmias; and, eventually, respiratory insufficiency and failure (as weakness of the chest muscles and diaphragm progresses).

Nursing Assessment

For a full description of the assessment phase of the nursing process, refer to the "Clinical Judgment and the Nursing Process" section earlier in the chapter. Assessment findings pertinent to Duchenne muscular dystrophy are discussed further on.

HEALTH HISTORY

Examine the health history for a family history of neuromuscular disorders. Note pregnancy and delivery history, as this information may be useful in ruling out a pregnancy problem or birth trauma as a cause of the motor dysfunction. Determine status of developmental milestone achievement. Children with Duchenne muscular dystrophy learn to walk but, over time, become unable to do so. If the child was previously diagnosed with muscular dystrophy, determine progression of the disease. Inquire about functional status and the need for assistive or adaptive equipment such as braces or wheelchairs. Determine skills related to ADLs. Note history of cough or frequent respiratory infections, which occur as the respiratory muscles weaken. While talking with the child and family, determine whether psychosocial issues such as decreased self-esteem, depression, alterations in socialization, or altered family processes might be present.

PHYSICAL EXAMINATION

Perform a thorough physical examination on the child with suspected muscular dystrophy or the child with known history of the disorder. Particular findings related to inspection, observation, auscultation, and palpation are presented in what follows.

Inspection and Observation

Observe the child's ability to rise from the floor. A hallmark finding of Duchenne muscular dystrophy is the presence of the Gowers sign: The child cannot rise from the floor in standard fashion because of increasing weakness (Fig. 22.24). Observe the child's gait. Determine effectiveness of cough.

Auscultation and Palpation

Auscultate the heart and lungs. Note tachycardia, which develops as the heart muscle weakens. Note adequacy of breath sounds, which may diminish with decreasing respiratory function. Note muscle strength with resistance testing. Palpate muscle tone.

LABORATORY AND DIAGNOSTIC TESTS

Electromyography (EMG) demonstrates that the problem lies in the muscles, not in the nerves. Serum creatine kinase levels are elevated early in the disorder, when

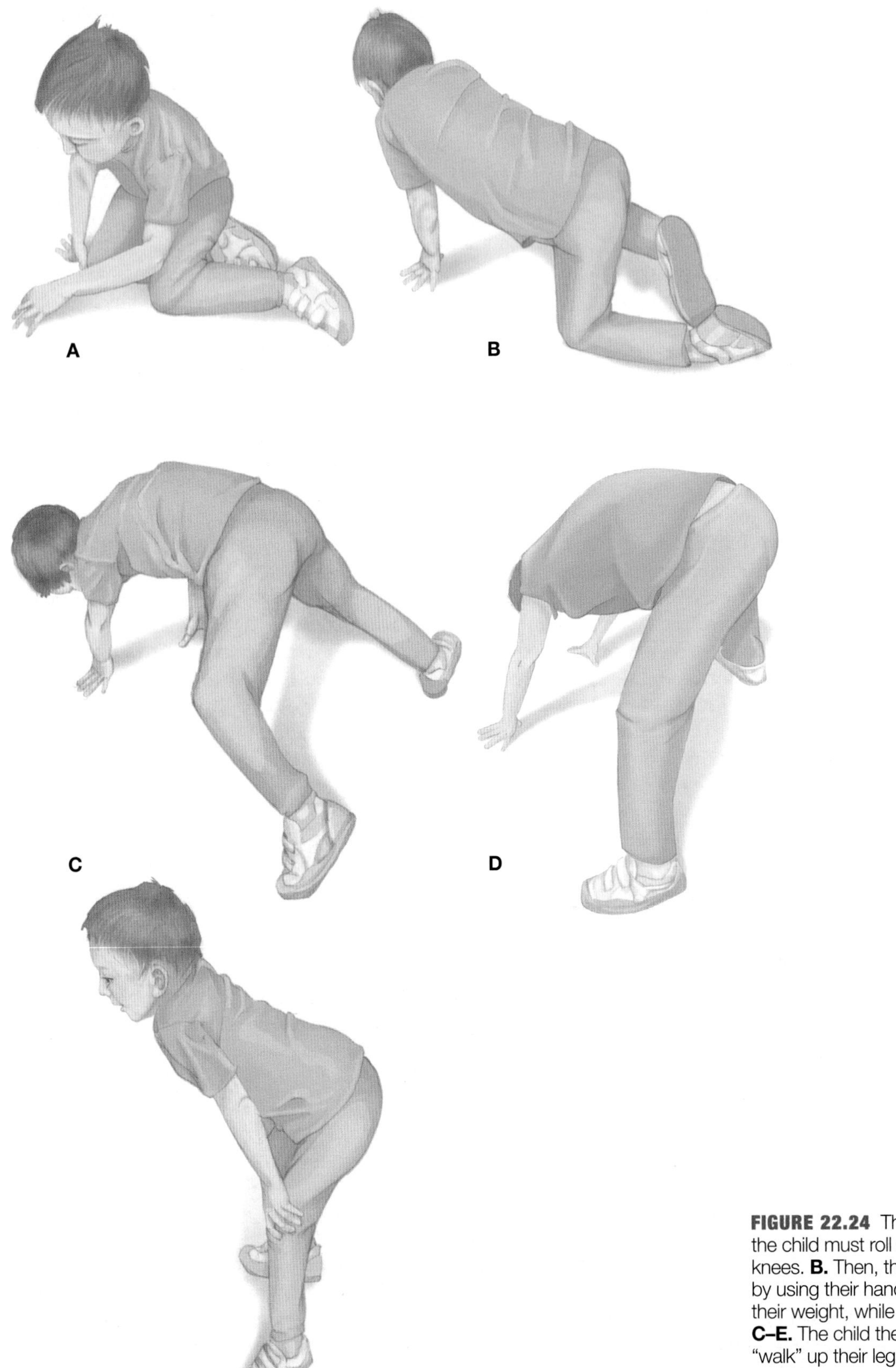

FIGURE 22.24 The Gower sign. **A.** First, the child must roll onto their hands and knees. **B.** Then, they must bear weight by using their hands to support some of their weight, while raising their posterior. **C–E.** The child then uses their hands to "walk" up their legs to assume an upright position.

significant muscle wasting is actively occurring. Muscle biopsy provides definitive diagnosis, demonstrating the absence of dystrophin. DNA testing reveals the presence of the gene.

Nursing Management

Nursing care is aimed at promoting mobility, maintaining cardiopulmonary function, preventing complications, and maximizing quality of life. Interventions directed at maintaining mobility and cardiopulmonary function also help to prevent complications. Refer to the "Clinical Judgment and the Nursing Process" section earlier in the chapter, and individualize nursing care based on the child's and family's response to the illness. Additional specifics related to care of the child with muscular dystrophy are discussed in the following sections.

PROMOTING MOBILITY

Administer glucocorticoids and calcium supplements as ordered. Encourage at least minimal weight bearing in a standing position to promote improved circulation, healthier bones, and a straight spine. Children with Duchenne muscular dystrophy may use a standing walker or standing frame to maintain an upright position. Perform passive stretching or strengthening exercises as recommended by the physical therapist. These exercises preserve mobility and may help to prevent muscle atrophy. Use orthotic supports such as hand braces or AFOs to prevent contractures of joints. Schedule activities during the part of the day when the child has the most energy. Teach parents the use of positioning, exercises, orthoses, and adaptive equipment. Use of a wheelchair full time typically occurs between 10 to 14 years of age (Bharucha-Goebel, 2020).

THINKING ABOUT **DEVELOPMENT**

You are caring for a 6-year-old child with Duchenne muscular dystrophy. How can you best help them meet developmental milestones? How would this differ if they were 12 years old?

MAINTAINING CARDIOPULMONARY FUNCTION

Assess respiratory rate, depth of respirations, and work of breathing. Auscultate the lungs to determine whether aeration is sufficient and to assess clarity of breath sounds. Position the child for maximum chest expansion, usually in the upright position. Teach the child and family deep-breathing exercises to strengthen or maintain respiratory muscles, and encourage coughing to clear the airways. Perform chest physical therapy or assist with chest percussion. Monitor the results of pulmonary function testing. Use of intermittent positive-pressure ventilation and mechanically assisted coughing will become necessary in adolescence for some, possibly later for others. Teach the parents monitoring of respiratory status and use of these modalities in conjunction with the respiratory therapist. Monitor cardiac status closely to identify heart failure early. Assess for edema, weight gain, or crackles. Strictly monitor fluid intake and output.

MAXIMIZING QUALITY OF LIFE

Long periods of bed rest may contribute to further weakness. Work with the family and child to develop a schedule for diversional activities that provide appropriate developmental stimulation, but avoid overexertion or frustration (related to inability to perform the activity). Periods of adequate rest must be balanced with activities. Walking or riding a stationary bike is appropriate for the child who has upper extremity involvement. For the child with lower extremity involvement, a wheelchair may become necessary for mobility, and the child may participate in crafts, drawing, and computer activities. Participating in the Special Olympics may be appropriate for some children. Do not place limits on the child, but encourage activities they are interested in that can be modified as needed to fit their abilities.

Provide emotional support to the child and family. Long-term direct care is stressful for families and becomes more complex as the child gets older. Families often need respite from continual caregiving duties. When a child is hospitalized, the caregiver may feel comfortable allowing nurses and other health care professionals to assume more of the child's daily care; this can be an opportunity for the caregiver to obtain respite from daily care. Respite care may also be offered in the home by various community services, so explore these resources with families.

Assess the child's educational status. Some children attend school; other families may opt for home schooling. Administer antidepressants as ordered; managing depression may increase the child's desire to participate in activities and self-care. Refer the child and family to the Muscular Dystrophy Association (MDA), which provides multidisciplinary care via clinics located throughout the United States. The association is also a clearinghouse for resources for people with muscular dystrophy. Ensure that families receive genetic counseling for family planning purposes as well as determining which family members may be carriers for muscular dystrophy.

Spinal Muscular Atrophy

SMA is a genetic motor neuron disease that affects the spinal nerves' ability to communicate with the muscles. It is inherited via an autosomal recessive mechanism. The motor neuron protein survival of motor neurons (SMNs) is deficient as a result of a faulty gene on chromosome 5. The motor neurons are located mostly in the spinal cord. Without adequate SMN, the signals from the neurons to the muscles instructing them to contract are ineffective, so the muscles lose function and atrophy over time. The proximal muscles, those closer to the body's center, are usually more affected than the distal muscles. Cognition is unaffected by this disease (Bodamer, 2023).

There are several types of SMA, classified as type 0 to type 4, based on age of onset, severity of weakness, and clinical course. SMA0 and SMA1 are the most common and most severe (Bodamer, 2023). Their usual progression and prognosis are compared in Table 22.4.

Respiratory muscle weakness may occur with all types of SMA and is usually the cause of death in type 1 SMA. Upper respiratory tract infections and aspiration related to dysphagia or gastroesophageal reflux often develop into pneumonia and eventual respiratory failure, as the affected child cannot effectively cough independently in order to clear the airway. Many children with severe type 1 SMA are ventilator dependent. Pectus excavatum develops in children with type 1 and type 2 SMA who exhibit paradoxical breathing (use of the diaphragm without intercostal muscle support). The chest becomes funnel shaped, and the xiphoid process is retracted (pectus excavatum), further restricting respiratory development. Inability to appropriately suck and swallow leads to difficulty feeding in the child with type 1 SMA. Weak back muscles affect the developing spine, resulting in the complication of scoliosis, kyphosis, or both.

Therapeutic management of SMA is supportive, aimed at promoting mobility, maintaining adequate nutrition and pulmonary function, and preventing complications. Spinal fusion may be performed in older children with significant scoliosis. Since the discovery of the disease-causing gene for SMA, further research and improved diagnostic techniques have occurred. Therapies, such as nusinersen (which is an intrathecally injected medication), and gene replacement, such as onasemnogene abeparvovec, have both shown promising results (Bodamer, 2023).

Nursing Assessment

Note history of attainment of developmental milestones, as well as loss of milestones. SMA should be suspected in a child showing symmetric, unexplained weakness that is more proximal than distal and greater in the legs than

TABLE 22.4 • Features of Spinal Muscular Atrophy

Features	Type 0 (Prenatal SMA)	Type 1 SMA (Werdnig–Hoffman Disease, Infantile SMA)	Type 2 SMA (Intermediate SMA)	Type 3 SMA (Kugelberg–Welander Disease, Juvenile SMA)	Type 4 SMA (Late Onset)
Onset	Prenatal	Less than 6 months of age	6–18 months of age	After 18 months of age; child has started walking or has taken at least five independent steps.	Age not strictly defined; typically, adult onset
Symptoms	• Loss of or decreased fetal movement later in pregnancy • At birth, severe hypotonia • Joint contractures may be present.	• Generalized weakness; cannot sit without support • Weak cry • Difficulty sucking, swallowing, and breathing	• Proximal muscles are more affected; that is, thighs are weaker than lower legs; legs tend to be weaker than arms. • Respiratory muscles may be involved. • Scoliosis may occur.	• Weakness that is most severe in the shoulders, hips, thighs, and upper back • Respiratory muscles may be involved. • Scoliosis may occur.	• Symptoms are mild, all motor milestones achieved. • Ambulation maintained
Progression	Rapidly progresses to early death by 6 months of age (typically by 1 month)	Rapidly progresses to early childhood death. Use of ventilators and gastrostomy feeding tubes may prolong life expectancy, but, typically, death occurs by age 2.	Slower progression; life expectancy related to age of onset (The younger the onset, the more severe the disease and the shorter the life expectancy.) Survival into adulthood common if respiratory status maintained appropriately	Slow progression Lifespan usually unaffected. Walking ability maintained until at least adolescence; may need wheelchair later in life	Normal lifespan

Data from Bodamer, O. A. (2023). Spinal muscular atrophy. *UpToDate*. Retrieved May 16, 2023, from https://www.uptodate.com/contents/spinal-muscular-atrophy

arms; diminished or absent tendon reflexes; history of difficulty with motor skills; or loss of motor skills (Bodamer, 2023). In the infant or child with known SMA, assess for recent hospitalizations or respiratory illness. Determine the respiratory support regimen used at home (if any). Note level of motor ability and identify the orthoses or adaptive equipment used. Elicit history related to feeding patterns at home. Assess for floppy appearance in the infant with SMA. Note decreased ability to initiate spontaneous muscle movement. In the infant or young child with SMA, note a narrow chest with decreased excursion, relatively protuberant abdomen, and paradoxical breathing pattern (Fig. 22.25). Observe the chest for formation of pectus excavatum. Auscultate the lungs for diminished or adventitious breath sounds. Monitor laboratory testing, which may include:

- Creatine kinase (CK): elevated when muscular damage is occurring
- Genetic testing: identifies presence of gene for SMA
- Muscle biopsy: shows the muscle abnormality
- Nerve conduction velocity test and electromyogram: to determine extent of involvement

Nursing Management

Nursing management of type 2 and type 3 SMA focuses on promoting mobility, maintaining pulmonary function, and preventing complications. Children with type 1 SMA need additional interventions related to prevention of complications from immobility and assistance with nutrition. Refer to the "Clinical Judgment and the Nursing Process" section earlier in the chapter for interventions related to these areas. Individualize the nursing plan of care based on the individual child's responses to the disorder.

Promote mobility through the use of range-of-motion exercises, lightweight orthotics, standing frames, and wheelchair use as appropriate. Support parents in their efforts to adhere to physical and occupational therapy regimens. Older children may exercise with assistance in a warm pool. Position the child in a fashion that maintains appropriate body alignment.

Provide airway clearance techniques such as manual or mechanical cough assistance, chest percussion, and postural drainage to assist with clearance of secretions. In collaboration with the respiratory therapy, teach the family the use of noninvasive ventilation support, in which positive pressure is delivered to the lungs through a mask or mouthpiece (Fig. 22.26). Provide routine tracheostomy care if the child has a tracheostomy (refer to "Tracheostomy" section of Chapter 18).

Administer gastrostomy tube feedings if ordered, and teach the family gastrostomy tube care. Use bracing as prescribed to prevent spinal curvature. Make frequent inspections for skin breakdown in areas affected by bracing.

Cerebral Palsy

Cerebral palsy is a term used to describe a range of nonspecific clinical symptoms characterized by abnormal motor pattern and postures caused by nonprogressive abnormal brain function. The majority of causes occur before delivery (80%) but can also occur in the natal and postnatal periods (Box 22.1) (Johnston, 2020). Often,

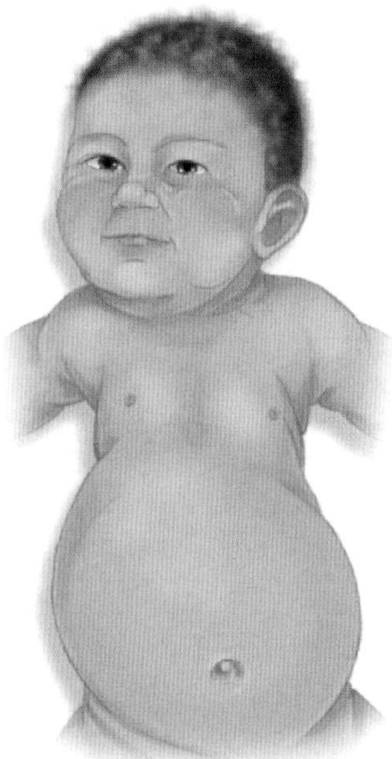

FIGURE 22.25 Note the very narrow chest, beginning xiphoid depression, and relatively enlarged appearance of the abdomen in this infant with type 1 spinal muscular atrophy (SMA).

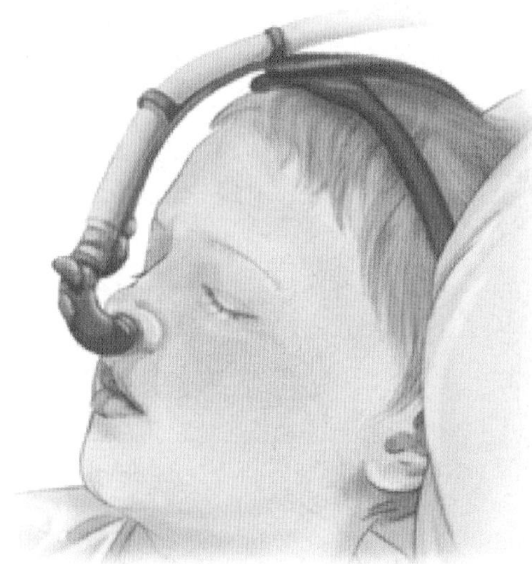

FIGURE 22.26 Use of noninvasive positive-pressure monitoring via nasal prongs can maximize respiration and may help prevent pulmonary complications.

BOX **22.1 Causes of Cerebral Palsy**

Prenatal

- Congenital malformation
- Hypoxia
- Fever in the pregnant parent
- Seizures in the pregnant parent
- Bleeding in the pregnant parent
- Exposure to radiation
- Environmental toxins
- Genetic abnormalities
- Metabolic disorders
- Intrauterine growth restriction
- Intrauterine infection, such as cytomegalovirus and toxoplasmosis
- Nutritional deficits
- Preeclampsia
- Multiple births
- Prematurity
- Low birth weight
- Malformation of brain structure
- Abnormalities of blood flow to the brain
- Abdominal insults
- Accidental injury to the pregnant parent
- Heavy alcohol consumption by the pregnant parent
- Smoking during pregnancy

Perinatal

- Prematurity (<32 weeks)
- Asphyxia
- Hypoxia
- Abnormal fetal presentation
- Sepsis or central nervous system infection
- Placental complications
- Electrolyte disturbance
- Cerebral hemorrhage
- Chorioamnionitis (infection of the placental tissues and amniotic fluid)

Postnatal

- Kernicterus (a type of brain damage that may result from neonatal hyperbilirubinemia)
- Asphyxia
- Head trauma (e.g., motor vehicle crashes, abuse)
- Seizures
- Toxins
- Viral or bacterial infection of the central nervous system (e.g., meningitis)
- Cerebral infarcts
- Intraventricular hemorrhage

no specific cause can be identified (Barkoudah & Aravamuthan, 2023). Cerebral palsy is the most common movement disorder of childhood; it is a lifelong condition and one of the more common causes of physical disability in children (Johnston, 2020). The incidence is about 2 in every 1,000 live births and is higher in premature and low–birth weight infants (Barkoudah & Aravamuthan, 2023). See the Healthy People 2030 box.

Most affected children will develop symptoms in infancy or early childhood. There is a large variation in symptoms and disability. For some children, it may be as mild as a slight limp; for others it may result in severe motor and neurologic impairments. Primary signs include motor impairments such as spasticity, muscle weakness, and **ataxia**, which is lack of coordination of muscle movements during voluntary movements such as walking or picking up objects. Complications include mental impairments, seizures, growth problems, impaired vision or hearing, abnormal sensation or perception, and hydrocephalus. Most children can survive into adulthood, but function and quality of life can vary from near expected to substantial impairments (Barkoudah, 2023).

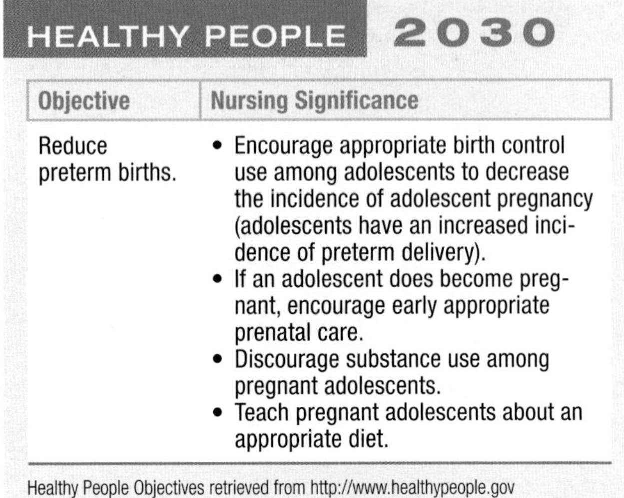

HEALTHY PEOPLE 2030

Objective	Nursing Significance
Reduce preterm births.	• Encourage appropriate birth control use among adolescents to decrease the incidence of adolescent pregnancy (adolescents have an increased incidence of preterm delivery). • If an adolescent does become pregnant, encourage early appropriate prenatal care. • Discourage substance use among pregnant adolescents. • Teach pregnant adolescents about an appropriate diet.

Healthy People Objectives retrieved from http://www.healthypeople.gov

Pathophysiology

Cerebral palsy is a disorder caused by abnormal development of, or damage to, the motor areas of the brain, resulting in a neurologic lesion. It is difficult to establish an exact location of the neurologic lesion, but it causes a disruption in the brain's ability to control movement and posture. The lesion itself does not change over time; thus, the disorder is considered nonprogressive since the brain injury does not progress. However, the clinical manifestations of the lesion change as the child grows. Some children may improve, but many either plateau in their attainment of motor skills or demonstrate worsening of motor abilities because it is difficult to maintain the ability to move over time.

Cerebral palsy is classified in several ways. One common way is by the type of movement disturbance (Table 22.5).

Therapeutic Management

Management of cerebral palsy involves multiple disciplines, including a primary health care provider, specialty health care providers such as a neurologist and an orthopedic surgeon, nurses, physical therapists, occupational therapists, speech therapists, dietitians, psychologists,

TABLE 22.5 • Classification of Cerebral Palsy

Types	Description	Characteristics
Spastic	Hypertonicity and permanent contractures; different types based on which limbs are affected: • Hemiplegia: both extremities on one side • Quadriplegia: all four extremities • Diplegia or paraplegia: lower extremities	• Most common form • Poor control of posture, balance, and movement • Exaggeration of deep tendon reflexes • Hypertonicity of affected extremities • Continuation of primitive reflexes • In some children, failure to progress to protective reflexes
Dyskinetic or athetoid	Abnormal involuntary movements	• The infant is limp and flaccid. • Uncontrolled, slow, worm-like writhing or twisting movements • Affects all four extremities with possible involvement of face, neck, and tongue • Movements increase during periods of stress. • Dysarthria and drooling may be present.
Ataxic	Affects balance and depth perception	• Poor coordination • Unsteady gait • Wide-based gait • Motor milestones and language skills delayed
Mixed	Combination of the foregoing	Most common is spastic and dyskinetic.

counselors, teachers, and parents. There is no standard treatment for all children. The overall focus of therapeutic management will be to assist the child to gain optimal development and function within the limits of the disease. Treatment is mainly preventive, symptomatic, and supportive. Spasticity management will be a primary concern and will be determined by clinical findings.

Medical management is focused on promoting mobility through the use of therapeutic modalities and medications. Surgical management is often required and is used to correct deformities related to spasticity.

PHYSICAL, OCCUPATIONAL, AND SPEECH THERAPY

The use of therapeutic modalities such as physical therapy, occupational therapy, and speech therapy will be essential in promoting mobility and development in the child with cerebral palsy. The earlier the treatment begins, the better chance the child has of overcoming developmental disabilities (National Institute of Neurological Disorders and Stroke, 2023).

Physical therapists work with children to assist in the development of gross motor movements such as walking and positioning, and they help the child develop independent movement. They also assist in preventing contractures, and they instruct children and caregivers in the use of assistive devices such as walkers and wheelchairs. Occupational therapists may be responsible for fashioning orthotics and splints. AFOs are the most common orthotic used by children with cerebral palsy (Fig. 22.27) (Barkoudah & Whitaker, 2022). AFOs help prevent deformity from conditions such as contractures and help reduce the effects of existing deformities. They can help improve a child's mobility by assisting in control of alignment and helping to increase the efficiency of the child's gait. Spinal orthotics such as braces are used by young children with cerebral palsy to combat scoliosis that develops due to spasticity. These braces are used to delay surgical management of the scoliosis until the child reaches skeletal maturity. Splinting is used to maintain muscle length. Serial casting may also be used to increase muscle and tendon length.

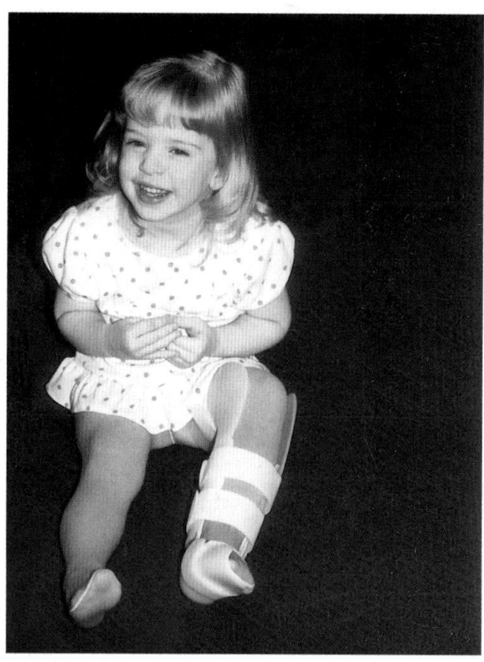

FIGURE 22.27 The child with cerebral palsy may benefit from wearing ankle–foot orthotics (AFOs) to provide support needed for independent or assisted walking.

Occupational therapy also assists in the development of fine motor skills and will help the child to perform optimal self-care by working on skills such as ADLs. Speech therapy assists in the development of receptive and expressive language and addresses the use of appropriate feeding techniques for the child who has swallowing problems. Speech therapists may teach augmented communication strategies to children who are nonverbal or who have articulation problems. Many children may not communicate verbally but can use alternative means such as communication books or boards and computers with voice synthesizers to make their desires known or to participate in conversation.

PHARMACOLOGIC MANAGEMENT

Various pharmacologic options are available to manage spasticity (see Drug Guide 22.1). Oral medications used to treat spasticity include baclofen, dantrolene sodium, and diazepam. Children with dyskinetic/athetoid cerebral palsy may be given anticholinergics to help decrease abnormal movements. Anticholinergic agents, such as scopolamine (also known as hyoscine) or glycopyrrolate, decrease saliva and are used to help control drooling.

TAKE NOTE!

Pathologic drooling is a problem for many children with cerebral palsy. It can lead to dehydration, dental enamel erosion, and maceration of the skin, and an odor can result, along with social stigmatization. Recent research has shown that intraglandular injection of botulinum toxin type A can improve drooling with few side effects in children with neurologic disorders (Barkoudah).

DOSAGE CALCULATION BOX 22.1

Child's weight: 87 lb

Medication order: Glycopyrrolate 0.8 mg per gastrostomy tube three times a day

Per the *Pediatric Dosage Handbook*, the recommended dose is 20 mcg/kg/dose three times daily and may titrate to a maximum dose of 100 mcg/kg/dose three times daily (not to exceed 1,500 to 3,000 mcg/dose)

Is this ordered dose safe?

Parenterally administered medications such as botulin toxins and baclofen are also used to manage spasticity. Botulinum toxin is injected into the spastic muscle to balance the muscle forces across joints and to decrease spasticity. It is useful in managing focal spasticity in which the spasticity is interfering with function, producing pain, or contributing to a progressive deformity. It can also help reduce drooling when injected into the salivary glands. Botulin toxin injection is performed by the health care provider or nurse practitioner and can be done in the clinic or outpatient setting. Phenol or ethanol block, a neurolytic agent that provides a temporary reduction in spasticity, may be used in conjunction with botulinum toxin or alone if botulinum toxin has been proved to be ineffective or contraindicated for the child (Barkoudah & Whitaker, 2022).

Intrathecal administration of baclofen has been shown to decrease tone, but it must be infused continuously due to its short half-life. Surgical placement of a baclofen pump will be considered in children with general spasticity that is limiting function, comfort, ADLs, and endurance. To test whether it is a suitable option, an intrathecal test dose of baclofen will be administered. If the trial is successful, a baclofen pump will be implanted. Once inserted, delivery of the drug can be individualized to meet the child's unique needs. The pump needs to be replaced every 5 to 7 years and must be refilled with medication approximately every 2 to 6 months, depending on the type of pump. Complications with baclofen pump placement include infection, rupture, dislodgement, and blockage of the catheter.

Medications are also used to treat seizure disorders in children with cerebral palsy (refer to Chapter 16 for information related to seizure management).

SURGICAL MANAGEMENT

Many children will require surgical procedures to correct deformities related to spasticity. Multiple corrective surgeries may be required; they are usually orthopedic or neurosurgical. Surgery may be used to correct contractures that are severe enough to cause movement limitations. Common orthopedic procedures include tendon lengthening procedures; correction of hip and adductor muscle spasticity; and fusion of unstable joints to help improve locomotion, correct bony deformities, decrease painful spasticity, and maintain, restore, or stabilize a spinal deformity. Neurosurgical interventions may include placement of a shunt in the child who has developed hydrocephalus or surgical interventions to decrease spasticity. Selective dorsal root rhizotomy is used to decrease spasticity in the lower extremities by reducing the amount of stimulation that reaches the muscles via the nerves.

Nursing Assessment

For a full description of the assessment phase of the nursing process, refer to the "Clinical Judgment and the Nursing Process" section earlier in the chapter. Assessment findings pertinent to cerebral palsy are discussed further on.

HEALTH HISTORY

Elicit a description of the present illness and chief complaint. Obtain a detailed account of gestational and perinatal events (refer to Box 22.1). Common signs and symptoms reported during the health history of the undiagnosed child might include:

- Intrauterine infections
- Prematurity with intracranial hemorrhage
- Difficult, complicated, or prolonged labor and delivery
- Multiple births
- History of possible anoxia during prenatal life or birth
- History of head trauma
- Delayed attainment of developmental milestones
- Muscle weakness or rigidity
- Poor feeding
- Hips and knees feel rigid and unbending when pulled to a sitting position
- Seizure activity
- Subnormal learning
- Abnormal motor performance, scoots on back instead of crawling on abdomen, walks or stands on toes

Children known to have cerebral palsy are often admitted to the hospital for corrective surgeries or other complications of the disease, such as aspiration pneumonia and urinary tract infections. The health history should include questions related to:

- Respiratory status: Has a cough, sputum production, or increased work of breathing developed?
- Motor function: Has there been a change in muscle tone or increase in spasticity?
- Presence of fever
- Feeding and weight loss
- Any other changes in physical state or medication regimen

PHYSICAL EXAMINATION

Observe the child's general appearance. Pay close attention to the neurologic assessment and motor assessment. Assess for delayed development, size for age, and sensory alterations such as strabismus, vision problems, and speech disorders. Abnormal postures may be present. While lying supine, the infant may demonstrate scissor crossing of the legs with plantar flexion. In the prone position, the infant may raise their head higher than normal due to arching of the back, or the opisthotonic position may be noted. The infant may also abnormally flex the arms and legs under the trunk. Primitive reflexes may persist beyond the point at which they disappear in a healthy infant. Evolution of protective reflexes may be delayed. Watch the infant or child play, crawl, walk, or climb to determine motor function and capability. Note any movement disorder. Infants with cerebral palsy may demonstrate abnormal use of muscle groups such as scooting on their back instead of crawling or walking.

Assess active and passive ROM. Pay particular attention to muscle tone. Although an increased or decreased resistance may be noted with passive movements, hypertonicity is most often seen. Increased resistance to dorsiflexion and passive hip abduction are the most common early signs. Sustained **clonus** (muscular spasm) may be present after forced dorsiflexion. Lift the child by placing your hands in the infant's or child's axillary area to assess shoulder girdle function and tone. Infants with cerebral palsy often demonstrate prolonged standing on their toes when supported in an upright standing position in this fashion. Lift the young child off the ground while the child holds your thumbs to test hand strength. Observe for presence of limb deformity, as decreased use of an extremity (as in the case of hemiparesis) may result in shortening of the extremity compared to the other one.

LABORATORY AND DIAGNOSTIC TESTS

A complete history, physical examination, and ancillary investigations are the primary modality for establishing a diagnosis of cerebral palsy. The following laboratory and diagnostic tests will help determine whether cerebral palsy is the likely cause or whether another condition may be the cause of the child's symptoms. These tests will also be important in evaluating the severity of the child's physical disabilities. Common supplementary laboratory and diagnostic tests ordered for the diagnosis and assessment of cerebral palsy include:

- Electroencephalogram: usually unexpected but the pattern is highly variable
- Cranial radiographs or ultrasound: may show cerebral asymmetry
- MRI or CT: may show area of damage or unexpected development but may be expected
- Screening for metabolic defects and genetic testing may be performed to help determine the cause of cerebral palsy.

Nursing Management

In addition to the patient problems and related interventions discussed in the "Clinical Judgment and the Nursing Process" section earlier in the chapter, nursing management focuses on promoting growth and development by promoting mobility and maintaining optimal nutritional intake. Providing support and education to the child and family is also an important nursing function.

PROMOTING MOBILITY

Mobility is critical to the development of the child with cerebral palsy. Treatment modalities to promote mobility include physiotherapy, pharmacologic management, and surgery. Surgical procedures are discussed earlier. Physical or occupational therapy as well as medications may be used to address musculoskeletal abnormalities, to facilitate ROM, to delay or prevent deformities such as contractures, to provide joint stability, to maximize activity, and to encourage the use of adaptive devices. The nurse's role in relation to the various therapies is to provide ongoing follow-through with prescribed exercises, positioning, or bracing.

When casting, splinting, or orthotics are used, assess skin integrity frequently. Pain management may also be necessary. Nursing care of children receiving botulin toxin focuses on assisting with the procedure and providing education and support to the child and family. Nursing interventions related to baclofen include assisting with the test dose and providing preoperative and postoperative care if a pump is placed, as well as providing support and education to the child and family. Teaching Guidelines 22.5 gives information related to baclofen pump insertion.

PROMOTING NUTRITION

Children with cerebral palsy may have difficulty eating and swallowing due to poor motor control of the mouth, tongue, and throat. This may lead to poor nutrition and problems with growth. The child may require a longer time to eat because of poor motor control. Special diets, such as soft or puréed, may make swallowing easier. Proper positioning during feeding is essential to facilitate swallowing and reduce the risk of aspiration. Speech or occupational therapists can assist in working on strengthening swallowing muscles as well as assisting in developing accommodations to facilitate nutritional intake. Consult a dietitian to ensure adequate nutrition for children with cerebral palsy. In children with severe swallowing problems or malnutrition, a feeding tube such as a gastrostomy tube may be placed.

PROVIDING SUPPORT AND EDUCATION

Cerebral palsy is a lifelong disorder that can result in severe physical and cognitive disability. In some cases, disability may require complete intensive daily care of the child. Adjusting to the demands of this multifaceted illness is difficult. Children are frequently hospitalized and need numerous corrective surgeries, which places strain on the family and its finances. From the time of diagnosis, the family should be involved in the child's care. It is important to include parents in the planning of interventions and care of this child. In most cases, they are the primary caregivers and will assist the child in development of functioning and skills as well as providing daily care. They will provide essential information to the health care team and will be advocates for their child throughout their life. It is important that nurses provide ongoing education for the child and family.

As the child grows, the needs of the family and child will change. Recognize and respect these needs. Providing daily intense care can be demanding and tiring. When a child with cerebral palsy is admitted to the hospital, this may serve as a time of respite for family and primary caregivers. Encourage respite care and provide support and encouragement. Because cerebral palsy is a lifelong condition, the child will need meaningful education programs that emphasize independence in the least restrictive educational environment. Refer caregivers to local resources, including education services and support groups.

Refer children younger than age 3 years to the local early intervention service. Early intervention provides case management of developmental services for children with special needs. Each state has a coordinator for early intervention. The office of the early intervention coordinator can then direct the health care professional to the local or district early intervention office.

TEACHING GUIDELINES 22.5 Baclofen Pump: Child/Family Education

- Check the incisions daily for redness, drainage, or swelling.
- Notify the health care provider or nurse practitioner if the child has a temperature greater than 101.5°F or if the child has persistent incision pain.
- Avoid tub baths for 2 weeks.
- Do not allow the child to sleep on their stomach for 4 weeks after pump insertion.
- Discourage twisting at the waist, reaching high overhead, stretching, or bending forward or backward for 4 weeks.
- When the incisions have healed, normal activity may be resumed.
- Wear loose clothing to prevent irritation at the incision site.
- Carry implanted device identification and emergency information cards at all times.

ACQUIRED DISORDERS

A number of neuromuscular and musculoskeletal disorders may be acquired during childhood or adolescence. These include rickets; slipped capital femoral epiphysis (SCFE); Legg–Calvé–Perthes disease; transient synovitis of the hip; and scoliosis (spinal curvature), which may occur as a result of a neuromuscular disorder or idiopathically.

Injuries throughout childhood are inevitable. Trauma or unintentional injury is a leading cause of childhood morbidity and mortality in the United States (Gill & Kelly, 2022). The child is at increased risk for trauma based on the developmental factors of physical and emotional immaturity; additionally, adolescents often display belief of invincibility. The developing neuromuscular system, if injured, may be irreparable, so the injury may result in life-threatening or lifelong effects. Neuromuscular trauma includes spinal cord injury and birth trauma. Younger children tend to suffer contusions, sprains, and simple upper extremity fractures; adolescents more frequently experience lower extremity trauma. As the number of children participating in youth sports increases and the intensity of training and the level of competition also increase, the incidence of injury is also likely to increase.

Many types of musculoskeletal injuries exist. This discussion will focus on fractures, sprains, overuse syndromes, and dislocated radial head.

Rickets

Rickets is a condition in which there is softening or weakening of the bones. Childhood rickets may occur as a result of nutritional deficiencies such as inadequate consumption of calcium or vitamin D or limited exposure to sunlight (required for adequate production of vitamin D). Rickets caused by vitamin D deficiency is a preventable condition, but cases continue to be reported in infants, children, and adolescents (Misra, 2022). Rickets may also occur if the body cannot regulate calcium and phosphorus in the appropriate balance, such as in chronic kidney disease. Gastrointestinal disorders in which fat absorption is altered (e.g., Crohn disease, celiac disease, and cystic fibrosis) may lead to rickets, as vitamin D is a fat-soluble vitamin.

Calcium is primarily laid down in the bones of the fetus during the third trimester. Premature infants miss this period of calcium accumulation and also suffer from inadequate calcium intake in the neonatal period. Thus, premature infants often demonstrate rickets of prematurity. Regardless of the underlying cause, rickets is most likely to occur during periods of rapid growth.

Vitamin D regulates calcium absorption from the small intestine and levels of calcium and phosphate in the bones. When calcium and phosphate levels in the blood are imbalanced, then calcium is released from the bones into the blood, resulting in loss of the supportive bony matrix.

Therapeutic Management

Treatment of rickets is aimed at correcting the calcium imbalance so that the skeleton may develop properly and without deformity. Calcium and phosphorus supplements are given, and some children also require vitamin D supplements. If rickets is not corrected while the child is still growing, permanent skeletal deformities and short stature may result.

TAKE NOTE!

The Academy of Pediatrics currently recommends that all infants have a minimum daily intake of 400 IU of vitamin D beginning soon after birth and that children 1 to 18 years of age have a minimum daily intake of 600 IU of vitamin D (Misra, 2022).

Nursing Assessment

Obtain a health history, determining risk factors such as:

- Limited exposure to sunlight
- Strict vegetarian diet or lactose intolerance (either one without milk product ingestion)
- Exclusive chest or breastfeeding by a person who has a vitamin D deficiency
- Dark-pigmented skin
- Prematurity
- Malabsorptive gastrointestinal disorder
- Chronic kidney disease

Note history of fractures or bone pain. Observe for dental deformities and bowlegs. Decreased muscle tone may also be present. Note low serum calcium and phosphate levels and high alkaline phosphatase levels. Radiographs may show changes in the shape and structure of the bone.

Nursing Management

Administer calcium and phosphorus supplements at alternate times to promote proper absorption of both of these supplements. Encourage exposure to moderate amounts of sunlight, and administer vitamin D supplements as prescribed. Teach the family that good dietary sources of vitamin D are fish, liver, and processed milk.

Slipped Capital Femoral Epiphysis

SCFE is a condition in which the femoral head dislocates from the neck and shaft of the femur at the level of the epiphyseal plate. The epiphysis slips downward and backward. The left hip is more often affected (Kienstra & Macias, 2022a; Sankar et al., 2020). The exact cause is unknown, but it is thought that during the adolescent growth spurt the femoral growth plate weakens and becomes less resistant to stressors. Hormonal alterations during this period may also play a role.

SCFE is classified based on its severity and whether the slip is acute or chronic. Chronic SCFE may lead to shortening of the affected leg and thigh atrophy.

Therapeutic Management

Promptly refer the child with SCFE to an orthopedic surgeon, as early surgical intervention will decrease the risk of long-term deformity. The goals of therapeutic management are to prevent further slippage, minimize deformity, and avoid the complications of cartilage necrosis (chondrolysis) and avascular necrosis of the femoral head. Surgical intervention may include in situ pinning, in which a pin or screw is inserted percutaneously into the femoral head to hold it in place. Osteotomy may be used for more severe cases. Osteoarthritis may be a long-term complication of SCFE.

Nursing Assessment

Elicit a health history, determining the onset and extent of pain. In acute SCFE, the pain is usually sudden in onset and results in inability to bear weight. Chronic SCFE may present with an insidious onset of pain and limp. Note risk factors for SCFE, including higher weight (significant risk factor), age 9 to 16 years, African American or Polynesian heritage, sedentary lifestyle, rapid growth spurt, and male sex (slightly higher incidence seen in males) (Kienstra & Macias, 2022a; Sankar et al., 2020). Observe ambulation, noting Trendelenburg gait. Assess for pain that is in the hip or that is referred to the groin, medial thigh, or knee. Note decreased ROM in the affected hip with external rotation. Radiographs will be obtained to confirm the diagnosis (anteroposterior and lateral frog-leg views of hips). Bone scan can rule out avascular necrosis, and CT scan helps define the extent of slippage.

TAKE NOTE!

Do not attempt to perform passive ROM to determine the extent of limitation in the child with SCFE; this may cause worsening of the condition.

Nursing Management

Enforce bed rest and activity restriction. If traction is used for a period before surgery, perform routine traction care and neurovascular assessments. Provide routine pre- and postoperative care. Assess pain and administer analgesics as needed. After in situ pinning, assist the child with crutch walking. Teach the family that weight bearing is usually resumed about a week after the surgery and that the pin will be removed later. Prolonged immobility may isolate the adolescent from usual peer interactions, so encourage phone calls or texting and visits with friends. Provide books, games, electronic devices, and magazines for distraction during the period of immobility. Provide education and support to the child and family.

Legg–Calvé–Perthes Disease

Legg–Calvé–Perthes disease is a self-limiting condition that involves avascular necrosis of the femoral head. It most often affects males between 4 and 8 years of age (Sankar et al., 2020). The etiology is unknown, but interruption of the blood supply to the femoral head results in bone death, and the spherical shape of the femoral head may be lost. Swelling of the soft tissues around the hip may occur. As new blood vessels develop, the area is supplied with circulation, allowing bone resorption and deposition to take place. During this period of revascularization, which takes 18 to 24 months, the bone is soft and more likely to fracture. Over time, the femoral head reforms.

Therapeutic Management

The goal of therapeutic management is to maintain normal femoral head shape and to restore appropriate motion. Treatment of Legg–Calvé–Perthes disease includes antiinflammatory medication to decrease muscle spasms around the hip joint and to relieve pain. Activity limitation may be prescribed, and sometimes bracing, casting, or traction is recommended to contain the femoral head. Serial x-ray follow-up determines progress of the disease. If surgery becomes warranted, which is rare, then osteotomy may be performed. Complications include joint deformity, early degenerative joint disease, persistent pain, loss of hip motion or function, and gait disturbance.

Nursing Assessment

Explore the health history for short stature, delayed bone maturation, related trauma, or a family history of Legg–Calvé–Perthes disease. Note painless limp, which may be intermittent over a period of months. Mild hip pain may result and may be referred to the knee or the thigh. Pain may be aggravated by exercise. Observe the child walking and note Trendelenburg gait. Perform ROM, noting internal rotation of the hip and limited abduction. Muscle spasm may result with hip extension and rotation. Hip radiographs are obtained to evaluate the extent of epiphyseal involvement. MRI or bone scan may also be used to differentiate Legg–Calvé–Perthes disease from other disorders. Ultrasound and arthrograms may also be useful.

Nursing Management

Nursing care of Legg–Calvé–Perthes disease is highly variable and depends on the stage of the disease and its severity. Administer antiinflammatory medications, noting their effect on pain. If activities are restricted, exercise the unaffected body parts. Assist the family with use of the brace if prescribed. The brace may be wiped with a damp cloth if it becomes dirty. Some children will be prescribed no treatment other than avoidance of contact or high-impact sports. Swimming and bicycle riding help to maintain ROM with little risk. If mobility equipment is needed, educate the child and family on its use. If osteotomy is performed, provide routine postoperative care, including education and support of the child and family.

Transient Synovitis of the Hip

Transient synovitis of the hip (also termed toxic synovitis) is a common cause of hip pain and limping in children in the United States, typically occurring in children between 3 and 8 years of age (Sankar et al., 2020). The exact cause is unclear, but it is thought to be associated with recent or active infection, trauma, or allergic hypersensitivity (Sankar et al., 2020). It is a self-limiting disease, and most cases resolve within a week, but it may last as long as 3 to 6 weeks.

Typically, it is a clinical diagnosis with laboratory and radiographic tests used to rule out other serious conditions. Therapeutic management involves nonsteroidal antiinflammatory medications, analgesics, and bed rest to relieve weight bearing on the affected hip joint.

Nursing Assessment

Explore the health history for risk factors such as antecedent trauma, concurrent or recent upper respiratory tract infection, pharyngitis, or otitis media. Note sudden acute onset of moderate to severe pain of one hip. Sometimes, pain is referred to the anterior thigh or knee. Pain is usually the worst on arising in the morning, and the child refuses to walk; pain then decreases throughout the day. The child's temperature will usually be normal or low grade (less than 38°C). Observe for a limp or for refusal to bear weight. Observe the position of the affected hip: it will be held in a flexed and externally rotated position. Note restricted ROM for abduction and internal rotation.

Nursing Management

Nursing care focuses on educating the family, including instructions on administering nonsteroidal antiinflammatory medications, analgesics, and bed rest. Parents are very concerned when their child refuses to walk; therefore, provide significant support, and reassure the child and family of the self-limiting nature of the disease.

Scoliosis

Scoliosis is a lateral curvature of the spine that exceeds 10 degrees. It may be congenital, associated with other disorders, or idiopathic. Table 22.6 explains the types of scoliosis. Idiopathic scoliosis, with the majority of cases occurring during adolescence, is the most common scoliosis (Mistovich & Spiegel, 2020b). Hence, this discussion will focus on adolescent idiopathic scoliosis. The etiology of idiopathic scoliosis is not known, but genetic factors; growth abnormalities; and bone, muscle, disk, or central nervous system disorders may contribute to its development. Early screening and detection of scoliosis result in improved outcomes.

TABLE 22.6 • Types of Scoliosis

Type	Associated Factors
Idiopathic	Unknown cause Infantile: occurs in the first 3 years of life Juvenile: diagnosed between age 4 and 10 years or prior to adolescence Adolescent: age 11–17 years
Neuromuscular	Associated with neurologic or muscular disease such as cerebral palsy, myelomeningocele, spinal cord tumors, spinal muscular atrophy, muscular dystrophies
Congenital	Results from anomalous vertebral development

Pathophysiology

In the rapidly growing adolescent, the involved vertebrae rotate around a vertical axis, resulting in lateral curvature, and asymmetry of the shoulder and waistline is evident. The vertebrae rotate to the convex side of the curve, with the spinous processes rotating toward the concave side, resulting in displacement of the ribs and rib asymmetry (Mistovich & Spiegel, 2020b). As the curve progresses, the shape of the thoracic cage continues to change, and respiratory and cardiovascular compromise may occur (the main complications of severe scoliosis).

Therapeutic Management

Treatment of scoliosis is aimed at preventing progression of the curve and decreasing the impact on pulmonary and cardiac function. Treatment is based on the age of the child, expected future growth, and severity of the curve. Observation with serial examinations and spine radiographs is used to monitor curve progression. For curves of 25 to 45 degrees, bracing may be sufficient to decrease progression of the curve (Mistovich & Spiegel, 2020b). Box 22.2 describes types of scoliosis braces, and Figure 22.28 shows examples of braces. The choice of brace will depend on the location and severity of the curve. Some curves will progress despite appropriate bracing and adherence.

Surgical correction is often required for curves greater than 45 degrees; it is achieved with rod placement and bone grafting (Mistovich & Spiegel, 2020b). Partial spinal fusion accompanies many of the corrective surgeries. Multiple surgical approaches and techniques with various instrumentation methods exist for fusion and rod placement. The surgical approach may be anterior, posterior, or both. Traditional rod placement (Harrington rod) involves a single rod fused to the vertebrae, resulting in curve correction but also a flat-backed appearance. Newer rod instrumentations allow for scoliosis curve correction with maintenance of normal back curvature. The rods are shorter, and several are wired or grafted to the appropriate vertebrae to achieve

BOX 22.2 Types of Braces Used to Treat Scoliosis

- Underarm (thoracolumbosacral orthosis [TLSO], Boston, Wilmington): for low thoracic and thoracolumbar curves; less conspicuous, no visible neckpiece
- Milwaukee: for thoracic or major double curves; traditional, standard, has a visible neckpiece with chin rest
- Nighttime bending (Charleston): creates a curve so severe that walking is not possible and brace can be worn only at night

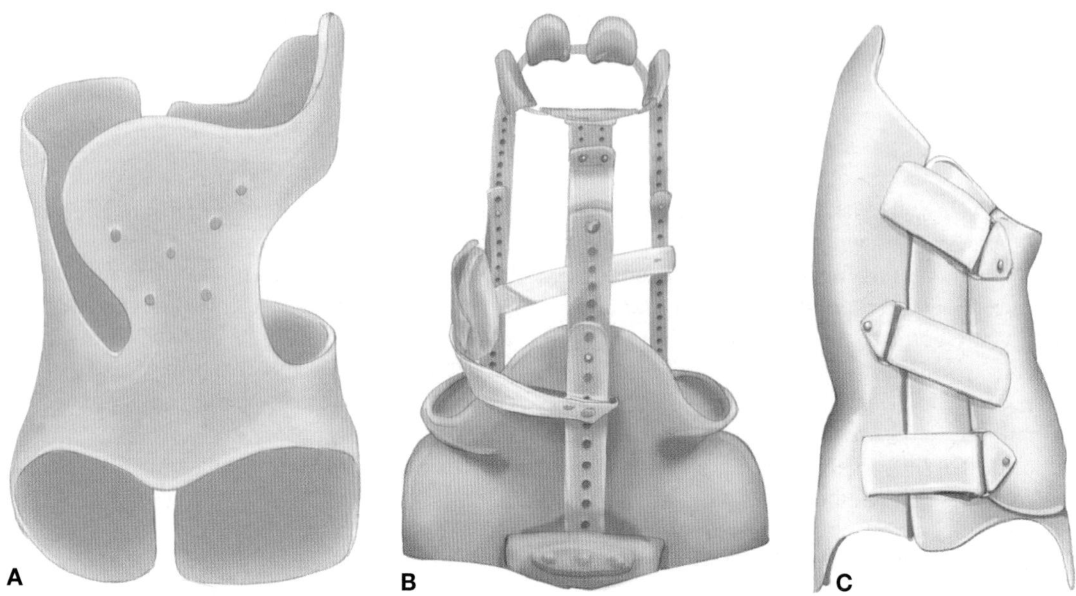

FIGURE 22.28 **A.** Boston brace. **B.** Milwaukee brace. **C.** Nighttime bending brace.

correction. Figure 22.29 shows one example of surgical rod instrumentation. Newer minimally invasive techniques such as growth modulation techniques also exist (Scherl & Hasley, 2023).

Nursing Assessment

For a full description of the assessment phase of the nursing process, refer to the "Clinical Judgment and the Nursing Process" section earlier in the chapter. Assessment findings pertinent to scoliosis are discussed following.

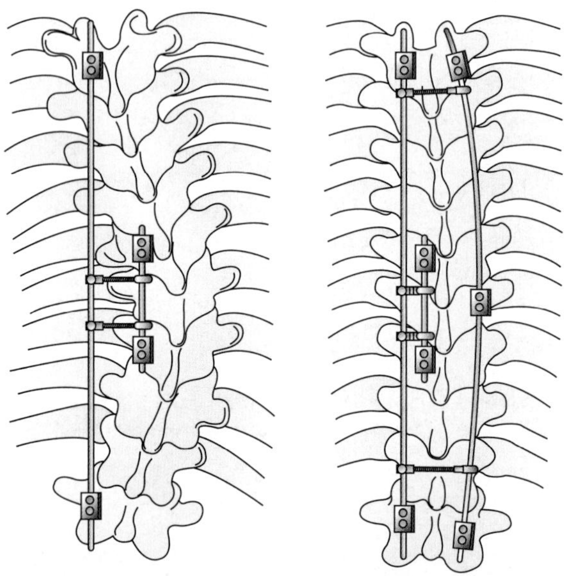

FIGURE 22.29 Rods are fused to the vertebrae and connected to a distracting rod to rotate the vertebral column (Cotrel–Dubousset method is shown).

HEALTH HISTORY

Determine why the child is presenting for evaluation for scoliosis. Commonly, the child or adolescent will not report back pain; only mild discomfort is associated with idiopathic scoliosis until the curve becomes severe. Often, the family recognizes asymmetry in the hips or shoulders, or the child is screened for scoliosis at school and determined to be at risk. Explore the child's current and past medical history for risk factors such as:

- Family history of scoliosis
- Recent growth spurt
- Physical changes related to puberty

Determine the age of development of secondary sex characteristics and the age of menarche, as these signs of pubertal development indicate the expected velocity and length of remaining growth.

PHYSICAL EXAMINATION

The physical assessment of a child with possible or actual scoliosis involves mainly inspection and observation. Auscultate the heart and lungs to determine compromise related to severe curvature.

Observe the child at rest, sitting, and standing for evidence of poor posture. Inspect the child's back in a standing position. Note asymmetries such as shoulder elevation, prominence of one scapula, uneven curve at the waistline, or a rib hump on one side. Measure shoulder levels from the floor to the acromioclavicular joints. Note the difference between the height of the high and low shoulder in centimeters. Measure the heights of anterior and posterior iliac spines, and note the difference in centimeters. View the child from the side, noting abnormalities in the spinal curve. With the child bending forward, arms hanging freely, note asymmetry of the back (pronounced hump on one side). Figure 22.30 shows scoliosis noted on visual inspection. Note leg-length discrepancy if present. During the neurologic examination, balance, motor strength, sensation, and reflexes should all be normal.

LABORATORY AND DIAGNOSTIC TESTS

Full-spine radiographs are necessary to determine the degree of curvature. The radiologist will determine the extent of the curve based on specific formulas and techniques of measurement.

Nursing Management

The "Clinical Judgment and the Nursing Process" section earlier in the chapter lists general interventions. Tailor nursing care based on the adolescent's response to the disease and its treatment. Additional nursing interventions specific to scoliosis are discussed here.

ENCOURAGING ADHERENCE TO BRACING

Bracing is intended to prevent progression of the curve but does not correct the current curve. Although modern braces display an improved appearance, with no visible neckpiece, and can be worn under clothes, many adolescents do not adhere to brace wear. The brace is recommended to be worn 18 hours per day to prevent curve progression, although recent studies have found 13 hours to be sufficient in some cases (Scherl & Hasley, 2023). Many factors may contribute to nonadherence, including the discomfort associated with brace wear such as pain, heat, and poor fit. The family environment may not be conducive to adherence to brace wear, and adolescents are concerned about body image.

Inspect the skin for evidence of rubbing by the brace that may impair skin integrity. Teach families appropriate skin care, and recommend they check the brace daily for fit and breakage. Encourage the adolescent to shower during the time of day that the brace is off and to ensure that the skin is clean and dry before putting the brace back on. Wearing a cotton T-shirt under the brace may decrease some of the discomfort associated with brace wear. Exercises to strengthen back muscles may prevent muscle atrophy from prolonged bracing and maintain spine flexibility.

PROMOTING POSITIVE BODY IMAGE

Encourage the adolescent to express their feelings or concerns about wearing the brace. Give the adolescent ways to explain scoliosis and its treatment to their peers. Wearing stylish baggy clothes may help the adolescent to conceal the brace if desired. Refer adolescents and their families to the National Scoliosis Foundation for additional support.

PROVIDING PREOPERATIVE CARE

If the curve progresses despite bracing or causes pulmonary or cardiac compromise, surgical intervention will be warranted. Before surgery, teach the adolescent the importance of turning, coughing, and deep breathing in the postoperative period. Explain the tubes and lines that

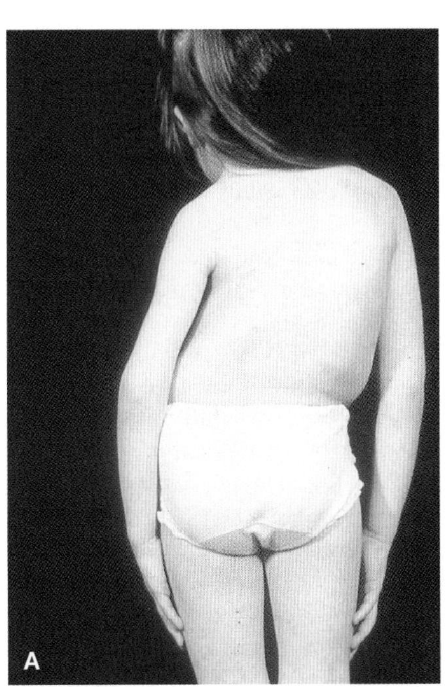

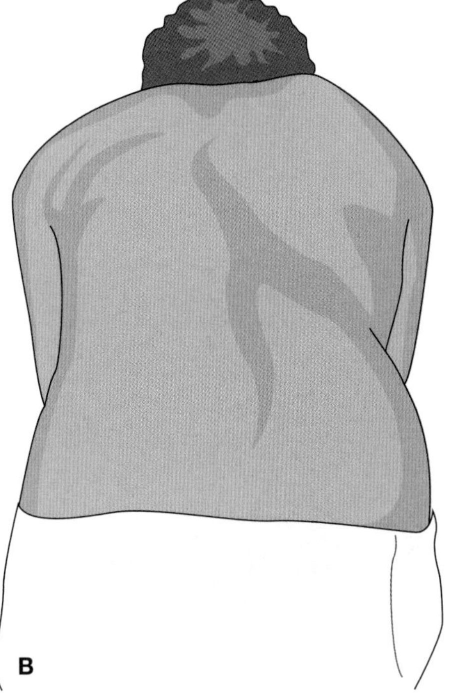

FIGURE 22.30 **A.** Note right shoulder, scapula, and hip elevation as well as discrepancy in waist curvature. **B.** Note right upper back hump.

will be present immediately after the surgery. Review positioning guidelines: Back flexion or extension will not be allowed. Introduce the child to the patient-controlled analgesia pump, and explain pain scales. There is a high risk of significant blood loss with spinal fusion and instrumentation, so, if possible, arrange for preoperative autologous blood donation.

PROVIDING POSTOPERATIVE CARE

The goal of nursing management in the postoperative period after spinal fusion with or without instrumentation is to avoid complications. Perform neurovascular checks with each set of vital signs. When turning the child, use the log-roll technique to avoid flexion of the back (Fig. 22.31). Provide proper pain management and medicate for pain before repositioning and ambulation. Administer prophylactic intravenous antibiotics if ordered. Assess for drainage from the operative site and for excess blood loss via the Hemovac or other drainage tube. Maintain Foley patency, as the child will be confined to bed for the first couple of days. Maintain strict recording of fluid intake and output. Administer transfusions of packed red blood cells if ordered. Ambulation, once ordered, should be done slowly to avoid orthostatic hypotension. Assist the family with arrangements to continue the adolescent's school work while hospitalized, and/or arrange for home tutoring during the several-week recovery period.

> **CONSIDER THIS!**
>
> I have been diagnosed with scoliosis, and the doctor told me I have to wear a brace at night. How did this happen? I will never be able to go to another sleepover; all the other kids will laugh at me.
>
> Thoughts: How would you respond to their concerns? What education will be necessary, and how can you promote adherence?
>
> What local resources could you refer them to?

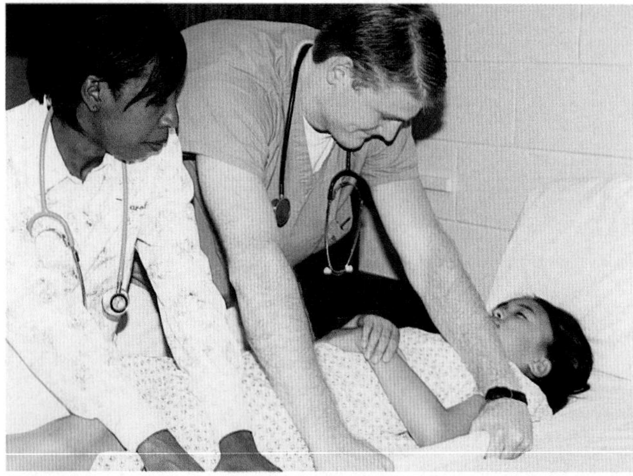

FIGURE 22.31 Logroll the postoperative spinal fusion child to prevent spine flexion.

Spinal Cord Injury

Spinal cord injury is damage to the spinal cord that results in loss of function. Frequent causes are trauma, such as car crashes, falls, diving into shallow water, gunshot or stab wounds, sports injuries, child abuse, or birth injuries. Spinal cord injuries are relatively uncommon in children, but when they do occur, they have a devastating impact on the child's physical and functional status, social and emotional development, and family functioning.

Spinal cord injury is a medical emergency, and immediate medical attention is required. Cervical traction is often used initially, and surgical intervention is sometimes necessary. Ongoing medical treatment will be based on the child's age and overall health and the extent and location of the injury. Therapeutic management focuses on rehabilitation and prevention of complications. Spinal cord injury in children is managed similarly to that in adults.

Nursing Assessment

Symptoms vary based on the location and severity of the injury. Common signs and symptoms associated with spinal cord injury include:

- Inability to move or feel extremities
- Numbness
- Tingling
- Weakness

Paralysis depends on the location of the injury to the spinal cord; the higher the injury in the spinal cord, the more extensive the damage and the greater the loss of function. High cervical injury will result in damage to the phrenic nerve, which innervates the diaphragm. Damage to this nerve will leave the child unable to breathe without assistance.

The diagnosis of spinal cord injury is made by clinical signs and diagnostic tests, which may include radiographs, CT scans, and MRI.

Nursing Management

Any child who requires hospitalization due to trauma should be considered at risk for a spinal cord injury. Immobilization of the spine is essential until full evaluation of the injury is complete and spinal cord damage is ruled out. Nursing management will be similar to management of the adult with a spinal cord injury and will focus on optimizing mobility, promoting bladder and bowel management, promoting adequate nutritional status, preventing complications associated with extreme immobility such as contractures and muscle atrophy, managing pain, and providing support and education to the child and family. Refer to the Myelomeningocele section of this chapter for information related to urinary and bowel elimination.

The nurse plays an important role not only in the acute care of children with spinal cord injury but also during rehabilitation. Recovery from a spinal cord injury requires long-term hospitalization and rehabilitation. An interdisciplinary team of health care providers, nurses, therapists, social workers, and case managers will work to manage the child's complex and long-term needs. Promoting communication among the interdisciplinary team is essential and will be a key nursing function. Rehabilitation will need to focus on the everchanging developmental needs of the child as they grow.

Prevention of spinal cord injuries is an important nursing consideration. Educate the public on vehicular safety, including seat belt use and the proper use of age-appropriate safety seats. Additional education topics include bicycle, sports, and recreation safety; prevention of falls; violence prevention, including gun safety; and water safety, including the risk of diving. This education can help decrease the incidence of spinal cord injury in children.

Birth Trauma

Birth traumas are injuries sustained by the newborn during the birthing process. They may result from the pressure of birth, especially in a prolonged or abrupt labor, abnormal or difficult presentation, cephalopelvic disproportion, or mechanical forces, such as forceps or vacuum used during delivery. Newborns at risk include multiple fetus deliveries, large-for-gestational-age infants, infants born extremely premature, infants with large heads, or newborns with congenital anomalies. Most injuries are minor and resolve without treatment. See Table 22.7 for common types of birth trauma.

Nursing Assessment

Assess the eyes and face for facial paralysis, observing for asymmetry of the face with crying or appearance of the mouth being drawn to the unaffected side. Ensure that the infant spontaneously moves all extremities. Note any absence of or decrease in deep tendon reflexes or abnormal positioning of extremities.

Nursing Management

Nursing management will be mainly supportive and will focus on assessing for resolution of the trauma or any associated complications, along with providing support and education to the parents. Provide the parents with an explanation and reassurance that these injuries are harmless. Parents are alarmed when their newborn cannot move an extremity or demonstrates asymmetric facial movement. Reassure the parents and offer support. Provide the parents with education regarding the length of time until resolution and when and if they need to seek further medical attention for the condition.

Fracture

Fractures occur frequently in children and adolescents; common sites include fingers, the forearm, and wrist (Baldwin et al., 2020). Most pediatric fractures heal well

TABLE 22.7 • Common Types of Birth Trauma

Types	Description
Brachial plexus injury	• Primarily in large babies and babies with shoulder dystocia or breech delivery • Results from stretching, hemorrhage within a nerve, or tearing of the nerve or the roots associated with cervical cord injury • Associated traumatic injuries include fracture of the clavicle or humerus and subluxations of the shoulder or cervical spine. • Erb palsy is an upper brachial plexus injury, and the involved extremity usually presents adducted, prone, and internally rotated. • Moro, biceps, and radial reflexes are absent, but the grasp reflex is usually present. • Treatment consists of prevention of contractures, which involves immobilization of the limb gently across the abdomen for the first week and then the use of passive range-of-motion exercises. • There is usually no associated sensory loss, and this condition usually improves rapidly. • In some cases, deficits may persist; therefore, observation is warranted.
Cranial nerve injuries	• Most common is facial palsy. • Frequently attributed to pressure resulting from forceps • May also result from to pressure on the nerve in utero, which may be due to fetal positioning such as the head lying against the shoulder • Physical findings include asymmetry of the face when crying; the mouth may be drawn toward the normal side. • The paralyzed side may be smooth with a swollen appearance. • Most infants begin to recover in the first week, but full resolution may take up to several months. • In most cases, treatment is not necessary, only observation. • In cases in which the eye is affected and unable to close, protection with the use of patches and synthetic tears may be necessary.

with minimal treatment (Baldwin et al., 2020). Midclavicular, humerus, or femur fractures can occur as a result of birth trauma. They typically heal well but may require limiting mobility or splinting. Several factors contribute to differences in pediatric fractures compared to adult fractures. Different fracture patterns are seen due to the anatomic, biomechanic, and physiologic differences in the pediatric immature skeleton (see the "Pathophysiology" section next) (Baldwin et al., 2020). When caring for children with fractures, the caregiver must consider their high activity level and their continued skeletal growth and development. Fractures in children result most frequently from accidental trauma (Baldwin et al., 2020). Nonaccidental trauma (child abuse) and other disease processes are the other causes of fractures.

CLINICAL REASONING ALERT!

Fracture in the newborn (with the exception of birth trauma) or infant should raise a high index of suspicion for abuse, as fractures are very unusual in children who cannot yet walk.

Pathophysiology

The growth plate is the most vulnerable portion of the child's bone and is frequently the site of injury. The Salter–Harris classification system is used to describe fractures involving the growth plate (Table 22.8). The thicker, more elastic periosteum in children yields to the force encountered with trauma, resulting more frequently in nondisplaced fractures in children. The increased vascularity and decreased mineral content make the child's bones more flexible. Plastic or bowing deformities and buckle and greenstick fractures are the result. Complete fractures do occur in children, but they tend to be more stable than in the adult, resulting in improved healing and function. Spiral, pelvic, and hip fractures are rare in children. Table 22.9 explains common types of fractures in children.

Fractures in children heal more rapidly and result in less disability and deformity than adults. The younger the child, the more quickly the bone heals. However, plastic deformity and Salter–Harris type IV fractures may result in an angular deformity. Although healing of fractures is usually quick and without incident in children,

TABLE 22.8 • The Salter–Harris Classification System

Type	Description	Illustration
I	The fracture is through the physis, widening it.	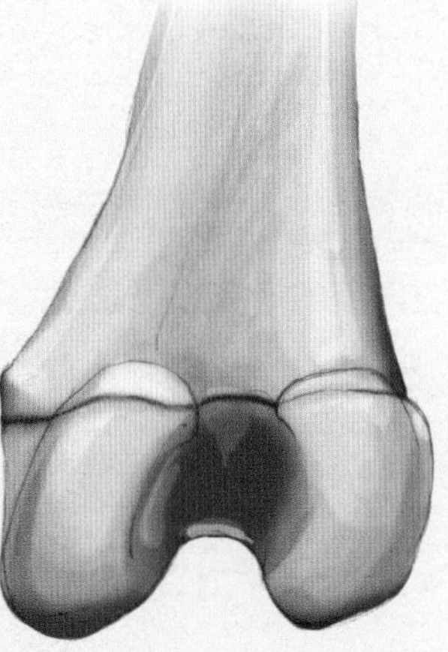
II	The fracture is partially through the physis, extending into the metaphysis.	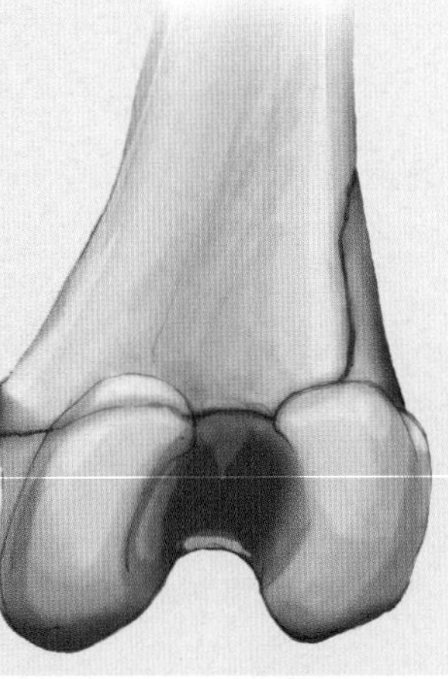

TABLE 22.8 • The Salter–Harris Classification System

Type	Description	Illustration
III	The fracture is partially through the epiphysis, extending into the epiphysis.	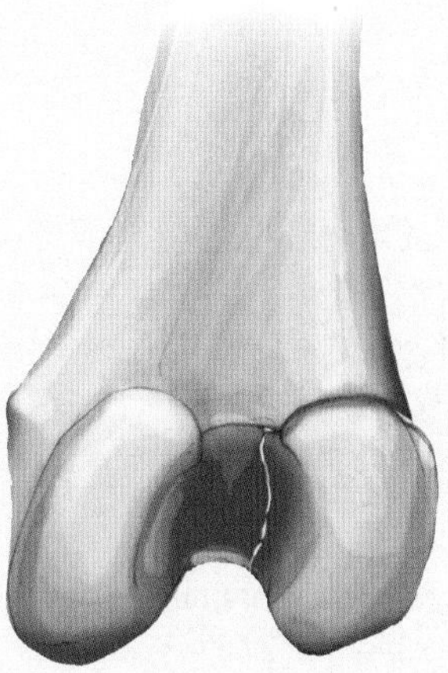
IV	The fracture is through the metaphysis, physis, and epiphysis.	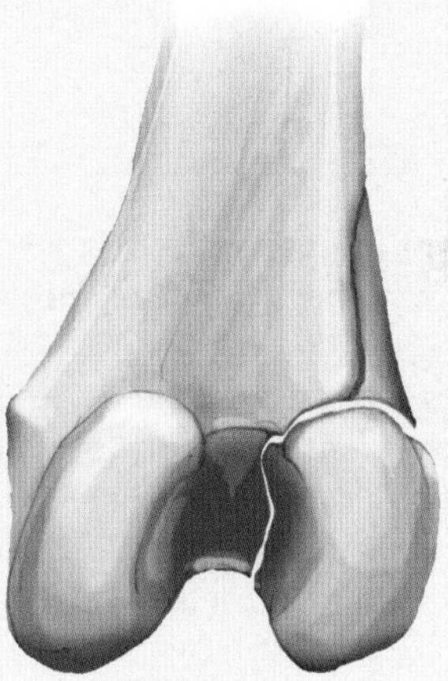
V	Crushing injury to the physis	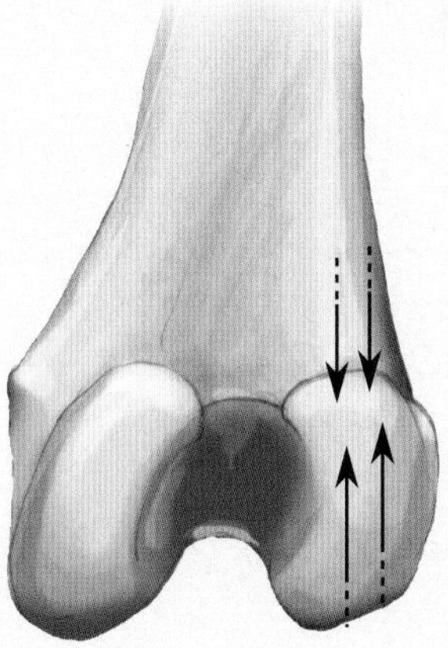

delayed union, nonunion, or malunion can occur. Additional complications include infection, avascular necrosis, bone shortening from epiphyseal arrest, vascular or nerve injuries, fat embolism, reflex sympathetic dystrophy, and compartment syndrome, which is an orthopedic emergency (Baldwin et al., 2020).

TAKE NOTE!

Any type of fracture can be the result of child abuse, but spiral femur fractures, rib fractures, and humerus fractures, particularly in the child younger than 2 years, should always be thoroughly investigated to rule out the possibility of abuse (Baldwin et al., 2020).

TABLE 22.9 • Types of Fractures in Children

Fracture Type	Description	Illustration
Plastic or bowing deformity	Significant bending without breaking of the bone	A
Buckle fracture	Compression injury; the bone buckles rather than breaks.	B
Greenstick fracture	Incomplete fracture of the bone	C
Complete fracture	The bone breaks into two pieces.	D

Therapeutic Management

The vast majority of childhood fractures would heal well with splinting only, but casting of these fractures is performed to provide further comfort to the child and to allow for increased activity while the fracture is healing. Displaced fractures require manual traction to align the bones, followed by casting. More severe fractures may require traction for a period of time, usually followed by casting. Severe or complicated fractures may alternatively require open reduction and internal fixation for healing to occur. Complex fractures are often treated with external fixation (Fig. 22.32).

TAKE NOTE!

Significant swelling may occur initially after immobilization with a splint. Delaying casting for a few days provides time for some of the swelling to subside, allowing for successful casting a few days after the injury.

Nursing Assessment

For a full description of the assessment phase of the nursing process, refer to the "Clinical Judgment and the Nursing Process" section earlier in the chapter. Assessment findings pertinent to fractures are discussed further on.

HEALTH HISTORY

Elicit a description of the present illness and chief complaint. Common signs and symptoms reported during the health history might include recent injury, trauma, or fall; complaint of pain; difficulty bearing weight; limp; or refusal to use an extremity. Young children often demonstrate sudden onset of irritability and refusal to bear weight. Ask about the mechanism of injury, and obtain a description of the traumatic event. Be alert to inconsistencies between the history and the clinical picture or mechanism of injury; inconsistency may be an indicator of child abuse. Explore the child's current and past medical history for risk factors such as:

- Rickets
- Renal osteodystrophy
- OI

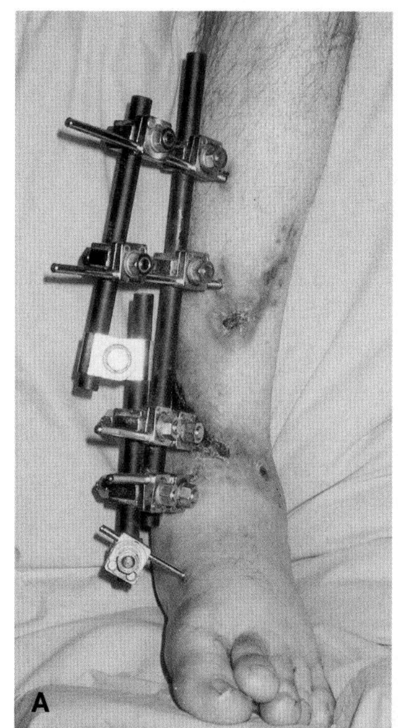

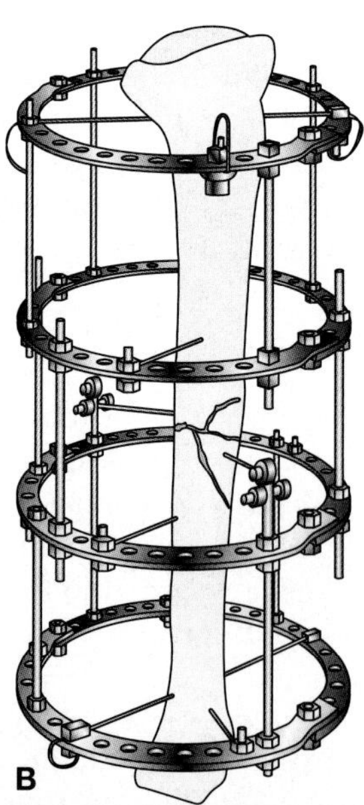

FIGURE 22.32 **A.** External fixation is required for complicated fractures. **B.** The Ilizarov fixator is a circular apparatus usually used for complicated lower extremity fractures. The pins are smaller in diameter, more like wires, than those used in other fixators.

- Participation in sports, particularly contact sports
- Failure to use protective equipment as recommended for various physical activities and sports (e.g., wrist guards while rollerblading)

PHYSICAL EXAMINATION

Perform the physical examination of the child with a potential fracture carefully so as not to cause further pain or trauma. The physical examination particular to fractures includes inspection, observation, and palpation.

TAKE NOTE!

Do not attempt to straighten or manipulate an injured limb.

Inspection and Observation

Inspect the skin for bruising, erythema, or swelling. Observe the extremities for deformity. Note neglect of an extremity or an inability to bear weight. If ambulating, note any limp.

Palpation

Carefully palpate the joint or injured part. Distract the young child with a toy or activity while palpating. Note point tenderness, which is a reliable indicator of fracture in children. Assess neurovascular status, noting distal extremity temperature, spontaneous movement, sensation, numbness, capillary refill time, and quality of pulses. The neurovascular assessment is critical to providing a baseline so that any changes associated with compartment syndrome can be identified quickly.

LABORATORY AND DIAGNOSTIC TESTS

Usually, plain x-ray films are all that are required to identify a simple fracture. Complicated fractures that require surgical intervention may require further evaluation with CT or MRI.

Nursing Management

Immediately after the injury, immobilize the limb above and below the site of injury in the most comfortable position with a splint. Use cold therapy to reduce swelling in the first 48 hours after injury. Elevate the injured extremity above the level of the heart. Perform frequent neurovascular checks.

CLINICAL REASONING ALERT!

Assess the injured, splinted, or casted extremity frequently for the "5 P's," which may indicate compartment syndrome: pain (increased out of proportion), pulselessness, pallor, paresthesia, and paralysis. Report these findings immediately.

Assess pain level and administer pain medications as needed. Utilize nonpharmacologic methods of pain relief as needed. Administer a tetanus vaccine to the child with an open fracture if they have not received a tetanus booster within the past 5 years. Additional nursing interventions include providing family education and teaching on fracture prevention.

PROVIDING FAMILY EDUCATION

Unless bed rest is prescribed, children with upper extremity casts and "walking" leg casts can resume increased levels of activity as the pain subsides. Children who require crutches while in a cast may return to school, but those in spica casts will be at home for several weeks. Providing distraction and finding ways to keep up with school work are important. Teach the family to care for the cast (see Teaching Guidelines 22.1).

PREVENTING FRACTURES

Discourage risky behavior such as climbing trees and performing tricks on bicycles. Provide appropriate supervision, particularly with outdoor activity. Encourage appropriate use of protective equipment, such as wrist guards with rollerblading and shin guards with soccer. Ensure that playground equipment is in good working order and intact; there should not be protruding screws or unbalanced portions of equipment, which may increase the risk of falling.

Sprains

Sprains result from a twisting or turning motion of the affected body part. The tendons and ligaments stretch excessively and may tear slightly. They are uncommon in young children as their growth plates are weaker than their muscles and tendons, making them more prone to fracture. Sprains may occur at any joint, but the most common are ankle and knee sprains. Therapeutic management of sprains includes rest, ice, compression, and elevation (RICE). Other treatment options may include activity restrictions, splints or casts, crutches or wheelchair, and physical therapy. On initial evaluation, sprains need to be differentiated from torn ligaments and meniscal tears, as those conditions are more serious and may require surgical intervention.

Nursing Assessment

Elicit a health history, determining the mechanism of injury (whether it occurred during sports or simply a misstep or fall). Determine what treatment the family has used so far. Inspect the affected body part for edema, which is frequently present, and bruising, which sometimes occurs. Note limp or inability to bear weight. Do not attempt to perform passive ROM on the affected body part. Assess neurovascular status distal to the injury (usually normal).

Nursing Management

Instruct the child and family in appropriate treatment of sprains, which includes:

- Rest: Limit activity.
- Ice: Apply cold packs for 20 to 30 minutes, remove them for 1 hour, and repeat (for the first 24 to 48 hours).
- Compression: Apply an Ace wrap or other elastic bandage or brace; check the skin for alterations when rewrapping.
- Elevation: Elevate the injured extremity above the level of the heart to decrease swelling (Fig. 22.33).

The child may require instruction in crutch walking as well. Teach the family that to prevent sprains during sports, it is important for the child to perform appropriate stretching and warm-up activities.

TAKE NOTE!

If the child's fingers or toes become increasingly swollen or discolored, remove the Ace wrap immediately.

Overuse Syndromes

The term "overuse syndrome" refers to a group of disorders that result from repeated force applied to normal tissue. The connective tissues fail in response to repetitive stress, leading to a small amount of tissue breakdown. Overuse syndromes develop over the course of weeks to months. There is usually no identifiable injury associated with overuse syndromes. Pain is usually associated with the activity and worsens with continued participation in the activity. The incidence of overuse injuries in the young athlete has increased as participation of youths in organized sports has grown along with children today participating in sports year-round and sometimes in multiple sports simultaneously, the increased competitive nature of youth sports, and the early specialization in a particular sport with inadequate periods of rest (Brenner & The Council on Sports Medicine and Fitness, 2007, reaffirmed 2021). The young athlete is at risk for more serious overuse injuries due to the following:

- The growing bones of the young athlete cannot handle as much stress as mature bones in adults. Growth patterns are often uneven. Bones grow faster than muscles, leaving the child more susceptible to injury.
- The child is just learning the proper mechanisms for skills, such as throwing a baseball.
- The child is unable to recognize vague signs of injury such as fatigue and poor performance (Brenner & The Council on Sports Medicine and Fitness, 2007, reaffirmed 2021).

Table 22.10 gives details on several common overuse syndromes. Therapeutic management is aimed at reassurance, pain management, and limiting rather than eliminating activity.

Nursing Assessment

Elicit a health history to determine the extent of involvement in sports. Note onset of pain, duration, intensity, aggravating factors, and treatments used at home. Examine the painful part, noting findings similar to those noted for each syndrome in Table 22.10.

RICE

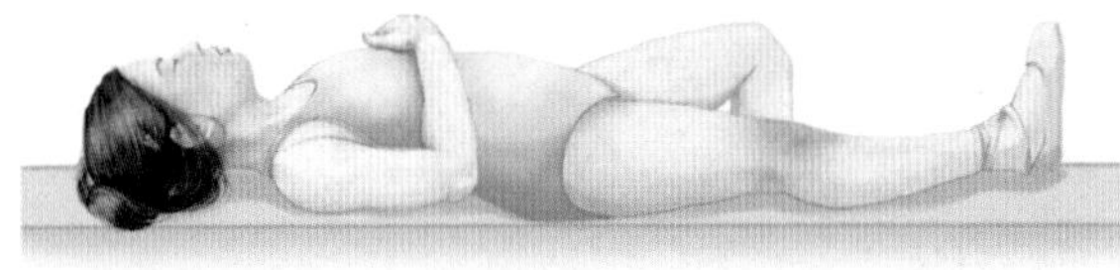

Rest

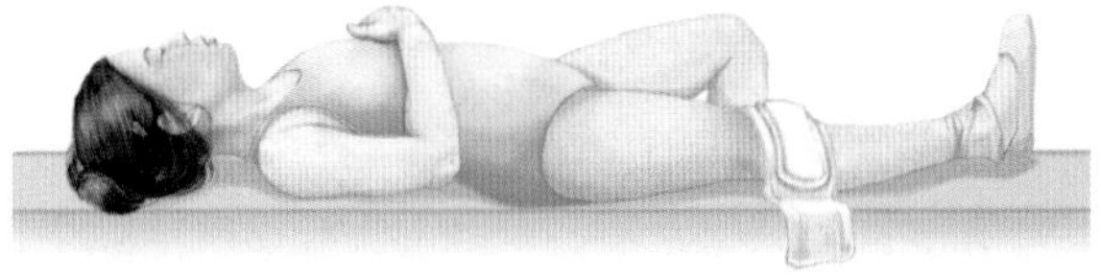

Ice

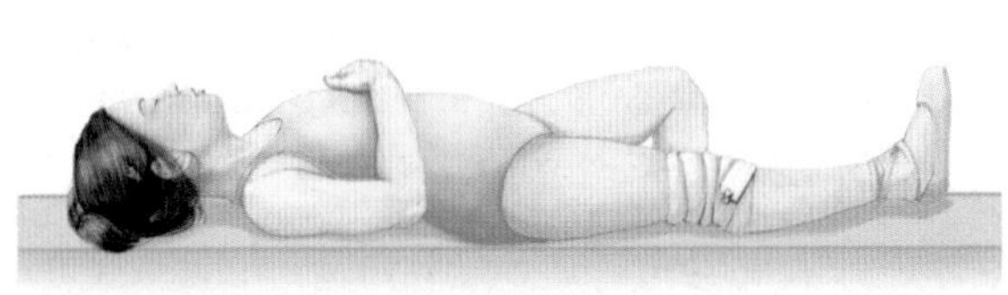

Compression

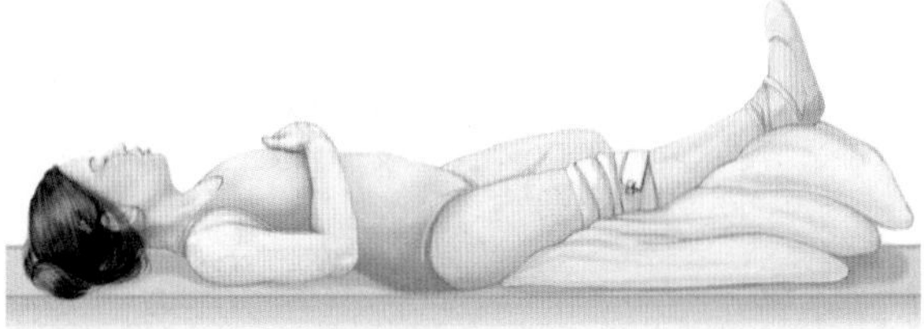

Elevation

FIGURE 22.33 RICE (rest, ice, compression, elevation) is the appropriate treatment for sprains.

TABLE 22.10 • Overuse Disorders

Disorder	Anatomic Area Affected	Most Commonly Occurs in	Symptoms
Osgood–Schlatter disease	Partial avulsion of the ossification center of the tibial tubercle	Active adolescents, most often males Most frequently during periods of rapid growth	• Mild to moderate pain, activity related • The tibial tubercle is tender when palpated. • Painful swelling or prominence of the anterior portion of the tibial tubercle
Epiphysiolysis of proximal humerus	Proximal humerus (widening of growth plate)	Occurs with rigorous upper extremity activity, such as baseball pitching	• Tenderness in the shoulder or proximal humerus • Pain with active internal rotation • Full shoulder ROM continues.
Epiphysiolysis of distal radius	Distal radius (widening of growth plate)	Occurs with overuse of the distal radius, such as in gymnasts	• Wrist pain that worsens with activity
Sever disease (calcaneal apophysitis)	Calcaneus (heel)	Usually in 9- to 14-year-olds	• Pain over the posterior aspect of the calcaneus • Limited active and passive dorsiflexion of foot
Shin splints	Refer to a variety of overuse syndromes associated with the shin (stress fracture, tibial stress, muscular issues).	Occur with activities that place repeated exertion on the lower leg, as in runners, ballerinas, elite soccer players	• Exercise-induced pain of the anterior aspect of the middle part of the lower leg • May be sharp pain • Worsens with exercise • With stress fracture, may have a limp that worsens with activity

Nursing Management

Initially, apply ice when pain is severe. Antiinflammatory medications such as ibuprofen may be helpful. Encourage the child to limit exercise and participate in a different activity. After a few weeks, most overuse syndromes resolve; at that point, the athlete may resume the prior activity. Osgood–Schlatter disease is the exception and may require 6 to 18 months to resolve (Kienstra & Macias, 2022b). Using pads or braces that are appropriate to the painful body part is also helpful. Supporting the arm with a sling may relieve stress on the proximal humerus when epiphysiolysis occurs. Heel cups used in athletic shoes help relieve stress on the heels associated with Sever disease. To prevent overuse syndromes, encourage athletes to perform appropriate stretching exercises during a 20- to 30-minute warm-up period before each practice or game. Also encourage several weeks of conditioning training before the season begins.

There is currently limited research pertaining to overuse injuries in the young athlete. The American Academy of Pediatrics has developed some guidelines to help prevent these injuries such as the following: Encourage 1 to 2 days off per week of competitive athletics, sports training, and competitive practice; encourage 2 to 3 months away from a specific sport during the year; and educate to increase weekly training time, number of repetitions, or total distance by no more than 10% a week. Participation in sports should be about fun, skill acquisition, sportsmanship, and safety (Brenner & The Council on Sports Medicine and Fitness, 2007, reaffirmed 2021). See Evidence-Based Practice 22.1.

TAKE NOTE!

"Energy healing" such as therapeutic touch and Reiki may provide a nonpharmacologic adjunct to pain management for musculoskeletal injuries.

Radial Head Subluxation

Subluxation of the radial head ("nursemaid's elbow") occurs when a pulling motion on the arm causes the annular ligament surrounding the radial head to stretch or tear, therefore displacing the radial head. The ligament becomes entrapped within the joint, preventing spontaneous reduction. It usually occurs in children younger than 5 years (Carrigan, 2020). In most cases, a parent, sibling, or caregiver inadvertently injures the child while holding or pulling on a pronated upper extremity. Radiologic examination may be done, especially if the mechanism of injury is not clear, to rule out fracture or dislocation. To reduce the injury, the elbow is flexed to

EVIDENCE-BASED PRACTICE 22.1

Are Overuse Injuries Associated With Sport-Specific Specialization and Sex of the Athlete?

Youth sports provide many benefits to children. In recent years, there has been an increased focus on scholarships and playing time that has resulted in youth focusing more training (more hours/week and months/year) on a single sport, referred to as sport specialization. Evidence exists that sport specialization is associated with an increased risk of overuse injuries in youth athletes. This study examined if the risks of overuse are sport specific, particularly sports that are more technical and repetitive, such as volleyball, compared with sports that have a broader movement profile, such as soccer. It also examined if the sex of an athlete influenced the risk of overuse injury associated with sport specialization.

STUDY

This was a cross-sectional study that used a self-administered, anonymous questionnaire given at club team tournaments in youth soccer, volleyball, and basketball. It included athletes aged 12 to 18 years of age, and 716 youth athletes completed the questionnaire.

Findings

The study found that the influence of sex, sport specialization, and excessive sport volume on overuse injury may be sport specific. The results showed that high levels of specialization were associated with overuse injury only in volleyball, not in basketball or soccer. Female basketball athletes were more likely than male athletes to report an overuse injury. In soccer athletes, the trend was toward more females with overuse injuries, but the association was not significant.

Nursing Implications

Nurses need to assess youth athletes' specialization level, including hours of training per week, months of training per year, and information on specific sport specialization. This study had limitations but does demonstrate the need for future research focused on sports that are more repetitive and limited in their movement profile, such as volleyball, along with examining the role of sex and the risk of overuse injuries. Nurses are in a unique position to counsel youth on the importance of diversified training and the benefits of being a well-rounded athlete. Educate youth and caregivers on the evidence that supports delayed specialization until late adolescence and that the sport an athlete plays and specializes in may influence their risk of overuse injuries.

Data from Post, E. G., Biese, K. M., Schaefer, D. A., Watson, A. M., McGuine, T. A., Brooks, M. A., & Bell, D. R. (2020). Sport-specific associations of specialization and sex with overuse injury in youth athletes. *Sports Health*, *12*(1), 36–42. https://doi.org/10.1177/1941738119886855

90 degrees, and then the forearm is fully and firmly supinated, causing the ligament to snap back into place. With appropriate reduction of the radial head, no complications result.

Nursing Assessment

Elicit a health history to help determine the mechanism of injury. Common precipitators of this injury include pulling on the child's arm while leading them in one direction, helping the child up the stairs, a child dropping or falling to the ground while an adult is holding the hand, or swinging or lifting the child by the hands. Assess neurovascular status and examine the extremity. The child will hold the arm slightly flexed at the side or across the abdomen and refuse to move it. When the arm is still, the child apparently has no discomfort. Neurovascular status is normally intact with no bruising or swelling present.

Nursing Management

After treatment, usually hyperpronation to reduce the dislocation, assess the child's ability to use the arm without pain. Typically, after reduction, the child will demonstrate less pain almost immediately. Educate the parents that once a radial head subluxation occurs, it may recur. Teach the parents to avoid excessive pulling or pulling up on the child's arm, particularly in an abrupt jerking fashion, to prevent recurrence. Encourage the parents and caregivers to always lift the child under the arms.

KEY CONCEPTS

- Muscles, tendons, ligaments, and cartilage are all present and functional at birth, although intentional, purposeful movement develops only as the infant matures.
- The spine is very mobile in the newborn and infant, especially the cervical spine region, resulting in a high risk of cervical spine injury.
- Rapid muscle growth in the adolescent years places the adolescent at increased risk for injury compared with other age groups.
- The bones of the infant and young child are more flexible and have a thicker periosteum and more abundant blood supply than the adult's; as a result, bending occurs more frequently than breaking of the bone, and the fractured bone heals more quickly.
- The epiphysis of long bones is the growth center of the bones in children. Injury to this area may result in long-term extremity deformity.
- The nurse's role in laboratory and diagnostic testing for neuromuscular or musculoskeletal disorders is mainly that of educating the child and family about and preparing the child for the test or procedure.
- Plain radiographs are usually sufficient for diagnosing injuries in children. If CT or MRI scans are required, the nurse may need to help the child stay calm and still during the procedure.
- Apply a pressure dressing following joint aspiration to prevent hematoma formation or fluid recollection.

- Perform frequent assessments of pain status and the effect of pain medication in the child with a musculoskeletal disorder.
- Diazepam may be helpful in relieving muscle spasm associated with traction.
- Maintain traction and the appropriate amount of weight as ordered.
- The bulk of cast care occurs in the home. Teach the family of a child with a cast to perform neurovascular assessments, prevent the cast from getting wet, and care for the skin appropriately.
- Assessment of ROM and muscle tone is critical in the child with a neuromuscular disorder. Hypertonia or hypotonia is an unexpected finding in the infant or child.
- Assessment of neurovascular status is an essential component of care for a child with a musculoskeletal disorder.
- Determining attainment of developmental milestones and subsequent progression or loss of those milestones is useful in distinguishing various neuromuscular disorders.
- The nurse reinforces and carries out the exercise plans and adaptive equipment use as prescribed by the physical or occupational therapist in order to maintain neuromuscular and musculoskeletal function and to prevent complications.
- Nursing management of myelomeningocele focuses on preventing infection; promoting bowel and urinary elimination; promoting adequate nutrition; preventing latex allergy reaction; maintaining skin integrity; providing education and support to the family; and recognizing complications, such as hydrocephalus or increased ICP, associated with the disorder.
- Cerebral palsy may result in significant motor impairment. Children with cerebral palsy require ongoing physical therapy as well as nutritional intervention.
- Children with Duchenne muscular dystrophy initially learn to walk but later lose this ability.
- Respiratory compromise occurs in muscular dystrophy and SMA and eventually leads to death.
- Children with chronic disorders such as OI may demonstrate slower or lesser growth than other children and may also be unable to participate in certain activities because of bone fragility.
- Congenital or developmental disorders such as DDH or clubfoot require bracing or casting for correction and to prevent deformity later in life.
- Torticollis may be treated by teaching the family to perform daily neck muscle–stretching exercises.
- To prevent complications after a spinal fusion for scoliosis correction, use the log-roll method for turning the child so that back flexion is avoided.
- Children with spinal cord injury require intense nursing care and lengthy rehabilitation to maintain or regain function.
- Children with neuromuscular disorders often suffer depression related to the chronic nature of the disorder.
- School attendance and participation in activities such as the Special Olympics are important for children with neuromuscular dysfunction.
- Fractures may occur as a result of unintentional or intentional injury or because the bones are fragile, as in rickets or OI.
- Sprains, fractures, and overuse syndromes occur frequently in young athletes. Appropriate warm-up and stretching may help prevent some of these injuries.
- Rest, ice, compression, and elevation are the appropriate treatment for sprains.

REFERENCES AND RECOMMENDED READINGS

American Academy of Pediatrics, Committee on Genetics. (1999, reaffirmed 2017). Policy Statement: Folic acid for the prevention of neural tube defects. *Pediatrics*, *104*(2), 325–327. https://doi.org/10.1542/peds.104.2.325

Balasubramanian, M. (2022). Osteogenesis imperfecta: An overview. *UpToDate*. Retrieved May 14, 2023, from https://www.uptodate.com/contents/osteogenesis-imperfecta-an-overview?search=osteogenesis%20imperfecta%20children&source=search_result&selectedTitle=1~77&usage_type=default&display_rank=1

Baldwin, K. D., Shah, A. S., Wells, L., & Arkader, A. (2020). Common fractures. In R. M. Kleigman, J. W. St. Geme III, N. J. Blum, S. S. Shah, R. C. Tasker, K. M. Wilson, & R. E. Behrman (Eds.), *Nelson textbook of pediatrics* (21st ed., pp. 19134–19180). Elsevier.

Barkoudah, E. (2023). Cerebral palsy: Overview of management and prognosis. *UpToDate*. Retrieved May 16, 2023, from https://www.uptodate.com/contents/cerebral-palsy-overview-of-management-and-prognosis?search=cerebral%20palsy&source=search_result&selectedTitle=2~150&usage_type=default&display_rank=2

Barkoudah, E., & Aravamuthan, B. (2023). Cerebral palsy: Epidemiology, etiology, and prevention. *UpToDate*. Retrieved May 16, 2023, from https://www.uptodate.com/contents/cerebral-palsy-epidemiology-etiology-and-prevention?search=cerebral%20palsy&source=search_result&selectedTitle=3~150&usage_type=default&display_rank=3

Barkoudah, E., & Whitaker, A. (2022). Cerebral palsy: Treatment of spasticity, dystonia, and associated orthopedic issues. *UpToDate*. Retrieved May 16, 2023, from https://www.uptodate.com/contents/cerebral-palsy-treatment-of-spasticity-dystonia-and-associated-orthopedic-issues?search=cerebral%20palsy&source=search_result&selectedTitle=5~150&usage_type=default&display_rank=5

Bharucha-Goebel, D. X. (2020). Muscular dystrophies. In R. M. Kleigman, J. W. St. Geme III, N. J. Blum, S. S. Shah, R. C. Tasker, K. M. Wilson, & R. E. Behrman (Eds.), *Nelson textbook of pediatrics* (21st ed., pp. 17216–17284). Elsevier.

Boas, S. R. (2020). Skeletal diseases influencing pulmonary function. In R. M. Kleigman, J. W. St. Geme III, N. J. Blum, S. S. Shah, R. C. Tasker, K. M. Wilson, & R. E. Behrman (Eds.), *Nelson textbook of pediatrics* (21st ed., pp. 12375–12398). Elsevier.

Bodamer, O. A. (2023). Spinal muscular atrophy. *UpToDate*. Retrieved May 16, 2023, from https://www.uptodate.com/contents/spinal-muscular-atrophy?search=Spinal%20muscular%20atrophy&source=search_result&selectedTitle=1~67&usage_type=default&display_rank=1

Bowman, R. M. (2022). Myelomeningocele (spina bifida): Management and outcome. *UpToDate*. Retrieved May 12, 2023, from https://www.uptodate.com/contents/myelomeningocele-spina-bifida-management-and-outcome?search=myelomeningocele&source=search_result&selectedTitle=1~126&usage_type=default&display_rank=1

Brenner, J. S., & The Council on Sports Medicine and Fitness. (2007, reaffirmed 2021). Overuse injuries, overtraining, and burnout in child and adolescent athletes. *Pediatrics, 119*(6), 1242–1245. https://doi.org/10.1542/peds.2007-0887

Carrigan, R. B. (2020). The upper limb. In R. M. Kleigman, J. W. St. Geme III, N. J. Blum, S. S. Shah, R. C. Tasker, K. M. Wilson, & R. E. Behrman (Eds.), *Nelson textbook of pediatrics* (21st ed., pp. 9075–9106). Elsevier.

Centers for Disease Control and Prevention. (2022a). *Folic acid recommendations*. http://www.cdc.gov/ncbddd/folicacid/recommendations.html

Centers for Disease Control and Prevention. (2022b). *Birth defects: Facts about upper and lower limb reduction defects*. http://www.cdc.gov/ncbddd/birthdefects/UL-LimbReductionDefects.html

Darras, B. T. (2021). Patient education: Overview of muscular dystrophies (Beyond the Basics). *UpToDate*. Retrieved May 16, 2023, from https://www.uptodate.com/contents/overview-of-muscular-dystrophies-beyond-the-basics?search=muscular%20dystrophy%20children&source=search_result&selectedTitle=4~150&usage_type=default&display_rank=4

Darras, B. T. (2022). Duchenne and Becker muscular dystrophy: Management and prognosis. *UpToDate*. Retrieved May 16, 2023, from https://www.uptodate.com/contents/duchenne-and-becker-muscular-dystrophy-management-and-prognosis?search=muscular%20dystrophy%20children&topicRef=6149&source=see_link

Darras, B. T. (2023). Duchenne and Becker muscular dystrophy: Glucocorticoid and disease-modifying treatment. *UpToDate*. Retrieved May 16, 2023, from https://www.uptodate.com/contents/duchenne-and-becker-muscular-dystrophy-glucocorticoid-and-disease-modifying-treatment?sectionName=GENETIC%20THERAPIES&search=muscular%20dystrophy%20children&topicRef=6181&anchor=H4007909118&source=see_link#H4007909118

Fischbach, F. T., Fischbach, M. A., & Stout, K. (2022). *A manual of laboratory and diagnostic tests* (11th ed.). Wolters Kluwer.

Gill, A. C., & Kelly, N. R. (2022). Pediatric injury prevention: Epidemiology, history, and application. *UpToDate*. Retrieved May 15, 2023, from https://www.uptodate.com/contents/pediatric-injury-prevention-epidemiology-history-and-application?search=Pediatric%20injury%20prevention:%20Epidemiology,%20history,%20and%20application&source=search_result&selectedTitle=1~150&usage_type=default&display_rank=1

Holmes, S. B., Brown, S. J., & Pin Site Care Expert Panel. (2005). Skeletal pin site care: National Association of Orthopaedic Nurses guidelines for orthopaedic nursing. *Orthopaedic Nursing, 24*(2), 99–107. https://doi.org/10.1097/00006416-200503000-00003

Iobst, C. A. (2017). Pin-track infections: Past, present, and future. *Journal of Limb Lengthening and Reconstruction, 3*(2), 78–84. https://doi.org/10.4103/jllr.jllr_17_17

Johnston, M. V. (2020). Cerebral palsy. In R. M. Kleigman, J. W. St. Geme III, N. J. Blum, S. S. Shah, R. C. Tasker, K. M. Wilson, & R. E. Behrman (Eds.), *Nelson textbook of pediatrics* (21st ed., pp. 16718–16741). Elsevier.

Kienstra, A. J., & Macias, C. G. (2022a). Evaluation and management of slipped capital femoral epiphysis (SCFE). *UpToDate*. Retrieved May 16, 2023, from https://www.uptodate.com/contents/evaluation-and-management-of-slipped-capital-femoral-epiphysis-scfe?search=Evaluation%20and%20management%20of%20slipped%20capital%20femoral%20epiphysis%20(SCFE).&source=search_result&selectedTitle=1~45&usage_type=default&display_rank=1

Kienstra, A. J., & Macias, C. G. (2022b). Osgood-Schlatter disease (tibial tuberosity avulsion). *UpToDate*. Retrieved May 16, 2023, from https://www.uptodate.com/contents/osgood-schlatter-disease-tibial-tuberosity-avulsion?search=Osgood-Schlatter%20disease%20&source=search_result&selectedTitle=1~147&usage_type=default&display_rank=1

Kinsman, S. L., & Johnston, M. V. (2020). Congenital anomalies of the central nervous system. In R. M. Kleigman, J. W. St. Geme III, N. J. Blum, S. S. Shah, R. C. Tasker, K. M. Wilson, & R. E. Behrman (Eds.), *Nelson textbook of pediatrics* (21st ed., pp. 16200–16290). Elsevier.

Lexicomp. (2023). Pediatric drug information. *UpToDate*. Retrieved May 10, 2023, from https://www.uptodate.com/contents/table-of-contents/drug-information/pediatric-drug-information

Marini, J. C. (2020). Osteogenesis imperfecta. In R. M. Kleigman, J. W. St. Geme III, N. J. Blum, S. S. Shah, R. C. Tasker, K. M. Wilson, & R. E. Behrman (Eds.), *Nelson textbook of pediatrics* (21st ed., pp. 19520–19539). Elsevier.

Mayer, O. H. (2022). Pectus excavatum: Treatment. *UpToDate*. Retrieved May 14, 2023, from https://www.uptodate.com/contents/pectus-excavatum-treatment?search=pectus%20excavatum&source=search_result&selectedTitle=2~56&usage_type=default&display_rank=2#H20

Misra, M. (2022). Vitamin D insufficiency and deficiency in children and adolescents. *UpToDate*. Retrieved May 17, 2023, from https://www.uptodate.com/contents/vitamin-d-insufficiency-and-deficiency-in-children-and-adolescents?search=Vitamin%20D%20insufficiency%20and%20deficiency%20in%20children%20and%20adolescents.%20&source=search_result&selectedTitle=1~150&usage_type=default&display_rank=1

Mistovich, R. J., & Spiegel, D. A. (2020a). The neck. In R. M. Kleigman, J. W. St. Geme III, N. J. Blum, S. S. Shah, R. C. Tasker, K. M. Wilson, & R. E. Behrman (Eds.), *Nelson textbook of pediatrics* (21st ed., pp. 19051–19074). Elsevier.

Mistovich, R. J., & Spiegel, D. A. (2020b). The spine. In R. M. Kleigman, J. W. St. Geme III, N. J. Blum, S. S. Shah, R. C. Tasker, K. M. Wilson, & R. E. Behrman (Eds.), *Nelson textbook of pediatrics* (21st ed., pp. 18972–19049). Elsevier.

National Institute of Neurological Disorders and Stroke. (2023). *Cerebral palsy*. https://www.ninds.nih.gov/Disorders/All-Disorders/Cerebral-Palsy-Information-Page

Neudauer, C. (2019). Cell and tissue characteristics. In T. L. Norris (Ed.), *Porth's pathophysiology: Concepts of altered health states* (10th ed., pp. 13–45). Wolters Kluwer Health.

Post, E. G., Biese, K. M., Schaefer, D. A., Watson, A. M., McGuine, T. A., Brooks, M. A., & Bell, D. R. (2020). Sport-specific associations of specialization and sex with overuse injury in youth athletes. *Sports Health, 12*(1), 36–42. https://doi.org/10.1177/1941738119886855

Sankar, W. N., Horn, B. D., Winell, J. J., & Wells, L. (2020). The hip. In R. M. Kleigman, J. W. St. Geme III, N. J. Blum, S. S. Shah, R. C. Tasker, K. M. Wilson, & R. E. Behrman (Eds.), *Nelson textbook of pediatrics* (21st ed., pp. 18924–18971). Elsevier.

Sarant, H. B. (2020). Evaluation and investigation of neuromuscular disorders. In R. M. Kleigman, J. W. St. Geme III, N. J. Blum, S. S. Shah, R. C. Tasker, K. M. Wilson, & R. E. Behrman (Eds.), *Nelson textbook of pediatrics* (21st ed., pp. 17070–17111). Elsevier.

Scherl, S. A., & Hasley, B.P. (2023). Adolescent idiopathic scoliosis: Management and prognosis. *UpToDate*. Retrieved May 17, 2023, from https://www.uptodate.com/contents/adolescent-idiopathic-scoliosis-management-and-prognosis?search=adolescent%20idiopathic%20scoliosis&topicRef=6286&source=see_link

Schweich, P. (2021). Patient education: Cast and splint care (Beyond the Basics). *UpToDate*. Retrieved May 11, 2023, from https://www.uptodate.com/contents/cast-and-splint-care-beyond-the-basics?search=cast%20and%20splint%20care&source=search_result&selectedTitle=9~150&usage_type=default&display_rank=9

Shields, D. W., Iliadis, A. D., Kelly, E., Heidari, N., & Jamal, B. (2022). Pin-site infection: A systematic review of prevention strategies. *Strategies in Trauma and Limb Reconstruction, 17*(2), 93–104. https://doi.org/10.5005/jp-journals-10080-1562

U.S. Department of Health and Human Services. (n.d.). *Healthy People 2030*. https://health.gov/healthypeople

U.S. Food and Drug Administration. (2014). *Recommendations for labeling medical products to inform users that the product or product container is not made with natural rubber latex. Guidance for industry and Food and Drug Administration staff.* https://www.fda.gov/media/85473/download

Walker, J. (2018). Assessing and managing pin sites in patients with external fixation. *Nursing Times [Online], 114*(1), 18–21. Retrieved May 11, 2023, from https://cdn.ps.emap.com/wp-content/uploads/sites/3/2017/12/171220-Assessing-and-managing-pin-sites-in-patients-with-external-fixation.pdf

Winell, J. J., Baldwin, K. D., & Wells, L. (2020). Torsional and angular deformities of the limb. In R. M. Kleigman, J. W. St. Geme III, N. J. Blum, S. S. Shah, R. C. Tasker, K. M. Wilson, & R. E. Behrman (Eds.), *Nelson textbook of pediatrics* (21st ed., pp. 18838–18871). Elsevier.

Winell, J. J., & Davidson, R. S. (2020). The foot and toes. In R. M. Kleigman, J. W. St. Geme III, N. J. Blum, S. S. Shah, R. C. Tasker, K. M. Wilson, & R. E. Behrman (Eds.), *Nelson textbook of pediatrics* (21st ed., pp. 18787–18837). Elsevier.

DEVELOPING CLINICAL JUDGMENT

PRACTICING FOR NCLEX

1. A child with Duchenne muscular dystrophy is admitted to the pediatric unit. They have an ineffective cough. Lung auscultation reveals diminished breath sounds. What is the priority nursing intervention?
   a. Apply supplemental oxygen.
   b. Notify the respiratory therapist.
   c. Monitor pulse oximetry.
   d. Position for adequate airway clearance.

2. A 7-year-old child with cerebral palsy has been admitted to the hospital. Which information is most important for the nurse to obtain in the history?
   a. Age that the child learned to walk
   b. Parents' expectations of the child's development
   c. Functional status related to eating and mobility
   d. Birth history to identify cause of cerebral palsy

3. The nurse is caring for a child with cerebral palsy who requires a wheelchair to attain mobility. Which intervention would help the child achieve a sense of normality?
   a. Encourage follow-through with physical therapy exercises.
   b. Restrict the child to a classroom equipped with functional aids.
   c. Encourage afterschool activities within the limits of the child's abilities.
   d. Ensure the school is aware of the child's capabilities.

4. The nurse is caring for children who are in the postoperative period following spinal fusion. What is the most appropriate activity to delegate to unlicensed assistive personnel?
   a. Ambulate the children twice daily to promote mobility.
   b. Encourage commode use to promote bowel function.
   c. Provide diversionary activities, as the children must stay flat on their backs.
   d. Assist with logrolling the children every 2 hours.

5. A 2-month-old infant with a history of a repaired myelomeningocele is seen in your clinic for a well-child check. The parents report the child has been irritable. Upon assessment, the nurse notes a _________ and _________, leading the nurse to assess the infant's _______________.
   Blanks 1 and 2:
   a. depressed fontanelle
   b. bulging fontanelle
   c. high-pitched cry
   d. HR 148 bpm

   Blank 3:
   a. weight
   b. head circumference
   c. respiratory rate
   d. heart rate

6. The nurse is teaching a family with a child newly diagnosed with muscular dystrophy. The nurse can determine teaching has been successful when the parents indicate that which are early symptoms of the condition? Select all that apply.
   a. "Our child did not walk until 20 months old."
   b. "Our child suffers from frequent respiratory infections."
   c. "Our child has higher body weight."
   d. "Our child has difficulty climbing stairs."
   e. "Our child has increased muscle strength."
   f. "Our child has difficulty getting up from the floor."

DOSAGE CALCULATION QUESTION

The nurse is caring for a child who is experiencing painful spasms. The child is 6 years old and weighs 42 lb. The medication order reads: Baclofen 25 mg per GT every 8 hours. Baclofen is supplied as 5 mg/mL.

How many milliliters will the nurse administer? Round to the nearest tenth.

CRITICAL THINKING EXERCISES

1. A 5-year-old child, diagnosed with myelomeningocele, is admitted to the hospital for a corrective surgical procedure. Choose four of the following questions that the nurse should ask when obtaining the health history that would assist in planning the child's care.
   a. What is the child's current mobility status?
   b. Is there a family history of myelomeningocele?
   c. What is the child's genitourinary and bowel function and regimen?
   d. Does this child have a history of hydrocephalus with presence of shunt?
   e. Does the child have known latex sensitivity?
   f. Were there any complications during the pregnancy or birth of this child?
   g. Did the birthing parent take prenatal folic acid supplementation?

2. Based on the case in the preceding question, develop a nursing plan of care or concept map for the child with myelomeningocele.

3. A 5-year-old child is admitted to the pediatric unit with a history of cerebral palsy sustained at birth. The child is admitted for a scheduled tendon lengthening procedure. Based on your knowledge about the effects of cerebral palsy, list three priorities to

focus on when planning their care. Compare this to a child admitted for surgical correction of a broken femur with no significant past medical history.

4. Develop a discharge teaching plan for a 2-year-old who will be in a hip spica cast for 10 more weeks at home.

5. Devise a developmental/education plan for a child who will be confined to traction for 6 weeks. Choose a child in the clinical area whom you have cared for, or choose a particular age group and develop the plan.

STUDY ACTIVITIES

1. In the clinical setting, compare the growth of a child with muscular dystrophy, SMA, or cerebral palsy to the growth of a similar-age child who has been healthy. What differences or similarities do you find? What are the explanations for your findings?

2. Identify the role of the registered nurse in the multidisciplinary care of the child with a debilitating neuromuscular disorder.

3. In the clinical setting, interview the parent of a child with Duchenne muscular dystrophy, myelomeningocele, SMA, or severe cerebral palsy. Determine the parent's feelings about the ongoing care that they are responsible for. Reflect on this interview in your clinical journal.

4. In the clinical setting, compare the cognitive abilities of two children with a severe neuromuscular disorder. What are the reasons for the similarities or differences that you find?

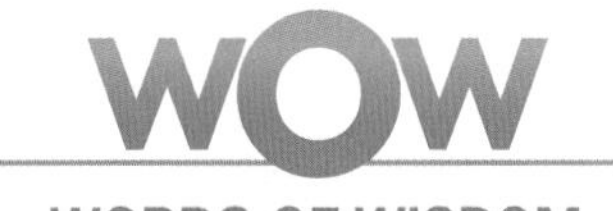

WORDS OF WISDOM

To a nurse the child's skin is life's gift wrapping, but to the child the skin is the space suit for life.

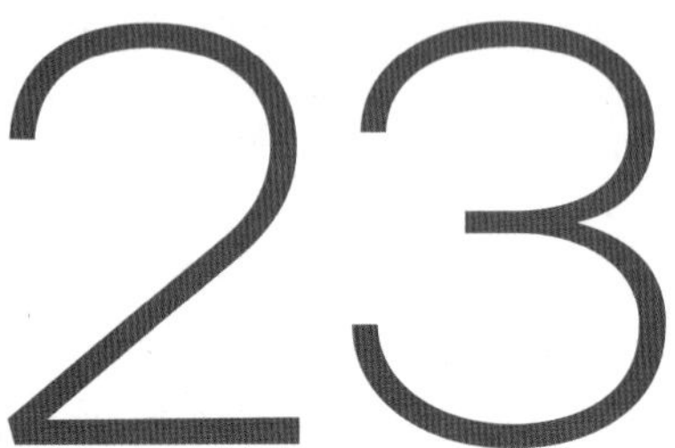

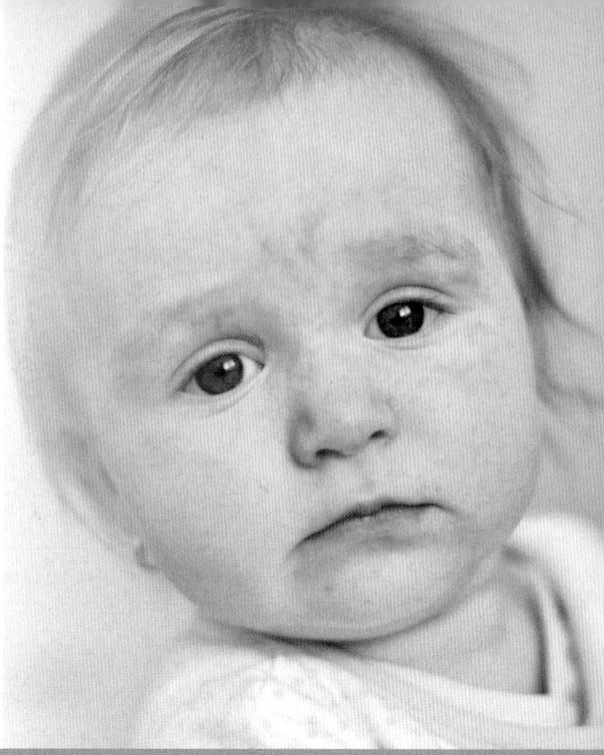

Nursing Care of the Child With an Alteration in Tissue Integrity/ Integumentary Disorder

LEARNING OBJECTIVES

Upon completion of the chapter, you will be able to:

1. Compare the anatomy and physiology of the integumentary system in infants and children to that of adults.
2. Describe nursing care related to common laboratory and diagnostic tests used in the medical diagnosis of integumentary disorders/ alterations in tissue integrity in infants, children, and adolescents.
3. Distinguish alterations in tissue integrity/integumentary disorders common in infants, children, and adolescents.
4. Identify appropriate nursing assessments and interventions related to pediatric integumentary disorders/alterations in tissue integrity.
5. Develop an individualized nursing care plan for the child with an alteration in tissue integrity integumentary disorder.
6. Describe the psychosocial impact of a chronic integumentary disorder on children or adolescents.
7. Develop child and family teaching plans for the child with an integumentary disorder/tissue integrity alteration.

KEY TERMS

annular (an´yŭ-lăr)
dermatitis
erythema (er´i-thē´mă)
macule
papule
pruritus (prū-rī´tŭs)
scaling
vesicle

Eva Lopez, aged 1 year, is brought to the clinic by her parent, who states, "Eva has dry patches of skin, her wrists bleed from her scratching, and she's having trouble sleeping at night."

INTRODUCTION

Tissue integrity refers to the ability of body tissues to maintain normal physiologic processes (Giddens, 2021). Nurses may encounter children with alterations in tissue integrity and should be familiar with various integumentary disorders that children experience. Alterations in tissue integrity or integumentary disorders occur often in children and are caused by exposure to infectious microorganisms, hypersensitivity reactions, hormonal influences, and injuries. Some integumentary disorders are as mild and self-limited as a minor abrasion. Others, such as atopic dermatitis (AD), are chronic and must be managed consistently. Finally, some tissue integrity alterations can be severe and even life-threatening, such as full-thickness burns. If the integumentary disorders are chronic or severe, they can have a major impact on the child's physiologic or psychological status (Teichgräber et al., 2021). Nurses who care for children need to be familiar with common skin disorders of infancy, childhood, and adolescence so they can effectively intervene with children and their families.

VARIATIONS IN PEDIATRIC ANATOMY AND PHYSIOLOGY

The skin is the largest organ of the body and serves to protect the underlying tissues from trauma and invasion by microorganisms. The skin's health reflects the internal well-being of the body. The skin is also important for the perception of pain, heat, and cold and for the regulation of body temperature.

Differences in the Skin Between Children and Adults

The infant's epidermis is thinner than the adult's, and the blood vessels lie closer to the surface because there is a decreased amount of subcutaneous fat. Thus, the infant loses heat more readily through the skin's surface than the older child or adult does. The thinness of the infant's skin also allows substances to be absorbed through the skin more readily than they would be in an adult. Bacteria can gain access via the infant's and younger child's skin more readily than they can through the adult's skin. The infant's skin contains more water than the adult's, and the epidermis is loosely bound to the dermis. This means that friction may easily cause separation of the layers, resulting in blistering or skin breakdown. The infant's skin is also less pigmented than that of the adult (in all races), placing the infant at increased risk of skin damage from ultraviolet (UV) radiation. Over time, the infant's skin toughens and becomes less hydrated and is thus less susceptible to microorganism invasion. The skin thickness and characteristics reach adult levels in the late teenage years.

Differences With Skin Tone

The increased pigmentation in children with darker skin influences the appearance of skin lesions (Armstrong, 2023). Pruritic dermatologic conditions may result in increased lichenification in darker skinned children as compared to lighter skinned children with the same disorders (Sangha, 2021). Dry, darker skin may look whitish or ashy (Armstrong, 2023). Additionally, in darker skin, erythema may be difficult to identify as it may appear as simply a darker area, an ashen gray color, or have a violaceous hue (Armstrong, 2023; Sangha, 2021). Hypopigmentation or hyperpigmentation in the affected area following healing of a dermatologic condition is exaggerated in children with darker skin (Armstrong, 2023). Hypertrophic scarring and keloid formation (Fig. 23.1) occur more often in darker skinned children (Heath et al., 2016).

Sebaceous and Sweat Glands

Sebaceous glands function immaturely at birth. The sebum secreted serves to lubricate the skin and hair. Sebum production increases in the preadolescent and adolescent years, which is why acne develops at that time. The infant's eccrine sweat glands are somewhat functional and will produce sweat as a response to emotional stimuli and heat. They become fully functional in the middle childhood years. Until that time, temperature regulation is less effective compared to older children and adults. The apocrine sweat glands are small and nonfunctional in the infant. They mature during puberty, at which time body odor develops in response to the fluid secreted by these glands.

COMMON MEDICAL TREATMENTS

A variety of medications as well as other medical treatments are used to treat integumentary disorders in children. Most of these treatments will require a health care provider's order when the child is in the hospital. The most common treatments and medications are listed in Common Medical Treatments 23.1 and Drug Guide 23.1. The nurse caring for the child with an integumentary disorder should be familiar with the procedures and medications, how they work, and common nursing implications related to their use.

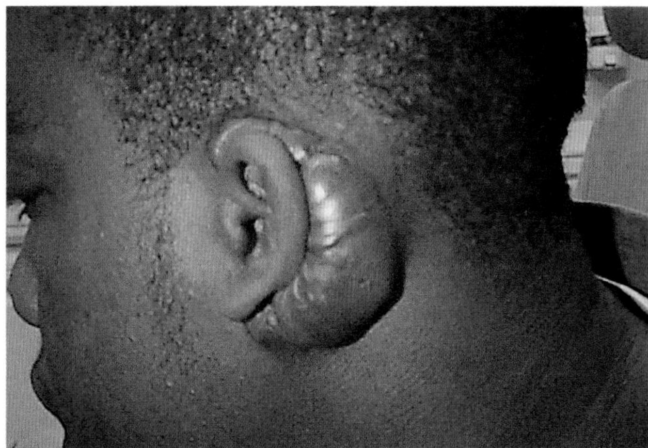

FIGURE 23.1 Keloid formation is more common in dark-skinned than light-skinned children.

COMMON MEDICAL TREATMENTS 23.1

Treatment	Explanation	Indications	Nursing Implications
Wet dressing	Dressing moistened with lukewarm water (sterile water may be required in certain cases.)	In the presence of itching, crusting, or oozing—helps to remove crusts	May use Burow, Domeboro, or saline solutions in certain cases Provide atraumatic care by giving premedication before dressing change.
Sunscreen	Lotion, gel, or cream with a sun-protective factor (SPF)	All children older than 6 months	Use a fragrance-free, para-aminobenzoic acid (PABA)–free preparation with an SPF of 15 or higher. Apply at least 30 minutes prior to sun exposure. Reapply at least every 2 hours while exposed (every 60–80 minutes while in the water). Sweat- and water-resistant preparations are available yet still require reapplication, as noted previously. Use daily in summer and in warm climates, even on overcast and cloudy days.
Bathing	Use of lukewarm water (with or without soap) to bathe	Itchy and irritating skin conditions	Recommend fragrance-free, dye-free soaps such as Dove, Aveeno, Basis, Lubriderm. Colloids (oatmeal baths) are especially helpful. Pat the child dry; do not rub the skin. Leave the child moist before applying medication, dressing, or moisturizer.

DRUG GUIDE 23.1

COMMON DRUGS FOR INTEGUMENTARY DISORDERS

Medication	Actions/Indications	Nursing Implications
Antibiotics (topical)	Decrease skin colonization with bacteria. Indicated for mild acne vulgaris, impetigo, folliculitis	Apply as prescribed to clean skin or a cleansed wound. Be alert for neomycin allergy.
Antibiotics (systemic)	Bactericidal or bacteriostatic against a variety of organisms, depending on the preparation Used for moderate to severe acne vulgaris, extensive impetigo, cellulitis, scalded skin syndrome	Check for medication allergies prior to administration. Teach families to finish entire course of antibiotics.
Corticosteroids (topical)	Antiinflammatory effect in atopic dermatitis and certain kinds of contact dermatitis	Do not use moderate- or high-potency corticosteroid preparations on the face or genitals. Do not cover with an occlusive dressing. Absorption is increased in the young infant.
Antifungals (topical)	Fungicidal used to treat tinea, candidal diaper rash	Apply a thin layer as prescribed. Adhere with length of treatment as prescribed to prevent reemergence of the rash.
Antifungals (systemic): griseofulvin, ketoconazole	Kill fungus; bind to human keratin, making it resistant to fungus Indicated for tinea capitis and severe or widespread fungal skin infections	Griseofulvin: give with fatty food to increase absorption. Requires minimum 4-week course Monitor liver function tests and CBC. May cause photosensitivity Ketoconazole: Administer with food to decrease GI upset.
Benzoyl peroxide	Decreases colonization of *Propionibacterium acnes* in mild acne vulgaris	Available in combination with topical antibiotics Apply sparingly. Shake before application. Avoid contact with eyes and mucous membranes.
Retinoids (topical): tretinoin, adapalene, tazarotene	Anticomedogenic activity in moderate to severe acne vulgaris	Adverse effects: dryness, burning, photosensitivity Instruct child to use SPF 15 or higher sunscreen.
Topical immune modulators (tacrolimus, pimecrolimus)	Inhibit T-lymphocyte action at the skin level. Used for moderate to severe atopic dermatitis, or in conditions resistant to topical steroids	Use only in children older than 2 years. Avoid sunlight exposure. May cause burning, pruritus, flulike symptoms, or headache

DRUG GUIDE 23.1

COMMON DRUGS FOR INTEGUMENTARY DISORDERS

Medication	Actions/Indications	Nursing Implications
Systemic immune modulators (dupilumab)	Inhibit interleukin-4 and interleukin-13 inflammatory processes.	Given by subcutaneous injection every 2 to 4 weeks in children 6 months of age or older
Antihistamines (diphenhydramine, chlorpheniramine, hydroxyzine)	Antihistaminic effect, results in sedation Indicated for hypersensitivity reactions, atopic dermatitis, or contact dermatitis that is severely pruritic	May give three or four times a day unless sedation effect interferes with activities of daily living or school
Systemic corticosteroids (prednisone, dexamethasone, methylprednisolone)	Antiinflammatory and immunosuppressive action Used in severe contact dermatitis	Administer with food to decrease GI upset. May mask signs of infection Monitor blood pressure, urine for glucose. Do not stop treatment abruptly, or acute adrenal insufficiency may occur. Monitor for Cushing syndrome. Doses may be tapered over time.
Isotretinoin	Reduces sebaceous gland size, decreases sebum production, and regulates cell proliferation and differentiation Indicated for cystic acne or severe acne that is resistant to 3 months of treatment with oral antibiotics	Ensure that the adolescent is not pregnant and does not become pregnant. Monitor CBC, lipid profiles, liver function tests, and beta-human chorionic gonadotropin monthly. Monitor for suicide risk.
Coal tar preparations	Antipruritic and antiinflammatory effect Useful in psoriasis, atopic dermatitis	May stain fabrics; strong and unpleasant odor Apply at bedtime and rinse off in the morning to improve adherence.
Silver sulfadiazine 1%	Bactericidal against Gram-positive and Gram-negative bacteria and yeasts Indicated for burns	Cover with occlusive dressing. Apply twice daily. Do not use in children with sulfa allergy. Forms a gel on the burn that is painful to remove May cause transient neutropenia Do not use on the child's face or on an infant younger than 2 months.

CBC, complete blood count; GI, gastrointestinal.

Source: UpToDate, Inc. (2024). *Lexi-comp* ® (Version 7.10.0) [Mobile app]. Wolters Kluwer. https://apps.apple.com/us/app/lexicomp/id313401238

COMMON LABORATORY AND DIAGNOSTIC TESTS 23.1

Test	Explanation	Indications	Nursing Implications
Complete blood count (CBC) with differential	Evaluates hemoglobin and hematocrit, white blood cell (WBC) count (particularly the percentage of individual WBCs), and platelet count	Infection or inflammatory process	Normal values vary according to age and sex. WBC differential is helpful in evaluating source of infection. May be affected by myelosuppressive drugs Eosinophils may be elevated in the child with atopic dermatitis.
Erythrocyte sedimentation rate (ESR)	Nonspecific test used to detect presence of infection or inflammation	Infection or inflammatory process	Send sample to laboratory immediately; if allowed to stand for longer than 3 hours, may result in falsely low result.
Potassium hydroxide (KOH) prep	Reveals branching hyphae (fungus) when viewed under microscope	To identify fungal infection	Place skin scrapings on a microscope slide, and add KOH 20% drop.
Culture of wound or skin drainage	Allows for microbial growth and organism identification	Identification of specific organism	Note sensitivities.
Immunoglobulin E (IgE)	Measurement of serum IgE	Atopic dermatitis	Often elevated in allergic or atopic disease, though this is a nonspecific finding; may be increased if the child takes systemic corticosteroids
Patch or skin testing	Needle prick testing with allergens	Atopic or contact dermatitis	Have emergency equipment available in the event of anaphylaxis (rare).

Data from Corbett, J. A., & Banks, A. D. (2019). *Laboratory tests and diagnostic procedures with nursing diagnoses* (9th ed.). Pearson Education Inc.

Clinical Judgment and the Nursing Process for the Child With an Integumentary Disorder

Nursing management of the child with an alteration in tissue integrity or integumentary disorder requires astute assessment skills, development of accurate patient problems and expected outcomes, implementation of appropriate interventions, and evaluation of the entire process. Many skin rashes may be associated with other, often serious illnesses, so the nurse must use comprehensive and excellent assessment skills when evaluating rashes in children. Certain integumentary conditions are chronic and require ongoing care related to health maintenance, education, and psychosocial needs.

Remember Eva, the 1-year-old with the dry patches, itching, and trouble sleeping? What additional health history and physical examination assessment information should the nurse obtain?

Assessment

Nursing assessment of the child with an integumentary disorder or tissue integrity alteration includes obtaining the health history and performing a physical examination. Assisting with or obtaining laboratory tests may also be necessary.

Health History

Determine the child's or parent's chief complaint, which is most often related to **pruritus** (sensation of itching), **scaling** (dry, flaky skin), or a cosmetic disruption. Document the history of the present illness, noting onset, location, duration, characteristics, other symptoms, and relieving factors, particularly as related to a rash or lesion. Also ask about the quantity and quality of any discharge from the rash or lesions. Document accompanying symptoms. Note the child's general state of health, history of chronic medical conditions, recent surgeries, hospitalizations, medications, or immunizations. Has there been a recent change in the child's food intake or environment? Is there a family history of chronic or acute skin conditions? Does anyone in the home have a similar concern at this time? Does the family have pets that go outdoors? Does the child play in the woods or garden? Note usual skin care routines, as well as types of soaps, cosmetics, or other skin care products used. Determine the amount of daily sun exposure and whether the child consistently uses sunscreen.

Physical Examination

Perform a complete physical examination, noting any abnormalities. Perform a focused and thorough examination of the skin. The best lighting for examination of the skin is natural daylight. Look at the skin, in general, noting distribution of any obvious rashes or lesions. Inspect the mucous membranes, noting and describing lesions if present. Examine all surfaces of the skin and scalp carefully. Note temperature, moisture, texture, and fragility of the skin. If a rash or lesions are present, note their location and provide a detailed description of them. Describe whether a rash is macular, papular, pustular, or vesicular.

Provide a description of vascular lesions if present. If lesions are present on the scalp, has hair loss in that region occurred? Describe lesions according to the following criteria:

- Linear: in a line
- Shape: are the lesions round, oval, or **annular** (ring around central clearing)?
- Morbilliform: a rosy, maculopapular rash
- Target lesions: like a bull's eye

If drainage is present, describe it as clear, purulent, honey colored, or otherwise. Note scaling or lichenification of the skin. Palpate for regional lymphadenopathy.

Laboratory and Diagnostic Testing

Common Laboratory and Diagnostic Tests 23.1 details the laboratory and diagnostic tests most commonly used when considering integumentary disorders. The tests can assist the health care provider or nurse practitioner in diagnosing the disorder or can be used as guidelines in determining ongoing treatment. Some of the tests are obtained by laboratory or nonnursing personnel, while others might be obtained by the nurse. In either instance, the nurse should be familiar with how the tests are obtained, what they are used for, and normal versus abnormal results. This knowledge will also be necessary when providing child and family education related to the testing.

Nursing Analysis

After recognizing and analyzing cues from a thorough assessment, the nurse might identify several patient problems, including:

- Impaired skin integrity
- Risk for infection
- Risk for fluid volume deficit
- Altered nutrition
- Disturbed body image
- Pain
- Interrupted family processes
- Risk for caregiver role strain

After completing an assessment of Eva, the nurse noted the following: hypopigmentation of the skin behind her knees, dry patches on her wrists and face, and slight wheezing heard bilaterally on auscultation. Based on these assessment findings, what would your top three patient problems be for Eva?

The foregoing patient problems provide suggestions for nursing care planning or concept mapping. Suggested interventions with rationales are provided further on. Care planning should be individualized, based on the child's and family's needs. Refer to Chapter 14 for the nursing process for pain management and to Chapter 11 for nursing interventions related to interrupted family processes and caregiver role strain risk. Additional information will be included later in the chapter as it relates to nursing management of children with specific disorders, as well as particular nursing interventions for deficient knowledge.

Nursing Analysis

Impaired skin integrity related to infectious process, hypersensitivity reaction, injury, or mechanical factors as evidenced by alteration in skin integrity (rash, inflammation, abrasion, laceration, or disrupted epidermis)

Goal/Outcome

Integrity of skin surface will be restored; rash, abrasion, laceration, or other skin disruption will heal.

Restoring Skin Integrity (interventions with *rationale*)

- Assess site of skin impairment *to determine extent of involvement and plan care.*
- Monitor skin impairment every shift for changes in color, warmth, redness, or other signs of infection *to identify problems early.*
- Determine the child's and family's skin care practices *to establish need for education related to skin care.*
- Individualize the child's skin care regimen depending on the child's particular skin condition *to care for skin most appropriately in light of the child's disorder.*
- In the immobile child, use a risk assessment tool (such as a modified Norton or Braden Q scale) *to identify risk for skin breakdown.*
- Position the child on the opposite side of the skin impairment *to avoid further skin breakdown.*
- Encourage appropriate nutritional intake *as adequate nutrients are necessary for appropriate immune function and skin healing.*
- Consult the wound and ostomy care nurse specialist *to determine the best approach for individualized wound care.*
- Provide dressing change and wound care as prescribed *to promote wound or burn healing.*

Nursing Analysis

Risk for infection related to alteration in skin integrity

Goal/Outcome

Child will remain free from local or systemic infection, will remain afebrile, without additional redness or warmth at skin disruption site.

Preventing Infection (interventions with *rationale*)

- Use appropriate hand hygiene *to decrease transmission of infectious organisms.*
- Assess the skin impairment site for increased warmth, redness, discharge, or new purulence *to identify infection early.*
- Assess temperature every 4 hours or more frequently if needed, *as children develop fever quickly in response to infection.*
- Note white blood cell (WBC) count and culture results, reporting unexpected values to the health care provider or nurse practitioner *so that appropriate treatment may be started.*
- Follow prescribed therapies for skin alteration *to maintain skin moisture and prevent further breakdown, which may lead to infection.*
- Encourage appropriate nutritional intake, *as adequate nutrients are necessary for appropriate immune function and skin healing.*

Nursing Analysis

Risk for deficient fluid volume related to fluid loss through abnormal route (burns)

Goal/Outcome

Fluid volume status will be balanced, child will maintain urine output of 1 to 2 mL/kg/h, oral mucosa will be moist and pink, heart rate will remain within age- and situation-specific parameters.

Promoting Fluid Balance (interventions with *rationale*)

- Assess fluid volume status at least every shift, more frequently if disrupted, *to obtain baseline for comparison.*
- Strictly monitor intake and output *to detect imbalance or need for additional fluid intake.*
- Weigh the child daily on the same scale, at the same time, in the same amount of clothing *as changes in weight are an accurate indicator of fluid volume status in children.*
- Provide intravenous (IV) fluid resuscitation in initial period, followed by encouragement of oral fluid intake in the burned child, *to compensate for fluid loss through burned areas.*

Nursing Analysis

Imbalanced nutrition, less than body requirements, related to insufficient dietary intake in relation to increased metabolic state (burns) as evidenced by poor wound healing, difficulty gaining or maintaining body weight

Goal/Outcome

Child will demonstrate balanced nutritional state, will maintain or gain weight as appropriate for situation, will demonstrate improvement in wound healing.

Promoting Nutrition (interventions with *rationale*)

- Assess the child's food preferences and ability to eat *to provide a baseline for planning nursing care.*
- Consult the nutritionist *because nutritional needs are increased related to altered metabolic state as a result of burns.*
- Collaborate with the nutritionist, child, and parents to plan meals that appeal to the child *to increase the child's intake.*
- Administer vitamin and mineral preparations as prescribed *to supplement nutrients.*
- Provide smaller, more frequent meals and snacks *to promote increased intake.*
- Weigh the child daily *to determine progress.*

Nursing Analysis

Disturbed body image related to injury or alteration in body function (chronic skin changes or burns) as evidenced by child's negative feeling about body or fear of reaction by others

Goal/Outcome

Child will verbalize or demonstrate acceptance of alteration in body, will return to previous level of social involvement.

Promoting Appropriate Body Image (interventions with *rationale*)

- Assess child or adolescent for feelings about alteration in skin *to determine baseline.*
- Acknowledge feelings of anger or depression related to skin changes *to provide an outlet for feelings.*
- Encourage the child or adolescent to participate in skin care *to give some sense of control over what is occurring.*
- Help the child or adolescent to accept self *as the perception of self is tied to knowing oneself and identifying self-values.*

Based on your top three nursing patient problems for Eva, describe appropriate nursing interventions.

INFECTIOUS DISORDERS

Infectious disorders of the skin include those caused by viral, bacterial, or fungal infection. The viral exanthems are discussed in Chapter 15. Bacterial and fungal infections of the skin are discussed in what follows.

Bacterial Infections

Bacterial infections of the skin include bullous and nonbullous impetigo, folliculitis, cellulitis, and staphylococcal scalded skin syndrome. These bacterial skin infections are often caused by *Staphylococcus aureus* and group A beta-hemolytic streptococcus, which are ordinarily normal flora on the skin. Impetigo, folliculitis, and cellulitis are usually self-limited disorders that rarely become severe.

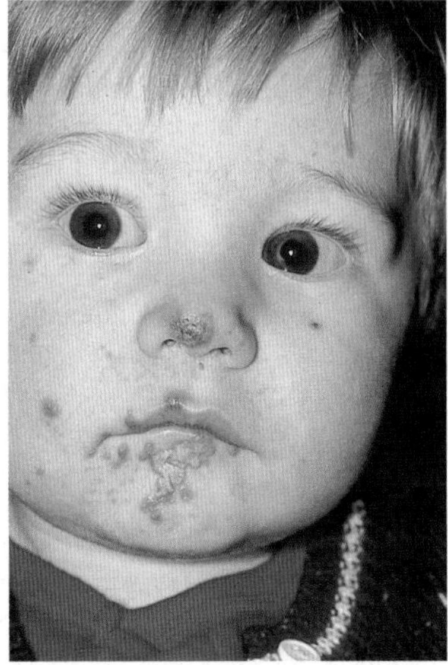

FIGURE 23.2 Note honey-colored crusting with impetigo.

Impetigo is a readily recognizable skin rash (Fig. 23.2). Nonbullous impetigo generally follows some type of skin trauma or may arise as a secondary bacterial infection of another skin disorder, such as AD. Bullous impetigo demonstrates a sporadic occurrence pattern and develops on intact skin, resulting from toxin production by *S. aureus.*

Folliculitis, infection of the hair follicle, most often results from occlusion of the hair follicle. It may occur as a result of poor hygiene, prolonged contact with contaminated water, maceration, a moist environment, or use of occlusive emollient products.

Cellulitis is a localized infection and inflammation of the skin and subcutaneous tissues and is usually preceded by skin trauma of some sort (Fig. 23.3). Periorbital

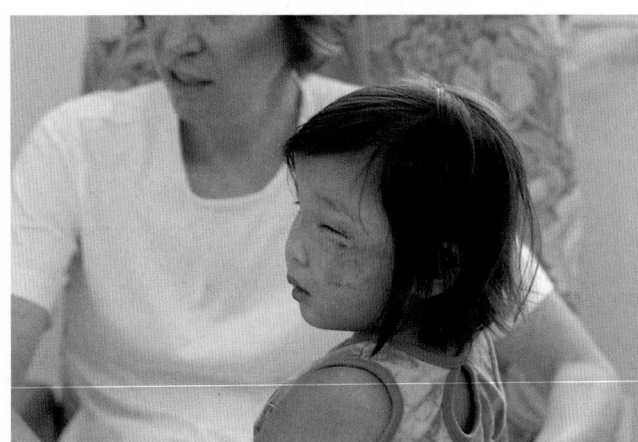

FIGURE 23.3 Note erythema and edema associated with cellulitis.

cellulitis is a bacterial infection of the eyelids and tissue surrounding the eye. The bacteria may gain entry to the skin via an abrasion, laceration, insect bite, foreign body, or impetiginous lesion. Periorbital cellulitis may also result from a nearby bacterial infection, such as sinusitis. *Staphylococcus aureus, Streptococcus pyogenes,* and *Streptococcus pneumoniae* are the most commonly implicated bacteria. The bacteria produce either an enzyme or endotoxins that initiate the inflammatory response. Redness, swelling, and infiltration of the skin by the inflammatory mediators occur.

Staphylococcal scalded skin syndrome results from infection with *S. aureus* that produces a toxin, which then causes exfoliation. It has an abrupt onset and results in diffuse **erythema** (reddening of the skin) and skin tenderness (Fig. 23.4). Scalded skin syndrome is most common in infancy and rare beyond 5 years of age (McMahon, 2022).

Of particular concern are community-acquired bacterial skin infections caused by methicillin-resistant *S. aureus* (CA-MRSA) (Baddour, 2022). CA-MRSA most commonly occurs as a skin or soft tissue infection, such as cellulitis or an abscess. Risk factors for CA-MRSA are turf burns, towel sharing, participation in team sports, or attendance at day care or outdoor camps. If the child presents with a moderate to severe skin infection or with an infection that is not responding as expected to therapy, it is important to culture the infected area for MRSA.

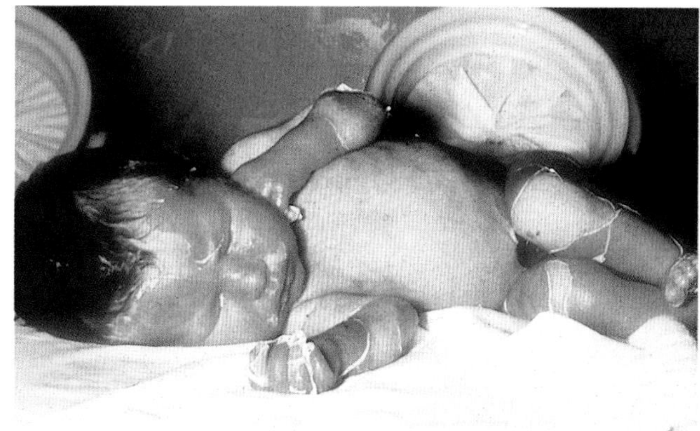

FIGURE 23.4 Staphylococcal scalded skin syndrome (SSSS) with ruptured bullae. (Reprinted with permission from Goodheart, H. P., & Gonzalez, M. E. [2016]. *Goodheart's photoguide to common pediatric and adult skin disorders* [4th ed.]. Wolters Kluwer.)

Therapeutic management of most bacterial skin infections includes topical or systemic antibiotics and appropriate hygiene (Table 23.1). Treatment of periorbital cellulitis focuses on IV antibiotic administration during the acute phase, followed by completion of the course with oral antibiotics. Complications of periorbital cellulitis include bacteremia and progression to orbital cellulitis, which is a more extensive infection involving the orbit of the eye.

TABLE 23.1 • Bacterial Skin Infections

Disorder	Skin Findings	Usual Treatment
Nonbullous impetigo	• Papules progressing to vesicles, then painless pustules with a narrow erythematous border • Honey-colored exudate when the vesicles or pustules rupture, which forms a crust on the ulcer-like base (see Fig. 23.2)	• Limited amount: treat topically with mupirocin ointment. • If numerous lesions, oral first-generation cephalosporin is indicated. • Clindamycin may be needed for MRSA. • Remove honey-colored crust with cool compresses twice daily.
Bullous impetigo	• Red macules and bullous eruptions on an erythematous base • Size may be from a few millimeters to several centimeters.	• Oral first-generation cephalosporin • Good hygiene
Folliculitis	Red, raised hair follicles	• Treat with aggressive hygiene: warm compresses after washing with soap and water several times a day. • Topical mupirocin is indicated; occasionally, oral antibiotics are required.
Cellulitis	Localized reaction: erythema, pain, edema, warmth at site of skin disruption (see Fig. 23.3)	• Mild cases are usually treated with cephalexin or amoxicillin/clavulanic acid. • More severe cases and periorbital or orbital cellulitis require IV cephalosporins.
Staphylococcal scalded skin syndrome	• Flattish bullae that rupture within hours • Red, weeping surface is left, most commonly on face, groin, neck, and axillary region (see Fig. 23.4)	• Mild to moderate cases are treated with oral cephalexin, dicloxacillin, or amoxicillin/clavulanic acid. • Severe cases are managed similar to burns with aggressive fluid management and IV oxacillin or clindamycin.

MRSA, methicillin-resistant *Staphylococcus aureus*

Data from Prok, L. D., & Torres-Zegarra, C. X. (2022). Chapter 15: Skin. In M. Bunik, W. W. Hay, M. J. Levin, & M. J. Abzug (Eds.), *Current diagnosis & treatment: Pediatrics* (26th ed.). McGraw-Hill Education; Baddour, L. M. (2022). Impetigo. *UpToDate*. Retrieved January 29, 2024, from http://www.uptodate.com/contents/impetigo

Nursing Assessment

Obtain the history as noted in the nursing process overview section. Note history of skin disruption such as a cut, scrape, or insect or spider bite (nonbullous impetigo and cellulitis). Note body piercing in the adolescent, which can lead to impetigo or cellulitis. Measure the child's temperature. Fever may occur with bullous impetigo or cellulitis and is common with scalded skin syndrome. Inspect the skin, noting abnormalities, documenting their location and distribution, and describing drainage if present. Table 23.1 gives specific clinical manifestations of the various bacterial skin infections. Assess for pain. In periorbital cellulitis, note marked eyelid edema as well as a purplish or red color of the eyelid (Fig. 23.5) and restricted movement of the eye area.

Palpate for regional lymphadenopathy, which may be present with impetigo or cellulitis. Blood cultures are indicated in the child with cellulitis with lymphangitic streaking and in all cases of periorbital or orbital cellulitis.

CLINICAL REASONING ALERT!

Notify the health care provider or nurse practitioner immediately if any of these signs of progression to orbital cellulitis occur: conjunctival redness, change in vision, pain with eye movement, eye muscle weakness or paralysis, or proptosis.

Nursing Management

Administer antibiotics topically or systemically as prescribed. Teach the family about antibiotic administration and care of the lesions or rash. Soak impetiginous lesions with cool compresses or Burow solution to remove crusts before applying topical antibiotics. Although impetigo is considered a contagious disorder among vulnerable populations, removal from school or day care is not necessary unless the condition is widespread or actively weeping. Prevent transmission of nosocomial MRSA by appropriately isolating children according to the institution's policy when the child is hospitalized. In children with scalded skin syndrome, reduce the risk of scarring by minimal handling, avoiding corticosteroids, and applying soothing ointments as the skin heals.

For periorbital cellulitis, apply warm soaks to the eye area for 20 minutes every 2 to 4 hours. Administer IV antibiotics as prescribed. Instruct parents to call the health care provider or nurse practitioner or have the child evaluated again if the child is not improving or cannot move their eye, if proptosis occurs, or if perceived visual acuity lessens.

Teach families the importance of completing the entire course of oral antibiotic treatment at home. Educate the family about prevention of bacterial skin infections. Stress the importance of cleanliness and hygiene. Teach the family to keep the child's fingernails cut short and to clean the nails with a nail brush at bath time. When a skin disruption such as a cut, scrape, or insect bite occurs, teach the family to clean the area well to prevent the development of cellulitis. Folliculitis may be prevented with diligent hygiene and avoidance of occlusive emollients. Table 23.1 gives additional information about specific treatments for bacterial skin infections. See Dosage Calculation Box 23.1.

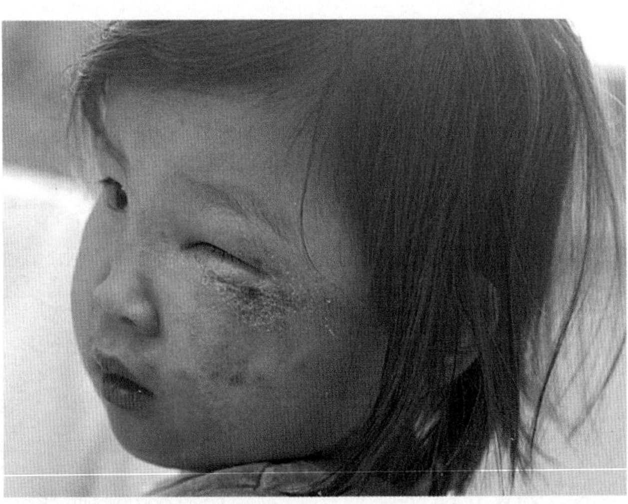

FIGURE 23.5 Periorbital cellulitis.

DOSAGE CALCULATION BOX 23.1

Child's weight: 13 lb 3 oz

Medication order: cephalexin 125 mg/5 mL, 4 mL PO every 6 hours.

Per the Pediatric Dosage Handbook, the recommended dose is 25–50 mg/kg/day divided every 6 to 8 hours daily.

Is the ordered dose safe?

Fungal Infections

Fungi also cause infections on children's skin. *Tinea* is a fungal disease of the skin occurring on any part of the body. The part of the body affected determines the second word in the name. Examples of tinea infections occurring on various parts of the body include:

- Tinea pedis: fungal infection on the feet
- Tinea corporis: fungal infection on the arms or legs
- Tinea versicolor: fungal infection on the trunk and extremities
- Tinea capitis: fungal infection on the scalp, eyebrows, or eyelashes
- Tinea cruris: fungal infection on the groin

The three organisms most often responsible for tinea are *Epidermophyton*, *Microsporum*, and *Trichophyton*,

TABLE 23.2 • Management of Fungal Infections

Disorder	Skin Findings	Usual Treatment
Tinea corporis (ringworm)	Annular lesion with raised peripheral scaling and central clearing (looks like a ring) (see Fig. 23.6)	Topical antifungal cream is required for at least 4 weeks.
Tinea capitis	• Patches of scaling in the scalp with central hair loss • Risk of kerion development (inflamed, boggy mass that is filled with pustules) (see Fig. 23.7)	• Oral griseofulvin for 4–6 weeks • Selenium sulfide shampoo may be used to decrease contagiousness (adjunct only). • No school or day care for 1 week after treatment initiated
Tinea versicolor	• Superficial tan or hypopigmented oval scaly lesions, especially on upper back and chest and proximal arms • More noticeable in the summer with tanning of unaffected areas (see Fig. 23.8)	• Apply selenium sulfide shampoo all over body (from face to knees) and allow to stay on skin overnight, rinsing in the morning, once a week for 4 weeks (this may cause skin irritation). • Topical antifungals in the imidazole family may be used instead.
Tinea pedis (athlete's foot)	Red, scaling rash on soles and between the toes (see Fig. 23.9)	• Topical antifungal cream, powder, or spray • Appropriate foot hygiene
Tinea cruris	Erythema, scaling, maceration in the inguinal creases and inner thighs (penis/scrotum spared)	Topical antifungal preparation for 4–6 weeks
Diaper candidiasis (also called monilial diaper rash)	Fiery red lesions, scaling in the skin folds, and satellite lesions (located further out from the main rash) (see Fig. 23.10)	• Topical nystatin with diaper changes for several days • See section on diaper dermatitis for additional information.

Data from Prok, L. D., & Torres-Zegarra, C. X. (2022). Chapter 15: Skin. In M. Bunik, W. W. Hay, M. J. Levin, & M. J. Abzug (Eds.), *Current diagnosis & treatment: Pediatrics* (26th ed.). McGraw-Hill Education.

although *Malassezia furfur* causes tinea versicolor. *Candida albicans* may cause an infection of the skin, particularly in a warm, moist area such as the diaper area. All fungal skin infections may occur year-round, but tinea versicolor is more common in warm weather.

Therapeutic management of fungal infections involves appropriate hygiene and administration of an antifungal agent. Table 23.2 gives further information about treatment.

Nursing Assessment

Elicit the health history, noting exposure to another person with a fungal infection or exposure to a pet (fungi are often carried by pets). Note onset of the rash and whether it is itchy. Determine if the child has recently visited the barber (tinea capitis). Note contact with damp areas such as locker rooms and swimming pools, use of nylon socks or nonbreathable shoes, or minor trauma to the feet (tinea pedis). Document a history of wearing tight clothing or participating in a contact sport such as wrestling (tinea cruris). Inspect the skin and scalp, noting the location, description, and distribution of the rash or lesions (Figs. 23.6 to 23.10). Table 23.2 describes the clinical findings associated with various types of tinea.

Scraping and KOH preparation show branching hyphae. For tinea capitis, the Wood lamp will fluoresce yellow-green if it is caused by *Microsporum*, but not with *Trichophyton*. A fungal culture of a plucked hair is more reliable for diagnosis of tinea capitis.

Nursing Management

Maintain appropriate hygiene and administer antifungal agents as prescribed (see Table 23.2). Additional specifics related to the individual fungal disorders are as follows:

- Tinea corporis is contagious, but the child may return to day care or school once treatment has begun. Identify and treat family members or other contacts.
- Counsel the child with tinea capitis and parents that hair will usually regrow in 3 to 12 months. Wash sheets

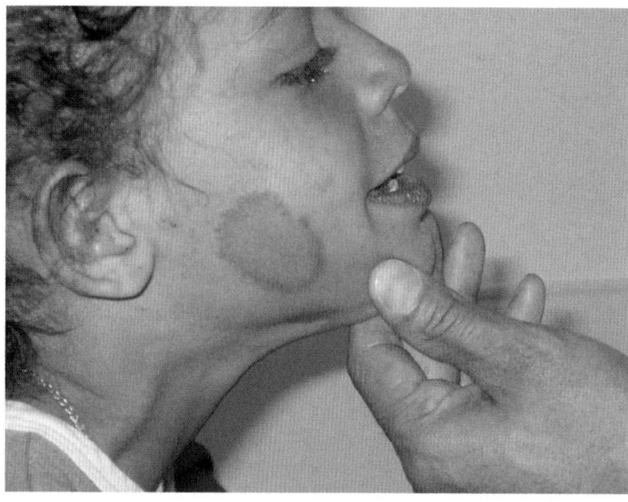

FIGURE 23.6 Tinea corporis: note raised scaly border with clearing in center.

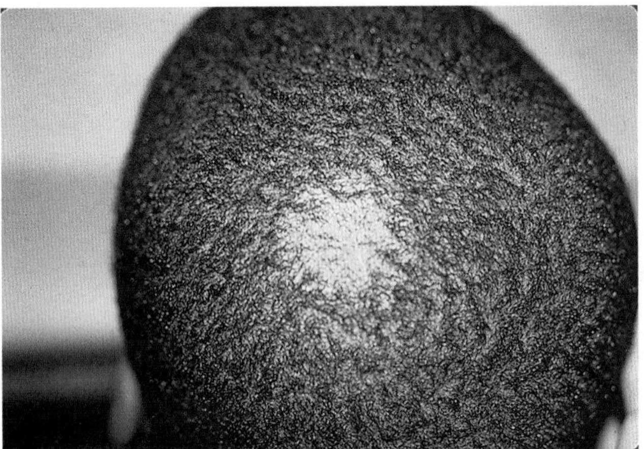

FIGURE 23.7 Note hair breakage and loss with tinea capitis.

and clothes in hot water to decrease the risk of the infection spreading to other family members.

- Instruct the child with tinea pedis to keep the feet clean and dry. Rinse feet with water or a water/vinegar mixture and dry them well, especially between the toes. Encourage the child to wear cotton socks and shoes that allow the feet to breathe. Going barefoot at home is allowed, but flip-flops should be worn around swimming pools and in locker rooms.
- Inform the child with tinea versicolor that return to normal skin pigmentation may take several months.
- Counsel the child or adolescent with tinea cruris to wear cotton underwear and loose clothing. It is important to maintain good hygiene, particularly after sports practice or a sporting event.
- For management of diaper candidiasis, follow the suggestions listed further on in the section on diaper dermatitis.

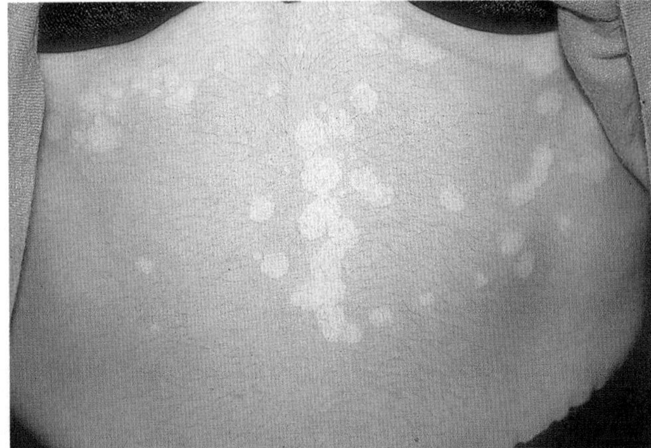

FIGURE 23.8 Tinea versicolor. Hypopigmented scaly lesions on the back of a darkly pigmented adolescent. (Reprinted with permission from Goodheart, H. P., & Gonzalez, M. E. [2016]. *Goodheart's photoguide to common pediatric and adult skin disorders* [4th ed.]. Wolters Kluwer.)

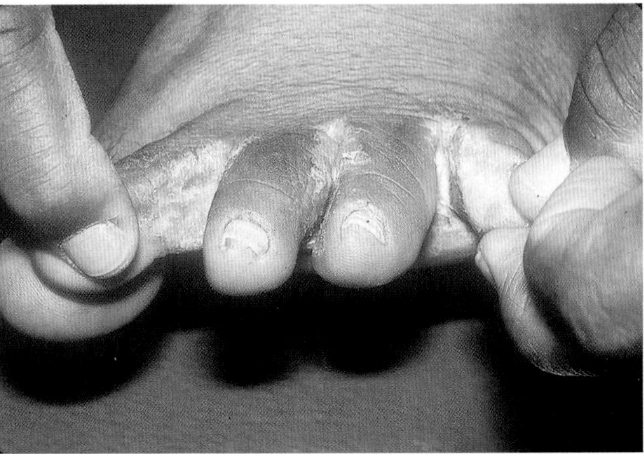

FIGURE 23.9 Tinea pedis. The interdigital pattern of tinea pedis is common. (Reprinted with permission from Goodheart, H. P. [2009]. *Goodheart's photoguide to common skin disorders* [3rd ed.]. Wolters Kluwer.)

INFLAMMATORY SKIN CONDITIONS

Inflammatory skin conditions (**dermatitis**) may be either acute or chronic. Acute hypersensitivity reactions may cause diaper dermatitis, contact dermatitis, erythema multiforme, and urticaria. AD is a chronic hypersensitivity disorder. Seborrhea and psoriasis are chronic inflammatory skin disorders that do not occur as a result of hypersensitivity.

Diaper Dermatitis

Dermatitis refers to an inflammatory reaction of the skin. Diaper dermatitis refers to an inflammatory reaction of the skin in the area covered by a diaper. It is a nonimmunologic response to a skin irritant that results in skin cell hydration disturbance. Prolonged exposure to urine and feces may lead to skin breakdown (Fig. 23.11). Diaper wearing increases the skin's pH, activating fecal enzymes that further contribute to skin maceration.

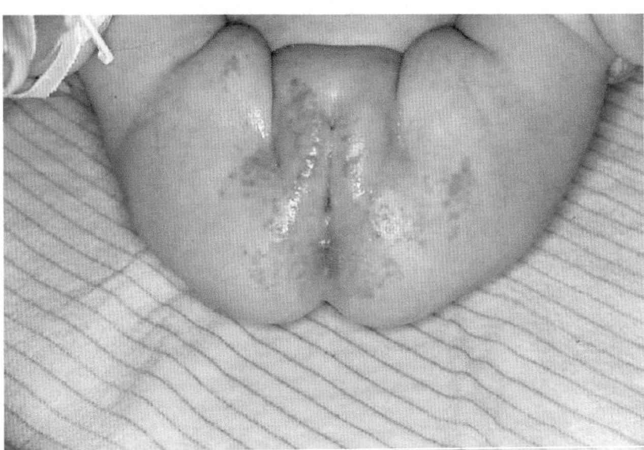

FIGURE 23.10 A bright red rash with satellite lesions occurs with diaper candidiasis.

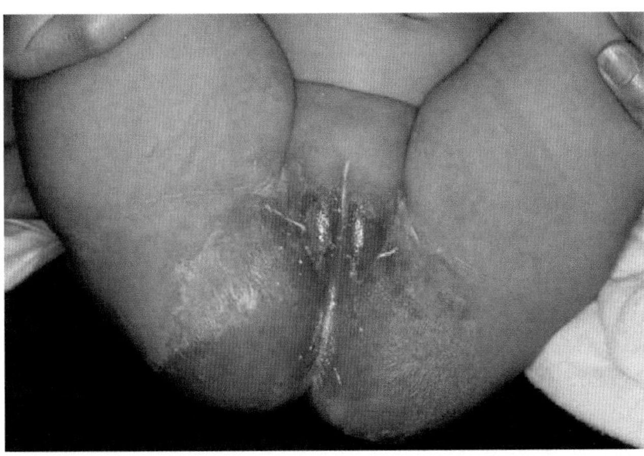

FIGURE 23.11 Diaper dermatitis.

Nursing Assessment

Determine from the history whether the infant or child wears diapers. Ask about the onset and progression of the rash, as well as any treatments and response. Inspect the skin in the diaper area for erythema and maceration (see Fig. 23.11). Ordinary diaper dermatitis does not usually result in a bumpy rash but starts as a flat red rash in the convex skin creases. It may appear red and shiny and may or may not also have **papules** (raised lesion). Untreated, it may become more widespread or severe. Some cases of diaper dermatitis are caused by overgrowth of *C. albicans* (see Fig. 23.9 and the "Fungal Infections" section).

Nursing Management

Prevention is the best management of diaper dermatitis. Topical products such as ointments or creams containing vitamins A, D, and E; zinc oxide; or petrolatum are helpful to provide a barrier to the skin. Teaching Guidelines 23.1 gives further information on prevention and management of diaper dermatitis. See earlier for treatment of diaper rash caused by *C. albicans* infection.

TEACHING GUIDELINES 23.1 Prevention and Management of Diaper Dermatitis

- Change diapers frequently. Change stool-soiled diapers as soon as possible.
- Avoid rubber pants.
- Gently wash the diaper area with a soft cloth, avoiding harsh soaps.
- Use baby wipes in most children, but avoid wipes that contain fragrance or preservatives.
- Once a rash has occurred, follow all the earlier prevention tips and add the following:
  - Allow the infant or child to go diaperless for some time each day to allow the rash to heal.
  - Blow-dry the diaper area/rash area with the dryer set on the warm (not hot) setting for 3 to 5 minutes.

TAKE NOTE!

Discourage parents from using any type of baby powder to avoid the risk of aspiration; inhalation of talcum-containing powders may result in pneumonitis (Hagan et al., 2017).

Atopic Dermatitis

Atopic dermatitis (AD; also called eczema) is one of the disorders in the atopy family (along with asthma and allergic rhinitis). AD affects 16% to 19% of US children (Howe, 2023). Onset of symptoms occurs usually before 2 years of age (Prok & Torres-Zegarra, 2022). AD is often associated with food allergies, allergic rhinitis, and asthma, although not all children with AD will develop one of those other disorders (Howe, 2023).

The chronic itching associated with AD causes a great deal of psychological distress. The child's self-image may be affected, particularly if the rash is extensive. Difficulty sleeping may occur because of the itching. The child is irritable and has difficulty concentrating, and family life is disrupted. Parents' stress related to the child's condition may increase the child's anxiety and lead to an increase in itching and scratching. The child may outgrow AD, its severity may decrease as the child approaches adulthood, or the child may continue to have difficulties into the adult years. Bacterial superinfection may occur as a complication.

Therapeutic management includes good skin hydration, application of topical corticosteroids or immune modulators, oral antihistamines for sedative effects, and antibiotics if secondary infection occurs.

Pathophysiology

AD is a chronic disorder characterized by extreme itching and inflamed, reddened, and swollen skin. It has a relapsing and remitting nature. The skin reaction occurs in response to specific allergens, usually food (especially eggs, wheat, milk, and peanuts) or environmental triggers (e.g., molds, dust mites, and cat dander). Other factors, such as high or low ambient temperatures, perspiring, scratching, skin irritants, or stress, may contribute to flare-ups. When the child encounters a triggering antigen, antigen-presenting cells stimulate interleukins to begin the inflammatory process. The skin begins to feel pruritic, and the child starts to scratch. The sensation of itchiness comes first, and then the rash becomes apparent. The scratching causes the rash to appear. Sweating causes AD to worsen, as does excessively humid or dry environments.

Nursing Assessment

For a full description of the assessment phase of the nursing process, refer to the "Clinical Judgment and the Nursing Process" section earlier in the chapter. Assessment findings pertinent to AD are discussed here.

HEALTH HISTORY

Elicit a description of the present illness and chief complaint. Common signs and symptoms reported during the health history might include:

- Wiggling or scratching
- Dry skin
- Scratch marks noticed by the parents
- Disrupted sleep
- Irritability

Explore the child's current and past medical history for risk factors such as:

- Family history of AD, allergic rhinitis, or asthma
- Child's history of asthma or allergic rhinitis
- Food or environmental allergies

Determine the onset of the rash; its location, progression, and severity; and response to treatments used so far. Note medications used to treat the rash, as well as other medications the child may be taking.

PHYSICAL EXAMINATION

Physical examination consists of inspection and observation and auscultation.

Inspection and Observation

Observe whether the infant is wiggling or the child is actively scratching. Carefully inspect the skin. Document dry, scaly, or flaky skin, as well as hypertrophy and lichenification (Fig. 23.12). If lesions are present, they may be dry lesions or weepy papules or **vesicles** (fluid-filled lesions). In children younger than 2 years, the rash is most likely to occur on the face, scalp, wrists, and extensor surfaces of the arms or legs. In older children, it may occur anywhere on the skin but is found more commonly on the flexor areas. Note erythema or warmth, which may indicate associated secondary bacterial infection. Document areas of hyperpigmentation or hypopigmentation, which may have resulted from a prior exacerbation of AD or its treatment. Inspect the eyes, nose, and throat for symptoms of allergic rhinitis.

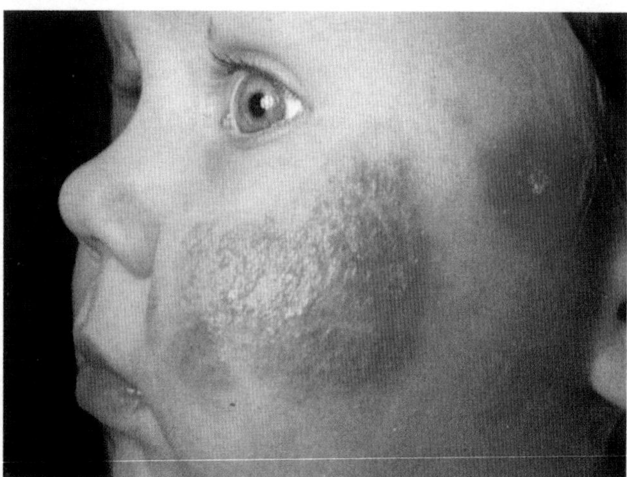

FIGURE 23.12 Atopic dermatitis rash is red, dry, and scaly.

Auscultation

Auscultate the lungs for wheezing (commonly found in the associated condition of asthma).

LABORATORY AND DIAGNOSTIC TESTS

Serum immunoglobulin E (IgE) levels may be elevated in the child with AD. Skin prick allergy testing may determine the food or environmental allergen to which the child is sensitive.

Nursing Management

Nursing management of the child with AD focuses on promoting skin hydration, maintaining skin integrity, and preventing infection.

PROMOTING SKIN HYDRATION

First and foremost, avoid hot water and any skin or hair product containing perfumes, dyes, or fragrance. Bathe the child twice daily in warm (not hot) water. Use a mild soap to clean only the dirty areas. Recommended mild soaps or cleansing agents include:

- Unscented Dove or Dove for sensitive skin
- Tone
- Caress
- Oil of Olay
- Cetaphil
- Aquanil

Slightly pat the child dry after the bath, but do not rub the skin with the towel. Leave the child moist. Apply prescribed topical ointments or creams such as corticosteroids or immune modulators (see Drug Guide 23.1) to the affected area. Apply fragrance-free moisturizer over the prescribed topical medication and all over the child's body. Recommended moisturizers include:

- Eucerin, Moisturel, Curel (cream or lotion)
- Aquaphor
- Vaseline
- Crisco

TAKE NOTE!

Vaseline or generic petrolatum is an inexpensive, readily available moisturizer.

Apply moisturizer multiple times throughout the day. Avoid clothing made of synthetic fabrics or wool. Avoid triggers known to exacerbate AD.

Herbal supplements and oils (such as evening primrose oil) have demonstrated mixed results for reduction in redness and scaling. If not initially recommended by the health care provider or nurse practitioner, the parent should consult with them first before starting these supplements. Headache and nausea are rare adverse effects of these supplements and, if they occur, are usually mild. Chamomile preparations for topical use help some children and are generally considered safe.

MAINTAINING SKIN INTEGRITY AND PREVENTING INFECTION

Cut the child's fingernails short and keep them clean. Avoid tight clothing and heat. Use 100% cotton bed sheets and pajamas. In addition to keeping the child's skin well moisturized, it is extremely important to prevent the child from scratching. Scratching causes the rash to appear, and further scratching may lead to secondary infection. Antihistamines given at bedtime may sedate the child enough to allow them to sleep without awakening because of itching.

During the waking hours, behavior modification may help to keep the child from scratching. Have the parent keep a diary for 1 week to determine the pattern of scratching. Help the parent to determine specific strategies that may raise the child's awareness of scratching. A handheld clicker or counter may help to identify the scratching episode for the child, thus raising awareness. The use of diversion, imagination, and play may help to distract the child from scratching. The parent and child may create a game together that results in the child participating in a behavior rather than scratching. Pressing the skin or clenching the fist may replace scratching. It is important for the child to stay active to distract their mind from the itching. It is important for the parent to positively reinforce and reward the desired behaviors. See Evidence-Based Practice 23.1.

Contact Dermatitis

Contact dermatitis is a cell-mediated response to an antigenic substance exposure. The first exposure is the sensitization phase. The antigen attaches to cells that migrate to regional lymph nodes and have contact with T lymphocytes, where recognition of antigen is developed. During the second phase, elicitation, contact with the antigen results in T-lymphocyte proliferation and release of inflammatory mediators. An allergic response occurs within 24 to 48 hours after contact with the substance.

Contact dermatitis may occur as a result of allergy to nickel or cobalt found in clothing hardware and dyes, and chemicals found in many hygiene products and cosmetics. One of the more common causes of contact dermatitis in children results from exposure to highly allergenic plants such as *Toxicodendron radicans* (poison ivy), *Toxicodendron quercifolium* (Eastern poison oak), *Toxicodendron diversilobum* (Western poison oak), and *Toxicodendron vernix* (poison sumac).

Direct or indirect contact with the plant's oleoresin found in the leaves, stems, and roots results in an allergic reaction. Even contact with dormant plants or plants perceived to be dead may cause an allergic response. The rash is extremely pruritic and may last for 2 to 4 weeks; lesions continue to appear during the illness. Contact dermatitis is not contagious and does not spread either to other parts of the affected child's skin or to other people. Scratching does not spread the rash, but it may cause skin damage or secondary infection. Complications of contact dermatitis include secondary bacterial skin infections and lichenification or hyperpigmentation, particularly in darker skin tones.

Therapeutic management is directed toward management of itching and the use of topical corticosteroids.

EVIDENCE-BASED PRACTICE 23.1

Phototherapy for Atopic Dermatitis

STUDY

Conventional medications do not always provide the relief children and their parents desire for atopic dermatitis. This review focused on the use of phototherapy (narrow-band ultraviolet B [NB-UVB] therapy) compared to placebo or other treatments for atopic dermatitis. The authors reviewed 32 studies with 1,219 participants aged 5 years and older.

Findings

Overall, the use of NB-UVB did result in modest improvements in signs of eczema as assessed by a health care professional, moderate to significant improvement as reported by the participants, and an increased number of participants reporting less severe itching. Confidence in the findings is limited, as the reviewed studies were quite disparate from each other.

Nursing Implications

The impact of phototherapy on AD has not been well studied. If parents wish to pursue alternative treatments, this study reported on a particular type of phototherapy, NB-UVB. Additional high-quality rigorous studies are needed to establish the benefit of NB-UVB therapy as well as other forms of phototherapy.

Data from Musters, A. H., Mashayekhi, S., Harvey, J., Axon, E., Lax, S. J., Flohr, C., Drucker, A. M, Gerbens, L., Ferguson, J., Ibbotson, S., Dawe, R. S., Garritsen, F., Brouwer, M., Limpens, J., Prescott, L. E., Boyle, R. J., & Spuls, P. I. (2021). Phototherapy for atopic eczema. *Cochrane Database of Systematic Reviews.* https://doi.org/10.1002/14651858.CD013870.pub2

Moderate-potency topical glucocorticoid cream or ointment is used for mild to moderate contact dermatitis, and high-potency preparations are used for more severe cases. Some severe cases of contact dermatitis may require the use of systemic steroids.

Nursing Assessment

Elicit the health history, noting onset, description, location, and progression of the rash, which may be intensely pruritic and vesicular if caused by allergenic plant exposure (Fig. 23.13). Rashes caused by other allergic exposure may be quite variable in their appearance and intensity of pruritus. Document treatment used thus far, and the child's response to it. Examine the skin, noting rash that may vary from maculopapular in nature to an erythematous papulovesicular rash at the site of contact. Some lesions may be weeping; others may erupt and form a crust. The lesions are often distributed in an asymmetric linear pattern on exposed body parts if caused by allergenic plant exposure. If the child's shirt came in contact with the plant and then the shirt was removed by pulling it over the head, widespread lesions might be found over both sides of the face. Lesions near the eyes often cause significant eyelid edema.

TAKE NOTE!

Nickel dermatitis may occur from contact with jewelry, eyeglasses, belts, or clothing snaps. Infants may display a small red circle with scaling at the site of contact with sleeper snaps.

Nursing Management

Contact dermatitis may be prevented by avoiding contact with the allergen. When the condition does occur, nursing management focuses on relieving the discomfort associated with the rash. Administer topical or systemic corticosteroids as prescribed, and teach the family about use of the medications. Teaching Guidelines 23.2 gives more information about the treatment and prevention of contact dermatitis.

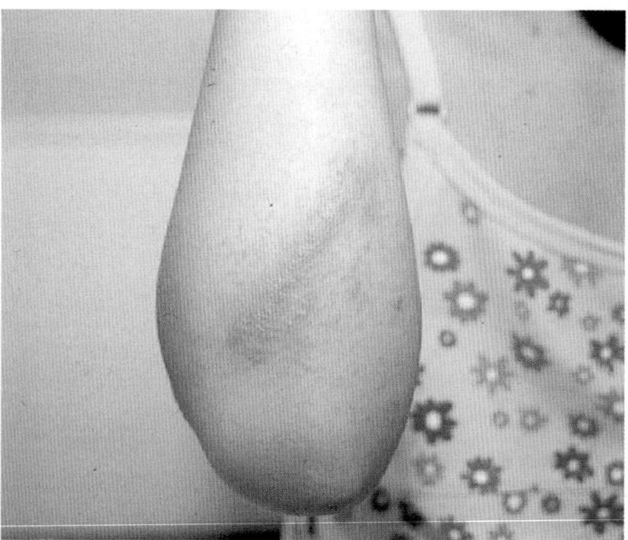

FIGURE 23.13 Note vesicular rash in linear formation characteristic of poison ivy.

Erythema Multiforme

Erythema multiforme, although uncommon in children, is an acute, self-limiting hypersensitivity reaction. It may occur in response to viral infections, such as adenovirus

TEACHING GUIDELINES 23.2 Prevention and Treatment of Contact Dermatitis

Prevention

- Wear long sleeves and long pants on outings in the woods.
- Identify and remove offending plants in the yard by using a commercial weed or underbrush killer.
- Vinyl gloves (not rubber or latex) are an effective barrier.
- The plant's oil residue may be on clothes, pets, garden and sports equipment, and toys; wash those well with soap and water.
- If contact occurs, wash vigorously with soap and water within 10 minutes of contact.
- Zanfel and Tecnu Oak-N-Ivy Outdoor Skin Cleanser (both soap mixtures) may prevent rash if used to wash the skin soon after exposure.
- Ivy Block (an organoclay) is a U.S. Food and Drug Administration–approved preventive treatment for contact dermatitis related to poison ivy, oak, or sumac. It is applied to the skin before possible exposure.

Treatment

- Wash lesions daily with mild soap and water.
- Mildly debride crusted lesions.
- Tepid baths (colloidal oatmeal such as Aveeno) are helpful to decrease itching.
- Avoid hot baths or showers, as they aggravate itching.
- Apply corticosteroid preparations topically as directed (if using high-potency preparations, do not cover with an occlusive dressing).
- Weeping lesions may be wrapped lightly; avoid occlusion.
- Burow or Domeboro solutions with a dressing applied twice daily for 20 minutes may help to dry weepy lesions.
- Over-the-counter preparations such as calamine lotion or Ivy Rest may reduce itching and help the lesions to dry.
- Do not use topical antihistamines, benzocaine, or neomycin because of the potential for sensitization.

BOX 23.1 Stevens–Johnson Syndrome and Toxic Epidermal Necrolysis

- High fever and flulike symptoms for 1 to 3 days prior to rash appearing
- Rash is characteristic of erythema multiforme with the addition of inflammatory bullae on at least two types of mucosa (lips, oral mucosa, bulbar conjunctivae, or anogenital region).
- Stevens–Johnson syndrome results in skin detachment of 10% or less, while toxic epidermal necrolysis involves 30% skin detachment.
- Mortality rate of 23% (Lee, 2024)
- Treatment: hospitalization, isolation, fluid and electrolyte support, treatment of secondary infection of the lesions
- Ophthalmologic consult to determine if corneal ulceration, keratitis, uveitis, or panophthalmitis is present

or Epstein–Barr virus; *Mycoplasma pneumoniae* infection; or a drug (especially sulfa drugs, penicillins, or immunizations) or food reaction. Stevens–Johnson syndrome and toxic epidermal necrolysis are the severest forms of erythema multiforme and most often occur in response to certain medications or to *Mycoplasma* infection (Box 23.1). Therapeutic management of erythema multiforme is generally supportive because it resolves on its own.

Nursing Assessment

Note history of fever, malaise, and achiness (myalgia). Determine onset and progression of rash, as well as presence of pruritus and burning. Document the child's temperature on assessment. Inspect the skin for lesions, which most commonly occur over the hands and feet and extensor surfaces of the extremities, with spread to the trunk. Lesions progress from erythematous **macules** (flat reddened areas) to papules, plaques, vesicles, and target lesions over a period of days (hence the name *multiforme*) (Fig. 23.14).

Nursing Management

Discontinue the medication or food if it is identified as the cause. Ensure that treatment for *Mycoplasma* is instituted if present. Encourage oral hydration. Administer analgesics and antihistamines as needed to promote comfort. If oral lesions are present, encourage soothing mouthwashes or use of topical oral anesthetics in the older child or adolescent. Oral lesions may be debrided with hydrogen peroxide.

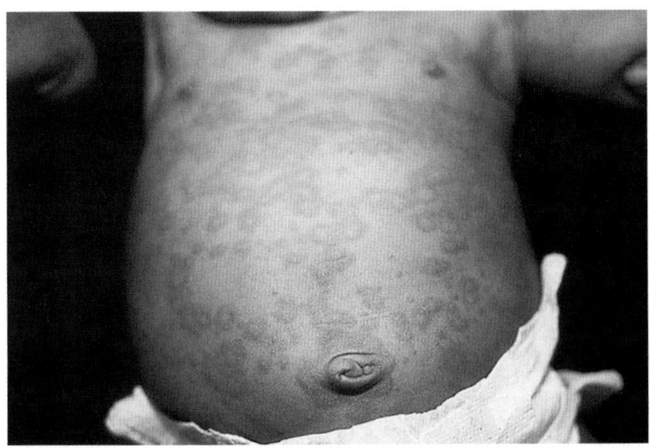

FIGURE 23.14 Erythema multiforme.

Urticaria

Urticaria, commonly called hives, is a type I hypersensitivity reaction caused by an immunologically mediated antigen–antibody response of histamine release from mast cells. Vasodilation and increased vascular permeability result, and erythema and wheals then occur. Urticaria usually begins rapidly and may disappear in a few days or may take up to 6 weeks to resolve. The most common causes of this reaction are foods, drugs, animal stings, infections, environmental stimuli (e.g., heat, cold, sun, tight clothes), and stress. Therapeutic management focuses on identifying and removing the cause as well as providing antihistamines or steroids.

Nursing Assessment

Obtain a detailed history of new foods, medications, symptoms of a recent infection, changes in environment, or unusual stress. Inspect the skin, noting raised, edematous hives anywhere on the body or mucous membranes (Fig. 23.15). The hives are pruritic, blanch when pressed, and may migrate. Angioedema may also be present and is identifiable as subcutaneous edema and warmth, occurring most frequently on the extremities, face, or genitalia. Carefully assess airway and breathing, as hypersensitivity reactions may affect respiratory status.

Nursing Management

Identify and remove the offending trigger. Discontinue antibiotics. Administer antihistamines, corticosteroids,

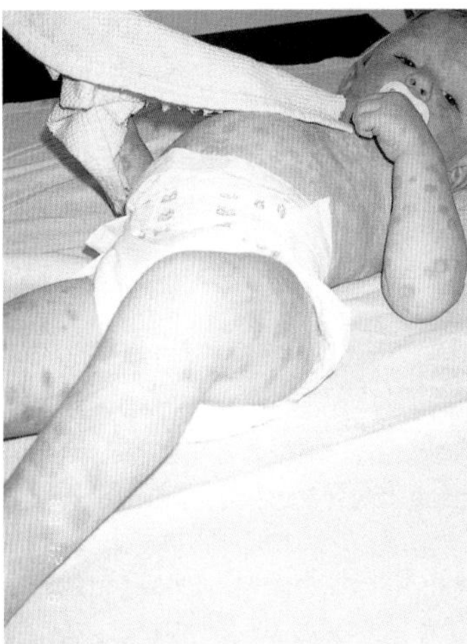

FIGURE 23.15 Ill-appearing child with urticaria. (Reprinted with permission from Fleisher, G. R., Ludwig, S., & Baskin, M. N. [2004]. *Atlas of pediatric emergency medicine* [p. 88]. Lippincott Williams & Wilkins.)

and topical antipruritics as prescribed. Inform the child and family that the episode should resolve within a few days. If it lasts up to 6 weeks, the child should be reevaluated (Covar et al., 2022). Advise the family to obtain a medical alert bracelet for the child if the reaction is severe.

TAKE NOTE!

In an emergency situation when airway and breathing are compromised, subcutaneous epinephrine followed by IV diphenhydramine and corticosteroids is necessary.

Seborrhea

Seborrhea is a chronic inflammatory dermatitis that may occur on the skin or scalp. In infants, it occurs most often on the scalp and is commonly referred to as cradle cap. Infants may also manifest seborrhea on the nose or eyebrows, behind the ears, or in the diaper area. It usually resolves over the course of weeks to months (Sasseville, 2023). Adolescents manifest seborrhea on the scalp (dandruff) and on the eyebrows and eyelashes, behind the ears, and between the shoulder blades.

It is thought that seborrhea is an inflammatory reaction to the fungus *Pityrosporum ovale* and is worsened by sebaceous involvement related to the birthing parent's hormones in the infant and androgens in the adolescent.

Therapeutic management includes treating the skin lesions with corticosteroid creams or lotions. Antidandruff shampoos containing selenium sulfide, ketoconazole, or tar are used to treat the scalp.

Nursing Assessment

Elicit the health history, determining onset and progression of skin and scalp changes. Note response to treatment used so far. In the infant, inspect the scalp and forehead, behind the ears, and the neck, trunk, and diaper area for thick or flaky greasy yellow scales (Fig. 23.16). In the adolescent, note mild flakes in the hair with yellow greasy scales on the scalp, forehead, and eyebrows; behind the ears; or between the scapulae.

Nursing Management

Wash or shampoo the affected areas with a mild soap. Apply antiinflammatory cream to skin lesions if prescribed. In the infant, apply mineral oil to the scalp, massage it well with a washcloth, and then shampoo 10 to 15 minutes later, using a brush to gently lift the crusts; do not forcibly remove the crusts. If needed, selenium sulfide shampoo may safely be used on the infant, following the aforementioned procedure. The adolescent may require daily shampooing with an antidandruff shampoo.

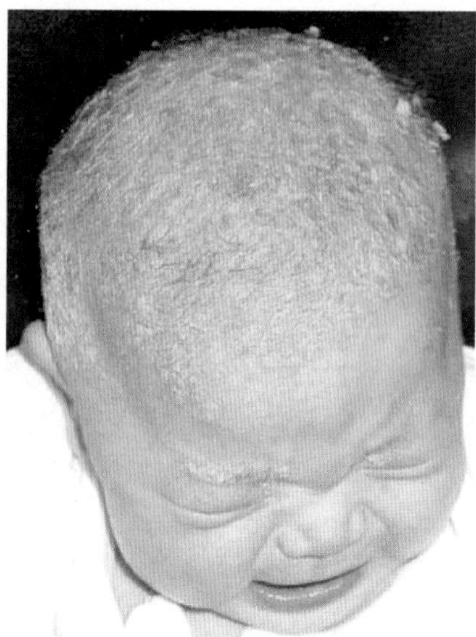

FIGURE 23.16 Severe cradle cap (yellow, greasy-appearing plaques).

Psoriasis

Psoriasis is a chronic inflammatory skin disease with periods of remission and exacerbation; control is possible with conscientious therapy. It is an immune-mediated disorder occurring in people with a genetic predisposition. About 30% of adults with this disorder experienced its onset prior to 2 years of age (Bender & Chiu, 2020).

Hyperproliferation of the epidermis occurs, with a rash developing at sites of mechanical, thermal, or physical trauma. Therapeutic management includes skin hydration with emollient creams, use of tar preparations, topical steroids, and UV light, among others. Narrow-band UV light has been used with some success in children with severe psoriasis.

Nursing Assessment

Note family history of psoriasis. Determine onset and progression of rash, as well as treatments used and the response to treatment. Question the child about pruritus, which is usually absent with psoriasis. Inspect the skin for erythematous papules that coalesce to form plaques, most frequently found on the scalp, elbows, genital area, and knees (Fig. 23.17). Facial plaques may also occur and are more common in children than in adults. The plaques have a silvery or yellow-white scale and sharply demarcated borders. Layers of scale may be present, which, when removed, result in pinpoint bleeding (referred to as the Auspitz sign). Plaques on the scalp may result in alopecia. Examine the palms and soles, noting fissures and scaling. Skin biopsy, although rarely needed for diagnosis, will show hyperplastic epidermis, with thinning of the papillary dermis.

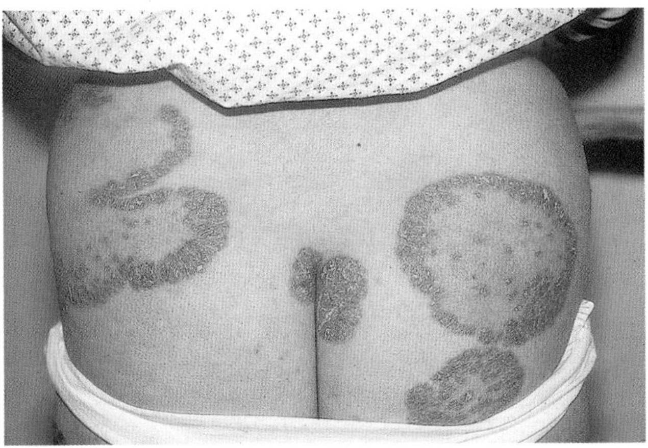

FIGURE 23.17 Psoriasis. (Reprinted with permission from Goodheart, H. P. [2009]. *Goodheart's photoguide to common skin disorders* [3rd ed.]. Wolters Kluwer.)

Nursing Management

Exposure to sunlight may promote healing, but take care not to allow the child to become sunburned. Apply skin moisturizers or emollients daily to prevent dry skin and flare-ups. Apply topical antiinflammatory creams as prescribed during flare-ups. Apply tar shampoos or skin preparations. Use mineral oil and warm towels to soak and remove thick plaques.

> THINKING ABOUT **DEVELOPMENT**
>
> Emily Wilson is a 15-year-old girl with a history of moderate psoriasis. She experiences significant scaling along her hairline, forehead, scalp, and arms. Hypopigmentation and striae are beginning to occur on her arms as a result of topical medication use. She is a talented ballerina but expresses increasing concerns about her skin alterations showing while she is performing.
>
> How does Emily's developmental stage affect self-care related to her psoriasis?
>
> What is the most appropriate approach for the nurse to take to educate Emily about control of her psoriasis?
>
> How will the nurse best promote an appropriate body image for Emily?

ACNE

Acne is a disorder that affects the pilosebaceous unit and is common in childhood (Prok & Torres-Zegarra, 2022). Acne that persists past the usual course of time for infantile or adolescent acne may be caused by endocrine abnormalities. It may also occur in response to the use of certain types of drugs such as corticosteroids, androgens, phenytoin, and others. The usual presentation and nursing management of neonatal acne and acne vulgaris are discussed in what follows.

Neonatal Acne

Neonatal acne occurs as a response to the presence of the birthing parent's androgens or to transient androgen production in the newborn. It may be present immediately after birth but often occurs between 2 and 4 weeks of age (Prok & Torres-Zegarra, 2022). Usually, no treatment is necessary, but in severe cases there is a risk of scarring, so a topical preparation may be prescribed.

Nursing Assessment

Note oily face or scalp. Examine the face (especially the cheeks), upper chest, and back for inflammatory papules and pustules. Document absence of fever.

Nursing Management

Instruct parents to avoid picking or squeezing the pimples; to do so places the infant at risk for secondary bacterial infection and cellulitis. Teach parents to wash the affected areas daily with clear water. Avoid using fragranced soaps or lotions on the area with acne. Inform the parents that as the newborn's hormones stabilize over time, the acne usually resolves without additional intervention.

Acne Vulgaris

Beginning as early as 7 to 10 years of age, acne vulgaris affects about 85% of adolescents, and endogenous androgens play a role in its development (Prok & Torres-Zegarra, 2022). It occurs most frequently on the face, chest, and back. Risk factors for the development of acne vulgaris include preadolescent or adolescent age, male sex (due to the presence of androgens), an oily complexion, Cushing syndrome, or another disease process resulting in increased androgen production.

Pathophysiology

The sebaceous gland produces sebum and is connected by a duct to the follicular canal that opens on the skin's surface. Androgens stimulate sebaceous gland proliferation and production of sebum. These hormones exhibit increased activity during the pubertal years. Abnormal shedding of the outermost layer of the skin (the stratum corneum) occurs at the level of the follicular opening, resulting in a keratin plug that fills the follicle. The sebaceous glands increase sebum production. Bacterial overgrowth of *Propionibacterium acnes* occurs because the presence of sebum and keratin in the follicular canal creates an excellent environment for growth. Inflammation occurs as the follicular wall perforates, allowing the contents to leak into nearby tissue.

Therapeutic Management

Therapeutic management focuses on reducing *P. acnes,* decreasing sebum production, normalizing skin shedding, and eliminating inflammation. Teach the adolescent to cleanse the skin gently twice a day. Medication therapy may include a combination of benzoyl peroxide, salicylic acid, retinoids, and topical or oral antibiotics. Isotretinoin may be used in severe cases. Drug Guide 23.1 gives further information on these medications. Oral contraceptives may help lessen acne by decreasing the effects of androgens on the sebaceous glands. Diode laser or blue UV light therapy may also be used. CO_2 lasers and dermabrasion may be used to treat pitted scarring.

Nursing Assessment

Note history of onset of acne lesions, as well as family history of acne. Determine medication use; certain medications may hasten the onset of acne or worsen it when already present. In particular, note use of corticosteroids, androgens, lithium, phenytoin, and isoniazid. Document history of an endocrine disorder, particularly one that results in hyperandrogenism. Note worsening of acne 2 to 7 days before the start of the menstrual period. Inspect the skin for lesions (particularly on the face and upper chest and back, which are the areas of highest sebaceous activity). Note presence, distribution, and extent of noninflammatory lesions, such as open and closed comedones, as well as inflammatory lesions such as papules, pustules, nodules, or cysts (open comedones are commonly referred to as blackheads and closed comedones as whiteheads; Fig. 23.18). Examine the skin for hypertrophic scarring resulting from inflammatory lesions. Table 23.3 explains the acne classification. Note oily skin and oily hair, which result from increased sebum production. Determine remedies that have been used and the extent of success of those treatments. Assess the child's or adolescent's feelings about the disorder.

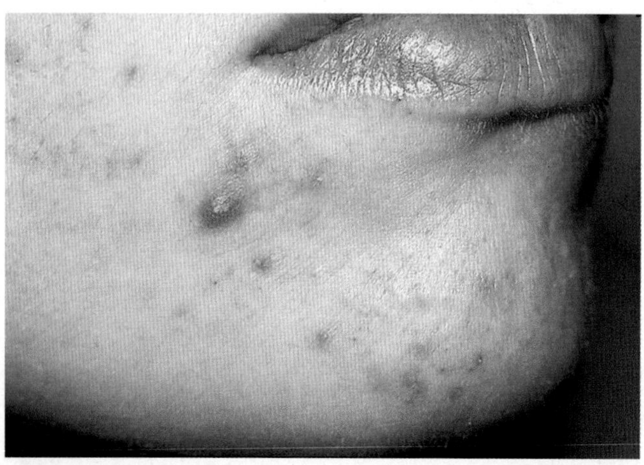

FIGURE 23.18 Acne vulgaris.

TABLE 23.3 • Classification of Acne

Classification	Manifestations
Mild acne	Primarily noninflammatory lesions (comedones)
Moderate acne	Comedones plus inflammatory lesions such as papules or pustules (localized to face or back)
Severe acne	Lesions similar to moderate acne, but more widespread, and/or presence of cysts or nodules; associated more frequently with scarring

Nursing Management

Avoid oil-based cosmetics and hair products, as their use may block pores, contributing to noninflammatory lesions. Look for cosmetic products labeled as noncomedogenic. Headbands, helmets, and hats may exacerbate the lesions by causing friction. Dryness and peeling may occur with acne treatment, so encourage the child to use a humectant moisturizer. Mild cleansing with soap and water twice daily is appropriate. Avoid excessive scrubbing and harsh chemical or alcohol-based cleansers. Avoid picking or squeezing the lesions. Using a noncomedogenic sunscreen with a sun-protective factor (SPF) of 30 or higher is recommended (Kim, 2020).

Teach adolescents that the prescribed topical medications must be used daily and that it may take 4 to 6 weeks to see results. Avoid the use of over-the-counter preparations because they are irritating and aggravate the drying effect of prescription acne treatments. Instruct adolescents who wish to remove facial hair to shave gently and avoid using dull razors, so as not to further irritate the condition. Adolescents taking isotretinoin who could become pregnant must be on a pregnancy prevention program because the drug causes defects in fetal development (Kim, 2020) (Box 23.2).

BOX 23.2 Decreasing Risk of Fetal Exposure to Isotretinoin: iPLEDGE

- As of 2006, health care providers, pharmacists, and patients are required to register in the iPLEDGE program before they prescribe, dispense, or receive isotretinoin.
- The iPLEDGE program is a central registry requiring monthly input as noted following in order to continue isotretinoin treatment.
- Monthly input includes the following:
  - Females of childbearing age are using two forms of contraception.
  - Pregnancy test results are negative.
  - Isotretinoin users do not donate blood during treatment or for 1 month after completion of treatment.
- Additional information available at https://www.ipledgeprogram.com/iPledgeUI/home.u

Data from iPledge. (2021). *iPledge: Committed to pregnancy prevention.* https://www.ipledgeprogram.com/iPledgeUI/home.u

If the acne is severe, depression may occur as a result of body image disturbances. Provide emotional support to adolescents undergoing acne therapy. Refer adolescents for counseling if necessary.

> **CONSIDER THIS!**
>
> Paxton Herman, age 16, comes to the clinic with complaints of acne on his face and back. He states, "I hate the way my face looks." "I'll never get a date looking like this." "I don't even want to take my shirt off at the beach, because there's bumps on my back."
>
> Think back to when you were an adolescent. How would you have felt if you had a skin condition that altered the way your face looked? As the nurse, how can you help Paxton in this situation?

INJURIES

Children, by their inquisitive natures, developmental immaturity, and skin's properties, are prone to experience a variety of skin injuries. Pressure injuries are most likely to occur in hospitalized or otherwise immobile children. Typical healthy, active children are likely to suffer cuts, abrasions, foreign-body penetration, burns and other thermal injuries, bites, and stings.

Pressure Injuries

Skin breakdown involves changes in intact skin, which may range from blanchable erythema to deep pressure injuries. The term pressure injury refers to damage to the skin resulting in skin loss and development of a crater that may range from mild to deep. Pressure injuries develop from a combination of factors, including immobility or decreased activity, decreased sensory perception, increased moisture, impaired nutritional status, inadequate tissue perfusion, and the forces of friction and shear. Common sites of pressure injuries in hospitalized children include the occiput and toes, while children who require wheelchairs for mobility have pressure injuries on the sacral or hip area more frequently.

Nursing Assessment

Note history of immobility (chronic, related to a condition such as paralysis) or lengthy hospitalization, particularly in intensive care. Inspect the skin for areas of erythema or warmth. Note ulceration of the skin. Use the facility's wound assessment scale to document the extent of the injury. Take a photo of the injury if possible.

Nursing Management

Position the child to alleviate pressure on the area of the injury. Use specialized beds or mattresses to prevent further pressure areas from developing. Perform prescribed wound care meticulously, noting the formation of granulation tissue as the injury begins to heal. Prevent pressure injuries in the child who is hospitalized for long periods by turning the child frequently, assessing the entire surface of the child's skin at least every shift, using pressure-alleviating beds and mattresses, and maintaining the child's nutritional status.

Minor Injuries

Children suffer minor injuries frequently. Because of their developmental immaturity and inquisitive nature, children often attempt tasks they are not yet capable of or take risks that an adult would not, often resulting in a fall or other accident. Minor injuries include minor cuts and abrasions, as well as skin penetration of foreign bodies such as splinters or glass fragments. The break in the skin allows an entry point for bacteria, and the complication of cellulitis may occur. Treatment is directed at cleaning the wound and preventing infection.

Nursing Assessment

Obtain the history from the child or caregiver to determine whether dirt or a foreign object may be present in the wound. Inspect the wound, noting depth of injury, a foreign body, and bleeding.

Nursing Management

Cleanse the wound with mild soap and water or with an antibacterial cleanser. Wet gauze helps to scrub away fine and large sand particles. Remove pieces of loose skin with sterile scissors, foreign particles with sterile forceps, and road tar with petrolatum. Small abrasions and minor, well-approximated cuts may be left open to the air. Apply a small amount of antibacterial ointment and cover large abrasions with a loose dressing. Change the dressing 12 hours later and redress after cleaning the wound. Leave it open to air after 23 hours have passed from the time of injury. Assess the wound daily for signs of infection, which include purulence, warmth, edema, increasing pain, and erythema that extends past the margin of the cut or abrasion.

Burns

Burns are a common preventable mechanism of injury among children and adolescents. Young children are at highest risk for burns, and the mortality rate from burns is highest in children younger than 5 years (Joffe, 2023). Most pediatric burn-related injuries do not result in death, but injuries from burns often cause extreme pain, and extensive burns can result in serious disfigurement. In young children, 85% of burns are scald burns, and 18% of pediatric burn injuries result from child abuse (Antoon, 2020). Fires in the home are often related to cooking and cigarette or other smoking materials. Carbon monoxide poisoning often occurs in conjunction with burns as a result of smoke inhalation, and infants and children are at greater risk for carbon monoxide poisoning than adults. Great advances have been made in the care of children with serious burns. As a result of improved burn care, children who in the past would have died as a result of burns over large body surface areas have a much greater chance of survival (Joffe, 2023). Conventional wisdom is that children with severe burns should be transferred to a specialized burn unit. The American Burn Association has developed the following criteria for referral of burned people to a specialized burn unit:

- Partial-thickness burns greater than 10% of total body surface area
- Burns that involve the face, the hands and feet, genitalia, perineum, or major joints
- Full-thickness burns of any size
- Chemical or electrical burns (including lightning injury)
- Inhalation injury
- Burn injury in children who have preexisting conditions that might affect their care
- People with burns and traumatic injuries
- People who will require special social, emotional, or long-term rehabilitative care
- Burned children in a hospital without qualified personnel or equipment for the care of children (Joffe, 2023)

Burns are classified according to the extent of injury, and the terminology used to describe each type includes superficial (formerly first degree), partial thickness (second degree), deep partial thickness (second degree), and full thickness (third and fourth degree) (Antoon, 2020). Superficial burns involve only epidermal injury and usually heal without scarring or other sequelae within 4 to 5 days. In partial-thickness burns, injury occurs not only to the epidermis but also to portions of the dermis. These burns usually heal within about 2 weeks and carry a minimal risk of scar formation. Deep partial-thickness burns take longer to heal, may scar, and result in changes in nail and hair appearance as well as sebaceous gland function in the affected area. They may require surgical intervention. Full-thickness burns result in significant tissue damage as they extend through the epidermis, dermis, and hypodermis. Extensive scarring results, as hair follicles and sweat glands are destroyed. Full-thickness burns require a significant time to heal. If underlying tendons and/or bone are involved, the burn may be termed fourth degree. Contractures and limited function may occur as a complication of full-thickness burns. Skin grafting is usually necessary. Full or partially circumferential burns may result in ischemia from loss of blood flow related to progressive swelling of the area.

Pathophysiology

Burned tissue begins to coagulate after the injury, and direct coagulation and microvascular reactions in the adjacent dermis may extend the burn. The blood vessels demonstrate increased capillary permeability, resulting in vasodilatation. This leads to increased hydrostatic pressure in the capillaries, causing water, electrolytes, and protein to leak out of the vasculature and result in significant edema. Edema forms rapidly in the first 18 hours after the burn, peaking at around 48 hours. Capillary permeability then returns to normal between 48 and 72 hours after the burn, and the lymphatics can reabsorb the edema fluid. Diuresis occurs, ridding the body of the excess fluid. Fluid loss from burned skin occurs at an amount that is five to 10 times greater than that from undamaged skin, and this fluid loss continues until the damaged surface is healed or grafted.

Initially, the severely burned child experiences a decrease in cardiac output, with a subsequent hypermetabolic response during which cardiac output increases dramatically. During this heightened metabolic state, the child is at risk for insulin resistance and increased protein catabolism. Children who are burned during an indoor or chemical fire are at an increased risk of respiratory injury. Children who have aspirated hot liquids are particularly at risk for airway-altering edema.

Therapeutic Management

Therapeutic management of burns focuses on fluid resuscitation, wound care, prevention of infection, and restoration of function. Burn infections are treated with antibiotics specific to the causative organism. If invasive burn damage occurs, surgery may be necessary.

Nursing Assessment

Refer to the "Clinical Judgment and the Nursing Process" section for a full description of the assessment phase of the nursing process. Upon arrival, evaluate the child with burns to determine if they will require intensive management. Remove any smoldering clothing. Obtain a brief history of the burn circumstances while you are assessing the child and providing care.

HEALTH HISTORY

If the burn is severe or there is a potential for respiratory compromise, obtain a brief history while simultaneously evaluating the child and providing emergency care. If the burn does not appear to pose an immediate life-threatening risk, obtain an in-depth history. Elicit a description of how the burn occurred, noting date, time, and cause. Determine if smoke inhalation or an associated fall may have occurred. Document treatment that the parent or caregiver has provided to the child's burn so far. Note the child's recent health status, current medications, recent or chronic illness, and immunization status, noting, in particular, the date of the most recent tetanus vaccination.

Determine whether the history being given sounds consistent with the type of burn injury that has occurred. Inquire about what caused the burn and whether the event was witnessed by anyone. Spatter-type burns resulting from the child pulling a source of hot fluid onto themselves usually yield a nonuniform, asymmetric distribution of injury. In contrast, intentional scald injuries usually yield a uniform "stocking" or "glove" distribution when the child's extremity is held under very hot water as punishment (Ford et al., 2022). It is important for the nurse to pick up on clues in the health history that may indicate that the burn is a result of child abuse rather than an accident (Box 23.3). Children are also burned by curling irons, gasoline, fireworks, room heaters, ovens, and ranges. Obtain a detailed history about the circumstances surrounding these types of burns. Ask the parent what the home hot water heater temperature is.

PHYSICAL EXAMINATION

Emergency examination of the burned child consists of a primary survey followed by a secondary survey. The primary survey includes evaluation of the child's airway, breathing, and circulation. The secondary survey focuses on evaluation of the burns and other injuries. Box 23.4 gives information about emergency assessment of the burned child. Inspect the child's skin, noting erythema, blistering, weeping, or eschar (charred skin).

Classify the burn according to its severity. Superficial burns are painful, red, dry, and possibly edematous (Fig. 23.19). Partial-thickness and deep partial-thickness burns are painful and edematous and have a wet appearance or blisters (Fig. 23.20). Full-thickness burns may be painful or numb or pain-free in some areas. They appear red, edematous, leathery, dry, or waxy and may display peeling or charred skin (Fig. 23.21). Note whether the burn is circumferential (encircling a body part) or partially circumferential.

BOX 23.3 Signs of Child Abuse–Induced Burns

- Inconsistent history given when caregivers are interviewed separately
- Delay in seeking treatment by caregiver
- Uniform appearance of the burn, with clear delineation of burned and nonburned area (as with a hot object applied to the skin)
- In the case of a scald-induced burn, lack of spattering of water but evidence of so-called "porcelain-contact sparing," where the portion of the child's skin that was in contact with the tub or sink is not burned (commonly seen with a forced immersion in extremely hot water used as punishment)
- Flexor-sparing burns or burns that involve the dorsum of the hand
- A stocking/glove pattern on the hands or feet (circumferential ring appearing around the extremity, resulting from a caregiver forcefully holding the child under extremely hot water)

Based on Ford, C. R., Chiesa, A., & Sirotnak, A. P. (2022). Chapter 8: Child abuse & neglect. In M. Bunik, W. W. Hay, M. J. Levin, & M. J. Abzug (Eds.), *Current diagnosis & treatment: Pediatrics* (26th ed.). McGraw-Hill Education.

BOX 23.4 Emergency Assessment of the Burned Child

Primary Survey

- Assess the child's airway, noting whether it is patent, maintainable, or unmaintainable.
- Suspect airway injury from burn or smoke inhalation if any of the following are present: burns around the mouth, nose, or eyes; carbonaceous (black-colored) sputum; hoarseness or stridor.
- Evaluate the child's skin color, respiratory effort, symmetry of breathing, and breath sounds.
- Determine the pulse strength, perfusion status, and heart rate. Note extent and location of edema.

Secondary Survey

- Determine burn depth.
- Estimate burn extent by determining the percentage of body surface area affected. Use a chart for estimation (see Fig. 23.21), or rapidly estimate by using the child's palm size, which is equivalent to about 1.25% of the child's body surface area.
- Inspect the child for other traumatic injuries (children who have jumped or fallen from a house fire may suffer cervical spine or internal injuries).

Based on Joffe, M. D. (2023). Moderate and severe thermal burns in children: Emergency Management. *UpToDate*. Retrieved January 29, 2024, from http://www.uptodate.com/contents/emergency-care-of-moderate-and-severe-thermal-burns-in-children.

TAKE NOTE!

Due to overlying blistering, it is difficult to accurately distinguish between partial- and full-thickness burns. In addition, in the case of third-degree burns, it is difficult to estimate burn depth during the initial evaluation.

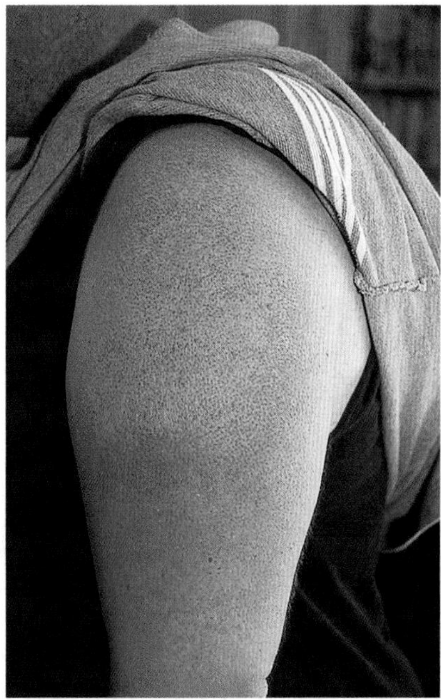

FIGURE 23.19 Superficial burn—painful but without blisters.

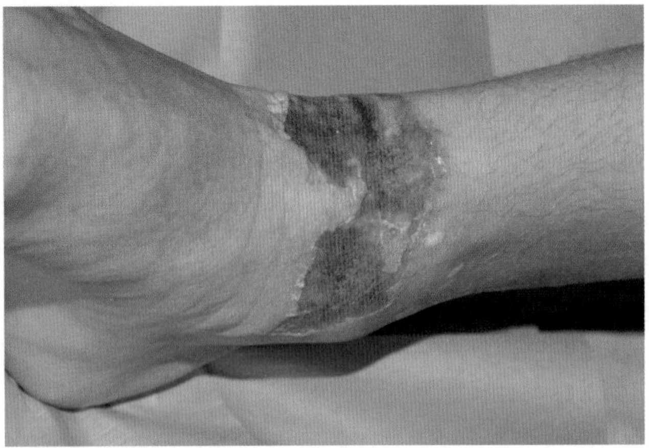

FIGURE 23.20 Partial-thickness burn—very painful, with blistering.

LABORATORY AND DIAGNOSTIC TESTS

In the child with more extensive burns, electrolytes and complete blood count are used to measure fluid and electrolyte balance and to determine the possibility of infection, respectively. If wound infection is suspected, culture of the drainage will determine the particular bacteria. Nutritional indices such as albumin, transferrin, carotene, retinol, copper, cholesterol, calcium, thiamine, riboflavin, pyridoxine, and iron may be evaluated when the child has severe or extensive burns. Pulmonary status may be evaluated via pulse oximetry and end-tidal CO_2 monitoring, arterial blood gases, carboxyhemoglobin levels, and chest radiography. Fiberoptic bronchoscopy and xenon ventilation–perfusion scanning may be used to evaluate inhalation injury. Electrocardiographic monitoring is important for the child who has suffered an electrical burn to identify cardiac dysrhythmias, which can be noted for up to 72 hours after a burn injury.

Nursing Management

Nursing management of the child who has been burned focuses first on stabilizing the child. Place the child on a cardiac/apnea monitor, measure the child with the Broselow tape, monitor pulse oximetry, and apply an end-tidal CO_2 monitor if the child is ventilated. Further management focuses on cleansing the burn, pain management, and prevention and treatment of infection. Fluid status and nutrition are important components of burn care, particularly in the early stages. Rehabilitation of the child with severe burns is also an important nursing function. Providing child and family education about the prevention of burns as well as care of burns at home is critical. The "Clinical Judgment and the Nursing Process" section gives additional interventions related to fluid and nutritional management.

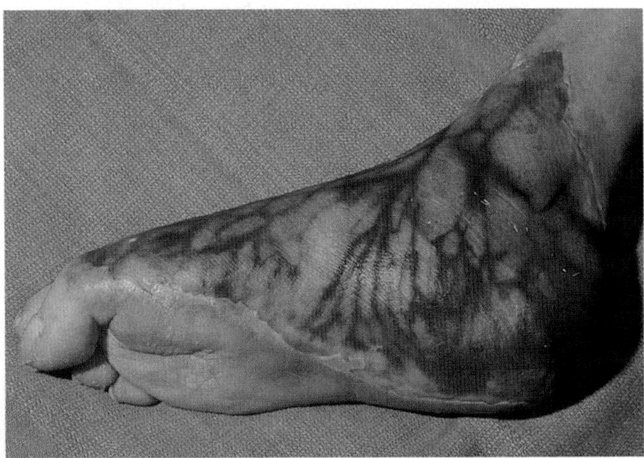

FIGURE 23.21 Full-thickness burn—color ranges from red to charred, or white, minimal pain, marked edema.

PROMOTING OXYGENATION AND VENTILATION

Institute emergency airway management as needed. If the child requires intubation, make sure that the tracheal tube is taped in a secure manner, as reintubation in these children will become increasingly difficult as the edema spreads. The burned child's respiratory status warrants vigilant evaluation and reevaluation, as airway edema that is secondary to a burn may not become evident until 2 days after the injury. Administer 100% oxygen via nonrebreather mask or bag–valve–mask ventilation to all children with severe burns. Continue to reassess the child's pulmonary status, adjusting the interventions as necessary (refer to Chapter 29 for further information about respiratory emergency care).

> **TAKE NOTE!**
>
> High levels of carboxyhemoglobin as a result of smoke inhalation may contribute to falsely high pulse oximetry readings (Mechem, 2024).

RESTORING AND MAINTAINING FLUID VOLUME

Several formulas are available for the calculation of resuscitative fluids in children. Most experts recommend that pediatric burn therapy include:

- Fluid calculation based on the body surface area burned (Fig. 23.22)
- Use of a crystalloid (Ringer's lactate) during the first 24 hours; in smaller children, a small amount of dextrose may be added
- Administration of most of the volume during the first 8 hours (amounts and timing of fluid volume resuscitation will vary from child to child)
- Reassessment of the child and adjustment of the fluid rate accordingly; fluid requirements greatly decrease after 24 hours and should be adjusted to reflect this.
- Administration of a colloid fluid later in therapy once capillary permeability is less of a concern
- Monitoring of the child's urine output as part of ongoing assessment of response to therapy, expecting at least 1 mL/kg/h

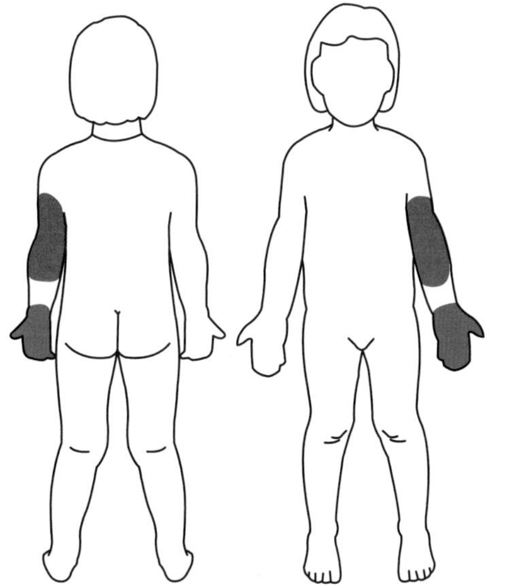

EXAMPLE

Calculating TBSA By Age (Total Body Surface Area)

Color Code
Red - 3° (full thickness)
Blue - 2° (partial thickness)

Area	Birth 1 yr	1–4 yrs	5–9 yrs	10–14 yrs	15 yrs	Adult	2	3	Total
Head	19	17	13	11	9	7	—	8	8.0
Neck	2	2	2	2	2	2	—	1	1.0
Ant. Trunk	13	13	13	13	13	13	1	12	13.0
Post. Trunk	13	13	13	13	13	13	—	—	—
R. Buttock	2 1/2	2 1/2	2 1/2	2 1/2	2 1/2	2 1/2	—	—	—
L. Buttock	2 1/2	2 1/2	2 1/2	2 1/2	2 1/2	2 1/2	—	—	—
Genitalia	1	1	1	1	1	1	—	—	—
R.U. Arm	4	4	4	4	4	4	—	3.5	3.5
L.U. Arm	4	4	4	4	4	4	1	2.5	3.5
R.L. Arm	3	3	3	3	3	3	—	3	3
L.L. Arm	3	3	3	3	3	3	—	3	3
R. Hand	2 1/2	2 1/2	2 1/2	2 1/2	2 1/2	2 1/2	—	2.5	2.5
L. Hand	2 1/2	2 1/2	2 1/2	2 1/2	2 1/2	2 1/2	—	2.5	2.5
R. Thigh	5 1/2	6 1/2	8	8 1/2	9	9 1/2	1	2	3
L. Thigh	5 1/2	6 1/2	8	8 1/2	9	9 1/2	—	2	2
R. Leg	5	5	5 1/2	6	6 1/2	7	—	—	—
L. Leg	5	5	5 1/2	6	6 1/2	7	—	—	—
R. Foot	3 1/2	3 1/2	3 1/2	3 1/2	3 1/2	3 1/2	—	—	—
L. Foot	3 1/2	3 1/2	3 1/2	3 1/2	3 1/2	3 1/2	—	—	—
						Total	3%	42%	45%

FIGURE 23.22 Calculate total body surface area (TBSA) affected by using the child's age and the area affected, as well as whether the burned area is second degree (partial thickness) or third degree (full thickness).

- Daily weights obtained at the same time each day (the best indicator of fluid volume status)
- Monitoring of electrolyte levels (particularly sodium and potassium) for their return to normal levels

PREVENTING HYPOTHERMIA

Due to the loss of the protective dermis, children who are burned are at high risk for hypothermia and secondary infection. Therefore, take care to keep the child warm. Warm intravenous fluids before administration. Maintain a neutral thermal environment, and monitor the child's temperature frequently.

CLEANSING THE BURN

Initially, it is important to stop the burning. Therefore, remove charred clothing. Wash and rinse the burn thoroughly with mild soap and cool water from the tap. Never apply ice. Children who are burned with tar require special care. Remove tar with cool water and mineral oil. Do not routinely remove blisters, because they provide a protective barrier; however, debridement is recommended in certain cases where large blisters impede wound care. Wounds that are open require debridement. Debridement involves the removal of loose skin and eschar (dead, charred skin). This procedure is usually performed with sterile scissors and a pair of forceps or with a gauze sponge. Gently cleanse the burned area; there is no advantage to aggressive scrubbing, and this technique only makes the pain more intense for the child. Wear a gown, mask, head covering, and gloves during dressing changes. Debridement is a necessary, but often excruciatingly painful, procedure. Thus, pain management needs of the child are of utmost importance (refer to the pain management section further on).

When children return for evaluation of a wound that was previously seen in your facility, remove the dressing. Soak the dressing in lukewarm tap water to ease the removal of gauze, which may be stuck to the wound. The nurse plays an important role in ensuring that the dressing change goes smoothly. Be sure to:

- Have all dressing supplies ready.
- Provide pain medication as ordered.
- Promote good infection control technique among your colleagues.
- Assist with restraining young children, using the positions of comfort previously discussed in relation to atraumatic care.
- Encourage participation by the child's parents.
- Talk soothingly to the child, explain what you are going to do, and provide distraction during the procedure.

PREVENTING INFECTION

Prevention of infection is critical to successful outcomes for burned children. If the child's immunization status is unknown or if it has been 5 years or longer since the last tetanus vaccine, administer the tetanus vaccine (Joffe, 2023). If the child has never received tetanus vaccination, also give 250 units tetanus human immunoglobulin intravenously. Apply antibiotic ointment in conjunction with burn dressing changes. Refer to Drug Guide 23.1 for information about topical antibiotics. Membrane dressings such as biosynthetic, hydrocolloid, and antibiotic-impregnated foam dressings are alternatives to topical antibiotics and sterile dressings. Evaluate the child's wound during dressing changes, looking for wound redness, swelling, odor, or drainage. Strictly adhere to infection control procedures and hand hygiene to decrease the risk of burn infection. Maximize the child's nutritional status to decrease their susceptibility to a burn infection. Monitor the child's temperature for the development of fever. Upon discharge, instruct the parents about the signs of a wound infection.

MANAGING PAIN

Pain management is of the utmost importance, and several options are available for the treatment of burn-related pain. Local anesthesia, sedatives, and systemic analgesics are commonly used. Children who have less severe burns that are managed at home can be given oral medications such as acetaminophen with codeine 30 to 45 minutes before dressing changes. In burns that result in more severe pain, the child should be hospitalized and given intravenous pain control with medications such as morphine sulfate. Midazolam (a sedative) may be used in conjunction with pain medication for pain reduction during dressing changes.

Pain may also occur at any time of the day or night, not just in relation to dressing changes. Assess the child's pain status frequently using an age-appropriate pain assessment scale. Administer pain medications as prescribed and/or use nonpharmacologic techniques to alleviate or decrease the child's perception of pain.

• • • ATRAUMATIC CARE • • •

Immersion in virtual reality computer games before and during burn dressing changes provides an exceptionally powerful form of cognitive distraction (Ahmadpour et al., 2019).

TREATING INFECTED BURNS

The potential for burn infection increases if the child has a large, open burn wound and if there are other sources of infection, such as multiple intravenous lines. In addition, children who are immunocompromised have an increased risk of burn infection. In burn wound cellulitis, the area around the burn becomes increasingly red, swollen, and painful early in the course of burn management. With invasive burn cellulitis, the burn develops a dark brown, black, or purplish color, with a discharge and foul odor. Burn impetigo is characterized by multifocal small superficial abscesses. Burn impetigo causes marked destruction of skin-grafted areas. Extensive infected burns may also become infected with a fungus.

When an infection is suspected, antibiotics are usually started, pending wound culture results. Administer antibiotics as prescribed or antifungals if necessary.

PROVIDING BURN REHABILITATION

Children who have suffered a significant burn injury face myriad physical and psychological challenges that extend well beyond the acute injury phase. Burned children may experience higher levels of anxiety than children who have never been burned, and they may display traumatic stress symptoms (Woolard et al., 2021). Skin grafting or special burn dressings are required for some children (Box 23.5). Children who have suffered extensive burns often require multiple skin-grafting surgeries. Figures 23.23 and 23.24 show healed skin grafts. Extensive burns may also result in the need for pressure garments to decrease the risk of extensive scarring. Pressure garments are not comfortable, and they must be worn continuously for at least 1 year, sometimes 2, but they have been shown to be effective in reducing hypertrophic scarring resulting from significant burn injury.

BOX 23.5 **Special Burn Care and Skin Grafting**

- To prevent infection and promote healing:
  - Biosynthetic skin coverings such as Biobrane (silicone film bonded to flexible nylon fabric and purified collagen peptides) and Mepilex Ag (soft silicone soaked with silver)
  - Kaltostat (calcium alginate dressing) is a brown seaweed extract that is spun into a fiber that is highly absorbent. It reacts with exudate on the wound to form a protective gel.
- Autograft allows for permanent coverage of a deep partial-thickness or full-thickness burn.
  - Consists of child's own skin
  - Split thickness consists of epidermis and superficial layers of dermis. The donor site heals completely.
  - Full thickness consists of full dermal thickness. Cover the donor site with fine-mesh gauze or synthetic wound coverings to allow the site to heal.

Based on Leon-Villapalos, J., & Dziewulski, P. (2022). Skin autografting. *UpToDate*. Retrieved January 29, 2024, from https://www.uptodate.com/contents/skin-autografting; and Tenenhaus, M., & Rennekampff, H.-O. (2023). Topical agents and dressings for local burn wound care. *UpToDate*. Retrieved April 26, 2023, from https://www.uptodate.com/contents/topical-agents-and-dressings-for-local-burn-wound-care

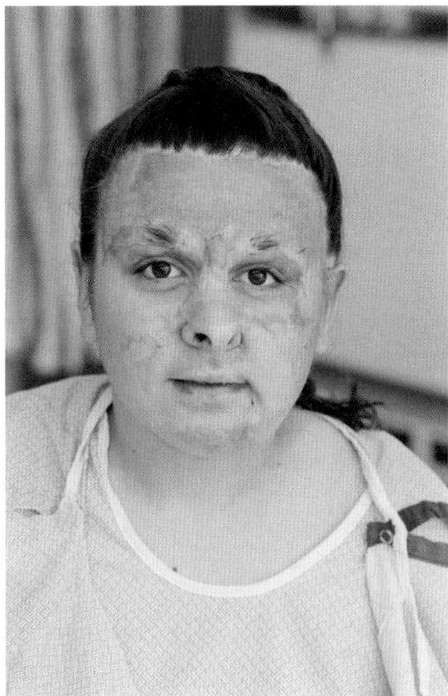

FIGURE 23.24 Extensive grafting to the face.

Physical therapy will usually be initiated in the critical care setting and will continue long after hospital discharge, sometimes throughout life. Positioning, exercise, and range of motion are necessary to maintain joint flexibility.

Nurses play a key role in smoothing the transition from the acute care phase of life-saving interventions and frequent dressing changes to normal activities such as school and play. Body image considerations may have a significant impact on the child when they return to school and should be addressed. Children with altered body image as a result of a burn might benefit from regular counseling and group therapy. Parents often need assistance with the behavioral challenges of caring for a child who is recovering from a burn injury. Various websites are available for support of people who are burned.

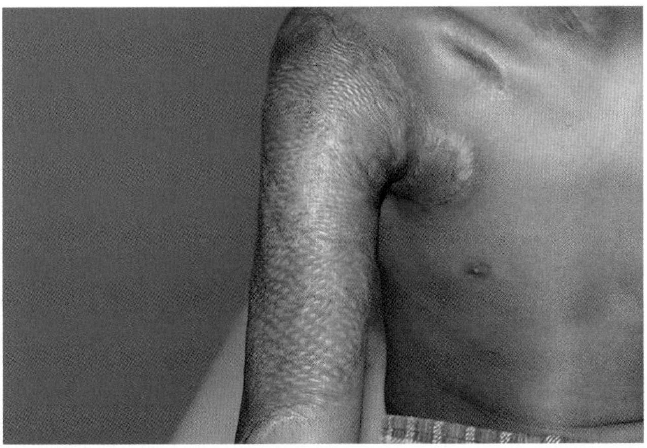

FIGURE 23.23 Healed mesh graft.

Navigating through life after suffering a serious burn injury can be difficult for the child and family, and a skilled nurse can provide valuable assistance to families during the equally important, but less acute, phase of the journey.

PREVENTING BURNS AND CARBON MONOXIDE POISONING

Instruct parents about prevention of burns. Explain that all homes should have working smoke detectors and that batteries should be changed yearly. Instruct families that all homes should be equipped with fire extinguishers and that adults and older teenagers should be taught how to operate them. Explain that children should sleep in fire-retardant sleepwear, parents should not smoke in the house or the car, and parents should keep lighters and matches out of children's reach. Young children are particularly susceptible to burns that occur in the kitchen, such as scalds from hot liquids and foods and burns from contact with hot burners or oven doors. Caution parents about the extreme danger that fireworks present to children. Teaching Guidelines 23.3 gives additional information for parents related to burn prevention. The booklet "Burn Prevention Tips," which includes a coloring book, is available from the Shriners Hospitals for Children.

Children are at significant risk for burns related to hot water. Scald burns can occur when hot water comes into contact with the child's skin, even for a relatively short time. Since hot water presents such a serious risk to children, the temperature on all hot water heaters should be 49°C (120°F) or lower. Figure 23.25 is a graph that

TEACHING GUIDELINES 23.3 Burn Prevention

- Keep hot water heater temperature lower than 49°C (120°F).
- Test bath water temperature before bathing children.
- Keep children away from open flames, stoves, and candles.
- Cook with pots on the inside of the stove with the handles turned in.
- Keep children away from the stove while cooking.
- Place hot liquids out of reach of children.
- Avoid drinking hot beverages while holding a child.
- Keep curling irons out of reach of children.
- Teach older children how to safely get out of the house in case of fire.
- Practice fire drills.
- Teach children to "stop, drop, and roll" if their clothes catch fire.

shows how long a child can be exposed to water of various temperatures before a burn occurs. For example:

- If the water is 66°C (150°F), a child can receive a third-degree burn within 2 seconds.
- If the water is 60°C (140°F), it takes 6 seconds of exposure to cause a significant burn.
- If the water is 54°C (130°F), a child can be burned significantly in only 30 seconds.
- At 49°C (120°F), the recommended maximal home hot water heater temperature, it takes as long as 5 minutes of exposure to burn a person (plenty of time to get out of the tub!) (Accurate Building Inspectors, 2024).

Instruct parents about prevention of carbon monoxide poisoning. All homes should have working carbon monoxide detectors, and batteries should be changed yearly. Teach parents the signs of carbon monoxide poisoning: headaches, dizziness, disorientation, and nausea. If the carbon monoxide detector sounds, turn off any potential sources of combustion, if possible, and evacuate all occupants immediately. Do not attempt to reenter the home until a qualified professional repairs the source of the carbon monoxide leak.

PROVIDING BURN CARE AT HOME

Teach parents about proper burn care in the home. Seek medical attention for burns when:

- The child has a second- or third-degree burn.
- Burns result from a fire, an electrical wire or socket, or chemicals.
- The child has a burn on the face, scalp, hands, feet, or genitals or over the joints.
- The burn appears to be infected.
- The burn is causing prolonged and significant pain.
- Concern exists that the burn was a result of abuse.

If the burn is extensive, even if it appears to be a first-degree burn, seek medical attention immediately. Teaching Guidelines 23.4 gives specific information about burn care at home.

Sunburn

Sunburn occurs as a result of overexposure to the UV rays of the sun. The erythema and eventual blisters occur

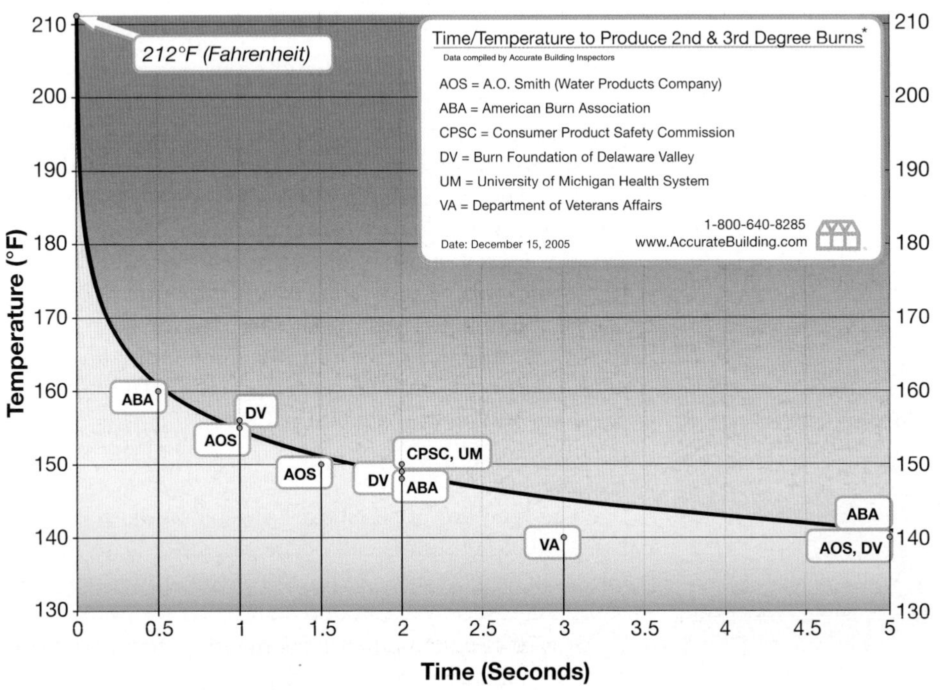

FIGURE 23.25 Length of hot water exposure that results in significant burns based on water temperature. (Used with permission from Accurate Building Inspectors. [2024]. *Water temperature thermometry.* http://www.accuratebuilding.com/services/legal/charts/hot_water_burn_scalding_graph.html)

TEACHING GUIDELINES 23.4 Providing Burn Care at Home

For First-Degree (Superficial) Burns

- Run cool water over the burned area until the pain lessens.
- Do not apply ice to the skin.
- Do not apply butter, ointment, or cream.
- Cover the burn lightly with a clean, nonadhesive bandage.
- Administer acetaminophen or ibuprofen for pain.
- Have the child seen by the health care provider or nurse practitioner within 24 hours.
- Ongoing care: clean in tub or shower with fragrance-free mild soap; pat or air dry.
  - Apply a thin layer of antibiotic ointment.
  - Cover with a nonadherent dressing such as Adaptic, and then cover with dry gauze.

For More Extensive Burns

- Remove clothing only if it comes off easily or if it is still smoldering.
- Check the child's ABCs (airway, breathing, and circulation) and perform cardiopulmonary resuscitation (CPR) if necessary.
- Do not apply butter, ointment, or any other type of cream.
- Cover the burn with a clean, lint-free bandage or sheet.
- Avoid applying large, wet sheets, as this can cause the child to become too cold.
- Do not attempt to break any blisters.
- If the child appears to be in shock, elevate the legs while protecting the burn and call 911.

as a result of the skin's blood flow changes as well as alterations in cell kinetics and pigment products in response to UV exposures. Erythema may occur within 4 hours and blisters within 6 hours. Sunburn is usually treated with cool compresses, cooling lotions, and oral nonsteroidal antiinflammatory agents (Pitone, 2023).

Nursing Assessment

Obtain the health history, noting recent sun exposure. Determine length of exposure and whether any type of sunscreen or sun block product was used. Note redness of the skin on the exposed areas. More severe areas will have a darker red, slightly purple hue. Blisters may be noted with more severe sunburn.

Nursing Management

Cool compresses may help to cool the burn. Aloe vera gel applied topically may provide significant soothing. Rarely are adverse effects reported with the use of aloe vera gel. Administer a nonsteroidal antiinflammatory such as ibuprofen. Discourage hot showers or baths. Instruct the child to wear loose clothing and to ensure that burned areas are covered when going outside (until they are healed). If skin flaking occurs, discourage the child from "peeling" the flaked skin in order to prevent further injury. Refer to Chapter 9 for further information about safe sun exposure.

Cold Injury

The term "frostbite" implies freezing of the tissues. It is described on a continuum from first to fourth degree. When a child is exposed to an extremely cold environment, changes in cutaneous circulation help to maintain the core body temperature. Because circulation is shunted to the core, the most peripheral body parts are those at highest risk for frostbite. Local damage occurs when the tissue temperature drops to 32°F (0°C). Initially, skin sensation is lost, the vasculature constricts, and plasma leakage occurs. Ice crystals develop in the extracellular fluid, and eventually, vascular stasis leads to endothelial cell damage, necrosis, and sloughing of dead tissue (Peters & Buchel, 2023).

Nursing Assessment

Note history of cold exposure. Inquire about pain or numbness. Examine the skin for indications of frostbite. First-degree frostbite results in superficial white plaques with surrounding erythema. Second-degree frostbite demonstrates blistering with erythema and edema. In third-degree frostbite, hemorrhagic blisters occur, progressing to tissue necrosis and sloughing in fourth-degree frostbite.

Nursing Management

Remove wet or tight clothing. Avoid vigorous massage to decrease the chance of damaging the skin further. Immerse the affected part in 40°C (104°F) water for 15 to 30 minutes. Thawing may cause significant pain, so administer analgesics. Keep the thawed part loosely covered, warm, and dry. Splinting may be used to help decrease associated edema. Consult the wound care specialist or plastic surgeon for further management.

Prevent frostbite by:

- Dressing warmly in layers and keeping warm and dry
- Avoiding exertion
- Not playing outside when wind chill advisories are in effect, and locking doors with high locks to prevent toddlers from going outside

Human and Animal Bites

Yearly, significant emergency room visits occur as a result of bites from mammals. In children, dog bites account for the majority of injuries, but human and cat bites account for the most infected bites (Hunstad, 2020). The hand and face are common locations for animal bites. A dog is most often provoked to bite a child when the child is playing with the dog or when the child hits, kicks, hugs, grabs, or chases the dog.

Therapeutic management involves cleansing and irrigating the wound, wound suturing or stapling if necessary, and administering topical and/or systemic antibiotic therapy. Rabies prophylaxis is indicated if the rabies status of the dog is unknown. Secondary bacterial infection of the bite wound with streptococci, staphylococci, or *Pasteurella multocida* may occur.

Nursing Assessment

Determine the history of the attack and whether it was provoked. Determine the child's tetanus vaccination status. Inspect the bite to determine the extent of laceration, avulsion, or crushing injury.

Nursing Management

Provide rabies immunoprophylaxis and a tetanus booster vaccination if indicated. Thoroughly cleanse the wound with soap and water or a povidone–iodine solution. Irrigate the wound well with normal saline after cleansing. If the animal may be rabid, cleanse the wound for at least 10 minutes with a virucidal agent such as povidone–iodine solution. Administer antibiotics as prescribed. Help children who have been bitten by talking about the incident or reading books about this type of event.

Prevention of animal bites is important. Teach children the following:

- Never provoke a dog with teasing or roughhousing.
- Get adult permission before interacting with a dog, cat, or other animal that is not your pet.
- Do not bother an eating, sleeping, or nursing dog.
- Avoid high-pitched talking or screaming around dogs.
- Display a closed fist first for the dog to sniff.
- Keep ferrets away from the face.
- If a cat hisses or lashes out with the paw, leave it alone.

Never leave a child younger than 5 years of age alone with a dog (American Veterinary Medical Association, 2023). Contact the local humane society for a dog bite prevention program that is appropriate for school-age children.

Insect Stings and Spider Bites

Members of the *Hymenoptera* class of insects sting. This class includes bees, wasps, imported fire ants, and yellow jackets. Other insects, such as mosquitos and fleas, bite. Spiders inject their venom when they bite. Stings and bites usually result in a local reaction. A systemic or anaphylactic reaction to a *Hymenoptera* sting may also occur, possibly resulting in airway compromise (refer to Chapter 29 for additional information on anaphylaxis). Serious reactions may occur with brown recluse or black widow spider bites. This discussion will focus on local reactions (Goddard & Steward, 2023).

Local reactions to insect stings and spider bites include pruritus, pain, and edema. A hypersensitivity reaction thought to be mediated by IgE occurs in response to the venom. This may be a physiologic response to the antigens present in the insect's or spider's saliva and other fluids that are transmitted during stinging or biting. Bacterial superinfection may occur as a complication and as a result of scratching. Therapeutic management includes antihistamines to decrease itching and in some cases corticosteroids to decrease inflammation and swelling (Freeman, 2024).

Nursing Assessment

Obtain the history of the bite or sting. Children are usually acutely aware when they have been stung by an insect, but spiders are generally not observed before the bite. Inspect the bite or sting, noting an urticarial wheal or papular reaction. A large local reaction may be mistaken for cellulitis. Note whether a stinger remains present. Assess the child's work of breathing to determine if a systemic reaction or anaphylaxis is occurring (refer to Chapter 29).

Nursing Management

Remove jewelry or constrictive clothing if the sting is on an extremity. Cleanse the wound with mild soap and water. If the stinger is present, scrape it away with your fingernail or a credit card. Apply ice intermittently to decrease pain and edema. Administer diphenhydramine as soon as possible after the sting in an attempt to minimize the reaction.

Prevent insect stings and spider bites by wearing protective clothing and shoes when outdoors. Use insect repellants (with a maximum concentration of 30% *N,N*-diethyl-meta-toluamide [DEET] in infants and children older than 2 months) (American Academy of Pediatrics, 2021). Teach children never to disturb a bee or wasp nest or an anthill.

KEY CONCEPTS

- The infant's epidermis is thinner, loses heat more readily, absorbs substances more easily, and is more accessible to bacterial invasion than the skin of the adult. The increased water content of the infant's skin compared with the adult's places the infant at increased risk of blister development and other skin alterations.
- The child's skin thickness and characteristics reach adult levels in the late teenage years.

- Children with dark skin tend to have more pronounced cutaneous reactions than children with lighter skin.
- Sebum production increases in the preadolescent and adolescent years, contributing to the development of acne at that time.
- Most bacterial skin infections are caused by *S. aureus* and group A beta-hemolytic streptococcus.
- Skin scrapings placed on a slide and prepared with potassium chloride may be evaluated microscopically to determine the presence of fungus.
- Fungal skin infections, referred to collectively as tinea, may require up to several weeks of treatment.
- Contact dermatitis and AD both present as pruritic rashes, whereas psoriasis is generally nonpruritic.
- Hypersensitivity responses may result in erythema multiforme or urticaria.
- Scaling may occur with AD and psoriasis, whereas honey-colored crusting is common with impetigo. Erythema is a common finding with many skin disorders in children.
- Burns may result in significant weeping and fluid loss.
- Keeping the skin well moisturized is a key intervention in the management of AD and psoriasis.
- Appropriate hygiene is of particular importance in integumentary disorders.
- Pain management, prevention of infection, and rehabilitation are the focus of nursing management for the burned child.
- The constant itch–rash–itch cycle of AD may have a considerable impact on the child's sleep, school functioning, and self-esteem.
- Acne vulgaris, particularly if moderate or severe, may have a significant negative effect on the adolescent's self-esteem.
- Teach children with chronic disorders such as AD, psoriasis, and acne (and their parents) to cleanse and moisturize the skin properly, avoid particular skin irritants, and use medications appropriately.
- Many skin disorders are preventable. Teach families how to prevent contact dermatitis, burns, sunburn, frostbite, and bites and stings.
- Educate children and families about the importance of good soap-and-water cleansing of all minor skin injuries.

REFERENCES AND RECOMMENDED READINGS

Accurate Building Inspectors. (2024). *Water temperature thermometry. Ubell Enterprises*. http://www.accuratebuilding.com/services/legal/charts/hot_water_burn_scalding_graph.html

Ahmadpour, N., Randall, H., Choksi, H., Gao, A., Vaughan, C., & Poronnik, P. (2019). Virtual reality interventions for acute and chronic pain management. *The International Journal of Biochemistry & Cell Biology, 114*, 105568. https://doi.org/10.1016/j.biocel.2019.105568

American Academy of Pediatrics. (2021). *American Academy of Pediatrics: Get kids outdoors and use these safety tips to ward off insects and prevent sunburn*. https://www.aap.org/en/news-room/news-releases/health--safety-tips/american-academy-of-pediatrics-get-kids-outdoors-and-use-these-safety-tips-to-ward-off-insects-and-prevent-sunburn/

American Veterinary Medical Association. (2023). *Dog bite prevention*. https://www.avma.org/public/Pages/Dog-Bite-Prevention.aspx

Antoon, A. Y. (2020). Chapter 92: Burn injuries. In R. M. Kliegman, J. W. St Geme, N. J. Blum, S. S. Shah, R. C. Tasker, & K. M. Wilson (Eds.), *Nelson textbook of pediatrics* (21st ed.). Elsevier.

Armstrong, C. A. (2023). Approach to the clinical dermatologic diagnosis. *UpToDate*. Retrieved April 12, 2024, from https://www.uptodate.com/contents/approach-to-the-clinical-dermatologic-diagnosis

Baddour, L. M. (2022). Impetigo. *UpToDate*. Retrieved April 12, 2024, from http://www.uptodate.com/contents/impetigo

Bender, N. R., & Chiu, Y. E. (2020). Chapter 676.1: Psoriasis. In R. M. Kliegman, J. W. St Geme, N. J. Blum, S. S. Shah, R. C. Tasker, & K. M. Wilson (Eds.), *Nelson textbook of pediatrics* (21st ed.). Elsevier.

Corbett, J. A., & Banks, A. D. (2019). *Laboratory tests and diagnostic procedures with nursing diagnoses* (9th ed.). Pearson Education Inc.

Covar, R. A., Fleisher, D. M., Cho, C., & Boguniewicz, M. (2022). Chapter 38: Allergic disorders. In M. Bunik, W. W. Hay, M. J. Levin, & M. J. Abzug (Eds.), *Current diagnosis & treatment: Pediatrics* (26th ed.). McGraw-Hill Education.

Ford, C. R., Chiesa, A., & Sirotnak, A. P. (2022). Chapter 8: Child abuse & neglect. In M. Bunik, W. W. Hay, M. J. Levin, & M. J. Abzug (Eds.), *Current diagnosis & treatment: Pediatrics* (26th ed.). McGraw-Hill Education.

Freeman, T. (2024). Bee, yellow jacket, wasp, and other Hymenoptera stings: Reaction types and acute management. *UpToDate*. Retrieved April 12, 2024, from https://www.uptodate.com/contents/bee-yellow-jacket-wasp-and-other-hymenoptera-stings-reaction-types-and-acute-management

Giddens, J. F. (2021). *Concepts for nursing practice* (3rd ed.). Elsevier.

Goddard, J., & Stewart, P. H. (2023). Insect and other arthropod bites. *UpToDate*. Retrieved April 12, 2024, from https://www.uptodate.com/contents/insect-and-other-arthropod-bites

Hagan, J. F., Shaw, J. S., & Duncan, P. M. (Eds.). (2017). *Bright futures: Guidelines for health supervision of infants, children, and adolescents* (4th ed.). American Academy of Pediatrics.

Heath, C. R., Mazza, J. M., & Silverberg, N. B. (2016). Chapter 84: Pediatrics. In A. P. Kelly, S. C. Taylor, H. W. Lim, & A. M. A. Serrano (Eds.), *Taylor and Kelly's dermatology for skin of color* (2nd ed.). McGraw-Hill Education.

Howe, W. (2023). Atopic dermatitis (eczema): Pathogenesis, clinical manifestations, and diagnosis. *UpToDate*. Retrieved April 12, 2024, from https://www.uptodate.com/contents/atopic-dermatitis-eczema-pathogenesis-clinical-manifestations-and-diagnosis

Hunstad, D. A. (2020). Chapter 743: Animal and human bites. In R. M. Kliegman, J. W. St Geme, N. J. Blum, S. S. Shah, R. C. Tasker, & K. M. Wilson (Eds.), *Nelson textbook of pediatrics* (21st ed.). Elsevier.

iPledge. (2021). *iPledge: Committed to pregnancy prevention*. https://www.ipledgeprogram.com/iPledgeUI/home.u

Joffe, M. D. (2023). Moderate and severe thermal burns in children: Emergency management. *UpToDate*. Retrieved April 12, 2024, from http://www.uptodate.com/contents/emergency-care-of-moderate-and-severe-thermal-burns-in-children

Kim, W. E. (2020). Chapter 689: Acne. In R. M. Kliegman, J. W. St Geme, N. J. Blum, S. S. Shah, R. C. Tasker, & K. M. Wilson (Eds.), *Nelson textbook of pediatrics* (21st ed.). Elsevier.

Lee, H. Y. (2024). Stevens-Johnson syndrome and toxic epidermal necrolysis: Pathogenesis, clinical manifestations, and diagnosis. *UpToDate*. Retrieved April 12, 2024, from http://www.uptodate.com/contents/stevens-johnson-syndrome-and-toxic-epidermal-necrolysis-pathogenesis-clinical-manifestations-and-diagnosis

Leon-Villapalos, J., & Dziewulski, P. (2022). *Skin autografting. UpToDate*. Retrieved April 12, 2024, from https://www.uptodate.com/contents/skin-autografting

McMahon, P. (2022). Staphylococcal scalded skin syndrome. *UpToDate*. Retrieved April 12, 2024, from https://www.uptodate.com/contents/staphylococcal-scalded-skin-syndrome

Mechem, C. C. (2024). Pulse oximetry. *UpToDate*. Retrieved April 12, 2024, from https://www.uptodate.com/contents/pulse-oximetry

Musters, A. H., Mashayekhi, S., Harvey, J., Axon, E., Lax, S. J., Flohr, C., Drucker, A. M, Gerbens, L., Ferguson, J., Ibbotson, S., Dawe, R. S., Garritsen, F., Brouwer, M., Limpens, J., Prescott, L. E., Boyle, R. J., & Spuls, P. I. (2021). Phototherapy for atopic eczema. *Cochrane Database of Systematic Reviews. 2021*(11). https://doi.org/10.1002/14651858.CD013870.pub2

Peters, B., & Buchel, E. W. (2023). *Cold injuries. Medscape*. https://emedicine.medscape.com/article/1278523-overview

Pitone, M. L. (2023). *How to handle sunburn*. https://kidshealth.org/en/parents/sunburn-sheet.html

Prok, L. D., & Torres-Zegarra, C. X. (2022). Chapter 15: Skin. In M. Bunik, W. W. Hay, M. J. Levin, & M. J. Abzug (Eds.), *Current diagnosis & treatment: Pediatrics* (26th ed.). McGraw-Hill Education.

Sangha, A. M. (2021). Dermatological conditions in skin of color: Managing atopic dermatitis. *Journal of Clinical and Aesthetic Dermatology*, *14*(3 Suppl. 1), S20–S22.

Sasseville, D. (2023). Cradle cap and seborrheic dermatitis in infants. *UpToDate*. Retrieved April 12, 2024, from http://www.uptodate.com/contents/cradle-cap-and-seborrheic-dermatitis-in-infants

Teichgräber, F., Jacob, L., Koyanagi, A., Shin, J. I., Seiringer, P., & Kostev, K. (2021). Association between skin disorders and depression in children and adolescents: A retrospective case-control study. *Journal of Affective Disorders*, *282*, 939–944. https://doi.org/10.1016/j.jad.2021.01.002

Tenenhaus, M., & Rennekampff, H.-O. (2023). *Topical agents and dressings for local burn wound care. UpToDate*. Retrieved April 12, 2024, from https://www.uptodate.com/contents/topical-agents-and-dressings-for-local-burn-wound-care

UpToDate, Inc. (2024). *UpToDate® Lexidrug™* (Version 8.2.0) [Mobile app]. Wolters Kluwer. https://apps.apple.com/us/app/lexicomp/id313401238

Woolard, A., Hill, N. T. M., McQueen, M., Martin, L., Milroy, H., Wood, F. M., Bullman, I., & Lin, A. (2021). The psychological impact of paediatric burn injuries: A systematic review. *BMC Public Health*, *21*(2281). https://doi.org/10.1186/s12889-021-12296-1

DEVELOPING CLINICAL JUDGMENT

PRACTICING FOR NCLEX

1. The nurse is teaching about skin care for AD. Which statement by the parent indicates that further teaching may be necessary?
   a. "I will use Vaseline or Crisco to moisturize my child's skin."
   b. "A hot bath will soothe my child's itching when it is severe."
   c. "I will buy cotton rather than wool or synthetic clothing for my child."
   d. "I will apply a small amount of the prescribed cream after the bath."
2. The nurse is caring for a child who has received significant partial-thickness burns to the lower body. What is the priority assessment in the first 24 hours after injury?
   a. Fluid balance
   b. Wound infection
   c. Respiratory arrest
   d. Separation anxiety
3. The nurse is caring for a child in the emergency department who was bitten by the family dog, who is fully immunized. What is the priority nursing action?
   a. Administer rabies immunoglobulin.
   b. Refer the child to a counselor.
   c. Assess the depth and extent of the wound.
   d. Administer a tetanus booster.
4. The nurse is caring for an infant on the pediatric unit who has a very red rash in the diaper area, with red lesions scattered on the abdomen and thighs. What is the priority nursing intervention?
   a. Administer griseofulvin with a fatty meal.
   b. Institute contact isolation precautions.
   c. Apply topical antibiotic cream.
   d. Apply topical antifungal cream.
5. A varsity high school wrestler presents with a "rug burn" type of rash on their shoulder that is not healing as expected, despite use of triple antibiotic cream. Two other wrestlers on the team have a similar abrasion. What infection should the nurse be most concerned about, based on the history?
   a. Tinea cruris
   b. Methicillin-resistant *Staphylococcus aureus* (MRSA)
   c. Impetigo
   d. Tinea versicolor
6. The nurse has taught the parent of a child with AD how to bathe the child. Which statement by the parent indicates the education was effective?
   a. "I should let my child play in the tub for 40 minutes every night."
   b. "I will be sure to use a moisturizing bubble bath."
   c. "When my child gets out of the tub, I will just pat the skin dry."
   d. "It is important that my child has a bath every night."
7. The nurse is teaching an adolescent about interventions to improve facial acne. What should the nurse include when educating the patient?
   a. Wash the face twice a day with mild soap and water.
   b. Remove whiteheads and blackheads after each face washing.
   c. Apply vitamin E ointment twice daily to each lesion.
   d. Expose the face to the sun after applying tretinoin in the morning.

DOSAGE CALCULATION QUESTION

The nurse is caring for a child who has tinea corporis. The child weighs 18 lb 11 oz. The medication order reads: griseofulvin 85 mg PO every day. Griseofulvin is supplied as 125 mg/5 mL. How many milliliters will the nurse administer? Round to the nearest tenth.

CRITICAL THINKING EXERCISES

1. A 4-year-old presents with their parent for evaluation of a yellowish, runny sore on the head. What questions would be most appropriate to ask the parent when taking the history? Should this child be placed in isolation? If so, why?
2. An 11-month-old comes to the primary care office with the parent for evaluation of a significant flaking red rash on both cheeks. The child is diagnosed with AD. What additional information should be obtained in the health history? What information should be included in the teaching plan for this family?

STUDY ACTIVITIES

1. Plan an educational activity:
   a. For parents of babies about the treatment and prevention of diaper dermatitis
   b. For parents of school-age children about prevention of contact dermatitis (related to poison ivy)
2. During your clinical rotation, spend a day with the wound and ostomy care nurse in a children's hospital. Report to the clinical group about what you learned that day.
3. Talk to adolescents with severe acne, AD, or psoriasis about their feelings about their skin's appearance. Reflect on this information in your clinical journal.

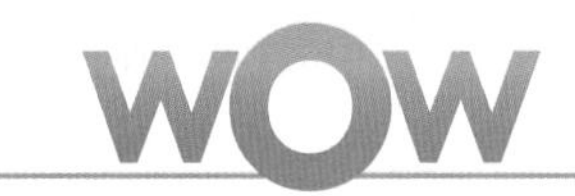

WORDS OF WISDOM

Be inspired by the courage of a child with cancer and reflect it in the care you provide.

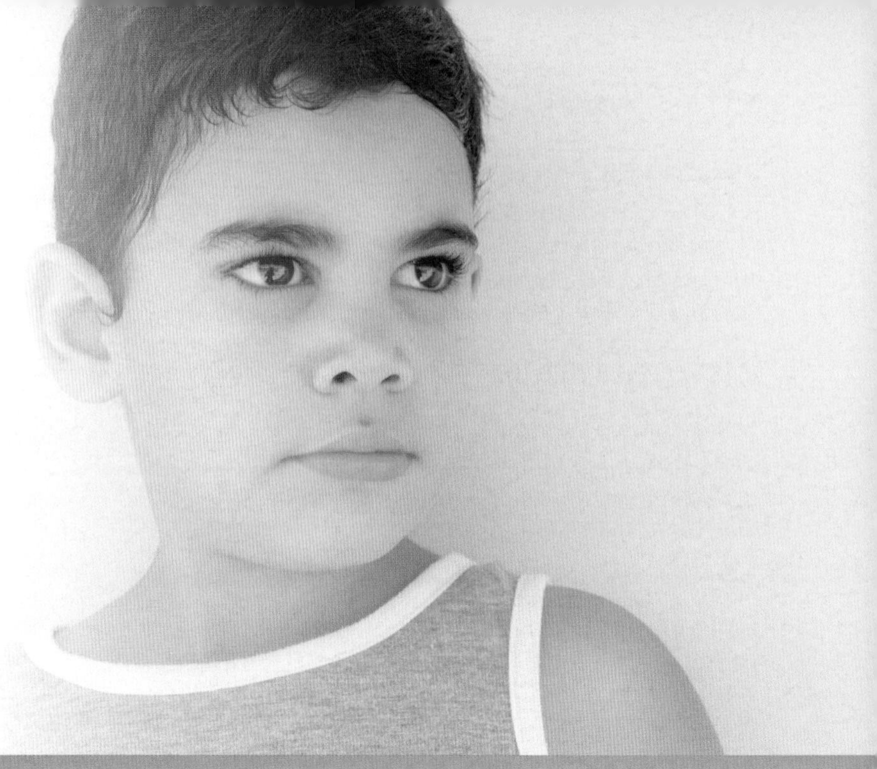

24

Nursing Care of the Child With an Alteration in Cellular Regulation/ Hematologic or Neoplastic Disorder

KEY TERMS

anisocytosis (an-ī´sō-sī-tō´sis)

chelation therapy (kē-lā´shŭn thār´ă-pē)

clinical trial

extravasation (eks-trav´ă-sā´shŭn)

hematocrit

hemoglobin

hemosiderosis (hē´mō-sid-ĕr-ō´sis)

hypochromic

macrocytic

malignant

metastasis (mĕ-tas´tă-sis)

microcytic

neoplastic

platelet count

poikilocytosis (poy´ki-lō-sī-tō´sis)

polycythemia

splenomegaly

staging

LEARNING OBJECTIVES

Upon completion of the chapter, you will be able to:

1. Identify major hematologic disorders that affect children.
2. Compare childhood and adult cancers.
3. Identify types of cancer common in infants, children, and adolescents.
4. Determine priority assessment information for children with alterations in cellular regulation/hematologic and neoplastic disorders.
5. Analyze laboratory data and describe nursing care related to common laboratory and diagnostic testing used in alterations in cellular regulation/hematologic and neoplastic disorders.
6. Develop an individualized nursing care plan or concept map for the child with cancer or a hematologic disorder.
7. Identify priority interventions for children with alterations in cellular regulation.
8. Develop a teaching plan for the family of children with hematologic disorders or cancer.
9. Devise a nutrition plan for the child with cancer.
10. Describe the psychosocial impact of cancer on children and their families.
11. Identify resources for children and families with hematologic disorders, or cancer.

Shaun O'Malley, 10 months old, is being admitted to the pediatric unit after being brought to the clinic by his parent for a small laceration that he thought needed stitches. His parent states, "I didn't think the cut was very deep. I was surprised by how long it bled."

INTRODUCTION

Cellular regulation is the process by which cells replicate, proliferate, and grow. The hematologic system is integrally involved in the process of cellular regulation. The hematologic system consists of the blood and blood-forming tissues of the body. These typically function together in a balance that affects the metabolism of the body. The three categories of cells are erythrocytes, or red blood cells (RBCs); thrombocytes, or platelets; and leukocytes, or white blood cells (WBCs). RBCs are responsible for transporting nutrients and oxygen to the body tissues and waste products from the tissues. The platelets are responsible for clotting. WBCs are responsible for fighting infection. WBCs are further divided into granulocytes (neutrophils, eosinophils, and basophils) and agranulocytes (lymphocytes and monocytes).

All blood cells originate from a single type of cell called a multipotent stem cell, which goes on to differentiate into the various types of blood cells. Thrombopoietin (TPO) and interleukin-7 (IL-7) act on the cell and differentiate the cell into either myeloid or lymphoid progenitor cells. The lymphoid cells either, under the influence of IL-6, become B lymphocytes or change directly into T lymphocytes. The myeloid cells are differentiated by the action of either erythropoietin (EPO) or granulocyte–monocyte colony-stimulating factor (GM-CSF). When the cell is acted upon by EPO, which is produced by the kidneys, the cell becomes the megakaryocyte, also known as the erythroid progenitor cell. The megakaryocyte is acted on by either EPO, to become the RBC, or TPO and IL-11, to become a megakaryocyte that goes on to form platelets. GM-CSF influences the cell to become the granulocyte, also known as the macrophage progenitor cell. These cells further differentiate under various influences to become the WBCs (Fig. 24.1).

Certain conditions may cause problems to develop within this system, resulting in an alteration in blood cellular regulation. These problems are related to either the production of the blood cells (too much or too little) or loss and destruction of these cells. Many factors are involved in the development of hematologic disorders, ranging from genetic causes to disorders resulting from injury, infection, or nutritional deficit.

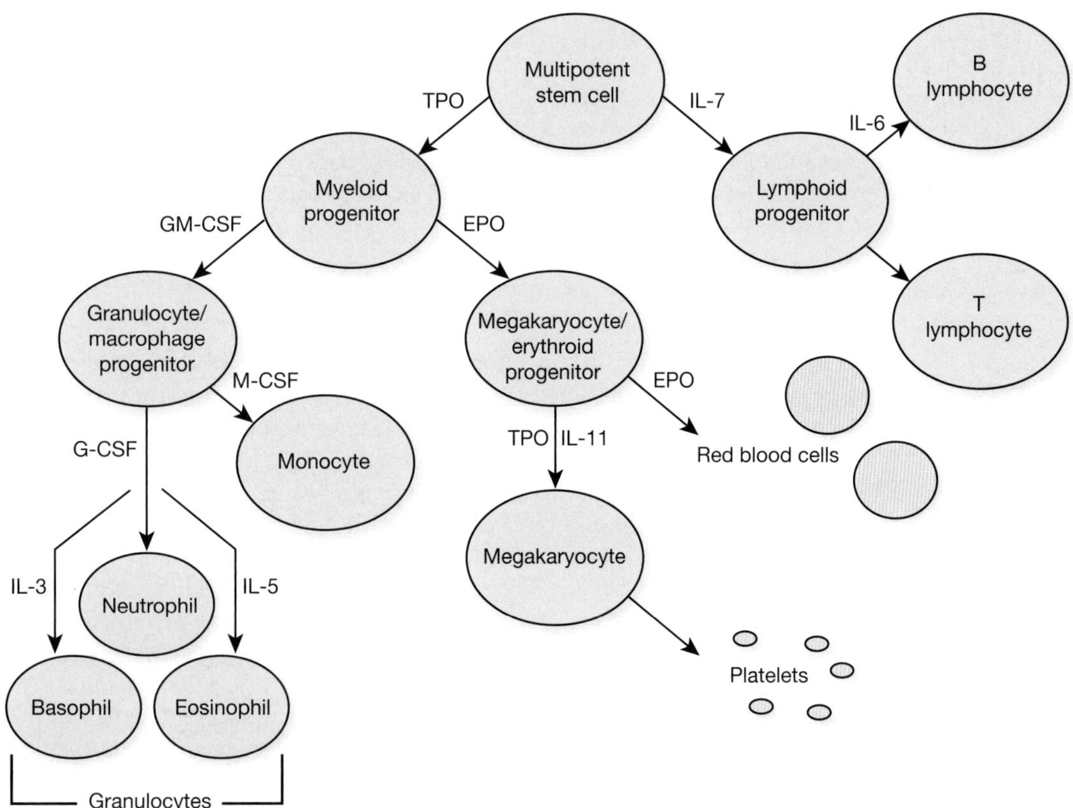

FIGURE 24.1 Process of blood cell formation. EPO, erythropoietin; GM-CSF, granulocyte–monocyte colony-stimulating factor; IL, interleukin; TPO, thrombopoietin.

Neoplastic (referring to cells that abnormally proliferate) disorders are also alterations in cellular regulation. Cancer results from an alteration in cellular regulation resulting in out-of-control cell growth. Cancer accounts for the most deaths from disease in children older than 1 year of age. Cure has been achieved in some children with childhood leukemia and other cancers, but there is no universal long-term cure available for any of the childhood cancers. However, the 5-year survival rate for all cancers in children is 85% (American Cancer Society [ACS], 2024a).

Cancer is a life-threatening illness that involves emotional distress, fear of the unknown, and changes in life priorities for the child and family. Initial and ongoing diagnostic testing and the adverse effects of treatment for cancer, including chemotherapy, radiation, surgery, or other treatments, are often painful as well. Management of cancer also has a significant psychosocial impact on the child or adolescent. Children with cancer are at risk for distress because they have a life-threatening illness and must undergo frequent and stressful tests and treatments (National Cancer Institute [NCI], 2023). In addition, the child often feels isolated from their peers, and the adolescent may have difficulty achieving independence, which is the core developmental task of the adolescent years. Children and adolescents with cancer often demonstrate poorer school performance compared to healthy peers.

Nursing care for the child with a hematologic disorder is often multifaceted. A child who has iron-deficiency anemia requires adequate oxygenation and may require packed red blood cells (PRBCs); a child with hemophilia requires factor replacement and monitoring for safety. Nursing care for the child with cancer is also complex. Nurses caring for children with cellular regulation alterations such as cancer and hematologic disorders need to be not only knowledgeable about the medical treatment of the disease (including adverse effects) but also able to effectively intervene with these children. Nurses need to be particularly aware of the psychosocial and emotional impact of cancer or a chronic hematologic disorder on the child and family.

VARIATIONS IN PEDIATRIC ANATOMY AND PHYSIOLOGY

In the absence of a congenital defect, the hematologic system is intact and functional at birth. RBC and hemoglobin production as well as iron stores undergo changes in the first few months of life; thereafter, hematologic function is stable.

RBC Production

The production of blood cells in the embryo begins by 8 weeks' gestation. In the embryo, blood cells form primarily in the liver; this continues until a few weeks before delivery. Some cell production, lymphoid cells, in particular, takes place in the spleen of the embryo, and the thymus is a site for some transient lymphocyte production. EPO, the hormone that regulates RBC production, is derived primarily from the liver in the fetus, and after birth, the kidneys take over this production.

Hemoglobin

Three types of normal hemoglobin (Hgb) are present at any given time in the blood: Hgb A, Hgb F or fetal hemoglobin, and Hgb A_2. After 6 months of age, Hgb A is the predominant type. In the neonatal period, the largest difference is with the RBCs. Fetal hemoglobin, which has a much shorter cell life, is present in higher quantities, putting the infant at risk for anemia and leading to problems with the oxygen-carrying capacity of the blood. As the production of the cells transfers from the liver to the bone marrow of the long and flat bones, the balance between oxygenation and production is affected.

Iron

The fetus receives iron through the placenta from the pregnant parent. The preterm infant misses out on the final weeks or months of transplacental iron transfer, putting them at increased risk for anemia (Cunningham et al., 2022). In the term infant, a period of physiologic anemia occurs between the ages of 2 and 6 months. This is because the infant demonstrates rapid growth and an increase in blood volume over the first several months of life, and maternally derived iron stores are depleted by 4 to 6 months of age. Sufficient iron intake is critical for the appropriate development of hemoglobin and RBCs. Therefore, the infant must ingest adequate quantities of iron either from breast milk or from iron-fortified formula in early infancy and other food sources in later infancy. Adolescence is also a time of rapid growth, and intake of iron must increase.

CHILDHOOD CANCER VERSUS ADULT CANCER

Cancers in children differ greatly from those in adults. Pediatric cancers most often arise from primitive embryonal (mesodermal) and neuroectodermal tissues, resulting in leukemias, lymphomas, sarcomas, or central nervous system (CNS) tumors (ACS, 2024a). This is in direct contrast to adult cancers, which arise mostly from epithelial cells, resulting in carcinomas. The most common childhood cancers, in order of frequency, are leukemia, CNS tumors, lymphoma, neuroblastoma, rhabdomyosarcoma, Wilms tumor, bone tumors, and retinoblastoma. Comparison Chart 24.1 explains how cancer is different in children versus adults.

In children, warning signs of cancer are most often related to changes in blood cell production or as a result of compression, infiltration, or obstruction caused by the tumor. Changes in blood cell production may result in fatigue, pallor, frequent or severe infection, or easy bruising. Infiltration, obstruction, or compression by a tumor

COMPARISON CHART 24.1 Childhood Cancer Versus Adult Cancer

	Childhood Cancer	Adult Cancer
Cancer usually affects	Tissues	Organs
Histologic type	Embryonal, leukemia, lymphoma	Epithelial in origin
Most common sites	Blood, lymph, brain, bone, kidney, muscle	Breast, lung, prostate, bowel, bladder
Environmental and lifestyle factors	Only a small amount of environmental influence proven	Strong influence on cancer development
Cancer prevention	Little known	80% preventable
Detection	Usually incidental or accidental	Very early detection possible if screening recommendations followed
Latent period	Relatively short	Can be very long (20 years or greater)
Extent of disease	Metastasis often present at diagnosis	Metastasis less often present at diagnosis
Response to treatment	Very responsive	Less responsive

Data from American Cancer Society. (2024a). *Cancer in children.* https://www.cancer.org/cancer/cancer-in-children.html

may result in bone or abdominal pain, pain in other parts of the body, swelling, or unusual discharge.

COMMON MEDICAL TREATMENTS

Various medications as well as other medical treatments are used to treat hematologic and neoplastic disorders in children. Most of these treatments will require a health care provider's or nurse practitioner's order when the child is in the hospital. Deciding on a course of medical treatment for cancer in a developing child is complicated. Some of the treatments can impair the child's growth and development. Many pediatric oncologists and cancer treatment centers are active members of the Children's Oncology Group (COG), an NCI-supported group that approves and administers clinical trials devoted exclusively to childhood and adolescent cancer research. A **clinical trial** is a carefully designed research study that assesses the effectiveness of a treatment as well as its acute and long-term effects on the child. Current cancer care in children is a result of the knowledge gained through clinical trials. A clinical trial may include existing medications or treatments in combination with new drugs or may involve a different approach to sequencing or dosing of medications and treatment (NCI, 2023).

To provide optimal outcomes, the child with cancer should be treated at an institution with multidisciplinary cancer care specialists that can provide the most advanced care available. Each case of pediatric cancer should be considered individually, with the oncology health care team and the family reaching treatment decisions together, whether the treatment plan is standard or involves enrollment in a clinical trial.

In the child with cancer, particularly advanced disease, the decision to provide treatment ("let's do everything we can") or to withhold treatment in the event of an extremely poor prognosis is extraordinarily challenging in an ethical sense. A mature older child or adolescent may have a strong desire to continue or discontinue treatment, and sometimes this desire conflicts with the parents' desires or choices. The American Academy of Pediatrics (AAP) Committee on Bioethics recommends that decision making for older children and adolescents should include the assent of the older child or adolescent (Box 24.1).

Commonly, chemotherapy and radiation therapy are used to treat childhood cancers. In some instances, hematopoietic stem cell transplantation (HSCT) is used. The nurse caring for the child with a hematologic disorder or cancer should be familiar with the procedures used, how the treatments and medications work, and common nursing implications related to use of these modalities. The most common treatments and medications are listed in Common Medical Treatments 24.1 and Drug Guide 24.1.

BOX 24.1 Pediatric Assent

- Give consideration to each child's developmental capacity, rationality, and autonomy.
- Help each child to achieve a developmentally appropriate understanding of the illness.
- Tell the child what they can expect regarding testing procedures and treatments.
- Assess the child's understanding of the situation and how they are responding.
- Note if there is inappropriate pressure to assent to testing or treatment.
- Seriously solicit the child's expression of willingness to accept the proposed plan of care.

Data from Spriggs, M. (2023). Children and bioethics: Clarifying consent and assent in medical and research settings. *British Medical Bulletin, 145*(1), 110. https://doi.org/10.1093/bmb/ldac038

COMMON MEDICAL TREATMENTS 24.1

Treatment	Explanation	Indications	Nursing Implications
Blood product transfusion	Intravenous administration of whole blood, packed red blood cells (PRBCs), platelets, or plasma	PRBCs: severe anemia, thalassemia, sickle cell disease Whole blood: acute hemorrhage or trauma Fresh-frozen plasma: hemophilia Platelets: thrombocytopenia	Follow institution's transfusion protocol. Double check blood type and product label with a second nurse. Use only leukodepleted, CMV-negative blood products in the child with a hemoglobinopathy or cancer. Monitor vital signs and assess child frequently to detect adverse reaction to blood transfusion. If adverse reaction is suspected, immediately discontinue transfusion, run normal saline IV, reassess the child, and notify the health care provider. Some children require premedication with diphenhydramine and/or acetaminophen before receiving blood products.
Leukapheresis	Whole blood is removed from the body, the WBCs are extracted, and then the blood is retransfused into the child.	Hyperviscosity with leukemia (WBC >100,000)	Performed by specially trained personnel Monitor blood pressure and other vital signs.
Hematopoietic stem cell transplantation	Bone marrow transplant: transfer of healthy bone marrow into a child with disease; the transplanted cells can then develop into functional cells. Stem cell transplant: Peripheral stem cells are removed from the donor via apheresis, or stem cells are retrieved from the umbilical cord and placenta. The stem cells are then transplanted into the recipient.	Leukemia, lymphoma, other cancers, sickle cell disease, aplastic anemias, thalassemia	Maintain medical asepsis and protective isolation to prevent infection. Monitor closely for graft-versus-host disease. Provide meticulous oral care. Avoid taking rectal temperatures and inserting suppositories. Encourage appropriate nutrition. Administer immunosuppressive medications as ordered.
Supplemental oxygen	Administration of oxygen via mask, cannula, or blow-by	Hypoxia associated with sickle cell crisis or severe anemia	Frequently monitor work of breathing, oxygen saturation via pulse oximetry, cardiopulmonary status, and level of consciousness.
Biopsy	A small piece of the tumor is removed with a needle or via an open incision.	Solid tumors	Monitor for bleeding at the needle biopsy site. Provide routine incision care for open biopsy site.
Splenectomy	Surgical removal of the spleen	Life-threatening or recurrent splenic sequestration of sickle cell disease; thalassemia	Provide immunization against the following organisms, because they place the child at risk for overwhelming infection: *Streptococcus pneumoniae*, *Neisseria meningitidis*, and *Haemophilus influenzae* type B. Monitor carefully for signs of infection. Administer prophylactic antibiotics. Instruct child or adolescent to wear medical alert bracelet. Teach families to seek medical treatment at first sign of infection or fever.
Surgical removal of tumor	The tumor is completely or partially resected surgically.	Solid tumors	Provide routine postoperative nursing care based on the location of the tumor excision.

COMMON MEDICAL TREATMENTS 24.1

Treatment	Explanation	Indications	Nursing Implications
Radiation therapy	Ionizing radiation (high-energy x-ray) is delivered to the cancerous area. The radiation damages all cells in the locally treated area (normal and cancerous), but the normal cells are able to repair themselves. Usually administered several times a week for several weeks. (A short rest between treatments allows the normal cells time to regenerate.) The lowest possible dose of radiation is used, and it is directed to a specific area.	Solid tumors, before or after surgical resection, leukemia, lymphoma	Do not wash off radiation marking. Keep skin clean and dry. Fatigue is a common side effect. Skin at the site of radiation may become red, dry, or pruritic or may peel; eventually, may become moist and red Mucositis, dry mouth, and loss of taste may occur if head or neck radiated. Radiation may also have adverse effects on the organ irradiated, such as the brain; monitor for changes.
Central venous catheter (see Image A)	IV catheters are inserted into the central circulation for the purpose of administering medications, total parenteral medication, or blood products. A Image A: The central venous access catheter is tunneled under the skin and secured with a cuff.	Any child with cancer who will require long-term IV medications or parenteral nutrition	Complaints of shortness of breath or chest pain may indicate air entry into the central venous catheter. Have child lie on left side and notify health care provider immediately. Keep dressing clean and dry. Perform sterile dressing change per institution policy or health care provider order. Monitor for fever. Monitor insertion site for erythema or drainage. Maintain sterile technique when accessing line, performing dressing change, or administering any fluid through catheter.
Implanted port (see Image B)	A needle-accessible port is implanted under the skin, usually on the chest. The port has a thin catheter exiting it that is tunneled under the skin into the superior vena cava or subclavian vein.	Any child with cancer who will require long-term IV medications or parenteral nutrition	Flush nonaccessed port with prescribed heparin dose per institution policy. Use sterile technique to access port with Huber needle. Monitor port site for erythema or warmth.

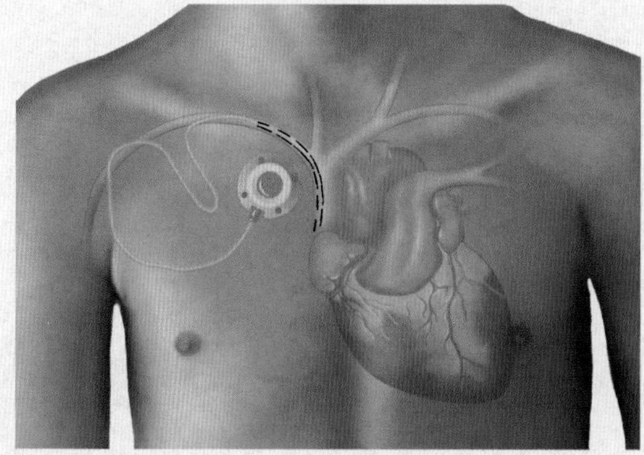

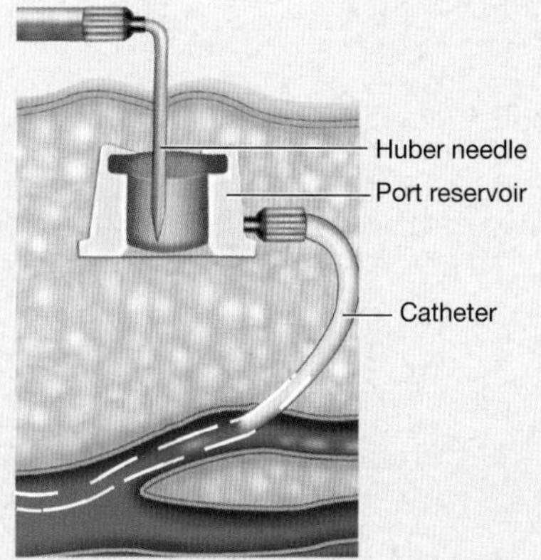

Image B: The implanted port consists of a reservoir under the skin for ready access. The catheter exiting the port is threaded into the subclavian vein or right atrium. Image C: A 90-degree Huber needle is used to access the port.

CMV, cytomegalovirus; WBC, white blood cells.

Based on Anzilotti, A. (2019). *Stem cell transplants.* https://kidshealth.org/en/parents/stem-cells.html; Blaney, S. M., Adamson, P. C., & Helman, L. J. (2021). *Pizzo & Poplack's pediatric oncology* (8th ed.). Wolters Kluwer; and Larson, S. D., Hebra, A., Raju, R., & Lee, S. (2020). Vascular access in children. *Medscape.* Retrieved on April 13, 2023, from https://emedicine.medscape.com/article/1018395-overview#a1

DRUG GUIDE 24.1

COMMON DRUGS FOR HEMATOLOGIC AND NEOPLASTIC DISORDERS

Medication	Actions/Indications	Nursing Implications
Iron supplements (ferrous sulfate, ferrous fumarate)	Supplemental iron in deficient child Iron-deficiency anemia	Dosage is based on milligrams of elemental iron. Give with vitamin C–containing foods to increase absorption. Do not administer with milk or milk products. May color stools and urine black. Liquid can stain the teeth; mix with a small amount of juice; drinking with straw decreases tooth staining. May cause constipation; increase fiber and fluid intake.
Deferasirox	Binds with iron, which is removed in the feces Iron toxicity (as in children chronically transfused)	Oral agent, should be taken at the same time daily, on an empty stomach Do not chew or swallow whole pills; disperse completely in orange juice, apple juice, or water. Monitor iron level, CBC, creatinine, hearing, and vision.
Deferoxamine	Binds with iron, which is removed via the kidneys Iron toxicity (as in children chronically transfused)	Rotate subcutaneous injection sites to decrease local reactions. Apply corticosteroid cream to irritation.
Factor (VIII or IX) replacement	Replaces deficient clotting factors Hemophilia	Use filter needle to draw up medication. Administer IV when bleeding occurs.
Penicillin VK	Kills susceptible bacteria Prophylaxis of infection in asplenia	Determine whether penicillin allergy is present. Monitor kidney and hematologic function during prolonged use.
Folic acid	Replaces the vitamin Folic acid deficiency; questionable use with sickle cell anemia	Administer without regard to meals. Monitor hematologic function.
Hydroxyurea	Stimulates the development of hemoglobin F in sickle cell anemia	Monitor for mild GI discomfort, modest neutropenia, hyperpigmentation of the skin and nails.
L-Glutamine	Conditionally essential amino acid whose production is decreased during times of stress	Decrease frequency of sickle cell disease (SCD) painful vaso-occlusive events.
Intravenous immune globulin (IVIG)	Provides exogenous IgG antibodies Idiopathic thrombocytopenic purpura	Do not mix with IV medications or with other IV fluids. Do not give IM or SQ. Monitor vital signs and watch for adverse reactions frequently during infusion. Child may require antipyretic or antihistamine to prevent chills and fever during infusion. Have epinephrine available during infusion.
Chelating agents: dimercaprol, edetate calcium disodium, succimer	Remove lead from soft tissues and bone, allowing for its excretion via the renal system. Used for blood lead levels >45 mcg/dL	Monitor intake and output closely to ensure adequacy of renal system. Encourage adequate oral hydration or provide IV hydration if required. Follow lead levels as prescribed. Ensure lead is being removed from the child's home.
Allopurinol	Decreases production of uric acid Used to treat secondary hyperuricemia occurring during leukemia or tumor treatment	Give PO after meals with plenty of food. Cardiovascular adverse effects may occur with IV administration. Maintain adequate hydration.
Antibiotics (oral, parenteral)	Treatment of documented bacterial infections Also used as prophylaxis of *Pneumocystis jirovecii* and in the neutropenic child	Check for antibiotic allergies. Should be given as prescribed for the length of time prescribed Start IV antibiotics as soon as possible in the neutropenic child admitted with fever.
Antiemetics: promethazine, metoclopramide, ondansetron	Act on the CNS transmitters to prevent vomiting.	May cause CNS side effects, such as drowsiness or irritability Ondansetron: may cause dry mouth

DRUG GUIDE 24.1

Medication	Actions/Indications	Nursing Implications
Antifungal agents: nystatin, amphotericin B (conventional and lipid complex)	Invade fungal cell wall, enabling its destruction. Indicated for mucositis, or systemic fungal infection	Nystatin: administer after meals Amphotericin B: may cause fever, chills, rigors, cardiovascular adverse effects; monitor child closely throughout infusion; note dose differences between conventional and lipid complex.
Immunosuppressant drugs: cyclosporine A (CyA), mycophenolate, tacrolimus	Inhibition of production and release of interleukin-2 (CyA) Inhibition of T- and B-cell proliferation (mycophenolate). Inhibition of T-cell activation (tacrolimus) Used for treatment of graft-versus-host disease (GVHD) after HSCT	Monitor CBC, serum creatinine, potassium, and magnesium. Monitor blood pressure and for signs of infection. Draw blood levels prior to morning dose. CyA: do not give with grapefruit juice. Mycophenolate: give on empty stomach; do not open capsule or crush tablet. Tacrolimus: give on empty stomach; monitor for anaphylaxis with first IV dose.
Mesna	Binds with and detoxifies cyclophosphamide and ifosfamide metabolites in the urinary bladder to prevent hemorrhagic cystitis	Maintain adequate hydration. Administer concurrently and after cyclophosphamide or ifosfamide. May cause hypotension
Methotrexate antidote: leucovorin	Reduces toxic effects of methotrexate	May cause skin disturbances, wheezing, thrombocytosis Dose depends on methotrexate level. Dose increases with increased creatinine levels.
Biotherapy		
Colony-stimulating factors: darbepoetin alfa, epoetin alfa, filgrastim, sargramostim	Stimulate production of red blood cells (epoetin) or granulocytes (filgrastim, sargramostim) Used to counteract myelosuppressive effects of chemotherapy	Administer SQ or IV. Filgrastim, sargramostim: may cause bone pain Sargramostim may cause hypotension and a first-dose reaction.
Interleukins: aldesleukin	Recombinant DNA interleukin-2 product that recruits T, B, and natural killer cells Indicated for non-Hodgkin lymphoma	Adverse effects are dose-dependent. May cause capillary leak syndrome within 2–12 hours of start of treatment: hypotension and decreased organ perfusion result.
Tumor necrosis factor (protein cytokine)	Increases effectiveness of immune cells, stops cancer cells from dividing, damages tumor blood vessels Used in a variety of cancer protocols	May cause fever, chills, rigors, nausea, vomiting
Monoclonal antibodies: rituximab, gemtuzumab	Bind to CD20 antigen on B lymphocytes Indicated in CD20-positive non-Hodgkin lymphoma, posttransplant lymphoproliferative disorder	Monitor blood pressure for hypotension. Monitor for anaphylaxis and infusion-related reaction. Have epinephrine, antihistamines, and steroids available at bedside for treatment of reaction.
Interferons: alpha, gamma	Alter cancer cell proliferation (alpha), stimulate macrophage production to fight bacteria and fungus (gamma) Indicated in a variety of cancer protocols	May cause flulike symptoms Maintain adequate hydration.
Chemotherapy		
Alkylating agents: busulfan, carboplatin, cisplatin, ifosfamide, temozolomide, thiotepa Nitrosoureas: carmustine, lomustine Nitrogen mustard: chlorambucil, cyclophosphamide, mechlorethamine, melphalan	Interfere with DNA replication and RNA transcription by alkylation (replacing the hydrogen ion with an alkyl group), cross-link DNA Cell cycle nonspecific The nitrosoureas are highly lipid soluble and easily cross the blood–brain barrier. Used in a variety of cancer protocols	Causes myelosuppression, nausea, vomiting, alopecia, mucositis Monitor for signs of infection. Provide adequate hydration. Cyclophosphamide, ifosfamide: Administer in the morning, provide adequate hydration, and have child void frequently during and after infusion to decrease risk of hemorrhagic cystitis. Cisplatin, mechlorethamine, melphalan: Avoid **extravasation** (leakage into surrounding tissues, potentially damaging them). Temozolomide: Avoid opening capsules. Thiotepa: If contact with skin occurs, wash thoroughly with soap and water.

(*continued*)

DRUG GUIDE 24.1 *(continued)*

Medication	Actions/Indications	Nursing Implications
Antitumor antibiotics: bleomycin, dactinomycin, daunorubicin, doxorubicin, idarubicin, mitomycin, mitoxantrone	Interfere with cellular metabolism, causing disruptions in DNA and/or RNA synthesis Cell cycle nonspecific Indicated in a variety of cancer protocols	May cause alopecia, nausea, vomiting, myelosuppression Bleomycin: Fever and chills may occur 20 hours after infusion Dactinomycin, mitomycin: Avoid extravasation. Daunorubicin, doxorubicin, idarubicin: May turn urine red-orange, monitor for arrhythmias, congestive heart failure; avoid extravasation. Mitoxantrone: May color urine, sweat, tears, skin, sclera blue-green; monitor for arrhythmias, congestive heart failure.
Antimetabolites: cladribine, cytarabine, fludarabine, fluorouracil, mercaptopurine, methotrexate, thioguanine	Substitute for a natural metabolite in the molecule, altering the cell's function and ability to replicate. Cell cycle specific (S phase); cladribine is cell cycle nonspecific. Used in a variety of cancer protocols	May cause alopecia, nausea, vomiting, mucositis, and myelosuppression Cladribine: Monitor for fever. Cytarabine: Use corticosteroid eye drops to prevent conjunctivitis with high doses. Fludarabine: Monitor for visual changes and neurotoxicity; maintain adequate hydration. Fluorouracil: Maintain adequate hydration; may cause photosensitivity. Mercaptopurine: Do not give oral doses with meals; may cause drug fever; avoid extravasation. Methotrexate: intensive hydration with high doses; may cause photosensitivity Thioguanine: Maintain hydration; administer on empty stomach.
Antimicrotubulars: paclitaxel	Inhibit mitotic cellular function in late G2 and M phases of cell cycle Indicated for refractory leukemia, recurrent Wilms tumor	May cause alopecia, nausea, vomiting, mucositis, myelosuppression May cause drowsiness Avoid extravasation.
Miscellaneous: asparaginase, pegaspargase	Inhibit protein synthesis by depriving tumor cells of the essential amino acid asparagine Used in acute lymphocytic leukemia, lymphomas	May cause alopecia, nausea, vomiting, and myelosuppression Monitor for vital signs during infusion and for signs of anaphylaxis. Have emergency equipment, oxygen, epinephrine, antihistamines, and steroids available at bedside.
Miscellaneous: dacarbazine, procarbazine	Inhibit DNA and RNA synthesis via cross-linking or suppression of mitosis Indicated in a variety of cancer protocols	May cause alopecia, nausea, vomiting, myelosuppression Monitor for flulike symptoms. Dacarbazine: Photosensitivity may occur; avoid extravasation.
Mitotic inhibitors: etoposide, vinblastine, vincristine	Inhibit mitotic activity by inhibiting DNA topoisomerase (etoposide) Cause metaphase arrest by binding to the mitotic spindle (vinblastine, vincristine) Used in a variety of cancer protocols	May cause alopecia, nausea, vomiting, myelosuppression (only minimal with vincristine) Etoposide: Monitor for anaphylaxis; have emergency equipment, oxygen, epinephrine, antihistamines, and steroids available at bedside. Vinblastine, vincristine: Maintain hydration; administer allopurinol; avoid extravasation.
Topoisomerase inhibitors: irinotecan, topotecan	Bind to DNA complex, preventing religation of single-strand DNA breaks. Indicated for refractory solid tumors	May cause alopecia, nausea, vomiting, myelosuppression, severe diarrhea (irinotecan), hypotension (topotecan) Maintain hydration. Avoid extravasation. Monitor blood pressure during topotecan infusion.
Corticosteroids: prednisone, dexamethasone	Suppress immune system by decreasing lymphatic activity and volume. Also decrease edema caused by tumor or tumor necrosis. Indicated for leukemia and some other cancers	Administer with food to decrease GI upset. May mask signs of infection Monitor blood pressure; monitor urine for glucose. Do not stop treatment abruptly or acute adrenal insufficiency may occur. Monitor for Cushing syndrome. Doses may be tapered over time.

CBC, complete blood count; CNS, central nervous system; GI, gastrointestinal; HSCT, hematopoietic stem cell transplantation; IgG, immunoglobulin G; IM, intramuscularly; IV, intravenous; SQ, subcutaneously.

Data from Blaney, S. M., Adamson, P. C., & Helman, L. J. (2021). *Pizzo & Poplack's pediatric oncology* (8th ed.). Wolters Kluwer; and UpToDate, Inc. (2024). *Lexi-comp®* (Version 8.1.0) [Mobile app]. Wolters Kluwer. https://apps.apple.com/us/app/lexicomp/id313401238

Chemotherapy

To understand how chemotherapy works to destroy cancer cells, it is necessary to review the normal cell cycle, through which all cells progress (Fig. 24.2). The cell cycle consists of five phases:

- G0 phase: the resting phase; lasts from a few hours to a few years; cells have not started to divide
- G1 phase: cell makes more protein in preparation for dividing; lasts 18 to 30 hours
- S phase: chromosomes are copied so that newly formed cells have the appropriate DNA; lasts 18 to 20 hours
- G2 phase: just before the cell splits into two cells; lasts 2 to 10 hours
- M phase: mitosis, the actual splitting of the cell into two new cells; lasts 30 minutes to 1 hour

Chemotherapy drugs work in two different ways in relation to the cell cycle. Cell cycle–specific agents exert their actions during a specific phase of the cell cycle. Cell cycle–nonspecific drugs exert their effect on the cells regardless of which phase the cell is in. Chemotherapy protocols often call for a combination of drugs that act on different phases of the cell cycle, thus maximizing the destruction of cancer cells.

Chemotherapy drugs are divided into classes that exert slightly different actions and have an effect on different portions of the cell cycle. Drug Guide 24.1 gives further explanation about the different classes of chemotherapy drugs.

Unfortunately, chemotherapeutic medications disrupt the cell cycle of not only cancer cells but also normal rapidly dividing cells. This results in a significant number of adverse effects. The cells most likely to be affected by chemotherapy are those in the bone marrow, the digestive tract (especially the mouth), the reproductive system, and hair follicles.

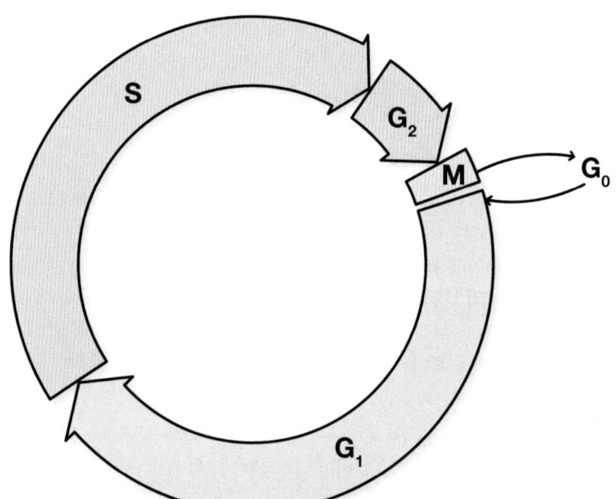

FIGURE 24.2 Phases of the cell cycle.

Adverse effects common to chemotherapeutic drugs include immunosuppression, infection, myelosuppression, nausea, vomiting, constipation, oral mucositis, alopecia, and pain. Long-term complications include microdontia and missing teeth as a result of damage to developing permanent teeth; hearing and vision changes; hematopoietic, immunologic, or gonadal dysfunction; endocrine dysfunction, including altered growth and precocious or delayed puberty; various alterations of the cardiorespiratory, gastrointestinal (GI), and genitourinary systems; and development of a second cancer as an adolescent or adult (ACS, 2024b).

TAKE NOTE!

Acupuncture as an adjunct therapy may help to decrease nausea, vomiting, and aversion to chemotherapy.

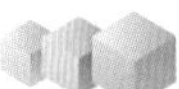 *Concept Mastery Alert*

Chemotherapeutic drugs that act as cell cycle–specific agents are classified as antimetabolites. Alkylating agents are not cell cycle–specific agents.

Radiation Therapy

Radiation therapy uses high-energy radiation to damage or kill cancer cells. Radiant energy in either a gamma or particle form is emitted during the treatment. Radiation affects not only cancer cells but also any rapidly growing cells with which they are in contact. It may be used as a curative, adjuvant, or palliative treatment, either alone or in combination with chemotherapy. Radiation therapy is also used to shrink a tumor prior to surgical resection. The area to be treated is marked carefully to minimize damage to normal cells.

Adverse effects of radiation therapy include fatigue, nausea, vomiting, oral mucositis, myelosuppression, and alterations in skin integrity at the site of irradiation. Long-term complications are related to the area of the body that was irradiated and include alterations in growth; hormone dysfunction; hearing and vision alterations; learning problems; cardiac dysfunction; pulmonary fibrosis; hepatic, sexual, or kidney dysfunction; osteoporosis; and development of secondary cancer (particularly at the site of irradiation) (Mitin, 2023).

Hematopoietic Stem Cell Transplantation

HSCT, also called bone marrow transplantation, is a procedure in which hematopoietic stem cells are infused intravenously into the child. This follows a period of purging of abnormal cells in the child that is accomplished through high-dose chemotherapy or irradiation. The use of high-dose chemotherapy and total body irradiation kills the tumor cells but also destroys the child's bone marrow. The transplanted cells migrate to the empty spaces in the child's bone marrow and reestablish normal hematopoiesis in the child.

HSCT is used for a variety of childhood cancers, including leukemia, lymphoma, brain tumors, neuroblastoma, and other solid tumors. For most pediatric cancers, it is not the first line of treatment but is used for refractory or advanced disease.

Autologous HSCT is achieved through harvest and treatment of the child's own bone marrow, followed by infusion of the treated stem cells. Risk of relapse of the original disease is highest in autologous HSCT. Allogenic HSCT refers to transplantation using stem cells from another individual that are harvested from the bone marrow, peripheral blood, or umbilical cord blood. Allogenic HSCT requires human leukocyte antigen (HLA) matching for antigen-specific sites on the leukocytes. Closely matched HLA donors may be difficult to find from a donor listing, and sibling donors are often the closest match. The degree of match is inversely related to the risk for graft rejection and the development of graft-versus-host disease (GVHD). In other words, the lesser the degree of HLA matching in the donor, the higher the risk of graft rejection and GVHD (Secola, 2022a).

In addition to graft rejection and GVHD, additional initial complications of HSCT are infection; electrolyte imbalance; bleeding; and organ, skin, and mucous membrane toxicities. Long-term complications include impaired growth and fertility related to endocrine dysfunction, developmental delay, cataracts, pulmonary and cardiac disease, avascular necrosis of the bone, and development of secondary cancers.

Palliative Care

Hospice or palliative care may be needed for the child with cancer. Children facing the end of life experience the same symptoms that adults do, including pain, fatigue, nausea, and dyspnea. All dying children have the right to die comfortably and with palliation of symptoms, as has been well established in adult hospice programs. The most recent guidelines for palliative care call for comprehensive assessment and planning by an interdisciplinary team, with care delivered in a culturally sensitive and developmentally appropriate manner (National Hospice and Palliative Care Organization [NHPCO], 2022). For further information related to nursing care of the dying child, refer to Chapter 12.

LABORATORY AND DIAGNOSTIC TESTING

The nurse must understand the main elements of the complete blood count (CBC; hemogram) to recognize critical values and intervene as appropriate. The components of the CBC are:

- RBC count: the actual number of counted RBCs in a certain volume of blood
- **Hemoglobin** (Hgb): measure of the protein made up of heme (iron surrounded by protoporphyrin) and globin, alpha- and beta-polypeptide chains, primarily responsible for the transport of nutrients and oxygen to the tissues
- **Hematocrit** (Hct): an indirect measure of RBCs (number and volume)
- RBC indices:
  - Mean corpuscular volume (MCV): average size of the RBC
  - Mean corpuscular hemoglobin (MCH): a calculated value of the oxygen-carrying capacity of the Hgb in the RBCs
  - Mean corpuscular hemoglobin concentration (MCHC): a calculated value that reflects the concentration of Hgb inside the RBC
  - Red cell distribution width (RDW): a calculated value that is a measure of the width of RBCs
- WBC count: actual count of the number of WBCs in a volume of blood
- **Platelet count:** number of platelets per blood volume
- Mean platelet volume (MPV): a measurement of the size of the platelets

Tables 24.1 and 24.2 provide age-related values for the CBC and leukocyte count. When evaluating the CBC, the nurse must take into account the presenting clinical picture of the child. For instance, the RBC count may be truly elevated (erythrocytosis or **polycythemia**) in certain diseases or in the case of dehydration from diarrhea or burns. When anemia is present, the RBC count is low. When the MCV is elevated, the RBCs are larger than normal (**macrocytic**). When the MCV is decreased, the RBCs are smaller than normal (**microcytic**). A decrease in the MCHC means that the Hgb is diluted in the cell and that less of the red color is present (**hypochromic**). When the Hgb concentration is increased in the RBC, then the pigmentation (red color) is increased (**hyperchromic**). Alterations in these RBC indices assist the health care provider or nurse practitioner with diagnosis.

WBCs are the body's defense against infection or injury. The specific types of WBCs are discussed in Chapter 15. Platelets are necessary for clot formation, and if changes occur, problems may develop. Elevations in platelet levels can indicate an increase in clotting, while decreases can put the child at risk for increased bleeding. Decreases can result if the platelets are being used up when bleeding is present, if an inherited disorder is present, or if the spleen holds them, as in hypersplenism. Platelets are larger when they are new; thus, an elevation in the MPV indicates that an increased number of platelets are being produced in the bone marrow.

TABLE 24.1 • Normal Hemogram Values

Age	WBC ($\times 10^3/mm^3$)	RBC ($\times 10^6/mm^3$)	Hgb (g/dL)	Hct (%)	MCV (fL)	MCH (pg/cell)	MCHC (g/dL)	Platelets ($\times 10^3/mm^3$)	RDW (%)	MPV (fL)
Birth–2 weeks	9.0–30.0	4.1–6.1	14.5–24.5	44–54	98–112	34–40	33–37	150–450	—	—
2–8 weeks	5.0–21.0	4.0–6.0	12.5–20.5	39–59	98–112	30–36	32–36	—	—	—
2–6 months	5.0–19.0	3.8–5.6	10.7–17.3	35–49	83–97	27–33	31–35	—	—	—
6 months–1 year	5.0–19.0	3.8–5.2	9.9–14.5	29–43	73–87	24–30	32–36	—	—	—
1–6 years	5.0–19.0	3.9–5.3	9.5–14.1	30–40	70–84	23–29	31–35	—	—	—
6–16 years	4.8–10.8	4.0–5.2	10.3–14.9	32–42	73–87	24–30	32–36	—	—	—
16–18 years	4.8–10.8	4.2–5.4	11.1–15.7	34–44	75–89	25–31	32–36	—	—	—
>18 years (males)	5.0–10.0	4.5–5.5	14.0–17.4	42–52	84–96	28–34	32–36	140–400	11.5–14.5	7.4–10.4
>18 years (females)	5.0–10.0	4.0–5.0	12.0–16.0	36–48	84–96	28–34	32–36	140–400	11.5–14.5	7.4–10.4

Hct, hematocrit; Hgb, hemoglobin; MCH, mean corpuscular hemoglobin; MCHC, mean corpuscular hemoglobin concentration; MCV, mean corpuscular volume; MPV , mean platelet volume; RBC, red blood cell; RDW, red cell distribution width; WBC, white blood cell.

Data from Fischbach, F. T., Fischbach, M. A., & Stout, K. (2022). *A manual of laboratory and diagnostic tests* (11th ed.). Wolters Kluwer Health.

TABLE 24.2 • Normal Differential for Leukocytes (White Blood Cell Differential)

Age	Bands/Stab (%)	Segs/Polys (%)	Eos (%)	Basos (%)	Lymphs (%)	Monos (%)
Birth–1 week	10–18	32–62	0–2	0–1	26–36	0–6
1–2 weeks	8–16	19–49	0–4	0	38–46	0–9
2–4 weeks	7–15	14–34	0–3	0	43–53	0–9
4–8 weeks	7–13	15–35	0–3	0–1	41–71	0–7
2–6 months	5–11	15–35	0–3	0–1	42–72	0–6
6 months–1 year	6–12	13–33	0–3	0	46–76	0–5
1–6 years	5–11	13–33	0–3	0	46–76	0–5
6–16 years	5–11	32–54	0–3	0–1	27–57	0–5
16–18 years	5–11	34–64	0–3	0–1	25–45	0–5
>18 years	3–6	50–62	0–3	0–1	25–40	3–7

Data from Fischbach, F. T., Fischbach, M. A., & Stout, K. (2022). *A manual of laboratory and diagnostic tests* (11th ed.). Wolters Kluwer Health.

Clinical Judgment and the Nursing Process for the Child With an Alteration in Cellular Regulation/ Hematologic or Neoplastic Disorder

Care of the child with a hematologic disorder or cancer includes assessment, nursing analysis, planning, interventions, and evaluation. Development of a plan of care will depend on which component of the blood is altered in the hematologic disorder. A decrease in hemoglobin will necessitate evaluation of oxygen-carrying capacity and effects of hypoxia on the tissues. A reduction in platelet production will lead the nurse to evaluate for prolonged bleeding, hemorrhage, and shock. An elevation in WBCs would require an evaluation for infection.

From a general understanding of the care involved for a child with cancer, the nurse can then individualize the care based on specifics for the particular child. Children with cancer often suffer many physical effects as a result of the disease and its treatment. The nurse must be diligent when assessing for these effects and should involve the parents as a reliable source for reporting the child's physical symptoms.

Assessment

Signs of changes in the hematologic system are often insidious and overlooked. Children with cancer often demonstrate similar signs. Skin color changes such as pallor, bruising, and flushing are often the first signs that a problem is developing. Changes in mental status such as lethargy can indicate a decrease in Hgb and a decreased amount of oxygen being delivered to the brain. Nursing assessment must include a thorough approach.

Health History

Elicit the birth and maternal history, noting low birth weight or gestational diabetes and ascertaining whether vitamin K was given after birth. The past medical history might be significant for recent illnesses that may contribute to a change in blood cell distribution. Determine the child's sleep/wake patterns and bowel elimination patterns, which may be affected by alterations in circulating blood volume or changes in oxygenation. Explore the family history for inherited disorders such as hemophilia, sickle cell disease, thalassemia, or history of cancer. Determine the presence of risk factors such as previous malignancy and treatment; synthetic chemical exposures; parental exposure to radiation, chemicals, or chemotherapeutic agents; and a family history of malignancy (especially childhood), immune disorders, or genetic disorders such as neurofibromatosis or Down syndrome. Evaluate the child's typical diet for nutritional deficits.

Determine risk for lead exposure based on the use of a standard questionnaire. Determine current medical history. When eliciting the history of the present illness, inquire about:

- Fatigue or malaise
- Pallor of the skin
- Unusual bruising or petechiae
- Excessive bleeding or difficulty stopping bleeding

- Pain: location, onset, duration, quality, and relieving factors
- Recurrent fever or frequent infections
- Early-morning headache with nausea or vomiting
- Gait or behavior changes
- Visual disturbances
- History of bone fractures unrelated to trauma

Physical Examination

A child's general appearance gives great insight into their health and can indicate problems such as malnutrition or lead poisoning. A complete physical examination should be performed on any child with, or suspected of having, cancer or a hematologic disorder. Note particular findings as discussed in what follows. Physical examination of the child with a hematologic or neoplastic disorder includes inspection and observation, palpation, and auscultation.

INSPECTION AND OBSERVATION

Observe the child's overall appearance and energy level. Note a thin or frail appearance, fatigue, or altered level of consciousness. Measure weight and height (or length) and plot on standardized growth charts. Examine the oral cavity for bleeding gums or pale mucous membranes. Document visible masses or asymmetry of the face, thorax, abdomen, or extremities. Observe the nail beds, palms, and soles for pallor. Evaluate the fingertips for clubbing, which occurs with chronic hypoxemia. Document the location and extent of bruises, petechiae, or purpura. Count the respiratory rate and observe for work of breathing. Obtain a pulse oximeter reading to determine oxygen saturation of tissues. Note conjunctival color as well as color and moisture of oral mucosa. Determine urinary output, which may be altered with decreases in circulatory blood volume or inadequate oxygenation. Note the child's responsiveness to stimuli and movement of extremities. Observe the child's gait, noting ataxia or limp. Note rectal bleeding or vaginal discharge.

AUSCULTATION

Auscultate breath sounds, noting adequacy of air movement and depth of respiration. Note adventitious sounds or absence of breath sounds (which would occur in an area of the lung filled with blood). Auscultate heart sounds, listening closely for murmurs (which can develop with changes in blood viscosity and volume). Note the rate and rhythm of the heart tones. Auscultate bowel sounds, noting presence and normalcy.

PERCUSSION

Percuss the abdomen, noting dullness over a mass if present.

PALPATION

Measure blood pressure, which may change with alterations in blood volume. Palpate the peripheral pulses for strength and equality. Palpate for lymphadenopathy; in particular, note nontender or firm lymph nodes. Determine capillary refill time, which may be prolonged when the circulating blood volume is decreased. Carefully palpate the abdomen for tenderness, hepatomegaly, **splenomegaly** (increased spleen size), or presence of a mass. Palpate any unusual area of swelling anywhere on the body, noting size and absence of tenderness. Note temperature of the skin. Determine elasticity of skin, noting decreased turgor. Palpate the joints for tenderness and determine if range of motion (ROM) is limited.

Psychosocial Assessment

Assess the child's and family's psychosocial status, using open-ended questions. It is particularly important to determine the child's self-esteem, level of anxiety or stress, and coping mechanisms. Determine the spiritual status of the child and family. Ongoing medical procedures and the fear of dying take a toll on the child and family when cancer is present. Ask the child how things are going at home; how do they get along with brothers, sisters, and parents? If the child is school-age, ask how school is going. Does the child have friends with whom they get to spend time? Ask the child what they do in their spare time; are there any hobbies? These types of queries will provide the nurse with information about how well the child is coping. Assess the parents' status as well. Ask about the parental relationship and how other children in the family are doing. Determine whether certain stressors may need to be addressed.

Laboratory and Diagnostic Testing

Common Laboratory and Diagnostic Tests 24.1 explains the most commonly used laboratory and diagnostic tests for children with hematologic and neoplastic disorders. The tests can assist the health care provider or nurse practitioner in diagnosing the disorder and/or be used as guidelines in determining ongoing treatment. Laboratory or nonnursing personnel obtain some of the tests, while the nurse might obtain others. In either instance, the nurse should be familiar with how the tests are obtained, what they are used for, and normal versus abnormal results. This knowledge will also be necessary when providing child and family education related to the testing.

Remember Shaun, the 10-month-old with the laceration and prolonged bleeding? What additional health history and physical examination assessment information should you obtain?

COMMON LABORATORY AND DIAGNOSTIC TESTS 24.1

Test	Explanation	Indications	Nursing Implications
Alpha-fetoprotein (AFP)	Produced by the fetal liver and yolk sac; normally decreases to very low levels by 1 year of age	May be elevated in Hodgkin disease and other cancers; used to determine tumor burden	No food or fluid restriction required.
Blood type and cross-match	Determines ABO blood type as well as presence of antigens. Cross-match is performed on RBC-containing products to avoid transfusion reaction.	Person who has sustained trauma or any person in whom blood loss is suspected, in preparation for transfusion	Avoid hemolysis of specimen. Appropriately sign and date specimen. Apply "type and cross" or "blood band" to child at the time of blood draw if indicated by the institution. Most type and cross-match specimens expire after 48–72 hours.
Bone marrow aspiration and biopsy	A needle is inserted through the cortex of the bone into the bone marrow (most often the iliac spine), bone marrow is aspirated, and the cells are evaluated.	Evaluation for leukemia or metastasis of other cancers to bone marrow	Use eutectic mixture of local anesthetic (EMLA) or lidocaine to decrease pain with procedure. Often performed under conscious sedation Apply a pressure dressing to arrest bleeding. Assess for tenderness or erythema. May require mild analgesia for postprocedure pain
Bone scan	Administration of IV radionuclide material, which is taken up by the bone and is visible on the scans	Identify metastasis to bone	Requires patent IV for injection Encourage fluid intake after injection to increase uptake of injected radionuclide. Scan will be performed 1–3 hours after injection.
Chest radiography	Radiograph of the chest	Identify tumor or metastasis in the thorax.	Chest must be held stationary for a brief time.
Clotting studies	Prothrombin time (PT), partial thromboplastin time (PTT), activated partial thromboplastin time (aPTT), international normalized ratio (INR)	Evaluation of common pathway in clotting mechanism PT, INR: evaluation of extrinsic system PTT, aPTT: evaluation of intrinsic system	Apply pressure to venipuncture site. Assess for bleeding (gums, bruising, blood in urine or stool).
Coagulating factor concentration	Measures concentration of specific coagulating factors in the blood	Hemophilia, disseminated intravascular coagulation (DIC)	Apply pressure to venipuncture site. Assess for bleeding (gums, bruising, blood in urine or stool). Deliver specimen to laboratory as soon as possible (unstable at room temperature).
Complete blood count (CBC) with differential	Evaluates hemoglobin and hematocrit, WBC count (particularly the percentage of individual WBCs), and platelet count	Anemia, infection, bleeding disorder, clotting disorder, immunosuppression, to determine neutropenia in myelosuppression	Normal values vary according to age and sex. WBC differential is helpful in evaluating source of infection. May be affected by certain medications
Computed tomography (CT) scan	Multiple films taken in successive layers to provide a 3D view of the body part being scanned	Identify tumor location or metastasis.	Some CT scans are done with oral or IV contrast (notify health care provider if child has iodine or shellfish allergy). May require a several-hour period of NPO if contrast is used (contrast may cause nausea). Encourage fluid intake after scan to facilitate excretion of contrast dye.
Hemoglobin electrophoresis	Measures percentage of normal and abnormal hemoglobin in the blood	Sickle cell anemia, thalassemia	Blood transfusions within the previous 12 weeks may alter test results.

COMMON LABORATORY AND DIAGNOSTIC TESTS 24.1

Test	Explanation	Indications	Nursing Implications
Iron	Evaluates iron metabolism	Iron-deficiency anemia, hemosiderosis with chronic transfusion or hemoglobinopathies	Recent blood transfusions increase level. Child should fast for 12 hours before the test. Avoid hemolysis (will falsely elevate result).
Lead	Measures level of lead in blood	Lead poisoning	Normal amount in blood is zero.
Lumbar puncture (LP)	A needle is placed in the subarachnoid space of the spinal column, below the base of the cord, and cerebrospinal fluid is withdrawn for analysis.	Evaluation of tumor or metastasis to brain or spinal cord; also used to administer intrathecal medications	Use EMLA before the procedure to decrease pain. May be performed under conscious sedation. Position child appropriately. Use distraction techniques in the older child or adolescent. Encourage child to recline for up to 12 hours after LP.
Magnetic resonance imaging (MRI)	Based on how hydrogen atoms behave in a magnetic field when disturbed by radiofrequency signals; does not require ionizing radiation; provides a 3D view of the body part being scanned	Identify extent of tumor or metastatic spread.	Remove all metal objects from the child. Child must remain motionless for entire scan; parent can stay in room with child. Younger children will require sedation to keep still. A loud thumping sound occurs inside the machine during the scan procedure; this can be frightening to children.
Reticulocyte count	Measures the number of reticulocytes (immature RBCs) in the blood	Indicates bone marrow's ability to respond to anemia with production of RBCs	Rises quickly in response to iron supplementation in the iron-deficient child
Serum ferritin	Measures the level of ferritin (the major iron storage protein) in the blood	Most sensitive test for determining iron-deficiency anemia	Elevated in hemolytic disease and if transfused recently Iron supplementation increases ferritin levels.
Urine catechol amines (VMA, HVA)	Catabolism of catecholamines causes elevated levels in urine.	Diagnosis of neuroblastoma (produces catecholamines)	24-hour urine collection Levels may be altered with certain foods and drugs or vigorous exercise.
Ultrasound	High-frequency sound waves are directed at internal organs and structures, and an image is made of the waves as they are reflected back through the tissues.	Identify tumor presence, especially in abdomen or on kidney.	Fasting for a few hours may be required when certain organs are to be visualized.

IV, intravenous; HVA, homovanillic acid; NPO, nothing by mouth; VMA, vanillylmandelic acid; RBC, red blood cell; WBC, white blood cell.

Data from Corbett, J. A., & Banks, A. D. (2019). *Laboratory tests and diagnostic procedures with nursing diagnoses* (9th ed.). Pearson Education Inc.

Nursing Analysis

After recognizing and analyzing cues from a thorough assessment, the nurse might identify several patient problems, including:

- Nausea
- Malnutrition risk
- Constipation
- Diarrhea
- Altered oral mucous membrane integrity
- Activity intolerance
- Impaired physical mobility
- Bleeding risk
- Infection risk
- Anxiety
- Altered body image perception
- Coping impairment
- Situational low self-esteem
- Grief
- Pain
- Interrupted family processes
- Caregiver role strain risk

Shaun's health history revealed he bled with all four of the teeth he has cut. Upon physical examination, numerous bruises are noted. Based on these assessment findings, what would your top three patient problems be for Shaun?

The preceding patient problems provide suggestions for nursing care planning or concept mapping. Suggested interventions with rationales are provided further on. Children's responses to alterations in cellular regulation and their treatments will vary; care planning should be individualized, based on the child's and family's needs. Other conditions may contribute to these patient problems and must also be considered when prioritizing care. Refer to Chapter 14 for the nursing process for pain management and to Chapter 11 for nursing interventions related to interrupted family processes and caregiver role strain risk. Additional information will be included later in the chapter as it relates to nursing management of children with specific disorders, as well as particular nursing interventions for deficient knowledge.

Nursing Analysis

Nausea related to exposure to toxin (adverse effects of chemotherapy or radiation therapy) as evidenced by aversion toward food, increase in salivation, increase in swallowing movements, gagging sensation, or sour taste

Goal/Outcome

Child will experience decreased nausea: will verbalize symptom relief and will be free from vomiting.

Alleviating Nausea and Vomiting (interventions with *rationale*)

- Administer antiemetics prior to chemotherapy and as needed thereafter *to decrease frequency of nausea.*
- Assess frequency of vomiting and level of hydration *to provide baseline data and recognize alterations early.*
- Offer frequent, smaller meals or snacks: *smaller amounts are less likely to be vomited.*
- Avoid spicy foods *to avoid stomach upset.*
- Allow bubbles to dissipate from carbonated beverages before they are ingested: *carbonation may contribute to nausea.*
- Remove cover from meal tray before entering child's room: *this will allow the food odor to dissipate outside of the room; food odors may trigger nausea and vomiting.*

Nursing Analysis

Malnutrition risk; risk factors include insufficient dietary intake, and food aversion.

Goal/Outcome

Child will improve nutritional intake, resulting in steady increase in weight and length/height.

Promoting Adequate Nutrition (interventions with *rationale*)

- Determine body weight and length/height norm for age or find out what the child's pretreatment measurements were *to determine goal to work toward.*
- Determine child's food preferences and provide favorite foods as able *to increase the likelihood that the child will consume adequate amounts of foods.*
- Administer antiemetics as ordered *to increase the likelihood that the child will retain the food they ingest.*
- Weigh child daily or weekly (according to health care provider order or institutional standard), and measure length/height weekly *to monitor for growth.*
- Offer highest-calorie meals at the time of day when the child's appetite is the greatest *to increase likelihood of increased caloric intake.*
- Provide increased-calorie shakes or puddings within diet restriction: *high-calorie foods increase weight gain.*
- Administer vitamin and mineral supplements as prescribed *to attain/maintain vitamin and mineral balance in the body.*
- Administer total parenteral nutrition and intravenous lipids as ordered *to provide adequate nutrition for healing.*

Nursing Analysis

Constipation related to decreased gastric motility (effects of vinca alkaloids, opioid use, decreased activity, dietary changes) as evidenced by decrease in stool frequency or volume or inability to defecate

Goal/Outcome

Child's bowel function will return to usual pattern: child will pass a formed, soft stool every day (or modify this criterion according to child's usual pattern).

Preventing or Managing Constipation (interventions with *rationale*)

- Ensure that child increases fluid *intake to provide enough water in the intestines for soft stool formation.*
- Increase fiber in the diet *to provide bulk for stool formation.*
- Administer stool softeners such as mineral oil or docusate sodium; *these help soften the stool, aiding in passage.*
- Provide motivator laxatives such as magnesium hydroxide, lactulose, or sorbitol *to stimulate stool passage.*
- Use stimulant laxatives such as senna or bisacodyl only intermittently rather than on a daily basis *to avoid dependency and diarrhea.*

Nursing Analysis

Diarrhea related to treatment regimen (effects of radiation therapy) as evidenced by bowel urgency, cramping, or loose, liquid stools

Goal/Outcome

Child's bowel function will return to usual pattern: child will pass a formed, soft stool daily (or modify this criterion according to child's usual pattern).

Managing Diarrhea (interventions with *rationale*)

- Assess frequency of diarrhea and level of hydration *to provide data about severity.*
- Obtain weight daily on same scale *to determine extent of fluid loss.*
- Maintain accurate intake and output records *to determine extent of fluid loss.*
- Administer oral rehydration solutions or intravenous fluids as ordered *to maintain or restore adequate hydration.*
- Restrict roughage and residue in diet *to decrease likelihood of diarrhea.*
- Avoid milk products during acute diarrheal phase: *lactose often worsens diarrhea.*
- Provide an elemental diet to relieve symptoms: *absorbed in the upper small bowel.*
- Provide meticulous perineal care *to avoid skin breakdown related to frequent or loose stools.*
- Administer antidiarrheal medications if ordered *to decrease frequency of stools.*
- If severe and related to radiation therapy, a 3- to 4-day rest period from radiation may be required *to begin recovery of normal absorptive capabilities of bowel.*

Nursing Analysis

Altered oral mucous membrane integrity related to chemotherapy, radiation therapy, immunosuppression, decrease in platelets, malnutrition, or dehydration as evidenced by oral discomfort, cheilitis, bleeding, hyperemia, stomatitis, or other oral lesions

Goal/Outcome

Child will maintain intact, moist mucosa free from redness, ulceration, or debris.

Restoring Healthy Oral Mucosa (interventions with *rationale*)

- Frequently assess oral cavity for redness, lesions, ulcers, plaques, or bleeding *to provide baseline for comparison and identify alterations early.*
- Offer ice chips frequently while child is nothing by mouth (NPO) *to maintain hydration of mucosa.*
- Use only a soft toothbrush or toothette for dental care, avoiding excessive pressure with brushing, *to decrease incidence of bleeding with mouth care.*
- Keep lips lubricated with petroleum jelly or fragrance-free lip balm *to maintain moist, hydrated lips.*
- Rinse with salt solution or mouthwash every 1 to 2 hours *to keep oral cavity clean and moist.*
- Administer glutamine and/or beta-carotene supplements, *which have been shown to decrease the incidence and severity of mucositis.*
- Have child swish and spit 1:1 Benadryl/Maalox solution *to decrease pain.*
- Administer antifungal solution *to prevent or treat oral candidiasis.*
- Avoid spicy, acidic, or very hot or very cold foods *to decrease pain.*
- Administer pain medication (usually acetaminophen or codeine) as ordered *to decrease pain.*

Nursing Analysis

Activity intolerance related to imbalance between oxygen supply and demand (treatment adverse effects, anemia) as evidenced by abnormal heart rate response to activity, exertional dyspnea, weakness, or fatigue

Goal/Outcome

Child will display increased activity tolerance: desire to play without developing symptoms of exertion.

Promoting Activity (interventions with *rationale*)

- Encourage activity or ambulation per health care provider's orders: *early mobilization results in better outcomes.*
- Observe child for symptoms of activity intolerance such as pallor, nausea, lightheadedness or dizziness, or changes in vital signs *to determine level of tolerance.*
- If child is on bed rest, perform ROM exercises and frequent position changes: *negative changes to the musculoskeletal system occur quickly with inactivity and immobility.*
- Cluster nursing care activities and plan for periods of rest before and after exertion *to decrease oxygen need and consumption.*
- Refer the child to physical therapy *for exercise prescription to increase skeletal muscle strength.*

Nursing Analysis

Impaired physical mobility related to pain (from sickle cell crisis or acute bleeds), or physical deconditioning as evidenced by discomfort, decreased motor skills, or slowed movement

Goal/Outcome

Child will be able to engage in activities within age parameters and limits of disease: child is able to move extremities, move about environment, and participate in exercise programs within limits of age and disease.

Promoting Physical Mobility (interventions with *rationale*)

- Encourage gross and fine motor activities as able within constraints of pain/bleed *to facilitate motor development.*
- Collaborate with physical therapy to strengthen muscles and promote mobility *to facilitate motor development.*
- Use passive and active ROM exercises, and teach the child and family how to perform them *to prevent*

contractures and facilitate joint mobility and muscle development (active ROM) to help increase mobility.
- Praise accomplishments and emphasize child's abilities *to improve self-esteem and encourage feelings of confidence and competence.*

Nursing Analysis

Bleeding risk; risk factors include decreased platelet count, deficient coagulation factor, treatment regimen effects.

Goal/Outcome

Child will not experience hemorrhage: will experience decreased bruising or episodes of prolonged bleeding.

Preventing Bleeding (interventions with *rationale*)

- Assess for petechiae, purpura, bruising, or bleeding *to provide baseline data for comparison; if present, may warrant intervention.*
- Encourage quiet activities or play *to avoid trauma with active play.*
- Avoid rectal temperatures and examinations. Post sign at head of bed "no rectal temperatures or medications" *to avoid rectal mucosa damage resulting in bleeding.*
- Avoid intramuscular injections and lumbar puncture if possible *to decrease risk of bleeding from a puncture site.*
- If bone marrow aspiration must be performed, apply pressure dressing to site *to prevent bleeding.*
- Teach families about preferred physical activities for the child with immune thrombocytopenia or hemophilia *to provide safe physical activities and decrease risk of injury.*

Nursing Analysis

Infection risk related to immunosuppression or leukopenia

Goal/Outcome

Child will not experience overwhelming infection; child will be free from infection or able to recover if they become infected.

Preventing Infection (interventions with *rationale*)

- Assess for fever, pain, cough, tachypnea, adventitious breath sounds, skin ulceration, stomatitis, and perirectal fissures *to identify potential infection.*
- Administer antibiotics for temperature greater than 38.4°C *to decrease likelihood of overwhelming sepsis.*
- Maintain meticulous hand hygiene (including family, visitors, staff) *to minimize spread of infectious organisms.*
- Maintain isolation as prescribed *to minimize exposure to infectious organisms.*
- Avoid rectal temperatures and examinations, intramuscular injections, and urinary catheterization when child is neutropenic *to decrease possibility of introducing microorganisms.*
- Educate family and visitors that child should be restricted from contact with known infectious exposures (in hospital and at home) *to encourage cooperation with infection control.*
- Strictly observe medical asepsis *to avoid unintentional introduction of microorganisms.*
- Promote nutrition and appropriate rest *to maximize body's potential to heal.*
- Inform family to contact the health care provider or nurse practitioner if child has known exposure to chickenpox or measles *so that preventive measures (e.g., varicella zoster immunoglobulin [VZIG]) can be taken.*
- Administer vaccines (not live) as prescribed (after clearance with oncologist) *to prevent common childhood communicable diseases.*
- Teach family to monitor for fever at home, and report temperature elevations to oncologist immediately *so that antibiotic therapy may be instituted as soon as possible.*

Nursing Analysis

Anxiety related to ineffective coping strategies, or insufficient knowledge to manage a situation, as evidenced by verbalization

Goal/Outcome

Child and/or parents will demonstrate control: child's anxiety/fear will be minimized (verbalization, decreased crying with procedures); parents (and child as developmentally able) will make decisions regarding care as appropriate.

Promoting a Sense of Control (interventions with *rationale*)

- Maintain a quiet and calm environment *to reduce the child's stress.*
- Educate the child, as appropriate, and the family regarding the need for laboratory specimens *to alleviate anxiety related to the unknown.*
- Identify the need for the specific test and explain the procedure before obtaining the specimen *to decrease the anxiety and time required for the procedure.*
- Use topical anesthetic creams or agents for nonemergency laboratory draws to decrease stress related *to needlesticks or venipunctures.*
- Encourage child and family to make decisions regarding care as appropriate, *to increase sense of control.*
- Provide developmentally appropriate activities for the child: *activities can reduce stress and also provide stimulus for children; serves as a model for the family.*

Nursing Analysis

Altered body image perception related to surgery or treatment regimen (amputation or hair loss), as evidenced by negative feeling about body

Goal/Outcome

Child or adolescent will display appropriate body image: will look at self in mirror and participate in social activities.

Promoting Body Image (interventions with *rationale*)

- Acknowledge the child's feelings of anger over body changes and illness: *venting feelings is associated with less body image disturbance.*
- Encourage the child or adolescent to choose a wig or hats and scarves *to involve the child in making decisions about appearance.*
- Support the child's or adolescent's choices of comfortable, fashionable clothing *to disguise weight loss or scarring while promoting self-esteem.*
- Involve the child in the decision-making process, *as a sense of control will improve body image.*
- Encourage the child to spend time with peers who have experienced hair, limb, or weight loss, *as peers' opinions are often better accepted than those of people in authority, such as parents or health care professionals.*

Nursing Analysis

Coping impairment related to prolonged disease (cancer or genetic disorder), or situational crisis as evidenced by protective behaviors incongruent with child's abilities or autonomy, or inadequate understanding/insufficient knowledge interfering with effective behaviors

Goal/Outcome

Child and/or family will demonstrate adequate coping skills: will verbalize feeling supported and demonstrate healthy family interactions.

Promoting Child and Family Coping (interventions with *rationale*)

- Provide emotional support to the child and family *to improve coping abilities.*
- Actively listen to the child's and family's concerns *to validate their feelings and establish trust.*
- Provide open communication with the child and siblings; *children appreciate honesty about their illness, and coping is improved.*
- Refer families to community resources, such as parent support groups and grief counseling, *to improve coping abilities.*
- Give terminally ill children permission to discuss their feelings about their illness, *allowing them to conquer fears and express love for their family and friends.*
- Encourage families to be honest with siblings about the treatment and prognosis of the child with cancer; *children often sense what is going on and cope better when they are prepared and are given an honest explanation of events.*
- Prepare siblings for the death of the child with cancer, using the child life specialist and chaplain as necessary; *the bereavement period is eased when siblings are prepared.*

Nursing Analysis

Situational low self-esteem related to decreased control over environment and developmental transition (inability to progress with quest for independence [adolescents])

Goal/Outcome

Child/adolescent will maintain or increase self-esteem: will display increased coping responses and verbalize control as appropriate as well as discuss plans for future.

Promoting Self-Esteem (interventions with *rationale*)

- Identify the adolescent's positive abilities *to promote self-esteem.*
- Give genuine and honest positive feedback, *as the child or adolescent desires honesty.*
- Explore strengths and weaknesses with the adolescent *to help the adolescent to see similarities and differences with healthy peers of the same age.*
- Encourage the adolescent to perform self-care as possible *to promote independence.*
- Offer emotional support *to reduce psychological distress and increase coping abilities.*
- Encourage participation in a support group *to allow adolescents to discuss body changes and the reactions they perceive in others.*
- When the adolescent is physically able, encourage attendance at camp or an adventure/wilderness event: *these programs have been shown to improve mental health and coping skills.*

Nursing Analysis

Grief related to anticipatory loss of child (diagnosis of cancer), as evidenced by psychological distress, anger, blame, or denial

Goal/Outcome

Family will express feelings of grief: seek help in dealing with feelings, plan for future one day at a time.

Supporting the Grieving Family (interventions with *rationale*)

- Use therapeutic communication with open-ended questions *to encourage an open and trusting relationship for better communication.*

- Actively listen to the family's expression of grief: *just being present and listening conveys support.*
- Encourage the family to cry and express feelings away from the child *to work through feelings while not upsetting the child.*
- Assess for spiritual distress and refer the family to the hospital chaplain or clergy of choice *for support.*
- Educate the family about the child's condition honestly: *knowing what is going on, what is to be expected, and what the treatment plan is gives the family a sense of control.*
- Support the family through discussions with the child about anticipated death when the illness is deemed terminal: *support is needed for this difficult discussion.*

Based on your top three patient problems for Shaun, describe appropriate nursing interventions.

CARING FOR THE CHILD WITH CANCER

Providing Education

Provide education to families of all children with cancer as outlined in Teaching Guidelines 24.1.

TEACHING GUIDELINES 24.1 Education for Families of Children With Cancer

- Obtain a printed or written copy of the child's treatment plan.
- Keep a calendar of all appointment times, blood count lab draw days, and phone numbers of all health care providers and nurse practitioners, home care companies, the laboratory, and the hospital.
- Seek medical care IMMEDIATELY if the child's temperature is 38.3°C (101°F) or higher.
- Call the oncologist or seek medical care if any of the following occur:
  - Cough or rapid breathing
  - Increased bruising, bleeding or petechiae, pallor, or increased levels of fatigue
  - Earache, sore throat, nuchal rigidity
  - Blisters, rashes, ulcers
  - Red, irritated skin on the child's buttocks
  - Abdominal pain, difficulty or pain with eating, drinking, or swallowing
  - Constipation or diarrhea
  - For children with central venous catheters:
    - Pus, redness, or swelling at the site
    - Breakage of the catheter
    - Do not give the child aspirin

Data from Kline, N. E. (2014). *Essentials of pediatric oncology nursing: A core curriculum* (4th ed.). Association of Pediatric Hematology/Oncology Nurses.

Administering Chemotherapy

All chemotherapy medications have the potential to cause toxicities in the child as well as in the people handling or preparing the medication. General guidelines related to the preparation and administration of chemotherapy include:

- Chemotherapy should be prepared and administered only by specially trained personnel.
- Personal protective equipment (PPE) in the form of double gloves and nonpermeable gowns should be worn when preparing or administering chemotherapy. If splashing is possible or a spill occurs, then a face shield and/or mask may also be necessary.
- Dispose of all equipment used in chemotherapy preparation and administration in a puncture-resistant container (Kline, 2014).

It is critical to calculate the chemotherapy dose correctly. Chemotherapy medication doses in children are based on body surface area (BSA). A nomogram is a commonly used device for determining BSA. To use the nomogram, draw a straight line between the child's height on the left and the child's weight on the right. The point at which the straight line crosses the center is the child's BSA expressed in meters squared (Fig. 24.3).

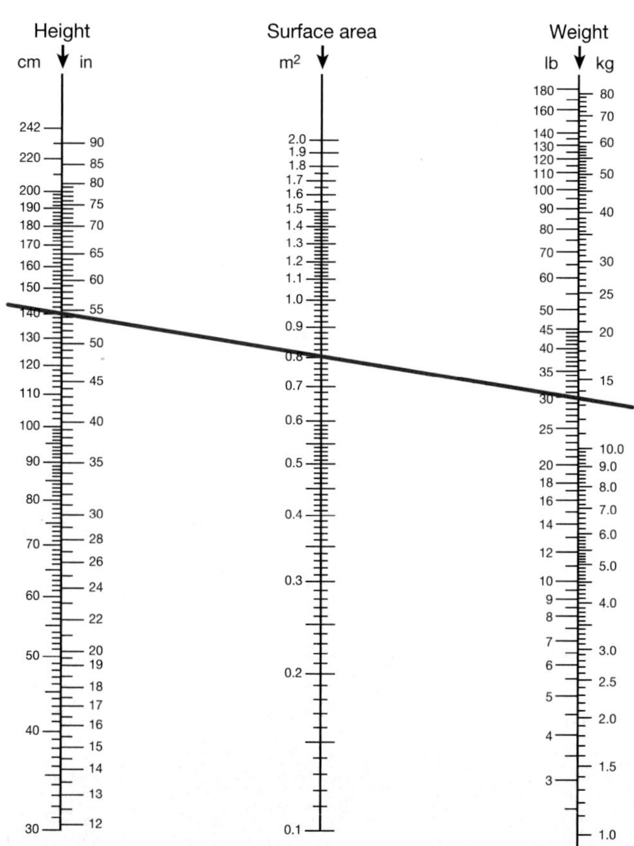

FIGURE 24.3 A child who weighs 13.2 kg and is 140 cm tall has a body surface area (BSA) of 0.80 m^2.

An alternative to using the nomogram is to use the following formula: BSA (m^2) = the square root of (height [in centimeters] × weight [in kilograms] divided by 3,600) (Kline, 2014). For example, for a child 140 cm tall and weighing 30 kg: 140 × 30 = 4,200; 4,200/3,600 = 1.167; and the square root of 1.167 is 1.08. The BSA would be 1.08.

Managing Adverse Effects of Chemotherapy

Chemotherapy can result in multiple adverse effects. Myelosuppression leads to low blood counts in all cell lines, placing the child at risk for infection, hemorrhage, and anemia. Nausea, vomiting, and anorexia may hinder the child's growth. Alopecia and facial changes may affect the child's self-esteem (Fig. 24.4). Nursing interventions related to the effects of myelosuppression, nausea, vomiting, and anorexia are discussed further on. Refer to the "Clinical Judgment and the Nursing Process" section for nursing interventions related to altered body image perception.

> ***TAKE NOTE!***
>
> Cooling the scalp during chemotherapy administration with the use of a cooling cap may decrease hair loss (Rugo & van den Hurk, 2023).

PREVENTING INFECTION

Many chemotherapeutic drugs cause significant bone marrow suppression and decreased amounts of circulating mature neutrophils ("segs," or segmented neutrophils). Administer granulocyte colony–stimulating factor (GCSF) as ordered to promote neutrophil growth and maturation (Ahmed & Flynn, 2022). Administer VZIG within 72 hours of exposure to active chickenpox. If the child is actively infected with chickenpox, administer intravenous acyclovir as ordered. Children receiving treatment for acute lymphoblastic leukemia (ALL) are at risk for opportunistic infection with *Pneumocystis jirovecii,* as most children are colonized with this fungus. Administer prophylactic antibiotics as ordered, and teach the parents to administer them at home. Teaching Guidelines 24.2 gives further information about infection prevention at home.

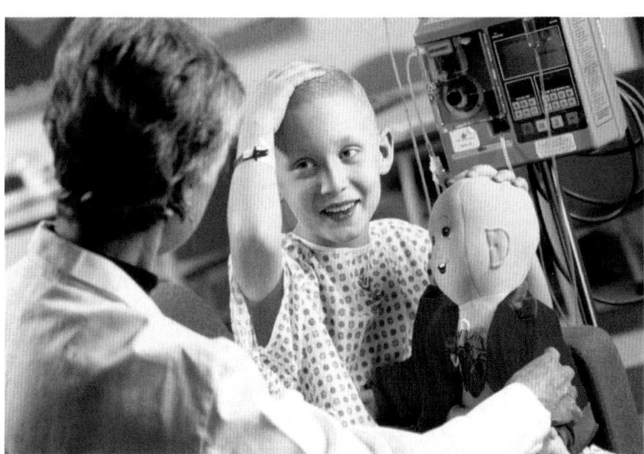

FIGURE 24.4 Chemotherapy often causes alopecia.

As neutrophils are the primary means of fighting bacterial infection, when the neutrophil count is low, the chance of developing an overwhelming bacterial infection is high. Each drug that causes bone marrow suppression has a point of nadir. *Nadir* is the time after administration of the drug when bone marrow suppression is expected to be at its greatest and the neutrophil count is expected to be at its lowest (neutropenia). Nadir is individual for each drug and ranges from 7 to 28 days after dosing. An absolute neutrophil count (ANC) below 500 places the child at greatest risk (Ahmed & Flynn, 2022). Refer to Box 24.2 for information related to calculating the ANC.

Depending on institutional policy, precautions for neutropenia will be followed if the ANC is depressed. These include the following:

- Place the child in a private room.
- Perform hand hygiene before and after contact with each child.
- Monitor vital signs every 4 hours.
- Assess for signs and symptoms of infection at least every 8 hours.
- Avoid rectal suppositories, enemas, or examinations; urinary catheterization; and invasive procedures.
- Restrict visitors with fever, cough, or other signs/symptoms of infection.
- Do not permit raw fruits or vegetables or fresh flowers or live plants in the room.
- Place a mask on the child when they are being transported outside of the room.
- Perform dental care with a soft toothbrush if the platelet count is adequate.

TEACHING GUIDELINES 24.2 Preventing Infection in Children Receiving Chemotherapy for Cancer

- Practice meticulous hygiene (oral, body, perianal).
- Avoid known ill contacts, especially people with chickenpox.
- Immediately notify the health care provider or nurse practitioner if exposed to chickenpox.
- Avoid crowded areas.
- Do not let the child receive live vaccines.
- Do not take the child's temperature rectally or give medications by the rectal route.
- Administer twice-daily trimethoprim–sulfamethoxazole for 3 consecutive days each week as ordered for prevention of Pneumocystis pneumonia.

Data from Kline, N. E. (2014). *Essentials of pediatric oncology nursing: A core curriculum* (4th ed.). Association of Pediatric Hematology/Oncology Nurses.

BOX **24.2 Calculating the ANC**

- Add together the percentage of banded and segmented neutrophils reported on the CBC with differential.
- Multiply the total number of WBCs reported on the CBC by the preceding sum. This yields the ANC (total number of neutrophils present).

Example: Bands 5%, Segs 15%, WBCs 2,500

5% + 15% = 20% (0.20)
2,500 × 0.20 = 500
ANC = 500

ANC, absolute neutrophil count; CBC, complete blood count; WBC, white blood cell.

Data from Children's Oncology Group. (2023). *Low white blood cell count (neutropenia)*. https://www.childrensoncologygroup.org/index.php/lowwhitebloodcellcount

Children with neutropenia and fever must be started on intravenous broad-spectrum antibiotics without delay to avoid overwhelming sepsis (Ahmed & Flynn, 2022).

PREVENTING HEMORRHAGE

Assess for petechiae, purpura, bruising, or bleeding. Determine changes from baseline that warrant intervention. Encourage quiet activities or play to avoid trauma. Avoid rectal temperatures and examinations to avoid rectal mucosal damage that results in bleeding. Post a sign at the head of the bed stating, "no rectal temperatures or medications." Avoid intramuscular injections and lumbar puncture, if possible, to decrease the risk of bleeding from a puncture site. If bone marrow aspiration must be performed, apply a pressure dressing to the site to prevent bleeding. For active or uncontrolled bleeding, transfuse platelets as ordered to control bleeding.

TAKE NOTE!

Administer acetaminophen for mild pain; avoid salicylate and NSAIDs due to increased risk for bleeding.

PREVENTING ANEMIA

To maintain blood volume, limit blood draws to the minimum volume required. Encourage the child to eat an appropriate diet that includes adequate iron. Administer EPO injections as ordered. Teach families to give the injections at home if prescribed.

MANAGING NAUSEA, VOMITING, AND ANOREXIA

Many chemotherapeutic drugs produce the adverse effect of nausea and vomiting, which often leads to anorexia. The cycle of nausea, vomiting, and anorexia is difficult to break once it begins. In addition, taste alterations are common in children who have received chemotherapy. During or after chemotherapy, children may develop an aversion to a food that was previously their favorite. Provide foods the child desires or asks for in order to increase the likelihood of eating.

Prevent nausea by administering antiemetic medications prior to the administration of chemotherapy and on a routine schedule around the clock for the first 1 to 2 days rather than on an as-needed (PRN) basis. Herbal or complementary therapies may provide another option for management of nausea.

TAKE NOTE!

Ginger capsules, ginger tea, and candied ginger have been used as a nausea remedy for centuries (ginger ale is usually artificially flavored, so it would not have the same effect). Although ginger is considered safe, instruct families to check with the oncologist before using this remedy.

Bright lights and noise may worsen nausea. Therefore, keep the child's environment dimly lit and calm. Relaxation therapy and guided imagery may also be helpful in preventing or treating nausea and vomiting. Refer to the "Clinical Judgment and the Nursing Process" section for additional interventions.

TAKE NOTE!

Foot massage may decrease the nausea and vomiting associated with chemotherapy (Asha et al., 2020).

Monitoring the Child Receiving Radiation Therapy

Assess the child's skin daily (particularly at the treatment site), as radiation causes damage to the cells in a localized area, which may include normal cells in addition to the cancerous cells. Teach parents not to scrub ink off the marked radiation field, and avoid adhesive tape in that area. Cleanse gently using a mild soap, and pat dry rather than rubbing, so as to avoid skin irritation. Moisturize the skin with aloe vera lotion or other aqueous cream. Administer diphenhydramine or apply hydrocortisone 1% cream to reduce itching and urge to scratch. Apply Silvadene cream once or twice a day to areas of desquamation related to radiation.

Avoid perfumed lotions or soaps, deodorants, heat, cold, or sun, as these will further irritate the skin in the irradiated area. Instruct the child and family that clothing should fit loosely so as not to irritate the site (ACS, 2024c). During the radiation treatment and for 8 weeks thereafter, the skin will be more photosensitive. Explain the importance of protecting the skin with a high-SPF (30 or higher) sunscreen.

Providing Care to the Child Undergoing HSCT

Stem cell transplantation is performed at limited specialty medical centers in the United States. In addition, special training is required for all personnel caring for the child who undergoes a stem cell transplant. The intent of this discussion is to provide only a brief introduction to, and overview of, nursing management related to HSCT.

Care for the child undergoing HSCT may be divided into three phases—the pretransplant phase, the posttransplant phase, and the lengthy supportive care phase. Nursing management of each phase is discussed briefly in what follows.

Nursing Management of the Child During the HSCT Pretransplant Phase

In the pretransplant phase, the child is being prepared to receive the transplant. The child's own bone marrow cells are eradicated through high-dose chemotherapy and total body irradiation. This phase usually occurs over 7 to 10 days. The child will be hospitalized because they are at extreme risk for serious infection. Maintain protective isolation in a positive-pressure room and limit visitors. Administer gamma globulin, acyclovir, or antibiotics as ordered to prevent or treat infection. Lymphohematopoietic rescue occurs with infusion of the donor or autologous cells (Kline, 2014).

Nursing Management of the Child During the HSCT Posttransplant Phase

The posttransplant phase is also a time of high risk for the child. Monitor closely for symptoms of GVHD such as severe diarrhea and maculopapular rash progressing to redness or desquamation of the skin (especially palms or soles) (Fig. 24.5). If GVHD occurs, administer immunosuppressive drugs such as cyclosporine, tacrolimus, or mycophenolate (which place the child at further risk for infection) (Secola, 2022b).

Providing Supportive Care Following the HSCT

During the supportive care phase, which lasts several months after the transplant, continue to monitor for and prevent infection. Administer PRBCs or platelets and GCSF as needed. Families and children who undergo HSCT need prolonged and extensive emotional and psychosocial support. A medical social worker and psychologist or counselor are usually members of the transplant team and are excellent resources for these families' needs (Nuuhiwa, 2022).

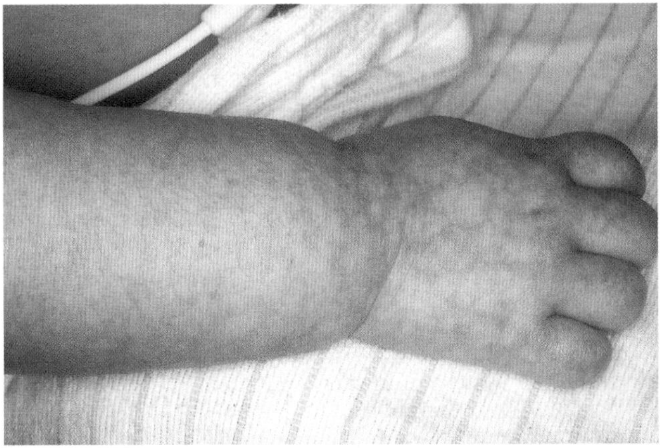

FIGURE 24.5 The first sign of graft-versus-host disease (GVHD) may be a maculopapular rash. (Courtesy of Mary L. Brandt, MD.)

Promoting a Normal Life

Children and adolescents want to be normal and to experience the things that other children of their age do. The child should attend school when they are well enough and the WBC counts are not dangerously low. Children, their families, and their teachers should be aware that cancer and its treatment can affect scholastic abilities. Learning disabilities, difficulty with memory, attention disorders, and cognitive deficits can occur (NCI, 2024).

Maintain other activities if the child is able and if platelet counts are within normal limits. Special camps are available for children with cancer. These camps offer an opportunity for children and adolescents to experience a variety of activities safely and to network with other children who are experiencing similar physical and emotional challenges. The Children's Oncology Camping Association and the American Childhood Cancer Foundation provide lists of camps throughout the United States and Canada and internationally for children and adolescents with cancer.

Promoting Growth

Promote growth in children with cancer by encouraging an appropriate diet and preventing nausea and vomiting and also by addressing concerns such as diarrhea and constipation. Chronic diarrhea related to radiation therapy may prevent the child from gaining weight and growing properly (see the "Clinical Judgment and the Nursing Process" section). The use of vinca alkaloids and opioids, as well as the decreased activity level of the child with cancer, may contribute to constipation. Constipation increases the pain experience, contributes to the child's malaise, and decreases quality of life. It directly affects the child's ability to grow by increasing anorexia, nausea, and vomiting (Kline, 2014). Detail for interventions related to preventing and managing constipation is provided in the "Clinical Judgment and the Nursing Process" section earlier in the chapter.

Preventing and Treating Oncologic Emergencies

Oncologic emergencies may occur as an effect of the disease process itself or from cancer treatment. As progress is made in chemotherapy and radiation treatment, children with cancer have an increased survival rate, but they still face the risk of developing an oncologic emergency. Nurses caring for children with cancer need to be familiar with signs and symptoms of oncologic emergencies as well as with their treatment. All of these problems warrant careful, frequent monitoring of respiratory, cardiovascular, neurologic, and kidney status. Table 24.3 provides information about oncologic emergencies.

TABLE 24.3 • Oncologic Emergencies

Emergency	Associated With	Signs and Symptoms	Laboratory or Diagnostic Test Findings	Management
Sepsis	Neutropenia resulting from bone marrow suppression due to chemotherapy	• Fever or low temperature • Respiratory distress • Poor perfusion • Altered level of consciousness	• ANC <500 • Positive blood culture • Increased BUN, creatinine, potassium, clotting times • Decreased platelet count • Metabolic acidosis	• Airway and ventilation maintenance • Fluid volume resuscitation • Inotropic support • Broad-spectrum antibiotics and antifungals • Dialysis if needed
Tumor lysis syndrome	ALL, lymphoma, neuroblastoma	• Nausea, vomiting, diarrhea, anorexia • Lethargy • Increased heart rate and blood pressure • Decreased or absent urine output • Altered level of consciousness	• Hyperuricemia • Hyperkalemia • Hyperphosphatemia • Hypocalcemia • Hypoxia	• Prevent by giving allopurinol for several days prior to chemotherapy (also treat with allopurinol) • Double IV fluid maintenance • Sodium bicarbonate
Typhlitis (neutropenic enterocolitis)	Inflammatory process of GI tract occurring with induction phase of leukemia chemotherapy	• Acute abdominal pain • Nausea, vomiting • Bloody diarrhea and emesis • Fever • Anorexia	• KUB: scarcity of bowel gas, possibly ileus • CT (abdominal): inflammation, bowel wall thickening, peritoneal fluid	• Bowel rest (NPO status) • IV nutrition • Assess for bowel perforation/shock • Broad-spectrum antibiotics and antifungals • Comfort measures
Superior vena cava (SVC) syndrome	Compression on the SVC by NHL or other mediastinal mass, such as neuroblastoma	• Dyspnea and cyanosis • Large cervical lymph nodes • Wheezing, diminished breath sounds	• Chest radiograph or CT shows mediastinal mass • Pleural effusion	• Intubation and ventilation • Comfort measures • Treat cause (usually, surgical removal of mass)
Spinal cord compression	Tumor or metastasis compresses spinal cord	• Back, neck, or leg pain • Sensory or autonomic dysfunction • Extremity weakness or paralysis	• MRI reveals location of tumor or metastasis to epidural space	• Dexamethasone • Careful assessment • Radiation therapy • Comfort measures
Increased intracranial pressure	Brain tumor or metastasis to brain causing compression of brain; may result in herniation	• Headache, visual disturbances • Morning vomiting • Infants: increased head circumference • Altered level of consciousness • Cushing triad • Seizure activity	• Head CT or MRI reveals extent of mass	• Frequent, careful neurologic assessment • Limit fluids • Dexamethasone • Anticonvulsants • Tumor resection, radiation, or chemotherapy • Comfort measures
Massive hepatomegaly	Obstruction caused by neuroblastoma filling a large portion of the abdominal cavity	• Distended, enlarged abdomen • Respiratory distress, hypoxia • Poor perfusion • Tachycardia, hypotension	• Abdominal CT reveals extent of tumor • Coagulopathy	• Tumor resection or debulking • Mechanical ventilation, inotropic support • Nasogastric decompression • Position to minimize abdominal pressure • Blood transfusions • Comfort measures

ANC, absolute neutrophil count; BUN, blood urea nitrogen; CT, computed tomography; GI, gastrointestinal; KUB, kidney, ureters, and bladder scan; MRI, magnetic resonance imaging; NPO, nothing by mouth.

Data from Keating, A. K., Knight-Perry, J., Maloney, K., Levy, J. M. M., Greffe, B. S., Franklin, A. R. K., & Garrington, T. P. (2022). Chapter 31: Neoplastic disease. In M. Bunik, W. W. Hay, M. J. Levin, & M. J. Abzug (Eds.), *Current diagnosis & treatment: Pediatrics* (26th ed, pp. 931–963). McGraw-Hill Education; Hibberd, C., Hibberd, O., Karageorgos, S., & Barnard, G. (2023). Ten oncology emergencies in kids. *Don't Forget the Bubbles.* https://doi.org/10.31440/DFTB.53725

Caring for the Dying Child

Cancer accounts for the most deaths per year from disease for children (CureSearch, 2022). A "do not resuscitate" (DNR) order for the child with progressive cancer is obtained in many situations. This order helps to optimize care in the terminal phase of cancer. Nurses serve as child and family advocates, clarifying terminology and providing support as needed during the discussion of DNR orders and throughout the rest of the terminal phase.

Children with terminal cancer often experience a great deal of pain, particularly when death is imminent. Pain is often accompanied by agitation and dyspnea, which further contribute to the child's discomfort. Whether the child has a DNR order or their status remains that of "full code," pain management is central to the nursing care of the child who is dying from cancer. A primary goal for the child dying of cancer is prevention and alleviation of pain. The health care team partners with the child and parents to manage the child's pain (NHPCO, 2022). Refer to Chapter 14 for further information related to pain assessment and management.

Further discussion related to care of the dying child is found in Chapter 12.

ANEMIA

Anemia is a condition in which the level of RBCs is lower than the age-appropriate normal value. Anemia may develop as a result of decreased production of RBCs or loss and destruction of RBCs. The loss of production can be related to lack of dietary intake of the nutrients needed to produce the cells, alterations in the cell structure, or malfunctioning tissues (e.g., bone marrow). Anemia related to nutritional deficiency includes iron deficiency, folic acid deficiency, and pernicious anemia. Anemia may also result from toxin exposure (lead poisoning) or as an adverse reaction to a medication (aplastic anemia). Blood loss may result from surgery or trauma. Alteration or destruction of cells occurs in certain genetic and cellular development disorders (Nuss et al., 2022).

Anemia caused by the alteration or destruction of the RBCs is termed hemolytic anemia. There are several types of hemolytic anemia, such as sickle cell disease (SCD) and thalassemia; these two disorders are discussed in the section on hemoglobinopathies.

Anemia related to insufficient intake of specific nutrients is the most common type of anemia in children. Nutrient intake may be reduced in children due to food dislikes or conditions that produce malabsorption.

Iron-Deficiency Anemia

Iron-deficiency anemia occurs when the body does not have enough iron to produce Hgb. In the United States, iron-deficiency anemia has a peak prevalence in children between the ages of 12 and 24 months and again during adolescence (Powers, 2023). Cow's milk consumption contributes to iron-deficiency anemia in older infants and young children due to its poor iron availability (Powers, 2023).

The heme portion of Hgb consists of iron surrounded by protoporphyrin. When not enough iron is available to the bone marrow, Hgb production is reduced. Adequate dietary intake of iron is required for the body to make enough Hgb. As Hgb levels decrease, the oxygen-carrying capacity of the blood is decreased, resulting in weakness and fatigue. In addition to delayed growth, iron-deficiency anemia has been associated with cognitive delays and behavioral changes.

TAKE NOTE!

For appropriate growth to occur in adolescence, increased amounts of iron must be consumed and absorbed.

Therapeutic Management

Iron supplements are usually provided in the form of ferrous sulfate or ferrous fumarate and are available over the counter. The recommended dose is 3 mg/kg of elemental iron daily (Nuss et al., 2022). In more severe cases, blood transfusions may be indicated. Transfusion of PRBCs is reserved for uncompensated anemia. When PRBC administration is warranted, follow specific blood bank guidelines for administration. Monitor subsequent laboratory results for improvement.

Nursing Assessment

For a full description of the assessment phase of the nursing process, refer to the "Clinical Judgment and the Nursing Process" section. Assessment findings pertinent to iron-deficiency anemia are discussed further on.

HEALTH HISTORY

Elicit a description of the current illness and chief complaint. Common signs and symptoms reported during the health history may include irritability, headache, dizziness, weakness, shortness of breath, pallor, and fatigue. Other symptoms may be subtle and difficult for the clinician to identify; these include difficulty feeding, pica, muscle weakness, or unsteady gait.

Explore the health history for risk factors such as:

- Maternal anemia during pregnancy
- Poorly controlled diabetes during pregnancy
- Prematurity, low birth weight, or multiple birth
- Cow's milk consumption before 12 months of age
- Excessive cow's milk consumption (greater than 24 oz a day)
- Infant consumption of low-iron formula

- Lack of iron supplementation after age 6 months in breastfed infants
- Excessive weight gain
- Chronic infection or inflammation
- Chronic or acute blood loss
- Restricted diets
- Use of medication interfering with iron absorption, such as antacids
- Low socioeconomic status
- Recent immigration from a developing country (Powers, 2023)

Evaluate the child's diet for adequate intake of iron-rich foods. Recommended dietary daily intake for iron in children is:

- 0 to 6 months: 0.27 mg
- 7 to 12 months: 11 mg
- 1 to 3 years: 7 mg
- 4 to 8 years: 10 mg
- 9 to 13 years: 8 mg
- Males 14 to 18 years: 11 mg
- Females 14 to 18 years: 15 mg (Diab et al., 2022)

PHYSICAL EXAMINATION

Observe the child for fatigue and lethargy. Inspect the skin, conjunctivae, oral mucosa, palms, and soles for pallor. Note spooning of the nails (concave shape) (Fig. 24.6). Obtain a pulse oximeter reading. Evaluate the heart rate for tachycardia. Auscultate the heart for a flow murmur. Palpate the abdomen for splenomegaly.

LABORATORY AND DIAGNOSTIC TESTS

Laboratory evaluation will reveal decreased Hgb and Hct, decreased reticulocyte count, microcytosis, hypochromia, decreased serum iron and ferritin levels, and an increased free erythrocyte protoporphyrin (FEP) level.

Nursing Management

Nursing management of the child with iron deficiency focuses on promoting safety, ensuring adequate iron intake, and educating the family.

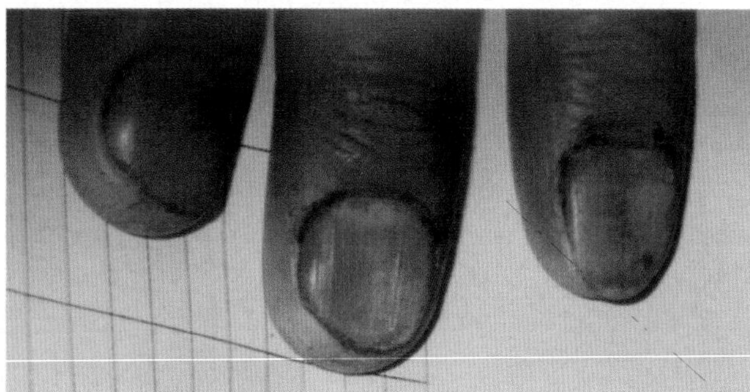

FIGURE 24.6 Note the concave shape of nails ("spooning") that occurs with iron-deficiency anemia.

PROMOTING SAFETY

The child with anemia is at risk for changes in neurologic functioning related to the decreased oxygen supply to the brain. This can lead to fatigue and inability to eat enough. Neurologic effects may be manifested when the child's ability to sit, stand, or walk is impaired. Provide close observation of the anemic child. Assist the older child with ambulation. Educate the parents on how to protect the child from injury due to an unsteady gait or dizziness.

PROVIDING DIETARY INTERVENTIONS

Ensure that iron-deficient infants are fed only formulas fortified with iron. Interventions for breast-fed infants include beginning iron supplementation around the age of 4 or 5 months. Iron supplementation may range from adding iron-fortified cereals to the child's diet to giving iron-containing drops. Encourage breastfeeding parents to increase their dietary intake of iron or take iron supplements when breastfeeding so that the iron may be passed on to the infant. For children over 1 year of age, limit cow's milk intake to 24 oz per day to decrease risk of microscopic GI bleeding and increase appetite for other foods. Limit fast-food consumption and encourage intake of iron-rich foods such as red meats (iron from red meat is the easiest for the body to absorb), tuna, salmon, eggs, tofu, enriched grains, dried beans and peas, dried fruits, leafy green vegetables, and iron-fortified breakfast cereals.

Teach the parents about dietary intake of iron. Encourage parents to provide a variety of foods for iron support and vitamins and other minerals necessary for growth. A big problem for toddlers is their picky eating. This often becomes a means of control for the child, and parents should guard against getting involved in a power struggle with their child. Referring parents to a developmental specialist who can assist them in their approach to diet may prove beneficial. Refer families who meet the financial limits and who have children aged 5 and younger to the Women, Infants, and Children (WIC) program, which provides for supplementation of infants' and children's diets. See the Healthy People 2030 box.

HEALTHY PEOPLE 2030

Objective	Nursing Significance
Reduce iron deficiency among children aged 1–2 years and females aged 12–49 years.	• Encourage use of iron-fortified formulas and infant cereal. • Encourage iron supplementation in the second half of infancy for the breastfed infant. • Educate parents about iron-containing foods. • Encourage adolescent females to consume a diet high in iron-rich foods.

Healthy People Objectives retrieved from http://www.healthypeople.gov

TEACHING ABOUT IRON SUPPLEMENT ADMINISTRATION

The use of iron supplements in infants begins with the use of formula fortified with iron in the formula-fed infant. Oral supplements may also be necessary if the baby's iron levels are extremely low. Oral supplements or multivitamin formulas that contain iron are often dark in color because the iron is pigmented. Teach parents to precisely measure the amount of iron to be administered. Parents should place the liquid behind the teeth, as iron in liquid form can stain the teeth. Iron supplementation can also cause constipation. In some cases, reducing the amount of iron can resolve this problem, but stool softeners may be necessary to control painful or difficult-to-pass stools. Encourage parents to increase their child's fluid intake and include adequate dietary fiber to avoid constipation.

TAKE NOTE!

Teach parents to keep iron-containing supplements out of the reach of young children in order to prevent accidental ingestion leading to overdose or poisoning.

Other Nutritional Causes of Anemia

Other forms of anemia related to nutritional deficit include folic acid deficiency and pernicious anemia. Comparison Chart 24.2 discusses the causes, assessment, and management of these disorders.

Lead Poisoning

Despite concerted efforts in the past few decades to screen for lead poisoning in young children, there are over 500,000 U.S. children between 1 and 5 years of age with elevated lead levels (Halmo & Nappe, 2023). Lead exerts toxic effects on the bone marrow, erythroid cells, nervous system, and kidneys. The presence of lead in the bloodstream interferes with the enzymatic processes of the biosynthesis of heme. The process results in hypochromic, microcytic anemia, and children may exhibit classic signs of anemia. Risk factors for lead poisoning are related to lead exposure in the home, school, or local environment. Sources of lead include:

- Paint in homes built before 1978, at which time lead was banned as an additive to paint used in houses
- Soil where cars that used leaded gas have been in the past (lead was removed from all gasoline in the United States as of 1996)
- Glazed pottery
- Stained glass products
- Lead pipes supplying water to the home
- On the clothing of parents who work in certain manufacturing jobs (battery makers, cable makers)
- Certain folk remedies, such as *greta* or *azarcon*
- Old painted toys or furniture (Centers for Disease Control and Prevention [CDC], 2024)

Complications of lead poisoning include behavioral problems and learning difficulties and, with higher lead levels, encephalopathy, seizures, and brain damage. Therapeutic management for high blood levels of lead involves **chelation therapy** (removal of heavy metals from the body via chelating agents), either orally or intravenously. Drug Guide 24.1 gives further information on chelating agents.

Nursing Assessment

Explore the health history for subtle signs such as anorexia, fatigue, or abdominal pain. Determine whether

COMPARISON CHART 24.2 Folic Acid Deficiency Versus Pernicious Anemia

	Folic Acid Deficiency	Pernicious Anemia
Cause	Low dietary intake of green leafy vegetables, liver, and citrus Malabsorption from medication such as phenytoin (Dilantin) or parasitic infection	Deficiency in vitamin B_{12}
Assessment	Determine risk factors such as prematurity, low socioeconomic status, and history of malabsorption disease. Determine dietary history, noting dislike of fresh vegetables or fruit, ingestion of overcooked foods, or lack of family purchase of fruits and vegetables. Note history of fatigue, headache, poor growth, anorexia, or diarrhea. Inspect the skin for pallor or jaundice, and note presence of a sore on the mouth or tongue.	Note history of anorexia, irritability, or chronic diarrhea. Observe the skin or conjunctivae for pallor and the tongue for smooth texture and bright-red color.
Laboratory analysis	RBC, Hgb, Hct	RBC, Hgb, Hct, low vitamin B_{12} level
Management	Encourage parents to include green leafy vegetables, liver, and citrus in diet. Ensure parents adhere with dietary changes.	Administer monthly injections of vitamin B_{12}. Inform parents that injections will be required throughout the child's life. Provide emotional support related to the chronic nature of this disorder.

Hct, hematocrit; Hgb, hemoglobin; RBC, red blood cell.

behavioral problems, irritability, hyperactivity, or lack of ability to meet developmental milestones have occurred in recent months. Screen children for risk of exposure to lead in the home. Refer to Chapter 9 for a simple screening questionnaire that can be used to determine the need for lead screening in young children. Blood levels of lead greater than 10 mcg/dL require conscientious follow-up. Note pallor of the skin.

Nursing Management

Prevention of elevated lead levels is critical. Screen children for lead exposure risk. The AAP recommends performing a risk assessment at 6, 9, 12, 18, and 24 months, and 3, 4, 5, and 6 years. If positive, the decision may be made to evaluate a blood lead level (Hagan et al., 2017). Table 24.4 gives recommendations for appropriate follow-up depending on lead levels.

Removing old paint is the best way to eliminate the most significant source of lead exposure for a large number of children. If the family rents or lives in public housing, the landlord or owner is responsible for following the guidelines set forth by local and state governmental agencies to correct the problem. Educate families about how to prevent exposure to lead, particularly in young children.

If the child is undergoing chelation therapy, ensure adequate fluid intake and monitor intake and output closely. Refer children with elevated lead levels and developmental or cognitive deficits to developmental centers. These children may need an early intervention program for further evaluation and treatment of developmental delays. See the Healthy People 2030 box.

TABLE 24.4 • Interventions Based on Blood Lead Level

Blood Lead Level (mcg/dL)	Recommended Action
<3.5	May require retesting if determined to be high risk
3.5–14	Repeat test in 1–3 months. Educate parents to decrease lead exposure. Repeat test again in 1–3 months.
15–44	Confirm with repeat test in 1–4 weeks. Educate parents to decrease lead exposure. Report to local health authorities for surveillance.
>44	Retest asymptomatic children with levels 45–69 within 48 hours. Begin chelation therapy and refer to health department as before. Hospitalize child if level ≥70 and begin chelation therapy. Ensure lead is removed from the home.

Data from Sample, J. A. (2024). *Childhood lead poisoning: Management.* Retrieved on February 17, 2024, from http://www.uptodate.com/contents/childhood-lead-poisoning-management

HEALTHY PEOPLE 2030

Objective	Nursing Significance
Reduce blood lead levels in children aged 1–5 years.	Appropriately screen infants and young children for lead exposure at each health care visit.

Healthy People Objectives retrieved from http://www.healthypeople.gov

Aplastic Anemia

Aplastic anemia (failure of the bone marrow to produce cells) is characterized by bone marrow aplasia and pancytopenia (decreased numbers of all blood cells). Most cases are acquired, but there are a few rare types of inherited aplastic anemias (Nuss et al., 2022). The inherited types present as congenital bone marrow failure; the best known is Fanconi anemia, an autosomal recessive disorder. Acquired aplastic anemia is thought to be an immune-mediated response. Most cases are idiopathic, meaning the trigger remains unidentified. Other causes include exposure to environmental toxins, viruses, myelosuppressive drugs, or radiation.

Complications of aplastic anemia include severe overwhelming infection, hemorrhage, and death. Therapeutic management of aplastic anemia in children involves HSCT from an HLA-matched sibling donor; if one is not available, immunosuppressive therapy or high-dose cyclophosphamide can be given.

Nursing Assessment

Determine history of exposure to myelosuppressive medications or radiation therapy. Obtain a detailed family, environmental, and infectious disease history. Note history of epistaxis, gingival oozing, or increased bleeding with menstruation. Anemia may lead to headache and fatigue. On physical examination, note ecchymoses, petechiae or purpura, oral ulcerations, tachycardia, or tachypnea. In addition to suppression of all blood cells, laboratory and diagnostic testing may reveal:

- Guaiac-positive stool
- Blood in the urine
- Severe decrease in or the absence of hematopoietic cells on bone marrow aspiration

Nursing Management

Safety is of the utmost concern in children with aplastic anemia. It is important to prevent injury in order to avoid hemorrhage. Stool softeners may be used to prevent anal fissures associated with constipation. Administer only irradiated and leukocyte-depleted PRBCs or platelet transfusions as necessary. This limits exposure to HLA should the child require bone marrow transplantation in the future. If the child requires HSCT, refer to the section earlier in this chapter for additional nursing management information.

Refer families whose child has only mild or moderate disease to the Aplastic Anemia and Myelodysplastic Syndrome International Foundation.

HEMOGLOBINOPATHIES

Hemoglobinopathy is a condition in which abnormal hemoglobin is present. A large percentage of the newborn's hemoglobin is fetal hemoglobin (Hgb F). Hgb F can exchange oxygen molecules at lower oxygen tensions compared to adult hemoglobin. Over the first several months of life, Hgb F levels fall as it is replaced with Hgb A (adult hemoglobin). The healthy older infant then displays Hgb AA. In hemoglobinopathies, this Hgb configuration is disturbed. Causes of hemoglobinopathies are genetic and include SCD, hemoglobin SC disease, alpha-thalassemia, and beta-thalassemia. This discussion will focus on SCD and beta-thalassemia (Cooley anemia).

Sickle Cell Disease

SCD is a group of inherited hemoglobinopathies in which the RBCs do not carry the normal adult hemoglobin but instead carry a less effective type. In the United States, the most common types of SCD are hemoglobin SS disease (termed sickle cell anemia [SCA]), hemoglobin SC disease, and hemoglobin sickle–beta-thalassemia. SCD is most common in individuals of African, Mediterranean, Middle Eastern, and Indian descent (CDC, 2023a).

The focus of this discussion will be on hemoglobin SS disease. Instead of Hgb AA, individuals with SCA have Hgb SS (Hgb A refers to adult hemoglobin, Hgb S refers to sickle hemoglobin). In hemoglobin S, glutamic acid is replaced with valine in the hemoglobin molecule. This results in an elongated RBC with a shortened lifespan. The elongated cell is more rigid than a normal cell and becomes sickled in shape (Fig. 24.7). One in 325 Black newborns has SCD (CDC, 2023a).

People with heterozygous representation (Hgb AS) are said to have sickle cell trait and are carriers for the disorder; about 1 in 13 Black newborns have sickle cell trait (CDC, 2023a). Generally, individuals with sickle cell trait have only minimal health problems.

SCA is transmitted via an autosomal recessive inheritance pattern. The recessive genes for sickle cell are passed on from both parents who have the gene for Hgb AS (sickle cell trait). Refer to Chapter 27 for further information on autosomal recessive gene transmission.

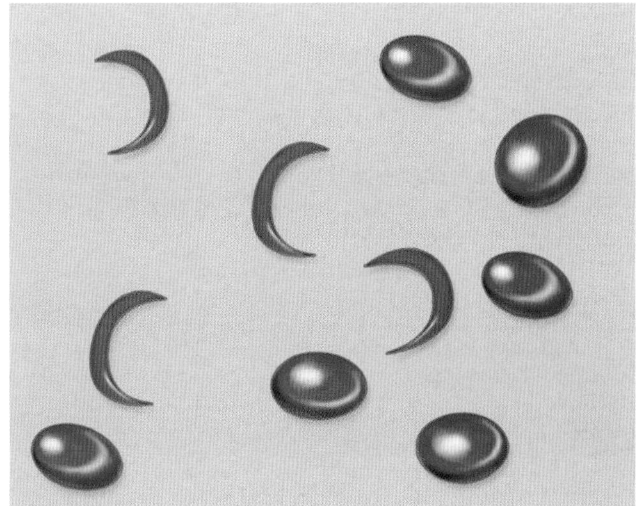

FIGURE 24.7 This peripheral blood smear demonstrates the elongated sickle-shaped red blood cell seen in sickle cell disease.

Figure 24.8 illustrates the inheritance probability with each reproductive event. Infants with SCA are usually asymptomatic until 3 to 4 months of age because Hgb F protects against sickling.

Complications of SCA include recurrent vaso-occlusive pain crises, stroke, sepsis, acute chest syndrome, splenic sequestration, reduced visual acuity related to decreased retinal blood flow, chronic leg ulcers, cholestasis and gallstones, delayed growth and development, delayed puberty, and priapism (the sickled cells prevent blood from flowing out of an erect penis). Children with SCA have an increased incidence of enuresis because the kidneys cannot concentrate urine effectively (Lerma & Vichinsky, 2023). As children reach adulthood, multiple organ dysfunction is common.

Pathophysiology

Significant anemia may occur when the RBCs sickle. Sickling may be triggered by any stress or traumatic

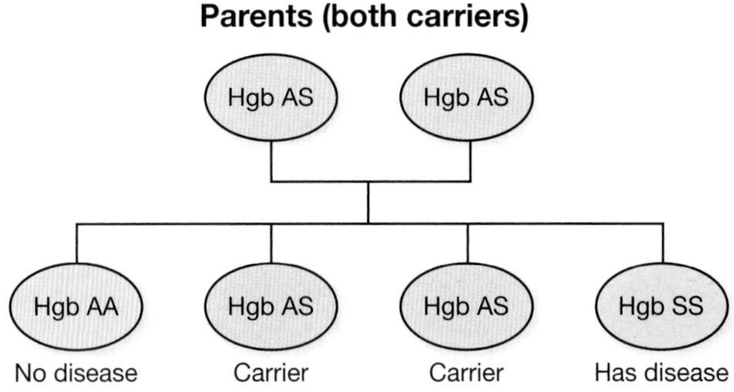

FIGURE 24.8 Simplified genetic scheme for sickle cell disease. *A* denotes adult hemoglobin; *S* denotes sickle hemoglobin. Hemoglobin AA, normal hemoglobin; hemoglobin AS, sickle cell trait; hemoglobin SS, sickle cell disease.

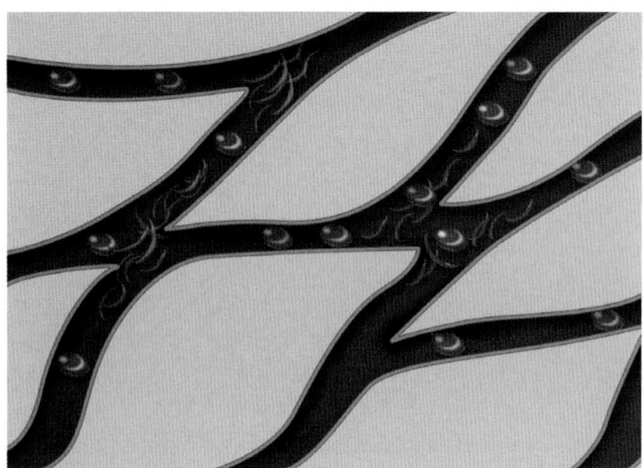

FIGURE 24.9 Clumping of sickle-shaped cells.

event, such as infection, fever, dehydration, physical exertion, excessive cold exposure, or hypoxia (Borhade & Kondamudi, 2022).

As the cells sickle, the blood becomes more viscous because the sickled cells clump together and prevent normal blood flow to the tissues of that area. The sickle-shaped RBCs cannot pass through the smaller capillaries and venules of the circulatory system (Fig. 24.9). This vaso-occlusive process leads to local tissue hypoxia, followed by ischemia and may result in infarction. Pain results as circulation is decreased to the area. Pain can occur in any part of the body but is most common in the joints. Pain causes increased metabolic need by resulting in tachycardia and sometimes tachypnea, which leads to further sickling.

Clumping of cells in the lungs (acute chest syndrome) results in decreased gas exchange, producing hypoxia, which leads to further sickling. Acute chest syndrome and multiorgan failure are the leading common causes of death in children with SCD (Vichinsky, 2023). Sequestration of blood in the spleen leads to splenomegaly and abdominal pain. Hemolysis follows sickling and leads to further anemia. The increased activity of the spleen related to RBC hemolysis leads to splenomegaly, then fibrosis and atrophy. Functional asplenia develops in early childhood (Vichinsky, 2023).

Therapeutic Management

The therapeutic management of children with SCA focuses on preventing vaso-occlusive episodes and infection as well as other complications. Functional asplenia (decrease in the ability of the spleen to function appropriately) places the child at significant risk for serious infection with *Streptococcus pneumoniae* or other encapsulated organisms. Prophylactic antibiotics in the young child and appropriate immunization in all children with SCA can reduce the risk of serious infection (Field & Vichinsky, 2023).

DOSAGE CALCULATION BOX 24.1

Child's weight: 50 lb

Medication order: hydroxyurea 450 mg oral daily

Per the Pediatric Dosage Handbook, the recommended dose is 20 mg/kg/dose, once daily.

Is the ordered dose safe?

Treatment of vaso-occlusive episodes focuses on pain control. Oxygen administration is necessary during episodes of crisis to prevent additional cell sickling. Adequate hydration with intravenous fluids is critical. Close monitoring of Hgb, Hct, and reticulocytes determines the point at which transfusion of PRBCs becomes necessary. Electrolyte analysis is also necessary to ensure that appropriate amounts of electrolytes are present in the serum. When RBCs are administered, there is the potential for hemolysis of the cells, thus increasing the potassium level in the serum. Antibiotic therapy is necessary when infection is present. Box 24.3 describes additional medical treatments that are needed in some children.

Nursing Assessment

Children with SCA experience a significant number of acute and chronic manifestations of the condition (Comparison Chart 24.3). For a full description of the assessment phase of the nursing process, refer to "Clinical Judgment and the Nursing Process" section. Assessment findings pertinent to SCA are discussed in here.

HEALTH HISTORY

Elicit the health history, noting growth and development, frequency and extent of vaso-occlusive crises, past hospitalizations, and treatment for pain crises. Note history of immunizations, including pneumococcal, flu, and meningococcal vaccinations. Determine history

BOX 24.3 Additional Medical Treatments for Some Children With Sickle Cell Anemia

- Cholecystectomy may become necessary if gallstones develop.
- Splenectomy may be performed to prevent recurrence of splenic sequestration if it is life threatening.
- Hydroxyurea increases the percentage of fetal hemoglobin (helping to decrease vaso-occlusive events).
- L-Glutamine in addition to hydroxyurea, or alone, decreases incidence of painful vaso-occlusive episodes.
- Blood transfusions, although not routinely given to children with sickle cell disease, are indicated in children with prolonged or widespread pain, aplastic crisis, or splenic sequestration.
- Partial exchange transfusion may be used to rapidly lower the circulating amount of Hgb SS in the event of stroke or acute chest syndrome.
- HSCT is usually reserved for children with an identical HLA-matched sibling (risk of death and incidence of graft-versus-host disease is high).

Hgb, hemoglobin; HLA, human leukocyte antigen; HSCT, hematopoietic stem cell transplantation.

COMPARISON CHART 24.3 Acute Versus Chronic Manifestations of Sickle Cell Anemia

Acute	Chronic
[a]Acute chest syndrome	Anemia
[a]Aplastic crisis	Avascular necrosis of the hip
[a]Bacterial sepsis or meningitis	Cardiomegaly, functional murmur
Bone infarction	Cholelithiasis
Dactylitis	Delayed growth and development
Hematuria	Delayed puberty
Recurrent pain episodes	Functional asplenia
Pain crisis	Hyposthenuria (low urine specific gravity) and enuresis
[a]Splenic sequestration	Jaundice
[a]Stroke	Leg ulcers
Priapism	Proteinuria [a]Pulmonary hypertension [a]Restrictive lung disease Retinopathy

[a]Often life threatening.

of blood transfusions. Document the current medication regimen. Note history of recurrent infections. Determine history of the present illness that results in a precipitating event, such as hypoxia, infection, or dehydration. Note onset, character, and quality of pain, as well as relieving factors.

PHYSICAL EXAMINATION

Perform a thorough physical examination, because sickling, hypoxia, and tissue ischemia affect most areas of the body (Fig. 24.10). In what follows, note the physical findings discussed that may be detected using inspection, observation, auscultation, and palpation.

Inspection and Observation

Inspect the conjunctivae, palms, and soles for pallor and the skin for pallor, lesions, or ulcers. Note jaundice of the skin or scleral icterus. Document color and moisture of oral mucosa. Measure temperature to evaluate for infection (which can precipitate a sickling crisis). Note blood pressure, which may be decreased with severe anemia or increased with sickle cell nephropathy. Determine baseline mental status. Perform a neurologic assessment frequently, as about 11% of children with SCA will experience an overt stroke (Nuss et al., 2022).

Auscultation

Auscultate heart sounds for a murmur. The heart rate is often elevated with pain, hyperthermia, or dehydration. Listen to breath sounds, noting the rate and depth of respiration as well as the adequacy of aeration. Adventitious breath sounds may be present if a respiratory infection has triggered the sickle cell crisis or in the case of acute chest syndrome. About half of the cases of acute chest syndrome occur in the child already hospitalized for a pain crisis.

Palpation

Palpate the joints for warmth, tenderness, and ROM. Palpate the abdomen for areas of tenderness. Note hepatomegaly or splenomegaly.

CLINICAL REASONING ALERT!

Immediately report symmetric swelling of the hands and feet in the infant or toddler. Termed dactylitis, aseptic infarction occurs in the metacarpals and metatarsals (Fig. 24.11).

LABORATORY AND DIAGNOSTIC TESTING

Newborn screening for SCA is required by law or rule across the United States (CDC, 2023b). Screening by Sickledex or sickle cell prep does not distinguish between SCD and sickle cell trait. If the screening test result indicates the possibility of SCD or sickle cell trait, Hgb electrophoresis is performed promptly to confirm the diagnosis. As the only accurate test for SCD, Hgb electrophoresis will demonstrate the presence of Hgb S and Hgb F only in the young infant; in the older infant or child, the result will be Hgb SS.

Common laboratory and diagnostic studies ordered for the assessment of SCA include:

- Hemoglobin: baseline is usually 7 to 10 mg/dL; will be significantly lower with splenic sequestration, acute chest syndrome, or aplastic crisis
- Reticulocyte count: greatly elevated
- Peripheral blood smear: presence of sickle-shaped cells and target cells
- Platelet count: increased
- Erythrocyte sedimentation rate: elevated
- Abnormal liver function tests with elevated bilirubin

X-ray studies or other scans may be performed to determine the extent of organ or tissue damage resulting from vaso-occlusion.

Nursing Management

Nursing care of the child with SCA focuses on preventing vaso-occlusive crises, providing education to the family and child, managing pain episodes, and providing psychosocial support to the child and family. All children

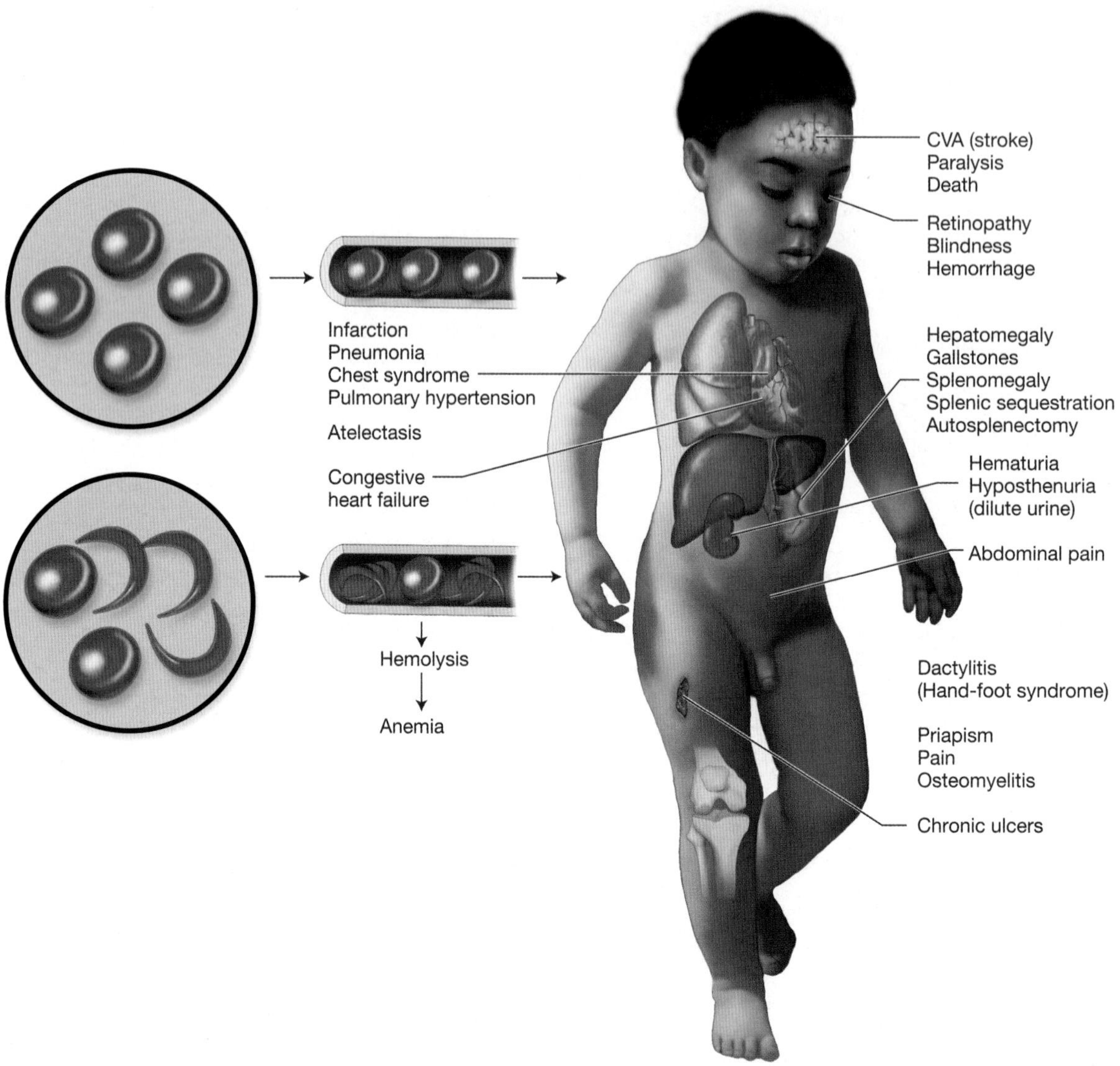

Infarction
Pneumonia
Chest syndrome
Pulmonary hypertension
Atelectasis
Congestive heart failure
Hemolysis
Anemia
CVA (stroke)
Paralysis
Death
Retinopathy
Blindness
Hemorrhage
Hepatomegaly
Gallstones
Splenomegaly
Splenic sequestration
Autosplenectomy
Hematuria
Hyposthenuria (dilute urine)
Abdominal pain
Dactylitis (Hand-foot syndrome)
Priapism
Pain
Osteomyelitis
Chronic ulcers

FIGURE 24.10 Effects of sickle cell anemia on various parts of the body. CVA, cerebrovascular accident

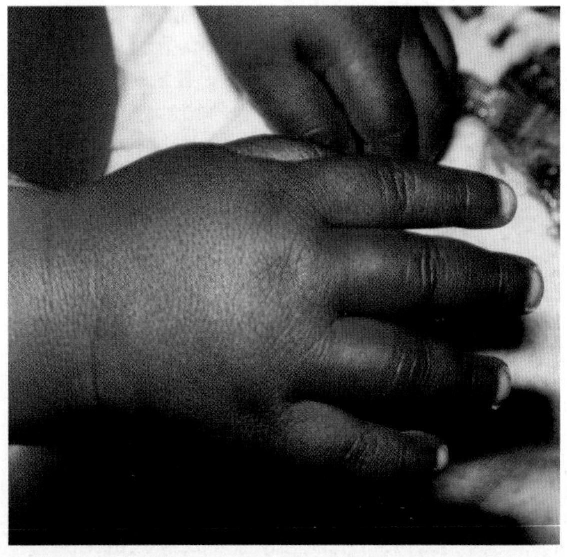

FIGURE 24.11 Swelling of the hands (dactylitis) in a toddler.

with SCA need ongoing evaluation of growth and development to maximize their potential in those areas. Monitor school performance to detect neurodevelopmental problems and seek intervention early. The patient problems and interventions provided in the "Clinical Judgment and the Nursing Process" section should be individualized based on the child's and family's response to the disorder. Specifics related to SCA are discussed further on.

EDUCATING THE FAMILY AND CHILD

Begin child and family education immediately after the diagnosis of SCA is confirmed. Initially, teach the family about the genetics of the disease, and encourage family members to be tested for carrier status. Educate families about the disease process. Emphasize the importance of regularly scheduled health maintenance visits and immunizations. Teach families how to administer prophylactic penicillin for infection prevention and hydroxyurea and/or L-glutamine for prevention of acute pain episodes. Encourage families to seek medical evaluation urgently for any febrile illness. Educate families about how to prevent and recognize vaso-occlusive events (Teaching Guidelines 24.3). Discuss complications such as delayed growth and development, delayed puberty, stroke, cholelithiasis, retinopathy, avascular necrosis, priapism, and leg ulcers.

• • • ATRAUMATIC CARE • • •

Teach the child with SCA age-appropriate distraction and coping skills to assist the child to relieve stress related to their disease and/or recurrent crises.

MANAGING PAIN DURING A VASO-OCCLUSIVE EPISODE

Adequate pain management helps to decrease the child's stress level; elevated stress may contribute to further sickling and additional pain. Initiate pain assessment with a standardized pain scale upon admission. Provide frequent evaluations of pain. Always believe the child's report of pain; only the person suffering the pain knows what it feels like. Moderate to severe pain usually requires opioid medication. To bring the pain under control, initially administer analgesics routinely rather than on an "as needed" (PRN) basis. Once the pain is better managed, medications may be moved to PRN status. Monitor patient-controlled analgesia (PCA) in the child or adolescent. In light of the opioid epidemic concerns, it is important to note that the rate of opioid misuse is lower in individuals with SCD than others with chronic pain syndromes (DeBaun, 2022). Ensure the child is adequately hydrated with hypotonic fluid.

Nonsteroidal antiinflammatory medications and acetaminophen are often used for less severe pain. Use distraction with nonpharmacologic pain management techniques such as relaxation or hypnosis, music, massage, play, guided imagery, therapeutic touch, or behavior modification to augment the pain medication regimen.

TEACHING GUIDELINES 24.3 Prevention or Early Recognition of Vaso-occlusive Events

- Seek immediate attention for ANY febrile illness.
- Obtain vaccinations and penicillin prophylaxis.
- Encourage adequate fluid intake daily.
- Avoid temperatures that are too hot or too cold.
- Avoid overexertion or stress.
- Have 24-hour access to health care provider, nurse practitioner, or facility familiar with sickle cell care.
- Contact medical provider promptly if you suspect a pain crisis is developing.
- Seek medical attention immediately if any of the following develop:
  - Child is pale and listless.
  - Abdominal pain
  - Limp or swollen joints
  - Cough, shortness of breath, chest pain
  - Increasing fatigue
  - Unusual headache, loss of feeling, or sudden weakness
  - Sudden vision change
  - Painful erection that won't go down (priapism)

TAKE NOTE!

Do not use meperidine for pain management during sickle cell crises because multiple dosing has been associated with an increased risk of seizures (DeBaun, 2022).

MANAGING VASO-OCCLUSIVE EPISODES

Treat any underlying conditions such as infection or injury. Deficient fluid volume occurs as a result of decreased intake, increased fluid requirements during vaso-occlusive episode, and the kidney's inability to concentrate urine. Increasing fluid intake will dilute the blood and decrease its viscosity. To promote hemodilution, provide 150 mL/kg of fluids per day or as much as double maintenance, either orally or intravenously. Maintain appropriate electrolyte and pH balance.

Risk of ineffective tissue perfusion related to the effects of RBC sickling and infarction of tissues is another concern. Frequently evaluate respiratory and circulatory status. Encourage incentive spirometry to decrease the incidence of acute chest syndrome. Administer supplemental oxygen if the pulse oximetry reading is 92%; oxygen supplementation in the absence of hypoxia is unnecessary and may inhibit erythropoiesis. Monitor level of consciousness and immediately report changes. See the Healthy People 2030 box.

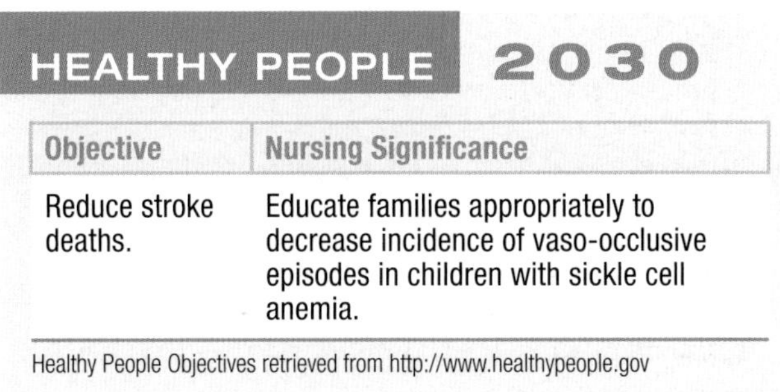

HEALTHY PEOPLE 2030

Objective	Nursing Significance
Reduce stroke deaths.	Educate families appropriately to decrease incidence of vaso-occlusive episodes in children with sickle cell anemia.

Healthy People Objectives retrieved from http://www.healthypeople.gov

PREVENTING INFECTION

To prevent severe infection in the child with SCA, a variety of interventions are necessary. By 2 months of age, begin administration of oral penicillin V potassium as prophylaxis against pneumococcal infection. In the penicillin-allergic child, erythromycin may be used. Continue prophylaxis until at least age 5 years. Administer childhood immunizations according to the currently recommended schedule. To prevent overwhelming sepsis or meningitis as a result of infection with *S. pneumoniae*, the child should receive not only the 7-valent pneumococcal vaccine series in infancy but also the 23-valent pneumococcal conjugate vaccine annually after age 2 years. Meningococcal vaccination is also warranted (refer to Chapter 9 for additional information on these vaccines). Provide influenza immunization annually before the onset of flu season (after 6 months of age) (Field & Vichinsky, 2023).

SUPPORTING THE FAMILY AND CHILD

As with any chronic illness, families of children with SCA need significant support. They often feel guilty or responsible for the disease. Reassure the family and provide education. Refer families to a regional SCD center for multidisciplinary care. See Evidence-Based Practice 24.1.

Thalassemia

Thalassemia is a genetic disorder that most often affects those of African descent, but it also affects individuals of Caribbean, Middle Eastern, South Asian, and Mediterranean descent (Benz & Angelucci, 2022). The genetics of thalassemia are similar to those of SCD in that it is inherited via an autosomal recessive process. Children with thalassemia have reduced production of Hgb.

There are two basic types of thalassemia, alpha and beta. In alpha-thalassemia, synthesis of the alpha chain of the hemoglobin protein is affected. Problems with the beta chain occur more often, and the condition beta-thalassemia can be divided into three subcategories based on severity:

- Thalassemia minor (also called beta-thalassemia trait): leads to mild microcytic anemia; often no treatment is required.
- Thalassemia intermedia: child requires blood transfusions to maintain adequate quality of life.
- Thalassemia major: to survive, the child requires ongoing medical attention, blood transfusions, and iron removal (chelation therapy).

The focus of this discussion will be on beta-thalassemia major (Cooley anemia).

In beta-thalassemia major, the beta-globulin chain in hemoglobin synthesis is reduced or entirely absent. A large number of unstable globulin chains accumulate, causing the RBCs to be rigid and hemolyzed easily. The result is severe hemolytic anemia and chronic hypoxia. In response to the increased rate of RBC destruction, erythroid activity is increased. The increased activity causes massive bone marrow expansion and thinning of the bony cortex. Growth retardation, pathologic fractures, and skeletal deformities (frontal and maxillary bossing) result.

Hemosiderosis (excessive supply of iron) is an additional complication of significant concern. It occurs as a result of rapid hemolysis of RBCs, the decrease in hemoglobin production, and the increased absorption of dietary iron in response to the severely anemic state. The excess iron is deposited in the body's tissues, causing bronze pigmentation of the skin, bony changes, and altered organ function, particularly in the cardiac system. Additional complications include splenomegaly, endocrine abnormalities, osteoporosis, liver and gallbladder

EVIDENCE-BASED PRACTICE 24.1
Comprehensive Clinic for Infants With Sickle Cell Disease

Children with sickle cell disease (SCD) require ongoing comprehensive medical care. Adherence with the medication regimen, infection prevention, and attempts to avoid triggering a vaso-occlusive event are critical to the short- and long-term health of the child. Parents of infants diagnosed with SCD require significant amounts of support and education.

STUDY

In a small convenience sample, parents of 100 children completed a telephone survey in order to determine the impact of the comprehensive clinic for infants with SCD and assess the families' experience with the clinic.

Findings

The results of the survey were mainly positive. One hundred percent of parents reported adherence with penicillin administration, while 78% knew for certain their child had received the meningococcal vaccine. Ninety-eight percent reported knowing to seek care when their child had a fever. A total of 73 of 75 parents participating in group sessions reported feeling comfortable sharing in those sessions, and 95% of parents reported satisfaction with the education received in the clinic.

Nursing Implications

Nurses are in an optimal position to educate and support families of infants with SCD. If high-quality education and support occur early in the child's life, there is potential to decrease the child's morbidity from the disease. Nurses should ensure infants diagnosed with SCD and their families are referred to a comprehensive sickle cell clinic.

Data from Martin, B. M., Thaniel, L. N., Speller-Brown, B. J., & Darbari, D. S. (2018). Comprehensive infant clinic for sickle cell disease: Outcomes and parental perspective. *Journal of Pediatric Health Care, 32*(5), 485–490.

disease, and leg ulcers. Left untreated, beta-thalassemia major is fatal usually by age 5 years, but the use of blood transfusions and chelation therapy has increased the life expectancy of these children (Benz & Angelucci, 2022).

Therapeutic Management

The therapeutic management for children with beta-thalassemia includes monitoring hemoglobin and Hct and transfusing PRBCs at regular intervals. Blood iron levels are also monitored, and iron chelation therapy is provided.

Nursing Assessment

Infants are usually diagnosed by 1 year of age and have a history of pallor, jaundice, failure to thrive, and hepatosplenomegaly (Benz & Angelucci, 2022). Determine the history of the present illness or whether the child is presenting for a routine blood transfusion. Note medications taken at home and any concerns that have arisen since the last visit. Inspect the skin, oral mucosa, conjunctivae, soles, and/or palms for pallor. Note icteric sclerae or jaundice of the skin. Measure weight and height (or length) and plot on an appropriate growth chart. Observe the child for bony deformities and frontal bossing (prominent forehead) (Fig. 24.12). Measure oxygen saturation via pulse oximetry. Evaluate neurologic status, determining level of consciousness and developmental abilities.

Laboratory testing may reveal the following:

- Hemoglobin and Hct are significantly decreased.
- Peripheral blood smear shows prominence of target cells, hypochromia, microcytosis, and extensive **anisocytosis** and **poikilocytosis** (variation in the size and shape of the RBCs, respectively).
- Bilirubin levels are elevated.
- Hgb electrophoresis shows the presence of Hgb F and Hgb A_2 only.
- Iron level is elevated.

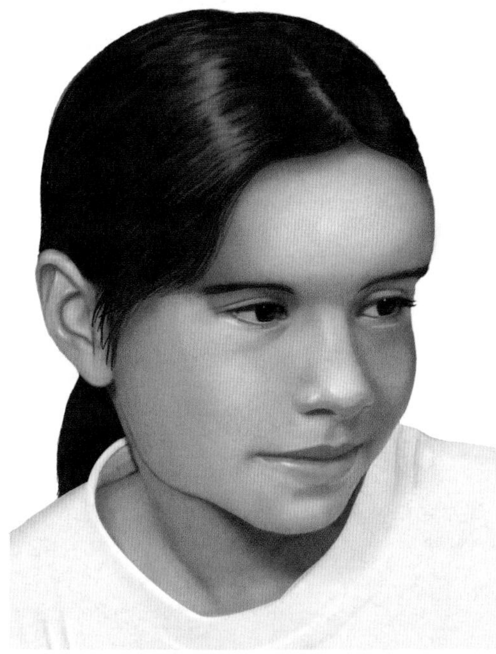

FIGURE 24.12 Iron overload related to thalassemia leads to bony changes such as frontal bossing and maxillary prominence.

Nursing Management

The nursing care of the child with thalassemia is primarily aimed at supporting the family and minimizing the effects of the illness. This includes administering blood transfusions and educating the family.

ADMINISTERING PACKED RBC TRANSFUSIONS

Administer PRBC transfusions as prescribed to maintain an adequate level of hemoglobin for oxygen delivery to the tissues and to suppress erythrocytosis in the bone marrow. Monitor for reactions to the transfusions.

Excess iron is removed by chelation therapy. Administer the chelating agent deferoxamine with the transfusion. Deferoxamine binds to the iron and allows it to be removed through the stool or urine. Oral deferasirox may also be prescribed and is generally well tolerated, with minimal GI side effects.

EDUCATING THE FAMILY

Educate the child and family about the recommended regimen. Ensure that families understand that adhering to the prescribed blood transfusion and chelation therapy schedule is essential to the child's survival. Chelation therapy must be maintained at home to continuously decrease the iron levels in the body. Teach family members to administer deferoxamine subcutaneously with a small battery-powered infusion pump over a period of several hours each night (usually while the child is sleeping). If oral deferasirox is prescribed, instruct the family to dissolve the tablet in juice or water and administer it once daily.

TAKE NOTE!

Have parents provide return demonstration of subcutaneous infusion of deferoxamine to ensure accuracy and independence in the home environment.

Refer the family for genetic counseling and family support as needed. A good resource for families of children with thalassemia is the Cooley's Anemia Foundation. A group of young adults with Cooley anemia started the Thalassemia Action Group (TAG) (a subgroup of the Cooley's Anemia Foundation) to provide a forum for communication and information, promote a positive outlook on living with the disease, and raise awareness on the importance of continuing therapy for the disease.

TAG is part of the Cooley's Anemia Foundation website, and more information about the group can be found by calling (360) 860–2023.

• • • ATRAUMATIC CARE • • •

When a child is receiving blood transfusion every few weeks, they must experience at least two venipunctures each time, one for the type and cross-match and other relevant laboratory tests on the day before transfusion and another for the intravenous (IV) insertion for the actual transfusion. Minimize trauma by teaching the parent to apply EMLA (eutectic mixture of local anesthetic) cream at home just before leaving for the blood draw or transfusion appointment.

Glucose-6-Phosphate Dehydrogenase Deficiency

Glucose-6-phosphate dehydrogenase (G6PD) is an enzyme that is responsible for maintaining the integrity of RBCs by protecting them from oxidative substances. G6PD deficiency is an X-linked recessive disorder that occurs when the RBCs have insufficient G6PD or the enzyme is abnormal and does not function properly. The RBCs are then affected by oxidative stress more easily. Triggers that may result in oxidative stress and hemolysis include bacterial or viral illness or exposure to certain substances such as medications (e.g., sulfonamides, sulfones, malaria-fighting drugs [such as quinine], or methylene blue [for treating urinary tract infections]), naphthalene (an agent in mothballs), or fava beans.

G6PD deficiency occurs most commonly in children of African, Mediterranean, or Asian descent (Nuss et al., 2022). Complications include prolonged neonatal jaundice and life-threatening acute episodes of hemolysis. Therapeutic management is primarily aimed at avoiding triggers that cause oxidative stress.

Nursing Assessment

Note health history, including fatigue. Determine the parents' understanding of the disorder and the medications and foods to avoid. Inspect the skin for pallor or jaundice. Evaluate neurologic status, which may also be affected. Measure heart rate and respiratory rate, noting elevations. Determine oxygen saturation via pulse oximeter or blood gas analysis. Note tea-colored urine. Palpate the abdomen for splenomegaly. Laboratory studies will reveal anemia.

Nursing Management

Administer oxygen and treat the symptoms. Once the triggering agent is removed or the child recovers from an illness, the child will improve. Provide further education to the child and family about triggers, and advise them that the child should avoid contact with these agents.

CLOTTING DISORDERS

Clotting of blood is a process that occurs after injury. The blood clotting system requires certain factors in the blood and platelets to perform adequately. Individuals with deficiencies of these factors or platelets tend to bleed; they do not bleed more easily than people without these conditions, but it is just more difficult for the clot to form, and bleeding cannot be stopped easily. Factors that are most often involved in problems with clotting include factor VIII, factor IX, and factor XI. Each plays a role in clot formation. Platelets also play a role in the clotting cascade and are necessary for clot formation. Some processes can lead to destruction of the platelets and may lead to a reduction in clotting. Bleeding times are prolonged when a clotting disorder is present. Table 24.5 provides usual values for clotting studies.

Conditions affecting clotting include immune thrombocytopenia (ITP), immunoglobulin A vasculitis, disseminated intravascular coagulation (DIC), and factor deficiencies such as hemophilia A (factor VIII deficiency), von Willebrand disease (vWD), hemophilia B (Christmas disease, factor IX deficiency), and hemophilia C (factor XI deficiency). Table 24.6 reviews the expected levels of proteins involved in coagulation.

Immune Thrombocytopenia

ITP is thought to be an immune response following a viral infection that produces antiplatelet antibodies. These antibodies destroy platelets, which then lead to the development of petechiae, purpura, and excessive bruising. Petechiae are pinpoint hemorrhages that occur anywhere on the body and do not blanch to pressure (Fig. 24.13).

TABLE 24.5 • Clotting Studies

Test	Measure
Prothrombin time (PT)	11.0–13.0 seconds (may vary by laboratory)
Partial thromboplastin time (PTT), activated partial thromboplastin time (aPTT)	21–35 seconds
International normalized ratio (INR) (used to evaluate coagulation)	2.0–3.0 usual target in thromboembolic conditions

Data from Fischbach, F. T., Fischbach, M. A., & Stout, K. (2022). *A manual of laboratory and diagnostic tests* (11th ed.). Wolters Kluwer Health.

TABLE 24.6 • Select Proteins Involved in Coagulation (Factors)

Protein	Synonym	Concentration in Plasma (mg/dL)
Fibrinogen	Factor I	200–400
Factor II	Prothrombin	10–15
Factor V	Proaccelerin; labile factor	0.5–1.0
Factor VII	Stable factor; proconvertin	0.2
Factor VIIIC	Antihemophilic factor; platelet cofactor I	1.0–2.0
Factor IX	Christmas factor; plasma thromboplastin component	0.3–0.4
Factor X	Stuart–Prower factor	0.6–0.8
Factor XI	Plasma thromboplastin antecedent	0.4
Factor XII	Hageman factor	2.9
Factor XIII	Fibrin-stabilizing factor; Laki–Lorand factor	2.5
Von Willebrand factor	Factor VIII–related antigen (VIII: VWD)	1.0

VWD, Von Willebrand disease.

Data from Fischbach, F. T., Fischbach, M. A., & Stout, K. (2022). *A manual of laboratory and diagnostic tests* (11th ed.). Wolters Kluwer Health.

Purpura are larger areas of hemorrhage in which blood collects under the tissues; they are purplish (see Fig. 24.13). ITP may develop within a few weeks after a viral infection. It is most common in young children, and most will recover spontaneously within a few months (Bussell, 2022a). Complications include severe hemorrhage, bleeding into vital organs, and intracranial hemorrhage, although these rarely occur.

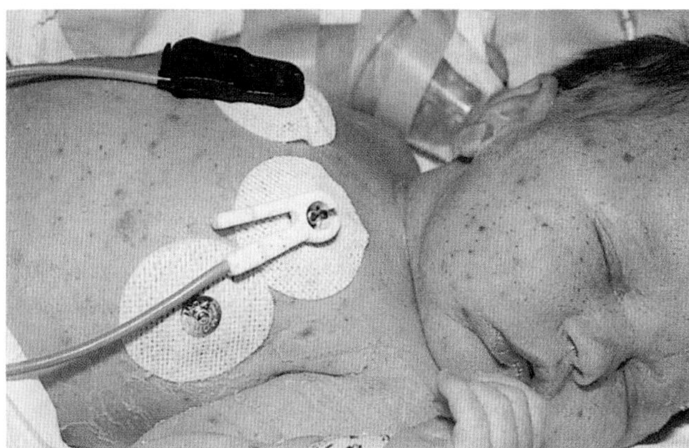

FIGURE 24.13 Pinpoint hemorrhages (petechiae) and large purplish areas of discoloration (purpura) in an infant with idiopathic thrombocytopenia purpura (ITP).

First-line treatment of ITP includes the use of corticosteroids and intravenous immunoglobulin (IVIG) (Bussell, 2022b). Platelet transfusions are not indicated unless life-threatening bleeding is present. ITP is usually self-limiting, but if it persists for a year or longer, splenectomy may be indicated.

Nursing Assessment

Elicit the child's health history (usually a previously healthy child who has recently developed increased bruising, epistaxis, or bleeding of the gums). Note history of blood in the stool. Note risk factors such as recent viral illness, recent measles, mumps, and rubella (MMR) immunization, or ingestion of medications that can cause thrombocytopenia. Inspect for petechiae, purpura, and bruising, which may progress rapidly within the first 24 to 48 hours of the illness. Document the size and location of each lesion. Inspect the lips and buccal mucosa for petechiae. The remainder of the physical examination is usually within normal limits.

Usual laboratory findings include an extremely low platelet count (less than 50,000), normal WBC count and differential, and Hgb and Hct unless hemorrhage has occurred (this is rare). Bone marrow aspiration may be performed to rule out leukemia.

Nursing Management

Many children require no medical treatment except observation and reevaluation of laboratory values. Educate the family about avoiding aspirin, nonsteroidal antiinflammatory drugs (NSAIDs), and antihistamines because these medications may precipitate the development of anemia in these children. The use of acetaminophen for pain control is more appropriate when necessary. Teach the family to prevent trauma by avoiding activities that may cause injury, such as contact sports. Instead, encourage activities, such as swimming, that provide physical activity with less risk of trauma. Explain to parents the signs and symptoms of serious bleeding and whom to call if it is suspected.

Immunoglobulin A Vasculitis (Henoch–Schönlein Purpura)

Immunoglobulin A vasculitis is a condition that affects mostly male young children and develops in association with a viral or bacterial infection (most often respiratory) (Nuss et al., 2022). The classic presentation is vasculitis with immunoglobulin A (IgA)–dominant immune deposits affecting small vessels. These small vessels are generally in the skin, gut, and kidney. In most children, the course of the disease is benign, and the prognosis is good. In a few children, however, ongoing nephrotic syndrome may occur as a result of kidney injury, and those children may have hypertension. Pulmonary, cardiac, and neurologic complications can also occur.

No specific treatment exists for IgA vasculitis since most of the cases resolve without treatment. Treatment with corticosteroids, such as prednisone, may be helpful in children with severe joint or GI manifestations (Nuss et al., 2022). If kidney injury occurs, children may require kidney function testing and evaluation for hypertension and treatment when present.

Nursing Assessment

Note history of viral or bacterial infection. Determine the onset of the complaint and how it has progressed or changed. Note history of joint or abdominal pain. Measure blood pressure. Inspect the skin for a purpuric palpable rash, and document the size and location of lesions. Palpate the rash to determine its extent (Fig. 24.14). Gently palpate the joints for tenderness. Palpate the abdomen for tenderness. Note visible or occult blood in the stool. Note cherry- or tea-colored urine, indicating the presence of blood in the urine; urinalysis can verify the amount of blood present in the urine. Serum IgA levels may be elevated.

Nursing Management

Treatment of the symptoms is the focus. In children with severe joint or abdominal pain, administer analgesics as prescribed, and note the response to pain medications. If the child has normal kidney function, maintaining hydration is the most important intervention. Monitor intake and output. Note the color of urine. Administer corticosteroids and anticoagulants, alone or together, if ordered to reduce kidney impairment. Teach the child and family about the therapy, such as management of hypertension with medications, and sodium restriction. Teach them about signs of kidney injury, such as blood in the urine and changes in weight, as well as frequency and volume of urine output.

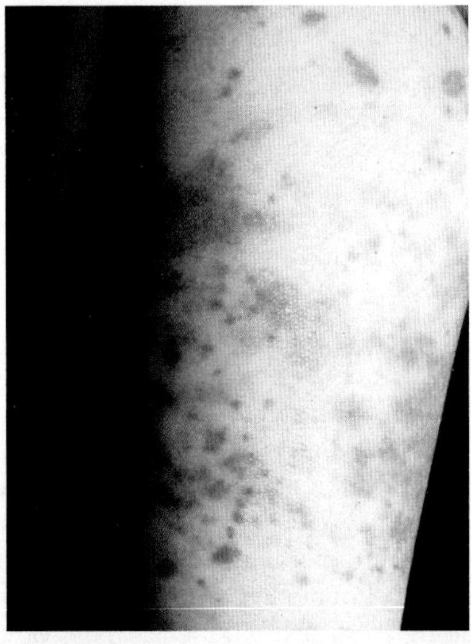

FIGURE 24.14 Palpable purpura on an adolescent's arm.

Disseminated Intravascular Coagulation

DIC is a complex condition that leads to activation of coagulation; it usually occurs in critically ill children. Common triggers of DIC include septic shock, presence of endotoxins and viruses, tissue necrosis or injury, and cancer treatment (Nuss et al., 2022). In DIC, thrombin is generated, fibrin is deposited in the circulation, and platelets are consumed. Deficiencies of coagulation and anticoagulation pathways occur. Hemorrhage and organ tissue damage result and can be irreversible if not recognized and treated immediately.

Therapeutic management of children with DIC requires careful consideration of the etiology. Initial treatment focuses on treating the underlying cause. For example, if DIC occurs secondary to an infection, appropriate antibiotics would be used to treat the infection. Heparin is also used at lower doses to counteract the deficiency in the coagulation/anticoagulation pathway. Heparin reduces consumption of the platelets, resulting in improved platelet counts. Since heparin is an anticoagulant, there is an increased risk of bleeding.

Nursing Assessment

Because DIC occurs as a secondary condition, it may occur in a child hospitalized for any reason. DIC may affect any body system, so a thorough physical examination is warranted. Inspect for signs of bleeding such as petechiae or purpura, blood in the urine or stool, or persistent oozing from venipuncture or from the umbilical cord in the newborn. Evaluate respiratory status, and determine the level of tissue oxygenation via pulse oximetry. Perform a complete circulatory assessment and note signs of circulatory collapse such as poor perfusion, tachycardia, prolonged capillary refill, and weak distal pulses. Note altered level of consciousness and decreased urine output. Careful abdominal palpation may reveal hepatomegaly or splenomegaly.

Laboratory testing may reveal prolonged prothrombin time (PT), partial thromboplastin time (PTT), activated partial thromboplastin time (aPTT), bleeding time, and thrombin time and decreased levels of fibrinogen; platelets; clotting factors II, V, VIII, and X; and antithrombin III. Increases will be noted in levels of fibrinolysin, fibrinopeptide A, positive fibrin split products, and D-dimers.

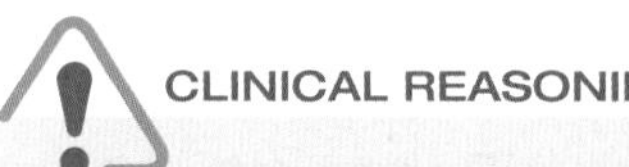

CLINICAL REASONING ALERT!

Diagnostic tests that indicate the development of DIC include increased fibrinogen/fibrin degradation products, decreased antithrombin III, increased fibrinopeptide A level, and an increased D-dimer assay.

Nursing Management

Continue to provide nursing care related to the triggering event. Assess the child's status frequently. If bleeding is observed, apply pressure to the area along with cold compresses. Elevate the affected body part if this does not affect the child's overall stability. If neurologic deficits are assessed, report the findings immediately so that treatment to prevent permanent damage can be started. Administer anticoagulation therapy (even though hemorrhage is a concern) to interrupt the coagulation process that is present in this condition. Provide ventilatory support as needed and provide continuous cardiac monitoring. Administer clotting factors, platelets, and cryoprecipitate as prescribed to prevent severe hemorrhage. Report changes in laboratory values to the health care provider or nurse practitioner. Changes can occur rapidly, and vigilance is necessary to prevent further tissue damage to the affected system.

Hemophilia

Hemophilia is a group of X-linked recessive disorders that result in deficiency in one of the coagulation factors in the blood. X-linked recessive disorders are transmitted by carrier female parents to their male children, so usually, only males are affected by hemophilia. The coagulation factors in the blood are essential for clot formation either spontaneously or from an injury, and when factors are absent, bleeding will be difficult to stop. There are several types of hemophilia, including factor VIII deficiency (hemophilia A), factor IX deficiency or Christmas disease (hemophilia B), and factor XI deficiency (hemophilia C). The most common, hemophilia A, will be the focus of this discussion (Nuss et al., 2022). Hemophilia A occurs when there is a deficiency of factor VIII in an individual. Factor VIII is essential in the activation of factor X, which is required for the conversion of prothrombin into thrombin, resulting in an inability of the platelets to be used in clot formation.

Hemophilia is classified according to the severity of the disease, ranging from mild to severe. The more severe the disease, the more likely it is that there will be bleeding episodes. When bleeding occurs, the vessels constrict and a platelet plug forms, but because of the deficient factor, the fibrin will not solidify and thus bleeding continues.

Therapeutic Management

The primary goal of managing hemophilia is to prevent bleeding. This is best accomplished by instructing the child to avoid activities with a high potential for injury (e.g., football, riding motorcycles, skateboarding). Instead, encourage the child to participate in activities with the least amount of contact (e.g., swimming, running, tennis). Limiting activities does not mean the child should do nothing; activities that promote health without increased exposure to injury are best.

If bleeding or injury occurs, factor administration is prescribed; this practice has been common in outpatient facilities or the child's home for many years. Once the deficient factor is replaced, clotting factors return to fairly normal levels for a period of time. Factor replacement should be given before any surgeries or other procedures that can lead to bleeding, such as intramuscular injections and dental care.

TAKE NOTE!

The Food and Drug Administration has approved a new long-acting form of factor XIII replacement to be used as routine prophylaxis for bleeding (Antihemophilic Factor (Recombinant), Fc-VWF-XTEN Fusion Protein-ehtl [ALTUVIIIO]) (Sanofi, 2023).

Nursing Assessment

For a full description of the assessment phase of the nursing process, refer to the "Clinical Judgment and the Nursing Process" section. Assessment findings pertinent to hemophilia in children are discussed further on.

HEALTH HISTORY

Elicit the health history, determining the nature of the bleeding episode or bruise. Include in the history any hemorrhagic episodes in other systems, such as the GI tract (e.g., black tarry stools, hematemesis) or caused by injury resulting in joint hemorrhage, or hematuria (Fig. 24.15). Inquire about length of bleeding and amount of blood loss. Because hemophilia A results in difficulty with clotting, the child may bleed for a longer period when injury occurs.

PHYSICAL EXAMINATION

Focus the physical examination on identification of any bleeding. This is of particular concern after injury, but a nosebleed or other spontaneous bleed can occur if factor levels are extremely low. Assess circulation by evaluating pulses and heart sounds if severe or prolonged bleeding is identified. Without intervention, hypovolemia could follow, leading to shock. Note chest pain or abdominal pain, which may indicate internal bleeding. Report these

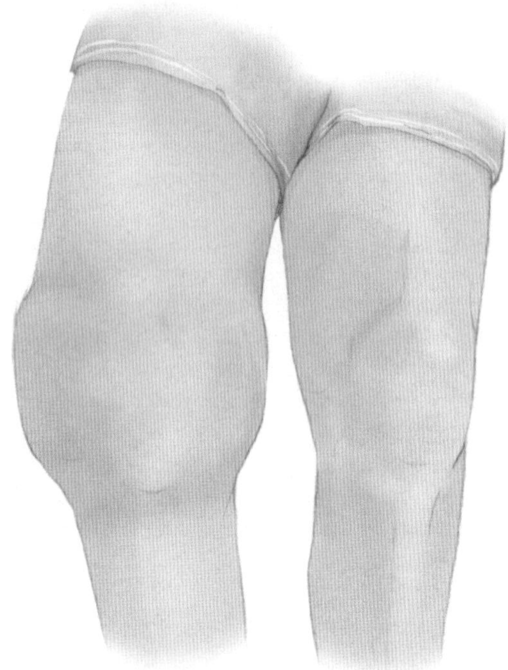

FIGURE 24.15 Significant swelling and discoloration associated with a bleeding episode in the knee of a person with hemophilia.

findings immediately so that the underlying condition can be diagnosed and treated rapidly.

LABORATORY AND DIAGNOSTIC TESTING

Laboratory findings may include decreased hemoglobin and Hct if bleeding is prolonged or severe. Factor levels may be quantified with blood testing.

Nursing Management

Nursing management includes preventing bleeding episodes, managing bleeding episodes, and providing education and support.

PREVENTING BLEEDING EPISODES

All children with hemophilia should attempt to prevent bleeding episodes. Recurrent bleeding into the joints (hemarthroses) may cause joint destruction, thereby limiting ROM and function over the long term (Nuss et al., 2022). Teach children and families that regular physical activity or exercise helps to keep the muscles and joints stronger and that children with stronger joints and muscles have fewer bleeding episodes (see Teaching Guidelines 24.4). Refer the child with moderate to severe hemophilia to a pediatric hematologist and/or a comprehensive hemophilia treatment center.

MANAGING A BLEEDING EPISODE

Administer factor VIII replacement as prescribed. Factor replacement is pooled from multiple blood donors, so families may be concerned about transmission of viruses via the product (specifically, hepatitis and human immunodeficiency virus [HIV]). Several methods of viral inactivation (solvent detergent, dry heat, and monoclonal purification) have been used to treat plasma-derived factors to eliminate the risk of HIV transmission via factor infusion (National Hemophilia Foundation [NHF], 2023).

Administer factor replacement by slow IV push. Document the product name, number of units, lot number, and expiration date. Doses are based on the severity of the bleeding and the weight of the child. Specific dosing guidelines can be obtained from the product insert. In mild cases of hemophilia A, desmopressin may be effective in stopping bleeding (see the nursing management section of VWD for additional information).

If external bleeding develops, apply pressure to the area until bleeding stops. If it is inside a joint, apply ice or cold compresses to the area and elevate any injured extremities, except when contraindicated by further injury. Make sure that all cases of bleeding are followed up to identify whether factor replacement is necessary.

TEACHING GUIDELINES 24.4 Preventing Bleeding in the Child With Hemophilia

- Protect toddlers with soft helmets, padding on the knees, carpets in the home, and softened or covered corners.
- Children should stay active: swimming, baseball, basketball, and bicycling (wearing a helmet) are good physical activities.
- Avoid intense contact sports such as football, wrestling, soccer, and high diving.
- Avoid trampoline use and riding all-terrain vehicles (ATVs).
- Arrange premedication with Amicar if oral surgery is indicated.

PROVIDING EDUCATION

Inform the family that the child should wear a medical alert bracelet. Families should notify the school nurse and teachers of the child's diagnosis and share precautions with them. Instruct all school personnel to call the parent immediately if the child sustains a head, abdominal, or orbit injury at school. Teach parents and caregivers how to administer the intravenous infusion of factor VIII. Administration in the home is the preferred method for factor infusion, as the child will be able to receive treatment in the most timely and efficient manner when a bleeding episode occurs. Alternatives to the parent giving the infusion are to arrange for a home care nursing visit or for the family to keep their own supply of factor VIII that they take to the local emergency room for infusion if bleeding occurs.

Involve children as developmentally appropriate in the infusion process. Young children may hold and apply the Band-Aid; older children may assist with dilution and mixing of the factor. Teach adolescents to administer their own factor infusions. Children with severe hemophilia may need factor infusions so often that implantation of a central venous access port is warranted. Teach the family access, care, and flushing of the implanted port.

TAKE NOTE!

Require a return demonstration of intravenous factor infusion by the parents to ensure independence in the home environment, as well as accuracy of infusion.

THINKING ABOUT DEVELOPMENT

Toby Henderson is an 18-month-old male with a history of moderate hemophilia. He is a very active child.

Considering Toby's developmental stage, how will his diagnosis impact his ability to accomplish toddler developmental milestones?

Develop a teaching plan for Toby's parents related to safety for Toby. Incorporate age-appropriate activities that would be safe for Toby in the plan.

How would the safety plan be different if Toby were 13 years old?

PROVIDING SUPPORT

Children with hemophilia may be able to lead a fairly normal life, with the exception of avoiding a few activities. However, accepting the diagnosis of a bleeding disorder in their child is very difficult for parents. They fear the worst (bleeding that won't stop) as well as complications such as infection with bloodborne viruses. Reassure parents that since factor replacement began to be treated, there have been no reports of HIV transmission from factor infusion. Educate and support the parents. Factor replacement is expensive, and bleeding episodes often cause parents to miss work, both of which create financial strains. Refer families to the NHF and NHF Youthworld, which offer support, education, youth leadership, scholarships, and a directory of camps for children with hemophilia and other bleeding disorders.

Von Willebrand Disease

vWD is a genetically transmitted bleeding disorder that may affect any sex or race. The disorder is a deficiency in von Willebrand factor (vWF). Under ordinary circumstances, vWF serves two functions: to bind with factor VIII, protecting it from breakdown, and to serve as the "glue" that attaches platelets to the site of injury. Deficiency in this factor results in a mild bleeding disorder. Children with vWD bruise easily, have frequent nosebleeds (epistaxis), and tend to bleed after oral surgery. Pubescent females often have menorrhagia.

Therapeutic management of vWD is similar to that of hemophilia. Prevention of injury is important. When bleeding or injury does occur, vWF is administered. Desmopressin may also be used to release the factors necessary for clotting. Desmopressin raises the plasma level from stores in the endothelium of blood vessels; this releases factor VIII and vWF from these stores into the bloodstream. These may also be administered before dental work or surgery.

Nursing Assessment

Nursing assessment of the child with vWD is similar to the assessment of the child with hemophilia, although severe bleeding occurs much less frequently.

Nursing Management

Nursing management is also similar to the management of the child with hemophilia. The major difference is the administration of desmopressin. Administer desmopressin nasal spray as prescribed when a bleeding episode occurs. Desmopressin may also be given via an intravenous infusion or subcutaneously (less common). Stimate is the only brand of desmopressin nasal spray that is used for controlling bleeding; the other brands are used for homeostasis and enuresis. Desmopressin is an antidiuretic hormone, so closely monitor fluid balance. Twenty-four hours should elapse between doses, as lessening of the response (tachyphylaxis) occurs with more frequent use (James, 2023). vWD may also be treated with intravenous infusion of vWF, similarly to factor VIII infusion for hemophilia A. Teach children and their families how to avoid or minimize bleeding episodes (see Teaching Guidelines 24.4).

LEUKEMIA

Leukemia is a primary disorder of the bone marrow in which the normal elements are replaced with abnormal WBCs. Normally, lymphoid cells grow and develop into lymphocytes, and myeloid cells grow and develop into RBCs, granulocytes, monocytes, and platelets. Leukemia may develop at any time during the usual stages of normal lymphoid or myeloid development.

Leukemia may be classified as acute or chronic, lymphocytic, or myelogenous. Acute leukemias are rapidly progressive diseases affecting the undifferentiated or immature cells; the result is cells without normal function. Chronic leukemias progress more slowly, permitting maturation and differentiation of cells so that they retain some of their normal function. Acute leukemias, including ALL and acute myelogenous leukemia (AML), occur much more commonly in children and adolescents than do chronic leukemias (Keating et al., 2022). Therefore, they will be the focus of the discussion that follows.

Complications of leukemia include **metastasis** (spread of cancer to other sites) to the blood, bone, CNS, spleen, liver, or other organs and alterations in growth. Late effects include problems with neurocognitive function and ocular, cardiovascular, or thyroid dysfunction. With advances in treatment over the past 50 years, most cases of childhood leukemia are curable. However, children who experience relapse or present with advanced disease have a poorer prognosis (Keating et al., 2022).

Acute Lymphoblastic Leukemia

ALL is the most common form of cancer in children. Eighty-five percent of cases of ALL occur in children between 2 and 10 years of age (Keating et al., 2022). It is more common in White children than in other races. ALL is classified according to the type of cells involved—T cell, B cell, early pre-B cell, or pre-B cell. Most children will achieve initial remission if appropriate treatment is given. The overall cure rate of ALL is over 70% (Keating et al., 2022).

Prognosis is based on the WBC count at diagnosis, the type of cytogenetic factors and immunophenotype, the age at diagnosis, and the extent of extramedullary involvement. Generally, the higher the WBC count at diagnosis, the worse the prognosis. Children between 1 and 9 years of age and with a WBC count of less than 50,000 at diagnosis have the best prognosis. When a child experiences a relapse, the prognosis becomes poorer. Complications include infection, hemorrhage, poor growth, and CNS, bone, or testicular involvement.

Pathophysiology

The exact cause of ALL remains unknown. Genetic factors and chromosome abnormalities may play a role in its development. In ALL, abnormal lymphoblasts abound in the blood-forming tissues. The lymphoblasts are fragile and immature, lacking the infection-fighting capabilities of the normal WBC. The growth of lymphoblasts is excessive, and the abnormal cells replace the normal cells in the bone marrow. The proliferating leukemic cells demonstrate massive metabolic needs, depriving normal body cells of needed nutrients and resulting in fatigue, weight loss or growth arrest, and muscle wasting. The bone marrow becomes unable to maintain normal levels of RBCs, WBCs, and platelets, so anemia, neutropenia, and thrombocytopenia result. As the bone marrow expands or the leukemic cells infiltrate the bone, joint and bone pain may occur. The leukemic cells may permeate the lymph nodes, causing diffuse lymphadenopathy, or the liver and spleen, resulting in hepatosplenomegaly. With spread to the CNS, vomiting, headache, seizures, coma, vision alterations, or cranial nerve palsies may occur (Keating et al., 2022).

CLINICAL REASONING ALERT!

Changes in behavior or personality, headache, irritability, dizziness, persistent nausea or vomiting, seizures, gait changes, lethargy, or altered level of consciousness may indicate CNS infiltration with leukemic cells. Immediately report these findings to the pediatric oncologist.

Therapeutic Management

Therapeutic management of the child with ALL focuses on giving chemotherapy to eradicate the leukemic cells and restore normal bone marrow function. Treatment is divided into three stages. CNS prophylaxis is provided at each stage in order to prevent metastasis to the CNS (Keating et al., 2022). The length of treatment and choice of medications are based on the child's age, risk category, and subtype determined by bone marrow analysis. Table 24.7 discusses the stages of leukemia treatment. For relapsed or less responsive leukemia, HSCT may be necessary.

Nursing Assessment

For a full description of the assessment phase of the nursing process, refer to the "Clinical Judgment and

TABLE 24.7 • Stages of Leukemia Treatment

Stage	Purpose	Length	Usual Medications
Induction	Rapid induction of complete remission	3–4 weeks	Oral steroids, IV vincristine, IM L-asparaginase, daunomycin (high risk)
Consolidation (intensification)	Strengthen remission, reduce leukemic cell burden	Varies	High-dose methotrexate, 6-mercaptopurine; possibly cyclophosphamide, cytarabine, asparaginase, thioguanine, epipodophyllotoxins
Maintenance	Eliminate all residual leukemic cells	2–3 years	Low dose: daily 6-mercaptopurine, weekly methotrexate, intermittent IV vincristine, and oral steroids
CNS prophylaxis	Reduce risk of development of CNS disease	Given periodically in all stages	Intrathecal chemotherapy; cranial radiation is used infrequently.

CNS, central nervous system; IM, intramuscular; IV, intravenous.

Data from Keating, A. K., Knight-Perry, J., Maloney, K., Levy, J. M. M., Greffe, B. S., Franklin, A. R. K., & Garrington, T. P. (2022). Chapter 31: Neoplastic disease. In M. Bunik, W. W. Hay, M. J. Levin, & M. J. Abzug (Eds.), *Current diagnosis & treatment: Pediatrics* (26th ed., pp. 931–963). McGraw-Hill Education; Horton, T. M., & McNeer, J. L. (2022). Treatment of acute lymphoblastic leukemia/lymphoma in children and adolescents. *UpToDate*. Retrieved on April, 26, 2023, from https://www.uptodate.com/contents/overview-of-the-treatment-of-acute-lymphoblastic-leukemia-in-children -and-adolescents

the Nursing Process" section. Assessment findings pertinent to ALL are discussed further on.

HEALTH HISTORY

Elicit a description of the present illness and chief complaint. Common signs and symptoms reported during the health history might include:

- Fever (may be persistent or recurrent, with unknown cause)
- Recurrent infection
- Fatigue, malaise, or listlessness
- Pallor
- Unusual bleeding or bruising
- Abdominal pain
- Nausea or vomiting
- Bone pain
- Headache (Keating et al., 2022)

Explore the child's current and past medical history for risk factors such as:

- Male sex
- Age 2 to 5 years
- White race
- Down syndrome (and many other genetic syndromes)
- Sibling with leukemia
- Radiation exposure
- Previous chemotherapy treatment American Cancer Society, 2024d

Determine the child's history of varicella zoster immunization or disease. Chickenpox infection in the leukemic child may lead to disseminated, overwhelming infection.

PHYSICAL EXAMINATION

Take the child's temperature (fever may be present), and look for petechiae, purpura, or unusual bruising (due to decreased platelet levels). Inspect the skin for signs of infection. Auscultate the lungs, noting adventitious breath sounds, which may indicate pneumonia (present at diagnosis or due to immunosuppression during treatment). Note location and size of enlarged lymph nodes. Palpate the liver and spleen for enlargement. Document tenderness on abdominal palpation.

TAKE NOTE!

Have the child lie flat for 30 minutes after a lumbar puncture, and increase fluid intake for 24 hours after the procedure to decrease incidence of headache.

LABORATORY AND DIAGNOSTIC TESTS

Common laboratory and diagnostic studies ordered for the assessment of ALL include:

- CBC: abnormal findings include low hemoglobin and Hct; decreased RBC count; decreased platelet count; and elevated, normal, or decreased WBC count
- Peripheral blood smear may reveal blasts.
- Bone marrow aspiration: stained smear from bone marrow aspiration will show greater than 25% lymphoblasts. Bone marrow aspirate is also examined for immunophenotyping (lymphoid versus myeloid and level of cancer cell maturity) and cytogenetic analysis (determines abnormalities in chromosome number and structure). Immunophenotyping and cytogenetic analysis are used in the classification of the leukemia, which helps guide treatment.
- Lumbar puncture will reveal whether leukemic cells have infiltrated the CNS.
- Liver function tests and blood urea nitrogen (BUN) and creatinine levels determine liver and kidney function, which, if abnormal, may preclude treatment with certain chemotherapeutic agents.
- Chest radiography may reveal pneumonia or a mediastinal mass.

ATRAUMATIC CARE

The child with leukemia undergoes frequent implantable port accesses for blood draws and chemotherapy, bone marrow aspirations for assessment of blood cell status, and lumbar punctures for laboratory studies and intrathecal medication administration. To decrease trauma produced by these repetitive painful procedures, utilize EMLA (eutectic mixture of local anesthetics) cream appropriately. Teach the child's primary caregiver to apply the cream to the implantable port site 30 minutes to 1 hour prior to the child's clinic appointment time. Apply EMLA cream to the posterior hip or lumbar spine, 1 to 3 hours prior to bone marrow aspiration or lumbar puncture.

Nursing Management

Nursing care of children with ALL focuses on managing disease complications such as infection, pain, anemia, bleeding, and hyperuricemia and the many adverse effects related to treatment. Many children require blood product transfusion for the treatment of severe anemia or low platelet levels with active bleeding.

Individualize nursing care based on the patient problems, interventions, and outcomes presented in the "Clinical Judgment and the Nursing Process" section earlier in the chapter, depending on the child's response to the disease and chemotherapy. Refer to that section for further information related to managing the adverse effects of chemotherapy.

TAKE NOTE!

Blood products administered to children with any type of leukemia should be irradiated, cytomegalovirus (CMV) negative, and leukodepleted. This treatment of blood products before transfusion will decrease the number of antibodies in the blood, an important factor in preventing GVHD if HSCT becomes necessary at a later date (Keating et al., 2022).

REDUCING PAIN

Children and adolescents with leukemia suffer pain related to the disease as well as the treatment. Chemotherapy drugs commonly used in leukemia may cause peripheral neuropathy and headache. Lumbar puncture and bone marrow aspiration, which are periodically performed throughout the course of treatment, also cause pain. The most common areas of pain are the head and neck, legs, and abdomen (probably from protracted vomiting with chemotherapy). Use distraction techniques, such as listening to music, watching TV, or playing games, to help take the child's mind off the pain. Administer mild analgesics such as acetaminophen for acute episodes of pain. Using EMLA cream prior to venipuncture, port access, lumbar puncture, and bone marrow aspiration may decrease procedure-related pain events. In addition, applying heat or cold to the painful area is usually acceptable. Administer narcotic analgesics, as prescribed, for episodes of acute severe pain or for palliation of chronic pain.

TAKE NOTE!

Administer medications as ordered using the least invasive method possible to avoid pain (intramuscular, subcutaneous, and rectal route should be avoided in the child with thrombocytopenia).

Acute Myeloid Leukemia

AML accounts for about 25% of leukemias in children, yet is responsible for about a third of deaths from leukemia in this age group (Keating et al., 2022). AML affects the myeloid cell progenitors or precursors in the bone marrow, resulting in **malignant** (invasive and fast-growing) cells. The French–American–British (FAB) classification system identifies eight subtypes of AML (M0 to M7), depending on myeloid lineage involved and the degree of cell differentiation. These subtypes are useful for determining treatment. The long-term survival rate for childhood AML is about 50% (Keating et al., 2022). Complications include treatment resistance, infection, hemorrhage, and metastasis. The induction phase of AML requires intense bone marrow suppression and prolonged hospitalization because AML is less responsive to treatment than ALL. Toxicity from treatment is more common in AML and is likely to be more serious than with ALL. Empiric broad-spectrum antibiotics and prophylactic platelet transfusions may be prescribed. After remission is achieved, children require intensive chemotherapy to prolong the duration of remission. HSCT is often required in children with AML, depending on the subtype (Keating et al., 2022).

TAKE NOTE!

At the time of diagnosis, some children with AML present with a WBC count of above 100,000 (hyperleukocytosis); this results in venous stasis and backup of blast cells in small vessels, causing hypoxia, hemorrhage, and lung or brain infarction. Hyperleukocytosis is a medical emergency. These children require leukapheresis to decrease hyperviscosity by quickly decreasing the number of circulating blasts (Keating et al., 2022).

Nursing Assessment

Explore the health history for common signs and symptoms, including recurrent infections, fever, or fatigue. Explore the medical history for risk factors, such as Hispanic background, previous chemotherapy, and genetic abnormalities, such as Down syndrome, Fanconi anemia, neurofibromatosis, Wiskott–Aldrich syndrome, and Diamond–Blackfan anemia.

Perform a thorough physical examination. Note skin pallor and salmon-colored or blue-gray papular lesions. Palpate the skin for subcutaneous rubbery nodules. Palpate for lymphadenopathy. Note headache, visual disturbance, or signs of increased intracranial pressure, such as vomiting, which may indicate CNS involvement. Upon diagnosis of AML, the child's WBC count is typically extremely elevated (Keating et al., 2022).

Nursing Management

Nursing management of the child with AML is similar to that of the child with ALL. Nursing interventions focus on managing the adverse effects of treatment and preventing infection. Refer to the "Clinical Judgment and the Nursing Process" section earlier in the chapter for appropriate interventions.

LYMPHOMAS

Lymphomas, or tumors of the lymph tissue (lymph nodes, thymus, spleen), account for about 10% to 15% of cases of childhood cancer (Keating et al., 2022). Lymphomas may be divided into two categories—Hodgkin disease (or Hodgkin lymphoma) and non-Hodgkin lymphoma (NHL), which includes more than a dozen types. Hodgkin disease tends to affect lymph nodes located closer to the body's surface, such as those in the cervical, axillary, and inguinal areas, whereas NHL tends to affect lymph nodes located more deeply inside the body.

Hodgkin Disease

In Hodgkin disease, malignant B lymphocytes grow in the lymph tissue, usually starting in one general area of lymph nodes. The presence of Reed–Sternberg cells (giant transformed B lymphocytes with one or two nuclei) differentiates Hodgkin disease from other lymphomas. As the cells multiply, the lymph nodes enlarge, compressing nearby structures, destroying normal cells, and invading other tissues. The cause of Hodgkin disease is still being researched, but there appears to be a link to Epstein–Barr virus infection American Cancer Society, 2024e. Hodgkin disease is rare in children younger than 5 years of age and is most common in adolescents and young adults; in preadolescents, it is more common in males than females (Keating et al., 2022).

In addition to the traditional **staging** (I through IV, depending on the amount of spread of the cancer; Table 24.8), Hodgkin is also classified as A (asymptomatic) or B (presence of symptoms of fever, night sweats, or weight loss of 10% or more). Prognosis depends on the stage of the disease, tumor bulk, and A or B classification (disease classified as A generally carries a better prognosis). Overall, children with Hodgkin disease have a 5- to 10-year survival rate of over 90% (Keating et al., 2022). Complications of Hodgkin disease include liver failure and secondary cancer such as acute nonlymphocytic leukemia and NHL.

Chemotherapy, usually with a combination of drugs, is the treatment of choice for children with Hodgkin disease. Radiation therapy may also be necessary. In the child with disease that does not go into remission or in the child who experiences relapse, HSCT may be an option.

Nursing Assessment

Explore the health history for common signs and symptoms, which may include recent weight loss, fever, drenching night sweats, anorexia, malaise, fatigue, or pruritus. Elicit the health history, determining risk factors such as prior Epstein–Barr virus infection, family history of Hodgkin disease, genetic immune disorder, or HIV infection.

Evaluate respiratory status, as the presence of a mediastinal mass may compromise respiration. Palpate for enlarged lymph nodes; they may feel rubbery and tend to occur in clusters (most common sites are cervical and supraclavicular) (Fig. 24.16). Palpate the abdomen for hepatomegaly or splenomegaly, which may be present with advanced disease. The chest radiograph may reveal a mediastinal mass. The CBC may be normal or reflect anemia. Tissue sampling will reveal Reed–Sternberg cells.

TAKE NOTE!

Pain and pruritus in the affected lymph node region has sometimes been noted after alcohol ingestion (Keating et al., 2022).

Nursing Management

Nursing management of the child with Hodgkin lymphoma focuses on addressing the adverse effects of chemotherapy or radiation. Refer to the "Clinical Judgment and the Nursing Process" section to develop an individualized nursing care plan based on the child's response to treatment.

Non-Hodgkin Lymphoma

NHL results from mutations in the B and T lymphocytes that lead to uncontrolled growth. NHL tends to affect lymph nodes located more deeply within the body. NHL spreads by the bloodstream and in children is a rapidly proliferating, aggressive malignancy that is very responsive to treatment. Prognosis depends on

TABLE 24.8 • Staging of Hodgkin Disease

Stage	Clinical Findings
I	Involves a single lymph node region
II	Two or more lymph node regions on the same side of the diaphragm are affected.
III	Lymph node regions or lymphatic structures above and below the diaphragm are affected.
IV	Metastasis to nonlymphatic organs such as the liver, bone, or lungs
A or B suffix	A—Absence of systemic symptoms at diagnosis B—Systemic symptoms present at diagnosis (fever, night sweats, weight loss)

Data from LaCasce, A. S., & Ng, A. K. (2022). Pretreatment evaluation, staging, and treatment stratification of classic Hodgkin lymphoma. *UpToDate*. Retrieved on April 26, 2023, from https://www.uptodate.com/contents/pretreatment-evaluation-staging-and-treatment-stratification-of-classic-hodgkin-lymphoma

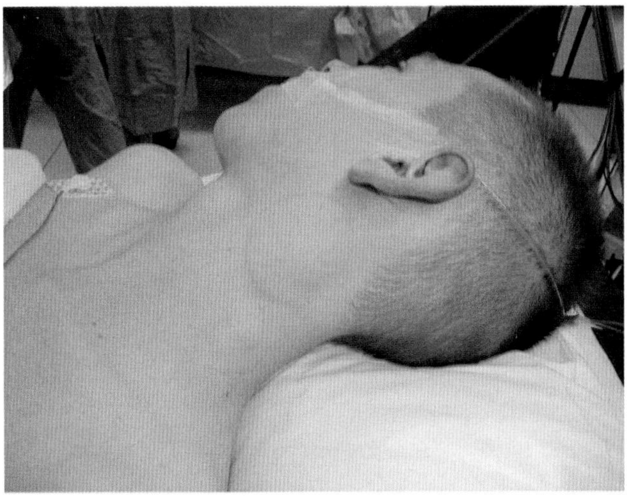

FIGURE 24.16 Hodgkin lymphoma. Large, fixed cervical masses in a 14-year-old with weight loss. (Reprinted with permission from Chung, E. K., Atkinson-McEvoy, L. R., Lai, N. L., & Terry, M. [2014]. *Visual diagnosis and treatment in pediatrics* [3rd ed.]. Wolters Kluwer.)

the cell type involved and the extent of the disease at diagnosis. Ninety percent of children with localized NHL have disease-free long-term survival after treatment (Keating et al., 2022). Complications include metastasis and the development of a secondary malignancy later in life.

Remission is induced with chemotherapy and followed with a maintenance phase of chemotherapy lasting about 2 years. NHL tends to spread easily to the CNS, so CNS prophylaxis similar to that used in leukemia is warranted (Keating et al., 2022). Autologous bone marrow transplantation may be used in some children.

Nursing Assessment

Children with NHL are usually symptomatic for only a few days or a few weeks before diagnosis because the disease progresses so quickly. Note onset and location of pain or lymph node swelling. Document history of abdominal pain, diarrhea, or constipation. Explore the health history for risk factors such as congenital or acquired immune deficiency.

Observe for increased work of breathing, facial edema, or venous engorgement (mediastinal mass). Palpate for the presence of lymphadenopathy, and palpate the abdomen for the presence of a mass. Lymph node biopsy and bone marrow aspiration determine the diagnosis. Computed tomography (CT) scan, chest radiography, and bone marrow results may be used to determine the extent of metastasis.

CLINICAL REASONING ALERT!

Assess for cough, dyspnea, orthopnea, facial edema, or venous engorgement in the child with possible NHL, as mediastinal NHL requires rapid treatment (Keating et al., 2022).

Nursing Management

As with Hodgkin lymphoma, nursing management of NHL is directed toward managing the adverse effects of chemotherapy. Refer to the "Clinical Judgment and the Nursing Process" section to plan nursing care for the child and family based on the responses they exhibit.

BRAIN TUMORS

Brain tumors are the most common form of solid tumor and the second most common type of cancer in children (Keating et al., 2022). Slightly more than half of brain tumors arise in the posterior fossa (infratentorial); the rest are supratentorial in origin. The cause of brain tumors in children is unknown. Some tumors are localized (low grade), while others are of higher grade and more invasive. The prognosis depends on the location of the tumor and extent of tumor. Low-grade tumors and those that are fully resectable have a better prognosis than tumors that are located deeper within the brain or that are more invasive, making them difficult to resect (Keating et al., 2022). There are many different types of childhood brain tumors; Table 24.9 explains the most common ones.

Complications of brain tumors include hydrocephalus, increased intracranial pressure, brain stem herniation, and negative effects of radiation such as neuropsychological, intellectual, and endocrinologic sequelae (Lau & Teo, 2024).

Pathophysiology

Although the cause of brain tumors is generally unknown, the effects of brain tumors are predictable. As the tumor grows within the cranium, it exerts pressure

TABLE 24.9 • Childhood Brain Tumors

Tumor	Location	Characteristics
Medulloblastoma (most common)	Cerebellum	Invasive, highly malignant, grows rapidly. Less favorable outcome with disseminated disease. Progresses quickly to increased intracranial pressure, seeds on CNS pathways. Peak incidence: 5–10 years old
Brain stem glioma	Brain stem	Aggressive, difficult to resect, resistant to chemotherapy. Spreads widely within the brain stem but rarely extends outside of brain stem area. Affects cranial nerve function
Ependymoma	Frequently arises from floor of fourth ventricle	Varying speed of growth. Often causes hydrocephalus. Usually diagnosed before it spreads to other parts of the brain or spinal cord
Astrocytoma	Cerebellum, cerebral hemispheres, thalamus, hypothalamus	Slow course with insidious onset. Responsive to chemotherapy, often resectable. Causes slowly increasing intracranial pressure. Low-grade tumor may be removed completely. High-grade tumors have poor prognosis.

CNS, central nervous system.

Data from Keating, A. K., Knight-Perry, J., Maloney, K., Levy, J. M. M., Greffe, B. S., Franklin, A. R. K., & Garrington, T. P. (2022). Chapter 31: Neoplastic disease. In M. Bunik, W. W. Hay, M. J. Levin, & M. J. Abzug (Eds.), *Current diagnosis & treatment: Pediatrics* (26th ed., pp. 931–963). McGraw-Hill Education.

on the brain tissues surrounding it. The tumor mass may compress vital structures in the brain, block cerebrospinal fluid flow, or cause edema in the brain. The result is an increase in intracranial pressure. Presenting symptoms vary according to location and type of tumor.

Therapeutic Management

The type of tumor may be identified at the time of surgery. The location of the tumor within the brain will determine the extent to which it can safely be resected. Children with hydrocephalus may require a ventriculoperitoneal shunt (see Chapter 16 for further information on hydrocephalus). Radiation is reserved for children older than age 3 years because it can have long-term neurocognitive effects (Lau & Teo, 2024). Chemotherapy is being used increasingly in the treatment of pediatric brain tumors in an attempt to avoid the use of radiation therapy.

Nursing Assessment

For a full description of the assessment phase of the nursing process, refer to "Clinical Judgment and the Nursing Process" section. Assessment findings pertinent to CNS tumors are discussed here.

Health History

Elicit a description of the present illness and chief complaint. Common signs and symptoms reported during the health history might include:

- Nausea or vomiting
- Headache
- Unsteady gait
- Blurred or double vision
- Seizures
- Motor abnormality or hemiparesis
- Weakness, atrophy
- Swallowing difficulties
- Behavior or personality changes
- Irritability, failure to thrive, or developmental delay (in very young children)

Explore the child's current and past medical history for risk factors such as history of neurofibromatosis, tuberous sclerosis, or prior treatment for CNS leukemia.

Physical Examination

Observe for strabismus or nystagmus, 'sunsetting' eyes, head tilt, alterations in coordination, gait disturbance, or alterations in sensation. Note alteration in gag reflex, cranial nerve palsy, lethargy, or irritability. Note the child's posture. Check pupillary reaction, noting size, equality, reaction to light, and accommodation.

Measure blood pressure, which may decrease with increasing intracranial pressure. In the infant, palpate the anterior fontanel for bulging. Assess deep tendon reflexes, noting hyperreflexia.

TAKE NOTE!

A fixed and dilated pupil is a neurosurgical emergency.

Laboratory and Diagnostic Tests

Common laboratory and diagnostic studies ordered for the assessment of CNS tumors are as follows:

- CT, magnetic resonance imaging (MRI), or positron emission tomography (PET) will demonstrate evidence of the tumor and its location within the intracranial cavity.
- Lumbar puncture with cerebrospinal fluid cell evaluation may show tumor markers or the presence of alpha-fetoprotein or human chorionic gonadotropin, which may assist in the diagnosis.

Nursing Management

Nursing management of the child with a brain tumor includes pre- and postoperative care, as well as interventions to manage adverse effects related to chemotherapy and radiation. Refer to the "Clinical Judgment and the Nursing Process" section for a discussion of nursing interventions related to chemotherapy adverse effects and for additional interventions that may be individualized depending on the child's response to the brain tumor and its treatment.

Providing Preoperative Care

Preoperatively, care focuses on monitoring for additional increases in intracranial pressure and avoiding activities that cause transient increases in intracranial pressure. Administer dexamethasone as prescribed to decrease intracranial inflammation. Prevent straining with bowel movements by use of a stool softener. Assess the child's pain level as well as level of consciousness, vital signs, and pupillary reaction to determine subtle changes as soon as possible. Provide a tour of the intensive care unit, which is where the child will wake up after the surgery. Instruct the child and family about the possibility of intubation and ventilation in the postoperative period. If a ventriculoperitoneal shunt will be placed for the treatment of hydrocephalus caused by the tumor, provide education about shunts to the child and family (see Chapter 16).

Shave the portion of the head as determined by the neurosurgeon. Some children may choose to have the entire head shaved. Sometimes, children with long hair may feel better about losing it if they donate it to Locks of Love, an organization that provides hairpieces for financially disadvantaged children who have long-term medical hair loss.

Providing Postoperative Care

Regulate fluid administration, as excess fluid intake may cause or worsen cerebral edema. Administer mannitol or hypertonic dextrose to decrease cerebral edema. Assess vital signs frequently, along with checking pupillary reactions and determining level of consciousness. Extreme lethargy or coma may be present for several days postoperatively. Increases in temperature may indicate infection or may be caused by cerebral edema or disturbance of the hypothalamus. Treat hyperthermia with antipyretics such as acetaminophen and with sponge baths, as increases in temperature increase metabolic need. Reduce the temperature slowly.

Monitor for signs of increased intracranial pressure. Headache is common in the postoperative period. Assess pain level and provide analgesics as prescribed. Minimize environmental stimuli, providing a calm and quiet atmosphere. Check the head dressing for cerebrospinal fluid drainage or bleeding. Assess for and document the extent of head, face, or neck edema. Administer eye lubricant if edema prevents complete closure of the eyelids. Apply cool compresses to the eyes to decrease swelling.

As the child begins to regain consciousness, they may be confused or combative. Restrain the child if needed to keep them in bed and prevent dislodging of tubes and lines.

POSITIONING THE CHILD IN THE POSTOPERATIVE PERIOD

Position the child on the unaffected side with the head of the bed flat or at the level prescribed by the neurosurgeon. Side positioning is usually preferred, as the child may have difficulty handling oral secretions if the level of consciousness is decreased. Do not elevate the foot of the bed, as this may increase intracranial pressure and contribute to bleeding. When changing the child's position, maintain the head in alignment with the remainder of the body. Children with paralyzed or spastic extremities will need additional positioning support.

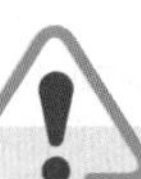

CLINICAL REASONING ALERT!

Observe pre- and postoperatively for signs of brain stem herniation such as opisthotonos (see Fig. 16.13 in Chapter 16), nuchal rigidity, head tilt, sluggish pupils, increased blood pressure with widening pulse pressure, change in respirations, bradycardia, irregular pulse, and changes in body temperature. Notify the health care provider immediately of these findings.

CONSIDER THIS!

Alice Tice, 8 years old, is scheduled to receive chemotherapy for a brain tumor. Alice states, "I'm scared!" A moment later she cries out, "And I don't want to go bald!" Think about when you were a school-age child—what things were important to you then? As the nurse caring for her, how can you prepare Alice for this?

NEUROBLASTOMA

Neuroblastoma, a tumor that arises from embryonic neural crest cells, is the most common extracranial solid tumor in children (Keating et al., 2022). It most frequently occurs in the abdomen, mainly in the adrenal gland, but it may occur anywhere along the paravertebral sympathetic chain in the chest or retroperitoneum. When diagnosed past infancy or early toddlerhood, by the time of diagnosis, the neuroblastoma has usually already metastasized. Neuroblastoma is the second most frequently occurring solid tumor in children; 90% of cases are diagnosed before the age of 5 years (Keating et al., 2022).

Staging of the tumor at diagnosis determines the course of treatment and prognosis. Table 24.10 discusses the staging of neuroblastomas. The 5-year survival rate for all children with neuroblastoma is about 80% (Shohet et al., 2024). Prognosis depends on the tumor stage, age at diagnosis, location of tumor, and location of metastasis. Metastasis to the bone is a worse prognostic factor than metastasis to the skin, liver, or bone marrow. Children who relapse after initial treatment also tend to have a dismal prognosis. In addition to metastasis, complications may include nerve compression, resulting in neurologic deficits.

The neuroblastoma must be removed surgically. Radiation and chemotherapy are administered to all

TABLE 24.10 • Staging of Neuroblastoma

Stage	Clinical Findings
I	Tumor confined to organ or structure of origin
II	Tumor extends beyond organ or structure, not beyond midline ("A" negative lymph nodes, "B" regional nodes on same side involved)
III	Tumor invasively extends beyond the midline with bilateral lymph node involvement
IV	Metastasis to bone, bone marrow, other organs, distant lymph nodes
IV-S	Tumor would have been considered a stage I or II, but remote metastasis to one or more sites (liver, skin, or bone marrow) has occurred without metastasis to the bone

Data from Keating, A. K., Knight-Perry, J., Maloney, K., Levy, J. M. M., Greffe, B. S., Franklin, A. R. K., & Garrington, T. P. (2022). Chapter 31: Neoplastic disease. In M. Bunik, W. W. Hay, M. J. Levin, & M. J. Abzug (Eds.), *Current diagnosis & treatment: Pediatrics* (26th ed., pp. 931-963). McGraw-Hill Education.

children with neuroblastoma except those with stage I disease, in whom the tumor is completely resected.

Nursing Assessment

For a full description of the assessment phase of the nursing process, refer to the "Clinical Judgment and the Nursing Process" section. Assessment findings pertinent to neuroblastoma are discussed here.

Health History

Presenting signs and symptoms of neuroblastoma depend on the location of the primary tumor and the extent of metastasis. Often, parents are the first to notice a swollen or asymmetric abdomen. Elicit the health history, documenting bowel or bladder dysfunction, especially watery diarrhea, neurologic symptoms (brain metastasis), bone pain (bone metastasis), anorexia, vomiting, or weight loss.

Physical Examination

Note neck or facial swelling, bruising above the eyes, or edema around the eyes (metastasis to skull bones). Inspect the skin for pallor or bruising (bone marrow metastasis) and document cough or difficulty breathing. Auscultate the lungs for wheezing. Palpate for lymphadenopathy, especially cervical. Palpate the abdomen, noting a firm, nontender mass. Palpate for and note hepatomegaly or splenomegaly if present.

Laboratory and Diagnostic Testing

Laboratory and diagnostic testing may reveal the following:

- CT scan or MRI to determine site of tumor and evidence of metastasis
- Chest radiograph, bone scan, and skeletal survey to identify metastasis
- Bone marrow aspiration and biopsy to determine metastasis to the bone marrow
- 24-hour urine collection for homovanillic acid (HVA) and vanillylmandelic acid (VMA); levels will be elevated.

Nursing Management

Postoperative nursing care depends on the site of tumor removal, which is most often the abdomen. Provide routine care after abdominal surgery. Refer to the "Clinical Judgment and the Nursing Process" section for nursing care related to the effects of chemotherapy and radiation. Provide emotional support and possible referrals to help children and families cope with a potentially poor prognosis (due to the fact that the disease has often metastasized significantly by the time of diagnosis).

• • • ATRAUMATIC CARE • • •

The child with cancer often undergoes many painful procedures related to laboratory specimens and treatment protocols. To assist the child to cope with these procedures, provide distraction in the form of reading a favorite book or playing a favorite movie or musical selection.

SARCOMAS

Sarcomas occur in bone and soft tissue in children. Bone tumors are most often diagnosed in adolescence, whereas soft tissue tumors tend to occur in younger children (Keating et al., 2022). This discussion will focus on the most common bone and soft tissue tumors occurring in childhood. The most common bone tumors in children are osteosarcoma and Ewing sarcoma (Keating et al., 2022). These bone tumors often initially go undiagnosed, as adolescents frequently seek care for traumatic events and the pain suffered with a bone tumor may initially be attributed to trauma. Rhabdomyosarcoma is the most common soft tissue tumor in childhood (Keating et al., 2022).

Osteosarcoma

Osteosarcoma accounts for 60% of bone cancer in children, occurring most frequently in adolescents and males (Keating et al., 2022). It presumably arises from the embryonic mesenchymal tissue that forms the bones. The most common sites are in the long bones, particularly the proximal humerus, proximal tibia, and distal femur. Complications include metastasis, particularly to the lungs and other bones, and recurrence of disease within 3 years, primarily affecting the lungs.

Surgical removal of the tumor is necessary. Chemotherapy is often administered before surgery to decrease the size of the tumor; it is usually administered after surgery to treat or prevent metastasis. Radiation is not helpful. The type of surgery performed depends on the tumor size, extent of disease outside of the bone, distant metastasis, and skeletal maturity. Radical amputation may be performed, but often, adolescents undergo a limb-sparing procedure (Keating et al., 2022).

Nursing Assessment

Obtain the health history, ascertaining when pain, limp, or limitation of motion was first noticed. Dull bone pain may be present for several months, eventually progressing to limp or gait changes. Inspect the affected limb for erythema and swelling. Palpate the affected area for warmth and tenderness and to determine the size of the soft tissue mass, if also present. As with other pediatric cancers, a thorough physical examination is warranted to detect other abnormalities that may indicate metastasis.

Laboratory and diagnostic testing may include:

- CT scan or MRI to determine the extent of the lesion and to identify metastasis
- Bone scan to determine the extent of malignancy

Nursing Management

The adolescent will generally be quite anxious about the possibility of amputation and even about the limb salvage procedure. Present preoperative teaching at the adolescent's developmental level, and ensure that they are included in planning treatment. Regardless of the type of surgery performed, provide routine orthopedic postoperative care. Educate the adolescent and parents on the care of the stump, if amputation is necessary, and ensure that the adolescent becomes competent in crutch walking. A prosthesis may be ordered. The adolescent will need time to adjust to these significant body image changes and may benefit from talking with another adolescent who has undergone a similar procedure. Support the adolescent in choosing clothing that may camouflage the prosthesis while still allowing the adolescent to appear fashionable. Provide emotional support, as the adolescent's maturity level allows them to understand the severity of the disease. Peer support groups are often helpful, as adolescents value their peers' opinions and enjoy being part of a group. Examples of comprehensive online support groups are Melissa's Living Legacy Foundation/Helping Teens Live with Cancer and The Wellness Community.

Ewing Sarcoma

Ewing sarcoma is a highly malignant bone tumor. It is rarer than osteosarcoma, accounting for about 30% of childhood bone tumors (Keating et al., 2022). It occurs most frequently in the long bones or pelvis (American Association of Orthopedic Surgeons, 2023). The prognosis for Ewing sarcoma depends on the extent of metastasis. Children with small, localized tumor have a 70% to 75% long-term survival rate, while those with metastasis have a poor survival rate (Keating et al., 2022).

Radiation, chemotherapy, and surgical excision are usually used in combination. Treatment varies depending on the site of the primary tumor and the extent of metastasis at diagnosis. Myeloablative chemotherapy (which destroys the child's marrow) may be used for metastatic disease, followed by a stem cell rescue transplant.

Nursing Assessment

Explore the history for intermittent pain that worsens progressively. Note a possible history of fever. Eventually, the pain becomes constant and severe, sometimes interrupting sleep.

Note the presence of swelling or erythema at the tumor site. CT scan or MRI of the affected area will reveal the extent of the tumor. Biopsy is necessary to establish the diagnosis. CT scan of the chest, bone scan, and bilateral bone marrow aspiration with biopsy determine the extent of metastasis.

Nursing Management

Before treatment begins, discourage active play or weight bearing on the affected extremity to avoid pathologic fracture at the tumor site. Nursing management focuses on addressing the adverse effects of treatment (refer to the "Clinical Judgment and the Nursing Process" section). Give honest and direct answers to adolescents with Ewing sarcoma who ask questions about their disease. These children will undergo intensive therapy and spend a great deal of time in the hospital. Depending on the age of the child, fantasy play, art or pet therapy, drama, writing, humor, and/or music may help the child to work through the psychological impact of this disease. Refer to the nursing process section earlier in the chapter for additional interventions, which should be individualized depending on the child's and family's response to the disease process and treatment.

> **THINKING ABOUT DEVELOPMENT**
>
> Serena Jameson is a 14-year-old cheerleader with newly diagnosed Ewing sarcoma. Her prescribed treatment protocol involves several medications known to cause severe alopecia. Considering Serena's developmental stage, how will this impact her ability and/or willingness to participate in future cheerleading exhibitions? Develop a list of ideas for assisting Serena to cope with the anticipated changes to her body image.

Rhabdomyosarcoma

Rhabdomyosarcoma is a soft tissue tumor that usually arises from the embryonic mesenchymal cells that would ordinarily form striated muscle. The most common locations for the tumor are the head and neck, genitourinary tract, and extremities (Fig. 24.17). The tumor is highly malignant and spreads via local extension or through the venous or lymphatic system, with the lung being the most common site for metastasis. Diagnosis is usually made between 2 and 5 years of age, with 70% of all rhabdomyosarcomas diagnosed by age 10 years (Keating et al., 2022). The prognosis is based on the stage of the disease at diagnosis. Box 24.4 explains the staging of rhabdomyosarcoma. Prognosis is generally favorable for stage I disease (Okcu & Hicks, 2023). Complications of rhabdomyosarcoma include metastasis to lung, bone, or

> **BOX 24.4 Staging of Rhabdomyosarcoma**
>
> - Stage I: completely resectable localized tumor
> - Stage II: after local tumor resection, microscopic residual disease remains (or spreads to regional lymph nodes)
> - Stage III: after local tumor resection, gross residual disease remains
> - Stage IV: distant metastasis present at diagnosis
>
> Data from Okcu, M. F., & Hicks, J. (2023). Rhabdomyosarcoma in childhood and adolescence: Clinical presentation, diagnostic evaluation, and staging. *UpToDate*. Retrieved on April 26, 2023, from https://www.uptodate.com/contents/rhabdomyosarcoma-in-childhood-and-adolescence-clinical-presentation-diagnostic-evaluation-and-staging

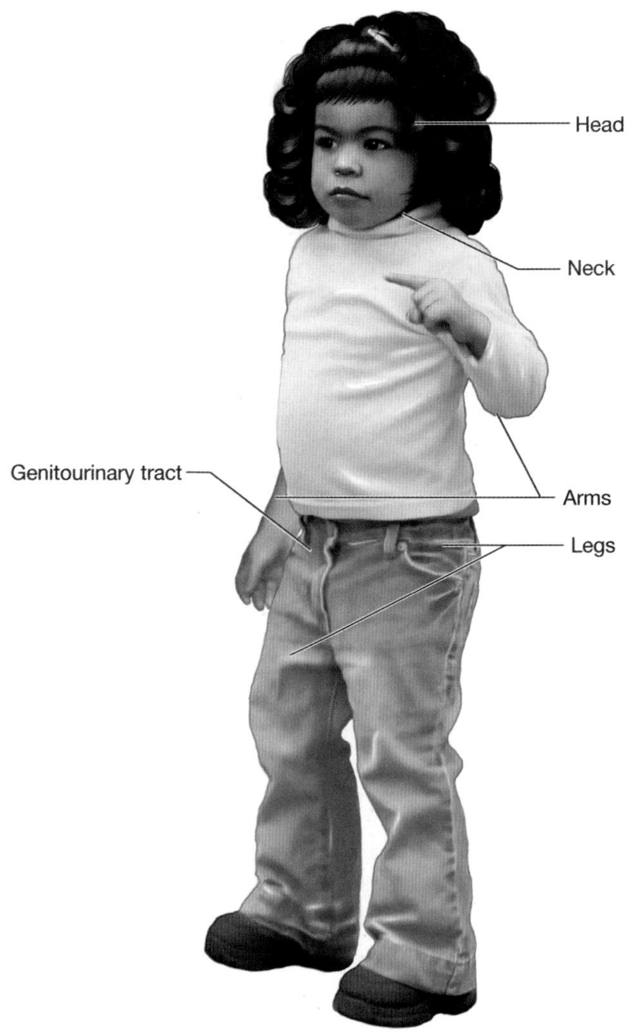

FIGURE 24.17 The most common sites of rhabdomyosarcoma.

bone marrow and direct extension into the CNS, resulting in brain stem compromise or cranial nerve palsy.

Surgical removal of the primary tumor is generally performed. At the time of the surgery, the lesion is biopsied, and the stage of disease determined. Depending on the site (especially head, neck, and pelvis) and size of the tumor, radiation and chemotherapy may be used to shrink the tumor to avoid disability.

Nursing Assessment

The child or parent will often discover an asymptomatic mass and seek medical attention at that time. Obtain a health history, noting recent illness, when the mass was discovered, and whether it has changed since first noted. Examine the history for risk factors such as parental smoking, exposure to environmental chemicals, family history of cancer, or neurofibromatosis. Note respiratory effort and cough, and auscultate the lungs for adventitious sounds. Palpate for lymphadenopathy. Palpate the abdomen for a mass or hepatosplenomegaly. Abnormalities found on physical examination depend on the location of the rhabdomyosarcoma (Table 24.11).

TABLE 24.11 • Presenting Signs and Symptoms Related to Location of Rhabdomyosarcoma

Location of Tumor	Presenting Signs and Symptoms
Orbit	Proptosis
Middle ear	Drainage, pain, facial nerve palsy
Sinuses	Discharge, pain, sinusitis, facial swelling
Nasopharynx	Pain, epistaxis, dysphagia, nasal quality to speech, airway obstruction
Neck	Dysphagia, hoarseness
Thorax, testicle, extremities	Enlarging mass, painless
Retroperitoneum	Gastrointestinal and urinary tract obstruction, pain, weakness, paresthesia
Bladder, prostate	Hematuria, urinary obstruction
Vagina	Mass, vaginal bleeding or chronic discharge

Data from Okcu, M. F., & Hicks, J. (2023). Rhabdomyosarcoma in childhood and adolescence: Clinical presentation, diagnostic evaluation, and staging. *UpToDate.* Retrieved on April 26, 2023, from https://www.uptodate.com/contents/rhabdomyosarcoma-in-childhood-and-adolescence-clinical-presentation-diagnostic-evaluation-and-staging

Laboratory and diagnostic testing may include:

- CT scan or MRI of primary lesion and the chest for metastasis
- Open biopsy of the primary tumor for definitive diagnosis
- Bone marrow aspiration and biopsy, bone scan, and skeletal survey to determine metastasis

CLINICAL REASONING ALERT!

Primary tumors arising in the neck region may compress the child's airway. Assess work of breathing and lung sounds.

Nursing Management

Provide routine postoperative care, depending on the site of surgery. Assess for adverse effects of high-dose radiation, which is generally used to treat the primary tumor as well as metastatic sites. Administer chemotherapy as ordered and assess for adverse effects. Refer to the "Clinical Judgment and the Nursing Process" section to determine an individualized plan of care based on the child's response to the treatment.

WILMS TUMOR

Wilms tumor is the most common kidney tumor and the second most common abdominal solid tumor in children and most commonly occurs between the ages of 2 and 5 years (Keating et al., 2022). It usually affects only one kidney (Fig. 24.18). The etiology is unknown, but some

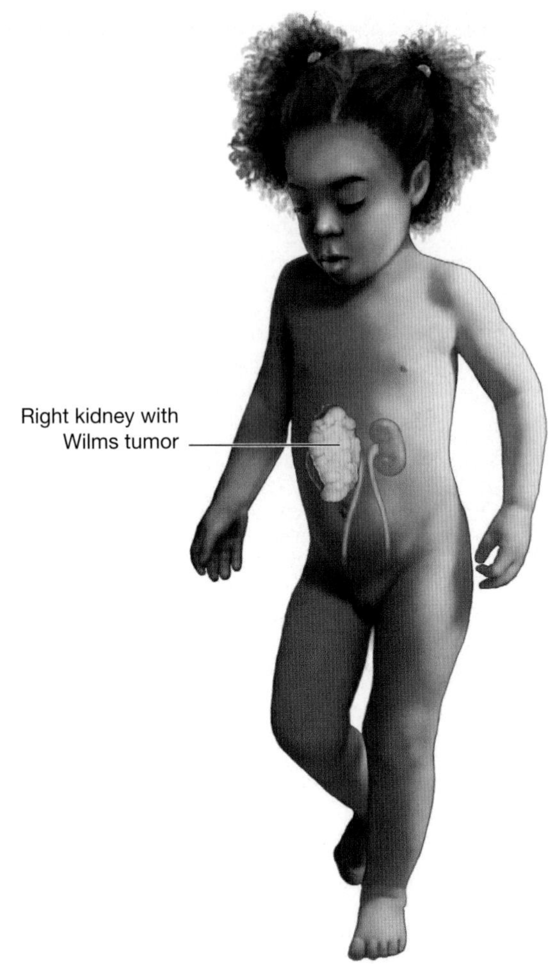

FIGURE 24.18 Wilms tumor is usually unilateral.

cases occur via genetic inheritance. Associated anomalies may occur with Wilms tumor. Wilms tumor demonstrates rapid growth and is usually large at diagnosis. Metastasis occurs via direct extension or through the bloodstream. Wilms tumor most commonly metastasizes to the perirenal tissues, liver, diaphragm, lungs, abdominal muscles, and lymph nodes.

Staging of Wilms tumor is provided in Box 24.5. The tumor is also additionally designated as having favorable histology (FH) or unfavorable histology (UH). UH is noted by the presence of anaplasia (focal or diffuse giant polypoid nuclei). The prognosis depends on staging at diagnosis and the extent of metastasis, with overall survival being more than 90% (Smith & Chintagumpala, 2023). Complications include metastasis or complications from radiation therapy such as liver or kidney damage, female sterility, bowel obstruction, pneumonia, or scoliosis.

Therapeutic Management

Surgical removal of the tumor and affected kidney (nephrectomy) is the treatment of choice and also allows for accurate staging and assessment of tumor spread. Radiation or chemotherapy may be administered either before or after surgery.

BOX 24.5 Staging of Wilms Tumor

- Stage I: unilateral, limited to kidney, completely resectable, renal capsule intact
- Stage II: unilateral, tumor extends beyond kidney but is completely resected
- Stage III: unilateral, tumor has spread outside of kidney, located in abdominal cavity only, not fully removed
- Stage IV: unilateral with metastasis in lung, liver, distant lymph node, bone, or brain
- Stage V: bilateral kidney involvement

Nursing Assessment

For a full description of the assessment phase of the nursing process, refer to "Clinical Judgment and the Nursing Process" section. Assessment findings pertinent to Wilms tumor are discussed further on.

Health History

Parents typically initially observe the abdominal mass associated with Wilms tumor and then seek medical attention. Elicit the health history, noting when the mass was discovered. Note abdominal pain, which may be related to rapid tumor growth. Document history of constipation, vomiting, anorexia, weight loss, or difficulty breathing. Determine risk factors such as hemihypertrophy of the spine, Beckwith–Wiedemann syndrome, genitourinary anomalies, absence of the iris, or family history of cancer.

Physical Examination

Measure blood pressure; hypertension occurs in 25% of children with Wilms tumor (Keating et al., 2022). Inspect the abdomen for asymmetry or a visible mass. Observe for associated anomalies, as noted previously. Auscultate the lungs for adventitious breath sounds associated with tumor metastasis. Palpate for lymphadenopathy.

TAKE NOTE!

Avoid palpating the abdomen after the initial assessment preoperatively. Wilms tumor is highly vascular and soft, so excessive handling of the tumor may result in tumor seeding and metastasis.

Laboratory and Diagnostic Testing

Laboratory and diagnostic testing may include:

- Kidney or abdominal ultrasound to assess the tumor and the contralateral kidney
- CT scan or MRI of the abdomen and chest to determine local spread to lymph nodes or adjacent organs, as well as any distant metastasis

- CBC, BUN, and creatinine: usually within normal limits
- Urinalysis: may reveal hematuria or leukocytes
- 24-hour urine collection for HVA and VMA to distinguish the tumor from neuroblastoma (levels will not be elevated with Wilms tumor)

Nursing Management

Postoperative care of the child with Wilms tumor resection is similar to that of children undergoing other abdominal surgery. Assessment of remaining kidney function is critical. The child may have adverse effects related to chemotherapy or radiation. Refer to the "Clinical Judgment and the Nursing Process" section to individualize care for the child based on the child's response to therapy.

TAKE NOTE!

To avoid injuring the remaining kidney, children with a single kidney should not play contact sports.

RETINOBLASTOMA

Retinoblastoma is a congenital, highly malignant tumor that arises from embryonic retinal cells. It accounts for 5% of cases of blindness in children (Keating et al., 2022). Most children are diagnosed by age 5, and the 5-year survival rate is 95% when the tumor is confined to the retina (Keating et al., 2022). Retinoblastoma may be hereditary or nonhereditary. Nonhereditary retinoblastoma may be associated with advanced paternal age and always presents with unilateral involvement. Hereditary retinoblastoma is inherited via the autosomal dominant mode. These cases may be unilateral or bilateral. The tumor may grow forward into the vitreous cavity of the eye or extend into the subretinal space, causing retinal detachment. The tumor may extend into the choroid, the sclera, and the optic nerve.

Complications include spread to the brain and the opposite eye, as well as metastasis to lymph nodes, bone, bone marrow, and liver. Secondary tumors, most often sarcomas, may also occur in children who have been treated for retinoblastoma. Table 24.12 explains the classification of retinoblastoma.

TABLE 24.12 • Classification of Retinoblastoma

Classification	Clinical Findings
A (very low risk)	Small discrete tumor distant from critical structures
B (low risk)	Discrete retinal tumor without subretinal or vitreous seeding
C (moderate risk)	Discrete retinal tumor with only focal subretinal or vitreous seeding
D (high risk)	Large nondiscrete eye tumor(s) and/or diffuse subretinal or vitreous seeding
E (very high risk)	Anatomic or functional destruction of eye by the tumor

Data from Berry, J. L. (2023). Retinoblastoma: Clinical presentation, evaluation, and diagnosis. *UpToDate*. Retrieved on April 26, 2023, from https://www.uptodate.com/contents/retinoblastoma-clinical-presentation-evaluation-and-diagnosis/print

The goals of treatment are to eradicate the tumor, preserve vision, and provide a good cosmetic outcome. Retinoblastoma may be treated with radiation, chemotherapy, laser surgery, cryotherapy, or a combination of these treatments. Moderate vision may be preserved for most children without advanced disease. In advanced disease or in the case of a massive tumor with retinal detachment, enucleation (removal of the eye) is necessary.

Nursing Assessment

Parents are often the first to notice the "cat's eye reflex" or "whitewash glow" to the child's affected pupil. Obtain the health history, determining when other associated symptoms such as strabismus, orbital inflammation, vomiting, or headache began. Inquire about risk factors such as a family history of retinoblastoma or other cancer, or the presence of chromosomal anomalies. Assess pupils for size and reactivity to light. Note the presence of leukocoria ("cat's eye reflex," a whitish appearance of the pupil) in the affected eye (Fig. 24.19). Assess the eyes for associated signs, which may include erythema, orbital inflammation, or hyphema.

Diagnostic evaluation includes an ophthalmologic examination under anesthesia. CT, MRI, or ultrasound of the head and eyes will help to visualize the tumor. The infant or toddler may also undergo lumbar puncture and bone marrow aspiration to determine the presence and extent of metastasis.

Nursing Management

Provide routine postoperative care to the infant or toddler. If the eye is enucleated, observe the large pressure dressing on

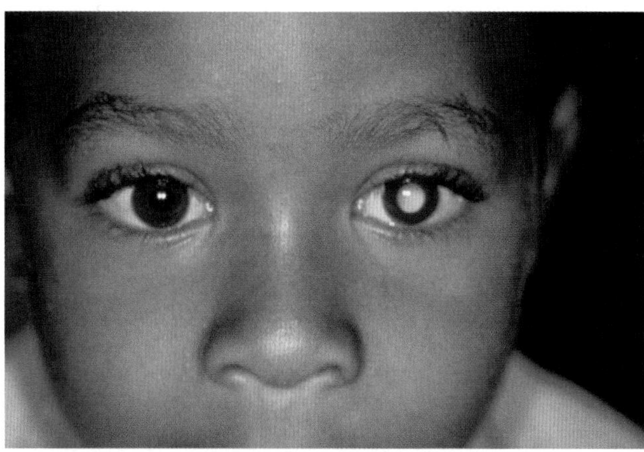

FIGURE 24.19 Note the whitish appearance of this child's pupil (leukocoria). (Reprinted with permission from Strayer, D. E., & Saffitz, J. E. [2019]. *Rubin's pathology: Mechanisms of human disease* [8th ed.]. Wolters Kluwer.)

the eye socket for bleeding. Dressing changes to the socket may include sterile saline rinses and/or antibiotic ointment application. If disease occurs outside of the eye or if metastasis is present, inform the parents that chemotherapy will be necessary. Monitor for side effects of chemotherapy (see the "Clinical Judgment and the Nursing Process" section).

Follow-up will include eye examinations every 3 to 6 months until age 6 and then annually to check for further tumor development. If the eye is enucleated, a prosthetic eye will be fitted several weeks after removal. Teach families use of the prosthetic eye; it does not require daily removal.

Provide parents with support and encouragement. Refer the family for genetic counseling. Children with a family history of retinoblastoma need ophthalmologic examination shortly after birth, at age 1 month, at age 2 months, every 3 months until age 3 years, and then at 4-to-6-month intervals until age 7 years (Berry, 2023).

TAKE NOTE!

Educate parents about protecting vision in the remaining eye: routine eye checkups, protection from accidental injury, use of safety goggles during sports, and prompt treatment of eye infections. Generally, children with one eye should not participate in contact sports.

SCREENING FOR REPRODUCTIVE CANCERS IN ADOLESCENTS

Increasingly, reproductive cancers are being diagnosed in adolescents. Cervical cancer and testicular cancer may be discovered early with appropriate screening, and earlier discovery leads to better outcomes. Starting screening in the adolescent years may also instill a lifelong healthy habit in the adolescent.

Cervical Cancer

Risk factors for cervical cancer include young age at first intercourse, infection with a sexually transmitted disease, and a history of multiple sex partners. More and more adolescents are presenting with these risk factors. Cervical cancer may be prevented through use of the human papillomavirus (HPV) vaccine, which is recommended to be given as a two-dose series to all children between 9 and 11 years of age (Fenton & Perkins, 2022). Despite the availability of the vaccine, not all children will receive it. Counsel all sexually active adolescents to seek reproductive care, which is available without parental consent in most states. The screening Papanicolaou (Pap) smear is efficient and reliable at determining abnormal cervical cells and is a key part of screening for cervical cancer (if cancer is present, the parent will have to be notified). Cervical cancer has a high response to therapy and rate of cure if treated in its early stages. Therefore, encourage adolescents to be responsible for their sexual health by seeking appropriate examination and screening. See the Healthy People 2030 box.

HEALTHY PEOPLE 2030

Objective	Nursing Significance
Increase the proportion of females who receive a cervical cancer screening based on the most recent guidelines.	When an adolescent female makes the decision to become sexually active, counsel them about the importance of getting annual Pap smears, which should begin within 3 years of becoming sexually active.

Healthy People Objectives retrieved from http://www.healthypeople.gov

Testicular Cancer

Although uncommon in adolescents, testicular cancer is most frequently diagnosed in young adult males (NCI, n.d.). It is one of the most curable cancers if diagnosed early. To get into the habit of screening for testicular lumps, encourage adolescents to begin performing testicular self-examinations monthly (Teaching Guidelines 24.5). See the Healthy People 2030 box.

TEACHING GUIDELINES 24.5 Testicular Self-Examination

- Perform the examination once a month, after a shower.
- Be familiar with the size and weight of your testicles.
- Roll the testicle between your fingers. The small rope-like structure is the epididymis; this is normal.
- Report any lump, swelling, or heaviness of one testicle to your health care provider or nurse practitioner.

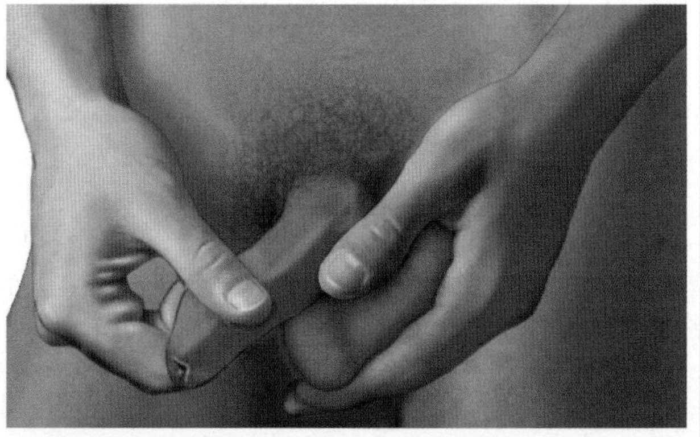

Based on Figueroa, T. E. (2021). *How to do a testicular self-exam*. http://kidshealth.org/teen/sexual_health/guys/tse.html

HEALTHY PEOPLE 2030

Objective	Nursing Significance
Reduce the overall cancer death rate. Increase the proportion of cancer survivors who are living 5 years or longer after diagnosis.	• Teach adolescents testicular self-examination. • Reinforce the importance of this self-screening measure at subsequent visits.

Healthy People Objectives retrieved from http://www.healthypeople.gov

Unfolding Patient Stories: Brittany Long • Part 2

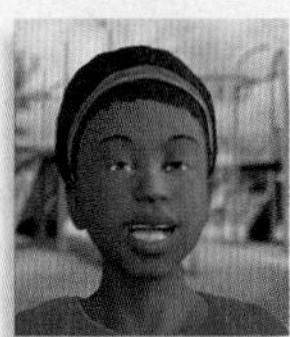

Think back to Brittany Long, whom you met in Chapter 13. Brittany is a 5-year-old Black child diagnosed with sickle cell anemia who lives with her parent, 7-year-old sister, and grandparent. Her pain crises are mostly managed at home, and she has been hospitalized three times. How can the nurse help Brittany and her family cope with a long-term illness and the management of acute crises? How can the reactions of family members influence Brittany's adjustment to sickle cell disease? What effect can a long-term illness have on the sister, and what actions can support her understanding and cooperation?

Care for Brittany and other patients in a realistic virtual environment: ***vSim** for Nursing* (thepoint.lww.com/vSimPediatric). Practice documenting these patients' care in DocuCare (thePoint.lww.com/DocuCareEHR).

KEY CONCEPTS

- The major forms of anemia affecting children are iron-deficiency anemia, lead poisoning, folic acid deficiency, pernicious anemia, sickle cell anemia, thalassemia, and G6PD deficiency.
- The major bleeding disorders affecting children are idiopathic thrombocytopenic purpura, immunoglobulin A vasculitis, DIC, hemophilia, and vWD.
- Childhood cancer tends to develop from embryonal tissue; in general, it is more responsive to therapy than adult cancers, which tend to be derived from epithelial tissue.
- In adults, cancer is influenced to a large extent by environmental factors. Cancer in children is most often not attributed to environmental factors, so generally, there are no routine screening measures or prevention strategies for childhood cancer.
- The pain associated with lumbar puncture or bone marrow aspiration may be minimized with the use of topical anesthetics or conscious sedation.
- CT scans and MRI are used extensively in the diagnosis and follow-up of childhood cancer. The young child may have difficulty holding still for these scans and may need short-term sedation.
- Assess for hypoxia, fatigue, and pallor in the child with anemia.
- Nursing assessment for the child with a bleeding disorder focuses on determining its extent and severity.
- Supplementation with iron is the key intervention for the child with iron-deficiency anemia.
- All young children should be screened for lead exposure.
- Prevention of infection and vaso-occlusive episodes takes priority in children with SCA.
- Multimodal pain management and astute physical assessment for serious complications are critical in the nursing care of the child having a sickle cell crisis.
- The priority intervention for management of thalassemia is chronic transfusion of PRBCs and chelation of iron.
- Idiopathic thrombocytopenic purpura and immunoglobulin A vasculitis are usually self-limiting diseases.
- Administration of factor VIII or desmopressin is the key nursing intervention when a bleeding episode occurs in the child with hemophilia A (desmopressin is also used for vWD).
- Significant anemia may result in hypoxia to the tissues.
- Prolonged bleeding times place the child at risk for hemorrhage.
- Prevention of injury is key for all children with hematologic disorders. Leukemia often presents in children with a history of fever, infection, and fatigue. Bone pain or CNS symptoms may be present if metastasis to the bone or brain has occurred.
- Lymphomas in children present similarly to those in adults, often with an enlarged, nontender lymph node.
- Symptoms of brain tumors depend on the location of the tumor; commonly, they present with signs and symptoms of increased intracranial pressure, such as headache, nausea, and vomiting.
- Neuroblastoma has often significantly metastasized at diagnosis. It most commonly presents as a mass in the abdomen.
- Shortness of breath or chest pain in the child with cancer is a medical emergency; it may indicate superior vena cava syndrome or a tumor in the mediastinal region.
- Retinoblastoma may be identified by the presence of leukocoria in one or both eyes. Retinoblastoma occurs in early infancy up until early childhood.
- Bone cancer does not necessarily require amputation; it may be treated with a combination of limb salvage procedure, radiation, and chemotherapy.
- The symptoms of rhabdomyosarcoma depend on the location of the tumor.

- Avoid abdominal palpation preoperatively in the child with Wilms tumor; palpation may cause seeding of the tumor and metastasis.
- Radiation therapy may result in fatigue, nausea, and vomiting, and long-term cognitive sequelae (if directed to the cranium).
- Nursing care of the child receiving treatment for cancer focuses on preventing or treating adverse effects such as fatigue, nausea, vomiting, alopecia, mucositis, and infection.
- The neutropenic child with fever should receive medical attention as soon as possible so that intravenous antibiotics may be started immediately.
- Cancer is a significant stressor for children and families. Families need support and education throughout the diagnostic process, treatment and cure, or palliative care.
- The child with cancer should lead as near normal a life as possible. When physically able and cleared by the oncologist, the child should resume usual activities such as school. Camps for children with cancer provide an excellent opportunity for children to enjoy everyday activities and meet children experiencing similar alterations in their lives.
- Nutrition may be optimized for children with cancer by managing nausea and vomiting with antiemetics, providing favorite foods, and possibly using total parenteral nutrition.
- Child and family teaching for anemias resulting from nutritional deficiencies focuses on promotion of a diet high in the deficient nutrients.
- Child and family teaching for bleeding disorders focuses on the prevention of injury.
- Numerous nationwide and local resources are available to children with hematologic disorders or nutritional deficits. These organizations offer a wide range of services, including education, support, multidisciplinary care (as appropriate), and financial assistance in caring for the disease.
- Teach adolescents appropriate screening techniques for reproductive cancers.
- Educate the child and family about the adverse effects of cancer treatments.
- Teach parents how to avoid infection in the child receiving chemotherapy, the signs and symptoms of infection, and when to seek medical treatment.

REFERENCES AND RECOMMENDED READINGS

Ahmed, N. M., & Flynn, P. M. (2022). Fever in children with chemotherapy-induced neutropenia. *UpToDate*. Retrieved on February 17, 2024, from https://www.uptodate.com/contents/fever-in-children-with-chemotherapy-induced-neutropenia

American Academy of Orthopedic Surgeons. (2023). *Ewing's sarcoma*. https://orthoinfo.aaos.org/en/diseases--conditions/ewings-sarcoma/

American Cancer Society. (2024a). *Cancer in children*. https://www.cancer.org/cancer/cancer-in-children.html

American Cancer Society. (2024b). *Chemotherapy*. https://www.cancer.org/treatment/treatments-and-side-effects/treatment-types/chemotherapy.html

American Cancer Society. (2024c). *Radiation therapy side effects*. https://www.cancer.org/treatment/treatments-and-side-effects/treatment-types/radiation/coping.html

American Cancer Society. (2024d). Risk factors for acute lymphocytic leukemia (ALL). https://www.cancer.org/cancer/types/acute-lymphocytic-leukemia/causes-risks-prevention/risk-factors.html

American Cancer Society. (2024e). *What causes Hodgkin lymphoma?* https://www.cancer.org/cancer/types/hodgkin-lymphoma/causes-risks-prevention/what-causes.html

Anzilotti, A. (2019). *Stem cell transplants*. https://kidshealth.org/en/parents/stem-cells.html

Asha, C., Manjini, K. J., & Dubashi, B. (2020). Effect of foot massage on patients with chemotherapy induced nausea and vomiting: A randomized clinical trial. *Journal of Caring Sciences*, *9*(3), 120–124. https://doi.org/10.34172/jcs.2020.018

Benz, E. J., & Angelucci, E. (2022). Diagnosis of thalassemia (adults and children). *UpToDate*. Retrieved on February 17, 2024, from https://www.uptodate.com/contents/diagnosis-of-thalassemia-adults-and-children

Berry, J. L. (2023). Retinoblastoma: Clinical presentation, evaluation, and diagnosis. *UpToDate*. Retrieved on February 17, 2024, from https://www.uptodate.com/contents/retinoblastoma-clinical-presentation-evaluation-and-diagnosis/print

Blaney, S. M., Adamson, P. C., & Helman, L. J. (2021). *Pizzo & Poplack's pediatric oncology* (8th ed.). Wolters Kluwer.

Borhade, M. B., & Kondamudi, N. P. (2022). Sickle cell crisis. *StatPearls*. https://www.ncbi.nlm.nih.gov/books/NBK526064/

Bussell, J. B. (2022a). Immune thrombocytopenia (ITP) in children: Clinical features and diagnosis. *UpToDate*. Retrieved on February 17, 2024, from https://www.uptodate.com/contents/immune-thrombocytopenia-itp-in-children-clinical-features-and-diagnosis

Bussell, J. B. (2022b). Immune thrombocytopenia (ITP) in children: Initial management. *UpToDate*. Retrieved on February 17, 2024, from https://www.uptodate.com/contents/immune-thrombocytopenia-itp-in-children-initial-management

Centers for Disease Control and Prevention. (2023a). *Data & statistics on sickle cell disease*. https://www.cdc.gov/ncbddd/sicklecell/data.html/

Centers for Disease Control and Prevention. (2023b). *State-based monitoring for selected hemoglobinopathies*. https://www.cdc.gov/ncbddd/hemoglobinopathies/features/keyfinding-state-based.html

Centers for Disease Control and Prevention. (2024). *Childhood lead poisoning prevention program*. https://www.cdc.gov/nceh/lead/

Children's Oncology Group. (2023). *Low white blood cell count (neutropenia)*. https://www.childrensoncologygroup.org/index.php/lowwhitebloodcellcount

Corbett, J. A., & Banks, A. D. (2019). *Laboratory tests and diagnostic procedures with nursing diagnoses* (9th ed.). Pearson Education Inc.

Cunningham, F. G., Leveno, K. J., Bloom, S. L., Dashe, J. S., Hoffman, B. L., Spong, C. Y., & Casey, B. M. (2022). *Williams obstetrics* (26th ed.). McGraw-Hill Education.

CureSearch. (2022). *Childhood cancer statistics*. https://curesearch.org/Childhood-Cancer-Statistics

DeBaun, M. R. (2022). Acute vaso-occlusive pain management in sickle cell disease. *UpToDate*. Retrieved on February 17, 2024, from https://www.uptodate.com/contents/vaso-occlusive-pain-management-in-sickle-cell-disease

Diab, L. K., Haemer, M., Primark, L. E., & Krebs, N. R. (2022). Chapter 11: Normal childhood nutrition & its disorders. In M. Bunik, W. W. Hay, M. J. Levin, & M. J. Abzug (Eds.), *Current diagnosis and treatment: Pediatrics* (26th ed., pp. 269–298). McGraw-Hill Education.

Fenton, R., & Perkins, R. (2022). *Here's why your preteen needs the HPV vaccine*. https://www.healthychildren.org/English/safety-prevention/immunizations/Pages/How-to-Talk-to-Your-Preteen-About-HPV-Vaccine.aspx

Field, J. J., & Vichinsky, E. P. (2023). Overview of the management and prognosis of sickle cell disease. *UpToDate*. Retrieved on February 17, 2024, from https://www.uptodate.com/contents/overview-of-the-management-and-prognosis-of-sickle-cell-disease

Figueroa, T. E. (2021). *How to do a testicular self-exam*. http://kidshealth.org/teen/sexual_health/guys/tse.html

Fischbach, F. T., Fischbach, M. A., & Stout, K. (2022). *A manual of laboratory and diagnostic tests* (11th ed.). Wolters Kluwer Health.

Hagan, J. F., Shaw, J. S., & Duncan, P. M. (Eds.). (2017). *Bright futures: Guidelines for health supervision of infants, children, and adolescents* (4th ed.). American Academy of Pediatrics.

Halmo, L., & Nappe, T. M. (2023). *Lead toxicity*. StatPearls. https://www.ncbi.nlm.nih.gov/books/NBK541097/

Hibberd, C., Hibberd, O., Karageorgos, S., & Barnard, G. (2023). Ten oncology emergencies in kids. *Don't Forget the Bubbles*. https://doi.org/10.31440/DFTB.53725

Horton, T. M., & McNeer, J. L. (2022). Treatment of acute lymphoblastic leukemia/lymphoma in children and adolescents. *UpToDate*. Retrieved on February 17, 2024, from https://www.uptodate.com/contents/overview-of-the-treatment-of-acute-lymphoblastic-leukemia-in-children-and-adolescents

James, P. (2023). Von Willebrand disease (VWD): Treatment of major bleeding and major surgery. *UpToDate*. Retrieved on February 17, 2024, from https://www.uptodate.com/contents/treatment-of-von-willebrand-disease

Keating, A. K., Knight-Perry, J., Maloney, K., Levy, J. M. M., Greffe, B. S., Franklin, A. R. K., & Garrington, T. P. (2022). Chapter 31: Neoplastic disease. In M. Bunik, W. W. Hay, M. J. Levin, & M. J. Abzug (Eds.), *Current diagnosis & treatment: Pediatrics* (26th ed., pp. 931–963). McGraw-Hill Education.

Kline, N. E. (2014). *Essentials of pediatric oncology nursing: A core curriculum* (4th ed.). Association of Pediatric Hematology/Oncology Nurses.

LaCasce, A. S., & Ng, A. K. (2022). Pretreatment evaluation, staging, and treatment stratification of classic Hodgkin lymphoma. *UpToDate*. Retrieved on February 17, 2024, from https://www.uptodate.com/contents/pretreatment-evaluation-staging-and-treatment-stratification-of-classic-hodgkin-lymphoma

Larson, S. D., Hebra, A., Raju, R., & Lee, S. (2020). Vascular access in children. *Medscape*. https://emedicine.medscape.com/article/1018395-overview#a1

Lau, C., & Teo, W-Y. (2024). Overview of the management of central nervous system tumors in children. *UpToDate*. Retrieved on February 17, 2024, from https://www.uptodate.com/contents/overview-of-the-management-of-central-nervous-system-tumors-in-children

Lerma, E. V., & Vichinsky, E. P. (2023). Sickle cell disease effects on the kidney. *UpToDate*. Retrieved April 16, 2024, from https://www.uptodate.com/contents/sickle-cell-disease-effects-on-the-kidney

Martin, B. M., Thaniel, L. N., Speller-Brown, B. J., & Darbari, D. S. (2018). Comprehensive infant clinic for sickle cell disease: Outcomes and parental perspective. *Journal of Pediatric Health Care, 32*(5), 485–490.

Mitin, T. (2023). Radiation therapy techniques in cancer treatment. *UpToDate*. Retrieved on February 17, 2024, from https://www.uptodate.com/contents/radiation-therapy-techniques-in-cancer-treatment

National Cancer Institute. (n.d.). *Cancer stat facts: Testicular cancer*. https://seer.cancer.gov/statfacts/html/testis.html

National Cancer Institute. (2023). *Childhood cancers*. https://www.cancer.gov/types/childhood-cancers

National Cancer Institute. (2024). *Late effects of treatment for childhood cancer (PDQ®)—Health professional version*. https://www.cancer.gov/types/childhood-cancers/late-effects-hp-pdq

National Hemophilia Foundation. (2023). *MASAC document 280—MASAC recommendations concerning products licensed for the treatment of hemophilia and selected disorders of the coagulation system*. https://www.hemophilia.org/healthcare-professionals/guidelines-on-care/masac-documents/masac-document-280-masac-recommendations-concerning-products-licensed-for-the-treatment-of-hemophilia-and-selected-disorders-of-the-coagulation-system

National Hospice and Palliative Care Organization. (2022). *Standards of practice for pediatric palliative care: Quality improvement resource*. https://www.nhpco.org/wp-content/uploads/Pediatric_Standards.pdf

Navin, M. C., & Wasserman, J. A. (2019). Capacity for preferences and pediatric assent implications for pediatric practice. *Hastings Center Report, 49*(1), 43–51.

Nuss, R., McKinney, C. & Wang, M. (2022). Chapter 30: Hematologic disorders. In M. Bunik, W. W. Hay, M. J. Levin, & M. J. Abzug (Eds.), *Current diagnosis and treatment: Pediatrics* (26th ed., pp. 931–963). McGraw-Hill Education.

Nuuhiwa, J. (2022). Module 9: Boundaries and self-care. In M. Evans, J. Nuuhiwa, R. L. Secola, & K. Wolownik, *Foundations of pediatric hematopoietic stem cell transplantation* (3rd ed.). Association of Pediatric Hematology/Oncology Nurses.

Okcu, M. F., & Hicks, J. (2023). Rhabdomyosarcoma in childhood and adolescence: Clinical presentation, diagnostic evaluation, and staging. *UpToDate*. Retrieved on February 17, 2024, from https://www.uptodate.com/contents/rhabdomyosarcoma-in-childhood-and-adolescence-clinical-presentation-diagnostic-evaluation-and-staging

Powers, J. M. (2023). Iron deficiency in infants and children <12 years: Screening, prevention, clinical manifestations, and diagnosis. *UpToDate*. Retrieved on February 17, 2024, from https://www.uptodate.com/contents/iron-deficiency-in-infants-and-children-less-than12-years-screening-prevention-clinical-manifestations-and-diagnosis

Rugo, H. S., & van den Hurk, C. (2023). Alopecia related to systemic cancer therapy. *UpToDate*. Retrieved on February 17, 2024, from https://www.uptodate.com/contents/chemotherapy-induced-alopecia

Sample, J. A. (2024). Childhood lead poisoning: Management. *UpToDate*. Retrieved on February 17, 2024, from http://www.uptodate.com/contents/childhood-lead-poisoning-management

Sanofi. (2023). *FDA approves once-weekly ALTUVIIIO™, a new class of factor VIII therapy for hemophilia A that offers significant bleed protection*. https://ml-eu.globenewswire.com/Resource/Download/23793006-c334-46f9-b225-27df9c8a9285

Secola, R. (2022a). Module 2—HSCT types, selections, stem cell/cellular therapy sources. In M. Evans, J. Nuuhiwa, R. L. Secola, & K. Wolownik, *Foundations of pediatric hematopoietic stem cell transplantation* (3rd ed.). Association of Pediatric Hematology/Oncology Nurses.

Secola, R. (2022b). Module 3—Hematopoietic stem cell transplant (HSCT) conditioning regimens. In M. Evans, J. Nuuhiwa, R. L. Secola, & K. Wolownik, *Foundations of pediatric hematopoietic stem cell transplantation* (3rd ed.). Association of Pediatric Hematology/Oncology Nurses.

Shohet, J. M., Nuchtern, J. G., & Foster, J. H. (2024). Treatment and prognosis of neuroblastoma. *UpToDate*. Retrieved on February 17, 2024, from https://www.uptodate.com/contents/treatment-and-prognosis-of-neuroblastoma

Smith, V., & Chintagumpala, M. (2023). Treatment and prognosis of Wilms tumor. *UpToDate*. Retrieved June 4, 2024, from https://www.uptodate.com/contents/treatment-and-prognosis-of-wilms-tumor

UpToDate, Inc. (2024). *Lexi-comp® (Version 8.1.0) [Mobile app]*. Wolters Kluwer. https://apps.apple.com/us/app/lexicomp/id313401238

U.S. Department of Health and Human Services. (n.d.). *Healthy People 2030*. https://health.gov/healthypeople

Vichinsky, E. P. (2023). Overview of the clinical manifestations of sickle cell disease. *UpToDate*. Retrieved on April 19, 2023, from https://www.uptodate.com/contents/overview-of-the-clinical-manifestations-of-sickle-cell-disease

DEVELOPING CLINICAL JUDGMENT

PRACTICING FOR NCLEX

1. A child on the pediatric unit has morning laboratory results of Hgb 10.0, Hct 30.2, WBC 24,000, and platelets 20,000. What is the priority nursing assessment?
   a. Assess for pallor, fatigue, and tachycardia.
   b. Monitor for fever.
   c. Assess for bruising or bleeding.
   d. Determine intake and output.
2. A child with hemophilia A fell while riding his bicycle. He was wearing a helmet and did not lose consciousness. He has a mild abrasion on his knee that is not oozing. He is complaining of abdominal pain. What is the priority nursing assessment?
   a. Perform neurologic checks.
   b. Assess ability to void frequently.
   c. Carefully assess his abdomen.
   d. Examine his knee frequently.
3. A 14-year-old with thalassemia asks for your assistance in choosing her afternoon snack. Which choice is the most appropriate?
   a. Peanut butter with rice cake
   b. Small spinach salad
   c. Apple slices with cheddar cheese
   d. Small burger on wheat bun
4. The nurse is caring for a child who has just been admitted to the pediatric unit with sickle cell crisis. He is complaining that his right arm and leg hurt. What is the priority nursing intervention?
   a. Administer pain medication every 3 hours intravenously until pain is controlled.
   b. Perform passive ROM of the arm and leg to maintain function.
   c. Try acetaminophen for pain first, moving up to opioids only if needed.
   d. Use narcotic analgesics and warm compresses as needed to control the pain.
5. A 5-year-old has been diagnosed with Wilms tumor. What is the priority nursing intervention for this child?
   a. Educate the parents about dialysis, as the kidney will be removed.
   b. Measure abdominal girth every shift.
   c. Avoid palpating the child's abdomen.
   d. Monitor BUN and creatinine every 4 hours.
6. A child with leukemia has the following AM laboratory results: Hgb 8.0, Hct 24.2, WBC 8,000, platelets 150,000. What is the priority nursing assessment?
   a. Monitor for fever.
   b. Assess for bruising or bleeding.
   c. Determine intake and output.
   d. Assess for pallor, fatigue, and tachycardia.
7. A child with leukemia received chemotherapy about 10 days ago. She presents today with a temperature of 100.4°F, an absolute neutrophil count of 500, and mild bleeding of the gums. What is the priority nursing intervention?
   a. Administer IV antibiotics as ordered.
   b. Provide vigorous oral care frequently with a firm toothbrush.
   c. Monitor pulse and blood pressure for changes.
   d. Administer packed RBC transfusion.
8. A child with cancer is receiving chemotherapy, and their parent is concerned that the nausea and vomiting associated with chemotherapy are reducing his ability to eat and gain weight appropriately. Which is the appropriate nursing action?
   a. Administer an antiemetic at the first hint of nausea.
   b. Offer the child's favorite foods to encourage him to eat.
   c. Start antiemetic drugs prior to the chemotherapy infusion.
   d. Maintain IV fluid infusion to avoid dehydration.
9. A child is admitted to the hospital with the diagnosis of acute lymphoblastic leukemia (ALL). Which clinical manifestations require the most urgent nursing intervention? Select all that apply.
   a. Anorexia
   b. Enlarged cervical lymph nodes
   c. Fatigue
   d. Fever
   e. Hepatomegaly
   f. Lethargy
   g. Petechiae
   h. Splenomegaly
10. A child has been newly diagnosed with leukemia, and the nurse has reviewed the child's laboratory report.

Test	Traditional Units	SI Units
Hgb	11.1 g/dL	6.89 mmol/L
Hct	35.6%	0.365
WBC	6,750 mm^3	6.75 * 109/L
Platelets	39,000 mm^3	39 * 109/L

The child is at risk for ________, related to ________.

Blank 1:
a. activity intolerance
b. bleeding
c. impaired tissue perfusion
d. infection

Blank 2:
a. hemoglobin level
b. hematocrit
c. platelet count
d. WBC count

DOSAGE CALCULATION QUESTION

The nurse is caring for a 4-year-old with acute lymphoblastic leukemia. The child weighs 38 lb. The medication order reads: ondansetron 2.6 mg IV every 8 hours for chemotherapy-related nausea/vomiting. Ondansetron is supplied as 4 mg/2 mL. How many milliliters will the nurse administer? Round to the nearest tenth.

CRITICAL THINKING EXERCISES

1. Develop a discharge teaching plan for the parent of a toddler who has just been diagnosed with hemophilia and received factor infusion treatment for a bleeding episode.
2. An 8-year-old has been diagnosed with iron-deficiency anemia. Formulate a nutrition plan for this child.
3. A 5-year-old with beta-thalassemia is resistant to nightly chelation therapy at home. Devise a developmentally appropriate teaching plan for this child.
4. Develop a nursing care plan for a child with sickle cell disease who experiences frequent vaso-occlusive crises.
5. Develop a discharge teaching plan for a child who has just completed the induction phase of chemotherapy for acute lymphocytic leukemia.
6. A 17-year-old female has recently been diagnosed with osteosarcoma. She is worried about how treatment will affect her plans for college, marriage, and children. How will you respond to her concerns?
7. A 3-year-old is going to be starting chemotherapy for rhabdomyosarcoma. Develop an age-appropriate teaching plan for this child.
8. Develop a nursing care plan for an adolescent with cancer who is undergoing radiation and chemotherapy and experiencing a significant number of adverse effects from the treatment.

STUDY ACTIVITIES

1. Visit your local WIC office. Meet with the staff and learn about the services offered for prevention of and nutritional support for anemia. Provide a written report of your learning experience or provide a presentation to your classmates.
2. In the clinical setting, compare the growth and development of a child with sickle cell disease to that of a similarly aged child who has been healthy.
3. Talk to an adolescent with hemophilia about their life experiences and feelings about their disease and their health. Reflect on this conversation in your clinical journal.
4. Visit a public health clinic that provides primary care to children. Spend time with the registered nurse (RN), the advanced practice nurse, and the unlicensed assistive personnel. Write a summary of the roles of the RN in screening for and managing hematologic disorders in children, noting roles that are reserved for the advanced practice nurse and activities that the RN would delegate to unlicensed assistive personnel.
5. While in the clinical area, care for a young child who has undergone therapy for a brain tumor. Compare this child's growth and development to those of a healthy child of similar age whom you know or have cared for.
6. During your clinical rotation, care for a child who has received several chemotherapy treatments. After establishing a therapeutic relationship, talk with the child about their understanding of the disease and the experience the child has had with diagnosis and treatment thus far. If time allows, ask the child to draw a picture describing this experience. Record your observations in your clinical journal, and reflect on the emotions you feel about this experience.
7. Attend the pediatric oncology clinic. Determine the role of the advanced practice nurse (nurse practitioner or clinical nurse specialist) compared to the role of the RN in the outpatient care of children with cancer. Determine which activities the nurse appropriately delegates to unlicensed assistive personnel in that setting.
8. Talk to the hospital chaplain about their experiences with dying children. Reflect on this conversation in your clinical journal.

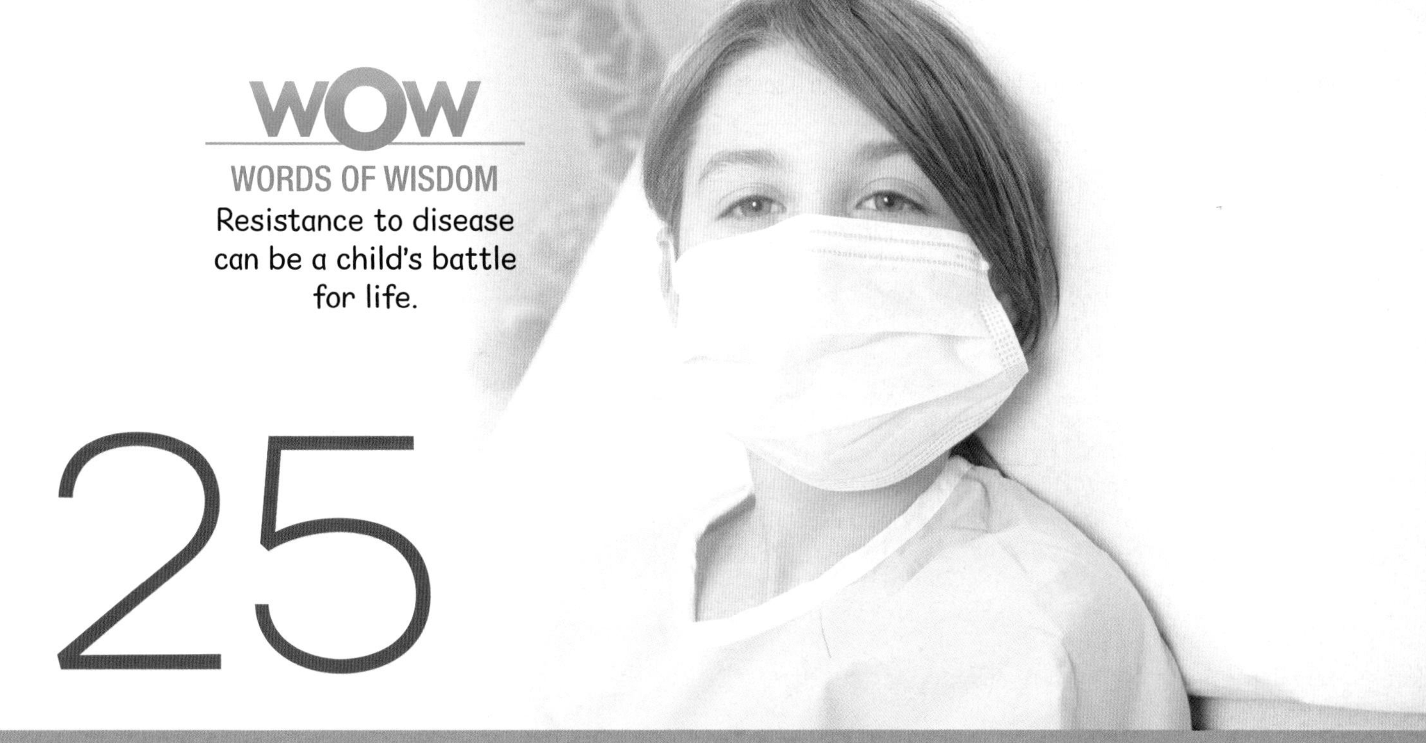
WOW
WORDS OF WISDOM
Resistance to disease can be a child's battle for life.
25

Nursing Care of the Child With an Alteration in Immunity or Immunologic Disorder

LEARNING OBJECTIVES

Upon completion of the chapter, you will be able to:

1. Explain the anatomic and physiologic differences of the immune systems of infants and children compared to that of adults.
2. Describe nursing care related to common laboratory and diagnostic testing used in the medical diagnosis of pediatric immune and autoimmune disorders.
3. Distinguish immune, autoimmune, and allergic disorders common in infants, children, and adolescents.
4. Identify appropriate nursing assessments and interventions related to medications and treatments for pediatric immune, autoimmune, and allergic disorders.
5. Develop an individualized nursing care plan or concept map for the child with an immune or autoimmune disorder.
6. Describe the psychosocial impact of chronic immune disorders on children.
7. Devise a nutrition plan for the child with immunodeficiency.
8. Develop child and family teaching plans for the child with an immune or autoimmune disorder.

KEY TERMS

antibodies
antigen
autoantibodies
cellular immunity
chemotaxis (kē′mō-tak′sis)
humoral immunity
immunodeficiency
immunoglobulins
immunosuppressive
opsonization (op′sŏ-nī-zā′shŭn)
phagocytosis (fāg′ō-sī-tō′sis)

Lakeisha Harris, 15 years old, is brought to the clinic by her parent. She presents with complaints of pain and swelling in her joints, weight gain, and fatigue. Lakeisha states, "I'm just very tired all the time, and my knees and ankles ache."

INTRODUCTION

Immunity refers to natural or induced resistance to infection. Nurses may encounter children with alterations in immunity and should be familiar with various immunologic disorders that children experience. **Immunodeficiency** (incapacity to mount an appropriate immune response), autoimmune, and allergic disorders have a significant impact on the lives of affected children. Infants and children are exposed to many infectious microorganisms and allergens and thus need a functional immune system to protect themselves.

Primary or secondary immune deficiencies are the focus of this discussion, along with allergy and anaphylaxis. These immune disorders are chronic, and affected children have more infections compared with healthy children. Recurrent viral or bacterial infections may cause the child to miss significant amounts of school or playtime with other children. Many immunodeficiencies require chronic and frequent clinic visits as well as daily medications. This can be a stress on the family as well. Autoimmune disorders are also chronic, causing significant disruption to the child's and family's life. Allergic disorders in some children may cause significant stress for the child and family. Nurses who care for children need to be familiar with common immunodeficiencies, autoimmune disorders, and allergies to intervene effectively with children and their families.

VARIATIONS IN PEDIATRIC ANATOMY AND PHYSIOLOGY

Normal immune function is a complex process involving **phagocytosis** (process by which phagocytes swallow up and break down microorganisms), **humoral immunity** (immunity mediated by antibodies secreted by B cells), **cellular immunity** (cell-mediated immunity controlled by T cells), and activation of the complement system. The lymphatic system and the white blood cells (WBCs) are the primary players in the immune response. Although these structures and cells are present at birth, the healthy full-term infant's immune system is still immature. The newborn exhibits a decreased inflammatory response to invading organisms, and this increases their susceptibility to infection. Cellular immunity is generally functional at birth, and as the infant is exposed to various substances over time, humoral immunity develops. Comparison Chart 25.1 provides more information on humoral and cellular immunity.

Lymph System

Lymph nodes in the newborn are relatively small, soft, and difficult to palpate. As the infant is exposed to various germs or illnesses, the lymph system passively filters plasma for bacteria or other foreign material before returning it to the bloodstream and back to the heart. As WBCs infiltrate the lymph nodes to attack the foreign substance, the nodes enlarge. Young children have frequent episodes of localized enlarged lymph nodes because of their repeated exposure to viral illnesses (Tosi, 2019). The spleen is functional at birth and also filters the blood for foreign cells. The thymus, responsible for the production of lymphocyte T cells as well as for the development and maturation of peripheral lymphoid tissue, is quite enlarged at birth and remains so until about 10 years of age. It then involutes slowly throughout adulthood. The tonsils are also often enlarged throughout early childhood. The bone marrow is functional at birth, producing stem cells capable of differentiating into various blood cells.

Phagocytosis

Under conditions of stress, the newborn and infant exhibit decreased phagocytic activity. The complement system, which is responsible for **opsonization** (process of making microorganisms more susceptible to phagocytosis) and **chemotaxis** (movement of neutrophils toward microorganisms),

COMPARISON CHART 25.1 Humoral Versus Cellular Immunity

Humoral Immunity (Antibody Protection)	Cellular Immunity (Cell-Mediated Immune Response)
• Lymphocytes: B cells	• Lymphocytes: T cells
• Secrete antibodies to viruses and bacteria; antibodies mark the antigen cell for destruction.	• Direct and regulate immune response (helper T cells).
• Recognize antigens.	• Do not recognize antigens.
• Do not destroy the foreign cell.	• Attack infected or foreign cells (killer T cells and natural killer cells).
• Cross the placenta in the form of IgG.	• Do not cross the placenta.

IgG, immunoglobulin G.

is immature in the newborn but reaches adult levels of activity by 3 to 6 months of age. The infant's phagocytic cells (neutrophils and monocytes) demonstrate decreased chemotaxis, reaching adult levels when the child is several years old. With complement levels being only 50% to 75% of adult levels in the full-term infant, decreased opsonization may be responsible for decreased phagocytic activity compared with adults.

Cellular Immunity

Maternal T cells do not cross the placenta, so the fetal thymus begins production of T cells early in gestation, and the newborn demonstrates a relative lymphocytosis compared with the adult, probably due to increased amounts of T-cell lymphocytes. Although cellular immunity does not cross the placenta, the fetal T cells may become sensitized to antigens that do cross the placenta. Viral infection, hyperbilirubinemia, and drugs taken by the pregnant parent late in pregnancy may contribute to depressed T-cell function in the newborn. Since delayed hypersensitivity reactions are mediated by T cells rather than antibodies, skin test responses (such as purified protein derivative [PPD] for tuberculosis detection) are diminished until about 1 year of age, probably due to the infant's decreased ability to mount an inflammatory response.

Humoral Immunity

The newborn's B cells do not respond as well to infection as do adults'. B cells are responsible for the formation of **antibodies** (specific immunity). The antibodies bind to the **antigen** (substance stimulating an immune response), thus disabling the specific toxin. The fetus is normally in an antigen-free environment and so produces only trace amounts of **immunoglobulins** (Ig; gamma globulin antibody proteins), specifically IgM. Most of the newborn's IgG is acquired transplacentally from the pregnant parent. Hence, the newborn exhibits passive immunity to antigens to which the pregnant parent had developed antibodies. These antibodies wane over the initial months of life as the transplacental IgG is catabolized, having a half-life of only about 25 days.

The newborn begins to make IgG but ordinarily experiences a physiologic hypogammaglobulinemia between 2 and 6 months of age until self-production of IgG reaches higher levels. The breastfed infant will acquire passive transfer of maternal immunity via the breast milk and will be better protected during the physiologic hypogammaglobulinemia phase. By 1 year of age, IgG is 50% of the adult level, and by 7 years of age it reaches the average adult level.

IgA, IgD, IgE, and IgM do not cross the placenta; they require an antigenic challenge for production. IgD and IgE constitute a very small percentage of the immunoglobulins in all ages. IgA increases slowly to about 30% of the adult level at 2 years of age, reaching near-adult levels by age 10 to 13 years. IgM is close to the adult level by 4 years of age (Mayo Foundation for Clinical Education and Research, 2024).

COMMON MEDICAL TREATMENTS

A variety of medications and other medical treatments are used to treat immune deficiencies and autoimmune problems in children. Most of these treatments will require a health care provider's or nurse practitioner's order when the child is in the hospital. The most common treatments and medications are listed in Common Medical Treatments 25.1 and Drug Guide 25.1. The nurse caring for the child with an immune deficiency or autoimmune disorder should be familiar with what the procedures and medications are, how they work, and common nursing implications related to use of these modalities.

COMMON MEDICAL TREATMENTS 25.1

Treatment	Explanation	Indications	Nursing Implications
Immunizations	Killed or modified microorganisms, or components of them, cause the immune system to develop antibodies to the microorganism without developing disease.	Prevention of certain viral and bacterial infections	Do not administer live vaccines to immunosuppressed people. Refer to the individual vaccine for method of administration and contraindications. Report adverse reactions via the vaccine adverse reaction (VAR) reporting system.
Bone marrow or stem cell transplantation	Bone marrow transplant: transfer of healthy bone marrow into the bones of a person with immune malfunction; the transplanted cells can then develop into functional B and T cells Stem cell transplant: Peripheral stem cells are removed from the donor via apheresis or stem cells are retrieved from the umbilical cord and placenta. The stem cells are then transplanted into the recipient	Wiskott–Aldrich syndrome, severe combined immune deficiency (SCID)	Administer immunosuppressive medications as ordered. Maintain medical asepsis and protective isolation to prevent infection. Monitor closely for graft-versus-host disease. Provide meticulous oral care. Avoid rectal temperatures and suppositories. Encourage appropriate nutrition.

DRUG GUIDE 25.1

COMMON DRUGS FOR IMMUNOLOGIC DISORDERS

Medication	Actions/Indications	Nursing Implications
Intravenous immune globulin (IVIG)	Provides exogenous IgG antibodies Indicated for primary immune deficiencies, human immunodeficiency virus (HIV) infection, myasthenia gravis	Do not mix with IV medications or with other IV fluids. Do not give IM or SQ. Monitor vital signs and watch for adverse reactions frequently during infusion. May require antipyretic or antihistamine to prevent chills and fever during infusion Have epinephrine available during infusion.
Nucleoside analog reverse transcriptase inhibitors (NRTIs): abacavir, lamivudine, zidovudine	Inhibit reverse transcription of the viral DNA chain. For treatment of HIV-1 infection as part of a three-drug regimen; zidovudine is also used to prevent perinatal transmission of HIV.	Notify health care provider of muscle weakness, shortness of breath, headache, insomnia, rash, or unusual bleeding. Give IV zidovudine over 1 hour. Fatal hypersensitivity reaction may occur with abacavir.
Nonnucleoside analog reverse transcriptase inhibitors (NNRTIs): efavirenz, nevirapine	Bind to HIV-1 reverse transcriptase, blocking DNA polymerase activity and disrupting the virus life cycle; used for treatment of HIV-1 infection as part of a three-drug regimen	*Nevirapine*: Avoid St. John's wort. Shake suspension gently before administration. Observe for symptoms of Stevens–Johnson syndrome. *Efavirenz*: May cause drowsiness
Protease inhibitors: amprenavir, atazanavir, indinavir, lopinavir, nelfinavir, ritonavir, saquinavir	Inhibit protease activity in the HIV-1 cell, resulting in immature, noninfectious viral particles; used for treatment of HIV-1 infection as part of a three-drug regimen	Multiple drug interactions; review specific medication for adverse effects and administration implications.
Nonsteroidal antiinflammatory drugs (NSAIDs): diclofenac, ibuprofen, naproxen, others	Inhibit prostaglandin synthesis, antiinflammatory action Indicated for juvenile idiopathic arthritis	Administer with food to decrease GI upset. May cause gastric bleeding, increased liver enzymes, decreased kidney function Monitor liver enzymes. Do not crush or chew extended-release or timed-release preparations.
Neuromuscular blocking agent: pyridostigmine	Cholinergic for myasthenia gravis—inhibits destruction of acetylcholine	Note muscle strength, heart rate, and respirations. Overdose may result in a cholinergic crisis. Monitor for sweating, salivation, urinary incontinence.
Corticosteroids	Antiinflammatory and immunosuppressive action; used for juvenile idiopathic arthritis, systemic lupus erythematosus (SLE), myasthenia gravis, and immunosuppression in children with bone marrow or stem cell transplants	Administer with food to decrease GI upset. May mask signs of infection Monitor blood pressure and urine for glucose. Do not stop treatment abruptly, or acute adrenal insufficiency may occur. Monitor for Cushing syndrome. Doses may be tapered over time. *Intravenous pulse:* Monitor for hypertension during infusion.
Cytotoxic drugs (cyclophosphamide)	Interfere with normal function of DNA by alkylation; for treatment of severe SLE	Cause bone marrow suppression; monitor for signs of infection. *Cyclophosphamide*: Administer in the morning. Provide adequate hydration and have child void frequently during and after infusion to decrease risk of hemorrhagic cystitis.
Immunosuppressant drugs (cyclosporine A [CyA], azathioprine)	Inhibition of production and release of interleukin II (CyA) Antagonize purine metabolism (azathioprine); used for severe steroid-resistant autoimmune disease	Monitor CBC, serum creatinine, potassium, and magnesium. Monitor blood pressure and watch for signs of infection. Draw blood levels before morning dose. *CyA*: Do not give with grapefruit juice.

DRUG GUIDE 25.1

COMMON DRUGS FOR IMMUNOLOGIC DISORDERS

Medication	Actions/Indications	Nursing Implications
Antimalarial drugs: hydroxychloroquine sulfate	Impair complement-dependent antigen–antibody reactions to prevent flares in SLE and juvenile arthritis	Funduscopic eye examination and visual field testing every year
Disease-modifying antirheumatic drugs (DMARDs): methotrexate, etanercept	Methotrexate: antimetabolite that depletes DNA precursors, inhibits DNA and urine synthesis Etanercept: binds to tumor necrosis factor (TNF), rendering it ineffective. Used for severe polyarticular juvenile arthritis	*Methotrexate*: Do not give oral form with dairy products. Approximate time to benefit in treatment of arthritis is 3–6 weeks. Salicylates may delay clearance. Protect IV preparation from light. Monitor CBC, kidney and liver function, and symptoms of infection. *Etanercept*: Monitor closely for infection. Do not give live vaccines. Give SQ, twice weekly; effect in 1 week to 3 months

CBC, complete blood count; GI, gastrointestinal; IM, intramuscularly; IV, intravenous; SQ, subcutaneously.

Data from UpToDate, Inc. (2024). *Lexi-comp®* (Version 8.1.0) [Mobile app]. Wolters Kluwer. https://apps.apple.com/us/app/lexicomp/id313401238

COMMON LABORATORY AND DIAGNOSTIC TESTS 25.1

Test	Explanation	Indications	Nursing Implications
Complete blood count (CBC) with differential	Evaluates hemoglobin and hematocrit, WBC count (particularly the percentage of individual WBCs), and platelet count	Infection, inflammatory process, immunosuppression	Normal values vary according to age and sex. WBC count differential is helpful in evaluating source of infection. May be affected by myelosuppressive drugs
Immunoglobulin electrophoresis	Determines level of individual immunoglobulins (IgA, IgD, IgE, IgG, IgM) in the blood	Immune deficiency, autoimmune disorders	Normal levels vary with age. IVIG administration and steroids alter levels.
IgG subclasses	Measure the levels of the four subclasses of IgG (1, 2, 3, and 4)	Determine immune deficiency.	Normal levels vary with age. IVIG administration and steroids alter levels.
Lymphocyte immunophenotyping T-cell quantification	Measures level of T cells (T helper [CD4], T suppressor [CD8]), B cells, and natural killer cells in the blood	Ongoing monitoring of progressive depletion of CD4 T lymphocytes in HIV disease	Do not refrigerate specimen. Steroids may elevate and immunosuppressive drugs may depress lymphocyte levels.
Delayed hypersensitivity skin test	Measures the presence of activated T cells that recognize certain substances	Immune disorders	Administered intradermally Read and document size of reaction at 48–72 hours (tuberculosis, mumps, Candida, tetanus).
Virologic assay (HIV RNA and DNA nucleic acid and polymerase chain reaction tests)	Used to detect HIV RNA and DNA	Diagnosis of HIV infection in children older than 2 weeks of age and ongoing monitoring of viral load	Sensitive and specific for presence of HIV in blood Sequential testing needed to determine perinatal transmission
CD4 count	Measures the number of CD4 T lymphocytes in the blood	Used in people with HIV to determine response to antiretroviral therapy	Normal is $\geq$1,500/mm^3 in the infant, $\geq$1,000/mm^3 in the 1–5-year-old, $\geq$500/mm^3 in children 6 years and older

(*continued*)

COMMON LABORATORY AND DIAGNOSTIC TESTS 25.1 (continued)

Test	Explanation	Indications	Nursing Implications
Complement assay (C3 and C4)	Measures the level of total complement in the blood, as well as levels of C3 and C4	Monitor SLE; determine complement deficiency	Send to laboratory immediately (unstable at room temperature). Usually sent out to a reference laboratory
Erythrocyte sedimentation rate (ESR)	Nonspecific test used to determine presence of infection or inflammation	Immune disorder initial workup, ongoing monitoring of autoimmune disease	Send to laboratory immediately; if allowed to stand >3 hours, falsely low result may occur.
Rheumatoid factor (RF)	Determines the presence of RF in the blood	Juvenile idiopathic arthritis, SLE	Positive RF is also sometimes seen in chronic infectious disorders.
Antinuclear antibody (ANA)	Tests for presence of autoantibodies that react against cellular nuclear material	SLE	Check for signs of infection at venipuncture site. Steroid use can cause false-negative result. May be weakly positive in about 20% of healthy individuals
RAST (radioallergosorbent test)	Measures minute quantities of IgE in the blood Carries no risk of anaphylaxis but is not as sensitive as skin testing	Asthma (food allergies)	Blood test that is usually sent out to a reference laboratory
Allergy skin testing	Suggested allergen is applied to skin via scratch, pin, or prick. A wheal response indicates allergy to the substance. Carries risk of anaphylaxis (Nursing note: Antihistamines must be discontinued before testing, as they inhibit the test.)	Allergic rhinitis, asthma	Close observation for anaphylaxis is necessary. Epinephrine and emergency equipment should be readily available. Some children react to the skin test almost immediately; others take several minutes.
Food-specific IgE antibody testing	Measures IgE antibody to specific food allergens	Accurately determine specific food allergy.	IVIG administration and steroids alter levels.

Ig, immunoglobulin; IVIG, intravenous immune globulin; SLE, systemic lupus erythematosus; WBC, white blood cell.

Data from Corbett, J. A., & Banks, A. D. (2019). *Laboratory tests and diagnostic procedures with nursing diagnoses* (9th ed.). Pearson Education Inc.

ATRAUMATIC CARE

When a child requires repeat injections related to an immune or allergic disorder, use a local anesthetic such as EMLA (eutectic mixture of local anesthetic) cream or a numbing spray to reduce the amount of associated pain.

Clinical Judgment and the Nursing Process for the Child With an Immunologic Disorder

Care of the child with an immunologic or allergic disorder includes assessment, analysis, planning, interventions, and evaluation. There are many general concepts related to the nursing process that may be applied to immunodeficiencies, autoimmune, and allergic disorders. From a general understanding of the care involved for a child with immune dysfunction, the nurse can then individualize the care based on the particular child's specifics.

Assessment

Assessment of children with immunodeficiency, autoimmune disorders, or allergy includes health history, physical examination, and laboratory and diagnostic testing.

Health History

The health history consists of past medical history, including the birthing parent's pregnancy history; family history; and history of present illness (when the symptoms started and how they have progressed), as well as medications and treatments used at home. The past medical history may be significant for:

- Maternal HIV infection
- Frequent, recurrent infections such as otitis media, sinusitis, or pneumonia
- Chronic cough
- Recurrent low-grade fever
- Two or more serious infections in early childhood
- Recurrent deep skin or organ abscesses
- Persistent thrush in the mouth
- Extensive eczema
- Growth failure

Family history may be positive for primary immune deficiency or autoimmune disorder. Document history of known allergy. Note the response that occurs when the child encounters the allergen.

Physical Examination

Physical examination of the child with immunodeficiency or autoimmune disorder includes inspection and observation, auscultation, percussion, and palpation.

INSPECTION AND OBSERVATION

Plot weight and length or height on appropriate growth charts. Inspect the oropharynx for tonsillar size. Note eczematous or other skin lesions, which may occur with allergic diseases or Wiskott–Aldrich syndrome. Document the presence of thrush, which occurs frequently in children with immunodeficiency. Observe gait for unexplained ataxia (neurologic alterations occur with HIV infection).

AUSCULTATION, PERCUSSION, AND PALPATION

Auscultate the lungs for adventitious sounds, which may be present with a concurrent respiratory infection. Note any wheezing that may occur with an allergic reaction. Percuss the abdomen and determine liver span. Palpate for unusually enlarged lymph nodes, particularly in nonadjacent locations. Palpate the abdomen for an enlarged spleen or liver.

Laboratory and Diagnostic Testing

Common Laboratory and Diagnostic Tests 25.1 explains the laboratory and diagnostic tests most commonly used when considering immune disorders. Results of these tests may assist the health care provider or nurse practitioner in diagnosing the disorder and/or be used as guidelines in determining ongoing treatment. Laboratory or nonnursing personnel obtain some of the tests, while the nurse might obtain others. In either instance, it is important for the nurse to be familiar with how the tests are obtained, what they are used for, and normal versus abnormal results. This knowledge will also be necessary when providing child and family education related to the testing.

Remember Lakeisha, the 15-year-old with joint pain and swelling, fatigue, and weight gain? What additional health history and physical examination assessment information should you obtain?

Nursing Analysis

After recognizing and analyzing cues from a thorough assessment, the nurse might identify several patient problems, including:

- Infection risk
- Malnutrition risk
- Impaired skin integrity risk
- Activity intolerance
- Delayed development risk
- Pain
- Interrupted family processes
- Caregiver role strain risk
- Knowledge deficiency

After completing an assessment of Lakeisha, you note the following: alopecia, abdominal tenderness, and oral ulcers. Based on these assessment findings, what would your top three patient problems be for Lakeisha?

The foregoing patient problems provide suggestions for nursing care planning or concept mapping for the child with an alteration in immunity. Suggested interventions with rationales for the child with an immunologic disorder, autoimmune disorder, or allergic response are provided next. Care planning should be individualized, based on the child's and family's needs. Refer to Chapter 14 for the nursing process for pain management and to Chapter 11 for nursing interventions related to interrupted family processes and caregiver role strain risk. Additional information will be included later in the chapter as it relates to nursing management of children with specific disorders, as well as particular nursing interventions for deficient knowledge.

Nursing Analysis

Infection risk; immunodeficiency is a risk factor.

Goal/Outcome

Child will not experience overwhelming infection: will be infection-free or able to recover if they become infected

Preventing Infection (interventions with *rationale*)

- Maintain meticulous handwashing procedures (include family, visitors, staff) *to minimize spread of infectious organisms.*
- Maintain isolation as prescribed *to minimize exposure to infectious organisms.*

- Clean frequently touched surfaces with an appropriate cleanser *to minimize spread of infectious organisms.*
- Educate family and visitors that child should be restricted from contact with known infectious exposures (in hospital and at home) *to encourage cooperation with infection control.*
- Strictly observe medical asepsis *to avoid unintentional introduction of microorganisms.*
- Promote nutrition and appropriate rest *to maximize body's potential to heal.*
- Educate family to contact health care provider or nurse practitioner if child has known exposure to chickenpox or measles *so that preventive measures (e.g., varicella zoster immunoglobulin [VZIG]) can be taken.*
- Administer vaccines (not live) as prescribed *to prevent common childhood communicable diseases.*
- Administer prophylactic antibiotics as prescribed *to prevent infection with opportunistic organisms.*

Nursing Analysis

Malnutrition risk; insufficient dietary intake is a risk factor.

Goal/Outcome

Child will consume adequate intake, demonstrating appropriate weight gain and growth of length/height and/or head circumference.

Promoting Adequate Nutritional Intake (interventions with *rationale*)

- Monitor growth (weight and height/length weekly) *to determine progress toward goal.*
- Determine realistic goal for weight gain for age (consulting dietitian if necessary) *to have a specific outcome to work toward.*
- Observe child's physical ability to eat *(if pain from candidiasis or motor impairment is present, will need additional interventions).*
- Provide nutrient-rich meals and snacks *to maximize caloric intake.*
- Supplement milkshakes with protein powder or other additives *to maximize caloric intake.*
- Provide child's favorite foods *to encourage increased intake.*
- Provide smaller, more frequent meals *to reduce sensation of fullness and increase overall intake.*
- If vomiting is an issue, administer antiemetics as ordered prior to meals *to provide optimal state for success at mealtime.*

Nursing Analysis

Impaired skin integrity risk; immunodeficiency is a risk factor.

Goal/Outcome

Skin integrity will be maintained: secondary infection will not occur; rash will not increase.

Preventing Skin Impairment (interventions with *rationale*)

- Assess and monitor extent and location of rash *to provide baseline information and evaluate success of interventions.*
- Keep skin clean and dry *to prevent secondary infection.*
- For the child with limited mobility, turn frequently and use specialty mattress or bed *to prevent pressure injuries.*
- Implement a written plan of care directed toward topical treatment of skin integrity impairment *to provide consistency of care and documentation.*
- Educate child and family to limit direct sun exposure and use sunscreen *to prevent sun damage.*

Nursing Analysis

Activity intolerance related to immobility (from joint pain) or physical deconditioning as evidenced by exertional discomfort, exertional dyspnea, fatigue, or generalized weakness

Goal/Outcome

Child will participate in activities: will demonstrate easy work of breathing and participate in daily routine and play.

Promoting Activity (interventions with *rationale*)

- Cluster care *to decrease disturbances and allow for longer uninterrupted rest periods.*
- Pace activities and encourage regular rest periods *to conserve energy.*
- Administer early morning warm bath *to ease morning stiffness (juvenile arthritis).*
- Use assistive devices such as splints and orthotics *to improve physical function.*
- Plan developmentally appropriate activities that the child can participate in while in bed *to encourage play and continued development.*
- Schedule activities for the time of day the child usually has the most energy *to encourage successful participation.*

Nursing Analysis

Delayed development risk; chronic illness is a risk factor.

Goal/Outcome

Development will be enhanced; child will make continued progress toward expected developmental milestones.

Enhancing Development (interventions with *rationale*)

- Screen for developmental capabilities *to determine child's current level of functioning.*

- Offer age-appropriate toys, play, and activities (including gross motor) *to encourage further development.*
- Encourage peer contact through telephone, e-mail, or letters *to promote/continue socialization.*
- Perform interventions as prescribed by physical or occupational therapist: *repeat participation in those activities helps child improve function and acquire developmental skills.*
- Provide support to families of children with developmental delay: *progress in achieving developmental milestones can be slow, and ongoing motivation is needed.*
- Encourage child to continue school work *so that child will not fall behind.*
- Reinforce positive attributes in the child *to maintain motivation.*

Based on your top three patient problems for Lakeisha, describe appropriate nursing interventions.

PRIMARY IMMUNODEFICIENCIES

Many primary immunodeficiencies have been identified. They are mostly hereditary or congenital. Primary immunodeficiencies may be related to humoral deficiencies, cellular immunity deficiencies, or a combination of the two; phagocytic system defects; or complement deficiencies. This discussion will focus on a few of the more common and/or severe primary immunodeficiencies in children. Box 25.1 lists 10 warning signs that a child may need further evaluation for the possibility of primary immunodeficiency.

BOX 25.1 10 Warning Signs of Primary Immunodeficiency

- Four or more new episodes of acute otitis media in 1 year
- Two or more episodes of severe sinusitis in 1 year
- Treatment with antibiotics for 2 months or longer with little effect
- Two or more episodes of pneumonia in 1 year
- Failure to thrive in the infant
- Recurrent deep skin or organ abscesses
- Persistent oral thrush or skin candidiasis after 1 year of age
- History of infections requiring IV antibiotics to clear
- Two or more serious infections such as sepsis
- Family history of primary immunodeficiency

Data from Abbott, J. K., Dutmer, C. M., & Hauk, P. J. (2022). Immunodeficiency. In M. Bunik, W. W. Hay, M. J. Levin, & M. J. Abzug (Eds.), *Current diagnosis & treatment: Pediatrics* (26th ed.). McGraw-Hill Education.

Hypogammaglobulinemia

Hypogammaglobulinemia refers to a variety of conditions in which the child does not form antibodies appropriately. It results in low or absent levels of one or more of the immunoglobulin classes or subclasses. Table 25.1 provides an overview of several types of hypogammaglobulinemia. Therapeutic management of most types of hypogammaglobulinemia is periodic administration of intravenous immunoglobulin (IVIG).

TABLE 25.1 • Types of Hypogammaglobulinemia

Type	Definition	Characteristics	Treatment
Selective IgA deficiency	Serum IgA <7 mg/dL, normal IgG and IgM	May be asymptomatic Child is more prone to allergies due to lack of the mucosal protection that IgA offers; recurrent infections of respiratory, gastrointestinal, and genitourinary tracts, development of autoimmune disorders	No specific gamma globulin treatment available Treat infections or autoimmune disorders. Severe anaphylactic reaction can occur if child receives transfusion of blood containing IgA and IgA antibodies.
X-linked agammaglobulinemia	Markedly reduced or absent IgG, IgM, and IgA; absence of B cells	Males only Recurrent respiratory and gastrointestinal infections	Routine IVIG infusions Treat infections.
X-linked hyper-IgM syndrome	Defect in protein found on T-cell surface, resulting in decreased IgG and IgA levels with significant increase in IgM levels	Males only Recurrent respiratory infections, diarrhea, malabsorption Neutropenia, autoimmune disorders	Routine administration of IVIG Subcutaneous granulocyte colony-stimulating factor (G-CSF) when neutropenic Bone marrow transplantation Treatment of autoimmune disorders
IgG subclass deficiency	Low levels of one or more of the subclasses of IgG	Recurrent respiratory infections; some children outgrow this condition.	Treatment of respiratory infections Administration of IVIG is helpful in some children.

Ig, immunoglobulin

Nursing Assessment

Note history of recurrent respiratory, gastrointestinal, or genitourinary infections. Palpate for enlarged lymph nodes and spleen in the child with X-linked hyper-IgM syndrome. In children presenting for routine administration of IVIG, determine whether any infections have occurred since the previous infusion.

Nursing Management

Nursing management of hypogammaglobulinemia involves IVIG administration and the provision of education and support to the child and family.

ADMINISTERING INTRAVENOUS IMMUNOGLOBULIN

Determine the amount of IVIG to be given, and reconstitute the product according to the manufacturer's directions (available on the package insert). Some IVIG preparations are provided as a solution, requiring no reconstitution (Fig. 25.1). Others are packaged as two vials, one of IVIG powder and one of sterile diluent. After the diluent is added to the powder, gently roll the vial between your hands to mix. Reconstituted IVIG may be refrigerated overnight but should be brought to room temperature prior to infusion. Assess baseline serum blood urea nitrogen (BUN) and creatinine, as acute renal insufficiency may occur as a serious adverse reaction. Although less common in children than adults, assess for risk factors associated with an increased risk of a thromboembolic event, such as history of atherosclerosis, hyperviscosity or hypercoagulability, stroke, hypertension, hypercholesterolemia, impaired cardiac output, immobility (Lexicomp®, 2024).

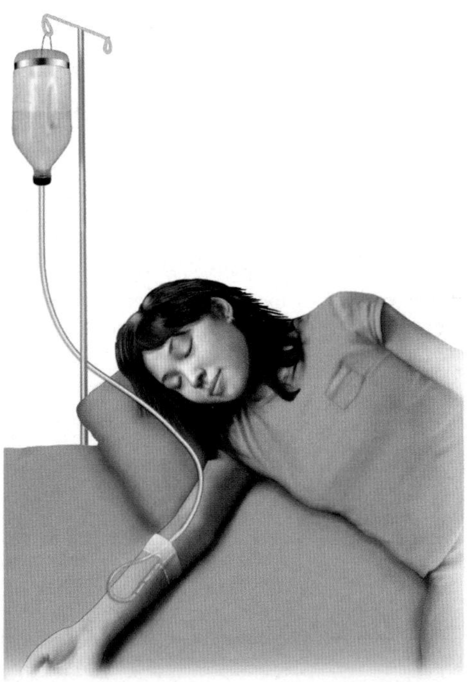

FIGURE 25.1 Intravenous administration of exogenous immunoglobulin every several weeks can decrease the frequency and severity of infections in children with various forms of hypogammaglobulinemia.

> **TAKE NOTE!**
>
> Do not shake the IVIG, as this may lead to foaming and may cause the immunoglobulin protein to degrade (Lexicomp®, 2024).

Ensure the child is well hydrated before the infusion to decrease the risk of rate-related reactions and aseptic meningitis after the infusion. Premedication with diphenhydramine or acetaminophen may be indicated in children who have never received IVIG, have not had an infusion in more than 8 weeks, have had a recent bacterial infection, have a history of serious infusion-related adverse reactions, or are diagnosed with agammaglobulinemia or hypogammaglobulinemia (Lexicomp®, 2024).

The rate for infusion of IVIG is generally prescribed as milligrams of IVIG per kilogram of body weight per minute. Carefully calculate the infusion rate. Obtain a baseline physical assessment and set of vital signs. Begin the infusion slowly, increasing to the prescribed rate as tolerated (see Fig. 25.1). Assess vital signs and check for adverse reactions every 15 minutes for the first hour, then every 30 minutes throughout the remainder of the infusion (the frequency of assessments may vary according to institutional protocol). IVIG is a plasma product, so observe closely for signs of anaphylaxis such as headache, facial flushing, urticaria, dyspnea, shortness of breath, wheezing, chest pain, fever, chills, nausea, vomiting, increased anxiety, or hypotension. If these symptoms occur, discontinue the infusion and notify the health care provider or nurse practitioner. The infusion may be restarted after the symptoms have subsided. Have oxygen and emergency medications such as epinephrine, diphenhydramine, and intravenous corticosteroids available in case of anaphylactic reaction. If the child complains of discomfort at the intravenous site, a cold compress may be helpful.

DOSAGE CALCULATION BOX 25.1

Child's weight: 33 lb

Medication order: intravenous immunoglobulin 6,000 mg IV today.

Per the *Pediatric Dosage Handbook*, the recommended dose is 300 to 600 mg/dose, IV, every 3 to 4 weeks. Infuse at 0.5 mL/kg/h for first 30 minutes, increasing rate every 30 minutes as tolerated, not to exceed 5 mL/kg/h.

Is the ordered dose safe?

IVIG is provided as 100 mg/mL. If the dose is safe, what will the infusion rate be for the first 30 minutes?

TAKE NOTE!

Many children who have had previous reactions to IVIG can tolerate the infusion without reaction if they are premedicated and if the infusion is given at a slower rate (Lexicomp®, 2024).

PROVIDING EDUCATION AND SUPPORT

Provide education and support to the child and family. An excellent book for children with an immune deficiency is *Our Immune System* (1993) by Sara le Bien (available from the Immune Deficiency Foundation).

Wiskott–Aldrich Syndrome

Wiskott–Aldrich syndrome is an X-linked genetic disorder that results in immunodeficiency, eczema, and thrombocytopenia. It affects males only. The defective gene responsible for this disorder is called the Wiskott–Aldrich syndrome protein (WASp). Complications include autoimmune hemolytic anemia, neutropenia, skin or cerebral vasculitis, arthritis, inflammatory bowel disease, and kidney disease (Ochs, 2022).

Autoimmune disease may require high-dose steroids, azathioprine, or cyclophosphamide. Splenectomy may be performed to correct thrombocytopenia. The only cure is hematopoietic cell transplantation, although gene therapy is currently under investigation.

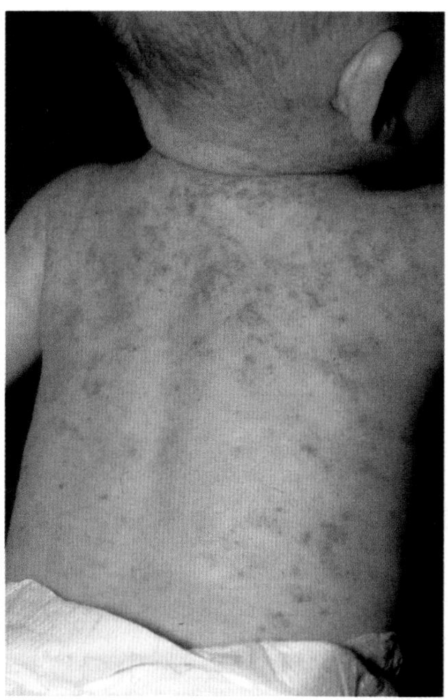

FIGURE 25.2 Children with Wiskott–Aldrich syndrome often have worsening of eczema over time.

Nursing Assessment

Note history of petechiae, bloody diarrhea, or bleeding episode in the first 6 months of life. Note any history of hematemesis or intracranial or conjunctival hemorrhages. Observe the skin for eczema, which usually worsens with time and tends to become secondarily infected (Fig. 25.2). Laboratory findings include low IgM concentration, elevated IgA and IgE concentrations, and normal IgG concentrations.

TAKE NOTE!

An episode of prolonged bleeding, such as at the umbilical stump or after circumcision, may be the first sign of Wiskott-Aldrich syndrome in the newborn (Ochs, 2022).

Nursing Management

Administer IVIG as ordered to help decrease the frequency of bacterial infections. Perform good skin care and frequently assess eczematous areas to detect secondary infection (refer to Chapter 23 for care of eczema). If the child undergoes splenectomy, in addition to providing routine postoperative care, be aware of the additional risk of development of infection in the asplenic child. Refer to Chapter 24 for information related to hematopoietic cell transplantation.

Severe Combined Immune Deficiency

Severe combined immune deficiency (SCID) is a rare X-linked or autosomal recessive disorder; it can occur in any sex. SCID is characterized by absent T-cell and B-cell function. There are at least five types of SCID, classified according to the exact genetic defect. SCID is a potentially fatal disorder requiring emergency intervention at the time of diagnosis. Gene therapy provides some promise for the future treatment of SCID, but until then, hematopoietic cell transplantation is necessary (Heimall, 2019).

TAKE NOTE!

Use only cytomegalovirus (CMV)-negative, irradiated blood or platelets if transfusion is necessary in the infant with SCID. CMV-positive blood could cause an infection in the infant, and T lymphocytes in blood products may cause fatal graft-versus-host disease (GVHD) to occur (Heimall, 2019).

IVIG infusions may help decrease the number of infections until bone marrow or stem cell transplantation can be done (Heimall, 2019). Certain children with SCID (adenosine deaminase enzyme deficiency) may benefit from lifelong subcutaneous adenosine deaminase enzyme replacement. In addition, long-term antibiotic therapy helps to contain chronic infections in some children with SCID.

Nursing Assessment

Note history of chronic diarrhea and failure to thrive. Note history of severe infections beginning early in infancy. Inspect the mouth for persistent thrush. Auscultate the lungs, noting adventitious sounds related to pneumonia. Laboratory findings include very low levels of all of the immunoglobulins.

Nursing Management

Preventing infection is critical. Teach the family to practice good handwashing. The child must not be exposed to people outside the family, particularly young children. Instruct families to administer prophylactic antibiotics if prescribed. Educate families that the child should not receive live vaccines. Encourage adequate nutrition; supplemental enteral feedings may be necessary in the child with poor appetite. Administer IVIG infusions as prescribed, and monitor for adverse reactions (refer to the nursing management section for hypogammaglobulinemia for further information related to IVIG administration). If the child receives a bone marrow transplant (human leukocyte antigen [HLA]–matched sibling is preferred), provide posttransplant care as outlined in Chapter 24. Teach the family that severe cutaneous human papillomavirus infection may occur after stem cell transplantation (even years later). Refer the family for genetic counseling. Provide ongoing support; this is a difficult disease for families to cope with, and the therapy required is lifelong.

TAKE NOTE!

Monitor the child who had a bone marrow or stem cell transplant closely for a maculopapular rash that usually starts on the palms and soles; this is an indication that GVHD is developing. GVHD is a life-threatening condition in which donor cells attack host cells (Wolownik, 2022).

SECONDARY IMMUNODEFICIENCIES

Secondary immunodeficiency may occur as a result of chronic illness, malignancy, use of **immunosuppressive** (lowering the immune response) medication, malnutrition or protein-losing state, prematurity, or HIV infection. This discussion will focus on HIV infection.

HIV Infection

In the United States, 53 children younger than 13 years old are infected with HIV annually, and 19% of all cases of HIV infection occur in people aged 13 to 24 years (National Institutes of Health [NIH], 2024a, 2024b). Children acquire HIV either vertically or horizontally. Vertical transmission refers to perinatal (in utero or during birth) transmission or via breast milk. Horizontal transmission refers to transmission via nonsterile needles (as in intravenous drug use or tattooing) or via intimate sexual contact. With nationwide screening of blood products, HIV transmission via transfused blood products has become rare (National Hemophilia Foundation, 2023). HIV infection in children may be further classified depending on severity of immune suppression. This classification may serve to guide health care planning.

Infants become infected primarily through their birthing parent, whereas adolescents contract HIV infection primarily through sexual activity or intravenous drug use. In the United States, perinatal transmission of HIV infection has declined dramatically due to improved maternal detection and treatment, as well as newborn treatment (Smith & McFarland, 2022). Currently, there is no cure for HIV infection, although survival has improved since the advent of antiretroviral therapy (ART). In addition to improved survival, improved growth, neurodevelopment, and immune function occur with ART (Panel on Antiretroviral Therapy and Medical Management of Children Living with HIV, 2024).

Pathophysiology

HIV affects immune function via alterations mainly in T-cell function, but it also affects B cells, natural killer cells, and monocyte/macrophage function. HIV infects the CD4 (T-helper) cells. The virus replicates itself via the CD4 cell and renders the cell dysfunctional. Immune deficiency results as the number of normal, functioning CD4 cells drops. Initially, as CD4 counts decrease, the T-suppressor (CD8) counts increase, but as the disease progresses, CD8 counts also fall. The helper T-cell function declines even in asymptomatic infants and children who have not experienced significant decreases in the CD4 cell count. The T cells lose response to recall antigens, and this loss is associated with an increased risk of serious bacterial infection (Smith & McFarland, 2022).

B-cell defects also occur in children with HIV, contributing to high rates of serious bacterial infections. The B cells demonstrate impaired response to mitogens and antigens. They also exhibit defective antibody production in response to antigen exposure or vaccination. Also, infants lack a pool of memory B cells for recall antigens (simply from lack of exposure). Natural killer cells also are affected by HIV infection, as they are dependent on cytokines secreted by the CD4 cells for development of functionality. Functional killer cells play a role in fighting viruses and are critical to immunity in the newborn while the T-cell line develops. Decreased function of the natural killer cells then contributes to increased severity of viral infection in the child or infant with HIV. Although the virus does not destroy monocytes and macrophages, their function is affected. Macrophages in the child with HIV exhibit decreased chemotaxis, and the antigen-presenting capability of the monocytes is defective.

Without appropriate T cell, B cell, natural killer cell, monocyte, and macrophage function, the infant's or child's immune system cannot fight infections it ordinarily could. Recurrent infection with ordinary organisms occurs more frequently in children with HIV infection, and the infections are more severe than in noninfected children. Opportunistic infections also occur in children with HIV, similarly to those in adults with HIV infection. Current guidelines related to prevention of opportunistic infection emphasize ART for prevention as well as ensuring appropriate immunization and antibiotic prophylaxis for certain organisms (Smith & McFarland, 2022).

HIV rapidly invades the central nervous system in infants and children and is responsible for progressive HIV encephalopathy. As a result of encephalopathy, acquired microcephaly, motor deficits, or loss of previously achieved developmental milestones may occur. In children with progressive HIV encephalopathy, neurologic symptoms may present before immune suppression.

Therapeutic Management

Current recommendations for treatment of HIV infection in children include the use of a combination of antiretroviral drugs (Smith & McFarland, 2022). Medication therapy ranges from single-drug therapy in the asymptomatic HIV-exposed newborn to highly active ART, consisting of a combination of antiretroviral drugs. Medications are prescribed based on the severity of the child's illness. One of the goals of ART is to prevent or arrest progressive HIV encephalopathy (Gillespie, 2023).

Nursing Assessment

For a full description of the assessment phase of the nursing process, refer to the "Clinical Judgment and the Nursing Process" section. Assessment findings pertinent to HIV infection in children are discussed further on.

HEALTH HISTORY

Elicit a description of the present illness and chief complaint. Common signs and symptoms reported during the health history might include:

- Failure to thrive
- Recurrent bacterial infections
- Opportunistic infections
- Chronic or recurrent diarrhea
- Recurrent or persistent fever
- Developmental delay
- Prolonged candidiasis

These signs and symptoms may be present in either the child who is undergoing initial diagnosis or the child with known HIV infection. Explore the child's current and past medical history for risk factors such as maternal HIV infection or acquired immunodeficiency syndrome (AIDS), receipt of blood transfusions in a developing country (without adequate screening measures), adolescent or childhood sexual abuse, substance use or misuse (including intravenous drug use), or participation in vaginal or anal sex without the use of a condom. Document who the primary caregiver is, as many children with HIV have lost their parents to the disease. In addition, for the child with known HIV infection, determine the child's medications and dosages as well as the outcome of any recent health care visits or hospitalizations.

PHYSICAL EXAMINATION

Perform a thorough and complete physical examination on the child with suspected or known HIV infection. Note presence of fever. Measure weight, height or length, and head circumference (in children younger than 3 years) and plot this information on standard growth charts, noting whether the measurements fall within the average or below the lower percentiles. Perform a developmental screening test to detect developmental delay. Inspect the oral cavity for candidiasis. Observe work of breathing (may be increased if pneumonitis or pneumonia is present). Determine level of consciousness (may be depressed if HIV encephalopathy is present).

Auscultate the lungs, noting adventitious breath sounds associated with pneumonia or pneumonitis. Palpate for the presence of enlarged lymph nodes (lymphadenopathy) or swollen parotid glands. Palpate the abdomen, noting hepatosplenomegaly.

LABORATORY AND DIAGNOSTIC TESTS

Common laboratory and diagnostic studies ordered for the assessment of HIV infection include:

- RNA or DNA—nucleic acid (NAT) or polymerase chain reaction (PCR) test: positive in infected infants who are not breastfed at 1 month of age and in all infected infants at 6 months of age. Box 25.2 gives information on timing of testing.
- CD4 counts (low in HIV infection)

Nursing Management

Nursing care of the child with HIV infection is directed at avoiding infection, promoting adherence with the

BOX 25.2 Virologic Assay Testing for HIV-Exposed Infants

- 14 to 21 days of age
- 1 to 2 months of age
- 4 to 6 months of age
- In the infant who was not breastfed, two or more negative tests (one at ≥1 month of age and one at ≥4 months of age) determine absence of HIV infection

From Panel on Antiretroviral Therapy and Medical Management of Children Living with HIV. (2024). *Guidelines for the use of antiretroviral agents in pediatric HIV infection.* Department of Health and Human Services. https://clinicalinfo.hiv.gov/en/guidelines/pediatric-arv/whats-new

medication regimen, promoting nutrition, providing pain management and comfort measures, educating the child and caregivers, and providing ongoing psychosocial support. Children with HIV infection may access health services through funding provided by the Ryan White Comprehensive AIDS Resources Emergency Act (Health Resources and Services Administration, the HIV/AIDS Program, 2022). This federal funding provides for primary health care and other services to people with HIV infection. The "Clinical Judgment and the Nursing Process" section lists appropriate patient problems and interventions. In addition, nursing management specific to HIV infection is covered in what follows.

PREVENTING HIV INFECTION IN CHILDREN

It is important to offer all pregnant people routine HIV counseling and voluntary testing. Depending on the stage of pregnancy, the pregnant person should be treated with an antiretroviral drug if they are HIV positive. Children born to HIV-positive birthing parents will receive ART at least until 6 weeks of age, depending on risk (Panel on Antiretroviral Therapy and Medical Management of Children Living with HIV, 2024). Discourage breastfeeding in the parent with HIV, and instruct them about safe alternatives. Early recognition of infection is crucial so that treatment can begin, HIV encephalopathy may be prevented, and progression to AIDS can be prevented. Educate sexually active adolescents about HIV transmission, and urge them to use condoms. Counsel adolescents about the increased risk of HIV transmission with all forms of sexual activity, explaining that vaginal and anal sex are even riskier than oral sex. Urge adolescents to limit the number of sexual partners. Discourage substance use, as the effects of drugs and alcohol often impair the adolescent's ability to make wise choices about sexual conduct. Warn adolescents of the risk of contracting HIV infection via shared needles (as with intravenous drug use or via unclean needles used in tattooing). See the Healthy People 2030 box.

HEALTHY PEOPLE 2030

Objective	Nursing Significance
Reduce the rate of vertically transmitted HIV infection.	• Encourage sexually active adolescents to seek appropriate reproductive health care and screening. • For the pregnant adolescent, encourage HIV testing to determine status. • Encourage the HIV-positive pregnant adolescent to adhere with HIV treatment as prescribed.
Reduce the number of new HIV infections.	• Discourage intravenous illicit drug use. Educate adolescents about the risk of contaminated tattoo needles. • Encourage abstinence in adolescents. • If adolescents are sexually active, educate them about the risks of HIV transmission; encourage condom use with all sexual activity.

Healthy People Objectives retrieved from http://www.healthypeople.gov

PROMOTING ADHERENCE WITH ART

Without treatment, progressive HIV encephalopathy will lead to developmental regression, motor spasticity, and possibly seizures (Gillespie, 2023). To prevent progression of HIV disease and prevent encephalopathy, adherence with the ART regimen is required. Educate the family about the importance of adhering with the medication regimen. Help the caregivers develop a schedule for medication administration that is compatible with the family's home routine. See the Healthy People 2030 box.

HEALTHY PEOPLE 2030

Objective	Nursing Significance
Increase the percentage of people 13 years and older with diagnosed HIV infection who are virally suppressed.	Educate families about the importance of adhering with medication therapy (highly active antiretroviral therapy [HAART]) and receiving regularly scheduled medical evaluations.

Healthy People Objectives retrieved from http://www.healthypeople.gov

REDUCING RISK FOR INFECTION

In the newborn whose birthing parent is infected with tuberculosis, syphilis, toxoplasmosis, CMV, hepatitis B or C, or herpes simplex virus, provide testing and treatment. To prevent infection with *Pneumocystis jirovecii,* administer prophylactic antibiotics as prescribed in any HIV-exposed infant in whom HIV infection has not yet been excluded. Provide tuberculosis screening and childhood immunization in accordance with national guidelines.

THINKING ABOUT DEVELOPMENT

Jasmine Smith is a 5-year-old female with HIV infection. She fights taking her antiretroviral medications because of the nausea and vomiting associated with them. Lucy Panco is a 15-year-old female also with HIV infection. She is noncompliant with her antiretroviral medications, also because of the associated nausea and vomiting.

How will the nurse teach Jasmine about the medications? How will she foster adherence in Jasmine?

What is the most appropriate approach for the nurse to take to educate Lucy about adherence with medications?

How will the approaches to education and encouragement of adherence be different for these two children? How will they be similar?

TAKE NOTE!

Do not administer live vaccines to the immunocompromised child without the express consent of the infectious disease or immunology specialist.

PROMOTING NUTRITION

For the infant, provide increased-calorie formula as tolerated. For the child, provide high-calorie, high-protein meals and snacks. Supplements may be added to milkshakes to increase the protein intake. Ensure that the child is able to choose foods that they prefer from the hospital menu. Document growth through weekly measurements of weight and height/length.

PROMOTING COMFORT

Children with HIV infection experience pain from infections, encephalopathy, adverse effects of medications, and the numerous procedures and treatments that are required, such as venipuncture, biopsy, or lumbar puncture. Refer to Chapter 14 for detailed information about pain assessment and management.

PROVIDING FAMILY EDUCATION AND SUPPORT

Educate caregivers about the medication regimen, the ongoing follow-up that is needed, and when to call the infectious disease provider. Families of children with HIV experience a significant amount of stress from many sources: the diagnosis of an incurable disease, financial difficulties, multiple family members with HIV, HIV-associated stigmas, desire to keep HIV infection confidential, and multiple medical appointments and hospitalizations. Parents of children with HIV often die of AIDS themselves, leaving care of the child to another relative or foster parent. The day care center or school that the child attends will need education about HIV, which can be provided only if the parent or caregiver consents to divulging the child's diagnosis to that agency. Provide education to the school or day care center about how the infection is transmitted (i.e., not through casual contact).

Disclosure of the diagnosis of HIV to the child is another source of stress for the family. The timing of this disclosure will vary considerably depending on the child's and family's situation. Generally, children older than 6 years of age will eventually need to have their diagnosis disclosed to them in an age-appropriate manner. They begin to ask questions and often seem to sense that something is going on other than what they've been told so far. When made aware of the diagnosis and educated about the disease, the child may exhibit a variety of reactions. Anger, depression, or school problems may occur. The child may experience a spiritual dilemma. The nurse should continue to provide emotional support to the child and family. If the disclosure results in significant emotional turmoil, refer the child and caregivers to a counselor, social worker, or psychologist. Anticipatory grieving may also occur. Parents or caregivers may express guilt or anger over the diagnosis of HIV infection. At the other end of the spectrum, families may use denial as their method of coping. Use therapeutic communication with open-ended questions to discover the family's thoughts and fears. Provide emotional support and allow for crying and verbalization. If needed, refer the caregivers to the appropriate professional for additional psychological and emotional intervention.

Many children with HIV have psychosocial, emotional, and cognitive problems. These contribute to a lower quality of life. They are affected by the stigma of their diagnosis and often by the social isolation associated with it. Children and adolescents with HIV infection often exhibit mental health concerns, including mood, anxiety, and substance use disorders (Gillespie, 2023). They may suffer multiple losses within the family related to deaths caused by HIV infection. Children with HIV infection need significant psychosocial support and intervention. Resources for families of children with HIV are listed in Box 25.3.

BOX **25.3** Resources for Children With HIV and Their Families

- www.pedaids.org: Elizabeth Glaser Pediatric AIDS Foundation—resources for children with HIV and their families
- www.avert.org/professionals/hiv-social-issues/key-affected-populations/children: Children page of Avert, Global Information and Education on HIV and AIDS
- www.vachss.com/help_text/hiv_aids_ped.html: Pediatric HIV infection and AIDS resources
- www.thewellproject.org/hiv-information/women-and-hiv: The Well Project: Women and HIV (includes Spanish resources)

AUTOIMMUNE DISORDERS

Autoimmune disorders result from the immune system's malfunction. The body manufactures T cells and antibodies against its own cells and organs (**autoantibodies**). The development of an autoimmune disorder is thought to be multifactorial. Potential influencing factors include heredity, hormones, self-marker molecules, and environmental influences such as viruses and certain drugs.

Systemic Lupus Erythematosus

Systemic lupus erythematosus (SLE) is a multisystem autoimmune disorder that affects both humoral and cellular immunity. SLE can affect any organ system, so the onset and course of the disease are quite variable. The presentation of SLE in childhood most commonly occurs in females 9 to 15 years of age (Soep, 2022). SLE is more common in people who are not White, and young people have a greater relative risk of death from SLE (Klein-Gitelman, 2022).

Pathophysiology

In SLE, autoantibodies react with the child's self-antigens to form immune complexes. The immune complexes accumulate in the tissues and organs, causing an inflammatory response resulting in vasculitis. Injury to the tissues and pain occur. Since SLE may affect any organ system, the potential for alterations or damage to tissues anywhere in the body is significant. In some cases, the autoimmune response may be preceded by a drug reaction, an infection, or excessive sun exposure. In children, the most common initial symptoms are hematologic, cutaneous, and musculoskeletal in origin. The disease is chronic, with periods of remission and exacerbation (flares). Common complications of SLE include ocular or visual changes, cerebrovascular accident (CVA), transverse myelitis, immune complex–mediated glomerulonephritis, pericarditis, valvular heart disease, coronary artery disease, seizures, and psychosis.

Therapeutic Management

Therapeutic management focuses on treating the inflammatory response. Nonsteroidal antiinflammatory drugs (NSAIDs), corticosteroids, and antimalarial agents are often prescribed for the child with mild to moderate SLE. The child with severe SLE or frequent flare-ups of symptoms may require high-dose (pulse) corticosteroid therapy or drugs. When end-stage kidney disease develops as a result of glomerulonephritis, dialysis becomes necessary.

Nursing Assessment

For a full description of the assessment phase of the nursing process, refer to the "Clinical Judgment and the Nursing Process" section. Assessment findings pertinent to SLE in children are discussed here.

HEALTH HISTORY

Elicit a description of the present illness and chief complaint. Common signs and symptoms reported during the health history are history of fatigue, fever, weight changes, pain or swelling in the joints, numbness, tingling or coolness of extremities, or prolonged bleeding. Assess for risk factors, which include female sex; family history; African, Native American, or Asian descent; recent infection; drug reaction; or excessive sun exposure.

PHYSICAL EXAMINATION

Measure temperature and document the presence of fever. Observe the skin for malar rash (a butterfly-shaped rash over the cheeks); discoid lesions on the face, scalp, or neck; changes in skin pigmentation; or scarring (Fig. 25.3). Document alopecia. Inspect the oral cavity for painless ulcerations and the joints for edema.

Measure blood pressure, as hypertension may occur with kidney involvement. Auscultate the lungs; adventitious breath sounds may be present if the pulmonary system is involved. Palpate the joints, noting tenderness. Palpate the abdomen and note areas of tenderness (abdominal involvement is more common in children with SLE than in adults). Box 25.4 lists common clinical findings in SLE.

LABORATORY AND DIAGNOSTIC FINDINGS

Laboratory findings may include decreased hemoglobin and hematocrit, decreased platelet count, and low WBC count. Complement levels, C3 and C4, will also be decreased. Although not specific to SLE, the antinuclear antibody (ANA) is usually positive in children with SLE.

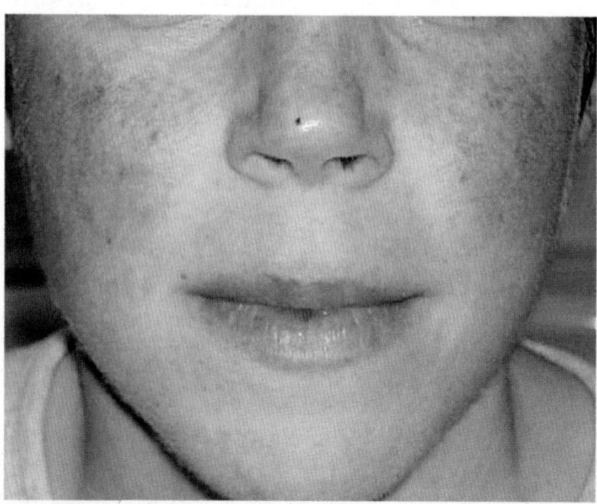

FIGURE 25.3 The malar or butterfly rash (erythema over the cheeks in the shape of a butterfly) is typical in systemic lupus erythematosus (SLE).

BOX 25.4 **Most Common Clinical Manifestations of Systemic Lupus Erythematosus**

- Alopecia
- Anemia
- Arthralgia
- Arthritis
- Fatigue
- Lupus nephritis
- Photosensitivity
- Pleurisy
- Raynaud phenomenon
- Seizures
- Skin rashes, including malar rash
- Stomatitis
- Thrombocytopenia

Nursing Management

Nursing management of the child or adolescent with SLE is long-term and supportive. Management focuses on preventing and monitoring for complications. Educate the child and family about the importance of a healthy diet, regular exercise, and adequate sleep and rest. Administer NSAIDs, corticosteroids, and antimalarial agents as ordered for the child with mild to moderate SLE and pulse corticosteroid therapy or immunomodulators to the child with severe SLE or frequent flare-ups. Assist families to deal with this chronic illness and adolescents with their struggles with body image and independence. Refer families to support services such as the Lupus Alliance of America and the Lupus Foundation of America.

PREVENTING AND MONITORING FOR COMPLICATIONS

Teach families to apply sunscreen (minimum SPF 15) to their child's skin daily to prevent rashes resulting from photosensitivity. Instruct the child and family to protect against cold weather by layering warm socks and wearing gloves when outdoors in the winter. If the child is outside for extended periods during the winter months, inspect the fingers and toes for discoloration. Watch for the development of nephritis by evaluating blood pressure, serum BUN and creatinine levels, and urine output and monitoring for hematuria or proteinuria. Ensure that yearly vision screening and ophthalmic examinations are performed to preserve visual function should changes occur.

TAKE NOTE!

Avascular necrosis (lack of blood supply to a joint, resulting in tissue damage) may occur as an adverse effect of long-term or high-dose corticosteroid use. Teach families to report new onset of joint pain, particularly with weight bearing, or limited range of motion to their health care provider or nurse practitioner (Patel, 2022).

Juvenile Idiopathic Arthritis

Juvenile idiopathic arthritis is an autoimmune disorder in which the autoantibodies target mainly the joints. Inflammatory changes in the joints cause pain, redness, warmth, stiffness, and swelling. Stiffness usually occurs after inactivity (as in the morning, after sleep). Some forms also affect the eyes or other organs. Table 25.2 explains the three types. Juvenile idiopathic arthritis is a chronic disease; the child may experience healthy periods alternating with flare-ups (Soep, 2022). Juvenile idiopathic arthritis was formerly termed "juvenile rheumatoid arthritis," but unlike adult rheumatoid arthritis, few types of juvenile arthritis actually demonstrate a positive RF.

Therapeutic management focuses on inflammation control, pain relief, promotion of remission, and maintenance of mobility. NSAIDs, corticosteroids, and antirheumatic drugs such as methotrexate and etanercept are prescribed, depending on the type and severity of the disease. NSAIDs are helpful with pain relief, but disease-modifying (antirheumatic) drugs are necessary to prevent disease progression (several of which are approved for use in children).

TABLE 25.2 • Types of Juvenile Idiopathic Arthritis

Type	Definition	Nonjoint Manifestations	Complications
Pauciarticular (oligoarticular)	Involvement of four or fewer joints; quite often, the knee is involved. Most common type	Eye inflammation, malaise, poor appetite, poor weight gain	Iritis, uveitis, uneven leg bone growth
Polyarticular	Involvement of five or more joints; frequently involves small joints and often affects the body symmetrically	Malaise, lymphadenopathy, organomegaly, poor growth	Often, a severe form of arthritis; rapidly progressing joint damage, rheumatoid nodules
Systemic	In addition to joint involvement, fever and rash may be present at diagnosis.	Enlarged spleen, liver, and lymph nodes; myalgia; severe anemia	Pericarditis, pericardial effusion, pleuritis, pulmonary fibrosis

Based on Soep, J. B. (2022). Rheumatic diseases. In M. Bunik, W. W. Hay, M. J. Levin, & M. J. Abzug (Eds.), *Current diagnosis & treatment: Pediatrics* (26th ed.). McGraw-Hill Education.

Nursing Assessment

Note history of irritability or fussiness, which may be the first sign of this disease in the infant or very young child. Note complaints of pain, although children do not always communicate this. Document history of withdrawal from play or difficulty getting the child out of bed in the morning (joint stiffness after inactivity). Inquire about history of fever (above 39.5°C for 2 weeks or more in systemic disease).

Measure temperature (fever is present with systemic disease). Inspect skin for evanescent, pale red, nonpruritic macular rash, which may be present at diagnosis of systemic disease. Observe the gait, noting limping or guarding of a joint or extremity. Document growth, which may be delayed. Inspect and palpate each joint for edema, redness, warmth, and tenderness (Fig. 25.4). Note positioning of joints (usually flexed in position of comfort). Mild to moderate anemia and an elevated erythrocyte sedimentation rate are common. Young children with the pauciarticular form may demonstrate a positive ANA, and adolescents with polyarticular disease may have a positive RF.

Nursing Management

Nursing management focuses on managing pain, maintaining mobility, and promoting a normal life. Refer the child to a pediatric rheumatologist to ensure that they receive the most up-to-date treatment. Administer disease-modifying medications and teach children and families how to do so. Refer families to Childhood Arthritis and Rheumatology Research Alliance for clinical research trial information. Encourage regular eye examinations and vision screening to allow for early treatment of visual changes and to prevent blindness.

MANAGING PAIN AND MAINTAINING MOBILITY

Administer medications as prescribed to control inflammation and prevent disease progression. Refer to Drug Guide 25.1 for information related to NSAIDs, corticosteroids, and disease-modifying antirheumatic drugs. Maintain joint range of motion and muscle strength via exercise (physical or occupational therapy). Swimming is a particularly useful exercise to maintain joint mobility without placing pressure on the joints. Teach families appropriate use of splints prescribed to prevent joint contractures. Monitor for pressure areas or skin breakdown with splint or orthotic use.

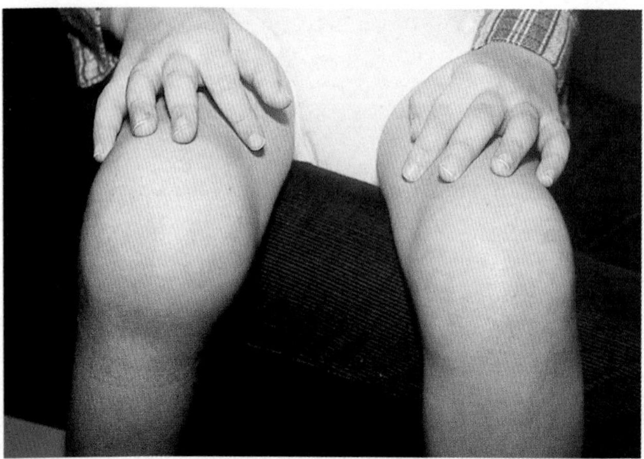

FIGURE 25.4 Note the swollen, reddened joints of this child with juvenile arthritis.

PROMOTING NORMAL LIFE

Chronic pain and decreased mobility may impact the child's psychological and emotional status significantly, during both childhood and adulthood. Providing adequate pain relief and promoting adherence with the disease-modifying medication regimen may allow the child to have a more normal life in the present as well as in the future. In addition to measures described in the previous section, encourage adequate sleep to improve the child's ability to cope with symptoms and with school function. Promote sleep with a warm bath at bedtime and warm compresses to affected joints or massage. To prevent social isolation, encourage the child to attend school and ensure that teachers, the school nurse, and classmates are educated about the child's disease and any limitations on activity. Having two sets of books (one at school and one at home) allows the child to do homework without having to carry heavy books home. Modifications such as allowing the child to leave the classroom early in order to get to the next class on time may seem small but can have a significant impact on the child's life.

Encourage children and families to become involved with local support groups so they can see that they are not alone. Assist children to set and achieve goals to increase their sense of hopefulness. Special summer camps for children with juvenile arthritis allow the child to socialize and belong to a group and have been shown to promote self-esteem in the child with chronic illness. Encourage appropriate family functioning and refer the family to support groups, such as those sponsored by the American Juvenile Arthritis Organization.

Guillain–Barré Syndrome

Guillain–Barré syndrome (GBS) (also called acute immune-mediated polyneuropathies) is a diverse group of syndromes with several forms. In the disorder occurring most often, an immune response within the body attacks the peripheral nervous system but does not usually affect the brain or spinal cord. GBS results in inflammation and demyelinization of the peripheral nerves. Weakness and paralysis occur in a progressive fashion. Progression is usually complete in 2 to 4 weeks, followed by a stable period leading to the recovery phase, which lasts for a few weeks to months in most cases but can take years. Severity of the disorder ranges from mild weakness to total paralysis.

Although not fully understood, it is believed to be an autoimmune condition that is most commonly triggered by a previous viral or bacterial infection, usually described as an upper respiratory tract infection or an acute gastroenteritis with fever. In rare cases, it has occurred after the child has had an immunization or surgery. GBS is more commonly seen in adults than in children (Yiu, 2023).

Therapeutic Management

Treatment of GBS is symptomatic and focuses on lessening the severity and speeding recovery. Management may include plasma exchange and administration of IVIGs, especially in severe cases. The goal of treatment is to keep the body functioning until the nervous system recovers. GBS is a life-threatening condition, and some children will die during the acute phase due to respiratory failure. Most children will make a full recovery, but a few may have residual damage.

Nursing Assessment

Early diagnosis and prompt treatment are essential since the disorder can quickly lead to respiratory failure and death from muscle paralysis. For a full description of the assessment phase of the nursing process, refer to the "Clinical Judgment and the Nursing Process" section. Assessment findings pertinent to GBS are discussed here.

HEALTH HISTORY

Elicit a description of the present illness and chief complaint. The clinical presentation of GBS is fairly similar in children and adults. Note onset of symptoms within a few days or weeks after the causative infection or event. Determine the presence of muscle weakness and paresthesias such as numbness and tingling which have a quick onset. Classically, GBS initially affects the legs and progresses in an ascending manner, but occasionally, it affects the arms or face first and proceeds in a descending manner. Ask about presence of paralysis, ataxia, or sensory disturbances.

PHYSICAL EXAMINATION AND LABORATORY AND DIAGNOSTIC TESTS

Note decreased or absent tendon reflexes, facial weakness, difficulty swallowing, or paralysis. Cerebrospinal fluid (CSF) analysis may reveal an increased level of protein, but this may not be evident until after the first week of the illness. Electrodiagnostic studies, such as electromyogram (EMG) and nerve conduction velocity, can assist in the diagnosis of GBS.

TAKE NOTE!

Tickling may be a successful technique for assessing the level of paralysis in the child with Guillain–Barré syndrome, either initially or in the recovery phase.

Nursing Management

Nursing management is supportive. In severe cases, the child may require intensive nursing care along with mechanical ventilation. Observe the child closely for the extent of paralysis, and monitor for respiratory involvement. Nursing care focuses on the same concerns as in any child with extreme immobility or paralysis.

Prevention of complications associated with immobility is a central concern and involves maintaining skin integrity, preventing respiratory complications and contractures, maintaining adequate nutrition, and managing pain. Turn and/or reposition the child every 2 hours, perform range-of-motion exercises, assess the skin for redness or breakdown, keep the skin clean and dry, encourage fluid intake to maintain hydration status, and encourage coughing and deep breathing every 2 hours and as needed. Provide enteral feeding or parenteral nutrition if swallowing becomes impaired. Perform physical therapy exercises as prescribed to help prevent complications and promote motor skill recovery. Provide support and education to the parent and child. Support the family as the rapid onset and long recovery can be difficult, causing strain on the family and its finances. If residual disability occurs, assist the family to adjust and to care for their child.

TAKE NOTE!

Serial measurement of tidal volumes may reveal respiratory deterioration in the child with Guillain–Barré syndrome.

Myasthenia Gravis

Myasthenia gravis is an autoimmune disease that may be inherited as a rare genetic disease (congenital), may be acquired by infants born to birthing parents with myasthenia gravis (neonatal), or may develop later in childhood (juvenile). The most common form seen is juvenile myasthenia gravis and will be covered here. See Comparison Chart 25.2 for further information on the less common forms, neonatal myasthenia gravis and congenital myasthenia gravis. Juvenile myasthenia gravis is a relatively rare autoimmune disorder (Lin et al., 2023). The child's antibodies attack the acetylcholine receptor (AchR) and other proteins at the neuromuscular junction, inhibiting normal neuromuscular transmission. The result is progressive weakness and fatigue of the skeletal muscles.

There is no cure for myasthenia gravis. Symptoms can be controlled, but it is a lifelong condition, with early detection being the key to managing the disorder successfully. The disease may be aggravated by stress, exposure to extreme temperatures, and infections, resulting in a myasthenic crisis. Myasthenic crisis is a medical

COMPARISON CHART 25.2 Types of Myasthenia Gravis

	Neonatal Myasthenia Gravis	Congenital Myasthenia Gravis
Definition	Transient form resulting from transplacental transfer of maternal antibodies that interfere with neuromuscular junction	A group of disorders resulting from a genetic mutation of components of the neuromuscular junction resulting in neuromuscular junction failure
Characteristics	Present within a few hours after birth; generalized weakness and hypotonia; bulbar and respiratory weakness leads to poor suck and swallow, weak cry, and possible respiratory failure. Neonate will be very ill. Prompt diagnosis and treatment is essential. Recovery usually occurs within a few weeks.	Apparent at birth; frequently have ptosis, ophthalmoplegia, bulbar, and respiratory muscle weakness; Fluctuating generalized weakness and hypotonia, life-threatening apnea; typically improves with age but spontaneous exacerbations seen. Exacerbations are also seen during periods of stress, increased activity, or febrile illness. Management depends on specific type.

emergency with symptoms including sudden respiratory distress, dysphagia, dysarthria, ptosis, diplopia, tachycardia, anxiety, and rapidly increasing weakness.

Therapeutic management generally involves the use of anticholinesterase medications such as pyridostigmine, which blocks the breakdown of acetylcholine at the neuromuscular junction and enhances neuromuscular transmission. If weakness is not controlled, additional medications may include corticosteroids and other immunosuppressants. Other treatments include plasmapheresis to remove antibodies from the blood, IVIG, and thymectomy (however, the role of the thymus gland in the disease process is unclear; therefore, this procedure may or may not improve the child's symptoms).

Nursing Assessment

Note history of fatigue and weakness; difficulty chewing, swallowing, or holding up the head; or pain with muscle fatigue. In the verbal child, note complaints of double vision. Observe the child for ptosis (droopy eyelids) or altered eye movements from partial paralysis. Note increased work of breathing. Laboratory testing may involve the edrophonium (Tensilon) test, in which a short-acting cholinesterase inhibitor is used. AchR antibodies may be present in elevated quantities in the serum.

Nursing Management

The goals of nursing management include prevention of respiratory problems and providing adequate nutrition. Administer anticholinergic or other medications as ordered, teaching children and families about the use of these drugs. Anticholinergic drugs should be given 30 to 45 minutes before meals, on time and exactly as ordered. Encourage families to seek prompt medical treatment for suspected infections. Encourage appropriate stress management and avoidance of extreme temperatures. Teach families that physical activities should be performed during times of peak energy; rest periods are needed for energy conservation. Teach families to call their neurologist immediately if signs and symptoms of myasthenic crisis or cholinergic crisis, which results from overmedication with anticholinergic medications, appear. Myasthenic crisis and cholinergic crisis have a similar presentation: rapidly increasing muscle weakness with resultant respiratory distress. Encourage children to wear a medical alert bracelet.

CLINICAL REASONING ALERT!

Signs and symptoms of myasthenic crisis include severe muscle weakness, respiratory difficulty, tachycardia, and dysphagia. Signs and symptoms of cholinergic crisis include severe muscle weakness, sweating, increased salivation, bradycardia, and hypotension.

Dermatomyositis

Juvenile dermatomyositis is an autoimmune disease that results in inflammation of the muscles or associated tissues. It occurs more often in females and is generally diagnosed between the ages of 5 and 10 years (Hutchinson & Feldman, 2024). The cause remains unclear, but it may be an autoimmune response triggered by exposure to a virus or to certain medications (Hutchinson & Feldman, 2024). As with other autoimmune diseases, a genetic predisposition is present. The inflammatory cells of the immune system cause a vasculitis that affects the skin, muscles, kidneys, retinas, and gastrointestinal tract.

Therapeutic management involving the use of high-dose glucocorticoid or other immunosuppressants is necessary to prevent the complications of painful calcium deposits under the skin, as well as joint contractures. Methotrexate, IVIG, and cyclosporine may also be used. With appropriate treatment, children may recover completely, although some children experience relapses (Hutchinson & Feldman, 2023).

Nursing Assessment

Elicit a health history, which commonly includes fever, fatigue, and rash, usually followed by muscle pain and weakness. Determine onset and progression of muscle weakness. Inspect the skin for the presence of rash involving the upper eyelids and extensor surfaces of the knuckles, elbows, and knees. The rash is initially a reddish-purplish color and then progresses to scaling, with resulting roughness of the skin. Test muscle strength, particularly noting weakness in the pelvic and shoulder girdles. Laboratory and diagnostic testing may include muscle enzyme levels, a positive ANA test, and an EMG to distinguish muscular weakness from other causes.

Nursing Management

Administer medications as ordered and teach families about their use; instruct them to monitor for side effects. Educate the family about the importance of maintaining the medication regimen in order to prevent calcinosis (calcium deposits) and joint deformity in the future. Encourage adherence with physical therapy regimens. Ensure that children are excused from physical education classes while the disease is active.

ALLERGY AND ANAPHYLAXIS

Allergy is an immune-mediated response resulting in an adverse physiologic event or reaction and affects up to 25% of population in developed countries (Covar et al., 2022). The extent of the allergic response is determined by the duration, rate, and amount of exposure to the allergen as well as environmental and host factors. IgE-mediated allergy will be the focus of this discussion. This type of allergic response is mediated by antigen-specific IgE antibodies. When the antibody is exposed to the antigen (allergen), rapid cell activation occurs, and potent mediators and cytokines are released, resulting in changes in the blood vessels, bronchi, and mucus-secreting glands. In addition to the atopic diseases (asthma, allergic rhinitis, and atopic dermatitis), urticaria, digestive allergy, and systemic anaphylaxis are also IgE-mediated. Although any allergen has the potential to trigger an anaphylactic response, food, drug, and insect sting allergies are most common (Campbell & Kelson, 2024).

Food Allergies

A true food hypersensitivity or allergy is defined as an immunologic reaction resulting from the ingestion of a food or food additive. This type of reaction is an IgE-mediated response to a particular food. Food allergy affects approximately 8% of children and can lead to significant medical complications (Covar et al., 2022). The most common food allergies include milk and dairy, eggs, fish and shellfish, peanuts and tree nuts, and wheat, soy, and sesame (American Academy of Allergy, Asthma & Immunology, 2024). Most reactions occur within minutes of exposure, but they may occur up to 2 hours after ingestion. Signs and symptoms of a food allergy reaction include hives, flushing, facial swelling, mouth and throat itching, and runny nose. Many children also have a gastrointestinal reaction, including vomiting, abdominal pain, and diarrhea. In extreme cases, swelling of the tongue, uvula, pharynx, or upper airway may occur. Wheezing can be an ominous sign that the airway is edematous. Rarely, cardiovascular collapse occurs. Although the risk of anaphylaxis is small, parents, caregivers, and health care providers and nurse practitioners should be vigilant when caring for children with food allergies.

Therapeutic Management

Therapeutic management involves verifying the food allergy, avoiding the allergen, and treating the reaction with medications, including antihistamines and epinephrine (in the case of an anaphylactic reaction). To verify the food allergy, a trial elimination diet may be indicated. If symptoms resolve without the food, true allergy may be present. On an elimination diet, the child stops eating all suspicious foods for 1 to 2 weeks and then retries the foods one at a time, over a period of several days, to see whether a similar reaction occurs. Oral challenge testing and retrying of foods after an elimination diet are often done in the health care provider's or nurse practitioner's office or hospital setting if severe reactions have occurred in the past. Food avoidance is recommended for those who have a highly predictive reaction to testing or a history of anaphylactic response. Prevention of food allergies is also important (see Evidence-Based Practice Box 25.1).

Discerning a true food allergy from intolerance to certain foods is an important part of therapeutic management. "Food intolerance" is a general term that describes an abnormal physiologic response to an ingested food or food additive that has not been proven to be immunologic. Often a milk allergy is confused with lactose intolerance. Therefore, a detailed dietary history is important when distinguishing a true allergy versus intolerance.

TAKE NOTE!

To prevent the development of food allergies, infants should be breastfed for at least the first 6 months of life.

Nursing Assessment

It is important to accurately assess children with food allergy reactions. In the initial nursing assessment, immediately assess the child for airway, breathing, or circulation problems (see Chapter 29). If the child's condition is stable, finish the assessment. Make sure that the health history includes a detailed food history and documentation of the reaction, including the food suspected of

EVIDENCE-BASED PRACTICE 25.1

Early Introduction of Peanuts for the Prevention of Allergy

STUDY

Infants with severe eczema and/or egg allergy are at high risk for peanut allergy. Multiple studies over the past couple of decades have indicated that developmentally appropriate food should be introduced at approximately 6 months of age in typical children. These studies have noted a decrease in peanut allergy when peanut exposure occurs during infancy. The researchers conducted a randomized controlled trial involving 640 infants. The infants were divided into two groups: those with positive skin-prick test for peanut allergy and those without. The groups were then further divided. Infants either consumed developmentally appropriate peanut food or they did not.

Findings

The authors noted additional questions remain in relation to the provision of developmentally appropriate peanut food to infants with severe eczema and/or egg allergy. The current recommendation for these infants is to introduce them to peanut food after sensitivity testing is negative.

Nursing Implications

The current recommendation to prevent the development of peanut allergy in typical children is early introduction of developmentally appropriate peanut food for infants once solid foods have been successfully introduced. Children with severe eczema and/or egg allergy may require sensitivity testing prior to the introduction of peanut food. Parents may be fearful of peanut allergy as the recommendation for decades was to avoid peanut foods until after age 12 months. Educate parents that current research demonstrates decreased allergy incidence with earlier introduction. Parents should discuss peanut food introduction with their baby's primary care provider, prior to trying it.

Data from Abrams, E. M., Chan, E. S., & Sicherer, S. (2020). Peanut allergy: New advances and ongoing controversies. *Pediatrics, 145*(5), e20192102. https://doi.org/10.1542/peds.2019-2102

causing the reaction, the quantity of food ingested, the length of time between ingestion and development of symptoms, the symptoms, what treatment has been administered, and the subsequent response. Note gastrointestinal symptoms such as:

- Burning in the mouth or throat
- Bloating
- Nausea
- Diarrhea

Assess for risk factors such as previous exposure to the food, history of poorly controlled asthma, or an increase in atopic dermatitis flare-ups in relation to food intake. Inspect the skin for color, rash, hives, or edema. Auscultate the heart and lungs to determine heart rate and to assess for wheezing.

Allergy skin-prick tests and radioallergosorbent blood tests (RASTs) are used widely by health care providers and nurse practitioners to look for allergic reactions. Food-specific IgE testing is recommended if the child has a history of food allergy. If the child has episodic symptoms, an oral challenge in a controlled setting may be appropriate. For an oral challenge, the child slowly eats a serving of the offending food over the period of 1 hour. Record vital signs and note the presence or absence of allergic symptoms.

Nursing Management

Initial nursing management is aimed at stabilizing the child's condition if an acute reaction to a food allergen is present (see Chapter 29). As stated previously, medications used in the treatment of a food allergy reaction include histamine blockers and, in anaphylactic reactions, epinephrine. Teach the child (if appropriate) and the parents how and when to use these medications during an allergic reaction. The child who has been prescribed an EpiPen should carry the pen with them at all times. Since these reactions can be so sudden (unknown ingestion of allergen) and severe, it is helpful for the family to have a written emergency plan in case of a reaction.

MANAGING THE CHILD'S DIET

Aim dietary teaching at educating the child and family on how to avoid the offending foods. Families should be extremely careful when reading food labels. A dietitian may be helpful in this teaching process. Teaching Guidelines 25.1 gives information about hidden allergens in food. Teach the parents what "safe" foods can be substituted for offensive ones (Box 25.5). Children with peanut allergy should also avoid tree nuts.

Having a child with a food allergy can be anxiety-producing for parents; they often live in fear that the child may accidentally ingest an allergen. Educate the child and family about allergic reactions to help decrease their anxiety. Teach the child and family how to recognize the signs and symptoms of an allergic reaction. It may be necessary to provide information to day

BOX 25.5 Food Substitutions

- Replace milk with water, fruit juice, rice milk, or soymilk.
- Replace each egg with 1.5 tablespoons each of water and oil and 1 teaspoon baking powder; OR 1 packet plain gelatin with 2 tablespoons warm water added at time of use; OR 1 teaspoon yeast and a quarter-cup warm water.
- Replace peanuts or tree nuts with raisins, dates, or crispy cereal.

Data from Winkels, K. (2023). *Allergy-free foods.* http://www.eatingwithfoodallergies.com/allergyfreesubstitutes.html

TEACHING GUIDELINES 25.1 Allergens Hidden in Food

If Child Is Allergic to	Teach Families to Avoid	Unexpected Locations of Common Ingredients
Milk	Artificial butter flavor, casein, lactalbumin, nougat, pudding, whey, yogurt, ghee	Some deli meats and hot dogs, nondairy products, coffee whiteners
Wheat	Cereal extract, couscous, durum, semolina, spelt	Some imitation crab meat and wheat flour shaped to look like shrimp, beef, or pork
Eggs	Albumin, globulin, ovalbumin	Some egg substitutes and foam toppings for drinks, commercially cooked pastas
Peanuts	Fast food cooked in peanut oil, baked goods with nuts, or foods processed on equipment that also processes peanuts	Brown gravy, barbeque sauce, meat sauce, egg rolls, enchilada sauce, hot chocolate

Based on Kids with Food Allergies. (2023). *Recipe substitutions*. https://kidswithfoodallergies.org/recipes-diet/recipe-substitutions/

care providers as well as schoolteachers, staff, and camp counselors. Refer families to the Food Allergy & Anaphylaxis Network.

CONSIDER THIS!

The parent of Mina Stepelman (6 years old) is distraught about the significance of Mina's peanut allergy. She has been prescribed an EpiPen and is comfortable with when and how to use it. Mina's parent says tearfully, "I'm just so scared she'll eat the wrong thing when she's not with me. I'm never letting her go to a party alone or spend the night at someone's house. Even though I've talked to her school nurse, I'm even scared about what she'll eat at school."

Think about if you or your child had this type of significant allergy, how would you feel? How would you deal with this perceived risk?

As a nurse, how should you respond to Mina's parent?

Anaphylaxis

Anaphylaxis is an acute IgE-mediated response to an allergen that involves many organ systems and may be life-threatening. In addition to nuts, shellfish, eggs, and bee or wasp stings, drugs such as beta-lactam antibiotics and NSAIDs, and latex (though rarer) are the leading causes of anaphylaxis (Linzer, 2024). The reaction is severe and usually starts within 5 to 10 minutes of exposure, although delayed reactions are possible. Histamines and secondary mediators are released from the mast cells and eosinophils in response to contact with an allergen. Cutaneous, cardiopulmonary, gastrointestinal, and neurologic symptoms occur. Vasodilation results in a rapid decrease in plasma volume, leading to the risk of circulatory collapse. Prolonged resuscitation may be needed, and death may occur.

Therapeutic management focuses on assessment and support of the airway, breathing, and circulation. Epinephrine is usually required, and intramuscular or intravenous diphenhydramine is used secondarily. Late-onset reactions can be prevented with corticosteroids.

Nursing Assessment

Assess patency of the airway and adequacy of breathing. Determine if circulation is sufficient. Note level of consciousness. Obtain a brief history, inquiring specifically about allergen exposure. Determine whether the child has received any medication (e.g., epinephrine or diphenhydramine) since the onset of the reaction and what effect the medication had on the symptoms. Table 25.3 gives additional signs and symptoms of anaphylaxis.

TABLE 25.3 • Clinical Manifestations of Anaphylaxis

Body Area or System	Manifestation
Oral	• Lip, tongue, or palate pruritus • Lip or tongue edema
Cutaneous	Urticaria (hives), flushing, pruritus, angioedema
Respiratory	• Nasal pruritus, congestion, sneezing, rhinorrhea • Stridor, tightness in the throat, dysphagia, dysphonia, hoarseness • Shortness of breath, dyspnea, tight chest, wheeze
Cardiovascular	Tachycardia, chest pain, arrhythmia, hypotension
Neurologic	Syncope, feeling faint, aura of doom, lethargy, disorientation
Gastrointestinal	Bloating, abdominal pain, diarrhea, vomiting

Based on Covar, R. A., Fleischer, D. M., Cho, C., & Boguniewicz, M. (2022). Allergic disorders. In M. Bunik, W. W. Hay, M. J. Levin, & M. J. Abzug (Eds.), *Current diagnosis & treatment: Pediatrics* (26th ed.). McGraw-Hill Education; Campbell, R. L., & Kelso, J. M. (2024). Anaphylaxis: Acute diagnosis. *UpToDate.* Retrieved April 16, 2024, from https://www.uptodate.com/contents/anaphylaxis-acute-diagnosis

Nursing Management

Nursing management initially focuses on supporting the airway, breathing, and circulation. Provide supplemental oxygen by mask or bag-valve-mask ventilation. Administer epinephrine as ordered to reverse the allergic process. Ensure that bronchodilator inhalation treatment (albuterol) is given if bronchospasm is present. Administer intravenous fluids to provide volume expansion. Observe the child for 4 to 6 hours in case of recurrent attack (Covar et al., 2022).

PREVENTING AND MANAGING FUTURE EPISODES

It is critical to educate the family about preventing and managing future episodes. Teach the family how to use injectable epinephrine in case of subsequent allergen exposure. Intramuscular epinephrine may be given via the EpiPen or EpiPen Jr. Dosage is based on the child's weight. The child should carry the pen with them at all times. Explain to the child and family that the gray safety release on the EpiPen should never be removed until just before use. In addition, teach the child and family that the thumb, fingers, or hand should not be placed over the black tip. Nursing Procedure 25.1 gives further instructions related to EpiPen use. Instruct the child and family to call 911 and seek immediate medical attention after using the EpiPen. Warn the child that the epinephrine may make them feel as if the heart is racing.

Day care providers, school nurses, teachers, and staff who interact with the child must know how to recognize an anaphylactic event. In 2004, Public Law No. 108-377, Asthmatic Schoolchildren's Treatment and Health Management Act, was passed by the U.S. Congress. This law is intended to ensure that students with severe allergies can carry prescribed medications (i.e., EpiPen) with them. All children with allergies should have an action plan in place at the school or day care center. Advise the child to wear a medical ID alert bracelet or necklace at all times.

Teach children and families to avoid known food allergens. Avoid stings from bees and wasps by being alert when eating outdoors, wearing long sleeves and pants when in fields, and having bee and wasp hives or nests removed from areas near the family's home. Immunotherapy (allergy shots) may be indicated in children with a hypersensitivity to stinging insects. Avoid use of cephalosporins in children with severe penicillin allergy. Desensitization is available for children with severe penicillin allergy. Desensitization involves administration of increasingly larger doses of penicillin over a period of hours to days in an intensive care setting.

Latex Allergy

Latex allergy is an IgE-mediated response to exposure to latex, a natural rubber product used in many common

NURSING PROCEDURE 25.1 Using the EpiPen or EpiPen Jr

1. Grasp the EpiPen or EpiPen Jr with the black tip pointing downward, forming a fist (Fig. 1).

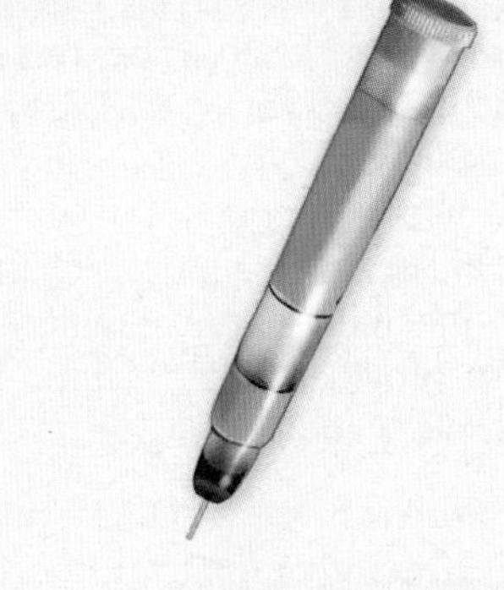

2. With the other hand, pull off the gray safety release.
3. Swing and jab the EpiPen firmly into the outer thigh at a 90-degree angle, and hold firmly there for 10 seconds (Figs. 2 and 3).

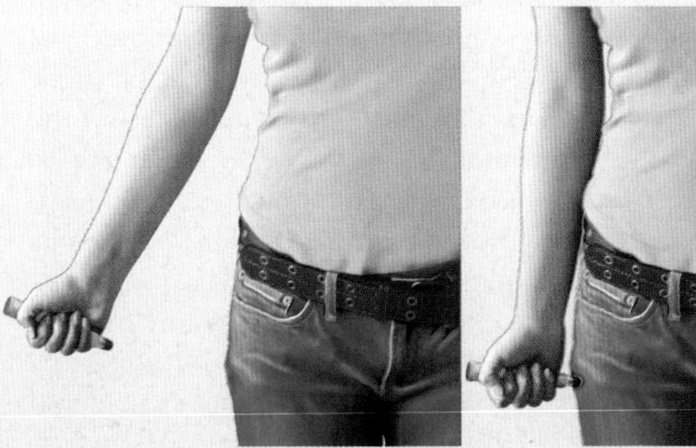

4. Remove the EpiPen and massage the thigh for 10 seconds.

Based on Viatris. (2023). *EpiPen: How to use.* https://www.epipen.com/en/about-epipen-and-generic/how-to-use-epipen

items (especially gloves in the health care setting). The pathophysiology of latex allergy is similar to that of food allergy. Avoidance of latex products is recommended for those who are allergic to it. An immediate allergic reaction may occur if a latex-allergic child comes into contact with latex. Latex allergy can also result in anaphylaxis (refer to previous section on anaphylaxis).

Nursing Assessment

Screen all children who visit a health care facility of any kind for latex allergy. Ask if the child is allergic to rubber gloves or has ever developed hives after exposure to them. Ask the parent if the child has symptoms such as coughing, wheezing, or shortness of breath after glove exposure. Has the child ever had swelling in the mouth or complained that the mouth itched after a dental examination? Determine whether the child has ever had allergic symptoms after eating foods with a known cross-reactivity to latex, such as pear, peach, passion fruit, plum, pineapple, kiwi, fig, grape, cherry, melon, nectarine, papaya, apple, apricot, banana, chestnut, carrot, celery, avocado, tomato, or potato. For the child who has come into contact with latex, assess for symptoms of a reaction such as hives; wheeze; cough; shortness of breath; nasal congestion and rhinorrhea; sneezing; nose, palate, or eye pruritus; or hypotension.

Nursing Management

Nursing management of latex allergy focuses on preventing exposure to latex products. Instruct children and their families to avoid foods with a known cross-reactivity to latex such as those listed earlier. If the child is exposed to latex, remove the irritating substance and cleanse the area with soap and water. Assess for the need for resuscitation and perform it if needed. Become familiar with your institution's latex allergy policy. Know which products contain latex and which do not. Document latex allergy on the chart, the child's identification band, the medication administration record, and the health care provider's order sheet. Refer families to resources for people with latex allergy.

Unfolding Patient Stories: Charlie Snow • Part 2

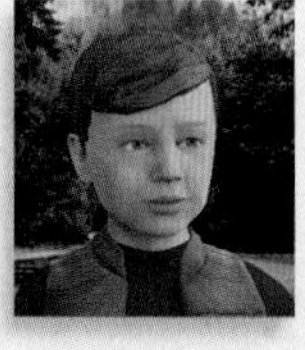

Recall Charlie Snow, a 6-year-old with a known hypersensitivity to dyes, perfumes, and peanuts whom you first met in Chapter 6. Since living with his aunt and uncle while his parents are in the military, he has been treated for a skin reaction and is now hospitalized with an anaphylactic reaction from peanut ingestion. How would the nurse determine if Charlie is at risk for maltreatment or neglect? What measures can the nurse take to ensure his safety at home?

Care for Charlie and other patients in a realistic virtual environment: ***vSim** for Nursing* (thepoint.lww.com/vSimPediatric). Practice documenting these patients' care in DocuCare (thePoint.lww.com/DocuCareEHR).

KEY CONCEPTS

- Waning of maternal antibodies in early infancy while humoral immunity is developing leads to physiologic hypogammaglobulinemia, placing the young infant at risk for overwhelming infection.
- Infants and young children have large lymph nodes, tonsils, and thymus compared with adults.
- Infants have decreased phagocytic activity, placing them at higher risk for serious infection.
- Children with immune disorders often show a decreased or absent response to delayed hypersensitivity skin testing (e.g., the tuberculosis test).
- Primary immune deficiencies such as SCID and Wiskott–Aldrich syndrome are congenital and serious; they can be cured only by bone marrow or stem cell transplantation.
- SLE is a chronic autoimmune disorder that can affect any organ system, primarily causing vasculitis.
- Juvenile idiopathic arthritis results in chronic pain and affects growth and development as well as school performance.
- Nasal, palatal, or throat pruritus and difficulty breathing may indicate an anaphylactic reaction.
- Various forms of hypogammaglobulinemia may be treated with exogenous immunoglobulin administered intravenously every several weeks, allowing children to lead a healthier life with fewer infections.
- Children with severe allergy or previous anaphylactic episodes must avoid contact with allergens.
- Nursing management of lupus focuses on preventing flare-ups and complications.
- Managing pain, maintaining mobility, and administering disease-modifying medications are key nursing interventions in the management of juvenile idiopathic arthritis.
- HIV infection may be prevented in infants by prenatal screening and maternal treatment, as well as postnatal treatment with zidovudine.
- HIV infection in children often results in encephalopathy and developmental delay.
- Spread of HIV infection can be prevented in adolescence by avoiding high-risk behaviors.
- For children with immune deficiency or autoimmune disease, prevention of infection is a primary nursing concern.
- A chronic illness such as immune deficiency, SLE, or juvenile arthritis has a significant impact on the family as well as the child.
- When planning care for the child with an immune deficiency or autoimmune disorder, the nurse should include the child and the family.
- To promote proper growth, encourage the child with an immune or autoimmune disorder to eat a balanced diet.
- Teach families of children with immune deficiencies about infection prevention.
- Teach the family of the child with juvenile arthritis about ways to decrease pain while increasing or maintaining the child's mobility.

- Teach families of children with severe allergy how to avoid allergens and how to use the EpiPen. Make sure that staff at the child's school or day care center are aware of the allergy.
- Explain to the child with severe allergy the importance of wearing a medical ID alert bracelet or necklace.

REFERENCES AND RECOMMENDED READINGS

Abbott, J. K., Dutmer, C. M., & Hauk, P. J. (2022). Chapter 33: Immunodeficiency. In M. Bunik, W. W. Hay, M. J. Levin, & M. J. Abzug (Eds.), *Current diagnosis & treatment: Pediatrics* (26th ed., pp. 976–994). McGraw-Hill Education.

Abrams, E. M., Chan, E. S., & Sicherer, S. (2020) Peanut allergy: New advances and ongoing controversies. *Pediatrics, 145*(5), e20192102. https://doi.org/10.1542/peds.2019-2102

American Academy of Allery, Asthma & Immunology. (2024). Food allergy. https://acaai.org/allergies/allergic-conditions/food/

Campbell, R. L., & Kelso, J. M. (2024). Anaphylaxis: Acute diagnosis. *UpToDate*. Retrieved April 16, 2024, from https://www.uptodate.com/contents/anaphylaxis-acute-diagnosis

Corbett, J. A., & Banks, A. D. (2019). *Laboratory tests and diagnostic procedures with nursing diagnoses* (9th ed.). Pearson Education Inc.

Covar, R. A., Fleischer, D. M., Cho, C., & Boguniewicz, M. (2022). Chapter 38: Allergic disorders. In M. Bunik, W. W. Hay, M. J. Levin, & M. J. Abzug (Eds.), *Current diagnosis & treatment: Pediatrics* (26th ed., pp. 1105–1147). McGraw-Hill Education.

Gillespie, S. L. (2023). Pediatric HIV infection: Classification, clinical manifestations, and outcome. *UpToDate*. Retrieved February 25, 2024, from https://www.uptodate.com/contents/pediatric-hiv-infection-classification-clinical-manifestations-and-outcome

Health Resources and Services Administration, the HIV/AIDS Program. (2022). *About the program*. https://ryanwhite.hrsa.gov/about

Heimall, J. (2019). Severe combined immunodeficiency (SCID): An overview. *UpToDate*. Retrieved February 25, 2024, from http://www.uptodate.com/contents/severe-combined-immunodeficiency-scid-an-overview

Hutchinson, C., & Feldman, B. M. (2023). Juvenile dermatomyositis and polymyositis: Treatment, complications, and prognosis. *UpToDate*. Retrieved February 25, 2024, from http://www.uptodate.com/contents/treatment-and-prognosis-of-juvenile-dermatomyositis-and-polymyositis

Hutchinson, C., & Feldman, B. M. (2024). Juvenile dermatomyositis and other idiopathic inflammatory myopathies: Epidemiology, pathogenesis and clinical manifestations. *UpToDate*. Retrieved February 25, 2024, from http://www.uptodate.com/contents/pathogenesis-and-clinical-manifestations-of-juvenile-dermatomyositis-and-polymyositis

Kids with Food Allergies. (2023). *Recipe substitutions*. https://kidswithfoodallergies.org/recipes-diet/recipe-substitutions/

Klein-Gitelman, M. S. (2022). Pediatric systemic lupus erythematous. *Medscape*. Retrieved April 28, 2023, from https://emedicine.medscape.com/article/1008066-overview#a6

Lexicomp®. (2024). *Lexi-Drugs/immune globulin (Version 8.1.0) [Mobile app]*. Wolters Kluwer. https://apps.apple.com/us/app/lexicomp/id313401238

Lin, Y., Kuang, Q., Li, H., Liang, B., Ly, J., Jiang, Q., & Yang., X. (2023). Outcome and clinical features in juvenile myasthenia gravis: A systematic review and meta-analysis. *Frontiers in Neurology, 14*. https://doi.org/10.3389/fneur.2023.1119294

Linzer, J. F. (2024). *Pediatric anaphylaxis*. Medscape. https://emedicine.medscape.com/article/799744-overview#a1

Mayo Foundation for Clinical Education and Research. (2024). *Pediatric test reference values*. http://www.mayomedicallaboratories.com/test-info/pediatric/refvalues/reference.php

National Hemophilia Foundation. (2023). *MASAC Document 280 - MASAC recommendations concerning products licensed for the treatment of hemophilia and selected disorders of the coagulation system*. https://www.hemophilia.org/healthcare-professionals/guidelines-on-care/masac-documents/masac-document-280-masac-recommendations-concerning-products-licensed-for-the-treatment-of-hemophilia-and-selected-disorders-of-the-coagulation-system

National Institutes of Health. (2024a). *HIV and adolescents and young adults*. https://hivinfo.nih.gov/understanding-hiv/fact-sheets/hiv-and-adolescents-and-young-adults

National Institutes of Health. (2024b). *HIV and children*. https://hivinfo.nih.gov/understanding-hiv/fact-sheets/hiv-and-children

Ochs, H. D. (2022). Wiskott-Aldrich syndrome. *UpToDate*. Retrieved February 25, 2024, from http://www.uptodate.com/contents/wiskott-aldrich-syndrome

Panel on Antiretroviral Therapy and Medical Management of Children Living with HIV. (2024). *Guidelines for the use of antiretroviral agents in pediatric HIV infection*. Department of Health and Human Services. https://clinicalinfo.hiv.gov/en/guidelines/pediatric-arv/whats-new

Patel, S. B. (2022). Avascular necrosis. *Medscape*. Retrieved February 25, 2024, from http://emedicine.medscape.com/article/333364-overview

Smith, C., & McFarland, E. J. (2022). Chapter 41: Human immunodeficiency virus infection. In M. Bunik, W. W. Hay, M. J. Levin, & M. J. Abzug (Eds., pp. 1224–1236), *Current diagnosis & treatment: Pediatrics* (26th ed.). McGraw-Hill Education.

Soep, J. B. (2022). Chapter 29: Rheumatic diseases. In M. Bunik, W. W. Hay, M. J. Levin, & M. J. Abzug (Eds.), *Current diagnosis & treatment: Pediatrics* (26th ed., pp. 865–874). McGraw-Hill Education.

Tosi, M. F. (2019). Chapter 2: Normal and impaired immunologic responses to infection. In J. Cherry, G. J. Harrison, W. J. Steinbach, S. L. Kaplan, & P. Hotez (Eds.), *Feigin & Cherry's textbook of pediatric infectious diseases* (8th ed., pp. 15–40). Elsevier.

U.S. Department of Health and Human Services. (n.d.). *Healthy People 2030*. https://health.gov/healthypeople

U.S. House of Representatives. (2004). *Public law No. 108-377 asthmatic schoolchildren's treatment and health management act of 2004*. Library of Congress.

UpToDate, Inc. (2024). *Lexi-comp® (Version 8.1.0) [Mobile app]*. Wolters Kluwer. https://apps.apple.com/us/app/lexicomp/id313401238

Viatris. (2023). *EpiPen®: How to use*. https://www.epipen.com/en/about-epipen-and-generic/how-to-use-epipen

Winkels, K. (2023). *Allergy-free foods*. http://www.eatingwithfoodallergies.com/allergyfreesubstitutes.html

Wolownik, K. (2022). Common HSCT complications. In M. Evans, J. Nuuhiwa, R. L. Secola, & K. Wolownik (Eds.), *Foundations of pediatric hematopoietic stem cell transplantation* (3rd ed.). Association of Pediatric Hematology/Oncology Nurses.

Yiu, E. (2023). Guillain-Barré syndrome in children: Epidemiology, clinical features, and diagnosis. *UpToDate*. Retrieved February 25, 2024, from http://www.uptodate.com/contents/epidemiology-clinical-features-and-diagnosis-of-guillain-barre-syndrome-in-children

DEVELOPING CLINICAL JUDGMENT

PRACTICING FOR NCLEX

1. The nurse is caring for a 6-year-old with juvenile idiopathic arthritis. The parent states they have trouble getting their child out of bed in the morning and believe the child's behavior is due to a desire to avoid going to school. What is the best advice by the nurse?
   - **a.** Refer them to a psychologist for evaluation of school phobia related to chronic illness.
   - **b.** Administer a warm bath every morning before school.
   - **c.** Give the child prescribed NSAIDs 30 minutes before getting out of bed.
   - **d.** Allow the child to stay in bed some mornings if they want.

2. A 14-year-old with SLE wants to know how to care for their skin. What should the nurse teach this adolescent?
   - **a.** Careful sun-tanning will give their skin an attractive color.
   - **b.** No special skin care is needed.
   - **c.** Use sunscreen daily to avoid rashes.
   - **d.** Use makeup to camouflage the butterfly rash on their face.

3. The parent of a child with hypogammaglobulinemia reports that their child had a fever and slight chills with an intravenous gamma globulin infusion last month. They want to know what other course of treatment might be available. What is the best response by the nurse?
   - **a.** Administration of acetaminophen or diphenhydramine prior to the next infusion may decrease the incidence of fever or chills.
   - **b.** Giving the gamma globulin intramuscularly is recommended to prevent a reaction.
   - **c.** Talk to the health care provider or nurse practitioner about alternative medications that may be used to boost the gamma globulin level in the blood.
   - **d.** If the child is no longer experiencing frequent infections, then the IV infusions may not be necessary.

4. A 4-month-old infant born to a parent with HIV infection is going into foster care because the birthing parent is too ill to care for the child. The foster parent wants to know if the infant is also infected. What is the best response by the nurse?
   - **a.** "It's too early to know; we have to wait until the infant has symptoms."
   - **b.** "Since the birthing parent is so ill, it's likely the child is also infected with HIV."
   - **c.** "The ELISA test is positive, so the child is definitely infected."
   - **d.** "The PCR test is positive; this indicates HIV infection, which may or may not progress to AIDS."

5. A parent has received instructions about avoiding wheat and soy allergens. Which response by the parent would indicate that further education is needed?
   - **a.** "I will not feed my child any breads made with wheat flour."
   - **b.** "I will allow my child to eat semolina pasta, the kind they love."
   - **c.** "I will not feed my child shakes made with soy protein."
   - **d.** "I will read labels to be sure I am avoiding wheat and soy."

6. The nurse is caring for a child in the acute phase of Guillain–Barré syndrome. What is the priority nursing action?
   - **a.** Perform range-of-motion exercises.
   - **b.** Take temperature every 4 hours.
   - **c.** Monitor respiratory status closely.
   - **d.** Assess skin frequently.

7. At a classmate's birthday celebration at school, a child with a known food allergy is coughing and exhibiting retractions when the school nurse assesses them. The child states they "don't feel right" and that they have an itchy throat.
   Place the nursing actions in priority order from first to last.
   - **a.** Administer the child's prescribed EpiPen.
   - **b.** Determine the child's vital signs.
   - **c.** Position the child to facilitate breathing.
   - **d.** Ask another adult to activate the Emergency Management Systems (EMS).
   - **e.** Notify the parents.

8. The charge nurse on the pediatric unit assigns an adolescent with HIV infection and poor growth to the licensed practical nurse (LPN). The LPN states, "I do not want to care for this adolescent." Which is the appropriate response by the charge nurse?
   - **a.** "Okay, I will check if the other LPN will care for them."
   - **b.** "So you are confident with the adolescent's care, I will help you."
   - **c.** "You seem worried about caring for this adolescent."
   - **d.** "Let's review blood and body fluid precautions you will using."

DOSAGE CALCULATION QUESTION

The nurse is caring for a term newborn born to a parent with HIV infection. The infant weighs 6 lb 5 oz. The medication order reads: zidovudine 25 mg PO twice daily. Zidovudine is supplied as 50 mg/5 mL. How many milliliters will the nurse administer? Round to the nearest tenth.

CRITICAL THINKING EXERCISES

1. Develop a discharge teaching plan for a 14-year-old with SLE who will be taking corticosteroids long term.
2. Devise a developmental stimulation plan for a 22-month-old with HIV infection and encephalopathy with developmental delay (to the level of a 9-month-old).
3. Determine an appropriate nursing plan of care for an infant who has undergone bone marrow transplantation for SCID.
4. Develop a prioritized list of patient problems for a child with HIV infection, candidiasis, poor growth, and pneumonia requiring oxygen.
5. A child with recurrent infections is being evaluated. Other than information about onset of symptoms and events leading up to this present episode, what other types of information would the nurse ask while obtaining the history?

STUDY ACTIVITIES

1. In the clinical setting, compare the growth and development of two children of the same age, one with HIV infection and one who has been healthy.
2. Attend an outpatient clinic that provides care to children with HIV infection. Observe the health care or nurse practitioner during office visits, and attend a multidisciplinary planning meeting. Identify the role of the registered nurse in providing family education, coordination of care, and referrals.
3. Conduct an internet search to determine the educational material available to children and their families related to immune deficiencies, autoimmune disorders, or allergies.
4. Research your clinical institution's policies related to latex allergy, alternative products available at the institution, and how to obtain them for a child with latex allergy. Provide a presentation to your clinical group about your findings.

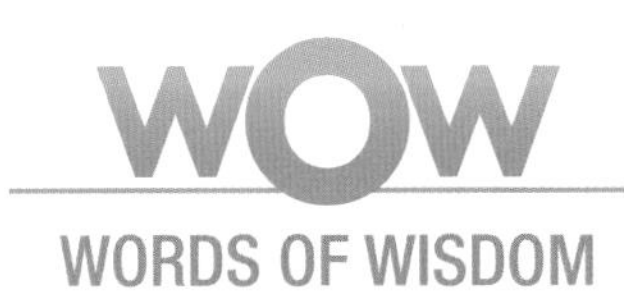
WORDS OF WISDOM
Endocrine disorders in children often elude the medical radar screen.

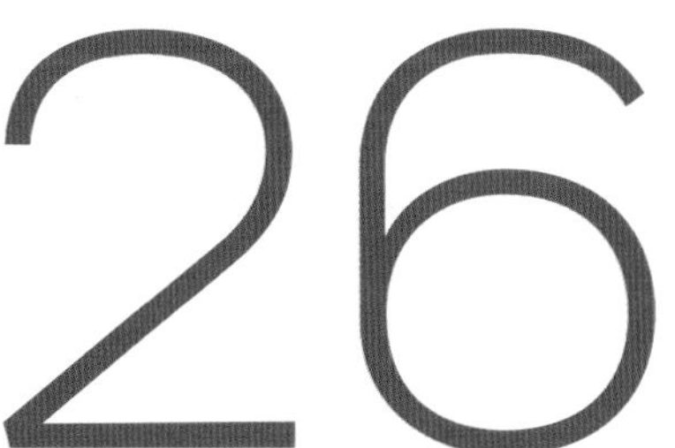

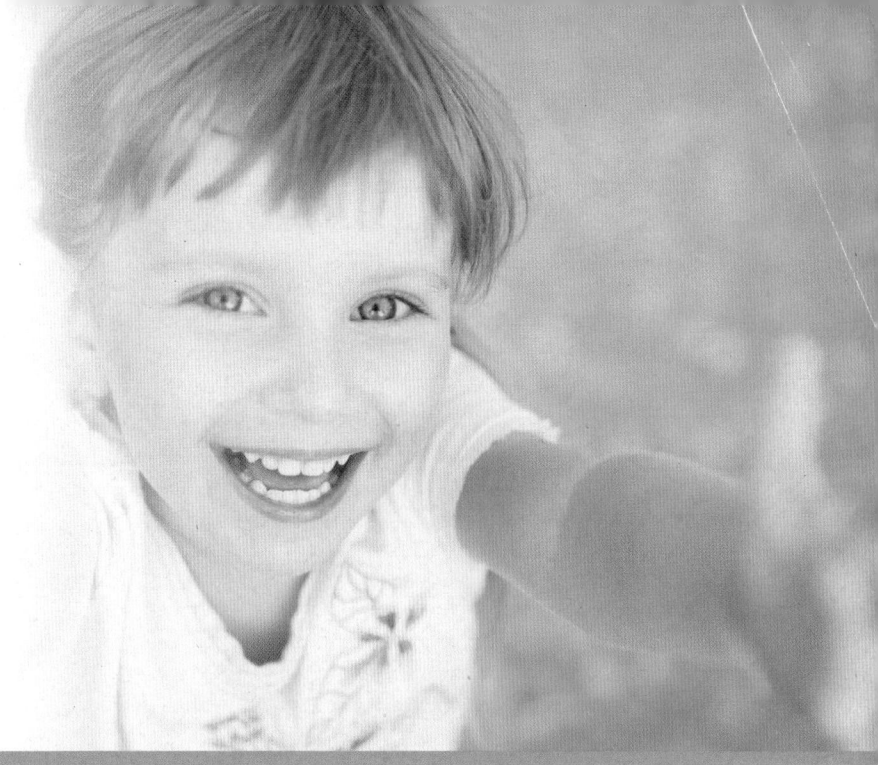

Nursing Care of the Child With an Alteration in Metabolism/Endocrine Disorder

KEY TERMS

adrenarche (ad-ren-ahr´kē)
constitutional delay
diabetic ketoacidosis (DKA)
exophthalmos (eks´of-thal´mos)
goiter
hemoglobin A1C
hirsutism (hir´sū-tizm)
hormone
hyperfunction
hypofunction
polydipsia
polyuria

LEARNING OBJECTIVES

Upon completion of the chapter, you will be able to:

1. Describe the major components and functions of a child's endocrine system.
2. Differentiate between the anatomic and physiologic differences of the endocrine system in children versus adults.
3. Identify the essential assessment elements, common diagnostic procedures, and laboratory tests associated with the diagnosis of endocrine disorders in children.
4. Identify the common medications and treatment modalities used for palliation of endocrine disorders in children.
5. Distinguish specific disorders of the endocrine system that affect children.
6. Associate the clinical manifestations of specific endocrine disorders with the appropriate patient problems.
7. Establish nursing outcomes, evaluative criteria, and interventions for children with specific disorders in the endocrine system.
8. Develop teaching plans for children and their families regarding endocrine disorders.

Carlos Rodriguez, a 12-year-old, is seen in the clinic today with complaints of weakness, fatigue, blurred vision, and headaches. His parent states, "Carlos's teacher has noticed mood changes and is concerned about his behavior at school. He's always been a good boy. I'm not sure what's going on."

INTRODUCTION

Metabolism refers to all physical and chemical reactions occurring in the body's cells that are necessary to maintain and sustain life. Nurses encounter potential and actual alterations in metabolism in all types of patients and must detect problems and intervene early to prevent life-threatening or long-term complications. The endocrine system consists of various glands, tissues, or clusters of cells that produce and release hormones. **Hormones** are chemical messengers that stimulate or regulate the actions of other tissues, organs, or other endocrine glands that have specific receptors for the hormone. Along with the nervous system, the endocrine milieu influences all physiologic effects such as growth and development, metabolic processes related to fluid and electrolyte balance and energy production, sexual maturation and reproduction, and the body's response to stress. The release patterns of hormones vary, but the level in the body is maintained within specified limits to preserve health.

Alterations in metabolism develop in the endocrine system when there is a deficiency (**hypofunction**) or excess (**hyperfunction**) of a specific hormone. In children, alterations in metabolism or endocrine conditions often develop insidiously and result from an insufficient production of hormones. If the problem is not diagnosed and treated early, delayed growth and development, cognitive impairments, or death may result. Generally, the treatment plan involves correction of the underlying reason for the dysfunction, such as surgical removal of a tumor, and supplementation of missing hormones or adjustment of specific hormone levels. This allows most children to live normal lives.

VARIATIONS IN ANATOMY AND PHYSIOLOGY

The organs or tissues of the endocrine system include the hypothalamus, pituitary gland, thyroid gland, parathyroid glands, adrenal glands, gonads, and islets of Langerhans located in the pancreas. Figure 26.1 shows the location of these organs or tissues involved in the endocrine system. Typically, most endocrine glands begin to develop during the first trimester of gestation, but their development is incomplete at birth. Thus, complete hormonal control is lacking during the early years of life, and infants cannot appropriately balance fluid concentration, electrolytes, amino acids, glucose, and trace substances.

Hormone Production and Secretion

The hypothalamic–pituitary axis produces a number of releasing and inhibiting hormones that regulate the function of many of the other endocrine glands, including the thyroid gland, the adrenal glands, and the male and female gonads. Some glands regulate their function in connection with the nervous system, such as the islets of Langerhans in the pancreas and the parathyroid glands. Many other cells in the body secrete hormones such as the pineal gland, the scattered epithelial cells in the gastrointestinal (GI) tract, and the thymus. Disorders related to these other cells are discussed in other chapters of this book.

Figure 26.1 shows the major glands, the hormones produced by these glands, and the effects each hormone has on the target cell, tissue, or organ. The process of hormone production and secretion involves the principle of feedback control. One gland produces a hormone that affects another endocrine gland. Once the physiologic effect is achieved, this gland, known as the target organ, inhibits the further release of the original hormone. The reverse occurs when the first gland detects low levels of the target gland hormone. If the original gland does not release enough of the hormone, the inhibition process stops so that the gland increases the production of the hormone. The endocrine system and the nervous system work closely together to maintain an optimal internal environment for the body, a state known as homeostasis.

COMMON MEDICAL TREATMENTS

Primarily, the treatment of endocrine disorders involves decreasing hormone production in cases of hypersecretion or replacing hormones in cases of hypofunction. The first step in treating many of these disorders is to screen for potential problems, especially when familial patterns are present. Since the proper functioning of the endocrine system is critical to growth and development, the child's growth is affected by endocrine dysfunction, and lack of treatment may lead to serious problems such as intellectual disability or even death. Early treatment is often associated with a better prognosis and prevention of long-term problems. The next step in treatment involves identifying underlying causes for the dysfunction (e.g., a tumor or growth that requires surgical removal or irradiation). The use of supplemental hormones in cases of hypofunction is generally successful in children, as is the use of inhibiting substances in cases of hyperfunction.

Common Medical Treatments 26.1 describes the common treatments used in children with endocrine disorders. The table explains and gives indications for each treatment, as well as relevant nursing implications. Advances in technology and our understanding of molecular biology continue to increase our knowledge of these disorders and the modalities needed to prevent them or improve quality of life for affected children. These advances are vital, since the whole body is influenced by the endocrine milieu.

Drug Guide 26.1 lists the medications most commonly used to treat endocrine disorders. The table gives the actions and indications of each drug, as well as pertinent nursing implications. Many of the medications are synthetic preparations of the actual hormones. It is important to maintain specific blood levels of the

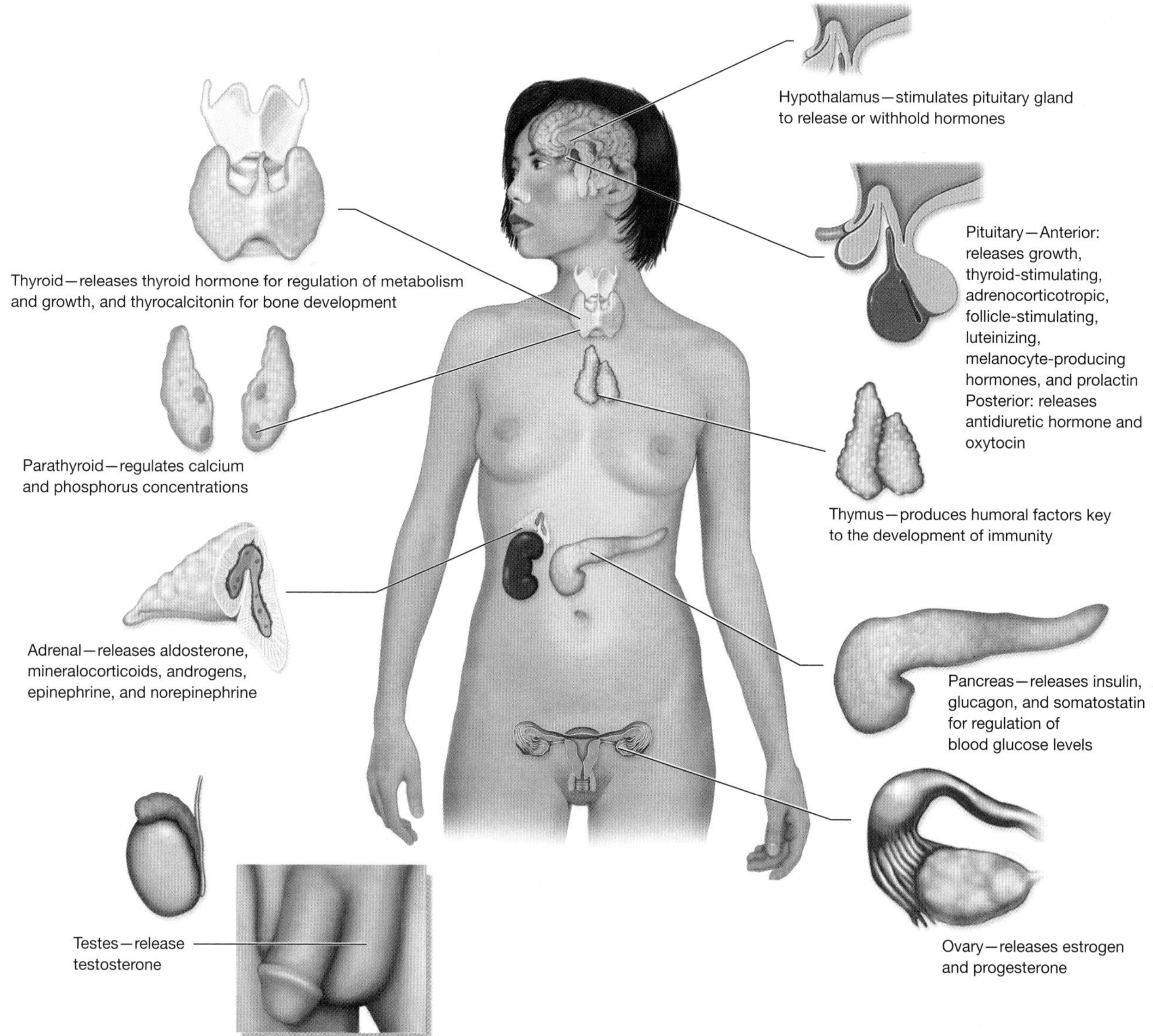

FIGURE 26.1 Location of the endocrine glands in the body, with the major effects of the glands listed.

COMMON MEDICAL TREATMENTS 26.1

Treatment	Explanation	Indications	Nursing Implications
Surgery	Surgical removal of tumors or cysts	Any endocrine malfunction caused by the presence of a mass	• Provide routine preoperative and postoperative care depending on location and extent of surgery. • Keep the family informed of choices.
Irradiation/radioactive iodine	Radiation is used to influence the hormone secretion of a gland; it is less invasive than surgery.	Hyperfunction of an endocrine gland; may be used when surgery is not possible	• Prepare the child for specific procedures following protocols. • Explain the procedure. • Check to ensure the child has no sensitivity to iodine preparations.
Glucose monitoring	Fingerstick blood sample several times per day	Monitoring of glucose control	• Teach the family appropriate procedure. • Refer family to sources for equipment and supplies. • Assist the family with developing a system of record-keeping that works for them.
Dietary interventions (medical nutritional therapy)	Restriction or manipulation of dietary intake	Diabetes mellitus (DM)	• Refer family to a dietitian specializing in pediatric DM. • Reinforce teaching related to special diets.

DRUG GUIDE 26.1

COMMON DRUGS FOR ENDOCRINE DISORDERS

Medication	Actions/Indications	Nursing Implications
Insulin	Used for diabetes mellitus (DM) to replace body's natural insulin, which is necessary for proper glucose use. Indicated for DM type 1 and, sometimes, DM type 2	• Monitor vital signs and blood glucose levels. • Educate the child and the family on proper techniques, actions, and adverse effects. • Rotate site of injections to prevent adipose hypertrophy.
Oral hypoglycemic drugs (glipizide, glyburide, metformin)	Assist the body's production of insulin by stimulating β cells to secrete more insulin. Indicated for type 2 DM	• Monitor vital signs and glucose levels. • Administer with food to minimize gastric upset. • Instruct the child and the family on the use of drug and its adverse effects. • Warn family that some over-the-counter or other drugs may increase hypoglycemic effect.
Growth hormone (GH)/somatropin	Stimulates linear bone, skeletal muscle, and organ growth Used for GH deficiency, growth failure related to inadequate pituitary hormone	• Monitor blood glucose and electrolyte levels. • Administer before epiphyses are fused. • Monitor growth with accurate measurements. • Instruct the child and the family on appropriate route and method of administration. • Periodic thyroid function tests will be needed. • May interact with glucocorticoid therapy • Monitor for limping or complaints in knee or hip related to slipped epiphysis.
Octreotide acetate	Suppresses GH release. Indicated for acromegaly	• Monitor for biliary tract abnormalities, glucose tolerance, and hypothyroidism. • Give subcutaneous injections between meals to decrease gastric effects (may alter absorption of fats). • May switch to intramuscular (IM) depot injection every 1–3 months once stabilized
Corticosteroids (dexamethasone or hydrocortisone)	Cortisol replacement in congenital adrenal hyperplasia, absence of adrenal glands. Also used to close epiphyseal plates in hyperpituitarism	• Give with milk or food. • May need to increase dose if the child is ill or runs fever • Monitor for edema, weight gain, glycosuria, signs of infection, and symptoms of peptic ulcer development. • Do not decrease dose or abruptly stop drug to avoid adrenal crisis.
Desmopressin acetate (DDAVP)	Synthetic antidiuretic hormone that promotes reabsorption of water by action on renal tubules Used to control arginine vasopressin deficiency (AVP-D)	• Monitor for water intoxication, signs and symptoms of hyponatremia, and adverse effects such as nasal irritation, headache, nausea, and increased blood pressure. • Record fluid intake and output and weigh the child daily. • Titrate dose until appropriate fluid output is obtained. • Instruct the child and the family on proper intranasal administration. • May need to be stored in refrigerator
Levothyroxine	Thyroid hormone replacement for hypothyroidism	• Monitor blood pressure and pulse. • Monitor fluid intake and output, daily weights, and thyroid function tests. • Watch for thyroid storm. • Report irritability or anxiety. • Instruct the child and the family to avoid over-the-counter preparations with iodine or foods such as soybeans, iodized salt, tofu, and turnips. If the infant must be on soy formula, administer it between feedings. • Do not administer within 4 hours of antacids (such as simethicone) and iron or calcium supplements. • Administer at same time each day.
Methimazole	Antithyroid drug; blocks synthesis of T_3 and T_4 Indicated for hyperthyroidism	• Monitor pulse and blood pressure. • Monitor input and output, daily weights, serum T_3 and T_4 levels; watch for edema, leukopenia, thrombocytopenia, or agranulocytosis. • Signs of overdose: periorbital edema, cold intolerance, mental depression • Signs of inadequate dose: tachycardia, diarrhea, fever, or irritability
Mineralocorticoid	Promotes reabsorption of Na and K, water from distal renal tubules Used in adrenal insufficiency	• Monitor daily weights, blood pressure, and intake and output. • Observe for potassium depletion. • Titrate dose to lowest effective dose. • Monitor for signs of infection. • Monitor for signs of edema.

T3, triiodothyronine; T4, thyroxine

Source: Lexicomp. (2023). Pediatric drug information. *UpToDate*. Retrieved May 20, 2023, from https://www.uptodate.com/contents/table-of-contents/drug-information

drugs to mimic the actual hormone levels in the body. Nurses must monitor for side effects of both too little and too much of the hormone in the child's system. Most endocrine disorders in children require treatment and follow-up with a pediatric endocrinologist, as well as a multidisciplinary team that includes a registered nurse who specializes in this area.

Clinical Judgment and the Nursing Process for the Child With an Endocrine Disorder

The nursing care of the child with an endocrine disorder requires astute assessment skills, accurate nursing analysis and expected outcomes, skilled interventions, and evaluation of the entire process. Children, especially very young ones, easily develop imbalances such as fluid and electrolyte disturbances that can cause further problems. Most of the endocrine disorders are chronic conditions that require ongoing care related to health maintenance, education, developmental issues, and psychosocial needs. These conditions are sometimes complex and range from mild to profound. Early diagnosis and treatment can improve the long-term outcomes for these children.

Assessment

Nursing assessment of a child with endocrine dysfunction includes obtaining a thorough health history, performing a physical assessment, and assisting with or obtaining laboratory and diagnostic tests. The clinical manifestations of endocrine disorders occur as a result of the altered control of the bodily processes normally regulated by the gland or hormone. These manifestations present in many areas of the body because of the diverse functions associated with the endocrine system.

Health History

The health history should include questions regarding any family history of an endocrine disorder or growth and development difficulties. Use a genogram or family tree to detail the information about the family history in a clear and concise manner.

Discuss prenatal history, including any maternal factors that may affect growth and development, such as substance misuse, use of tobacco or alcohol, and Graves disease; address birth history, including trauma during delivery, birth size, feeding difficulties, and neonatal screening and results. Additionally, consider past medical history, such as any chronic childhood diseases, treatment for endocrine problems, recent gastroenteritis or viral syndromes, or exposures to exogenous steroids or gonadotropins. Finally, evaluate growth and development patterns, including the presence of any delays, learning disabilities, and early or late development of secondary sexual characteristics.

Discuss present complaints or illness. Note the onset of symptoms, whether gradual or sudden. Endocrine disorders often cause problems in normal growth and development, as well as behavioral changes. Question the parent or caregiver about prior growth patterns, achievement of developmental milestones, and the child's behavior. Inquire about recent increases or decreases in weight and height, changes in physical appearance, sleep patterns, muscle weakness, cramps, twitching, or headaches. Have the child and family describe the child's activities on a typical day, including school performance, to identify subtle variations in the child's behavior or moods. For example, a child who is typically quiet might ordinarily be less active than average children of that age, and a child with decreased endocrine function often displays inactivity and fatigue. By having the family and child describe a typical day, the nurse can distinguish between what is appropriate for that child and what may be a change related to endocrine dysfunction.

In addition, obtain a history of dietary and elimination habits. Note any extreme thirst, excessive appetite, vomiting, or frequent voiding. Children with endocrine disorders may exhibit some of these symptoms.

Physical Examination

Physical examination of the child with an endocrine disorder includes inspection and observation, auscultation, percussion, and palpation. Table 26.1 lists key physical examination findings that may be present in children with endocrine dysfunction.

INSPECTION AND OBSERVATION

Note a fatigued appearance, poor muscle tone, sweatiness, faintness, nervousness, or confusion. Inspect the head and face, and note hair texture and growth, a protuberant tongue, drooping eyelids, or **exophthalmos** (protrusion of the eyeballs). Plot the child's height and weight on growth charts to determine abnormal growth velocity, which occurs in many of these disorders.

AUSCULTATION

Auscultate the heart and lungs. Note heart rate and rhythm. During auscultation of the lungs, note labored respiratory effort, such as Kussmaul breathing, which occurs in diabetic ketoacidosis (DKA). Document blood pressure.

PERCUSSION AND PALPATION

Percuss and then palpate the abdomen. Dull (nontympanic) sounds or the presence of masses may indicate constipation or a tumor of the ovaries.

Laboratory and Diagnostic Testing

Common Laboratory and Diagnostic Tests 26.1 describes the diagnostic tests and procedures frequently used in identifying and monitoring endocrine disorders in

TABLE 26.1 • Key Physical Examination Findings Related to Endocrine Problems

Height and weight	Below third percentile or above 90th percentile (pituitary, thyroid, adrenal, or diabetes mellitus)
Hair	Coarse, brittle, excessive (hypothyroidism) Abnormal distribution (adrenal disorders)
Face	Round with hair growth (Cushing syndrome) Deformities or abnormal features (hypoparathyroidism)
Eyes	Blurred or changes in vision (diabetes mellitus, pituitary tumors, precocious puberty)
Mouth	Delayed dentition (hypocalcemia, hypopituitarism) Fruity breath (ketoacidosis)
Neck	Goiter (hyperthyroidism)
Skin	Cool to touch, dry (hypothyroidism) Changes in color or texture (pituitary disorders) Easy bruising, striae (Cushing syndrome)
Chest	Tachycardia (hyperthyroidism) Palpitations, sweating (thyroid disorders) Deep, labored breathing (ketoacidosis) Hypertension (Cushing syndrome)
Abdomen	Extreme weight loss (diabetes mellitus) Extreme fat (Cushing syndrome) Changes in bowel habits (SIADH, AVP-D, diabetes mellitus)
Fingers	Trembling (hyperthyroidism, parathyroid disorders)
Genitals	Excessive growth (adrenogenital syndrome) Early growth (precocious puberty) Delayed growth (hypopituitarism)

AVP-D, arginine vasopressin deficiency; SIADH, syndrome of inappropriate antidiuretic hormone.

COMMON LABORATORY AND DIAGNOSTIC TESTS 26.1

Diagnostic Test or Procedure	Explanation	Indications	Nursing Implications
Newborn metabolic screening programs (refer to Chapter 9 for further information)	Newborn blood testing to identify certain harmful or potentially fatal disorders that are otherwise not apparent at birth. Disorders tested vary by state.	Identify newborns so that treatment can begin early to prevent impact of disorder, such as severe cognitive impairment or death.	• Refer to each state's protocol for fetal or newborn screening for endocrine disorders. • Explain to the family the rationale and procedure. • Collect blood sample accurately. • Collect prior to blood transfusion if possible. • Ensure screening is done for early discharges. • Screening typically between 24 and 48 hours after birth • If collected before 24 hours of age, a repeat test is needed within 14 days. Some states now require a repeat screen at 2 weeks of age.[a]
Random serum hormone levels	Serum levels of various hormones; immunoassay measures levels with very small amounts of blood	High or low levels are used to evaluate the function of specific gland.	• May need to draw specimens at specific times • Keep the child NPO after midnight before test if ordered. • Diurnal variations and episodic secretion of many hormones may require special directions or further testing.
Self-monitoring blood glucose (SMBG)	Fingerstick (monitors that utilize alternative sites, such as the forearm, are available); blood sample several times per day Noninvasive methods available[b]	Monitor glucose level and effectiveness of treatment.	• Teach the family appropriate procedure. • Refer the family to sources for equipment and supplies. • Assist the family with developing a system of record-keeping that works for them. • Refer to Teaching Guidelines 26.2.

COMMON LABORATORY AND DIAGNOSTIC TESTS 26.1

Diagnostic Test or Procedure	Explanation	Indications	Nursing Implications
Fasting plasma glucose	Fasting forces the body to produce glucagon, which causes the release of glucose. In a healthy child, the body will respond by releasing insulin, therefore lowering blood glucose and preventing hyperglycemia.	Detect hyperglycemia related to diabetes or other conditions, such as Cushing syndrome or liver or kidney disease. Can detect prediabetes	• The child should not have had any caloric intake for at least 8 hours. • Draw sample prior to insulin or oral diabetes medications. • Normal value in children 2–18 years of age, 60–100 mg/dL; in children 0–2 years of age, 60–110 mg/dL; impaired fasting glucose or prediabetes is between 100 and 125 mg/dL; diabetes is considered with a result ≥126 mg/dL on two separate occasions.
Two-hour plasma glucose test (2-h PG)	Oral glucose tolerance test Oral glucose is ingested and in a healthy child, insulin will respond and return blood glucose to normal levels.	Usually performed to detect diabetes, often gestational diabetes Can also detect prediabetes	• The child should not have taken any insulin or oral diabetes medication before the test. • Time of oral glucose ingestion needs to be noted. • Specimen to be drawn at specified time interval from ingestion • May have limited value in diagnosing children
Urine or serum ketone testing	Ketones are the result of the metabolism of fat and in a healthy child are present in insignificant amounts.	Screening for ketones in urine is regularly performed in children, people with diabetes, hospitalized patients, preoperatively, and in pregnant people. In children, ketones found in urine during routine urinalysis can detect undiagnosed diabetes. In children with diabetes, the presence of ketones in serum or urine is a sign that their diabetes is not well controlled and can be an early sign of diabetic ketoacidosis (DKA).	• Urine ketone testing can be performed using dipsticks at the bedside and at home (follow manufacturer's directions; time reaction accurately and compare the strip to the control chart on the bottle). • Encourage testing for ketones when blood glucose is elevated, when therapy regimen is changing, or during times of stress or illness.
Hemoglobin A1C (glycated hemoglobin)	Glycated hemoglobin reflects the percentage of hemoglobin to which glucose is attached. In the case of hyperglycemia, an increase in glycohemoglobin leads to an increase in hemoglobin A1C. This test shows the average blood glucose level for the past 2–3 months.	Diagnose diabetes. Indicated for children with diabetes. Provides information regarding long-term glycemic control and effectiveness of therapy.	• Elevated levels seen in newly diagnosed diabetes or poorly controlled diabetes. • Levels can be elevated in children without diabetes with certain conditions such as blood loss, hemolysis, iron-deficiency anemia, sickle cell anemia, and lead toxicity.
Genetic testing	Tests for the presence of the gene for disease or carrier status	Determine genetic involvement of any disorder.	• Explain the procedure and the expense involved. • Refer for genetic counseling if needed.
Serum chemistry levels	Serum blood urea nitrogen (BUN), creatinine, sodium, potassium, glucose, calcium, phosphorus, alkaline phosphatase, etc.	Rule out chronic kidney disease or other chronic illnesses; monitor effects of treatment.	• BUN levels may be elevated with high-protein diet or dehydration and may be decreased with overhydration or malnutrition. • A diet high in meat may cause a transient but not pronounced increase in creatinine. There are also slight diurnal variations in levels. • Avoid hemolysis of specimen, as this may cause elevation in potassium levels. • Calcium and phosphorus: avoid prolonged tourniquet use during blood draw, as this may falsely increase levels. The child should be NPO past midnight prior to the morning of the blood draw.

(*continued*)

COMMON LABORATORY AND DIAGNOSTIC TESTS 26.1 (*continued*)

Diagnostic Test or Procedure	Explanation	Indications	Nursing Implications
Growth hormone (GH) stimulation	Stimulate release of GH in response to administration of insulin, arginine, clonidine, or glucagon.	Evaluate and diagnose GH deficiency.	• Keep the child NPO for specified time. • Limit stress and physical activity at least 30 minutes before test. • Obtain serial blood samples at specific times. • Monitor blood glucose levels during study. • Observe for signs of hypoglycemia, diaphoresis, and somnolence. • Provide a snack, such as cookies and juice at end of test.
Water deprivation study	The child is deprived of fluids for several hours, and serum sodium and urine osmolality are monitored.	Diagnose AVP-D or AVP-R (previously known as diabetes insipidus [DI]) and distinguish between AVP-D and AVP-R (previously known as central or nephrogenic DI).	• Stop the test if the child exhibits extreme weight loss or changes in vital signs or neurologic status. • Weigh child before, during, and after test. • Rehydrate the child after test. • Monitor for orthostatic hypotension.
Bone age radiograph	Radiographic study of wrist or hand to determine bone maturation compared to national standards	Determine if bone age is consistent with chronologic age to rule out GH deficiency or excess or hypothyroidism.	• Explain the procedure to the child because they need to hold still for the radiograph. • Allow the family to accompany the child. • Enlist the family's help if needed to calm the child during radiography.
Other nuclear medicine studies	Contrast media uptake is assessed with serial radiographs.	Visualize an ectopic, enlarged, absent, or nodular gland.	• Assess the child for allergy to iodine or shellfish. • Explain the procedure to the child.
CT	Noninvasive x-ray study that looks at tissue density and structures. Images a "slice" of tissue	Evaluate the presence of tumors, cysts, or structural abnormalities that may affect specific gland or structure.	• Machine is large and can be frightening to children. • Scan may be lengthy and the child must remain still, so sedation may be necessary. • If contrast medium is to be used, assess for allergy. • Encourage fluids after procedure if not contraindicated.
MRI	Based on how hydrogen atoms behave in a magnetic field when disturbed by radiofrequency signals. Does not require ionizing radiation. Provides a 3D view of the body part being scanned	Evaluate the presence of tumors, cysts, or structural abnormalities that may affect specific gland or structure.	• Remove all metal objects from the child. • The child must remain motionless for entire scan; the parent can stay in room with the child. Younger children will require sedation in order to be still. • A loud thumping sound occurs inside the machine during the procedure, which can be frightening to children.
Ultrasonography	Noninvasive sound waves are used to visualize structures, such as thyroid or pelvic region.	Evaluate the presence of tumors or cysts in a specific gland, such as the adrenal glands or ovaries, to rule out disorders.	• Requires full bladder if in pelvic region. • It is better tolerated by nonsedated children than CT or MRI. • Can be performed with a portable unit at bedside.

AVP-D, arginine vasopressin deficiency; AVP-R, arginine vasopressin resistance; CT, computed tomography; MRI, magnetic resonance imaging; NPO, nothing by mouth.

[a]Kemper, A. R. (2021). Newborn screening. *UpToDate*. Retrieved May 20, 2023 from https://www.uptodate.com/contents/newborn-screening

Data from Fischbach, F. T., Fischbach, M. A., & Stout, K. (2022). *A manual of laboratory and diagnostic tests* (11th ed.). Wolters Kluwer.

children. Serum and urine hormone and other levels are used to determine whether amounts are adequate, deficient, or excessive. Radiographic studies are used to evaluate bone maturation, growth potential, and density or tissue calcification. Genetic studies may be used to determine enzyme deficiencies or chromosome defects. Stimulation studies provide a more accurate or definitive test for identifying the disorder after preliminary serum levels are abnormal. Serial blood sampling identifies peak or trough levels of hormones. Computed tomography (CT) scans, magnetic resonance imaging (MRI), nuclear medicine studies, and ultrasonography are used to look for tumors, cysts, or structural defects. These tests can assist the health care provider or nurse practitioner in diagnosing disorders and guiding ongoing treatment. Laboratory or nonnursing personnel perform some of the tests, while the nurse might perform others. In either instance, the nurse should be familiar with how the tests are performed, what they are used for, and normal versus abnormal results. This knowledge will also be necessary when providing children and family education related to the testing.

Remember Carlos, the 12-year-old, with weakness, fatigue, blurred vision, headaches, and mood changes? What additional health history and physical examination assessment information should the nurse obtain?

Nursing Analysis

After recognizing and analyzing cues from a thorough assessment, the nurse might identify several patient problems, including the following:

- Malnutrition risk
- Dehydration or fluid overload risk
- Delayed development risk
- Altered body image perception
- Knowledge deficiency
- Altered health maintenance
- Interrupted family processes
- Risk for caregiver role strain

After completing an assessment of Carlos, the nurse noted the following: history reveals Carlos has had episodes of bedwetting over the past month and has polydipsia and polyphagia. His weight continues to be above the 95th percentile on the growth chart. Based on these assessment findings, what would be your top three patient problems for Carlos?

The previously listed patient problems or concerns provide suggestions for developing a nursing plan of care or concept mapping. The nurse will then generate solutions by planning interventions (suggested with rationales further on). The plan of care should be individualized, based on the child's and family's needs.

Refer to Chapter 11 for nursing interventions related to interrupted family processes and risk for caregiver role strain. Additional information will be included later in the chapter as it relates to specific disorders. Because of the gradual, insidious onset of many of these disorders, the child may first be seen in an acute situation. It may be easier for the child and family to work with short-term goals until they accept the chronic situation. A major goal will be to achieve adherence to medical management. The goals for the child with a disorder of the endocrine system generally include reestablishing homeostasis, promoting adequate growth and development, establishing appropriate body image, promoting health-seeking behaviors, and providing education so the family can manage the condition.

A key element to include in any plan of care or concept map for a child with an endocrine disorder involves preparing the child, based on their developmental needs, for invasive procedures and tests. Provide an opportunity for the family and child to express their concerns and fears during diagnosis and treatment. Reinforce realistic expectations for treatment and prospects for improvement with the family and child. The plan of care or concept map also needs to address developmental, acute, chronic, and home care issues, as well as child and family education. Families will need assistance with managing the condition from a multidisciplinary team.

Nursing Analysis

Malnutrition risk related to biologic factors, as evidenced by growth parameters less than expected for age

Goal/Outcome

The child's nutritional status is balanced. The child adheres to nutritional guidelines and demonstrates adequate growth (weight and height) patterns within the normal range for age and sex, or shows a progressive increase over time if has growth difficulties.

Maintaining Adequate Nutrition (interventions with *rationale*)

- Determine the body weight and length/height norm for age or what the child's pretreatment measurements were *to determine goal to work toward.*
- Weigh daily or weekly (according to health care provider's order or institutional standard) and measure length/height weekly *to monitor for appropriate growth.*
- Determine the child's food preferences and provide favorite foods when possible *to increase the likelihood of the child consuming appropriate amounts of foods.*

- Instruct the child and family about nutritional requirements *so that they are involved and are prepared for home care.*
- Refer to a dietitian *for more detailed information and assistance.*
- Offer the highest-calorie meals at the time of day when the child's appetite is greatest *to increase the likelihood of increased caloric intake.*
- Provide increased-calorie shakes or puddings within dietary restrictions, *as high-calorie foods increase weight gain.*
- Administer vitamin and mineral supplements as prescribed *to attain/maintain vitamin and mineral balance in the body.*

Nursing Analysis

Dehydration or fluid overload risk related to compromised regulatory function (pathophysiology of endocrine dysfunction), as evidenced by signs and symptoms of dehydration or edema and excessive urine output (fluid overload)

Goal/Outcome

The child will maintain adequate fluid volume, as evidenced by elastic skin turgor, absence of edema, moist and pink oral mucosa, presence of tears, urine output of 1 mL/kg/h or more, vital signs within the normal range for age, and normal electrolyte/hormone serum levels.

Maintaining Adequate Fluid Volume (interventions with *rationale*)

- Assess hydration status (skin turgor, oral mucosa, presence of tears) every 4 to 8 hours *to evaluate the maintenance of adequate fluid volume.*
- Assess the adequacy of urine output *to evaluate end-organ perfusion.*
- Maintain a strict intake and output record *to evaluate the effectiveness of rehydration.*
- Weigh the child daily: *accurate weight is one of the best indicators of fluid volume status in children.*
- Administer specific hormone, fluid, and electrolyte requirements as ordered *to aid in fluid balance.*
- For fluid volume deficit: Maintain the intravenous (IV) line and administer IV fluid as ordered *to maintain fluid volume.*
- For fluid volume excess: Maintain fluid restriction as ordered *to restore homeostasis.*

Nursing Analysis

Delayed development risk (risk factors include chronic illness [endocrine disorder], treatment regimen, and inadequate nutrition)

Goal/Outcome

The child's development will be enhanced. The child will not suffer regression in abilities and will make continued progress toward the attainment of developmental milestones within age parameters and limits of disease. Also, the child expresses interest in the environment and people around them and interacts with the environment appropriately for their developmental level.

Promoting Development (interventions with *rationale*)

- Encourage adherence to hormone supplementation to enhance the ability *to achieve appropriate growth and development.*
- Screen for developmental capabilities *to determine the child's current level of functioning.*
- Offer age-appropriate toys, play, and activities (including gross motor) *to encourage further development.*
- Provide support to families; *due to disability and deficits, the child's progress toward developmental milestones may be slow.*
- Use therapeutic play and adaptive toys *to facilitate developmental functioning.*
- Provide a stimulating environment whenever possible *to maximize the potential for growth and development.*
- Praise accomplishments and emphasize the child's abilities *to improve self-esteem and encourage feeling of confidence and competence.*

Nursing Analysis

Altered body image perception related to an alteration in self-perception (abnormal growth and development or changes in physical appearance due to hormone dysfunction), as evidenced by verbalization of dissatisfaction with the child's or adolescent's looks

Goal/Outcome

The child demonstrates appropriate self-esteem in relation to body image by expressing positive feelings about themselves and participating in social activities.

Promoting Healthy Body Image (interventions with *rationale*)

- Provide opportunities for the child to explore feelings related to appearance; *venting feelings is associated with less body image disturbance.*
- Relate to child on their age level, not appearance level; *"babying" a child who looks younger due to their small size may reduce their self-image.*
- Involve the child, especially the adolescent, in the decision-making process; *a sense of control will improve body image.*
- Encourage the child to spend time with peers who have similar endocrine disorders; *peers' opinions are often better accepted than those of people in authority, such as parents or health care professionals.*
- Refer the child to counseling or support groups *to further support them.*

Nursing Analysis

Knowledge deficiency related to insufficient information (regarding therapeutic regimen), as evidenced by questions about the endocrine disorder and self-management

Goal/Outcome

The child and family will demonstrate sufficient understanding and skills for self-management: verbalize information about disorder, complications/adverse effects, home care regimen, and long-term needs, and provide return demonstrations of medication administration or other procedures.

Promoting Knowledge Required for Self-Management (interventions with *rationale*)

- Assess the child's developmental level and the family's ability to absorb instruction, as well as their willingness to learn, *to determine how to approach teaching sessions; the child and family must be willing to learn for teaching to be effective.*
- Provide the family with time to adjust to the diagnosis *to facilitate their adjustment and ability to learn and participate in the child's care.*
- Establish a teaching plan with the child and family *to gain their cooperation and involvement.*
- Use multiple modes of learning involving many senses (provide written, verbal, demonstration, and videos) when possible; *the child and family are more likely to retain information when it is presented in different ways using multiple senses.*
- Teach and provide printed instructions on disorder, complications, home care, and follow-up requirements *so the family has a reference to use at home.*
- Repeat information *to allow the family and child time to learn and understand.*
- Teach in short sessions: *many short sessions are more helpful than one long session.*
- Gear teaching to the level of understanding of the child and family (depends on age of child, physical condition, memory) *to ensure understanding.*
- Provide reinforcement and rewards *to facilitate the teaching and learning process.*
- Evaluate teaching through return demonstrations *to determine whether the child/family is skilled enough for home management of the disorder.*

For children with diabetes mellitus (DM), include the following:

- First teach "survival skills" (e.g., glucose and urine testing, administering insulin, record-keeping, food guidelines, when to call health care provider) *to provide an initial base of knowledge for self-management.*
- Implement a second-phase home management program with more extensive instruction; *providing additional teaching over time is necessary for managing a significant chronic illness.*
- Monitor the outcomes of teaching with every contact *to ensure progress with child and family education.*

Nursing Analysis

Altered health maintenance related to difficulty managing a complex treatment regimen or insufficient knowledge of the therapeutic regimen, as evidenced by difficulty with the prescribed regimen or failure to include the treatment regimen in daily living

Goal/Outcome

The child and family will adhere to the treatment regimen. They will list treatment expectations, agree to follow through, and keep appointments with providers.

Encouraging Adherence (interventions with *rationale*)

- Listen nonjudgmentally while the child and family describe reasons for nonadherence; *assessment of the problem should begin with a nonthreatening discussion.*
- Help the child and family develop a schedule for medication administration and other home regimens that works best for them; *involving the child and family in planning care will increase adherence by making them feel respected and valued.*
- Work with the child and family to develop a written treatment plan or schedule that best suits their needs *to provide support for the maintenance of the treatment plan.*
- Establish follow-up visits to fit the family's situation *to promote adherence.*
- Encourage monitoring with a pediatric endocrinologist and specialists; *multidisciplinary involvement has been shown to increase adherence.*
- Recognize that behavioral change comes slowly; *allow time for the child and family to adjust to chronic nature of the illness.*

Based on your top three patient problems for Carlos, describe appropriate nursing interventions.

PITUITARY DISORDERS

Because of the close anatomic and functional relationships between the hypothalamus and pituitary gland, we will discuss them together. The hypothalamus affects the pituitary by releasing and inhibiting hormones and may be the cause of pituitary disorders. In general, disorders of the pituitary fall into two major groups: anterior pituitary hormones and posterior pituitary hormones. Anterior pituitary primary disorders in children include growth hormone (GH) deficiency, hyperpituitarism, and precocious puberty. Posterior pituitary disorders include arginine vasopressin deficiency (AVP-D; previously known as diabetes insipidus [DI]) and syndrome of inappropriate antidiuretic hormone (SIADH) secretion.

CLINICAL REASONING ALERT!

Infants with congenital defects of the pituitary gland or hypothalamus may present with symptoms that include apnea, cyanosis, severe hypoglycemia with possible seizures, and prolonged jaundice and should be treated as an emergency (Patterson & Felner, 2020).

GH Deficiency

GH deficiency, also known as hypopituitarism or dwarfism, is characterized by poor growth and short stature. GH is vital for postnatal growth. It is released throughout the day, with most secreted during sleep. GH stimulates linear growth, bone mineral density, and growth in all body tissues.

GH deficiency occurs in approximately one in 4,000 to one in 10,000 children (Patterson & Felner, 2020). Often, this condition is first identified when the health care provider or nurse practitioner assesses growth patterns. Children may start with a normal birth weight and length, but within a few years, their growth falls below the third percentile on the growth chart.

Possible complications related to GH deficiency and its treatment include altered carbohydrate, protein, and fat metabolism; hypoglycemia; glucose intolerance or diabetes; slipped capital femoral epiphysis; pseudotumor cerebri; leukemia; recurrence of central nervous system (CNS) tumors; infection at the injection site; edema; and sodium retention.

Pathophysiology

GH deficiency generally results from the failure of the anterior pituitary or hypothalamic stimulation on the pituitary to produce sufficient GH. This lack of GH impairs the body's ability to metabolize protein, fat, and carbohydrates.

Primary causes of GH deficiency include injury to or destruction of the anterior pituitary gland or hypothalamus. Causes include a tumor (e.g., craniopharyngioma), infection, infarction, CNS irradiation, abnormal formation of these organs in utero, or damage or trauma during birth or afterward. It may also be part of a genetic syndrome, such as Prader–Willi syndrome or Turner syndrome, or the result of a genetic mutation or deletion.

In some cases, the cause of GH deficiency may be idiopathic, such as nutritional deprivation or psychosocial issues, and reversible. Psychosocial dwarfism results from emotional deprivation, which suppresses the production of pituitary hormones, resulting in decreased GH levels. Children with psychosocial dwarfism may exhibit withdrawal, bizarre eating and drinking habits, such as drinking from toilets, and primitive speech. Treatment involves removing the child from the dysfunctional environment and providing normal dietary intake. With normalized eating and behavioral habits, pituitary secretion is restored, and the child experiences dramatic catch-up growth.

Therapeutic Management

Treatment of primary GH deficiency involves the use of supplemental GH and should be started as soon as possible. (See Dosage Calculation Box 26.1.) Secondary GH deficiency requires removal of any tumors that might be the underlying problem, followed by GH therapy. Biosynthetic GH, derived from recombinant DNA, is given by subcutaneous injection. Treatment continues until near-final height is achieved. This can be determined by the child deciding they are tall enough, a growth rate of less than 0.8 to 1 in/year, or bone age greater than 16 years in males and greater than 14 years in females (Patterson & Felner, 2020; Rogol & Richmond Padilla, 2023).

DOSAGE CALCULATION BOX **26.1**

Child's weight: 30 lb

Medication order: Somatropin 0.5 mg subcutaneously once a day

Per the *Pediatric Dosage Handbook*, the recommended dose is 0.18–0.3 mg/kg weekly, divided into 6–7 doses.

Is the ordered dose safe?

Nursing Assessment

The focus of the evaluation for GH deficiency is to rule out chronic illnesses such as kidney disease, liver disorders, and thyroid dysfunction. For a full description of the assessment phase of the nursing process, refer to the "Clinical Judgment and the Nursing Process" section earlier in the chapter. Assessment findings pertinent to GH deficiency are discussed further on.

HEALTH HISTORY

The health history may reveal a familial pattern of short stature or a prenatal history of maternal disorders such as malnutrition. The past history may be significant for birth history of intrauterine growth restriction or past history of severe head trauma or a brain tumor such as craniopharyngioma. Evaluate previous and current growth patterns. Note history of chronic illnesses such as cardiac, kidney, or intestinal disorders that may contribute to a decreased growth pattern. Also, assess the child's feelings about their height.

PHYSICAL EXAMINATION

In addition to linear height being at or below the third percentile on standard growth charts, physical assessment findings may show that the child has a higher weight-to-height ratio (Fig. 26.2). Other physical findings may include prominent subcutaneous deposits of abdominal fat; a child-like face with a large, prominent forehead; a high-pitched voice; delayed sexual maturation (e.g., micropenis and undescended testes in males); delayed dentition; delayed skeletal maturation; and decreased muscle mass.

TAKE NOTE!

Growth measurements are often inaccurate and unreliable in children. An important anthropometric measurement is body height, and improved accuracy could yield earlier detection and diagnosis of growth disorders (Warrier et al., 2022). According to the Centers for Disease Control and Prevention (CDC), the stadiometer is the preferred tool for assessing height in children >3 years of age (Warrier et al., 2022) (see Fig. 26.2). To improve and ensure accuracy, the CDC has implemented standardized procedures for measuring body height.

LABORATORY AND DIAGNOSTIC TESTING

The child will undergo laboratory tests to rule out chronic illnesses such as kidney disease, liver dysfunction, and thyroid dysfunction. Laboratory and diagnostic tests used in children with suspected GH deficiency include the following:

- Bone age (as shown by radiographs) will be two or more deviations below normal.
- CT or MRI scans are used to rule out tumors or structural abnormalities.
- Pituitary function testing confirms the diagnosis. This test consists of providing a GH stimulant such as glucagon, clonidine, insulin, arginine, or L-dopa to stimulate the pituitary to release a burst of GH. Peak GH levels below 7 to 10 mcg/mL in at least two tests confirm the diagnosis.

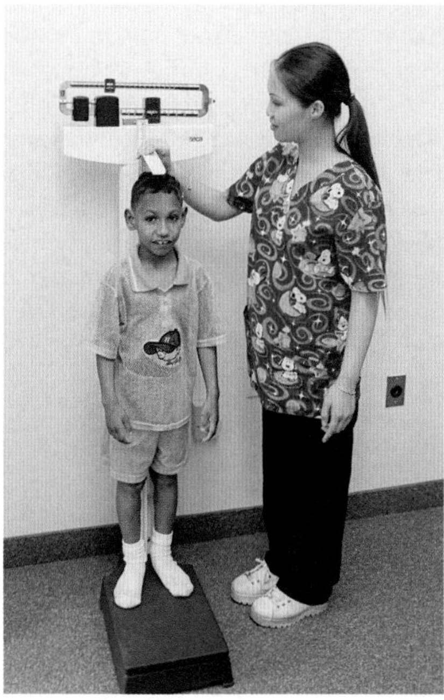

FIGURE 26.2 The child with growth hormone deficiency displays short stature.

Nursing Management

Nursing management for the child with GH deficiency focuses on promoting growth, enhancing the child's self-esteem related to short stature, and providing appropriate education about the disorder.

PROMOTING GROWTH

The goal of growth promotion is for the child to demonstrate an improved growth rate, as evidenced by at least 3 to 5 inches in linear growth in the first year of treatment without complications. With early diagnosis and treatment, the child has a better prognosis for reaching a normal adult height. Growth is usually excellent in the first year of therapy compared to later years (Patterson & Felner, 2020). Treatment stops when the epiphyseal growth plates fuse.

At the beginning of treatment, monitor for height increase and possible side effects related to the medications. Measure the child's height at least every 3 to 6 months and plot growth over time on standardized growth charts. Provide information to the child and family about normal development and growth rates, bone age, and growth potential. Discuss with the family and child their expectations and understanding of what is normal, so they will have realistic expectations of treatment. Consult a dietitian if the child and family need assistance in providing adequate nutrition for growth and development.

ENHANCING THE CHILD'S SELF-ESTEEM

The child with GH deficiency often exhibits younger-looking features and is shorter than their peers. Encourage the child to express positive feelings about their self-image, as shown by comments during health care visits and involvement with peers. Encourage the child to voice any concerns they have. Emphasize the child's strengths and assets. Provide information about community support groups or websites related to GH deficiency. Evaluate for long-term learning problems that may develop if the child had a tumor and underwent surgery or irradiation to remove it. Unidentified learning problems can have a negative impact on the child's self-esteem. Treat and communicate with the child in an age-appropriate manner, even though they may appear younger.

EDUCATING THE FAMILY

GH is available as a powder that is mixed with packaged diluents. Most are available in multidose pen delivery systems, with some systems not requiring reconstitution (Rogol & Richmond Padilla, 2023). Explain how to prepare the medication and give the correct dosage. Encourage rotation of injection sites in the subcutaneous tissue to prevent skin irritation. Have the family provide a return demonstration to make sure they understand the correct dilution and administration of GH. Continue to provide periodic evaluation and ongoing support.

Instruct the family to report any headaches, rapid weight gain, increased thirst or urination, or painful hip or knee joints as possible adverse reactions. Explain to the family that the child will need to visit the pediatric endocrinologist every 3 to 6 months to monitor growth, potential adverse effects, and adherence to therapy. Stress the importance of complying with GH replacement therapy and frequent supervision by a pediatric endocrinologist. Emphasize that the success of the treatment is dependent on adherence to the regimen prescribed. Educate the family about the financial costs of therapy, which may be high, and assist them in obtaining assistance through referral to social services if needed.

Guide the family and child in setting realistic goals and expectations based on age, personal abilities, strengths, and the effectiveness of GH replacement therapy. For example, encourage the family to consider sports that are not dependent on height and to dress the child according to age, not size. Refer the child and family to counseling if indicated. Also, inform families about support groups such as the Human Growth Foundation and the Magic Foundation.

Precocious Puberty

In precocious puberty, the child develops sexual characteristics before the usual age of pubertal onset. Puberty, also known as sexual maturation, occurs when the gonads produce increased amounts of sex hormones. Typically, this occurs around 10 to 12 years of age for females and 11 to 14 years of age for males. In precocious puberty, secondary sex characteristics develop in females before the age of 8 years and in males younger than 9 years (Harrington & Palmert, 2022). The disorder is more common in females, and the majority of the time the cause is unknown in females, while in males, a structural CNS abnormality is often present (Garibaldi & Chemaitilly, 2020). Other causes include benign hypothalamic tumor, brain injury or radiation, a history of infectious encephalitis or meningitis, congenital adrenal hyperplasia (CAH), and tumors of the ovary, adrenal gland, pituitary gland, or testes.

Pathophysiology

Central precocious puberty, the most common form, develops as a result of premature activation of the hypothalamic–pituitary–gonadal axis that results in the production of gonadotropin-releasing hormone (GnRH), which stimulates the pituitary to produce luteinizing hormone (LH) and follicle-stimulating hormone (FSH). These hormones, in turn, stimulate the gonads to secrete the sex hormones (estrogen or testosterone). The child develops sexual characteristics, shows increased growth and skeletal maturation, and has reproductive capability. Peripheral precocious puberty presents with no early secretion of gonadotropin or maturation of gonads but rather early overproduction of sex hormones. The condition results in increased end-organ sensitivity to low levels of circulating sex hormones and leads to premature pubic hair and breast development.

If left untreated, the child may reach fertility. In addition, the hormones stimulate rapid growth. Therefore, the child may appear taller than peers but will reach skeletal maturity and closure of the epiphyseal plates early, which will result in overall short stature.

Therapeutic Management

The clinical treatment for precocious puberty first involves determining the cause. For example, if the etiology is a tumor of the CNS, the child undergoes surgery, radiation, or chemotherapy. The treatment for central precocious puberty involves administering a GnRH analog. This is available as a subcutaneous injection given daily, an intranasal compound administered two or three times daily, a depot injection given every 3 to 4 weeks, a depot injection administered quarterly, or a subcutaneous implant yearly. This analog stimulates gonadotropin release initially, but when given long-term, it suppresses gonadotropin release. With this treatment, the growth rate slows, and secondary sexual development stabilizes or regresses. Medroxyprogesterone injections (Depo-Provera) or tablets (Cycrin) reduce secretion of gonadotropins and prevent menstruation. When treatment is discontinued, puberty resumes according to appropriate developmental stages. The overall aim of treatment is to halt or even reverse sexual development and rapid growth, as well as promote psychosocial well-being.

Nursing Assessment

For a full description of the assessment phase of the nursing process, refer to the "Clinical Judgment and the Nursing Process" section earlier in the chapter. Pertinent assessment findings related to precocious puberty are discussed further on.

HEALTH HISTORY

The health history may reveal complaints of headaches, nausea, vomiting, and visual difficulties due to circulating hormones. Psychosocial development is typical for the child's age, but they may exhibit emotional lability, aggressive behavior, and mood swings. Additional information gathered from the child and family may also reveal risk factors such as exposure to exogenous hormones, a history of CNS trauma or infection, or a family history of early puberty.

PHYSICAL EXAMINATION

The physical examination may reveal acne and an adult-like body odor. The child will present with an accelerated rate of growth. Tanner staging of breasts, pubic hair, and genitalia may indicate advanced maturation for the child's age, although the child typically does not display sexual behavior.

LABORATORY AND DIAGNOSTIC TESTING

Radiologic examinations and pelvic ultrasound can identify advanced bone age, increased uterus size, and development of ovaries consistent with the diagnosis of precocious puberty. Laboratory studies include screening radioimmunoassays for LH, FSH, estradiol, or testosterone. The child's response to GnRH stimulation confirms the diagnosis of central precocious puberty versus gonadotropin-independent puberty. This test involves administering synthetic GnRH intravenously (IV) and drawing serial blood levels, about every 2 hours, of LH, FSH, and estrogen or testosterone. A positive result is defined as pubertal or adult levels of these hormones in response to the GnRH administration. Also, CT, MRI, or skull radiography can reveal any lesions in the CNS or tumors or cysts present in the abdomen, pelvic area, or testes.

Nursing Management

In general, nursing management of a child with precocious puberty focuses on educating both the child and their family about the physical changes the child is experiencing and how to correctly use the prescribed medications and helping the child to deal with self-esteem issues related to the accelerated growth and development of secondary sexual characteristics. Goals of nursing management include appropriate physical development and pubertal progression appropriate for the child's age. Refer to the "Clinical Judgment and the Nursing Process" section earlier in the chapter, and individualize care based on the child's and family's response to this disorder.

PROVIDING EDUCATION

Nursing care involves assessing and documenting the physical changes the child is experiencing, as well as administering medications. Demonstrate correct administration of medication and observe for potential adverse effects (teach this information to the family as well). Encourage families to comply with follow-up appointments, typically scheduled every 6 months, which may include stimulation tests. Inform families that pharmacologic intervention stops when the child reaches the age appropriate for pubertal development. Also, provide appropriate sex education.

DEALING WITH SELF-ESTEEM ISSUES

Due to the body image changes that differ from their peers, these children may develop self-esteem issues. The goal is to foster normal psychosocial development and help the child understand the physical and emotional changes that occur with early onset of puberty. Communicate with the child on an age-appropriate level, even when physical characteristics make the child appear older. Maintain a calm, supportive atmosphere and provide for privacy during examinations. Refer the child and family for counseling as needed. Since the child may have issues with self-image and may be self-conscious, encourage them to express their feelings about the changes, and use role-playing to show the child how to handle teasing from other children. Let the child know that everyone develops sexual characteristics in their own time.

Delayed Puberty

Delayed puberty is a condition of delayed secondary sexual development. In females, it is identified if the breasts have not developed by ages 12 to 13. In males, it is identified when there is no testicular enlargement or scrotal changes by ages 13 to 14 (Crowley & Pitteloud, 2023).

The most common cause for delayed puberty is a hereditary pattern of growth and development known as **constitutional delay** of growth and puberty (or a "late bloomer") (Crowley & Pitteloud, 2023). In these cases, there is a familial pattern of late-onset puberty; affected adolescents typically develop normally, just at a later time than their peers. Hypogonadism may also result when there is decreased stimulation of the gonads due to dysfunction or tumors in the hypothalamus or pituitary gland. Other causes include irradiation, infection, trauma, or genetic syndromes such as Turner or Klinefelter syndrome. Also, chronic conditions, such as anorexia or cystic fibrosis, lead to delayed puberty.

Therapeutic management involves administering testosterone (males) or estradiol-conjugated estrogen (females) in low dosages if there is no underlying medical condition to address. This is usually necessary for only a short time to get puberty started.

Nursing Assessment

Assessment involves obtaining a health history to identify the indications for this condition. Assessment of the growth pattern using correct techniques and standards for comparison is essential. On physical assessment, note the absence of secondary sex characteristics, as noted earlier. Laboratory and diagnostic testing rules out other potential causes for delayed puberty. Blood levels of reproductive hormones may also be evaluated.

Nursing Management

In addition to the general interventions presented in the "Clinical Judgment and the Nursing Process" section earlier in the chapter, instruct the child and family about the medication therapy. Educate them about the different stages of puberty. Help the family develop a home management schedule for the administration of medication. Address any questions the family may have about the condition or potential complications (e.g., infertility), depending on the underlying cause of the condition.

Arginine Vasopressin Resistance (AVP-R) and Arginine Vasopressin Deficiency (AVP-D)

AVP-R (previously referred to as nephrogenic DI) and AVP-D (previously referred to as central DI) are both major causes of polyuria in children (Working Group for Renaming Diabetes Insipidus et al., 2022). AVP-R can be transmitted genetically (e.g., sex-linked, autosomal dominant or recessive forms) or be acquired due to chronic kidney disease, hypercalcemia, hypokalemia, or use of certain drugs such as lithium, amphotericin, methicillin, and rifampin (Breault & Majzoub, 2020a). AVP-R is not associated with the pituitary gland and is related to decreased renal sensitivity to antidiuretic hormone (ADH). Therapeutic management for AVP-R involves diuretics, high fluid intake, restricted sodium intake, and a high-protein diet. Desmopressin acetate (DDAVP) is usually ineffective in the treatment of nephrogenic DI.

AVP-D is a disorder of the posterior pituitary gland and is the most common form of AVP dysfunction (Mutter et al., 2021). Therefore, AVP-D (central DI) will be the focus of the remainder of this discussion. It is characterized by excessive thirst (**polydipsia**) and excessive urination (**polyuria**) that is not affected by decreasing fluid intake. Typically, this disorder occurs in children as a result of complications from head trauma or after cranial surgery to remove hypothalamic–pituitary tumors, such as craniopharyngioma. Some cases can be hereditary; however, 10% of AVP-D cases in children are idiopathic (Breault & Majzoub, 2020a). Other causes include genetic mutations, granulomatous disease, infections such as meningitis or encephalitis, vascular anomalies, congenital malformations, infiltrative disease such as leukemia, or administration of certain drugs that are associated with inhibition of vasopressin release, such as phenytoin (Breault & Majzoub, 2020a). AVP-D is usually permanent and requires treatment throughout life.

Pathophysiology

AVP-D (central DI) results from a deficiency in the secretion of ADH. This hormone, also known as vasopressin, is produced in the hypothalamus and stored in the pituitary gland. ADH is involved in concentrating urine from the kidneys by stimulating the reabsorption of water in the renal collecting tubules through increased membrane permeability. This mechanism conserves water and helps maintains normal osmolality. With a deficiency in ADH, the kidneys lose massive amounts of water and retain sodium in the serum.

Therapeutic Management

Unless a tumor is present (in which case it is removed by surgery), the usual treatment for AVP-D (central DI) involves a low-solute diet (low sodium and low protein), daily replacement of ADH, and possibly the use of a thiazide diuretic (Bichet, 2023). The drug of choice for home treatment is DDAVP, a long-acting vasopressin analog (Breault & Majzoub, 2020a). In children, it is typically given intranasally. However, it can also be administered subcutaneously, orally, or buccally. The dose depends on the child's age, urine output, and urine specific gravity. Treatment of AVP-D and the use of DDAVP in infants and small children can be challenging and complicated due to their inability to access fluids and articulate thirst (Bichet, 2023). In neonates and young infants, treatment often focuses solely on fluid therapy due to their high volume requirements of nutritive fluid (i.e., the drive behind an infant's fluid intake is hunger rather than thirst) (Breault & Majzoub, 2020a). However, some experts suggest that subcutaneously administered DDAVP may be more effective than oral or intranasal therapy in infants and small children due to variable absorption and the challenge of administering accurate doses via these routes (Bichet, 2023).

In the hospital, the child may receive aqueous vasopressin or 8-arginine vasopressin (Pitressin) IV (Breault & Majzoub, 2020a). This is a short-acting drug, so the dosage can be adjusted quickly.

Both the long- and short-acting forms of the medication decrease urinary output and thirst, and the dosages of both forms of these drugs need to be titrated to achieve the desired effect.

> **TAKE NOTE!**
>
> A metered nasal spray form of DDAVP is available, but the prescribed dose must be >10 mcg/0.1 mL for the child to use the spray (Bichet, 2023).

Nursing Assessment

For a full description of the assessment phase, refer to the "Clinical Judgment and the Nursing Process" section earlier in the chapter. Assessment findings pertinent to AVP-D are discussed further on.

HEALTH HISTORY

Nursing assessment involves obtaining a history of any conditions that may have led to the development of the disorder. This review includes information about the neonatal period as well as a current history of infections such as meningitis, diseases such as leukemia, or familial patterns. Although most symptoms of endocrine disorders develop slowly, the onset of this disorder is often abrupt. The health history usually elicits the cardinal symptoms, as well as complaints representing the early signs of dehydration.

The most commonly reported initial symptoms are polyuria and polydipsia (Bichet, 2023; Breault & Majzoub, 2020a). Except for unconscious children, the child typically maintains adequate perfusion by drinking water. Parents or the child may report frequent trips to the bathroom, nocturia, or enuresis. When the child cannot compensate for the excessive loss of water by increasing fluid intake, other symptoms will be reported, such as weight loss or signs of dehydration. For example, irritability may be due to the early signs of dehydration or the frustration the child feels at being unable to quench their thirst. Other signs may include intermittent fever, vomiting, and constipation.

PHYSICAL EXAMINATION

Observation and inspection may reveal weight loss or failure to thrive in young infants. Inspection may also reveal signs of dehydration, such as dry mucous membranes or decreased tears. The child may excrete more than 3 L/m^2 of urine per day. On auscultation, tachycardia or an increased respiratory rate may indicate compensation for the decrease in fluid volume. Palpation may reveal slightly depressed fontanels or decreased skin turgor.

LABORATORY AND DIAGNOSTIC TESTING

Diagnostic tests used to evaluate AVP-D include the following:

- Radiographic studies such as CT scan, MRI, or ultrasound of the skull and kidneys can determine whether a lesion or tumor is present.
- Urinalysis: urine is dilute, osmolality is less than 3,000 mOsm/L, specific gravity is less than 1.005, and sodium level is decreased.
- Serum osmolality is greater than 300 mOsm/L.
- Serum sodium is elevated.
- A fluid deprivation test measures vasopressin release from the pituitary in response to water deprivation. Normal results will show decreased urine output, increased urine specific gravity, and no change in serum sodium levels.

TAKE NOTE!

During a fluid deprivation test, the child may be irritable and frustrated because fluid is being withheld. Don't drink in front of the child.

Nursing Management

Refer to the "Clinical Judgment and the Nursing Process" section earlier in the chapter, and individualize the plan of care based on the child's and family's response to the illness. Specific interventions related to nursing care of the child with AVP-D are discussed further on.

PROMOTING HYDRATION

The goal of treatment is to achieve an hourly urine output of 1 to 2 mL/kg and a urine specific gravity of at least 1.010.

CLINICAL REASONING ALERT!

Notify the health care provider or nurse practitioner if the urine output exceeds 1,000 mL/h for two consecutive voids.

Maintain fluid intake regimens as ordered. Monitor fluid status by measuring vital signs, fluid intake and output, and daily weights (using the same scale at the same time of day). If fluids are stopped too soon, the child may become hypernatremic, which can lead to seizures. Feed infants more frequently, since they excrete more dilute urine, consume larger volumes of free water, and secrete lower amounts of vasopressin than older children. Monitor for signs and symptoms of dehydration during the fluid deprivation test and when starting the treatment regimen.

TAKE NOTE!

Monitor blood pressure closely when initiating vasopressin.

If the child is unconscious or has brain injury, maintain hydration and nutrition by administering nasogastric or gastrostomy feedings.

PROMOTING ACTIVITY

Establish appropriate activity levels for the child, and allow time for them to regain strength and the desire to increase their level of activity. Assess the child's abilities daily, schedule frequent bathroom breaks, and ensure that fluids the child enjoys are available at all times. Tailor the treatment plan to fit the child's daily activities.

EDUCATING THE FAMILY

Involve the family in developing fluid intake regimens. A journal or daily log is essential for maintaining the fluid regimen and identifying problems. Children with intact thirst centers can self-regulate their need for fluids, but if this is not the situation, help the family develop a 24-hour fluid replacement plan. This may require instruction on nasogastric or gastrostomy feedings. Infants will need fluid intake at night. Educate the family about the symptoms of water intoxication (drowsiness, listlessness, headache, confusion, sudden weight gain, and anuria) and dehydration. Help the family develop a plan to inform the school and other people in the child's life about the need for liberal bathroom privileges and extra fluids to prevent accidents or dehydration. Teaching Guidelines 26.1 provides tips on educating the family about the medication regimen. Recommend that the family obtain a medical ID alert bracelet or necklace for the child. Encourage adherence to follow-up appointments, which will probably be every 6 months.

TEACHING GUIDELINES 26.1 DDAVP Intranasal Administration

- Keep desmopressin acetate (DDAVP) in the refrigerator at all times (if directed; some products no longer require refrigeration—refer to product insert).
- Clear the nostrils (medication may be poorly absorbed if the child has nasal congestion).
- Insert the measuring tube into the bottle.
- Fill to the proper dosage and hold the top of the tube closed while inserting the medication-filled end into the nostril.
- Blow the liquid out of the tubing into the nostril.
- When using a metered nasal spray, the spray must be primed before first use.
- If the child sneezes, repeat the dosage.
- Measure urine specific gravity to monitor effectiveness of the drug.
- Monitor for signs and symptoms of overdosage such as confusion, headache, drowsiness, and rapid weight gain due to fluid retention.

Syndrome of Inappropriate Antidiuretic Hormone

SIADH occurs when ADH (vasopressin) is secreted in the presence of low serum osmolality because the feedback mechanism that regulates ADH does not function properly. ADH continues to be released, and this leads to water retention, decreased serum sodium levels due to hemodilution, and extracellular fluid volume expansion. SIADH can be caused by CNS infections such as meningitis, head trauma, brain tumors, intracranial surgery, and certain medications such as analgesics, barbiturates, or chemotherapy. SIADH is rare in children; however, when observed, it is often related to excessive administration of vasopressin during the treatment of AVP-D (central DI) (Breault & Majzoub, 2020b).

The therapeutic management of SIADH includes correcting the underlying disorder, in addition to fluid restriction and intravenous sodium chloride administration to correct hyponatremia and increase serum osmolality.

Nursing Assessment

Obtain a health history, noting a history of CNS infection or tumor, intracranial surgery, head trauma, use of the aforementioned medications, or a history of AVP-D or AVP-R. Note symptoms such as decreased urine output and weight gain, or GI symptoms such as anorexia, nausea, and vomiting. Assess neurologic status, noting lethargy, behavioral changes, headache, altered level of consciousness, seizure, or coma. Neurologic signs develop as the sodium level decreases. Diagnostic tests reveal low serum sodium and osmolality, as well as decreased levels of urea, creatinine, uric acid, and albumin. Urine samples demonstrate elevated osmolality, high sodium concentrations, and specific gravity greater than 1.030. Adrenal, thyroid, and kidney function studies may be used to rule out other causes of hyponatremia.

Comparison Chart 26.1 lists the differences between AVP-D and SIADH.

COMPARISON CHART 26.1 Arginine Vasopressin Deficiency Versus Syndrome of Inappropriate Antidiuretic Hormone

AVP-D (Central DI)	SIADH
• "High and dry"	• "Low and wet"
• Increased urination	• Decreased urination
• Hypernatremia	• Hyponatremia
• Serum osmolality >300 mOsm/kg	• Serum osmolality <280 mOsm/kg
• Urine specific gravity <1.005	• Urine specific gravity >1.030
• Decreased urine osmolality	• Increased urine osmolality
• Dehydration, thirst	• Fluid retention, weight gain, and hypertension

Nursing Management

Nursing goals focus on restoring fluid balance and preventing injury. Institute safety precautions if altered levels of consciousness, confusion, or seizures are present. Notify the health care provider or nurse practitioner if headache or irritability is present. Monitor fluid intake and output and weigh the child daily. An indwelling urinary catheter may be needed to allow for hourly monitoring of urine volume and specific gravity. Help the child cope with fluid restriction by offering sugarless candy, a wet washcloth, or, perhaps, ice chips. Administer electrolyte replacement as necessary to correct imbalances.

DISORDERS OF THYROID FUNCTION

Disorders of the thyroid gland are seen in infancy and childhood and are broadly classified as hypothyroidism and hyperthyroidism. These disorders can be serious because thyroid hormones are important for growth and development; they regulate metabolism of nutrients and energy production.

Congenital Hypothyroidism

Congenital hypothyroidism usually results from a defect in the thyroid gland during fetal development or a defect in thyroid hormone synthesis (Connelly & LaFranchi, 2023a). This results in malformation or malfunction of the thyroid gland, which leads to insufficient production of the thyroid hormones that are required to meet the body's metabolic, growth, and development needs. Congenital hypothyroidism leads to low concentrations of circulating thyroid hormones (triiodothyronine [T_3] and thyroxine [T_4]).

Congenital hypothyroidism occurs in one in 2,000 to 4,000 live births (Connelly & LaFranchi, 2023a). It affects a wide range of populations, though less frequently among African Americans, and is more common in females than males (Connelly & LaFranchi, 2023a). Complications include intellectual disability if untreated, short stature, growth failure, and delayed physical maturation and development (Wassner & Smith, 2020). Congenital hypothyroidism is one of the most common preventable causes of intellectual disability. The later it is diagnosed, the greater the disability is (Connelly & LaFranchi, 2023a). Most newborns have few, if any, symptoms, and the occurrence is sporadic, not typically hereditary; therefore, most cases of congenital hypothyroidism are detected via newborn screening programs.

Pathophysiology

Congenital hypothyroidism is due to a defect in the development of the thyroid gland in the fetus, owing to a spontaneous gene mutation, an inborn error of thyroid hormone synthesis resulting from an autosomal recessive trait, pituitary dysfunction, or failure of the CNS–thyroid feedback mechanism to develop. Transient primary hypothyroidism may also occur; it results from transplacental transfer of maternal medications, maternal thyroid-blocking antibodies, iodine deficiency, or fetal or neonatal exposure to excessive iodine (such as the use of iodine antiseptics during delivery or procedures, or excess ingestion of iodine by the birthing parent) (Connelly & Lafranchi, 2023a).

Therapeutic Management

To prevent intellectual disability and restore normal growth and motor development, thyroid hormone replacement with sodium L-thyroxine (Synthroid, synthetic thyroxine, or Levothroid) is given. The recommended starting dosage is 10 to 15 mcg/kg/day (Connelly & LaFranchi, 2023b). There are no adverse effects with physiologic doses, but thyroid function tests are initially performed every 2 weeks to closely monitor for effects and ensure proper dosing. Since thyroid hormone is vital to the infant's developing CNS, the goal is to normalize thyroid function as quickly as possible. This treatment will be needed lifelong to maintain normal metabolism and promote normal physical and mental growth and development.

Nursing Assessment

Nursing assessment of the child with congenital hypothyroidism includes health history, physical examination, and laboratory testing.

HEALTH HISTORY

Inquire whether the neonatal metabolic screening test was performed and if results were obtained. Determine if the test was conducted less than 24 to 48 hours after birth. If so, a repeat test may be warranted (see the "Laboratory and Diagnostic Testing" section). Inquire about maternal history that may indicate a connection to hypothyroidism, such as maternal exposure to iodine. Additional history findings may include sensitivity to cold, constipation, feeding problems, or lethargy. Since parents prefer babies to sleep well, they may not complain that the baby is sleeping too much; rather, they may remark that it is difficult to keep the baby awake.

PHYSICAL EXAMINATION

Most infants do not show symptoms until the first month when they begin to develop clinical signs. Inspection and observation reveal a lethargic baby or a child with hypotonia, hypoactivity, and a dull expression. A combination of lethargy and irritability may exist, with overall delayed mental responsiveness. Measurements of weight and height may reveal delayed growth. Other findings may include a persistent open posterior fontanel, coarse facies with a short neck and limbs, periorbital puffiness, enlarged tongue, and poor sucking response (Fig. 26.3). The skin may appear pale with mottling or yellow from prolonged jaundice, or it may be cool, dry, and scaly to the touch, with sparse hair development on older children. Auscultation of the chest might reveal bradycardia. Signs of respiratory distress and decreased pulse pressure may also be present. On palpation of the abdomen, there may be evidence of an umbilical hernia or a mass due to constipation.

LABORATORY AND DIAGNOSTIC TESTING

Every infant should have a newborn screen for thyroid hormone levels before discharge from the hospital or

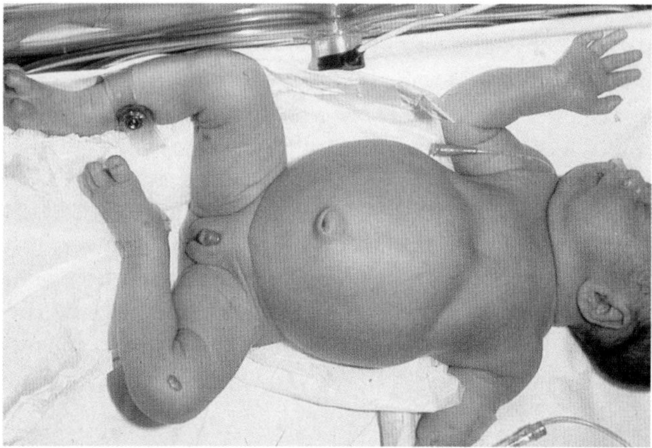

FIGURE 26.3 Newborn with congenital hypothyroidism.

2 to 4 days after birth (Connelly & LaFranchi, 2023a). When the test is performed within the first 24 to 48 hours along with other metabolic screenings, the result may be inaccurate because of the immediate increase in thyroid-stimulating hormone (TSH) shortly after birth (Connelly & LaFranchi, 2023a). Radioimmunoassay is used to measure levels of T_4, which accurately reflect the child's thyroid status. If the T_4 level is low, then a second confirming laboratory test is performed, as well as determining whether the TSH is elevated. A thyroid scan may also be used to check for the absence or ectopic placement of the gland. In addition to serum measurement of T_4, other diagnostic tests include serum T_3, radioiodine uptake, thyroid-bound globulin, and ultrasonography.

Nursing Management

The overall goal of nursing management for infants or children with congenital hypothyroidism is to establish a normal growth pattern without complications such as intellectual disability or failure to thrive. Individualize the nursing care plan based on the infant's responses to the illness.

PROMOTING APPROPRIATE GROWTH

Measure and record growth at regular intervals. Thyroid levels are measured at recommended intervals, such as every 2 weeks until the target range is reached on a stabilized dose of medication, then every 1 to 2 months until the child is 1 year old, every 1 to 3 months until the child is 3 years old, and less frequently as the child gets older (Connelly & LaFranchi, 2023b). A trial off the medication may be performed around the age of 3, under a health care provider's or nurse practitioner's supervision, to confirm the diagnosis (Connelly & LaFranchi, 2023b). Monitor for signs of hypo- or hyperfunction, including changes in vital signs, thermoregulation, and activity level. Provide adequate rest periods and meet thermoregulation needs. If the infant's tongue is unusually large, observe feeding ability, prevent airway obstruction, and position the infant on their side. Fluid restrictions or a low-salt diet may be ordered.

TAKE NOTE!

Observe for signs of thyroid hormone overdose (irritability, rapid pulse, dyspnea, sweating, and fever) or ineffective treatment (fatigue, constipation, and decreased appetite).

EDUCATING THE FAMILY

Since many infants do not show symptoms, the diagnosis may be unexpected, so reassure and convey realistic expectations to the family. Developmental screening may be required if the child showed any symptoms initially or as the child gets older, to ensure that drug therapy is appropriate. Educate the family about the disorder, the medication and method of administration, and adverse effects such as increased pulse rate (which may indicate an overdose of thyroid hormone).

L-Thyroxine is an oral medication. The pill form must be crushed for infants and young children. It can be mixed with a small amount of formula or breast milk and placed in the nipple, but it should not be placed in a full bottle of formula or breast milk because the infant will not ingest all the medication if they do not finish the bottle. The medication can also be mixed with a small amount of liquid and given with a dropper. Medication absorption is affected by soy-based formulas, fiber, and iron preparations (Connelly & LaFranchi, 2023b). Therefore, carefully evaluate the formula the infant is on before administering L-thyroxine.

Inform the family that this medication will be needed throughout the child's life. Explain that missed doses may lead to developmental delays and poor growth. Tell them that frequent blood tests will be needed to evaluate thyroid function and the child's growth rate; genetic counseling may be needed. Clinical examination, including growth and development assessment, should occur every few months until the child is 3 years old. Serum T_4 and TSH should be evaluated often, and more frequent monitoring may be needed if nonadherence occurs, if abnormal values occur, or with any changes in medication dosage or treatment regimen. The nurse may need to help the family to find a nearby laboratory or to handle financial issues related to therapy. Educate the family about infant stimulation programs if the child shows cognitive problems, retarded physical growth, or slow intellectual development. Some information may need to be reinforced during the school-age or adolescent stages of development. Finally, encourage the family to obtain a medical ID bracelet or necklace for the child.

CONSIDER THIS!

Asha Virani, 1 week old, is brought to the clinic. Her newborn screening test was positive for hypothyroidism. Her parents are shocked and upset by the news. Her parent states, "My daughter's been doing so well since she came home from the hospital. She seems to be doing everything she should be. I just can't believe anything's wrong with her. I felt so blessed to have a baby that slept so much but she could have died. What kind of parent will I be?"

Thought: How would you respond to this parent?

Acquired Hypothyroidism

Hypothyroidism also occurs as an acquired condition. This disorder most commonly results from an autoimmune chronic lymphocytic (Hashimoto) thyroiditis (LaFranchi, 2022a). As a genetic condition, antibodies develop against the thyroid gland, causing the gland to become inflamed, infiltrated, and progressively destroyed. It occurs more often in females during childhood and adolescence (LaFranchi, 2022a). Less common etiologies include hypothyroidism associated with pituitary or hypothalamic disease; exposure to drugs or substances such as antithyroid medications, anticonvulsants, lithium, and amiodarone that interfere with thyroid hormone synthesis; thyroid injury such as radiation, thyroidectomy, and hemangiomas; and iodine deficiency or excess (LaFranchi, 2022a).

Therapeutic management is the same as for congenital hypothyroidism. Management involves oral sodium L-thyroxine, which is given at 2 to 6 mcg/kg/day based on age to maintain T_4 in the upper half of the normal range and to suppress TSH (LaFranchi, 2022a).

Nursing Assessment

Interview the family and child to determine activity tolerance and behavior changes. The symptoms may develop over a period of time and may be subtle. Note vague complaints of fatigue, weakness, weight gain, cold intolerance, constipation, and dry skin. The severity of symptoms depends on the length of time that the hormone deficiency has existed and its extent. Reviewing the growth pattern may reveal a slowed or arrested growth rate (height) and increased weight.

Physical examination may reveal a **goiter** (enlargement of the thyroid gland). Deep tendon reflexes may be sluggish, and the face, eyes, and hands may be edematous. Note thinning or coarse hair, muscle hypertrophy with muscle weakness, and signs of delayed or precocious puberty. The diagnostic evaluation involves serum thyroid function studies (TSH, T_3, and T_4), as well as serum thyroid antibodies to confirm autoimmune thyroiditis. MRI and a thyroid uptake test and scan may also be necessary.

Nursing Management

Work with the family to establish a daily schedule for administering L-thyroxine, which should be taken 30 to 60 minutes before a meal for optimal absorption. Explain to the family that growth is related to the child's response to the treatment, and there are no specific strategies to aid in this growth. The family should understand the diagnosis, should be able to recognize signs and symptoms of thyroid hypo- and hyperfunction, and should know when to notify the health care provider or nurse practitioner. The family and child may need assistance in accepting the therapy, as well as the experience of catch-up growth that may occur at the beginning of therapy. The child with chronic or severe hypothyroidism may be at risk for adverse effects such as restlessness, insomnia, or irritability. The child's thyroid levels should be evaluated at recommended intervals, such as every 3 to 6 months, by a pediatric endocrinologist.

Hyperthyroidism

Hyperthyroidism is the result of hyperfunction of the thyroid gland. This leads to excessive levels of circulating thyroid hormones. This condition is uncommon in children, with its peak incidence occurring during adolescence, often due to Graves disease (LaFranchi, 2022b). Graves disease is an autoimmune disorder that causes excessive amounts of thyroid hormone to be released in response to human thyroid stimulator immunoglobulin (TSI). It affects females five times more frequently than males (LaFranchi, 2022b) and a goiter usually develops in this condition. There is a strong genetic factor, with the majority of children having a positive family history of autoimmune thyroid problems (LaFranchi, 2022b). A congenital form of hyperthyroidism, neonatal thyrotoxicosis, occurs in infants of birthing parents with Graves disease. This neonatal condition, which can be life-threatening, is a self-limiting disorder lasting 2 to 4 months. Less common causes of hyperthyroidism are thyroiditis, thyroid hormone–producing tumors, and pituitary adenomas.

Therapeutic management is aimed at decreasing thyroid hormone levels. Current treatment involves antithyroid medication, radioactive iodine therapy, and subtotal thyroidectomy. First-line treatment involves methimazole (MTZ, Tapazole), which blocks the production of T_3 and T_4 (Wassner & LaFranchi, 2021). Adjunct therapy, with beta-adrenergic blockers (such as propranolol or atenolol), may also be used if the child has marked symptoms. Radioactive iodine therapy is restricted to children older than 10 years as a long-term therapy (Wassner & LaFranchi, 2021). This therapy is administered orally and leads to tissue damage and destruction of the thyroid gland within 6 to 18 weeks, but it can result in hypothyroidism. Subtotal thyroidectomy is used when drug therapy is not possible or other treatments have failed. Risks include hypothyroidism, hypoparathyroidism, or laryngeal nerve damage.

Nursing Assessment

Initially, symptoms of hyperthyroidism are mild and can often be overlooked. Many children with hyperthyroidism are first seen in outpatient settings with a history of problems with sleep, school performance, and distractibility. They may become easily frustrated, overheated, and fatigued during physical education classes. Also, the child may complain of diarrhea, excessive perspiration, and muscle weakness. Further, the history may reveal signs of hyperactivity, heat intolerance, emotional lability, and insomnia.

During physical examination, older children may reveal an increased rate of growth, weight loss despite an excellent appetite, hyperactivity, warm and moist skin, tachycardia, fine tremors, an enlarged thyroid gland or goiter, and ophthalmic changes (exophthalmos, which is less pronounced in children; proptosis; lid lag and retraction; staring expression; periorbital edema; and diplopia) (Fig. 26.4). Elevated pulse and blood pressure may also be noted. Laboratory and diagnostic tests reveal that serum T_4 and T_3 levels are markedly elevated, while TSH levels are suppressed.

CLINICAL REASONING ALERT!

The sudden release of high levels of thyroid hormones results in thyroid storm, which progresses to heart failure and shock. Immediately report the signs of thyroid storm, which include the sudden onset of severe restlessness and irritability, fever, diaphoresis, and severe tachycardia (Smith & Wassner, 2020).

Nursing Management

Once the treatment plan is initiated, educate both the family and the child about the medication, its potential adverse effects, the goals of treatment, and possible complications. Monitor for adverse drug effects such as rash, mild leukopenia, loss of taste, sore throat, GI disturbances, and arthralgia. If the medication needs to be taken two or three times a day, teach the family to use a pill dispenser and set alarms. Inform the family of the need for routine blood tests and follow-up visits with the pediatric endocrinologist every 2 to 4 months until normal hormone levels are achieved; then, visits may be decreased to once or twice a year. Instruct the parents to contact the health care provider or nurse practitioner if the child has tachycardia or extreme fatigue.

Help the child and family to cope with symptoms such as heat intolerance, emotional lability, or eye problems. Explain these symptoms to the school or day care personnel and make sure that they understand that the child may require more frequent rest breaks in a cool environment and should refrain from participating in physical education classes until normal hormone levels are attained. Encourage the family to ensure the child maintains a healthy diet with an appropriate level of calories; they may need to eat five or six meals a day. Provide community referrals such as to the Graves Disease and Thyroid Foundation. Also, encourage the family to obtain a medical ID bracelet or necklace for the child.

If surgical intervention is chosen, provide appropriate preoperative teaching and postoperative care. Provide supportive measures such as fluid maintenance, nutritional support, and electrolyte correction. Monitor red blood cell count and liver function tests. Close monitoring for signs and symptoms of hypothyroidism is important.

Comparison Chart 26.2 compares hypothyroidism and hyperthyroidism.

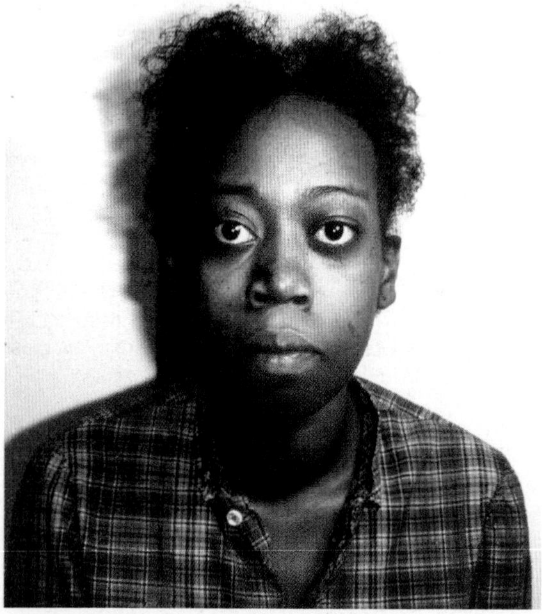

FIGURE 26.4 Adolescent with Graves disease.

COMPARISON CHART 26.2 Hypothyroidism Versus Hyperthyroidism

Hyperthyroidism	Hypothyroidism
• Nervousness/anxiety • Diarrhea • Heat intolerance • Weight loss • Smooth, velvety skin	• Tiredness/fatigue • Constipation • Cold intolerance • Weight gain • Dry, thick skin; edema of face, eyes, and hands • Decreased growth

DISORDERS RELATED TO PARATHYROID GLAND FUNCTION

The parathyroid glands secrete parathyroid hormone (PTH). This hormone, along with vitamin D and calcitonin, regulates calcium and phosphate homeostasis by increasing osteoclastic activity, promoting calcium absorption in the kidneys, and enhancing calcium absorption in the GI tract while facilitating phosphate excretion by the kidneys. The two primary disorders associated with parathyroid gland dysfunction are hypoparathyroidism and hyperparathyroidism, both of which are rare in children. Refer to Table 26.2, for further information.

DISORDERS RELATED TO ADRENAL GLAND FUNCTION

Disorders of the adrenal gland include both acute and chronic adrenal insufficiency (hypofunction) as well as disorders of hyperfunction like Cushing syndrome (Fig. 26.5). The adrenal cortex is the site of production of glucocorticoids (for blood glucose regulation), mineralocorticoids (for sodium retention), and androgenic and estrogenic steroid compounds (for phallic and secondary sex development). The adrenal medulla is the site of production of the catecholamines (dopamine, norepinephrine, and epinephrine) and is under neuroendocrine control. When production of these compounds is altered, disease results. Pediatric adrenocortical insufficiency is similar to adults, exception for CAH, which will be discussed later. Refer to Table 26.3, for an overview of other disorders of the adrenal gland.

Congenital Adrenal Hyperplasia

CAH is a group of autosomal recessive inherited disorders in which there is an insufficient supply of the enzymes required for the synthesis of cortisol and aldosterone. More than 90% of the CAH cases are caused

TABLE 26.2 • Parathyroid Disorders

Parathyroid Disorder	Cause	Nursing Assessment	Nursing Management
Hypoparathyroidism (deficiency of PTH)	Most common is accidental removal or destruction of the parathyroid gland during thyroidectomy or radial neck dissection; may also be congenital (result of aplasia or hypoplasia of the parathyroid gland)	Hypocalcemia Hyperphosphatemia Hyperexcitability of neuromuscular function, uncontrolled spasms, and hypocalcemic tetany (general muscular hypertonia); positive Chvostek sign (facial muscle spasm elicited by tapping the facial nerve); positive Trousseau sign (carpopedal spasm that results from oxygen deficiency) Laryngeal spasm, stridor Poor eating Lethargy	• Administer intravenous calcium gluconate for acute or severe tetany, then intramuscular or oral calcium as prescribed. • Monitor the child for the development of cardiac arrhythmias. Ensure that the intravenous site is patent; if extravasation occurs, tissue damage or cardiac arrhythmias may result. • Monitor fluid and electrolyte status, weigh the child daily, and measure urinary calcium excretion to prevent nephrocalcinosis. • Institute seizure precautions and reduce environmental stimuli (e.g., loud or sudden noises, bright lights, or stimulating activities). • Observe for signs and symptoms of laryngospasm (e.g., stridor, hoarseness, or a feeling of tightness in the throat). Teach the child and family about the need for continuous daily administration of calcium salts and vitamin D. Have the family observe for vitamin D toxicity by observing for signs such as weakness, fatigue, lassitude, headache, nausea and vomiting, and diarrhea.
Hyperparathyroidism (hypersecretion of PTH)	Parathyroid adenoma is the most common cause; secondary hyperparathyroidism is primarily due to kidney disease.	Hypercalcemia Hypophosphatemia Depression of neuromuscular function, the child may trip and drop objects, general fatigue, failure to thrive, headaches, poor school performance, and irritability, somnolence, stupor, or difficulty concentrating. Irregular heart rate, possibly related to cardiac dysrhythmias. Skeletal pain, fractures, formation of bone tumors, or flank pain related to renal calculi	• Administer IV fluids and diuretics as prescribed to increase urinary excretion of calcium in children without kidney disease. • Administer prescribed medication to treat hypercalcemia, such as oral phosphate (antihypercalcemic agent), pamidronate, calcitonin, or etidronate disodium (by inhibiting bone resorption of calcium). • Increase the child's fluid intake to minimize renal calculi formation. Provide fruit juices to maintain low urinary pH, acidity of body fluids, and calcium absorption. Strain the urine for renal casts. • Dietary calcium is restricted. • Monitor for safety by assessing the child's level of muscular weakness, preventing falls or injury, and checking for fractures. • If the child develops renal rickets (osteodystrophy), long-term braces may be required, so provide family education and encourage adherence. • Surgery may be performed to remove abnormal parathyroid tumor. • Keep the diet low in phosphorus and watch for hypocalcemia and onset of tetany after surgery.

IV, intravenous; PTH, parathyroid hormone.

Doyle, D. A. (2020a). Chapter 589: Hypoparathyroidism. In R. M. Kleigman, J. W. St. Geme III, N. J. Blum, S.S. Shah, R.C. Tasker, K.M. Wilson, & R. E. Behrman (Eds.), *Nelson textbook of pediatrics* (21th ed., pp. 15565-15579). Elsevier;

Doyle, D. A. (2020b). Chapter 591: Hyperparathyroidism. In R. M. Kleigman, J. W. St. Geme III, N. J. Blum, S.S. Shah, R.C. Tasker, K.M. Wilson, & R. E. Behrman (Eds.), *Nelson textbook of pediatrics* (21th ed., pp. 15587-15601). Elsevier.

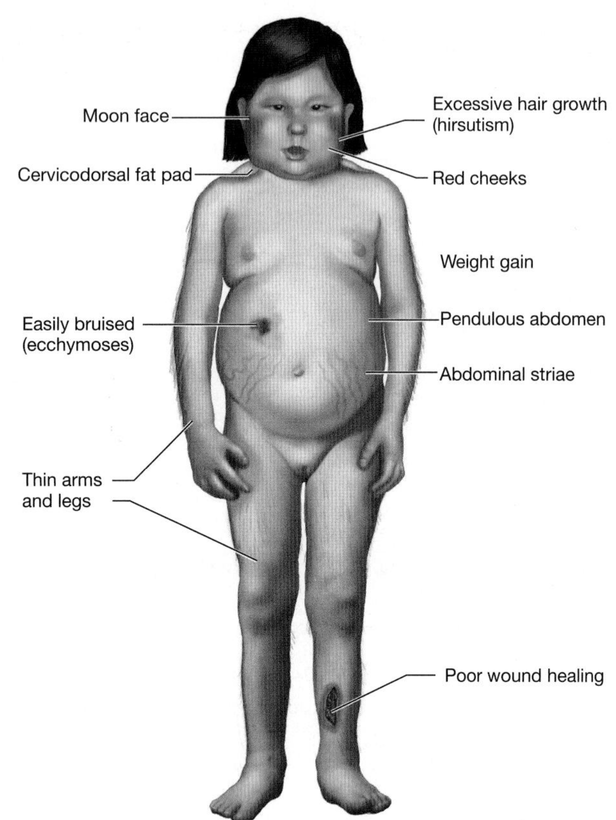

FIGURE 26.5 Cushing syndrome.

by a deficiency of the 21-hydroxylase (21-OH) enzyme (White, 2020b). It is the most common type of adrenocortical insufficiency seen in children with an incidence of about one in 15,000 to 20,000 live births (White, 2020b). Therefore, our discussion will focus on this type. This condition can be life-threatening and requires prompt diagnosis and treatment after birth (White, 2020b). Complications of CAH include hyponatremia, hyperkalemia, hypotension, shock, hypoglycemia, short adult stature, and adult testicular tumor in males.

Pathophysiology

Classic 21-OH enzyme deficiency results in blocking the production of adrenal mineralocorticoids and glucocorticoids. A reduction of cortisol occurs, which leads to increased adrenocorticotropic hormone (ACTH) production by the anterior pituitary to stimulate adrenal gland production. Prolonged oversecretion of ACTH causes enlargement or hyperplasia of the adrenal glands and excess production of androgens, leading to male characteristics appearing early or inappropriately.

In males, the enzyme deficiency of 21-OH with excessive androgen secretion leads to a slightly enlarged penis, which may become adult size by school age, and a hyperpigmented scrotum. Males do not have obvious signs at birth but may enter puberty by 2 to 3 years of age. The female fetus develops male secondary sexual characteristics; thus, CAH causes ambiguous genitalia (Merke & Auchus, 2022; White, 2020b). The clitoris is enlarged and may resemble the penis, the labia have a rugated appearance, and the labial folds are fused, but the internal reproductive organs, including the ovaries, fallopian tubes, and uterus, are typical.

A milder form of 21-OH deficiency becomes evident later (genitals are typical in appearance at birth), in the toddler or preschool years, with premature **adrenarche** (early sexual maturation), pubic hair development, accelerated growth velocity, advanced bone age, early closure of the epiphyseal plates resulting in short stature as an adult, acne, and **hirsutism** (excessive body hair growth). Males usually have typical fertility, while females may have lower fertility.

Aldosterone insufficiency also leads to fluid and electrolyte imbalances, such as hyponatremia, hyperkalemia, and hypotension due to depletion of extracellular fluid. Cortisol insufficiency leads to hypoglycemia.

Therapeutic Management

The goal of treatment is to stop excessive adrenal secretion of androgens while maintaining normal growth and development. Most children with 21-OH deficiency will take a glucocorticoid such as hydrocortisone and the mineralocorticoid fludrocortisone for life. Infants may also require sodium supplementation. When the medications are taken at physiologic doses, there are no adverse effects, but if the drug levels become elevated, hypertension, growth impairment, and acne become a problem. Regular follow-up care and appropriate titration maintain the dose at appropriate levels to allow normal growth and development.

Often when females are born with ambiguous genitalia, standard medical treatment is to correct the external genitalia and establish adequate sexual functioning. Sex can be assigned by karyotyping chromosomes. Typically, a reduction of the clitoris and opening of the labial folds are done within 2 to 6 months of life, with further surgeries at puberty (White, 2020b). Some argue that surgery should be delayed until the child is old enough to decide what kind of correction (if any) should be performed (White, 2020b). The decision to intervene immediately or to delay treatment is a complex one that raises many concerns for the family. The medical team needs to be sensitive to this and provide psychosocial support to the parents and family (Merke, 2022).

Nursing Assessment

Nursing assessment of the child with CAH includes health history, physical examination, and laboratory and diagnostic testing. Specific findings related to CAH are presented further.

TABLE 26.3 • Other Disorders of the Adrenal Gland

Disorder	Cause	Nursing Assessment	Nursing Management
Addison disease (deficiency in the adrenal steroids, glucocorticoids [cortisol], and mineralocorticoids [aldosterone])	It results from damage or destruction of the adrenal glands caused by infections such as tuberculosis, fungal infections, or HIV-related infections; hemorrhage or surgical removal of both glands; or dysfunction of the hypothalamus or pituitary gland. Generally, the etiology in children is an autoimmune process that is familial or sporadic.[a]	Hyponatremia Hyperkalemia Water loss, dehydration, muscular weakness, fatigue, weight loss, anorexia, syncope, nausea, vomiting, and diarrhea Hypoglycemia Hypotension Hyperpigmentation of skin Adrenal crisis, also referred to as Addisonian crisis, can occur (refer to section on CAH for more information)	Similar to that of congenital adrenal insufficiency
Cushing syndrome (excess levels of one or all the hormones [glucocorticoids, mineralocorticoids, and adrenal androgens] but most commonly glucocorticoid excess)	Usually, this condition is due to a small ACTH-producing pituitary adenoma. The most common cause in older children is prolonged or excessive use of corticosteroid therapy.[b]	Note history of rapid weight gain, decreased velocity of linear growth, muscle weakness, fatigue, irritability, sleep disturbance, and hypertension. History of long-term corticosteroid use, water retention, poor wound healing, frequent infections, and missed menstrual periods Refer to Figure 26.5. Skin may be thin and fragile; acne may be present.	• Management varies depending on the cause. • The goal is to restore hormone balance and reverse Cushing syndrome. • If the cause is an adrenal or pituitary tumor, then surgical removal of the tumor alone or the entire adrenal gland is performed. • If the cause is long-term steroid therapy, then the corticosteroid dose is reduced to the lowest dose that is effective in treating the underlying disorder. • Cortisol synthesis–inhibiting medications may be used. • Counsel the family that the cushingoid appearance is reversible with appropriate treatment. • Be alert for signs of adrenal insufficiency if the child has surgery or if corticosteroid withdrawal occurs quickly.

ACTH, adrenocorticotropic hormone; CAH, congenital adrenal hyperplasia; HIV, human immunodeficiency virus.

[a]White, P. C. (2020a). Chapter 593: Adrenocortical insufficiency. In R. M. Kleigman, J. W. St. Geme III, N. J. Blum, S. S. Shah, R. C. Tasker, K. M. Wilson, & R. E. Behrman (Eds.), *Nelson textbook of pediatrics* (21st ed., pp. 15636–15689). Elsevier.

[b]White, P. C. (2020b). Chapter 597: Cushing syndrome. In R. M. Kleigman, J. W. St. Geme III, N. J. Blum, S. S. Shah, R. C. Tasker, K. M. Wilson, & R. E. Behrman (Eds.), *Nelson textbook of pediatrics* (21st ed., pp. 15753–15766). Elsevier.

HEALTH HISTORY AND PHYSICAL EXAMINATION

Obtain the health history, noting any history of atypical genitalia at birth in the infant. For toddlers or preschoolers, take note of any history of accelerated growth velocity and signs of premature adrenarche. During inspection of the infant's genitalia, observe for the presence of a large penis or ambiguous genitalia (Fig. 26.6). When observing toddlers or preschoolers, note pubic hair development, acne, and hirsutism.

LABORATORY AND DIAGNOSTIC TESTING

The most common type of CAH, 21-OH enzyme deficiency, is detected by newborn metabolic screening. If this test has not been done or the results are unavailable, obtain random hormone levels or levels associated with ACTH stimulation. Radiographs reveal advanced bone age and premature closure of epiphyseal plates of the long bones.

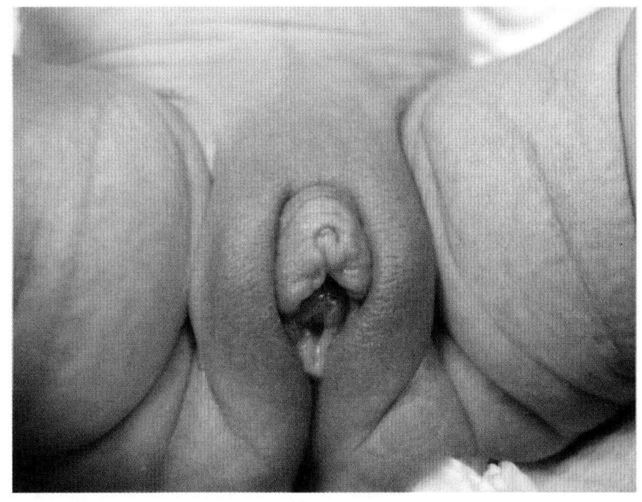

FIGURE 26.6 Newborn with ambiguous genitalia.

Nursing Management

In addition to the common interventions associated with endocrine disorders in childhood (see "Clinical Judgment and the Nursing Process" section earlier in the chapter), nursing management of infants or children with CAH focuses on preventing and monitoring for acute adrenal crisis, helping the family to understand the disease, educating both the child and the family about the importance of maintaining hormone supplementation, and providing emotional support to the family.

PREVENTING AND MONITORING FOR ACUTE ADRENAL CRISIS

Providing continuous assessment of an ill or hospitalized child with a history of CAH is crucial to recognize the development of life-threatening acute adrenal crisis. Signs and symptoms of acute adrenal crisis include persistent vomiting, dehydration, hyponatremia, hyperkalemia, hypotension, tachycardia, and shock. Closely monitor children with CAH and notify the health care provider or nurse practitioner if adrenal crisis is suspected. If signs and symptoms of adrenal crisis develop, the child will receive intravenous steroids, such as hydrocortisone, and aggressive fluid resuscitation, often using 5% dextrose in normal saline (D5NS), to correct electrolyte imbalances.

CLINICAL REASONING ALERT!

Adrenal crisis in newborns is often unrecognized. It presents within the first few days to weeks of life, with vomiting, lethargy, and feeding difficulties.

EDUCATING THE FAMILY ABOUT THE MEDICATION REGIMEN

Medication will be required throughout the child's life because cortisone is necessary for sustaining life. Educate the family on the appropriate oral dosages of hydrocortisone and fludrocortisone. It is critical to maintain tight control over the levels of these medications in the bloodstream. Underdosing or overdosing can lead to short adult stature, while low levels of the hormones may also result in adrenal crisis (as discussed previously). These drugs are usually given orally, but in some instances, will need to be given via intramuscular injections. Teach families how to administer hydrocortisone intramuscularly if the child is vomiting and unable to tolerate oral medication. If the child becomes ill, is under stress, or needs surgery, additional doses of medications may be required. Encourage the family to obtain a medical ID bracelet or necklace for the child.

TAKE NOTE!

Families must keep extra steroids in an injectable form, such as Solu-Cortef or Decadron, at home to administer during emergencies.

PROVIDING FAMILY SUPPORT

Make sure the family of a newborn with ambiguous genitalia feels comfortable asking questions and exploring their feelings. There are many factors to consider, including whether the family will opt to reassign the child's sex, raise the child according to the original assignment at birth, or allow for ambiguity until the child expresses their own gender identification. The birth certificate may pose a problem if the state requires identification of sex. Cultural attitudes, parental expectations, and the extent of family support influence the family's response to the child and the decision-making process related to sex assignment and surgical correction. If corrective surgery is immediately decided upon, then typical surgical concerns for newborns will need to be addressed.

In general, laypeople do not understand adrenal function and what this diagnosis may mean to the family. Provide families with privacy to discuss these issues, and offer emotional support. When referring to infants, use terms such as "your baby" instead of the pronouns "he," "she," or "it," and describe the genitals as "sex organs" instead of "penis" or "clitoris." Refer families to the CARES Foundation (Congenital Adrenal Hyperplasia Research, Education, and Support) and the Magic Foundation, for additional support and resources. Local parent-to-parent support groups are also helpful.

POLYCYSTIC OVARY SYNDROME

Polycystic ovary syndrome (PCOS), also referred to as functional ovarian hyperandrogenism or ovarian androgen excess, is an endocrine disorder that produces a variety of symptoms in adolescent and adult females. The exact cause is unknown. Testosterone production by the ovaries and adrenal cells is excessive, causing hirsutism, balding, topical treatment resistant acne, increased muscle mass, and decreased breast size. Polycystic ovaries may or may not be present.

Complications of excess androgen production in females include infertility, insulin resistance, and hyperinsulinemia, leading to DM, increased risk for endometrial carcinoma, and cardiovascular disease (Shaw & Rosenfield, 2022). Therapeutic management involves the administration of oral contraceptives for their hormonal effects, as well as insulin-sensitizing medications such as metformin (Glucophage).

Nursing Assessment

Explore the health history for oligomenorrhea (irregular, infrequent periods) or amenorrhea. Symptoms typically emerge at or soon after puberty but often go undiagnosed. Note weight in relation to standardized growth charts, and calculate body mass index (BMI) to determine if overweight or higher weight is present. Inspect the skin for acne, acanthosis nigricans (darkened, thickened pigmentation, particularly around the neck or in the axillary region), and hirsutism (excess body hair growth). Assist with collection of timed blood specimens for glucose and insulin levels (which will often show unexpectedly elevated insulin levels in relation to the glucose level). Laboratory tests may show elevated levels of free testosterone and other androgenic hormones.

Nursing Management

One of the most important functions of the nurse in relation to PCOS is to assist with early recognition and treatment. Educate the adolescent about the use of oral contraceptives to normalize hormone levels, which will decrease androgenic effects. Support the adolescent in their efforts to develop nutrition and physical activity habits to maintain a healthy weight. Oral insulin-sensitizing drugs such as metformin (Glucophage) may be prescribed. Encourage the adolescent to comply with the medication regimen. Routinely measure weight to determine progress with weight loss. Monitor blood pressure to screen for hypertension, which may develop as a complication of PCOS. Also, online support groups and education resources are available.

DIABETES MELLITUS

DM is a common chronic disease seen in children and adolescents. In DM, carbohydrate, protein, and lipid metabolism are impaired. The cardinal feature of DM is hyperglycemia. The major forms of diabetes are classified as follows:

- Type 1, which is caused by a deficiency of insulin secretion due to pancreatic beta-cell damage
- Type 2, which is a consequence of insulin resistance that occurs at the level of skeletal muscle, liver, and adipose tissue with different degrees of beta-cell impairment (Weber & Jospe, 2020)
- Other types of diabetes secondary to certain conditions such as cystic fibrosis, glucocorticoid use (as in Cushing syndrome), infections, autoimmune syndromes, and certain genetic syndromes such as Down syndrome, Klinefelter syndrome, and Turner syndrome (Weber & Jospe, 2020)
- Gestational diabetes (diabetes during pregnancy)

The discussion for this chapter will focus on type 1 and type 2 diabetes as these are the most common types seen in children.

Every year, approximately 18,000 children and adolescents are diagnosed with type 1 DM and approximately 5,700 with type 2 DM (CDC, 2020). Historically, diabetes in childhood was assumed to be type 1, and type 2 DM occurred mostly in adults. However, in recent years, type 2 DM has been reported in U.S. children and adolescents at an increasing rate (American Diabetes Association Professional Practice Committee, 2022). This increase in incidence of type 2 DM among children and adolescents can be attributed to factors such as increasing rates of higher weight and decreased physical activity in young people, as well as exposure to diabetes in utero. Many children with type 2 diabetes have a family history of the condition or are overweight. See the Healthy People 2030 box.

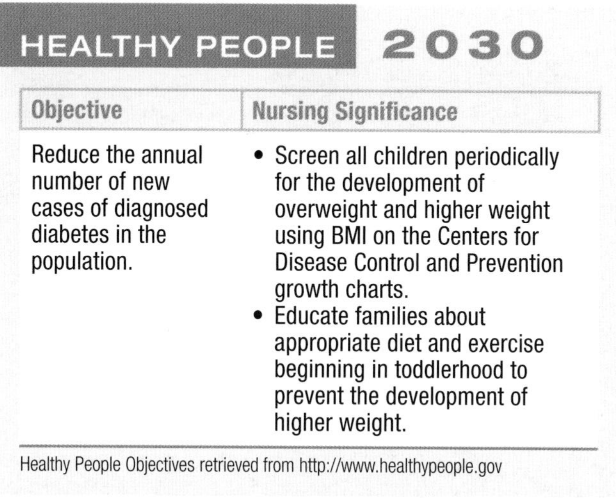
HEALTHY PEOPLE 2030

Objective	Nursing Significance
Reduce the annual number of new cases of diagnosed diabetes in the population.	• Screen all children periodically for the development of overweight and higher weight using BMI on the Centers for Disease Control and Prevention growth charts. • Educate families about appropriate diet and exercise beginning in toddlerhood to prevent the development of higher weight.

Healthy People Objectives retrieved from http://www.healthypeople.gov

Care of children with diabetes differs from that of adults due to physiologic and developmental differences. In children, insulin sensitivity varies as the child grows and goes through sexual maturation. Children are dependent on others for their care, and self-management ability varies among children based on factors such as age, developmental level, and unique differences. Care will be needed in a variety of settings, such as schools, daycares, and extracurricular activities. Therefore, teaching and education will need to involve parents and other caregivers throughout childhood and adolescence. Refer to Table 26.4, which discusses developmental issues related to DM.

Pathophysiology

Type 1 DM is an autoimmune disorder that occurs in genetically susceptible people who may also be exposed to one of several environmental or acquired factors, such as chemicals, viruses, or other toxic agents implicated in the development process. As the genetically susceptible person is exposed to environmental factors, the immune system begins a T lymphocyte–mediated process that damages and destroys the beta cells of the pancreas, resulting in inadequate insulin secretion. This deficiency of insulin leads to an inability of cells to take up glucose, resulting in hyperglycemia, glucose accumulation in the blood, and the body's inability to use its main source of fuel efficiently. The kidneys try to lower blood glucose, resulting in glycosuria and polyuria, and protein and fat are broken down for energy. The metabolism of fat leads to a buildup of ketones and acidosis (see discussion of DKA that follows).

TABLE 26.4 • Developmental Issues Related to Diabetes Mellitus

Age Group	Child and Family Implications	Nursing Implications
Infants	Management falls on parents or caregivers. Infant is unable to communicate hypo/hyperglycemic symptoms; signs and symptoms are sometimes difficult to assess. Increased risk of hypoglycemia due to inconsistent feeding times and amounts. Developing brain may experience adverse consequences to severe hypo/hyperglycemia.	Prevent extreme fluctuations in blood glucose. Prevent hypoglycemia and, if present, treat promptly. Attempt to achieve consistent dietary intake. Establish rituals/routines with home management. Provide support for parents and caregivers.
Toddlers	Management falls on parents or caregivers. Increased risk of hypoglycemia due to inconsistent food intake (picky eaters). Developing brain may experience adverse consequences to severe hypo/hyperglycemia. Discipline and temper tantrums common in this age group; may be hard to distinguish between normal toddler behavior and hypoglycemia symptoms. Parents may be overcautious and hinder child's ability to explore and develop normally.	Prevent hypoglycemia and, if present, treat promptly. Assist parents in managing a picky eater. Let toddler choose foods. Get toddler to find a word or phrase to use to describe feelings when hypoglycemic. Help parents provide appropriate discipline and protection while continuing to promote normal development. Establish rituals and routines with home management.
Preschoolers	Increased motor maturity. Widening social circle, so the child will notice that they are "different." Magical thinking presents some issues. Developing brain may experience more adverse consequences to severe hypo/hyperglycemia than older children. Preschooler wants to be an active participant in diabetes care but may lack some of the developmental skills (such as fine motor and cognitive skills). Some children can begin to perform blood glucose testing with the newer devices. Increased risk of hypoglycemia due to varied food intake and activity	Prevent hypoglycemia and if present, treat promptly. Use simple explanations and play therapy when instructing or preparing for a procedure. Encourage the child's participation as appropriate.
School-age children	Can begin to participate in more of the daily diabetes care; may be able to perform self-monitoring blood glucose testing, record glucose levels, choose injection sites and give injections, perform ketone testing, count carbohydrates, recognize need to eat, and treat for hypoglycemia. Begin to rely on others (such as school nurse, child care provider, preschool teacher) to provide diabetes care. Children may feel different from their peers and struggle socially. Must incorporate management into school day and plan for field trips.	Use concise and concrete terms when instructing. Allow the child to proceed at their own rate. Assist the family with incorporating the testing and injections into school day and plan for field trips. Involve the school nurse in helping with the school plan. Encourage the child's participation but emphasize importance of continued adult supervision. Encourage regular attendance at school and participation in extracurricular activities. Assist in the development of a care schedule that is flexible enough to allow for participation in school activities. Assist with education of other care providers as needed.
Adolescents	Undergoing rapid physical, emotional, and cognitive growth. Working toward separate identity from parents and the demands of diabetes care can hinder this. This struggle for independence can lead to nonadherence of diabetes care regimen. Conflicts develop with self-management, body image, and peer group acceptance. They acquire the skills to perform tasks related to diabetes care but may lack decision-making skills needed to adjust treatment plan. Adolescents do not always foresee the consequences of their activity.	Slowly, care is turned over to the adolescent with minor supervision from the family. Encourage parents and adolescent to find the right balance of shared management. Encourage parents to continue to provide guidance and supervision and be actively involved in the plan of care. Assess adherence to diabetes care regimen. Assess for signs and symptoms of depression, eating disorders, or evidence of risky behaviors. In later adolescence, assist the adolescent in transitioning to independent self-management and adult diabetes health care provider or nurse practitioner.

In type 2 DM, the pancreas usually produces insulin, but the body is resistant to the insulin or there is an inadequate insulin secretion response (the body can produce insulin but not enough to meet the body's needs). Eventually, insulin production decreases (resulting from the pancreas working overtime to produce insulin), with a result similar to type 1 DM.

If DM goes unrecognized or is inadequately treated (especially type 1 DM), **diabetic ketoacidosis (DKA)** or fat catabolism develops (a deficiency or ineffectiveness of insulin results in the body using fat instead of glucose for energy), resulting in anorexia, nausea and vomiting, lethargy, stupor, altered level of consciousness, confusion, decreased skin turgor, abdominal pain, Kussmaul respirations and air hunger, fruity (sweet-smelling) or acetone breath odor, presence of ketones in urine and blood, tachycardia, and, if left untreated, coma and death.

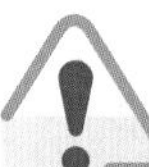

CLINICAL REASONING ALERT!

DKA is a medical emergency. It requires early recognition and prompt intervention. Be alert to the increased chance of DKA during times of stress, such as illness, infection, and surgery, as hormones produced by the body in times of stress result in decreased insulin sensitivity and increased glucose production.

Prolonged exposure to high blood glucose levels results in damage to blood vessels and nerves. Long-term complications of DM include failure to grow, delayed sexual maturation, poor wound healing, recurrent infections (especially of the skin), retinopathy, neuropathy, vascular complications, nephropathy, cerebrovascular disease, peripheral vascular disease, and cardiovascular disease. Consistent, well-controlled blood glucose levels can prevent these complications from developing for many years. On the other hand, poorly controlled DM can lead to complications much earlier.

Therapeutic Management

Treatment for DM must occur as part of a multidisciplinary health care team, with the family and child as a central part of that team. In the past, children would be admitted to the hospital for 3 to 5 days for stabilization and education, but today the trend is toward treating children on an outpatient basis. Established glucose control is essential in reducing the risk of long-term complications associated with DM. Therefore, general goals for therapeutic management include the following:

- Achieving normal growth and development
- Promoting optimal serum glucose control, including fluid and electrolyte levels and near-normal **hemoglobin A1C** (glycosylated hemoglobin, which is hemoglobin that glucose is bound to, a measure of long-term control of blood glucose and diabetes) levels
- Preventing complications
- Promoting positive adjustment to the disease, with ability to self-manage in the home

The key to success is educating the child and family so they can self-manage this chronic condition. Therapeutic management involves blood glucose monitoring, daily insulin injections or administration of oral hypoglycemic medications, following a realistic and well-balanced diet, participating in an exercise program, and developing self-management and decision-making skills.

Research is ongoing to develop alternative medications, including alternative routes for insulin administration and therapies to monitor and treat diabetes.

Monitoring Glycemic Control

Maintain consistent glycemic control leads to fewer long-term diabetes-related complications. Two important methods for monitoring glycemic control include blood glucose monitoring and monitoring hemoglobin A1C (HgbA1C) levels.

BLOOD GLUCOSE MONITORING

Blood glucose monitoring evaluates short-term glycemic control. It allows for tight glucose control because supplemental insulin can be used to correct or prevent hyperglycemia; it also enables children and their parents and their health care providers or nurse practitioners to provide better management of the disease (refer to Common Laboratory and Diagnostic Tests 26.1). The frequency of blood glucose monitoring is based on the individual goals. Children hospitalized for management of their DM or on insulin therapy require blood glucose monitoring before meals and at bedtime, if not more frequently. Additional glucose checks may be necessary if glycemic control has not occurred, during times of illness, during episodes of hypoglycemic or hyperglycemic symptoms, or when there are changes in therapy. Children receiving noninsulin therapy may check their blood glucose levels less frequently, but it can remain a useful guide to their therapy and its effectiveness. The procedure for blood glucose monitoring will vary based on the equipment used but often involves a fingerstick, a reagent strip, and a glucometer.

SMBG at home is essential to improve glycemic control, to provide self-management of this disease, and to help prevent complications such as severe hypoglycemia or hyperglycemia. The child and caregiver need to be aware of the importance of checking blood glucose regularly, and more frequently when needed. Documenting blood glucose values is necessary to provide information on glucose control. This allows their health care provider or nurse practitioner to evaluate the effectiveness of their treatment regimen. Accuracy of SMBG is dependent on proper user technique; therefore, assessment of technique and education reinforcement are important at each visit (see Teaching Guidelines 26.2).

Real-time continuous glucose monitoring should be considered for children with type 1 diabetes. This may be helpful in children with hypoglycemic unawareness or frequent hypoglycemic episodes. A sensor is placed under the skin that measures interstitial glucose. These systems provide valuable information regarding glycemic control. For example, time in range, which is the time in the past 14 days that the child's blood glucose was in the desired range, correlates well with HgbA1C. Additionally, some monitors can provide an estimated HgbA1C (Levitsky & Misra, 2023b).

MONITORING HEMOGLOBIN A1C LEVELS

Hemoglobin A1C (HgbA1C) provides the health care provider or nurse practitioner with information regarding

TEACHING GUIDELINES 26.2 Blood Glucose Monitoring

- Obtain blood glucose levels multiple times daily (up to 6–10 times per day by blood glucose meter or continuous glucose monitoring), including before meals and snacks, at bedtime, and as needed for safety in specific situations such as exercise, driving, or the presence of symptoms of hypoglycemia.
- Perform monitoring more often during prolonged exercise, if you are ill, if you have eaten more food than usual, or if you suspect nighttime hypoglycemia.
- Use the manufacturer's recommendations and perform quality control measures as directed.
- Look for patterns. For example, 3–4 days of a consistent pattern of glucose values above 200 mg/dL before dinner indicates a need to adjust the insulin dose.
- Blood glucose measurements are the best way to determine daily insulin dosages.
- Normal levels are as follows: for children without diabetes: 70–110 mg/dL; target levels should be individualized; time in range is considered 70–180 mg/dL, time below target is <70 mg/dL, time above target is 180 mg/dL.

(American Diabetes Association Professional Practice Committee, 2022).

the long-term control of glucose levels (refer to Common Laboratory and Diagnostic Tests 26.1). In children, especially infants and children younger than 6 years, hypoglycemia poses some unique risks and can be hard to recognize. Therefore, the HgbA1C goals in children need to take into account the risks of severe hypoglycemia, and glycemic control goals need to be individualized (American Diabetes Association Professional Practice Committee, 2022) However, recent data have shown that lower HgbA1C levels lead to reduced long-term complications; therefore, the targets for HgbA1C in children have become lower in recent years. Currently, the American Diabetes Association Professional Practice Committee (2022) recommends that children and adolescents have a target HgbA1C lower than 7.0%.

Insulin Replacement Therapy

Insulin replacement therapy is the cornerstone of management of type 1 DM. Insulin is administered daily by subcutaneous injections into adipose tissue over large muscle masses using a traditional insulin syringe or a subcutaneous injector (Fig. 26.7). U-100 insulin may also be administered using a portable insulin pump (see discussion later). The frequency, dose, and type of insulin are based on how much the child needs to achieve a normal, average blood glucose concentration and to prevent hypoglycemia. Typically, two to four daily injections are commonly used, with dosage depending on the needs of the child. The dose may need to be increased during the pubertal growth spurt, as well as during times of illness or stress.

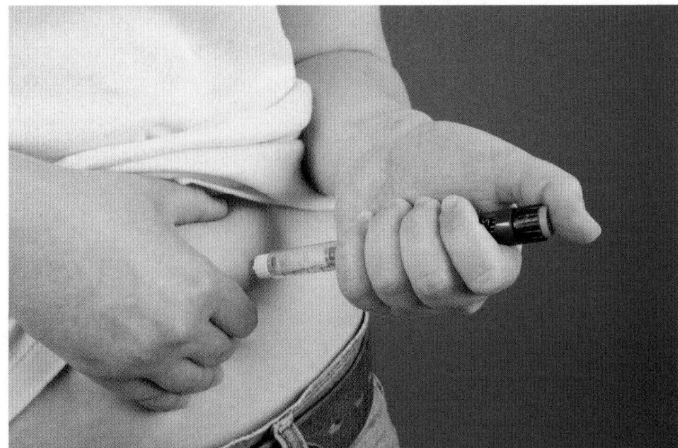

FIGURE 26.7 The subcutaneous injector uses pressure jets to deliver insulin safely and accurately.

An insulin pump is a device that administers a continuous infusion of rapid-acting insulin. It consists of a computer, a reservoir of rapid-acting insulin, thin tubing through which the insulin is delivered, and a small needle inserted into the abdomen. Insulin pumps attempt to mimic the physiologic insulin release by delivering small continuous infusions of insulin with additional bolus units administered at mealtimes, for planned carbohydrate intake, and if glucose testing results show it is needed. Many insulin pumps have a built-in sensor to monitor blood glucose continuously. Advantages of this kind of therapy include the following:

- There are fewer injections and less trauma.
- Children's food intake can be unpredictable, so insulin delivery can occur after a meal and be adjusted based on actual intake.
- Children can be sensitive to insulin and require only minute doses, which the pump can deliver with precision.
- The pumps can store different basal rates for different times during the day and days of the week. For example, a higher basal rate may be needed in the morning when the child is sitting at their desk and a lower rate may be necessary during the afternoon when the child is more active with recess and physical education classes. In addition, rates can be programmed differently for school days versus weekend days, when the child may sleep later and have differing activity levels.

The use of an insulin pump does require a commitment from the child and caregiver to achieve success and improved glycemic control. The child and caregiver must be able to count carbohydrates, monitor glucose levels frequently, and work closely with the health care provider or nurse practitioner.

TAKE NOTE!

Hybrid closed loop systems (artificial pancreas) will automatically decrease, increase, or stop insulin delivery in response to readings from the continuous glucose monitor. Studies have found these systems to improve glycemic control and decrease hypoglycemic episodes. More advanced closed loop systems are in development (Levitsky & Misra, 2023c).

Types of insulin include ultra rapid-acting, rapid-acting, short-acting, intermediate-acting, and long-acting (Table 26.5). Each type works at a different pace, and most children will use more than one type. Neutral protamine Hagedorn (NPH) and regular insulin are no longer recommended in the routine care of children with type 1 diabetes, but in some cases, premixed combinations of intermediate-acting and short- or rapid-acting, such as 70% NPH and 30% regular, may be used (Levitsky & Misra, 2023c). Again, this depends on the needs of the child. Insulin can be kept at room temperature (insulin that is administered cold may increase discomfort with injection) but should be discarded 1 month after opening even if refrigerated. Any extra, unopened vials should be stored in the refrigerator.

TAKE NOTE!

Do not mix long-acting insulin with other insulins.

TAKE NOTE!

New insulins, including orally absorbed or inhaled insulin, are being developed (Levitsky & Misra, 2023c).

Oral Diabetes Medications

Oral diabetes medications, also referred to as hypoglycemic, antidiabetic, or antihyperglycemic medications, are used in type 2 diabetes if glycemic control cannot be achieved by diet and exercise. The largest clinical trial to date, the Treatment Options for Type 2 Diabetes in Adolescents and Youth (TODAY) study, found that monotherapy with oral diabetes medication did not result in lasting glycemic control in the majority of youth with type 2 diabetes (Laffel & Svoren, 2023). Therefore, children and adolescents with type 2 diabetes need a combination of nonpharmacologic and pharmacologic interventions along with close monitoring and follow-up.

Oral diabetes medications work in a variety of ways. Metformin is the first line of therapy (Laffel & Svoren, 2023). It is an example of a biguanide and is an effective initial therapy unless significant liver or kidney impairment is present. It works by reducing glucose production from the liver and makes the body more sensitive to insulin by increasing insulin-mediated glucose uptake.

Common adverse effects of oral diabetes medications include headache, dizziness, flatulence and GI distress, edema, and liver enzyme elevation. If the oral hypoglycemics fail to maintain a normal glucose level, then insulin injections will be required to manage type 2 diabetes.

Diet and Exercise

Other therapies involve diet and exercise protocols. Medical nutritional therapy (MNT) can be initiated to prevent type 2 diabetes in children showing signs of prediabetes, to help glycemic control in existing diabetes, and to help

TABLE 26.5 Insulin Type, Action, and Duration

Type	Generic (Brand) Name	Onset	Peak	Duration (hours)
Ultra-rapid-acting	Faster aspart Insulin lispro-aabc	6–12 minutes	1–3 hours	3–5
Rapid-acting	Aspart (NovoLog) Lispro (Humalog) Glulisine (Apidra)	Within 15–20 minutes	1–3 hours	3–5
Short-acting	Regular (Humulin R, Novolin R)	0.5–1 hour	2–4 hours	5–8
Intermediate-acting	NPH (Humulin N, Novolin N)	2–4 hours	4–12 hours	12–24
Basal long-acting	Glargine (Lantus) Detemir (Levemir) Glargine 300U Degludec (Tresiba)	2–4 hours 1–2 hours 2–6 hours 0.5–1.5 hours	8–12 hours 4–7 hours None None	22–24 20–24 30–36>42

NPH, neutral protamine Hagedorn

Data from Levitsky, L. L., & Misra, M. (2023c). Insulin therapy for children and adolescents with type 1 diabetes mellitus. *UpToDate*. Retrieved May 23, 2023, from https://www.uptodate.com/contents/insulin-therapy-for-children-and-adolescents-with-type-1-diabetes-mellitus

slow the development of complications associated with diabetes. MNT can be complex and must be individualized to each child, incorporating the child's food preferences, activity level, cultural preferences, and family habits and schedule. Enlisting the help of a registered dietician who has expertise in diabetes management is recommended (American Diabetes Association Professional Practice Committee, 2022).

The appropriate diet for a child or adolescent with diabetes is a balanced, healthy diet that meets the child's growth and development needs. The child and family need to understand the effect that food has on the child's glucose levels. Monitoring carbohydrate intake is an important component of diet management and assists with glycemic control. Nutritional recommendations for a child with diabetes or prediabetes include the following: limit sweets, ensure consistent food intake (eat often and try to avoid skipping meals), monitor carbohydrate intake, eat whole grains and plenty of fruits and vegetables, and limit fat (Gray & Threlkeld, 2019).

It has been shown that regular exercise can improve glycemic control and can prevent the development of type 2 diabetes (American Diabetes Association Professional Practice Committee, 2022). Also, exercise has an important influence on the hypoglycemic effects of insulin (by causing the release of glucagon, which will result in increased blood glucose). Therefore, it is important for the child to maintain or increase their activity levels. Exercise can lead to both hyperglycemia or hypoglycemia; therefore, frequent glucose monitoring before, during, and after exercise is important (American Diabetes Association Professional Practice Committee, 2022). If the child is taking insulin, the family must know how to adjust the medication dosage or add food to maintain blood glucose control. The child needs to have access to rapid-acting carbohydrates, and the child and family should ensure preexercise blood glucose levels of 126 to 180 mg/dL (exact recommendations should be individualized based on the child and the activity) (American Diabetes Association Professional Practice Committee, 2022). Children with type 2 diabetes often are overweight, so the exercise plan is very important in helping the child to lose weight, as well as assisting with the hypoglycemic effects of the medications.

THINKING ABOUT **DEVELOPMENT**

Jayda Jones, a 12-year-old, is recently diagnosed with type 2 diabetes.

Based on her developmental age, how will you instruct her and her caregivers on ways to manage her diabetes at home?

How would your instructions change if she was 16 years old?

Management of Complications

Another important aspect of therapeutic management includes monitoring and managing complications. The American Diabetes Association Professional Practice Committee (2022) has developed recommendations for standards of medical care to help monitor complications and reduce risk. These include the following:

- Retinopathy:
  - Type 1 diabetes: eye examination by ophthalmologist (with expertise in diabetes) once the child is 11 years old or puberty has started (whichever is earlier) and has had diabetes for 3 to 5 years; eye examinations every 2 years unless different recommendation by professional
  - Type 2 diabetes: eye examination by ophthalmologist (with expertise in diabetes) shortly after diagnosis; annual examinations unless different recommendation by professional
- Nephropathy:
  - Type 1 diabetes: annual screening for microalbuminuria (which occurs when the kidneys leak small amounts of albumin into the urine) once the child is 10 years old or puberty has started (whichever is earlier) and has had diabetes for 5 years; if normal then annually
  - Type 2 diabetes: screen at diagnosis and annually thereafter for microalbuminuria
- Neuropathy:
  - Type 1 diabetes: annual foot examination once the child has reached puberty or is 10 years or older (whichever is earlier) and has had diabetes for 5 years, then annually
  - Type 2 diabetes: foot examination at diagnosis and annually
- Dyslipidemia:
  - Type 1 diabetes: Obtain a lipid profile in children above 2 years old at the time of diagnosis (once glucose levels have been stabilized); if normal, repeat at 9 to 11 years of age, and then repeat every 3 years.
  - Type 2 diabetes: Obtain a fasting lipid panel at diagnosis (once glucose levels have been stabilized), then annually.
- Hypertension: blood pressure measured at each routine visit
- In addition, children with type 1 diabetes should be screened for additional autoimmune disorders such as celiac disease (screen after diagnosis and then after 2 years, and again after 5 years, screen more often if symptoms or family history are present) and hypothyroidism (screen after diagnosis, and every 1 to 2 years or sooner if symptoms are present). Children with type 2 diabetes should be screened for nonalcoholic fatty liver disease at diagnosis and annually, and obstructive sleep apnea and PCOS at diagnosis and every visit.

EVIDENCE-BASED PRACTICE **26.1**

What is the Prevalence of Diabetes-Specific Eating Disorder (DSED) in Adolescents With Type 1 Diabetes and Are There Associated Psychopathologies, Such as Anxiety and Depression?

STUDY

Adolescents with type 1 diabetes are at an increased risk for eating disorders and disturbed eating behaviors (DEBs) such as fasting, extreme dieting, binge eating, and omitting or underdosing insulin to cause weight loss (newly referred to as diabulimia). This may be linked to the constant focus on food and its effect on blood glucose and the weight gain related to insulin. This study used cross-sectional data of 92 adolescents aged 12 to 18 years with type 1 diabetes for at least 1 year. It evaluated the frequency of DSED risk and its relationship with metabolic, anthropometric, and socio-demographic parameters and parenting styles, as well as accompanying psychopathologies. The Diabetes Eating Problem Survey-Revised (DEPS-R) was used to determine the risk of DSED along with the Eating Disorder Examination Questionnaire (EDE-Q), Child Anxiety and Depression Scale—Child version, and Parenting Style Scale to help detect if accompanying psychopathologies were present.

In this study, 23.9% of adolescents were found to be at risk for DSED. A weak correlation was found between a higher risk of DSED and higher HgbA1C levels. DEPS-R scores were higher in adolescents with increased BMI. Adolescents with divorced parents were more likely to have DSED, and anxiety and depression scores were higher in adolescents who had a positive DEPS-R.

Nursing Implications

DEBs often are not recognized by clinicians and parents, but the risk of DEBs and eating disorders remains high in children with type 1 diabetes. This study supports the importance of routinely screening people at risk and referring them to child psychiatry services. The American Diabetes Association Professional Practice Committee (2022) recommends screening children with type 1 diabetes for eating disorders beginning between 10 and 12 years of age. The DEPS-R is a reliable, valid, and short screening tool (American Diabetes Association Professional Practice Committee, 2022).

Data from Tarçın, G., Akman, H., Güneş Kaya, D., Serdengeçti, N., İncetahtacı, S., Turan, H., Doğangün, B., & Ercan, O. (2023). Diabetes-specific eating disorder and possible associated psychopathologies in adolescents with type 1 diabetes mellitus. *Eating and Weight Disorders: EWD, 28*(1), 36. https://doi.org/10.1007/s40519-023-01559-y

- Assess for psychosocial and diabetes-related distress generally starting around 7 to 8 years old.
- Screen for eating disorders starting at 10 to 12 years old. Refer to Evidence-Based Practice 26.1.

Nursing Assessment

Assessment involves understanding the everchanging needs of children as they grow and develop. The first phase of assessment involves identifying children who may have diabetes. The second phase involves recognizing problems that may develop in children with diabetes. It is important to always be aware of this when observing for possible complications or management problems. In addition, always be alert for opportunities to provide education that will enhance the understanding and skills related to managing of DM for both the child and the family.

Health History and Physical Examination

During the initial diagnosis of DM, obtain a detailed family history and inquire about any school-related issues that may indicate mental and behavioral changes associated with hyperglycemic state (e.g., weakness, fatigue, mood changes). The child or parent may report unusual or excessive thirst (polydipsia) coupled with frequent urination (polyuria). The child may also complain of blurred vision, headaches, or bedwetting. The child with type 1 diabetes may have a history of poor growth. Comparison Chart 26.3 gives information about common history and physical examination findings in children with type 1 diabetes versus type 2 diabetes.

In a child known to have diabetes, the health history should include any problems related to hyperglycemia or hypoglycemia, dietary habits, activity and exercise patterns, types of medications (insulin or oral diabetes medications) and dose and times of administration, ability to monitor blood glucose levels, and ability to administer insulin. Perform a thorough physical examination, noting any abnormal findings.

Laboratory and Diagnostic Testing

Refer to Common Laboratory and Diagnostic Tests 26.1. A fasting glucose level equal to or greater than 126 mg/dL, a 2-hour plasma glucose level equal to or greater than 200 mg/dL during an oral glucose tolerance test, a random glucose level equal to or greater than 200 mg/dL (accompanied by typical symptoms of diabetes), or a HgbA1C greater than 6.5% are laboratory criteria for the diagnosis of DM (Levitsky & Misra, 2023a). For each of these tests, if hyperglycemia is not explicit, the results should be confirmed with a repeat test on a different day (Levitsky & Misra, 2023a). Other laboratory and diagnostic tests include serum measurements of islet cell antibodies, urea nitrogen, creatinine, calcium, magnesium, phosphate, and electrolytes such as potassium and sodium. Additional tests include a complete blood count, urinalysis, and immunoassay to measure levels of C-peptides after a glucose challenge to verify endogenous insulin secretion.

The American Diabetes Association Professional Practice Committee (2022) recommends screening for type 2 DM if a child presents with overweight or higher

COMPARISON CHART 26.3 Type 1 Versus Type 2 Diabetes Mellitus

History and Physical Findings Usually Present at Diagnosis	Type 1	Type 2
Family history	Less tendency than type 2	Yes
Prone ethnicity	All	Native American, African descent, Hispanic/Latino descents
Polydipsia, polyuria, polyphagia	Yes	Yes, may be mild or absent
Weight	Possibly, weight loss	Usually, higher weight
Age of onset	Usually, younger children	Usually, pubertal children
Incidental finding on screening urinalysis	Rare	Common
Antecedent flulike illness/symptoms	Common	Possible
Autoimmune antibodies	Yes	No
Diabetic ketoacidosis	Common	Possible
Hypertension	No	Common
Acanthosis nigricans	No	Common
Dyslipidemia	No	Common

Data from Weber, D. R., & Jospe, N. (2020). Chapter 607: Diabetes mellitus. In R. M. Kleigman, J. W. St. Geme III, N. J. Blum, S. S. Shah, R. C. Tasker, K. M. Wilson, & R. E. Behrman (Eds.), *Nelson textbook of pediatrics* (21st ed., pp. 15955–16147). Elsevier.

weight after the onset of puberty or at age 10 years or older, along with one of the following risk factors:

- Family history: a parent or relative with type 2 diabetes
- Ethnic background: Native American, African American, Latino, Asian American, or Pacific Islander
- Conditions associated with insulin resistance such as acanthosis nigricans, hypertension, dyslipidemia, or PCOS
- History of maternal diabetes or a birthing parent with gestational diabetes when the child was in utero (Weber & Jospe, 2020).

Nursing Management

Individualize the general nursing care discussed in the "Clinical Judgment and the Nursing Process" section earlier in the chapter, based on the child's and family's response to illness. Additional nursing care topics related to DM are discussed later, including regulating glucose control, monitoring for complications, providing education to the child and family, and offering support to both the child and family.

Regulating Glucose Control

Consistent and established glucose control can reduce the risk of long-term complications associated with diabetes. Therefore, regulating glucose is an important nursing function.

Typically, in children with type 1 diabetes and sometimes in cases of type 2 diabetes, glucose is regulated by subcutaneous insulin via injection or insulin pump. Often, the regimen consists of three injections of intermediate-acting insulin, with the addition of rapid-acting insulin before breakfast and dinner, or three injections of short-acting insulin with a long-acting injection at bedtime. Insulin doses are typically ordered on a sliding scale related to the serum glucose level and how the insulin works. Insulin doses and frequency are based on the needs of the child, utilizing information gained from blood glucose testing. Regulating glucose can be challenging in children due to continual growth, onset of puberty, varying activity levels with unpredictable schedules, unpredictable eating habits, and the inability to always verbalize the way they are feeling. Thus, close monitoring of changing glucose levels through SMBG is essential in determining adjustments needed in insulin therapy, food intake, and activity levels. Adjustment of insulin dosing based on carbohydrate intake is essential for managing blood glucose levels. The use of carbohydrate counting can help children enjoy more freedom to choose their type or amount of food and allow them to vary their mealtime and snack times. It allows them to predict the rise in blood glucose that will occur after eating a specific amount or type of carbohydrate and take into account recent or expected activity levels. It requires knowledge of carbohydrate amounts and calculations with each dose of short-acting insulin. Each scale will vary per child as the insulin per carbohydrate serving is calculated based on the child's specific requirement. See the Dosage Calculation Question under Developing Clinical Judgment at the end of the chapter for an example. Parents will need extensive education and continual follow-up to ensure the successful use of this method.

TAKE NOTE!

Blood glucose level should never be the only factor considered when calculating insulin dosing. Food intake and recent or expected activity/exercise must also be factored.

Teach the child and family to use proper subcutaneous injection techniques to avoid injecting into muscle or vascular spaces. Figure 26.8 shows appropriate sites for subcutaneous injection of insulin. Teach the child and family to rotate sites to avoid adipose hypertrophy (fatty lumps that absorb insulin poorly). If the child is using an insulin pump, additional education will be needed.

• • • ATRAUMATIC CARE • • •

Children with diabetes experience numerous finger pricks and injections. Providing atraumatic care remains important. Allow the child to choose the prick or injection site when possible. Use positioning that is comforting to the child. Encourage participation in care as developmentally appropriate.

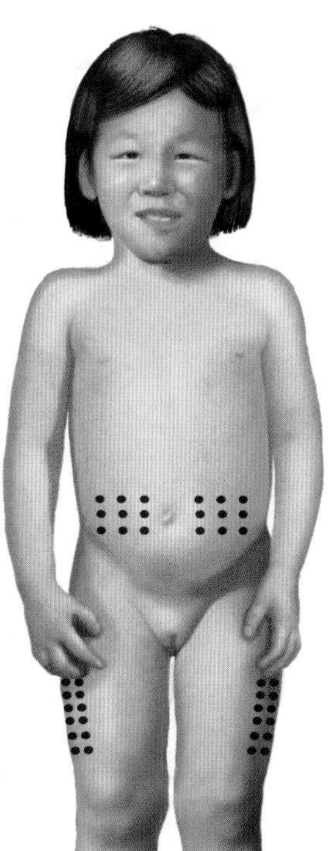

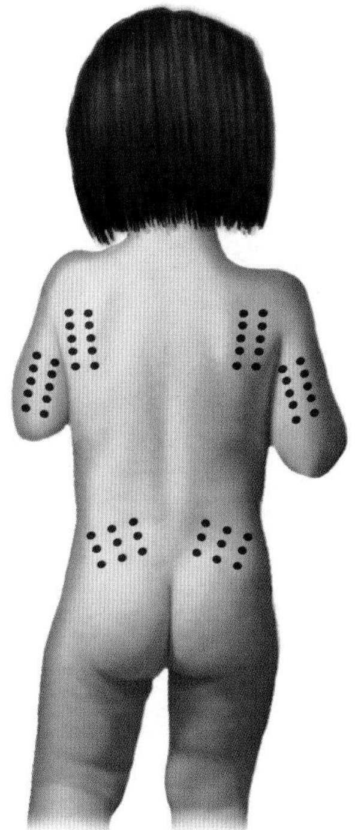

FIGURE 26.8 Insulin injection sites.

In children with type 2 diabetes, glucose levels can be controlled by diet, exercise, oral diabetes medications, or a combination of all three.

Monitoring for and Managing Complications

While the child is in the hospital, monitor for signs of complications such as acidosis, coma, hyperkalemia, hypokalemia, hypocalcemia, cerebral edema, or hyponatremia. Assess for the development of hypoglycemia or hyperglycemia every 2 hours (Comparison Chart 26.4). Monitor the child's status closely during peak times of insulin action. Perform blood glucose testing as ordered or as needed if the child develops symptoms.

COMPARISON CHART 26.4 Hypoglycemia Versus Hyperglycemia

Hypoglycemia	Hyperglycemia
Behavioral changes (tearfulness, irritability, naughtiness), confusion, slurred speech, belligerence	Mental status changes, fatigue, weakness
Diaphoresis	Dry, flushed skin
Tremors	Blurred vision
Palpitations, tachycardia	Abdominal cramping, nausea, vomiting, fruity breath odor

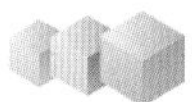
Concept Mastery Alert

Manifestations of hypoglycemia include behavioral changes, confusion, slurred speech, diaphoresis, tremors, palpitations, and tachycardia. In contrast, manifestations of hyperglycemia include blurred vision; dry, flushed skin; and a fruity odor to the breath.

If the child has a severe hypoglycemic reaction, administer glucagon (a hormone produced by the pancreas and stored in the liver) either subcutaneously or intramuscularly. Children under 20 kg receive 0.5 mg; children over 20 kg receive 1 mg (Weber & Jospe, 2020). Dextrose (50%) may be given IV if needed. If the child is not having a severe reaction and is coherent, glucose paste or tablets may be used. Offer 10 to 15 g of a simple carbohydrate, such as orange juice, if the child feels some symptoms of low blood glucose and glucose monitoring indicates a drop in blood glucose level. Follow this with a more complex carbohydrate, such as peanut butter and crackers, to maintain the glucose level.

The child with severe hyperglycemia resulting in DKA is usually treated in the pediatric intensive care unit. In the case of a child presenting with DKA to the hospital, monitor the glucose level hourly to prevent it from falling more than 100 mg/dL/h. A too-rapid decline in blood glucose predisposes the child to cerebral edema. Fluid therapy is given to treat dehydration, correct electrolyte imbalances (sodium and potassium due to osmotic diuresis), and improve peripheral perfusion. Administration of regular insulin, given IV, is preferred during DKA (only regular insulin may be given IV).

Any child exhibiting signs and symptoms of hyperglycemia requires insulin. The dosage is usually based on a sliding scale or determined after consultation with the health care provider or nurse practitioner.

TAKE NOTE!

Double check all insulin doses against the order sheet and with another nurse to ensure accuracy.

Educating the Family

Education is the priority intervention for DM because it will enable the child and family to self-manage this chronic condition. Allow the child and family time to adjust to the diagnosis of a chronic illness that will require self-management. DM is a lifelong condition that requires regular follow-up visits (three or four times a year) to a diabetes specialty clinic. Because approximately 210,000 children and adolescents younger than the age of 20 have diabetes, this becomes a health issue for the community, especially for the schools (CDC, 2020). Daily management of the child with diabetes is complex and dynamic. It will require frequent monitoring of blood glucose levels, medications (including oral diabetes medications and insulin injections), and personalized meal plans, including snacks, while the child is at school. The school nurse will be a principal contact person for both staff and family. With appropriate management, community involvement, and confidence and adherence by the family, the child can maintain a happy, productive life. See the Healthy People 2030 box.

HEALTHY PEOPLE 2030

Objective	Nursing Significance
Increase the proportion of people with diagnosed diabetes who ever receive formal diabetes education.	• Begin diabetes education with the child and family upon knowledge of diagnosis. • Use developmentally appropriate education with children. • Increase the self-management skills taught as the child progresses in age and cognitive development.

Healthy People Objectives retrieved from http://www.healthypeople.gov

Challenges related to educating children with diabetes include the following:

- Children lack the maturity to understand the long-term consequences of this serious chronic illness.
- Children do not want to be different from their peers; having to make lifestyle changes may result in anger or depression.
- Families with limited resources may not be able to afford appropriate food, medication, transportation, and telephone service.
- Families may demonstrate unhealthy behaviors, making it difficult for the child to initiate change because of the lack of supervision or role modeling.
- Family dynamics are affected because management of diabetes must occur all day, every day.

TAKE NOTE!

Children with diabetes have higher rates of depression and may have other comorbid conditions, such as eating disorders, adjustment disorders, or anxiety disorders (American Diabetes Association Professional Practice Committee, 2022; Weber & Jospe, 2020).

The initial goal of education is for the family to develop basic management and decision-making skills. Assess the family's ability to learn the basic concepts and offer psychological support. Teach about specific topics in sessions lasting 15 to 20 minutes for the children and 45 to 60 minutes for the caregivers. Teaching must be geared toward the child's level of development and understanding (see Table 26.4).

Among the topics to include when teaching children and their families about diabetes management are as follows:

- Self-measurement of blood glucose (Fig. 26.9)
- Urine ketone testing

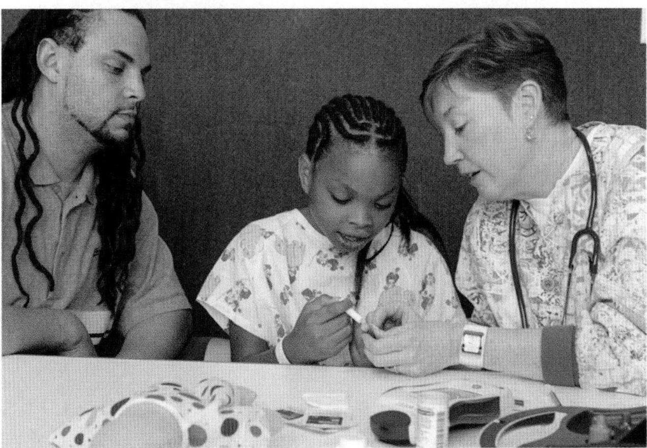

FIGURE 26.9 The school-age child has developed the psychomotor skills needed for blood glucose monitoring and insulin injection.

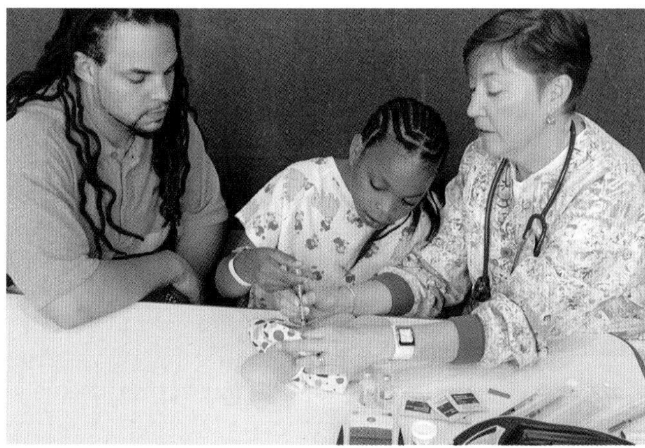

FIGURE 26.10 The school-age child may first practice insulin injections on a doll.

- Medication use (Fig. 26.10)
  - Oral diabetes agents
  - Subcutaneous insulin injection or insulin pump use
  - Subcutaneous site selection and rotation
  - When to alter insulin dosages
  - Use of glucagon to treat severe hypoglycemia
- Signs and symptoms of hypoglycemia and hyperglycemia (refer to Comparison Chart 26.4)
- Treatment for hypoglycemia and hyperglycemia at home or other setting such as school
- Monitoring for and managing complications (see earlier)
- Sick-day instructions
- Laboratory testing and follow-up care
- Diet and exercise as part of DM management (see earlier)

Teaching Guidelines 26.2 presents information to cover when teaching the family about SMBG. Teach families how to give insulin, how to use the insulin pump, and how to rotate injection sites.

Good glucose control is dependent on accurate monitoring and medication administration by the child or caregiver. Assessment of the child's or parent's technique and review of procedure and instructions should occur with each visit. Treatment of hypoglycemia and hyperglycemia may have to occur at home or in another setting such as school. In either case, someone trained to check the child's blood glucose level must be available. In the case of hypoglycemia, early recognition is key. Therefore, all caregivers need to be educated on the causes of hypoglycemia (such as increased physical activity, delayed meals or snacks, insulin, oral diabetes medication, illness, stress, and hormonal fluctuations) along with the signs and symptoms. The child also needs access to glucose tablets or a rapidly absorbing carbohydrate such as orange juice, as well as a snack with complex carbohydrates and protein within 30 to 60 minutes of the hypoglycemic episode. Injectable glucagon should be available in the case that the hypoglycemia is severe and the child is unconscious. In the event of hyperglycemia, the child needs immediate access to rapid-acting insulin injection.

Sick-day instructions may include the following:

- Contact the health care provider or nurse practitioner.
- Perform SMBG more often.
- Check for ketones in the urine, especially if blood glucose is elevated.
- Use a sliding scale to calculate the insulin dosage.

A dietitian can help the family with detailed meal planning and dietary guidelines. Review basic nutritional information with the child and family and provide sample meals. Encourage the child and family to keep a food diary. For the child who needs to lose weight, suggest low-carbohydrate snacks. Encourage all children with diabetes to incorporate physical activity daily (Teaching Guidelines 26.3).

Supporting the Child and Family

Children with diabetes and their families may have difficulty coping if they lack confidence in their self-management skills. Assess the ability of the child and family to handle situations. Role play specific situations

TEACHING GUIDELINES 26.3 Diet and Exercise for Children With Diabetes

- Provide sufficient calories and good nutrition for normal growth and development. The diet should be low in saturated fats and concentrated carbohydrates.
- Learn to identify carbohydrate, protein, and fat foods.
- Make adjustments during periods of rapid growth and for issues such as travel, school parties, and holidays.
- Consult a dietitian with expertise in diabetes education as needed.
- Provide three meals per day and midafternoon and bedtime snacks. Consistency of intake can help prevent complications and maintain near-normal blood glucose levels.
- Encourage the child to exercise routinely to help the body use insulin efficiently, thus reducing the insulin requirement.
- Encourage the child to participate in age-appropriate sports.
- When exercising, monitor insulin dose and nutritional and fluid intake, and observe for hypoglycemic reactions. Add an extra snack containing 15–30 g carbohydrate for each 45–60 minutes of exercise. Avoid exercising excessively when insulin is peaking.

related to symptoms or complications to help them see different ways to solve problems. Work with the child and family to enhance their conflict resolution skills. Provide opportunities for them to express their feelings. Observe for signs of depression, especially in adolescents.

To enhance the child's confidence and promote feelings of mastery and inclusion, refer them to a special camp for children with diabetes. Also refer families to local support groups, parent-to-parent networks, or one of many national support resources and foundations.

KEY CONCEPTS

- The endocrine system consists of cells, tissues, and glands that produce hormones (chemical messengers) and secrete them in response to a negative feedback system involving the hypothalamus and nervous system.
- Hormones (chemical messengers), along with the nervous system, play an intricate role in reproduction, growth and development, energy production and use, and maintenance of the internal homeostasis.
- The pituitary, along with the hypothalamus connection, is considered the "control center," producing hormones that stimulate many glands to produce other hormones or to inhibit the process.
- Hormonal control is immature at birth; this is partly why the infant has trouble maintaining an appropriate balance of fluid concentration, electrolytes, amino acids, glucose, and trace substances.
- Linear growth and cognitive development may be impaired by untreated endocrine dysfunction in the infant or child.
- A thorough health history of the child with a known or potential endocrine disorder often reveals poor growth, school or learning problems, and inactivity or fatigue.
- Serial measurement of growth parameters is a key part of the physical assessment for children with endocrine dysfunction.
- Close monitoring of the child's status is critical during a hormone stimulation test or water deprivation study.
- Hormone supplementation is required lifelong for many of the endocrine disorders.
- The key nursing functions related to hormone supplementation are educating the child and family about medication use and monitoring for therapeutic results and adverse effects.
- Children with adrenocortical dysfunction will require additional hormone supplementation during times of stress such as fever, infection, or surgery.
- GH deficiency is characterized by poor growth and short stature as a result of failure of the anterior pituitary to produce sufficient GH. Early treatment enables the child to reach normal growth.
- Precocious puberty involves early development of secondary sex characteristics as a result of premature activation of the hypothalamic–pituitary–gonadal axis.
- AVP-D is characterized by water intoxication as a result of a deficiency in the ADH that leads to the cardinal signs of polyuria and polydipsia, resulting in hypernatremic dehydration.
- Key findings in congenital hypothyroidism are a thickened protuberant tongue, an enlarged posterior fontanel, feeding difficulties, hypotonia, and lethargy.
- Early diagnosis and treatment of hypothyroidism can prevent impaired growth and severe cognitive impairment.
- CAH results from a genetic defect that causes a breakdown in steroid synthesis and an overproduction of androgens that can lead to ambiguous genitalia in females.
- DM is the most common endocrine disorder now seen in children.
- Type 1 DM is an autoimmune disorder resulting from damage and destruction of the beta cells in the islets of Langerhans in the pancreas; the end result is insulin insufficiency. Peak onset occurs in childhood.
- Type 2 DM results in an insensitivity or resistance to insulin. The incidence of type 2 DM has risen dramatically. It is occurring at an alarming rate in children, especially in those with higher weight and those from certain ethnicity.
- DKA is a medical emergency. The child will usually be admitted to a pediatric intensive care unit.
- The focus of DM management is regulation of glucose control, which is accomplished by medications, diet, and exercise.
- DM education involves instruction in glucose monitoring, administration of insulin or oral hypoglycemics, meal planning, and promotion of a healthy lifestyle.
- Critical areas in the nursing management of children with endocrine dysfunction include maintaining appropriate nutrition and fluid balance and promoting growth and development.
- The nurse provides ongoing assessment and education of the child and family, imparting to them the knowledge and skills required for self-management.
- Encouraging the child to have a healthy body image and working with the family in establishing healthy family processes are also key nursing functions.

REFERENCES AND RECOMMENDED READINGS

American Diabetes Association Professional Practice Committee. (2022). 14. Children and adolescents: Standards of medical care in diabetes—2022. *Diabetes Care*, *45*, (Suppl._1), S208–S231. https://doi.org/10.2337/dc22-S014

Bichet, D. G. (2023). Arginine vasopressin deficiency (central diabetes insipidus): Treatment. *UpToDate*. Retrieved May 23, 2023, from https://www.uptodate.com/contents/arginine-vasopressin-deficiency-central-diabetes-insipidus-treatment

Breault, D. T., & Majzoub, J. A. (2020a). Diabetes insipidus. In R. M. Kleigman, J. W. St. Geme III, N. J. Blum, S. S. Shah, R. C. Tasker, K. M. Wilson, & R. E. Behrman (Eds.), *Nelson textbook of pediatrics* (21st ed., pp. 15266–15279). Elsevier.

Breault, D. T., & Majzoub, J. A. (2020b). Other abnormalities of arginine vasopressin metabolism and action. In R. M. Kleigman, J. W. St. Geme III, N. J. Blum, S. S. Shah, R. C. Tasker, K. M. Wilson, & R. E. Behrman (Eds.), *Nelson textbook of pediatrics* (21st ed., pp. 15280–15292). Elsevier.

Centers for Disease Control and Prevention. (2020). *National diabetes statistics report, 2020: Estimates of diabetes and its burden in the United States*. U.S. Department of Health and Human Services. https://www.cdc.gov/diabetes/pdfs/data/statistics/national-diabetes-statistics-report.pdf

Connelly, K., & LaFranchi, S. (2023a). Clinical features and detection of congenital hypothyroidism. In *UpToDate*. Retrieved May 23, 2023, from https://www.uptodate.com/contents/clinical-features-and-detection-of-congenital-hypothyroidism

Connelly, K., & LaFranchi, S. (2023b). Treatment and prognosis of congenital hypothyroidism. *UpToDate*. Retrieved May 23, 2023, from https://www.uptodate.com/contents/treatment-and-prognosis-of-congenital-hypothyroidism

Crowley, W. F., & Pitteloud, N. (2023). Approaches to the patient with delayed puberty. *UpToDate*. Retrieved May 23, 2023, from https://www.uptodate.com/contents/approach-to-the-patient-with-delayed-puberty

Doyle, D. A. (2020a). Hypoparathyroidism. In R. M. Kleigman, J. W. St. Geme III, N. J. Blum, S. S. Shah, R. C. Tasker, K. M. Wilson, & R. E. Behrman (Eds.), *Nelson textbook of pediatrics* (21st ed., pp. 15565–15579). Elsevier.

Doyle, D. A. (2020b). Hyperparathyroidism. In R. M. Kleigman, J. W. St. Geme III, N. J. Blum, S. S. Shah, R. C. Tasker, K. M. Wilson, & R. E. Behrman (Eds.), *Nelson textbook of pediatrics* (21st ed., pp. 15587–15601). Elsevier.

Fischbach, F. T., Fischbach, M. A., & Stout, K. (2022). *A manual of laboratory and diagnostic tests* (11th ed.). Wolters Kluwer.

Garibaldi, L., & Chemaitilly, W. (2020). Disorders of pubertal development. In R. M. Kleigman, J. W. St. Geme III, N. J. Blum, S. S. Shah, R. C. Tasker, K. M. Wilson, & R. E. Behrman (Eds.), *Nelson textbook of pediatrics* (21st ed., pp. 15324–15382). Elsevier.

Gray, A., & Threlkeld, R. J. (2019). Nutritional recommendations for individuals with diabetes. In K. R. Feingold, B. Anawalt, M. R. Blackman, A. Boyce, G. Chrousos, E. Corpas, W. W. de Herder, K. Dhatariya, K. Dungan, J. Hofland, S. Kalra, G. Kaltsas, N. Kapoor, C. Koch, P. Kopp, M. Korbonits, C. S. Kovacs, W. Kuohung, B. Laferrère, . . . , D. P, Wilson (Eds.), *Endotext [Internet]*. https://www.ncbi.nlm.nih.gov/books/NBK279012/

Harrington, J., & Palmert, M. R. (2022). Definition, etiology, and evaluation of precocious puberty. *UpToDate*. Retrieved May 23, 2023, from https://www.uptodate.com/contents/definition-etiology-and-evaluation-of-precocious-puberty

Kemper, A. R. (2021). Newborn screening. *UpToDate*. Retrieved May 20, 2023 from https://www.uptodate.com/contents/newborn-screening

Laffel, L., & Svoren, B. (2023). Management of type 2 diabetes mellitus in children and adolescents. *UpToDate*. Retrieved May 23, 2023, from https://www.uptodate.com/contents/management-of-type-2-diabetes-mellitus-in-children-and-adolescents

LaFranchi, S. (2022a). Acquired hypothyroidism in childhood and adolescence. *UpToDate*. Retrieved May 23, 2023, from https://www.uptodate.com/contents/acquired-hypothyroidism-in-childhood-and-adolescence

LaFranchi, S. (2022b). Clinical manifestations and diagnosis of Graves disease in children and adolescents. *UpToDate*. Retrieved May 23, 2023, from https://www.uptodate.com/contents/clinical-manifestations-and-diagnosis-of-graves-disease-in-children-and-adolescents

Levitsky, L. L., & Misra, M. (2023a). Epidemiology, presentation, and diagnosis of type 1 diabetes mellitus in children and adolescents. *UpToDate*. Retrieved May 23, 2023, from https://www.uptodate.com/contents/epidemiology-presentation-and-diagnosis-of-type-1-diabetes-mellitus-in-children-and-adolescents

Levitsky, L. L., & Misra, M. (2023b). Overview of the management of type 1 diabetes mellitus in children and adolescents. *UpToDate*. Retrieved May 23, 2023, from https://www.uptodate.com/contents/overview-of-the-management-of-type-1-diabetes-mellitus-in-children-and-adolescents

Levitsky, L. L., & Misra, M. (2023c). Insulin therapy for children and adolescents with type 1 diabetes mellitus. *UpToDate*. Retrieved May 23, 2023, from https://www.uptodate.com/contents/insulin-therapy-for-children-and-adolescents-with-type-1-diabetes-mellitus

Lexicomp. (2023). Pediatric drug information. *UpToDate*. Retrieved April 5, 2023, from https://www.uptodate.com/contents/table-of-contents/drug-information

Merke, D. P. (2022). Treatment of classic congenital adrenal hyperplasia due to 21-hydroxylase deficiency in infants and children. *UpToDate*. Retrieved May 23, 2023, from https://www.uptodate.com/contents/treatment-of-classic-congenital-adrenal-hyperplasia-due-to-21-hydroxylase-deficiency-in-infants-and-children

Merke, D. P., & Auchus, R. J. (2022). Clinical manifestations and diagnosis of classic congenital adrenal hyperplasia due to 21-hydroxylase deficiency in infants and children. *UpToDate*. Retrieved May 23, 2023, from https://www.uptodate.com/contents/clinical-manifestations-and-diagnosis-of-classic-congenital-adrenal-hyperplasia-due-to-21-hydroxylase-deficiency-in-infants-and-children?

Mutter, C. M., Smith, T., Menze, O., Zakharia, M., & Nguyen, H. (2021). Diabetes insipidus: Pathogenesis, diagnosis, and clinical management. *Cureus, 13*(2), e13523. https://doi.org/10.7759/cureus.13523

Patterson, B. C., & Felner, E. I. (2020). Hypopituitarism. In R. M. Kleigman, J. W. St. Geme III, N. J. Blum, S. S. Shah, R. C. Tasker, K. M. Wilson, & R. E. Behrman (Eds.), *Nelson textbook of pediatrics* (21st ed., pp. 15230–15265). Elsevier.

Rogol, A. D., & Richmond Padilla, E. J. (2023). Treatment of growth hormone deficiency in children. *UpToDate*. Retrieved May 22, 2023, from https://www.uptodate.com/contents/treatment-of-growth-hormone-deficiency-in-children

Shaw, N., & Rosenfield, R. L. (2022). Definition, clinical features, and differential diagnosis of polycystic ovary syndrome (PCOS) in adolescents. *UpToDate*. Retrieved May 23, 2023, from https://www.uptodate.com/contents/definition-clinical-features-and-differential-diagnosis-of-polycystic-ovary-syndrome-in-adolescents

Smith, J. R., & Wassner, A. J. (2020). Thyrotoxicosis. In R. M. Kleigman, J. W. St. Geme III, N. J. Blum, S. S. Shah, R. C. Tasker, K. M. Wilson, & R. E. Behrman (Eds.), *Nelson textbook of pediatrics* (21st ed., pp. 15478–15510). Elsevier.

Tarçın, G., Akman, H., Güneş Kaya, D., Serdengeçti, N., İncetahtacı, S., Turan, H., Doğangün, B., & Ercan, O. (2023). Diabetes-specific eating disorder and possible associated psychopathologies in adolescents with type 1 diabetes mellitus. *Eating and Weight Disorders: EWD, 28*(1), 36. https://doi.org/10.1007/s40519-023-01559-y

U.S. Department of Health and Human Services. (n.d.). *Healthy People 2030*. https://health.gov/healthypeople

Warrier, V., Krishan, K., Shedge, R., & Kanchan, T. (2022). Height assessment. In *StatPearls* [Internet]. StatPearls Publishing. https://www.ncbi.nlm.nih.gov/books/NBK551524/

Wassner, A. J., & LaFranchi, S. (2021). Treatment and prognosis of Graves disease in children and adolescents. *UpToDate*. Retrieved May 23, 2023, from https://www.uptodate.com/contents/treatment-and-prognosis-of-graves-disease-in-children-and-adolescents

Wassner, A. J., & Smith, J. R. (2020). Hypothyroidism. In R. M. Kleigman, J. W. St. Geme III, N. J. Blum, S. S. Shah, R. C. Tasker, K. M. Wilson, & R. E. Behrman (Eds.), *Nelson textbook of pediatrics* (21st ed., pp. 15401–15445). Elsevier.

Weber, D. R., & Jospe, N. (2020). Diabetes mellitus. In R. M. Kleigman, J. W. St. Geme III, N. J. Blum, S. S. Shah, R. C. Tasker, K. M. Wilson, & R. E. Behrman (Eds.), *Nelson textbook of pediatrics* (21st ed., pp. 15955–16147). Elsevier.

White, P. C. (2020a). Adrenocortical insufficiency. In R. M. Kleigman, J. W. St. Geme III, N. J. Blum, S. S. Shah, R. C. Tasker, K. M. Wilson, & R. E. Behrman (Eds.), *Nelson textbook of pediatrics* (21st ed., pp. 15636–15689). Elsevier.

White, P. C. (2020b). Congenital adrenal hyperplasia and related disorders. In R. M. Kleigman, J. W. St. Geme III, N. J. Blum, S. S. Shah, R. C. Tasker, K. M. Wilson, & R. E. Behrman (Eds.), *Nelson textbook of pediatrics* (21st ed., pp. 15690–15735). Elsevier.

White, P. C. (2020c). Cushing syndrome. In R. M. Kleigman, J. W. St. Geme III, N. J. Blum, S. S. Shah, R. C. Tasker, K. M. Wilson, & R. E. Behrman (Eds.), *Nelson textbook of pediatrics* (21st ed., pp. 15753–15766). Elsevier.

Working Group for Renaming Diabetes Insipidus, Arima, H., Cheetham, T., Christ-Crain, M., Cooper, D., Gurnell, M., Drummond, J. B., Levy, M., McCormack, A. I., Verbalis, J., Newell-Price, J., & Wass, J. A. H. (2022). Changing the name of diabetes insipidus: a position statement of The Working Group for Renaming Diabetes Insipidus. *Endocrine Connections, 11*(11), e220378. https://doi.org/10.1530/EC-22-0378

DEVELOPING CLINICAL JUDGMENT

PRACTICING FOR NCLEX

1. A young parent brings their new baby, diagnosed with congenital hypothyroidism, to the clinic so they can learn how to administer levothyroxine. The nurse should include which of the following instructions?
   a. Crush the medication and place it in a full bottle of formula to disguise the taste.
   b. Administer the medication every other day.
   c. Use an oral dispenser syringe or nipple to give the crushed medication mixed with a small amount of formula.
   d. The medication will not be needed after the age of 7.
2. During a well-child examination, which of the following comments made by the parent would indicate the possibility of a GH deficiency?
   a. "I have to buy my child new clothes every 2 to 3 months."
   b. "I have to buy my child much larger shirts than pants but then the sleeves are too long."
   c. "My child wears out their clothes before they outgrow them."
   d. "I can hand down my child's clothes to their younger brother."
3. The nurse is caring for a 14-year-old child with type 1 diabetes. The child takes Lantus insulin every morning at 7:30 a.m. Which assessment data will the nurse use to evaluate the therapeutic effectiveness of the medication?
   a. Presence of signs and symptoms of hypoglycemia or hyperglycemia during the morning physical assessment
   b. Blood glucose level at 1,630
   c. Appetite and food intake at lunch
   d. Blood glucose level before breakfast
4. When monitoring the blood glucose level of a 12-year-old child with type 2 diabetes, your reading is 50 mg/dL. Which is the most appropriate action?
   a. Encourage the child to get out of bed and increase activity.
   b. Take the child's vital signs.
   c. Ask the child about frequent urine output.
   d. Give the child 4 oz of orange juice.
5. The nurse is caring for a 13-year-old recently diagnosed with Hashimoto disease. Which assessment findings may the nurse find upon examination? Select all that apply.
   a. Fatigue
   b. Weight loss
   c. Constipation
   d. Goiter
   e. Diarrhea
   f. Thinning hair
   g. Nervousness
6. You are the school nurse, and a student recently diagnosed with type 1 diabetes is brought to your office after recess stating they did not eat breakfast and are not feeling well. Which clinical manifestations suggest the student is hypoglycemic? Select all that apply.
   a. Flushed skin
   b. Slurred speech
   c. Diaphoresis
   d. Nausea
   e. Vomiting

DOSAGE CALCULATION QUESTION

The school nurse is caring for a child with type 1 diabetes. The child weighs 56 lb. The sliding scale corrective dose order reads: Insulin aspart before meals: (blood glucose − 120 divided by 70) + (total carbohydrate expected intake divided by 13 carbohydrates per unit). This is the corrective dose + carbohydrate consumption correction. Her blood glucose before lunch is 139 with an expected intake of 47 carbohydrates at lunch and regular activity level the rest of the day. Calculate the insulin dose to be administered. Round to the nearest unit.

CRITICAL THINKING EXERCISES

1. A 12-year-old with type 1 diabetes has the flu. His parent calls the diabetes clinic to report that he stayed home from school and does not have an appetite, so he is not eating. The parent asks the nurse how much insulin the child should take. He is currently taking three injections daily with regular and NPH in the morning before breakfast, regular and NPH in the evening after dinner, and regular before bedtime. What questions should the nurse ask before answering the parent's question? Based on the answers to these questions, how would you instruct the parent?
2. The parent of Robin, a 5-year-old, reports that Robin has a body odor. She is developing breasts and some pubic hair and was teased when she had a sleepover with friends. The review of her growth charts reveals that Robin went from the 50th percentile to the 93rd percentile in the past 6 months. Based on this information, what are the major nursing analyses to begin establishing a plan of care for the child and family? What are the expected outcomes and major interventions associated with the patient problem of knowledge deficit?

3. A parent brings their baby to the clinic after receiving a phone message from the clinic saying there was a problem with the baby's thyroid test. The parent says the trip on the bus took a long time, but the infant slept the entire way, and the baby is sleeping much of the time and does not want to eat very much. The baby was discharged from the hospital 2 weeks ago. The birth was without difficulty and there were no problems during labor. Why is this visit urgent? What would the test show if the disorder was due to a pituitary gland problem and not the thyroid gland?

STUDY ACTIVITIES

1. During your clinical experiences, ask to be on an inpatient unit that provides care for children with alterations in endocrine function. Compare and contrast the health histories, assessments, laboratory tests, diagnostic procedures, and plans of care for these children with those for the care of children on other units. Participate in the teaching plan for these children and their families.
2. Attend an outpatient clinic that provides care to children with endocrine disorders. Identify the role of the registered nurse in providing coordination of care, health teaching, and referrals for these children and their families.
3. Shadow a diabetes nurse educator to observe the teaching methods and strategies they use to provide an education plan for a child with diabetes. Observe how the nurse educator includes the family in the plan. Are there any differences between the teaching plans for type 1 DM and type 2 DM?
4. Conduct a literature review for one of the common endocrine disorders to research current management practices. Are there evidence-based practice guidelines for nursing interventions?
5. Conduct an internet search to research the information that is available to children and their families related to DM.

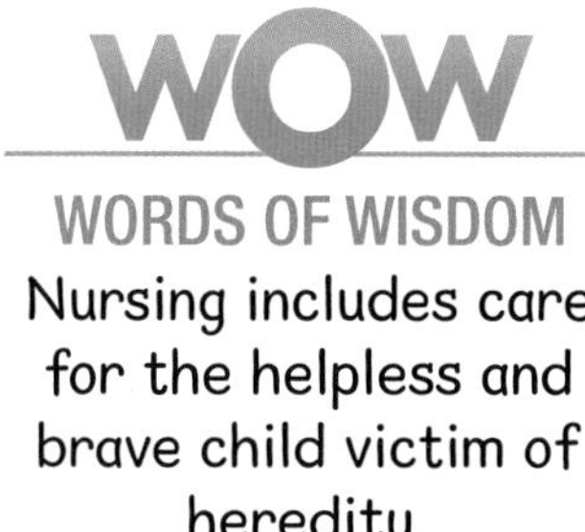

WOW
WORDS OF WISDOM
Nursing includes care for the helpless and brave child victim of heredity.

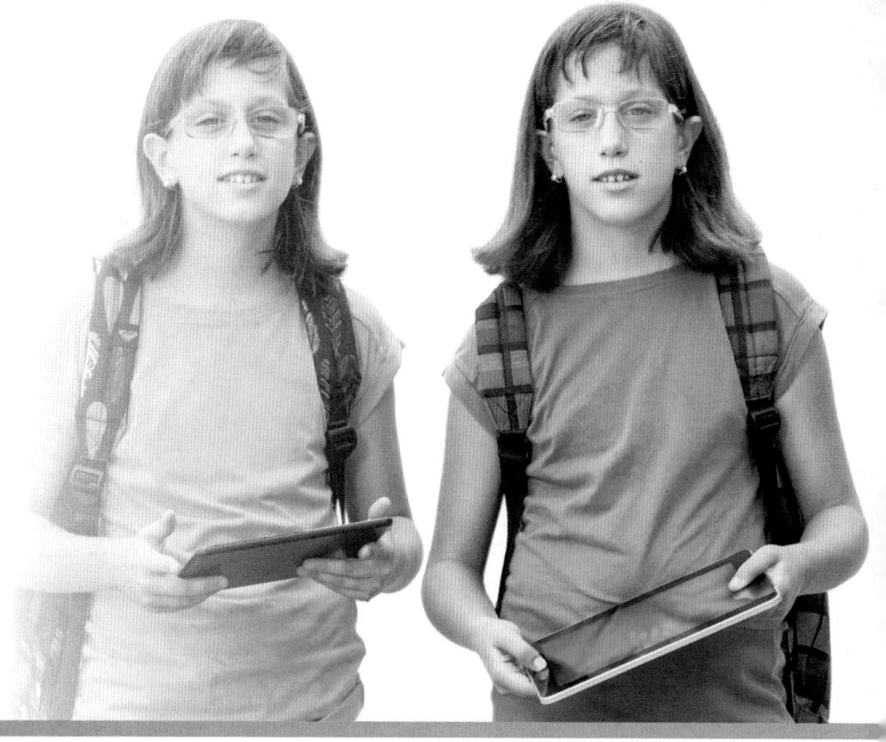

27 Nursing Care of the Child With an Alteration in Genetics

KEY TERMS

allele (ă-lēl)
chromosome
gene
genome
genotype
heterozygous (het′ĕr-ō-zī′gŭs)
homozygous (hō′mō-zī′gŭs)
karyotype (kar′ē-ō-tīp)
nondisjunction
phenotype (fē′nō-tīp)
translocation

LEARNING OBJECTIVES

Upon completion of the chapter, you will be able to:

1. Identify various inheritance patterns, including nontraditional patterns of inheritance.
2. Discuss ethical and legal issues associated with genetic testing.
3. Explain genetic counseling and the role of the nurse.
4. Discuss the nurse's role and responsibilities when caring for a child diagnosed with a genetic disorder and their family.
5. Identify nursing interventions related to common laboratory and diagnostic tests used in the diagnosis and management of genetic conditions.
6. Distinguish various genetic disorders occurring in childhood.
7. Devise an individualized nursing concept map or plan of care for the child with a genetic disorder.
8. Develop child/family teaching plans for the child with a genetic disorder.

Julie Woods, a 5-year-old, is brought to the clinic for her annual examination. Her parent states, "She's so much smaller than all of the other kindergartners."

INTRODUCTION

Genetics refers to the study of heredity—its transmission and characteristic variation. Nurses encounter potential or actual alterations in genetics in all types of patients and must detect problems and intervene early to prevent complications. A genetic disorder is a disease caused by an abnormality in a person's genetic material or genome. Some genetic disorders occur in multiple family members (via inheritance of abnormal genes). Other disorders may occur in only a single family member (via spontaneous mutation).

A genetic disorder is caused by completely or partially altered genetic material. In contrast, a familial disorder is more common in relatives of the affected person but may be caused by environmental influences, not genetic alterations.

Many chronic disorders of childhood have a genetic or inherited cause. Common disorders suspected to be caused or influenced by genetic factors include birth defects, chromosomal abnormalities, neurocutaneous disorders, intellectual disability, many types of short stature disorders, connective tissue disorders, and inborn errors of metabolism. Genetic disorders can present at any age, but the most obvious and severe disorders are present in childhood (Scott & Lee, 2020a).

Our ability to diagnose genetic conditions is far superior to our ability to cure or treat them. However, accurate diagnosis does lead to improved treatment and outcomes. Nurses should have a basic knowledge of genetics, common genetic disorders in children, genetic testing, and genetic counseling so that they can provide support and information to families and can promote an improved quality of life.

TAKE NOTE!

Genetic science has the potential to revolutionize health care with regard to national screening programs, predisposition testing, detection of genetic disorders, and pharmacogenetics.

ADVANCES IN GENETICS

Recent advances in genetic knowledge and technology have affected all areas of health. Genetic testing can identify presymptomatic conditions in children and adults and can provide carrier screening, prenatal diagnostic testing, newborn screening, confirmation of a diagnosis, forensic and identity testing, preimplantation genetic diagnosis, and pharmacogenetic testing, which provides information on how a person will respond to certain medications based on genetic variability (Scott & Lee, 2020a). Thousands of genetic tests are available for diseases such as Duchenne muscular dystrophy/Becker muscular dystrophy, cystic fibrosis, and sickle cell disease (Lee, 2020). Gene therapy can be used to replace or repair defective or missing genes with normal ones. It is a promising treatment option for many inherited and incurable diseases; however, it remains an experimental and risky treatment option (Lee, 2020). Clinical trials continue to test gene therapy for diseases that have no other cures, with some treatments gaining U.S. Food and Drug Administration (FDA) approval (Lee, 2020).

The Human Genome Project (HGP) and continued research by the National Human Genome Research Institute have helped foster much of this progress. The **genome** of an organism is its entire hereditary information encoded in the DNA. The HGP, an international effort to produce a comprehensive sequence of the human genome, was coordinated by the U.S. Department of Energy and the National Institutes of Health. It began in October 1990 and was completed in May 2003.

The HGP has led to the discovery of the genetic basis for hundreds of disorders and has advanced our understanding of basic genetic processes at the molecular level.

One goal of the HGP was to translate the findings into new and more effective strategies for the prevention, diagnosis, and treatment of genetic disorders. Current and potential applications for the HGP to health care include rapid and more specific diagnosis of disease, with hundreds of genetic tests available in research or clinical practice; earlier detection of genetic predisposition to disease; less emphasis on treating the symptoms of a disease and more emphasis on seeking the fundamental causes of the disease; new classes of drugs; avoiding environmental conditions that may trigger disease; and repair or replacement of defective genes using gene therapy. This knowledge, along with the commercialization of the technology, can change both professional and parental understanding of genetic disorders.

The potential benefits of these discoveries are vast, but so is the potential for misuse. These advances challenge all health care professionals to consider the many ethical, legal, and social ramifications of genetics in human lives. In the near future, risk profiling based on a person's unique genetic makeup will be used to tailor prevention, treatment, and ongoing management of health conditions. This profiling will raise issues associated with privacy and confidentiality related to workplace discrimination and access to health insurance. Issues of autonomy are equally problematic as society considers how to address the injustices that will inevitably surface when disease risk can be determined years in advance of its occurrence. People are currently protected from genetic discrimination by health insurers and employers through the Genetic Information Nondiscrimination Act of 2008, but this does not extend to providers of life, disability, or long-term care insurance (Scott & Lee, 2020a). Nurses will play an important role in developing policies and providing direction and support in this arena. In order to fulfill this important role, nurses need a basic understanding of genetics, including inheritance and inheritance patterns.

INHERITANCE

A **gene** is the basic unit of heredity of all traits. Genes occupy a specific location on a **chromosome** (a long, continuous strand of DNA that carries genetic information) and determine the organism's physical and mental characteristics. In humans, each somatic cell (a cell forming the body of an organism) has 46 chromosomes: 22 pairs of nonsex chromosomes (autosomes) and one pair of sex chromosomes. The **genotype** is the specific genetic makeup of a person; it is the internally coded inheritable information and refers to the particular **allele** (one of two or more alternative versions of a gene at a given position on a chromosome that imparts the same characteristic of that gene). For example, each human has a gene that controls height, but there are variations of these genes (alleles) that can produce a height of 5 ft or one of 6 ft, 2 in. A gene that controls eye color may have an allele that can produce blue eyes or an allele that produces brown eyes. The genotype, together with environmental variation that influences the person, determines the **phenotype** (the outward characteristics of the person).

A human inherits two genes, one from each parent; therefore, one allele comes from the female parent and one from the male parent. These alleles may be the same for the characteristic (**homozygous**) or different (**heterozygous**). If the two alleles differ, the dominant one will usually be expressed in the person's phenotype.

Patterns of Inheritance

Patterns of inheritance demonstrate how genetic abnormalities can be passed on to offspring. Although the diagnosis of a genetic disorder is usually based on clinical signs and symptoms or on laboratory confirmation of an altered gene associated with the disorder, accurate diagnosis can be aided by identifying the pattern of inheritance within a family. In addition, nurses must understand the patterns of inheritance so they can teach and counsel families about the risks of genetic disorders occurring in future pregnancies.

Mendelian or Monogenic Laws of Inheritance

The principles of inheritance of single-gene disorders are the same that govern the inheritance of other traits, such as eye and hair color. These are known as Mendel's laws of inheritance, named for Gregor Mendel, an Austrian naturalist who conducted genetic research. These patterns occur because a single gene is defective, and the disorders that result are referred to as monogenic or, sometimes, mendelian disorders. If the defect occurs on the autosome, the genetic disorder is termed autosomal; if the defect is on the X chromosome, the genetic disorder is termed X linked. The defect can also be classified as dominant or recessive. Monogenic disorders include autosomal dominant, autosomal recessive, X-linked dominant, and X-linked recessive. Not all single-gene disorders follow typical mendelian inheritance, as the pattern of inheritance can be complicated by other genes, epigenetic changes, or environmental factors (Raby, 2021). These nontraditional inheritance patterns are discussed.

AUTOSOMAL DOMINANT INHERITANCE

Autosomal dominant inheritance occurs when a single gene in the heterozygous state is capable of producing the phenotype. In these instances, the abnormal or mutant gene overshadows the normal gene, and the person will demonstrate signs and symptoms of the disorder. The affected person usually has one affected parent. However, there are varying degrees of presentation among individuals in a family. For example, a parent with a mild form of the disorder could have a child with a more severe form (termed variable expression). In some autosomal dominant disorders, there may be no history of an affected family member. This can be due to the child representing a new mutation or the result of incomplete or reduced penetrance, which means that a person with the genetic mutation does not develop phenotypic features of the disorder. Incomplete or reduced penetrance may result from a combination of genetic, environmental, and lifestyle factors; age; and sex.

Offspring of an affected parent will have a 50% chance of inheriting two normal genes (disorder free) and a 50% chance of inheriting one normal and one abnormal gene (and, thus, the disorder; Scott & Lee, 2020b; Fig. 27.1). Females and males are equally affected by autosomal dominant disorders, and an affected male can pass the disorder on to their male offspring (Scott

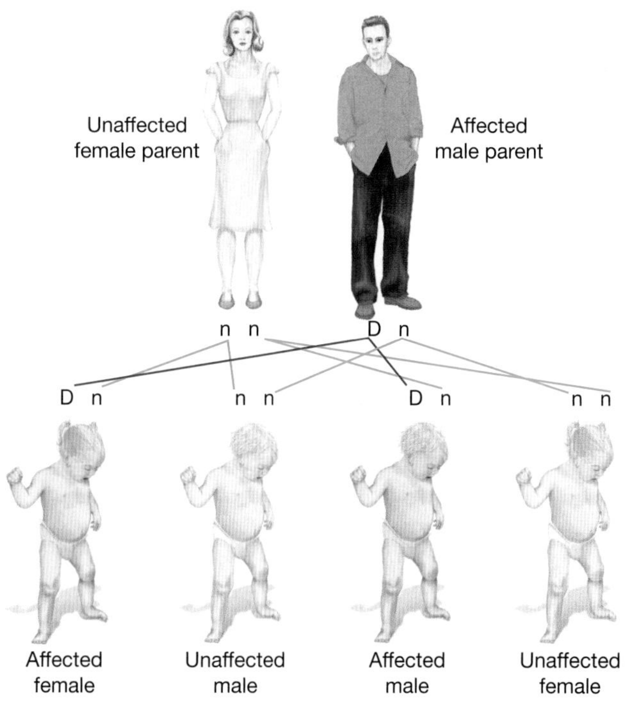

FIGURE 27.1 Autosomal dominant inheritance pattern.

& Lee, 2020b). This male-to-male transmission is important in distinguishing autosomal dominant inheritance from X-linked inheritance. Common types of genetic disorders that follow the autosomal dominant pattern of inheritance include achondroplasia, neurofibromatosis, Huntington disease, Marfan syndrome, and osteogenesis imperfecta type 1 (Breilyn & Levy, 2023).

AUTOSOMAL RECESSIVE INHERITANCE

Autosomal recessive inheritance occurs when two copies of the mutant or abnormal gene in the homozygous state are necessary to produce the phenotype. In other words, two abnormal genes are needed for the person to demonstrate signs and symptoms of the disorder. Both parents of the affected person must be heterozygous carriers of the gene (clinically normal, but carriers of the gene). Offspring of two carriers of the abnormal gene have a 25% chance of inheriting two normal genes, a 50% chance of inheriting one normal gene and one abnormal gene (carrier), and a 25% chance of inheriting two abnormal genes (and, thus, the disorder; Scott & Lee, 2020b; Fig. 27.2).

Affected people are usually present in only one generation of the family. Females and males are equally affected, and a male can pass the disorder on to their male offspring (Scott & Lee, 2020b). The chance that any two parents will both be carriers of the mutant gene is increased if the couple has consanguinity (relationship by blood or common ancestry; Scott & Lee, 2020b). Common types of genetic disorders that follow the autosomal recessive inheritance pattern include cystic fibrosis and sickle cell disease (Breilyn & Levy, 2023).

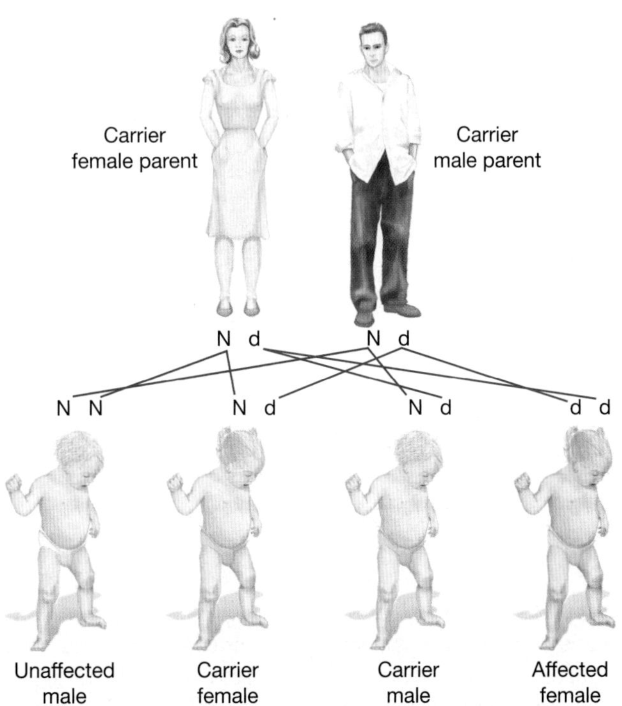

FIGURE 27.2 Autosomal recessive inheritance pattern.

X-LINKED INHERITANCE

X-linked inheritance disorders are those associated with altered genes on the X chromosome. They differ from autosomal disorders. If a male inherits an X-linked altered gene, they will express the condition. This is because a male has only one X chromosome and, therefore, all the genes on their X chromosome will be expressed (the Y chromosome carries no normal allele to compensate for the altered gene). Because females inherit two X chromosomes, they can be either heterozygous or homozygous for any allele. Therefore, X-linked disorders in females express similarly to autosomal disorders.

> **TAKE NOTE!**
>
> The distinction between X-linked recessive and X-linked dominant inheritance is not clear and should not be made per some experts' opinions. This is because it is possible for females with uneven X-inactivation to demonstrate clinical features of X-linked conditions (Raby, 2021).

X-Linked Recessive Inheritance

Most X-linked disorders demonstrate recessive inheritance (Breilyn & Levy, 2023). In the X-linked recessive pattern of inheritance, there are more affected males than females because all the genes on a male's X chromosome will be expressed since a male has only one X chromosome (Raby, 2021). On the other hand, a female will usually need two abnormal X chromosomes to exhibit the disease and one normal and one abnormal X chromosome to be a carrier of the disease. There is no male-to-male transmission (since no X chromosome from the male is transmitted to male offspring), but any male who is affected by an X-linked recessive disorder will have carrier female offspring. If a female is a carrier, there is a 50% chance their male offspring will inherit the trait and a 50% chance their female offspring will be a carrier (Breilyn & Levy, 2023; Fig. 27.3). Common types of genetic disorders that follow X-linked recessive inheritance patterns include hemophilia and Duchenne muscular dystrophy (Breilyn & Levy, 2023).

X-Linked Dominant Inheritance

X-linked dominant inherited disorders are not very common (Breilyn & Levy, 2023). X-linked dominant inheritance occurs when a male has an abnormal X chromosome or a female has one abnormal X chromosome. All of the female offspring and none of the male offspring of an affected male will inherit the condition, while both male and female offspring of an affected female have a 50% chance of inheriting the condition (Raby, 2021; Fig. 27.4). Males are more severely affected than females. Many X-linked dominant disorders have lethal results in

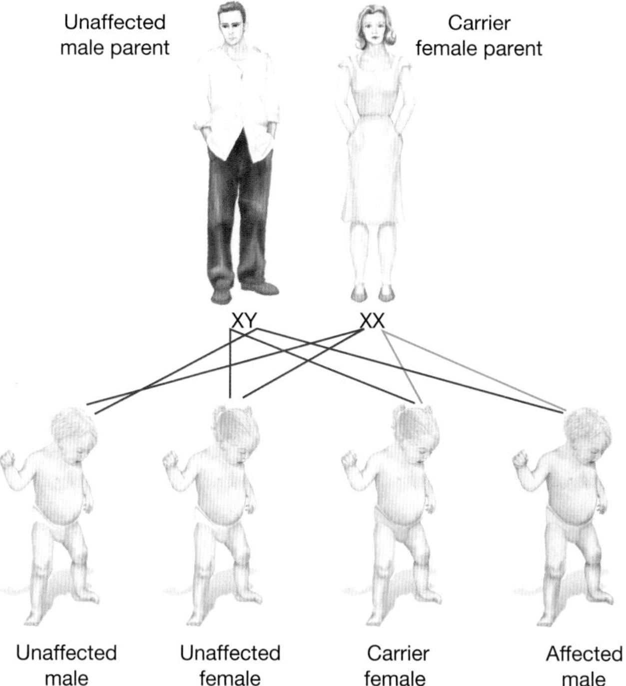

FIGURE 27.3 X-linked recessive inheritance pattern.

males (Raby, 2021). In females, even though the gene is dominant, having a second normal X gene offsets the effects of the dominant gene to some extent, resulting in decreasing severity of the disorder. X-linked dominant disorders are rare; an example is hypophosphatemic (vitamin D-resistant) rickets (Raby, 2021).

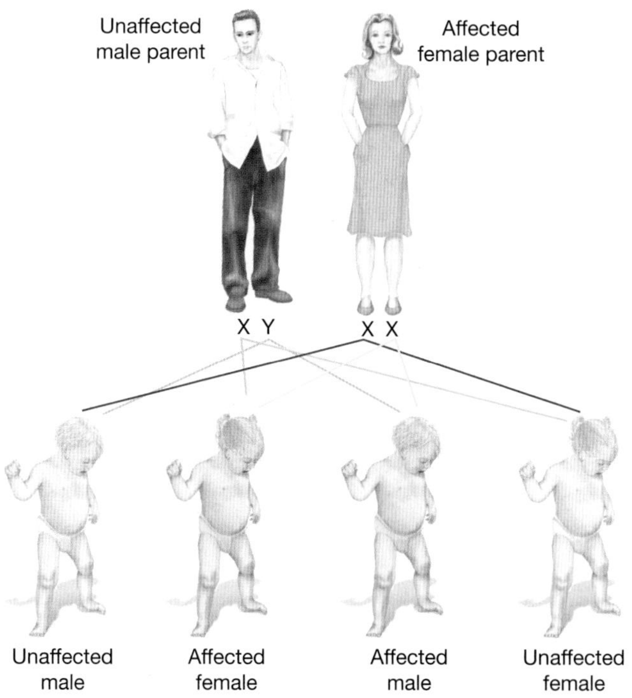

FIGURE 27.4 X-linked dominant inheritance pattern.

Multifactorial Inheritance

Many of the common congenital malformations, such as cleft lip, cleft palate, neural tube defects, pyloric stenosis, clubfoot, congenital hip dysplasia, and cardiac defects, are attributed to multifactorial inheritance (Scott & Lee, 2020b). These conditions are thought to be caused by inherited and environmental factors. That is, a combination of genes from both parents, along with unknown environmental factors, produces the trait or condition. A person may inherit a predisposition to a particular anomaly or disease. The anomalies or diseases vary in severity, and often a sex bias is present. For example, pyloric stenosis is seen more often in males, while congenital hip dysplasia is much more likely to occur in females. Multifactorial conditions tend to run in families, but the pattern of inheritance is not as predictable as with single-gene disorders. The chance of recurrence is also less than in single-gene disorders, but the degree of risk is related to the number of genes in common with the affected person. The closer the degree of relationship, the more genes a person has in common with the affected family member, and thus the higher the risk that the person's offspring will have a similar defect. In multifactorial inheritance, the likelihood that both identical twins will be affected is not 100%, indicating that there are nongenetic factors involved.

Nontraditional Inheritance Patterns

Molecular studies have revealed that some genetic disorders are inherited in ways that do not follow the typical patterns of dominant, recessive, X-linked, or multifactorial inheritance. Examples of nontraditional inheritance patterns include mitochondrial inheritance and genomic imprinting. As the science of molecular genetics advances and we learn more about inheritance patterns, other nontraditional patterns of inheritance may be discovered or may be found to be relatively common.

MITOCHONDRIAL INHERITANCE

Certain diseases result from mutations in the mitochondrial DNA. Mitochondria (the part of the cell responsible for energy production) are inherited almost exclusively from the female parent. Therefore, mitochondrial inheritance is usually passed from the female parent to the offspring, regardless of the offspring's sex (differentiating mitochondrial inheritance from X-linked recessive inheritance). These mutations are often deletions and abnormalities and are often seen in one or more organs, such as the brain, eye, and skeletal muscle. They are often associated with energy deficits in cells with high energy requirements, such as nerve and muscle cells. These disorders tend to be progressive, and the age of onset can vary from infancy to adulthood. There is an extreme amount of variability in symptoms within a family. Examples of disorders that follow mitochondrial inheritance include Kearns–Sayre syndrome (a neuromuscular disorder) and Leber hereditary optic neuropathy (which causes progressive visual impairment; Scott & Lee, 2020b).

GENETIC IMPRINTING

Another nontraditional inheritance pattern results from a process called genetic imprinting. Genetic imprinting plays a critical role in fetal growth and development and placental functioning. It is a phenomenon in which the expression of a gene is determined by its parental origin. In genomic imprinting, both the maternal and paternal alleles are present, but only one is expressed; the other is inactive. Genetic imprinting does not alter the genetic sequence itself but affects the phenotype observed. In these instances, the altered genes in a certain region of the genome have very different expressions depending on whether they were inherited from the female or male parent. Several human syndromes are known to be associated with defects in gene imprinting. Disorders that result from a disruption of imprinting usually involve a growth phenotype and include varying degrees of developmental problems. Common examples include Prader–Willi syndrome (a condition resulting in severe hypotonia and hyperphagia, leading to higher weight and intellectual disability), Angelman syndrome (a neurodevelopmental disorder associated with intellectual disability, jerky movements, and seizures), and Beckwith–Wiedemann syndrome (characterized by somatic overgrowth, congenital malformations, and a predisposition to embryonic neoplasia; Scott & Lee, 2020b).

Chromosomal Abnormalities

In some cases of genetic disorders, the abnormality occurs due to problems with the chromosomes. Chromosomal abnormalities do not follow straightforward patterns of inheritance. Although some chromosomal disorders can be inherited, most others occur due to random events during the formation of reproductive cells or in early fetal development.

Sperm and egg cells each have 23 unpaired chromosomes. When they unite during conception, they form a fertilized egg with 46 chromosomes. Sometimes, before pregnancy begins, an error occurs during the process of cell division, leaving an egg or sperm with too many or too few chromosomes. If this egg or sperm cell joins with a normal egg or sperm cell, the resulting embryo has a chromosomal abnormality. Chromosomal abnormalities can also occur due to an error in the structure of the chromosome. Small pieces of the chromosome may be deleted, duplicated, inverted, misplaced, or exchanged with part of another chromosome.

Most chromosomal abnormalities occur due to an error in the egg or sperm. Therefore, the abnormality is present in every cell of the body. Some abnormalities can happen after fertilization, during mitotic cell division, and result in mosaicism. Mosaicism or the mosaic form is when the chromosomal abnormalities do not show up in every cell; only some cells or tissues carry the abnormality. In mosaic forms of the disorder, the symptoms are usually less severe than if all the cells were abnormal.

Chromosomal abnormalities occur in about 1% to 2% of live births (Bacino & Lee, 2020). There is a much higher frequency of chromosomal abnormalities in spontaneous abortions and stillbirths (Bacino & Lee, 2020). Congenital anomalies and intellectual disability are often associated with chromosomal abnormalities (Bacino & Lee, 2020). These abnormalities occur on autosomal or nonsex chromosomes as well as sex chromosomes and can result from abnormalities of either chromosome number or chromosome structure.

A **karyotype** is a pictorial analysis of chromosomes. It depicts a systematic arrangement of the chromosomes of a single cell in pairs (Fig. 27.5). Karyotyping is often used in prenatal testing to diagnose or predict genetic diseases.

ABNORMALITIES OF CHROMOSOME NUMBER

Chromosomal abnormalities of number often result due to **nondisjunction** (failure of separation of the chromosome pair) during cell division, meiosis, or mitosis. Few chromosomal numerical abnormalities are compatible with full-term development, and most result in spontaneous abortion (Bacino & Lee, 2020). Some numerical abnormalities, however, can support development to term because the chromosome on which the abnormality is present carries relatively few genes (e.g., chromosome 13, 18, 21, or X).

Two common abnormalities of chromosome number are monosomies or trisomies. In monosomies, there is only one copy of a particular chromosome instead of the usual pair; in these instances, all fetuses spontaneously abort in early pregnancy. Survival occurs only in mosaic forms of these disorders. In trisomies, there are three of a particular chromosome instead of the usual two. The most common trisomies include trisomy 21 (Down syndrome [DS]), trisomy 18, and trisomy 13 (see "Common Chromosomal Abnormalities" section for further discussion). Trisomies may be present in every cell or may present in the mosaic form.

ABNORMALITIES OF CHROMOSOME STRUCTURE

Abnormalities of chromosome structure usually occur when there is a breakage and loss of a portion of one or more chromosomes, and during the repair process, the broken ends are rejoined incorrectly. Structural abnormalities usually lead to having too much or too little genetic material. Altered chromosome structure can take on several forms. Deletions occur when a portion of the chromosome is missing, resulting in a loss of that portion of the chromosome. Duplications are seen when a

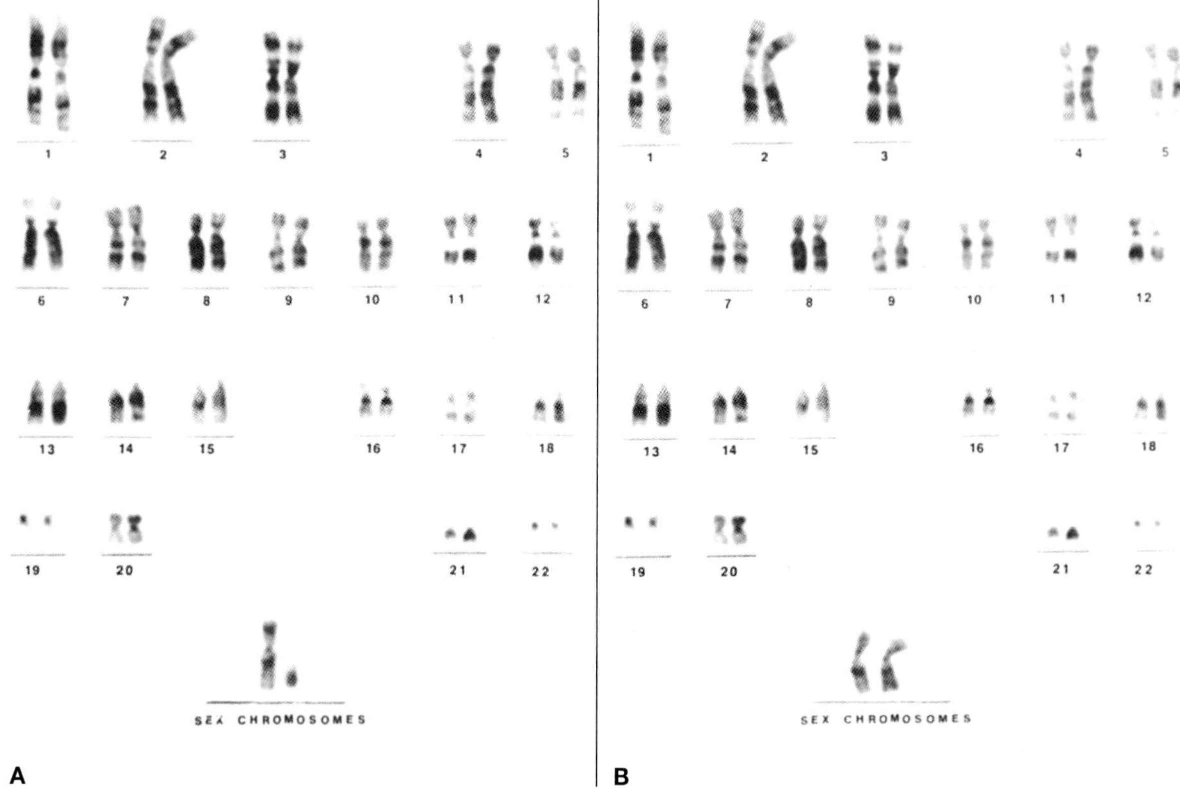

FIGURE 27.5 Chromosomes in a karyotype are arranged and numbered by size, from largest to smallest. The normal human karyotype has 46 chromosomes: 22 pairs of autosomes and two sex chromosomes. **A.** A normal male. **B.** A normal female.

portion of the chromosome is duplicated and an extra chromosomal segment is present. Clinical findings vary depending on how much chromosomal material is involved. Inversions occur when a portion of the chromosome breaks off at two points and is turned upside down and reattached; therefore, the genetic material is inverted. With inversion, there is no loss or gain of chromosomal material and carriers are phenotypically normal, but they do have an increased risk for miscarriage and having chromosomally abnormal offspring (Bacino & Lee, 2020). Ring chromosomes are seen when a portion of a chromosome has broken off in two places and has formed a circle or ring. The most clinically significant structural abnormality is a **translocation**. This occurs when a portion of one chromosome is transferred to another chromosome and an abnormal rearrangement is present.

Structural abnormalities can be balanced or unbalanced. Balanced abnormalities involve the rearrangement of genetic material with neither an overall gain nor loss. People who inherit a balanced structural abnormality are usually phenotypically normal but are at a higher risk for miscarriages and having chromosomally abnormal offspring. Examples of structural rearrangements that can be balanced include inversions, translocations, and ring chromosomes. Unbalanced structural abnormalities are similar to numerical abnormalities because genetic material is either gained or lost. Unbalanced structural abnormalities can encompass several genes and result in severe clinical consequences.

SEX CHROMOSOME ABNORMALITIES

Chromosomal abnormalities can also involve sex chromosomes. These cases usually have milder clinical effects than autosomal chromosomal abnormalities (Bacino & Lee, 2020). Sex chromosome abnormalities are sex specific and involve a missing or extra sex chromosome. They affect sexual development and may cause infertility, growth abnormalities, and, possibly, behavioral and learning problems. However, many affected people lead essentially normal lives. Examples are Turner syndrome in females and Klinefelter syndrome in males (see discussion later in this chapter).

GENETIC EVALUATION AND COUNSELING

Genetic counseling is a communication and educational process where the genetic influence of health is explained along with information regarding a specific genetic disorder, its transmission, its inheritance, and options available in testing, management, and family planning (Raby & Kohlmann, 2022). There are a variety of reasons a person should be referred for genetic counseling (Box 27.1). In many cases, geneticists and genetic

BOX **27.1** **Those Who May Benefit From Genetic Counseling**

- Age of the birthing parent 35 years or older when the baby is born
- Paternal age 40 years or older
- Previous child, parents, or close relatives with an inherited disease, congenital anomalies, metabolic disorders, developmental disorders, or chromosomal abnormalities
- Consanguinity or incest
- Pregnancy screening abnormality, including alpha-fetoprotein, triple/quadruple screen, amniocentesis, or ultrasound
- Stillborn with congenital anomalies
- Two or more pregnancy losses
- Teratogen exposure or risk
- Concerns about genetic defects that occur frequently in their ethnic or racial group (e.g., those of African descent are most at risk for having a child with sickle cell anemia)
- Abnormal newborn screening
- Child born with one or more major malformations in a major organ system
- Child with abnormalities of growth
- Child with developmental delay, intellectual disability, blindness, or deafness

Data from Lee, B. (2020). Integration of genetics into pediatric practice. In R. M. Kleigman, J. W. St. Geme III, N. J. Blum, S. S. Shah, R. C. Tasker, K. M. Wilson, & R. E. Behrman (Eds.), *Nelson textbook of pediatrics* (21st ed., pp. 3789–3820). Elsevier.

counselors provide information to families regarding genetic diseases. However, an experienced primary provider, nurse practitioner, or nurse who has received special training in genetics may also provide the information. A genetic consultation involves the evaluation of a person or a family. Its purpose is to confirm, diagnose, or rule out genetic conditions; identify medical management issues; calculate and communicate genetic risks to a family; discuss ethical and legal issues; and assist in providing and arranging psychosocial support. Genetic counselors serve as educators and resource people for other health care providers and the general public.

The ideal time for genetic counseling is before conception. Preconception counseling allows couples to identify and reduce potential pregnancy risks, plan for known risks, and establish early prenatal care. Genetic counseling is particularly important if a congenital anomaly or genetic disease has been diagnosed prenatally or when a child is born with a life-threatening congenital anomaly or genetic disease. In these cases, families need urgent information because they need to make immediate decisions. If a diagnosis with genetic implications is made later in life, if a couple with a family history or a previous child with a genetic disorder is planning a family, or if there is suspected teratogen exposure, the urgency of information is not such an issue. In these situations, the family needs to take in all the information and explore all their options. This may occur during several meetings over a longer period of time.

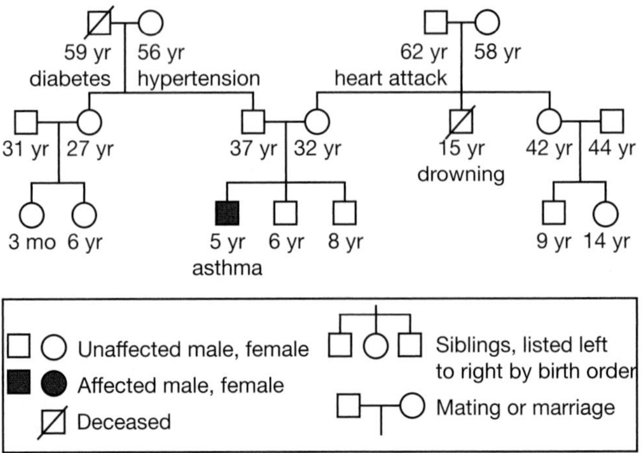

FIGURE 27.6 A pedigree is a diagram that shows the links between family members and includes medical information for each relative.

Genetic counseling involves gathering extensive information about birth history, past medical history, and current health status. A detailed family history is imperative and in most cases will include the development of a pedigree, which is like a family tree (Fig. 27.6). Information is ideally gathered on three generations, but if the family history is complicated, information from more distant relatives may be needed. Families receiving genetic counseling should be told that this information will be necessary so that they can discuss these sensitive issues with family members in advance. When necessary, medical records may be requested for family members, especially those who have a genetic disorder. Sometimes the process of preparing a pedigree may reveal information that is not known by all family members, such as an adopted child, a child conceived through in vitro fertilization, or a husband not being the parent of a baby. Therefore, it is extremely important to take steps to maintain confidentiality.

Medical genetic knowledge has increased dramatically over the past few decades. This has greatly expanded the role of the genetic counselor. It is possible not only to detect specific diseases with genetic mutations but also to test for a genetic predisposition to various diseases or conditions and certain physical characteristics. This leads to complex ethical, moral, and social issues. Health care providers need to maintain privacy and confidentiality and administer care in a nondiscriminatory manner while maintaining sensitivity to cultural differences. It is essential to respect the child's autonomy and present information in a nondirective manner.

NURSE'S ROLE AND RESPONSIBILITIES

Pediatric nurses will encounter children with genetic disorders in every clinical specialty area. This includes clinics, hospitals, schools, and community-based centers.

Talking with families who have recently been diagnosed with a genetic disorder or who have had a child born with congenital anomalies is very difficult. Many times, the nurse is the one who has first contact with these parents and will be the one to provide follow-up care. Genetic disorders are significant, life-changing, and possibly life-threatening situations. The information is highly technical, and the field is still evolving. Therefore, it is important to refer the family to a primary provider or nurse practitioner who specializes in genetics. The nurse should understand who will benefit from genetic counseling and should be able to discuss the role of the genetic counselor with families. Inform families at risk that genetic counseling is available before they attempt to have another baby.

The nurse is in an ideal position to help families review what has been discussed during the genetic counseling sessions and to answer any additional questions they might have. Nurses play an essential role in providing emotional support to the family throughout this challenging time. Nurses should also refer the family to appropriate agencies, support groups, and resources, such as a social worker, a chaplain, or an ethicist.

COMMON MEDICAL TREATMENTS

A variety of medications and other medical treatments are used to treat the symptoms of genetic disorders in children. Genetic disorders do not have specific treatments, and there is no cure, so treatment focuses on the specific symptoms of each disorder. Genetic disorders often involve multiple organ systems, and children with these disorders have complex medical needs. Thus, a multidisciplinary approach and good communication are imperative. See the following for a discussion on common genetic disorders and their management.

Clinical Judgment and the Nursing Process for the Child With a Genetic Disorder

Care of the child with a genetic disorder includes assessment, analysis, planning, interventions, and evaluation. There are a number of general concepts related to the nursing process that may be applied to the care of children with genetic disorders. From an overall understanding of the care involved for a child with an alteration in genetics, the nurse can then individualize the care based on specifics for the particular child.

Assessment

Assessment of the child with a genetic disorder includes health history, physical examination, and laboratory and diagnostic testing.

Health History

The health history consists of past medical history, including the birthing parent's pregnancy history; family history; neonatal history; and history of present illness (when the symptoms started and how they have progressed), as well as treatments used at home. Explore the child's current and past medical history for risk factors such as:

- Family history of genetic disorders
- Any complications during the prenatal, perinatal, or postnatal periods
- Changes in developmental status or delays in developmental milestones

The pregnancy history can be extremely relevant when identifying a genetic disorder. The pregnancy history may be significant for maternal age older than 35 years or paternal age older than 40 years, repeated premature births, breech delivery, congenital hip dysplasia, abnormalities found on ultrasound, abnormalities in prenatal blood screening tests (e.g., triple/quadruple screen, alpha-fetoprotein [AFP]), amniotic fluid abnormalities (polyhydramnios, oligohydramnios), multiple births, exposure to medications and known teratogens, and decreased fetal movement.

A focused neonatal history can also help identify a genetic problem. The neonatal history may be significant for symmetric intrauterine growth restriction, large for gestational age without a reason, hard of hearing, persistent hyperbilirubinemia, poor adaptation to the extrauterine environment (demonstrated by temperature and heart rate instability and poor feeding), hypotonia or hypertonia, seizures, and abnormal newborn screening results.

The family history plays a critical role in identifying genetic disorders. Gather data for three generations. If there is a positive family history, the likelihood of a genetic disorder in the child is increased. It is helpful to create a family pedigree (refer to the Genetic Evaluation and Counseling section). The family history may be significant for major congenital anomalies, intellectual disability, genetic diseases, metabolic disorders, multiple miscarriages or stillbirths, developmental delays, significant learning disabilities, psychiatric problems, consanguinity, and chronic serious illness (e.g., diabetes, hypertension, kidney disease, hearing impairment, blindness, asthma, seizures, and unexplained death).

When eliciting the history of the present illness, inquire about:

- Developmental delay
- Seizures
- Hypotonia or hypertonia
- Feeding problems
- Lethargy
- Failure to thrive
- Septic appearance
- Vomiting

Children known to have a genetic disorder are often admitted to the hospital for other health-related issues or complications and management of the genetic disorder. The health history should include questions related to:

- Age when the disorder was diagnosed
- Developmental delay
- Complications of the disorder (e.g., thyroid problems, cardiac problems, respiratory problems, leukemia, seizures, cognitive impairment)
- Medications the child takes for complications associated with the disorder
- Dietary restrictions
- Adherence to management regimen

Once complications have been identified, further investigation into their severity, frequency, and management is essential to the care of this child while in the hospital.

Physical Examination

Physical examination of the child with a genetic disorder includes inspection and observation, palpation, and auscultation.

INSPECTION AND OBSERVATION

Inspect and observe for congenital anomalies, either major or minor. A major anomaly is an anomaly or malformation that creates significant medical or cosmetic problems and requires surgical or medical management (Bacino, 2023; Box 27.2). Minor anomalies are features that vary from those seen in the general population but do not cause an increase in morbidity in and of themselves (Bacino, 2023; Box 27.3).

TAKE NOTE!

Low-set ears are a minor anomaly that is associated with numerous genetic dysmorphisms. If noted, assess thoroughly for other abnormalities.

BOX 27.2 Examples of Major Congenital Anomalies

- Cleft lip
- Cleft palate
- Congenital heart disease, structural and conduction disorders
- Neural tube defects, such as myelomeningocele
- Chromosomal abnormalities
- Omphalocele; gastroschisis
- Renal agenesis/hypoplasia
- Absent or limb deficiencies
- Generalized dysmorphism
- Ambiguous genitalia

Data obtained from Bacino, C. A. (2023). Birth defects: Epidemiology, types and pattern. *UpToDate*. Retrieved May 26, 2023, from https://www.uptodate.com/contents/birth-defects-epidemiology-types-and-patterns

BOX 27.3 Examples of Minor Congenital Anomalies

- Flat occiput
- Prominent occiput
- Triple hair whorl
- Flat-bridged nose
- Nostrils anteverted
- Ear lobe crease
- Ear lobe notched
- Cup-shaped ears
- Small ears
- Cleft uvula
- Webbed neck
- Short neck
- Extra nipples
- Sacral dimple
- Tapered fingers
- Overlapping digits
- Syndactyly
- Hemangioma
- Nevi

Data from Bacino, C. A. (2023). Birth defects: Epidemiology, types and pattern. *UpToDate*. Retrieved May 26, 2023, from https://www.uptodate.com/contents/birth-defects-epidemiology-types-and-patterns

As the number of minor anomalies present increases, the probability of the presence of a major anomaly increases. In fact, when three or more minor anomalies are present, the risk for a major anomaly or intellectual disability is approximately 19% to 26% (Bacino, 2023). Assess for a recognized pattern of anomalies that may be associated with certain syndromes.

TAKE NOTE!

Cleft lip and cleft palate are associated with many syndromes. If noted, assess for other anomalies.

Inspect and observe for an abnormal or foul odor of the child's excretions. Certain metabolic disorders or inborn errors of metabolism are associated with specific odors (Table 27.1).

AUSCULTATION

Physical examination includes auscultation of the heart. Murmurs or dysrhythmias may have a genetic cause. In a child with a congenital heart problem (e.g., ventricular septal defect) and a strong family history of cardiac structural problems, a genetic cause needs to be considered.

PALPATION

Palpation can be used to detect hepatosplenomegaly (an enlarged spleen and liver). However, primary providers or nurse practitioners usually perform this assessment because it requires skill and experience. Hepatosplenomegaly may indicate a metabolic disorder.

TABLE 27.1 • Inborn Errors of Metabolism and Associated Odor

Inborn Error of Metabolism	Associated Odor
Phenylketonuria	Mousy or musty
Maple syrup urine disease	Maple syrup, burnt sugar, or curry
Tyrosinemia	Cabbagelike, rancid butter
Trimethylaminuria	Rotting fish

Data from Shchelochkov, O. A., & Venditti, C. P. (2020). An approach to inborn errors of metabolism. In R. M. Kleigman, J. W. St. Geme III, N. J. Blum, S. S. Shah, R. C. Tasker, K. M. Wilson, & R. E. Behrman (Eds.), *Nelson textbook of pediatrics* (21st ed., pp. 404–408). Elsevier.

Laboratory and Diagnostic Testing

Common Laboratory and Diagnostic Tests 27.1 explains the laboratory and diagnostic tests used most commonly to detect genetic disorders. The tests can assist the primary provider or nurse practitioner in diagnosing the disorder or can be used as guidelines in determining treatment. Laboratory or nonnursing personnel obtain some of the tests, while the nurse might obtain others. In either instance, the nurse should be familiar with how the tests are obtained, what they are used for, and normal versus abnormal results. This knowledge will also be necessary when providing child and family education related to the testing. Due to the nature of the information, a referral to genetic counseling before testing may be appropriate. Advances in genetic technology have led to dramatic increases in the number of diagnostic and screening tests.

COMMON LABORATORY AND DIAGNOSTIC TESTS 27.1

Test	Explanation	Indications	Nursing Implications
Amniocentesis	Ultrasound-guided (to determine placental location) insertion of a needle through the abdomen and into the uterine cavity of a pregnant person to obtain a sample of amniotic fluid. The fluid contains skin cells that have been shed by the fetus and can be isolated and grown in the laboratory to provide enough genetic material for testing.	Test for chromosomal abnormality, neural tube defects, or specific genetic conditions of the fetus. Performed if considered high risk for a genetic disorder or abnormal ultrasound. The most common prenatal test used to diagnose chromosomal and congenital anomalies	Usually not performed until after 15 weeks' gestation Complications include miscarriage, fetal injury, amniotic fluid leakage, infection, premature labor, maternal hemorrhage, amniotic fluid embolism, abruptio placentae, and damage to the bladder or intestines. Results are usually not available for 7–10 days or longer, but this varies by laboratory. Monitor the fetus before and after the procedure.
Chorionic villi sampling (CVS)	Involves the removal of a small amount of tissue directly from the chorionic villi (minute vascular projections of the fetal chorion that combine with maternal uterine tissue to form the placenta). In the laboratory, the chromosomes of the fetal cells are analyzed for number and type. Extra chromosomes, such as are present in Down syndrome, can be identified. Additional laboratory tests can be performed to look for specific disorders.	Test for chromosomal abnormality, fetal metabolic or blood disorders, or specific genetic conditions of the fetus. Performed if considered high risk for a genetic disorder or abnormal ultrasound. CVS cannot detect alpha-fetoprotein levels; therefore, it does not detect neural tube defects	Performed at 7–11 weeks of gestation, so provides early detection of genetic abnormalities Complications include miscarriage, infection, bleeding, amniotic fluid leakage, and fetal limb deformities. Results can be available within 24 hours, but this varies depending on the laboratory and location of the procedure (results are usually available sooner than with an amniocentesis). Monitor the fetus before and after the procedure.
Triple/quadruple screen	A maternal serum laboratory screening test that measures the level of three substances made by the developing baby and placenta: alpha-fetoprotein (AFP), human chorionic gonadotropin (hCG), and unconjugated estriol (uE3). Dimeric inhibin A has been added to make the "quadruple test." The addition of dimeric inhibin A increases the detection rate of Down syndrome and trisomy 18 in the quadruple screen.	A screening test for low-risk pregnant people to determine pregnancies at an increased risk for open neural tube defects, Down syndrome, and trisomy 18	Performed between 15 and 21 weeks of gestation Educate parents that a normal test does not guarantee a healthy baby. Conversely, an abnormal result does not guarantee the baby has a problem. Additional testing will be necessary to confirm or rule out a specific genetic condition.

(continued)

COMMON LABORATORY AND DIAGNOSTIC TESTS 27.1 (*continued*)

Test	Explanation	Indications	Nursing Implications
Fetal nuchal translucency (FNT); may be combined with pregnancy-associated plasma protein (PAPP-A) and beta-hCG to increase the detection rate	Ultrasound prenatal screening to help identify higher risks of Down syndrome, trisomy 13, trisomy 18, and Turner syndrome. The ultrasound assesses the amount of fluid behind the neck of a fetus (known as the nuchal fold). Increased fluid increases the risk of a chromosomal abnormality. During this early ultrasound, other markers may be looked at, such as the presence of nasal bones (in Down syndrome, hypoplasia or absence of the nasal bones may be noted); short femur or humerus increases the risk of trisomy, echogenic foci (bright spots) in the heart can increase the risk of Down syndrome, and echogenic bowel (bowel looks bright and white) can be associated with chromosomal abnormalities. A serum blood test is performed to determine the level of two hormones, PAPP-A and beta-hCG. Using a combination of the results of the ultrasound and the blood test, the risk of having a baby with Down syndrome is predicted.	Any pregnant person presenting by 11–13 weeks' gestation can be screened. Particularly for people with increased risk or desired screening for Down syndrome, trisomy 13, trisomy 18, or Turner syndrome	Must be performed between 11 and 13 weeks Genetic counseling before testing may be warranted. Positive tests require follow-up tests and genetic counseling.
Ultrasound	Safe, noninvasive, accurate investigation of the fetus. A transducer is placed in contact with the pregnant person's abdomen, and high-frequency sound waves are directed at the fetus. The sound waves are reflected back through the tissues and recorded and displayed in real time on a screen.	Screen for structural malformations	Usually performed at 18–20 weeks of gestation; routinely done Early ultrasound can be performed at 11–14 weeks to evaluate for Down syndrome and other chromosomal abnormalities.
Cell-free fetal DNA testing	Fetal circulating cell-free DNA is taken from a sample of maternal blood. It is an advanced screening test that can detect fetal aneuploidies for chromosomes 21, 18, and 13. It can also detect X or Y chromosomes.	Indicated for higher risk pregnancies: • Pregnant people 35 or older at the time of delivery • Prior testing reveals increased risk of trisomy 21, 18, or 13. • History of previous pregnancy with a trisomy • Parental balanced-Robertsonian translocation	Can be performed as early as 10 weeks Results usually available in 1 week Not recommended for low-risk pregnancies at this time due to lack of evaluation on this population Positive test results require more invasive testing and genetic counseling. High detection rates with low false positives
Percutaneous umbilical blood sampling	An ultrasound-guided needle is inserted through the abdominal and uterine wall to the umbilical cord, and a sample of blood is retrieved and sent to the laboratory for analysis. Used to detect disorders such as hemophilia, hemoglobinopathies, infections, drug levels, chromosomal abnormalities, and cord blood pH. The procedure is similar to amniocentesis but requires a higher level of expertise and experience. Less risk than fetoscopy	Detects chromosome abnormalities; usually done when diagnostic information cannot be obtained through amniocentesis, CVS, or ultrasound or the results of these tests were inconclusive	Performed at or after 18 weeks. Complications include miscarriage, blood loss, infection, and premature rupture of membranes. The risk to the pregnancy is greater than with amniocentesis and CVS. Beginning to replace fetoscopy

COMMON LABORATORY AND DIAGNOSTIC TESTS 27.1

Test	Explanation	Indications	Nursing Implications
Fetoscopy	Endoscopic procedure that allows direct visualization of the fetus through the insertion of a tiny flexible instrument called a fetoscope. It is inserted through the abdominal wall and into the uterine cavity. Ultrasound is used to guide the placement of the scope. Direct visualization can evaluate the fetus for severe congenital anomalies such as neural tube defects. Fetal blood samples from the umbilical cord can be obtained and tested for congenital blood disorders such as hemophilia and sickle cell anemia. Fetal tissue samples (usually skin) can be collected and tested for genetic diseases.	Indicated for any pregnant person at risk for delivering a baby with significant congenital anomalies; can be used to perform corrective surgery (e.g., shunt placement) on the fetus	Performed during or after the 18th week of pregnancy Complications include miscarriage, premature delivery, premature rupture of membranes, amniotic fluid leak, intrauterine fetal death, and infection. Monitor the fetus before and after the procedure.
Gene testing	Gene testing is currently available for many inherited diseases. It involves analysis of DNA, RNA, chromosomes, proteins, metabolites, and biochemical agents. Specimens for gene testing can be obtained from numerous sources; leukocytes from blood are the most common and easily obtained site; during pregnancy, amniocentesis, and CVS; and fetal tissue or products of conception after a miscarriage The most common use is DNA or chromosomes isolated from blood. Direct detection of abnormalities in genes and chromosomes is performed using DNA-based test or cytogenetic tests (which look at chromosome) and other methods. Cytogenetic tests also include FISH to assist in detecting chromosomal abnormalities such as duplication, deletion, rearrangements, and translocations; newer testing, known as array comparative genomic hybridization (aCGH), or microarray, analyzes small duplications or deletions across all of the chromosomes.	To detect abnormalities that may indicate actual disease or predict future disease. Indicated in the evaluation of congenital anomalies, intellectual disability, growth retardation, and recurrent miscarriage to determine the reason for the loss of a fetus, and prenatal diagnosis of genetic disease	Provide support, information, and resources to the family. Refer to genetic counseling before and after the test.
Newborn screening (refer to Chapter 9 for further information)	Blood screening performed shortly after birth is used to identify many life-threatening genetic illnesses that have no immediate visible effects but can lead to physical problems, intellectual disability, and even death. Every U.S. state routinely screens all newborns, but each state dictates which disorders to screen for, so components of the screening vary from state to state.	Identification of newborns so that treatment can begin early to prevent the impact of disorders, such as severe cognitive impairment or death	Refer to each state's protocol for fetal/newborn screening for endocrine disorders. Explain to the family the rationale and procedure. Collect blood sample accurately. Collect prior to blood transfusion if possible. Ideally performed after 24 hours of age; obtain specimen as close to the time of discharge from newborn or labor and delivery unit as possible and no later than 7 days of age. Screening typically between 24 and 48 hours after birth The test is less accurate if done before 24 hours of age and should be repeated by 2 weeks of age if the newborn is younger than 24 hours old. Some states now require a repeat screen at 2 weeks of age.[a] Ensure appropriate follow-up with newborn screening results; results are available in 2 to 3 weeks.

FISH, fluorescence in situ hybridization.

[a]Kemper, A. R. (2021). Newborn Screening. *UpToDate*. Retrieved May 25, 2023, from https://www.uptodate.com/contents/newborn-screening

Data from Fischbach, F. T., Fischbach, M. A., & Stout, K. (2022). *A manual of laboratory and diagnostic tests* (11th ed.). Wolters Kluwer.

Remember Julie, the 5-year-old brought in for her annual examination? What additional health history and physical examination information should you obtain?

Nursing Analysis

After recognizing and analyzing cues from a thorough assessment, the nurse might identify several patient problems, including:

- Delayed development risk
- Knowledge deficiency (specify)
- Decisional conflict
- Fear
- Interrupted family processes
- Caregiver role strain

After completing an assessment of Julie, the nurse noted the following: short stature for age and a low posterior hairline. Based on these assessment findings, what would your top three patient problems be for Julie?

The previously listed patient problems or concerns provide suggestions for developing a nursing plan of care or concept mapping. The nurse will then generate solutions by planning interventions (suggested following with rationales). The plan of care should be individualized based on the child's and family's needs.

Refer to Chapter 11 for nursing interventions related to interrupted family processes and risk for caregiver role strain. Additional information will be included later in the chapter as it relates to specific disorders.

Nursing Analysis

Delayed development risk; risk factors include genetic disorder and treatment regimen.

Goal/Outcome

Child's development will be enhanced: The child will not suffer regression in abilities and will make continued progress toward the attainment of developmental milestones within age parameters and limits of disease. Child expresses interest in the environment and people around them and interacts with the environment appropriately for developmental level.

Promoting Development (interventions with *rationale*)

- Screen for developmental capabilities *to determine the child's current level of functioning.*
- Offer age-appropriate toys, play, and activities (including gross motor) *to encourage further development.*
- Perform exercises or interventions as prescribed by physical or occupational therapist: *these activities promote function and developmental skills.*
- Provide support to families: *due to disability and deficits, the child's progress toward developmental milestones may be slow.*
- Use therapeutic play and adaptive toys *to facilitate developmental functioning.*
- Provide a stimulating environment when possible *to maximize potential for growth and development.*
- Praise accomplishments and emphasize the child's abilities *to improve self-esteem and encourage feelings of confidence and competence.*

Nursing Analysis

Knowledge deficiency related to insufficient information (regarding complex, technical medical condition, prognosis, and medical needs) as evidenced by insufficient knowledge or inaccurate follow-through of instruction

Goal/Outcome

Child and family will verbalize accurate information and understanding about the condition, prognosis, and medical needs: child and family demonstrate knowledge of the condition, prognosis, and medical needs, including possible causes, contributing factors, and treatment measures.

Providing Child and Family Teaching (interventions with *rationale*)

- Assess the child's and family's willingness to learn; the *child and family must be willing to learn for teaching to be effective.*
- Provide family with time to adjust to diagnosis *to facilitate adjustment and ability to learn and participate in child's care.*
- Repeat information *to allow family and child time to learn and understand.*
- Teach in short sessions; *many short sessions are more helpful than one long session.*
- Gear teaching to the child and family's level of understanding (depends on the age of the child, physical condition, and memory) *to ensure understanding.*
- Provide reinforcement and rewards *to facilitate the teaching/learning process.*
- Use multiple modes of learning involving many senses (written, verbal, demonstration, and videos) when possible; *the child and family are more likely to retain information when it is presented in different ways using many senses.*
- Refer the child and family to a genetics specialist; *genetic information is highly technical, the field is advancing at a rapid pace, and information needs to be the most current and accurate. A genetic specialist can provide this along with expertise, support, and resources.*

Nursing Analysis

Decisional conflict related to conflict with moral obligation, moral principle, rule, and value supports mutually inconsistent actions (treatment options; conflicting values; and ethical, legal, and social issues surrounding genetic testing) as evidenced by verbalization of uncertainty about choices or undesired consequences of alternative actions being considered, delay in decision making, and physical signs of distress.

Goal/Outcome

Family will state they are able to make an informed decision: The family will state the advantages and disadvantages of choices and share fears and concerns regarding choices.

Providing Decision-Making Support (interventions with *rationale*)

- Give the family time and encourage them to express their feelings associated with decision making; *the decision-making process becomes more difficult if feelings are not expressed.*
- Encourage the family to list the advantages and disadvantages of each alternative *to aid in problem solving and help the family recognize all alternatives.*
- Initiate health teaching and referral to a genetic specialist when needed; *genetic testing information is often technical and complex. Families need accurate and up-to-date information to aid in decision making.*
- Maintain a nondirective manner; *this is a difficult decision that the family must make for themselves, and the nurse should provide all the necessary information while maintaining an unobtrusive role.*
- Validate the family's feelings regarding the decisional conflict; *validation is a therapeutic communication technique that promotes the nurse–family relationship.*

Nursing Analysis

Fear related to learned response to threat (outcome of genetic testing) as evidenced by apprehensiveness and increased tension

Goal/Outcome

Family will state they can cope with the results of the genetic testing or demonstrate reduced fear: The family accurately discusses the chances of offspring having genetic disease, demonstrates positive coping, and asks questions about genetic testing and the meaning of results.

Managing Fear (interventions with *rationale*)

- Empathize with the family and avoid false reassurances; be truthful *to allow the family to recognize that fear is a reasonable response. Giving false information or reassurance will actually increase fear.*
- Explore coping skills used previously by the family to cope with fear. Reinforce these skills and explore other outlets, such as relaxation, breathing, and physical activity *to encourage the use of coping mechanisms that help control fear.*
- Encourage verbalization of feelings and concerns about genetic testing. Allow time for questions *to provide a safe outlet to express feelings and encourage open communication between the family members.*
- Explain all procedures and review results as available; *knowledge deficit contributes to fear.*
- Refer the family to appropriate support groups and genetic counseling; *talking with families who have gone through similar situations can help decrease fear and provide methods of coping. Genetic counseling provides information along with support and additional resources.*

No matter what the genetic abnormality is, the news may be shattering to the family. It is difficult for nurses to even begin to understand what the family is going through. When providing support and education to families of children with serious genetic abnormalities, use these guiding principles:

- Build a trusting relationship.
- Stress the authenticity of the parents' feelings.
- Reject your own personal biases.
- Recognize that people cope in various ways; the family's behavior may not be what you would expect.
- Help the family to identify their own strengths and supports, building on those as able.
- Know that the family's emotions may exhaust and disorganize them.
- Assist the family members to maintain open communication among themselves.
- Provide referrals to local parent groups or other families with a child with a similar disorder.
- Allow the family to verbalize their emotions and ask questions.
- Always ask the parents how *they* are doing (Lashley, 2005).

Based on your top three patient problems for Julie, describe appropriate nursing interventions.

COMMON CHROMOSOMAL ABNORMALITIES

Major chromosomal abnormalities are seen in about one in 140 live births (Giersch, 2022). Many children with chromosomal abnormalities have associated intellectual disabilities, learning disabilities, behavioral problems, and distinct features, including physical birth defects. The most common chromosomal abnormalities will be discussed next. Refer to Table 27.2 for less common chromosomal abnormalities identified in children.

TABLE 27.2 • Less Common Chromosomal Abnormalities

Chromosomal Abnormality	Features
Prader–Willi syndrome (abnormality on chromosome 15)	Affects one in 10,000–30,000 babies[a] Severe hypotonia, higher weight, short stature, small hands and feet, hypogonadism, hyperphagia, and intellectual disability (varies from mild to severe)
Angelman syndrome (abnormality on chromosome 15)	Affects one in 12,000–20,000 babies[b] Microcephaly with flatness on the back of the head, fair skin and light hair, large mouth with tongue protrusion, seizures, jerky ataxic movements (resembling a puppet gait), uncontrolled bouts of laughter/smiling, happy demeanor, easily excitable personality, developmental delay and speech impairment, and severe intellectual disability
Cri du chat syndrome (abnormality on chromosome 5)	Affects one in 15,000–50,000 babies[c] Hypotonia; short stature; slow growth; low birth weight; failure to thrive; characteristic weak, catlike cry during infancy; microcephaly with protruding metopic suture; moonlike round face; bilateral epicanthal folds (folds of skin over the eyelids); high-arched palate; wide and flat nasal bridge; micrognathia (small receding chin); wide-set eyes (hypertelorism); low-set malformed ears; intellectual disability and developmental delay
Wolf–Hirschhorn syndrome (abnormality on chromosome 4)	Affects one in 50,000 babies[d] Hypotonia, intellectual disability, delayed growth and development, seizures, and characteristic facial features (broad, flat nose bridge; high forehead; widely spaced, protruding eyes; microcephaly)
Williams syndrome (abnormality on chromosome 4)	Affects one in 7,500–75,000 children[e] Affects multiple systems. Cardiovascular disease (supravalvular aortic stenosis most common, hypertension also seen); distinct facial features often described as elfinlike, such as broad forehead, flat nasal bridge, short nose with a broad tip, full cheeks, and a wide mouth with full lips; small, wide-spaced teeth with occlusal abnormalities; hypercalcemia; early puberty for both males and females; structural abnormalities of the kidneys, delayed bladder training and urinary frequency, hypotonia, and joint laxity; learning disabilities and intellectual disability, attention deficit disorder, problems with anxiety and phobias such as fears of sounds and tactile issues; unique personality characteristics, such as outgoing and engaging personality; other medical problems involving eyes and vision and digestive tract
Beckwith–Wiedemann syndrome (abnormality on chromosome 11)	Affects one in 10,300–13,700 babies[f] Infants are considerably larger than normal and grow at an unusual rate in childhood, growth slows in later childhood with adults not unusually tall, and specific parts of the body may grow larger leading to asymmetric appearance; abdominal wall defects such as omphalocele, umbilical hernia; infants present with abnormally large tongue that may interfere with breathing, swallowing, and speaking; abnormally large abdominal organs; crease or pits in skin near ears, hypoglycemia, and kidney abnormalities; increased risk of developing cancerous and noncancerous tumors, such as Wilms tumor, neuroblastoma.
22q11 deletion syndrome (DiGeorge syndrome; abnormality of chromosome 22)	Affects one in 4,000–6,000 babies[g] Hypoplasia or agenesis of the thymus and parathyroid glands; hypocalcemia; hypoplasia of auricle and external auditory canal; cardiac anomalies; immune system abnormalities; cleft palate; short stature; distinctive facial appearance (elongated face, almond-shaped eyes, wide nose, small ears); developmental delays; and learning, speech, feeding, and behavioral problems

[a]Duis, J., & Scheimann, A. O. (2023). Prader–Willi syndrome: Clinical features and diagnosis. *UpToDate.* Retrieved May 29, 2023, from https://www.uptodate.com/contents/prader-willi-syndrome-clinical-features-and-diagnosis?

[b]Madaan, M., & Mendez, M. D. (2023). *Angelman syndrome.* StatPearls Publishing. https://www.ncbi.nlm.nih.gov/books/NBK560870/

[c]Ajitkumar, A., Jamil, R. T., & Mathai, J. K. (2023). *Cri du chat syndrome.* StatPearls Publishing. https://www.ncbi.nlm.nih.gov/books/NBK482460/

[d]Genetic and Rare Diseases (GARD) Information Center. (2023). *Wolf–Hirschhorn syndrome.* https://rarediseases.info.nih.gov/diseases/7896/wolf-hirschhorn-syndrome

[e]Wilson, M., & Carter, I. B. (2022). *Williams syndrome.* StatPearls Publishing. https://www.ncbi.nlm.nih.gov/books/NBK544278/

[f]Hon-Yin, B. C., Shuman, C., Choufani, S., & Weksberg, R. (2022). Beckwith-Wiedemann syndrome. *UpToDate.* Retrieved May 29, 2023, from https://www.uptodate.com/contents/beckwith-wiedemann-syndrome

[g]Lackey, A. E., & Muzio, M. R. (2023). *DiGeorge syndrome.* StatPearls Publishing. https://www.ncbi.nlm.nih.gov/books/NBK549798/

Trisomy 21 (Down Syndrome)

Trisomy 21 (DS) is a genetic disorder caused by the presence of all or part of an extra 21st chromosome. It is the most common chromosomal abnormality associated with intellectual disability (Ostermaier, 2022b). Trisomy 21 is seen in all ages, races, and socioeconomic levels, but a higher incidence is found with a maternal age older than 35 years (Bacino & Lee, 2020). This is partly explained by the fact that 90% of cases with an extra chromosome 21 originate from the female parent (Giersch, 2022). The likelihood of having a baby with DS is around one in 1,000 in females younger than age 30, one in 350 at age 35, one in 85 at age 40, and one in 35 at age 45 (Giersch, 2022).

Trisomy 21 is associated with some degree of intellectual disability, characteristic facial features (e.g., slanted eyes and depressed nasal bridge), and other health problems (e.g., cardiac defects, visual and hearing impairment, intestinal malformations, and an increased susceptibility to infections). The severity of these problems varies.

The prognosis has been improving over the past few decades. Fundamental changes in the care of these children have resulted in longer life expectancy (around 55 to 56 years of age) and an improved quality of life (Ostermaier, 2022b).

Pathophysiology

Trisomy 21 is a disorder caused by nondisjunction or translocation before, at, or after conception. Each egg and sperm cell normally contain 23 chromosomes. When they join, this results in 23 pairs or 46 chromosomes. Sometimes an extra chromosome originates in the development of either the egg or the sperm, resulting in an embryo with three chromosome 21s in *all* cells (Fig. 27.7). This results in the characteristic features and birth defects of DS. This type and timing of nondisjunction, resulting in the presence of three chromosome 21s in all cells, is responsible for about 96% of the cases of DS (Bull et al., 2022).

In approximately 1% to 2% of cases of DS, the nondisjunction occurs *after* fertilization, and a mixture of two cell types is seen (Bull et al., 2022). In these instances, some cells have 47 chromosomes (due to three chromosome 21s), while others have the normal 46 chromosomes (with the normal two chromosome 21s present). This is referred to as the mosaic form of DS. Children with mosaic DS may have a milder form of the disorder, but this is not a general finding.

About 3% to 4% of DS cases involve a translocation, in which part of the number 21 chromosome breaks off during cell division *before or at* conception and attaches (or translocates) to another chromosome (usually chromosome 14; Bull et al., 2022). The cells will remain with 46 chromosomes, but this extra portion of the number 21 chromosome results in the clinical findings of DS. Cases of translocation are not associated with advanced maternal age, as is the situation with nondisjunction errors (Giersch, 2022).

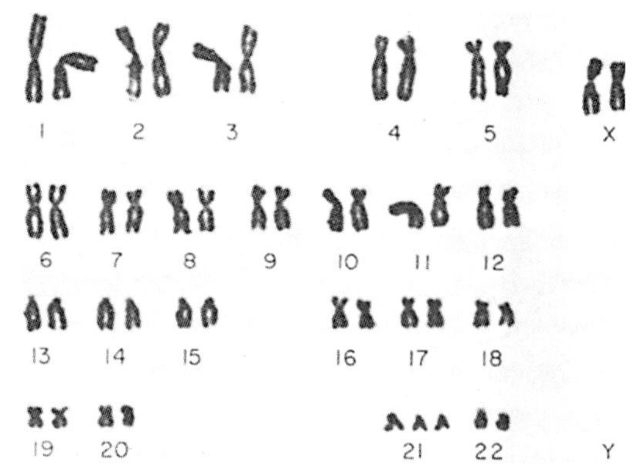

FIGURE 27.7 Down syndrome karyotype. Note the third chromosome located at chromosome 21.

Therapeutic Management

Management of DS will involve multiple disciplines, including a primary provider; specialty primary providers such as a cardiologist, ophthalmologist, and gastroenterologist; nurses; physical therapists; occupational therapists; speech therapists; dietitians; psychologists; counselors; teachers; and, of course, the parents. There is no standard treatment for all children, and there is no prevention or cure. Treatment is mainly symptomatic and supportive. The overall focus of therapeutic management will be to promote the child's optimal growth and development and function within the limits of the disease.

MANAGING COMPLICATIONS

Children with DS need the usual immunizations, well-child care, and screening recommended by the American Academy of Pediatrics. In addition, medical management will focus on complications associated with DS.

Congenital heart disease occurs in 40% to 50% of children with DS (Bull et al., 2022). Cardiac problems vary from minor defects that respond to medication therapy to major defects that require surgical intervention. Children with DS also have an increased incidence of gastrointestinal disorders (Bull et al., 2022). These disorders vary from those that can be managed by dietary manipulation, such as celiac disease and constipation, to intestinal malformations such as Hirschsprung disease and imperforate anus, which require surgical intervention.

Hearing and vision impairments also are common. More than 75% of children with DS have hearing loss (Bull et al., 2022). Otitis media is a common problem affecting 50% to 70% of children with DS and is often the cause of hearing loss (Ostermaier, 2022a). Of children with DS, 60% to 80% have vision problems (Bull et al., 2022). Therefore, regular evaluation of vision and hearing is essential.

Obstructive sleep apnea is present in 50% to 79% of children with DS (Bull et al., 2022). Often parents are unaware their child is having sleep disturbances, so baseline testing in young children may be warranted.

Children with DS have a higher incidence of thyroid disease, which can affect growth and cognitive function (Bull et al., 2022). Most of these children have hypothyroidism (an underactive thyroid), but sometimes hyperthyroidism (an overactive thyroid) occurs. Periodic thyroid testing may be warranted. Children with DS are also at a higher risk for higher weight and delayed dental eruptions or hypodontia (Bull et al., 2022). Some studies have found an increased risk of type 1 diabetes in children with DS (Ostermaier, 2022a).

DOSAGE CALCULATION 27.1

Child's age: 4 years old

Child's weight: 30 lb

Medication order: Levothyroxine (Synthroid) 75 μg by mouth once a day

Per the *Pediatric Dosage Handbook*, the recommended dose for a child 1 to 5 years of age is 5 to 6 μg/kg/day.

Is the ordered dose safe?

Children with DS are at an increased risk for atlantoaxial instability (increased mobility of the cervical spine at the first and second vertebrae; Bull et al., 2022). In most cases, these children are without symptoms, but symptoms may appear if spinal cord compression occurs (Ostermaier, 2022b). Screening for signs and symptoms of atlantoaxial instability is important, especially if the child is involved in sports.

CLINICAL REASONING ALERT!

If neck pain, unusual posturing of the head and neck (torticollis), change in gait, loss of upper body strength, abnormal reflexes, or change in bowel or bladder functioning is noted in the child with DS, immediate attention is required.

Children with DS are at an increased risk for certain hematologic problems, such as anemia, transient leukemia (mostly during the newborn period), leukemia (later onset), and polycythemia during infancy (Bull et al., 2022). Children with DS also have a higher susceptibility to infection and a higher mortality rate from infectious diseases (Ostermaier, 2022b). Precautions to prevent and monitor for infection are needed. Other potential complications include alopecia, communication disorders, and seizures.

Due to their increased risk for certain congenital anomalies and diseases, children with DS will need to be monitored closely, and regular medical care is essential. Children with DS have a higher incidence of autism and behavioral problems (Bull et al., 2022). Screening for autism spectrum disorder (ASD) may be appropriate. Discuss and assess behavioral and social development and refer children with autism, attention-deficit/hyperactivity disorder, or other behavioral or psychiatric issues appropriately. See Evidence-Based Practice 27.1.

EARLY INTERVENTION THERAPY

Early intervention refers to a variety of specialized programs and resources available to young children with developmental delay or other impairment. These programs may involve an array of health care professionals such as physical, occupational, and speech therapists; special educators; and social workers. The programs focus on providing stimulation and encouragement to children with DS. They help encourage and accelerate development and may help to prevent some developmental delays. The earlier the intervention can begin, the

EVIDENCE-BASED PRACTICE 27.1

What Are the Experiences of Families of Children With a Dual Diagnosis of Down Syndrome (DS) and Autism Spectrum Disorder (ASD; DS-ASD)?

The prevalence rate of ASD is much higher in children with DS compared to the general population. They are often diagnosed later and, in some cases, may go undiagnosed due to the difficulty identifying ASD-associated impairments versus DS-related impairments. Earlier identification of ASD is associated with greater efficacy of interventions. This study aimed to learn about caregiver's perspectives, observations, and experiences when caring for a child with DS-ASD.

STUDY

This was a qualitative study where caregivers, in a closed online community for families who care for a child with DS-ASD, completed a survey with open-ended questions.

Findings

Data analysis found a 4.65-year gap from when a caregiver first noticed symptoms to the time of diagnosis. Caregivers expressed feelings that their concerns over their child's behaviors were initially dismissed, which contributed to a delay in ASD diagnosis. Caregivers expressed feelings of social isolation, frustration, and increased levels of stress, mainly related to providers' lack of knowledge surrounding DS-ASD.

Nursing Implications

It can be challenging to identify children with DS and ASD due to the developmental impairments and behaviors that accompany DS. ASD can contribute to comorbidity of the child with DS, and research has shown children with ASD and DS have lower cognitive, language, and adaptive levels and increased behavioral problems. Providers and educators need training in recognizing ASD-like symptoms. They need to assess for the presence of multiple signs and symptoms of ASD, listen to parental concerns, and consider referral for evaluation by a specialist. Identification and intervention are imperative. Nurses need to utilize appropriate valid and reliable screening tools. Continued research into appropriate screening tools, particularly for children younger than 3 years of age, is warranted. Providers need to provide parental support and resources to minimize feelings of social isolation, frustration, and stress. This study has limitations, including its small sample size. Further research is needed relating to how children with DS-ASD differ from those with DS alone.

Data from Spinazzi, N. A., Velasco, A. B., Wodecki, D. J., & Patel, L. (2023). Autism spectrum disorder in Down syndrome: Experiences from caregivers. *Journal of Autism and Developmental Disorders, 54*, 1171–1180. https://doi.org/10.1007/s10803-022-05758-x

more beneficial it will be. The programs are individualized to meet the specific needs of each child.

Children with DS progress through the same developmental stages as typical children, but they do so on their own timetable (refer to Table 27.3 for the average age of skill acquisition in children with DS). For example, children with DS will learn to walk, but the average child with DS walks at 24 months (versus 12 months for a child without DS). Conditions such as hypotonia, ligament laxity, decreased strength, enlarged tongue, and short arms and legs are common in children with DS, and early intervention can help in the development of gross and fine motor skills, language, and social and self-care skills.

Parents also benefit from early intervention programs in terms of support, encouragement, and information. Early intervention programs teach parents how to interact with their child while meeting the child's specific needs and encouraging development.

Nursing Assessment

For a full description of the assessment phase of the nursing process, refer to the "Clinical Judgment and the Nursing Process" section earlier in the chapter. Assessment findings pertinent to DS are discussed next.

HEALTH HISTORY

DS is often diagnosed prenatally using perinatal screening and diagnostic tests. If not diagnosed prenatally, most cases are diagnosed in the first few days of life based on the physical characteristics associated with DS. Identify high-risk deliveries. Explore the pregnancy history and past medical history for risk factors such as:

- Lack of prenatal care or screening
- Abnormal prenatal screening or diagnostic tests for DS (e.g., fetal nuchal translucency, triple/quadruple screen, ultrasound, amniocentesis)
- Maternal age older than 35 years

The older infant or child known to have DS is often admitted to the hospital for corrective surgeries or other complications of the disease, such as infections. Elicit a description of the present illness and chief complaint. In an infant or child returning for a clinic visit or hospitalization, the health history should include questions related to:

- Cardiac defects or disease (treatment regimen, surgical repair)
- Hearing or vision impairment (last hearing and vision evaluation, any corrective measures)
- Developmental delays (speech, gross and fine motor skills)
- Sucking or feeding problems
- Cognitive abilities (degree of intellectual disability)
- Gastrointestinal disorders such as vomiting or absence of stools (special dietary management, surgical interventions)
- Thyroid disease
- Hematologic problems, such as anemia, leukemia
- Atlantoaxial instability
- Seizures
- Infections such as recurrent or chronic respiratory infections, otitis media

TABLE 27.3 • Average Age Range of Skill Acquisition in Children With Down Syndrome

Developmental Milestone	Age Range of Acquisition, Children With Down Syndrome	Age Range of Acquisition, Typical Children
Smile	1–5 months	1–3 months
Sit alone	6–36 months	5–9 months
Crawl	8–22 months	6–12 months
Stands	1–3.25 years	8–17 months
Walk	1–4 years	8–17 months
First word	1–4 years	1–2 years
Speak in sentences	2–7.5 years	15–32 months
Feed self with fingers	10–24 months	7–15 months
Use spoon	13–39 months	12–20 months
Bowel training	2–7 years	16–42 months
Put on clothes	3.5–8.5 years	3.25–5 years

Data from National Down Syndrome Society. (2023). *Early intervention.* https://www.ndss.org/resources/early-intervention/

- Growth (height and weight changes, feeding problems, unexplained weight gain)
- Signs and symptoms of sleep apnea, such as snoring, restlessness during sleep, daytime sleepiness
- Any other changes in physical state or medication regimen

PHYSICAL EXAMINATION

The initial assessment after birth may reveal certain physical features characteristic of DS (Box 27.4 and Fig. 27.8).

Observe the child's general appearance. Note the lack of muscle tone and loose joints; this is usually more pronounced in infancy, and the infant has a floppy appearance. Observe growth and development. Plot growth on appropriate growth charts. Because children with DS grow at a slower rate, special growth charts have been developed. Refer to the Centers for Disease Control and Prevention (CDC) website for clinical growth charts for children with DS.

When assessing the achievement of developmental milestones in children with DS, it may be more useful to look at the sequence of milestones rather than the age at which they were achieved. Each milestone represents a skill that is needed for the next stage of development.

BOX 27.4 Common Clinical Manifestations of Down Syndrome

- Hypotonia
- Short stature
- Flattened occiput
- Small (brachycephalic) head
- Flat facial profile
- Depressed nasal bridge and small nose
- Oblique palpebral fissures (an upward slant to the eyes)
- Brushfield spots (white spots on the iris of the eye)
- Low-set, small ears
- Abnormally shaped ears
- Small mouth
- Protrusion of tongue; tongue is large compared to mouth size.
- Arched, narrow palate
- Hands with broad, short fingers
- A single deep transverse crease on the palm of the hand (simian crease)
- Congenital heart defect
- Short neck, with excessive skin at the nape
- Hyperflexibility and looseness of joints (excessive ability to extend the joints)
- Dysplastic middle phalanx of fifth finger (one flexion furrow instead of two)
- Epicanthal folds (small skin folds on the inner corner of the eyes)
- Excessive space between large and second toe

Data from Ostermaier, K. K. (2022a). Down syndrome: Clinical features and diagnosis. *UpToDate*. Retrieved May 23, 2023, from https://www.uptodate.com/contents/down-syndrome-clinical-features-and-diagnosis; Bull, M. J., Trotter, T., Santoro, S. L., Christensen, C., Grout, R. W.; The Council on Genetics. (2022). Health supervision for children and adolescents with Down syndrome. *Pediatrics, 149*(5), e2022057010. https://doi.org/10.1542/peds.2022-057010

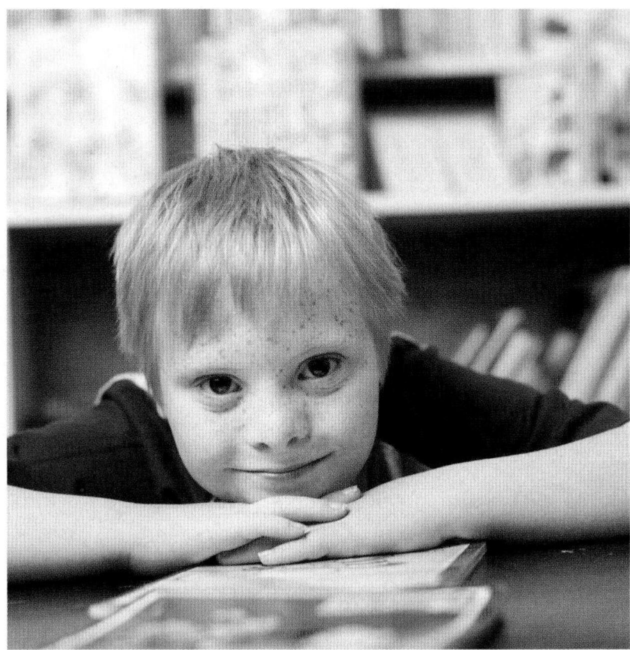

FIGURE 27.8 Child with Down syndrome.

Perform a subjective assessment of hearing and refer the child for further evaluation if indicated. Assess vision, especially for cataracts. Assess respiratory status and cardiac status. Auscultate for murmurs and pulmonary changes, which can indicate congenital heart disease. Chronic or recurrent respiratory infections, such as pneumonia and otitis media, may be found.

LABORATORY AND DIAGNOSTIC TESTS

A variety of screening tests are available using maternal serum and ultrasound. In recent years, noninvasive cell-free fetal DNA testing has become available and provides a high sensitivity and specificity (Bull et al., 2022). DS risk screening can be calculated incorporating maternal age prenatally between 11 and 14 weeks using ultrasound and blood tests (nuchal translucency and pregnancy-associated plasma protein A [PAPP-A] and human chorionic gonadotropin [hCG]), and around 16 and 18 weeks using triple/quadruple blood tests to detect AFP, hCG, estriol, and/or inhibin A levels (Bullet al., 2022). Ultrasound and amniocentesis or chorionic villi sampling (CVS) to detect chromosomal abnormalities can also be done prenatally. DS can be confirmed after birth using chromosome analysis (see Common Laboratory and Diagnostic Tests 27.1).

Common laboratory and diagnostic studies ordered for the diagnosis and assessment of complications associated with DS include:

- Echocardiogram: to detect cardiac defects
- Vision and hearing screening: to detect vision and hearing impairments
- Thyroid hormone level: to detect thyroid disease

- Cervical radiographs: to assess for atlantoaxial instability
- Ultrasound: to assess for gastrointestinal malformations

These tests will be important in evaluating the severity of the child's physical disabilities.

Nursing Management

Due to the high incidence of DS and the complex medical needs of these children, most pediatric nurses are likely to care for these children in their practice. Nursing management focuses on providing supportive measures such as promoting growth and development, preventing complications, promoting nutrition, and providing support and education to the child and family. In addition to the patient problems and related interventions discussed in the "Clinical Judgment and the Nursing Process" section earlier in the chapter, additional considerations are reviewed next.

ATRAUMATIC CARE

When planning atraumatic care interventions when caring for a child with DS, be sure to individualize interventions based on the child's developmental level.

PROMOTING GROWTH AND DEVELOPMENT

Children with DS tend to grow more slowly, learn more slowly, have shorter attention spans, and have trouble with reasoning and judgment. Their personality tends to be one of genuine warmth and cheerfulness along with patience, gentleness, and a natural spontaneity. Growth and developmental milestones for children with DS have been developed as a guide for primary providers and nurse practitioners. Table 27.3 gives examples of the average age range at which these children reach selected milestones versus typical children.

THINKING ABOUT DEVELOPMENT

As a nurse in a primary provider's office, how will your education on safety differ when caring for an infant with DS compared to a toddler or adolescent?

Nurses play a key role in connecting families with appropriate resources that can facilitate the child's growth and development. The sooner early intervention programs can begin, the better for the child (see the earlier discussion on early intervention). Speech and language therapy, occupational therapy, and physical therapy will be important in promoting the child's growth and development. Special education should fit the child's individual needs, and the child should be integrated into mainstream education whenever possible.

Preventing Complications

Children with DS are at risk for certain health problems (see "Managing Complications" section). Even though most nurses will encounter a child with DS in their practice, only a few nurses will become experts in their care. The needs of these children are complex, and the American Academy of Pediatrics has developed guidelines that can help the nurse care for these children and their families. Nurses play a key role in educating parents and caregivers about how to prevent the complications of DS (see Teaching Guidelines 27.1).

TEACHING GUIDELINES **27.1** Health Guidelines for Children With Down Syndrome

- Have your child evaluated by a pediatric cardiologist, including an echocardiogram.
- Take your child for routine vision and hearing tests. By 6 months, have your child seen by a pediatric ophthalmologist.
- Make sure your child gets regular medical care, including recommended immunizations and a thyroid test at birth, then every 5–7 months until 1 year, then yearly.
- Have your child follow a regular diet and exercise routine.
- Make sure all family members perform proper hand hygiene to prevent infection.
- Monitor for signs and symptoms of respiratory infections, such as pneumonia, and otitis media.
- Discuss with your primary provider the use of pneumococcal, respiratory syncytial virus, and influenza vaccines.
- Begin early interventions, therapy, and education as soon as possible.
- Make sure your child brushes their teeth regularly. They should visit the dentist every 6 months.
- Report any changes in gait or use of arms and hands, weakness, changes in bowel or bladder function, complaints of neck pain or stiffness, head tilt, torticollis, or generalized changes in function. Ensure cervical spine positioning precautions (to avoid overextending or flexing of the neck) are utilized during procedures, such as those involving anesthetic, surgery, or radiographs.

Adapted from Bull, M. J., Trotter, T., Santoro, S. L., Christensen, C., Grout, R. W.; The Council on Genetics. (2022). Health supervision for children and adolescents with Down syndrome. *Pediatrics*, *149*(5), e2022057010. https://doi.org/10.1542/peds.2022-057010

Promoting Nutrition

Children with DS may have difficulty sucking and feeding due to lack of muscle tone. They tend to have small mouths; a smooth, flat, large tongue; and due to the underdeveloped nasal bone, chronically stuffy noses. This may lead to poor nutritional intake and problems with growth. These problems usually improve as the child gains tongue control. Use of a bulb syringe, humidification, and changing the infant's position can lessen the problem. Breastfeeding a baby with DS is usually possible, and the antibodies in breast milk can help the infant fight infections. The caregiver's hand can be used to provide additional support for the chin and throat. Speech or occupational therapists can work on strengthening muscles and assisting in feeding accommodations. Other feeding problems and failure to thrive can be related to cardiac defects and usually improve after medical management is initiated or corrective surgery is performed.

Children with DS do not need a special diet unless an underlying gastrointestinal disease is present, such as celiac disease. A balanced, high-fiber diet and regular exercise are important. Research has suggested that children with DS have lower basal metabolic rates, which can lead to problems with higher weight, so it is important in the early years to develop appropriate eating habits and a regular exercise routine. High fiber intake is important for children with DS because their lack of muscle tone may decrease gastric motility, leading to constipation.

PROVIDING SUPPORT AND EDUCATION FOR THE CHILD AND FAMILY

DS is a lifelong disorder that can result in health problems and cognitive disability. The diagnosis is usually made prenatally or shortly after birth. Parents and caregivers will need support and education during this difficult time. The range of mental impairment varies from mild to moderate; severe deficits occur occasionally. Some families may see having a child with DS as a lifelong tragedy; others may view it as a positive growing experience. Evaluate how the family defines and manages this experience. Base the plan of care on each family's values, beliefs, strengths, and resources.

Family members may have trouble meeting the demands of caring for a child with DS. These children have complex medical needs, which place strain on the family and its finances. From the time of diagnosis, the family should be involved in the child's care. Include parents in planning interventions and care for the child. In most cases, they are the primary caregivers and will provide daily care as well as assisting the child in the development of functioning and skills. They can provide essential information to the health care team and will be advocates for their child throughout their life.

As the child grows, the needs of the family and child will change. Recognize and respect these needs, and provide ongoing education and support for the child and family. Children with DS will need meaningful education programs. Many children with DS begin formal education in infancy and continue through high school.

The outlook is brighter than it once was for children with DS. Many go on in adulthood to obtain jobs, to receive secondary education, and to live on their own or in semi-independent housing. Be familiar with local and national resources for families of children with DS so that you can help these children fulfill their potential.

CONSIDER THIS!

"The day after my son was born, I was told they suspected he had DS. Once the diagnosis was confirmed, I felt devastated. I grieved the loss of all the dreams I had for him and felt alone and scared. I wonder 'why us.'"

Thoughts: How will you respond to this parent?

Trisomy 18 and Trisomy 13

Trisomy 18 (also known as Edwards syndrome) and trisomy 13 (also known as Patau syndrome) are two other common trisomies. These trisomies are much more severe and debilitating than trisomy 21. The incidence of trisomy 18 (the presence of three number 18 chromosomes) is one in 6,000 births; the incidence of trisomy 13 (the presence of three number 13 chromosomes) is one in 10,000 births (Bacino & Lee, 2020). Like DS, trisomy 13 and trisomy 18 usually result from nondisjunction during cell division. Trisomy 18 and trisomy 13 can be present in all cells or may occur in mosaic forms. Both are associated with a characteristic set of anomalies and severe intellectual disability (Bacino & Lee, 2020).

The prognosis for trisomy 18 and trisomy 13 is usually poor; these children usually do not survive beyond the first year of life. There is no cure for trisomy 18 or trisomy 13. Therapeutic management will focus on managing the various congenital anomalies and health issues associated with the disorders.

Nursing Assessment

Nursing assessment will include a general observation for characteristic anomalies (Table 27.4; Figs. 27.9 and 27.10).

Prenatal screening and diagnostic tests for trisomy 18 and trisomy 13 exist. If not diagnosed during the prenatal period, most cases are diagnosed in the first few days of life based on the physical characteristics associated with the disorders.

Nursing Management

Nursing management will be mainly supportive. This will be a difficult time for the family, so providing support and resources for the family will be an important nursing function. SOFT is a support organization for families who have had a child with a chromosome abnormality.

TABLE 27.4 • Clinical Manifestations of Trisomy 18 and Trisomy 13

Chromosomal Abnormality	Clinical Manifestations
Trisomy 18	Prominent occiput, low-set ears, short eyelid fissures, severe intellectual disability, severe hypotonia, webbing, clenched fist with index finger over third digit and fifth digit overlapping the fourth, hypoplasia of fingernails, narrow hips with limited abduction, short sternum, congenital cardiac defects
Trisomy 13	Microcephalic head, wide sagittal suture and fontanels, malformed ears, small eyes, extra digits, severe hypotonia, severe intellectual disability, congenital heart defects, cleft lip, cleft palate

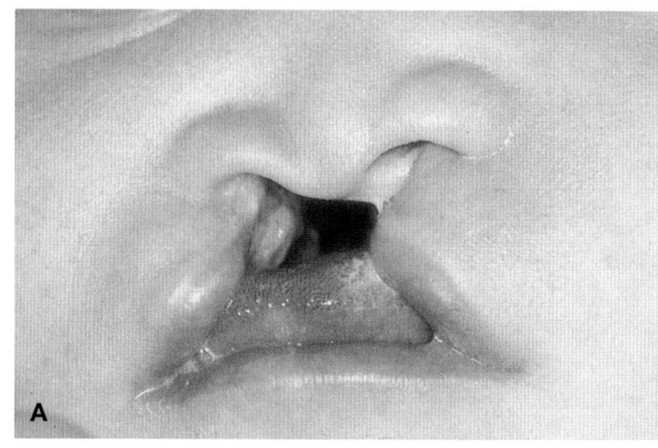

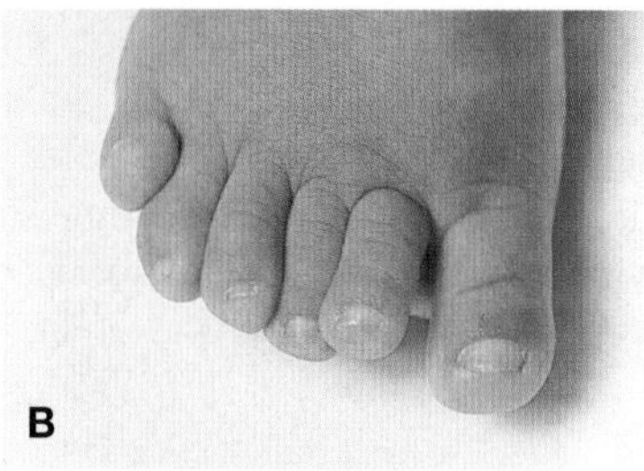

FIGURE 27.10 Trisomy 13. **A.** Note cleft lip and palate. **B.** Note extra digits (polydactyly).

Turner Syndrome

Turner syndrome is a common abnormality of the sex chromosome. The phenotype is female. It occurs in about one in 2,500 live female births (Bacino, 2023c). The abnormality is due to a loss of all or part of one of the sex chromosomes. About half of the affected people have only one X chromosome; the other half have a variety of abnormalities of one of their sex chromosomes and may present with the mosaic form.

There is no cure for Turner syndrome. Therapeutic management will focus on managing the health issues associated with the syndrome. Children with Turner syndrome are more prone to cardiovascular problems, kidney and thyroid problems, skeletal disorders such as scoliosis and osteoporosis, hearing and eye disturbances, learning disabilities, and higher weight (Bacino & Lee, 2016; Backelijauw, 2022). Infertility is usually present, but a few spontaneous pregnancies have been reported (Backelijauw, 2022). Growth hormone administration is a standard of care and usually begins when the child's height falls below the fifth percentile for healthy females. Hormone replacement therapy may also be given to initiate puberty and complete growth.

Nursing Assessment

On assessment, note patterns of growth; short stature and slow growth will be a characteristic finding and often the first indication. Other physical characteristics include a webbed neck, low posterior hairline, wide-spaced nipples, edema of the hands and feet, amenorrhea, no development of secondary sex characteristics, sterility, and perceptual and social skill difficulties (Fig. 27.11).

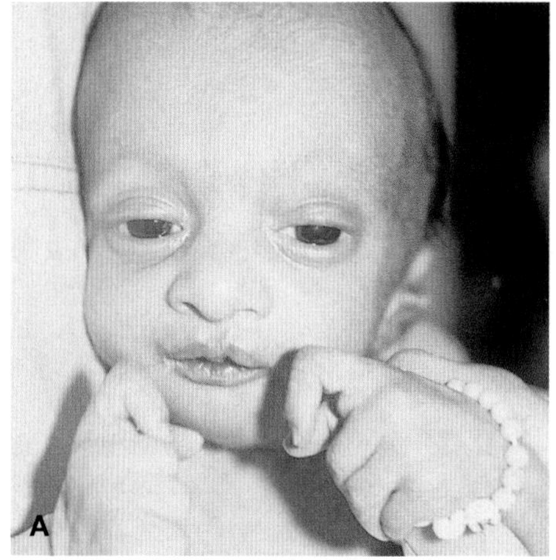

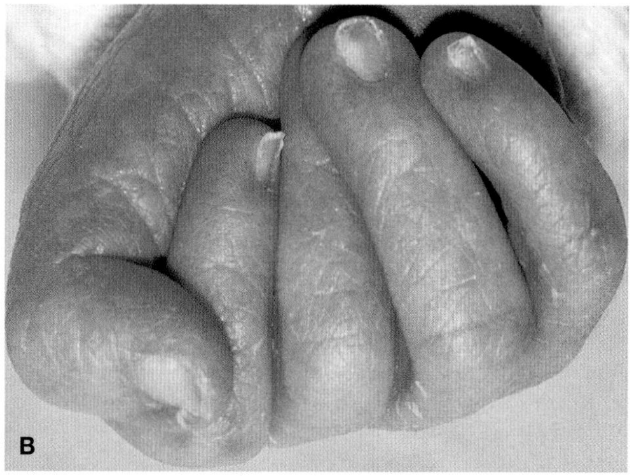

FIGURE 27.9 Trisomy 18. **A.** Note prominent occiput, low set ears and short eyelid fissures. **B.** Note clenched fist with index finger over third digit and fifth digit overlapping the fourth, hypoplasia of the fingernails.

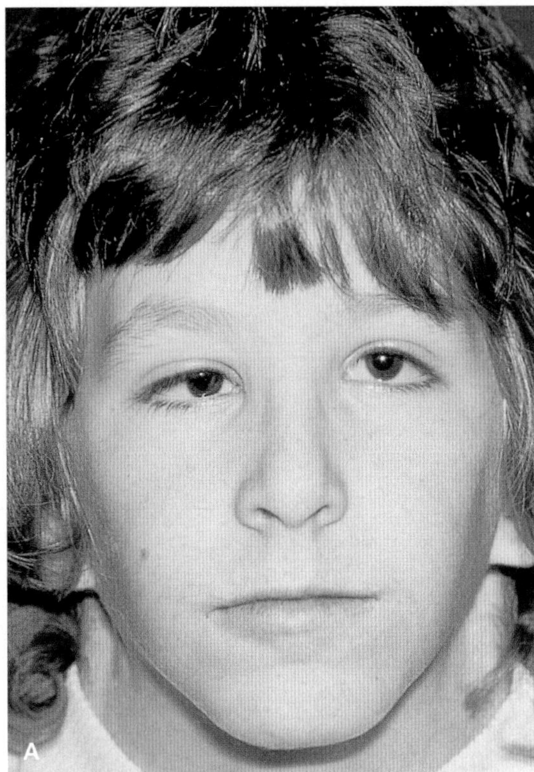
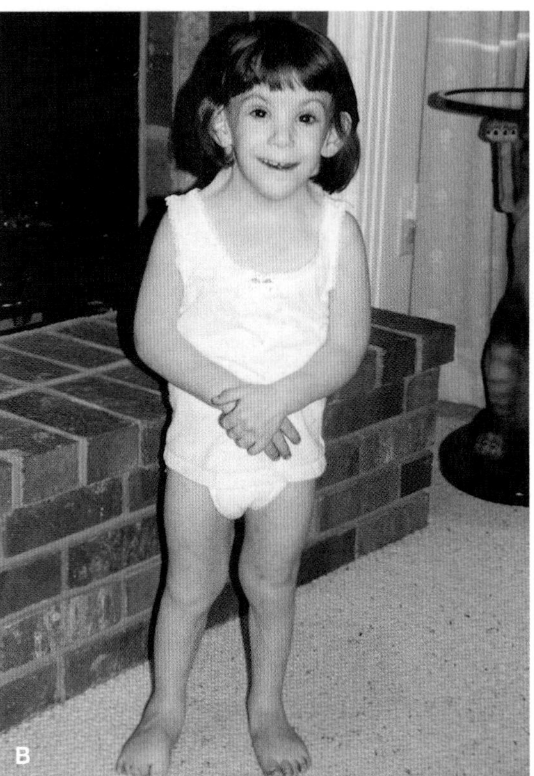

FIGURE 27.11 Note the webbed neck of the child with Turner syndrome. **A.** Note the webbed neck, ocular and ear lobe abnormalities. **B.** Note short stature, webbed neck, genu valgum.

Turner syndrome can be suspected prenatally by ultrasound findings such as fetal edema or redundant nuchal skin (Backelijauw, 2022). It can be diagnosed by chromosomal analysis, either prenatally or after birth. Most children are diagnosed at birth or in early childhood when slow growth or growth failure is noted. Some cases will not be diagnosed until the pubertal growth spurt does not occur.

Nursing Management

Nursing management is mainly supportive. Provide education and support to the family; they need to understand that short stature and infertility are likely. Explain that intellectual disability is unlikely, but some learning disabilities may be present. Emphasize that with medical supervision and support, people with Turner syndrome may lead healthy, satisfying lives. Counseling about infertility is important. Parents may be upset that their child will not be able to reproduce, so explain that many alternatives for reproduction, such as in vitro fertilization and adoption, are available.

Providing resources for the family is an important nursing function. The Turner Syndrome Society of the United States provides assistance, support, and education to people with Turner syndrome and their families.

Klinefelter Syndrome

Klinefelter syndrome is the most common sex chromosomal abnormality (Bacino & Lee, 2016). The karyotype and phenotype are male, but one or more extra X chromosomes are present. The abnormality is usually caused by nondisjunction during meiosis, but mosaic forms do present. The incidence of Klinefelter syndrome is one in 500 to 1,000 males (Bacino, 2023c). Males present with some femalelike physical features that are caused by testosterone deficiency. The risk of recurrence in future pregnancies is not increased.

There is no cure for Klinefelter syndrome. Therapeutic management will focus on interventions to enhance masculine characteristics, such as testosterone replacement. Early recognition and hormonal treatment are important to improve quality of life and prevent serious consequences. Cosmetic surgery may be performed to minimize female characteristics such as gynecomastia (increased breast size).

Nursing Assessment

Due to nonspecific findings during childhood, the diagnosis is not usually made until adolescence or adulthood. Prenatal diagnosis is rare unless amniocentesis is performed for genetic testing. Many males with Klinefelter syndrome reach adulthood without being diagnosed (Bacino & Lee, 2020). The diagnosis is confirmed by chromosomal analysis.

On assessment, a lack of development of secondary sex characteristics may be found. The person may have decreased facial hair, gynecomastia, decreased pubic hair, and hypogonadism or underdeveloped testes, which leads to infertility. The person may be taller than

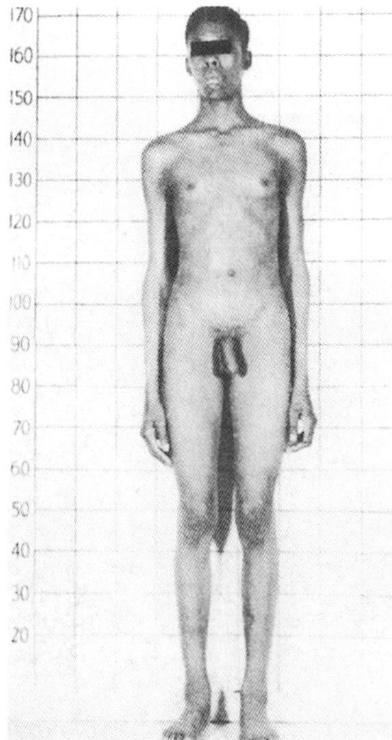

FIGURE 27.12 Klinefelter syndrome.

average by 5 years of age, with long legs and a short torso (Fig. 27.12). Intellectual disability is not present, but cognitive impairments of varying degrees, such as motor delay, speech or language difficulties, attention deficits, and learning disabilities, may be found.

Nursing Management

Nursing management will be mainly supportive. Provide education and support to the family, and make them aware of the American Association for Klinefelter Syndrome and the Association for X and Y Chromosome Variations.

Counseling about infertility is important. Educate children and families that marriage and sexual relations are possible. Parents may be upset that their child will not be able to reproduce, so explain that many alternatives for reproduction are available and technology is advancing in the field of infertility.

Fragile X Syndrome

Fragile X syndrome is the most common inherited cause of intellectual disability (Van Esch, 2022). It is the outcome of a mutation of a gene (FMR1 [fragile X mental retardation]) on the X chromosome. This mutation essentially "turns off" the gene, triggering fragile X syndrome. Males and females are both affected, but it is more commonly seen in males, and affected females usually have milder symptoms (Van Esch, 2022). The incidence is approximately 1 in 8,000 females and 1 in 4,000 males (Stone et al., 2023). The inheritance of fragile X is complex and is less straightforward than single-gene or mendelian inheritance. Some carrier females are affected, and not all males with the gene abnormality show symptoms. Males and females are both fertile and can transmit the disorder to their offspring, so genetic counseling is appropriate. The prognosis for people with fragile X is good, and they tend to live a normal lifespan.

There is no cure for fragile X syndrome. Therapeutic management will be multidisciplinary and aimed at interventions to improve cognitive, emotional, and behavioral impairments.

Nursing Assessment

During childhood, clinical manifestations are subtle, with minor dysmorphic features and developmental delays. Problems with sensation, emotion, and behavior are often the first signs. A delay in attaining developmental milestones will most likely be the first clue found on assessment. Intellectual impairment can range from subtle learning disabilities to severe intellectual disability and autismlike behaviors. In adolescence, males tend to present with characteristic features such as an elongated face; prominent jaw; large, protruding ears; large size; macroorchidism (large testes); and a range of behavioral abnormalities and cognitive deficits (Fig. 27.13). There is a characteristic pattern to the cognitive deficits, with problems in abstract reasoning, sequential processing, and mathematics. Typical behavior problems include attention deficits, hand flapping and biting, hyperactivity, shyness, social isolation, low self-esteem, and gaze aversion. In females, the clinical manifestations are similar but are more varied and often present in a milder form.

Diagnosis is confirmed by molecular genetic testing. Fragile X can be diagnosed prenatally if inheritance is suspected.

Nursing Management

Nursing management will be mainly supportive. Early diagnosis and intervention with developmental therapies and an individualized education plan are ideal. Care of these children will be the same as care of other children with intellectual disability (see Chapter 28 for further information on intellectual disability).

Provide education and support to the family. The National Fragile X Foundation provides education and emotional support and works to increase awareness and advance research for fragile X.

NEUROCUTANEOUS DISORDERS

Neurocutaneous disorders, also referred to as hamartoses, are a group of disorders characterized by abnormalities of both the skin and the central nervous system. Many neurologic conditions are associated with cutaneous manifestations since the skin and the nervous system share a common embryologic origin. They are complex

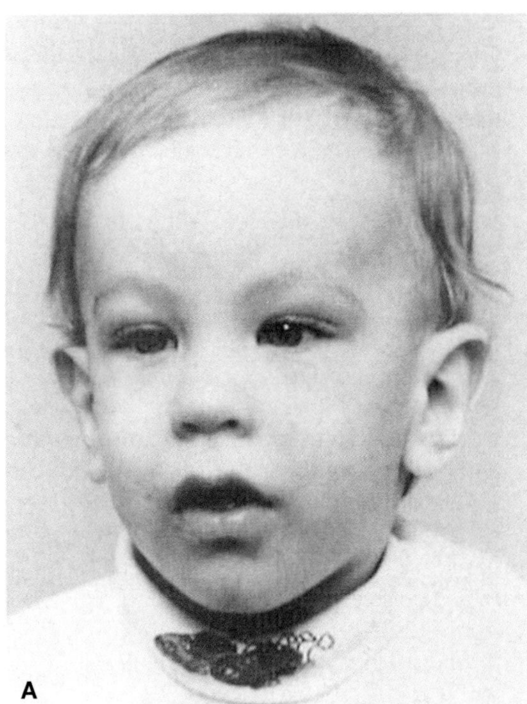

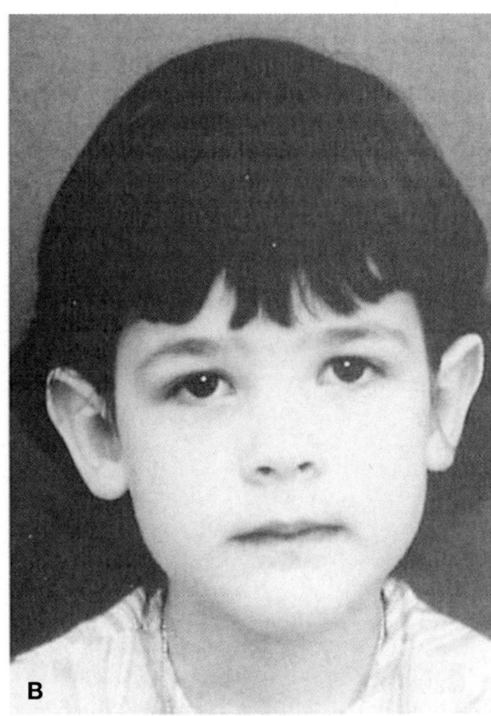

FIGURE 27.13 Fragile X syndrome. **A** and **B.** Note the subtle minor dysmorphic features such as large and protruding ears.

conditions and most also affect other organ systems such as eyes, bones, heart, and kidneys. Most are hereditary and follow an autosomal dominant inheritance pattern or sporadic occurrence. Neurofibromatosis is a common neurocutaneous syndrome and will be discussed in detail next. Table 27.5 provides information on other neurocutaneous syndromes.

Neurofibromatosis

Neurofibromatoses are neurocutaneous genetic disorders of the nervous system that primarily affect the development and growth of neural cell tissues. There are distinct types: neurofibromatosis 1, *NF2*-related schwannomatosis (NF2, formerly neurofibromatosis type 2), and schwannomatosis (Korf et al., 2023).

Neurofibromatosis 1 (von Recklinghausen disease) is the more common type and is discussed here (Korf et al., 2023). This disorder causes tumors to grow on nerves and produce other abnormalities such as skin changes and bone deformities. Although many affected people inherit the disorder, nearly half of the cases are due to a new mutation (Korf et al., 2023). The inheritance pattern is autosomal dominant; therefore, the offspring of affected people have a 50% chance of inheriting the altered gene and presenting with symptoms. Neurofibromatoses are due to a mutation of the neurofibromin gene on chromosome 17. The estimated prevalence is one in 2,600 to 3,000 live births (Korf et al., 2023).

Complications associated with neurofibromatosis include headaches; hydrocephalus; scoliosis; cardiac defects; hypertension; seizures; vision and hearing loss; neurocognitive deficits, including learning disabilities, attention deficit disorder, fine and gross motor delays, ASD, and behavior and psychosocial issues; abnormalities of speech; and a higher risk for neoplasms.

There is no cure for neurofibromatosis. Therapeutic management is aimed at controlling symptoms and managing complications. Surgical intervention can help reduce some of the bone malformations and remove painful or disfiguring tumors. These children should have a yearly physical examination, including blood pressure and cardiovascular examination, scoliosis screening, ophthalmology examination, developmental screening, and a neurologic examination.

The disease is progressive and symptoms usually worsen over time, but it is difficult to predict the course. Most affected people develop mild to moderate symptoms, with non–life-threatening complications, and live a normal, productive life. Recent studies have shown a decreased life expectancy compared to the general population (Korf et al., 2023).

Nursing Assessment

On assessment, the nurse may find café-au-lait spots (light-brown macules), which are the hallmark of neurofibromatosis (Korf et al., 2023; Fig. 27.14). These are usually present at birth but can appear during the first year of life and usually increase in size, number, and pigmentation. They are present all over the body, particularly the trunk and extremities, while usually sparing the face. Pigmented nevi, axillary freckling, and slow-growing cutaneous, subcutaneous, or dermal neurofibromas, which are

TABLE 27.5 • Other Neurocutaneous Syndromes

Disorder	Incidence	Clinical Manifestations	Nursing Considerations
Tuberous sclerosis	1 in 6,000–10,000[a]	Benign tumors present in the brain and skin. Presents most often as a generalized seizure disorder. Tumors can also involve heart, kidney, eyes, lung, and bones. Developmental delay and behavioral problems may be noted. Usually evident in early childhood. Wide clinical spectrum from severe intellectual disability with incapacitating seizures to normal intelligence and no seizures	Treatment will be mainly symptomatic with goal to prevent and treat associated complications. Seizure control will be a primary concern. Provide support and education to the family. Referral for genetic counseling (it follows an autosomal dominant inheritance pattern and half the cases are due to a new mutation) and appropriate resources www.tsalliance.org: Tuberous Sclerosis Alliance
Sturge–Weber syndrome	1 in 20,000–50,000[a]	Facial nevus (port wine stain) most often seen on the forehead and on one side of the face, seizures, hemiparesis, and intracranial calcifications. In many cases, intellectual disability, behavioral and emotional problems, and learning disabilities are present. Seizures usually begin in infancy and may worsen with age. Convulsions are usually noted on the side of the body opposite the facial nevus. Muscle weakness may be present on the same side. Most affected people have glaucoma at birth or will develop it later in life.	Treatment will be mainly symptomatic. Seizure control will be a primary concern (use of anticonvulsants or surgery). Seizures due to Sturge–Weber are often difficult to control. Laser treatment may be used to lighten or remove the facial nevus. Surgery may be performed on more serious cases of glaucoma. Physical therapy should be considered for infants and children with muscle weakness. Educational therapy is often prescribed for those with an intellectual disability or developmental delays. Provide support and education to the family. Refer to appropriate resources. Genetic counseling may be appropriate (inheritance is unclear and sporadic). www.sturge-weber.org: Sturge–Weber Foundation

[a]Sahin, M., Ullrich, N., Srivastava, S., & Anna Pinto, A. (2020). Neurocutaneous syndromes. In R. M. Kleigman, J. W. St. Geme III, N. J. Blum, S. S. Shah, R. C. Tasker, K. M. Wilson, & R. E. Behrman (Eds.), *Nelson textbook of pediatrics* (21st ed., pp. 16593–16642). Elsevier.

benign tumors, are other signs of neurofibromatosis. Many children with neurofibromatosis have a larger than normal head circumference and are shorter than average. The severity of symptoms varies greatly, but the diagnosis is made if two or more of the clinical signs in Box 27.5 are present.

TAKE NOTE!

If more than six café-au-lait spots are present, neurofibromatosis should be suspected.

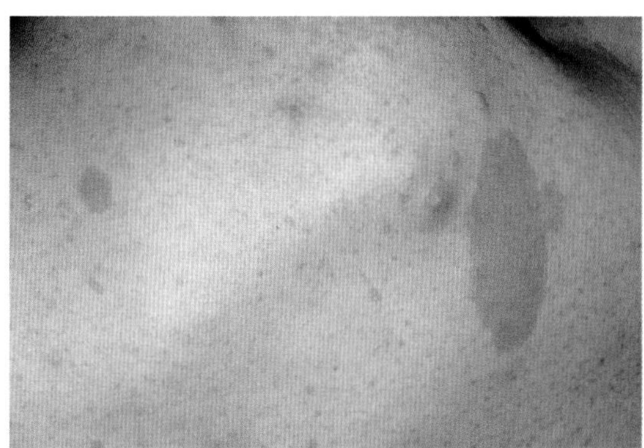

FIGURE 27.14 Café-au-lait spots associated with neurofibromatosis.

Nursing Management

Nursing management will be mainly supportive. Early detection of treatable conditions and complications is a priority. Provide support and education to the child and

BOX 27.5 Clinical Signs of Neurofibromatosis

Diagnosis is made if two or more of the following are present in a child without a parent with a diagnosis of NF1, or if one of the following is present in a child with a parent with a diagnosis of NF1:

- Six or more café-au-lait macules (light-brown spots) >5 mm in diameter in children and >15 mm in diameter in adolescents and adults
- Two or more neurofibromas (benign tumors) or one plexiform neurofibroma (tumor that involves many nerves)
- Freckling in the armpit or groin
- Presence of an optic glioma (a tumor on the optic nerve)
- Two or more growths on the iris of the eye (Lisch nodules or iris hamartomas)
- Presence of a specific osseous lesion such as sphenoid dysplasia, anterolateral bowing of the tibia, or pseudarthrosis of a long bone
  - Genetic testing showing NF1 variant

Data from Korf, B. R., Lobbous, M., & Metrock, L. K. (2023). Neurofibromatosis type 1 (NF1): Pathogenesis, clinical features, and diagnosis. *UpToDate*. Retrieved May 29, 2023, from https://www.uptodate.com/contents/neurofibromatosis-type-1-nf1-pathogenesis-clinical-features-and-diagnosis

family. Discuss genetic counseling with the family. Referral to appropriate resources is essential, such as the Children's Tumor Foundation.

OTHER GENETIC DISORDERS

Thousands of genetic disorders are known, and new ones are being discovered, but most of them are rare. Table 27.6 lists other genetic disorders that the pediatric nurse may encounter. Nursing management of these disorders will be mainly supportive and will focus on providing support and education to the family and child, with an emphasis on developmental and educational needs. Referral to genetic counseling and appropriate resources is an important nursing function.

TAKE NOTE!

Children with VATER syndrome who have only one kidney should not play contact sports.

TABLE 27.6 • Other Genetic Disorders, Syndromes, and Associations

Disorder	Inheritance/Cause	Signs and Symptoms	Management
CHARGE syndrome (a recognizable pattern of congenital anomalies seen) C: *C*oloboma H: *H*eart disease A: *A*tresia (choanal) R: *R*etarded growth and development and/or CNS anomalies G: *G*enital anomalies, hypogonadism E: *E*ar anomalies and deafness Incidence is one in 10,000 live births.[a]	Autosomal dominant inheritance possible, but most instances are due to new mutation in the gene *CDH7*. Occurs during fetal development and affects multiple organ systems	Coloboma is a lesion or defect of the eye, usually a fissure or cleft in the iris, ciliary, or choroid; can also see microphthalmos (small eyes) and cryptophthalmos (absent eye). Can lead to vision impairments Heart anomaly can include any type, but the most common are aortic arch anomalies and tetralogy of Fallot. Atresia (choanal) is blocked or narrowed passages from the nose to the throat, which can lead to aspiration. Retarded growth or cognitive development can range from mild to severe. Genital anomaly may include micropenis, undescended testes, and hypoplastic labia. Ear anomalies include short, wide ears with little or no lobe, prominent inner fold, floppy appearance, asymmetry; can have hearing impairment Each feature occurs in a spectrum from absent to severe; no single feature is present in all people.	Focus is on identifying and treating all defects; early diagnosis is important. www.chargesyndrome.org: CHARGE Syndrome Foundation
Marfan syndrome: disorder of connective tissue Incidence is one in 3,000–5,000.[b]	Autosomal dominant inheritance; in most instances caused by a mutation in the gene *fibrillin-1*, which results in changes in connective tissue	Primarily involves the skeletal, cardiovascular, and ocular systems. Tall stature with long slim limbs, minimal subcutaneous fat, muscle hypotonia, loose joints, long and narrow face, abnormalities of the skeletal system (e.g., pectus excavatum [funnel chest] or pectus carinatum [pigeon breast]), ocular system (e.g., enlarged cornea or lens subluxation), and cardiovascular system (e.g., dilation of the aorta or mitral valve prolapse) Delayed achievement of gross and fine motor milestones may occur.	Focus is on preventing complications. www.marfan.org: National Marfan Foundation
VATER association (not a diagnosis, but refers to a nonrandom association of defects found to occur together) V: *V*ertebral defects A: *A*nal atresia TE: *T*racheo*e*sophageal fistula with esophageal atresia R: *R*adial and *r*enal dysplasia May also occur as VACTERL association, with C: *C*ardiac anomalies L: *L*imb abnormalities added	Sporadic inheritance; cause is unknown. Can occur with other chromosomal abnormalities such as trisomy 18	One anomaly is present in three body parts (limb, thorax, lower abdomen/pelvis). Anomalies seen include hypoplastic (small) vertebrae or hemivertebra (only half the bones are formed). These anomalies lead to an increased risk of scoliosis. With imperforate anus or anal atresia, the anus does not open to the outside of the body. Tracheoesophageal fistula and/or esophageal atresia leads to an increased risk for aspiration, feeding, and swallowing problems. Incomplete formation of one or more kidneys, obstruction of urine flow out of kidneys, or severe reflux back into kidneys can all lead to kidney failure later in life.	Focus is on identifying and treating all defects. www.eatef.org: EA/TEF Child and Family Support Connection, Inc.

TABLE 27.6 • Other Genetic Disorders, Syndromes, and Associations

Disorder	Inheritance/Cause	Signs and Symptoms	Management
		Cardiac anomalies: most common are ventricular septal defects, atrial septal defects, and tetralogy of Fallot. Absent or displaced thumb, polydactyly (extra digits), syndactyly (fusion of digits) A single umbilical artery at birth is often present. Failure to thrive and slow development in early infancy due to anomalies Usually normal intelligence	
Apert syndrome (named for the French physician who described the syndrome) Incidence is 6–15.5 out of 1 million live births.[c]	Autosomal dominant inheritance. Cases are sporadic.	Craniosynostosis and maxillary hypoplasia resulting in a flat recessed forehead and flat midface, bilateral symmetric syndactyly, and craniofacial anomalies such as high-arched palate and associated clefting, short anteroposterior diameter, protruding eyes, down-slanting eyelids, and low-set ears Small nasopharynx can lead to upper airway obstruction and sleep apnea. Acne vulgaris, strabismus, and hearing loss Learning disabilities and mental deficiency	Early surgery for craniosynostosis when increased intracranial pressure is noted. Vigorous early management should occur with a multidisciplinary approach to address multiple anomalies. aboutface-usa.org: About Face USA www.ccakids.com: Children's Craniofacial Association www.faces-cranio.org: National Craniofacial Association
Achondroplasia (most common chondrodysplasia [diseases resulting in disordered growth]) Incidence is one in 20,000.[d]	Autosomal dominant inheritance pattern. Caused by mutations in fibroblast growth factor receptor 3 (FGFR3). 80% new gene mutation[d]	Characterized by abnormal body proportion Small stature (average adult height is 4 ft for all sexes), short limbs with normal-size torso, low nasal bridge with prominent forehead. Midface hypoplasia, caudal narrowing of spinal canal, megalocephaly, small foramen magnum; hands are short and stubby with separation between middle and ring fingers ("trident hand"). Delayed motor skills, problems with persistent middle ear dysfunction and infections, and bowing of lower legs Less common complications include hydrocephalus, craniocervical junction compression, upper airway obstruction, and thoracolumbar kyphosis. Usually present with normal intelligence and lead independent, productive lives	Medical management of symptoms Monitor height, weight, and head circumference. Manage and prevent complications (careful and thorough neurologic examination, assessment for sleep apnea) Growth hormone therapy is controversial and currently not recommended. New treatments such as, vosoritide, a recombinant C-type natriuretic peptide analog, may be used. Limb-lengthening surgeries may be performed. www.lpaonline.org/: Little People of America

CNS, central nervous system.

[a]Usman, N., & Sur, M. (2023). *CHARGE syndrome.* StatPearls Publishing. https://www.ncbi.nlm.nih.gov/books/NBK559199/

[b]Wright, M. J., & Connolly, H. M. (2022). Genetics, clinical features, and diagnosis of Marfan syndrome and related disorders. *UpToDate*. Retrieved May 29, 2023, from https://www.uptodate.com/contents/genetics-clinical-features-and-diagnosis-of-marfan-syndrome-and-related-disorders

[c]Firth, H. V. (2023). Craniosynostosis syndromes. *UpToDate.* Retrieved May 29, 2023, from https://www.uptodate.com/contents/craniosynostosis-syndromes

[d]Bacino, C. A. (2023). Achondroplasia. *UpToDate.* Retrieved May 29, 2023, from https://www.uptodate.com/contents/achondroplasia

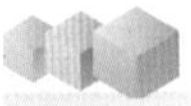
Concept Mastery Alert

Assessment findings in a child with achondroplasia are a trident hand (separation between the middle and ring fingers) and persistent otitis media caused by middle ear dysfunction. In contrast, a child with Marfan syndrome would have slim stature, hypotonia, and a narrow face.

INBORN ERRORS OF METABOLISM

Inborn errors of metabolism are a group of hereditary disorders. They are collectively common, but individually rare, with most having an incidence of less than one in 100,000 (Sutton, 2022). Most follow an autosomal recessive inheritance pattern. They are caused by gene mutations that result in abnormalities in the synthesis or catabolism of proteins, carbohydrates, or fats. The body cannot convert food into energy as it normally would. Most inborn errors are due to a defect in an enzyme or transport protein that results in a block in the metabolic pathway. The blocked metabolic pathway allows for the accumulation of the damaging byproduct of the impaired metabolic process or may be responsible for a deficiency or absence of a necessary product. Presentation can occur at any time, even in adulthood, but many affected people exhibit signs in the newborn period or shortly after. Most inborn errors of metabolism presenting in the neonatal period are lethal if specific treatment is not initiated immediately.

Newborn screening is used to detect these disorders before symptoms develop. It began in the early 1960s with screening for phenylketonuria (PKU). Technical advances and developments in screening techniques (such as tandem mass spectrometry) now allow dozens of metabolic disorders to be detected from a single drop of blood (Kemper, 2021). A child who tests positive will require additional testing to confirm the diagnosis (see Chapter 9 for more information on newborn screening for inborn errors of metabolism).

Therapeutic management of these disorders varies depending on the cause of the error of metabolism, but dietary management is often a key component.

Nursing Assessment

Clinical signs and symptoms vary with each disorder. Table 27.7 gives information on some common inborn errors of metabolism seen in children.

TABLE 27.7 • Inborn Errors of Metabolism

Disorder/Explanation	Clinical Manifestations	Management
Phenylketonuria (PKU): deficiency in a liver enzyme leading to inability to process the essential amino acid phenylalanine properly. Phenylalanine accumulation can lead to brain damage unless PKU is detected soon after birth and treated.	No symptoms at birth. Most instances are identified before symptoms are present due to newborn screening (PKU is screened for in all states). If undiagnosed, most common sign is developmental delay along with vomiting, irritability, eczemalike rash, mousy odor to urine, microcephaly, seizures, and behavioral abnormalities	Low-phenylalanine diet Can be difficult to follow for entire life so new treatments are being developed such as administrations of large neutral amino acids Phenylalanine is found mostly in protein-containing foods such as meat and milk (including breast milk and formula) www.pkunetwork.org: Children's PKU Network www.pkunews.org: National PKU News
Galactosemia: deficiency in the liver enzyme needed to convert galactose, the breakdown product of lactose, which is commonly found in dairy products, into glucose. Galactose accumulation leads to damage to vital organs.	No symptoms at birth. If undiagnosed, newborn will have jaundice, feeding intolerance, diarrhea, and vomiting and will not gain weight. Signs and symptoms of sepsis and cataracts are often seen. If untreated, can lead to liver disease, blindness, severe intellectual disability, and death	Ingestion of galactose can produce sepsis in an affected child; therefore, septic workup and antibiotics may be necessary in a child if galactose ingestion has occurred. Elimination of galactose and lactose from the diet is the only treatment. Therefore, milk and dairy products will be eliminated for life. www.galactosemia.org: Parents of Galactosemic Children
Maple sugar urine disease: affects the metabolism of amino acids. A deficiency in the enzyme that metabolizes leucine, isoleucine, and valine, which are components of protein often referred to as the branch chain amino acids. These amino acids then accumulate in the blood and cause damage to the brain.	No symptoms at birth, but if untreated, newborns soon begin to show neurologic signs, vomiting, poor feeding, hypertonicity, increased reflex action, and seizures. Lower intake of protein (as occurs with breastfeeding) may delay presentation of symptoms. If untreated, can lead to life-threatening neurologic damage	Special low-protein diet; will vary based on severity of symptoms; limited natural protein requires a medical food product supplement such as branched-chain amino acid-free protein. Thiamine supplements may be given. Diet must be continued throughout life. Liver transplant has been performed with good results (child on normal diet posttransplant). www.msud-support.org: Maple Syrup Urine Disease Family Support Group

TABLE 27.7 • Inborn Errors of Metabolism

Disorder/Explanation	Clinical Manifestations	Management
Biotinidase deficiency: lack of the enzyme biotinidase results in biotin deficiency.	Typically no symptoms at birth; in first weeks or months of life, symptoms such as hypotonia, uncoordinated movement, seizures, developmental delay, alopecia, seborrheic dermatitis, hearing loss, optic nerve atrophy, and intellectual disability develop. Metabolic acidosis can lead to death.	Daily oral free biotin
Medium-chain acyl-CoA dehydrogenase deficiency (MCAD): lack of an enzyme required to metabolize fatty acids	Classic presentation is a child 3 months to 5 years with vomiting and lethargy after a period of not eating (fasting typically associated with a viral illness). Recurrent episodes of metabolic acidosis and hypoglycemia, lethargy, seizures, liver failure, brain damage, coma, and cardiac arrest. Can lead to serious and fatal illness in children not eating well	Avoid fasting; have frequent meals. Special considerations during illness. If unable to tolerate food, IV dextrose is required. www.fodsupport.org: Fatty Oxidation Disorders (FOD) Family Support Group
Homocystinuria: deficiency in the enzyme needed to digest a component of food called methionine (an amino acid)	Typically, no symptoms at birth. In the first few months of life, symptoms including vomiting, poor feeding, failure to thrive, hypotonia. If undetected and untreated, can lead to intellectual disability, psychiatric disturbances, developmental delays, displacement of the lens of the eye, abnormal thinning and weakness of bones, and formation of thrombi in veins and arteries that can lead to life-threatening complications such as stroke	Vitamin B_6 and B_{12} supplements and possibly other supplements, such as betaine and folic acid; methionine-restricted diet and cystine supplements; aspirin and dipyridamole to decrease thromboembolic events www.rarediseases.org: National Organization for Rare Disorders
Tyrosinemia: deficiency in an enzyme essential in the metabolism of tyrosine; accumulation of the byproducts results in liver and kidney damage.	Symptoms usually appear in the first months of life: fever, failure to thrive, poor weight gain, vomiting, diarrhea, cabbagelike odor, enlarged liver and spleen, increased bleeding tendency, distended abdomen, jaundice, cirrhosis, and liver failure	Treatment of choice is administration of nitisinone. Diet low in phenylalanine and tyrosine www.liverfoundation.org: American Liver Foundation
Tay–Sachs (one of GM_2 gangliosidoses) caused by insufficient activity of an enzyme called hexosaminidase A, which is necessary for the breakdown of certain fatty substances in brain and nerve cells	Occurs more frequently among people of Ashkenazi Jewish descent (with one in every 25 being a carrier)[a] Infants appear normal and healthy for the first few months of life. Then, as harmful quantities of the fatty substances (called gangliosides) build up in tissues and nerve cells and cause damage, mental and physical deterioration occur. The child becomes blind, deaf, and unable to swallow; muscles begin to atrophy; and paralysis sets in. Dementia, seizures, and an increased startle reflex may be seen. There is a late-onset type of Tay–Sachs seen in people in their 20s and early 30s, but this is much rarer.	No treatment or cure. Medical management will focus on managing symptoms and maintaining comfort. Anticonvulsants may be given to control seizures. Death usually occurs in early childhood, by age 4 or 5. Carriers can be identified by a blood test and prenatal testing is available. www.ntsad.org: National Tay–Sachs & Allied Diseases Association

[a]McGovern, M. M., & Desnick, R. J. (2020). Lipidoses (lysosomal storage disorders). In R. M. Kleigman, J. W. St. Geme III, N. J. Blum, S. S. Shah, R. C. Tasker, K. M. Wilson, & R. E. Behrman (Eds.), *Nelson textbook of pediatrics* (21st ed., pp. 4446–4484). Elsevier.

Data from Shchelochkov, O. A., & Venditti, C. P. (2020a). An approach to inborn errors of metabolism. In R. M. Kleigman, J. W. St. Geme III, N. J. Blum, S. S. Shah, R. C. Tasker, K. M. Wilson, & R. E. Behrman (Eds.), *Nelson textbook of pediatrics* (21st ed., pp. 4054–4087). Elsevier; Shchelochkov, O. A., & Venditti, C. P. (2020b). Defects in metabolism of amino acids. In R. M. Kleigman, J. W. St. Geme III, N. J. Blum, S. S. Shah, R. C. Tasker, K. M. Wilson, & R. E. Behrman (Eds.), *Nelson textbook of pediatrics* (21st ed., pp. 4053–4330). Elsevier; Kishnani, P. S., & Chen, Y. T. (2020). Defects in metabolism of carbohydrates. In R. M. Kleigman, J. W. St. Geme III, N. J. Blum, S. S. Shah, R. C. Tasker, K. M. Wilson, & R. E. Behrman (Eds.), *Nelson textbook of pediatrics* (21st ed., pp. 4488–4614). Elsevier; Stanley, C. A., & Bennett, M. J. (2020). Disorders of mitochondrial fatty acid beta oxidation. In R. M. Kleigman, J. W. St. Geme III, N. J. Blum, S. S. Shah, R. C. Tasker, K. M. Wilson, & R. E. Behrman (Eds.), *Nelson textbook of pediatrics* (21st ed., pp. 4331–4357). Elsevier; McGovern, M. M., & Desnick, R. J. (2020). Lipidoses (lysosomal storage disorders). In R. M. Kleigman, J. W. St. Geme III, N. J. Blum, S. S. Shah, R. C. Tasker, K. M. Wilson, & R. E. Behrman (Eds.), *Nelson textbook of pediatrics* (21st ed., pp. 4446–4484). Elsevier; McGovern, M., & Desnick, R. J. (2016). Lipidoses (lysosomal storage disorders). In R. M. Kleigman, B. F. Stanton, J. W. St. Geme III, N. F. Schor, & R. E. Behrman (Eds.), *Nelson textbook of pediatrics* (20th ed., pp. 705–714). Saunders.

Because of newborn screening and early identification and management, it is rare to see an untreated newborn with clinical signs and symptoms of disease caused by one of the inborn errors of metabolism disorders. If seen, a newborn who was healthy at birth will often present with lethargy, poor feeding, apnea or tachypnea, recurrent vomiting, altered consciousness, failure to thrive, seizures, septic appearance, or developmental delay. Physical changes that may be seen include dysmorphology, cardiomegaly, rashes, cataracts, retinitis, optic atrophy, corneal opacity, deafness, skeletal dysplasia, macrocephaly, hepatomegaly, jaundice, or cirrhosis.

TAKE NOTE!

When a previously healthy newborn presents with a history of deterioration, suspect an inborn error of metabolism.

The diagnostic workup usually requires a variety of specific laboratory studies and may include:

- Glucose: may be elevated
- Ammonia: may be elevated
- Blood gases: may have low bicarbonate and low pH, metabolic acidosis (respiratory alkalosis may also be seen, especially when high ammonia levels are present)

Early diagnosis is the key to saving and improving the lives of these children.

TAKE NOTE!

If an inborn error of metabolism is suspected, feedings will usually be stopped until the test results are received.

When a child who has previously been diagnosed with an inborn error of metabolism is hospitalized, the nurse must determine the prescribed diet and medications so these may be continued while in the hospital setting.

Nursing Management

Ensure that the diet prescribed for the infant or child is followed. For amino acid disorders (e.g., PKU), urea cycle defects (e.g., tyrosinemia type I), and organic acidemia (e.g., maple syrup urine disease), nutritional therapy is the major intervention. Dietary intake of specific amino acids is restricted according to the disorder. Ensure that overall protein and calorie needs are still met, as children need sufficient calories for proper growth. In children with urea cycle defects and organic acidemia, anorexia is common and severe, and the child may need gastrostomy tube feeding supplementation. In fatty acid oxidation disorders (e.g., medium-chain acyl-coenzyme A [CoA] dehydrogenase deficiency), the goal is to avoid prolonged periods of fasting and to provide frequent feeds when the child is sick. Supplementation with specific vitamins may also be important in the treatment of these disorders. Strict adherence to the diet is necessary and will require close supervision by registered dietitians, primary providers, and nurses and the cooperation of both the parent and child.

Nursing management will focus on education and support for the family, who will need thorough knowledge about the child's disease and management. Refer the child and family to a dietitian and appropriate resources, including support groups. In addition, monitor the child's developmental progress and begin therapies as soon as a concern arises.

KEY CONCEPTS

- Nurses must understand the pattern of inheritance (which demonstrates how a genetic disorder can be passed onto offspring) so they can teach and counsel families about the risks of future pregnancies.
- If the defect occurs on the autosome, the genetic disorder is termed autosomal; if the defect is on the X chromosome, the genetic disorder is termed X linked. The defect also can be classified as dominant or recessive. Monogenic disorders include autosomal dominant, autosomal recessive, X-linked dominant, and X-linked recessive patterns.
- Many of the common congenital malformations, such as cleft lip, cleft palate, spina bifida, pyloric stenosis, clubfoot, congenital hip dysplasia, and cardiac defects, are attributed to multifactorial inheritance. These conditions are thought to be caused by multiple gene and environmental factors.
- Molecular studies have revealed that some genetic disorders are inherited in ways that do not follow the typical patterns of dominant, recessive, X-linked, or multifactorial inheritance. Examples of nontraditional inheritance patterns include mitochondrial inheritance and genomic imprinting.
- In some instances of genetic disorders, the abnormality occurs due to problems with the chromosomes. Chromosomal abnormalities do not follow straightforward patterns of inheritance.
- Medical genetic knowledge has increased dramatically over the past few decades. It is possible not only to detect specific diseases with genetic mutations but also to test for a genetic predisposition to various diseases or conditions and certain physical characteristics. This leads to complex ethical, moral, and social issues.
- Primary providers and nurse practitioners need to maintain privacy and confidentiality and administer care in a nondiscriminatory manner while maintaining

sensitivity to cultural differences. It is essential to respect the child's autonomy and present information in a nondirective manner.

- The purpose of a genetic consultation is to confirm or rule out genetic conditions, identify medical management issues, calculate and communicate genetic risks to a family, discuss ethical and legal issues, and provide psychosocial support.
- Nurses play an important role in the counseling process. Many times, the nurse is the one who has first contact with these parents and is the one to provide follow-up care.
- The nurse must be able to identify those who could benefit from genetic counseling and must be able to discuss the role of the genetic counselor with families. Families at risk must be aware that genetic counseling is available before they attempt to have another baby.
- Nurses play an essential role in providing emotional support and referrals to appropriate agencies, support groups, and resources when caring for families with suspected or diagnosed genetic disorders.
- Referral for genetic counseling prior to genetic testing may be appropriate.
- Many children with chromosomal abnormalities have intellectual disability, learning disabilities, behavioral problems, and distinct features, including birth defects.
- Trisomy 21 (DS) is associated with some degree of intellectual disability, characteristic facial features (e.g., slanted eyes and depressed nasal bridge), and other health problems, such as cardiac defects, visual and hearing impairments, intestinal malformations, and an increased susceptibility to infections.
- In Turner syndrome, short stature and slow growth are characteristic findings.
- Klinefelter syndrome is usually diagnosed in adolescence or adulthood due to a lack of development of secondary sex characteristics.
- Fragile X syndrome's clinical manifestations are subtle during childhood, with minor dysmorphic features and developmental delay. Problems with sensation, emotion, and behavior often are the first signs.
- Café-au-lait spots (light-brown macules) are the hallmark of neurofibromatosis (Korf et al., 2023).
- Inborn errors of metabolism are caused by gene mutations that result in abnormalities in the synthesis or catabolism of proteins, carbohydrates, or fats. Most inborn errors of metabolism presenting in the neonatal period are lethal if specific treatment is not initiated immediately.
- Nurses should have a basic knowledge of genetics, common genetic disorders in children, genetic testing, and genetic counseling so they can provide support and information to families and can help improve their quality of life.
- Genetic disorders usually result in a lifelong complex medical condition. Nurses must provide ongoing education and support for the child and family about the disorder, treatment, and management as well as available resources.

REFERENCES AND RECOMMENDED READINGS

Ajitkumar, A., Jamil, R. T., & Mathai, J. K. (2023). *Cri du chat syndrome*. StatPearls Publishing. https://www.ncbi.nlm.nih.gov/books/NBK482460/

Bacino, C. A. (2023a). Achondroplasia. *UpToDate*. Retrieved May 29, 2023, from https://www.uptodate.com/contents/achondroplasia

Bacino, C. A. (2023b). Congenital anomalies: Epidemiology, types and pattern. *UpToDate*. Retrieved May 26, 2023, from https://www.uptodate.com/contents/congenital-anomalies-epidemiology-types-and-patterns

Bacino, C. A. (2023c). Sex chromosome abnormalities. *UpToDate*. Retrieved May 29, 2023, from https://www.uptodate.com/contents/sex-chromosome-abnormalities

Bacino, C. A., & Lee, B. (2020). Cytogenetics. In R. M. Kleigman, J. W. St. Geme III, N. J. Blum, S. S. Shah, R. C. Tasker, K. M. Wilson, & R. E. Behrman (Eds.), *Nelson textbook of pediatrics* (21st ed., pp. 3903–3999). Elsevier.

Backelijauw, P. (2022). Clinical manifestations and diagnosis of Turner syndrome. *UpToDate*. Retrieved May 29, 2023, from https://www.uptodate.com/contents/clinical-manifestations-and-diagnosis-of-turner-syndrome

Breilyn, M. S., & Levy, P. A. (2023). Human genetics and dysmorphology. In K. J. Marcdante, R. M. Kleigman, & A. M. Schuh (Eds.), *Nelson essentials of pediatrics* (9th ed., pp. 177–199). Elsevier.

Bull, M. J., Trotter, T., Santoro, S. L., Christensen, C., Grout, R. W., & The Council on Genetics. (2022). Health supervision for children and adolescents with Down syndrome. *Pediatrics, 149*(5), e2022057010. https://doi.org/10.1542/peds.2022-057010

Duis, J., & Scheimann, A. O. (2023). Prader–Willi syndrome: Clinical features and diagnosis. *UpToDate*. Retrieved May 29, 2023, from https://www.uptodate.com/contents/prader-willi-syndrome-clinical-features-and-diagnosis

Firth, H. V. (2023). Craniosynostosis syndromes. *UpToDate*. Retrieved May 29, 2023, from https://www.uptodate.com/contents/craniosynostosis-syndromes

Fischbach, F. T., Fischbach, M. A., & Stout, K. (2022). *A manual of laboratory and diagnostic tests* (11th ed.). Wolters Kluwer.

Genetic and Rare Diseases (GARD) Information Center. (2023). *Wolf–Hirschhorn syndrome*. https://rarediseases.info.nih.gov/diseases/7896/wolf-hirschhorn-syndrome

Giersch, A. (2022). Congenital cytogenetic abnormalities. *UpToDate*. Retrieved May 27, 2023, from https://www.uptodate.com/contents/congenital-cytogenetic-abnormalities

Hon-Yin, B. C., Shuman, C., Choufani, S., & Weksberg, R. (2022). *Beckwith-Wiedemann syndrome*. *UpToDate*. Retrieved May 29, 2023, from https://www.uptodate.com/contents/beckwith-wiedemann-syndrome

Kemper, A. R. (2021). Newborn screening. *UpToDate*. Retrieved May 25, 2023, from https://www.uptodate.com/contents/newborn-screening

Kishnani, P. S., & Chen, Y. T. (2020). Defects in metabolism of carbohydrates. In R. M. Kleigman, J. W. St. Geme III, N. J. Blum, S. S. Shah, R. C. Tasker, K. M. Wilson, & R. E. Behrman (Eds.), *Nelson textbook of pediatrics* (21st ed., pp. 4488–4614). Elsevier.

Korf, B. R., Lobbous, M., & Metrock, L. K. (2023). Neurofibromatosis type 1 (NF1): Pathogenesis, clinical features, and diagnosis. *UpToDate*. Retrieved May 29, 2023, from https://www.uptodate.com/contents/neurofibromatosis-type-1-nf1-pathogenesis-clinical-features-and-diagnosis

Lackey, A. E., & Muzio, M. R. (2023). *DiGeorge syndrome*. StatPearls Publishing. https://www.ncbi.nlm.nih.gov/books/NBK549798/

Lashley, F. R. (2005). *Clinical genetics in nursing practice*. Springer Publishing.

Lee, B. (2020). Integration of genetics into pediatric practice. In R. M. Kleigman, J. W. St. Geme III, N. J. Blum, S. S. Shah, R. C. Tasker, K. M. Wilson, & R. E. Behrman (Eds.), *Nelson textbook of pediatrics* (21st ed., pp. 3789–3820). Elsevier.

Madaan, M., & Mendez, M. D. (2023). *Angelman syndrome*. StatPearls Publishing. https://www.ncbi.nlm.nih.gov/books/NBK560870/

McGovern, M. M., & Desnick, R. J. (2020). Lipidoses (lysosomal storage disorders). In R. M. Kleigman, J. W. St. Geme III, N. J. Blum, S. S. Shah, R. C. Tasker, K. M. Wilson, & R. E. Behrman (Eds.), *Nelson textbook of pediatrics* (21st ed., pp. 4446–4484). Elsevier.

National Down Syndrome Society. (2023). *Early intervention*. https://www.ndss.org/resources/early-intervention/

Ostermaier, K. K. (2022a). Down syndrome: Clinical features and diagnosis. *UpToDate*. Retrieved May 23, 2023, from https://www.uptodate.com/contents/down-syndrome-clinical-features-and-diagnosis

Ostermaier, K. K. (2022b). Down syndrome: Management. *UpToDate*. Retrieved May 27, 2023, from https://www.uptodate.com/contents/down-syndrome-management

Raby, B. A., & Kohlmann, W. (2022). Genetic counseling: Family history interpretation and risk assessment. *UpToDate*. Retrieved June 20, 2019, from https://www.uptodate.com/contents/genetic-counseling-family-history-interpretation-and-risk-assessment

Raby, B. A. (2021). Inheritance patterns of monogenic disorders (Mendelian and non-Mendelian). *UpToDate*. Retrieved May 26, 2023, from https://www.uptodate.com/contents/inheritance-patterns-of-monogenic-disorders-mendelian-and-non-mendelian

Sahin, M., Ullrich, N., Srivastava, S., & Anna Pinto, A. (2020). Neurocutaneous syndromes. In R. M. Kleigman, J. W. St. Geme III, N. J. Blum, S. S. Shah, R. C. Tasker, K. M. Wilson, & R. E. Behrman (Eds.), *Nelson textbook of pediatrics* (21st ed., pp. 16593–16642). Elsevier.

Scott, D. A., & Lee, B. (2020a). The genetic approach in pediatric medicine. In R. M. Kleigman, J. W. St. Geme III, N. J. Blum, S. S. Shah, R. C. Tasker, K. M. Wilson, & R. E. Behrman (Eds.), *Nelson textbook of pediatrics* (21st ed., pp. 3821–3837). Elsevier.

Scott, D. A., & Lee, B. (2020b). Patterns of genetic transmission. In R. M. Kleigman, J. W. St. Geme III, N. J. Blum, S. S. Shah, R. C. Tasker, K. M. Wilson, & R. E. Behrman (Eds.), *Nelson textbook of pediatrics* (21st ed., pp. 3862–3902). Elsevier.

Shchelochkov, O. A., & Venditti, C. P. (2020a). An approach to inborn errors of metabolism. In R. M. Kleigman, J. W. St. Geme III, N. J. Blum, S. S. Shah, R. C. Tasker, K. M. Wilson, & R. E. Behrman (Eds.), *Nelson textbook of pediatrics* (21st ed., pp. 4054–4087). Elsevier.

Shchelochkov, O. A., & Venditti, C. P. (2020b). Defects in metabolism of amino acids. In R. M. Kleigman, J. W. St. Geme III, N. J. Blum, S. S. Shah, R. C. Tasker, K. M. Wilson, & R. E. Behrman (Eds.), *Nelson textbook of pediatrics* (21st ed., pp. 4053–4330). Elsevier.

Spinazzi, N. A., Velasco, A. B., Wodecki, D. J., & Patel, L. (2023). Autism spectrum disorder in Down syndrome: Experiences from caregivers. *Journal of Autism and Developmental Disorders*, *54*, 1171–1180. https://doi.org/10.1007/s10803-022-05758-x

Stanley, C. A., & Bennett, M. J. (2020). Disorders of mitochondrial fatty acid beta oxidation. In R. M. Kleigman, J. W. St. Geme III, N. J. Blum, S. S. Shah, R. C. Tasker, K. M. Wilson, & R. E. Behrman (Eds.), *Nelson textbook of pediatrics* (21st ed., pp. 4331–4357). Elsevier.

Stone, W. L., Basit, H., Shah, M., & Los, E. (2023). *Fragile X syndrome*. StatPearls Publishing. https://www.ncbi.nlm.nih.gov/books/NBK459243/

Sutton, V. R. (2022). Inborn errors of metabolism: Epidemiology, pathogenesis, and clinical features. *UpToDate*. Retrieved May 29, 2023, from https://www.uptodate.com/contents/inborn-errors-of-metabolism-epidemiology-pathogenesis-and-clinical-features

Usman, N., & Sur, M. (2023). *CHARGE syndrome*. StatPearls Publishing. https://www.ncbi.nlm.nih.gov/books/NBK559199/

Van Esch, H. (2022). Fragile X syndrome: Clinical features and diagnosis in children and adolescents. *UpToDate*. Retrieved May 29, 2023, from https://www.uptodate.com/contents/fragile-x-syndrome-clinical-features-and-diagnosis-in-children-and-adolescents

Wilson, M., & Carter, I. B. (2022). *Williams syndrome*. StatPearls Publishing. https://www.ncbi.nlm.nih.gov/books/NBK544278/

Wright, M. J., & Connolly, H. M. (2022). Genetics, clinical features, and diagnosis of Marfan syndrome and related disorders. *UpToDate*. Retrieved May 29, 2023, from https://www.uptodate.com/contents/genetics-clinical-features-and-diagnosis-of-marfan-syndrome-and-related-disorders

DEVELOPING CLINICAL JUDGMENT

PRACTICING FOR NCLEX

1. The nurse is counseling a couple, one of whom is affected by neurofibromatosis, an autosomal dominant disorder. They want to know the risk of transmitting the disorder. The nurse should tell them that each offspring has what chance of getting the disease?
   a. One in four (25%)
   b. One in eight (12.5%)
   c. One in one (100%)
   d. One in two (50%)
2. The nurse working in a women's health clinic determines that genetic counseling may be appropriate for people with which criteria? Select all that apply.
   a. Just had their first miscarriage at 10 weeks
   b. Is 30 years old and planning to conceive
   c. Has a close relative with fragile X syndrome
   d. Is 18 weeks pregnant and triple screen came back normal
   e. Reports a history of three miscarriages
   f. Reports their first-born child had a cleft lip
3. A child born with a single transverse palmar crease, a short neck with excessive skin at the nape, a depressed nasal bridge, and cardiac defects is most likely to have which autosomal abnormality?
   a. Trisomy 21
   b. Trisomy 18
   c. Trisomy 14
   d. Trisomy 13
4. A parent brings their 4-day-old infant to the clinic with vomiting and poor feeding. The newborn was healthy at birth. What should the nurse suspect?
   a. Sturge–Weber syndrome
   b. An inborn error of metabolism
   c. Trisomy 18
   d. Turner syndrome
5. The nurse is caring for a child with Down syndrome. What should the nurse's focus be?
   a. Teaching hygiene skills to the child in order to increase self-esteem
   b. Screening for anomalies and teaching about the prevention of respiratory infection
   c. Finding opportunities to increase socialization for the child and family
   d. Expecting walking at age 1 year and toilet training completion at age 2 years
6. The nurse is caring for a child with Turner syndrome admitted to the unit for treatment of a kidney infection. What characteristics associated with this syndrome may the nurse expect to find upon assessment? Select all that apply.
   a. Microcephaly
   b. Polydactyly
   c. Short stature
   d. Gynecomastia
   e. Taller than average
   f. Webbed neck
   g. Low posterior hair line
   h. Cleft lip

DOSAGE CALCULATION QUESTION

The nurse is caring for a child with Down syndrome. The child weighs 26 lb. The primary provider orders intravenous (IV) maintenance fluids. What would be the expected maintenance IV fluid rate? (Round to the nearest milliliter.)

CRITICAL THINKING EXERCISES

1. An 8-month-old is seen in the clinic. On assessment, the nurse finds eight café-au-lait spots on the child's trunk and extremities. What other assessment findings may be pertinent?
2. A child's newborn screen came back positive for PKU. After further testing, the diagnosis is confirmed. What instructions would you give the parents regarding the care of their child?
3. A 6-year-old with Down syndrome is admitted to the hospital with pneumonia. What three pieces of information should the nurse seek when obtaining the health history?
   a. Presence of cardiac defects or disease
   b. Last hearing and vision evaluation
   c. Birthing parent's pregnancy history
   d. Presence of thyroid disease
   e. Birthing parent's immunization history

STUDY ACTIVITIES

1. Develop a nursing plan of care for a child with Down syndrome.
2. Shadow a genetic counselor. Identify ways they help families understand and cope with genetic disorders.
3. Attend a meeting of an ethics committee at a local hospital. Identify some of the ethical, legal, and social issues in health care that they discuss, particularly related to genetic testing and genetic disorders.

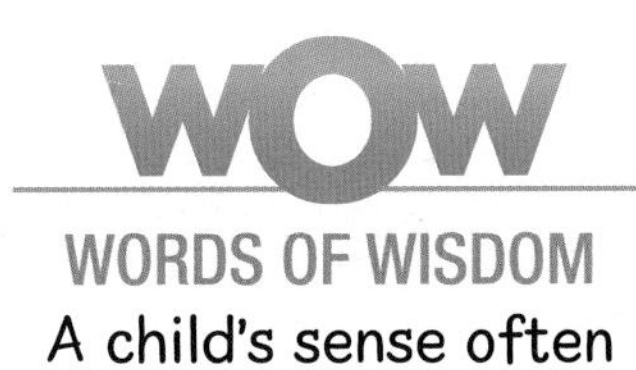

WORDS OF WISDOM

A child's sense often exceeds all human intellect.

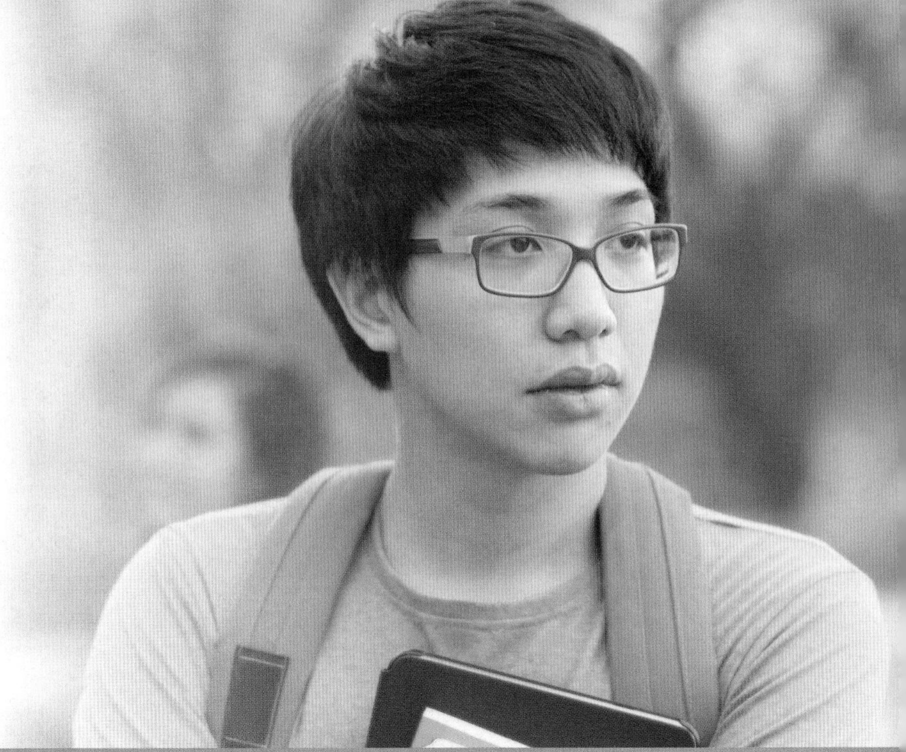

28

Nursing Care of the Child With an Alteration in Behavior, Cognition, or Development

LEARNING OBJECTIVES

Upon completion of the chapter, you will be able to:

1. Discuss the impact of alterations in mental health on the growth, development, and future health of infants, children, and adolescents.
2. Describe techniques used to evaluate the status of mental health in children.
3. Identify appropriate nursing assessments and interventions related to therapy and medications for the treatment of childhood and adolescent mental health disorders.
4. Distinguish mental health disorders common in infants, children, and adolescents.
5. Devise an individualized nursing care plan or concept map for the child with a mental health disorder.
6. Develop child and family teaching plans for the child with a mental health disorder.

KEY TERMS

affect
bingeing
comorbid
neglect
purging
suicide
violence

John Howard, age 6 years, is brought to the clinic for his annual examination. His parent states, "John has frequent emotional outbursts, and his mood seems to switch from happy to sad rather quickly. His teachers have said his performance at school has been poor."

INTRODUCTION

Mental health issues make up the bulk of the "new morbidity" of children. Such issues include developmental and behavioral disorders, eating disorders, mood disorders, anxiety disorders, and abuse and **violence** (acts of aggression) directed toward children. As many as 14% to 20% of children may be suffering from mental health–related problems (Kelsay et al., 2022). Failure to receive appropriate treatment may lead to further academic and social difficulties. Mental illness manifested in the early years increases the risk of adolescent emotional issues, use of firearms, reckless driving, substance misuse, and risky sexual activity. Some cognitive or neurobehavioral disorders may have a genetic or physiologic cause, whereas others result from family or environmental stressors.

Usually, children with cognitive or mental health disorders are treated in the community or on an outpatient basis, but sometimes, a disorder can have such a significant impact on the child and family that hospitalization is required. Many hospitalized children also experience cognitive or mental health disorders. When a child is diagnosed with a cognitive or mental health disorder, the family may become overwhelmed by the multifaceted services that they require.

Over the past several years, the extensive scope of mental health issues among children, adolescents, and their families has become more apparent, leading the American Academy of Pediatrics (AAP) to create initiatives that address the needs of these children and their families (AAP, 2023). Mental health problems in children are real and painful and can be severe. For affected children to have a chance at a healthy future, nurses must participate in the early identification and referral of children with potential cognitive deficits or other mental health issues.

EFFECTS OF MENTAL HEALTH ISSUES ON DEVELOPMENT AND FUTURE HEALTH

Children's behavior is influenced by biologic or genetic characteristics, nutrition, physical health, developmental ability, environmental and family interactions, the child's individual temperament, and the parents' or caregivers' responses to the child's behavior. The changes that occur with normal growth and development are often a source of stress for children, and in some children, they may lead to dysfunction. Children progress at different rates, so it is often difficult to identify subtle abnormalities. When stress, fatigue, or pain occurs in children, they may quickly regress to earlier patterns of behavior. These regressive behaviors may continue if a mental health concern is present. It is possible that stress placed on developing neurons leads to decreased coping abilities later in life. Children learn through their experiences. Therefore, they may develop maladaptive behaviors through life interactions (Kelsay et al., 2022).

Adverse childhood experiences (ACEs) in childhood are linked to negative long-term adolescent and adult health (Goddard, 2021). ACEs may include abuse, neglect, or other traumatic events experienced by the child. These events trigger the complex stress response humans experience, and when repetitive or chronic, these elevated stress hormones lead to long-term morbidities such as severe obesity, diabetes, and heart disease. Additionally, chronic, toxic stress negatively affects brain development, leading to maladaptive behavioral responses as well as learning difficulties. In order to build resilience during the childhood years, regular screening for ACEs and appropriate referrals may make a difference in the long-term outcome for these children (Goddard, 2021).

COMMON MEDICAL TREATMENTS

A variety of medications and other medical and psychological treatments are used to treat mental health disorders in children. Most of these treatments will require a health care provider's or nurse practitioner's order when the child is in the hospital. The most common medications are listed in Drug Guide 28.1. The nurse caring for the child with a mental health disorder should become familiar with how the treatments and medications work, as well as medication adverse effects for which to monitor. Many mental health disorders are treated with some type of therapy, including behavioral, play, family, and cognitive therapies. Table 28.1 reviews the types of therapies commonly used. These therapies are generally carried out only by specially trained personnel.

Behavior management techniques are also used to help children alter negative behavior patterns. The methods may be used outside of therapy sessions, in the hospital, clinic, classroom, or home. Behavior management techniques include:

- Set limits with the child, holding them responsible for their own behavior.
- Do not argue, bargain, or negotiate about the limits once established.
- Provide consistent caregivers (unlicensed assistive personnel and nurses for the hospitalized child), and establish the child's daily routine.
- Use a low-pitched voice and remain calm.
- Redirect the child's attention when needed.
- Ignore inappropriate behaviors.
- Praise the child's self-control efforts and other accomplishments.
- Use restraints only when necessary.

DRUG GUIDE 28.1

DRUGS USED FOR PEDIATRIC MENTAL HEALTH DISORDERS

Medication	Actions/Indications	Nursing Implications
Psychostimulants: methylphenidate, dextroamphetamine, lisdexamfetamine, pemoline, long-acting methylphenidate, long-acting dextroamphetamine	Increase synaptic levels of dopamine and norepinephrine ADHD	• Methylphenidate has a short half-life; give TID (am, midday at school, at home after school). • Long-acting preparations are given once daily in the morning. • Adverse effects include decreased appetite, headache, abdominal pain, difficulty sleeping, irritability, social withdrawal, and motor tics. If the dose is too high, the child may have a flat affect. • Lisdexamfetamine—If chest pain and fainting occur, notify the provider at once. • Pemoline is only rarely used because of hepatotoxicity.
Antianxiety agent: buspirone	Highly blocks reuptake of dopamine Anxiety, rage, mania, psychosis, depression, Tourette syndrome	• Administer in consistent relation to food (either with or without). • May cause drowsiness • Monitor for disinhibition, agitation, confusion, and depression.
Antimanic agent: lithium	Influences reuptake of serotonin and/or norepinephrine Bipolar disorder, depression, hyperaggression	• Monitor closely. • May cause polyuria, polydipsia, tremor, nausea, weight gain, diarrhea
Selective serotonin reuptake inhibitors: fluoxetine, paroxetine, sertraline	Potentiate serotonin activity in the brain Depression, obsessive-compulsive disorder, anxiety	• Observe for irritability, insomnia, GI distress, nausea, or headache. • Monitor BP for increases.
Atypical antidepressants: trazodone	Inhibit reuptake of serotonin Depression	• Monitor BP for postural hypotension. • Observe for sedation and drowsiness; avoid alcohol use. • Administer after meals or with a snack.
Nonstimulant norepinephrine reuptake inhibitors: atomoxetine	Enhance norepinephrine activity ADHD	• Administer without regard to food once or twice daily. • Monitor weight, height, BP, and heart rate. • May cause dizziness, dry mouth
Alpha-agonist antihypertensive agents: clonidine, guanfacine	Activate inhibitory neurons in the brain stem ADHD, Tourette syndrome, self-harm, aggression	• Clonidine is strongly sedating. • Monitor BP and pulse. • Observe for dry mouth, confusion, depression, urinary retention, and constipation.
Antipsychotic agents: thioridazine, chlorpromazine, haloperidol	Reversibly block type 2 dopamine receptors in the central nervous system Psychosis, mania, self-harm, violent or destructive behavior	• May cause drowsiness • Monitor for anticholinergic effects, drowsiness and dystonia (extrapyramidal effects), and dizziness. • Evaluate for the development of orthostatic hypotension and tachycardia. • Observe closely for the development of tardive dyskinesia, particularly early in treatment.
Atypical antipsychotics: risperidone, clozapine, olanzapine	Reversibly block type 2 dopamine receptors in the central nervous system Psychosis, bipolar disorder, autism spectrum disorder, Tourette syndrome	• Monitor for seizures, agitation, headache, nausea, and sedation. • Olanzapine may cause weight gain. • Note WBC count.
Tricyclic antidepressants: amitriptyline, desipramine, imipramine, nortriptyline	Enhance synaptic concentration of serotonin and/or norepinephrine Depression, ADHD, tics, anxiety	• Monitor for anticholinergic effects or weight loss. • Check blood levels. • Monitor ECG for arrhythmias.

ADHD, attention-deficit/hyperactivity disorder; BP, blood pressure; ECG, electrocardiogram; GI, gastrointestinal; TID, three times a day; WBC, white blood cell.

Data from Halter, M. J., & Fratena, C. A. (2023). *Varcarolis' manual of psychiatric nursing care planning: An interprofessional approach* (7th ed.). Elsevier; UpToDate, Inc. (2024). *UpToDate Lexidrug* (Version 8.2.0) [Mobile app]. Wolters Kluwer. https://apps.apple.com/us/app/lexicomp/id313401238

TABLE 28.1 • Types of Therapy

Treatment	Explanation
Behavioral therapy	Uses stimulus and response conditioning to manage or alter behavior; reinforces desired behaviors, replacing the inappropriate ones; consistency is of utmost importance.
Play therapy	Designed to change emotional status; encourages the child to act out feelings of sadness, fear, hostility, or anger
Cognitive behavioral therapy	Teaches children to change reactions so that automatic negative thought patterns are replaced with alternative ones
Dialectical behavioral therapy	Group and individual sessions to treat chronic suicidal thoughts in borderline personality disorder; individuals learn responsibility for their problems and to better deal with negative emotions.
Family therapy	Exploration of the child's emotional issue and its effect on family members; helps the family focus in more constructive ways
Group therapy	May be conducted in a school, hospital, treatment facility, or neighborhood center; feelings are expressed and participants gain hope, feel a part of something, and benefit from role modeling. Takes advantage of peer relationships as developmental focus in preadolescent and adolescent groups
Milieu therapy	A specially structured setting designed to promote the child's adaptive and social skills; a safe and supportive environment for those at risk for self-harm or those who are very ill or aggressive
Individual therapy	The child and therapist work together to resolve the conflicts, emotions, or behavior problems. Trust is central. Structured based on the child's developmental level (e.g., may use play therapy for a younger child)
Hypnosis	Deep relaxation with suggestibility remarks

Data from American Academy of Child and Adolescent Psychiatry. (2019). *Psychotherapy for children and adolescents: Different types.* https://www.aacap.org/AACAP/Families_and_Youth/Facts_for_Families/FFF-Guide/Psychotherapies-For-Children-And-Adolescents-086.aspx; Halter, M. J., & Fratena, C. A. (2023). *Varcarolis' manual of psychiatric nursing care planning: An interprofessional approach* (7th ed.). Elsevier; and Swick, S. D., & Jellinek, M. S. (2022). Demystifying psychotherapy. *Pediatric News, 56*(10), 18.

Clinical Judgment and the Nursing Process for the Child With a Mental Health Disorder

Care of the child with mental health disorder includes assessment, nursing analysis, planning, interventions, and evaluation. It is important to individualize each step of this process for each child.

Assessment

A careful and thorough health history forms the basis of the nursing assessment of a child with a mental health or cognitive disorder. The physical examination may yield clues to the type of disorder, but the physical examination often yields expected findings (except in cases of physical or sexual abuse).

CLINICAL REASONING ALERT!

Observe a child's play or drawings; if the manner or theme of play or nature of the drawings leads you to suspect cognitive or psychological issues, refer the child for further mental health evaluation.

Health History

Elicit the health history, noting the child's prenatal and birth history, past medical history (including previously diagnosed cognitive or mental health disorders), history of neurologic injury or disease, and family history of mental health disorders. Perform a developmental history, noting age of attainment (or loss) of milestones. Question the child and/or parent about behavior changes such as:

- Altered sleep
- Difference in eating patterns, weight loss or gain, change in appetite
- Problems at school
- Participation in risk-taking behaviors
- Alterations in friendships
- Changes in extracurricular activity participation

A number of tools are available for screening for mental health disorders in children and adolescents. Use one of these tools as needed. Note results of any developmental testing performed. Ask the family about progression of the child's skills. Note any unusual deficits or capabilities. Question the family about recent stress, trauma, or change in family structure. Ask if any family members are chronically ill. Note medications the child takes routinely, and ask about any allergies to food, drugs, medications, or environmental agents.

Interview the child at an age-appropriate level to determine their self-perception, future plans, and stressors and how they cope with them. Determine the child's perception of their relationships with parents, siblings, friends, peers, pets, inanimate objects, and transitional or security objects. What is the child's predominant mood? Determine whether the child likes themselves, asking such questions as "What do you like most about yourself?" and "What would you like to change about yourself?" Determine whether the child has a sense of pride in their accomplishments. Has the child developed an appropriate conscience (understanding right and wrong)? Determine the child's gender identity status.

Document whether the child displays any of the following during the health interview:

- Hallucinations
- Aggression
- Impulsivity
- Distractibility
- Intolerance to frustration
- Lack of sense of humor or fun
- Inhibition
- Poor attention span
- Potential cognitive or learning disabilities
- Unusual motor activities

Note history of physical complaints that may be associated with physical abuse such as burns or other injuries or with sexual abuse situations, such as sore throat, difficulty swallowing, or genital burning or itching.

Physical Examination

Observe the child's clothing, noting whether it is appropriate for age, developmental level, and setting. Note the child's facial expression and response to the parent or caregiver and the nurse. Does the child make appropriate eye contact? Determine the child's level of consciousness and extent of interest in and interaction with surroundings. Note the child's posture, **affect** (facial emotional display), and mood. How appropriate to the situation are the child's emotional reactions? Does the child communicate well?

Measure the child's weight and height/length, as well as head circumference if they are younger than 3 years old. Perform a thorough physical examination, noting any physical abnormalities or signs of other physical health disorders. Note abnormal findings that may be associated with particular mental health disorders, such as bruising, burns, contusions, cuts, abrasions, unusual skin marks, soft/sparse body hair, split fingernails, inflamed oropharynx, eroded tooth enamel, reddened gums, or genitourinary discharge or bleeding.

Laboratory and Diagnostic Testing

Mental health disorders are generally diagnosed based on clinical features. However, brain imaging such as computed tomography or magnetic resonance imaging may be used to evaluate for a congenital abnormality or alterations in the brain tissue that may lead to developmental delay. A blood or urine toxicology panel is useful in the diagnosis of substance misuse or overdose, or instances of bizarre behavior.

Remember John, the 6-year-old brought in for his annual examination? What additional health history and physical examination assessment information should the nurse obtain?

Nursing Analysis and Related Interventions

The overall goal of nursing management of cognitive and mental health disorders in children is to help the child and family reach an optimal level of functioning. This may be achieved through interventions designed to decrease the impact of stressors on the child's life. After recognizing and analyzing cues from a thorough assessment, the nurse might identify several patient problems, including:

- Malnutrition risk
- Delayed development risk
- Impulsivity
- Impaired social interaction
- Coping impairment
- Hopelessness
- Caregiver role strain risk
- Knowledge deficiency

These patient problems provide suggestions for nursing care planning or concept mapping for the child with a mental health disorder or an alteration behavior, cognition, or development. Suggested interventions with rationales are provided as follows. Care planning should be individualized, based on the child's and family's needs. Refer to Chapter 14 for the nursing process for pain management and to Chapter 11 for nursing interventions related to caregiver role strain risk. Additional information will be included later in the chapter as it relates to nursing management of children with specific disorders, as well as particular nursing interventions for deficient knowledge.

After completing an assessment of John, the nurse noted difficulty sitting still for the examination, that he was easily distracted and frustrated, and demonstrated a labile mood. Based on the assessment findings, what would your top three patient problems be for John?

See the Healthy People 2030 box.

HEALTHY PEOPLE 2030

Objective	Nursing Significance
Increase the proportion of children with mental health problems who receive treatment and increase the number of children receiving preventive mental health care in school.	• Screen all children and adolescents for mental health problems. • Support families with finding and following up on appropriate treatment. • Assist schools with mental health screenings (either physically or through educating others).

Healthy People Objectives retrieved from http://www.healthypeople.gov

Nursing Analysis

Malnutrition risk; risk factors include insufficient dietary intake, insufficient interest in food, body mass index (BMI) of less than the 5th percentile for age, satiety immediately upon ingesting food, or weight loss with adequate food intake.

Goal/Outcome

The child or adolescent will demonstrate appropriate growth, making gains in weight and stature as appropriate.

Improving Nutritional Intake (interventions with *rationale*)

- Provide favorite foods *to encourage the child with poor appetite to eat more.*
- Assist families with choosing nutrient-rich foods *so that the food the child does eat is most beneficial.*

For the child with an eating disorder:

- Mutually establish a contract related to treatment *to promote the child's sense of control.*
- Provide mealtime structure, *as clear limits let the child know what the expectations are.*
- Encourage the child to choose foods and timing of meals *to develop independence in eating habits.*
- Ensure the eating environment is pleasant and relaxed with minimal distractions *to minimize the child's anxiety and guilt about not eating.*
- Withdraw attention if the child refuses to eat; *secondary gain is minimized if refusal to eat is ignored.*
- Provide continuous supervision during the meal and for 30 minutes following it *so that the child cannot conceal or dispose of food or induce vomiting.*

Nursing Analysis

Delayed development risk; risk factors include inadequate nutrition, presence of abuse, behavioral disorder, chronic (mental) illness.

Goal/Outcome

The child will demonstrate progress toward developmental milestones; the child expresses interest in the environment and people around them and interacts with the environment in an age-appropriate way.

Promoting Development (interventions with *rationale*)

- Use therapeutic play and adaptive toys *to facilitate developmental functioning.*
- Provide stimulating environment when possible *to maximize potential for growth and development.*
- Praise accomplishments and emphasize the child's abilities *to improve self-esteem and encourage feelings of confidence and competence.*
- Follow through with physical, occupational, and speech therapists' recommendations *to maximize exposure to exercises designed to increase the child's skills.*
- Determine parents' expectations of the child's future achievement *to help them work toward these goals.*

Nursing Analysis

Impulsivity related to alteration in cognitive functioning or development, or mood or personality disorder as evidenced by acting without thinking, irritability, sensation seeking, temper outbursts, or violence

Goal/Outcome

Child's impulse control will improve: The child will improve in ability to control impulses, remain free from physical harm, and participate in usual activities as able.

Reducing Impulsivity (interventions with *rationale*)

- Observe for causes of impulsivity *to provide a baseline for assessment and intervention.*
- Perform an age-appropriate mental status examination *to determine the extent of altered thinking.*
- Work together with the child and family to develop a plan for controlling impulses; *individualization will be necessary.*
- Listen carefully and seek clarification *to determine the basis for the child's agitation or other behaviors.*
- Provide validation of the child's thoughts and feelings *to improve trust in the relationship.*
- Establish a daily routine *to provide the child with a sense of security.*

Nursing Analysis

Impaired social interaction related to disturbance in self-concept or thought processes or insufficient skill so as to enhance mutuality as evidenced by dysfunctional interaction or impaired social functioning

(impulsivity, intrusive behavior, feelings of unattractiveness or unworthiness)

Goal/Outcome

The child will demonstrate socially acceptable skills, interacting successfully with peers and in the educational setting, completing tasks as required.

Promoting Appropriate Social Interaction (interventions with *rationale*)

- Identify factors that may aggravate the child's performance *to minimize stimuli that exacerbate the child's undesired behaviors.*
- Modify the environment to decrease distracting stimuli *as the child's ability to deal with external stimuli may be impaired.*
- Ensure that the child hears their name and makes eye contact prior to conversing or receiving instructions *so that the child is engaged and has increased ability to follow through.*
- State expectations for tasks or behaviors clearly *as understanding is necessary to ensure completion.*
- Provide positive feedback for appropriate behaviors or task completion, *encouraging the child to adopt expectations into their behaviors and routine.*

Nursing Analysis

Coping impairment related to inadequate confidence in ability to deal with a situation, insufficient sense of control, or situational crisis as evidenced by alteration in confidence, destructive behavior toward self or others, substance misuse, or ineffective coping strategies

Goal/Outcome

The child will demonstrate improved coping, verbalize feelings, socially engage, and demonstrate problem-solving skills.

Promoting Coping Skills (interventions with *rationale*)

- Encourage discussion of thoughts and feelings, *as this is an initial step toward learning to deal with them appropriately.*
- Provide positive feedback for appropriate discussion, *as this increases the likelihood of continuing performance.*
- Demonstrate unconditional acceptance of the child as a person *to increase self-esteem in the child who has been feeling rejected.*
- Set clear limits on behavior as needed *so the child has a structure to adhere to.*
- Teach the child problem-solving skills *as an alternative to acting-out behaviors.*
- Role model appropriate social and conversational skills *so the child can see what is expected in a nonthreatening manner.*

Nursing Analysis

Hopelessness related to chronic stress (due to mental, behavioral, or developmental disorder), social isolation, or history of abandonment, as evidenced by passivity, decrease in affect, alteration in sleep pattern, or despondent verbal cues

Goal/Outcome

Child will display a sense of hope; they will verbalize feelings, participate in care, and make positive statements.

Promoting Hope (interventions with *rationale*)

- Monitor and document potential for suicide, *as hopelessness often leads to suicidal ideation.*
- Assist the child to identify reasons for hope and for living *so the nurse is aware of the child's values.*
- Help the child set goals that are important to them *to allow the child to see possibilities.*
- Encourage simple decision making on a daily basis, *as hopelessness often occurs as a response to loss of control.*
- Assist the child in identifying positive qualities in themselves and their life *to facilitate the development of hope.*
- Involve parents or others the child loves in the child's care *as social support is critical to the development of hope.*

For each of your top three patient problems for John, choose the top three nursing interventions.

DEVELOPMENTAL AND BEHAVIORAL DISORDERS

Developmental and behavioral disorders make up a large proportion of mental health disorders in children. They include learning disabilities, intellectual disability, autism spectrum disorder (ASD), and attention-deficit/hyperactivity disorder (ADHD).

Learning Disabilities

Up to 15% of children and adolescents have learning disabilities, and in children with chronic illness, learning disabilities are two times more common than in the general population (von Hahn, 2023a). The essential characteristic of learning disability is an innate cognitive difficulty resulting in lower academic achievement than would be expected for the child's intellectual potential (von Hahn, 2023a). Learning disabilities become evident when a child of average intelligence has difficulty mastering basic academic skills. Learning disabilities can affect the child's ability to listen, speak, read, write, and perform mathematics. For example:

- Children with dyslexia have difficulty with reading, writing, and spelling.
- Children with dyscalculia have problems with mathematics and computation.
- Children with dyspraxia have problems with manual dexterity and coordination.
- Children with dysgraphia have difficulty producing the written word (composition, spelling, and writing).

TAKE NOTE!

Sensory processing disorder may be mistaken for a learning disability, but it is not and should be treated differently (Box 28.1).

Therapeutic Management

Therapeutic management may involve remedial or compensatory approaches or may use interventions directed toward social–emotional problems. The focus of the remedial approach is to improve specific skills. The compensatory approach helps the child compensate for the disability, rather than attempting to directly correct it (von Hahn, 2023b). Social–emotional problems may result from frustration or low self-esteem related to capabilities. These may respond to supportive interventions and improvement in coping.

CONSIDER THIS!

Victor Johnson, a third grader with learning disabilities, tells the nurse, "I get made fun of at school." He begins to sniffle and says, "Everybody calls me stupid. It hurts my feelings." Victor's parent adds, "I really just don't know how to help." How should the nurse reply? What would be the most therapeutic response?

BOX 28.1 Sensory Processing Disorder (Also Called Sensory Integration Dysfunction)

- A neurologic disorder in which the child cannot organize sensory input used in daily living
- Hyposensitivity or hypersensitivity to sensory input
- Results in overreaction to different textures, decreasing the child's ability to participate in the world
- Preterm and low-birth-weight infants are at increased risk compared with other infants.
- Occupational and other therapies may increase the child's ability to function.

Data from Star Center Foundation. (2024). *Understanding sensory processing disorder*. https://www.spdstar.org/basic/understanding-sensory-processing-disorder

Nursing Assessment

Elicit the health history, noting risk factors such as a family history of learning disability, problems during pregnancy or birth, prenatal alcohol or drug exposure, low birth weight, premature or prolonged labor, head injury, poor nutritional status or failure to thrive, or lead poisoning. Obtain detailed information about the educational difficulties the child is experiencing (e.g., they seem to do fine in math but always reverse letters when reading). A thorough physical examination may reveal clues to **comorbid** (simultaneously existing) conditions. Ensure the child has undergone a comprehensive education evaluation with assessment testing to diagnose the specific learning disability. Testing may be performed by a school, educational, developmental, or clinical psychologist; occupational therapist; speech and language therapist; or other developmental specialist, depending on the areas of learning with which the child is experiencing difficulty.

CLINICAL REASONING ALERT!

If a child cannot speak in sentences by 30 months of age; does not have understandable speech 50% of the time by age 3 years; cannot sit still for a short story by 3 to 5 years of age; or cannot tie shoes, cut, button, or hop by 5 to 6 years of age, refer the child to be evaluated for a learning disability.

Nursing Management

Ensure families are aware of their child's rights under the Individuals with Disabilities Education Act (IDEA), which was reapproved in 2004 (108th Congress, 2004). IDEA offers protection from discrimination and the right to assistance in the school or workplace. Each child will need an individualized education plan (IEP) that reflects their particular needs, which must then be provided through the school system. Offer encouragement and support to families as they advocate for their child. Follow up at subsequent health care visits to determine if the child is receiving the services they need to optimize their potential for success. Refer families for additional resources through the National Center for Learning Disabilities, Learning Disabilities Online, or the Center for Learning Differences.

Intellectual Disability

Intellectual disability refers to a functional state in which significant limitations in intellectual status and adaptive behavior (functioning in daily life) develop before the age of 18 to 22 years. Intellectual disability occurs in about 1% to 2% of the population (Pivalizza, 2024). The range of impairments associated with the intellectual disability is variable. Impairments in the adaptive domains of conceptual, social, or practical assist with determining the severity of intellectual disability (from mild to profound) (Pivalizza, 2024).

In the past, people with intellectual disability were confined to institutions and were thought to be harmful to society. In the early 21st century, most children with intellectual disability are receiving their education in public schools with their peers and living at home with their families or elsewhere in the community. Only the most severely affected individuals require separate classrooms or schools.

Pathophysiology

In many instances of intellectual disability, the exact cause remains unknown. Prenatal errors in central nervous system development may be responsible. Other potential causes include an insult or damage to the brain during the prenatal, perinatal, or postnatal period. Prenatal exposure to alcohol or other drugs may impact cognitive development as well. Motor problems such as hypertonia or hypotonia, tremor, ataxia, or clumsiness, or visual motor problems may occur concomitantly with intellectual disability. In addition, functioning at a higher level may be prevented when a learning disability or sensory processing impairment is also present. Intellectual disability may be categorized according to severity of impairment across domains. See Table 28.2.

Therapeutic Management

The primary goal of therapeutic management of children with intellectual disability is to provide appropriate educational experiences that allow the child to achieve a level of functioning and self-sufficiency needed for existence in the home, community, work, and leisure settings. A multidisciplinary approach may be used, and the child's conceptual, social, practical, and intellectual abilities will drive school placement and the focus of the educational experience. The majority of individuals with intellectual disability require only minimal support in the school or home setting, and these individuals are able to achieve some level of self-sufficiency. Only some children and adults with intellectual disability require extensive support and require long-term caregiving.

Nursing Assessment

Perform developmental screening at each health care visit to identify developmental delays early. Elicit the health history, determining the mental and adaptive capacities of the child's parents and other family members. Obtain a detailed pregnancy and birth history. Document sequence and age of attainment of developmental milestones. Note history of motor, visual, or language difficulties. Assess the child's health history for risk factors such as preterm or postterm birth, low birth weight, birth injury, prenatal or neonatal infection, prenatal alcohol or drug exposure, genetic syndrome, chromosomal alteration, metabolic disease, exposure to toxins (e.g., lead), head injury or other trauma, nutritional deficiency, cerebral malformation, and other brain diseases or mental health disorders. Note history of or concomitant seizure disorder, orthopedic problems, speech problems, or vision or hearing deficit.

For the child with known intellectual disability, assess language, sensory, and psychomotor functioning. Determine the child's ability to toilet, dress, and feed themselves. Ask the parents about involvement with school and community services and support.

On physical examination, note dysmorphic features (possibly mild) consistent with certain syndromes (e.g., fetal alcohol syndrome; Box 28.2). Evaluate the newborn or metabolic screening results. Computed tomography

TABLE 28.2 Severity of Intellectual Disability

Severity	Level of Support	Conceptual	Social	Practical
Mild	Intermittent	Requires academic supports	Immature social skills and personal judgment	Usually independent in activities of daily living
Moderate	Limited	Complex tasks require substantial support.	Social cues, judgment, and life decisions need regular support	Independent self-care with moderate supports
Severe	Extensive	Little understanding of written language, time; require extensive supports	Benefit from healthy supportive interactions	Require significant and ongoing supervision for activities of daily living
Profound	Pervasive	May use objects in a goal-directed fashion	May understand gestures and emotional cues; use nonverbal expression	Dependent upon support for all activities of daily living

BOX 28.2 Fetal Alcohol Syndrome

- Results from in utero alcohol exposure
- Typical facial features include low nasal bridge with short upturned nose, flattened midface, long philtrum with narrow upper lip.
- Poor coordination, skeletal abnormalities
- Microcephaly
- Failure to thrive
- Hearing loss

Data from Reynolds, A., Angulo, A., Breheney, M., Green, J., & Goldson, E. (2022). Child development and behavior. In M. Bunik, W. W. Hay, M. J. Levin, & M. J. Abzug (Eds.), *Current diagnosis & treatment: Pediatrics* (26th ed.). McGraw-Hill Education.

or magnetic resonance imaging of the head may be performed to evaluate the brain structure. Thyroid function tests may be ordered to rule out thyroid problems leading to developmental delay.

TAKE NOTE!

Due to the extent of cognition required to understand and produce speech, the most sensitive early indicator of intellectual disability is delayed language development.

Nursing Management

When children with intellectual disability are admitted to the hospital (usually for some other physical or medical condition), it is important for the nurse to continue the child's usual home routine. Follow through with feeding and motor supports that the child uses. Ensure that the child is closely supervised and remains free from harm. Allow parents time to verbalize frustrations or fears. For some families, the caregiving burden is extensive and lifelong; arrange for respite care as available. Support the child's strengths, and assist the child and family with following through with therapy or treatment designed to enhance the child's functioning. Assist with the development of the child's IEP as appropriate.

Autism Spectrum Disorder

ASD has its onset in infancy or early childhood and affects one in 68 children (Reynolds et al., 2022). Brain development and function and, ultimately, social behavior and communication are affected (Sohl, 2022). The spectrum ranges from mild to severe. Some children with ASD may be intellectually disabled, requiring lifelong supervision, but the majority will display expected to high intelligence levels (Reynolds et al., 2022). ASD behaviors may be first noticed in infancy as developmental delays or between the ages of 12 and 36 months, when the child exhibits regression or loses previously acquired skills. Parental concerns about development may be sensitive indicators of the development of ASD.

Pathophysiology

Although the exact etiology of ASD continues to be unknown, genetic factors have been well studied in these children, and ASD is considered to be mainly a genetic disorder; however, there may also be issues with brain connectivity (Reynolds et al., 2022). Children with ASD display impaired social interactions and communication as well as perseverative or stereotypic behaviors. They may have difficulty developing interpersonal relationships and experience social isolation.

Therapeutic Management

There are no medications or treatments available to cure ASD. The goal of therapeutic management is for the child to reach optimal functioning within the bounds of the disorder. Each child's treatment is individualized; behavioral and communication therapies are important. Children with ASD respond well to highly structured educational environments, so early, intensive behavioral interventions are necessary. Stimulants may be used to control hyperactivity, and antipsychotic medications are sometimes helpful in children with repetitive and aggressive behaviors.

Some families may be drawn to the use of complementary and alternative medical therapies in attempts to treat a child with ASD. They may use vitamins and nutritional supplements, herbs or restrictive diets, music therapy, art therapy, and sensory integration techniques. The effectiveness of these therapies has not been shown by studies to be beneficial, and herbal and other supplements may interact with prescribed medications (Weissman & Harris, 2022). However, music therapy used within a comprehensive behavioral program has no harmful effects and may improve ASD severity and the child's quality of life (Weissman & Harris, 2022). See Evidence-Based Practice Box 28.1.

Nursing Assessment

Elicit the health history, noting delay or regression in developmental skills, particularly speech and language abilities. Failure to point at objects and to gaze at an object jointly with another by 18 months are concerning signs. The most common early characteristics are a consistent failure to orient to one's name, regard people directly, use gestures, and develop speech (Reynolds et al., 2022). The child may be nonverbal, utter only sounds (not words), or repeat words or phrases over and over. The parent may report that the infant or toddler spends hours in repetitive activity and demonstrates bizarre motor and stereotypic behaviors. The infant may resist cuddling, lack eye contact, be indifferent to touch or affection, and show little change in facial expression. Toddlers may display hyperactivity, aggression, temper

EVIDENCE-BASED PRACTICE 28.1

Early Behavioral Intervention for Autism Spectrum Disorder

STUDY

As the incidence of ASD continues to rise, it is necessary to evaluate the efficacy of interventions for ASD. Early intensive behavioral intervention (delivered at 20 to 40 hours per week) is a commonly used therapy for ASD. The authors reviewed one randomized controlled trial and four clinical control trials with a total of 219 participants under the age of 6 years.

Findings

The Vineland Adaptive Behavioral Scales was used to assess adaptive behavior following treatment. The authors noted that early intensive behavioral intervention resulted in an improvement in adaptive behavior, although it did not change the severity score.

Nursing Implications

Caring for a child with ASD can be challenging for families. If adaptive behaviors can be improved, both the child and the parents will benefit. Assist families with finding schools or centers utilizing early intensive behavioral intervention. Support and encourage parents to encourage interventions in the home setting as prescribed.

Data from Reichow, B., Hume, K., Barton, E. E., & Boyd, B. A. (2018). Early intensive behavioral intervention (EIBI) for young children with autism spectrum disorders (ASD). *Cochrane Database of Systematic Reviews*, (5), CD009260. https://doi.org/10.1002/14651858.CD009260.pub3

tantrums, or self-injurious behaviors, such as head banging or hand biting. The history may also reveal hypersensitivity to touch or hyposensitivity to pain.

Assess the child's functional status, including behavior, nutrition, sleep, speech and language, education needs, and developmental or neurologic limitations. Assist with screening, using an approved ASD screening tool such as the Modified Checklist for Autism in Toddlers-Revised (M-CHAT-R), which is recommended for administration at 18 months of age, and then again at 24 to 30 months of age. Additional screening tools include the Social Communication Questionnaire (SCQ) and the Pervasive Developmental Disorders Screening Test-II (PDDST-II).

Perform a thorough physical examination. Observe the infant or toddler for lack of eye contact, failure to look at objects pointed to by the examiner, failure to point to themselves, failure to let their needs be known, perseverative play activities, and unusual behavior such as hand flapping or spinning. Measure growth parameters, noting, in particular, head circumference (macrocephaly or microcephaly may be associated with ASD). Note the presence of large, prominent, or posteriorly rotated ears. Examine the skin for hypopigmented or hyperpigmented lesions. Note asymmetry of nerve function or palsy, hypertonia, hypotonia, alterations in deep tendon reflexes, toe-walking, loose gait, or poor coordination. Obtain hearing screening results and ascertain that lead screening has been performed.

TAKE NOTE!

Screen all infants and toddlers for warning signs of ASD:

- *Does not imitate*
- *Lack of interest in joint attention*
- *Avoiding eye contact*
- *Delayed language development*
- *Failure to develop symbolic-imaginative play (pretending)*
- *Difficulty with minor changes or transitions* (Augustyn & von Hahn, 2023)

Additional signs at specific ages include:

- At 12 months, does not respond to name
- At 14 months, does not show interest in items by pointing
- At 18 months, does not participate in pretend play (Sohl, 2022)

Nursing Management

When children are initially diagnosed with ASD, provide parents with an extensive amount of emotional support, professional guidance, and education about the disorder while they are attempting to adjust to the diagnosis. Assess the fit between the child's developmental needs and the treatment plan. Help parents overcome barriers to obtaining appropriate education, developmental, and behavioral treatment programs. Ensure that the child younger than 36 months of age receives services via the local early intervention program and that children 3 years and older have an IEP in place if enrolled in the public school system. Stress the importance of rigid, unchanging routines, as children with ASD often have difficulty when their routine changes (which is likely to occur if the child must be hospitalized for another condition). Many specialized schools exist for children with significant developmental disorders, although some are extremely expensive. Assess the parents' need for respite care and make referrals accordingly. Provide positive feedback to parents for supporting their child's unique needs.

ATRAUMATIC CARE

Provide family-centered care, being sure to treat the family and not just the child. Minimize parent–child separation.

Attention-Deficit/Hyperactivity Disorder

ADHD is the most common neurodevelopmental disorder of childhood, estimated to affect 9% to 15% of school-aged children (Krull & Chan, 2023). It is characterized by inattention, impulsivity, distractibility, and hyperactivity. Three subtypes of ADHD exist: hyperactive–impulsive, inattentive, and combined. The child with ADHD has a disruption in learning ability, socialization, and adherence, placing demands on the child, parents, teachers, and community. Children with ADHD often have a comorbidity (disorder accompanying the primary illness) such as oppositional defiant disorder, conduct disorder, an anxiety disorder, depression, a less severe developmental disorder, an auditory processing disorder, or learning or reading disabilities (Krull & Chan, 2023). Comparison Chart 28.1 gives information about oppositional defiant disorder and conduct disorder to distinguish them from ADHD.

Pathophysiology

Although the exact cause of ADHD remains unidentified, an alteration in the catecholamine neurotransmitter system may be responsible, but genetics, environmental exposures, and structural brain abnormalities may play a role (Krull & Chan, 2023). The symptoms of impulsivity, hyperactivity, and inattention begin before 7 years of age and persist longer than 6 months. Symptoms exist in the school and home settings, impairing family and social interactions. Children and adolescents with ADHD may experience frustration, labile moods, emotional outbursts, peer rejection, poor school performance, and low self-esteem. They may also have difficulty with metacognitive skills like organization, time management, and the ability to break a project down into a series of smaller tasks. Box 28.3 provides criteria for the diagnosis of ADHD (Reynolds et al., 2022).

BOX 28.3 Diagnosis of Attention-Deficit/Hyperactivity Disorder

Presence of six or more of the following findings in the child 17 years of age and younger:

- Failure to pay close attention
- Careless mistakes on school work
- Difficulty paying attention to tasks or play
- Doesn't listen
- Doesn't follow through
- Doesn't complete tasks
- Doesn't understand instructions
- Difficulty with organization
- Avoids, dislikes, or fails to engage in activities requiring mental effort
- Loses things needed for task completion
- Easily distracted
- Forgetful
- Fidgety or squirmy
- Often out of seat
- Activity inappropriate to the situation
- Cannot engage in quiet play
- Always on the go
- Talks excessively
- Blurts out answers
- Has difficulty waiting their turn
- Often interrupts or intrudes on others

Additionally, symptoms have been present in two or more settings, and at least two of the symptoms occurred prior to age 12; symptoms have persisted beyond 6 months and to a degree inconsistent with developmental level or negatively interfere with social or academic performance. Symptoms are not associated with purely oppositional behavior or as a component of a psychotic disorder and cannot be explained by the diagnosis of a different mental health disorder.

Data from Reynolds, A., Angulo, A., Breheney, M., Green, J., & Goldson, E. (2022). Child development and behavior. In M. Bunik, W. W. Hay, M. J. Levin, & M. J. Abzug (Eds.), *Current diagnosis & treatment: Pediatrics* (26th ed.). McGraw-Hill Education.

COMPARISON CHART 28.1 Oppositional Defiant Disorder Versus Conduct Disorder

Oppositional Defiant Disorder	Conduct Disorder
• Excessive arguing with adults • Frequent temper tantrums • Active defiance • Revenge-seeking behaviors • Frequent resentment or anger • Touchiness; easily annoyed • Nonadherence with adult requests or limits • Blaming of others for misbehavior or mistakes	• Bullying and threatening of others • Initiation of physical fights • Weapon use to cause others harm • Physical cruelty to animals or people • Destruction of property or arson • Lying and stealing • Serious violation of rules, like staying out past curfew, truancy, running away • Use of force in sexual activity

Based on Kelsay, K., Glaze, K., & Talmi, A. (2022). Child & adolescent psychiatric disorders & psychosocial aspects of pediatrics. In M. Bunik, W. W. Hay, M. J. Levin, & M. J. Abzug (Eds.), *Current pediatric diagnosis and treatment* (26th ed.). McGraw-Hill Education.

Therapeutic Management

Medication management of ADHD includes the use of psychostimulants, nonstimulant norepinephrine reuptake inhibitors, and/or alpha-agonist antihypertensive agents. These medications are not a cure for ADHD but help increase the child's ability to pay attention and decrease the level of impulsive behavior. The child's activity level is not usually affected. Behavior therapy and classroom restructuring may be useful as part of the therapeutic management plan. Concomitant disorders, such as anxiety, should also be treated (see the discussion of anxiety disorders that follows).

Nursing Assessment

For a full description of the assessment phase of the nursing process, refer to the "Clinical Judgment and the Nursing Process" section. Assessment findings pertinent to ADHD are discussed here.

HEALTH HISTORY

Elicit a description of the behavioral issue or school performance problem. Explore the child's history for risk factors such as head trauma, lead exposure, cigarette smoke exposure, prematurity, and low birth weight. The past history may also reveal a larger than usual number of accidents. Determine if there is a family history of ADHD. Question the parent about school behavior. The school-aged child may be unable to stay on task, talk out of turn, leave their desk frequently, and either neglect to complete in-class and homework assignments or forget to turn them in. The adolescent may be inattentive in school, poorly organized, and forgetful.

Several behavioral checklists are available that may assist in the diagnosis of ADHD. They may be completed by the child's teacher and/or parent and focus on behavior patterns related to conduct or learning problems, social competence, anxiety, activity level, and attention. Obtain the completed behavioral checklists (usually one from the parent and one from the teacher) as well as any school records or testing performed.

PHYSICAL EXAMINATION

Perform vision and hearing screening to rule out difficulty with vision or hearing as the cause of poor school performance. Observe the preschool child's behavior, noting quickness, agility, fearlessness, and the desire to touch or explore everything in the room. The older child or adolescent may have difficulty staying on task during the examination or change the subject frequently while conversing.

LABORATORY AND DIAGNOSTIC TESTS

No definitive laboratory or diagnostic test is available for the identification of ADHD. A complete blood count may be performed to rule out anemia, and thyroid hormone levels may be drawn to determine whether they are within the expected range.

Nursing Management

The child's inattention, high activity level, impulsivity, and distractibility can be challenging for caregivers. Parents may doubt their ability to be effective parents or may view their child in a negative light. Children with ADHD may also feel bad about themselves. Provide emotional support, allowing enough time for the family to air their concerns. Work with the child and family to develop goals such as completion of homework, improved communication, and increasing independence in self-care.

Assist the family in advocating for their child's needs through the public school system. The child is entitled to a developmentally appropriate education via an IEP as necessary (refer to Chapter 12 for additional information about special education). The IEP should be updated as needed. Ensure coordination of health and school services. Flag the child's chart and set up a schedule for systematic communication with the family and school. Teach families and school personnel to use behavioral techniques such as time-out, positive reinforcement, reward or privilege withdrawal, or a token system. The token system rewards appropriate behavior with a token and results in a token being taken away if inappropriate behavior occurs. At the end of a specified period of time, the tokens may be exchanged for a prize or privilege. Refer families to local support groups and the national ADHD support group.

Explain that stimulant medications should be taken in the morning to mitigate the risk of the adverse effect of insomnia. Some children may experience decreased appetite, so giving the medication with or after the meal may be beneficial. The child may feel "different" from their peers if they have to visit the school nurse for a lunchtime dose of ADHD medication; this may lead to nonadherence and a subsequent increase in ADHD symptoms with deterioration in school work. In this situation, encourage the family to explore with their provider the option of one of the newer extended-release or once-daily ADHD medications. See Dosage Calculation Box 28.1.

DOSAGE CALCULATION BOX 28.1

Child's weight: 50 lb

Medication order: Start methylphenidate 10 mg PO now.

Per the *Pediatric Dosage Handbook*, for initial dosing, the recommended dose is 0.3 mg/kg/dose.

Is the ordered dose safe?

TOURETTE SYNDROME

Tourette syndrome consists of multiple motor tics and one or more vocal tics occurring either simultaneously or at different times. Children are not tic-free for longer than 3 months. Tics are defined as sudden, rapid, recurrent stereotypical movements and/or sounds over which the child appears to have no control. Tourette syndrome affects about 0.5% of children with onset before 21 years of age (Jankovic, 2023).

Comorbid conditions such as ADHD, obsessive-compulsive disorder (OCD), and others may occur in up to 60% of children with Tourette syndrome (incidence depending upon the comorbid condition) (Jankovic, 2023). The exact pathophysiologic mechanism of Tourette syndrome has yet to be identified, although genetics does seem to play a part. Therapeutic management is highly individualized and involves psychopharmacology and behavioral therapies. Habit reversal training may help in some children.

Nursing Assessment

Evaluate the health history for the occurrence of tics. The child may be embarrassed about or ashamed of the tics, and the parents may feel fearful, angry, or guilty. Determine the presence of symptoms of comorbid conditions. Elicit the child's past health history, noting a family history of tics. Assess the child's psychosocial history to determine the extent to which the tics interfere with friendship, school performance, and self-esteem. Observe the child for simple or complex motor tics. Vocal tics such as sniffling, grunting, clicking, or word utterance may occur. Perform a thorough physical examination, which is usually as expected.

Nursing Management

Inform families that the tics may become more noticeable or severe during times of stress and less pronounced when the child is focused on an activity such as watching TV, reading, or playing a video game. Help the family build on the child's functional behaviors and adaptive skills to improve the child's self-esteem. Encourage the family to pursue classroom accommodations such as allowing for "tic breaks," taking untimed tests or tests in another room, or using note takers or tape recording. Support the family's decisions related to medication use and therapy, and provide appropriate education about the particular drugs and therapies. *Teaching the Tiger* by M. P. Dornbush and S. K. Pruitt (Hope Press) is useful for teachers of children with Tourette syndrome. For additional support, refer families to Tourette Syndrome Association, Tourette Syndrome Foundation of Canada, or Tourette Syndrome Plus.

EATING DISORDERS

Eating disorders include pica, rumination, anorexia nervosa, and bulimia. They affect a significant number of children, especially adolescents. Pica, which occurs most frequently in 2- to 3-year-olds, is an eating disorder in which the child ingests (over at least a 1-month period) a nonnutritive material such as paint, clay, or sand. Rumination is an eating disorder occurring in infants in which the baby regurgitates partially digested food or formula and expels or swallows it. The numbers of children affected by pica and rumination are not known. This discussion will focus on anorexia nervosa and bulimia, as they are more commonly encountered.

Anorexia nervosa and bulimia are common eating disorders affecting primarily adolescents, although younger children may also be affected. In American society, thinness is highly valued, compounding the problem. The lifetime prevalence rate for eating disorders is about 8% for females and 2% for males, and these problems often arise in childhood, particularly adolescence (Guarda, 2023). Anorexia nervosa is characterized by dramatic weight loss as a result of decreased food intake and sharply increased physical exercise. Bulimia refers to a cycle of normal food intake, followed by binge eating and then purging. Typically, the adolescent with bulimia remains around an expected weight. Complications of anorexia and bulimia include fluid and electrolyte imbalance, decreased blood volume, cardiac dysrhythmias, esophagitis, rupture of the esophagus or stomach, tooth loss, and menstrual problems.

Therapeutic management may occur in either the inpatient or outpatient setting. In either case, a multidisciplinary approach including individual and family therapy as well as nutritional therapy is needed for the best chance at successful treatment. Typically, medications are not an initial or primary treatment for eating disorders (Yager, 2022).

Nursing Assessment

Determine the health history, noting risk factors such as family history, female sex, White race, preoccupation with appearance, obsessive traits, and low self-esteem. Adolescents with anorexia may have a history of constipation, syncope, secondary amenorrhea, abdominal pain, and periodic episodes of cold hands and feet. Parents usually note the chief complaint as weight loss. Note history of depression in the child with bulimia. Evaluate the child's self-concept, and pay attention to multiple fears, high need for acceptance, disordered body image, and perfectionism.

Perform a thorough physical examination. The child with anorexia is usually severely underweight, with a BMI of less than 17. Note cachectic appearance, dry sallow skin, thinning scalp hair, soft sparse body hair, and nail pitting. Measure vital signs, noting low temperature, bradycardia, or hypotension. Auscultate the heart, noting murmur as a result of mitral valve prolapse (occurs in about one third of adolescents with anorexia).

The adolescent with bulimia will be of expected weight or slightly overweight. Inspect the hands for calluses on the backs of the knuckles and split fingernails. Inspect the mouth and oropharynx for eroded dental enamel, red gums, and inflamed throat from self-induced vomiting.

Careful laboratory and diagnostic evaluation of serum electrolytes and an electrocardiogram are needed in adolescents with anorexia and bulimia due to severe electrolyte disturbances, and cardiac arrhythmias often occur.

TAKE NOTE!

An adolescent with anorexia nervosa may experience amenorrhea, hypothermia, low blood pressure, and bradycardia. The nurse may also note soft hair on the individual's back and arms.

Nursing Management

Most children with eating disorders can be treated successfully on an outpatient basis, although this treatment may require many months. Those with anorexia who display severe weight loss, unstable vital signs, food refusal, or arrested pubertal development or who require enteral nutrition will need to be hospitalized. Refeeding syndrome (involving cardiovascular, hematologic, and neurologic complications) may occur in the adolescent with severe malnourishment with anorexia if rapid nutritional replacement is given. Therefore, slow refeeding is essential to avoid complications. Give phosphorus supplements as ordered. Assess vital signs frequently for orthostatic hypotension, irregular and decreased pulse, or hypothermia.

Consult the nutritionist for assistance with calculating caloric needs and determining an appropriate diet. Aim for a weight gain goal of 0.5 to 2 lb per week. Instruct the child and family to keep a daily journal of intake, **bingeing** (excessive consumption) and **purging** (forced vomiting) behaviors, mood, and exercise. The journal may be used as an assessment tool as well as to document progress toward recovery. Assist the child and family in planning a suitably structured routine for the child that includes meals, snacks, and appropriate physical activity.

Use the physical findings associated with anorexia to educate the child about the consequences of malnutrition and how they can be remedied with adequate nutrient intake. Refer the adolescent, as appropriate, to behavior or group therapy. Assess the child's need for medical intervention for concomitant depression or anxiety (some also require psychotropic medications). Provide emotional support and positive reinforcement to the child and family. Refer the family to local support groups or online resources such as the Academy for Eating Disorders or the National Eating Disorders Association.

MOOD DISORDERS

Mood disorders in children include depressive disorders and bipolar disorder. It is difficult to quantify the incidence of depression in children under age 5 years due to lack of sophistication of communication skills. In prepubertal children, about 1% to 3% are diagnosed with depression compared to 9% of adolescents (Kelsay et al., 2022). Children may experience major depressive disorder or dysthymic disorder. Females are twice as likely to be affected as males, particularly during adolescence. Bipolar disorder refers to a condition of alternating manic and depressive episodes, and its incidence in children is unknown (Birmaher, 2023). During the manic episode, mood is significantly elevated, and the child displays excess energy.

Depression may cause significant alterations in school performance and social relationships. Anxiety disorders and disruptive behavior may occur together with depression. Substance misuse may also occur concurrently with depression. Divorce and serious family issues may contribute to the development of depression because of the ongoing stress they place on the child and their strong psychological impact.

Children and adolescents experiencing depressive episodes may harm themselves purposefully without intent to kill themselves (**suicide**). They may hit, cut, or burn themselves. Additionally, children with depression are at risk for suicide (Birmaher, 2023). The Centers for Disease Control and Prevention (CDC) Youth Risk Behavior Surveillance 2011-2021 Report revealed that in 2021, the percentage of adolescents who had seriously considered suicide increased to 22%; 18% made a suicide plan, and 10% had attempted suicide (CDC, 2023).

Pathophysiology

Depression in children is likely multifactorial in nature. It may result from neuroendocrine changes (particularly serotonin), genetic transmission, adverse early life events, and/or family factors. Family factors include abuse, parental early-onset mood disorder, parental substance misuse or criminality, or lack of family cohesion and increased incidence of discord (Brent & Maalouf, 2019).

Therapeutic Management

Children with mood disorders usually benefit from psychotherapy, often paired with pharmacologic antidepressants (Brent & Maalouf, 2019). This helps the child deal with the psychosocial consequences of their behavior on their interpersonal relationships with others. Crisis management; parental counseling; and individual, group, or family therapy may be useful. Bipolar disorder may be treated with second-generation antipsychotics for mania and antidepressants for depression, ideally combined with psychotherapy (Axelson, 2022).

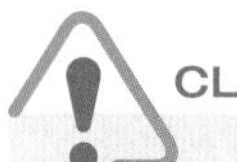

CLINICAL REASONING ALERT!

Closely observe children taking antidepressants for the development of suicidal ideation.

Nursing Assessment

Children with untreated depression are at high risk for suicide as well as the development of comorbid disorders such as anxiety disorders, substance misuse, eating disorders, self-harm, and disruptive behavioral disorders (such as conduct disorder or ADHD) (Kelsay et al., 2022). The nurse must screen all children for the development of depression.

Health History

Obtain a health history from the child and separately from the parent. Evaluate the child for history of recent changes in behavior, changes in peer relationships, alterations in school performance, withdrawal from previously enjoyed activities, sleep disturbances, changes in eating behaviors, increase in accidents, or risky sexual behavior. If possible, use a standardized depression screening questionnaire, many of which are available.

Ask about potential stressors such as school concerns, conflicts with parents, dating issues, and abuse (physical or sexual). When bipolar disorder is suspected, the history may reveal rapid, pressured speech; increased energy; decreased sleep; flamboyant behavior; or irritability during manic episodes.

Note history of weight loss, failure to thrive, or increased incidence of infections in the infant. For the toddler, note delay or regression in developmental skills, increase in nightmares, or parental reports of clinginess. The preschooler may have a history of loss of interest in newly acquired skills; manifest encopresis, enuresis, anorexia, or binge eating; or make frequent negative self-statements. The parents of a school-aged child may report that they have a depressed, irritable, or aggressive mood.

Assess for risk factors for suicide, which include:

- Previous suicide attempt
- Change in school performance, sleep, or appetite
- Loss of interest in formerly favorite school or other activities
- Feelings of hopelessness or depression
- Statements about thoughts of suicide

Physical Examination

Observe the infant for weepiness, withdrawn behaviors, or a frozen facial expression. Note a sad or expressionless face in the toddler or preschooler. In any age child, observe for apathy. Inspect the entire body surface for self-inflicted injuries (such as cuts or burns), which may or may not be present. The remainder of the physical examination is generally normal unless the child with depression also has a chronic medical condition.

Nursing Management

Nursing management of children and adolescents with mood disorders focuses on education and support and prevention of depression and suicide.

Educating and Supporting the Child and Family

Teach families that mood disorders are biologic conditions, not personality flaws. They will need to understand how to administer antidepressant medications and to monitor for adverse effects. Encourage and praise the child's and family's efforts at following through with cognitive and behavioral therapies. Support the family throughout the process, as treatment may sometimes be lengthy. Refer parents to local support resources or to the Depression and Bipolar Support Alliance or the Child and Adolescent Bipolar Foundation.

ATRAUMATIC CARE

Promote a family's sense of control through effective communication and teaching and providing the family with appropriate resources and referrals.

Preventing Depression and Suicide

Establish a trusting relationship with the children and adolescents with whom you interact, particularly in the primary care setting, school, or clinic. This trusting relationship may encourage children or adolescents to confide feelings or problems earlier than they may do with their parents. Screen all preadolescents and adolescents for the development of depression (Kelsay et al., 2022). Use standardized screening tools such as those listed in Box 28.4. When a potential problem is identified, immediately refer the child for mental health assessment and intervention. It is important to identify depression early so that treatment can start. When a grief-inducing event is impending (such as the death of

BOX **28.4** Screening Tools for Depression

The following tools are used to screen for depression:
- Children's Depression Rating Scale-Revised (CDRS-R)
- Center for Epidemiological Studies Depression Scale Modified for Children (CES-DC)
- Weinberg Depression Scale for Children and Adolescents (WDSCA)
- Children's Depression Inventory (CDI)
- Beck Depression Inventory for Youth (BDI-Y)

a family member), begin preventive intervention to help the child to deal with it. Provide appropriate observation for any child exhibiting suicidal ideation. See the Healthy People 2030 box.

HEALTHY PEOPLE **2030**

Objective	Nursing Significance
Reduce suicide attempts by adolescents.	• Screen all children and adolescents for the development of depression. • When depression or excess stress is present, refer the child to the appropriate support.

Healthy People Objectives retrieved from http://www.healthypeople.gov

ANXIETY DISORDERS

Anxiety disorders are the most commonly diagnosed psychiatric conditions among children and adolescents (Bennett & Walkup, 2022). Anxiety often occurs together with other mental health disorders, especially depression. All children experience fear, worry, and shyness. Infants fear loud noises, being startled, and strangers. Toddlers are afraid of the dark and of separation. Preschoolers fear imaginary creatures and body mutilation. School-aged children worry about injury and natural events, and adolescents are anxious about school and social performance. These normal fears produce a certain level of anxiety that is tolerated by most children, but it is important to distinguish developmentally appropriate anxiety from an anxiety disorder.

Anxiety is considered to be a reaction to a perceived or actual threat. The threat may or may not be distorted by the child, and the emotional distress leads to behavioral responses.

THINKING ABOUT **DEVELOPMENT**

Consider the issue of military deployment of a parent. How might a toddler or preschooler react to the parent's absence and return as contrasted with the response of an adolescent? What types of mental health concerns might be manifested in either group?

Types of Anxiety Disorders

Generalized anxiety disorder (GAD) is characterized by unrealistic concerns over past behavior, future events, and personal competence. Social phobia is a disorder characterized by the child or adolescent demonstrating a persistent fear of speaking or eating in front of others, using public restrooms, or speaking to authorities. Selective mutism refers to a persistent failure to speak. Separation anxiety is more common in children than adolescents. In this disorder, the child may need to remain close to the parents, and the child's worries focus on separation themes. OCD is characterized by compulsions (repetitive behaviors such as cleaning, washing, or checking something), which the child performs to reduce anxiety about obsessions (unwanted and intrusive thoughts). Posttraumatic stress disorder (PTSD) is an anxiety disorder that occurs after a child experiences a traumatic event, later experiencing physiologic arousal when a stimulus triggers memories of the event.

Pathophysiology

Anxiety disorders are thought to occur as a result of disrupted modulation within the central nervous system. Underactivation of the serotonergic system and overactivation of the noradrenergic system are thought to be responsible for dysregulation of physiologic arousal and the resulting emotional experience. Disruption of the gamma-aminobutyric acid (GABA) system may also play a role. Genetic factors may also play a role in the development of anxiety disorders, as may family and environmental influences. Additionally, abnormal thoughts or behaviors may have been learned through observation or conditioning (Bennett & Walkup, 2022).

Therapeutic Management

Therapeutic management of anxiety disorders generally involves the use of pharmacologic agents and psychological therapies. Anxiolytics or antidepressants are the most common pharmacologic approaches. Cognitive behavioral therapy; individual, family, or group psychotherapy; and other behavioral interventions such as relaxation techniques such as yoga may also be useful (Shreve et al., 2021).

Nursing Assessment

Children and adolescents do not always directly express anxiety. Therefore, it is important for the nurse to evaluate somatic complaints and perform a careful health history.

Health History

Explore the child's current and past medical history for risk factors such as depression, anxious temperament, family history of anxiety disorders, certain environmental or life experiences (such as parental dysfunction or significant stressful event or trauma), or unstable parental attachment. Elicit the health history, noting history of social inhibition, panic, or "heart racing." Young children may display overactivity, acting out, sleep difficulties, or separation issues. Older children may describe feelings of nervousness, anger, fear, or tension and may display disruptive behavior. Ask the child to choose a number on a scale from 0 to 10 to describe how much they worry about things. Have the parent rank the child's worry in the same fashion, and ask the parent what the child worries about most. Determine frequency of headaches and stomachaches. Use a standardized screening tool such as the Multidimensional Anxiety Scale for Children (MASC), Spence Children's Anxiety Scale (SACS), Preschool Anxiety Scale, and Beck Anxiety Inventory for Youth.

Physical Examination

Perform a complete physical examination to rule out physiologic causes of the child's symptoms. Note patches of hair loss that occur with repetitive hair twisting or pulling associated with anxiety. Evaluate for evidence of nail biting, sucking blisters, or skin erosion from finger rubbing. Inspect the entire body for signs of self-injury, which may or may not be present.

Nursing Management

Screen children at well-child or other health care visits as well as upon admission to the hospital for anxiety symptoms. If an anxiety disorder is suspected, refer the child to the appropriate mental health provider for further evaluation. When the child is diagnosed with an anxiety disorder and medication is prescribed, teach families about medication administration and any adverse effects. Encourage and praise them for follow-through related to cognitive and behavioral therapy or psychotherapy. Provide emotional support to the child and family. Assess the family for the presence of parental anxiety or insecure attachment. Note parenting style and parent–child interactions. Both the child and the family will benefit from interventions that improve parent–child relationships, decrease parental anxiety, and foster parenting skills that promote autonomy in the child. Thus, refer the child and family to concurrent family therapy if needed.

ABUSE AND VIOLENCE

Abuse and violence contribute significantly to mental illness in children. Children may suffer from child maltreatment, medical child abuse, or substance misuse.

Child Maltreatment

Child maltreatment includes physical abuse, sexual abuse, emotional abuse, and neglect. Physical abuse refers to injuries that are intentionally inflicted on a child and result in morbidity or mortality. Sexual abuse refers to involvement of the child in any activity meant to provide sexual gratification to an adult. Emotional abuse may be verbal denigration of the child or may occur as a result of the child witnessing domestic violence. **Neglect** is defined as failure to provide a child with appropriate food, clothing, shelter, medical care, and schooling (Ford et al., 2022).

Statistics related to family violence as well as child physical and sexual abuse are difficult to determine, as the perpetrator usually forces the victim into silence. Children usually do not want to admit that their parent or relative has hurt them, partly from feelings of guilt and partly because they do not want to lose that person. In 2019, 4.4 million referrals to child protective services were made, alleging child maltreatment in 7.9 million children; however, this may be an underestimate of the prevalence of child abuse (Ford et al., 2022). Abuse and violence occur across all socioeconomic levels but are more prevalent among people with limited resources, and the largest percentage of those affected are under 3 years of age. Despite the lack of complete statistics, it is well known that the problem of abuse and violence is widespread. Parents or caregivers are the most frequent perpetrators of abuse against children (Ford et al., 2022).

A history of childhood abuse is associated with the development of anxiety and depressive disorders, suicidal ideation and attempts, and alcohol and drug misuse. Child maltreatment may result in significant physical injury, poor physical health, and, in some cases, impaired brain development. Abuse places children at risk for developmental and behavioral problems, decreased cognitive functioning, poor academic achievement, and deficits in relationships (Child Welfare Information Gateway, 2019).

Therapeutic management of victims of abuse and violence involves physical treatment of injuries, palliative care in some cases, and intervention to preserve or restore the child's mental well-being as well as family functioning. To protect children, all states legally require health care professionals to report suspected cases of child abuse or neglect (Child Welfare Information Gateway, 2023).

Nursing Assessment

Elicit the health history, noting the chief complaint and timing of onset. Assess for appropriateness of the parent–child attachment (often altered in the case of neglect). Pay particular attention to statements made by the child's parent or caregiver. Is the history given consistent with the child's injury? Identify abuse and violence by screening all children and families using these questions:

- Questions for children:
  - Are you afraid of anyone at home?
  - Whom could you tell if someone hurt you or touched you in a way that made you uncomfortable?
  - Has anyone hurt you or touched you in that way?
- Questions for parents:
  - Are you afraid of anyone at home?
  - Do you ever feel like you may hit or hurt your child when frustrated?

Assess for risk factors in children and parents or caregivers. Risk factors for abuse in children include poverty, prematurity, cerebral palsy, chronic illness, or intellectual disability. Risk factors for parents or caregivers becoming abusive include a history of being abused themselves, alcohol or substance misuse, and extreme stress.

Determine if the child has a history of hurting themselves (e.g., cutting) or others, running away, attempting suicide, or being involved in high-risk behaviors. Note inappropriate sexual behavior for developmental age as this may indicate sexual abuse. Note history of chronic sore throat or difficulty swallowing, which may occur with forced oral sex or sexually transmitted infections. Document history of genital burning or itching (associated with sexual abuse). Note nonspecific symptoms of emotional abuse such as low self-confidence, sleep disturbance, hypervigilance, headaches, or stomachaches.

TAKE NOTE!

A delay in seeking medical treatment, a history that changes over time, or a history of trauma that is inconsistent with the observed injury all suggest child abuse.

Physical Examination

Perform a gentle but thorough physical examination, using a soft touch and calm voice. Observe the parent–child interaction, noting fear or an excessive desire to please. Note the infant's level of consciousness. Vigorous shaking in the infant can lead to intracranial hemorrhage and brain injury. Inspect the skin for bruises, burns, cuts, abrasions, contusions, scars, and any other unusual or suspicious marks. Current or healed scratches or cuts may be found on parts of the body ordinarily covered by clothing in the child who self-mutilates. Burns that occur in a stocking or glove pattern, or only to the soles or palms, are highly suspicious for inflicted burns. Injuries in various stages of healing are also indicative of abuse. Bruises on the chest, head, neck, or abdomen are suspicious for abuse.

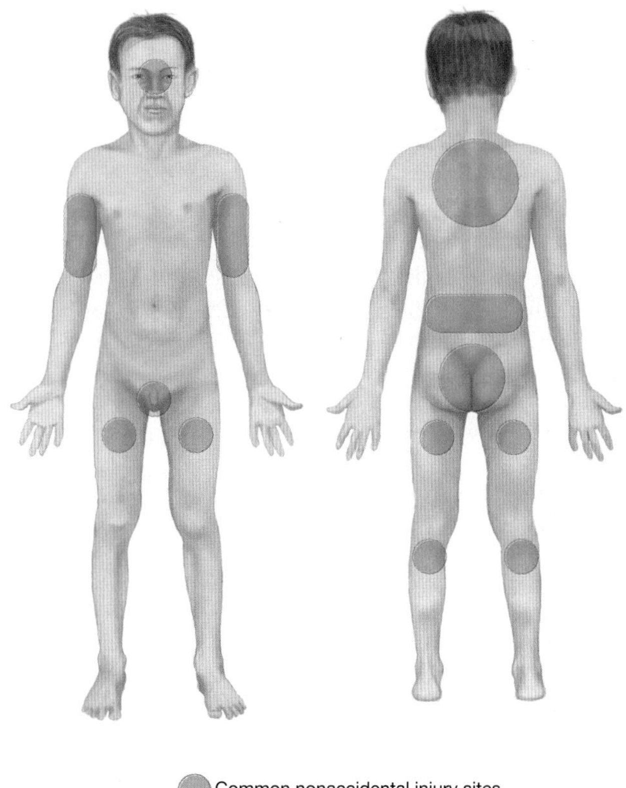

FIGURE 28.1 Injury sites that are suspicious for abuse.

Nonambulatory children infrequently experience bruises or fractures. Figure 28.1 shows injury sites usually indicative of abuse; Figure 28.2 is a photograph of a child who was beaten with an electric cord. Observe for inflammation of the oropharynx. Inspect the anus and penis or vaginal area for bleeding or discharge.

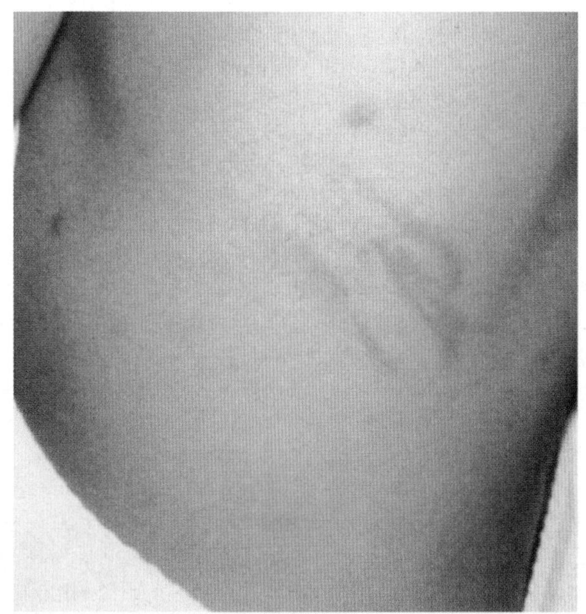

FIGURE 28.2 Note the mark left from a looped electric cord.

Laboratory and Diagnostic Tests

Common laboratory and diagnostic studies ordered for the assessment of abuse include:

- Radiographic skeletal survey or bone scan may reveal current or past fractures.
- Computed tomography scan of the head may reveal intracranial hemorrhage.
- Rectal, oral, vaginal, or urethral specimens may reveal sexually transmitted infections such as gonorrhea or chlamydia.

Nursing Management

Refer suspected cases of neglect or abuse to the local child protection agency. When abusive activity is identified in the hospital, notify the social services and risk management departments. In addition to physical or palliative care needed for the injuries, abused children need to redevelop a sense of trust in adults. Provide consistent care to the abused child by assigning a core group of nurses. Child abuse requires a multidisciplinary approach that will include psychological therapy for the child and the family.

Role model appropriate caregiving activities to the parent or caregiver. Call attention to normal growth and development activities noted in the infant or child, as parents sometimes have expectations of child behavior that may be unrealistic based on the child's age, leading to the abuse. Praise parents and caregivers for taking appropriate steps toward getting help and for providing appropriate care to the child. Refer parents to Parents Anonymous, an organization dedicated to the prevention of child abuse through strengthening of the family (see https://parentsanonymous.org).

When it is determined by the child protective team that the child would be in danger by continuing to live in the current situation, the child may be removed from the home. If the child is removed from the family temporarily or permanently, provide the foster or adoptive family with education necessary to assume the child's care.

Medical Child Abuse

Medical child abuse was historically termed Munchausen syndrome by proxy. It is a type of child abuse in which the parent or caregiver creates physical and/or psychological symptoms of illness or impairment in the child. The adult meets their own psychological needs by having an ill child. Medical child abuse is difficult to detect and may remain hidden for years. In most cases, the birthing parent is the perpetrator (Roesler & Jenny, 2022). Therapeutic management focuses on ensuring the safety and well-being of the child, as well as providing psychotherapy for the perpetrator.

Nursing Assessment

Take a thorough and detailed health history of the child's illness or illnesses. Use quotations to document the parent's responses. Warning signs of medical child abuse include:

- Child with one or more illnesses that do not respond to treatment or that follow a puzzling course; a similar history in siblings
- Symptoms that do not make sense or that disappear when the perpetrator is removed or not present; the symptoms are witnessed only by the caregiver (e.g., cyanosis, apnea, seizure)
- Physical and laboratory findings that do not fit with the reported history
- Repeated hospitalizations failing to produce a medical diagnosis, transfers to other hospitals, discharges against medical advice
- Parent who refuses to accept that the diagnosis is not medical (Roesler & Jenny, 2022)

Observe the parent's behavior with the child, spouse or partner, and staff. Use of covert video surveillance may reveal actions causing illness in the child when the nurse, health care provider, or nurse practitioner is not in the room. Perform a thorough physical examination, noting where the physical examination findings differ from the reported health history.

Nursing Management

Management of medical child abuse is complex. When abusive activity is identified, notify the social services and risk management departments of the hospital. Ensure that the local child protection team and the caregiver's family or support system is present when the caregiver is confronted. Inform the caregiver of the plan of care for the child and of the availability of psychiatric assistance for the caregiver.

Substance Misuse

Substance misuse most often begins before age 20. In 2021, in the United States, 23% of students reported they currently drink alcohol and 16% that they currently use cannabis (CDC, 2023). In addition to alcohol, youths also use cocaine, heroin, methamphetamines, inhalants, ecstasy, nonprescribed steroids, and prescription drugs outside of their intended use (CDC, 2023).

Nursing Assessment

Note risk factors for substance misuse, such as family history of substance use disorder, current parental substance misuse, dysfunctional family relationships, concurrent mental health disorder, aggressive behaviors, low self-esteem or poor academic performance, negative life events, poor social skills, or peers who misuse substances.

Determine the child's history, noting altered school performance or attendance, changes in peer group participation, frequent mood swings, changes in physical appearance, or an altered relationship with or perception of parents. Document history of insomnia, appetite loss, excessive itching, sleepiness or extreme fatigue, dry mouth, or shakiness. Note violent behavior, drunkenness, stupor, blank expression, drowsiness, lack of coordination, confusion, incoherent speech, extremes in emotions, aggressive behavior, silly behavior, or rapid speech. A screening assessment recommended by the AAP is the CRAFFT Screening Tool (Boston Children's Hospital, 2018). Perform a complete physical examination. Observe for an odor of alcohol or cannabis smoke. Assess the eyes, noting wateriness or dilated pupils. Inspect the nares, noting rhinorrhea or absence of nasal hair. Inspect the fingers for glue smears or discoloration and the skin for needle marks or tracks. Palpate the hands and feet for coolness.

Laboratory and diagnostic tests include toxicology studies, such as urine screening, to determine the presence of stimulants, sedative–hypnotics, barbiturates, hallucinogens, opiates, cocaine, and cannabis.

Nursing Management

Help the adolescent acknowledge that they have a problem. Explain the negative consequences of substance misuse, and raise the adolescent's awareness of risks. Remain empathetic while leaving responsibility with the adolescent. Key nursing interventions include promoting participation in treatment programs and preventing substance misuse.

PROMOTING PARTICIPATION IN TREATMENT PROGRAMS

Refer the adolescent to a substance misuse program. Outpatient or day treatment programs are useful in most situations. Family-based programs produce the highest level of recovery. Self-help or 12-step groups are an important element in the recovery process. Serious addiction, the presence of one or more comorbid psychiatric conditions, or suicidal ideation requires residential treatment or hospitalization. See the Healthy People 2030 box.

HEALTHY PEOPLE 2030

Objective	Nursing Significance
Increase the proportion of people with co-occurring substance misuse and mental disorders who receive treatment for both disorders.	• Screen all children and adolescents with mental health disorders for the coexistence of substance misuse (and vice versa). • Refer children and adolescents to appropriate treatment programs and therapy.

Healthy People Objectives retrieved from http://www.healthypeople.gov

PREVENTING SUBSTANCE MISUSE

Establish a trusting relationship with children and adolescents in order to improve acceptance of education about substance misuse and to provide a safe environment for confiding about their problems. Screen all children and adolescents for risk factors. During routine psychosocial screening, be alert to alterations as noted earlier. Teach all children, beginning at the elementary school level (or earlier if appropriate), that all chemicals have the potential to be harmful to the body, including tobacco, alcohol, and illicit drugs. Educate children and adolescents that no matter which administration route is used, the drug still enters the body and affects it negatively. Help children learn problem-solving skills that they can call upon in the future rather than relying on drugs or other substances to avoid their problems. Teach children to "just say no." Reinforce that they are the ones who have control over their bodies and what they expose them to. Encourage children to participate in the local community Drug Abuse Resistance Education (DARE) program, and praise them for completing it. Teach parents that being involved in their child's social life and knowing where they are and with whom when they are outside of the home is an important step toward limiting substance exposure.

KEY CONCEPTS

- Mental health and behavioral disorders account for the bulk of the "new morbidity" among children and adolescents.
- The child with behavioral problems or mental health issues often has difficulty with school, peer relationships, and family, all of which may worsen the child's self-concept, further hindering their emotional health.
- Developmental screening is a key component in the evaluation of a child's mental health.
- Various screening tools are available for depression, ADHD, and anxiety.
- Children with ASD often have impaired social interactions as well as altered communication.
- Learning disabilities and ADHD can have a significant negative impact on the child's education.
- IEPs help children with learning disabilities, intellectual disability, and ADHD receive the educational support they require to optimize their educational capacity.
- Provide support and education to children with mood or anxiety disorders and their families.
- Educating parents about medication administration and any adverse side effects is a critical aspect of nursing management of the child with a mental health disorder.
- Provide nutritional replacement at the appropriate pace in the child with anorexia nervosa. Monitor

the child closely for the development of refeeding syndrome.

- A key nursing function is screening all children and their families for abuse and violence.
- Report suspected cases of child abuse to the appropriate authorities.
- Educate children about the dangers associated with substance misuse. Reward and praise children and adolescents who do not experiment with or use alcohol or illicit drugs.

REFERENCES AND RECOMMENDED READINGS

108th Congress. (2004). *Individuals with Disabilities Education Improvement Act of 2004*. https://www.govinfo.gov/app/details/CRPT-108hrpt779/CRPT-108hrpt779

American Academy of Child and Adolescent Psychiatry. (2019). *Psychotherapy for children and adolescents: Different types*. https://www.aacap.org/AACAP/Families_and_Youth/Facts_for_Families/FFF-Guide/Psychotherapies-For-Children-And-Adolescents-086.aspx

American Academy of Pediatrics. (2023). *Mental health initiatives*. https://www.aap.org/en/patient-care/mental-health-initiatives/

Augustyn, M., & von Hahn, L. E. (2023). Autism spectrum disorder in children and adolescents: Clinical features. *UpToDate*. Retrieved March 22, 2024, from https://www.uptodate.com/contents/autism-spectrum-disorder-in-children-and-adolescents-clinical-features

Axelson, D. (2022). Pediatric bipolar disorder: Overview of choosing treatment. *UpToDate*. Retrieved March 22, 2024, from www.uptodate.com/contents/pediatric-bipolar-disorder-overview-of-choosing-treatment

Bennett, S., & Walkup, J. T. (2022). Anxiety disorders in children and adolescents: Epidemiology, pathogenesis, clinical manifestations, and course. *UpToDate*. Retrieved March 22, 2024, from http://www.uptodate.com/contents/anxiety-disorders-in-children-and-adolescents-epidemiology-pathogenesis-clinical-manifestations-and-course

Birmaher, B. (2023). Pediatric bipolar disorder: Clinical manifestations and course of illness. *UpToDate*. Retrieved March 22, 2024, from https://www.uptodate.com/contents/pediatric-bipolar-disorder-clinical-manifestations-and-course-of-illness#H2995284799

Boston Children's Hospital. (2018). *CRAFFT*. http://crafft.org

Brent, D. A., & Maalouf, F. (2019). Depressive disorders (in childhood and adolescence). In M. H. Ebert, J. F. Leckman, & I. L. Petrakis (Eds.), *Current diagnosis & treatment: Psychiatry* (3rd ed.). McGraw-Hill Education.

Centers for Disease Control and Prevention. (2023). *Youth risk behavior survey: Data summary & trends report 2011-2021*. https://www.cdc.gov/healthyyouth/data/yrbs/pdf/YRBS_Data-Summary-Trends_Report2023_508.pdf

Child Welfare Information Gateway. (2019). *Long-term consequences of child abuse and neglect*. U.S. Department of Health and Human Services. https://www.childwelfare.gov/pubpdfs/long_term_consequences.pdf

Child Welfare Information Gateway. (2023). *Mandatory reporting of child abuse and neglect*. U.S. Department of Health and Human Services. https://www.childwelfare.gov/resources/mandatory-reporting-child-abuse-and-neglect/

Ford, C. R., Chiesa, A., & Sirotnak, A. P. (2022). Child abuse & neglect. In M. Bunik, W. W. Hay, M. J. Levin, & M. J. Abzug (Eds.), *Current diagnosis & treatment: Pediatrics* (26th ed.). McGraw-Hill Education.

Goddard, A. (2021). Adverse childhood experiences and trauma-informed care. *Journal of Pediatric Health Care, 35*(2), 145–155. https://doi.org/10.1016/j.pedhc.2020.09.001

Guarda, A. (2023). Eating disorders: Overview of epidemiology, clinical features, and diagnosis *UpToDate*. https://www.uptodate.com/contents/eating-disorders-overview-of-epidemiology-clinical-features-and-diagnosis

Halter, M. J., & Fratena, C. A. (2023). *Varcarolis' manual of psychiatric nursing care planning: An interprofessional approach* (7th ed.). Elsevier.

Jankovic, J. (2023). Tourette syndrome: Pathogenesis, clinical features, and diagnosis. *UpToDate*. Retrieved March 22, 2024, from https://www.uptodate.com/contents/tourette-syndrome-pathogenesis-clinical-features-and-diagnosis#H5

Kelsay, K., Glaze, K., & Talmi, A. (2022). Child & adolescent psychiatric disorders & psychosocial aspects of pediatrics. In M. Bunik, W. W. Hay, M. J. Levin, R. R. Deterding, & M. J. Abzug (Eds.), *Current pediatric diagnosis and treatment* (26th ed.). McGraw-Hill Education.

Krull, K. R., & Chan, E. (2023). Attention deficit hyperactivity disorder in children and adolescents: Epidemiology and pathogenesis. *UpToDate*. Retrieved March 22, 2024, from http://www.uptodate.com/contents/attention-deficit-hyperactivity-disorder-in-children-and-adolescents-epidemiology-and-pathogenesis

Pivalizza, P. (2024). Intellectual disability (ID) in children: Clinical features, evaluation, and diagnosis. *UpToDate*. Retrieved March 22, 2024, from https://www.uptodate.com/contents/intellectual-disability-id-in-children-clinical-features-evaluation-nd-diagnosis

Reichow, B., Hume, K., Barton, E. E., & Boyd, B. A. (2018). Early intensive behavioral intervention (EIBI) for young children with autism spectrum disorders (ASD*). Cochrane Database of Systematic Reviews*, (5), CD009260. https://doi.org/10.1002/14651858.CD009260.pub3

Reynolds, A., Angulo, A., Breheney, M., Green, J., & Goldson, E. (2022). Child development and behavior. In M. Bunik, W. W. Hay, M. J. Levin, & M. J. Abzug (Eds.), *Current diagnosis & treatment: Pediatrics* (26th ed.). McGraw-Hill Education.

Roesler, T. A., & Jenny, C. (2022). Medical child abuse (Munchausen syndrome by proxy). *UpToDate*. Retrieved March 22, 2024, from http://www.uptodate.com/contents/medical-child-abuse-munchausen-syndrome-by-proxy

Shreve, M., Scott, A., McNeill, C., & Washburn, L. (2021). Using yoga to reduce anxiety in children: Exploring school-based yoga among rural third- and fourth-grade students. *Journal of Pediatric Health Care, 35*(1), 42–52. https://doi.org/10.1016/j.pedhc.2020.07.008

Sohl, K. T. (2022). Understanding physician practice patterns for autism spectrum disorder. *Pediatric News*, 1–8.

Star Center Foundation. (2024). *Understanding sensory processing disorder*. https://www.spdstar.org/basic/understanding-sensory-processing-disorder

Swick, S. D., & Jellinek, M. S. (2022). Demystifying psychotherapy. *Pediatric News, 56*(10), 18.

UpToDate, Inc. (2024). *UpToDate Lexidrug* (Version 8.2.0) [Mobile app]. Wolters Kluwer. https://apps.apple.com/us/app/lexicomp/id313401238

U.S. Department of Health and Human Services. (n.d.). *Healthy People 2030*. https://health.gov/healthypeople

von Hahn, L. E. (2023a). Specific learning disorders in children: Clinical features. *UpToDate*. Retrieved March 22, 2024, from http://www.uptodate.com/contents/specific-learning-disabilities-in-children-clinical-features

von Hahn, L. E. (2023b). Specific learning disorders in children: Role of the primary care provider. *UpToDate*. Retrieved March 22, 2024, from http://www.uptodate.com/contents/specific-learning-disabilities-in-children-role-of-the-primary-care-provider

Weissman, L., & Harris, H. K. (2022). Autism spectrum disorder in children and adolescents: Complementary and alternative therapies. *UpToDate*. Retrieved March 22, 2024, from https://www.uptodate.com/contents/autism-spectrum-disorder-in-children-and-adolescents-complementary-and-alternative-therapies

Yager, J. (2022). Eating disorders: Overview of prevention and treatment. *UpToDate*. Retrieved March 22, 2024, from https://www.uptodate.com/contents/eating-disorders-overview-of-prevention-and-treatment

DEVELOPING CLINICAL JUDGMENT

PRACTICING FOR NCLEX

1. The nurse is caring for a child with ADHD. Which behaviors would the nurse expect the child to display? Select all that apply.
   a. Interruptions
   b. Inability to take turns
   c. Moody, morose behavior
   d. Forgetfulness
   e. Easy distractibility
   f. Pouting
   g. Excessive motor activities
   h. Fidgeting
2. An adolescent who has been receiving treatment for anorexia nervosa has failed to gain weight over the past week despite eating all meals and snacks. What is the priority nursing intervention?
   a. Increase the adolescent's daily caloric intake by at least 500 calories.
   b. Ensure the adolescent's entire fluid intake includes calories.
   c. Supervise the adolescent for 2 hours after all meals and snacks.
   d. Assess the adolescent's anxiety level to determine need for medication.
3. A 15-year-old has been making demands all day, exaggerating every need. They are now crying, saying they have nothing to live for and threatening to kill themselves. What is the priority nursing action?
   a. Ignore the continued exaggerated and melodramatic behavior.
   b. Consult with the health care provider or nurse practitioner to increase the antidepressant dose.
   c. Leave the adolescent alone for a little while until they compose themselves.
   d. Take the suicidal threat seriously and provide close supervision.
4. When trying to manage aggressive or impulsive behaviors in children or adolescents, what is the best nursing intervention?
   a. Train the child to be assertive.
   b. Provide consistency and limit setting.
   c. Allow the child to negotiate the rules.
   d. Encourage the child to express feelings.
5. The nurse is caring for an adolescent who says, "I'm sick of this. I wish I weren't alive anymore." What is the best response by the nurse?
   a. "I often feel sad and sick of things."
   b. "Have you thought about hurting yourself?"
   c. "Are you trying to escape your problems?"
   d. "Do your parents know about this feeling?"
6. The nurse is assessing an adolescent being admitted for an eating disorder. The physical examination reveals temperature 96.7°F oral, heart rate 54 bpm, and blood pressure 88/54 mm Hg. Which eating disorder do these clinical manifestations suggest?
   a. Pica
   b. Bulimia nervosa
   c. Binge eating disorder
   d. Anorexia nervosa
7. The nurse is caring for an adolescent whose physical examination reveals chipped teeth, calluses on the knuckles, and dental enamel erosion. The adolescent is at risk for ____ as related to ______.
   Blank 1:
   a. bradycardia
   b. dysrhythmia
   c. esophagitis
   Blank 2:
   a. decreased oral intake
   b. vomiting
   c. food avoidance

DOSAGE CALCULATION QUESTION

The nurse is caring for a 10-year old diagnosed with depression. The child weighs 72 lb. The medication order reads: fluoxetine 10 mg PO daily. The child refuses to swallow pills. Fluoxetine is supplied as 20 mg/5 mL. How many milliliters will the nurse administer? Round to the nearest tenth.

CRITICAL THINKING EXERCISES

1. A parent tells you that their child's behavior is unmanageable and that they are having difficulty coping with it. The child is argumentative and is bullying others. They are struggling with their school work because they have difficulty staying on task, get out of the chair often, and frequently distract others. What additional assessments should you obtain? What interventions would be helpful in managing the child's behavior?
2. A 14-year-old with moderate intellectual disability is able to feed themselves but is incontinent. Discuss the issues with which the family must deal.

STUDY ACTIVITIES

1. Explore several of the websites related to child abuse prevention. Develop a list of resources for families in your local area.
2. Attend a group therapy session during your pediatric clinical rotation. Observe the children's verbal and nonverbal communication, noting inconsistencies or other interesting observations.
3. Visit a school for children with ASD. Spend time with the various specialists who work with the children, determining their roles and the effect the treatment they are providing has on the children. Report your findings to your classmates.
4. Attend a local Children and Adults with ADHD (CHADD) meeting. Talk to parents about having a child with ADHD.

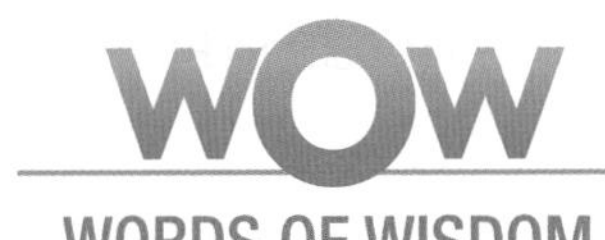

WORDS OF WISDOM

A nurse must possess the knowledge and skills to aid an acutely ill child.

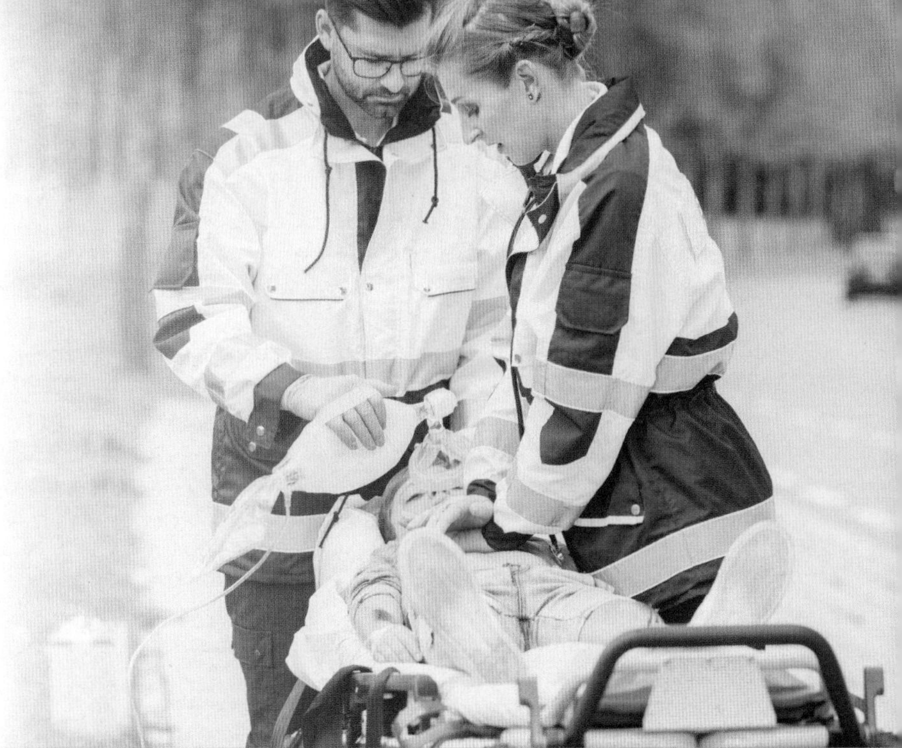

29

Nursing Care During a Pediatric Emergency

LEARNING OBJECTIVES

Upon completion of the chapter, you will be able to:

1. Identify various factors contributing to emergency situations among infants and children.
2. Discuss common treatments and medications used during pediatric emergencies.
3. Conduct a health history of a child in an emergency situation, specific to the emergency.
4. Perform a rapid cardiopulmonary assessment.
5. Discuss common laboratory and other diagnostic tests used during pediatric emergencies.
6. Integrate the principles of the American Heart Association and Pediatric Advanced Life Support in the comprehensive management of pediatric emergencies, such as respiratory arrest, shock, cardiac arrest, near drowning, poisoning, and trauma.
7. Devise an individualized nursing care plan or concept map for the child experiencing a pediatric emergency.

KEY TERMS

asystole (ā-sis´tō-lē)
barotrauma (bar´ō-traw´mă)
bradycardia
cardioversion
defibrillation (dē-fib´ri-lā´shŭn)
hyperventilation
hypocapnia (hī´pō-kap´nē-ă)
hypoventilation
intubation
periodic breathing
tachycardia

Alma Anderson, age 8 years, has been admitted to the pediatric unit. Her parent calls the nurse into the room, stating, "Alma's having trouble breathing!"

INTRODUCTION

Children are uniquely vulnerable to a range of emergency situations. These situations are often life-threatening if not treated quickly and effectively. Because of their developmental level, children are at a greater risk for submersion injury, poisoning, and traumatic injury compared to adults. Most pediatric cardiopulmonary arrests result from respiratory failure or shock. Data suggest that children who have a cardiopulmonary arrest requiring resuscitative measures rarely fare well. For these reasons, the American Heart Association (AHA) has delineated two distinct chains of survival, one for adults and one for children, which should be followed during a life-threatening situation.

The adult chain of survival is:

- Early emergency medical system (EMS) activation
- Early cardiopulmonary resuscitation (CPR)
- Early defibrillation
- Early access to advanced care
- Integrated postcardiac arrest care

In contrast, the pediatric chain of survival is:

- Prevention of cardiac arrest and injuries
- Early CPR
- Early access to emergency response system
- Early advanced care (pediatric advanced life support [PALS])
- Integrated postcardiac arrest care (AHA & American Academy of Pediatrics [AAP], 2020)

Considering the special risks that threaten children, the AHA has also developed specific guidelines for PALS. Courses in PALS are offered for health care professionals so that they can provide expert care for children in emergencies. This chapter emphasizes the principles of PALS in its discussion of the nurse's role in the management of pediatric emergencies.

TAKE NOTE!

The current pediatric basic life support guidelines define an infant as between 0 and 12 months of age, and a child as age 1 year up until puberty. Children in this range should be managed using the PALS guidelines rather than those for adults (AHA & AAP, 2020).

COMMON MEDICAL TREATMENTS

A variety of medications and other medical treatments are used in pediatric emergencies. Most of these treatments will require a health care provider's order when the child is in the hospital, though some emergency departments and pediatric units may have standing orders for pediatric emergencies. The most common medical treatments and medications used in pediatric emergencies are listed in Common Medical Treatments 29.1 and Drug Guide 29.1, respectively. The nurse should be familiar with these procedures and medications, how they work, and nursing implications.

COMMON MEDICAL TREATMENTS 29.1

Treatment	Explanation	Indications	Nursing Implications
Suctioning (oropharyngeal, nasopharyngeal, ET, or tracheostomy)	Removal of secretions via bulb syringe or suction catheter	Excessive airway secretions affecting airway patency	Use caution and suction only as far as recommended for age, ET tube size, or tracheostomy tube size or until coughing or gagging occurs.
Oxygen	Supplementation via mask, nasal cannula, hood, or tent or via ET/nasotracheal tube	Hypoxemia, respiratory distress, shock, trauma	Monitor response via color, work of breathing, respiratory rate, oxygen saturation levels via pulse oximetry, and level of consciousness.
Bag-valve-mask ventilation	Provision of ventilation via a bag-valve-mask device, manual ventilation	Apnea, ineffective ventilation and oxygenation with spontaneous breaths, extremely slow respiratory rate	Ensure adequate chest rise with ventilation. Do not overventilate or bag aggressively to avoid barotrauma. Maintain a seal on the child's face with the appropriate-sized mask. Ensure the oxygen supply tubing is connected to 100% oxygen.
Intubation	Insertion of a tube into the trachea to provide artificial ventilation	Apnea, airway that is not maintainable, need for prolonged assisted ventilation	Determine adequacy of breath sounds with bagging immediately upon insertion of the ET tube. Assess for symmetric chest rise. Tape the tube securely in place and note the number marking on the tube. Connect to ventilator when available.

(*continued*)

COMMON MEDICAL TREATMENTS 29.1 (*continued*)

Treatment	Explanation	Indications	Nursing Implications
Needle thoracotomy	Insertion of a needle between the ribs into the pleural space to remove air	Tension pneumothorax	There should be a rush of air as the needle reaches the air space. Monitor breath sounds, work of breathing, and pulse oximetry. Ensure patency of IV catheter.
IV fluid therapy	Administration of crystalloid or colloid solutions to provide hydration or improve perfusion	Altered perfusion states such as respiratory distress, shock, trauma, cardiac disturbances	Use intraosseous route if a peripheral IV cannot be obtained quickly in the young child in shock. Reassess respiratory and circulatory status frequently after each IV fluid bolus and during continuous infusion.
Blood product transfusion	Administration of whole blood, packed red blood cells, platelets, or plasma intravenously	Trauma, hemorrhage	Follow the institution's transfusion protocol. Double-check blood type and product label with a second nurse. Monitor vital signs and assess the child frequently to identify adverse reaction to blood transfusion. If adverse reaction is suspected, immediately discontinue transfusion, infuse normal saline solution IV, reassess the child, and notify the health care provider.
Cervical stabilization	Maintenance of the cervical spine in an immobile position	Trauma, near drowning	Use the jaw-thrust maneuver without head tilt to open the airway. Maintain cervical stabilization until the cervical spine radiographs are cleared by the health care provider or radiologist.
Defibrillation and synchronized cardioversion	Provision of electrical current to alter the heart's electrical rhythm	Defibrillation: ventricular fibrillation and pulseless ventricular tachycardia Synchronized cardioversion: supraventricular tachycardia and ventricular tachycardia with a pulse	In the pulseless child, always ensure CPR is ongoing while the defibrillator is being readied. Ensure adequate oxygenation. Provide lidocaine or epinephrine if indicated before defibrillation. Sedate the child if time allows.

CPR, cardiopulmonary resuscitation; ET, endotracheal; IV, intravenous.

DRUG GUIDE 29.1

COMMON MEDICATIONS USED IN PEDIATRIC EMERGENCIES

Medication	Actions/Indications	Nursing Implications
Adenosine (antiarrhythmic)	Slows conduction through AV node, restoring normal sinus rhythm Supraventricular tachycardia (SVT)	• Administer IV at a dose ranging from 0.05 to 0.1 mg/kg for neonates and 0.1 to 0.2 mg/kg. • Administer very rapidly (1–2 seconds) followed by a rapid, generous saline flush. • Repeat every 1–2 minutes, increasing by 0.05–0.1 mg/kg with each dose (maximum dose 0.3 mg/kg). • Monitor for shortness of breath, dyspnea, and worsening of asthma.
Amiodarone (antiarrhythmic)	Prolongs repolarization of action potential, thus slowing the heart rate Ventricular tachycardia, ventricular fibrillation	• Administer IV or IO at a dose of 5 mg/kg over 20–60 minutes. • Avoid use with procainamide.
Atropine (anticholinergic)	Increases cardiac output, dries secretions, inhibits serotonin and histamine Sinus bradycardia, asystole, pulseless electrical activity	• Administer via IV, IO, or ET route at a dose of 0.02 mg/kg (maximum dose 0.5 mg for a child, 1 mg for an adolescent). • Repeat every 5 minutes PRN. • Give undiluted over 30 seconds for IV or IO route. • Dilute with 3–5 mL normal saline for ET route; follow with five positive-pressure ventilations. • Do not mix with sodium bicarbonate (incompatible).

DRUG GUIDE 29.1

COMMON MEDICATIONS USED IN PEDIATRIC EMERGENCIES

Medication	Actions/Indications	Nursing Implications
Dobutamine (adrenergic agent)	Beta-adrenergic agent primarily affecting beta-1 receptors; increases myocardial contractility and heart rate Ongoing short-term management of shock (hypovolemic and cardiogenic)	• Administer via IV or IO route at 2–20 μg/kg/min via a continuous infusion. Monitor for the development of ventricular dysrhythmias • Expect to titrate infusion rate based on cardiac output and BP. • Administer via central line if possible due to the risk of extravasation. • Monitor child closely, preferably in an ICU setting.
Dopamine (inotropic)	Increases cardiac output, BP, and renal perfusion (beta-adrenergic agonist) Bradycardia, hypotension, and poor cardiac output	• Administer via IV or IO route at a dose of 2–20 μg/kg/min via continuous infusion. • Ensure that child has received adequate fluid resuscitation prior to administration. • Due to risk of extravasation, give via central line if possible. • Monitor child closely, preferably in an ICU setting. • Assess for ventricular dysrhythmias
Epinephrine (vasopressor, inotropic)	Stimulates alpha- and beta-adrenergic receptors, increasing heart rate and systemic vascular resistance Bradycardia, anaphylaxis	• Administer via IV or IO route at a dose of 0.01 mg/kg (0.1 mL/kg of 1:10,000 solution) or via ET route at 0.1 mg/kg (0.1 mL/kg of 1:1,000 solution). • During CPR, repeat every 3–5 minutes. • Monitor for ventricular dysrhythmias • High doses may cause tachycardia in newborns. • Due to risk of extravasation and subsequent tissue necrosis, give through a central line if possible. • May also be used as a bronchodilator IV or via inhalation (racemic epinephrine).
Glucose	Increases blood glucose level Hypoglycemia	• Administer via IV or IO route at a dose of 1–2 mL/kg (D50%); maximum dose 2–4 mL/kg. • When administering via a peripheral IV line, dilute 1:1 with sterile water to make D25%. Monitor IV site for infiltration and tissue extravasation. • Monitor blood glucose levels closely.
Lidocaine (anti-dysrhythmic)	Decreases automaticity of conduction tissues of the heart Ventricular dysrhythmias	• Administer via IV or IO route at a dose of 1 mg/kg; administer via ET route at dose two times IV dose diluted with 3–5 mL normal saline, followed by positive-pressure ventilation. Maximum dose 5 mg/kg or 100 mg/dose. • Monitor ECG continuously. • Contraindicated in complete heart block. • With larger than normal doses, monitor for hypotension or seizures.
Naloxone (opioid receptor antagonist)	Antagonizes action of narcotic agents Reversal of respiratory depression related to narcotic effects	• Administer via IV, IO, SQ, or ET route at a dose of 0.01–0.1 mg/kg in children younger than 5 years or <20 kg or at a dose of 2 mg in children older than 5 years or >20 kg. Onset of action is within 2–5 minutes. • May repeat dose as necessary; narcotic effects outlast therapeutic effects of naloxone.

AV, atrioventricular; BP, blood pressure; ECG, electrocardiogram; ET, endotracheal; ICU, intensive care unit; IO, intraosseous; IV, intravenous; PRN, as needed; SQ, subcutaneous.

Data from American Heart Association & American Academy of Pediatrics. (2020). *Pediatric advanced life support provider manual.* American Heart Association; UpToDate, Inc. (2024). UpToDate Lexidrug (Version 8.2.0) [Mobile app]. Wolters Kluwer. https://apps.apple.com/us/app/lexicomp/id313401238

TAKE NOTE!

Certain emergency drugs for children may be given via an endotracheal tube. Use the mnemonic LEAN (lidocaine, epinephrine, atropine, and naloxone) to remember which drugs may be given via the endotracheal route. These drugs should be followed by sterile normal saline flush and positive-pressure ventilations to ensure that the drugs are delivered (AHA & AAP, 2020).

Clinical Judgment and the Nursing Process for the Child in an Emergency Situation

The nurse may encounter a pediatric emergency in a variety of settings. As a member of a trauma team at a pediatric hospital, the nurse may participate in the stabilization of a child who has suffered a near drowning or trauma. The emergency department nurse may encounter a child who has just been injured, such as from a fall, an accident, or sports. On the hospital unit, a child with asthma may suffer respiratory distress or stop breathing. Regardless of the setting or how the emergency developed, the principles for managing pediatric emergencies are the same.

Care of the child in an emergency includes all components of the nursing process: assessment, analysis, planning, interventions, and evaluation. In an emergency, the nurse must act quickly. It is important to intervene immediately when an abnormality is determined upon assessment. When evaluating a child who presents emergently, always follow the AHA's guidelines for basic life support, which includes evaluating the child's:

- Airway
- Breathing
- Circulation

After evaluating the child's airway, breathing, and circulation, provide care as necessary, including rescue breathing or CPR. Once the child's cardiopulmonary status is stabilized or the child is resuscitated, assessment and management will vary depending on the cause of the emergency.

Assessment

Nursing assessment of the child who presents emergently includes health history, physical examination, and laboratory and diagnostic testing. However, the initial history may be focused and very brief if the child is critically ill; the nurse may need to proceed immediately to rapid cardiopulmonary assessment. Once a child is stabilized, a more comprehensive history is obtained. Laboratory tests, while often important, should never take priority over cardiopulmonary and hemodynamic stabilization.

Health History

Obtain the health history rapidly while simultaneously evaluating the child and providing lifesaving interventions. A brief history is needed initially, followed by a more thorough history after the child is stabilized. The parents or caregiver will provide information about the child's chief complaint. Record the information using the caregiver's own words. For example, the caregiver might say, "He's been having trouble breathing" if the child is presenting in respiratory distress. If the child was injured in a bicycle accident, the caregiver might say, "She was riding her bike down the hill and lost control." This brief statement provides guidance for obtaining more in-depth information about the emergency.

Ask about any significant past history that may affect the care of the child. For example, children who are medically fragile, who were born prematurely, or who have a significant genetically linked disease (e.g., sickle cell anemia) may require special consideration when planning and implementing care.

CLINICAL REASONING ALERT!

When caring for a child injured in an accident, the nurse must always remember that assessment is the first step in the nursing process. So initial questions would relate to how the accident happened. The nurse could then go on to ask other questions such as medication allergies and chronic diseases.

Physical Examination

In an emergency, the nurse must perform a rapid cardiopulmonary assessment and intervene immediately if alterations are noted. The remainder of the physical examination then follows.

RAPID CARDIOPULMONARY ASSESSMENT

As the brief history is being obtained, begin the rapid cardiopulmonary assessment. Most pediatric arrests are related primarily to airway and breathing, and usually only secondarily to the heart. Supported breathing may be all that is needed if the child has a strong, adequate pulse. Always perform the assessment and interventions in that order. In most circumstances, if a child's airway is properly managed and breathing is assisted, the child may not experience a full arrest requiring chest compressions.

Airway Evaluation and Management First, evaluate the airway. Assess its patency. Position the airway in a manner that promotes good airflow. If secretions are obstructing the airway, suction the airway to remove them. If the child is unconscious or has just been injured, open the airway using the head tilt–chin lift maneuver. Place the fingertips on the bony prominence of the child's chin and lift the chin to open the airway. Simultaneously, place one hand on the forehead and tilt the child's head back (Fig. 29.1). If the airway is not maintainable, reposition the airway for appropriate airflow. Place the child immediately on oxygen at 100% and apply a pulse oximeter to monitor oxygen saturation levels.

TAKE NOTE!

If cervical spine injury is a possibility, do not use the head tilt–chin lift maneuver; use only the jaw-thrust technique for opening the airway (see "Trauma" section for explanation and illustration).

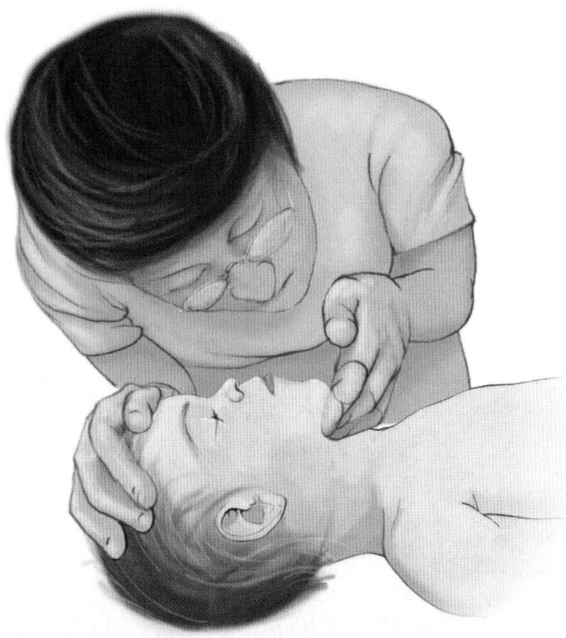

FIGURE 29.1 Head tilt–chin lift maneuver in a child.

Breathing Evaluation and Management After establishing an open airway, look for signs of respiration. Turn your head and place your ear over the child's mouth to "look, listen, and feel" for spontaneous respirations. Look to see if the child's chest is rising, listen for air escaping, and note if you feel any air coming out of the child's nose or mouth. If the child is breathing, evaluate the quality of the respirations: Is ventilation effective, or is the child simply gasping ineffectively for air? Count the respiratory rate. Observe the child's color. Note the depth of respiration, chest rise, adequacy of airflow in all lung fields, and presence of adventitious sounds. Evaluate for increased work of breathing and the use of accessory muscles.

When signs of respiratory distress are noted, immediately place the child on oxygen at 100% and apply a pulse oximeter to monitor oxygen saturation levels. If the child is breathing shallowly and has poor respiratory effort, attempt to reposition the airway to promote better airflow.

For the child receiving 100% oxygen who does not improve with repositioning, begin assisted ventilation with a bag-valve-mask (BVM) device. A need for ongoing BVM ventilation may require airway intubation (process by which an endotracheal [ET] tube is inserted into a child's airway to assist with breathing). See "Respiratory Arrest" section for information on assisting with ventilation using the BVM device and airway intubation.

Circulation Evaluation and Management Next, evaluate circulation. During this phase, evaluate the heart rate (HR), pulse, perfusion, skin color and temperature, blood pressure (BP), cardiac rhythm, and level of consciousness. Determine HR via direct auscultation or palpation of central pulses. Radial and brachial pulses are more difficult to palpate, especially in infants and young children. If perfusion is poor, such as with shock or cardiac arrest, the child may have a weak pulse or no pulse. In the young infant, check the brachial artery for a pulse. In the child and adolescent, evaluate the carotid pulse.

CLINICAL REASONING ALERT!

ALWAYS evaluate the presence of HR by auscultation of the heart or by palpation of central pulses. NEVER use the cardiac monitor to determine if the child has an HR. The presence of a cardiac rhythm is not a reliable method for evaluation of the ability to perfuse the body. In certain circumstances, a rhythm continues but there is no pulse (pulseless electrical activity [PEA]).

If the child has no HR (pulse), begin cardiac compressions. See later for information on performing CPR. High-quality chest compressions of adequate rate and depth are essential (AHA & AAP, 2020). If there is a pulse, note its quality: Is it barely palpable or weak? Is it strong or bounding? Compare the strength and quality of central and peripheral pulses. Assess capillary refill time.

Evaluate the child's perfusion by noting skin temperature and color. Is the skin pink? Is it warm to the touch? The child's skin may be cool to the touch and may appear pale, mottled, or cyanotic. As the child's condition worsens with developing shock and cardiovascular compromise, note a line of demarcation of skin temperature. In this situation, the distal extremities will feel cooler than the proximal regions of the body. Measure the BP and place the child on a cardiac monitor to evaluate the cardiac rhythm. Note the child's sensorium or level of consciousness; if circulation is poor, the child will demonstrate an altered level of consciousness as perfusion to the brain becomes diminished.

If the circulation or perfusion is compromised, then fluid resuscitation is necessary. Establish large-bore intravenous (IV) access immediately and administer isotonic fluid rapidly. Provide 20 mL/kg of normal saline (NS) or lactated Ringer's (LR) as an IV bolus (if the infant is younger than 1 month old, administer 10 mL/kg). If peripheral IV access cannot be obtained in the child with altered perfusion within three attempts or 90 seconds, assist with the insertion of an intraosseous needle for fluid administration (refer to "Shock" section for further information about intraosseous access). Central venous lines or cutdown access may also be used, but these measures take longer to accomplish.

Remember Alma, the 8-year-old with breathing trouble? What additional health history and physical examination assessment information should the nurse obtain?

ADDITIONAL PHYSICAL EXAMINATION COMPONENTS

In addition to assessing and stabilizing the child's airway, breathing, and circulation, perform a thorough physical examination and assess pain.

Neurologic Evaluation Quickly evaluate the sensorium in an older child. Ask the child to state their name. Ask what happened to the child. Does the child know what day it is? Is the child aware of where they are?

If the child is an infant, evaluate their interest in the environment and response to parents. An infant who is not interested in the environment or seems unable to recognize their parents is a cause for concern. In contrast, an infant who enjoys sucking on a finger and making eye contact with the nurse during the assessment is reassuring.

TAKE NOTE!

Use the mnemonic AVPU to quickly determine the level of consciousness:
A–Alert
V–Responsive to voice
P–Responds to pain
U–Unresponsive

Evaluate the child's head. In the infant or young toddler, palpate the anterior fontanel to determine if it is normal (soft and flat), depressed, or full. A sunken fontanel is associated with volume depletion from dehydration or blood loss. If the fontanel is full, note if it is bulging or tense, which may indicate increased intracranial pressure. Next, assess the eyes. Are they open or closed? If closed, do they open spontaneously, to voice, to pain? Does the child focus on and follow the nurse's movements? Evaluate the pupils for equality and reactivity. Sluggish pupillary reaction may occur with increased intracranial pressure.

Evaluate the child's face. Does the child smile or cry? Does the child react to playfulness with a laugh? Does the young infant cry vigorously? Are facial movements equal? In a child, a normal or near-normal neurologic examination can be a reassuring sign. Conversely, obtunded or muted responses to environmental stimuli are a cause for concern.

Next, evaluate for spontaneous movement of the extremities. Young infants cannot walk, so assess their ability to move their arms and legs, and grossly evaluate the tone of their extremities. Does the infant vigorously and equally move the arms and legs? Is the muscle tone normal, or does the infant appear floppy or flaccid? When evaluating the older child, note whether they are ambulatory independently, ambulatory with assistance, or unable to walk. Note whether the child has use of the upper extremities. In the case of trauma, the child may arrive immobilized on a backboard. In this scenario, evaluate the child's motor responsiveness and sensation in each extremity, comparing findings bilaterally while the child is in the supine position. Ask the child if they feel you touching each extremity. Ask the child to squeeze your fingers and to wiggle the toes. This will provide information about cerebral integrity and perfusion, cerebellar health, and spinal cord integrity.

The Pediatric Glasgow Coma Scale may also be used to evaluate the neurologic status in children. Chapter 16 provides a more in-depth discussion of this scale.

TAKE NOTE!

A nonreactive pupil is an ominous sign indicating a need for immediate relief of increased intracranial pressure.

Skin and Extremity Evaluation Remove the child's clothing and thoroughly examine the skin for bruising, lesions, or rashes. If the child has a rash, note the size, shape, color, configuration, and location. Apply pressure to the rash with the fingertips to see whether it blanches. Inspect the trunk, abdomen, and extremities for abrasions or deformities.

CLINICAL REASONING ALERT!

Rashes that do not blanch may be classified as petechiae or purpura. This type of rash may be associated with certain serious conditions, such as meningococcemia. Report this finding to the health care provider or nurse practitioner immediately.

Pain Assessment In emergencies, children may experience pain as a direct result of the injury or disease, and lifesaving interventions such as resuscitation, insertion of IV lines, and administration of medications may cause further pain. The child's pain may also be exaggerated by light, noise, movement of the stretcher or bed, and the sensations of cold or heat. Nurses play a key role in minimizing the child's pain, and this may decrease the child's future distress (Ring et al., 2023). If the child is awake and verbal, use an age-appropriate pain assessment scale to determine the child's pain level. If the child is sedated or unconscious, assess pain with a standardized scale that relies on physiologic measurements as well as behavioral parameters. Refer to Chapter 14 for additional information on pain assessment in children.

Laboratory and Diagnostic Testing

A number of laboratory and diagnostic tests may be ordered in a pediatric emergency. Laboratory tests can help to distinguish the cause of the emergency or additional problems that need to be treated. Standard laboratory tests obtained in most emergency departments include:

- Arterial blood gases (ABGs), obtained initially and then serially to assess for changes
- Electrolytes and glucose levels
- Complete blood count (CBC)
- Blood cultures
- Urinalysis

If ingestion is suspected, then a toxicology panel will be obtained. In suspected sepsis, erythrocyte sedimentation rate (ESR), C-reactive protein (CRP), and urine and spinal fluid cultures may also be obtained. The pediatric trauma victim may have additional laboratory tests performed, including amylase, liver enzymes, and blood type and cross-match.

Diagnostic tests may include radiologic tests, computed tomography (CT) scanning, and magnetic resonance imaging (MRI). One advantage of radiologic diagnostic testing is that the tests are relatively noninvasive. A disadvantage of CT and MRI scans is that before they can be performed, the child must be stabilized. Common Laboratory and Diagnostic Tests 29.1 discusses the tests most commonly used in pediatric emergencies.

COMMON LABORATORY AND DIAGNOSTIC TESTS 29.1

Test	Explanation	Indications	Nursing Implications
Chest radiograph	Radiograph used to evaluate heart and lung structures	To identify: • Infections (e.g., pneumonia) • Foreign body • Injury • Endotracheal tube placement • Central line placement • Pneumothorax • Reevaluation of lungs after chest tube placement	• Radiographs can be obtained quickly during resuscitation, usually available in the emergency department. • Assist the child to lie still if necessary.
Computed tomography (CT)	Use of high radiation (equivalent to about 100–150 chest x-rays) with computer processing targeting specific body areas	Rapid evaluation of tissues and skeletal areas Superior test for the evaluation of internal bleeding	• Expect the child to be transported out of the area for the study. • Accompany the child to provide continued observation and management, especially if child's condition is unstable.
Magnetic resonance imaging (MRI)	Incorporation of responses of hydrogen protons to a dynamic magnetic field	Superior test for the evaluation of the spinal cord and the cerebrospinal fluid spaces; less useful in emergency situations	• Administer sedation as ordered. • Assist child in remaining still; MRI requires child to remain still for a longer period than for a CT. • Assist the conscious child to deal with fear related to loud banging noise of the machine.
Arterial blood gases (ABGs)	Evaluation of blood pH and arterial blood levels of oxygen and carbon dioxide	Evaluation of quality of respiration and evaluation of acid–base balance	• Anticipate serial ABGs to assess for status changes. • Never delay resuscitation efforts pending blood gas results.
Serum electrolytes	Evaluation of electrolyte levels, such as sodium, potassium, and chloride, in the blood	Useful for determining baseline and if dehydration is hypertonic or isotonic	Hemolysis of specimen may lead to falsely elevated potassium levels.
Glucose	Evaluation of glucose level in the blood	Valuable for determining the need for supplementation, as in the case of hypoglycemia	• Use a rapid glucose test at the bedside or obtain serum blood specimen. • Elevated glucose levels can be associated with stress or with the use of corticosteroids.
Toxicology panel (blood and/or urine)	Determination of most commonly misused mood-altering medications, as well as commonly ingested drugs	Drug misuse, overdose, or poisoning	• Standard toxicology panel varies with the agency. • Follow agency protocol; may require special handling or labeling of specimen. • Use a blood specimen that is best for determining overdose or poisoning.
Complete blood count (CBC)	Evaluation of hemoglobin and hematocrit, white blood cell count, and platelet count	Any condition in which anemia, infection, or thrombocytopenia is suspected Trauma if blood loss is suspected	• Be aware of normal values and how they vary with age and sex. • Hemoglobin and hematocrit may be elevated secondary to hemoconcentration in the case of hypovolemia.
Blood type and cross-match	Determination of ABO blood typing as well as the presence of antigens Cross-match is performed on RBC-containing products to avoid transfusion reaction.	Trauma victim or any person with suspected blood loss as preparation for transfusion	• Handle the specimen gently to avoid hemolysis. • Ensure that specimen request and label are appropriately signed and dated. • Apply "type and cross" or "blood band" to child at the time of specimen collection if required by agency. • Most type and cross-match specimens expire after 48–72 hours.

(*continued*)

COMMON LABORATORY AND DIAGNOSTIC TESTS 29.1 (*continued*)

Test	Explanation	Indications	Nursing Implications
Urinalysis	Evaluation of color, pH, specific gravity, and odor of urine Assessment for protein, glucose, ketones, blood, leukocyte esterase, RBCs, WBCs, bacteria, crystals, and casts	Children with fever, dysuria, flank pain, urgency, or hematuria or those who have experienced trauma to provide information about the urinary tract	• Many drugs can affect urine color; notify the laboratory if the child is taking one. • Notify the laboratory and document on the laboratory form if the child or adolescent is menstruating. • Refrigerate the specimen if it is not processed promptly. • Specimen may be obtained by catheterization, clean-catch voiding sample, or a U-bag.

RBCs, red blood cells; WBCs, white blood cells.

Data from Corbett, J. A., & Banks, A. D. (2019). *Laboratory tests and diagnostic procedures with nursing diagnoses* (9th ed.). Pearson Education Inc.

Nursing Analysis and Related Interventions

After completing a thorough assessment and initial stabilization of the child, the nurse might identify several patient problems, including:

- Ineffective airway clearance
- Altered breathing pattern
- Impaired gas exchange
- Hypovolemia
- Decreased cardiac output (CO)
- Altered tissue perfusion
- Fear
- Interrupted family processes
- Knowledge deficiency

After completing an assessment of Alma, the nurse noted the following: a patent airway, anxious but able to speak in short sentences, and skin temperature cool on the extremities. Based on these assessment findings, what would your top three patient problems be for Alma? Describe appropriate nursing interventions.

Specific nursing goals, interventions, and evaluation for the child in an emergency are based on the patient's problems. Additional information about nursing management will be included later in the chapter as it relates to specific disorders.

Providing Cardiopulmonary Resuscitation

Check for pulse. In the child, the carotid or femoral pulses are easiest to assess. In the infant, check the femoral pulse. Carefully assess for signs of a pulse, but do not spend more than 10 seconds checking the pulse. If there is not a pulse or if the HR is less than 60 beats/min (bpm), begin chest compressions.

Evaluate and manage the airway. Call for help and assign someone to obtain the automatic external defibrillator (AED). Open the airway and assess for adequate breathing. If the child is not breathing, begin rescue breathing.

TAKE NOTE!

When a cardiac arrest occurs in a child out of the hospital and is a witnessed, sudden collapse, initial management is slightly different than that for other arrests. In these sudden, witnessed events, call 9-1-1 or the local emergency number for help first, get the AED, and return to start CPR (AHA & AAP, 2020).

Table 29.1 presents the AHA's most recent recommendations for ratios of breaths and compressions. These recommendations stress the importance of properly performed chest compressions. Therefore, several changes have been made to the guidelines:

- Rescuers must provide compressions of adequate rate and depth.
- Chest recoil should be allowed.
- Minimal interruption of chest compressions should be the goal.
- For infant CPR, two-person infant CPR can be performed by encircling the chest with two thumbs and simultaneously using the hands to provide a thoracic squeeze.
- For two-person CPR, no pauses should occur for ventilation, with the compressing health care provider giving continuous compressions (AHA & AAP, 2020).

Providing Defibrillation or Synchronized Cardioversion

In some cases, the child has an abnormal life-threatening cardiac rhythm or an dysrhythmia that does not respond to pharmacologic therapy or leads to hemodynamic instability. In these cases, electrical therapy, in the form of defibrillation or synchronized cardioversion, may be needed.

Defibrillation is the use of electrical energy to depolarize the cells of the myocardium to terminate an abnormal life-threatening cardiac rhythm, such as ventricular fibrillation (VF). Defibrillation is used in

TABLE 29.1 • Ratios of Breaths to Compressions

Age	One-Person CPR	Two-Person CPR
Infant	• 30 compressions to two breaths • Hand placement: two fingers, placed one fingerbreadth below the nipple line	• 15 compressions to two breaths • Hand placement: two thumbs encircling the chest at the nipple line
Child	• 30 compressions to two breaths • Hand placement: heel of hand or two hands (adult position in larger child), pressing on the sternum at the nipple line	• 15 compressions to two breaths • Hand placement: heel of one hand or two hands (adult position in larger child), pressing on the sternum at the nipple line

Data from American Heart Association & American Academy of Pediatrics. (2020). *Pediatric advanced life support provider manual.* American Heart Association.

conjunction with oxygen, CPR, and medications. The effects of defibrillation are enhanced in an oxygen-rich environment coupled with good artificial circulation (CPR).

Cardioversion, another means of applying electrical current to the heart, is delivered in a synchronized fashion—that is, the electrical current is applied on the R wave of the electrocardiogram (ECG). Cardioversion is used when the child has supraventricular tachycardia (SVT) or ventricular tachycardia with a pulse. Cardioversion may also be enhanced with medications.

The basic defibrillator is equipped with adult- and pediatric-sized paddles. A switch turns the machine on, and controls are used to select the amount of energy (joules). Typically, the initial energy amount is 2 J/kg; it can be increased up to 4 J/kg for defibrillation. Energy for cardioversion is delivered at 0.5 to 1 J/kg.

When the defibrillator is being used in an acute care setting, the leader of the code team will take charge of defibrillator use. The leader is responsible for ensuring that only the child receives the energy from the defibrillator. The code team leader will count to 4 before delivering a shock to the child to ensure that all personnel and other equipment are clear of the bed to avoid accidental shock.

Using Automated External Defibrillation

In cases of sudden, witnessed, out-of-hospital collapse, a dysrhythmia is often the cause. Therefore, the AHA has revised its recommendations about the use of an AED in children (AHA & AAP, 2020). An AED is an alternative to manually defibrillating an individual. The AED device consists of electrodes that are applied to the chest. These electrodes are used to monitor the heart rhythm and deliver the electrical current. AED devices are readily available in a variety of locations, such as airports, sports facilities, and businesses. Traditionally, the AED was designed for use in adults, but newer AEDs with smaller pads and the ability to alter energy delivery are now more readily available. Therefore, the AHA has recommended that an AED be used for children who are older than age 1 year who have no pulse and have suffered a sudden, witnessed collapse (AHA & AAP, 2020).

The AED is designed for people to use it in the prehospital setting. Once the AED is turned on, the machine uses auditory commands to guide laypeople and health care professionals alike through the correct placement of the electrodes and the administration of energy. The AED periodically evaluates the victim's cardiac rhythm and instructs the user about checking the pulse, continuing CPR, and delivering shocks. Nurses who care for children should be able to operate an AED and be prepared to use it in nontraditional settings.

TAKE NOTE!

Currently, the American Academy of Pediatrics (AAP) recommends the placement of AEDs in all secondary schools, in order to improve outcomes should sudden arrest occur in the school (Fuch, 2018).

Determining Medication Doses and Equipment Sizes

Many pediatric acute care facilities prepare code reference sheets when a child is admitted. This sheet uses the child's actual weight to determine medication doses and equipment sizes. The reference sheet is kept on a clipboard at the child's bedside or taped on the wall at the head of the bed. An additional copy is placed in the child's chart.

Ambulatory care providers often use the Broselow tape to estimate the child's weight based on the child's length (Fig. 29.2). The tape is color coded, and emergency equipment for a child of that size is stored in corresponding color-coded packages or in color-coded drawers on the pediatric emergency cart. Medication doses and equipment sizes are also located on the tape. The most accurate calculation for code medications is based on the child's weight, but use of the Broselow tape for estimating the weight has been shown to be successful in children weighing less than 25 kg (Jones, 2023).

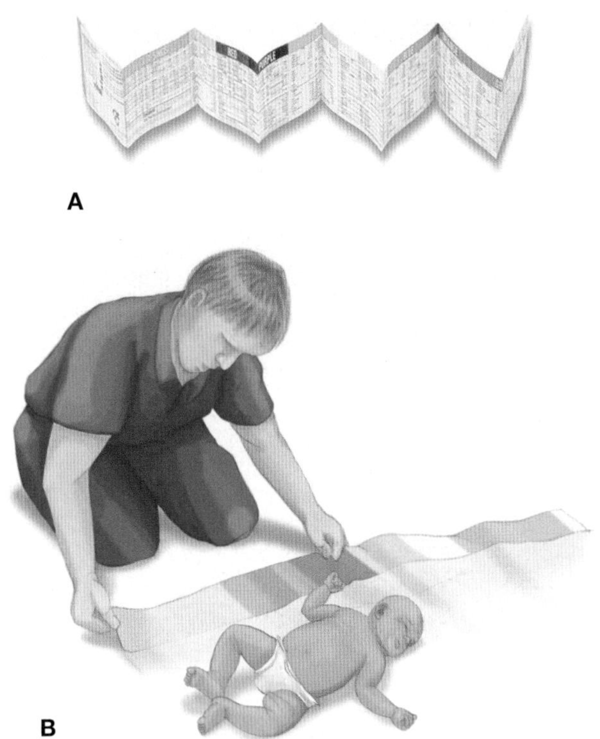

FIGURE 29.2 A. Broselow tape. B. Measure the child's length with the Broselow tape to determine medication doses and endotracheal tube size.

Managing Pain

Depending on the child's status and pain level, individualize pain management interventions. For the alert child, nonpharmacologic measures may be used in addition to medications. Provide atraumatic care for procedures and use aggressive pharmacologic treatments to manage pain as the child's condition allows. Refer to Chapter 14 for additional information on pain management strategies.

Ensuring Stabilization

After a child has been resuscitated, the nurse plays a key role in stabilization and transport. Thoroughly document the interventions that were performed as well as the ongoing assessment of the child's response to the interventions. Provide continued monitoring of the child while awaiting transport. Copy and assemble any pertinent documentation, such as the resuscitation record, nurse's notes, and laboratory test results, which will be given to the receiving institution. Ensure that all lines are taped securely and that vascular access sites are dressed and labeled with the date and time of insertion. As soon as possible, bring the child's family in to visit with the child. Provide explanations about the IV lines, monitoring equipment, and other medical equipment and devices. Encourage the family to talk to and touch the child.

Providing Support and Education to the Child and Family

The experience of respiratory distress, oxygen deprivation, and an emergency situation is a frightening one for people of all ages. The lifesaving interventions that take place during an emergency can be especially intimidating and upsetting to children. Infants and young children cannot understand explanations about these interventions, and older children and adolescents may feel frightened and angry about the loss of control. The caregivers may feel fear, anger, guilt, and sadness. They may be concerned about the very real possibility that their child might die.

Resuscitation of a child is often a perplexing and frightening event for laypeople to observe. Therefore, traditionally, family members have been excluded during the resuscitation of children. Recently, however, there has been a trend to allow family members to be present during pediatric resuscitation. Studies have shown that family presence during resuscitation may assist with family coping (Bush & Woodley, 2022).

Considering the highly technical nature of resuscitation, the rapidity with which interventions occur, and the fear associated with a life-threatening event, nurses can play a crucial role in providing understandable explanations to families, coupled with empathic support. During the acute phase, the nurse should give brief explanations as lifesaving interventions are being provided. Examples of these types of explanations include:

- When applying the pulse oximeter sensor: "I need to put this light on your child to check his oxygen level; it won't hurt."
- When connecting the child to the cardiac monitor: "We're going to put these sticky patches on your child and connect them so we can monitor her heart rate on this screen."
- When preparing for intubation and ventilation: "Your child can't breathe on their own right now, so we're going to give them some extra help with this tube. This tube will go through their breathing passage and this machine will help them to breathe" (see Evidence-Based Practice 29.1).

The nurse plays a key role in providing empathy and support. Do not provide false reassurance and say, for example, "Your child is going to be alright." The outcome is never certain. Rather, communicate empathically. For example, say, "This must be very difficult for you. We're doing everything we can to help your child." Provide honest answers in a reassuring manner. Respect each family's diversity and observe their strengths and weaknesses. Be nonjudgmental in all interactions with families, even when the child's emergency situation may have resulted from family neglect.

EVIDENCE-BASED PRACTICE **29.1**

Quality of Pediatric Emergency Care

Children and adolescents comprise a large percentage of the emergency care population, particularly with respect to being seen for injuries and infections. While intervening quickly is often necessary in an emergency situation, it is also important to respect and support children and their parents.

STUDY

Janhunen et al. (2019) conducted a descriptive study of 98 children (ages 7 to 15 years) and their parents from four emergency departments. The authors utilized a survey to compare perceptions of quality of care in the emergency room.

Findings

Overall, parents and children were satisfied with the care received in the emergency room. Interestingly, compared with their parents' scores, children reported the least satisfaction with nursing staff professionalism, ability to talk privately with staff, and ability to participate in planning their own care. Importantly, both parents and children ranked alleviation of the child's pain and fear lowest for all satisfaction items.

Nursing Implications

Though this was a small study, it highlights two important components of care: respect and pain/fear alleviation. When able, nurses should consider speaking with children privately and involve them in care planning, as the situation allows. In all instances, nurses must be vigilant about alleviating fears in children undergoing an emergency situation as well as proactively assessing and managing children's pain.

Data from Janhunen, K., Kankkunen, P., & Kvist, T. (2019). Quality of pediatric emergency care as assessed by children and their parents. *Journal of Nursing Care Quality, 34*(2), 180–184. https://doi.org/10.1097/NCQ.0000000000000346

Parents often feel helpless when their child is in a high-tech environment. Suddenly overwhelmed with the equipment and monitoring devices, they no longer are the people who are the most skilled in caring for their child. Integrate the child's parents into the health care team. Suggest ways the parents can make the hospital experience more normal for their child. For example, simply allowing a parent to read a story to their child or encouraging a parent to hold their child's hand is therapeutic for both the child and the parents. Be aware of this dramatic change and how it affects the parents. Always ensure that they feel like they are a welcome part of their child's care.

Providing the child with familiar comfort objects helps to decrease stress. Once the intubated child is alert and stabilized, assist them with communication. Some children can lift one finger for yes and two fingers for no. If the child is old enough to write, provide paper and pencil. Play is essential to the work of the child, and even if they are immobile, play is still possible. Puppets at the bedside and books help give the child a more normal experience in a scary situation that is far from the norm. Adolescents may enjoy listening to music through headphones. Even children who are comatose should be talked to and allowed to listen to familiar music.

Even if the outcomes are serious, the nurse can provide critical support to children and families. Whether hugging a crying parent or playing "peek-a-boo" with an intubated child, the nurse will be the one who can make a difference during a frightening experience.

• • • ATRAUMATIC CARE • • •

In the conscious child, ensure proximity of the caregiver during the postresuscitation phase to provide security and assist with keeping the child calm.

NURSING MANAGEMENT OF CHILDREN IN EMERGENCIES

Nurses must be adept at identifying the beginning stages of an emergency so they can quickly and appropriately intervene to prevent deterioration to cardiopulmonary arrest. Assessment and management of the most common types of emergencies in children are discussed following. The topics covered include respiratory arrest, shock, cardiac dysrhythmias and arrest, near drowning, poisoning, and traumatic injury.

Respiratory Arrest

Respiratory emergencies may lead to respiratory failure and eventual cardiopulmonary arrest in children. Infants and young children are at greater risk for respiratory emergencies than adolescents and adults because they have smaller airways and underdeveloped immune systems, resulting in a diminished ability to combat serious respiratory illnesses. Young children often lack coordination, making them susceptible to choking on foods and small objects, which may also lead to cardiopulmonary arrest. In addition, sudden unexplained infant death (SUID), also called sudden infant death syndrome (SIDS), is a leading cause of cardiopulmonary arrest in young infants and thus is the leading cause of postneonatal mortality in the United States (Graham & Peoples, 2019). For these reasons, nurses must be skilled at recognizing the signs of pediatric respiratory distress so they can prevent progression to cardiopulmonary arrest. Table 29.2 lists some of the more common causes of pediatric respiratory arrest.

TABLE 29.2 • Causes of Respiratory Arrest in Children

Condition	Cause
Upper airway	Burns Croup Epiglottitis Foreign-body aspiration Reflux Strangulation or near strangulation Tracheomalacia Vascular ring
Lower airway	Asthma Bronchiolitis Burns Foreign-body aspiration Pertussis infection Pneumonia Pneumothorax Reflux
Nonrespiratory origins	Septic shock HIV
Neurologic	CNS infection Guillain–Barré syndrome Poliomyelitis Seizures Sleep apnea Spinal cord trauma Sudden infant death
Chronic illness	Complications of severe prematurity Cystic fibrosis Bone marrow transplant Neutropenia
Metabolic/endocrine disorders	Diabetic ketoacidosis Mitochondrial disorders
Cardiac conditions	Dysrhythmia Congenital cardiac problems Acquired cardiac problems
Traumatic/unintentional/intentional injury	Asphyxia Child abuse/"shaken baby syndrome" Drowning Electrocution Gunshot wound Toxic ingestion Vehicle-related trauma

CNS, central nervous system; HIV, human immunodeficiency virus.

Data from Shaw, K. N., & Bachur, R. G. (Eds.). (2020). *Fleisher and Ludwig's textbook of pediatric emergency medicine* (8th ed.). Wolters Kluwer.

Nursing Assessment

If the child has severe respiratory compromise, obtain a brief history while simultaneously providing respiratory interventions. To obtain the history, use the following questions as a guide:

- When did the symptoms begin and when do they occur?
- Did the symptoms have a sudden onset (as with a foreign-body aspiration)?
- How have the symptoms progressed?
- Is the cough continual, intermittent, or worse at night or with exercise?
- Has there been any stridor? (Stridor is heard upon inhalation and may be associated with swelling of the trachea [as with croup] or with a foreign body in the upper airway.)
- Is there wheezing? If so, is the wheezing on inspiration, on expiration, or both?
- What makes the symptoms better and what makes them worse?
- Does drinking from a bottle induce the symptoms (as with gastroesophageal reflux–induced aspiration)?
- Is the child taking any medication for the symptoms? Does the child or do any members of the immediate family have a history of chronic respiratory disease, such as asthma?
- Are the child's immunizations up to date?
- Was the child born prematurely? If so, did the child require mechanical ventilation? For how long?
- Were there any respiratory problems during the first few days of life?
- When did the child last eat? (This question is important because a recent meal will increase the child's risk of aspiration in the event of a respiratory arrest. In addition, the presence of food in the stomach will increase the risk of aspiration during tracheal intubation.)

If the child can communicate, ask how they are feeling. Are they short of breath? Does their chest hurt? Observe the child while speaking. Children who are in respiratory distress may speak in short sentences with gasping between words.

PHYSICAL EXAMINATION

In an emergency, physical examination is often limited to inspection, observation, and auscultation. First, quickly survey the respiratory status. Determine if the child is breathing.

Inspection and Observation

Establish if the airway is patent, maintainable, or unable to be maintained. The child with a patent airway is breathing without signs of obstruction. The maintainable airway remains patent independently by the child or with interventions such as a towel roll under an infant's neck or the insertion of a nasal trumpet. The airway that cannot be maintained does not remain patent unless a more aggressive intervention, such as the insertion of a tracheal tube, is performed.

Look at the child's posture. Is the child sitting up, leaning forward, and drooling, as with epiglottitis? Observe the child's face: Do they appear anxious or relaxed? Children in respiratory distress often appear anxious. Look at the nose and mouth. Are the nares patent? Is there noticeable nasal congestion or mucus coming from the nose? Note nasal flaring or mouth breathing. Observe for head bobbing. Listen for audible expiratory grunting or inspiratory stridor. Note the child's color. Does the child appear pale, mottled, dusky, or cyanotic? Children may appear mottled in response to poor oxygenation, hypothermia, or stress. Children with severe respiratory compromise may appear dusky. Look for cyanosis around the mouth or on the trunk. Cyanosis is a late and often ominous sign of respiratory distress. Central cyanosis is more likely to be associated with respiratory or cardiac compromise. In contrast, peripheral cyanosis is more likely to be associated with circulatory alteration.

TAKE NOTE!

Closely inspect the color of the area around the mouth. Circumoral pallor is a sign of poor oxygenation.

Evaluate the pattern and quality of respiration, noting the respiratory rate. Tachypnea (increased respiratory rate) is often noted in children in respiratory distress. However, seriously ill children grunt and may have normal or subnormal respiratory rates. **Hypoventilation**, a decrease in the depth and rate of respirations, is noted in very ill children or in children who have central respiratory depression secondary to narcotics. If the child is a young infant (younger than 2 months) or premature, periodic breathing may occur. **Periodic breathing** is regular breathing with occasional short pauses (brief periods of apnea). After the apneic pause, the infant will breathe rapidly (up to 60 breaths/min) for a short period and then will resume a normal respiratory rate. In general, the infant who has periodic breathing looks pink and has a normal HR. Observe for the use of accessory muscles in the neck or retractions in the chest, determining the extent and severity of the retractions.

Auscultation

Auscultate the lungs with the diaphragm of the stethoscope. Breath sounds over the tracheal region are higher pitched and are described as vesicular, while breath sounds over the peripheral lung fields tend to be lower pitched, known as bronchial. Instruct the child to take deep breaths with the mouth open. To encourage the young child to exhale strongly, instruct them to "blow out" the penlight (as with a candle) or to blow on a tissue. Encourage the child not to breathe more rapidly than normal (to prevent **hyperventilation** [increased depth and rate of respirations]) and to avoid making any noises with the mouth.

TAKE NOTE!

Significant upper respiratory congestion often interferes with the assessment of the lower airways because the sound is easily transmitted throughout the chest. Differentiate between the upper and lower airway noises by listening with the stethoscope over the nose. The nurse may be able to determine whether the noise is nasal or bronchial by using this technique.

Auscultate the child's chest systematically. Listen in all anterior, axillary, and posterior regions, comparing the left to the right sides. Note any decreased or absent breath sounds, which may be the result of bronchial obstruction (as with mucous infection) or air trapping (as in children with asthma). Unilateral absent breath sounds are associated with foreign-body aspiration and pneumothorax.

TAKE NOTE!

Sometimes a child's respiratory status is so severely compromised that little or no air movement is noted. This commonly occurs during a severe asthma exacerbation. Minimal or no air movement requires immediate intervention.

Note the presence and location of adventitious breath sounds such as crackles, wheezes, or rhonchi. Document the presence of a pleural friction rub (a low-pitched, grating sound), a sound resulting from inflammation of the pleura.

Palpation

Palpate the chest for any abnormalities. In the older, less severely ill, and cooperative child, assess for tactile fremitus. Using the palm of the hand, palpate over the lung regions in the same manner as for auscultation and percussion while the child says "ninety-nine." Increased vibrations elicited during this maneuver are associated with consolidating conditions, such as pneumonia.

Percussion

Percuss the interspaces of the chest between the ribs in the same systematic fashion as with auscultation. Normally, percussion over an air-filled lung reveals resonant sounds. Note the presence of hyperresonance, which may indicate an acute problem such as a pneumothorax or a chronic disease such as asthma. In contrast, percussion sounds will be dull over a lobe of the lung that is consolidated with fluid, infectious organisms, and blood cells, as in the case of pneumonia.

LABORATORY AND DIAGNOSTIC TESTING

Use continuous pulse oximetry if respiratory status is a concern. Note and report oxygen saturation levels below 95% (see Chapter 18 for additional information about the use of the pulse oximeter).

Additional tests may reveal:

- Arterial or capillary blood gases: hypoxemia, hypercarbia, altered pH
- Chest radiograph: alterations in normal anatomy or lung expansion, or evidence of pneumonia, tumor, or foreign body
- Metal detector: evidence of coins (Gilger & Jain, 2022)

> **TAKE NOTE!**
>
> Children with cardiac conditions resulting in cyanosis often have baseline oxygen saturations that are relatively low because of the mixing of oxygenated with deoxygenated blood.

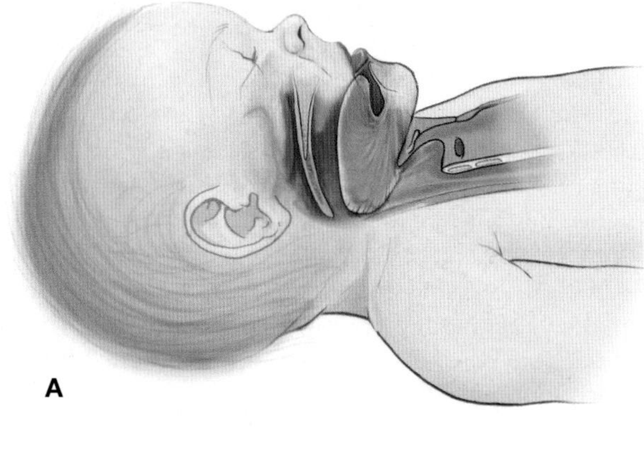

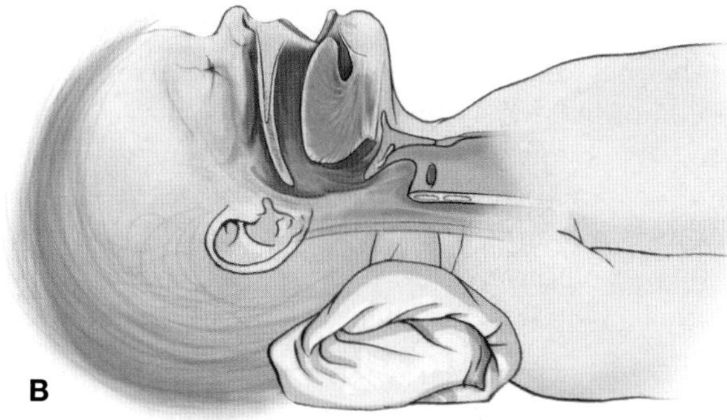

FIGURE 29.3 **A.** The infant and young child's prominent occiput encourages flexion of the neck and may result in airway occlusion. **B.** Putting a towel roll under the shoulders or neck helps to open the infant's or young child's airway by placing it in the neutral or "sniff" position.

Nursing Management

The basic principle of pediatric emergency care and PALS is the prevention of cardiopulmonary arrest (AHA & AAP, 2020). Therefore, the nurse must rapidly assess and appropriately manage children who have signs of respiratory distress. Nursing management of the child in respiratory distress involves maintaining a patent airway, providing supplemental oxygen, monitoring for changes in status, and in some cases assisting ventilation. In addition to providing these lifesaving measures and monitoring the child's progress, offer support and education to the child and family.

MAINTAINING A PATENT AIRWAY

When a child exhibits signs of respiratory distress, make a quick decision about whether it will be safe to allow the child to stay with the parent or whether the child must be placed on the examination table or bed. For example, in the case of croup, the child will often breathe more comfortably and experience less stridor while in the comfort of the parent's lap. Many children in respiratory distress often are most comfortable sitting upright, as this position helps to decrease the work of breathing by allowing appropriate diaphragmatic movement. In contrast, a child with a decreasing level of consciousness may need to be placed in the supine position to facilitate positioning of the airway.

The infant may benefit from a small towel folded under the shoulders or neck (Fig. 29.3). Avoid neck flexion or hyperextension, which may completely occlude the infant's airway. In children older than age 1 year, the optimal method for opening the airway is to hyperextend the neck (AHA & AAP, 2020). If a cervical spine injury is not suspected, use the head tilt–chin lift technique to open the airway. If the child has suffered head or neck trauma and cervical spine instability is a concern, use the jaw-thrust maneuver by placing three fingers under the child's lower jaw and lifting the jaw upward and outward (Fig. 29.4). In either case, never place the hand under the neck to open the airway.

Often the nurse encounters an acutely ill child who cannot maintain an airway independently but may be able to do so with some assistance. For example, sometimes simply opening the airway and moving the tongue

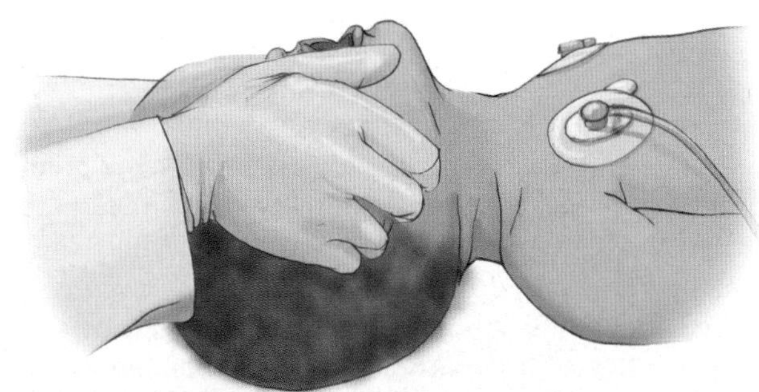

FIGURE 29.4 Jaw-thrust technique for opening the airway.

COMPARISON CHART 29.1 Oropharyngeal Versus Nasopharyngeal Airways

Oropharyngeal airway (used only in unconscious children)	• Consists of a simple plastic curved body that has a central air channel to allow for aeration • Is used when an unconscious child has difficulty maintaining airway patency due to upper airway obstruction, such as from the tongue • Allows for oral suction • Determine the correct size of the airway by placing it next to the child's cheek with the tip pointing down. An airway that is too large will extend past the angle of the child's mandible and can obstruct the glottic opening when inserted. • Choose the airway that best fits the child to decrease the risk of injury to the structures of the mouth.
Nasopharyngeal airway (may be used in conscious children and children who have an intact gag reflex)	• Consists of a flexible curved tube that is inserted nasally • Is used when the child has difficulty maintaining airway patency due to tongue obstruction or palate problems, when neurologic impairment causes poor pharyngeal tone, or in the child with impaired consciousness • Allows for nasopharyngeal suction • When selecting this airway, keep in mind that the diameter of the airway should not be so large that it puts too much pressure on the internal nasal tissue. There are two common methods for measuring this airway: (a) measure the distance from the end of the child's nose to the tragus of the ear; (b) look at the child's fifth digit, which is usually the approximate diameter of the nasopharyngeal airway. • Monitor for mucosal irritation, nasal septum swelling, and laceration of the adenoids. • Do not use this type of airway in children with a history of bleeding disorders and basilar skull fractures. • This airway's small diameter can easily become obstructed with secretions and blood.

away from the tracheal opening is all that is required to regain airway patency. In certain conditions, a nasopharyngeal or oropharyngeal airway may be necessary for airway maintenance. Comparison Chart 29.1 provides additional information about these types of airways.

ASSISTING VENTILATION USING A BVM

The child in respiratory distress may ventilate poorly, hypoventilate, or tire and become apneic. In this case, the child may require assistance with ventilation through BVM ventilation. Refer to Table 29.3 for additional information on BVM ventilation, tracheal **intubation** (the insertion of a tube into the trachea for the purposes of ventilation), the use of an anesthesia bag or flow-inflating ventilation system, and laryngeal mask airways.

BVM ventilation is used in the management of children who cannot ventilate or oxygenate effectively on their own. This technique is a more efficient way of

TABLE 29.3 • Airway and Ventilation Methods

Method	Description	Comments
Anesthesia bag or flow-inflating ventilation systems	A small, collapsible bag that consists of a reservoir bag, an overflow port, and a fresh gas inflow port	• Adjustment of the oxygen flow and of the outlet control valve is necessary. • Useful in providing positive end-expiratory pressure (PEEP) or continuous positive airway pressure (CPAP) • Adequate training and significant skill are needed to properly operate this device. • Hypercapnia and barotrauma may result with improper use. • Used more commonly in the postanesthesia care unit (PACU) and in the neonatal intensive care unit
Bag-valve-mask device or manual resuscitator	A self-inflating oxygen delivery bag that does not require an oxygen source for resuscitation and ventilation. The bag can be connected to oxygen to provide higher oxygen levels than room air. When the child exhales, the nonrebreathing valve closes, allowing exhaled, deoxygenated air to escape.	• Effective in providing oxygen to a child who is in severe respiratory distress or who has suffered a respiratory arrest • A more efficient method of respiratory resuscitation than mouth-to-mouth resuscitation; decreased rescuer exposure to communicable disease • Most medical personnel can be trained to perform resuscitation with this method • Possibly tiring for the rescuer when used to ventilate a child for long periods of time (see discussion on bag-mask ventilation)

(continued)

TABLE 29.3 • Airway and Ventilation Methods (*continued*)

Method	Description	Comments
Laryngeal mask airway	An inflatable silicone mask and rubber connecting tube that is inserted blindly into the airway, forming a seal	• The airway is introduced into the pharynx and advanced until it meets resistance; balloon cuff is then inflated. • Easier insertion than an endotracheal tube • Usually used in the unconscious child who benefits from bag-valve-mask ventilation but does not require intubation • Improvement in child comfort
Endotracheal intubation	A plastic tube inserted in the trachea to establish and maintain an airway when the airway cannot be maintained effectively using other measures (e.g., nasal trumpet or bag-valve-mask ventilation)	• Skilled medical professional (health care provider, nurse practitioner, respiratory specialist, emergency medical technician, or health care provider's assistant) necessary for insertion • The nurse acts as a valuable assistant during the intubation procedure.

ensuring ventilation than using only supplemental oxygen. In addition, resuscitating a child in this manner is superior to mouth-to-mouth resuscitation as it provides higher oxygen concentrations and protects the nurse from exposure to oral secretions (AHA & AAP, 2020). However, this technique requires proper training and practice. The proper procedure involves appropriate opening of the airway followed by providing breaths with the BVM.

Ventilation with the BVM may be performed with either one or two rescuers. First, choose an appropriate-sized bag and a corresponding facemask that fits the infant or child. Self-inflating bags are usually available in neonatal, infant, child, and adult sizes. Corresponding masks are available. Choose a facemask that properly fits the child's face and that provides a seal over the nose and mouth and excludes the eyes, thus preventing any pressure on the eyes (Fig. 29.5).

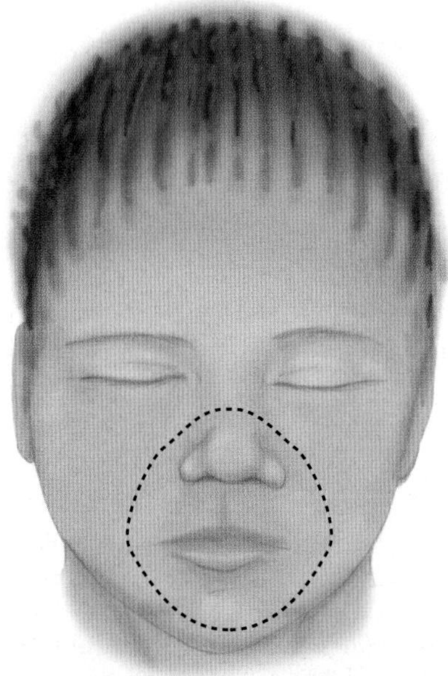

FIGURE 29.5 The mask should form a seal over the nose and mouth, across the chin and nose bridge.

TAKE NOTE!

Facemasks should be clear so that the nurse can see the child's lip color and identify any emesis during resuscitation.

Connect the BVM via the tubing to the oxygen source and turn on the oxygen. When resuscitating infants and children, set the flow rate at approximately 10 L/min. For an adolescent who is adult sized, set the flow rate at 15 L/min or higher to compensate for the larger volume bag. Check to make sure that the oxygen is flowing through the tubing to the bag. Self-inflating bags do not provide free-flow oxygen out of the facemask; manual pumping of the bag is necessary. However, the bags have a corrugated plastic tail that allows oxygen to freely flow. Therefore, check over the tail for oxygen flow through the bag.

After opening the airway appropriately (see earlier), place the mask over the child's face. When one rescuer is providing ventilation (commonly referred to as "bagging"), the person must provide a seal with the mask over the child's face with one hand and use the other hand to manipulate the resuscitator bag. The hand used to provide the mask seal will simultaneously maintain the airway in an open position. Generally, use the left thumb and index finger to hold the mask on the child's face. While maintaining a good seal with the mask, use upward pressure on the jaw angle while pressing downward on the mask below the child's mouth to keep the mouth open (Fig. 29.6). Take care not to put pressure on the neck with the fourth and fifth fingers.

If adequate personnel are available, a more desirable situation involves one person standing behind the child's head to maintain an open airway and to provide a seal of the mask over the face with a hand on each side (usually the thumbs and second fingers). A second rescuer stands on one side of the child and compresses the bag to ventilate the child using both hands. If the child is more difficult to ventilate, the two-rescuer method allows the ventilating nurse to provide better ventilation

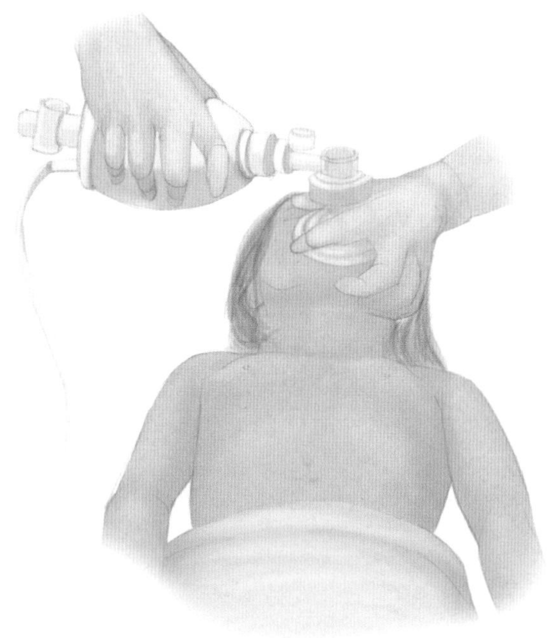

FIGURE 29.6 Proper hand placement for maintaining airway and adequate mask seal using one-rescuer technique.

than with the one-rescuer method. In addition, the two-rescuer method ensures the best possible mask seal, as the rescuer holding the mask can use both hands to maintain the seal.

Regardless of the number of people present, proper placement of the facemask is critical, and a good seal must be maintained throughout the resuscitation. In addition, during ventilation, use only the force and tidal volume necessary to cause a chest rise, no more. If a good chest rise is not observed, attempt to open the airway again. It may be necessary to adjust the position of the airway a few times to achieve a patency conducive to ventilation.

Compress the bag to deliver breaths at the amount recommended in infants and children. Initially, provide two rescue breaths and observe for a chest rise. Rescue breaths should not overinflate the lungs. Breaths should be delivered over 1 second. After the first two rescue ventilations, perform rescue breathing at a rate of one breath every 3 to 5 seconds or about 12 to 20 breaths/min. Delivering each breath should be a steady, one-inhalation-to-one-exhalation ratio. This means that the amount of time delivering the inspiratory ventilation is equal to the amount of time that expiration is allowed. While ventilating the infant or child, work with, not against, any spontaneous respiratory effort; in other words, if the child is breathing out, do not attempt to force air in at the same time.

Monitoring Effectiveness of Ventilation

During the resuscitation, continually reassess the child's response to the resuscitative efforts, noting:

- Adequacy of chest rise
- Absence or minimal presence of abdominal distention
- Improved HR and pulse oximetry readings
- Improved color
- Capillary refill less than 3 seconds with strengthening pulses

If the child's status deteriorates and they become pulseless, then CPR must be started. In addition, periodically and briefly stop ventilating to evaluate for spontaneous respirations.

Preventing Complications Related to BVM Ventilation

During resuscitation, health care personnel usually exhibit high-energy levels, a normal physiologic response that facilitates resuscitative efforts as the rescuers act quickly. However, this heightened state can lead to overzealousness while ventilating an infant or child. Health care providers may inadvertently ventilate the child too rapidly using too much tidal volume, leading to excessive ventilation volume and increased airway pressure. This poor technique can be detrimental to the child, causing:

- Reduced CO (due to increased intrathoracic pressure and increased cardiac afterload)
- Air trapping
- **Barotrauma** (trauma caused by changes in pressure)
- Air leak (thus reducing the oxygen delivered to the child)

Thus, nurses must be mindful of their technique during bagging, not exceeding the recommended respiratory rate or providing too much tidal volume to the child. Ventilate the child in a controlled and uniform manner, providing just enough volume to result in a chest rise.

Assisting With Ventilation Using Tracheal Intubation

ET intubation is needed if the infant or child does not have a maintainable airway or will require artificial ventilation for a prolonged time (see Table 29.3). Intubation of infants and children is a procedure that requires great skill and therefore should be performed by only the most qualified and experienced personnel. Children are most commonly intubated orally, rather than nasally, in acute situations.

Nurses are an essential part of the intubation team, usually assisting a health care provider, nurse practitioner, respiratory therapist, or health care provider's assistant during the intubation procedure (Nursing Procedure 29.1). The nurse may set up the equipment, prepare and administer intubation medications, or assist with suctioning the oral secretions and preparing the tape to secure the ET tube. In a child in full arrest, the nurse might be responsible for performing ongoing chest compressions while other team members manage the child's airway.

NURSING PROCEDURE 29.1 Assisting With Endotracheal Intubation

1. Prepare equipment and supplies.
2. Draw up medications (for rapid sequence intubation).
3. Turn up the volume on the cardiac monitor so that members of the team can easily hear the audible QRS indication of the child's heart rate and note any bradycardia with the procedure.
4. Turn on the suction. Make sure that suction is working by placing your hand over the tubing before you attach the suction catheter.
5. Continue to ventilate the child with the bag-valve-mask (BVM) and 100% oxygen as the team prepares to intubate the child.
6. When there is no suspected cervical spine injury, in the child older than age 2 years, place a small pillow under the child's head to facilitate opening of the airway; this step is unnecessary in children younger than age 2 due to the prominence of their occiput.
7. When assisting with the intubation, stand beside the child's head and prepare to assist with suctioning of oral secretions, providing BVM ventilation as needed, and assisting with securing the tube with tape.
8. Before the initial intubation attempt and after each subsequent attempt to intubate, provide several inhalations of 100% oxygen via the BVM ventilation method (optimally for a few minutes).
9. Administer premedication and medications for sedation.
10. Administer paralyzing medication.
11. Observe as the health care professional who is intubating the child follows the recommended procedure for intubation using the laryngoscope to visualize the vocal cords.

Setting Up Equipment

Appropriate setup and preparation of equipment is essential (Table 29.4). The ET tube size used depends on the child's size. To calculate ET tube size, divide the child's age by 4 and add 4. The resulting number will indicate the size of the ET tube in millimeters. For example, if the child is 2 years old, the proper-sized tube would be 4.5 ([2/4] + 4 = 4.5). Always have one size smaller ready also, so have a 4.0 and a 4.5 ET tube for this child.

TABLE 29.4 • Equipment and Supplies for Endotracheal Intubation

Laryngoscope blades	Straight blades (Miller) are usually used for infants and young children. A curved-blade laryngoscope (Macintosh) may be used for older children and adolescents. The blade has a little light bulb attached to it for visualization of the trachea. The light bulb should be bright and attached securely.
Endotracheal tubes	Three sizes should be readily available: the estimated size, a size smaller, and a size larger. A stylet may be used to guide the tube through the child's vocal cords (it is then removed after the intubation procedure).
Oxygen	100% oxygen is provided using a bag-valve-mask before intubation and after unsuccessful intubation attempts.
Suction	Properly working wall or portable suction with appropriate-sized suction catheters (that fit the endotracheal tube) should be prepared; the package is opened, leaving the sterile-tipped end inside the package, and connecting the other end to the suction tubing. A Yankauer suction catheter (large catheter) should also be available if copious secretions are present in the mouth that interfere with the ability to visualize the airway.
Monitors	Pulse oximeter and cardiac monitor with an audible tone indicating the QRS complex should be in place. Exhaled CO_2 device is needed to detect increased CO_2 levels after the intubation.
Nasogastric (NG) tube	Placing an NG tube will help to mitigate abdominal distention. Children who are manually ventilated typically have some abdominal distention as some air passes into the stomach.
Personal protective equipment	Usually, just gloves, goggles, and a mask are necessary to protect health care workers. In the case of copious bleeding, health care workers should wear gowns also.
Tape, etc.	Tape should be prepared for securing the tube. Benzoin, a sticky substance, is usually applied under the tape for enhanced security of the tape. For children who have had multiple intubations, a protective barrier (as used to protect the skin around an ostomy) may be applied under the tape to protect the skin. Gauze pads should be available to clean up excess secretions that may interfere with taping the endotracheal tube.

Administering Medications

Several medications are often used to facilitate intubation of children. Premedicating a child before passing an ET tube aids in:

- Reducing pain and anxiety (consistent with the concept of atraumatic care)
- Minimizing the effects of passing the ET tube down the airway (vagal stimulation leading to **bradycardia** [decrease in HR])
- Preventing hypoxia
- Reducing intracranial pressure
- Preventing airway trauma and aspiration of stomach contents

The use of medications during the intubation process is known as rapid sequence intubation (Table 29.5). Typically, these medications are used in controlled settings such as the emergency department or the intensive care unit (ICU). Rapid sequence intubation is done only in children who are not experiencing cardiac arrest. If the intubation is expected to be particularly difficult, paralyzing medication should not be used.

The nurse must be aware of the differences in the various medication classes, their advantages, their disadvantages, and adverse effects. The nurse must also be able to distinguish between medications that produce sedation and ones that produce analgesia. Children who are paralyzed and sedated may be suffering severe pain. The pain control needs of children who are acutely ill are of paramount importance and cannot be overstated. Do not mistake a child who is immobilized as a result of sedative and paralytic medications for a child who is pain free.

TABLE **29.5** • Medications for Rapid Sequence Intubation

Medications	Desired Effects	Undesirable Effects
Anticholinergic: atropine	Decreases respiratory secretions and mitigates the vagal effects of intubation, thus decreasing the risk of bradycardia	Doses that are too low (<0.1 mg) can cause a paradoxical bradycardia. Young infants are more prone to the bradycardic effects of atropine, so its use is generally contraindicated in this population.
Sedatives: barbiturates—thiopental (short-acting barbiturate)	Has very rapid onset and short duration of action; reduces intracranial pressure and oxygen demand	Hypotensive effects of this drug are more severe in the dehydrated child. When given in combination with narcotics, respiratory depression is potentiated.
Sedatives: benzodiazepines—midazolam	Has a slightly slower onset than thiopental but is associated with fewer adverse effects Also causes amnesia Can be titrated up or down (at lower doses, it causes conscious sedation; at higher doses, it can induce anesthesia)	When given in combination with narcotics, respiratory depression is potentiated.
Anesthetic agent: ketamine	Has a rapid onset with sedative, amnesic, and analgesic effects. Can be dissociative (child is awake but unaware). May improve BP and cause bronchodilation (helpful for children with status asthmaticus)	Ketamine can cause increased intracranial pressure and increased ocular pressure. Therefore, children who have suffered head trauma or globe injury should not receive this medication. Because of ketamine's sympathetic effects, hypertension can result from its use. Ketamine tends to cause increased secretions, often necessitating the concomitant use of atropine to counteract this adverse effect. May cause hallucinations and is therefore contraindicated in children with psychiatric problems.
Anesthetic agent: lidocaine	Can decrease intracranial pressure at higher doses Has an advantage when used in the management of hypovolemia because it is less likely to cause hypotension	Lidocaine can cause adverse cardiac effects (bradycardia, hypotension, dysrhythmias) in high doses. May be associated with CNS depression and seizures
Narcotic analgesic: fentanyl citrate	A highly concentrated opioid that causes fewer adverse effects (e.g., pruritus) than other opioids Also exerts a less hypotensive effect	Constipation and urinary retention (as is common with opioids) may occur. Increases risk for respiratory depression, increased intracranial pressure, and hypotension Chest wall rigidity is common with this drug and may cause difficulty with ventilation.

(*continued*)

TABLE 29.5 • Medications for Rapid Sequence Intubation (*continued*)

Medications	Desired Effects	Undesirable Effects
Paralyzing or neuromuscular blocking agents: rocuronium, succinylcholine, vecuronium	Used for short-term paralysis during the intubation process. May be used for extended paralysis in the ICU for children in whom movement would be detrimental. For example, a child with epiglottitis has a very precarious airway and must remain intubated until the epiglottis decreases in size. In certain respiratory conditions, spontaneous respiratory effort would interfere with the ventilation of a child, and therefore prolonged paralysis is desirable.	Succinylcholine (a depolarizing agent) has always been the gold standard for paralysis because it has a relatively rapid onset and is short acting. However, it has a greater risk of adverse effects (bradycardia, hyperkalemia, hypertension, increased intracranial, and ocular pressure) and is contraindicated in a variety of clinical conditions. The contemporary approach to paralysis involves the use of longer acting agents, such as rocuronium and vecuronium, because children have fewer adverse effects with these medications. In addition, rocuronium and vecuronium may be used for extended paralysis (not an option with succinylcholine).

BP, blood pressure; CNS, central nervous system; ICU, intensive care unit.

Data from American Heart Association & American Academy of Pediatrics. (2020). *Pediatric advanced life support provider manual.* American Heart Association; UpToDate, Inc. (2024). *UpToDate Lexidrug* (Version 8.2.0) [Mobile app]. Wolters Kluwer. https://apps.apple.com/us/app/lexicomp/id313401238

TAKE NOTE!

Attempts to insert an ET tube should last no longer than 20 to 30 seconds each. After each attempt, the child should receive multiple ventilations by the BVM method using 100% oxygen (AHA & AAP, 2020).

Ensuring and Maintaining Correct Tube Placement

To assess for correct placement once the ET tube is inserted, apply the end-tidal CO_2 monitor to check for placement. Also observe for symmetric chest rise and auscultate over the lung fields for equal breath sounds. Inspect the ET tube for the presence of water vapor on the inside, indicating that the tube is in the trachea. To rule out accidental esophageal intubation, auscultate over the abdomen while the child is being ventilated: There should not be breath sounds in the abdomen. Note improvement in the oxygen saturation level via pulse oximetry.

Once ET tube placement is verified, mark the tube with an indelible pen at the level of the child's lip and secure it with tape. Document the number on the ET tube at the level of the child's mouth. Anticipate a chest radiograph to confirm the correct placement of the ET tube.

After placement is confirmed, the ET tube is connected to the ventilator by respiratory personnel. The ventilator will provide continuous artificial ventilation and oxygenation. Exhaled CO_2 monitoring is recommended as it provides an indication of appropriate ventilation (Box 29.1); the exhaled CO_2 should register yellow.

The nurse plays a key role in ensuring that the ET tube remains taped securely in place by doing the following:

- Using soft wrist restraints if necessary to prevent the child from removing the ET tube
- Providing sedative and/or paralyzing medications
- Using caution when moving the child for radiographs, changing linens, and performing other procedures

Monitoring the Child Who Is Intubated

Provide ongoing and frequent monitoring of the intubated child to determine the adequacy of oxygenation and ventilation as noted earlier. Once the child is intubated, the ventilatory support being provided should result in improvement in oxygen saturation and vital signs. If the child begins to exhibit signs of poor oxygenation, perform a quick assessment. Auscultate the lungs for equal air entry and determine the HR. Are the breath sounds equal? Is the HR normal for age? Perform a quick survey of the equipment and look for any disconnected tubes or kinks in the tubing. Determine oxygen saturation levels via pulse oximeter and evaluate the end-tidal

BOX 29.1 Exhaled CO_2 Monitoring or End-Tidal CO_2 Monitoring

- Device that connects to the child's ventilator circuit to detect CO_2 in the tubing. CO_2 should be noted in the tubing after six ventilations.
- Devices are usually color coded. In the case of endotracheal intubation, observe the color on the device change from purple to tan to yellow.
- Colors on the end-tidal CO_2 device correspond with endotracheal tube placement:
  - Purple = little or no CO_2 detected, <3 mm Hg
  - Tan = 3 to 15 mm Hg exhaled CO_2
  - Yellow = >15 mm Hg exhaled CO_2 (Krauss et al., 2024)
- NOTE: Colorimetric end-tidal CO_2 devices may at times fail to detect the presence of exhaled carbon dioxide, so continue to rely upon visualization of tube placement, symmetric chest rise, and bilateral breath sounds.

(AHA & AAP, 2020)

CO_2 color (see Box 29.1). Use the mnemonic "DOPE" for troubleshooting when the status of a child who is intubated deteriorates:

- D = Displacement. The ET tube is displaced from the trachea.
- O = Obstruction. The ET tube is obstructed (e.g., with a mucous plug).
- P = Pneumothorax. Usually, a pneumothorax results in a sudden change in the child's assessment. The signs of a pneumothorax include decreased breath sounds and decreased chest expansion on the side of the pneumothorax. Subcutaneous emphysema may be noted over the chest. In the case of tension pneumothorax, there may be a sudden drop in HR and BP.
- E = Equipment failure. Relatively simple problems as previously discussed, such as a disconnected oxygen supply, can cause the child to deteriorate. Culprits such as a leak in the ventilator circuit or a loss of power are other types of equipment failure that may be responsible (AHA & AAP, 2020).

Make sure all equipment is appropriately connected and functional. When obstruction with secretions is suspected, suction the ET tube. If the ET tube is displaced from the trachea, remove the tube if it remains in the child's mouth and begin BVM ventilation. In the case of pneumothorax, prepare to assist with needle thoracotomy.

Preparing the Intubated Child for Transport

Once the child is stabilized with a secure ET tube in place, prepare to transport the child. The child will be moved by stretcher to an ICU in the acute care facility or by air or land ambulance to another facility that specializes in the care of acutely ill children. Make sure that all tubes are taped securely. During transport, use portable oxygen and ventilate manually with the BVM. As the sending nurse, ensure that all laboratory results are obtained and provided to the receiving nurse. If the child is going to another facility, complete a detailed summary of the resuscitation or provide a copy of the nurse's and/or progress notes. Complete the appropriate transfer forms as determined by the institution.

If the child is being transported by ambulance, the parents may not be able to accompany their child. In this case, find out as much as possible about the transport and assist the parents by giving directions to the receiving institution.

SHOCK

Shock may be defined as an inability for blood flow and oxygen delivery to meet the metabolic demands of tissue (Herchline & Gaw, 2023). If shock is left untreated, cardiopulmonary arrest will result. Shock, which may be classified as compensated or decompensated, is due to a variety of clinical problems. Compensated shock occurs when poor perfusion exists without a decrease in BP. In decompensated shock, inadequate perfusion is accompanied by a drop in BP. Unchecked decompensated shock leads to cardiac arrest and death. The principles of PALS stress the early evaluation and management of children in compensated shock with the goal of preventing decompensated shock (Herchline & Gaw, 2023). Once the child in shock is hypotensive, organ perfusion is dramatically impaired, and a dire clinical scenario ensues.

Pathophysiology

Shock is the result of dramatic respiratory or hemodynamic compromise. Impaired CO, impaired systemic vascular resistance (SVR), or a combination of both causes shock. CO is equal to HR times ventricular stroke volume (SV) (CO = HR × SV). SV is how much blood is ejected from the heart with each beat. SV is related to left ventricular filling pressure, the impedance to ventricular filling, and myocardial contractility. Left ventricular filling pressure is also known as preload, and the impedance to ventricular filling is commonly called afterload. Young children and infants have relatively small SVs compared to older children and adults. Therefore, infants and young children differ from their adult counterparts in that their CO depends on their HR, not their SV. Clinically, in cases of circulatory compromise and compensated shock in infants and children, HR is increased. The exception to this is a paradoxical phenomenon in neonates, who may have bradycardia rather than tachycardia.

SVR or afterload is the impediment to the heart's ventricular ejection. Increased SVR will result in a decrease in blood flow unless the ventricular pressure increases. Increased vascular resistance is a common problem in shock. In children who have shock-related increased SVR, CO will fall unless the ventricle can compensate by increasing pressure. In cardiac insufficiency, the child's heart will have an impaired ability to compensate for the increased afterload.

Altered microcirculatory status is common in all types of shock. Compensatory mechanisms are activated in response to decreased blood flow. Sympathetic nervous system response results in marked contraction of larger vessel sphincters and arterioles. This compression results in dramatically impaired capillary blood flow. Blood is redirected away from less important body systems, such as the skin and the kidneys, to the vital organs (the heart and brain).

During compensated shock, the body can maintain some level of blood flow to the vital organs. Peripheral vasoconstriction, the body's compensatory response to diminished blood flow, often results in the child's ability to maintain a normal or near-normal BP. As shock continues, capillary beds become obstructed by cellular debris, and platelets and white blood cells aggregate. Endothelial damage occurs as a result of capillary congestion. Poor blood flow to the capillaries results in anaerobic metabolism. Lactic acid accumulates, and this can lead to acidosis. In addition, children with septic shock sustain marked endothelial damage as a result of exposure to bacterial toxins.

The cumulative effect of capillary obstruction and dramatically impaired blood flow is tissue ischemia. As tissue ischemia progresses, the child will show signs of altered perfusion to vital organs. For example, as blood flow to the brain is diminished, the child will demonstrate an altered level of consciousness. Altered blood flow to the kidneys will result in decreased urine output or absence of urine output (oliguria). Commonly, HR will increase in the early stages of shock, but as the heart becomes compromised as a result of poor perfusion, the child will become bradycardic. The child will demonstrate an increased respiratory rate in the initial phase of shock. Tachypnea is seen in septic shock as well. In fact, the child may demonstrate marked hyperventilation in an effort to blow off carbon dioxide in response to the acidosis that is associated with septic shock.

Types of Shock

The most common types of shock are hypovolemic, septic, cardiogenic, and distributive. Hypovolemic shock, the most common type of shock in children, occurs when systemic perfusion decreases as a result of inadequate vascular volume (Peterson & Schuh, 2023). Children commonly have hypovolemic shock that occurs in association with fluid losses. For example, hypovolemic shock may occur with gastroenteritis that results in vomiting and diarrhea, medications such as diuretics, and heat stroke. Other causes of hypovolemia in children include blood loss, such as from a major injury, and third spacing of fluid, such as with burns.

Septic shock is related to a systemic inflammatory response in which there may be increased CO with a low SVR, known as warm shock. More commonly in children, septic shock results in a decrease in CO with an increase in SVR, known as cold shock.

Cardiogenic shock results from an ineffective pump, the heart, with a resultant decrease in SV. Children with structural heart disease and resultant dysrhythmia are at risk for cardiogenic shock (Peterson & Schuh, 2023).

Distributive shock is the result of a loss in the SVR. A relative hypovolemia occurs, most often with neurogenic injury–related shock and anaphylaxis. In relative hypovolemia, the vascular compartment expands due to systemic vasodilation. This results in a relatively larger vasculature requiring more fluid to maintain CO despite no actual loss of fluid.

Finally, toxic drug ingestions may also lead to shock.

Nursing Assessment

Nursing assessment of the child in shock includes the health history and physical examination as well as laboratory and diagnostic testing. The nursing assessment must be performed quickly and accurately so that resuscitation can be expedited.

Health History

In shock, the health history is based on the child's presentation. Children with shock are critically ill and require emergent intervention. Therefore, the history is obtained as lifesaving interventions are provided. Determine when the child first became ill and treatments that have been given thus far. Inquire about sources of volume loss, such as:

- Vomiting
- Diarrhea
- Decreased oral intake
- Blood loss

Ask when the child last urinated. Investigate for other related symptoms such as behavioral changes or lethargy. Has the child had a fever or rash, complained of headache, or been exposed to anyone with similar symptoms? Inquire about day care attendance and whether the family has recently traveled outside of the country. Determine if the child has a history of a congenital heart defect or other heart condition or if the child has severe allergies. Ask the parent about accidental ingestion of medications or other substances and, for the older child or adolescent, about the possibility of illicit substance use.

Physical Examination

The key to successful shock management is early recognition of the signs and symptoms. Obtain vital signs, noting any alterations. Measure BP, although this is not a reliable method of evaluating for shock in children. Children tend to maintain a normal or slightly less than normal BP in compensated shock while sacrificing tissue perfusion until the child suffers a cardiopulmonary arrest. Therefore, other components of the circulatory evaluation will be more valuable when assessing a child.

TAKE NOTE!

Bradycardia is a serious sign in neonates and may occur with respiratory compromise, circulatory compromise, and/or overwhelming sepsis (Aziz et al., 2021).

As with any emergency, determine the presence of a central pulse, if not present begin compressions. Evaluate the airway; is it patent? Then determine if the child is breathing. The child in shock will often demonstrate signs of respiratory distress, such as grunting, gasping, nasal flaring, tachypnea, and increased work of breathing. Auscultate breath sounds to determine the adequacy of air entry and airflow. If the child shows signs of respiratory distress, manage the airway and breathing problem first, as discussed earlier in the chapter.

Assess the skin color. Palpate the skin temperature and determine the quality of pulses. Except in special cases, such as distributive shock, the child in shock will generally have darker and cooler extremities with delayed capillary refill. Note the line of demarcation if present. This refers to the point on the distal extremity where cool temperature begins (the proximal portion of the extremity may continue to be warm). In distributive shock, the initial assessment will reveal full and bounding pulses and warm, erythemic skin. Evaluate the pulse quality. Distal pulses will likely be weaker than central pulses.

Evaluate the child's hydration state and check skin turgor. Decreased elasticity is associated with hypovolemic states, though this is usually a late sign. Observe the child's face; in compensated shock, the child may be awake but obtunded and demonstrate signs of distress. The child in decompensated shock may have their eyes closed and may be responsive only to voice or other stimulation. Evaluate pupillary responses. Determine urinary output, which will be decreased in the child with shock.

After having evaluated and provided initial lifesaving management for airway, breathing, and circulation, evaluate the child's entire body for other disabilities. Injuries warrant vigilant evaluation for ongoing blood loss, although they may also produce internal blood loss (e.g., a femur fracture). Look for signs of malformation, swelling, redness, or pain of the extremities, which may suggest internal blood loss. Also inspect for any open wounds and active sites of bleeding. Children with abdominal injuries also may lose copious amounts of blood internally. Inspect the abdomen for redness, skin discoloration, or distention. Auscultate for bowel sounds in all four quadrants.

Laboratory and Diagnostic Testing

As the child is being resuscitated, laboratory tests and radiographs will be ordered and obtained. However, no diagnostic test should replace the priority of respiratory support, vascular access, and fluid administration. Laboratory results will guide ongoing management. Common laboratory and diagnostic tests used for children with shock include:

- Blood glucose levels: usually performed at the bedside using a glucose meter to obtain a rapid result
- Electrolytes: to evaluate for electrolyte abnormalities
- CBC with differential: to assess for viral or bacterial infection (septic shock) and to evaluate for anemia and platelet abnormalities
- Blood culture: to evaluate for sepsis; preliminary results will not be available for 1 to 2 days
- CRP: to evaluate for infection
- ABGs: to assess oxygen and carbon dioxide levels and to provide information about acid–base balance
- Toxicology panel (if ingestion is suspected)
- Lumbar puncture: to evaluate the cerebrospinal fluid for meningitis
- Urinalysis: to evaluate for glucose, ketones, and protein; concentration (specific gravity) is increased in dehydration states.
- Urine culture: to evaluate for urinary tract or kidney infection
- Radiographs: to evaluate heart size; to evaluate the lungs for pneumonia or pulmonary edema (present with cardiogenic shock)

Nursing Management

Signs of shock in children warrant an emergent response.

Managing the Child's ABCs

Always evaluate and manage the airway and breathing and check for pulses. Initiate CPR if the child is pulseless. All children who have signs and symptoms of shock should receive 100% oxygen via mask. If the child has poor respiratory effort or is apneic, administer 100% oxygen via BVM or ET tube (refer to the "Respiratory Arrest" section for more specific information about the management of airway and breathing). As part of ongoing monitoring, institute cardiac and apnea monitoring and assess oxygen saturation levels via pulse oximetry.

Obtaining Vascular Access

Once the airway and breathing are addressed, nursing management of shock focuses on obtaining vascular access and restoring fluid volume. Children with signs of shock should receive generous amounts of isotonic IV fluids rapidly. However, obtaining vascular access in critically ill children can be challenging. Vascular access must be obtained using the quickest route possible in children whose condition is markedly deteriorated, such as those in decompensated shock.

Various forms of vascular access available for the management of the critically ill child include:

- Peripheral IV route: a large-bore catheter is used to give large amounts of fluid. This route may not be feasible in children with significant vascular compromise.
- Central IV route: central lines can be inserted into the jugular vein and threaded into the superior vena cava.

The femoral route is best for obtaining central venous access while CPR is in progress because the insertion procedure will not interfere with lifesaving interventions involving the airway and cardiac compressions. The subclavian vein, located under the clavicle, is an alternative route for central access.

- Saphenous vein: the saphenous vein (found in the ankle) is an alternative route for venous access that is obtained using a surgical incision.
- Intraosseous access: intraosseous access, obtained by cannulating the bone marrow, is recommended in cases of decompensated shock or cardiac arrest if IV access cannot be attained rapidly. The preferred site is the anterior tibia. Special intraosseous needles are used (generally a 15-gauge needle for older children, 18-gauge for younger children). The needle is inserted using a firm twisting motion slightly away from the growth plate. Any medications or fluids that can be administered using an IV site can be given using this route. Alternative sites include the femur, the iliac crest, the sternum, and the distal tibia.

Restoring Fluid Volume

Administer IV isotonic fluids, such as LR or NS (the isotonic fluids of choice) rapidly. Administer 20 mL/kg of the prescribed fluid as a bolus, infusing the fluid as rapidly as possible. In general, a large-bore syringe, such as a 35- to 60-mL syringe attached to a three-way stopcock, is the preferred method for rapid fluid delivery in children. Infusing the fluid via gravity is too slow. The fluid bolus may be repeated up to two times (for a total of three times) if required.

TAKE NOTE!

Dextrose solutions are contraindicated in shock because of the risk of complications such as osmotic diuresis, hypokalemia, hyperglycemia, and worsening of ischemic brain injury (AHA & AAP, 2020).

Children in septic shock will often require larger volumes of fluid as a result of the increased capillary permeability. Children in shock due to trauma will usually receive a colloid, such as blood, when there is an inadequate response to crystalloid isotonic fluid. After each fluid bolus, reassess the child for signs of positive response to the fluid administration.

Insert an indwelling urinary catheter to allow for accurate and frequent measurement of urine output.

Indicators of improvement include:

- Improved cardiovascular status: The central and peripheral pulses are stronger. The line of demarcation of extremity coolness is diminishing and capillary refill is improved (time is decreased). BP is improved.
- Improved mental status: The child is more alert. For example, the child's eyes are open and watching personnel. If the child is younger, they may be pulling at the IV line.
- Improved urine output: This may not be noted initially but should be noted over the next few hours; the goal is 1 to 2 mL/kg/hour.

The process of fluid resuscitation involves giving the fluid, assessing, and reassessing the child, and documenting findings. Children in shock may require as much as 100 to 200 mL/kg of resuscitative fluid during the initial hours of shock management. Most children in shock need and can tolerate this large volume of fluid. Continued reassessment will determine if the child is beginning to experience fluid overload in the form of pulmonary edema (this is rare but may occur in children with preexisting cardiac conditions or severe chronic pulmonary disease) (AHA & AAP, 2020; Herchline & Gaw, 2023).

CLINICAL REASONING ALERT!

Do not focus solely on the child's circulatory status; you may overlook signs and symptoms of respiratory deterioration.

Administering Medications

In some circumstances, such as septic shock or distributive shock, fluid alone does not adequately improve the child's status and adjunctive medications may be ordered. Vasoactive medications are used either alone or in combination to improve CO and to increase or decrease SVR. The selection of medications is dictated by the child's cardiac and vascular status. For example, dobutamine is a medication with significant beta-adrenergic effects and thus can improve cardiac contractility. Epinephrine, which affects the heart muscle, is also a powerful vasoconstrictor. Dopamine affects the heart at lower doses but increasingly affects the vasculature with increased doses. These medications may be given as a loading dose, followed by a continuous infusion. When vasoactive drugs are administered, monitor for improvement in HR, BP, perfusion, and urine output. Refer to Drug Guide 29.1 for additional information.

CARDIAC DYSRHYTHMIAS AND ARREST

Unlike adults, in whom cardiopulmonary arrest is most often caused by a primary cardiac event, children typically have healthy hearts and thus rarely experience primary cardiac arrest. More commonly, they experience cardiopulmonary arrest from gradual deterioration of respiration and/or circulation (Peterson & Schuh, 2023). In particular, children experiencing a respiratory emergency or shock may deteriorate and eventually demonstrate cardiopulmonary arrest. Thus, the standard of care for managing a child in this situation is vastly different from that for an adult.

Nurses should be skilled in evaluating and managing respiratory alterations and shock in children, as discussed in previous sections. Overwhelming evidence suggests that if primary respiratory compromise or shock is identified and treated in the critically ill child, a secondary cardiac arrest can be prevented.

Rare exceptions do exist, however. For example, electrolyte abnormalities and toxic drug ingestions are primary insults to the cardiovascular system that may lead to a sudden cardiac arrest rather than a gradual progression. Other exceptions in which the child is at risk for a primary and sudden cardiac arrest include:

- History of a serious primary congenital or acquired cardiac defect
- Potentially lethal dysrhythmias such as prolonged QT syndrome
- Hypertrophic cardiomyopathy
- Traumatic cardiac injury or a sharp blow to the chest, known as "commotio cordis" (e.g., when a high-velocity ball hits the chest)

The overwhelming majority of children rarely experience cardiac dysrhythmias so it is beyond the scope of this chapter to discuss the myriad of possible complex rhythm disturbances. Therefore, this discussion will be limited to the management of emergent cardiac conditions that are more typically found in children.

Pathophysiology

The AHA and AAP (2020) have simplified the nomenclature used to describe pediatric cardiac compromise and has established three major categories of cardiac rhythm disturbances:

- Slow: bradydysrhythmia
- Fast: tachydysrhythmia
- Absent: pulseless, cardiovascular collapse

The pathophysiology, causes, and therapeutic management of each of the categories of rhythm disturbances are discussed later.

Bradydysrhythmias

Bradycardia is HR significantly slower than the normal HR for that age. Bradycardia in children is most commonly sinus bradycardia. In other words, there is not a cardiac nodal abnormality associated with the slowed HR. In sinus bradycardia, the P waves and QRS complex remain normal on the ECG. Brief dips in HRs can be normal, such as when the child sleeps. Children are also susceptible to brief drops in HR that are associated with vagal stimulation. For example, passing an orogastric tube down the esophagus of a young infant may induce a temporary bradycardic response. These normal decreases in the child's HR should recover with or without stimulation and are not normally associated with signs of altered perfusion.

Less commonly, children manifest bradycardia as a result of cardiac abnormalities and heart block. Infants with bradycardia related to heart block may exhibit poor feeding and tachypnea, whereas older children may demonstrate fatigue, dizziness, and syncope. Comparison Chart 29.2 compares the causes of sinus bradycardia and heart block in children.

In contrast, the child with a serious and possibly life-threatening bradydysrhythmia will have an HR below 60 bpm, with signs of altered perfusion. The most common causes of profound bradycardia in children are respiratory compromise, hypoxia, and shock. Sustained bradycardia is commonly associated with arrest. It is an ominous sign and should be taken seriously.

Tachydysrhythmias

Children normally have faster HRs than adults, and fever, fear, and pain are common explanations for significant increases in the HR of a child (**tachycardia**). This normal elevation in HR is known as sinus tachycardia. However, once the fever is reduced, the child is comforted, or the pain is managed, the HR should return close to the child's baseline. Hypoxia and hypovolemia are pathologic reasons for tachycardia in the child. If the child has sinus tachycardia that results from any of these causes, the focus is on the underlying cause. It is inappropriate and dangerous to treat sinus tachycardia with medications aimed at decreasing the HR or with a defibrillation device.

Tachydysrhythmias in children that are associated with cardiac compromise have unique characteristics that present differently from sinus tachycardia. Examples of these include SVT and ventricular tachycardia. SVT is a cardiac conduction problem in which the HR is extremely rapid, and the rhythm is very regular, often described as "no beat-to-beat variability." Comparison Chart 29.3 explains the differences between SVT and

COMPARISON CHART 29.2 Causes of Sinus Bradycardia Versus Heart Block

	Sinus Bradycardia	Heart Block
Causes	• Pathologic: medications such as digoxin, hypoxia, hypothermia, head injury • Nonpathologic: well-conditioned athlete	• Congenital: associated with cardiac anomalies • Acquired: endocarditis, rheumatic fever, Kawasaki disease

COMPARISON CHART 29.3 Distinguishing Supraventricular Tachycardia (SVT) From Sinus Tachycardia

	SVT	Sinus Tachycardia
Rate (bpm)	Infants >220, children >180	Infants <220, children <180
Rhythm	Abrupt onset and termination	Beat-to-beat variability
P waves	Flattened	Present and normal
QRS	Narrow (<0.08 seconds)	Normal
History	Usually, no significant history	Fever, fluid loss, hypoxia, pain, fear

sinus tachycardia. The most common cause of SVT is a reentry problem in the cardiac conduction system. Commonly, SVT is the result of a genetic cardiac conduction problem such as Wolff–Parkinson–White syndrome. SVT may also be associated with medications such as caffeine and theophylline. Children often can tolerate the characteristically higher HR that is associated with SVT for short periods of time. However, the increased demand that is placed on the cardiovascular system usually overtaxes the child and results in signs of congestive heart failure if the SVT continues unchecked for a prolonged time.

Ventricular tachycardia is a rhythm involving an elevation of the HR and a wide QRS (greater than 0.08 seconds) that is the result of an abnormal, rapid firing of one or both of the ventricles. Ventricular tachycardia is a rare dysrhythmia in children and usually is associated with a congenital or acquired cardiac abnormality. In addition, prolonged QT syndrome is a conduction abnormality that can result in ventricular tachycardia and sudden death in children. Less commonly, ingestion of medications and toxins, acidosis, hypocalcemia, abnormalities of potassium, and hypoxemia have been associated with the development of ventricular tachycardia in children.

Collapsed Rhythms (Pulseless Rhythms)

A collapsed rhythm, as defined by PALS, is one that produces cardiac arrest with no palpable pulse and no signs of perfusion (cardiac arrest) (AHA & AAP, 2020). Typically, the most common pulseless arrest rhythms in children are asystole and PEA. **Asystole** occurs when there is no cardiac electrical activity, commonly referred to as "a straight line" on the ECG. The child with PEA has some appreciable rhythm on the ECG but no palpable pulses. PEA may be caused by hypoxemia, hypovolemia, hypothermia, electrolyte imbalance, tamponade, toxic ingestion, tension pneumothorax, or thromboembolism. Ventricular tachycardia may also present as pulseless. VF, once thought to be rare in children, occurs in serious cardiac conditions in which the ventricle is not pumping effectively. It may develop from ventricular tachycardia. VF is characterized by variable, high-amplitude waveforms (coarse VF) or a finer, lower-amplitude waveform with no discernible cardiac rhythm (fine VF). In either case, CO is insufficient.

Nursing Assessment

Nursing assessment of the child with a cardiac emergency includes the health history and physical examination as well as laboratory and diagnostic testing. The nursing assessment must be performed quickly and accurately so that resuscitation can be instituted if needed.

Health History

Obtain a brief health history of the child with a cardiac emergency while simultaneously assessing the child and providing lifesaving interventions. Key areas to inquire about include:

- History of cardiac problems, asthma, chromosomal anomaly, delayed growth
- Symptoms such as syncope, dizziness, palpitations or racing heart, chest pain, coughing, wheezing, increased work of breathing
- Activity tolerance with play or feeding: Does the child get out of breath, turn blue, or squat during play? Can the child keep up with playmates? Does the infant tire with feedings?
- Precipitating illness, fever, unexplained joint pains, ingested medications
- Participation in a sport before the cardiac event occurred or injury to the chest
- Family history of cardiac problems, sudden death from a cardiac condition, heart attacks at a young age, chromosomal abnormalities
- Treatment measures performed at the scene: Was CPR initiated? Was an AED used?

Physical Examination

Quickly establish the child's status. A child who is obviously in distress or is arresting must receive emergent lifesaving interventions. Briefly perform the assessment while simultaneously providing lifesaving interventions.

INSPECTION AND OBSERVATION

Assess the child's airway patency and efficiency of breathing. Observe the child's color, noting circumoral pallor or duskiness or central pallor, mottling, duskiness, or cyanosis. Note any increased work of breathing, grunting, head bobbing, or apnea. Inspect the chest for barrel shape, which may be associated with chronic pulmonary or cardiac disease. Observe the pericardium for the presence of lifts or heaves. Note diaphoresis, anxious appearance, or dysmorphic features (almost 50% of children with Down syndrome also have a congenital cardiac defect [Marion & Levy, 2023]). Determine if neck vein distention is present. Inspect the fingertips for clubbing, which is indicative of chronic tissue hypoxemia.

AUSCULTATION

Auscultate the breath sounds, noting any crackles or wheezes. Auscultate the HR. If the child does not have an adequate pulse, initiate CPR. If the child has a strong, perfusing pulse, complete the cardiac assessment. Auscultate with the diaphragm of the stethoscope first and then listen with the bell. Evaluate all of the auscultatory areas, listening first over the second right interspace (aortic valve) and then over the second left interspace (pulmonic valve); next move to the left lower sternal border (tricuspid area); and finally auscultate over the fifth interspace, midclavicular line (mitral area). Evaluate the rate and rhythm of the heart. Listen for any extra sounds or murmurs. Note and describe the quality, intensity, and location of any cardiac murmurs.

TAKE NOTE!

Murmurs are most often systolic and can be benign or associated with pathology.

PERCUSSION AND PALPATION

Percuss between the costal interspaces and note the heart's size. Palpate the heart to find the point of maximal impulse (PMI) and to evaluate for an associated thrill. A thrill feels like a fluttering under the fingers and is associated with cardiac pathology. Palpate and note the quality of the pulses. Evaluate each of the pulses bilaterally and note whether they are absent, faint, normal, or bounding. Compare the quality of pulses on each side of the body and also those of the upper and lower body. Note the skin temperature and evaluate the capillary refill.

Laboratory and Diagnostic Testing

The major diagnostic test used is the ECG. Identify the dysrhythmia according to the ECG reading (Fig. 29.7).

Nursing Management

Provide oxygen at 100%. Institute cardiac monitoring and assess oxygen saturation levels via pulse oximetry. Obtain the child's preprinted code drug sheet or use the Broselow tape to obtain the child's height to estimate the ET tube sizes and medication dosages that are appropriate for the child. Always remember to intervene in this order: first airway, then breathing, then circulation. The remainder of this discussion will assume that the nurse has initiated interventions for airway and breathing as discussed earlier in the chapter.

TAKE NOTE!

Pay attention to the rhythm on the monitor, but continually monitor the child's pulse. If the child does not have a pulse or has a pulse of less than 60 bpm, perform cardiac compressions despite the monitor reading (AHA & AAP, 2020).

MANAGING BRADYDYSRHYTHMIAS

The management of sinus bradycardia is focused on remedying the underlying cause of the slow HR. Since hypoxia is the most common cause of sustained bradycardia, oxygenation and ventilation are necessary. The newborn is particularly susceptible to bradycardia in relation to hypoxemia. Continue to reassess the child to determine if the bradycardia improves with adequate oxygenation and ventilation. If bradycardia persists, administer epinephrine and/or atropine as ordered. Epinephrine is the drug of choice for the treatment of persistent bradycardia.

Other causes of bradycardia such as hypothermia, head injury, and toxic ingestion are managed by addressing the underlying condition. Warming the hypothermic child may restore a normal sinus rhythm. Children with head injury may have bradycardia without any cardiac involvement, and with successful management of the head injury, the bradycardia will resolve. Antidotes to toxins may be necessary in children whose bradycardia is the result of a toxic ingestion.

MANAGING TACHYDYSRHYTHMIAS

The tachydysrhythmias include SVT (stable or unstable) and ventricular tachycardia with a pulse. Examine the ECG to determine if the child is experiencing ventricular tachycardia or SVT. Clinically, determine whether the child in SVT is showing signs that require emergent intervention or if the child is stable. In compensated SVT, the child will appear to be alert, breathing comfortably, and well perfused. The child who is demonstrating signs of compromise, such as a change in consciousness, respiratory status, and perfusion, is considered to be in uncompensated SVT. Uncompensated SVT requires emergent intervention. The child who has ventricular tachycardia with a pulse will have poor perfusion and also require immediate intervention. The evaluation and approaches to the tachydysrhythmias are discussed in Table 29.6.

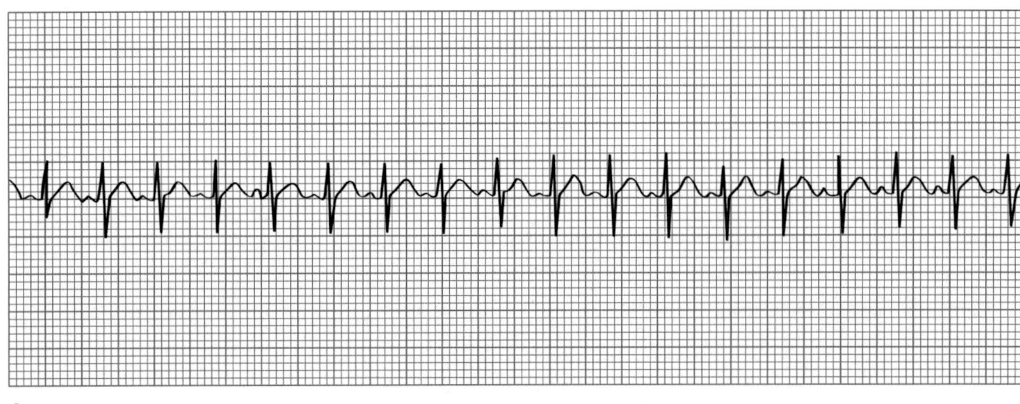

A

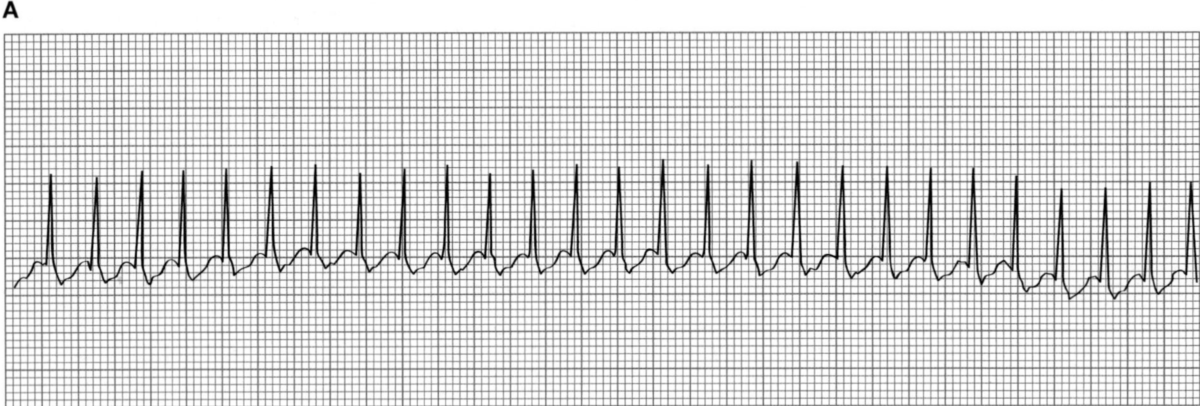

B

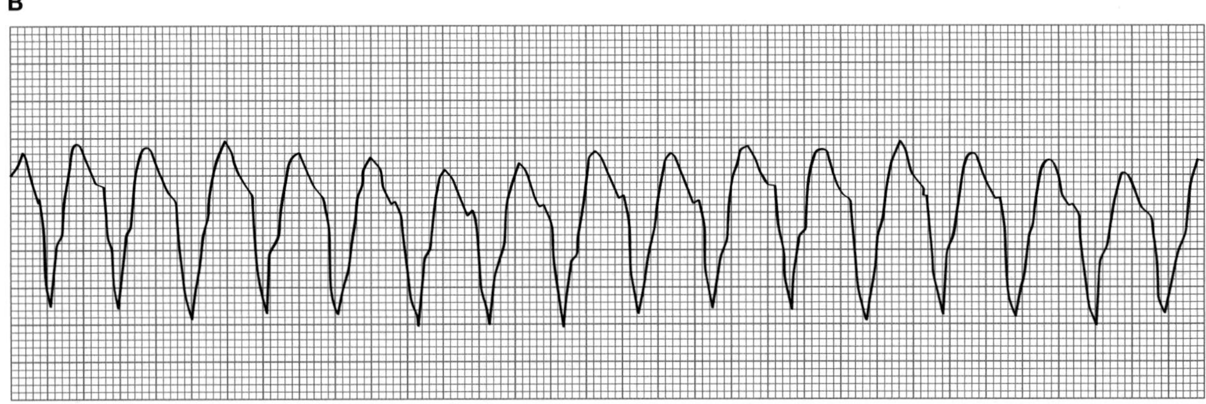

C

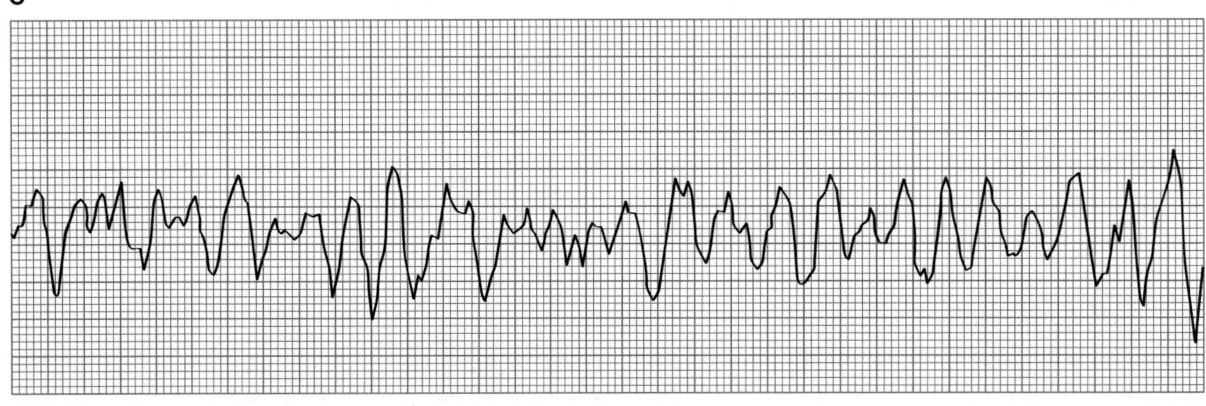

D

FIGURE 29.7 Dysrhythmias **A.** Sinus tachycardia: normal QRS and P waves, mild beat-to-beat variability. **B.** Supraventricular tachycardia: note rate above 220, abnormal P waves, no beat-to-beat variability. **C.** Ventricular tachycardia: rapid and regular rhythm, wide QRS without P waves. **D.** Coarse ventricular fibrillation: chaotic electrical activity.

TABLE 29.6 • Managing tachydysrhythmias

Tachydysrhythmia	Signs and Symptoms	Management
Compensated SVT	• Tachycardia, heart rate >220 • Abnormal P waves • Alert, well-perfused child • Possible complaints of headache and dizziness in older children	• Vagal maneuvers such as ice to face or blowing through a straw that is obstructed • Adenosine if vagal maneuvers fail
Uncompensated SVT	• Tachycardia, heart rate >220 • Abnormal P waves • Signs of shock: altered level of consciousness, poor perfusion, weak pulses	• Adenosine or synchronized cardioversion
Ventricular tachycardia	• Rate may range from normal to 200 bpm. • Wide QRS • No P waves • Pulse present, poor perfusion	• Synchronized cardioversion • IV amiodarone • Treatment of underlying causes

bpm, beats/min; IV, intravenous; SVT, supraventricular tachycardia.

Data from American Heart Association & American Academy of Pediatrics. (2020). *Pediatric advanced life support provider manual.* American Heart Association.

TAKE NOTE!

Adenosine has a rapid onset of action and an extremely short half-life. Administer it extremely rapidly with a generous amount of IV flush; otherwise, it will be ineffective (AHA & AAP, 2020).

MANAGING COLLAPSED RHYTHMS

As in any pediatric emergency, support the ABCs. Manage the airway, provide oxygen, and give fluids. In addition, if the child is pulseless or has HR less than 60 bpm, initiate cardiac compressions (see "Providing Cardiopulmonary Resuscitation" section earlier in the chapter). In addition, some children may require medications and/or defibrillation or synchronized cardioversion. The pulseless rhythms include ventricular tachycardia, VF, asystole, and PEA. ECG characteristics and management of these rhythms are summarized in Table 29.7. Also treat the underlying causes of the dysrhythmia if known.

The AHA emphasizes the importance of cardiac compressions in pulseless individuals with dysrhythmias (AHA & AAP, 2020). Give compressions before and

TABLE 29.7 • ECG Characteristics and Management of Pulseless Rhythms

Pulseless dysrhythmia	ECG Characteristics	Management
Ventricular tachycardia	Wide QRS, no P waves	• CPR • Defibrillation • Epinephrine; also possibly amiodarone, lidocaine, or magnesium • Treat underlying causes
Ventricular fibrillation	• Chaotic ventricular activity • No P waves, no QRS, no T waves	• CPR • Defibrillation • Epinephrine; also possibly amiodarone, lidocaine, or magnesium • Treat underlying causes
Asystole	Flat line	• Check lead placement • CPR if no pulse • Epinephrine
Pulseless electrical activity	Electrical activity that is not consistent with ventricular tachycardia or ventricular fibrillation.	• Check lead placement • CPR if no pulse • Treat underlying cause • Epinephrine

CPR, cardiopulmonary resuscitation; ECG, electrocardiogram.

Data from American Heart Association & American Academy of Pediatrics. (2020). *Pediatric advanced life support provider manual.* American Heart Association.

immediately after defibrillation (see "*Providing Defibrillation or Synchronized Cardioversion*" section earlier in the chapter). Administer medications such as epinephrine, lidocaine, or amiodarone as ordered. In the past, it was recommended that individuals who required defibrillation be given three shocks in a row, but recent research findings have shown that the individual should be defibrillated only once, followed by five cycles of CPR. For defibrillation to be most effective, cardiac compressions must be performed effectively with minimal interruptions (AHA & AAP, 2020).

DOSAGE CALCULATION BOX 29.1

Child's weight: 55 lb

Medication order: epinephrine 100 mg intravenous (IV) STAT

Per the *Pediatric Dosage Handbook*, the recommended dose is 0.01 mg/kg (0.1 mL/kg of 1:10,000 solution) per dose.

Is the ordered dose safe?

SUBMERSION INJURY

Water can be a great source of fun and exercise for children and adolescents, but drowning is the third-leading cause of preventable death in children and adolescents in the United States and worldwide (World Health Organization [WHO], 2023). In warm-weather states where swimming pools are more common, drowning is the primary cause of death in young people. Most drowning deaths are preventable, and the WHO (2023) notes that among younger children, lapse in adult supervision is associated with drowning.

Survival and neurologic outcome of drowning depend on early and appropriate resuscitation. In recent years, with appropriate resuscitation efforts and treatment, children have demonstrated better neurologic outcomes (Chandy & Richards, 2024).

Pathophysiology

Typically, a child who is drowning will struggle to breathe and eventually will aspirate water. Aspiration of relatively small amounts of water leads to poor oxygenation, with retention of carbon dioxide. Alveolar surfactant is depleted during the drowning event and pulmonary edema commonly occurs. Hypoxemia results in increased capillary permeability and resultant hypovolemia. Even small amounts of aspirated water may lead to pulmonary edema within an 8-hour period after the drowning episode (Chandy & Richards, 2024). A drowning survivor is also at risk for renal complications due to altered renal perfusion during the hypoxemic state.

Nursing Assessment

Nursing assessment of the drowning survivor is crucial and must take place quickly and accurately.

Health History

Obtain the history rapidly while providing lifesaving interventions. Ask about the circumstances of the event:

- Where did the incident occur? Was the child in a lake, river, ocean, or swimming pool? Was the child submerged in a toilet, bucket, or bathtub?
- Did someone witness the child's entry into the water?
- Was the water fresh or salty? Cold or warm?
- Is it likely the water was contaminated?
- Were there any extenuating circumstances, such as a diving or automobile accident, associated with the near drowning?
- What was the approximate length of time of the submersion? Was the child conscious or unconscious when rescued?
- What was done at the scene? Was CPR initiated? If so, when?
- If a cervical spine injury was suspected, was the cervical spine immobilized?
- Was an AED used?
- When did the child last eat (to prepare for possible intubation)?

Physical Examination

Evaluate airway patency and breathing. Auscultate all lung fields for signs of pulmonary edema, such as coarseness or crackles. Evaluate the HR, pulse, and perfusion. Note the cardiac rhythm on the monitor and report evidence of dysrhythmias. Evaluate the child's neurologic status. Use a pen light to determine the pupillary reaction. Use the pediatric coma score to further assess the neurologic status. Does the child open the eyes spontaneously, to stimuli, or not at all? Is there any spontaneous movement? Is the younger child crying? Can the older child speak? Measure the child's temperature, as hypothermia often occurs with near drowning.

Laboratory and Diagnostic Testing

While awaiting laboratory and diagnostic testing results, continue resuscitative efforts as addressed following. Laboratory and diagnostic tests typically include the following:

- ABGs: hypoxemia, acidosis
- ECG: cardiac dysrhythmias
- Chest radiography: pulmonary edema, infiltrates
- Serum electrolytes: imbalance related to development of shock

Nursing Management

Because of the potentially devastating effects that drowning-related hypoxia has on the child's brain, airway interventions must be initiated immediately after retrieving a child from the water. Every second counts. Initial interventions for a drowning victim are always focused on the ABCs; commonly, resuscitative efforts have begun before the child arrives at the acute care facility.

If a cervical spine injury is suspected (as in the case of a diving accident), provide stabilization either manually or with a cervical collar. As with any suspected neck injury, do not remove the cervical collar until injury to the cervical spine has been ruled out through a radiograph and clinical evaluation. Suction the airway to ensure airway patency. The child may have aspirated particles from a contaminated water source or emesis, a relatively common complication associated with drowning. A large-bore suction catheter (e.g., Yankauer) is an effective tool for clearing the upper airway. Administer supplemental oxygen at 100%. Children who have poor or absent respiratory effort most likely will require intubation. Insert an orogastric or nasogastric tube to decompress the stomach and prevent aspiration of stomach contents. Initiate chest compressions if a pulse is not present.

Usually, the child exhibits some degree of hypothermia and will require warming. Generally, the core body temperature should be raised slowly, as warming a drowning victim too quickly may have deleterious effects. Remove any wet clothing, dry the child, and cover them with warmed blankets. Warm IV fluids and use other warming methods as prescribed.

CONSIDER THIS!

A parent says to you, "I can't believe my toddler almost drowned. I turned away for a few minutes to check the hamburgers on the grill. I feel terrible. I'll never be able to let her go near a swimming pool again."

Thoughts: What will your response be to this parent? How can you best support them and assist them to work through their emotions?

POISONING

Emergency care of the pediatric poisoning victim consists of rapid nursing assessment and prompt management.

TAKE NOTE!

If a normally healthy child (particularly a young child) suddenly deteriorates without a known cause, suspect a toxic ingestion.

Nursing Assessment

Nursing assessment of the poisoning victim focuses on a thorough health history, followed by physical examination and laboratory and diagnostic testing.

Health History

Obtain the health history from the parents or caregiver or, in the case of an older child or adolescent, from the child. Inquire about the approximate time of poisoning and the nature of the toxin. Was the toxin ingested, inhaled, or applied to the skin? In the case of pill ingestion, does the caregiver have the medication bottle? Did the child experience nausea, vomiting, anorexia, abdominal pain, or neurologic changes such as disorientation, slurred speech, or altered gait? Determine the progression of the symptoms. Did the parent or caregiver call the National Poison Control Center Hotline? Has any treatment been given? In the case of older children and adolescents, inquire about any history of depression or threatened suicide.

TAKE NOTE!

The National Poison Control Center Hotline number is 1-800-222-1222.

Physical Examination

Ingestion of medications or chemicals may result in a wide variety of clinical manifestations. Perform a thorough physical examination, noting alterations that may occur with particular ingestions, such as:

- Hyper- or hypotension
- Hyper- or hypothermia
- Respiratory depression or hyperventilation
- Miosis (pupillary contraction) or mydriasis (pupillary dilatation)

Pay particular attention to the child's mental status, skin moisture and color, and bowel sounds (Velez et al., 2022).

Laboratory and Diagnostic Testing

The suspected poison may direct the laboratory and diagnostic testing. A variety of blood tests may be performed:

- Chemistry panel: to detect hypoglycemia or metabolic acidosis and assess kidney function
- ECG: to identify dysrhythmias or conduction delay
- Liver function tests: to assess for liver injury
- Urine and blood toxicology screens (available for a limited number of medications; may vary per institution)
- Specific drug levels if the substance ingested is known or highly suspected

Nursing Management

When poisoning occurs, give priority to the child's ABCs. Treat alterations as discussed earlier in this chapter. Monitor vital signs frequently and provide supportive care. Few specific antidotes are available for medications or other toxins. Activated charcoal may be administered to bind with the chemical substance in the bowel. Alternatively, whole bowel irrigation with polyethylene glycol electrolyte solutions may be necessary. Occasionally, dialysis is required to lower the level of toxin in the bloodstream. The intervention is based on the source of the ingestion. For example, activated charcoal is an effective method for preventing the absorption of many medications but is not effective in the case of an iron overdose.

If opiate or other narcotic ingestion is suspected, administer naloxone to reverse the respiratory depression or altered level of consciousness. Treatment of seizures and alterations in thermoregulation may also be needed.

Specific treatment of the poisoning will be determined when the toxin is identified, and poison control is queried. Maintain ongoing assessment of the poisoned child because many toxins exhibit very late effects.

TAKE NOTE!

Syrup of ipecac is not recommended for home treatment to induce vomiting after an accidental ingestion (AAP, 2021).

TRAUMA

The leading cause of death in children and adolescents is unintentional injuries (Centers for Disease Control and Prevention [CDC], n.d.). Automobile accidents continue to be a top cause of death in all child age groups (CDC, n.d.). Childhood trauma also results from pedestrian accidents, sporting and bicycling injuries, and firearm use. Children of varying ages are susceptible to various forms of injury due to their developmental level as well as their environmental exposure. Young children rely on their caregivers to promote their safety. Young children also are not developmentally equipped to be able to recognize dangerous situations. Because pediatric injury is so common, nurses must become adept at assessment and intervention in the pediatric trauma victim.

Nursing Assessment

The trauma survey includes a brief health history as the child is being assessed and lifesaving measures are being instituted.

Health History

Begin the health history by asking when the injury happened. If the child sustained a motor vehicle–related injury, ask how fast the vehicle was going. Determine if the child was appropriately restrained in the automobile. If the child was riding a bicycle, was skateboarding, or using in-line skates, were they wearing a helmet, kneepads, and wrist guards? Determine what interventions were performed at the scene. Was the child immobilized on a backboard to protect the cervical spine? If the child is bleeding, ask the person who transported the child to estimate the amount of blood lost.

If the child experienced a fall, ask if the fall was witnessed and the height from which the child fell. Did the child fall onto a hard surface such as concrete? How did the child land: on the head or back, or did the child catch themselves with the hands? Males are at higher risk for injuring their heads (CDC, 2023). Did the child lose consciousness at the scene? What kind of behavior did the child exhibit after the fall? Since the fall, has the child complained of a headache or been vomiting?

While obtaining a detailed history of the fall, think about the child's developmental stage. For example, does it seem plausible that a toddler might fall down the stairs? In contrast, what is the likelihood that a 2-month-old would suffer a fractured femur from a fall? Keep in mind the possibility of child abuse. Critically evaluate the reported circumstances and try to determine if the history, developmental stage of the child, and type of injury sustained match. In addition, evaluate the type of injury that the child sustained, and the history given by the caregiver. For example, children who fall from significant heights often suffer skeletal fractures, but abdominal and chest injuries rarely result from falling from significant heights.

Physical Examination

Physical examination of the child with a traumatic injury should be approached with an evaluation of the ABCs (primary survey) first. Assess the patency of the airway and establish the effectiveness of breathing (as discussed earlier in the chapter). Examine the child's respiratory effort, breath sounds, and color. Next, evaluate the circulation. Note the pulse rate and quality. Observe the color, skin temperature, and perfusion. If bleeding has occurred, the child's circulation may become compromised.

After assessing and intervening for the child's ABCs, proceed to the secondary survey. Assess for disability (D). Rapidly assess critical neurologic function. Determine the level of consciousness, pupillary reaction, and verbal and motor responses to auditory and painful stimuli. If the child is a young infant, palpate the anterior fontanel: A full and bulging fontanel signals increased intracranial pressure. The traumatized child's neurologic status may range from completely normal to comatose.

TAKE NOTE!

Unequal pupils or a fixed and dilated pupil is considered a neurosurgical emergency. Immediately report this finding.

Following the ABCs and D (disability) is E (exposure). Expose the child to observe the entire body for signs of injury, whether blunt or penetrating. Perform a systematic, thorough inspection of the child's body. Note active bleeding and extremity deformity, as well as any lacerations and abrasions. Observe for movement and any complaints of immobility or pain with movement. Inspect the abdomen for redness, skin discoloration, or distention. Auscultate for bowel sounds in all four quadrants. If the child is verbal, ask if they have any pain in the stomach. If the child is younger, ask, "Do you have a tummy ache?" If the child reports abdominal pain, ask the child to point to where it hurts. Note any guarding of the abdomen, which is an indication of abdominal pain. If bowel injury is a possibility, only light palpation is acceptable. Always assess the least tender areas first and palpate the more sensitive areas last.

Laboratory and Diagnostic Testing

As in other pediatric emergencies, never delay lifesaving measures to wait for laboratory or diagnostic test results. In addition to routine laboratory tests, common laboratory and diagnostic tests for the pediatric trauma victim include:

- Type and cross-match: to assess the child's blood type before blood products are given
- Prothrombin time and partial thromboplastin time: to evaluate for clotting dysfunction
- Amylase and lipase: to identify pancreatic injury
- Liver function tests: to assess for liver injury
- Pregnancy test (as appropriate)
- CT scan, ultrasound, or MRI of the head, abdomen, or extremities: to evaluate the extent of the injury

Nursing Management

Nursing management of the pediatric trauma victim focuses initially on the ABCs.

Providing Immediate Care

If head or spinal injury is suspected, open the airway using the jaw-thrust maneuver with cervical spine stabilization (see Fig. 29.4). The guidelines for basic life support recommend that if the airway cannot be opened using the jaw-thrust maneuver, it may be opened using the head tilt–chin lift maneuver since opening the airway is a priority (AHA & AAP, 2020). The head and neck of a trauma victim should be stabilized manually.

TAKE NOTE!

Infants and young children require unique cervical spine management because they have prominent occiputs that result in flexion of the neck in the supine position. To maintain the optimal neutral spinal position in the young child, use a special pediatric backboard with a head indentation, or use a folded towel to elevate the child's torso.

Clear the airway of obstruction using a large-bore suction device such as a Yankauer. If the child is breathing on their own, give oxygen at the highest flow possible (such as with a nonrebreathing mask). If the child is not breathing on their own, intervene with basic life support discussed earlier in this chapter (AHA & AAP, 2020).

If a BVM device is available, connect it to the oxygen source and use the bag to ventilate the child. Observe the chest rise and be careful not to overventilate, as this results in abdominal distention. Deliver breaths at a rate of one breath every 3 seconds (AHA & AAP, 2020). Do not hyperventilate. In the not-too-distant past, head injury in children was managed using hyperventilation. This resulted in **hypocapnia** (decreased amounts of carbon dioxide in the blood). The physiologic effect of hypocapnia is the induction of vasoconstriction, which in turn results in tissue ischemia. Therefore, current management of head injury in children does not use hyperventilation. The only exception to this rule is in an acute situation, if the child is showing signs of a possible brain stem herniation, hyperventilation may be used initially and briefly.

Assess the child for a strong central pulse. If the child has no pulse, initiate CPR immediately. When perfusion is compromised, administer IV fluid resuscitation. Trauma victims are more likely to require colloids or blood products due to blood loss from the injury.

KEY CONCEPTS

- Young children's smaller airways and immature respiratory and immune systems place them at higher risk for respiratory distress than older children and adults. Children generally have healthy hearts and cardiovascular systems and thus rarely present with primary cardiac arrest. Younger children and adolescents are at higher risk for injury due to normal development at those ages.
- Children present with a variety of emergencies and injuries and must be evaluated and treated in an appropriate and timely fashion to achieve a positive outcome. The health history is obtained rapidly while lifesaving measures are performed simultaneously.

- Assess the airway, then breathing, then circulation, providing interventions for alterations before moving on to the next assessment. Provide continuous reassessment, as children respond quickly to interventions and deteriorate quickly as well.
- Pulse oximetry and capnometry can be useful tools for evaluating respiratory status. Never delay intervention pending laboratory results if the child's clinical status warrants immediate action.
- Provide support and education to the child and family involved in an emergency. Teach families why certain procedures are being done, explaining technical medical interventions in simple terms and, for the child, at their developmental level.
- Small amounts of edema or secretions can contribute to significant respiratory effort in infants and young children.
- Children dehydrate more quickly than adults and experience alterations in perfusion related to hypovolemia.
- Children in respiratory distress and shock require supplemental oxygen. Intubation is necessary for the apneic child or the child whose airway is not maintainable.
- Accurate assessment of perfusion status and appropriate fluid resuscitation are critical in the prevention and treatment of shock in children.
- Life-threatening dysrhythmias in children, though uncommon, often must be quickly treated with defibrillation or synchronized cardioversion in addition to CPR.
- In the case of near drowning, maintain ongoing assessment and intervention of pulmonary status.
- Maintain airway, breathing, and circulation in the child who has experienced an accidental ingestion and prepare for gastric lavage or administration of activated charcoal.
- In addition to intervening for airway, breathing, and circulation problems in the pediatric trauma victim, assess for altered neurologic status and extent of bleeding or injury.

REFERENCES AND RECOMMENDED READINGS

American Academy of Pediatrics. (2021). *Using over-the-counter medicines with your child.* https://www.healthychildren.org/English/safety-prevention/at-home/medication-safety/Pages/Using-Over-the-Counter-Medicines-With-Your-Child.aspx

American Heart Association & American Academy of Pediatrics. (2020). *Pediatric advanced life support provider manual.* American Heart Association.

Aziz, K., Lee, H. C., Escobedo, M. B., Hoover, A. V., Kamath-Rayne, B. D., Kapadia, V. S., Magid, D. J., Niermeyer, S., Schmölzer, G. M., Szyld, E., Weiner, G. M., Wyckoff, M. H., Yamada, N. K., & Zaichkin, J. (2021). Part 5: Neonatal resuscitation 2020 American Heart Association guidelines for cardiopulmonary resuscitation and emergency cardiovascular care. *Pediatrics, 147*(Supplement 1), e2020038505E. https://doi.org/10.1542/peds.2020-038505E

Bush, R. N., & Woodley, L. (2022). Increasing nurses' knowledge of and self-confidence with family presence during pediatric resuscitation. *Critical Care Nurse, 42*(4), 27–37. https://doi.org/10.4037/ccn2022898

Centers for Disease Control and Prevention. (2023a). *QuickStats: percentage of children and adolescents aged ≤17 years who had ever received a diagnosis of concussion or brain injury,† by sex and age group—National Health Interview Survey,§ United States, 2022.* https://www.cdc.gov/mmwr/volumes/72/wr/mm7233a5.htm#suggestedcitation

Centers for Disease Control and Prevention. (n.d.). *10 leading causes of death, United States, 2021, both sexes, all ages, all races.* https://wisqars.cdc.gov/pdfs/leading-causes-of-death-by-age-group_2021_508.pdf

Chandy, D., & Richards, D. (2024). Drowning (submersion injuries). *UpToDate.* Retrieved April 10, 2024, from https://www.uptodate.com/contents/drowning-submersion-injuries

Corbett, J. A., & Banks, A. D. (2019). *Laboratory tests and diagnostic procedures with nursing diagnoses* (9th ed.). Pearson Education Inc.

Fuch, S. M. (2018). *AAP policy says more people need access to life support training, AEDs.* https://www.aappublications.org/news/2018/05/23/lifesupport052318

Gilger, M. A., & Jain, A. K. (2022). Foreign bodies of the esophagus and gastrointestinal tract in children. *UpToDate.* Retrieved April 10, 2024, from http://www.uptodate.com/contents/foreign-bodies-of-the-esophagus-and-gastrointestinal-tract-in-children

Graham, J., & Peoples, M. (2019). Nursing student knowledge and compliance with SIDS prevention strategies. *Infant, 15*(1), 29–32. https://www.infantjournal.co.uk/pdf/inf_085_ude.pdf

Herchline, D. J., & Gaw, C. E. (2023). Shock and sepsis. In R. Tenney Soerio & E. P. Devon (Eds.), *Netter's pediatrics* (2nd ed.). Elsevier.

Janhunen, K., Kankkunen, P., & Kvist, T. (2019). Quality of pediatric emergency care as assessed by children and their parents. *Journal of Nursing Care Quality, 34*(2), 180–184. https://doi.org/10.1097/NCQ.0000000000000346

Jones, M. A. (2023). Preparing an office practice for pediatric emergencies. *UpToDate.* Retrieved April 10, 2024, from https://www.uptodate.com/contents/preparing-an-office-practice-for-pediatric-emergencies

Krauss, B., Falk, J. L., & Ladde, J. G. (2024). Carbon dioxide monitoring (capnography). *UpToDate.* Retrieved April 10, 2024, from https://www.uptodate.com/contents/carbon-dioxide-monitoring-capnography

Marion, R. W., & Levy, P. A. (2023). Human genetics and dysmorphology. In K. J. Marcdante, R. M. Kliegman, & A. M Schuh (Eds.), *Nelson's essentials of pediatrics* (9th ed.). Elsevier.

Peterson, T. L., & Schuh, A. M. (2023). The acutely ill or injured child. In K. J. Marcdante, R. M. Kliegman, & A. M. Schuh (Eds.), *Nelson's essentials of pediatrics* (9th ed.). Elsevier.

Ring, L. M., Rana, M. S., & Deutsch, N. (2023). Implementation of a non-sedated procedural pain management practice guideline and order set. *Pediatric Nursing, 49*(1), 12–20.

Shaw, K. N., & Bachur, R. G. (Eds.). (2020). *Fleisher and Ludwig's textbook of pediatric emergency medicine* (8th ed.). Wolters Kluwer.

UpToDate, Inc. (2024). *UpToDate Lexidrug* (Version 8.2.0) [Mobile app]. Wolters Kluwer. https://apps.apple.com/us/app/lexicomp/id313401238

Velez, L. I., Shepherd, J. G., & Goto, C. S. (2022). Approach to the child with occult toxic exposure. *UpToDate.* Retrieved April 10, 2024, from http://www.uptodate.com/contents/approach-to-the-child-with-occult-toxic-exposure

World Health Organization. (2023). *Drowning.* https://www.who.int/en/news-room/fact-sheets/detail/drowning

DEVELOPING CLINICAL JUDGMENT

PRACTICING FOR NCLEX

1. An unresponsive toddler is brought to the emergency department. Assessment reveals mottled skin color, respiratory rate of 10 breaths/min, and a brachial pulse of 52 bpm. What is the priority nursing action?
   a. Prepare the defibrillator and draw up code medications.
   b. Provide 100% oxygen with a bag-valve-mask and start chest compressions.
   c. Start chest compressions and provide 100% oxygen via a nonrebreather mask.
   d. Begin an IV fluid infusion and administer epinephrine IV.
2. A 10-year-old child in respiratory distress requires intubation. Which sizes of endotracheal tubes will the nurse prepare?
   a. 9.5 mm and 10.0 mm
   b. 8.5 mm and 9.0 mm
   c. 6.0 mm and 6.5 mm
   d. 6.5 mm and 7.0 mm
3. A preschooler presents to the emergency department with a history of vomiting, diarrhea, and fever over the past few days. She is receiving 100% oxygen via a nonrebreather mask. Vital signs are temperature 104.5°F, pulse 144 bpm, respiratory rate 22 breaths/min, and BP 70/50 mm Hg. She is listless and difficult to arouse and has weak peripheral pulses and prolonged capillary refill. What nursing intervention takes priority?
   a. Administering acetaminophen rectally for the high fever
   b. Administering IV antibiotics for the infection
   c. Preparing the child for endotracheal intubation
   d. Giving an IV bolus of NS 20 mL/kg
4. Assessment of a 12-year-old who crashed his bicycle without a helmet reveals the following: temperature 99.2°F, pulse 100 bpm, respiratory rate 24 breaths/min with easy work of breathing, and BP 102/70 mm Hg. What is the priority action by the nurse?
   a. Assess neurologic status while observing for obvious injuries.
   b. Administer IV fluid bolus of NS at 20 mL/kg.
   c. Remove the cervical collar if he complains that it bothers him.
   d. Listen for bowel sounds while assessing for pain.
5. An 18-month-old child is brought to the emergency department via ambulance after an accidental ingestion. What is the priority nursing action?
   a. Take the child's vital signs.
   b. Give oral syrup of ipecac.
   c. Insert a nasogastric tube.
   d. Start an IV line.

DOSAGE CALCULATION QUESTION

The nurse is caring for an infant with SVT who is symptomatic and has an IV line in place. The infant weighs 16½ lb. The medication order reads: adenosine 0.01 mg/kg IV STAT followed by rapid flush. Adenosine is supplied as 6 mg/2 mL. How many milliliters will the nurse administer? Round to the nearest hundredth.

CRITICAL THINKING EXERCISES

1. A school-age child presents to the emergency department for evaluation. He had been feeling faint off and on and today fainted at school. On the cardiac monitor, an abnormal cardiac rhythm is noted. At present, the child is stable. What questions would be most appropriate for the nurse to ask when obtaining the child's health history? What objective assessments should the nurse make?
2. A 2-year-old is admitted to the hospital after accidentally ingesting a medication. The parent who brought their child to the hospital is upset and crying. How does this child's age and stage of development affect the child's risk for accidental ingestion? How should the nurse respond to the parent's distress? Develop a discharge teaching plan for this child and family related to poison prevention.
3. A 7-month-old is brought to the acute care facility with a chief complaint of difficulty breathing. The infant's parent says that the cold has gotten worse, and the infant won't eat. What additional questions should the nurse ask about the infant's health history? How would the nurse appropriately manage this infant's airway?

STUDY ACTIVITIES

1. Spend a day in the pediatric emergency department or urgent care center and document the role of the triage nurse.

2. Observe the pediatric emergency medical team at work or observe a pediatric code in the hospital. Compare and contrast the measures performed for the child with those that would be performed for an adult in a similar emergency situation.
3. Develop a teaching project related to injury prevention and present it at a local elementary, middle, or high school. Ensure that the education is geared toward the children's developmental level.
4. Interview the parents of a child who has experienced an emergency situation about how they felt during and after the emergency. Present the information to your classmates.
5. When providing care to a child in an emergency, the nurse performs the following assessments. Place them in the proper sequence.
   a. Pupillary reaction
   b. Presence of cough or sputum
   c. Heart rate and capillary refill
   d. Presence of bruises and abrasions
   e. Work of breathing

APPENDIX A

Growth Charts

Birth to 24 months: Boys
Length-for-age and Weight-for-age percentiles

NAME ______________________

RECORD # __________

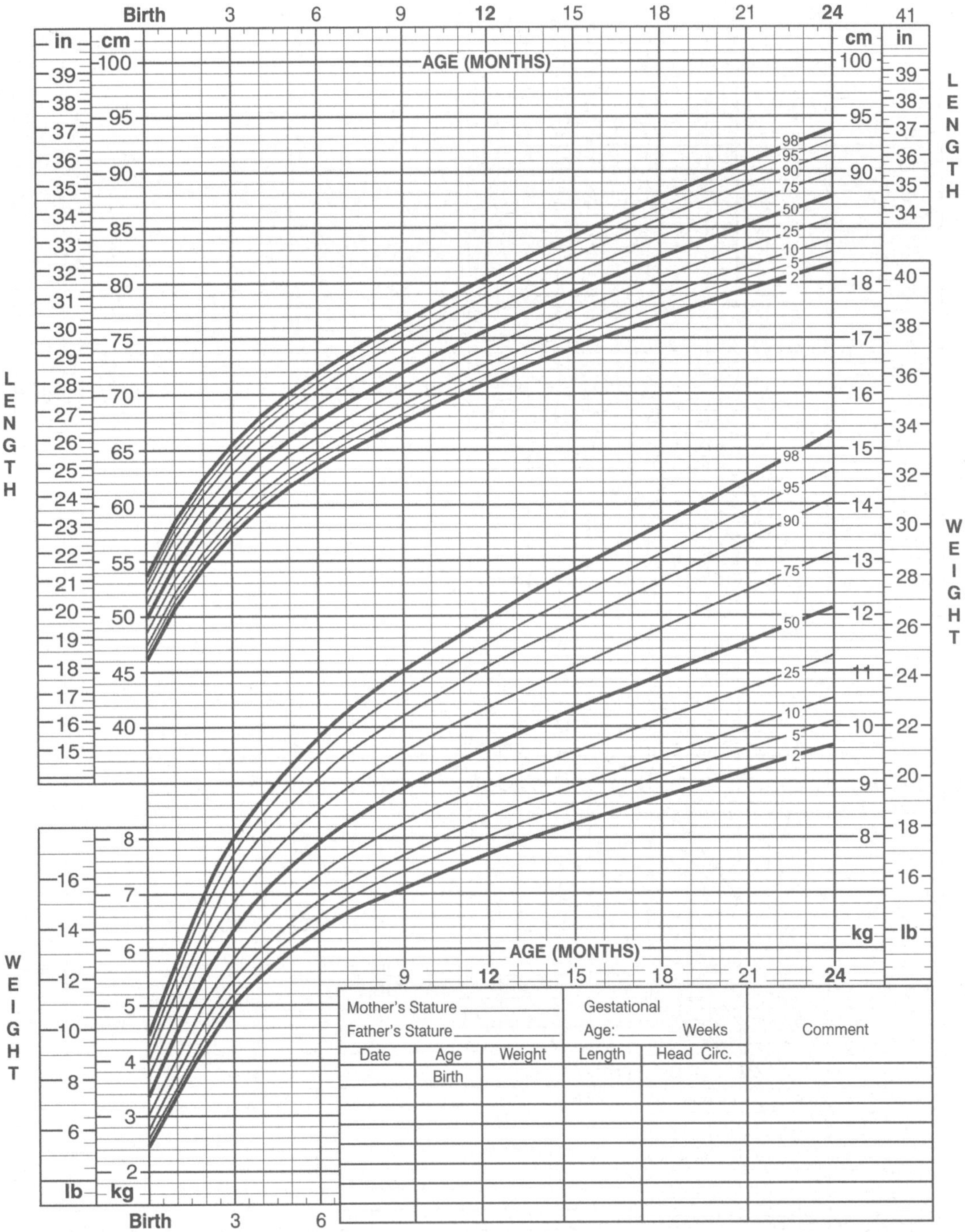

AGE (MONTHS): Birth, 3, 6, 9, 12, 15, 18, 21, 24

LENGTH (cm): 40–100; (in): 15–41

Percentiles: 2, 5, 10, 25, 50, 75, 90, 95, 98

WEIGHT (kg): 2–18; (lb): 6–40

Mother's Stature ____________

Father's Stature ____________

Gestational Age: ______ Weeks

Date	Age	Weight	Length	Head Circ.	Comment
	Birth				

Published by the Centers for Disease Control and Prevention, November 1, 2009
SOURCE: WHO Child Growth Standards (http://www.who.int/childgrowth/en)

SAFER • HEALTHIER • PEOPLE™

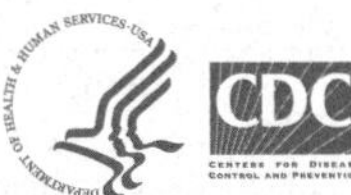

Birth to 24 months: Girls
Length-for-age and Weight-for-age percentiles

NAME ____________________

RECORD # ____________

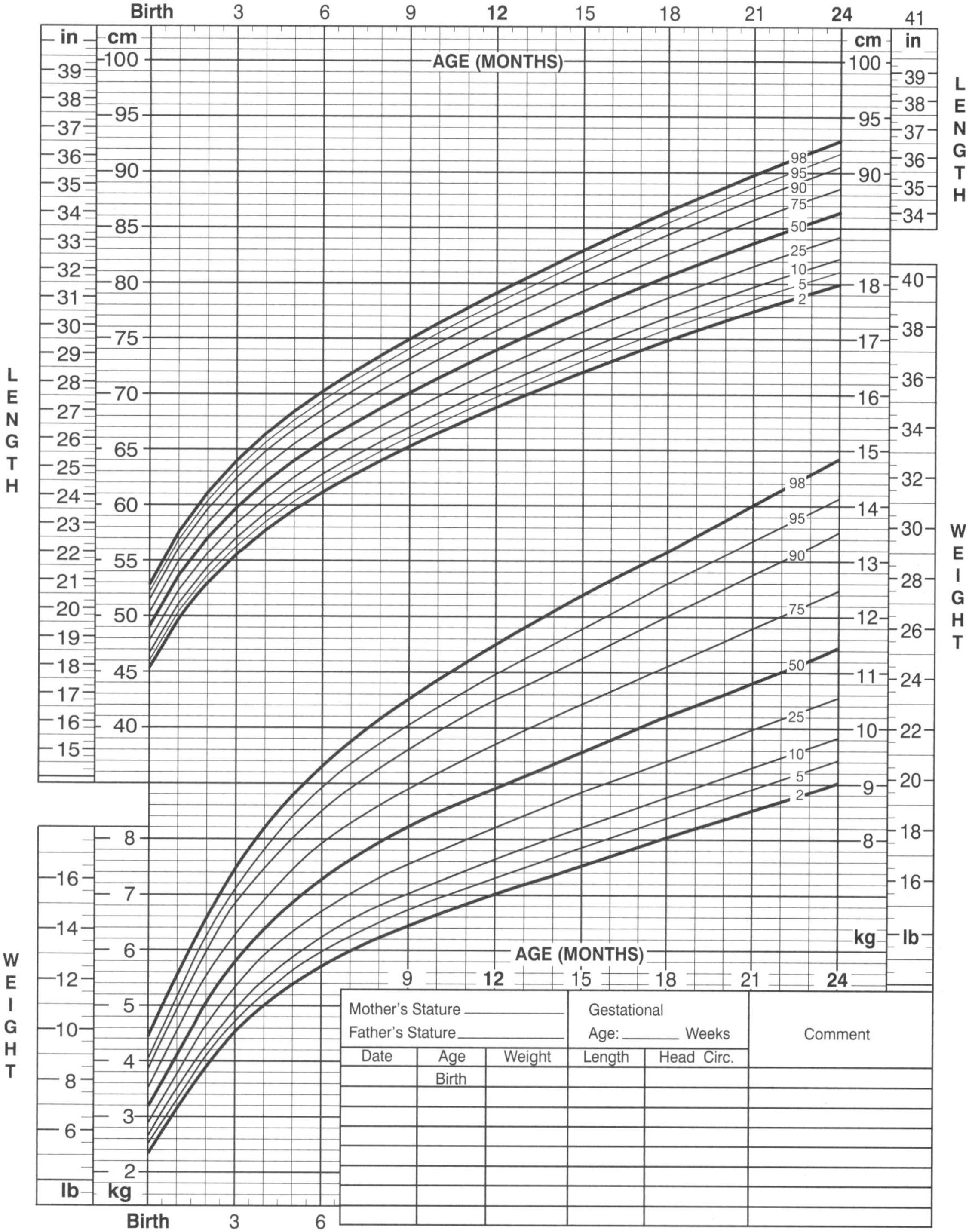

Birth 3 6 9 12 15 18 21 24

AGE (MONTHS)

in | cm — LENGTH: cm 40, 45, 50, 55, 60, 65, 70, 75, 80, 85, 90, 95, 100; in 15–39, 41

Length percentiles: 98, 95, 90, 75, 50, 25, 10, 5, 2

WEIGHT: kg 2–18; lb 6–40

Weight percentiles: 98, 95, 90, 75, 50, 25, 10, 5, 2

AGE (MONTHS) 9 12 15 18 21 24

Birth 3 6

Mother's Stature ____________			Gestational		Comment
Father's Stature ____________			Age: ________ Weeks		
Date	Age	Weight	Length	Head Circ.	
	Birth				

Published by the Centers for Disease Control and Prevention, November 1, 2009
SOURCE: WHO Child Growth Standards (http://www.who.int/childgrowth/en)

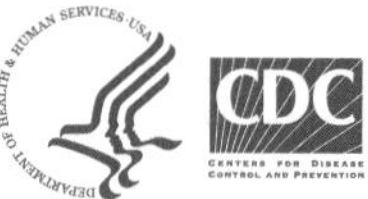

Birth to 24 months: Boys
Head circumference-for-age and Weight-for-length percentiles

NAME ______________________

RECORD # ____________

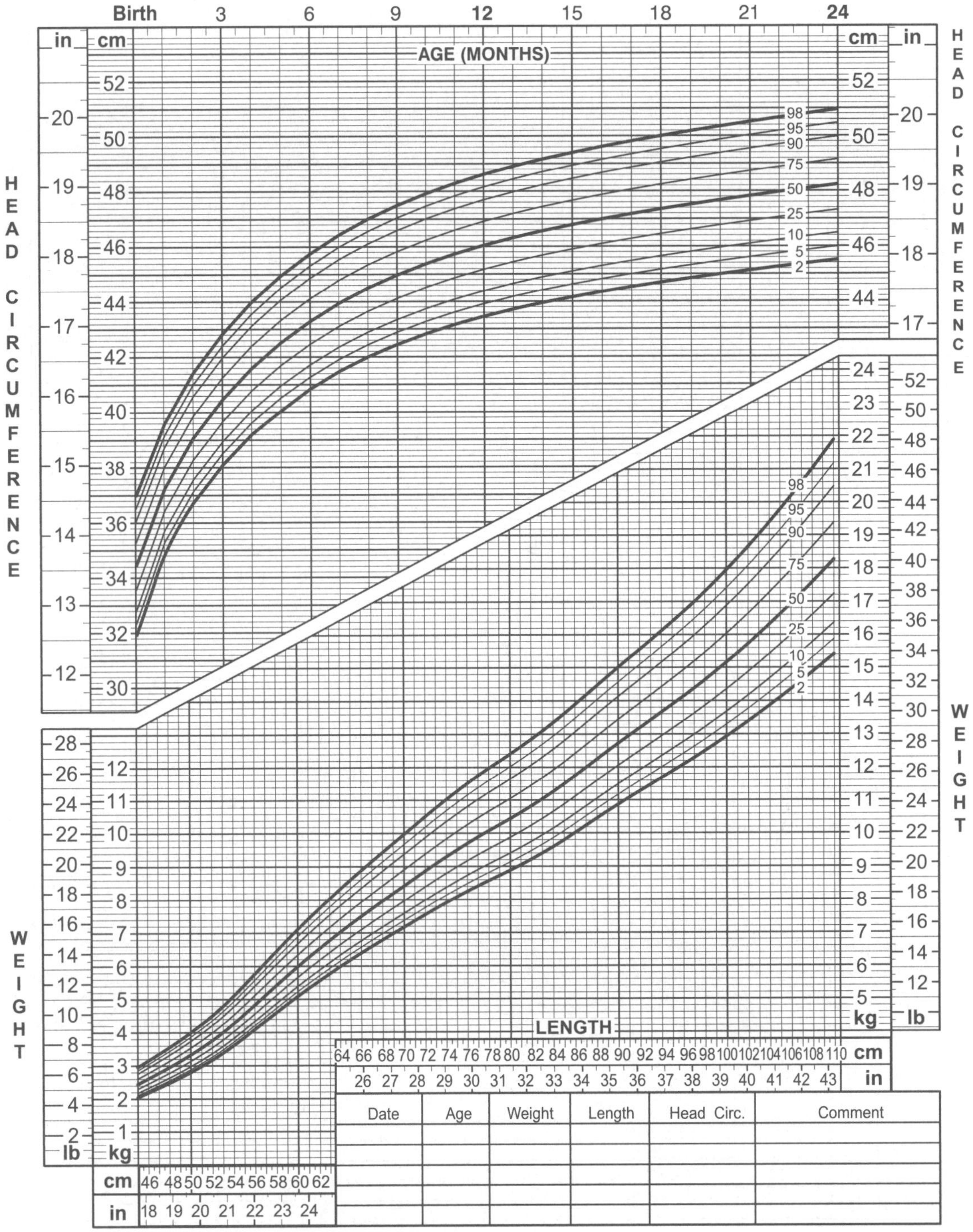

Birth 3 6 9 12 15 18 21 24

AGE (MONTHS)

HEAD CIRCUMFERENCE

in: 12 13 14 15 16 17 18 19 20

cm: 30 32 34 36 38 40 42 44 46 48 50 52

Percentiles: 98 95 90 75 50 25 10 5 2

WEIGHT

kg: 1 2 3 4 5 6 7 8 9 10 11 12 13 14 15 16 17 18 19 20 21 22 23 24

lb: 2 4 6 8 10 12 14 16 18 20 22 24 26 28 30 32 34 36 38 40 42 44 46 48 50 52

LENGTH

cm: 46 48 50 52 54 56 58 60 62 64 66 68 70 72 74 76 78 80 82 84 86 88 90 92 94 96 98 100 102 104 106 108 110

in: 18 19 20 21 22 23 24 26 27 28 29 30 31 32 33 34 35 36 37 38 39 40 41 42 43

Date	Age	Weight	Length	Head Circ.	Comment

Published by the Centers for Disease Control and Prevention, November 1, 2009
SOURCE: WHO Child Growth Standards (http://www.who.int/childgrowth/en)

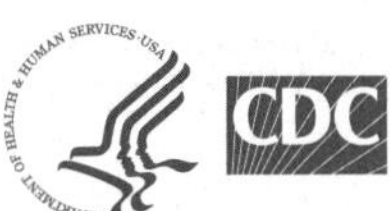

Birth to 24 months: Girls
Head circumference-for-age and
Weight-for-length percentiles

NAME ____________________

RECORD # ____________

Birth 3 6 9 12 15 18 21 24

AGE (MONTHS)

HEAD CIRCUMFERENCE

in: 12 13 14 15 16 17 18 19 20

cm: 30 32 34 36 38 40 42 44 46 48 50 52

Percentiles: 98 95 90 75 50 25 10 5 2

WEIGHT

kg: 1 2 3 4 5 6 7 8 9 10 11 12 13 14 15 16 17 18 19 20 21 22 23 24

lb: 2 4 6 8 10 12 14 16 18 20 22 24 26 28 30 32 34 36 38 40 42 44 46 48 50 52

LENGTH

cm: 46 48 50 52 54 56 58 60 62 64 66 68 70 72 74 76 78 80 82 84 86 88 90 92 94 96 98 100 102 104 106 108 110

in: 18 19 20 21 22 23 24 25 26 27 28 29 30 31 32 33 34 35 36 37 38 39 40 41 42 43

Date	Age	Weight	Length	Head Circ.	Comment

Published by the Centers for Disease Control and Prevention, November 1, 2009
SOURCE: WHO Child Growth Standards (http://www.who.int/childgrowth/en)

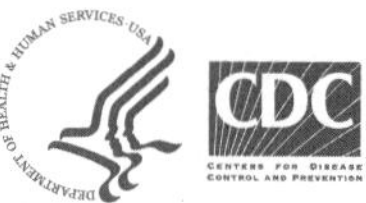

2 to 20 years: Boys
Stature-for-age and Weight-for-age percentiles

NAME ______________________

RECORD # ______________

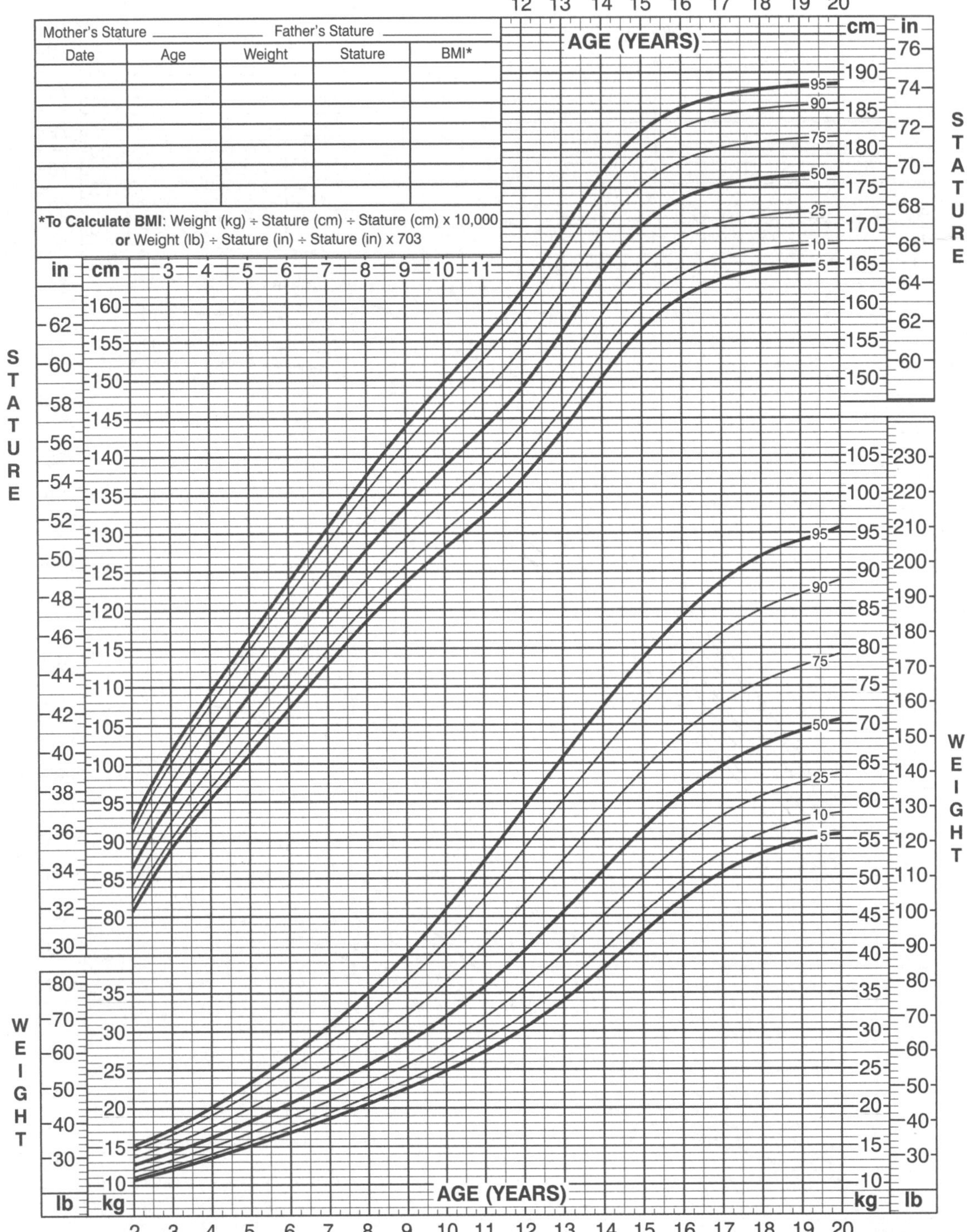

Published May 30, 2000 (modified 11/21/00).
SOURCE: Developed by the National Center for Health Statistics in collaboration with the National Center for Chronic Disease Prevention and Health Promotion (2000).
http://www.cdc.gov/growthcharts

CDC
SAFER • HEALTHIER • PEOPLE™

2 to 20 years: Girls
Stature-for-age and Weight-for-age percentiles

NAME ______________________

RECORD # ____________

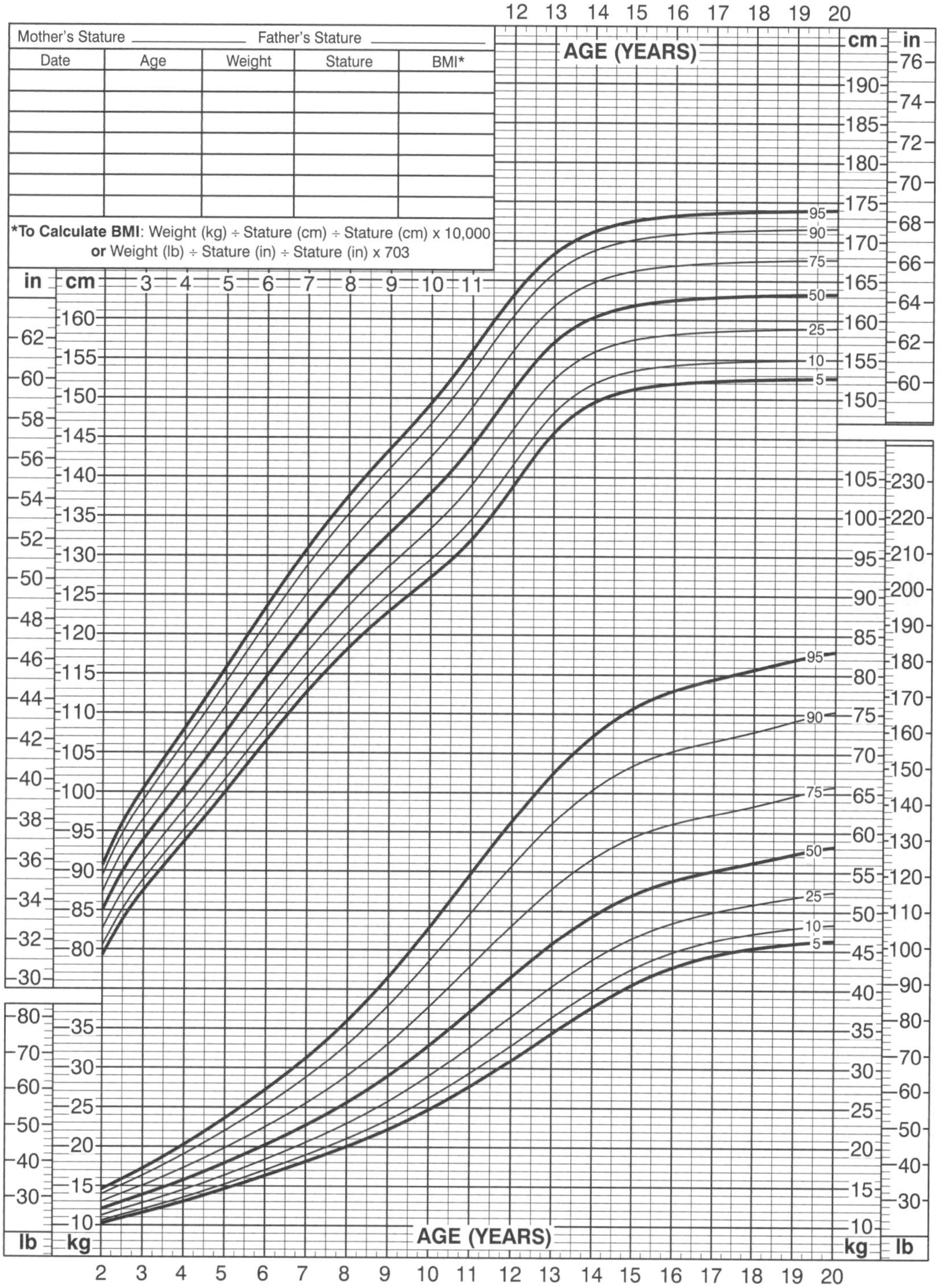

Mother's Stature ____________ Father's Stature ____________

Date	Age	Weight	Stature	BMI*

*To Calculate BMI: Weight (kg) ÷ Stature (cm) ÷ Stature (cm) x 10,000
or Weight (lb) ÷ Stature (in) ÷ Stature (in) x 703

Published May 30, 2000 (modified 11/21/00).
SOURCE: Developed by the National Center for Health Statistics in collaboration with
the National Center for Chronic Disease Prevention and Health Promotion (2000).
http://www.cdc.gov/growthcharts

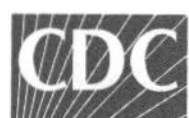

SAFER • HEALTHIER • PEOPLE™

2 to 20 years: Boys
Body mass index-for-age percentiles

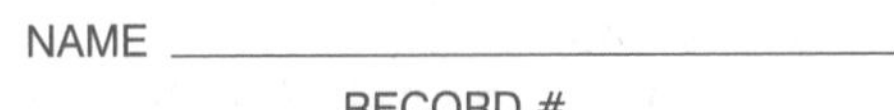
NAME ____________________

RECORD # ____________

Date	Age	Weight	Stature	BMI*	Comments

***To Calculate BMI**: Weight (kg) ÷ Stature (cm) ÷ Stature (cm) x 10,000
or Weight (lb) ÷ Stature (in) ÷ Stature (in) x 703

BMI

35 34 33 32 31 30 29 28 27 26 25 24 23 22 21 20 19 18 17 16 15 14 13 12

95 90 85 75 50 25 10 5

kg/m²

AGE (YEARS)

2 3 4 5 6 7 8 9 10 11 12 13 14 15 16 17 18 19 20

Published May 30, 2000 (modified 10/16/00).

SOURCE: Developed by the National Center for Health Statistics in collaboration with the National Center for Chronic Disease Prevention and Health Promotion (2000).
http://www.cdc.gov/growthcharts

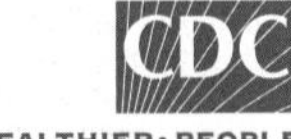

SAFER • HEALTHIER • PEOPLE™

2 to 20 years: Girls
Body mass index-for-age percentiles

NAME ____________________

RECORD # ____________

Date	Age	Weight	Stature	BMI*	Comments

***To Calculate BMI**: Weight (kg) ÷ Stature (cm) ÷ Stature (cm) x 10,000
or Weight (lb) ÷ Stature (in) ÷ Stature (in) x 703

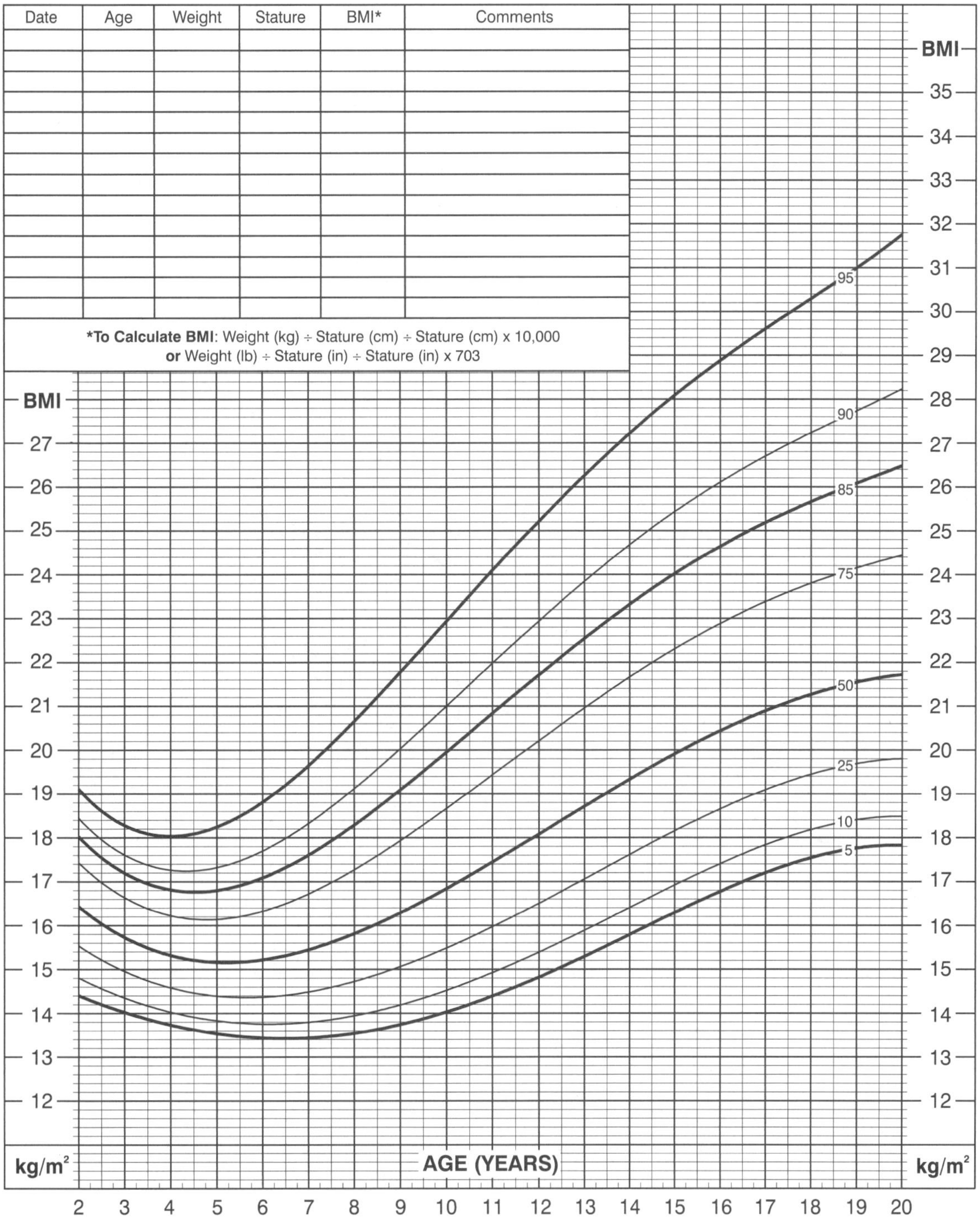

BMI

35 34 33 32 31 30 29 28 27 26 25 24 23 22 21 20 19 18 17 16 15 14 13 12

95 90 85 75 50 25 10 5

kg/m²

AGE (YEARS)

2 3 4 5 6 7 8 9 10 11 12 13 14 15 16 17 18 19 20

Published May 30, 2000 (modified 10/16/00).
SOURCE: Developed by the National Center for Health Statistics in collaboration with the National Center for Chronic Disease Prevention and Health Promotion (2000).
http://www.cdc.gov/growthcharts

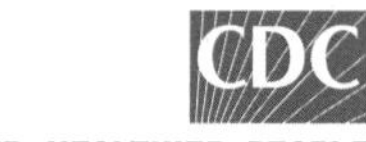

APPENDIX B

Blood Pressure Charts for Children and Adolescents

APPENDIX B.1 • Blood Pressure Levels for Males by Age and Height Percentile

Age (years)	BP Percentile ↓	SBP (mm Hg) ← Height Percentile or Measured Height →							DBP (mm Hg) ← Height Percentile or Measured Height →						
		5%	*10%*	*25%*	*50%*	*75%*	*90%*	*95%*	*5%*	*10%*	*25%*	*50%*	*75%*	*90%*	*95%*
1	Height (in)	30.4	30.8	31.6	32.4	33.3	34.1	34.6	30.4	30.8	31.6	32.4	33.3	34.1	34.6
	Height (cm)	77.2	78.3	80.2	82.4	84.6	86.7	87.9	77.2	78.3	80.2	82.4	84.6	86.7	87.9
	50th	85	85	86	86	87	88	88	40	40	40	41	41	42	42
	90th	98	99	99	100	100	101	101	52	52	53	53	54	54	54
	95th	102	102	103	103	104	105	105	54	54	55	55	56	57	57
	95th + 12 mm Hg	114	114	115	115	116	117	117	66	66	67	67	68	69	69
2	Height (in)	33.9	34.4	35.3	36.3	37.3	38.2	38.8	33.9	34.4	35.3	36.3	37.3	38.2	38.8
	Height (cm)	86.1	87.4	89.6	92.1	94.7	97.1	98.5	86.1	87.4	89.6	92.1	94.7	97.1	98.5
	50th	87	87	88	89	89	90	91	43	43	44	44	45	46	46
	90th	100	100	101	102	103	103	104	55	55	56	56	57	58	58
	95th	104	105	105	106	107	107	108	57	58	58	59	60	61	61
	95th + 12 mm Hg	116	117	117	118	119	119	120	69	70	70	71	72	73	73
3	Height (in)	36.4	37	37.9	39	40.1	41.1	41.7	36.4	37	37.9	39	40.1	41.1	41.7
	Height (cm)	92.5	93.9	96.3	99	101.8	104.3	105.8	92.5	93.9	96.3	99	101.8	104.3	105.8
	50th	88	89	89	90	91	92	92	45	46	46	47	48	49	49
	90th	101	102	102	103	104	105	105	58	58	59	59	60	61	61
	95th	106	106	107	107	108	109	109	60	61	61	62	63	64	64
	95th + 12 mm Hg	118	118	119	119	120	121	121	72	73	73	74	75	76	76
4	Height (in)	38.8	39.4	40.5	41.7	42.9	43.9	44.5	38.8	39.4	40.5	41.7	42.9	43.9	44.5
	Height (cm)	98.5	100.2	102.9	105.9	108.9	111.5	113.2	98.5	100.2	102.9	105.9	108.9	111.5	113.2
	50th	90	90	91	92	93	94	94	48	49	49	50	51	52	52
	90th	102	103	104	105	105	106	107	60	61	62	62	63	64	64
	95th	107	107	108	108	109	110	110	63	64	65	66	67	67	68
	95th + 12 mm Hg	119	119	120	120	121	122	122	75	76	77	78	79	79	80
5	Height (in)	41.1	41.8	43.0	44.3	45.5	46.7	47.4	41.1	41.8	43.0	44.3	45.5	46.7	47.4
	Height (cm)	104.4	106.2	109.1	112.4	115.7	118.6	120.3	104.4	106.2	109.1	112.4	115.7	118.6	120.3
	50th	91	92	93	94	95	96	96	51	51	52	53	54	55	55
	90th	103	104	105	106	107	108	108	63	64	65	65	66	67	67
	95th	107	108	109	109	110	111	112	66	67	68	69	70	70	71
	95th + 12 mm Hg	119	120	121	121	122	123	124	78	79	80	81	82	82	83
6	Height (in)	43.4	44.2	45.4	46.8	48.2	49.4	50.2	43.4	44.2	45.4	46.8	48.2	49.4	50.2
	Height (cm)	110.3	112.2	115.3	118.9	122.4	125.6	127.5	110.3	112.2	115.3	118.9	122.4	125.6	127.5
	50th	93	93	94	95	96	97	98	54	54	55	56	57	57	58
	90th	105	105	106	107	109	110	110	66	66	67	68	68	69	69
	95th	108	109	110	111	112	113	114	69	70	70	71	72	72	73
	95th + 12 mm Hg	120	121	122	123	124	125	126	81	82	82	83	84	84	85

APPENDIX B.1 • Blood Pressure Levels for Males by Age and Height Percentile

Age (years)	BP Percentile ↓	SBP (mm Hg)							DBP (mm Hg)						
		← *Height Percentile or Measured Height* →							← *Height Percentile or Measured Height* →						
		5%	*10%*	*25%*	*50%*	*75%*	*90%*	*95%*	*5%*	*10%*	*25%*	*50%*	*75%*	*90%*	*95%*
7	Height (in)	45.7	46.5	47.8	49.3	50.8	52.1	52.9	45.7	46.5	47.8	49.3	50.8	52.1	52.9
	Height (cm)	116.1	118	121.4	125.1	128.9	132.4	134.5	116.1	118	121.4	125.1	128.9	132.4	134.5
	50th	94	94	95	97	98	98	99	56	56	57	58	58	59	59
	90th	106	107	108	109	110	111	111	68	68	69	70	70	71	71
	95th	110	110	111	112	114	115	116	71	71	72	73	73	74	74
	95th + 12 mm Hg	122	122	123	124	126	127	128	83	83	84	85	85	86	86
8	Height (in)	47.8	48.6	50	51.6	53.2	54.6	55.5	47.8	48.6	50	51.6	53.2	54.6	55.5
	Height (cm)	121.4	123.5	127	131	135.1	138.8	141	121.4	123.5	127	131	135.1	138.8	141
	50th	95	96	97	98	99	99	100	57	57	58	59	59	60	60
	90th	107	108	109	110	111	112	112	69	70	70	71	72	72	73
	95th	111	112	112	114	115	116	117	72	73	73	74	75	75	75
	95th + 12 mm Hg	123	124	124	126	127	128	129	84	85	85	86	87	87	87
9	Height (in)	49.6	50.5	52	53.7	55.4	56.9	57.9	49.6	50.5	52	53.7	55.4	56.9	57.9
	Height (cm)	126	128.3	132.1	136.3	140.7	144.7	147.1	126	128.3	132.1	136.3	140.7	144.7	147.1
	50th	96	97	98	99	100	101	101	57	58	59	60	61	62	62
	90th	107	108	109	110	112	113	114	70	71	72	73	74	74	74
	95th	112	112	113	115	116	118	119	74	74	75	76	76	77	77
	95th + 12 mm Hg	124	124	125	127	128	130	131	86	86	87	88	88	89	89
10	Height (in)	51.3	52.2	53.8	55.6	57.4	59.1	60.1	51.3	52.2	53.8	55.6	57.4	59.1	60.1
	Height (cm)	130.2	132.7	136.7	141.3	145.9	150.1	152.7	130.2	132.7	136.7	141.3	145.9	150.1	152.7
	50th	97	98	99	100	101	102	103	59	60	61	62	63	63	64
	90th	108	109	111	112	113	115	116	72	73	74	74	75	75	76
	95th	112	113	114	116	118	120	121	76	76	77	77	78	78	78
	95th + 12 mm Hg	124	125	126	128	130	132	133	88	88	89	89	90	90	90
11	Height (in)	53	54	55.7	57.6	59.6	61.3	62.4	53	54	55.7	57.6	59.6	61.3	62.4
	Height (cm)	134.7	137.3	141.5	146.4	151.3	155.8	158.6	134.7	137.3	141.5	146.4	151.3	155.8	158.6
	50th	99	99	101	102	103	104	106	61	61	62	63	63	63	63
	90th	110	111	112	114	116	117	118	74	74	75	75	75	76	76
	95th	114	114	116	118	120	123	124	77	78	78	78	78	78	78
	95th + 12 mm Hg	126	126	128	130	132	135	136	89	90	90	90	90	90	90
12	Height (in)	55.2	56.3	58.1	60.1	62.2	64	65.2	55.2	56.3	58.1	60.1	62.2	64	65.2
	Height (cm)	140.3	143	147.5	152.7	157.9	162.6	165.5	140.3	143	147.5	152.7	157.9	162.6	165.5
	50th	101	101	102	104	106	108	109	61	62	62	62	62	63	63
	90th	113	114	115	117	119	121	122	75	75	75	75	75	76	76
	95th	116	117	118	121	124	126	128	78	78	78	78	78	79	79
	95th + 12 mm Hg	128	129	130	133	136	138	140	90	90	90	90	90	91	91

(continued)

APPENDIX B.1 • Blood Pressure Levels for Males by Age and Height Percentile (*continued*)

Age (years)	BP Percentile ↓	SBP (mm Hg) ← Height Percentile or Measured Height →							DBP (mm Hg) ← Height Percentile or Measured Height →						
		5%	*10%*	*25%*	*50%*	*75%*	*90%*	*95%*	*5%*	*10%*	*25%*	*50%*	*75%*	*90%*	*95%*
13	Height (in)	57.9	59.1	61	63.1	65.2	67.1	68.3	57.9	59.1	61	63.1	65.2	67.1	68.3
	Height (cm)	147	150	154.9	160.3	165.7	170.5	173.4	147	150	154.9	160.3	165.7	170.5	173.4
	50th	103	104	105	108	110	111	112	61	60	61	62	63	64	65
	90th	115	116	118	121	124	126	126	74	74	74	75	76	77	77
	95th	119	120	122	125	128	130	131	78	78	78	78	80	81	81
	95th + 12 mm Hg	131	132	134	137	140	142	143	90	90	90	90	92	93	93
14	Height (in)	60.6	61.8	63.8	65.9	68.0	69.8	70.9	60.6	61.8	63.8	65.9	68.0	69.8	70.9
	Height (cm)	153.8	156.9	162	167.5	172.7	177.4	180.1	153.8	156.9	162	167.5	172.7	177.4	180.1
	50th	105	106	109	111	112	113	113	60	60	62	64	65	66	67
	90th	119	120	123	126	127	128	129	74	74	75	77	78	79	80
	95th	123	125	127	130	132	133	134	77	78	79	81	82	83	84
	95th + 12 mm Hg	135	137	139	142	144	145	146	89	90	91	93	94	95	96
15	Height (in)	62.6	63.8	65.7	67.8	69.8	71.5	72.5	62.6	63.8	65.7	67.8	69.8	71.5	72.5
	Height (cm)	159	162	166.9	172.2	177.2	181.6	184.2	159	162	166.9	172.2	177.2	181.6	184.2
	50th	108	110	112	113	114	114	114	61	62	64	65	66	67	68
	90th	123	124	126	128	129	130	130	75	76	78	79	80	81	81
	95th	127	129	131	132	134	135	135	78	79	81	83	84	85	85
	95th + 12 mm Hg	139	141	143	144	146	147	147	90	91	93	95	96	97	97
16	Height (in)	63.8	64.9	66.8	68.8	70.7	72.4	73.4	63.8	64.9	66.8	68.8	70.7	72.4	73.4
	Height (cm)	162.1	165	169.6	174.6	179.5	183.8	186.4	162.1	165	169.6	174.6	179.5	183.8	186.4
	50th	111	112	114	115	115	116	116	63	64	66	67	68	69	69
	90th	126	127	128	129	131	131	132	77	78	79	80	81	82	82
	95th	130	131	133	134	135	136	137	80	81	83	84	85	86	86
	95th + 12 mm Hg	142	143	145	146	147	148	149	92	93	95	96	97	98	98
17	Height (in)	64.5	65.5	67.3	69.2	71.1	72.8	73.8	64.5	65.5	67.3	69.2	71.1	72.8	73.8
	Height (cm)	163.8	166.5	170.9	175.8	180.7	184.9	187.5	163.8	166.5	170.9	175.8	180.7	184.9	187.5
	50th	114	115	116	117	117	118	118	65	66	67	68	69	70	70
	90th	128	129	130	131	132	133	134	78	79	80	81	82	82	83
	95th	132	133	134	135	137	138	138	81	82	84	85	86	86	87
	95th + 12 mm Hg	144	145	146	147	149	150	150	93	94	96	97	98	98	99

BP, blood pressure; DBP, diastolic blood pressure; SBP, systolic blood pressure. ≥90th to ≤95th percentile, or 120/80 or ≤95th percentile (whichever is lower): elevated blood pressure; ≥95th to ≤95th percentile + 12 mm Hg, or 130/80 to 139/89 mm Hg (whichever is lower): stage 1 hypertension; ≥95th percentile + 12 mm Hg, or ≥140/90 mm Hg (whichever is lower): stage 2 hypertension.

APPENDIX B.2 • Blood Pressure Levels for Females by Age and Height Percentile

Age (years)	BP Percentile ↓	SBP (mm Hg)							DBP (mm Hg)						
		← *Height Percentile or Measured Height* →							← *Height Percentile or Measured Height* →						
		5%	*10%*	*25%*	*50%*	*75%*	*90%*	*95%*	*5%*	*10%*	*25%*	*50%*	*75%*	*90%*	*95%*
1	Height (in)	29.7	30.2	30.9	31.8	32.7	33.4	33.9	29.7	30.2	30.9	31.8	32.7	33.4	33.9
	Height (cm)	75.4	76.6	78.6	80.8	83	84.9	86.1	75.4	76.6	78.6	80.8	83	84.9	86.1
	50th	84	85	86	86	87	88	88	41	42	42	43	44	45	46
	90th	98	99	99	100	101	102	102	54	55	56	56	57	58	58
	95th	101	102	102	103	104	105	105	59	59	60	60	61	62	62
	95th + 12 mm Hg	113	114	114	115	116	117	117	71	71	72	72	73	74	74
2	Height (in)	33.4	34	34.9	35.9	36.9	37.8	38.4	33.4	34	34.9	35.9	36.9	37.8	38.4
	Height (cm)	84.9	86.3	88.6	91.1	93.7	96	97.4	84.9	86.3	88.6	91.1	93.7	96	97.4
	50th	87	87	88	89	90	91	91	45	46	47	48	49	50	51
	90th	101	101	102	103	104	105	106	58	58	59	60	61	62	62
	95th	104	105	106	106	107	108	109	62	63	63	64	65	66	66
	95th + 12 mm Hg	116	117	118	118	119	120	121	74	75	75	76	77	78	78
3	Height (in)	35.8	36.4	37.3	38.4	39.6	40.6	41.2	35.8	36.4	37.3	38.4	39.6	40.6	41.2
	Height (cm)	91	92.4	94.9	97.6	100.5	103.1	104.6	91	92.4	94.9	97.6	100.5	103.1	104.6
	50th	88	89	89	90	91	92	93	48	48	49	50	51	53	53
	90th	102	103	104	104	105	106	107	60	61	61	62	63	64	65
	95th	106	106	107	108	109	110	110	64	65	65	66	67	68	69
	95th + 12 mm Hg	118	118	119	120	121	122	122	76	77	77	78	79	80	81
4	Height (in)	38.3	38.9	39.9	41.1	42.4	43.5	44.2	38.3	38.9	39.9	41.1	42.4	43.5	44.2
	Height (cm)	97.2	98.8	101.4	104.5	107.6	110.5	112.2	97.2	98.8	101.4	104.5	107.6	110.5	112.2
	50th	89	90	91	92	93	94	94	50	51	51	53	54	55	55
	90th	103	104	105	106	107	108	108	62	63	64	65	66	67	67
	95th	107	108	109	109	110	111	112	66	67	68	69	70	70	71
	95th + 12 mm Hg	119	120	121	121	122	123	124	78	79	80	81	82	82	83
5	Height (in)	40.8	41.5	42.6	43.9	45.2	46.5	47.3	40.8	41.5	42.6	43.9	45.2	46.5	47.3
	Height (cm)	103.6	105.3	108.2	111.5	114.9	118.1	120	103.6	105.3	108.2	111.5	114.9	118.1	120
	50th	90	91	92	93	94	95	96	52	52	53	55	56	57	57
	90th	104	105	106	107	108	109	110	64	65	66	67	68	69	70
	95th	108	109	109	110	111	112	113	68	69	70	71	72	73	73
	95th + 12 mm Hg	120	121	121	122	123	124	125	80	81	82	83	84	85	85
6	Height (in)	43.3	44	45.2	46.6	48.1	49.4	50.3	43.3	44	45.2	46.6	48.1	49.4	50.3
	Height (cm)	110	111.8	114.9	118.4	122.1	125.6	127.7	110	111.8	114.9	118.4	122.1	125.6	127.7
	50th	92	92	93	94	96	97	97	54	54	55	56	57	58	59
	90th	105	106	107	108	109	110	111	67	67	68	69	70	71	71
	95th	109	109	110	111	112	113	114	70	71	72	72	73	74	74
	95th + 12 mm Hg	121	121	122	123	124	125	126	82	83	84	84	85	86	86

(*continued*)

APPENDIX B.2 • Blood Pressure Levels for Females by Age and Height Percentile (*continued*)

Age (years)	BP Percentile ↓	SBP (mm Hg) ← Height Percentile or Measured Height →							DBP (mm Hg) ← Height Percentile or Measured Height →						
		5%	10%	25%	50%	75%	90%	95%	5%	10%	25%	50%	75%	90%	95%
7	Height (in)	45.6	46.4	47.7	49.2	50.7	52.1	53	45.6	46.4	47.7	49.2	50.7	52.1	53
	Height (cm)	115.9	117.8	121.1	124.9	128.8	132.5	134.7	115.9	117.8	121.1	124.9	128.8	132.5	134.7
	50th	92	93	94	95	97	98	99	55	55	56	57	58	59	60
	90th	106	106	107	109	110	111	112	68	68	69	70	71	72	72
	95th	109	110	111	112	113	114	115	72	72	73	73	74	74	75
	95th + 12 mm Hg	121	122	123	124	125	126	127	84	84	85	85	86	86	87
8	Height (in)	47.6	48.4	49.8	51.4	53	54.5	55.5	47.6	48.4	49.8	51.4	53	54.5	55.5
	Height (cm)	121	123	126.5	130.6	134.7	138.5	140.9	121	123	126.5	130.6	134.7	138.5	140.9
	50th	93	94	95	97	98	99	100	56	56	57	59	60	61	61
	90th	107	107	108	110	111	112	113	69	70	71	72	72	73	73
	95th	110	111	112	113	115	116	117	72	73	74	74	75	75	75
	95th + 12 mm Hg	122	123	124	125	127	128	129	84	85	86	86	87	87	87
9	Height (in)	49.3	50.2	51.7	53.4	55.1	56.7	57.7	49.3	50.2	51.7	53.4	55.1	56.7	57.7
	Height (cm)	125.3	127.6	131.3	135.6	140.1	144.1	146.6	125.3	127.6	131.3	135.6	140.1	144.1	146.6
	50th	95	95	97	98	99	100	101	57	58	59	60	60	61	61
	90th	108	108	109	111	112	113	114	71	71	72	73	73	73	73
	95th	112	112	113	114	116	117	118	74	74	75	75	75	75	75
	95th + 12 mm Hg	124	124	125	126	128	129	130	86	86	87	87	87	87	87
10	Height (in)	51.1	52	53.7	55.5	57.4	59.1	60.2	51.1	52	53.7	55.5	57.4	59.1	60.2
	Height (cm)	129.7	132.2	136.3	141	145.8	150.2	152.8	129.7	132.2	136.3	141	145.8	150.2	152.8
	50th	96	97	98	99	101	102	103	58	59	59	60	61	61	62
	90th	109	110	111	112	113	115	116	72	73	73	73	73	73	73
	95th	113	114	114	116	117	119	120	75	75	76	76	76	76	76
	95th + 12 mm Hg	125	126	126	128	129	131	132	87	87	88	88	88	88	88
11	Height (in)	53.4	54.5	56.2	58.2	60.2	61.9	63	53.4	54.5	56.2	58.2	60.2	61.9	63
	Height (cm)	135.6	138.3	142.8	147.8	152.8	157.3	160	135.6	138.3	142.8	147.8	152.8	157.3	160
	50th	98	99	101	102	104	105	106	60	60	60	61	62	63	64
	90th	111	112	113	114	116	118	120	74	74	74	74	74	75	75
	95th	115	116	117	118	120	123	124	76	77	77	77	77	77	77
	95th + 12 mm Hg	127	128	129	130	132	135	136	88	89	89	89	89	89	89
12	Height (in)	56.2	57.3	59	60.9	62.8	64.5	65.5	56.2	57.3	59	60.9	62.8	64.5	65.5
	Height (cm)	142.8	145.5	149.9	154.8	159.6	163.8	166.4	142.8	145.5	149.9	154.8	159.6	163.8	166.4
	50th	102	102	104	105	107	108	108	61	61	61	62	64	65	65
	90th	114	115	116	118	120	122	122	75	75	75	75	76	76	76
	95th	118	119	120	122	124	125	126	78	78	78	78	79	79	79
	95th + 12 mm Hg	130	131	132	134	136	137	138	90	90	90	90	91	91	91

APPENDIX B.2 • Blood Pressure Levels for Females by Age and Height Percentile

Age (years) ↓	BP Percentile ↓	SBP (mm Hg) ← Height Percentile or Measured Height →							DBP (mm Hg) ← Height Percentile or Measured Height →						
		5%	*10%*	*25%*	*50%*	*75%*	*90%*	*95%*	*5%*	*10%*	*25%*	*50%*	*75%*	*90%*	*95%*
13	Height (in)	58.3	59.3	60.9	62.7	64.5	66.1	67	58.3	59.3	60.9	62.7	64.5	66.1	67
	Height (cm)	148.1	150.6	154.7	159.2	163.7	167.8	170.2	148.1	150.6	154.7	159.2	163.7	167.8	170.2
	50th	104	105	106	107	108	108	109	62	62	63	64	65	65	66
	90th	116	117	119	121	122	123	123	75	75	75	76	76	76	76
	95th	121	122	123	124	126	126	127	79	79	79	79	80	80	81
	95th + 12 mm Hg	133	134	135	136	138	138	139	91	91	91	91	92	92	93
14	Height (in)	59.3	60.2	61.8	63.5	65.2	66.8	67.7	59.3	60.2	61.8	63.5	65.2	66.8	67.7
	Height (cm)	150.6	153	156.9	161.3	165.7	169.7	172.1	150.6	153	156.9	161.3	165.7	169.7	172.1
	50th	105	106	107	108	109	109	109	63	63	64	65	66	66	66
	90th	118	118	120	122	123	123	123	76	76	76	76	77	77	77
	95th	123	123	124	125	126	127	127	80	80	80	80	81	81	82
	95th + 12 mm Hg	135	135	136	137	138	139	139	92	92	92	92	93	93	94
15	Height (in)	59.7	60.6	62.2	63.9	65.6	67.2	68.1	59.7	60.6	62.2	63.9	65.6	67.2	68.1
	Height (cm)	151.7	154	157.9	162.3	166.7	170.6	173	151.7	154	157.9	162.3	166.7	170.6	173
	50th	105	106	107	108	109	109	109	64	64	64	65	66	67	67
	90th	118	119	121	122	123	123	124	76	76	76	77	77	78	78
	95th	124	124	125	126	127	127	128	80	80	80	81	82	82	82
	95th + 12 mm Hg	136	136	137	138	139	139	140	92	92	92	93	94	94	94
16	Height (in)	59.9	60.8	62.4	64.1	65.8	67.3	68.3	59.9	60.8	62.4	64.1	65.8	67.3	68.3
	Height (cm)	152.1	154.5	158.4	162.8	167.1	171.1	173.4	152.1	154.5	158.4	162.8	167.1	171.1	173.4
	50th	106	107	108	109	109	110	110	64	64	65	66	66	67	67
	90th	119	120	122	123	124	124	124	76	76	76	77	78	78	78
	95th	124	125	125	127	127	128	128	80	80	80	81	82	82	82
	95th + 12 mm Hg	136	137	137	139	139	140	140	92	92	92	93	94	94	94
17	Height (in)	60.0	60.9	62.5	64.2	65.9	67.4	68.4	60.0	60.9	62.5	64.2	65.9	67.4	68.4
	Height (cm)	152.4	154.7	158.7	163.0	167.4	171.3	173.7	152.4	154.7	158.7	163.0	167.4	171.3	173.7
	50th	107	108	109	110	110	110	111	64	64	65	66	66	66	67
	90th	120	121	123	124	124	125	125	76	76	77	77	78	78	78
	95th	125	125	126	127	128	128	128	80	80	80	81	82	82	82
	95th + 12 mm Hg	137	137	138	139	140	140	140	92	92	92	93	94	94	94

BP, blood pressure; DBP, diastolic blood pressure; HTN, hypertension; SBP, systolic blood pressure; elevated BP: ≥90th percentile; stage 1 HTN: ≥95th percentile; stage 2 HTN: ≥95th percentile + 12 mm Hg.

INDEX

Note: Page numbers followed by *f*, *t*, and *b* denote figures, tables, and boxes, respectively.

B

C

D

E

M

O

R

S

T

U